Blaustein's Pathology of the Female Genital Tract

Robert J. Kurman, Lora Hedrick Ellenson and Brigitte M. Ronnett (Eds.)

Blaustein's Pathology of the Female Genital Tract

Sixth Edition

With 1446 Figures and 125 Tables

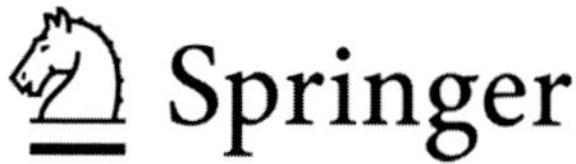

Springer

Editors
Robert J. Kurman
Richard W. TeLinde Distinguished Professor of Gynecologic Pathology
Departments of Gynecology, Obstetrics, Pathology and Oncology
The Johns Hopkins University School of Medicine and Director of Gynecologic Pathology,
The Johns Hopkins Hospital
401 N. Broadway, Weinberg Building Room 2242
Baltimore
MD, 21231
USA
rkurman@jhmi.edu

Brigitte M. Ronnett
Department of Pathology
Johns Hopkins University School of Medicine
401 N. Broadway, Weinberg Building 2242
Baltimore
MD, 21231
USA
bronnett@jhmi.edu

Lora Hedrick Ellenson
Department of Pathology and Laboratory Medicine
Weill Cornell Medical College and New York Presbyterian Hospital
525 East 68th Street, Starr 1015
New York
NY, 10065
USA
lora.ellenson@med.cornell.edu

ISBN 978-1-4419-0488-1 e-ISBN 978-1-4419-0489-8
Print and electronic bundle ISBN 978-1-4419-0490-4
DOI 10.1007/978-1-4419-0489-8
Springer New York Dodrecht Heidelberg London

Library of Congress Control Number: 2010928122

[illegible] free paper

Springer is part of Springer Science+Business Media (www.springer.com)

To Carole C. Kurman for her constant support and encouragement
To my ultimate mentors, Donald Ward Hedrick and Pauline Gray Hedrick
In memory of my parents, Alexander and Helga Ronnett, for their value of education

Preface

The advances in the field of gynecologic pathology since the publication of the last edition of this text in 2001 have been significant and the progress that the senior editor has witnessed since the first edition of this book appeared in 1977 has been truly remarkable. To cite just one example, in the first edition, Herpes virus type 2 was thought to cause cervical cancer and the nomenclature for cervical cancer precursors was cervical dysplasia and carcinoma in situ (CIS), with the emphasis placed on the distinction of severe dysplasia from CIS since a diagnosis of severe dysplasia resulted in a cone biopsy whereas the diagnosis of CIS resulted in a hysterectomy. Since then, the terminology and, in turn, the management of the precursor lesions has evolved to cervical intraepithelial neoplasia 1-3 (CIN 1-3) with treatment of all grades of CIN, to low- and high-grade squamous intraepithelial lesions (LSIL and HSIL respectively) in which LSIL is generally not treated, as it is recognized as a manifestation of human papillomavirus (HPV) infection, whereas HSIL is managed by LEEP excision, as it is recognized as the immediate precursor of cervical cancer. Along with these changes in terminology and treatment, the recognition that high-risk human HPVs represent the etiologic agents that cause essentially all cervical and vaginal cancers and a substantial fraction of vulvar carcinomas led to the development of prophylactic vaccines in preventing HPV infections. As a consequence the management of this disease will change again. In fact, the efficacy of these vaccines in preventing cervical cancer precursors has the potential, in the future, of eradicating a cancer that affects over 500,000 women yearly worldwide and the recent award of the Nobel Prize in Medicine to Professor zur Hausen for his identification of HPV 16 DNA in cervical cancer specimens is testimony to this truly remarkable achievement.

Examination of the trajectory of advances in gynecologic pathology over the last 35 years since the first edition of *Blaustein's Pathology of the Female Genital Tract* highlights the significant contributions made by a number of different disciplines including molecular biology and epidemiology. In fact, the application of molecular biologic methods in conjunction with histopathologic classifications based on the natural history of disease ushers in a new approach for surgical pathology in general and gynecologic pathology in particular, which undoubtedly will continue to evolve in the future. Thus, the publication of this 6th edition of the Blaustein text marks the transition in diagnosis from a largely morphological activity to one based upon an integrated assessment using microscopy, immunohistochemistry and molecular biology. Finally, the emerging role of digital technology that makes an ever-increasing amount of data available at our fingertips will undoubtedly change the way we access information in the future. It is not difficult to envision that the next edition of this text will be on an electronic reader of some type instead of in the form of a textbook.

As with previous editions of the Blaustein text, the 6th edition maintains our commitment to producing a comprehensive text that covers the field of gynecologic pathology in depth while not sacrificing its utility as a "desk-side" text that can be referred to in every day practice. Accordingly, significant changes have been made to inform the reader of advances in research that have occurred since the last edition while at the same time enhancing its usefulness in the everyday practice of gynecologic pathology. To accomplish this latter goal we have increased the number of photomicrographs, nearly all of which are now in color. Discussions of differential diagnosis have also been significantly expanded. Both the text and the photomicrographs emphasize the importance of immunohistochemistry and newly emerging molecular techniques as adjuncts to morphology in routine clinical diagnosis. To avoid the text becoming too ponderous we have reduced its size by asking contributors to delete sections they deemed no longer relevant while retaining older material that they regarded as "classic" or that described large series of cases with clinicopathologic data that are still relevant today. Similarly, given the ability to obtain references easily on the Internet, many older references have been deleted with emphasis on including those published since 2000. Unlike the last edition in which embryology, anatomy, epidemiology, immunohistochemistry, molecular biology and gross processing were separate chapters, these subjects have been incorporated into the individual chapters by organ site. This has resulted in a more streamlined format that integrates these various disciplines with the histopathology. Finally, two separate chapters, one on soft tissue tumors and the other on hematologic disorders involving the female reproductive organs, have been added because these are subspecialty areas in their own right and are authored by experts in these fields.

The publication of this text has depended on the assistance of many individuals to whom the authors are greatly indebted. In particular, in an effort to achieve a degree of uniformity in the quality of the images among the various chapters, Mr. Norman Barker, Associate Professor and Director of Pathology, Digital Imaging and Computer Graphics at Johns Hopkins reviewed and digitally edited all of the photomicrographs, many of which required his considerable expertise (particularly those images that were scanned from Kodachrome slides). We feel this has been successfully accomplished and are grateful for his efforts. Finally, there are many people, including fellows, our colleagues in the Divisions of Gynecologic Pathology at Johns Hopkins and Cornell and individuals from other disciplines who, through our collaboration with them, have enhanced our understanding of the pathobiology of neoplasms of the female reproductive organs. They are far too numerous to specifically mention but their influence on us has been considerable. To all these people we wish to express our thanks.

Robert J. Kurman, MD
Lora Hedrick Ellenson, MD
Brigitte M. Ronnett, MD

Table of Contents

Editors-in-Chief

Robert J. Kurman
Richard W. TeLinde Distinguished Professor of Gynecologic Pathology
Departments of Gynecology, Obstetrics, Pathology and Oncology
The Johns Hopkins University School of Medicine and Director of Gynecologic Pathology
The Johns Hopkins Hospital
401 N. Broadway, Weinberg Building Room 2242
Baltimore
MD 21231
USA
rkurman@jhmi.edu

Lora Hedrick Ellenson
Department of Pathology and Laboratory Medicine
Weill Cornell Medical College and
New York Presbyterian Hospital
525 East 68th Street, Starr 1015
New York
NY 10065
USA
lora.ellenson@med.cornell.edu

Brigitte M. Ronnett
Department of Pathology
Johns Hopkins University School of Medicine
401 N. Broadway, Weinberg Building 2242
Baltimore
MD 21231
USA
bronnett@jhmi.edu

List of Contributors

Kathleen R. Cho
Department of Pathology
University of Michigan Medical School
Room 1506 BSRB 109 Zina Pitcher Place
Ann Arbor, MI 48109-2200
USA
kathcho@umich.edu

Philip B. Clement
Department of Pathology
Vancouver Hospital and Health Sciences Center
910 W. 10th Avenue, Room 1302
Vancouver, BC V5Z 4E3
Canada
phil.clement@vch.ca

Lora Hedrick Ellenson
Department of Pathology and Laboratory Medicine
Weill Cornell Medical College and
New York Presbyterian Hospital
525 East 68th Street, Starr 1015
New York, NY 10065
USA
lora.ellenson@med.cornell.edu

Alex Ferenczy
Jewish General Hospital
McGill University
3755 Côte St. Catherine Road
Montreal, QC H3T 1E2
Canada
alex.ferenczy@mcgill.ca

Judith A. Ferry
Department of Pathology
Massachusetts General Hospital
Fruit Street
Boston, MA 02114
jferry@partners.org

John F. Fetsch
Department of Soft Tissue Pathology
Armed Forces Institute of Pathology
14th Street & Alaska Ave.
NW, Washington, DC 20306-6000
USA
John.Fetsch@us.army.mil

Deborah J. Gersell
Department of Laboratory Medicine
St. John's Mercy Medical Center
615 South New Ballas Road
St. Louis, MO
USA
deborah.gersell@mercy.net

Michael R. Hendrickson
Department of Surgical Pathology
Stanford University Medical Center
300 Pasteur Drive, Room L-235
Stanford, CA 94305
USA
hendrickson@stanford.edu

Julie A. Irving
Department of Laboratory Medicine, Pathology, and
Medical Genetics
Royal Jubilee Hospital
1952 Bay Street, Room DT 5821
Victoria BC V8R 1J8
Canada
Julie.Irving@viha.ca

Frederick T. Kraus
Adjunct Professor, Perinatal Biology Laboratory,
Department of Obstetrics and Gynecology
Washington University School of Medicine
St. Louis, MO
USA
krasf@msnotes.wustl.edu

Robert J. Kurman
Departments of Gynecology, Obstetrics, Pathology and Oncology, Division of Gynecologic Pathology
Johns Hopkins University School of Medicine
Weinberg Building Room 2242 401 N. Broadway
Baltimore, MD 21231
USA
rkurman@jhmi.edu

William B. Laskin
Department of Pathology
Northwestern Memorial Hospital
251 East Huron Street
Chicago, IL 60611
USA
wbl769@northwestern.edu

Melinda F. Lerwill
Department of Pathology
Massachusetts General Hospital and Harvard Medical School
55 Fruit Street
Boston, MA 02114
USA
mlerwill@partners.org

Nicole A. Massoll
College of Medicine, Department of Pathology
University of Arkansas for Medical Sciences
4301 W. Markham St. #517
Little Rock, AR 72205-7199
USA
NAMassoll@uams.edu

Michael T. Mazur
Pathology Associates of Syracuse
SUNY Upstate Medical University
600 E. Genesee St., Suite 305
Syracuse, NY 13202
USA
mazpath@pol.net

W. Glenn McCluggage
Department of Pathology
Royal Group of Hospitals Trust
Grosvenor Road
Belfast BT12 6BA
Northern Ireland
glenn.mccluggage@belfasttrust.hscni.net

Marisa Nucci
Brigham Women's Hospital
Women's Department of Pathology
75 Francis Street
Boston, MA 02115
USA
mnucci@partners.org

Brigitte M. Ronnett
Department of Pathology, Division of Gynecologic Pathology
Johns Hopkins University School of Medicine
Weinberg Building 2242, 401 N. Broadway
Baltimore, MD 21231
USA
bronnett@jhmi.edu

Jeffrey D. Seidman
Department of Pathology and Laboratory Medicine
Washington Hospital Center
110 Irving St.
Washington, DC N.W. 20010
USA
Jeffrey.D.Seidman@medstar.net

Ie-Ming Shih
Department of Pathology, Division of Gynecologic Pathology
Johns Hopkins University School of Medicine
1550 Orleans Street, CRB2, Room 305
Baltimore, MD 21231
USA
ishih@jhmi.edu

Robert A. Soslow
Department of Pathology
Memorial Sloan-Kettering Cancer Center
1275 York Avenue
New York, NY 10065
USA
soslowr@mskcc.org

Aleksander Talerman
Department of Surgical Pathology
Thomas Jefferson University Hospital
Room 285Q Main Building 11th and Walnut Streets
Philadelphia, PA 19107-5244
USA
mtalerman@aol.com

Russell Vang
Department of Pathology, Division of Gynecologic Pathology
The Johns Hopkins Medical Institutions
401 N. Broadway, Weinberg Building, Room 2242
Baltimore, MD 21231
USA
rvang1@jhmi.edu

James E. Wheeler
130 Llanfair Rd.
Ardmore, PA 19003-2501
USA
jewheele@mail.med.upenn.edu

Edward J. Wilkinson
Department of Pathology, Division of Anatomic Pathology
University of Florida College of Medicine
1600 S.W. Archer Road, Room 3110
Gainesville, FL 32610-0275
USA
wilkinso@pathology.ufl.edu

Agnieszka K. Witkiewicz
Department of Pathology
Thomas Jefferson University
Main Building Rm 285 D
Philadelphia, PA 19107
USA
nieszka@mac.com

Thomas C. Wright
Department of Pathology
Columbia Presbyterian Medical Center
630 W. 168th Street, Room 16404
New York, NY 10032
USA
tcw1@columbia.edu

Robert H. Young
Anatomic Pathology
James Homer Wright Pathology Laboratories, Massachusetts General Hospital, Harvard Medical School
55 Fruit Street, Warren Bldg. 2nd Floor
Boston, MA 02114
USA
rhyoung@partners.org

Richard J. Zaino
Department of Pathology, H179
M.S. Hershey Medical Center
500 University Drive
Hershey, PA 17033–0850
USA
rzaino@psu.edu

Charles J. Zaloudek
Department of Pathology
University of California, San Francisco
505 Parnassus Avenue, M563
San Francisco, CA 94122
USA
chuckz@itsa.ucsf.edu

1 Benign Diseases of the Vulva

Edward J. Wilkinson · Nicole A. Massoll

R. J. Kurman, L. Hedrick Ellenson, B. M. Ronnett (eds.), *Blaustein's Pathology of the Female Genital Tract (6th ed.)*, DOI 10.1007/978-1-4419-0489-8_1,

Anatomy

The external female genitalia include the mons pubis, labia majora and minora, prepuce, frenulum, clitoris, and vestibule. The orifices of the paraurethral (Skene) and Bartholin glands, as well as those of the minor vestibular glands and the urethral meatus, open into the vestibule (➋ *Fig. 1.1*). After menarche, the mons pubis and lateral aspects of the labia majora acquire increased amounts of subcutaneous fat and develop the coarse, curly pubic hair. During adolescence, the labia develop pigmentation and the clitoris undergoes some enlargement. Histologically, the entire vulva, with the exception of the vulvar vestibule, is covered by keratinized, stratified squamous epithelium [245]. The labia majora contain both smooth muscle and fat, whereas the labia minora are devoid of adipose tissue but are rich in elastic fibers and blood vessels [167]. Within the lateral aspects of the labia majora, sebaceous glands are associated with hair follicles but open directly to the surface epithelium toward the medial aspect. Similar sebaceous glands are seen on the perineum posterior to the vestibule. The labia minora typically do not contain glandular elements, except sebaceous glands near the junction with the interlabial sulcus and near the inferior and lateral aspects. The apocrine glands of the labia majora, prepuce, posterior vestibule, and perineal body, like the apocrine glands of the axilla, are activated at menarche, whereas the eccrine sweat glands, primarily involved in heat regulation, function before puberty [189]. The vestibule is bounded medially by the external portion of the hymen ring, posteriorly and laterally by the line of Hart, and anteriorly by the frenulum of the clitoris. The mucosa of the vestibule is glycogenated in women of reproductive age, or under estrogen influence, and resembles vaginal mucosa. The linea vestibularis, seen in approximately one quarter of newborn female infants, is located in the posterior portion of the vestibule, and is a white streak or spot in the midline of the posterior vestibule extending nearly to the posterior commissure [109]. The squamous epithelium of the vestibule merges with the transitional epithelium at the urethral meatus, and with the duct openings of the paraurethral glands (Skene), the major vestibular (Bartholin) glands, and the minor vestibular glands.

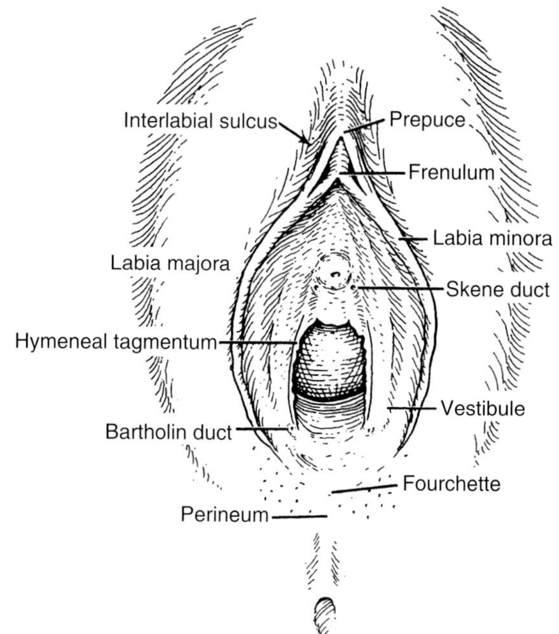

■ Fig. 1.1
External anatomy of the vulva and the Hart's line. **The line of Hart is the junction between the nonkeratinized mucous membrane epithelium of the vestibule, the thinly keratinized epithelium of the medial aspects of the labia minora, the posterior aspects of the labia majora, and the perineal body**

The paired Skene's glands, homologous of the prostate in females [80], are composed of pseudostratified mucus-secreting columnar epithelium, open to the external surface on both sides of the urethral meatus and along the posterior and lateral aspects of the urethra itself. The ducts are lined by transitional epithelium. The major vestibular glands of Bartholin are bilateral racemose, tubuloalveolar glands, with acini composed of simple, columnar, mucus-secreting epithelium (➋ *Fig. 1.2*). Each gland is drained just external to the hymen ring of the vestibule posterolaterally. The Bartholin duct, approximately 2.5 cm in length, has three types of epithelial linings depending on the location within the duct. It is lined proximally by mucus-secreting epithelium, distally by transitional epithelium, and, at its exit, by squamous epithelium. The minor vestibular glands are composed of acini lined by simple columnar mucus-secreting epithelium. They lie within 1–2.5 mm of the superficial epithelium and communicate with the vestibular surface. Squamous metaplasia often occurs within these glands and may obliterate them completely, resulting in the formation of a vestibular cleft. These minor glands ring the vestibule and extend from the frenulum on both sides of the meatus, around the external base of the hymenal ring, to the fourchette [38]. Specialized anogenital sweat glands (mammary-like) have been found within the vulvar interlabial sulcus, in the medial aspects of the labia majora, and in lesser numbers within the perineum and about the anus. These glands, with long and wide coiled ducts that

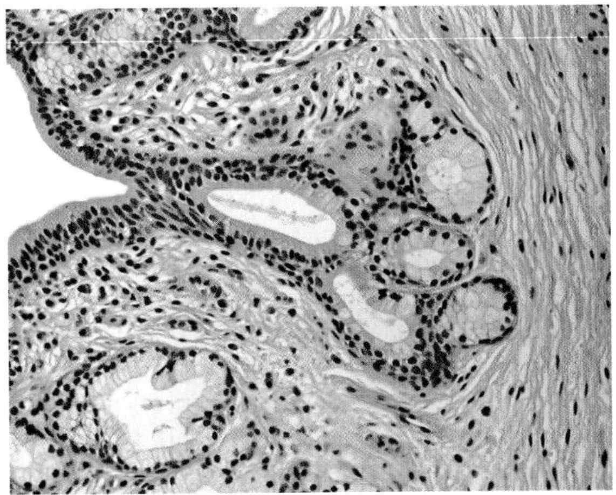

Fig. 1.2
Bartholin duct and gland. **The terminal Bartholin duct has a transitional epithelial-type lining that merges with the simple columnar mucus-secreting epithelium of the Bartholin gland acini. The glands are tubuloalveolar and racemose and the surrounding fibrous stroma is somewhat more cellular than the peripheral stroma**

open to the surface, have a simple columnar epithelium with apical snouts and myoepithelium beneath the glandular epithelium [232, 233].

The clitoris, which has no glands, is covered by thinly keratinized stratified squamous epithelium. Within the stroma of the clitoris are two conjoined corpora cavernosa, which branch near the base of the clitoris and lie along the pubic rami as divided crura. They are invested in a loose fibrous sheath containing abundant nerves and with an incomplete center septum. The dermis, subepithelium, and stroma of the vulva are rich in collagen, blood vessels, and myofibroblastic-type cells that are frequently immunoreactive for desmin [242]. Myxoid-like changes are present within the subepithelial stroma and have been reported extending from the ectocervix to the vulva. Atypical-appearing multinucleated cells may be observed in this subepithelial myxoid area [1]. Sparse numbers of inflammatory cells including lymphocytes, a few plasma cells, and mast cells are normally present in the perivascular spaces and interstitium.

The femoral and inguinal lymph nodes receive lymphatic drainage from the entire vulva except the clitoris, which has a minor secondary lymphatic pathway [97, 135]. Delicate intercommunicating lymphatic vessels extend to the labia minora, clitoral prepuce, and vestibule, bypassing the clitoris. The lymphatic bed of the labia majora drains in an anterosuperior direction toward the mons, joining the lymphatic vessels from the labia minora and prepuce, and then into the ipsilateral inguinal and femoral nodes. Some contralateral flow also may occur into the superior medial nodes of the femoral group. The superficial inguinal lymph nodes, consisting of 8–10 nodes on each side, divided into a superior oblique and an inferior ventral group, are the major nodes that drain the vulva and therefore are included in a radical vulvectomy [150]. The superior oblique group is found about the Poupart ligament, and the inferior ventral group lies above the junction of the saphenous vein and fascia lata. Lymphatic drainage from the clitoris and midline perineum proceeds bilaterally in more than 67% of cases and may bypass the superficial nodes [94]. A second minor lymphatic pathway from the glans clitoris joins the lymphatics of the urethra, traverses the urogenital diaphragm, and merges with the lymphatic plexus on the anterior surface of the bladder. From there, drainage is into the internal iliac, obturator, and external iliac nodes. No direct pathway of lymphatic flow from the clitoris to the pelvic nodes could be demonstrated by in vivo colloid injection [94]. Lymphatic flow from other sites on the vulva usually proceeds to the ipsilateral groin and pelvic lymph nodes. This finding correlates with the observation that in cases of clitoral carcinoma, in which the inguinofemoral lymph nodes are free of tumor, it is highly unlikely that the pelvic nodes are involved.

The superficial and deep external pudendal arteries branch from the femoral artery. The internal pudendal arteries branch from the internal iliac arteries. These branches from the femoral and internal iliac arteries provide the major blood supply to the vulva via the anterior and posterior labial branches. The clitoris, including the crura and corpora cavernosa, is supplied separately by the deep arteries of the clitoris, whereas the anterior vaginal artery supplies blood flow to the vestibule and the Bartholin glands. The venous return parallels the arterial supply. The nerve supply to the vulva includes sensory nerves, special receptors, and autonomic nerves to the vessels and various glands. The major nerves of the vulva derive from the anterior (ilioinguinal) and posterior (pudendal) labial nerves [123]. The clitoris is innervated by the dorsal nerve of the clitoris and the cavernous nerves of the clitoris, which also supply the vestibule [212].

Developmental Abnormalities

The clitoris in an adult women measures 16.064 mm in length, with a transverse diameter of 3.46 mm and longitudinal diameter of 5.161.4 mm. It is slightly larger in parous women. Height and weight do not influence clitoral size [236]. Clitoral hypertrophy may occur as an isolated finding or in association with generalized vulvar enlargement. Clitoral enlargement in a newborn suggests adrenogenital syndrome, exogenous maternal androgen therapy, or some form of hermaphroditism. A clitoral mass from an infant has been identified with chromosomal mosaicism in which the clitoral skin had a hyperdiploid chromosomal abnormality with normal chromosomes being found in the ovary; this is an example of ambiguous genitalia resulting from a somatic cell mutation with maldevelopment of the clitoris [211]. Clitoral enlargement also has been reported associated with lipodystrophy (Lawrence–Seip syndrome) [193]. In addition to developmental abnormalities, a variety of tumors including granular cell tumors, hemangiomas, and vascular, neural, and smooth muscle tumors may cause clitoral enlargement [171, 220].

Hypertrophy and asymmetry of the labia minora may occur without demonstrable etiology and, in some cases, may be associated with chronic irritation, as may be seen in women wearing indwelling urethral catheters. True hypoplasia occurs infrequently and may be a sign of defective steroidogenesis. Slight fusion of the labia minora may be seen in infants without apparent cause and typically responds to topical estrogen cream. Labial fusion, like clitoral hypertrophy, also may be present with intersex disorders. In these situations, the defect is developmental, but such fusion also may be acquired secondary to lichen sclerosus (LS), lichen planus (LP), or inflammatory conditions, with subsequent adhesion formation [107]. A low transverse vaginal septum may occlude the vaginal lumen and result in hematocolpos with the onset of menstruation. Excision of the septum is the usual therapy of choice. Imperforate hymen is remarkably rare, with a reported frequency of 0.014%, and usually is discovered at the onset of menarche between 10 and 18 years of age. Limited surgical excision of the hymen is the usual treatment. Duplication of the vulva is extremely rare and usually is associated with duplication of the internal müllerian system and rectum as well. In müllerian agenesis, the hymen and vagina usually are represented by only a depression in the vestibular area. Congenital absence of the clitoris and external genitalia has also been described. The urethra may open into the vagina rather than into the vestibule. Ectopic urethral orifices are seen occasionally adjacent to the hymen [107].

Inflammatory Diseases of Vulvar Skin

Inflammatory diseases of vulvar skin can be generally categorized into infectious and noninfectious groups (➋ *Table 1.1*). Further classification of infectious diseases according to etiologic agents is summarized in ➋ *Table 1.2*. The most prevalent infectious diseases of the vulva in North America include human papillomavirus (HPV), typically manifested as condyloma acuminatum,

Table 1.1
Inflammatory disorders of the vulva

Infectious diseases	Noninfectious dermatoses
Viral	Papulosquamous disorders
Fungal	Noninfectious bullous dermatoses
Bacterial	Miscellaneous
Parasitic	

Table 1.2
Infectious diseases of vulva skin

Viral infection
Human papillomavirus (HPV) (genital subtype)
Herpes virus (simplex and zoster)
Molluscum contagiosum
Others (rare)
Human papillomavirus (nongenital subtype)
HIV-associated plaques and ulcers
Cytomegalovirus (CMV)
Epstein–Barr virus (EBV)-associated ulcer
Coxsackie virus (hand-foot-mouth disease)
Bacterial infection
Syphilis
Granuloma inguinale
Lymphogranuloma venereum (LGV)
Chancroid
Malakoplakia
Others
Tuberculosis
Erythrasma
Fungal infections
Dermatophytosis
Candidiasis
Parasitic infection
Scabies
Pubic lice
Others
Enterobius vermicularis
Schistosomiasis
Demodex

HIV, human immunodeficiency virus.

Table 1.3
Infectious diseases of the vulva

Disease	Causative microorganism	Salient features	Diagnostic methods
Condyloma acuminatum	Papillomavirus	Acanthosis, hyperkeratosis, parakeratosis, papillomatosis, perinuclear halo (koilocyte)	Histopathology, Immunohistochemistry, Molecular hybridization
Herpes genitalis	Herpes simplex hominis type II	Intranuclear inclusions	Cytopathology, culture, serology, Immunohistochemistry
Syphilitic chancre	*Treponema pallidum*	Ulceration, chronic inflammation, vasculitis	Dark-field, fluorescence, silver stain, serology
Condyloma lata	*Treponema pallidum*	Like chancre, with epithelial hyperplasia	Same as syphilitic chancre
Molluscum contagiosum	DNA poxvirus group	Intracytoplasmic inclusions	Cytopathology, histopathology
Granuloma inguinale	*Calymmatobacterium granulomatis*	Donovan bodies, granulomatous reaction without caseation, pseudoepitheliomatous hyperplasia	Giemsa stain, silver stain
Lymphogranuloma venereum	Chlamydia (TRIC agent)	Granulomatous reaction without caseation	Serology
Tuberculosis	Mycobacterium tuberculosis	Acid-fast bacilli (AFB), granulomatous reaction with caseation	AFB stain, AFB culture, PCR
Chancroid	*Hemophilus ducreyi*	Granulomatous reaction without caseation	Culture, Gram stain

herpes genitalis, syphilis, and molluscum contagiosum (*Table 1.3*). Clinical diagnosis does not necessarily require specific organism characterization in all these conditions.

Human Papillomavirus Infection

General Features

Human papillomavirus (HPV) infection is responsible for benign tumors, that is, condylomata acuminata and precursor lesions of certain types of vulvar carcinoma (i.e., vulvar intraepithelial neoplasia, VIN) [56, 118, 185]. (The latter types are described in Chap. 2, Premalignant and Malignant Tumors of the Vulva.) Condylomata acuminata (genital warts) are predominately sexually transmitted benign neoplasms that may involve the vulva, vagina, cervix, urethra, anal canal, and perianal skin [164]. The prevalence of HPV infection varies greatly, depending on the population studied. In most studies, clinically evident vulvar involvement is less common than cervical HPV infection [69, 124]. Molecular biologic methods have identified HPV-6 as the most common HPV type in typical genital condylomata acuminata. HPV-11 has been found in approximately one fourth of genital warts [25, 255]. These two HPV types are responsible for over 90% of condyloma acuminata.

Clinical Features

Condylomas present as papillary, verrucous, or papular lesions of the skin and mucous membrane that are nearly always multiple and frequently confluent (*Fig. 1.3*). Most lesions are asymptomatic unless secondarily infected. Condylomata acuminata are commonly associated with vaginitis, pregnancy, diabetes mellitus, oral contraceptive use, poor perineal hygiene, immunosuppression, and sexual activity with multiple partners or a partner exposed to other partners [8, 39, 151, 169]. Approximately 30–50% of women with vulvar condyloma acuminatum have associated cervical HPV infection [240]. The presence of vulvar condyloma acuminatum in children may be related to sexual abuse [58, 163, 254].

Approximately 40–60% of children with laryngeal papillomatosis are born from mothers with a history of genital HPV infection [70]. However, the true incidence of infection of the larynx of the newborn infant, from a mother with genital papillomavirus infection is

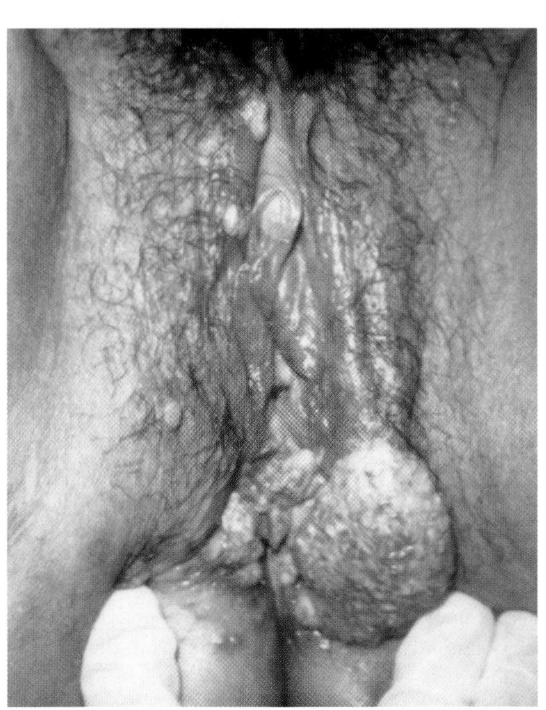

◘ Fig. 1.3
Condylomata acuminata. **Involvement of vulva and perianal region**

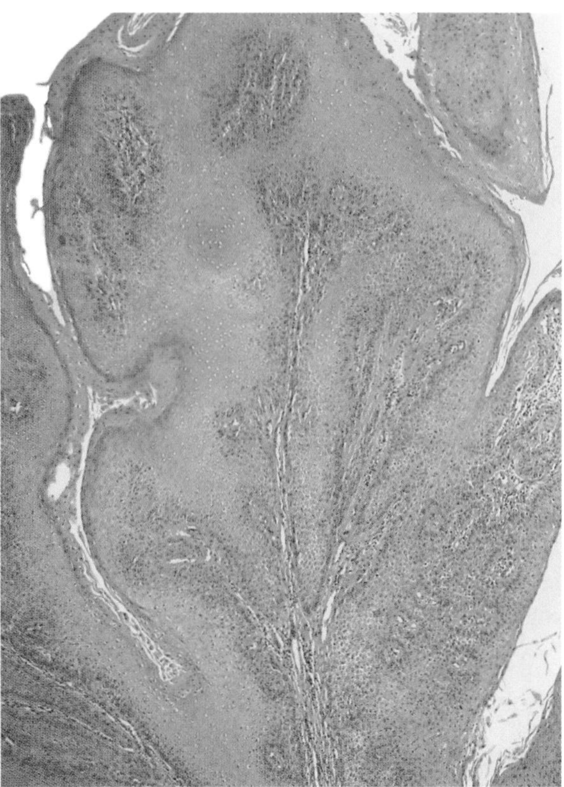

◘ Fig. 1.4
Condyloma acuminatum. **Verrucous epidermal hyperplasia with broad rounded papillation**

unknown but is probably low. No correlation has been shown between the volume of maternal wart tissue and occurrence of infantile laryngeal papillomatosis. Employing DNA hybridization techniques, it has been observed that approximately one half of laryngeal papillomas contain HPV-11 [59, 216]. This finding supports the view that laryngeal papillomas of infancy and childhood are acquired at the time of vaginal delivery.

Gross Findings

Condylomata acuminata usually present as discrete papillary growths, with a central stalk or as large sessile lesions. On the cervix, vagina, or vulva, condyloma acuminata may present as slightly raised rough areas with irregular borders. Small lesions are best appreciated with application of 3–5% acetic acid for 3–5 min on colposcopic examination. Lesions that are detectable by colposcopic magnification only, or by performing HPV testing on the tissue in question, are considered subclinical [48, 91].

Microscopic Findings

Acanthosis, dyskeratosis, parakeratosis, hyperkeratosis, and a prominent granular layer are seen. A superficial chronic inflammatory infiltrate often is present in the dermis. Typical perinuclear cytoplasmic "halos," with "raisinoid" pyknotic nuclei or slightly enlarged nuclei (koilocytosis), are commonly present in the superficial epithelial cells, and binucleated and multinucleated squamous cells often are found (➲ *Figs. 1.4* and ➲ *1.5*). Parabasal hyperplasia with accentuated intracellular bridges may be seen. Enlarged parabasal cells with "foamy" or "ground glass"-appearing nuclear chromatin may be present. In situ hybridization studies on cervical tissue have demonstrated the presence of HPV DNA in condylomata [159].

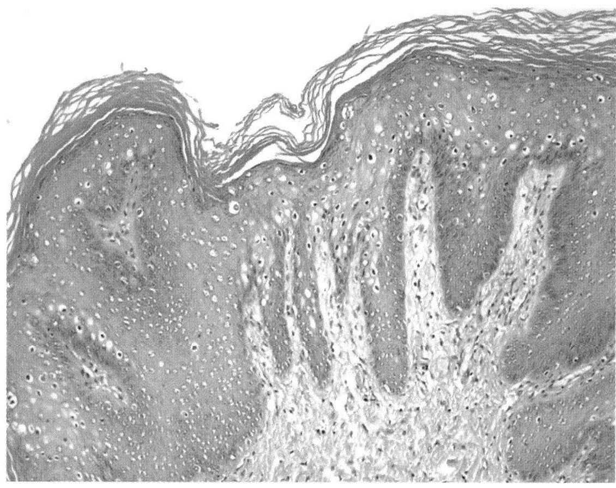

Fig. 1.5
Condyloma acuminatum. **Parabasal hyperplasia is present. Above the basilar layer, koilocytotic cells with prominent perinuclear halos are found in the more superficial epithelium**

Differential Diagnosis

Condylomata acuminata at times may be difficult to distinguish from VIN. Condylomata typically are verrucous or papillary and display koilocytosis, parabasal hyperplasia, accentuated intracellular bridges, dyskeratosis, accentuation of the granular layer, and hyperkeratosis. Mitotic figures are infrequently found. In contrast, the presence of flat macular growth, abnormal mitoses, cytologically atypical nuclei, marked variation in nuclear size and shape, and hyperchromasia are characteristics of VIN lesions. Unlike VIN, condylomas usually are diploid; however, atypia may be seen related to tetraploidy or octoploidy. Unlike VIN, this atypia is characterized by large nuclei, with moderate nuclear pleomorphism and some degree of hyperchromasia, but without abnormal mitosis. A high-grade VIN lesion induced by oncogenic HPV often correlates with aneuploidy [153, 194], which is rare in common condyloma.

Typical condylomas will be HPV antigen positive by immunoperoxidase techniques in approximately 50% of cases, whereas VIN will be immunoreactive in less than 10% of cases; however, such testing is not of value in distinguishing these two entities [98]. In a given case of VIN, a spectrum may be found from typical VIN 3 to adjacent changes that may have the morphologic changes of condyloma acuminatum. As a matter of practice, the first diagnosis given on the pathology report is that of the most serious lesion identified, with subsequent diagnosis following. In our present state of understanding, it is acceptable to classify flat condylomata acuminata (condyloma plana) of the vulva as VIN 1 (see Vulvar Intraepithelial Neoplasia in Chap. 2). Regressing or early flat condylomata acuminata also may resemble lichen simplex chronicus (LSC) or squamous cell hyperplasia; however, the prominent granular layer, accentuated intracellular bridges, parabasal hyperplasia, and koilocytosis are typically lacking. If this cannot be resolved by histopathologic examination, molecular biologic methods such as Hybrid Capture 2, polymerase chain reaction (PCR), or in situ hybridization, to detect HPV, may be applicable and are of value in establishing the diagnosis of HPV-associated changes when virus is identified [86].

Vulvar vestibular papilloma is differentiated from condylomata in that the epithelium lacks hyperkeratosis and other typical microscopic features of condyloma. Moreover, vestibular papilloma are confined to the vulva vestibule [17, 77]. Fibroepithelial polyps may have the shape of large condylomas; however, the epithelium also lacks the microscopic features of condyloma. Condylomata lata may resemble condylomata acuminata clinically; however, on biopsy, the deep inflammatory infiltrates with plasma cells and the presence of spirochetes on a Warthin–Starry silver stain distinguishes these lesions.

Clinical Behavior and Treatment

The natural history of HPV infection of the vulva usually is one of a long protracted course and may be influenced by immunologic factors [6]. Regression has been noted after pregnancy. Presentation following radiation therapy has been observed [169]. Progression of condyloma acuminatum of the vulva to VIN and malignant transformation to squamous cell carcinoma have been observed [227]. Oncogenesis secondary to papillomavirus is well recognized in experimental animals. The association of vulvar and vaginal condylomata acuminata with invasive squamous cell carcinoma has been documented in women with immunosuppressive conditions such as Fanconi anemia and Hodgkin disease [242] (see Chap. 2, Premalignant and Malignant Tumors of the Vulva).

The topical application of dilute podophyllin [21] or the judicious application of concentrated halogenated acetic acid (trichloroacetic acid) is the common approach to the treatment of small vulvar condylomata. Electrodesiccation, surgical excision, cryosurgery, hot wire electroloop excision, laser ablation, and interferon have been used for large lesions [6, 23, 49, 116, 206, 239].

Herpesvirus Infection

General Features

The causative agent is the herpes simplex virus (HSV) (var. hominis type 2), although in some instances the type I virus may be involved. The incidence of herpesvirus infection in the USA has been reported as 126 per 100,000; approximately 600,000 new cases of genital herpes occur each year in the USA. The prevalence of the HSV-2 antibody among women in the USA is 26%, although genital herpes has been diagnosed in only a small proportion (10–25%) of individuals with HSV-2 antibodies. Herpes simplex virus type I is becoming a more frequent cause of genital herpes, especially among young women. Although approximately 20% of the US population has been infected by HSV 2, the frequency of vulvar involvement is unknown [3, 127, 137, 161].

Clinical Features

The initial clinical presentation frequently includes dysuria or urinary retention with vulvar pain that may be incapacitating. Systemic symptoms, including generalized malaise and fever, are frequently seen along with a mild inguinal lymphadenopathy. The sequential appearance of vesicles, pustules, and painful shallow ulcers that often are infected secondarily with bacteria characterize the clinical findings. The vesicles usually are asymptomatic, whereas the ulcers are extremely painful (➋ *Fig. 1.6*). The lesions can involve the anus, urethra, bladder, cervix, and vagina, as well as the vulva. The acute ulcers heal in approximately 16 days [137, 234]. Of the women who are culture positive for HSV, diagnostic genital vesicles and ulcers are present in approximately two thirds; the remainder of the women have nondetectable or atypical lesions or are asymptomatic [122, 234].

Microscopic Findings

An early intact herpes simplex vesicle extends deeply into the epidermis. The histologic transformation of the HSV-infected epithelial cell begins with a homogenization of the nuclear chromatin resulting in a "ground glass" appearance, which then progresses to the more typical eosinophilic intranuclear inclusion body [75]. The characteristic intranuclear inclusions are seen at the periphery of the lesion (➋ *Figs. 1.7* and ➋ *1.8*). Subsequently, the cells undergo karyorrhexis and lysis. A biopsy taken in the late ulcerative phase, therefore, does not always show the intranuclear inclusions. Cytologic evaluation of the scraping of the base and edges (Tzank preparation) of a fresh ulcer, or freshly opened vesicle, usually will show the multinucleated cells with viral cytopathic effects characteristic of HSV infection. Cytologic examination of vesicular aspirate is an effective method of identifying the cytopathic changes of HSV and is almost as sensitive

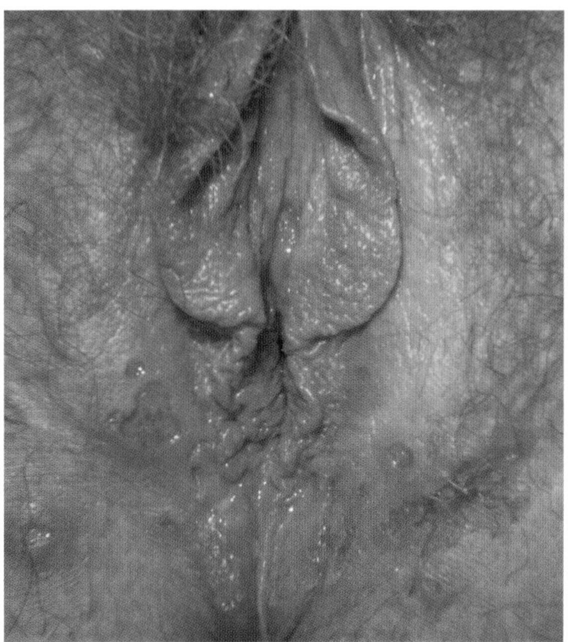

Fig. 1.6
Herpes simplex ulcer. **Herpes simplex virus (HSV) infection, untreated, 7 days after the onset of symptoms. Multifocal ulceration is present**

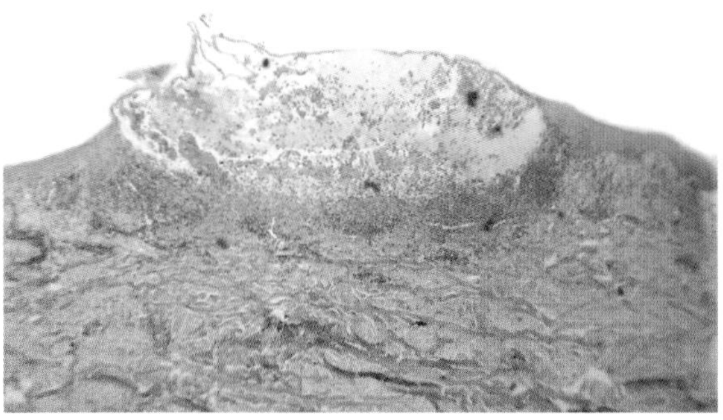

Fig. 1.7
Herpes simplex ulcer. **Sharply circumscribed crater**

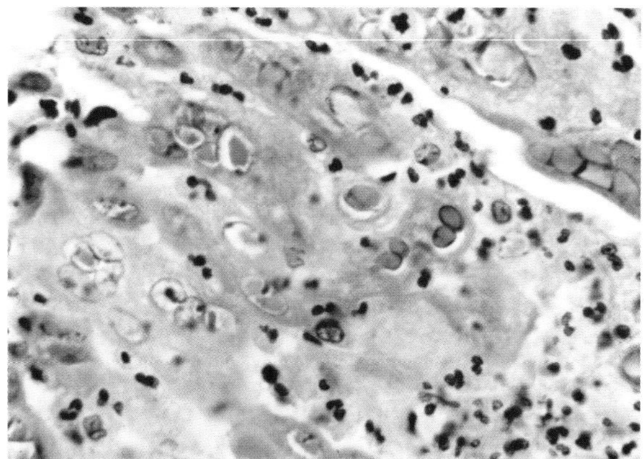

Fig. 1.8
Herpes simplex. **High-power view of viral-infected cells with multinucleation and homogenized "ground glass" intranuclear viral inclusions**

as virus isolation. Moistening the ulcer with a saline-soaked sponge and then scraping the ulcer with a wooden spatula may improve the diagnostic yield from ulcerative lesions. Whether the sample is from an ulcer or a freshly opened vesicle, the specimen should be smeared on a clean slide, rapidly fixed in 95% ethanol, or with spray fixative, and stained with Papanicolaou stain. Morphologic changes seen with HSV infection are not reliable in separating primary from secondary infection or in distinguishing HSV type I from type II infection. Development of serologic assays to detect antibodies to herpes simplex virus (HSV) glycoproteins (g)G1 and (g)G2 has allowed accurate definition of the seroprevalence of HSV-2 from HSV-1. Furthermore, herpes zoster can involve the vulva and may have similar cytologic findings.

Adjunctive Methods

HSV-specific fluorescein conjugated antiserum may be placed on smears of ulcers or vesicles to identify HSV antigens. Immunoperoxidase techniques, employing HSV-specific antibodies, may be of value if the histopathologic findings are nonspecific and can be employed on paraffin-embedded tissue. Isolation of HSV, whether type I or type II, can be achieved by the inoculation of tissue culture monolayers, such as WI-38 human embryonic lung fibroblasts or monkey kidney cells. Both types of HSV produce characteristic cytopathic changes on these cell lines, which are confirmed by direct immunofluorescence employing monoclonal antibodies to HSV [122]. Virus isolation can be achieved within 4 days [249]. Rapid viral culture over 24 h, followed by a search for HSV antigen using an immunoperoxidase technique, can give results in less than 2 days.

Polymerase chain reaction (PCR) technique, employing HSV-specific primers, is another approach to the positive identification of HSV infections [52, 199, 225]. Serologic studies on acute and convalescent serum samples are of value in distinguishing primary from recurrent infection. In primary infection, significant rises (more than fourfold dilution) are found. In recurrent infection, the patient is seropositive at presentation and antibody titers will not rise consistently. Serologic methods are not reliable in separating HSV type I from type II [249]. Asymptomatic viral shedding of HSV has been documented in 1.5–3% of women who are seropositive for HSV type II [122]. HSV infection may have some oncogenic potential; however, this relationship remains to be defined [100, 117].

Clinical Behavior and Treatment

Recurrent episodes of herpatic vulvitis are common after primary infection; recurrences decrease in frequency over time, whether or not acyclovir is given prophylactically. Acyclovir may reduce the severity of infection if given early in the course of illness [107, 137].

Varicella (Herpes Zoster) (Vulvar Shingles)

Varicella infection of the vulva is rare. The prodromal pain within the vulva, without apparent physical findings, may simulate vestibulitis. The subsequent development of vesicles and ulcers assists in making the distinction because vestibulitis is not associated with vesicles and ulcers. The patients usually are postmenopausal or immunosuppressed, and the vesicles are characteristically unilateral [11, 111]. The cytologic findings from scrapings of opened vesicles, as well as the histologic findings, are those of a herpesvirus infection. Therapy with famciclovir is reported to reduce pain significantly if begun within 48 hours of the presentation of the rash [175, 230]. The protracted neuralgia and recurrent bouts of vesicles are as described for shingles.

Cytomegalovirus Infection

Cytomegalovirus (CMV) vulvitis, like herpes type II vulvitis, presents with an ulcerated vulvovaginitis.

The histopathologic findings are similar, although the viral inclusions are both intranuclear and intracytoplasmic. Viral inclusions also may be seen involving vascular endothelial cells, as well as the epithelial cells. CMV infection has been associated with vulvar ulcers in a woman with acquired immunodeficiency syndrome (AIDS). Culture or immunoperoxidase studies using specific antibodies to CMV, or PCR employing CMV-specific primers, are necessary to establish the diagnosis [71].

Epstein–Barr Virus Infection

Epstein–Barr virus (EBV) has been cultured from painful ulcers on the labia minora during primary infection of infectious mononucleosis. The ulcers slowly healed over a few weeks [223]. EBV infection may be a sexually transmitted disease [223].

Molluscum Contagiosum

Molluscum contagiosum is a moderately contagious viral disease that, in adults, is often related to intimate or sexual contact [67]. Molluscum contagiosum usually is asymptomatic; however, perianal lesions frequently become pruritic or secondarily infected. The lesions are small, smooth papules (3–6 mm in diameter) with a central punctum or umbilication. They generally are multiple and separate, although they may be single. Rare plaque formations, made up of 50–100 individual clustered lesions, also have been described. The incubation period varies between 14 and 50 days. Clinical diagnosis usually does not require biopsy.

Cytologic identification of the typical eosinophilic intracytoplasmic inclusion bodies (Henderson–Paterson bodies) within scrapings from the interior of the molluscum papule is adequate to confirm the diagnosis. Histologic examination demonstrates marked acanthosis and the characteristic intracytoplasmic viral inclusions in recent infections (*Figs. 1.9* and *1.10*). With aging, the cytoplasmic bodies take on a more basophilic appearance preceding lysis of the cell [67]. The central dimple of the lesion is seen histologically if the lesion is carefully bisected. Within the dermis, there often is a marked vascular response with endothelial proliferation and perivascular inflammation. Electron microscopy has demonstrated that the virus is spherical, ellipsoidal, or brick shaped and contains a DNA core with a two-layered protein coat measuring 210–300 nm [148]. Most lesions regress spontaneously; untreated lesions may persist for

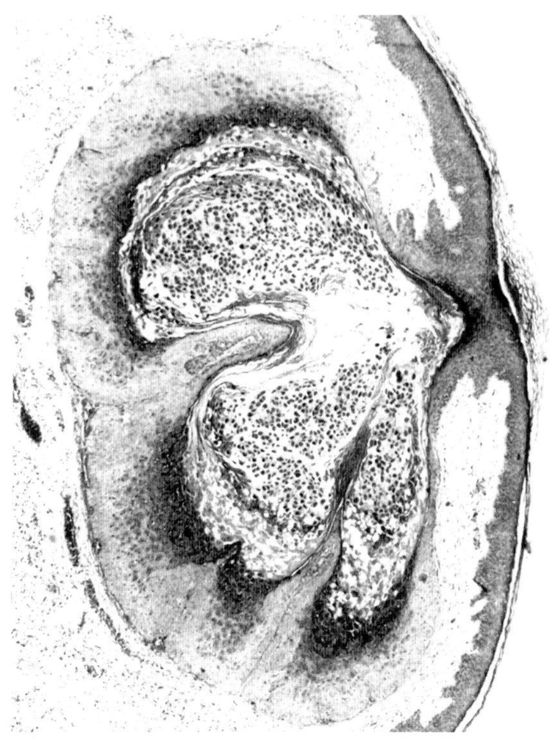

Fig. 1.9
Molluscum contagiosum. **Cup-shaped papule under low power shows exo- and endophytic epidermal acanthotic hyperplasia with increasing density of intracytoplasmic inclusions as the surface umbilication is approached**

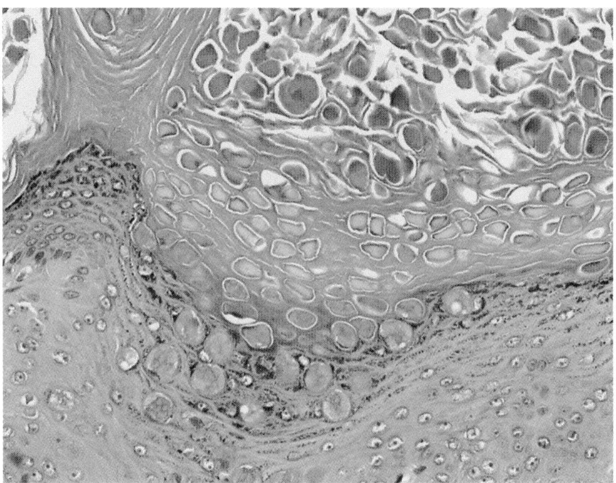

Fig. 1.10
Molluscum contagiosum. **High-power view of intracytoplasmic inclusions (molluscum bodies)**

years, during which time they may be spread by close contact or autoinoculation.

Syphilis

Clinical Features

Syphilis is a venereal disease caused by the spirochete *Treponema pallidum*. The primary lesion is the chancre, a painless, indurated, shallow, clean-based ulcer with raised edges. The chancre usually presents within 3 weeks after initial contact; the range, however, is 7–90 days. If secondarily infected, the chancre may become soft and painful and show an ulcerated surface. Although chancres are generally single, they may be multiple. Chancres may occur on inconspicuous surfaces, such as the cervix, anal mucosa,.or oral pharynx. In approximately 50% of women and 30% of men the primary lesion is never seen. Lymphadenopathy presents 3–4 days after the chancre. The nodes are nontender, freely movable, and rubbery [27]. Left untreated in the primary phase, the chancre will heal within 2–6 weeks and typically does not leave a scar [155, 244]. The secondary stage of the disease will become evident within 6 weeks to 6 months. At this point, the patient may present with a skin rash that often involves mucous membranes as well as the palms of the hands and soles of the feet [27]. On occasion, the secondary lesions are papular, especially about the vulva, presenting as elevated plaques up to 3 cm in diameter. These are known as condylomata lata, which clinically may mimic condylomata acuminata (➋ *Fig. 1.11*). Such lesions also may occur on other mucocutaneous borders. The tertiary gumma of syphilis is rarely seen on the vulva.

Microscopic Findings

If syphilis were not considered in the clinical differential diagnosis, the diagnosis may be quite difficult from histologic material alone. The primary chancre is characterized by ulceration of the epidermis with acute and chronic inflammation within the dermis. There is a marked perivascular inflammatory response, characterized by the presence of large numbers of plasma cells. Histologic examination of condylomata lata reveals marked acanthosis and hyperkeratosis (➋ *Figs. 1.12* and ➋ *1.13*). The inflammatory response within the dermis is similar to that in the primary chancre with a marked, predominantly plasma cell inflammatory infiltrate. The arteritis in both lesions may be sufficiently severe to result in obliteration of the smaller vessels. Dieterle, Warthin–Starry, or Steiner stains for spirochetes are always of value if there is any suspicion of syphilis (➋ *Fig. 1.14*), but may be negative with active infection. Serologic studies for syphilis should be performed if syphilis is considered clinically or from the pathologic findings [165].

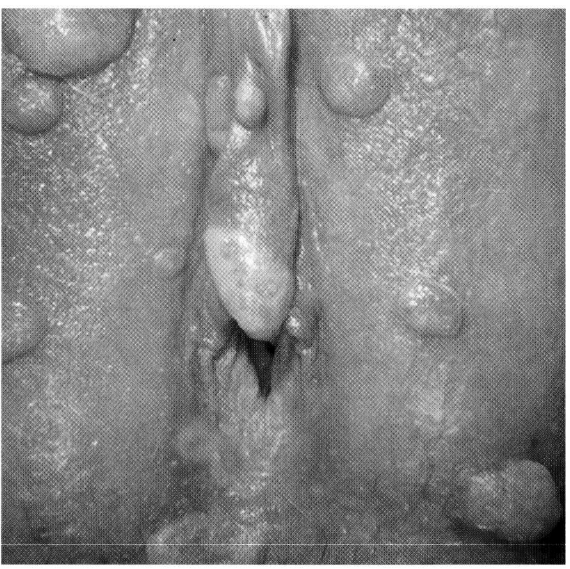

■ Fig. 1.11
Condyloma lata. **Multiple papules are present**

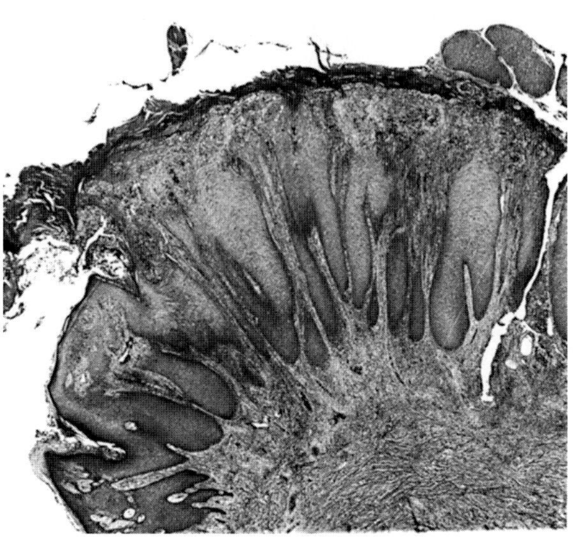

■ Fig. 1.12
Condyloma lata. **Marked psoriasiform epidermal hyperplasia with scales in the cornified layer. (Courtesy of R.J. Kurman, M.D., Baltimore, MD.)**

Adjunctive Methods

The primary chancre, as well as the condyloma latum and other secondary lesions, are rich in spirochetes. Therefore, when a chancre or secondary lesion of syphilis is suspected, an attempt to identify spirochetes within the lesion should be made. This examination is accomplished either through dark-field examination of serum expressed from the base of the ulcer or by the fluorescent conjugated antibody technique, which employs a dried smear preparation. The organism measures up to 15 mm in length and 0.20 mm in thickness; it is spiral in shape, with 6–14 coils. Motility, characterized by flexion, rotation about the long axis, and random movement are noted on dark-field examination of fresh sera from an active lesion. These methods for identification of spirochetes are far more sensitive and specific than is silver stain on paraffin-embedded tissue. The chancre may be present for weeks before serologic tests become reactive. More than 70% of patients with dark-field-positive lesions have a reactive serology at the time of initial diagnosis. The most common serologic testing methods are based on the identification of reagin. These tests become positive approximately 1 month after the disease is contracted. Common reagin testing methods employ microflocculation testing and include the Venereal Disease Research Laboratory (VDRL) and rapid plasma reagin (RPR) [252]. These two tests have similar specificity and can be quantitated to evaluate the course of the disease and response to therapy. The fluorescent treponemal antibody-absorbed (FTA-ABS) test, still the "gold standard," is highly sensitive and is ordered if the reagin tests are nonreactive, weakly reactive, or if there is a possibility of a false-positive result. Biologic false positives can occur in lupus erythematosus, virus infection, cirrhosis of the liver, pregnancy, malaria, and other inflammatory or autoimmune diseases. Treponemal enzyme immunoassays (EIAs) are an appropriate alternative to the use of combined Venereal Disease Research Laboratory/rapid plasma

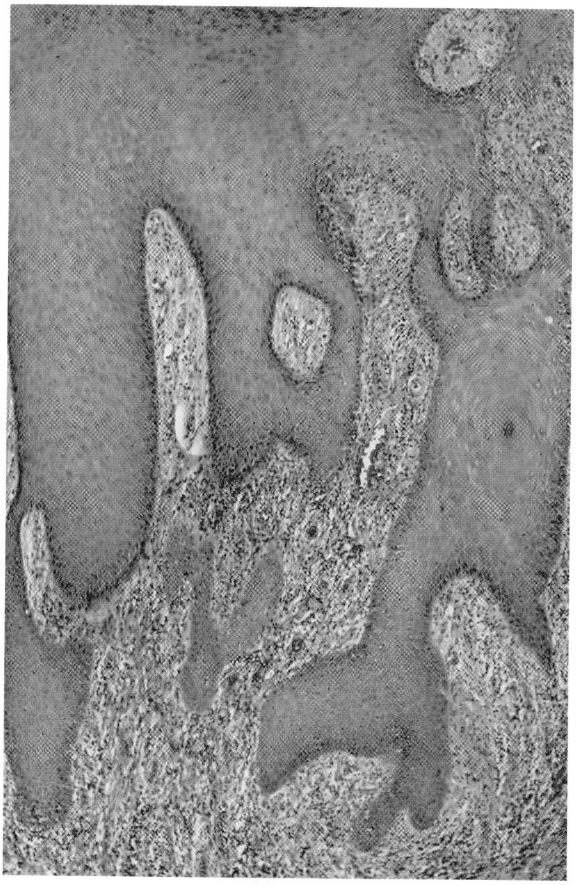

Fig. 1.13
Condyloma latum. **Prominent acanthosis is present with a marked dermal perivascular inflammatory cell infiltrate that consists primarily of plasma cells and lymphocytes, with some neutrophils**

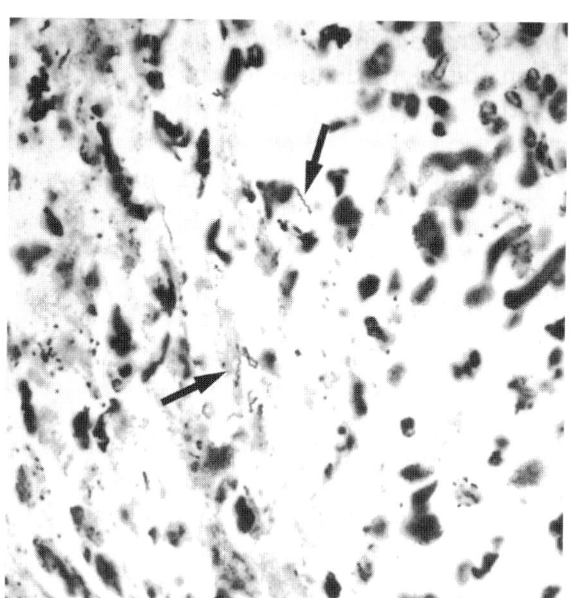

Fig. 1.14
Secondary syphilis. **Warthin–Starry stain shows spirochetes in the dermis**

reagin and Treponema pallidum hemagglutination assay (TPHA) tests for screening for syphilis. If a treponemal EIA is used for screening an alternative treponemal test, such as TPHA, should be used for confirmatory testing. The fluorescent treponemal antibody-absorbed test is probably best reserved for specimens giving discrepant results [64].

Once the FTA-ABS becomes positive, it can remain so forever in the life of the patient. Although newer technologies, such as PCR and immunoblotting, have been used in detection of syphilis, serologic tests with RPR/VDRL and FTA-ABS are still the current tests of choice [252]. If the FTA-ABS is positive, spinal fluid serologic evaluation will be necessary to rule out neurosyphilis. A false-positive FTA-ABS is rare and, if detected, requires *T. pallidum* mobilization testing and careful follow-up [155].

Clinical Behavior and Treatment

Approximately 30% of patients with primary syphilis will undergo spontaneous remission of the disease. Those who are not treated or who do not achieve spontaneous remission may progress to tertiary syphilis with its well-recognized cardiovascular and central nervous system effects. Untreated syphilis may prove fatal in 10% of those afflicted. Penicillin or another appropriate systemic antibiotic is the treatment of choice.

Granuloma Inguinale

Granuloma inguinale (donovanosis; granuloma venereum) is caused by Calymmatobacterium granulomatous, a gram-negative, heavily encapsulated rod considered to be in the bacterial family Enterobacteriaceae. Granuloma inguinale occurs with approximately equal frequency in men and women. Primary lesions may occur on the vulva, vagina, or cervix and may present as painless papules or necrotizing ulcers with rolled borders and a friable base. Inguinal adenopathy usually is absent [26]. The lesions usually appear within 1 week to 1 month of exposure; anal coitus or fecal contamination of the vulva or vagina has been incriminated as the mode of transmission [155, 244]. Granuloma inguinale extends primarily by local infiltration, although lymphatic permeation may occur during later stages of the disease. Chronic lymphatic infiltration and fibrosis frequently result in a massive brawny edema of the external genitalia. There is controversy as to the true origin of the edema, because dye injection studies suggest that the lymphatic drainage is intact. With involvement of the cervix, the disease may advance via the cervical lymphatics to involve parametrial tissue [191].

The clinical diagnosis of granuloma inguinale depends on the identification of the Donovan bodies within the tissue; this is best accomplished by preparing smears or a biopsy from the edge of the ulcer and pressing this biopsy tissue between two slides. The tissue imprints are air dried, fixed in methanol, and stained with Giemsa stain. Any antibiotic treatment may obscure the diagnosis, necessitating biopsy at a later date to identify organisms. Histologically, the main portion of the lesion consists of granulation tissue associated with an extensive chronic inflammatory cell infiltrate and endarteritis. An ulcer usually is covered with a fibrinous exudate, and necrosis may be present. The surface epithelium, adjacent to the ulcer, may show prominent pseudoepitheliomatous hyperplasia. Necrosis and microabscesses may be seen within the epidermis [191]. Within the granulation tissue there is a dense mixed inflammatory cell infiltrate, consisting predominantly of plasma cells and mononuclear cells with few lymphocytes, which extends into the dermis. Large vacuolated histiocytes that contain the characteristic encapsulated bacilli, Donovan bodies, within their cytoplasm frequently are present (➲ *Fig. 1.15*); they can be demonstrated with a Warthin–Starry stain or Giemsa stain. The Donovan bodies may be found extracellularly, as well as intracellularly, and may appear coccoid, coccobacillary, or bacillary [26, 191]. Ultrathin plastic-embedded sections, as well as electron microscopy, may be of value in diagnosis [26, 191].

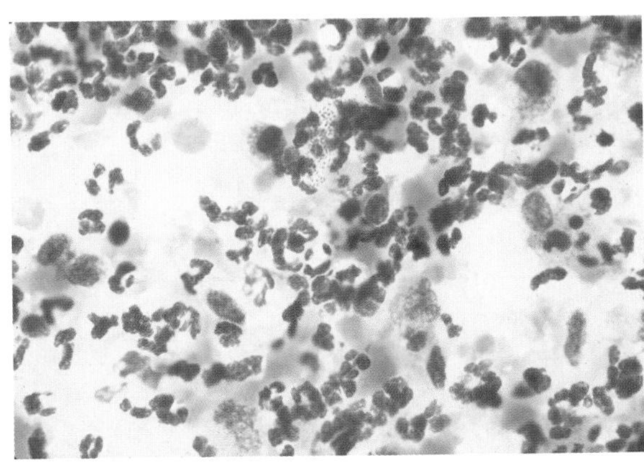

Fig. 1.15
Granuloma inguinale. **Giemsa stain shows intracytoplasmic Donovan bodies with characteristic halo around the organisms**

Calymmatobacterium granulomatous may be cultured by special techniques. The diagnosis depends on the clinical findings and documenting the organism within a tissue specimen or by culture. Syphilis, chancroid, and herpesvirus infection usually are included in the differential diagnosis [113].

Lymphogranuloma Venereum

Lymphogranuloma venereum (LGV) is caused by Chlamydia, and occurs approximately three times more frequently in men than in women. The disease has three phases: (1) erosion of the skin, (2) adenitis, and (3) fibrosis and destruction [26]. Lympho-granuloma venereum is spread primarily via the lymphatics. The initial ulcers, which generally are not tender or painful, often are ignored. Adenitis may evolve into painful superficial groin nodes, or buboes, that frequently rupture through the skin with exudation of a purulent discharge. The third phase of the disease often results in stricture and fibrosis of the vagina and rectum [246]. During this phase, chronic lymphatic obstruction is responsible for the characteristic nonpitting edema of the external genitalia. The histology of LGV is not diagnostic and reveals no characteristic identifiable organisms by the usual modes of investigation. Smears and biopsy specimens should be evaluated for organisms (spirochetes, Donovan bodies, etc.) to rule out other diseases with a similar presentation. Histologically, giant cells may be seen along with lymphocytes and plasma cells (➋ *Fig. 1.16*). Older lesions may exhibit extensive fibrosis of the dermis and sinus tracts. The diagnosis is based on the typical clinical presentation, along with positive complement fixation tests. Culture, as well as other specific immunohistochemical tests, can assist in the diagnosis of LGV. Treatment is systemic tetracycline or doxycycline [155, 244].

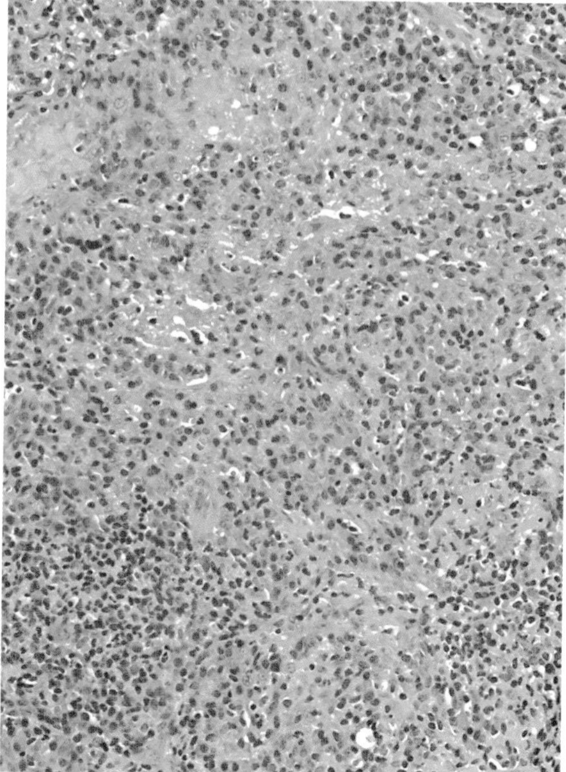

Fig. 1.16
Lymphogranuloma venereum (LGV). **An intense superficial and deep chronic inflammatory infiltrate is present, composed predominantly of lymphocytes and plasma cells**

Chancroid

Chancroid is relatively rare and presents with a genital ulcer that usually is tender, nonindurated, and has a friable purulent erythematous base. Primary lesions may be single or multiple and tend to be small, measuring approximately 1–2 mm in diameter. Coalescence of the lesions leads to ulcers approaching 3 cm in diameter. Tender inguinal adenopathy with flocculent nodes may be present. The incubation period may be as short as 10 days [228]. The clinical differential diagnosis includes herpesvirus infection and primary syphilis [113, 228]. Chancroid is caused by the organism *Haemophilus ducreyi*, a gram-negative, nonmotile bacillus, which in culture grows in pairs and parallel chains. Skin tests and biopsies may not be diagnostic. Identification of the organism by culture is necessary for accurate diagnosis [228]. Selective agar medium has been developed for the organism, which has improved culture isolation. Recent advances in nonculture diagnostic tests using PCR have enhanced our ability to diagnose chancroid [170, 228]. Histologic examination of the tissue demonstrated a granulomatous-type reaction with chronic inflammatory cells consisting primarily of lymphocytes and plasma cells, and the presence of the gram-negative organisms, which may be present in large numbers and in parallel chains [112].

HIV-Associated Vulva Ulcers

Human immunodeficiency virus (HIV) infection-associated vulva ulcers are usually painful and multiple. A recent study revealed that about 60% of vulva ulcerations have no proven etiologic agent. The rest of the patients are positive for HSV II, unusual or mixed bacteria, and rarely cytomegalovirus, *Chlamydia trachomatis*, and *Gardnerella vaginalis*. Human immunodeficiency virus may play a local role in causation or exacerbation [126].

Vulvar Apthosis

Vulvar apthus ulcers have been reported, but are rare. Vulvar apthosis manifests as painful, shallow ulcers typically with a gray-white base. Most ulcers are less than 5 mm and heal within 7 to 10 days. These ulcers as with oral aphthae, have a much higher predilection for white adolescents who are not sexually active. As with oral apthosis, the etioology is unclear. Risk factors for these ulcers include stress, infections, vitamin deficiency, and family history [95].

Tuberculosis

Tuberculosis of the vulva is rare. It usually is associated with tuberculosis of other genital sites, primarily the fallopian tube, and endometrium. Genital involvement usually is associated with pulmonary tuberculosis. Autoinoculation by hematogenous or direct spread therefore is the most common method of transmission to the vulva. Primary inoculation or sexual transmission of tuberculosis is very uncommon. Immunosuppression may play a role in susceptibility, as a case of vulvar tuberculosis has been described in a renal transplant patient [224]. The usual organism is *Mycobacterium tuberculosis*; however, atypical mycobacteria also have been incriminated. Diagnosis usually can be made by biopsy of the involved tissues. Caseating granulomas with Langhans giant cells are found, and acid-fast stains usually reveal the mycobacterium (➋ *Fig. 1.17*). Confirmation of the diagnosis can be made by culture techniques. Appropriate long-term systemic antibiotics are the recommended therapy. Giant cells of the foreign body type are encountered frequently in vulvar tissues in which a previous biopsy has been performed. These giant cells, associated with noncaseating granulomas, often result from embedded suture occasionally seen in prior biopsied areas, and should not be confused with tuberculosis. Vulvar ulceration, secondary to sarcoidosis, has been reported and should be included in the differential diagnosis of granulomatous ulcerations of the vulva [54, 114].

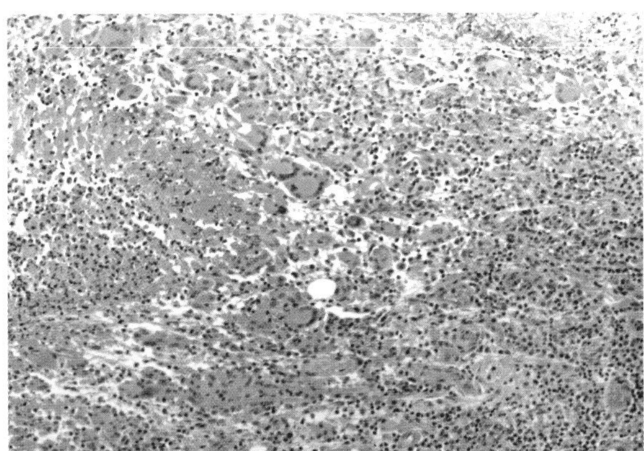

Fig. 1.17
Vulvar tuberculosis. **Caseating granulomas with Langhans giant cells**

Fungal Infection and Miscellaneous Infectious Diseases

Chronic inflammatory conditions of the vulvar and perianal skin without concomitant ulceration often are caused by fungal infections, although a variety of irritants, unrelated to infection, may be responsible [144]. Candida and dermatophytes are frequent pathogens. Such conditions rarely require biopsy, and accurate diagnosis generally can be accomplished by microscopic examination of skin scrapings placed in 10% potassium hydroxide, or by appropriate culture methods. Topical antifungal creams are the usual therapy. Chronic and acute vaginitis related to trichomonas, Chlamydia, Candida species, or other infectious agents may be associated with inflammation of the vulva, especially the vulvar vestibule. The histologic findings usually are not diagnostic. Vulvar candidiasis usually can be diagnosed by employing silver stains for fungus, with recognition of the fungal organisms within the keratin, or superficial epithelium. Bacterial infections may produce clinical findings similar to those seen with fungal infections.

Erythrasma is a chronic bacterial infection of the genitocrural area that shows a coral-red fluorescence under Wood's light. The disease is most common in obese diabetes. Scrapings of these lesions, when stained with Gram stain, demonstrate the causative gram-positive bacteria, *Corynebacterium minutissimum*, in rods, filaments, and coccoid forms [113].

Parasitic Infections

Enterobius vermicularis (pinworm, seatworm) is a relatively common intestinal parasite. The female worm measures 8–13 mm in length and 0.5 mm in diameter. The male is approximately one fourth as long as the female, with the same diameter. Infected children frequently present with complaints of severe vulvovaginal pruritus, which may awaken them at night. Other complaints include lower abdominal pain, diarrhea, restlessness, and nocturia. Studies for fungus and bacteria are not diagnostic, and examination of the vulvar vestibule and vagina reveals marked inflammation. Occasionally, an adult female helminth found on the vestibule or perineal areas is brought to the laboratory. More commonly, the pathologist is presented with a cellulose-tape-slide preparation for identification of the typical embryonated eggs of *E. vermicularis.* A granuloma secondary to Enterobius eggs has been reported involving the vulva [222]. Vulvar schistosomiasis, usually Schistosoma mansoni, is well documented, and primary skin lesions on the vulva from penetration of the infective cercariae may be seen. When biopsied, the parasite may be found within the epidermis [146]. Cutaneous myiasis of the vulva, secondary to infestation of the larval form of the muscoid fly and sarcophaga, has been reported. Recognition of the larva extracted from the vulvar tissues is diagnostic [43, 119].

Noninfectious Papulosquamous Dermatoses

Papulosquamous dermatoses often have a common component of epidermal hyperplasia in which the hyperplasia is somewhat psoriasiform. ➋ *Table 1.4* summarizes most of the entities in this group.

To establish a standardized system of nomenclature based on histopathological findings, the International Society for the Study of Vulvovaginal Disease (ISSVD) and International Society of Gynecological Pathologists (ISGP) recommended that all lesions be classified as nonneoplastic epithelial disorders or as lichen sclerosus, or other dermatoses. Diagnoses as kraurosis vulvae, leukoplakia, and atrophic vulvitis have generally been abandoned. Historically, the term dystrophy was proposed to describe a clinically related group of disorders of vulvar epithelium, which presented as white lesions, and that microscopically were characterized by benign alterations of the epithelial and dermal architecture. Two basic clinical varieties of dystrophy were recognized by the ISSVD in 1976: lichen sclerosus and hyperplastic dystrophy. When both clinical varities coexisted on different areas of the same vulva, it was recommended that the lesion be classified as a mixed dystrophy. The term mixed dystrophy is now recognized to refer to lichen sclerosus associated with variable lichen simplex chronicus and this reflects the spectrum of changes seen in lichen sclerosus, rather than the presentation of two distinctive epithelial disorders. The various forms of nonneoplastic epithelial disorders of the vulva cannot be reliably distinguished on the basis of their clinical appearance alone; all may be white, scaly, and fissured (➋ *Fig. 1.18*). Although biopsy may not be necessary in all cases, especially in children with typical findings of lichen sclerosus, one or more biopsies to sample the entire lesion usually are very informative. On the basis of the histologic findings, the pathologist can separate white lesions of a neoplastic type from nonneoplastic epithelial disorders.

Table 1.4
Noninfectious papulosquamous disorder

Psoriasis
Seborrheic dermatitis
Spongiotic dermatitis
Acute, subacute, and chronic atopic/contact dermatitis
Irritant contact dermatitis
Eczema
Nutritional deficiency
Vitamin deficiency-associated dermatitis
Glucagonoma (necrolytic migratory erythema)
Nonneoplastic epithelial disorders
Lichen simplex chronicus (LSC)
Lichen planus (LP) (hypertrophic form)
Lichen sclerosis (hypertrophic form)
Acanthosis nigricans

Lichen Sclerosus (Lichen Sclerosus et Atrophicus)

Clinical Features

The term Lichen Sclerosus Atrophicus is now referred to as Classic Lichen Sclerosus [102].

In children, symptoms include dysuria, painful defecation, and rectal bleeding [20, 181]. Lichen sclerosus can lead to anal fissures and strictures and to genital and perianal ulcers, which may resemble evidence of child sexual abuse. In adult women, the clinical findings typically include thinned and whitened epithelium, which usually is symmetric and involves the labia minora, clitoris, prepuce, frenulum, perineal body, and vulvar vestibule. Perirectal involvement is common. In advanced cases, loss and agglutination of the labia minora, frenulum, prepuce, and adhesions of the clitoris are found [181]. Stenosis of the introitus is common. In men, the glans penis and prepuce frequently are involved, and distal urethral stricture and phimosis may occur. Under these circumstances, the condition is clinically known as balanitis xerotica obliterans.

Gross Findings

The vulvar lesions of lichen sclerosus typically are pale white, flat, plaque-like areas that in advanced cases may be associated with thinned parchment-like epithelium and focal areas of ecchymosis and superficial ulceration (see *Fig. 1.18*). The vaginal mucosa is not involved.

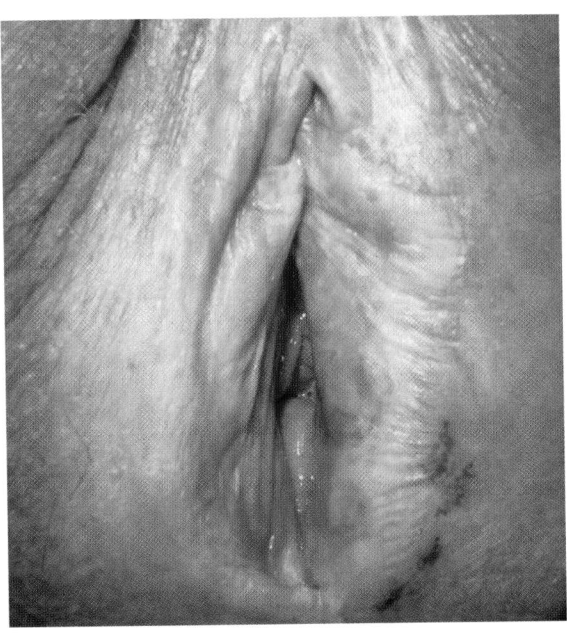

Fig. 1.18
Lichen sclerosus (LS). **White epithelium with focal subcutaneous ecchymosis is seen. The labia minora are somewhat atrophic**

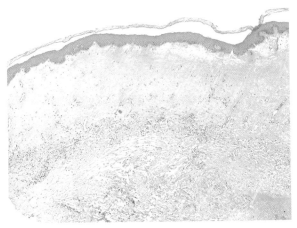

Microscopic Findings

The microscopic findings of lichen sclerosus can vary considerably, related to age of the lesion, excoriation, and treatment [32, 158]. The principal histologic changes show a sandwich appearance, including epidermis with blunting or loss of the rete ridges, a zone of homogeneous collagenized subepithelial edema of variable thickness, and a band of lymphocytic infiltration beneath this zone (*Fig. 1.19*). The homogeneous zone usually shows a reduction or absence of elastic fibers. The epithelium is thinned, but hyperkeratosis may be present in some cases and is believed to be superimposed lichen simplex chronicus [102]. The basal cell layer often is disorganized, and spongiosis may be evident. There is both an absence of melanosomes in the keratinocytes and a disappearance of the melanocytes. The lack of pigment, as well as edema, contributes to the white clinical appearance. Mitotic figures are rare or absent. In some cases, the mechanical trauma of rubbing and scratching will have produced bullous areas of lymph edema and subepithelial lacunae filled with erythrocytes. Areas of ulceration and acute inflammation also may be seen.

Differential Diagnosis

See Differential under "Lichen planus".

Fig. 1.19
Lichen sclerosus. **Hyperkeratosis is present along with loss of rete pegs and homogenization of the dermis**

Ultrastructural Findings

Ultrastructural studies have shown that collagen metabolism is abnormally active and the number of capillaries is reduced. The basal lamina is thickened and discontinuous. Degenerate dermal and collagenous material and formation of a hybrid of elastocollagenous bundles can be found between the cells of the epidermis, and melanocytes are rare [149].

Immunohistochemical and Related Studies

The presence of an elastase-type protease in vulvar fibroblasts from lichen sclerotic tissue has been reported that may be responsible for the loss of elastic tissue [84]. An increased concentration of collagenase inhibitor also has been reported. Tissue studies of glucose metabolism as well as alkaline phosphatase and adenosine triphosphatase have shown a surprisingly high rate of activity, equal to that seen in hyperplastic specimens and greater than that found in normal menopausal skin. The cell cycle protein Ki-67 is present in the basal and many parabasal epithelial cells involved by lichen sclerosus [209]. An apparent premature maturation of all cells above the basal layer has been reported, based on their high concentration of involucrin [32]. There is a growing body of evidence that an autoimmune mechanism may be involved. Patients with lichen sclerosus have been noted to have an increased number of organ-specific antibodies and more autoimmune disease than the normal population [29, 30]. However, the correlation is inconclusive [208]. On a histologic level, direct immunofluorescence studies have shown a deposit of fibrin along the dermoepidermal junction in 75% of the specimens studied [84, 208]. With an indirect fluorescent technique, IgM and C3 were concentrated along the basal lamina of the epithelium [84, 208]. Studies of the T cells within lichen sclerosus have identified monoclonal T cells that are predominantly cytotoxic CD8+ responsible for the destruction of basal keratinocytes [188].

Clinical Behavior and Treatment

Lichen sclerosus sometimes is associated with vulvar squamous carcinoma; however, it is not considered to be a premalignant intraepithelial neoplasm (see ➋ Chap. 2, Premalignant and Malignant Tumors of the Vulva). In a report of vulvar squamous cell carcinoma, 61% of the patients had lichen sclerosus. Until the time of the tumor diagnosis, 43 of the 47 cases with lichen sclerosus were not recognized to have vulvar lichen sclerosus [128]. Among patients with symptomatic vulvar lichen sclerosus, 9% developed VIN lesions and 21% invasive squamous cell carcinoma. Symptomatic lichen sclerosus preceded the carcinoma by a mean of 4 years. Squamous cell carcinomas associated with lichen sclerosus were located more commonly on the clitoris in an older age group, and were of the conventional squamous cell carcinoma type [32, 33]. Aneuploidy has been reported, which correlates with elevated p53 expression [31, 32]. In cases where lichen sclerosus is associated with vulvar squamous cell carcinoma, squamous cell hyperplasia usually is observed adjacent to the carcinoma [198]. Differentiated (simplex) type VIN and non-HPV-related squamous cell carcinoma have been associated with vulvar lichen sclerosus [250].

Traditional management has relied on the long-term topical application of testosterone or progesterone. Recent studies have reported good results with topical, superpotent corticosteroids for a short period [30, 53, 134]. In children, clearing or improvement of the anogenital lesions has been reported at puberty. However, this improvement has not been associated with menarche or pregnancy [93, 133]. Topical testosterone had been reported to arrest the symptoms and progress of the disease; however, it cannot be used in children because it is systemically absorbed. It is rarely used today. The recommended and accepted treatment according to the Guidelines for the management of lichen sclerosus as published on behalf of the British Association of Dermatologists is the ultrapotent topical corticosteroid ointment clobetasol propionate [160]. Current therapy using high-potency topical corticosteroids produces symptomatic relief and, in some cases, resolution of lichen sclerosus [36]. Opinion varies as to the ideal long-term therapy; most dermatologists advocate high-potency topical corticosteroids, but with reduced frequency. Lichen sclerosus is not a disease that requires vulvectomy or is cured by local excision or ablative treatment, however, some patients with persistent itch unresponsive to topical treatment, have responded to laser therapy or cryotherapy [160]. Women with lichen sclerosus, however, require continued therapy and follow-up because, over time, it is associated with a small but significant risk of vulvar differentiated (simplex) type VIN and squamous cell carcinoma in postmenopausal women. In these cases, tumor development occurs in the field of lichen sclerosus, and typically is associated with visible tumor or hyperplastic changes that indicate biopsy to establish the diagnosis of tumor. With improved therapy, it is expected that the frequency of tumor may be decreased.

Lichen Simplex Chronicus (Formerly Squamous Cell Hyperplasia or Hyperplastic Dystrophy)

Lichen simplex chronicus (LSC) is now considered to be equivalent to squamous cell hyperplasia by the International Society for the Study of Vulvovaginal Disease (ISSVD) and dermatopathologists [136, 178]. The microscopic diagnosis of lichen simplex chronicus, however, includes the finding of a superficial dermal chronic inflammatory infiltrate with vertical collagen streaks in the papillary dermis (➋ *Fig. 1.20*). A recent study revealed that the expression of retinoid acid receptor-alpha, a modulator of epithelial cell proliferation and differentiation, is decreased and the distribution of the receptor is changed in lichen sclerosus and squamous cell hyperplasia [16].

Gross Findings

The involved vulvar area usually is symmetric, and may be confined to a focal area, usually involving the labia majora. The involved area appears gray-white or reddened. The skin markings often are accentuated, a sign of intradermal edema and chronic rubbing; excoriation and fissures frequently bear witness to the intensity of the itching. There is shrinkage, stenosis, and agglutination of the labia.

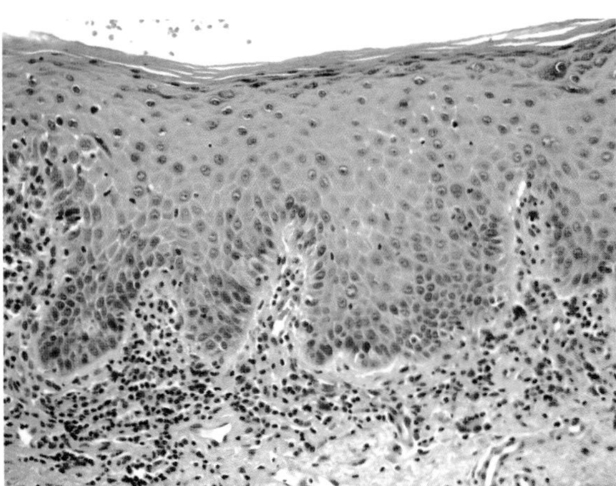

Fig. 1.20
Lichen simplex chronicus (LSC). **The epithelium is slightly thickened; however, no hyperkeratosis is present. Within the superficial dermis, there is a prominent chronic inflammatory cell infiltrate. In this example, there is minimal fibrosis within the superficial dermis**

Microscopic Findings

The histopathologic features of lichen simplex chronicus are epidermal acanthosis with superficial dermal fibrosis and variable superficial dermal chronic inflammation (➋ *Fig. 1.20*). Hyperkeratosis and parakeratosis may be present. There is typically an inflammatory infiltrate, predominately of lymphocytes in the superficial dermis. The changes are otherwise nonspecific, and the diagnosis is arrived at by exclusion of other dermatoses. The individual squamous cells are regular with distinct intercellular bridges. The nuclei are round to oval and contain finely distributed chromatin. Nucleoli may be prominent; however, there is progressive maturation of the cells as they approach the superficial layers. Mitotic figures, if present, are normal and confined to the basal layer. Hyperkeratosis may be seen associated with accentuation of the granular layer. Although parakeratosis may be present in otherwise typical areas of hyperplasia, its presence should prompt a careful search for cellular atypia and VIN of the differentiated type (see ➋ Vulvar Intraepithelial Neoplasia in Chap. 2). In the absence of atypia or lichen sclerosus, there is no evidence of risk of carcinoma from this process. The diagnosis of lichen simplex chronicus is one of exclusion.

Differential Diagnosis

The differential diagnosis of LSC includes chronic candidiasis or dermatophyte infection of the vulva that usually can be differentiated by a silver stain for fungus or periodic acid–Schiff (PAS) stain for the organisms. The fungal organisms usually are present in the keratin layer. The finding of inflammatory exocytosis, with neutrophils within the epithelium, is a clue for fungal infection. Regressing or early flat condylomata acuminata also may resemble LSC. However, the prominent granular layer, accentuated intracellular bridges, parabasal hyperplasia, and koilocytosis typically are lacking. If this cannot be resolved by histopathologic examination, molecular biologic methods, such as PCR or in situ hybridization, may be helpful in establishing the diagnosis of HPV-associated changes when virus is identified. Psoriasis or lichen planus may be included in the differential diagnosis; however, they represent distinct entities that are clinically and histologically identifiable.

Clinical Behavior and Treatment

Treatment is based on limiting or preventing exposure of the vulva to potential irritants in conjunction with the use of topical corticosteroids and antipruritics. Symptoms usually abate within 2–3 weeks [36]. Occasionally, local excision or laser ablation of the hyperplastic area may be effective in unresponsive cases. Combined treatment of 0.1% tacrolimus ointment and psoralen plus (PUVA) may be a good option in extensive cases of lichen sclerosus or when other treatment options have failed, and has a good tolerability and safety profile [231].

Lichen Planus

General Features

Lichen planus (LP) has a wide age distribution; however, it presents most commonly in women more than 40 years of age [130, 141]. Vulvar pruritus and burning are common symptoms; however, the patient may be asymptomatic. White, lacelike plaques (Wickham's striae) involving the oral and vaginal mucosa also may be present. Involvement of all three sites is referred to as the vulvovaginal-gingival syndrome reported by Pelisse. The syndrome is recognized as an erosive form of LP [173]. Patients with this condition experience vulvar pain, dyspareunia, and burning. Postcoital bleeding also has been reported [138, 173]. LP can result in severe introital and vaginal adhesions, scarring, and stenosis.

Gross Findings

The clinical appearance may be highly variable on the vulva, ranging from delicate reticulated papules to an erosive desquamative process involving the vagina and vulva. Within the vulva, the erosive process is typically confined to the vulvar vestibule and commonly involves the vagina. With advancing disease, there is loss and agglutination of the labia minora and prepuce, associated with thinned epithelium, postinflammatory hypopigmentation, and shrinkage with stenosis of the vaginal introitus. In advanced stages, it may be difficult to distinguish LP from advanced lichen sclerosus (LS). Vaginal involvement with adhesions and synechiae clinically characterizes LP, as does the finding of mucous membrane lesions outside the vulva.

Microscopic Findings

The histopathologic features may be highly variable depending on the age of the lesion as well as its location. Mucous membrane lesions may differ considerably from those occurring on vulvar skin [113]. In the skin, there are two important microscopic features: a bandlike chronic inflammatory infiltrate that is predominantly lymphocytic, with no or rare plasma cells. The inflammation is lichenoid, involving the upper dermis and immediate overlying epidermis (➲ *Fig. 1.21*). Liquefaction necrosis of the basal epithelial cells is seen, and these cells typically are admixed with chronic inflammatory cells. Degenerated keratinocytes result in the formation of colloid bodies (civatte bodies). Within the vulvar skin, the involved epithelium may show acanthosis, wedge-shaped hypergranulosis, and hyperkeratosis. Usually, parakeratosis is not present. Immunofluorescent studies often reveal fibrin deposition at the dermal–epidermal junction and, occasionally, granular IgM; rarely C3 and IgG deposits are also present. The cluster of necrotic keratinocytes (colloid bodies) positive for IgM in up to 87% of cases and, sometimes, C3 and IgG deposits may be helpful for the diagnosis [226]. The epithelial changes are variable within mucous membranes and include thinning

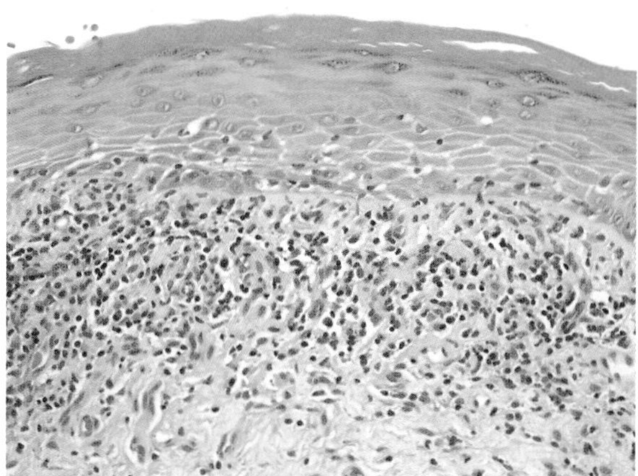

Fig. 1.21
Lichen planus (LP). **The epithelium is somewhat thinned with loss of rete ridges. A prominent granular layer is evident without significant hyperkeratosis in this example. There is a prominent bandlike chronic inflammatory infiltrate consisting almost entirely of lymphocytes, which is lichenoid and involves the basal layer**

of the epithelium, with ulceration and bullous formation. In contrast to the findings within the skin, plasma cells may be evident with mucosal involvement.

Differential Diagnosis

Well-developed lichen sclerosus (LS) can be distinguished from LP by the absence of the lichenoid inflammatory infiltrate at the dermal–epidermal junction in LS. Colloid bodies also are common in LP. LP typically involves mucosal as well as nonmucosal sites, whereas LS typically does not involve the vagina or oral mucosa. In advanced cases, mucosal involvement may be the most important distinguishing feature. Cicatricial pemphigoid and LP may both cause scarring and stenosis of the vulvar vestibule and vagina. Lichen planus has the characteristic lichenoid inflammatory pattern with colloid bodies within the epithelium. Cicatricial pemphigoid forms subepithelial blisters and has abundant eosinophils in the vesicles and in the dermis. Immunofluorescence demonstrates linear IgG and C3 deposits, which are usually absent in LP. Morphea (scleroderma) may be included in the differential diagnosis in that a band-like chronic inflammatory infiltrate may be seen with epithelial thinning; however, the inflammation is typically perivascular and around skin adnexa in the deep dermis, frequently with plasma cells. The interface liquefaction changes seen in LP typically are not seen in morphea. Morphea usually involves other sites, especially the trunk. Sclerosus of the dermis in morphea results in dermal thickening and loss of fat about skin appendages, as well as loss of skin appendages.

Clinical Behavior and Treatment

Adhesion formation can lead to scarring and agglutination of the labia minora [130]. The cause of erosive LP is unknown, although increasing evidence suggests that LP is a T-cell–mediated disease, representing an autoimmune response to altered self antigens or heterogeneous foreign antigens. C Topical cortical steroids are the usual form of treatment; fluorinated corticosteroids may be needed initially to provide relief. The most frequent first-line treatment was an ultrapotent topical corticosteroid, 0.05% clobetasol propionate ointment, which led to symptomatic improvement in 84 (94%) of 89 women, with 63 (71%) being symptom free while receiving treatment [51]. Additional therapy may include topical or oral cyclosporine, oral dapsone, and oral griseofulvin [61, 130].

Psoriasis

Psoriasis is inherited as an autosomal dominant trait (diathesis) with incomplete penetrance. Psoriasis affects approximately 2% of the population of the USA. On the vulva, the disease typically involves the lateral aspects of the labia majora and genitocrural areas [192]. The lesions present as sharply demarcated, silvery-topped erythematous papules and plaques on skin. When this loose silvery scale is removed, several punctuate bleeding points can be seen (Auspitz sign). In the vulva and other intertriginous areas, the silvery scales are lost. The sharply demarcated, bright red erythematous plaques are the main clinical finding. The lesions frequently are symmetric and may persist for years. At times, new psoriatic lesions develop at sites of trauma within 7–30 days after the trauma. This is referred to as Koebner phenomenon. Reiter's syndrome of the vulva, which is in the spectrum of psoriasis, rarely affects women [62].

Microscopic Findings

Hyperkeratosis, parakeratosis, uniform psoriasiform hyperplasia (elongation of the rete ridges to an even length) with club-shaped tips of rete ridges, diminution of the granular layer, and collections of polymorphonuclear leukocytes within the epidermis (Munro abscesses) are the epidermal changes (➋ *Fig. 1.22*). Mitotic activity increases within the epidermis above the basal layer, reflecting the significantly increased rate of epithelial turnover. The dermal papillae are clubbed and edematous. Prominent tortuous vessels are seen within the papillae, and there is a minimal chronic inflammatory cell infiltrate with the dermis [113].

Differential Diagnosis

The major differential diagnosis includes seborrheic dermatitis and chronic eczema. The latter two conditions also show psoriasiform hyperplasia; however, the rete ridges typically are not elongated to an even length as in the psoriasis. In seborrheic dermatitis, the subcorneal neutrophils are typically distributed around follicular ostia. Because psoriasis and seborrheic dermatitis have a similar clinical presentation, the differential diagnosis between these two diseases can be very difficult [192].

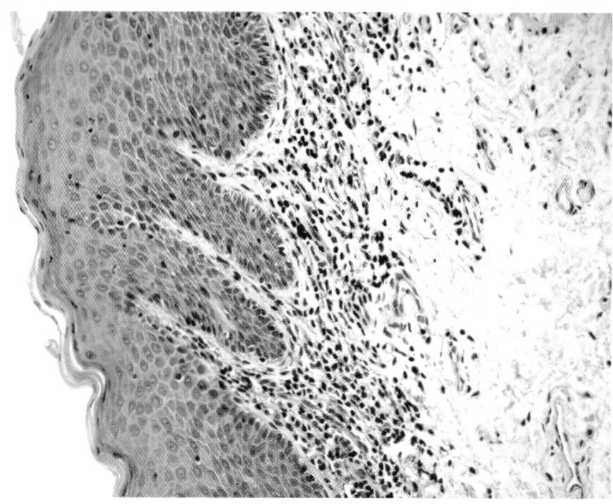

Fig. 1.22
Psoriasis. **Prominent uniform acanthosis is present. An intracorneal neutrophil collection (Munro abscess) is evident. The dermal papillae are clubbed and infiltrated by chronic inflammatory cells**

Contact Dermatitis

Vulvar contact dermatitis may be of an allergic type, which is a cell-mediated response to sensitizing agents such as nickel or rubber, or an irritant related to exposure to chemical or physical agents that damage the skin. Urinary incontinence is a common cause of irritation. Irritant dermatitis is the more common of the two. The lesions typically are confined to the area of exposure and usually persist for some time after the exposure [179]. The pathologic findings may be quite variable, depending on the severity and duration of the process and whether there is an associated allergic response. The most constant histopathologic findings are spongiosis with microvesiculation. The superficial perivascular inflammatory response consists predominantly of lymphocytes and histiocytes; eosinophils may be present. Superficial erosion or ulceration may be present and, in long-standing contact dermatitis, epithelial thickening with parakeratosis, and hyperkeratosis simulating lichen simplex chronicus also occurs.

Atopic Dermatitis

Women with atopic dermatitis may have involvement of the vulva, with associated pruritus and burning [179]. The physical findings may be limited to dryness and scaling, but thickening of the skin with localized excoriation may be evident if the vulva has been irritated by scratching. Vulvar biopsies are rarely performed on these patients. The pathologic findings often are typically squamous cell hyperplasia or are nonspecific. Spongiosis can at times be present. Within the dermis, lymphocytes and macrophages are present and the density of the infiltrate tends to correlate with the severity and chronicity of the process. Eosinophils and mast cells also may be identified. Immunofluorescent studies have demonstrated IgE on epidermal Langerhans cells [166, 221].

Fixed Drug Eruption (Dermatitis Medicamentosa)

Fixed drug eruptions constitute a complex group of cutaneous manifestations of drug-hypersensitive reactions that are subclassified as types I through IV. Type I is mediated through IgE antibodies and usually presents as urticaria. Type II is mediated through IgG and IgM antibodies and may be manifested as drug purpura or a bullous drug eruption. Type III is related to immune complexes and may be expressed as a maculopapular eruption, exanthem, urticaria, or vasculitis. Type IV is cell mediated and may be manifested as contact dermatitis, an exanthem, or a maculopapular eruption.

Fixed drug eruptions usually appear at the same place on reexposure to the same drug. Multiple reexposure may elicit lesions at new places in addition to the original locations. After discontinuation of the drug, the lesion may heal with prominent postinflammatory hyperpigmentation of the skin; however, this does not appear on the mucosa. The most common histopathologic findings of a fixed drug reaction are similar to erythema multiforme, that is, interface vacuolar changes with necrotic keratinocytes and scattered eosinophils in the dermis. Histologic findings in drug eruption are usually nonspecific and are only suggestive or supportive of a drug eruption. Patch testing, indirect and direct Coombs tests, and other specific laboratory testing, as well as a detailed clinical history, are necessary to precisely diagnose such cases [156].

Miscellaneous Inflammatory Dermatoses

A few special dermatoses, which are not classified into other categories in this chapter, are summarized in *Table 1.5*.

Table 1.5
Miscellaneous inflammatory dermatoses (noninfectious)

Miscellaneous inflammatory dermatoses (noninfectious)
Plasma cell vulvitis
Granulomatous diseases Sarcoidosis Vulvitis (chelitis) granulomatosa Crohn disease
Behçet syndrome
Pyoderma gangrenosum
Vulvodynia (Vulvar vestibulitis, Vulvar vestibular syndrome)
Fox–Fordyce disease
Fixed drug eruption (drug-induced erythema multiforme)

Plasma Cell Vulvitis (Vulvitis of Zoon)

Plasma cell vulvitis usually presents with symptoms of pruritus and burning. It is characterized by erythematous macules that usually have focal hemorrhagic areas and may appear orange in color. The lesions may be multiple [104, 251]. On microscopic examination the epithelium is thinned, with flattening of rete ridges and lack of a granular layer or keratinized surface. Parabasal keratinocytes have a horizontal orientation with marked spongiosis. The inflammatory infiltrate is lichenoid in type, consisting predominantly of plasma cells. Prominent dermal blood vessels are evident with associated intradermal hemorrhage and hemosiderin [113, 146]. The differential diagnosis includes syphilis, because of the perivascular plasma cell infiltrate, as well as lichen planus and other chronic dermatoses. The etiology is unknown; however, local irritation and poor hygiene may be contributing factors. Perineal hygiene, supportive care, and topical and intralesional corticosteroids are the usual treatment [251]. Use of etretinate has been reported in plasma cell vulvitis [196]. At present, topical tacrolimus can be considered an alternative treatment for plasma cell vulvitis only in cases resistant to conventional therapies [238].

Fox–Fordyce Disease

Fox–Fordyce disease is a disorder of the apocrine glands; 90% of cases occur in women. The disease generally begins at puberty and presents as a pruritic papular eruption usually involving the axilla, vulva, and perianal regions.

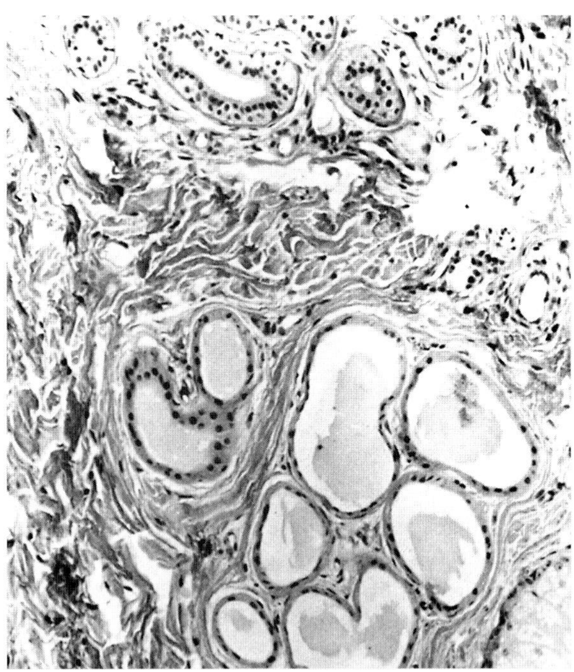

Fig. 1.23
Fox–Fordyce disease. **Dilated apocrine glands show inspissated secretion**

On microscopic examination, the center of the papule often contains a hair follicle and an apocrine sweat gland duct plugged by keratin. There may be an associated rupture of the intraepithelial portion of the duct with subsequent vesicle formation within the epidermis caused by spongiosis. These vesicles can be seen when serial sections are performed [187]. Transverse histologic sections to make the diagnosis have also been reported [218]. Chronic inflammatory changes are present in the dermis, and there is dilatation of the apocrine gland acini (*Fig. 1.23*). In addition, there is epidermal acanthosis and spongiosis. Deposition of mucin may be found in the ducts, glands, and tissues surrounding the skin appendages. Fox–Fordyce disease is a chronic condition that may progress somewhat during pregnancy or after menopause; however, no definite therapy is known. In women of reproductive age, oral contraceptives may relieve symptoms and reduce somewhat the severity of the process. Systemic antibiotics and topical, as well as locally injected, corticosteroids and antipruritics relieve symptoms. Isotretinoin has been used in treating this condition [152]. Hidradenitis suppurativa as well as folliculitis may complicate the clinical course.

Vulvodynia (Formerly Known as Vulvar Vestibulitis or Vulvar Vestibular Syndrome)

General Features

Vulvodynia formerly known as, Vulvar vestibulitis, was renamed at the ISSVD Terminology and Classification Consensus Among Health Care Providers in 2003. Vulvodynia is described as "vulvar discomfort, . . . a burning pain, occurring in the absence of relevant visible findings or a specific, clinically identifiable, neurologic disorder." Vulvodynia is divided into two categories: (1) vulvar pain related to a specific disorder and (2) vulvodynia, a condition in which the vulva has a normal appearance other than some erythema (*Table 1.6*).

Microscopic Findings

As seen in the table, vulvar pain related to a specific disorder, can be infectious, inflammatory, neoplastic or neurologic. This group has histopathologic features that include areas of mild to moderate inflammatory response, characterized by a superficial chronic inflammatory infiltrate that is composed predominantly of lymphocytes resembling female urethral syndrome [80]. Many cases also have plasma cells within the infiltrate, but leukocytes and eosinophils are rare. The stromal tissue beneath the vestibular epithelium is involved most prominently, and the inflammatory process may surround the minor vestibular glands. Inflammatory cells occasionally are found within the glandular epithelium or within the acini or ductal lumina [184]. These patients rarely have clinically or morphologically evident condyloma acuminatum or VIN [243]. The group under vulvodynia has essentially histologically unremarkable tissues.

Table 1.6
ISSVD 2003 terminology and classification of vulvar pain

Vulvar pain related to a specific disorder
Infectious (candidiasis, herpes, etc.)
Inflammatory (lichen planus, immuno-bullous disorders etc.)
Neoplastic (Paget disease, squamous cell carcinoma etc.)
Neurologic (herpes neuralgia, spinal nerve compression etc.)
Vulvodynia
Generalized
Provoked (sexual, nonsexual or both)
Unprovoked
Mixed (provoked and unprovoked)
Localized
Provoked (sexual, nonsexual or both)
Unprovoked
Mixed (provoked and unprovoked)

Clinical Behavior and Therapy

The natural history of vulvodynia is poorly understood, and no long-term controlled prospective studies have been reported to date [90]. Local excision of the vestibule has been advocated; however, the recurrence rate, with follow-up for as long as 5 years, reveals that recurrent symptoms after surgery are relatively common, occurring in more than one half the cases in some series. Biofeedback therapy appears effective in many patients as does cognitive-behavioral therapy [18, 81]. Antibiotics produce no response, nor can the symptoms be reliably alleviated by corticosteroids. Nonvaporization laser ablation of the superficial submucosal ectatic blood vessels has been proposed, especially in cases having recurrent symptoms after surgery [142]. Interferon has been advocated, with some response [24]. The administration of interferon and biofeedback training of the lower pelvic muscles are treatments used as a first choice before more aggressive treatment [24]. A low-oxalate diet has been proposed but has not been proven to be of value. More than one half of these patients initially obtain some relief from topical therapy. Management of symptoms is long term and supportive.

Vulvitis Granulomatosa (Chelitis Granulomatosa)

Vulvitis granulomatosa is of unknown etiology, related to cheilitis granulomatosa (Miescher–Melkersson–Rosenthal syndrome) and Crohn's disease [88, 89]. Clinically, the labia majora are indurated, swollen, and erythematous without tenderness. The labia minora, as well as the perineum and perianal areas, also may be involved. Mild regional lymphadenopathy typically is present. The process remains localized but is slowly progressive. Histopathologic findings include dermal edema and a chronic granulomatous inflammatory infiltrate composed of histiocytes and giant cells, as well as lymphocytes and plasma cells. The infiltrate involves the dermis and extends to the epithelium. The differential diagnosis includes other granulomatous inflammatory processes [89]. Treatment of this condition is with intralesional steroids.

Factitial Vulvitis

Factitial vulvitis is an uncommon disorder that may present as a mild chronic inflammatory process, often with associated superficial ulceration [179]. The pathologic findings often are nonspecific.

Behçet Syndrome

Behçet syndrome refers to the triad of oral aphthous ulcers, genital ulcers, and ophthalmologic inflammation [203]. Ocular changes may be absent in mild cases. Other findings include acne, cutaneous nodules, thrombophlebitis, encephalopathy, and colitis [203]. Behçet syndrome causes deep ulcerations on the vulva that may result in fenestration of the labia and lead to gangrene of the labia. The ulcerations characteristically heal and relapse, and are associated with simultaneous oral ulcers. Histologically, necrotizing arteritis frequently is seen and can be considered a cardinal pathologic finding. A chronic inflammatory infiltrate may be perivascular or involve the vessel wall with homogenization of the arterial media [113]. Endothelial cell swelling also occurs and may result in arteriolar occlusion as well as venous thrombosis.

Crohn's Disease

Crohn's disease is a chronic noncaseating granulomatous disease of unknown etiology that can involve, besides the gastrointestinal tract, the vulva and the perineum in adults and children [229, 237]. Cutaneous ulcerations occur in areas where there is close apposition of skin, such as the vulva and inframammary areas. When Crohn's disease involves the vulva, the resulting ulcers often are slit shaped, multiple, deep, and secondarily infected. Vulvar and perianal erythema, induration, or ulceration may be the presenting signs [172, 237]. Involvement of the colon, rectum, or small bowel is not always present when the vulva is involved. Perianal fistulas, as well as fistulas to other sites in the female genital tract, are complications. When perianal draining sinuses and abscesses occur, they often drain fluid resembling small bowel contents.

Microscopically, the disease is characterized by a noncaseating granulomatous inflammation within the dermis, which usually is deep and associated with fissures and sinus tracts. Studies for acid-fast bacteria and fungi are negative. A marked granulation tissue response frequently is seen surrounding the ulcers, but significant lymphadenitis is rare [113].

Pyoderma Gangrenosum

Pyoderma gangrenosum is a progressive necrotic and ulcerative condition of the skin, of uncertain etiology. Most case reports of pyoderma gangrenosum occur on the legs and are associated with idiopathic bowel disease such as chronic ulcerative colitis. Other associations include hematologic malignancy, connective tissue disease, and liver disease. Pyoderma gangrenosum of the vulva may present some time after treatment for colitis, ileostomy, or abdominal perineal resection of the colon and rectum.

The microscopic findings reveal epithelial ulceration with severe acute and chronic inflammation. If the biopsy is from the ulcer edge, the sharply demarcated ulcer is adjacent to hyperplastic squamous epithelium. Organisms are not identified within the inflammatory process. Systemic corticosteroid therapy with aggressive local excision, followed by skin grafting, may be necessary in addition to the treatment of the underlying disease [180].

Necrotizing Fasciitis (Includes Synergistic Bacterial Infection)

Postoperative, posttraumatic, or necrotizing fasciitis is a life-threatening condition that usually is secondary to a polymicrobial infection after episiotomy or other types of vaginal, vulvar, or abdominal surgery [13, 219]. Diabetes mellitus, arteriosclerosis, obesity, hypertension, and prior irradiation predispose to necrotizing fasciitis [4]. The clinical presentation is that of a rapidly progressing inflammatory process that may initially appear as mild cellulitis or edema with inflammation. Delay in diagnosis without therapy carries a nearly 50% mortality. Prompt radical excision of the infected tissue and broad-spectrum systemic antibiotic therapy offers the only chance of cure [219].

Hidradenitis Suppurativa

Hidradenitis suppurativa is a chronic inflammatory disorder of the apocrine glands [85]. Deep-seated, painful, subcutaneous nodules are found in areas containing apocrine glands, especially the axilla and vulva. The lesions commonly progress subcutaneously, producing confluent masses that subsequently ulcerate the epidermis and result in draining sinuses and extensive scarring. The condition may coexist with Fox–Fordyce disease. Total excision of involved areas may be necessary in advanced cases, although laser ablation and unroofing the sinuses has been reported to be effective [213]. Long-term isotretinoin therapy also has been reported to be effective in some cases [99]. Histologically, in the early stage hidradenitis suppurativa demonstrates a perifolliculitis with an acute and chronic inflammatory infiltrate within the dermis. The later stages of the disease result in destruction of the epithelial appendages with sinus tract formation [113] (➋ *Fig. 1.24*).

Mites and Lice

A variety of mites are capable of producing local and limited chronic skin infections of the perineal area, including scabies [41, 154]. Mites must be specifically considered, because definitive diagnosis sometimes is difficult [41]. Mites are small arachnids and belong to the order Acarina; they differ from lice, which are insects. Mites have a fused head and thorax, devoid of primary segmentation, and four pairs of legs. Mites burrow within the subcorneal area of the epidermis, inducing severe pruritus. The overt skin lesions are papular and, when examined under a magnifying lens, reveal an adjacent burrow. Scrapings from the burrow or specimens obtained from the patient's clothing can be fixed in an alcohol-ether-acetic acid-formalin mixture and analyzed microscopically for mites, eggs, and fecal material. Lice are associated with irritation of the skin from secondary infection of feeding sites. The pubic louse, Phthirus pubis, class Insecta, is the usual offender and can be diagnosed by identifying the louse and nits on the hair shaft.

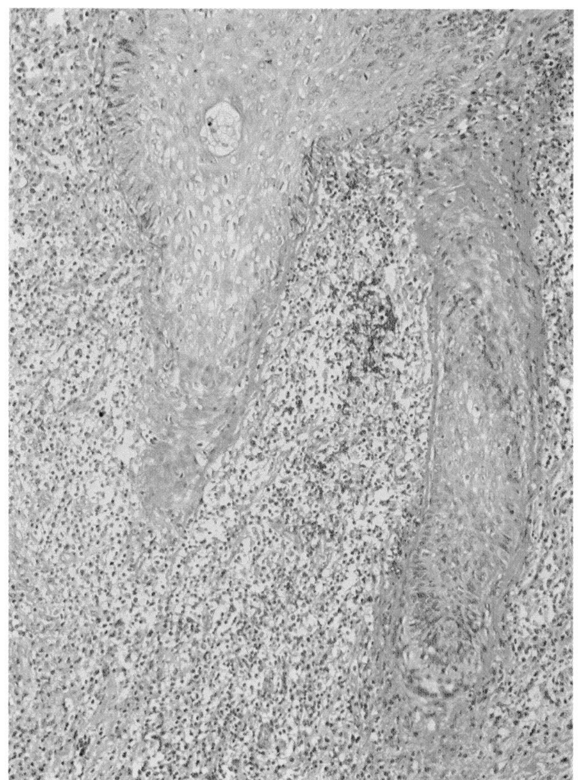

Fig. 1.24
Hidradenitis suppurativa. **There is a severe acute and chronic inflammatory cell infiltrate within the dermis with involvement and destruction of the skin appendages**

Spider Bite

A brown recluse (Loxosceles reclusa) spider bite on the vulva has been reported, associated with ulceration and infection of the vulva. Although secondary protracted infection may occur with such ulcers, slow and progressive healing over several months is the usual clinical course [139].

Bullous Diseases

Although virtually any dermatologic disease can involve the vulva, the following bullous diseases bear discussion, as they may first be observed and biopsied by the gynecologist. Definitive diagnosis of most bullous diseases requires clinical and pathologic correlation, and in some cases the clinical findings are essential in distinguishing these cutaneous diseases that otherwise have very similar or identical histopathologic findings. Some of the bullous diseases have immunologic components, and others are nonspecific (➋ *Table 1.7*). The key histopathologic features and differential diagnosis of bullous and bullous-like diseases are summarized in (➋ *Table 1.8*).

Pemphigus (Pemphigus Vulgaris)

Pemphigus vulgaris initially may present on the vulva as recurrent superficial ulcers and erosions. Associated oral lesions usually are present in these patients, and rectal and vaginal lesions may occur [15, 179]. The disease was life threatening before the era of steroid treatment. Biopsy of a fresh vulvar vesicle usually is diagnostic. Microscopic

Table 1.7
Noninfectious bullous dermatoses

Immunobullous dermatoses	Nonimmunobullous dermatoses
Bullous pemphigoid	Benign familial pemphigus (Hailey–Hailey)
Cicatricial pemphigoid	Darier disease (keratosis follicularis)
Pemphigus	Erythema multiforme
Dermatitis herpetiformis	Lichen planus and lichenoid vaginitis
Linear IgA dermatosis	Lichen sclerosus (LS)
Herpes gestationis	Pruritus, urticaria, papules and plaques of pregnancy (PUPPP)
Bullous lupus erythematosus	

findings include acantholysis with suprabasal vesicle formation and eosinophils in the vesicular fluid and the superficial dermis (*Fig. 1.25*). Direct immunofluorescent studies of perilesional skin demonstrate IgG deposited at the epidermal intercellular junctions. Circulating antibodies to epidermal intercellular spaces can be detected with indirect immunofluorescent method against monkey esophageal epithelium; the titer correlates with the clinical activity of the disease. Therapy includes high systemic doses of corticosteroids and cytotoxic agents, plasma pheresis, and supportive measures [28, 87, 217].

Pemphigus Vegitans

This rare variant of pemphigus may present as a localized, indurated, inflamed area with vesicles. The pathologic as well as immunofluorescent and immunologic findings are similar to pemphigus vulgaris, although intraepidermal eosinophilic abscesses and verrucous epidermal hyperplasia are prominent [179, 248]. The presence of eosinophils, as well as the localized and self-limited character of the disease, distinguish it from pemphigus vulgaris.

Pemphigoid (Bullous Pemphigoid)

Pemphigoid can involve the vulva and is characterized by moist, tender ulcers that involve the labia minora, majora, and perianal areas. At times, fluid-filled tense bullae also are present. Biopsies of fresh ulcers, including normal adjacent skin, typically show the characteristic subepidermal bullae (see *Table 1.8*). In advanced stages, biopsy of ulcerated areas may show only granulation tissue [120].

Cicatricial pemphigoid, unlike bullous pemphigoid, results in scarring and stenosis. Both bullous pemphigoid and cicatricial pemphigoid can be the result of a drug hypersensitivity reaction [235]. The disease presents as erosions, erythema, and small blisters of the vulva, perianal, and anal mucosa associated with chronic burning pain and painful ulcers. The origin of the recurrent scarring of the vulva may not be apparent until the presentation of ocular involvement secondary to cicatricial pemphigoid [74]. Severe cicatrization with shrinkage, suggesting advanced vulvar lichen sclerosus or lichen planus, characterizes the process. In contrast to lichen sclerosus or lichen planus, cicatricial pemphigoid is associated with small blisters and a positive Nikolsky phenomenon (slippage and detachment of the superficial epidermis from the underlying dermis when the examining finger is slid over the skin surface).

Microscopically, there is subepidermal blister formation with a mixed inflammatory cell infiltrate within the dermis (*Fig. 1.26*). Eosinophils are prominent. Direct immunofluorescence demonstrates linear IgG, and complement C3, along the basement membrane. Immunoglobulins IgA and IgM may or may not be present [76, 120]. Systemic corticosteroids and immunosuppressive drugs may be of value [87, 121]. If the condition is drug related, the offending medication should be discontinued.

Herpes Gestationis

This vesiculobullous disease is unique to pregnant women, with an estimated incidence of approximately 0.6 per 100,000 pregnancies. Patients have a strong association with HLA-DR3 and -DR4. Presenting signs and symptoms often are severe pruritus and a macular erythematous rash that leads to blistering and superficial ulcerations. The lesions may involve the vulva and pubic area in addition to the trunk and upper thigh. The process usually presents in the second trimester, and spontaneous regression follows soon after delivery, although regression may occur in the late third trimester.

Histopathologic findings include a subepidermal blister that may contain eosinophils, neutrophils, lymphocytes, and histiocytes. There is a perivascular superficial dermal inflammatory infiltrate that also is rich in lymphocytes and eosinophils. Immunofluorescent studies

Table 1.8

Differential diagnosis of vesicular bullous and bullous-like diseases of the vulva

Disease	Location of vesicle		Acantholysis of suprabasal cells	Significant systemic manifestations	ImmvLnoflvLOresce.nl localization
	Subepidermal	Intraepidermal suprabasal			
Pemphigus vulgaris	No	Yes	Yes	Yes	IgG Intercellular
Pemphigus vegitans	No	Yes	Yes	No	IgG Intercellular
Pemphigoid (bullous) (cicatricial pemphigoid)	Yes	No	No	Yes, localized scarring (sometimes debilitating)	IgG linear along basement membrane IgA, IgM, C_3, C_5 may be in basement membrane
Herpes gestationis	Yes	No	No	Yes	C_3 Linear along basement membrane. IgG may also be present. IgM, IgA is rare
Polymorphic eruption of pregnancy, pruritic urticarial plaques and papules in pregnancy (PUPPP)	Yes	No	No	Yes	Negative
Darier disease	No	Yes Yes Yes,	Yes, 3+ dyskeratosis	Yes	Negative
Warty dyskeratoma	No	necrotic	Yes	No	Negative
Erythema multiforme (Stevens-Johnson syndrome)	No	keratinocytes, Hydropic degeneration of basal keratinocytes	No	Yes	IgM Complement in and about superficial dermal vessels in some cases
Hailey-Hailey	No	Yes	Yes, 4+ No dyskeratosis	No	Negative
Localized acantholytic disease of the vulva	No	Yes	Yes	No	Negative
Benign chronic bullous disease of childhood (linear IgA disease)	Yes	No	Microabscesses in dermal papillae	No, flu-like symptoms may precede presentation	IgA linear along basement membrane (C_3, IgA, IgG, IgM also may be present)
Dermatitis herpetiformis	Yes	No	No	No, severe pruritus in some cases	IgA deposits in the tips of dermal papillae and/or along the basement

demonstrate C3 as a linear basement membrane deposit. Serologic studies demonstrate circulating complement-fixing IgG antibodies in 25% of the cases. The antibodies bind to 180-kDa hemidesmosome antigen (BPAg2) [214]. The main differential diagnosis is bullous pemphigoid, which is usually not associated with pregnancy. Prurigo of pregnancy, pruritic folliculitis of pregnancy, and polymorphic eruption of pregnancy may be included in the differential of dermatosis associated with pregnancy, but these are not bullous diseases, and the immunofluorescent studies are negative [146].

Darier Disease (Keratosis Follicularis)

Darier disease is inherited as an autosomal dominant trait with the gene locus mapped to chromosome 12q, although

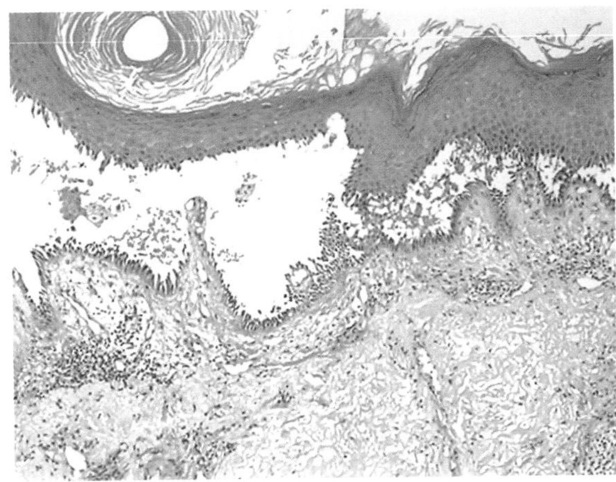

■ Fig. 1.25
Pemphigus (pemphigus vulgaris). **Suprabasal vesicle formation is evident with prominent acantholysis. (Courtesy of B. Smoller, Little Rock, AR)**

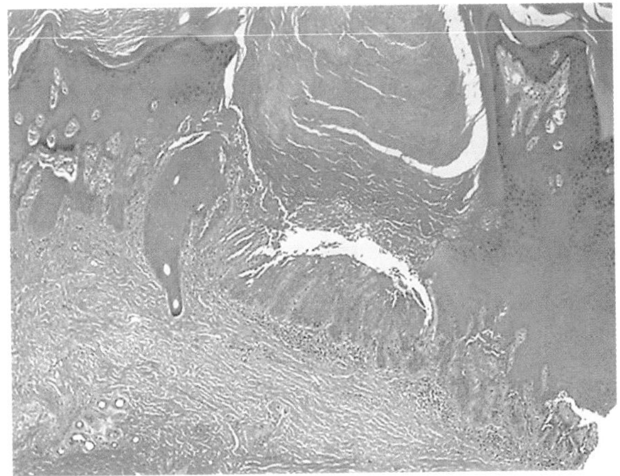

■ Fig. 1.27
Warty dyskeratoma. **Acantholysis of the suprabasal epithelial cells, with intraepithelial clefts extending from the basal layer through the granular layer. (Courtesy of B. Smoller, Little Rock, AR)**

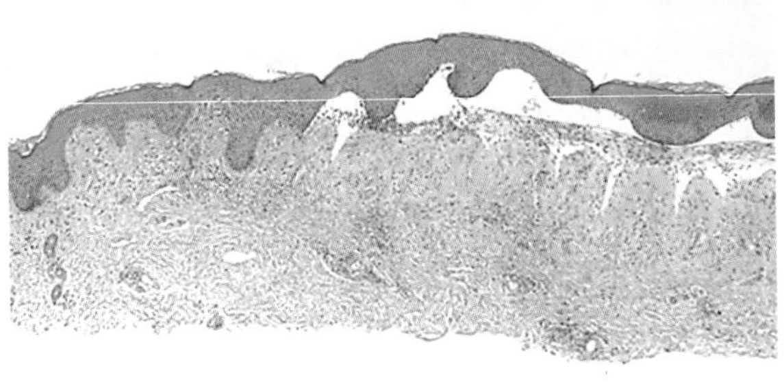

■ Fig. 1.26
Bullous pemphigoid. **A subepidermal bulla is evident, with intact epithelium separated from the underlying dermis. An intense inflammatory infiltrate of lymphocytes, neutrophils, and eosinophils is seen within the dermis with some inflammatory cells within the bulla (Courtesy of B. Smoller, Little Rock, AR)**

spontaneous cases also may occur. This disease affects anytime after late childhood. The disease has a seborrheic distribution and frequently involves the vulva. Although it usually is not considered a bullous disease, it is listed herein because microscopic intraepidermal acantholysis is a common observation. On clinical examination, the lesions are crusted, hyperkeratotic papules that often appear darker than the surrounding skin. The papules may be secondarily infected [113, 192].

Histologically, acantholysis of the suprabasal epithelial cells results in clefts that extend from the basal layer through the granular layer. Acantholytic cells are seen within the clefts. Corps ronds and nuclear grains can be found in the granular layer along microscopic findings with individual dyskeratotic cells. Hyperkeratosis, acanthosis, and papillomatosis are seen along with keratotic plugs. Rarely, epithelial basal cell budding into the adjacent dermis may be seen. The inflammatory cell infiltration within the dermis usually is minimal, unless the lesions are secondarily infected [113]. The main differential diagnosis is warty dyskeratoma, Hailey–Hailey disease, and localized acantholytic disease of the vulva (see ➋ *Table 1.8*).

Warty Dyskeratoma

Warty dyskeratoma of the vulva typically presents with a histologic picture essentially identical to that of Darier disease. Unlike Darier disease, which is multifocal and may involve the trunk and extremities as well as the face, warty dyskeratoma typically involves the head, neck, or vulva as a solitary lesion. Histologically, warty dyskeratoma has more prominent villous-like projections into the acantholytic space (➋ *Fig. 1.27*). Other distinguishing clinical features are that Darier disease usually is congenital, and is carried as an autosomal dominant, whereas warty dyskeratoma is not (see ➋ *Table 1.8*) [50].

Erythema Multiforme (Stevens–Johnson Syndrome)

Vulvar involvement has been reported in association with Stevens–Johnson syndrome, which is the severe form of erythema multiforme. Involvement of the mouth, eyes, and skin, with associated high fever and other systemic symptoms, characterizes the syndrome. The most common cause of the Stevens–Johnson syndrome is drug therapy. Herpesvirus infection is typically associated with a recurrent minor form of erythema multiforme in which the recurrence may be prevented by prophylactic use of systemic antiviral therapy (e.g., Valtrex). Other causes include mycoplasma infection, malignancy, or radiotherapy [202].

The histopathologic features are complex, depending on the age of the lesion. Major features include interface vacuolar dermatitis with necrotic keratinocytes and intraepithelial vesicle formation. Separation of the epithelium from the dermis is associated with hydropic degeneration of the basal keratinocytes (see *Table 1.8*). Within the dermis, there is a prominent chronic inflammatory infiltrate consisting of lymphocytes and histiocytes. Extravasated red blood cells may be present within the dermal inflammatory process, as well as within the epidermis. Nonspecific intravascular complement C3 and IgM deposits may be seen within the superficial dermal vessels by immunofluorescent staining [146]. There are case reports of "introital adenosis" occurring 1–3 years after the diagnosis of Stevens–Johnson syndrome, characterized clinically by erosions within the vulvar vestibule and medial aspects of the labia minora. On histopathologic examination, glandular epithelium has been identified within these areas, associated with submucosal inflammation [22, 143]. The epithelium was described in one case as columnar epithelium of tuboendometrial type, having secretory and ciliated-type cells [143]. The term mucinous metaplasia of the vulva has been used to describe these changes, which is consistent with columnar cell metaplasia [46, 60].

Hailey–Hailey Disease (Familial Benign Pemphigus)

Hailey–Hailey disease is inherited as an autosomal dominant trait with the gene locus mapped to chromosome 3q; approximately one third of patients, however, have no family history of the disease. Onset of the disease often occurs during adolescence. Intertriginous areas usually are involved, but several cases in which the lesions are confined exclusively to the vulva have been reported [241]. The usual clinical presentation is recurrent clusters of vesicles that develop, rupture, and result in crusted, moist papules that later coalesce to form plaques.

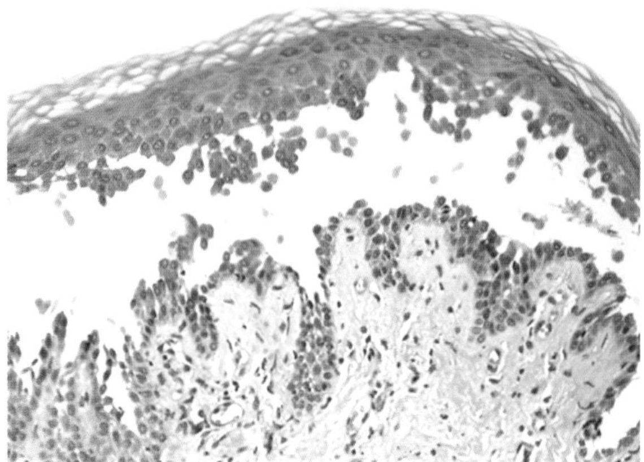

Fig. 1.28
Hailey–Hailey disease (benign familial pemphigus). **Acantholysis is present in the suprabasal area and lower dermis. The mid- and upper epidermis remain intact, although some acantholysis is present (Courtesy of B. Smoller, Little Rock, AR)**

Histologically, there is acantholysis with resultant suprabasalar lacunae. Acantholytic cells that maintain their nuclear details remain attached to each other in the acantholytic space, giving a dilapidated brick-wall appearance. The acantholysis is more marked than in Darier disease (*Fig. 1.28*) [113]. Basal cells maintain their orientation to the basement membrane. Rarely, corps ronds are seen in the granular layer. In contrast to Darier disease there is minimal, if any, dyskeratosis in Hailey–Hailey disease. Strands of epidermal cells may proliferate into the dermis, but little dermal inflammatory infiltrate exists unless secondary infection is present. *Table 1.8* summarizes the major distinguishing features of Darier disease, Hailey–Hailey disease (familial benign pemphigus), pemphigus vulgaris, pemphigus vegetans, and warty dyskeratoma. Recently, squamous cell carcinoma arising in Hailey–Hailey disease of the vulva has been reported [45].

Benign Chronic Bullous Disease of Childhood (Linear IgA Disease)

This disease commonly involves the lower abdominal, pelvic, inguinal, and genital areas, presenting as clusters of annular lesions or "clusters of jewels" that usually are pruritic and typically evolve over the course of 24 h. The annular lesions evolve to tense bullae that, if ruptured, ulcerate and become crusted. Patients may have fever and anorexia. In some cases the eruption is preceded by a bacterial or viral infection [63, 247], and other cases are drug induced, vancomycin being one of the more common offenders [115]. Because of the location and abrupt appearance of the lesions, they may be mistaken for evidence of child abuse. Biopsy of an early bullous lesion reveals subepithelial vesicles that contain predominantly neutrophils within the vesicular fluid. Microabscesses may occur within the epidermis. The diagnostic finding is the identification of a linear deposition of IgA in the basement membrane (see *Table 1.8*). Other immunoglobulins and complement C3 also may be found [113]. The antigen of the linear IgA disease is a 97-kDa molecule, which is identical to the carboxyl terminal of 180-kDa (BPAg2), located at the basement membrane [96]. The differential diagnosis includes dermatitis herpetiformis and bullous pemphigoid. Dermatitis herpetiformis is distinguished by having granular IgA at the dermal papillae, whereas bullous pemphigoid has linear IgG basement membrane deposits [113]. Therapy includes systemic antiinflammatory drugs including dapsone, colchicine, and intravenous immunoglobulin therapy [5, 112, 183].

Depigmentation and Hypopigmented Disorders

In adult women, the vulvar skin, especially that of the perineal body and lateral labia majora, usually is more pigmented than the general body surface. Biopsies of the normal vulva show dendritic melanocytes scattered along the basal layer of the epithelium as well as squamous keratinocytes containing variable concentrations of melanin granules. Areas of the vulvar skin that appear hypopigmented therefore are clinically remarkable. Three basic conditions result in vulvar hypopigmentation: vitiligo, albinism, and postinflammatory depigmentation (leukoderma).

Vitiligo

Vitiligo is an inherited disorder in which the melanocytes are lost from areas of skin that were previously normally pigmented. This condition frequently affects the vulva, and biopsies from vitiliginous areas show a remarkable absence of both basilar melanocytes and melanin granules. A Fontana stain for melanin pigment in the basal keratinocytes can be used to support the diagnosis [113].

Albinism

Albinism, an inherited genetic disorder, is characterized by an inability of the melanocytes to produce pigment. There is an absence of melanin granules in the keratinocytes. Large pale cells may be present within the basal layer, representing incompetent melanocytes.

Postinflammatory Depigmentation (Leukoderma)

In areas of previous ulceration, recently healed skin will temporarily lack a normal population of melanocytes, a condition referred to as postinflammatory depigmentation, or leukoderma. This disorder is common after herpes infection, syphilitic ulceration, burns, and deep laser or cryotherapy. Histologically, the skin appears thinned, metabolically active, and lacks the usual amount of pigment. On careful microscopic inspection, some melanin usually is evident.

Pigment Disorders of Melanocytic Origin and Nevi

In a prospective study of 301 women, 37 (12%) were found to have a pigmented lesion of the vulva. All these women were white, and only 26% of the patients were aware that they had a pigmented lesion. More than 50% of the pigmented lesions were lengito simplex (lentigines); seven patients had nevi, of which one had the histologic features of a dysplastic nevus, five patients had post-inflammatory hyperpigmentation, two cases represented hemangiomas, and one patient had a pigmented lesion that proved to be VIN with ulceration [197].

Lentigo Simplex

The most common hyperpigmented lesion occurring on the vulva is lentigo simplex (lentigines), which may occur on the mucous membranes as well as on the skin. The lesion is typically small, 4 mm or less in diameter, flat, and uniformly pigmented. Clinically, lentigines closely resemble junctional nevi and, therefore, are frequently biopsied. Except for the rare leopard syndrome, in which thousands of lentigines are present all over the body, lentigo simplex is essentially devoid of clinical significance. In contrast to lentigo simplex, solar lentigines usually are seen on sun-exposed areas only [12].

Histologically, lentigo simplex is a localized circumscribed area of slightly hyperplastic epidermis that contains an increased number of normal-appearing melanocytes along the side and tips of the elongated rete ridges associated with basilar hyperpigmentation. Extreme degrees of epidermal pigmentation may be present, with numerous squamous cells exhibiting cytoplasmic melanin granules, usually in highest concentration near the epithelial–stromal junction (➋ *Fig. 1.29*). There may be mild acanthosis and slight clubbing of the rete ridges, and heavily pigmented melanophages may be present in the upper dermis. At times, a minimal superficial dermal inflammatory cell infiltrate is noted, but this is by no means constant.

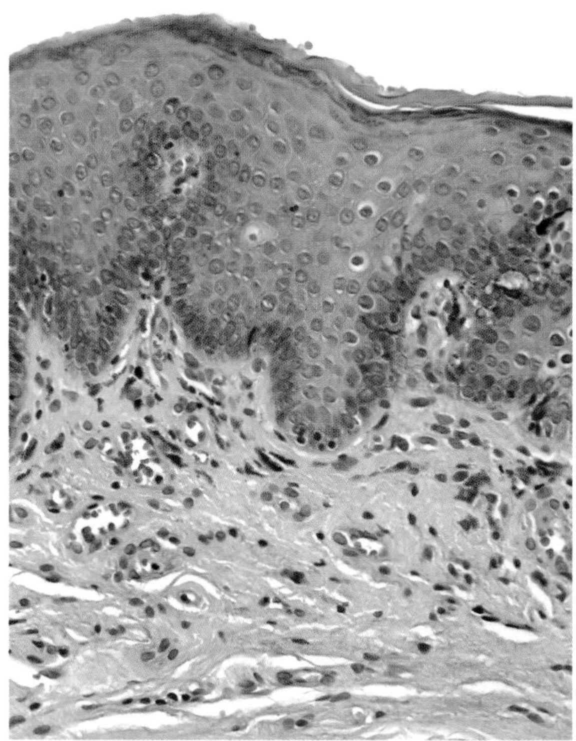

Fig. 1.29
Lentigo simplex. **Note the heavy concentration of deeply pigmented basalar keratinocytes at the tips of the accentuated rete ridges. Increased solitary melanocytes along the site of the retes are present (Taken from Atlas of Vulvar Disease [244])**

Vulvar Melanosis

Vulvar melanosis is characterized by prominent brown to black pigmented macular areas with irregular borders that may be solitary or multiple, located on the labia minora or labia majora as well as on the vaginal introitus and perineum. The pigmented areas vary in size and may cover much of the vulva skin. Vulvar melanosis typically occurs in women of reproductive age and is more common on the squamous mucosa portion of the vulva [68, 201].

The microscopic findings are essentially similar to lentigo simplex, with intense basilar keratinocytic hyperpigmentation, although epithelial hyperplasia usually is not seen. The lesions typically are larger than those of lentigo, which characteristically are not more than 4 mm in diameter. The pigmentation may be intense within the basal layer with slight or no increase in the number of melanocytes. The melanocytes are typically arranged in single solitary units within the dermal–epidermal junction [68, 201].

Congenital and Giant Nevomelanocytic Nevi

Congenital nevi are found in approximately 10% of newborns and usually are less than 4 mm in diameter. Giant nevomelanocytic nevi (20 cm or more in diameter) (garment type), although rare, carry an increased risk of developing malignant melanoma in prepubertal individuals.

Junctional, Compound, and Intradermal Nevi

Vulvar melanocytic nevi may be junctional, compound, or intradermal. These nevomelanocytic types occur on the vulva with nearly equal distribution [42]. Clinically they usually are well defined, papular, uniformly pigmented, and typically less than 10 mm in diameter [197]. Nevus cells are somewhat larger than melanocytes and have round or ovoid nuclei. Dendrites are not present, and intercellular connections are not visible. The cells may lie singly within the dermis, but more commonly they tend to form nests. Unless they contain melanin, their cytoplasm is clear without granules or fibrils.

In pure junctional nevi, which are identified relatively infrequently on the vulva, the nevus cells are located within the epidermis and at the dermal–epidermal junction. Individual cells, or cell nests, bulge downward from the tips of the rete ridges. There is no connective tissue noted between the nevus cells and the adjacent squamous keratinocytes. Such nevi are young and somewhat undifferentiated.

With age, the nevus becomes a compound nevus with melanocytes located in the epidermis and the dermis. The basement membrane of the epidermis surrounding the nests disappears, and collagen and elastic fibers envelop the nests, pushing the epidermis upward. During this process, the lesion is clinically elevated above the level of the surrounding skin. Further differentiation results in complete enclosure of the nevus cells and nests by connective tissue elements such that they are entirely intradermal; no activity is seen at the dermoepidermal junction. These nevi are referred to as intradermal (➋ *Fig. 1.30*). Most nevi biopsied on the vulva are either compound or intradermal in type. With time, nevi may regress completely or may result in a fibrous papule or acrochordon [177].

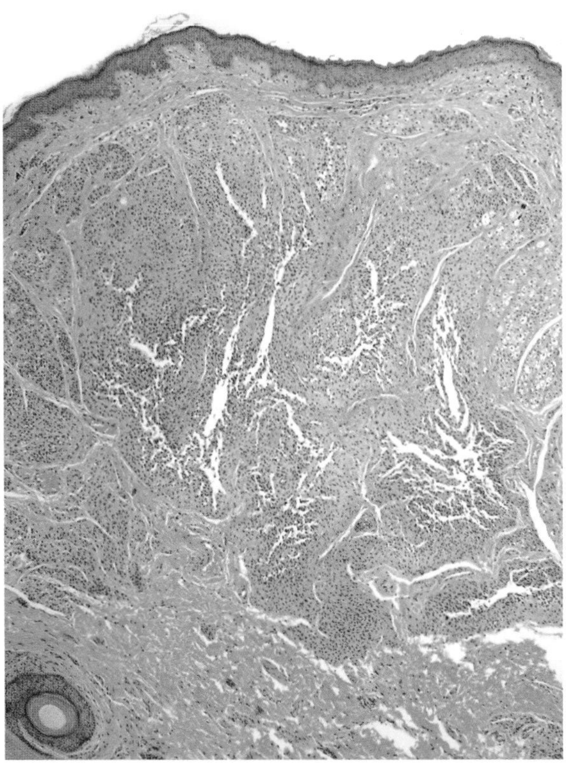

Fig. 1.30
Intradermal nevus. Nests of nevus cells are evident within the dermis

Atypical Vulvar Nevi

The so-called atypical vulvar nevus has many clinical and histopathologic features in common with acquired dysplastic nevi. The atypical vulvar nevus occurs in young women ranging from 20 to 30 years of age. Although not considered specifically as dysplastic by some authors, or associated with dysplastic nevi in other sites, the atypical vulvar nevus demonstrates prominent variable-sized junctional melanocytic nests and lentiginous spread. Because of their intertriginous location, vulvar nevi are subjected to chronic irritation and rubbing, and therefore some of the atypicality is probably reactive. Although some features may suggest a diagnosis of melanoma, the lesion is small, well circumscribed, has maturation toward the dermis and lacks pagetoid spread, necrosis, or mitotic activity in the dermis [2, 44] (➋ *Fig. 1.31*). A zone of eosinophilic fibrosis may be present in the superficial dermis [82].

Dysplastic Nevi

Dysplastic melanocytic nevi are seen most often in young women of reproductive age. Rare on the vulva, they present as pigmented, elevated lesions greater than 0.5 cm in diameter with irregular borders. Microscopic examination reveals large epithelioid or spindle-shaped nevus cells with nuclear pleomorphism and prominent nucleoli. The nevus cells are clustered in intraepithelial nests and are present in skin appendages, including hair shafts and the ducts of sweat glands [2, 44, 177]. They often have a low-power microscopic appearance of a large junctional nevus, with a dermal component that has spindle- or epithelioid-type nevus cells in nests or isolated within the papillary and reticular dermis. Three features distinguish a dysplastic nevus from melanoma. (1) Symmetric growth, which is evident on microscopic examination of a full cross section of the nevus, can be determined by visualizing a line drawn perpendicular to the surface of the center of the nevus. The halves should be mirror images of each other. (2) The most atypical cells are present in the superficial levels of the nevus, with smaller and more uniform cells in the deeper areas. (3) Rare pagetoid spread of single melanocytes with little or no involvement of the upper one third of the epithelium is seen and is usually present at the center of the lesion [2, 44, 177, 190]. In addition to malignant melanoma, a lesion of the dysplastic nevus syndrome should be included in the differential diagnosis. Individuals with dysplastic nevus syndrome have multiple large nevi, usually more than 0.5 cm in diameter, which may be found on the vulva and on the trunk and

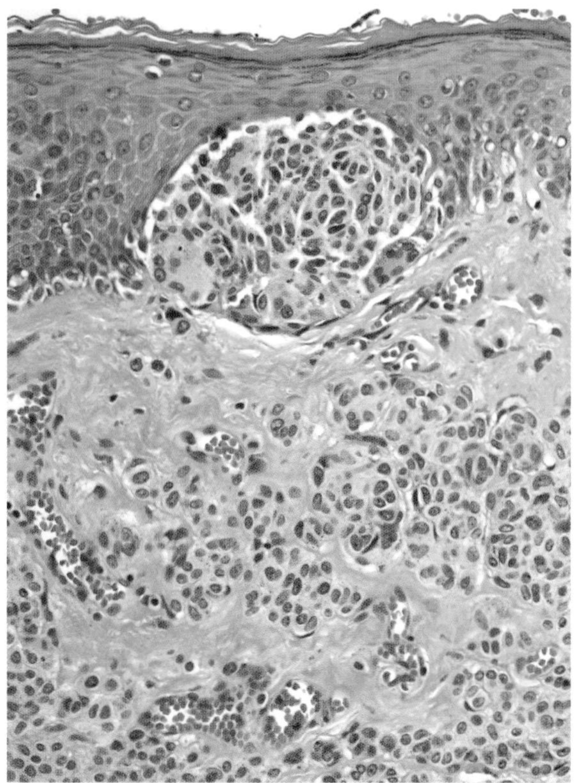

Fig. 1.31
Atypical vulvar nevus. **This acquired atypical nevus has marked variation in size and shape of the nests at the dermal epidermal junction with cytologic atypia characterized by hyperchromasia at this power. Small, benign-appearing nevus cells are present within the dermis, superficial and junctional areas (Taken from Atlas of Vulvar Disease [244])**

extremities. Individuals with dysplastic nevus syndrome have a high risk of subsequent malignant melanoma, whereas women with isolated atypical nevi of the vulva do not. Vulvar nevi are influenced by hormonal changes. They appear more active or atypical during pregnancy. Quite a few nevi are removed during pregnancy or at the time of the delivery because of the changes in color or size induced by pregnancy.

Acanthosis Nigricans and Pseudoacanthosis Nigricans

Acanthosis nigricans has been reported involving the vulva, although other sites where skin folds are found, including the axilla and submammary area, are more commonly involved. The clinical presentation is a diffuse, velvet-like, brown to gray-black skin change that is characteristically symmetric and may involve all the keratinized epithelium of the vulva, including the inguinal gluteal folds as well as the medial aspects of the upper thighs. Within the vulva, the pigmentation usually involves the labia majora and the lateral labia minora as well as the pubis [146]. In adults, acanthosis nigricans may be associated with adenocarcinoma of the stomach or other visceral malignancies. Its presentation should prompt the search for gastric and other tumors, especially if it occurs with sudden onset and is associated with pruritus and the appearance of multiple seborrheic keratosis (Leser–Trelet syndrome) [125].

A second variant of this type of skin change recognized in adults is pseudoacanthosis nigricans. This lesion has been reported in obese individuals as well as those with autoimmune or endocrine disorders or lipodystrophy.

A third variant of acanthosis nigricans occurs in children. It is not associated with any of the disorders described in adult variants [207]. The microscopic features are characterized by prominent papillomatosis with acanthosis and hyperkeratosis. Keratinous horn cysts may be seen within the epidermis. Increased melanin typically is seen within the basal layer. No significant inflammation or distinctive dermal changes are found.

Cysts

Bartholin Cyst and Abscess

The Bartholin ducts are prone to obstruction at their vestibular orifice. Such obstruction results in subsequent accumulation of secretion with associated cystic dilatation of the duct [176, 204]. The content of an uninfected Bartholin cyst is a mucoid, clear, translucent liquid that, when cultured, fails to grow bacteria. The secretion stains with mucicarmine, PAS before and after diastase digestion, and Alcian blue at pH 2.5, consistent with sialomucin. The epithelium lining the cyst may be squamous, transitional, or low cuboidal mucinous epithelium. In some cases it is flattened and otherwise not classifiable (➲ *Fig. 1.32*). Generally, there is minimal, if any, inflammatory response within the adjacent tissue. The epithelium of the cyst is immunoreactive for carcinoembryonic antigen (CEA). Bartholin cysts may be recurrent, and occasionally are associated with primary infection of the Bartholin gland, in which case they require marsupialization. In postmenopausal women, recurrent cysts or a palpable mass after cyst drainage may require excision of the gland because of the possibility of associated carcinoma of the Bartholin gland (see Chap. 2, Premalignant and Malignant Tumors of the Vulva). Bartholin adenocarcinomas, when present, tend to be in the tissues adjacent to the cyst wall.

Bartholin abscess is an acute process often associated with Neisseria gonorrheal infection, although it may be related to Staphylococcus or to other anaerobic organisms. The patient presents with tenderness and swelling in the Bartholin gland area. Microscopically, the Bartholin duct abscess demonstrates a striking acute inflammatory reaction within the stroma surrounding the duct. A purulent exudate is present within the lumen of the abscess wall. Excision, drainage, and antibiotics are the treatments of choice. Occasionally, the infection subsides without abscess formation or becomes chronic. Bartholin duct cysts, resulting from distal obstruction of the duct secondary to chronic inflammation and scarring, may be a late sequela of chronic infection. Mucocele-like changes have been reported in the Bartholin glands.

Keratinous Cyst (Epithelial Inclusion Cyst)

Keratinous cysts frequently are seen on the vulva; generally, these cysts are located on the labia majora and may involve the clitoris. Typically, they are superficial and range in size from 2 to 5 mm, but may be larger. They may occur at any age, even in newborns. Milium, a type of small keratinous cyst, has been reported in the vulva [105]. Keratinous cysts usually contain a white to pale yellow, grumous or cheesy material without hair. Foreign body-type giant cells may be seen in the tissue adjacent to the cyst wall, secondary to keratinous material leaking into the adjacent dermis. The lining of the cyst is characterized by a relatively flattened, stratified squamous epithelium that is immunoreactive for high molecular weight keratin (*Fig. 1.33*). Whether these cysts represent primary keratinous cysts, unrelated to sebaceous glands, or are actually occluded sebaceous glands that have undergone squamous metaplasia is debatable. Step sections through the cysts may show communication with the surface epithelium or underlying or adjacent sebaceous glands in some cases. An unusually high frequency of vulvar keratinous cyst has been reported in Nigerian children, related to female circumcision [92]. Such cysts are not considered premalignant, although carcinoma may arise in keratinous cysts. Treatment of asymptomatic small cysts usually is not necessary; however, surgical excision may be necessary for diagnosis or if the cyst is enlarging, symptomatic, or secondarily infected.

Mucous Cyst

Mucous cysts usually are seen within the vestibule and are lined by mucus-secreting, cuboidal to columnar epithelium without peripheral muscle fibers or evidence of myoepithelial cells (*Fig. 1.34*). Squamous metaplasia may be present. Histochemical studies demonstrate that

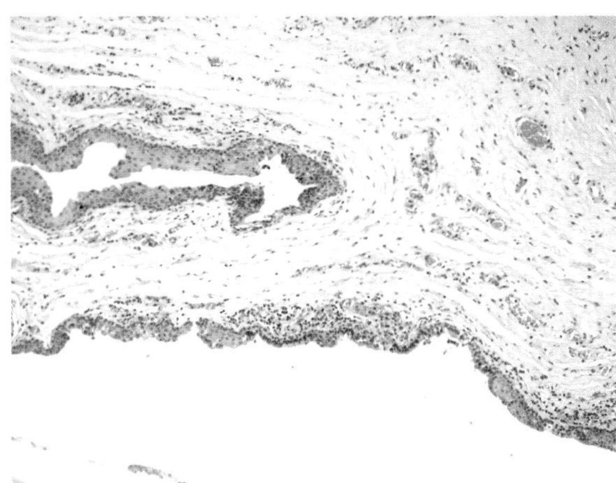

Fig. 1.32
Bartholin cyst. **The dilated duct has a flattened transitional type epithelial lining**

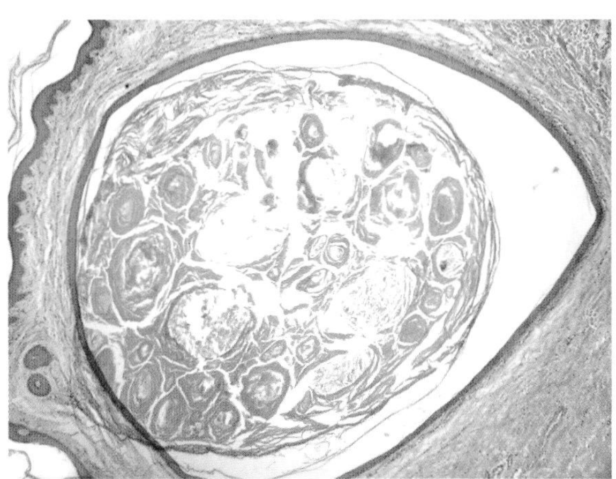

Fig. 1.33
Keratinous cyst. **Stratified squamous epithelial lining is evident**

the epithelial cells lining the cyst stain with both Alcian blue and Mayer mucicarmine, whereas the epithelial lining of cysts of mesonephric origin does not exhibit these reactions [72, 162]. The cysts probably develop from occlusion of minor vestibular glands [72]. Electron microscopic studies of mucinous cysts of the vestibule have demonstrated that these cysts have an epithelium consistent with an origin from urogenital sinus endoderm [195]. Because the vulvar vestibule arises embryologically primarily from the urogenital sinus, the origin of these cysts from minor vestibular glands is not inconsistent with a urogenital sinus origin.

Mucinous metaplasia of the vulva has been described, presenting as a solitary depressed red area of the labium minus [46]. In one reported case, this condition responded to topical estrogen cream. The finding of columnar cell metaplasia of the nonkeratinized squamous epithelium of the vulva vestibule or vagina, to columnar epithelium of mucinous or tuboepithelial type, also has been described after Stevens–Johnson syndrome as well as after laser and 5-fluorouracil (5-FU) therapy [143].

Apocrine Hidrocystoma/Cystadenoma of the Vulva

Apocrine hidrocystoma is a well-circumscribed cyst, lined by epithelium with apocrine differentiation. The lining cells have abundant pink cytoplasm with apical snoutlike secretion. When the lining cells form micropapillary projections into the cystic space, the lesion is termed apocrine cystadenoma (Fig. 1.35). The lesion typically arises in the apocrine gland-rich region, which includes the vulva [83].

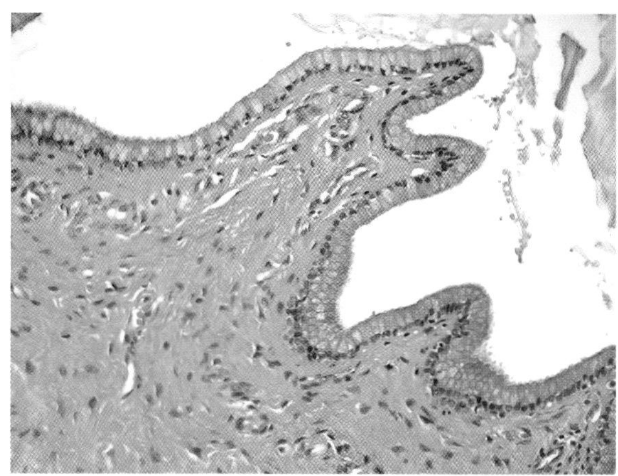

Fig. 1.34
Mucous cyst of the vestibule. **Simple columnar mucus-secreting cells rest on the basement membrane. Note absence of underlying smooth muscle layer (Courtesy of R.J. Kurman, M.D., Baltimore, MD)**

Ciliated Cysts of the Vulvar Vestibule: Vestibular Adenosis

Cysts lined with tuboendometrial epithelium resembling mullerian-type epithelium have been reported in the vulvar vestibule in women with chronic inflammation associated with Stevens–Johnson syndrome or with extensive laser or 5-FU therapy [106, 143, 210]. The cysts are believed to be acquired as the müllerian system does not contribute to the development of the vestibule. They are distinguished from endometriosis by the absence of

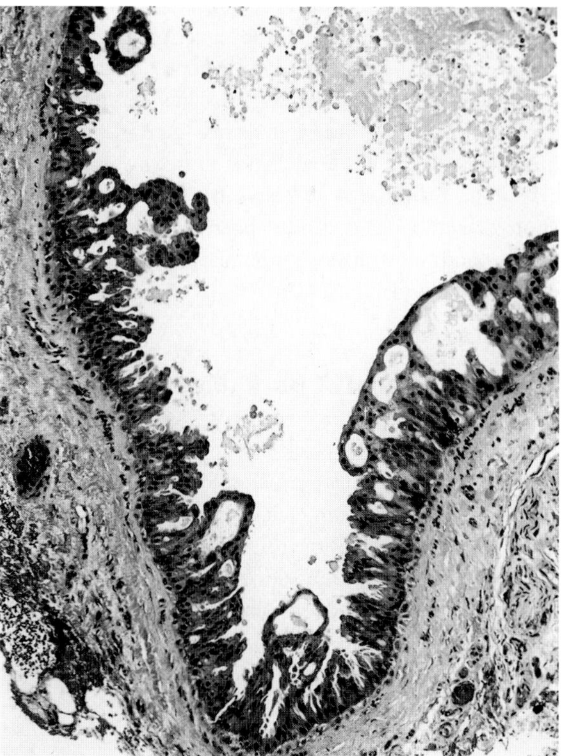

Fig. 1.35
Apocrine cystadenoma. **A well-circumscribed cystic space lined by epithelium with apocrine differentiation. The epithelial cells form micropapillary projections into the cystic lumen (Courtesy of R.J. Kurman, M.D., Baltimore, MD)**

associated endometrial stroma or hemosiderin-laden macrophages. In the vagina, such changes, when associated with 5-FU, slowly regress over time by a process of squamous metaplasia. In the vestibule, such cysts may be followed; if persistent or symptomatic, they can be excised.

Mesonephric-like Cyst (Wolffian-like Duct Cyst)

Mesonephric-like cysts are encountered occasionally on the lateral aspects of the vulva and the vagina. They are thin walled, translucent, and contain clear fluid. The lining epithelium is cuboidal to columnar and is not ciliated. Immunohistochemical techniques show smooth muscle in the submucosal area [103].

Mammary-like Cysts (Hidrocystoma)

Hidrocystoma originates in mammary-like glands involving the main collecting duct of anogenital mammary-like sweat glands. It is characterized by a peripheral basal layer of myoepithelial cells and a luminal layer of cuboidal to columnar cells. The luminal layer has discrete apical decapitation secretion. Cutaneous glands, including mammary-like glands, and dartos muscles surround the cysts. The mammary-like cysts may have similar alterations resembling eccrine, apocrine, and mammary glands, and most likely represent involution cysts of mammary-like glands [233].

Cyst of the Canal of Nuck (Mesothelial Cyst)

Cysts of the canal of Nuck are generally found in the superior aspect of the labia majora or inguinal canal and are believed to arise from inclusions of the peritoneum at the inferior insertion of the round ligament into the labia majora. As such, they are analogous to the hydrocele of the spermatic cord. These cysts can achieve substantial size and must be distinguished from an inguinal hernia, with which they are associated in approximately one third of cases [205].

Benign Solid Tumors and Tumor-like Lesions

Benign solid tumors of the vulva are rare. They may be divided into those that are of epithelial origin (squamous and glandular) and those that originate from vulvar soft tissue (mesenchymal origin).

Benign Squamous Epithelial Tumors

Fibroepithelial Polyp (Acrochordon)

A fibroepithelial polyp, or "skin tag," is a relatively uncommon benign polypoid tumor of the vulva. In contrast to the vestibular papilloma, the fibroepithelial polyp occurs on the hair-bearing skin of the vulva. These tumors vary in their clinical appearance from small, flesh-colored or hyperpigmented, papillomatous growths resembling condylomata to large pedunculated tumors that often are hypopigmented. On cut section, fibroepithelial polyps are soft and fleshy. Small tumors may resemble intradermal nevi; large lesions may present cosmetic problems but generally are clinically insignificant. They usually arise in hair-bearing skin but may be found on the labia minora [35]. The origin is most probably from a regressing nevus.

Histologically, fibroepithelial polyps may be of two types, one that is predominantly epithelial and another that is primarily stromal. The epithelial surface varies from a thickened layer with papillomatosis, hyperkeratosis, to an attenuated flattened layer exhibiting multiple primary folds (*Fig. 1.36*). The connective tissue stalk is composed of loose bundles of collagen with a moderate number of blood vessels. The stroma may be edematous and hypocellular. The stromal cells usually have relatively uniform nuclei; however, marked atypia may be seen in some cases [35].

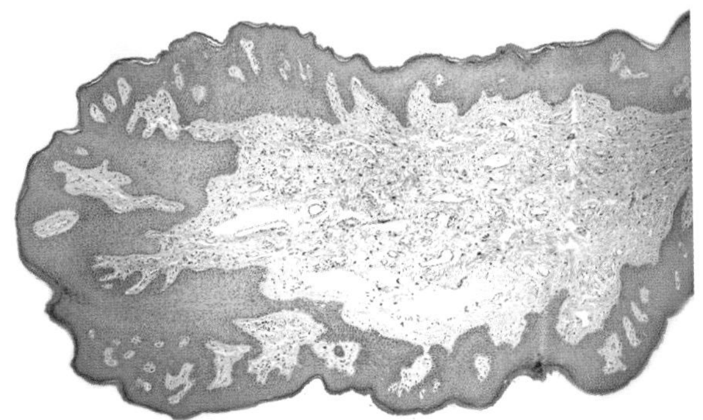

Fig. 1.36
Fibroepithelial polyp. **This polyp is primarily stromal, with prominent vessels within the central stalk. The epithelial surface is keratinized, stratified squamous epithelium. No inflammation or glandular elements are evident**

Vulvar Vestibular Papilloma (Micropapilloma Labialis)

The vestibular papilloma is a benign papillary lesion that is composed of a delicate fibrovascular connective tissue core covered by squamous epithelium, histologically similar to a fibroepithelial polyp. In contrast to a fibroepithelial polyp, vestibular papilloma typically occurs on the vestibule and may be single or multiple. They are relatively common lesions. When multiple, they also may involve the medial aspects of the labia minora and posterior medial labia majora, forming clusters of papules. They occur almost exclusively in women of reproductive age. Vestibular papillae are small, usually less than 5 mm in length, with a diameter of 1–2 mm. Solitary lesions usually are seen adjacent to the hymen, whereas multiple papillomas typically occur in clusters, usually on the lateroposterior aspects of the vestibule. They may be asymptomatic and associated with pruritus. In some cases, they may be seen in women with vulvar vestibulitis. Vulvar vestibular papilloma, associated with vestibular pruritus, burning, or dyspareunia, has been identified as a clinical complexity. The etiology of vestibular papillomatosis is unknown in most cases. No significant association with HPV has been demonstrated [17, 55, 157]. These papillae may be an anatomic variant, the female homologue of pearly penile papules.

On microscopic examination, vestibular papillae typically have features of an angiofibroma with stratified nonkeratinized squamous epithelium, which is glycogen-rich in women of reproductive age. They may have a thin keratin layer. The papillae have a fibrovascular core, often with a prominent central vessel. Usually inflammation is not present. The glycogen-rich squamous epithelium should be distinguished from HPV changes by having normal-sized nuclei whereas the koilocytes have enlarged atypical nuclei. Other features of HPV infection, including dyskeratosis, parabasal hyperplasia, accentuation of intracellular bridges, and multinucleation, are not identified in glycogen-rich epithelium. In situ hybridization and PCR for HPV may be performed if the findings are equivocal.

Seborrheic Keratosis

Seborrheic keratosis is a benign epithelial growth characterized by acanthosis, papillomatosis, hyperkeratosis, and epithelial invaginations forming horn cysts. The lesions are raised with irregular borders occurring on hair-bearing skin of the vulva. They vary from pale brown to brownish black and appear to be stuck onto the skin surface. Although clinically insignificant, their gross appearance often mimics that of a nevus or melanoma. Seborrheic keratosis of genital skin has been associated in a few studies with human papillomavirus (HPV) infection but is not generally considered a lesion caused by HPV [9, 131]. Multiple seborrheic keratosis presenting over a short period of time may be associated with internal malignancy (Leser–Trelat syndrome) [125]. This association is especially strong when associated with acanthosis nigricans.

On low-power examination, the entire lesion appears to be above a straight line drawn from the normal epidermis at one side of the lesion to the normal epidermis at the other side. Both mature squamous cells and basal type cells are noted in strands and cords surrounding numerous horny keratin cysts (*Fig. 1.37*). Varying degrees of hyperpigmentation may be present.

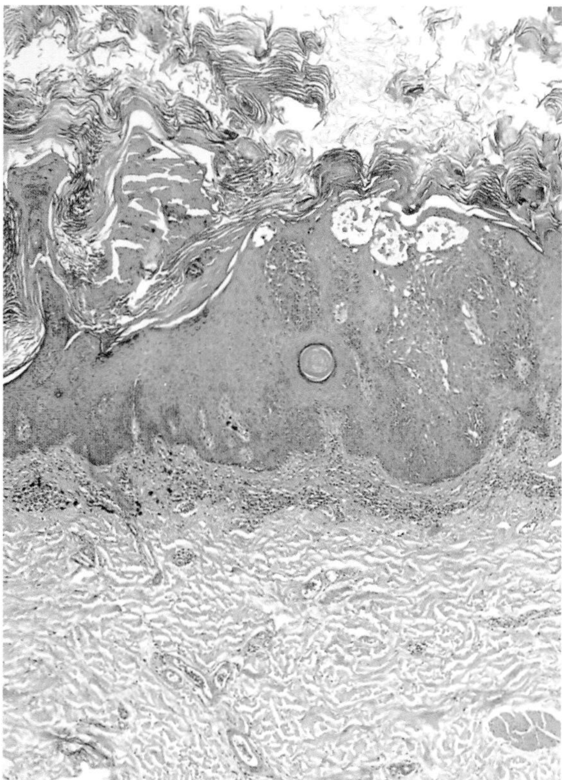

Fig. 1.37
Seborrheic keratosis, pigmented. **When pigmented, these lesions may mimic vulvar intraepithelial neoplasia (VIN) or melanoma on the vulva. The melanocytic hyperplasia and hyperpigmentation are present primarily in the basal layers. A keratin pearl is present**

Keratoacanthoma

Keratoacanthoma is composed of glassy squamous epithelial proliferation in which horny masses of keratin are pushed upward while tongues of squamous epithelium invade the dermis, resembling squamous cell carcinoma. These tumors commonly occur on sun-exposed skin and may arise on hair-bearing skin of the vulva. They are rapidly growing but are usually self-limited. Keratoacanthoma is generally accepted as a well-differentiated squamous cell carcinoma, keratoacanthoma type. Metastasis of keratoacanthoma has been reported [113, 78]. Complete excision with a clear histologic margin is the treatment of choice.

Glandular Tumors

Papillary Hidradenoma (Hidradenoma Papilliferum)

Clinical Features

Papillary hidradenoma is a benign tumor of apocrine sweat gland origin, composed of epithelial and myoepithelial cells lining complex delicate fibrovascular branching stalks. Papillary hidradenoma usually presents as a small, dome-shaped tumor less than 2 cm in size. The lesion generally arises from the interlabial sulci, or from the lateral surface of the labia minora. The tumors usually are asymptomatic; however, ulceration of the overlying surface may produce bleeding. Papillary hidradenomas have not been described before puberty, and almost all cases have occurred in Caucasian women [14]. There is evidence that they arise from specialized anogenital mammary-like "sweat" glands [232].

Microscopic Findings

Histologically, under low-power examination, the tumor simulates a well-differentiated adenocarcinoma (Fig. 1.38). Stromal compression often results in the formation of a well-circumscribed pseudocapsule. At times, epithelial cells become entrapped within the compressed connective tissue, creating a pseudoinfiltrative appearance. The tumor is composed of numerous tubules and acini lined by a single or double layer of cuboidal cells, the outer layer representing myoepithelial cells (Fig. 1.39). At times, the cells lining the lumen of the adenomatous structures are large and pale. An inflammatory reaction is unusual unless secondary infection is present. Mitotic figures are rare, and only mild degrees of cellular and nuclear pleomorphism are present.

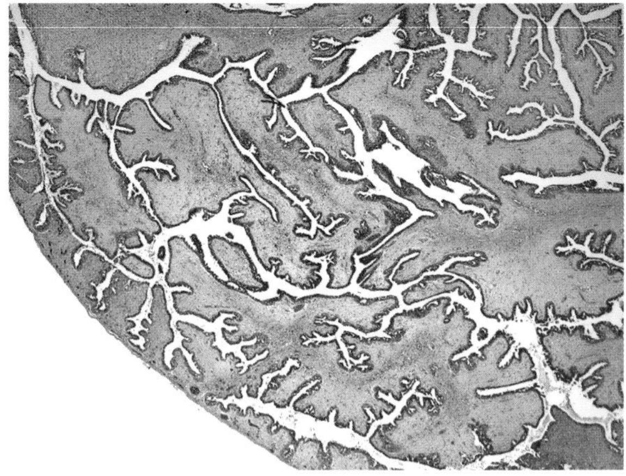

Fig. 1.38
Papillary hidradenoma. **This well-circumscribed adenomatous dermal tumor has no connection to skin surface. At low magnification, this benign tumor can be misinterpreted as adenocarcinoma**

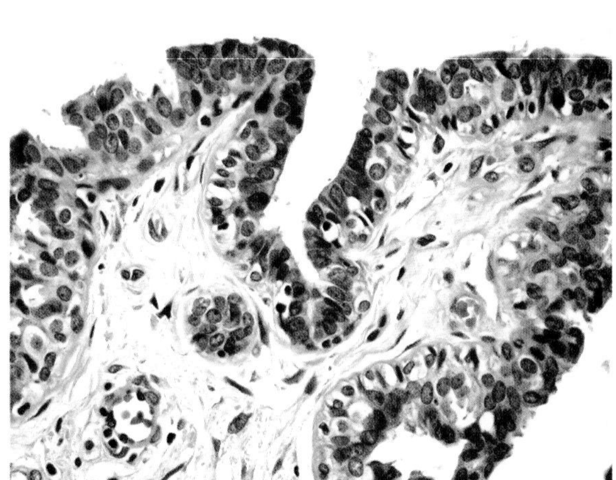

Fig. 1.39
Papillary hidradenoma. **High-power examination shows tubules and acini lined with a single or double layer of bland cuboidal to columnar cells with underlying myoepithelial cells**

Clinical Behavior and Treatment

Clinically, the hidradenoma is benign; however, an intraductal carcinoma resembling mammary-type apocrine epithelium has been described arising in a hidradenoma [174]. Local excision, including the base of the mass, is a sufficient therapy.

Nodular Hidradenoma

Many names, including clear cell hidradenoma, clear cell myoblastoma, solid cystic hidradenoma, eccrine acrospiroma, eccrine sweat gland adenoma of clear cell type, and apocrine hidradenoma, have all been used for this entity [113]. Nodular hidradenoma is generally considered a tumor of eccrine sweat gland origin because it contains eccrine enzymes. Isolated examples of this tumor have been reported on the vulva [57].

Histologically, nodular hidradenoma is composed of a well-circumscribed lobulated mass with occasional cystic spaces. Tubular structures, sometimes branching, are often found in the solid areas. The cells are usually the mixtures of pink polyhedral cells and clear cells. The proportion of these two types of cells varies. In addition, secretory cells, dermal and epidermal ductal cells, and immature basaloid cells can be found in this tumor. The relatively small nucleus is round to oval and may exhibit an irregular outline. The chromatin frequently is clumped, and a single small nucleolus often is seen. Mitotic figures are not uncommon (*Fig. 1.40*) [113]. Wide local excision is considered adequate therapy.

Syringoma

The syringoma is a benign tumor of eccrine duct origin characterized by multiple, small, relatively uniform epithelial-lined tubules and cysts within a fibrous stroma. It is assumed to be an adenoma of the eccrine ducts. These lesions occur on the vulva as well as the eyelids, cheeks, axillae, and abdomen. Clinically, multiple clustered flesh-colored papules are noted within the deeper skin layers of the labia majora bilaterally. They often are asymptomatic, although pruritus may occur [34].

Histologically, the tumor lacks a clearly defined border. Within the dermis, numerous small, dilated duct spaces are seen. These spaces usually are lined by two rows of epithelial cells that appear flat, secondary to pressure atrophy. The comma-like formation of these glandular spaces is characteristic (*Fig. 1.41*). The stroma has a desmoplastic appearance.

Mixed Tumor of the Vulva (Pleomorphic Adenoma, Chondroid Syringoma)

Mixed tumor of the vulva is a rare neoplasm that usually presents as a solid, subcutaneous tumor involving the labia majora or the Bartholin gland area or both. The histopathologic findings are similar to those of mixed tumors of the parotid and other salivary glands. The tumor consists of epithelial cells arranged in tubules or nests, mixed with a fibrous stroma containing chondromatous, osseous, and myxoid elements. These stromal-like elements are believed to arise from pluripotential myoepithelial cells that, in the vulva, are found in the Bartholin glands, sweat glands, and accessory breast tissue [200]. These tumors are benign, but local recurrence may occur. Malignant mixed tumors have

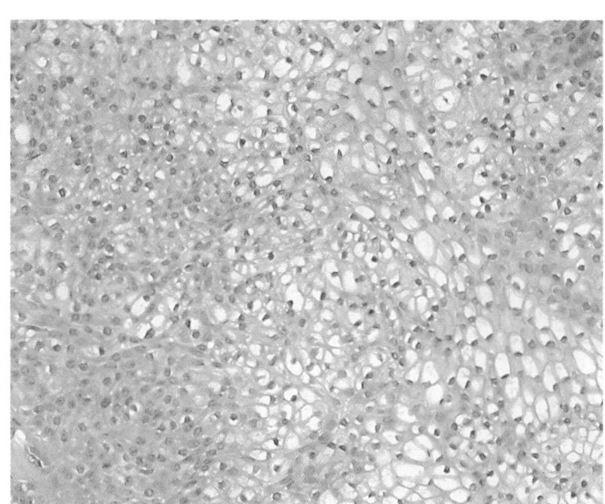

Fig. 1.40
Nodular hidradenoma (clear cell hidradenoma). **High power view of the sheets of large clear cells**

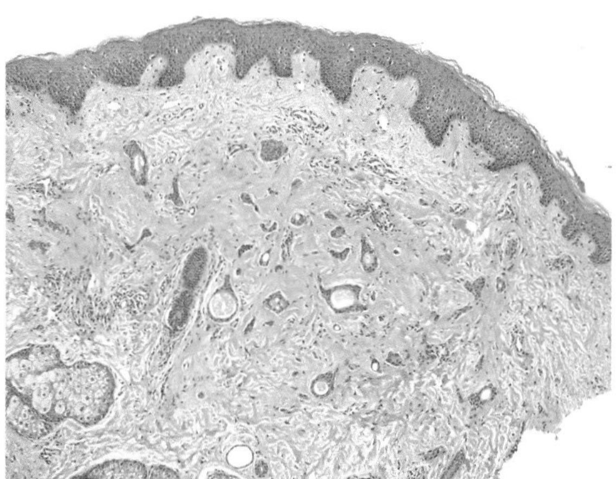

Fig. 1.41
Syringoma. **The comma pattern of the eccrine structures is easily appreciated (Courtesy of V. Vincek, Gainesville, FL)**

been reported [168]. When metastasis occurs from a malignant mixed tumor, it is usually composed of only epithelial elements. There are insufficient cases of vulvar mixed tumors to determine its natural history in this site. Wide local excision, with free margins, is the recommended therapy of choice for both the primary tumor and local recurrences.

Trichoepithelioma

Trichoepithelioma is a benign tumor of follicular origin that is rare in the vulva [40]. The tumor presents as single or multiple cutaneous nodules with normal-appearing overlying epithelium. On microscopic examination, the tumor is composed of complex interconnected nests of basaloid cells, which form small cysts containing keratin "horn cysts." The cells in trichoepithelioma are monomorphic without hyperchromasia or nuclear atypia. Occasionally, a granulomatous reaction with giant cells is present next to ruptured horn cysts. Hair or hair-forming elements are rare. Trichoepithelioma is distinguished from basaloid carcinoma or basal cell carcinoma in that it is not infiltrative, contains "horn cysts" and granulomas, may exhibit hair-forming elements, and is not associated with an intraepithelial neoplastic component. Local excision is therapeutic.

Proliferating Trichilemmal Tumor/Cyst (Pilar Tumors)

Proliferating trichilemmal tumor/cyst is rare on the vulva, occurring in the dermis of the labium majus, where it presents as a slowly growing solid mass that may have a cystic cavity in the center of the tumor [7, 186]. It is thought to arise from the cells of the outer root sheath of a hair follicle. Microscopic examination reveals a lobulated proliferation of squamous epithelium with a pushing border. The tumor may show no connection with the overlying epithelium. An eosinophilic glassy layer of collagen (vitreous layer) may surround some of the lobules. The tumor cells are palisaded peripherally and have increased cytoplasm in the cells toward the center of the lobules with abrupt changes into eosinophilic amorphous keratin, resembling keratinization of the follicular infundibulum (trichilemmal keratinization). Some degree of nuclear pleomorphism and cytologic atypia, as well as individual cell keratinization, forming squamous "eddies" may be present. Focal calcification within the amorphous keratin may occur.

Trichoblastic fibroma also has been described on the vulva [79]. Local excision is therapeutic.

Adenoma of Minor Vestibular Glands

Adenoma of minor vestibular glands is a rare benign tumor. These lesions are small, ranging from 1–2 mm to 1 cm. The tumor is composed of multiple lobular clusters of small glands lined by mucin-secreting columnar epithelium. Some may represent a nodular hyperplasia. Most cases have been found incidentally in vestibulectomy specimens excised for vulvar vestibulitis [73, 182].

Endometriosis

Vulvar endometriomas develop from ectopic endometrial epithelium. Endometrium implanted in an episiotomy incision at the time of delivery, as well as menstrual endometrium implanting in a small area of trauma, has been implicated in the etiology of this condition (see ➋ Chap. 13, Diseases of the Peritoneum). The clinical appearance is variable, ranging from bluish-red cystic masses to amorphous deep-seated nodules. Endometriomas of the vulva usually are located near the posterior fourchette. Cyclic enlargement and regression often are noted. Fine-needle aspiration may be of value in the diagnosis, demonstrating benign glandular and stromal cellular elements [140].

Histologically, both endometrial glands and stroma are present with a fibrotic response. A foreign body–giant cell reaction and hemosiderin-laden macrophages may be noted, especially in cases in which the onset was preceded by recent surgery.

Angiokeratoma

Angiokeratoma is a variant of hemangioma and occurs almost exclusively on the scrotum and vulva; however, it has been described as presenting as an ulcerated tumor of the clitoris [147]. Somewhat larger than senile hemangioma, these lesions often are purple to brown-black in color and occur primarily in women of childbearing age. Their peculiar appearance often prompts excisional diagnostic biopsy, although they usually have no clinical significance [47]. Multiple lesions may be associated with Fabry's disease [244].

Histologically, the dilated endothelial-lined channels are separated by strands and cords of squamous epithelial cells representing downgrowth from the overlying epithelium, which is often hyperkeratotic (➋ *Fig. 1.42*). Varying degrees of acanthosis and papillomatosis are present, along with a mild inflammatory reaction in the deep dermis. Angiosarcomas and Kaposi sarcoma are included

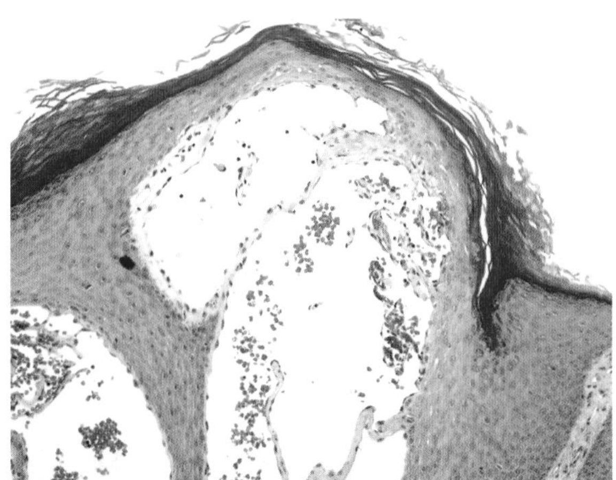

Fig. 1.42
Angiokeratoma. **Strands of squamous epithelium surround endothelial-lined vascular spaces**

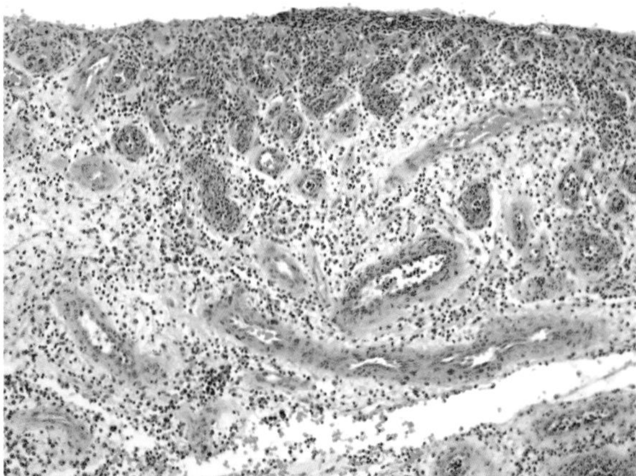

Fig. 1.43
Pyogenic granuloma. **Superficial ulceration of the mucosa is present, with a chronic inflammatory infiltrate. Within the submucosa, multiple endothelial-lined vascular spaces are seen surrounded by a delicate fibrous stroma, resembling granulation tissue**

in the differential diagnosis of vascular tumors [132]. These malignant tumors typically are more cellular and have greater cellular atypia. In addition, they have less well-formed vascular spaces that are usually slitlike and which are infiltrative with poorly defined margins.

Pyogenic Granuloma (Granuloma Pyogenicum)

Pyogenic granuloma is a variant of hemangioma that may occur anywhere on the skin. It is analogous to the epulis tumor of pregnancy. Most of the pyogenic granulomas that occur on the vulva do so during gestation. Although previously thought to be secondary to a superficial wound infection, this tumor is recognized as a form of hemangioma characterized by rapid growth. Because the surface is easily traumatized, the lesion often is secondarily infected. Histologically, a thin ulcerated epidermis is noted covering a mass of granulation tissue. Capillaries are numerous, and secondary inflammatory changes frequently are found within the stroma (*Fig. 1.43*). Around the periphery of the lesion, there may be a downward growth of the epidermis producing a "collarette." The overall architecture appears lobulated (lobular capillary hemangioma) with a few thickened fibrous septae separating the vascular proliferation.

Lymphangioma Circumscriptum

Lymphangioma circumscriptum is a relatively rare condition that is benign and thought to be secondary to a localized developmental defect of the dermal lymphatics or a malformation. Initial presentation may be in childhood; however, vulvar cases have been described initially presenting in women in their thirties. The lesion is characterized by multiple clustered blebs and vesicles that are white to purple. The lesions may be small, but may exceed 2 cm in diameter [37, 101, 215]. The blebs of lymphangioma circumscriptum may become secondarily infected, ulcerated, and macerated, resulting in pain and cellulitis. The diagnosis usually is made by the clinical appearance and by biopsy.

The microscopic findings reveal distinctive subepidermal cystic spaces containing lymph that is eosinophilic and acellular. These endothelial-lined cysts, which may be multiloculated, are located immediately beneath the basal epithelial layer in the papillary dermis (*Fig. 1.44*). Dilated lymphatic spaces can be found in the reticular dermis. Some of these deeper lymphatics may be surrounded by a prominent peripheral smooth muscle layer. The overlying epithelium usually is unremarkable but may be eroded or hyperkeratotic. Treatment includes surgical excision or laser therapy [101].

Miscellaneous Tumors and Tumor-like Lesions

Verruciform Xanthoma

Verruciform xanthoma is a benign lesion that clinically mimics a malignant tumor. It is a tumor of mucosal origin and is most commonly seen in oral cavity and, rarely, in anogenital mucosa as well as in the vulvar mucosa. Histologically, the lesion has verruciform hyperplasia with the expended dermal papillae/submucosa, which is filled with foamy histiocytes [129]. Patients with verruciform xanthoma may have autoimmune diseases.

Nevis Lipomatous Superficialis

This distinctive benign tumor of adipose tissue presents as a nodule within the dermis with normal overlying epithelium. This tumor has been considered a hamartoma of fat. Microscopic examination reveals adipose tissue within the superficial dermis, distinct from the underlying adipose tissue.

Mammary-like Tissue Within the Vulva

The findings of mammary-like tissue in the vulva is not well understood, but it is currently considered to be ectopic in nature [232, 233]. Clinically, mammary-like tissue in the vulva may present as an amorphous enlargement of the labia, usually first noted in association with pregnancy [232]. Benign cystic disease (fibrocystic disease), as well as fibroadenomas, lactating adenomas, and intraductal papillomas, have been described [232]. Cystosarcoma phyllodes, a tumor arising in these mammary-like tissues of the vulva is rare (➔ *Figs. 1.45* and ➔ *1.46*). Adenocarcinoma of the mammary-like tissue of the vulva has been reported [110, 232]. Surgical removal of symptomatic mammary-like tissue is advocated except when such tissue is discovered during pregnancy, in which case therapy should be deferred until after puerperal regression is complete.

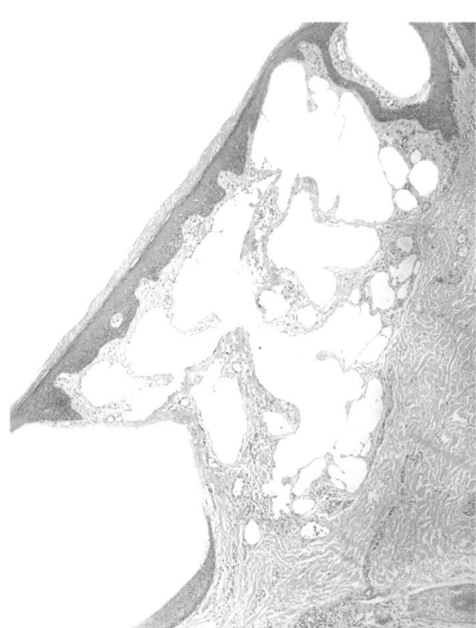

Fig. 1.44
Lymphangioma circumscriptum. **Subepidermal multiloculated cystic spaces filled with acellular lymph. Some slightly dilated deeper lymphatic channels are evident in the deeper dermis (Courtesy of G. Segal, M.D., Gainesville, FL)**

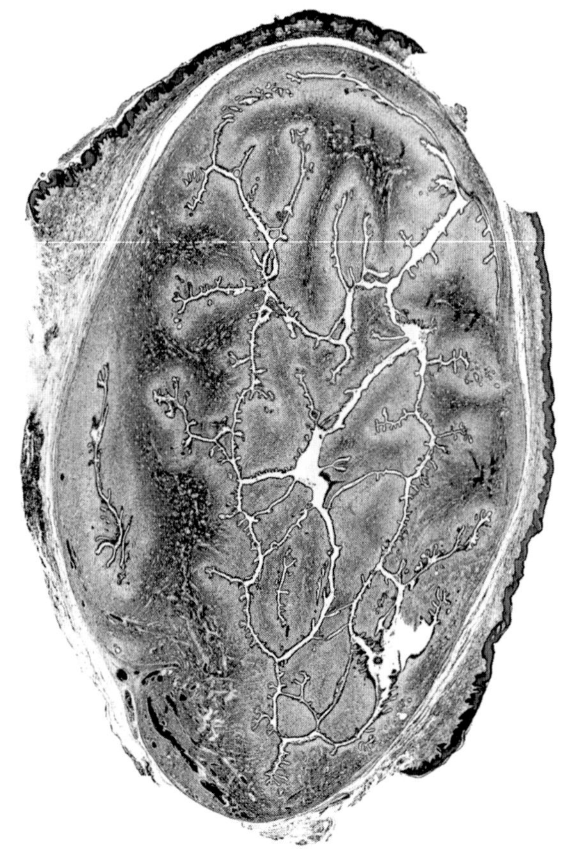

Fig. 1.45
Phyllodes tumor of vulva. **The tumor is well demarcated. The tumor displays a leaflike pattern identical to phyllodes tumor of breast (Courtesy of R.J. Kurman, M.D., Baltimore, MD)**

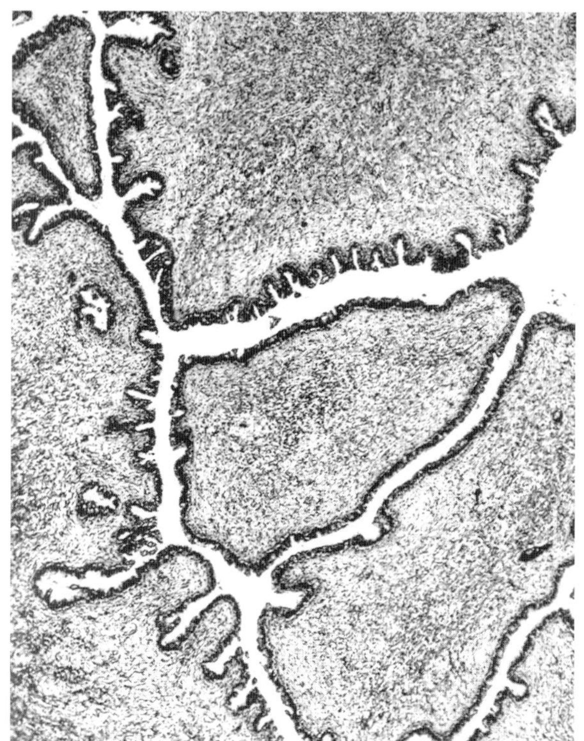

■ Fig. 1.46
Phyllodes tumor of the vulva. **Marked stromal expansion with spindle cells and proliferation of epithelial cells forming papillary structures (Courtesy of R.J. Kurman, M.D., Baltimore, MD)**

Salivary Glandlike Tissue

Salivary glandlike tissue has been observed in the vulva [145].

Idiopathic Vulvar Calcinosis

Although not a cystic condition, vulvar calcinosis may resemble keratinous cysts on clinical presentation, presenting as small (usually 2 mm or less), firm, subcutaneous nodules involving the majora and fourchette. The vulvar cases reported have occurred predominantly in adolescent women. Histologic examination demonstrates normal-appearing overlying epithelium with basophilic acellular superficial subcutaneous nodules measuring from less than 0.1 mm to approximately 2 mm, associated with a chronic inflammatory infiltrate, mast cells, and foreign body giant cells. The acellular material stains with Von Kossa stain and contains acid mucopolysaccharides [10]. The process is rare, benign, and of uncertain etiology but appears similar to idiopathic scrotal calcinosis [19].

Vulvar Amyloidosis

Nodules within the vulva have been described related to involvement of the vulva in a woman with systemic amyloidosis, which may mimic giant condyloma.

Benign Lesions of the Urethra

Urethra Prolapse

Prolapse of the urethral mucosa may occur at any age, but it is most common in premenarchal children and in postmenopausal women. Redundancy of the mucosa and laxity of the supporting periurethral fascia contribute to the formation of prolapse, which is aggravated by increased abdominal pressure; it may be related to relative lack of estrogen. The prolapsed urethra may present as a large red polypoid mass covered with urethral mucosa with edematous vascular submucosa, protruding from the urethra and mimicking a urethral neoplasm. Histologically, the urethral mucosa may exhibit ulceration, and the underlying connective tissue is generally filled with an inflammatory infiltrate. Vascular engorgement usually is present. Cryosurgery is an effective method of treatment [107].

Urethral Caruncles

Caruncles are sessile or polypoid masses that arise at the urethral meatus in postmenopausal women. They may represent localized areas of prolapse, and are by far the most common lesions of the urethra. Caruncles often are asymptomatic but may cause bleeding or dysuria. Clinical differentiation from urethral carcinoma may be impossible; therefore, excision is indicated for diagnosis. Recurrences may be observed [253]. Histologically, the submucosa of the urethral caruncle may contain large venous channels that often are dilated and engorged. A myxomatous or granulomatous pattern may be present in the supporting tissue, which often is densely infiltrated with chronic inflammatory cells. Excision, with hemostatic control of the base of the lesion, is the treatment of choice.

Malacoplakia of the Urethra

Malacoplakia is a chronic granulomatous inflammatory process that usually involves the bladder if the urethra is involved. The lesion presents as a polypoid mass at the urethral meatus.

On microscopic examination the lesion contains foamy histiocytes, lymphocytes, granulocytes, and plasma cells. The diagnostic Michaelis–Gutmann bodies are seen within the cytoplasm of the histiocytes as inclusions having a blue-gray color (➋ *Fig. 1.47*). The inclusions may appear laminated or targetoid. With PAS stains, the Michaelis–Gutmann bodies usually stain pink to red (see ➋ Chap. 3, Diseases of the Vagina). Many of the adjacent histiocytes also contain PAS-positive cytoplasmic material. Excision may be diagnostic and curative for small lesions within the urethra, although recurrences are not uncommon. Antibiotics also may be of value.

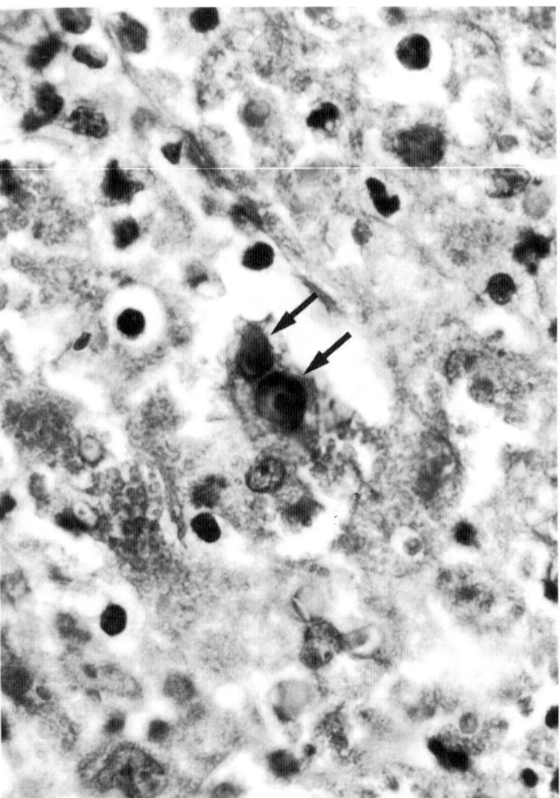

Fig. 1.47
Malacoplakia of the urethra. **Round inclusions are present in some of the histiocytes (Michaelis–Gutmann bodies), which are approximately the size of the nuclei of the histiocytes and have a dark periphery and pale center (Courtesy of R.J. Kurman, M.D., Baltimore, MD)**

Periurethral Cysts

Periurethral cysts can be subclassified according to their epithelial lining, and are similar to cysts of the vulvar vestibule. The cysts can be classified into four types: epithelial inclusion, mucous, mesonephric-like, and urothelial.

Epithelial Inclusion (Keratinous) Cysts

Epithelial inclusion cysts have a squamous epithelial lining, and may arise secondary to trauma or surgical procedures that entrap epithelium (see vulvar keratinous cysts).

Mucous Cysts

Mucous cysts have a columnar, endocervical-type epithelial lining and may have associated squamous epithelium, secondary to squamous metaplasia. The cytoplasm of the columnar epithelium contains mucin. These cysts appear essentially identical to the mucous cysts of the vulvar vestibule, although they have been referred to as müllerian cysts.

Mesonephric-like Cysts

Mesonephric-like cysts have a low cuboidal epithelium that does not stain with mucin.

Urothelial Cysts

Urothelial cysts usually are seen in infants and are rare in adults. They are believed to arise from the Skene ducts or from proximal urothelial ducts. These cysts have a urothelial epithelial lining, although those near the urethra meatus may have a squamous epithelial lining.

Suburethral Diverticulum

Suburethral diverticula originate from the upper two thirds of the posterior urethral wall and may extend cephalic to involve the region beneath the vesicle neck. Although a congenital etiology has been proposed for some cases, most are thought to begin as an infection in one of the tubular periurethral glands, followed by abscess formation with eventual breakthrough into the urethral lumen.

Urethral Condyloma Acuminatum

Urethral condyloma acuminatum may present like a caruncle or urethral carcinoma, and usually is seen in women of reproductive age and not in older individuals. In children, urethral and periurethral condylomata may be polypoid and clinically may suggest sarcoma botryoides. In adult women, they usually are associated with other lower genital infections, especially vulvar vestibular condyloma acuminatum. Some patients may have symptoms of urethritis associated with urethral condyloma acuminatum. In these patients, the condylomas may be in the mid- or upper urethra. On biopsy they have a stratified squamous epithelium within which typical features of mucosal HPV infection are seen, including koilocytosis, multinucleation, and parabasal hyperplasia. HPV types 6 and 16 have been observed in urethral condylomas.

References

1. Abdul-Karim FW, Cohen RE (1990) Atypical stromal cells of lower female genital tract. Histopathology 17:249–253
2. Ackerman AB, Mihara I (1985) Dysplasia, dysplastic melanocytes, dysplastic nevi, the dysplastic nevus syndrome, and the relation between dysplastic nevi and malignant melanomas. Hum Pathol 16:87–91
3. ACOG Committee on Practice Bulletins – Gynecology ACOG practice bulletin: clinical management guidelines for obstetrician-gynecologists, number 57, November 2004. Gynecologic herpes simplex virus infections
4. Adelson MD, Joret DM, Gordon LP, Osborne NG (1991) Recurrent necrotizing fasciitis of the vulva. A case report. J Reprod Med 36: 818–822
5. Ang P, Tay YK (1999) Treatment of linear IgA bullous dermatosis of childhood with colchicine. Pediatr Dermatol 16:50–52
6. Arany I, Tyring SK (1996) Status of local cellular immunity in interferon-responsive and -nonresponsive human papillomavirus-associated lesions. Sex Transm Dis 23:475–480
7. Avinoach I, Zirfkin HJ, Glezerman M (1989) Proliferating trichilemmal tumor of the vulva. Case report and review of the literature. Int J Gynecol Pathol 8:163–168
8. Aziz DC, Ferre F, Robitaille J, Ferenczy A (1993) Human papillomavirus testing in the clinical laboratory. Part II: Vaginal, vulvar, perineal, and penile squamous lesions. J Gynecol Surg 9:9–15
9. Bai H, Cviko A, Granter S, Yuan L, Betensky RA, Crum CP (2003) Immunophenotypic and viral (human papillomavirus) correlates of vulvar seborrheic keratosis. Hum Pathol 34(6): 559–564
10. Balfour FJT, Vincenti AC (1991) Idiopathic vulvar calcinosis. Histopathology (Oxf) 18:183–184
11. Balfour HH Jr (1991) Varicella-zoster virus infections in the immunocompromised host. Natural history and treatment. Scand J Infect Dis Suppl 80:69–74
12. Barnhill RL, Albert LS, Shama SK, Goldenhersh MA, Rhodes AR, Sober AJ (1990) Genital lentiginosis: a clinical and histopathologic study. J Am Acad Dermatol 22:453–460
13. Basoglu M, Gul O, Yildirgan I, Balik AA, Ozbey I, Oren D (1997) Fournier's gangrene: review of fifteen cases. Am Surg 63: 1019–1021
14. Basta A, Madej JG Jr (1990) Hydradenoma of the vulva. Incidence and clinical observations. Eur J Gynecol Oncol 11:185–189
15. Batta K, Munday PE, Tatnall FM (1999) Pemphigus vulgaris localized to the vagina presenting as chronic vaginal discharge. Br J Dermatol 140:945–947
16. Berger J, Telser A, Widschwendter M, Muller-Holzner E, Daxenbichler G, Marth C, Zeimet AG (2000) Expression of retinoic acid receptors in non-neoplastic epithelial disorders of the vulva and normal vulvar skin. Int J Gynecol Pathol 19:95–102
17. Bergeron C, Ferenczy A, Richart RM, Guralnick M (1990) Micropapillomatosis labialis appears unrelated to human papillomavirus. Obstet Gynecol 76:281–286
18. Bergeron S, Binik YM, Khalife S, Pagidas K, Glazer HI, Meana M, Amsel R (2001) A randomized comparison of group cognitive–behavioral therapy, surface electromyographic biofeedback, and vestibulectomy in the treatment of dyspareunia resulting from vulvar vestibulitis. Pain 1:297–306
19. Bernardo BD, Huettner PC, Merritt DF, Ratts VS (1999) Idiopathic calcinosis cutis presenting as labial lesions in children: report of two cases with literature review. J Pediatr Adolesc Gynecol 12: 157–160
20. Berth-Jones J, Graham-Brown RA, Burns DA (1991) Lichen sclerosus et atrophicus: a review of 15 cases in young girls. Clin Exp Dermatol 16:14–17
21. Beutner KR, von Krogh G (1990) Current status of podophyllotoxin for the treatment of genital warts. Semin Dermatol 9:148–151
22. Bonafe JL, Thibaut I, Hoff J (1990) Introital adenosis associated with the Stevens-Johnson syndrome. Clin Exp Dermatol 15: 356–357
23. Bonnez W, Oakes D, Bailey-Farchione A, Choi A, Hallahan D, Pappas P, Holloway M, Corey L, Barnum G, Dunne A, Stoler MH, Demeter LM, Reichman RC (1995) A randomized, double-blind, placebo- controlled trial of systemically administered interferon-alpha, -beta, or -gamma in combination with cryotherapy for the treatment of condyloma acuminatum. J Infect Dis 171:1081–1089
24. Bornstein J, Goldik Z, Alter Z, Zarfati D, Abra-movici H (1998) Persistent vulvar vestibulitis: the continuing challenge. Obstet Gynecol Surv 53:39–44
25. Brown DR, Bryan JT, Cramer H, Fife KH (1993) Analysis of human papillomavirus types in exophytic condylomata acuminata by hybrid capture and Southern blot techniques. J Clin Microbiol 31:2667–2673
26. Brown TJ, Yen-Moore A, Tyring SK (1999) An overview of sexually transmitted diseases. Part I. J Am Acad Dermatol 41:511–532
27. Buntin DM, Rosen T, Lesher JL Jr, Plotnick H, Brademas ME, Berger TG (1991) Sexually transmitted diseases: bacterial infections. Committee on Sexually Transmitted Diseases of the American Academy of Dermatology. J Am Acad Dermatol 25(pt 1):287–299

28. Bystryn JC, Steinman NM (1996) The adjuvant therapy of pemphigus. An update. Arch Dermatol 132:203–212
29. Carli P, Bracco G, Taddei G, Sonni L, De Marco A, Maestrini G, Cattaneo A (1994) Vulvar lichen sclerosus. Immunohistologic evaluation before and after therapy. J Reprod Med 39:110–114
30. Carli P, Cattaneo A, Pimpinelli N, Cozza A, Bracco G, Giannotti B (1991) Immunohistochemical evidence of skin immune system involvement in vulvar lichen sclerosus et atrophicus. Dermatologica (Basel) 182:18–22
31. Carlson JA, Grabowski R, Chichester P, Paunovich E, Malfetano J (2000) Comparative immunophenotypic study of lichen sclerosus epidermotrophic CD57[1] lymphocytes are numerous–implications for pathogenesis. Am J Dermatopathol 22(1):7–16
32. Carlson JA, Ambros R, Malfetano J, Ross J, Grabowski R, Lamb P, Figge H, Mihm MC Jr (1998) Vulvar lichen sclerosus and squamous cell carcinoma: a cohort, case control, and investigational study with historical perspective; implications for chronic inflammation and sclerosis in the development of neoplasia. Hum Pathol 29: 932–948
33. Carlson JA, Lamb P, Malfetano J, Ambros RA, Mihm MC Jr (1998) Clinicopathologic comparison of vulvar and extragenital lichen sclerosus: histologic variants, evolving lesions, and etiology of 141 cases. Mod Pathol 11:844–854
34. Carter J, Elliott P (1990) Syringoma—an unusual cause of pruritus vulvae. Aust NZ J Obstet Gynaecol 30:382–383
35. Carter J, Elliott P, Russell P (1992) Bilateral fibroepithelial polypi of labium minus with atypical stromal cells. Pathology 24:37–39
36. Cattaneo A, Bracco GL, Maestrini G, Carli P, Taddei GH, Colafranceschi M, Marchionni M (1991) Lichen sclerosus and squamous hyperplasia of the vulva. A clinical study of medical treatment. J Reprod Med 36:301–305
37. Cecchi R, Bartoli L, Brunetti L, Pavesi M, Giomi A (1995) Lymphangioma circumscriptum of the vulva of late onset. Acta Derm Venereol 75:79–80
38. Chadha S, Gianotten WL, Drogendijk AC, Weijmar Schultz WC, Blindeman LA, van der Meijden WI (1998) Histopathologic features of vulvar vestibulitis. Int J Gynecol Pathol 17:7–11
39. Chiasson MA, Ellerbrock TV, Bush TJ, Sun XW, Wright TC Jr (1997) Increased prevalence of vulvovaginal condyloma and vulvar intraepithelial neoplasia in women infected with the human immunodeficiency virus. Obstet Gynecol 89(pt 1):690–694
40. Cho D, Woodruff JD (1988) Trichoepithelioma of the vulva. A report of two cases. J Reprod Med 33:317–319
41. Chosidow O (2000) Scabies and pediculosis. Lancet 355:819–826
42. Christensen WN, Friedman KJ, Woodruff JD, Hood AF (1987) Histologic characteristics of vulvar nevocellular nevi. J Cutan Pathol 14:87–91
43. Cilla G, Pico F, Peris A, Idigoras P, Urbieta M, Perez-Trallero E (1992) Human genital myiasis due to Sarcophaga. Rev Clín Esp 190:189–190
44. Clark WH Jr, Hood AF, Tucker MA, Jampel RM (1998) Atypical melanocytic nevi of the genital type with a discussion of reciprocal-parenchymal-stromal interactions in the biology of neoplasia. Hum Pathol 29(suppl 1):S1–S24
45. Cockayne SE, Rassl DM, Thomas SE (2000) Squamous cell carcinoma arising in Hailey-Hailey disease of the vulva. Br J Dermatol 142:540–542
46. Coghill SB, Tyler X, Shaxted EJ (1990) Benign mucinous metaplasia of the vulva. Histopathology (Oxf) 17:373–375
47. Cohen PR, Young AW Jr, Tovell HM (1989) Angiokeratoma of the vulva: diagnosis and review of the literature. Obstet Gynecol Surv 44:339–346
48. Cone R, Beckmann A, Aho M, Wahlstrom T, Ek M, Corey L, Paavonen J (1991) Subclinical manifestations of vulvar human papillomavirus infection. Int J Gynecol Pathol 10:26–35
49. Congilosi SM, Madoff RD (1995) Current therapy for recurrent and extensive anal warts. Dis Colon Rectum 38:1101–1107
50. Cooper PH (1989) Acantholytic dermatosis localized to the vulvocrural area. J Cutan Pathol 16:81–84
51. Cooper SM, Wojnarowska F (2006) Influence of treatment of erosive lichen planus of the vulva on its prognosis. Arch Dermatol 142(3):289–294
52. Coyle PV, Desai A, Wyatt D, McCaughey C, O'Neill HJ (1999) A comparison of virus isolation, indirect immunofluorescence and nested multiplex polymerase chain reaction for the diagnosis of primary and recurrent herpes simplex type 1 and type 2 infections. J Virol Meth 83:75–82
53. Dalziel KL, Mallard R, Wojnarowska F (1991) The treatment of vulvar lichen sclerosus with very potent topical steroid (clobetasol propionate 0.05% cream). Br J Dermatol 124:461–464
54. Decavalas G, Adonakis G, Androutsopoulos G, Gkermpesi M, Kourounis G (2007) Sarcoidosis of the vulva: a case report. Arch Gynecol Obstet 275(3):203–205
55. de Deus JM, Focchi J, Stavale JN, de Lima GR (1995) Histologic and biomolecular aspects of papillomatosis of the vulvar vestibule in relation to human papillomavirus. Obstet Gynecol 86:758–763
56. Della Torre G, Donghi R, Longoni A, Pilotti S, Pasquini G, De Palo G, Pierotti MA, Rilke F, Della Porta G (1992) HPV DNA in intraepithelial neoplasia and carcinoma of the vulva and penis. Diagn Mol Pathol 1:25–30
57. El Demellawy D, Daya D, Alowami S (2008) Clear cell hidradenoma: an unusual vulvar tumor. Int J Gynecol Pathol 27(3):457–460
58. Derksen DJ (1992) Children with condylomata acuminata. J Fam Pract 34:419–423
59. Dickens P, Srivastava G, Loke SL, Larkin S (1991) Human papillomavirus 6, 11, and 16 in laryngeal papillomas. J Pathol 165(3):243–246
60. Dungar CF, Wilkinson EJ (1995) Vaginal columnar cell metaplasia. An acquired adenosis associated with topical 5–fluorouracil therapy. J Reprod Med 40:361–366
61. Edwards L (1992) Desquamative vulvitis. Dermatol Clin 10:325–337
62. Edwards L, Hansen RC (1992) Reiter's syndrome of the vulva. The psoriasis spectrum. Arch Dermatol 128:811–814
63. Egan CA, Zone JJ (1999) Linear IgA bullous dermatosis. Int J Dermatol 38:818–827
64. Egglestone SI, Turner AJ (2000) Serological diagnosis of syphilis. PHLS Syphilis Serology Working Group. Commun Dis Public Health 3(3):158–162
65. Elchalal U, Gilead L, Vardy DA, Ben-shachar I, Anteby SO, Schenker JG (1995) Treatment of vulvar lichen sclerosus in the elderly: an update. Obstet Gynecol Surv 50:155–162
66. Elgart ML (1992) Sexually transmitted diseases of the vulva. Dermatol Clin 10:387–403
67. Epstein WL (1992) Molluscum contagiosum. Semin Dermatol 11:184–189
68. Estrada R, Kaufman R (1993) Benign vulvar melanosis. J Reprod Med 38:5–8
69. Ferenczy A, Mitao M, Nagai N, Silverstein SJ, Crum CP (1985) Latent papillomavirus and recurring genital warts. N Engl J Med 313:784–788

70. Fletcher JL Jr (1991) Perinatal transmission of human papillomavirus. Am Fam Physician 43:143–148
71. Friedmann W, Schafer A, Kretschmer R, Lobeck H (1991) Disseminated cytomegalovirus infection of the female genital tract. Gynecol Obstet Invest 31:56–77
72. Friedrich EG Jr, Wilkinson EJ (1973) Mucous cysts of the vulvar vestibule. Obstet Gynecol 42:407–414
73. Friedrich EG Jr (1987) Vulvar vestibulitis syndrome. J Reprod Med 32:110–114
74. Frith P, Charnock M, Wojnarowska F (1991) Cicatricial pemphigoid diagnosed from ocular features in recurrent severe vulvae scarring. Two case reports. Br J Obstet Gynecol 98:482–484
75. Galloway DA, McDougall JK (1990) Alterations in the cellular phenotype induced by herpes simplex viruses. J Med Virol 31: 36–42
76. Gately LE III, Nesbitt LT Jr (1994) Update on immunofluorescent testing in bullous diseases and lupus erythematosus. Review Dermatol Clin 12:133–142
77. Gentile G, Formelli G, Pelusi G, Flamigni C (1997) Is vestibular micropapillomatosis associated with human papillomavirus infection? Eur J Gynaecol Oncol 18:523–525
78. Gilbey S, Moore DH, Look KY, Sutton GP (1997) Vulvar keratoacanthoma. Obstet Gynecol 89(Pt 2):848–850
79. Gilks CB, Clement PB, Wood WS (1989) Trichoblastic fibroma. A clinicopathologic study of three cases. Am J Dermatopathol 11:397–402
80. Gittes RF, Nakamura RM (1996) Female urethral syndrome. A female prostatitis? West J Med 164:435–438
81. Glazer HI, Rodke G, Swencionis C, Hertz R, Young AW (1995) Treatment of vulvar vestibulitis syndrome with electromyographic biofeedback of pelvic floor musculature. J Reprod Med 40:283–290
82. Gleason BC, Hirsch MS, Nucci MR, Schmidt BA, Zembowicz A, Mihm MC Jr, McKee PH, Brenn T (2008) Atypical genital nevi. A clinicopathologic analysis of 56 cases. Am J Surg Pathol 32(1): 51–57
83. Glusac EJ, Hendrickson MS, Smoller BR (1994) Apocrine cystadenoma of the vulva. J Am Acad Dermatol 31(pt 1):498–499
84. Godeau G, Frances C, Hornebeck W, Brechemier D, Robert L (1982) Isolation and partial characterization of an elastase-type protease in human vulva fibroblasts: its possible involvement in vulvar elastic tissue destruction of patients with lichen sclerosus et atrophicus. J Invest Dermatol 78:270–275
85. Goldberg JM, Buchler DA, Dibbell DG (1996) Advanced hidradenitis suppurativa presenting with bilateral vulvar masses. Gynecol Oncol 60:494–497
86. Gravitt PE, Burk RD, Lorincz A, Herrero R, Hildesheim A, Sherman ME, Bratti MC, Rodriguez AC, Helzlsouer KJ, Schiffman M (2003) A comparison between real-time polymerase chain reaction and hybrid capture 2 for human papillomavirus DNA quantitation. Cancer Epidemiol Biomark Prev 12(6):477–484
87. Groisser DS, Griffiths CE, Ellis CN, Voorhees JJ (1991) A review and update of the clinical uses of cyclosporine in dermatology. Dermatol Clin 9:805–817
88. Guerrieri C, Ohlsson E, Ryden G, Westermark P (1995) Vulvitis granulomatosa: a cryptogenic chronic inflammatory hypertrophy of vulvar labia related to cheilitis granulomatosa and Crohn's disease. Int J Gynecol Pathol 14:352–359
89. Hackel H, Hartmann AA, Burg G (1991) Vulvitis granulomatosa and anoperineitis granulomatosa. Dermatologica (Basel) 182:128–131
90. Haefner HK, Collins ME, Davis GD, Edwards L, Foster DC, Hartmann EH, Kaufman RH, Lynch PJ, Margesson LJ, Moyal-Barracco M, Piper CK, Reed BD, Steward EG, Wilkinson EJ (2005) The Vulvodynia Guideline. J Low Genit Tract Dis 9(1): 40–51
91. Handsfield HH (1997) Clinical presentation and natural course of anogenital warts. Am J Med 102(5A):16–20
92. Hanly MG, Ojeda VJ (1995) Epidermal inclusion cysts of the clitoris as a complication of female circumcision and pharaonic infibulation. Cent Afr J Med 41:22–24
93. Helm KF, Gibson LE, Muller SA (1991) Lichen sclerosus et atrophicus in children and young adults. Pediatr Dermatol 8:97–101
94. Horowitz IR, Copas P, Majmudar B (1995) Granular cell tumors of the vulva. Am J Obstet Gynecol 173:1710–1713
95. Huppert JS, Gerber MA, Dietch HR, Mortensen JE, Staat MA, Adams Hillard PJ (2006) Vulvar ulcers in young females: a manifestation of aphthosis. J Pediatr Adolesc Gynecol 19(3): 195–204
96. Ishiko A, Shimizu H, Masunaga T, Yancey KB, Giudice GJ, Zone JJ, Nishikawa T (1998) 97-kDa linear IgA bullous dermatosis antigen localizes in the lamina lucida between the NC16A and carboxyl terminal domains of the 180 kDa bullous pemphigoid antigen. J Invest Dermatol 111:93–96
97. Iversen T, Aas M (1983) Lymph drainage from the vulva. Gynecol Oncol 16:179–189
98. Iwasaki T, Sata T, Sugase M, Sato Y, Kurata T, Suzuki K, Ohmoto H, Iwamoto S (1992) Detection of capsid antigen of human papillomavirus (HPV) in benign lesions of female genital tract using anti-HPV monoclonal antibody. J Pathol 168: 293–300
99. Jemec GB (1999) Long-term results of isotretinoin in the treatment of 68 patients with hidradenitis suppurativa. J Am Acad Dermatol 41:658
100. Jha PK, Beral V, Peto J, Hack S, Hermon C, Deacon J, Mant D, Chilvers C, Vessey MP, Pike MC (1993) Antibodies to human papillomavirus and to other genital infectious agents and invasive cervical cancer risk. Lancet 341:1116–1118
101. Johnson TL, Kennedy AW, Segal GH (1991) Lymphangioma circumscriptum of the vulva. A report of two cases. J Reprod Med 36:808–812
102. Jones RW, Scurry J, Neill S et al (2008) Guidelines for the follow-up of women with vulvar lichen sclerosus in specialist clinics. Am J Obstet Gynecol 198:496.e1–496.e3
103. Junaid TA, Thomas SM (1981) Cysts of the vulva and vagina: a comparative study. Int J Gynecol Obstet 19:239–243
104. Kamarashev JA, Vassileva SG (1997) Dermatologic diseases of the vulva. Clin Dermatol 15:53–65
105. Kanekura T, Kanda A, Higo A, Kanzaki T (1996) Multiple milia localized to the vulva. J Dermatol 23:427–428
106. Kang IK, Kim YJ, Choi KC (1995) Ciliated cyst of the vulva. J Am Acad Dermatol 32:514–515
107. Kaufman RH (1994) Benign diseases of the vulva and vagina, 4th edn. Mosby, St. Louis
108. Kellogg ND, Parra JM (1991) Linea vestibularis: a previously undescribed normal genital structure in female neonates. Pediatrics 87:926–929
109. Kellogg ND, Parra JM (1993) Linea vestibularis: follow-up of a normal genital structure. Pediatrics 92:453–456
110. Kennedy DA, Hermina MS, Xanos ET, Schink JC, Hafez GR (1997) Infiltrating ductal carcinoma of the vulva. Pathol Res Pract 193:723–726

111. Kent HL, Wisniewski PM (1990) Interferon for vulvar vestibulitis. J Reprod Med 35:1138–1140
112. Khan IU, Bhol KC, Ahmed AR (1999) Linear IgA bullous dermatosis in a patient with chronic renal failure: response to intravenous immunoglobulin therapy. J Am Acad Dermatol 40:485–848
113. Kirkham N (1997) Tumors and cysts of the epidermis. In: Elder D, Elenitsas R, Jaworsky C, Johnson B Jr (eds) Lever's histopathology of the skin, 8th edn. Lippincott-Raven, Philadelphia, pp 685–746
114. Klein PA, Appel J, Callen JP (1998) Sarcoidosis of the vulva: a rare cutaneous manifestation. J Am Acad Dermatol 39(pt 1):281–283
115. Klein PA, Callen JP (2000) Drug-induced linear IgA bullous dermatosis after vancomycin discontinuance in a patient with renal insufficiency. J Am Acad Dermatol 42(Pt 2):316–323
116. Klutke JJ, Bergman A (1995) Interferon as an adjuvant treatment for genital condyloma acuminatum. Int J Gynaecol Obstet 49: 171–174
117. Koffa M, Koumantakis E, Ergazaki M, Tsatsanis C, Spandidos DA (1995) Association of herpesvirus infection with the development of genital cancer. Int J Cancer 63:58–62
118. Kondi-Paphitis A, Deligeorgi-Politi H, Liapis A, Plemenou-Frangou M (1998) Human papilloma virus in verrucus carcinoma of the vulva: an immunopathological study of the cases. Eur J Gynaecol Oncol 19:319–320
119. Koranantakul O, Lekhakula A, Wansit R, Koranantakul Y (1991) Cutaneous myiasis of vulva caused by the muscoid fly (Chrysomyia genus). Southeast Asian J Trop Med Public Health 22:458–460
120. Korman NJ (1998) Bullous pemphigoid. The latest in diagnosis, prognosis, and therapy. Arch Dermatol 134(9):1137–1141
121. Korman NJ (2000) New and emerging therapies in the treatment of blistering diseases. Dermatol Clin 18(127–137):ix–x
122. Koutsky LA, Stevens CE, Holmes KK, Ashley RL, Kiviat NB, Critchlow CW, Corey L (1992) Underdiagnosis of genital herpes by current clinical and viral isolation procedures. N Engl J Med 326:1533–1539
123. Krantz KE (1958) Innervation of the human vulva and vagina. Obstet Gynecol 12:382
124. Kulski JK, Demeter T, Rakoczy P, Sterrett GF, Pixley EC (1989) Human papillomavirus coinfections of the vulva and uterine cervix. J Med Virol 27:244–251
125. Kurzrock R, Cohen PR (1995) Cutaneous paraneoplastic syndromes in solid tumors. Am J Med 99:662–671
126. LaGuardia KD, White MH, Saigo PE, Hoda S, McGuinness K, Ledger WJ (1995) Genital ulcer disease in women infected with human immunodeficiency virus. Am J Obstet Gynecol 172(pt 1): 553–562
127. Lehtinen M, Hakama M, Aaran RK, Aromaa A, Knekt P, Leinikki P, Maatela J, Peto R, Teppo L (1992) Herpes simplex virus type 2 infection and cervical cancer: a prospective study of 12 years of follow-up in Finland. Cancer Causes Control 3:333–338
128. Leibowitch M, Neill S, Pelisse M, Moyal-Baracco M (1990) The epithelial changes associated with squamous cell carcinoma of the vulva: a review of the clinical, histological and viral findings of 78 women. Br J Obstet Gynaecol 97:1135–1139
129. Leong FJ, Meredith DJ (1998) Verruciform xanthoma of the vulva. A case report. Pathol Res Pract 194:661–665; 666–667
130. Lewis FM (1998) Vulval lichen planus. Br J Dermatol 138:569–575
131. Li J, Ackerman AB (1994) "Seborrheic keratoses" that contain human papillomavirus are condylomata acuminata. Am J Dermatopathol 16:398–405
132. LiVolsi VA, Brooks JJ (1987) Soft tissue tumors of the vulva. In: Wilkinson EJ (ed) Contemporary issues in surgical pathology, Pathology of the vulva and vagina, vol 9. Churchill Livingstone, New York, pp 209–238
133. Loening-Baucke V (1991) Lichen sclerosus et atrophicus in children. Am J Dis Child 145:1058–1061
134. Lorenz B, Kaufman RH, Kutzner SK (1998) Lichen sclerosus. Therapy with clobetasol propionate. J Reprod Med 43:790–794
135. Luesley DM (ed) (1999) Cancer and pre-cancer of the vulva. Oxford University Press, New York
136. Lynch PJ, Moyal-Barrocco M, Bogliotto F (2007) ISSVD classification of vulvar dermatoses: pathologic subsets and their clinical correlates. J Reprod Med 52(1):3–9
137. Maccato ML, Kaufman RH (1992) Herpes genitalis. Dermatol Clin 10:415–422
138. Mann MS, Kaufman RH (1991) Erosive lichen planus of the vulva. Clin Obstet Gynecol 34:605–613
139. Magrina JR, Masterson BJ (1981) Loxosceles reclusa spider bite: a consideration in the differential diagnosis of chronic, nonmalignant ulcers of the vulva. Am J Obstet Gynecol 140:341–343
140. Mahmud N, Kusuda N, Ichinose S, Gyotoku Y, Nakajima H, Ishimaru T, Yamabe J (1992) Needle aspiration biopsy of vulvar endometriois. A case report. Acta Cytol 36:514–516
141. Mann MS, Kaufman RH (1991) Erosive lichen planus of the vulva. Clin Obstet Gynecol 34:605–613
142. Marinoff SC, Turner MLC (1991) Vulvar vestibulitis syndrome: an overview. Am J Obstet Gynecol 165:1228–1233
143. Marquette GP, Su B, Woodruff JD (1985) Introital adenosis associated with Stevens-Johnson syndrome. Obstet Gynecol 66:143–145
144. Marren P, Wojnarowska F (1996) Dermatitis of the vulva. Semin Dermatol 15:6–41
145. Marwah S, Bergman ML (1980) Ectopic salivary gland in the vulva (choristoma): report of a case and review of the literature. Obstet Gynecol 56:389–391
146. McKee PH, Marsden RA, Santa Cruz DJ (1996) Pathology of the skin: with clinical correlations, 2nd edn. Mosby-Wolfe, London, pp 4.1–4.80
147. McNeely TB (1992) Angiokeratoma of the clitoris. Arch Pathol Lab Med 116:880–881
148. Mihara M (1991) Three-dimensional ultrastructural study of molluscum contagiosum in the skin using scanning-electron microscopy. Br J Dermatol 125:557–560
149. Mihara Y, Mihara M, Hagari Y, Shimao S (1994) Lichen sclerosus et atrophicus. A histological, immunohistochemical and electron microscopic study. Arch Dermatol Res 286:434–442
150. Milbrath JR, Wilkinson EJ, Friedrich EG Jr (1975) Xerographic evaluation of radical vulvectomy specimens. Am J Roentgenol Radiat Ther Nucl Med (AJR) 125:486–488
151. Mindel A (ed) (1995) Genital warts: human papillomavirus infection. Arnold, London
152. Monk BE (1993) Fordyce spots responding to isotretinoin therapy. Br J Dermatol 129:355
153. Monsonego J, Valensi P, Zerat L, Clavel C, Birembaut P (1997) Simultaneous effects of aneuploidy and oncogenic human papillomavirus on histological grade of cervical intraepithelial neoplasia. Br J Obstet Gynaecol 104:723–727
154. Moreland AA (1994) Vulvar manifestations of sexually transmitted diseases. Semin Dermatol 13:262–268
155. Morse SA, Moreland AA, Holmes KK (1996) Atlas of sexually transmitted diseases and AIDS, 2nd edn. Mosby-Wolfe, London

156. Moschella SL, Hurley HJ (1992) Dermatology, 3rd edn. Saunders, Philadelphia
157. Moyal-Barracco M, Leibowitch M, Orth G (1990) Vestibular papillae of the vulva. Lack of evidence for human papillomavirus etiology. Arch Dermatol 126:1594–1598
158. Mullins DL, Wilkinson EJ (1994) Pathology of the vulva and vagina. Curr Opin Obstet Gynecol 6:351–358
159. Multhaupt HA, Rafferty PA, Warhol MJ (1992) Ultrastructural localization of human papilloma virus by nonradioactive in situ hybridization on tissue of human cervical intraepithelial neoplasia. Lab Invest 67:512–518
160. Neill SM, Tatnall FM, Cox NH (2002) Guidelines for the management of lichen sclerosus. Br J Dermatol 147:640–649
161. Nettina SM (1998) Herpes genitalis. Lippincotts Prim Care Pract 2:303–306
162. Newland JR, Fusaro RM (1991) Mucinous cysts of the vulva. Nebr Med J 76:307–310
163. Obalek S, Misiewicz J, Jablonska S, Favre M, Orth G (1993) Childhood condyloma acuminatum: association with genital and cutaneous human papillomaviruses. Pediatr Dermatol 10:101–106
164. Ogunbiyi OA, Scholefield JH, Robertson G, Smith JH, Sharp F, Rogers K (1994) Anal human papillomavirus infection and squamous neoplasia in patients with invasive vulvar cancer. Obstet Gynecol 83:212–216
165. Olansky S (1972) Serodiagnosis of syphilis. Med Clin N Am 56:1145–1150
166. Olivry T, Moore PF, Affolter VK, Naydan DK (1996) Langerhans cell hyperplasia and IgE expression in canine atopic dermatitis. Arch Dermatol Res 288:579–585
167. O'Rahilly R, Müller F (1996) Human embryology & teratology, 2nd edn. Wiley-Liss, New York
168. Ordonez NG, Manning JT, Luna MA (1981) Mixed tumor of the vulva: a report of two cases probably arising in Bartholin's gland. Cancer (Phila) 48:181–186
169. Oriel JD (1990) Identification of people at high risk of genital HPV infections. Scand J Infect Dis Suppl 69:169–172
170. Orle KA, Gates CA, Martin DH, Body BA, Weiss JB (1996) Simultaneous PCR detection of Haemophilus ducreyi, *Treponema pallidum*, and herpes simplex virus types 1 and 2 from genital ulcers. J Clin Microbiol 34:49–54
171. Ortiz-Hidalgo C, de la Vega G, Moreno-Collado C (1997) Granular cell tumor (Abrikossoff tumor) of the clitoris. Int J Dermatol 36:935–937
172. Patton LW, Elgart ML, Williams CM (1990) Vulvar erythema and induration. Extraintestinal Crohn's disease of the vulva. Arch Dermatol 126:1351–1354
173. Pelisse M (1996) Erosive vulvar lichen planus and desquamative vaginitis. Semin Dermatol 15:47–50
174. Pelosi G, Martignoni G, Bonetti F (1991) Intraductal carcinoma of mammary-type apocrine epithelium arising within a papillary hidradenoma of the vulva. Report of a case and review of the literature. Arch Pathol Lab Med 115:1249–1254
175. Perry CM, Faulds D (1996) Valaciclovir. A review of its antiviral activity, pharmacokinetic properties and therapeutic efficacy in herpesvirus infections. Drugs 52:754–772
176. Peters WA III (1998) Bartholinitis after vulvovaginal surgery. Am J Obstet Gynecol 178:1143–1144
177. Pierson KK (1987) Malignant melanomas and pigmented lesions of the vulva. In: Wilkinson EJ (ed) Contemporary issues in surgical pathology, Pathology of the vulva and vagina, vol 9. Churchill Livingstone, New York, pp 155–179
178. Pincus SH, Stadecker MJ (1987) Vulvar dystrophies and noninfectious inflammatory conditions. In: Wilkinson EJ (ed) Contemporary issues in surgical pathology, vol 9, Pathology of the vulva and vagina. Churchill Livingstone, New York, pp 11–24
179. Pincus SH (1992) Vulvar dermatoses and pruritus vulva. Dermatol Clin 10:297–308
180. Powell FC, Su WP, Perry HO (1996) Pyoderma gangrenosum: classification and management. J Am Acad Dermatol 34(395–409):410–412
181. Powell JJ, Wojnarowska F (1999) Lichen sclerosus. Lancet 353: 1777–1783
182. Prayson RA, Stoler MH, Hart WR (1995) Vulvar vestibulitis. A histopathologic study of 36 cases, including human papillomavirus in situ hybridization analysis. Am J Surg Pathol 19:154–160
183. Pulimood S, Ajithkumar K, Jacob M, George S, Chandi SM (1997) Linear IgA bullous dermatosis of childhood: treatment with dapsone and co-trimoxazole. Clin Exp Dermatol 22:90–91
184. Pyka RE, Wilkinson EJ, Friedrich EG Jr, Croker BP (1988) The histopathology of vulvar vestibulitis syndrome. Int J Gynecol Pathol 7:249–257
185. Quan MB, Moy RL (1991) The role of human papillomavirus in carcinoma. J Am Acad Dermatol 25:698–705
186. Ramesh V, Iyengar B (1990) Proliferating trichilemmal cysts over the vulva. Cutis 45:87–189
187. Ranalletta M, Rositto A, Drut R (1996) Fox-Fordyce disease in two prepubertal girls: histopathologic demonstration of eccrine sweat gland involvement. Pediatr Dermatol 13:294–297
188. Regauer S, Liegl B, Reich O (2005) Early vulvar lichen sclerosus: a histopathological challenge. Histopathology 47(4):340–347
189. Requena L, Kiryu H, Ackerman AB (1998) Series: Ackerman's histologic diagnosis of neoplastic skin diseases: neoplasms with apocrine differentiation, with analogues in the breast by Darryl Carter. Lippincott-Raven, Philadelphia, pp 9–28
190. Rhodes AR, Mihm MC Jr, Weinstock MA (1989) A reproducible histologic definition emphasizing cellular morphology. Dysplastic melanocytic nevi. Mod Pathol 2:306–319
191. Richens J (1991) The diagnosis and treatment of donovanosis (granuloma inguinale). Genitourin Med 67:441–452
192. Ridley CM, Neill SM (1999) Non-infective cutaneous conditions of vulva. In: Ridley CM, Neill SM (eds) The vulva, 2nd edn. Blackwell, Oxford, pp 121–186
193. Ridley CM, Neill SM (1999) The vulva, 2nd edn. Blackwell, Oxford, pp 1–36
194. Rihet S, Lorenzato M, Clavel C (1996) Oncogenic human papillomaviruses and ploidy in cervical lesions. J Clin Pathol 49:892–896
195. Robboy SJ, Ross JS, Prat J, Keh PC, Welch WR (1978) Urogenital sinus origin of mucinous and ciliated cysts of the vulva. Obstet Gynecol 51:347–351
196. Robinson JB, Im DD, Simmons-O'Brien E, Rosenshein NB (1998) Etretinate: therapy for plasma cell vulvitis. Obstet Gynecol 92(pt 2):706
197. Rock B, Hood AF, Rock JA (1990) Prospective study of vulvar nevi. J Am Acad Dermatol 22:104–106
198. Rodke G, Friedrich EG Jr, Wilkinson EJ (1988) Malignant potential of mixed vulvar dystrophy (lichen sclerosis associated with squamous cell hyperplasia). J Reprod Med 33:545–550
199. Rogers BB, Josephson SL, Mak SK, Sweeney PJ (1992) Polymeras chain reaction amplification of herpes simplex virus DNA from clinical samples. Obstet Gynecol 79:464–469
200. Rorat E, Wallach RC (1984) Mixed tumors of the vulva: clinical outcome and pathology. Int J Gynecol Pathol 3:323–328

201. Rudolph RE (1990) Vulvar melanosis. J Am Acad Dermatol 23: 982–984
202. Saitoh A, Ohya T, Yoshida S, Hosoya R, Nishimura K (1995) A case report of Stevens-Johnson syndrome with Mycoplasma infection. Acta Paediatr Jpn 37:113–115
203. Sakane T, Takeno M, Suzuki N, Inaba G (1999) Behçet's disease. N Engl J Med 341:1284–1291
204. Sarrel PM, Steege JF, Maltzer M, Bolinsky D (1983) Pain during sex response due to occlusion of the Bartholin gland duct. Obstet Gynecol 62:261–264
205. Schneider CA, Festa S, Spillert CR, Bruce CJ, Lazaro EJ (1994) Hydrocele of the canal of Nuck. N J Med 91:37–38
206. Schoenfeld A, Ziv E, Levavi H, Samra Z, Ovadia J (1995) Laser versus loop electrosurgical excision in vulvar condyloma for eradication of subclinical reservoir demonstrated by assay for 2959-oligosynthetase human papillomavirus. Gynecol Obstet Invest 40:46–51
207. Schwartz RA, Janniger CK (1995) Childhood acanthosis nigricans. Cutis 55:337–341
208. Scrimin F, Rustja S, Radillo O, Volpe C, Abrami R, Guaschino S (2000) Vulvar lichen sclerosus: an immunologic study. Obstet Gynecol 95:147–150
209. Scurry J, Beshay V, Cohen C, Allen D (1998) Ki67 expression in lichen sclerosus of vulva in patients with and without associated squamous cell carcinoma. Histopathology 32:399–404
210. Sedlacek TV, Riva JM, Magen AB, Mangan CE, Cunnane MF (1990) Vaginal and vulvar adenosis. An unsuspected side effect of CO_2 laser vaporization. J Reprod Med 35:995–1001
211. Seely JR, Bley R Jr, Altmiller CJ (1984) Localized chromosomal mosaicism as a cause of dysmorphic development. Am J Hum Genet 36:899–903
212. Shafik A, Doss S (1999) Surgical anatomy of the somatic terminal innervation to the anal and urethral sphincters: role in anal and urethral surgery. J Urol 161:85–89
213. Sherman AL, Reid R (1991) CO_2 laser for suppurative hidradenitis of the vulva. J Reprod Med 36:113–117
214. Shornick JK (1993) Herpes gestationis. Dermatol Clin 11: 527–533
215. Sims SM, McLean FW, Davis JD, Morgan LS, Wilkinson EJ (2010) Vulvar lymphangioma circumscriptum: a report of 3 cases, 2 associated with vulvar carcinoma and 1 with hidradenitis suppurativa. J Low Genit Tract Dis 14(3):234–237
216. Soler C, Allibert P, Chardonnet Y, Cros P, Mandrand B, Thivolet J (1991) Detection of human papillomavirus types 6, 11, 16 and 18 in mucosal and cutaneous lesions by the multiplex polymerase chain reaction. J Virol Meth 35:143–157
217. Sondergaard K, Carstens J, Zachariae H (1997) The steroid-sparing effect of long-term plasmapheresis in pemphigus: an update. Ther Apher 1:155–158
218. Stashower LM, Krivda MS, Turiansky LG (2000) Fox-Fordyce disease: diagnosis with transverse histologic sections. J Am Acad Dermatol 42(pt 1):89–91
219. Stephenson H, Dotters DJ, Katz V, Droegemueller W (1992) Necrotizing fasciitis of the vulva. Am J Obstet Gynecol 166:1324–1327
220. Strayer SA, Yum MN, Sutton GP (1992) Epithelioid hemangioendothelioma of the clitoris: a case report with immunohistochemical and ultrastructural findings. Int J Gynecol Pathol 11:234–239
221. Sugiura H, Uehara M, Maeda T (1990) IgE-positive epidermal Langerhans cells in allergic contact dermatitis lesions provoked in patients with atopic dermatitis. Arch Dermatol Res 282:295–299
222. Sun T, Schwartz NS, Sewell C, Lieberman P, Gross S (1991) Enterobius egg granuloma of the vulva and peritoneum: review of the literature. Am J Trop Med Hyg 45:249–253
223. Taylor S, Drake SM, Dedicoat M, Wood MJ (1998) Genital ulcers associated with acute Epstein-Barr virus infection. Sex Transm Infect 74:296–297
224. Tham SN, Choong HL (1992) Primary tuberculous chancre in a renal transplant patient. J Am Acad Dermatol 26:342–344
225. Thomas CA, Smith SE, Morgan TM, White WL, Feldman SR (1994) Clinical application of polymerase chain reaction amplification to diagnosis of herpes virus infection. Am J Dermatopathol 16:268–274
226. Toussaint S, Kamino H (1997) Noninfectious erythemotous, papular and squamous diseases. In: Elder D (ed) Lever's histopathology of the skin, 8th edn. Lippincott-Raven, Philadelphia, pp 151–184
227. Traiman P, Bacchi CE, De Luca LA, Uemura G, Nahas Neto J, Nahas EA, Pontes A (1999) Vulvar carcinoma in young patients and its relationship with genital warts. Eur J Gynaecol Oncol 20: 191–194
228. Trees DL, Morse SA (1995) Chancroid and Haemo-philus ducreyi: an update. Clin Microbiol Rev 8:357–375
229. Tuffnell D, Buchan PD (1991) Crohn's disease of the vulva in childhood. Br J Clin Pract 45:159–160
230. Tyring SK (1998) Advances in the treatment of herpesvirus infection: the role of famciclovir. Clin Ther 20:661–670
231. Valdivielso-Ramos M, Bueno C, Hernanz JM (2008) Significant improvement in extensive lichen sclerosus with tacrolimus ointment and PUVA. Am J Clin Dermatol 9(3):175–179
232. van der Putte SCJ (1994) Mammary-like glands of the vulva and their disorders. Int J Gynecol 13:150–160
233. van der Putte SC, van Gorp LH (1995) Cysts of mammarylike glands in the vulva. Int J Gynecol Pathol 14:184–188
234. Vanderhooft S, Kirby P (1992) Genital herpes simplex virus infection: natural history. Semin Dermatol 11:190–199
235. Vassileva S (1998) Drug-induced pemphigoid: bullous and cicatricial. Clin Dermatol 16:379–387
236. Verkauf BS, Von Thron J, O'Brien WF (1992) Clitoral size in normal women. Obstet Gynecol 80:41–44
237. Vettraino IM, Merritt DF (1995) Crohn's disease of the vulva. Am J Dermatopathol 17:410–413
238. Virgili A, Mantovani L, Lauriola MM, Marzola A, Corazza M (2008) Tacrolimus 0.1% ointment: is it really effective in plasma cell vulvitis? Report of four cases. Dermatology 216(3): 243–246
239. Volz LR, Carpiniello VL, Malloy TR (1994) Laser treatment of urethral condyloma: a five-year experience. Urology 43:81–83
240. Walker PG, Colley NV, Grubb C, Tejerina A, Oriel JD (1983) Abnormalities of the uterine cervix in women with vulvar warts. A preliminary communication. Br J Vener Dis 59:120–123
241. Wieselthier JS, Pincus SH (1993) Hailey-Hailey disease of the vulva. Arch Dermatol 129:1344–1345
242. Wilkinson EJ (1992) Normal histology and nomenclature of the vulva, and malignant neoplasms, including VIN. Dermatol Clin 10:283–296
243. Wilkinson EJ, Guerrero E, Daniel R, Shah K, Stone IK, Hardt NS, Friedrich EG Jr (1993) Vulvar vestibulitis is rarely associated with human papillomavirus infection types 6, 11, 16 or 18. Int J Gynecol Pathol 12:344–349
244. Wilkinson EJ, Stone IK (2008) Atlas of vulvar disease, 2nd ed. Lippincott Williams & Wilkins, Baltimore

245. Williams PL (ed) (1995) Gray's anatomy: the anatomical basis of medicine and surgery, 38th edn. Churchill Livingstone, New York
246. Wisdom A (1989) A colour atlas of sexually transmitted diseases, 2nd edn. Wolfe, London
247. Wojnarowska F, Frith P (1997) Linear IgA disease. Dev Ophthalmol 28:64–72
248. Wong KT, Wong KK (1994) A case of acantholytic dermatosis of the vulva with features of pemphigus vegetans. J Cutan Pathol 21:453–456
249. Woods GL (1995) Update on laboratory diagnosis of sexually transmitted diseases. Clin Lab Med 15:665–684
250. Yang B, Hart WR (2000) Vulvar intraepithelial neoplasia of the simplex (differentiated) type: a clinicopathologic study including analysis of HPV and p53 expression. Am J Surg Pathol 24:429–441
251. Yoganathan S, Bohl TG, Mason G (1994) Plasma cell balanitis and vulvitis (of Zoon). A study of 10 cases. J Reprod Med 39:939–944
252. Young H (1998) Syphilis: serology. Dermatol Clin 16:691–698
253. Young RH, Oliva E, Garcia JA, Bhan AK, Clement PB (1996) Urethral caruncle with atypical stromal cells simulating lymphoma or sarcoma – a distinctive pseudoneoplastic lesion of females. A report of six cases. Am J Surg Pathol 20:1190–1195
254. Yun K, Joblin L (1993) Presence of human papillomavirus DNA in condylomata acuminata in children and adolescents. Pathology 25:1–3
255. Zhu WY, Leonardi C, Penneys NS (1992) Detection of human papillomavirus DNA in seborrheic keratosis by polymerase chain reaction. J Dermatol Sci 4:166–171

2 Premalignant and Malignant Tumors of the Vulva

Edward J. Wilkinson

R. J. Kurman, L. Hedrick Ellenson, B. M. Ronnett (eds.), *Blaustein's Pathology of the Female Genital Tract (6th ed.)*, DOI 10.1007/978-1-4419-0489-8_2,

Squamous Tumors

Vulvar Intraepithelial Neoplasia

(Vulvar Squamous Intraepithelial Lesion, Dysplasia, Carcinoma In Situ)

General Features

The incidence of vulvar intraepithelial neoplasia (VIN) (dysplasia, carcinoma in situ) has nearly doubled when comparing recorded cases between 1973–1976 and 1985–1986 and is becoming more frequent in young women 20–35 years of age (30, [87]). The true incidence of VIN probably is higher, because generally only a subset, carcinoma in situ (VIN 3) cases, is reported. Approximately 50% of these women have other neoplasia involving the genital tract, most often cervical intraepithelial neoplasia (CIN). Approximately one half of these women have a history of a preexisting or concomitant sexually transmitted disease, of which condylomata acuminata is the most frequent. There is an association between VIN and cigarette smoking. Most patients are symptomatic, often with pruritus. Current terminology for squamous intraepithelial lesions (dysplasia, carcinoma in situ, vulvar intraepithelial neoplasia (VIN), as proposed by the World Health Organization [WHO]) is summarized in ➲ *Table 2.1* [175]. Lesions of the vulva that are pigmented and papular or verrucoid have been clinically termed bowenoid papulosis by some authors [166], but they are histologically indistinguishable from other forms of intraepithelial neoplasia and behave in a similar fashion. The separate term bowenoid papulosis therefore is not included in the WHO classification.

◘ Table 2.1
Classification of squamous intraepithelial lesions of the vulva (vulvar intraepithelial neoplasia [VIN]/dysplasia, carcinoma in situ)

Low-grade vulvar intraepithelial neoplasia (VIN 1) (Mild dysplasia) (Low-grade squamous intraepithelial lesion (LSIL)0: a squamous intraepithelial lesion in which nuclear abnormalities are confined to the lowest one third of the epithelium
High-grade vulvar intraepithelial neoplasia (VIN 2) (Moderate dysplasia) (High-grade squamous intraepithelial lesion (HSIL)): a squamous intraepithelial lesion in which nuclear abnormalities involve the lower two thirds of the epithelium
High-grade vulvar intraepithelial neoplasia (VIN 3) (Severe dysplasia)) (High-grade squamous intraepithelial lesion (HSIL)): a squamous intraepithelial lesion in which nuclear abnormalities extend into the upper third of the epithelium, but not involving the full thickness
High-grade vulvar intraepithelial neoplasia (VIN 3) (Carcinoma in situ); includes differentiated (simplex) type VIN (High-grade squamous intraepithelial lesion (HSIL, differentiated type)): a squamous intraepithelial lesion in which nuclear abnormalities involve the full thickness of the epithelium or in which the lower portion of the epithelium is replaced by a lesion resembling grade 1 squamous cell carcinoma

Source: From ref. [92].

Clinical Features

Vulvar pruritus and irritation are the most common presenting symptoms. In some cases, the patients observe the lesion and seek medical assistance. Approximately one third of the patients are asymptomatic [174]. The lesions of VIN typically have a raised surface and are macular or papular (➲ *Figs. 2.1–2.4*). The most common sites of VIN on presentation are the labia minora and the perineum. Aproximately one third of VIN cases have perianal involvement, and such lesions may extend into the anus. Approximately two thirds of VIN lesions are multifocal [174].

Although the clinical appearance of VIN lesions can be highly variable, at presentation, approximately one half of patients with VIN have white lesions, or lesions that are distinctly aceto-white, after the application of topical 3–5% acetic acid. Approximately one quarter of the lesions are pigmented (➲ *Figs. 2.3* and ➲ *2.4*). VIN 3 is, in fact, the second most common pigmented vulvar lesion. Pigmented VIN usually occurs in keratinized vulvar skin. The remainder of VIN lesions may be pink, gray, or red. Lesions involving the nonkeratinized mucous membrane of the vestibule appear red. Such red lesions have been called erythroplasia of Queyrat, but like bowenoid, papulosis are not designated separately and are included within the VIN category. The lesions may be macular (➲ *Fig. 2.1*) or papular (➲ *Fig. 2.2*). In approximately three quarters of cases, they are multiple, and in the majority of the remainder of cases, VIN is a solitary lesion. Solitary lesions appear to be more common in older women and are more commonly associated with invasive squamous carcinoma [24]. Confluent growth of VIN is relatively uncommon [148,174] (see ➲ *Figs. 2.1* and ➲ *2.4*). The anal skin and squamous mucosa of the anal canal are the most frequently involved secondary sites.

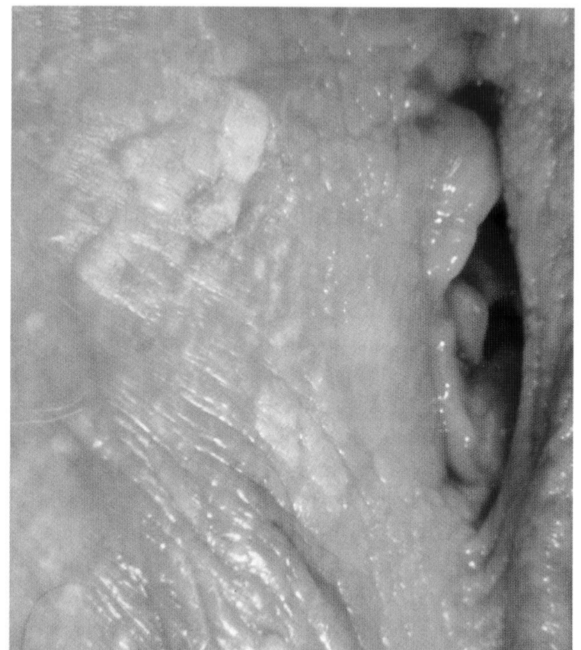

Fig. 2.1
Vulvar intraepithelial neoplasia (VIN). **Multiple macular and plaquelike aceto-white areas are present on the labia majora**

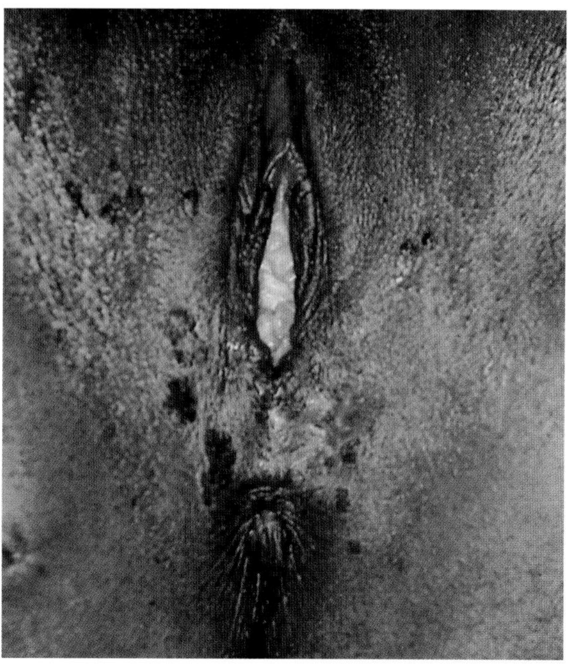

Fig. 2.3
Vulvar intraepithelial neoplasia (VIN). **Multiple warty pigmented macular papular VIN lesions are present on the vulva and perianal area**

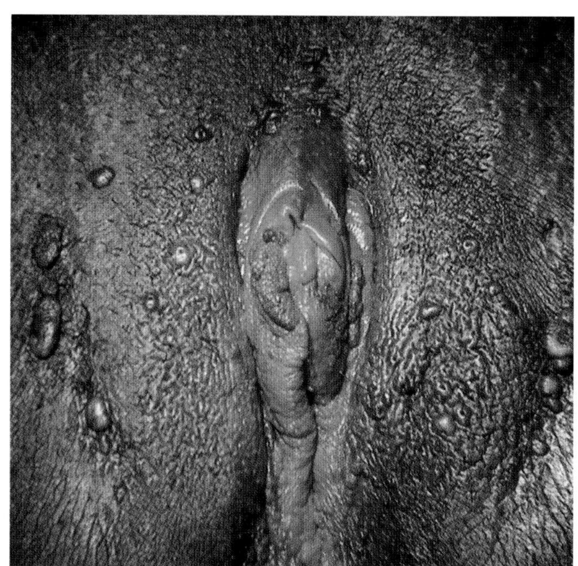

Fig. 2.2
Vulvar intraepithelial neoplasia (VIN). **Multiple pigmented papules are present on the labia majora**

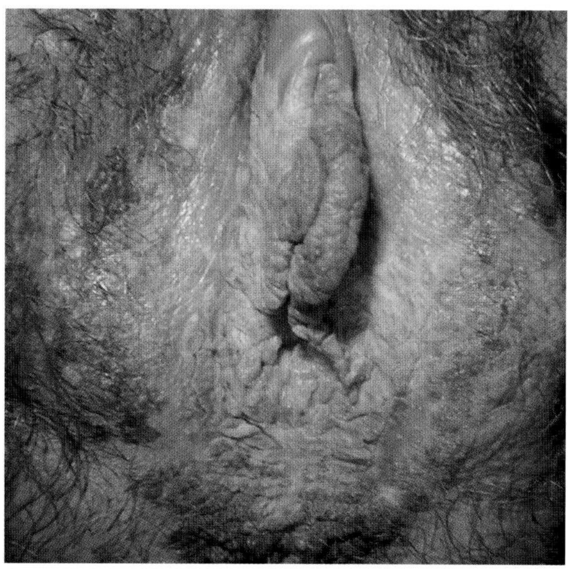

Fig. 2.4
Vulvar intraepithelial neoplasia (VIN). **Confluent distribution of pigmented, slightly raised, rough-surfaced areas involving the labia majora and minora**

Microscopic Findings

The epithelial cells of VIN have a high nuclear: cytoplasmic ratio and lack cytoplasmic maturation above the basal and parabasal layers. Mitotic activity is present above the basal layer, and the mitotic figures are often abnormal in appearance. Multinucleation and dyskeratosis, including formation of intraepithelial squamous pearls, may be seen (➲ *Figs. 2.5* and ➲ *2.6a, b*). Nuclear pleomorphism and hyperchromasia are present; however, nucleoli are uncommon. Radial dispersion of nuclear chromatin and coarse nuclear chromatin are seen in the epithelial cells of VIN, corresponding to an increased number of interchromatinic and perichromatinic granules. The so-called individual cell keratinization seen within the epithelium is attributed to the presence of aggregated intracytoplasmic tonofilaments that may be produced in the process of abnormal cell division.

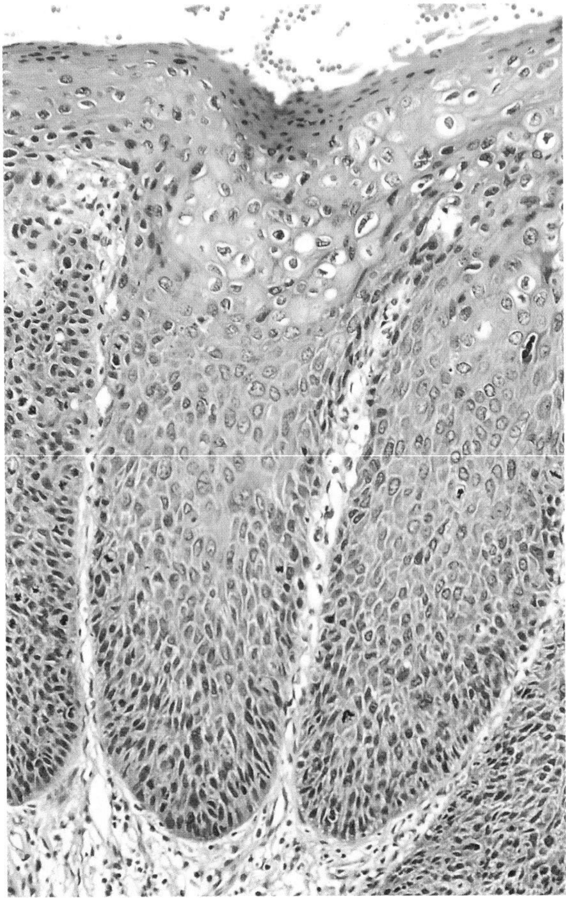

■ Fig. 2.5
VIN 2, warty type. **In the lower two thirds of the epithelium cells are crowded and lack maturation. Nuclei are hyperchromatic and pleomorphic. Within the upper third of the epithelium there is cellular maturation with prominent koilocytosis**

Parakeratosis is seen when keratinocytes fail to form granules of prekeratin and retain nuclear material at the epithelial surface. Both intracellular and extracellular pigment granules may be distributed throughout the epidermis. In pigmented VIN lesions, dermal melanophages are often prominent beneath the basal layer and within the dermal papillae. VIN involves the skin appendages in more than 50% of the cases studied. Skin appendage involvement by VIN should be differentiated from early invasion (compare ➲ *Fig. 2.6b, c* to ➲ *Fig. 2.7*). Skin appendages as deep as 2.7 mm in hair-bearing areas may be involved with VIN [144]. In non-hair-bearing areas, the skin appendages and minor vestibular glands are more superficial. The thickness of the epithelium involved by VIN may range from 0.10 to 1.90 mm, with a mean of 0.52 mm [12].

Microscopic Grading

The World Health Organization classification of vulva intraepithelial neoplasia is subdivided into three grades: VIN 1 mild dysplasia, VIN 2 moderate dysplasia, VIN 3 severe dysplasia, and carcinoma in situ/VIN 3. Differentiated (simplex) VIN is included in the VIN 3 category [92]. In this chapter, and in the most recent American Registery of Pathology Fascicle on cervix, vagina and vulva, the term "high-grade VIN" encompasses VIN 2 and VIN 3, and "low-grade VIN" encompasses VIN 1 and flat condylomas [92,175]. This terminology is relatively commonly used and is applicable provided one's clinicians understand its use and appropriate ICD9 coding is used.

Grading of VIN lesions should be performed based on the findings in the most severe, highest grade area. When the cellular epithelial abnormalities of VIN are confined to the lower third of the epithelium, low-grade VIN (VIN 1) is reported (➲ *Fig. 2.8*). Flat condyloma acuminatum of the vulva may be included in the low-grade VIN category because the biologic difference between low-grade VIN and flat condyloma is unknown and the morphologic distinction is unreliable. Flat condyloma acuminatum with koilocytosis and minimal evidence of proliferation or atypia, with atypia limited to the lower one third of the epithelium, are classified as "low-grade VIN." This practice eliminates the need for such terms as "atypical condyloma acuminatum, or flat condyloma acuminatum" that are not recommended. In the occasional case with

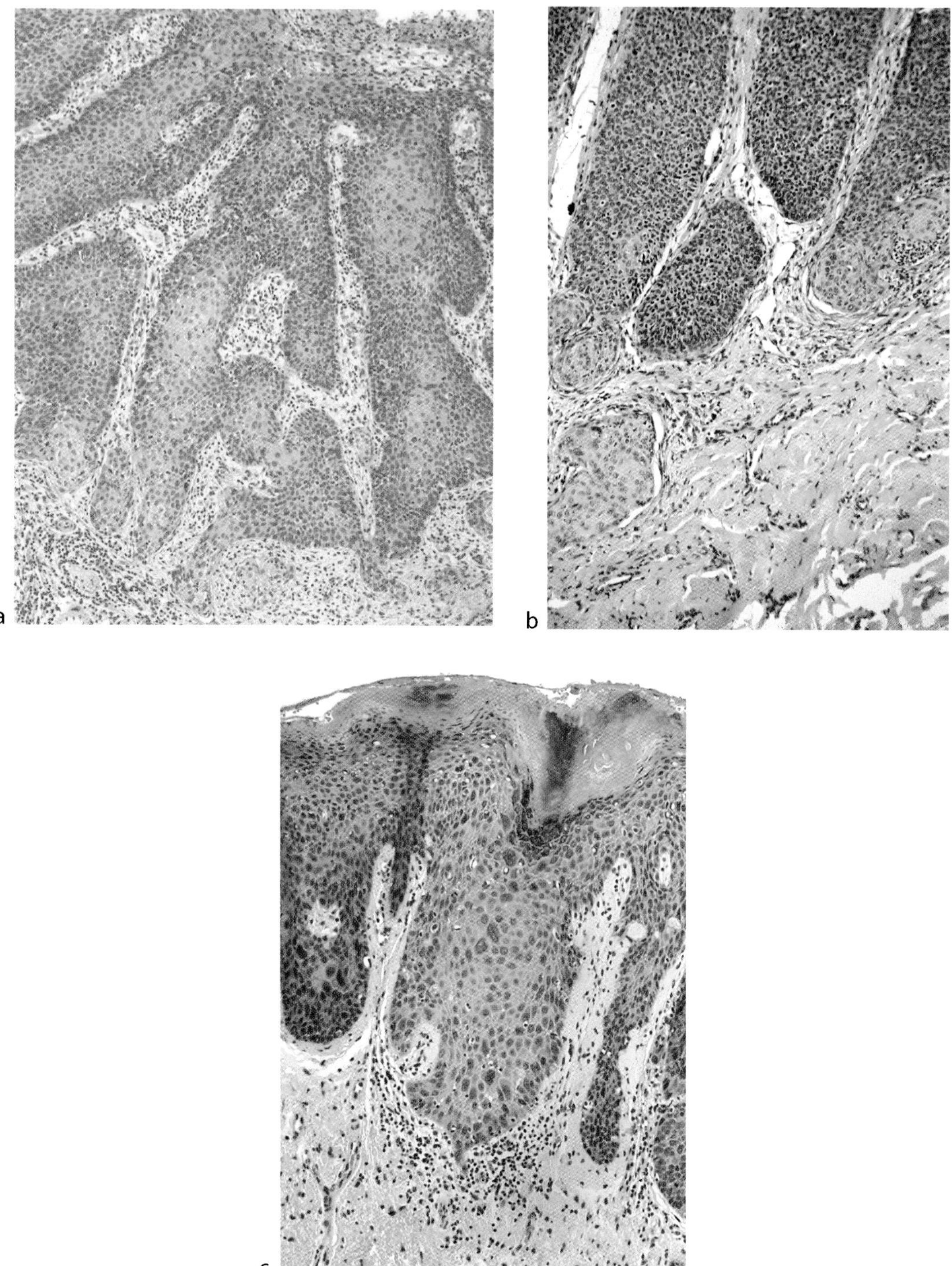

Fig. 2.6
VIN 3 with superficial invasion. (**a**) Squamous differentiation within the VIN is manifested by rounded foci of cells with eosinophilic cytoplasm near the basal layer. This is a useful feature in identifying early invasion. (**b**) Small clusters of invasive squamous cell carcinoma are present in the superficial dermis. (**c**) A small tongue of invasive squamous carcinoma is noted at the base of the dermal papillae. Note the loss of palisading of the basal cells, as compared to those in the adjacent dermal papillae

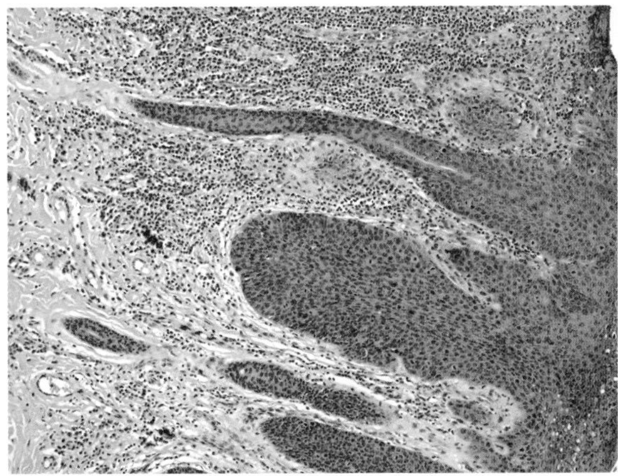

Fig. 2.7
VIN 3, involving a skin appendage. **Increased cellularity and disarray with lack of maturation is seen within the epithelium**

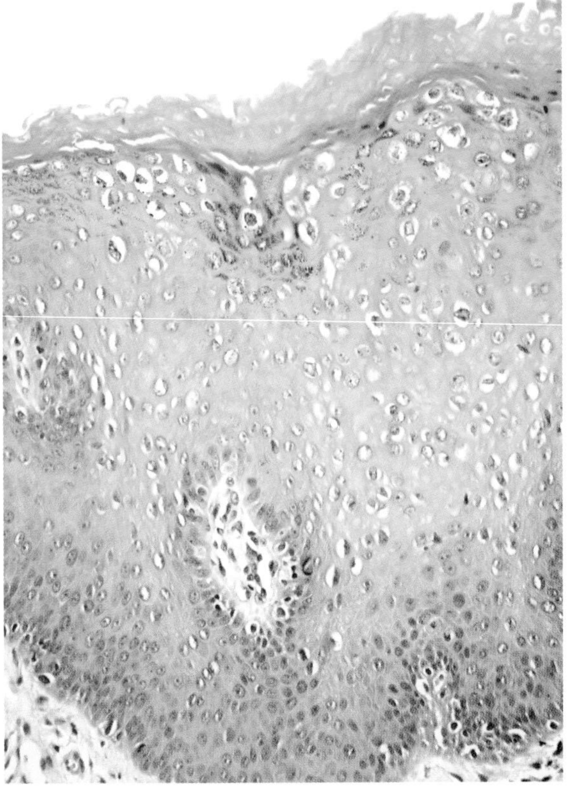

Fig. 2.8
VIN 1, warty type. **Crowding of the basal and parabasal cells with some cellular disarray and loss of maturation within the lower one third of the epithelium. Koilocytotic cells are present on the surface**

typical condyloma acuminatum associated with low- or high-grade VIN, a diagnosis of "low-grade VIN, with condyloma acuminatum, or 'high-grade VIN (VIN 2–3)' with condyloma acuminatum" is appropriate.

A lesion is classified as high-grade VIN (encompassing VIN 2 and VIN 3) if the cellular abnormalities extend through at least one half of the epithelium and may involve essentially the full thickness of the epithelium, not including the surface layers above the granular zone (*Figs. 2.5*, *2.9* and *2.10*). Abnormal mitoses are nearly always present in high-grade VIN lesions and may be seen in all but the most superficial layers of the epithelium. Lack of abnormal mitoses, or lack of mitosis above the basal layer, should raise the question as to whether a lesion belongs to the high-grade VIN. VIN lesions are predominately VIN 2 or 3; VIN 1 lesions are relatively rare. Ki-67 (MIB-1) demonstrates nuclear reactivity throughout most of the epithelium (*Fig. 2.9b*).

Differentiated VIN is a relatively rare lesion associated with prominent eosinophilic cytoplasm with nuclear chromatin changes including chromatin clearing and prominent nucleoli. Differentiated VIN is classified as a high-grade VIN lesion (*Fig. 2.11*). Differentiated VIN is commonly seen adjacent to invasive squamous cell vulvar carcinoma and may be associateed with lichen sclerosus (see *Fig. 2.6*) (see following, Histologic Subtypes of VIN).

The International Society for the Study of Vulvovaginal disease (ISSVD) has proposed that VIN not be graded, and used only to describe high-grade VIN lesions only (VIN 2 or VIN 3). The ISSVD has also recommended that the term low-grade VIN (VIN 1, or mild dysplasia) not be used and that such lesions be classified as flat condyloma acuminatum, or given an appropriate descriptive term [147]. Issues regarding the recommendation to not use the term VIN 1 are challenged by evidence that low-grade VIN lesions are associated with high-risk human papillomavirus (HPV) in approximately 40% of cases studied, and prospective studies on such cases regarding clinical behavior remain to be performed [152].

Histologic Subtypes of VIN

VIN has been subclassified into at least three types – warty (condylomatous), basaloid, and differentiated (simplex) on the basis of cellular features. Interobserver reproducibility for subtyping VIN lesions is fair (kappa, 0.31–0.42) [160]. An individual patient may have more than one histologic type in different VIN lesions, and occasionally both basaloid and warty types may be seen in a single

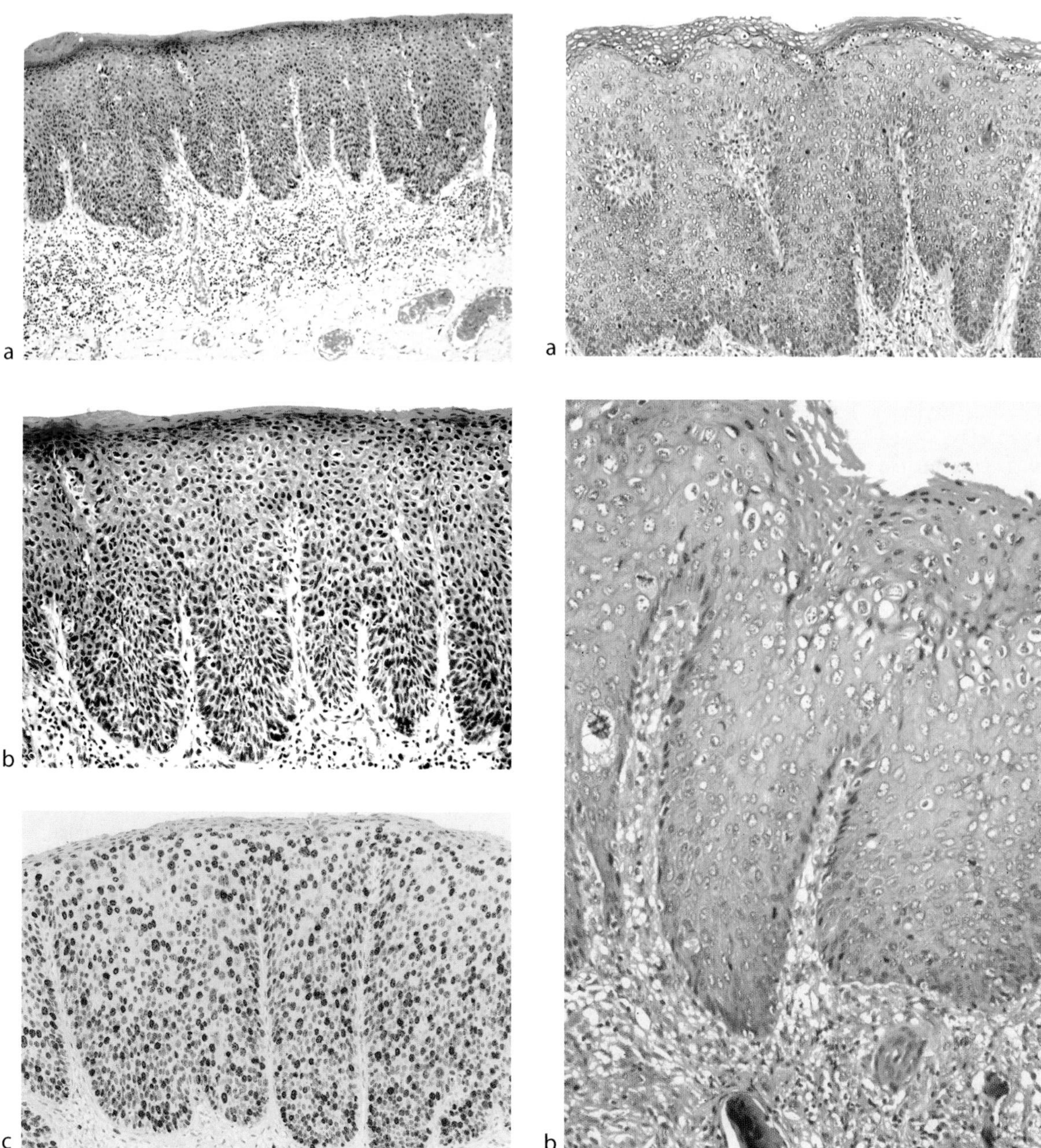

■ Fig. 2.9
VIN 3, basaloid type. (**a**) Prominent acanthosis and basaloid type neoplastic keratinocytes involve the full thickness of the epithelium. VIN 3 (carcinoma in situ), basaloid type. (**b**) Complete replacement of the epithelium with overlying parakeratosis resembles carcinoma in situ of the cervix. (**c**) Immunohistochemical study for Ki-67 demonstrates full epithelial thickness reactivity

■ Fig. 2.10
VIN 3, warty (condylomatous) type. (**a**) The surface shows hyperkeratosis. A prominent granular layer is evident. (**b**) Marked cellular disarray with prominent nuclear pleomorphism. Several multinucleated keratinocytes are present

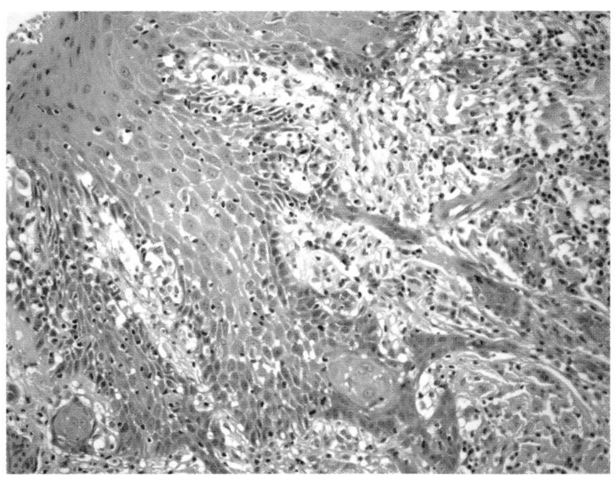

Fig. 2.11
VIN 3, differentiated type with invasive squamous carcinoma. The epithelium is composed of keratinocytes with abundant cytoplasm. The nuclei are enlarged and contain prominent nucleoli

lesion. Mixtures of basaloid and warty patterns are particularly frequent, and in some cases, both patterns may be seen in a single excised lesion. These "mixed" cases can be classified according to the predominant component or simply as VIN, basaloid/warty type. A rare pagetoid type of VIN is also recognized [125]. Some VIN lesions are not readily classifiable into one of these groups.

Warty (condylomatous) VIN lesions have an epithelial surface that is typically undulating or "spiked" surface with a warty/condylomatous appearance and is often keratinized with hypergranulosis and parakeratosis. There is usually prominent acanthosis with rete pegs that are relatively wide and extend deeply into the dermis. Dermal papillae are thinned and may be seen close to the surface. The cells show evidence of maturation with prominent parabasal hyperplasia. The epithelial cells have well-defined cell membranes and prominent eosinophilic cytoplasm. Individual cell keratinization and small cells with eosinophilic cytoplasm or "corps ronds" are often identified. Multinucleated epithelial giant cells are often observed. The nuclei are enlarged and pleomorphic, with coarsely granular chromatin and increased nuclear-cytoplasmic ratio. Nucleoli are not prevalent. Koilocytes, are cells with hyperchromatic, shrunken nuclei surrounded by a clear halo separating the nucleus from the cytoplasm cytoplasm, are characteristic (see ➋ *Figs. 2.5* and ➋ *2.10*). The warty type of VIN has larger cells with greater nuclear pleomorphism than basaloid VIN. Abnormal mitosis usually can be identified [117] (see ➋ *Fig. 2.10b*).

The basaloid type of VIN has a thickened epithelium with a relatively smooth and flat surface without the undulated and spiked appearance of warty VIN. Hyperkeratosis is often present, but less extensive than that is seen in warty VIN. The epithelium lacks cellular maturation and is typically nearly entirely composed of atypical parabasal type cells. These cells are relatively small, uniform cells with hyperchromatic and coarse nuclear chromatin. Nucleoli are rare, and mitosis is common;abnormal mitoses are usually found. Although there is little or no maturation of the keratinocytes, some keratinization or parakeratosis, as well as koilocytosis may be seen near the surface (see ➋ *Fig. 2.9*).

Both warty and basaloid VIN may have intraepithelial growth that extends into adjacent hair follicles and other skin adnexal structures. This is a relatively frequent finding and should be distinguished from invasive squamous cell carcinoma. Both basaloid and warty VIN may be identified adjacent to, and associated with, invasive squamous cell carcinomas. The invasive carcinoma may be of the basaloid or warty types corresponding to the VIN type, although the converse may occur with basaloid VIN adjacent to warty carcinoma or warty VIN adjacent to basaloid carcinoma (see ➋ Invasive Squamous Cell Carcinoma). Although basaloid VIN and basaloid carcinoma are often related to oncogenic HPV, nine (7%) of reported "differentiated" VIN cases in one study were basaloid VIN lesions that were negative for HPV and did not express p16INK4a, but did express p53 [60].

Differentiated VIN (VIN 3, differentiated/simplex type) has a thickened epithelium that is typically associated with elongation and anastomosis of rete ridges. Parakeratosis is usually present, associated with prominent intracellular bridges. The keratinocytes of differentiated VIN are large and pleomorphic with relatively large amounts of eosinophilic cytoplasm, as compared to the other two types of VIN (➋ *Fig. 2.11*). Keratin pearl formation within the rete may be seen. The nuclear chromatin is vesicular rather than coarse, and the nuclei have prominent nucleoli, usually most prominently in the basal and parabasal keratinocytes. A distinctive feature is the prominent increased eosinophilic cytoplasm within the keratinocytes in the basal and parabasal layers that is sometimes limited to the base of rete ridges [71,94,175,183]. Keratin pearl formation is common in differentiated VIN but is not common in other VIN lesions. In a study of 12 patients with differentiated VIN, 10 had squamous cell hyperplasia in the epithelium adjacent to the tumor, and four patients had associated lichen sclerosus. In this study, only one of the 12 patients had evidence of human papillomavirus (HPV); however, p53 was expressed in the suprabasal cells in ten of the 12 patients [183]. All the patients in this study were postmenopausal; three had a prior history of vulvar squamous cell carcinoma, and one patient had concurrent superficially invasive vulvar squamous cell carcinoma.

Pagetoid VIN is a very rare lesion with reports limited to a few cases [125]. It is characterized by a pagetoid growth pattern of neoplastic intraepithelial epithelial cells in groups and nests within otherwise normal-appearing epithelium. The cells of pagetoid VIN may resemble Paget disease of cutaneous type, or superficially spreading melanoma, having relatively pale cytoplasm and larger nuclei than the adjacent normal keratinocytes with relatively clear chromatin and evident nucleoli. Pagetoid VIN can be distinguished from Paget disease or melanoma in situ by immunohistochemical study in that unlike Paget disease, or melanoma in situ, the cells are not immunoreactive for CK 20, carcinoembryonic antigen (CEA), S-100 or Melan A but are immunoreactive for cytokeratin-7 [125].

Differential Diagnosis

The differential diagnosis of warty or basaloid VIN includes basal cell carcinoma, superficial spreading malignant melanoma, Paget disease, pagetoid urothelial intraepithelial neoplasia, and multinucleated atypia of the vulva.[30, 103,172]

Immunohistochemical methods to assist in distinguishing melanoma and Paget disease from VIN are summarized in *Table 2.2*. Multinucleated atypia of the vulva

Table 2.2

Immunohistochemical studies to differentiate vulvar Paget disease of skin or rectal origin, pagetoid urothelial intraepithelial neoplasia (PUIN), and melanoma

	CK7	CK20	GCDFP-15	CEA	S-100, HMB-45, and Melan-A	UPK
As a primary skin neoplasm	+	0	+	+	0	0
Related to anorectal carcinoma	0	+	0	+	0	0
PUIN related to urothelial carcinoma	+	+(0)	0	0	0	+
Melanoma	0	0	0	0	+	0

CK 7, cytokeratin 7; CK 20, cytokeratin 20; GCDFP-15, gross cystic disease fluid protein-15; CEA, carcinoembryonic antigen; UPK, Uroplakin III

Source: From refs. [173].

is characterized by multinucleated keratinocytes, without significant nuclear atypia, within the lower to middle epithelial layers. The possibility that a podophyllin effect on condylomata acuminata of the vulva could result in these lesions being misinterpreted as VIN is highly improbable because the changes from a single application of podophyllin regress within 1–2 weeks. Mitotic arrest with cells in metaphase seen after podophyllin contrasts with the abnormal mitotic figures seen in VIN. Nuclear karyorrhexis is rarely present in VIN, whereas it is found in most of the condyloma cases. In VIN, in contrast to the podophyllin effect, nuclear size tends to be vary, and the nuclear chromatin is usually coarse with little cellular swelling (see Chap. 1, Benign Diseases of the Vulva).

Differentiated VIN should be differentiated from repair or reaction related to erosion or superficial ulceration including pseudoepitheliomatous (pseudocarcinomatous) hyperplasia, trapped epithelium at a prior biopsy site, or granulomatous or decidual change in the immediately adjacent underlying epithelium. A similar lesion to differentiated VIN, but lacking the distinctive increased eosinophilic cytoplasm of the base of the rete ridges, has been designated by some as atypical squamous cell hyperplasia because this lesion has similar nuclear atypia but histologically resembles squamous cell hyperplasia more closely than it does in VIN[93] (see Chap. 1, Benign Diseases of the Vulva). Despite the association with keratinizing squamous cell carcinoma, there are no longitudinal studies demonstrating that squamous cell hyperplasia alone, as already defined here, is a precursor of squamous cell carcinoma. When associated with lichen sclerosus, follow-up studies suggest that associated squamous cell hyperplasia is probably a precursor to squamous cell carcinoma in some cases; however, the association between differentiated VIN, squamous cell hyperplasia, and squamous cell carcinoma requires further study [132]. Squamous cell hyperplastic-type lesions do not express p53, and this in part distinguishes these otherwise benign lesions from differentiated VIN [88,183].

Adjunctive Studies

Evidence for HPV, nearly always type 16, in VIN is predominately found in the warty and basaloid types, based on molecular biologic studies, and has been demonstrated in most cases [134]. In differentiated VIN, HPV is infrequent [134,148]. Alterations in the p16/pRb/Cyclin D1 pathway occur in VIN lesions as demonstrated by immunohistochemical methods. Epigenetic silencing of p16INK4a has been reported in approximately two thirds of basaloid or warty VIN lesions [137]. Immunohistochemical expression of p16INK-4a was demonstrated in 92% of high-grade VIN lesions in one study, and these cases had nearly the full thickness expression of p16INK in the involved epithelium. In low-grade VIN lesions, two of ten were immunoreactive, and in these cases, the reactivity was limited to the intraepithelial neoplastic predominately within in the lower half of the epithelium [133]. Oncogenic HPV is usually present in high-grade warty and basaloid VIN lesions, with type 16 being the usual type identified. Oncogenic HPV is significantly less common in VIN of differentiated type [94,134,148]. Approximately a third of cases demonstrated overexpression of Cyclin D1 in a series or 13 cases of VIN. None of these cases demonstrated lack of pRb protein [93]. Differentiated VIN lesions usually express p53 in the basal and some parabasal cells and are not associated with oncogenic HPV [88,183]. Cellular proliferation analysis employing immunohistochemical studies for BCL 2 and Ki – 67 (MIB – 1) does not appear to be of much value in the diagnosis of VIN lesions although Ki-67 may have some value in grading and identifying low-grade lesions [96].

Most high-grade VIN lesions contain DNA aneuploid populations of cells [59,178]. DNA analysis by microspectrophotometry of multifocal lesions suggests that separate lesions arise from separate stem cells, forming distinguishable clones. Large confluent lesions may result from centrifugal growth from a single cell line or by confluence of separate and distinct clones [178]. In single VIN lesions, approximately half have different stem cells by DNA microspectrophotometry, suggesting that such lesions may undergo clonal evolution[178]. The cells of VIN are immunoreactive for some low and high molecular-weight keratins and keratin expression provides some evidence of lack of cellular maturation in VIN [53].

Immunohistochemical studies for cellular proliferation employing BCL 2 and Ki-67 (MIB-1) have not been demonstrated to be of significant value in the diagnosis of VIN lesions.

Clinical Behavior and Treatment

The clinical course of VIN following treatment has been well studied; however, there are relatively few long-term studies of untreated VIN [85,86]. There is evidence that untreated VIN 3 will progress to invasive squamous cell carcinoma, and this has been reported with invasion being observed within 8 years of the diagnosis of VIN [85,86]. VIN associated with vulvar invasive squamous cell carcinoma diagnosed within excised VIN lesions is reported in 2–20% of larger series that have specifically looked for this association [24,80]. In evaluation of epithelial changes adjacent to vulvar squamous cell carcinoma, 60–80% of superficially invasive carcinomas and 25% of deeply invasive carcinomas have adjacent VIN [184]. Differentiated (simplex) VIN was reported associated with vulvar squamous cell carcinoma in seven of 12 (58%) patients in one study [183]. This study suggests that there is a stronger association between differentiated VIN and squamous cell carcinoma than there is between the other recognized VIN types and invasion. There are no known differences in clinical behavior between warty and basaloid VIN. Squamous cell carcinoma, in the other VIN types, also occurs most commonly in postmenopausal women, although it may occur in women of reproductive age [69]. Spontaneous regression of VIN has been observed in young women; however, no long-term controlled prospective studies have evaluated this event specifically [30,58]. Regression appears to be most common in young women and those who are pregnant, whereas women of advanced age, those who are severely immunosuppressed, and women with Fanconi anemia are at a greater risk for invasion [23,179].

Conservative therapy is now recommended for VIN, and most cases are managed with local excision; laser ablation also may be appropriate for selected patients, especially when the VIN lesion involves the non-hairy skin or mucous membrane areas (e.g., the vulvar vestibule and perianal areas). Topical imiquimod has gained some application in the treatment of vulvar condyloma acuminatum and VIN lesions [156,163]. Women who are cigarette smokers appear to have a higher frequency of recurrence of VIN lesions, and cessation of smoking is recommended [176].

Squamous Cell Carcinoma

Approximately 95% of malignant tumors of the vulva are squamous cell carcinomas. Vulvar squamous cell carcinoma has an overall incidence of approximately 1.5 per 100,000 women in the USA; this rate increases with advancing age to as high as 20 per 100,000 in older women [155]. The American Cancer Society reports over 3,400 new cases of vulvar squamous cell carcinoma in the USA annually [4]. Unlike VIN, the incidence of vulvar squamous cell carcinoma in the USA has not increased significantly since 1973 [155]. The mean age at presentation is 60–74 years [92,155]. Vulvar carcinoma may occur in younger women and adolescents, and has been described in a 12 year old [2,124].

Epidemiologic studies of women with vulvar carcinoma have identified an increased risk with prior or current vulvar VIN, condyloma acuminatum, and cervical carcinoma. In these cases, oncogenic human papillomavirus is usually a significant factor. Vulvar lichen sclerosus is also associated with an increased life-time risk of vulvar carcinoma, which does not appear directly related to oncogenic HPV. In addition, factors including older age, number of life-time sexual partners, cigarette smoking, immunodeficiency, chronic granulomatous disease, most notably granuloma inguinale, diabetes mellitus, achlorhydria, poor perineal hygiene, and genital granulomatous disease have been associated [128,146]. Occupational risk is reported in women cotton mill workers, and women with industrial exposure to industrial oils, as well as those working in the dyeing and cutlery industries. Topical exposure to arsenicals also increases risk. A possible increased frequency has been suggested for women with blood group A, but findings remain inconclusive [128]. Vulvar carcinoma may occur during pregnancy, although parity does not appear to be a significant risk factor.

Current evidence supports the view that women at risk for vulvar carcinoma can be separated into two groups: those who have associated HPV squamous lesions, specifically VIN, and those with vulvar disease not associated with HPV including known vulvar dermatoses (especially lichen sclerosus) and those related to other conditions, such as chronic granulomatous disease. One case related to hidradenitis suppurativa has been reported [146]. The frequency of oncogenic HPV associated vulvar squamous cell carcinoma is different between young and older women. HPV, usually type 16, is reported in less than one fifth of vulvar carcinomas in older women (mean age 77 years), whereas approximately four fifths of the vulvar squamous carcinomas identified in younger women (mean age 50 years) are HPV associated. The histopathologic type of invasive carcinoma also differs. In the older women vulvar squamous cell carcinomas are usually well differentiated and highly keratinized. In younger women, the tumors are usually warty or basaloid carcinomas [43,93,157].

Older women with vulvar carcinoma (mean age, 77 years) typically do not have associated VIN or a history of heavy cigarette smoking. Their tumors rarely contain HPV, and typically they are well-differentiated keratinizing squamous cell carcinomas (*Table 2.3*) [91,93,157]. Suppressed immunocompetence is recognized as a risk factor in these women [23,179]. Women with HPV-related cervical neoplasia with low CD 4 counts who are treated with triple combination antiretroviral therapy can have decreased plasma human immunodeficiency virus-1 (HIV-1) levels, increased CD 4 cell counts, and partially restored immune function. This restored immune function is associated with regression of cervical lesions in these women [74].

Table 2.3
Histologic subtypes of squamous vulvar carcinoma

Histologic subtypes
Basaloid carcinoma
Warty (condylomatous) carcinoma
Verrucous carcinoma
Giant cell carcinoma
Spindle cell carcinoma
Acantholytic squamous cell carcinoma (adenoid squamous carcinoma)
Lymphoepithelioma-like carcinoma
Plasmacytoid squamous cell carcinoma
Basal cell carcinoma
Metatypical basal cell carcinoma (basosquamous carcinoma)
Adenoid basal cell carcinoma
Sebaceous cell carcinoma
NOS, not otherwise specified.

Women with differentiated, non-HPV-related, vulvar squamous cell carcinoma often have associated vulvar dermatoses, especially lichen sclerosus [20]. Primary evidence based on p53 mutation analysis and clonal studies suggests that squamous cell hyperplasia of the vulva is probably not a precursor of non-HPV-related vulvar squamous cell carcinomas [88]. Women with vulvar lichen sclerosus who develop squamous cell carcinoma tend to be older; their primary tumors more commonly involve the clitoris and are typically not associated with VIN of the warty or basaloid types. VIN was identified in 5% of the cases in one series [20]. It is recognized that there is an under reporting of skin diseases related to vulvar carcinoma. Squamous carcinomas associated with lichen sclerosus express tumor suppressor gene product p53 in nearly one half the cases and cytokine transforming growth factor-beta (TGF-b) in one third of the cases as compared to 19% and 9%, respectively, for nonlichen sclerosus-related tumors. Approximately one half of these lichen sclerosus-associated tumors are associated with a prominent fibromyxoid stromal response, as compared to nonlichen sclerosus-related tumors [20]. From a literature review of a cohort of symptomatic women with vulvar lichen sclerosus, it was reported that 9% subsequently presented with VIN and 21% with vulvar squamous cell carcinoma. The carcinoma presented 1–23 years (mean, 4 years) after the onset of symptoms [20].

Stage IA Invasive Squamous Cell Carcinoma (AJCC T1a, M0, N0; FIGO Stage IA)

General Features

The majority of vulvar squamous cell carcinomas in the USA are stage 1, being 2 cm or less in diameter and clinically confined to the vulva without evidence of extension to other sites or lymph node metastasis. Stage 1 vulvar carcinomas are divided into two subgroups based on depth of invasion. A stage IA vulvar carcinoma is a superficially invasive squamous cell carcinoma with a depth of invasion of 1 mm or less and a diameter of 2 cm or less. The staging of vulvar carcinoma as recommended by the American Joint Committee on Cancer (AJCC) is as summarized in *Tables 2.4* and *2.5* (American Joint Committee on Cancer 2010) [5].

A stage IA (FIGO Stage IA; AJCC T1a) carcinoma of the vulva is defined as a single lesion measuring 2 cm or less in diameter with a depth of invasion of 1 mm or less regardless of the presence of vascular invasion. Tumors with more than one site of invasion are not included in this stage [89,180]. It is recommended that the term "microinvasive carcinoma" not be used in reporting vulvar carcinoma because there is no agreement on the definition of the term. When the term is used, it usually refers to vulvar squamous cell carcinomas with a depth on invasion or thickness of 5 mm or less. In a multivariate

Table 2.4

American Joint Committee on Cancer (AJCC) staging of vulvar carcinoma when pathologic staging is performed, it is designated "pT"; clinical staging is designated "T"

TX: Primary tumor cannot be assessed
T0: No evidence of primary tumor
Tis: Carcinoma in situ (preinvasive carcinoma)
T1: Tumor confined to the vulva or vulva and perineum, 2 cm or less in greatest dimension. (Stage T1 N0 M0)
T1a: Tumor confined to the vulva or vulva and perineum, 2 cm or less in greatest dimension, and with stromal invasion no greater than 1 mm.[a]
T1b: Tumor confined to the vulva or vulva and perineum, 2 cm or less in greatest dimension, and with stromal invasion greater than 1 mm.[a]
T2: Tumor of any size with extension to adjacent perineal structures (lower/distal1/3 urethra, lower/distal1/3 vagina, anal involvement, with negative nodes (FIGO uses the classification T2/T3. This is defined as T2 in TNM)
T3: Tumor of any size with extension to any of the following: upper/proximal 2/3 of urethra, upper/proximal 2/3 vagina, bladder mucosa, rectal mucosa, or fixed to pelvic bone (FIGO uses the classification T4 for this group. This is defined as T3 in TNM)

[a]The depth of invasion is defined as the measurement of the tumor from the epithelial–stromal junction of the adjacent most superficial dermal papilla to the deepest point of invasion.

Source: From *AJCC Cancer Staging Manual*, 7th ed. Springer, New York, Dordrecht, Heidelberg, London, 2010 [5].

Table 2.5

FIGO staging: carcinoma of the vulva 2009

Stage I	Tumor confined to the vulva (Stage I, T1 N0 M0).
	Stage IA: Lesions 2 cm or less in size, confined to the vulva or perineum, and with stromal invasion of 1.0 mm or less, no nodal metastasis.[a] (Stage T1a)
	Stage IB T1b: Lesions greater than 2 cm in size, with stromal invasion greater than 1.0 mm, confined to the vulva or perineum, with negative nodes.[a] (Stage T1b)
Stage II	Tumor of any size with extension to adjacent perineal structures (1/3 lower urethra, 1/3 lower vagina, anus, with negative nodes (Stage T2 N0 M0)
Stage III	Tumor of any size with or without extension to adjacent perineal structures (1/3 lower urethra, 1/3 lower vagina, anus) with positive inguinal–femoral nodes
IIIA	(i) with 1 lymph node metastasis (of 5 mm or less) or
IIIA	(ii) 1–2 lymph node metastasis(es) (<5 mm)
IIIB	(i) With two or more lymph node metastasis (of 5 mm or > 5 mm), or
IIIB	(ii) With three or more lymph node metastasis (<5 mm)
IIIC	With positive nodes with extracapsular spread.
Stage IV	Tumor invades other regional (2/3 upper urethra, 2/3 upper vagina) or distant structures
IA	Tumor involves any of the following:
IVA (i)	Upper urethra and/or vaginal mucosa, bladder mucosa, rectal mucosa, or fixed to pelvic bone; or,
IIVA (ii)	Fixed, or ulcerated inguinal–femoral lymph nodes;
IVB	Any distant metastasis including pelvic lymph nodes

[a]The depth of invasion is defined as the measurement of the tumor from the epithelial–stromal junction of the adjacent most superficial dermal papilla to the deepest point of invasion.

FIGO ref: Pecorelli S, Denny L, Ngan H, Pecorelli S, Hacker N, Bermudez A, Mutch D, Revised FIGO staging for carcinoma of the vulva, cervix, and endometrium. *Int J Gynecol Obstet.* 2009;105:103–104.

retrospective analysis of 78 cases of "microinvasive" vulvar squamous carcinoma fulfilling this 5 mm criteria, 28 (36%) were pathologic stage IA, 40 (51%) pathologic stage 1B, six (8%) pathologic stage II, and four (5%) pathologic stage III [184]. The term "microinvasion" is not recommended by the World Health Organization, the International Society for the Study of Vulvovaginal Disease (ISSVD), or the AJCC. Reporting the diameter of the tumor, the depth of invasion, the thickness of the tumor, the presence or absence of vascular space involvement, and the status of surgical margins clearly defines the tumor and its extent. These findings will influence treatment options and are included in the College of American Pathologists Vulvar Cancer protocol for synoptic reporting [31,171].

Gross Findings

Stage 1 invasive vulvar squamous cell carcinoma may present as an ulcer, a red, brown, or black macule or papule, or a white hyperkeratotic plaque. The invasive carcinoma may be associated with VIN and clinically present as a VIN lesion. Although the presence of invasion associated with VIN may be heralded by the finding of an associated ulcer, irregularly contoured elevated mass, abnormal vascularity, or marked hyperkeratosis, no specific clinical findings definitively separate VIN from VIN with squamous carcinoma [24].

Tumor diameter alone in stage 1 vulvar carcinoma is not a reliable predictor of lymph node status. In a study of 190 patients with vulvar carcinomas 2 cm in diameter or smaller, 36 (19%) had lymph node metastasis. Of those with node metastasis, the relative 5-year survival was 78.6%, compared with 97.9% survival at 5 years for those with negative nodes [78].

Microscopic Findings

The identification of a squamous cell carcinoma arising in VIN lesion, or in differentiated VIN, includes (1) Isolated neoplastic squamous cells with increased eosinophilic cytoplasm and atypical nuclei with prominent nucleoli within the adjacent dermis. (2) Loss of the orderly palisaded orientation of the basal keratinocytes of the dermal papillae. (3) Irregular nests of neoplastic squamous cells with disorderly orientation within the dermis. (4) Dyskeratosis and keratin pearl formation in the basal and parabasal layers. (5) Focal dermal reaction with fibrosis (dermal desmoplasia) or edema locally evident in the area of invasion [92,139]. Immunohistochemical study of laminin may also be of some value in that continuous reactive laminin is usually seen about nests of VIN, but discontinuous reactivity of laminin is identified about invasive squamous epithelium [48,92].

In a study of 78 cases of vulvar squamous cell carcinoma with invasion of 5 mm or less, of 40 patients with inguinal lymph node dissections, five had concurrent lymph node metastases. Concurrent lymph node metastases were compared to tumor depth of invasion, tumor thickness, tumor horizontal spread, estimated tumor volume, tumor histologic squamous tumor type, tumor grade, primary pattern of invasion, multi-focality of tumor of the vulva, presence of perineural invasion, presence of angiolymphatic invasion, histologic type of VIN, as well as the presence of lichen sclerosus. In this detailed study, only tumor depth of invasion was statistically significant in correlating with the presence of lymph node metastases ($p = 0.027$, $n = 78$, *ANOVA*). All additional correlations between these findings and lymph node metastasis were not statistically significant ($p > 0.05$) [184].

In that the staging of a stage IA invasive vulvar carcinoma is based upon the "depth of invasion of the tumor" (➲ *Fig. 2.12*). This measurement requires a calibrated ocular or comparable measuring device, as does the measurement of the thickness of the tumor. The measurement of the "depth of invasion" for staging stage 1 vulvar carcinoma is defined as the measurement from the epithelial dermal (stromal) junction of the most superficial adjacent dermal papillae to the deepest point of invasion (➲ *Fig. 2.12*). The measurement from the surface of the tumor, or from the base of the granular layer if a keratin layer is present, to the deepest point of invasion is defined as the "thickness of the tumor." Both measurements are valuable, because in cases in which the tumor is ulcerated the thickness may be 1 mm or less and the depth of invasion may be well beyond 1 mm, and a thickness measurement alone would underestimate the depth of invasion (➲ *Fig. 2.12*). Methods of measurement require a description along with the measurement within the pathology report [31,171,174].

There can be some difficulties in measuring the depth of invasion in some cases, especially if there is tangential sectioning of the specimen, or the surface epithelium is distorted, disrupted, or folded. In some cases, the depth of invasion can be more readily calculated by measuring the thickness of the tumor and subtracting the epithelial measurement from the surface to the epithelial–dermal (stromal) junction of the immediately adjacent dermal papillae. The measurement should be made from "...the epithelial-stromal junction of the adjacent most superficial dermal papilla," and in some cases, the immediately

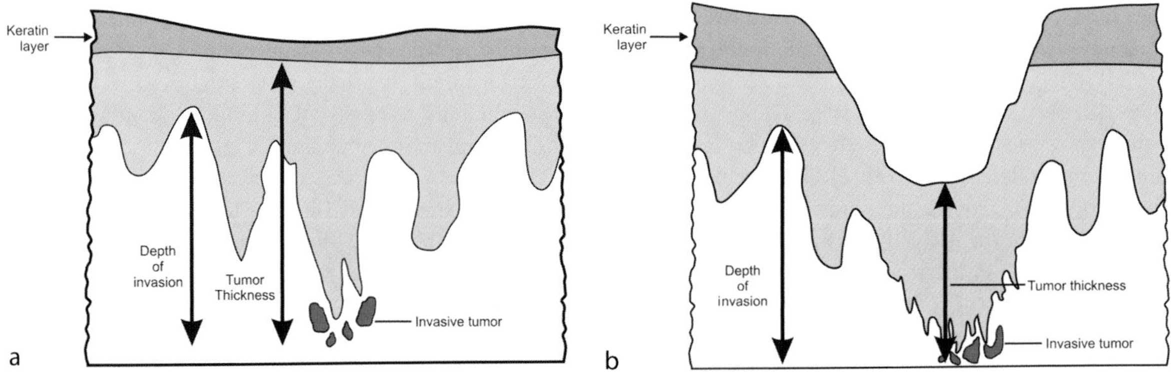

Fig. 2.12
Squamous cell carcinoma; measurement for the depth of invasion. **(a) The depth of invasion is measured from the epithelial–dermal junction of the adjacent-most superficial dermal papillae to the deepest point of invasion. This measurement is applicable whether or not the surface epithelium is ulcerated or keratinized. This is the AJCC recommended method of measuring vulvar squamous cell carcinomas in determining if a tumor is Stage T1a, or T1b (From *AJCC Cancer Staging Manual*, 6th ed. New York: Lippincott, Williams & Wilkins; 2002, with permission. Figure © E.J. Wilkinson, 2007). If the tumor is keratinized, the thickness of tumor is measured from the granular layer to the deepest point of invasion. For squamous cell carcinomas the convention is to measure from the bottom of the granular layer. For melanoma the convention is to measure from the top of the granular layer. If the epithelium is not keratinized the thickness of the tumor is measured from the surface of the tumor to the deepest point of invasion (Figure © E.J. Wilkinson, 2007.). (b)** Melanoma and squamous cell carcinoma; measurements for tumor thickness when the tumor is ulcerated. **The tumor thickness is measured from the surface of the ulcerated tumor to the deepest point of invasion. For melanomas, the level of invasion is measured and expressed as Clark's Levels. For squamous cell carcinoma the depth of invasion is a more accurate measurement of the true depth of the tumor, as measured from the epithelial dermal junction of the adjacent dermal papillae to the deepest point of invasion (Figure © E.J. Wilkinson, 2007.) (from Wilkinson EJ and Stone IK, Atlas of Vulvar Disease. Wolters Kluwer/ Lippincott-Williams Wilkins, 2008 (ref: 174)**

adjacent dermal papillae is not applicable for various reasons, including that it is not the most superficial dermal papillae, which may be the second papillae over on either side of the tumor. The issue is also not of such importance when the depth of invasion is obviously over 1 mm. In some cases, levels of the block containing the section of tumor with the apparent deepest point of invasion may be worth obtaining to identify the best-orientated section with the deepest point of invasion. In rare cases, the involved epithelium may not have dermal papillae, and in such cases, a measurement from the epithelial–dermal (stromal) junction of the adjacent epithelium uninvolved by tumor should be representative. In general, with a well-oriented specimen with a tumor less than 3 mm in depth, and totally excised with intact noninvolved epithelium adjacent to the tumor, the measurements of depth of invasion and tumor thickness can be made reliably (➋ *Figs. 2.12* and ➋ *2.13*). In larger tumors, the diameter and dimensions of the tumor may be too great to include an adjacent dermal papillae; however, this often can be overcome by appropriate sectioning. With a partially excised tumor, or when the tumor is superficially biopsied, these tumor measurements cannot be made reliably. When marked acanthosis is present, the thickness of the epithelium may give an overestimate of the depth of invasion. If the tumor is ulcerated, the thickness measurement may underestimate the true tumor size. The College of American Pathologists has recommended that the following information be included in the surgical pathology report [31,171].

1. Depth of invasion of the tumor in millimeters and thickness of the tumor in millimeters
2. Method of measurement of the depth of invasion and thickness
3. Presence or absence of vascular space involvement by tumor
4. Diameter of the tumor (as measured from the gross surgical specimen)
5. Clinical measurement of the tumor diameter, when available.

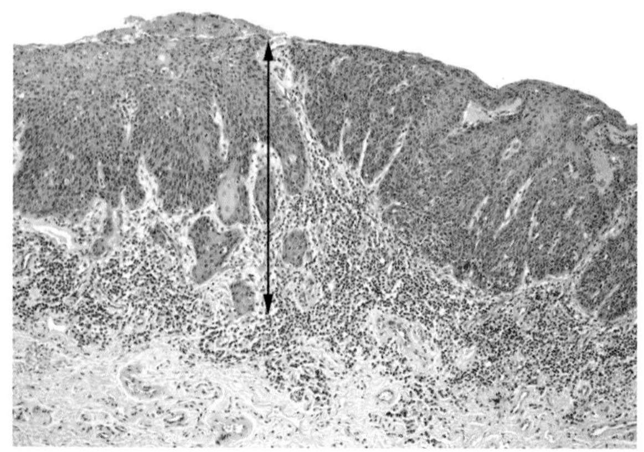

Fig. 2.13
Squamous cell carcinoma. **The depth of invasion is 0.7 mm from the most superficial adjacent dermal papillae to the deepest point of invasion**

When there is a question as to whether invasion is present and additional sectioning does not resolve the question, it is recommended that invasion not be diagnosed.

Clinical Behavior and Treatment

Patients who have had stage 1A invasive vulvar squamous cell carcinoma that was treated who have recurrence, or have a second primary squamous cell carcinoma of the vulva, risk regional lymph node metastasis and death from recurrence. In a study of 28 women with Stage 1A vulvar carcinoma, none had recurrence of squamous cell carcinoma 240 months of follow-up [184]. In a series of 26 women with VIN and associated superficially invasive squamous cell carcinoma, ten (38%) of these patients experienced recurrence of VIN or superficially invasive squamous cell carcinoma, all within 36 months of treatment [76]. Three of these ten women subsequently presented with frankly invasive vulvar squamous cell carcinoma. Of the patients without recurrence of VIN or superficially invasive carcinoma, none had regional lymph node or distant metastases and none died of tumor. In another study of 40 patients with T1a (stage 1A) vulvar carcinomas, none had regional lymph node metastasis; however, two patients had vulvar recurrence, and one of them had a groin node metastasis associated with the recurrence [100].

There are relatively limited data specifically evaluating tumors with a depth of invasion of 1.1 mm to 2 mm. In two relatively small studies specifically examining tumors with invasion of 1–2 mm, without vascular space involvement, none had node metastasis [13,122,184]. In a multivariate analysis performed by Yoder et al., six of 19 (31%) of cases with 1.1–2.0 mm depth of invasion had recurrence of vulvar squamous cell carcinoma [184]. Of these cases, however, recurrence did not influence survival and those women with tumors having a depth of invasion of 2.0 mm or less of invasion had 100% overall survival at 240 months [184]. Until more data are available on tumors that invade between 1 and 2 mm, the evidence that women with such tumors have limited risk of regional lymph node metastasis should be considered when node assessment is considered in such patients. Recurrence is a recognized risk, and treatment with wide local excision/partial vulvectomy in these patients is generally accepted.

Women with tumors having a depth of invasion of 2.1–3 mm or less have significant risk of regional lymph node metastasis, recurrence of tumor, and reduced survival. With this depth of invasion, there is inguinal lymph node metastasis in approximately 10% of cases. In one study on women with tumors having a depth of invasion between 2.1 and 3.0 mm, five of 16 (31%) cases had recurrent squamous cell carcinoma. These women had a 93% survival at 258 months, whereas women with tumors greater than 3.1 mm of invasion had 79% survival at 231 months [184]. Selected patients with tumors with a depth of invasion of 2.1–3 mm may be treated by wide local excision with ipsilateral regional node dissection [63].

Vulvar squamous cell carcinomas with a depth of invasion exceeding 3.1 mm are associated with an increased risk of recurrence and death. In one study of tumors exceeding 3 mm invasion, five of 15 (33%) cases had recurrence of tumor with an overall survival of 79% at 231 months [184]. In a study evaluating both depth of invasion and tumor thickness, more than 40% of the cases had groin metastasis when the thickness of the tumor exceeded 4 mm [13]. Women with vulvar squamous carcinomas with a 5 mm depth of invasion, have been found to have inguinal lymph node metastasis in approximately 15% of cases (*Fig. 2.14*).

The type of surgery for vulvar squamous cell carcinomas with a depth of invasion less that 5 mm does not appear to influence recurrence of squamous cell carcinoma. In a study of 78 patients with tumors of 5 mm in depth of invasion or less, 44 (56%) underwent wide local excision (partial vulvectomy), of which three had adjuvant radiation, seven (9%) had total (simple) vulvectomy, and 27 (35%) had total vulvectomy with inguinal–femoral lymph node dissection (radical vulvectomy); one of whom had adjuvant radiation therapy. No association was identified between recurrent squamous cell carcinoma and the type of surgical procedure performed [184].

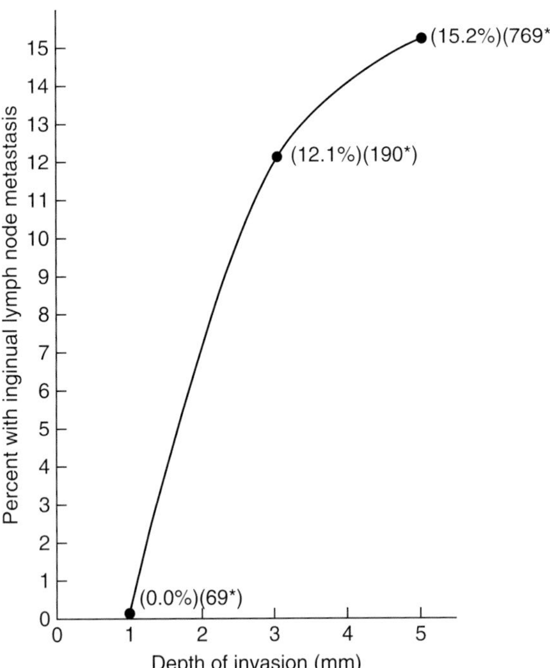

Fig. 2.14
Percent of women who underwent lymphadenectomy with inguinal lymph node metastasis plotted against the depth of invasion of their tumor. **The frequency of lymph node metastasis rises rapidly with depth of invasion beyond 1 mm (Reprinted by permission of E.J. Wilkinson)**

Surgical margin assessment correlates with recurrence in women treated with vulvar squamous cell carcinoma. The presence of VIN at a surgical margin has borderline statistical significance related to recurrence of VIN. Of 19 cases with VIN at a surgical margin, six (58%) had recurrence of VIN. In contrast, only four of 59 (91%) women with margins free of VIN or squamous cell carcinoma had recurrence of VIN. In this study, two cases had invasive squamous cell carcinoma at a surgical margin, and both had recurrence, or persistent, squamous cell carcinoma [184]. This study identified a strong association between the type of surgery performed and surgical margin involvement by either VIN or invasive squamous cell carcinoma. Of 19 cases with VIN at the margin of excision, 15 (79%) were found in cases treated with wide local excision. Of the 78 cases in this study, 44 cases were treated by wide local excision and of these, 15 had VIN at a surgical margin, and two had invasive squamous cell carcinoma at the margin [184].

For now, it is safe to say there is a diminishing small risk of inguinal lymph node metastasis with tumors that are stage IA (T1a1) with a depth of invasion of 1 mm or less. For patients with stage IA carcinoma of the vulva, the recommended therapy is wide local excision without vulvectomy. Total excision of a lesion suspected of being a stage IA invasive carcinoma is necessary to assure that an associated deeper squamous carcinoma is not immediately adjacent to the apparently superficially invasive focus. The surgical specimen typically encompasses the apparent VIN lesion and any associated hyperkeratotic or ulcerative lesions. The specimens are usually not more than 2–3 cm in greatest dimension, usually with 1 cm or less clinically negative margins. Sampling of the ipsilateral groin nodes, or bilateral groin nodes if the tumor is midline, has been suggested. For stage IA (T1a) vulvar carcinomas, the probability of node metastasis is extremely small, and node sampling or resection is not contributory in most cases [92,170,184]. Based on analysis of published series, the current treatment of these patients is partial deep vulvectomy (deep local excision) without lymphadenectomy [67,68,100,184].

Invasive Squamous Cell Carcinoma

Clinical Features

Women presenting with vulvar carcinoma may have a wide variety of presenting complaints relevant to the vulvar tumor, especially if the tumor is more advanced. Pruritus, burning, pain, bleeding, discharge, dyspareunia, dysuria, unpleasant odor, or palpation or observation of a mass have all been reported. A past medical history of vulvar intraepithelial neoplasia (VIN), condyloma acuminatum, lichen sclerosus, or other chronic inflammatory diseases of the vulva may be present. Mental confusion and disorientation related to hypercalcemia have been reported associated with vulvar squamous cell carcinoma. After the ovary, the vulva is the second most common gynecologic tumor site associated with hypercalcemia. Vulvar squamous carcinomas with associated hypercalcemia usually are large, well differentiated, and without bony metastasis [112]. Surgical excision of the tumor results in the serum calcium levels returning to normal, and if mental symptoms related to the hypercalcemia were present, these also regress. The hypercalcemia results from secretion by the tumor of parathyroid hormone (PTH) or PTH-like substance.

Invasive squamous carcinoma may present as a lesion associated with VIN, as a focal ulcer or hyperkeratotic area in a field of vulvar lichen sclerosus, an exophytic papillomatous mass, or as an endophytic ulcer. The tumor is usually located on the labium minus or majus; however, the clitoris is primarily involved in less than one fifth of cases. Typically, the tumor is solitary (*Figs. 2.15* and *2.16*); less than 10% are multifocal.

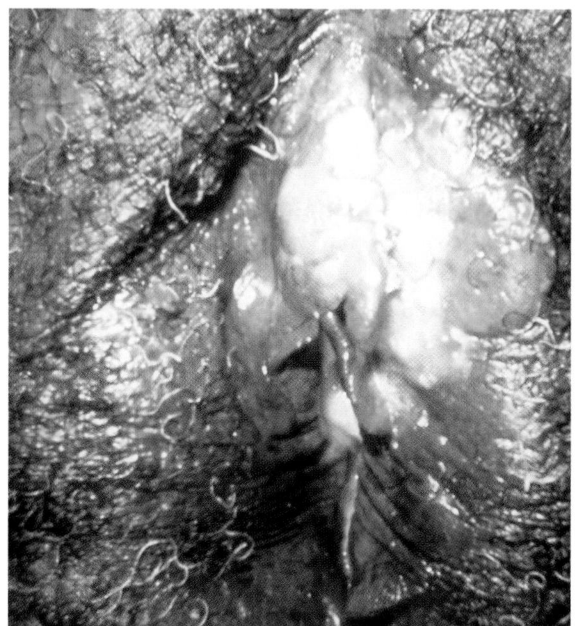

■ Fig. 2.15
Squamous cell carcinoma. **The tumor involves the medial aspect of the left anterior labium majus and clitoris**

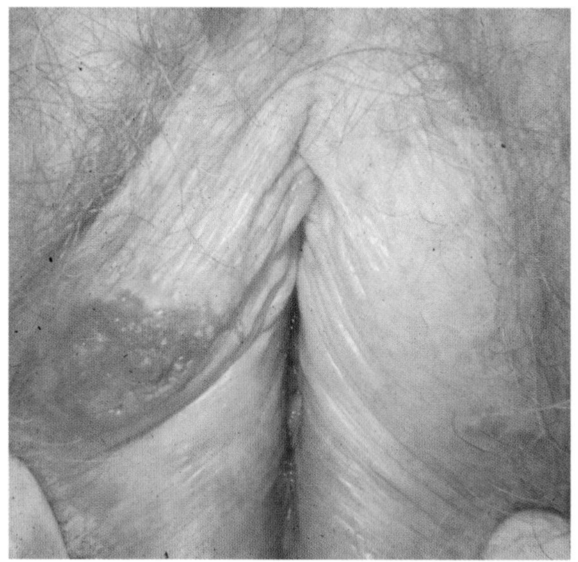

■ Fig. 2.16
Squamous cell carcinoma. **The tumor presents as a nodular mass on the right posterior labia majus. There is associated lichen sclerosus**

Microscopic Findings

Vulvar squamous cell carcinoma is typically contiguous with adjacent vulvar skin or mucosa, and that epithelium may be involved with VIN, lichen sclerosus, chronic inflammation, or other changes [28]. The invasive tumor typically lacks the usually orderly palisaded orientation of the basal epithelial cells with the underlying dermis. The adjacent dermis often has edema, desmoplastic change, and/or an associated inflammatory cell infiltrate that is typically not in direct contact with the invasive epithelial cells, but within the reactive dermis immediately below and adjacent to the tumor. Some prominent vascularity may be present within the dermis immediately below the tumor. The tumor may invade with a broad pushing pattern, or have variable degrees of "finger-like" growth within the dermis, including single tumor cells within dermis. The tumor growth pattern influences the risk of regional metastasis in tumors exceeding 1 mm in depth of invasion [184]. A grading system for infiltrative patterns of vulvar carcinoma has been proposed [184]. Capillary-like vascular space invasion by the tumor may be evident and in such cases the tumor can usually be found attached to the lining of the capillary-like space. The tumor is composed of neoplastic squamous epithelial cells that may have variable eosinophilic cytoplasm with nuclei that exhibit variable degrees of anisonucleocytosis with nuclear chromatin abnormalities including clumped and radially dispersed chromatin. Nucleoli are usually present, and mitotic figures including abnormal mitotic figures may be evident, especially near the epithelial–dermal junction.

A number of grading systems for vulvar squamous cell carcinomas have been proposed. However, to date no uniform grading system has been unanimously accepted. An effective grading system must reflect clinical behavior, preferably include three grades only as applied in most other grading systems in gynecologic pathology, and be applicable to the various subtypes of vulvar squamous carcinoma including warty, basaloid, and keratinizing types. The difficulty is that with current systems, basaloid carcinomas would be graded G3 or G4, which would not necessarily predict behavior. The American Joint Committee on Cancer (AJCC) recommends that histopathologic grading of vulvar carcinoma be recorded as follows: GX, grade cannot be assessed; G1, well differentiated; G2, moderately differentiated; G3, poorly differentiated; and G4, undifferentiated (American Joint Committee on Cancer 2010) [5]. The Gynecologic Oncology Group (GOG) advocates a system according to the percentage of undifferentiated cells. The latter are small cells with scant cytoplasm showing little or no differentiation and infiltrating the stroma in either elongated cords or small clusters [78]. Grade 1 tumors have no undifferentiated cells (➋ *Figs. 2.16–2.18*), grade 2 tumors contain less than 50% undifferentiated cells, grade 3 tumors (➋ *Fig. 2.19*) have greater than 50% but less than 100%, and grade 4 is essentially entirely composed of undifferentiated cells. The risk of recurrence is reportedly higher with increasing grade [78,81,142].

In addition to tumor staging (as summarized in ➋ *Tables 2.4*, ➋ *2.5*, and ➋ *2.6*), the AJCC staging system reports regional lymph node status (as N) and the presence or absence of metastases (as M) (➋ *Table 2.6*). All lymph node tissues should be submitted for microscopic analysis. The microscopic evaluation of lymph nodes for detection of metastatic cell squamous carcinoma may be augmented by immunohistochemistry using a polyclonal cytokeratin antibody. Pathologic findings included in the College of American Pathologists (CAP) guidelines for evaluation of vulvar squamous cell carcinoma are the same for deep and superficial invasive squamous cell carcinomas (see ➋ Stage 1a Invasive Squamous Cell Carcinoma, ➋ Microscopic Findings) [31,171]. The CAP Surgical Pathology Cancer Case Summary/Checklist provides a synoptic approach to reporting vulvar cancer cases for either excisional biopsies or resections. In addition to tumor staging, the checklist includes macroscopic observations including specimen type, type of lymphadenectomy if performed, specific tumor site, and tumor size. Microscopic features to record include the histological type of tumor, the histologic grade, the pathologic stage (pTNM/FIGO), tumor depth of invasion, tumor border features, surgical margin status, presence or absence of venous/lymphatic invasion by tumor. Additional pathologic findings, including the pathologic findings in the adjacent vulvar skin or mucosa, and any additional comments can be added [31,171].

Chromosomal and Immunohistochemical Studies

Cytogenetic studies on vulvar carcinomas have demonstrated that they are genetically complex with multiple chromosomal rearrangements [175]. Nonetheless, they remain karyotypically stable in culture. The tumors typically are heterogeneous with multiple, but closely related, clonal populations. Both development and progression are apparent sequelae of altered gene expression. A study of vulvar carcinomas employing flow cytometry and image analysis demonstrated a high frequency of aneuploidy with a predominance of tumors within the hypotetraploid range [44].

Immunohistochemical studies employing monoclonal antibodies to MIB-1 (Ki-67), a proliferation-associated marker, have demonstrated two distinct tumor labeling patterns, diffuse and localized, that appear to be associated with prognosis; the diffuse pattern is associated with poor prognosis [75]. Quantitation of Ki-67 (MIB-1) and Ag-NOR do not appear to predict the presence or absence of inguinal-femoral lymph node metastasis, although a correlation was found between the mitotic index and the Ki-67 expression [50]. In vulvar squamous cell carcinoma associated with lichen sclerosus, it has been observed

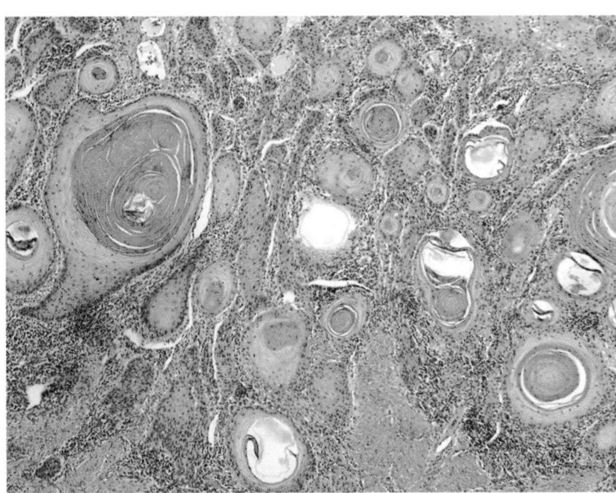

Fig. 2.17
Invasive keratinizing squamous cell carcinoma, well differentiated. Tongues of well-differentiated squamous epithelium with keratinization are evident

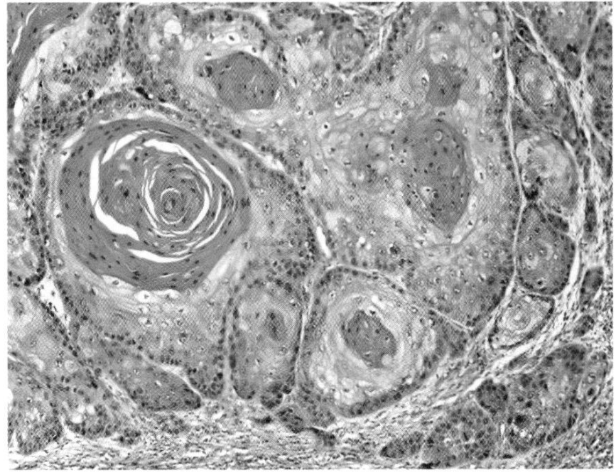

Fig. 2.18
Invasive keratinizing squamous cell carcinoma, well differentiated. The cells have abundant cytoplasm and large, round nuclei with prominent nucleoli

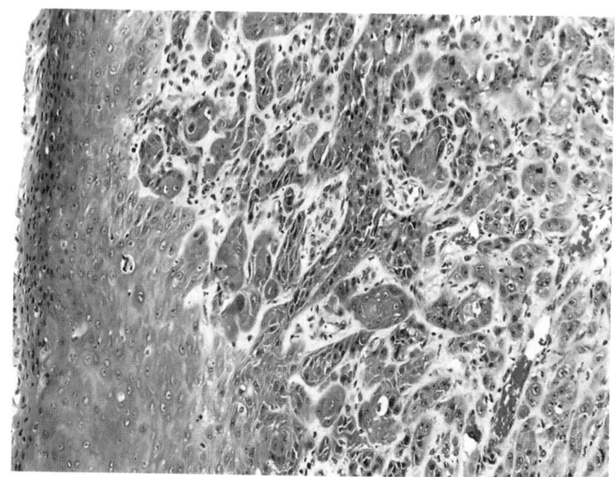

Fig. 2.19
Invasive squamous cell carcinoma, moderately to poorly differentiated. **Small nests and cords of invasive squamous cell carcinoma are present without keratinization**

Table 2.6
Lymph node status and metastasis staging using the American Joint Commission on Cancer (AJCC) staging system

pNX: Regional lymph nodes cannot be assessed
pN0: No regional lymph node metastasis
pN1: Regional lymph node metastasis with the following features:
pN1a: One or two (1 or 2) lymph node metastasis each less than 5 mm (FIGO IIIA)
pN1b: One (1) lymph node metastases 5 mm or greater (FIGO IIIA)
pN2: Regional lymph node metastasis with the following features:
pN2a: Three or more or more lymph node metastases each less than 5 mm (FIGO IIIB)
pN2b: Two or more lymph node metastases 5 mm or greater (FIGO IIIB)
pN2c: Lymph node metastasis with extracapsular spread (FIGO IIIC)
pN3: Fixed or ulcerated regional lymph node metastasis (FIGO IVA)
Distant Metastasis (pM)
pMX: Distant metastasis cannot be assessed
pM0: No distant metastasis
pM1: IVB Distant metastasis (includes pelvic node metastasis) (FIGO IVB)

Source adapted from ref. American Joint Committee on Cancer 2010.

that Ki-67 expression is increased in squamous hyperplasia adjacent to the squamous cell carcinoma. These findings may imply premalignancy or a reactive process related to the carcinoma [140]. In addition, p53 is expressed in the neoplastic component when differentiated VIN is also associated [183]. Immunohistochemical expression of p16INK-4a is commonly expressed in vulvar squamous tumors and VIN associated with oncogenic HPV [129,133].

Histologic Subtypes of Vulvar Squamous Cell Carcinoma

Squamous cell carcinoma of the vulva can be subdivided into several morphologically distinct subtypes (*Table 2.3*). Histologically, invasive squamous cell carcinomas that are not otherwise specified (NOS) usually are well-differentiated tumors, but moderately and poorly differentiated varieties are found in 5–10% of the cases (see *Figs. 2.13* and *2.16–2.19*).

Basaloid Carcinoma

An increased prevalence of human papillomavirus (HPV), mainly type 16, has been observed with certain types of invasive squamous carcinomas of the vulva. Among these are basaloid carcinomas, which occur in younger women (mean age, 54 years), compared with typical keratinizing squamous cell carcinomas (mean age, 77 years). HPV-associated vulvar squamous cell carcinomas can be distinguished histopathologically from non-HPV-related tumors, with agreement between observers noted in 67% of cases [160]. Basaloid carcinomas frequently are associated with adjacent VIN, usually of the basaloid type. In contrast to typical keratinizing squamous cell carcinomas, basaloid carcinomas are associated with synchronous or metachronous squamous neoplasms of the cervix and vagina [93]. On gross examination, basaloid carcinomas are similar to typical keratinizing squamous cell carcinomas. Microscopically, they are characterized by variable-sized nests of immature squamous cells with little, if any, squamous maturation. Some tumors are composed of small, irregularly shaped nests and cords of cells surrounded by a densely hyalinized stroma. The basal-type cells within the nests and cords resemble those in the classic type of carcinoma in situ of the cervix (*Figs. 2.20–2.22*). Characteristically, the cells are ovoid and relatively uniform in size, with scant cytoplasm and a high nuclear cytoplasmic ratio, and therefore they appear undifferentiated. Nuclei contain evenly distributed coarsely granular chromatin, creating a stippled appearance. A moderate degree of

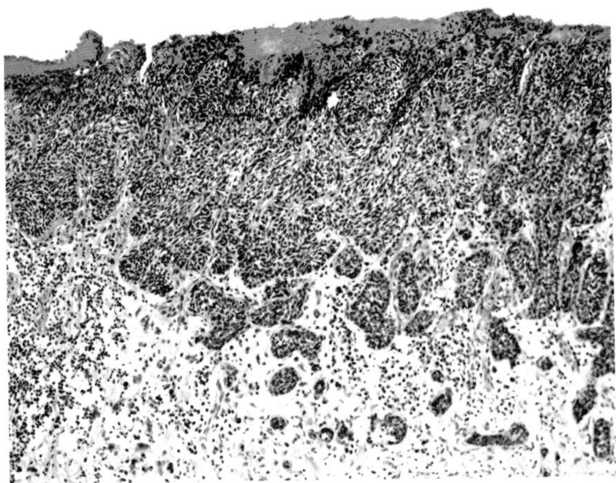

Fig. 2.20
Basaloid carcinoma. **A prominent desmoplastic stroma is present**

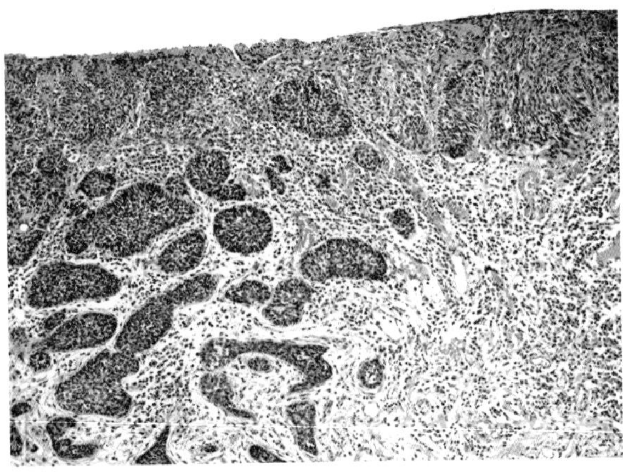

Fig. 2.21
Basaloid VIN with basaloid carcinoma. **The basaloid VIN within the overlying epithelium has similar cellular features to the basaloid invasive tumor within the superficial and deep dermis. The tumor is composed of immature-appearing keratinocytes without significant maturation or keratinization**

mitotic activity usually is evident. Occasionally, the cells in the center of a nest show evidence of maturation and contain more abundant cytoplasm. Small foci of keratinization may be evident in the center of the nests, and keratin pearls occasionally are present. Desmosomes usually are not evident. HPV-16 can be detected in approximately 70% of basaloid squamous carcinomas (*Fig. 2.22*) [93]. Although basaloid carcinoma is reported to be associated with decreased survival in one age-controlled study [118], no evidence of decreased survival was observed in relatively large study [93].

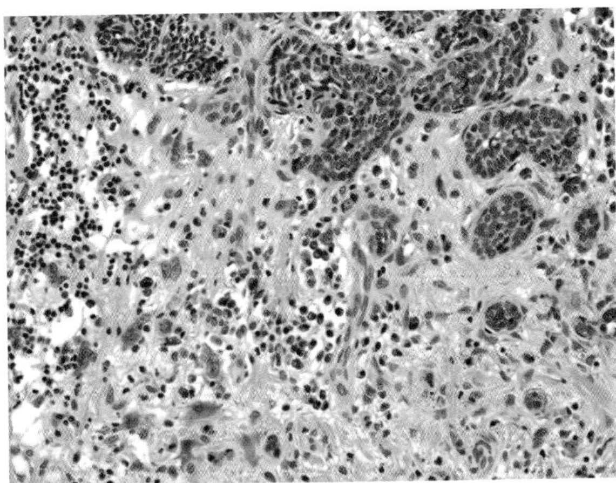

Fig. 2.22
Basaloid carcinoma. **The tumor is composed of relatively small cells with hyperchromatic, nuclei**

Basaloid squamous carcinoma must be distinguished from basal cell carcinoma, but at times this may be difficult. In contrast to basaloid carcinoma, basal cell carcinomas tend to be more circumscribed and have a lobular appearance. The characteristic palisading of the outermost layer of cells in the nests of basal cell carcinoma is lacking in basaloid carcinoma. The differential diagnosis of basaloid carcinoma also includes metastatic small cell carcinoma and Merkel cell tumor. These tumors have a more diffusely infiltrative pattern characterized by poorly defined nests, trabeculae, and individual cells invading the stroma rather than the broad anastomosing bands and well-defined nests typical of basaloid carcinoma. Small cell tumors usually are immunoreactive for neuroendocrine markers; Merkel cell tumors have a characteristic perinuclear cytoplasmic "dot" demonstrated by immunohistochemical study with cytokeratins.

Warty Carcinoma (Condylomatous Carcinoma)

Warty carcinoma is found predominantly in younger women (mean age, 55 years) and presents clinically as a verrucoid or papillary tumor that may resemble condyloma acuminatum. Occasionally warty carcinoma or verrucous carcinoma may arise in association with condyloma acuminatum [42,43]. On microscopic examination, warty carcinoma has multiple papillary projections with a keratinized epithelial surface and fibrovascular cores (*Figs. 2.23* and *2.24*). Cytologic atypia is seen,

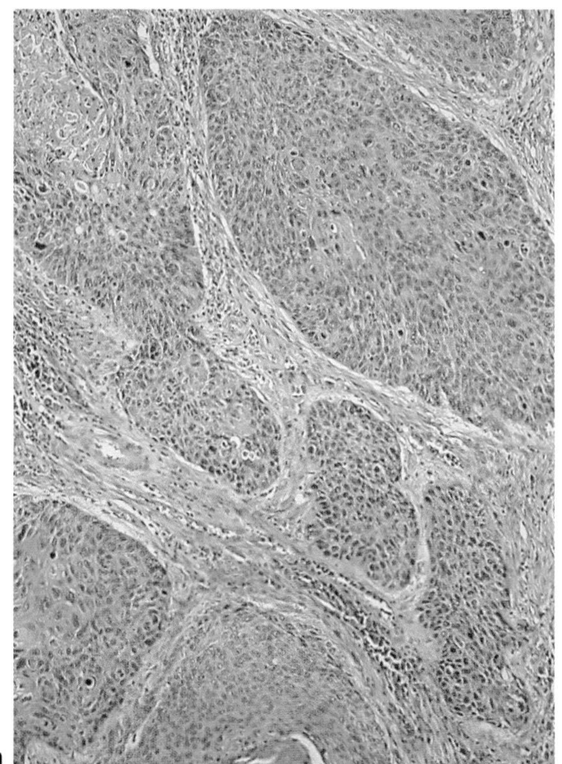

especially within the basal and parabasal cells, where there is nuclear pleomorphism and nuclear hyperchromasia. Multinucleation may be present. Mitotic figures usually can be found and sometimes may be atypical. Cytoplasmic perinuclear clearing similar to koilocytosis in VIN is present in a substantial number of cells; it is the most characteristic feature. At the junction between the exophytic portion of the tumor and the underlying stoma, irregularly shaped nests of epithelium are present that may be associated with keratin pearls and dyskeratotic cells. In this area, the tumor resembles a keratinized squamous cell carcinoma. In some cases, these areas are small and focal. Warty carcinoma is frequently associated with HPV type 16 [42,93,157].

The clinical course of warty carcinoma appears generally good; however, lymph node metastasis may occur. The prognosis appears intermediate between that of verrucous carcinoma and squamous cell carcinoma of the usual type [157]. Approximately 80% of warty and basaloid carcinomas have adjacent warty or basaloid VIN. About one quarter of the warty and basaloid carcinomas are associated with other genital tract squamous neoplasias[93].

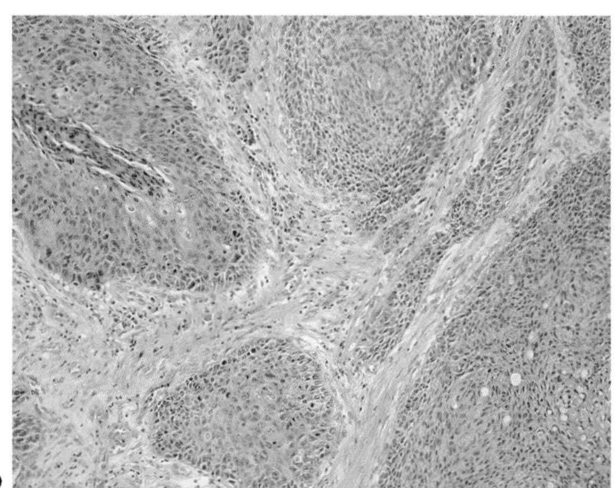

Fig. 2.23
Warty (condylomatous) carcinoma. **(a) The tumor has well-differentiated neoplastic keratinocytes with keratinization. At the deep margin, the tumor is composed of irregularly shaped, varying sized nests that infiltrate the stroma in a haphazard fashion. (b) The cords of neoplastic cells are separated by a fibrovascular stroma. Keratinization is present**

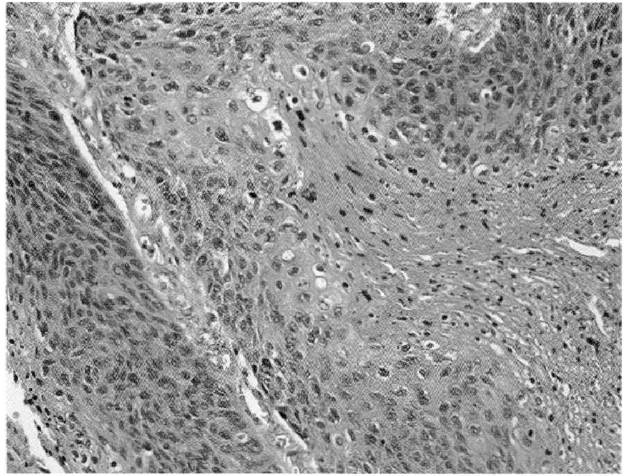

Fig. 2.24
Warty (condylomatous) carcinoma. **Cells with pleomorphic nuclei and vacuolated cytoplasm resembling koilocytes are present within the neoplastic epithelium (Courtesy of R.J. Kurman, M.D., Baltimore, MD.)**

Verrucous Carcinoma

Verrucous carcinoma is a highly differentiated squamous carcinoma that has a verrucous pattern and invades with a pushing border in the form of bulbous pegs of neoplastic cells [17]. The term giant condyloma of Buschke–Lowenstein is considered to be a synonym for verrucous carcinoma, but it is confusing and therefore is not recommended [175]. Squamous cell carcinomas at times may have some of the architectural features of verrucous carcinoma, but if they lack a high degree of differentiation, or have a nonpushing pattern of invasion, they should not be designated verrucous carcinoma. Verrucous carcinoma is a papillary exophytic growth that may have the appearance of an exophytic, broad-based condyloma acuminatum, and distort or completely obscure the vulva (➲ *Fig. 2.25*). Secondary infection may be associated with a malodorous discharge. Regional lymph nodes usually are not enlarged. Condyloma acuminatum may be adjacent to verrucous carcinoma, and rarely the tumor may merge into a typical squamous cell carcinoma [42,43]. "Vulvar acanthosis with altered differentiation" has been proposed as a probable precursor of vulvar verrucous carcinoma. It is characterized as a noninvasive squamous lesion with variable verrucoid growth with acanthosis and parakeratosis. There is associated loss of the granular layer and pale cytoplasm of the superficial keratinocytes. These changes were reported adjacent to vulvar verrucous carcinoma in seven cases in a study of nine verrucous carcinomas from seven patients. Neither this lesion nor the verrucous carcinomas in this study was associated with human papillomavirus [110]. Verrucous carcinoma may be associated with HPV, typically type 6 or variants of type 6.

The microscopic features of verrucous carcinoma include prominent acanthosis with a pushing tumor–dermal interface and bland cytologic features (➲ *Fig. 2.26*)

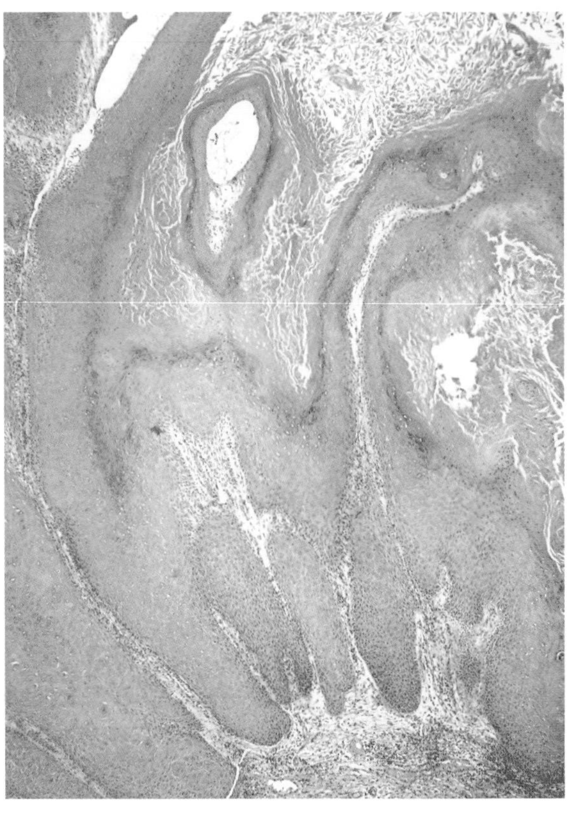

Fig. 2.25
Verrucous carcinoma. **At the stromal interface the tumor displays rounded, bulbous tongues of very well differentiated squamous epithelium**

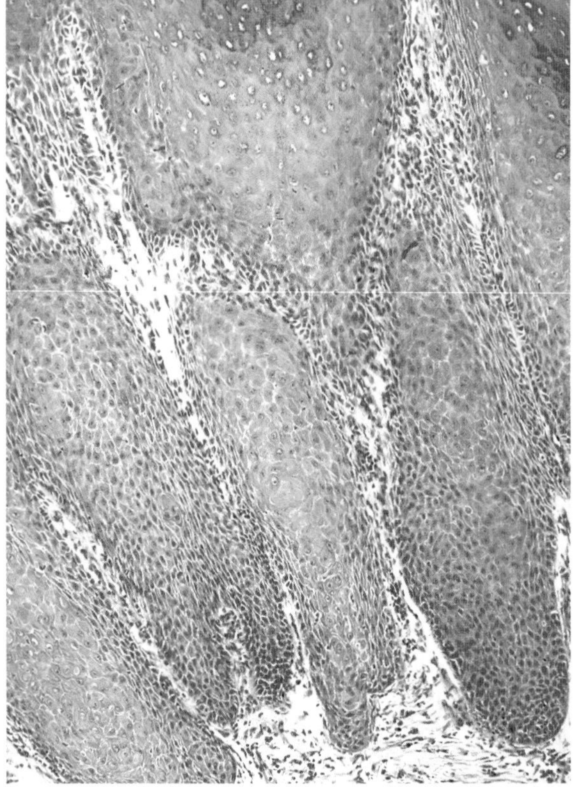

Fig. 2.26
Verrucous carcinoma. **There is a well-defined tumor–stromal interface with a pushing, growth pattern. The keratinocytes are very well differentiated**

(see Chap. 3, Diseases of the Vagina). Large bulbous nests of squamous epithelium characterize the deep margin. There is minimal nuclear pleomorphism, with the greatest degree of nuclear atypia nearest the dermal interface. The nuclei may have coarse chromatin and variable-sized nucleoli, distinguishing them from normal adjacent keratinocytes. Mitotic figures are rare and when present are normal. The abundant cytoplasm of the tumor cells is eosinophilic, without dyskeratosis. Koilocytosis is not a feature of this tumor. Parakeratosis or hyperkeratosis usually is present and may be prominent. There is an absence of fibrovascular cores separating the bulbous epithelial downgrowths. An inflammatory infiltrate within the dermis usually is present. These tumors typically are diploid.

The differential diagnosis includes the typical variety of squamous cell carcinoma, warty carcinoma, and condyloma acuminatum. Squamous cell carcinoma of the usual type (keratinizing squamous carcinoma) has greater nuclear pleomorphism and a more irregular pattern of infiltration of the stroma compared with the bulbous nests of verrucous carcinoma. Warty carcinoma, despite its verruciform appearance, has fibrovascular cores within the papillary fronds, unlike verrucous carcinoma. In addition, these tumors display greater nuclear atypia, "koilocytosis," and, at their deep margin, invade like typical squamous cell carcinomas. Condyloma acuminatum is characterized by a complex branching papillary architecture with vascular papillae, lacks bulbous downgrowths, and typically shows koilocytosis, although in vulvar condylomas koilocytosis may be quite subtle.

Verrucous carcinomas may recur locally after excision. Lymph node metastasis is extremely rare, and its presence should prompt reevaluation of the lesion for areas of the usual type of squamous cell carcinoma. Wide local excision and total vulvectomy without lymph node dissection are the most common methods of therapy. If the tumor is excised completely, the prognosis is excellent. The role of radiotherapy in vulvar verrucous carcinomas is not well studied, but it may be applicable in very advanced cases.

Giant Cell Squamous Carcinoma

Squamous cell carcinoma with tumor giant cells is a variant of squamous cell carcinoma characterized by multinucleated tumor giant cells, large nuclei with prominent nucleoli, and prominent eosinophilic cytoplasm (*Fig. 2.27*). This tumor variant is relatively rare and is associated with a poor prognosis. The most important differential diagnosis is malignant amelanotic melanoma, which commonly forms multinucleated tumor giant cells [177]. Melanomas typically have intranuclear inclusions and prominent nucleoli. Unlike giant cell carcinoma, melanomas are typically immunoreactive for S-100, melanoma antigen (HMB 45), and Melan-A and negative for cytokeratin [177].

Spindle Cell Squamous Cell Carcinoma

Spindle cell carcinoma of the vulva/sarcomatoid squamous cell carcinoma may mimic a sarcoma or be associated with sarcoma-like stroma (*Fig. 2.28*) [32,33,153].

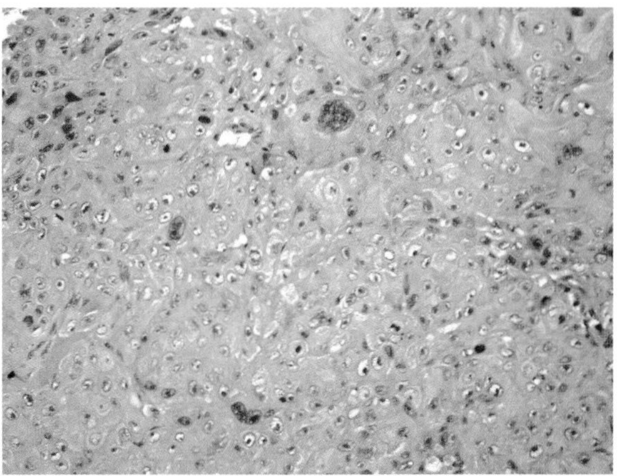

Fig. 2.27
Giant cell carcinoma of the vulva. **Multinucleated tumor giant cells are evident. The cells contain nuclei with prominent nucleoli and abundant eosinophilic cytoplasm**

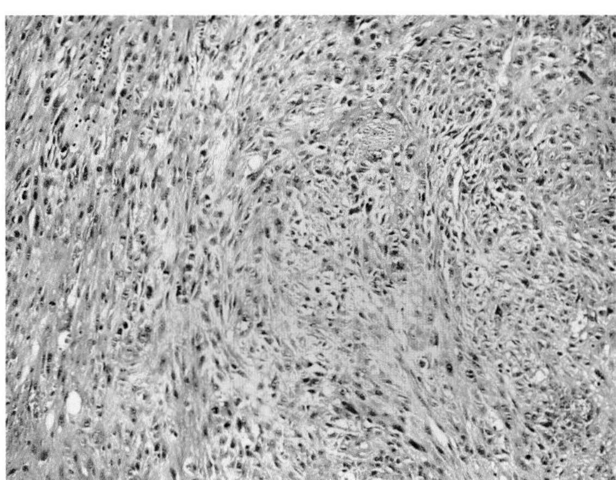

Fig. 2.28
Spindle cell (sarcomatoid) squamous cell carcinoma. **The tumor is composed of fascicles of spindle-shaped neoplastic squamous cells, showing moderate nuclear pleomorphism**

These tumors must be distinguished from mesenchymal spindle cell tumors, including leiomyosarcoma, malignant fibrous histiocytoma, and fibrosarcoma, as well as spindle cell malignant melanoma and transitional cell carcinoma with spindle cell features. The neoplastic cells of spindle cell carcinoma, unlike all the mesenchymal tumors and melanoma, are immunoreactive for keratin [135]. Spindle cell carcinoma may be associated with tumor giant cells, which are also immunoreactive for keratin [135].

Acantholytic Squamous Cell Carcinoma (Adenoid Squamous Carcinoma; Pseudoangiomatous Carcinoma)

The acantholytic squamous tumor forms rounded spaces, or pseudoacini, lined with a single layer of squamous cells. Dyskeratotic and acantholytic cells are sometimes present in the central lumen (*Fig. 2.29*). These changes are focal in most cases and may occur within otherwise well-differentiated squamous tumors. Acantholytic squamous cell carcinomas have been reported to have a prognosis similar to squamous carcinoma of the usual type; however, some recent reports describe a more aggressive behavior for this tumor type [79,136].

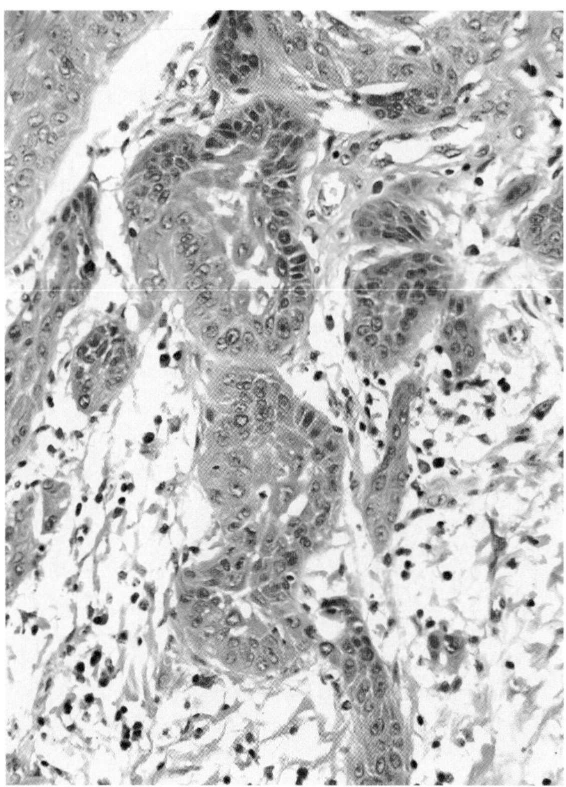

Fig. 2.29
Acantholytic squamous cell carcinoma. **Nests of poorly differentiated squamous cell carcinoma are arranged in a crude acinar manner. Some of the central acini are vacuolated**

Adenosquamous carcinoma, is a term used sometimes for acantholytic squamous cell carcinoma but may be better considered as a distinct tumor in that adenosquamous carcinoma should have a distinct secretory, glandular cell component. It has been reported as being associated with a poorer prognosis that the usual squamous cell carcinomas, but in one case had arisen in a hidradenoma [10]. As with Bartholin gland adenosquamous carcinomas, such tumors in the Bartholin gland have a poorer prognosis than squamous cell carcinomas. In the Bartholin gland, this is considered partly because of the higher frequency of lymph node metastasis (see Bartholin Gland Tumors).

Papillary Squamous Cell Carcinoma

This tumor is rare and has similar morphologic features to papillary squamous cell carcinoma of the cervix. The tumor is exophytic with an expansile and deep pushing infiltrative pattern within the dermis. Although there is very limited experience with this tumor, with negative nodes it can be managed by deep wide excision [97].

Lymphoepithelioma-Like Carcinoma

These tumors may occur rarely on the vulva in older individuals. They are composed of nests or syncytial groups of epithelioid-appearing cells mixed with, and surrounded by, a dense lymphocytic infiltrate (*Fig. 2.30*) (see Chap. 6, Carcinoma and Other Tumors of the Cervix). The epithelial cells are immunoreactive for high molecular–weight cytokeratins, which distinguishes them from inflammatory processes and malignant large cell lymphomas. Lymphomas, including Ki-1 lymphomas, which are immunoreactive for lymphocytic markers, contain an immunophenotypic monoclonal population of neoplastic lymphocytic cells. The therapy is wide local excision with or without local radiation therapy [22].

Plasmacytoid Squamous Carcinoma

Plasmacytoid squamous carcinoma is a rare tumor of the vulva, with one case reported in a 92-year-old woman who had been treated previously for multiple

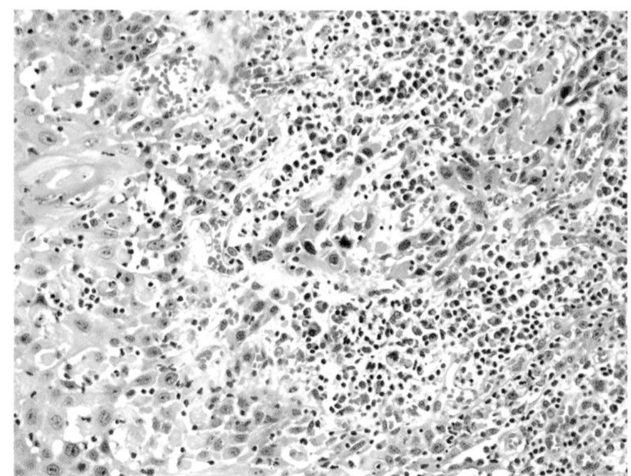

Fig. 2.30
Lymphoepithelial like carcinoma. **The tumor cells are small, uniform and lack maturation. The cells are in nests and syncytial groups mixed with, and surrounded by a prominent lymphocytic infiltrate**

vulvar squamous and verrucous carcinomas. The patient's prior tumors were all treated by local excision. The plasmacytoid tumor presented as a 3 cm polypoid vulvar mass superior but adjacent to the urethra. The surface of the tumor was ulcerated [158]. On gross examination, the tumor was submucosal, somewhat yellow in color, and abutted the overlying epithelium. No evidence of VIN or other related HPV changes were identified adjacent to the tumor. On microscopic examination, approximately 60% of the tumor cells had plasmacytoid features with cells having epithelioid differentiation. These cells lacked the nuclear characteristic "clock face" appearance of plasma cells, but did have prominent amphophilic cytoplasm with an eccentrically placed nucleus. In addition, these cells were more than twice the size of normal plasma cells. The tumor cells were immunoreactive for cytokeratin 5, AE3, and high molecular–weight cytokeratin 903. Some cells expressed AE1. In addition, the cells were reactive for p63, CD138, and VS38, but negative for Kappa or Lambda light chains. Other immunohistochemical studies performed were negative.

The differential diagnosis of vulvar plasmacytoid squamous cell carcinoma includes metastatic or primary melanoma, myoepithelial tumors, neuroendocrine tumors, or plasmacytoma. In addition metastatic plasmacytoid urothelial carcinoma and lobular breast carcinoma must be considered. These tumors can be distinguished by immunohistochemical studies, and clinical history is often contributory in metastatic cases.

The treatment was deep partial vulvectomy. Within 6 months postoperative the patient presented with a right inguinal enlarged lymph node with several pulmonary nodules. The patient died with metastatic tumor in less than 1 year of diagnosis [158].

Clinical Behavior and Treatment of Vulvar Squamous Cell carcinoma

Factors that may be of significance in prognosis and in the probability of lymph node metastasis include the diameter of the tumor, the presence of vascular space invasion, and tumor ulceration. Confluent growth, defined as anastomosing cords or tumor, or tumor in the dermis exceeding 1 mm^3, does not correlate with the occurrence of node metastasis but is not found in tumors having 1 mm or less of invasion [170]. When controlled for age, survival with vulvar carcinoma decreased with advancing age, higher stage and grade, increasing tumor thickness, prominent fibromyxoid dermal response, infiltrative pattern of growth, and basaloid tumor type [118].

Inguinofemoral lymph node status and the diameter of the tumor are independent prognostic factors. The overall 5-year relative survival, related to stage, as reported in a series of 588 patients with vulvar carcinoma is as follows: stage I, 98%; stage II, 87%; stage III, 75%; and stage IV, 29% [78]. The distance between the tumor and the surgical margin is a significant predictor of local recurrence. A surgical margin of 8 mm or less from the invasive carcinoma is associated with a 50% risk of local recurrence [73]. In a GOG study of 121 patients with stage I vulvar carcinoma with a tumor thickness of 5 mm or less, without vascular space invasion, and with negative lymph nodes, 19 patients (15.7%) experienced recurrence, and there were seven deaths (5.8%) from tumor. Of the seven deaths, five were related to recurrence in the groin nodes [154]. Tumors with a depth of invasion greater than 1 mm require more extensive surgery, including groin node dissection [63,67,170]. Terminology for surgical procedures and characterization of depth of invasion of vulvar tumors has been developed by the International Society for the Study of vulvovaginal Disease (ISSVD) and is shown in *Table 2.7* [84].

Vulvar carcinoma typically spreads by direct extension and lymphatic metastasis and tends to recur locally. Although distant metastasis is less common. Direct extension may include involvement of bone and metastasis may include bone metastasis. The reliability of clinical evaluation in the determination of whether tumor is present in inguinal nodes has a false-positive rate less than 10% but a false-negative rate of approximately 20% [16]. It is recognized that pathologic evaluation of lymph nodes for metastasis also may be falsely negative.

Table 2.7
Surgical procedures and characterization of depth of invasion of vulvar tumors

Vulvectomy
Partial vulvectomy: Removal of a part of the vulvar/perineal integument independent of depth
Total vulvectomy: Removal of the whole vulva and appropriate integument of the perineum independent of depth
Depth of excision
Superficial: Removal of the most superficial layer with a variable amount of dermis and subcutaneous tissue
Deep: removal of the vulva to the superficial aponeurosis of the urogenital diaphragm and/or pubic periosteum

Developed by the International Society for the Study of Vulvovaginal Disease (ISSVD) [84].

In assessing groin nodes, fine-needle aspiration may be the first step if clinically suspicious nodes are present because the technique is rapid, safe, cost-effective, and will detect gross metastasis. Current therapy attempts to define high- and low-risk groups and requires individualization of therapy [81]. Sentinel lymph node identification methods employing technetium-99 m-labeled noncolloid have been employed to attempt to select and sample sentinel lymph nodes and possibly avoid inguinofemoral lymph node resection if the sentinel lymph node, or nodes, are free of metastatic tumor [1,39,105]. Many patients are now offered immediate reconstructive surgery as part of the initial procedure [63]. Radiation techniques are now available that allow skin-sparing treatment of the groin nodes and have been used successfully in both primary and adjunctive treatment.

Basal Cell, Adenoid Basal Cell, Metatypical Basal Cell, and **Sebaceous Cell Carcinoma of the Vulva**.

Basal Cell Carcinoma

Although basal cell carcinomas of the skin are extremely common, they account for only 5–7% of vulvar carcinomas [56,119]. They are found primarily in elderly white women (mean age, 70–76 years), whose symptomatology consists of pruritus, irritation, soreness, or bleeding. The tumors usually present as an ulcer, an area of pigmentation or depigmentation, or as a mass [56,107,170].

Most of these tumors are confined to the labia majora, and approximately one half are of infiltrative type. Basal cell carcinomas are not associated with human papillomavirus.

The histologic pattern resembles that of basal cell carcinomas occurring elsewhere on the skin (Fig. 2.31).

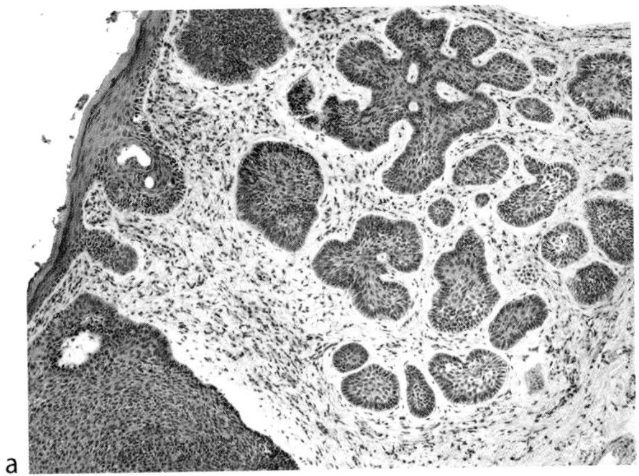

a

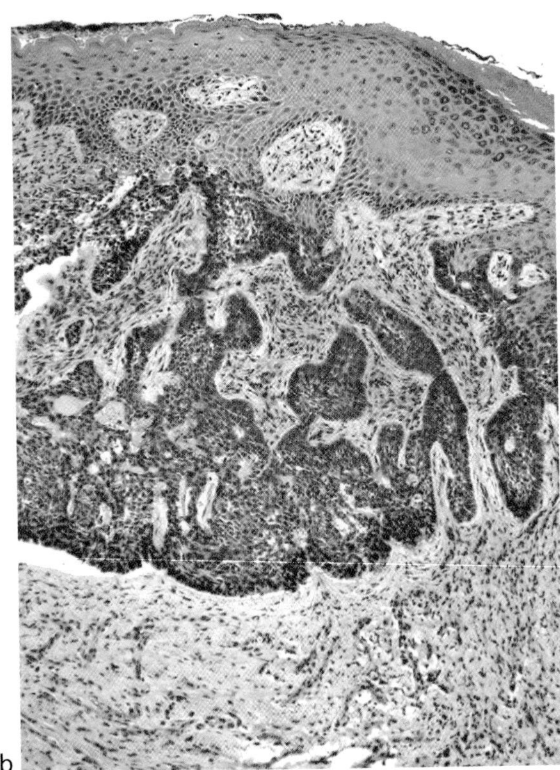

b

Fig. 2.31
Basal cell carcinoma. **(a) The tumor is composed of relatively small uniform cells in club shaped nests with a palisade orientation of the cells at the tumor-stromal interface. (b) The basal cell carcinoma has an infiltrative pattern, with focal cribriform formation (Courtesy of R.J. Kurman, M.D., Baltimore, MD.)**

The tumor is composed of small elongated cells with deeply basophilic nuclei and may have a large variety of architectural patterns, ranging from slight palisading of the basal layer of the epidermis to the formation of large club-shaped

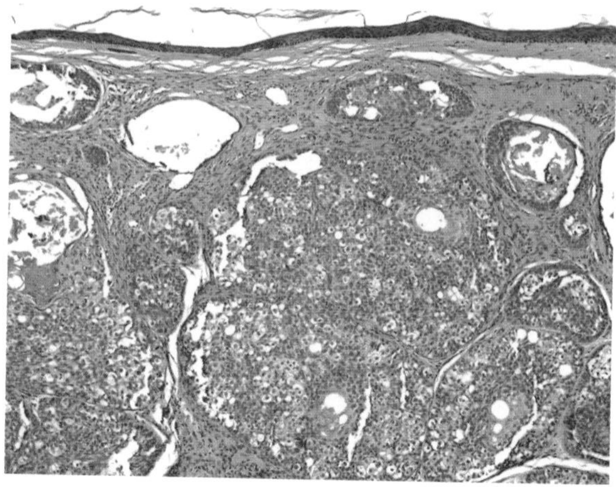

Fig. 2.32
Sebaceous carcinoma. **The tumor is composed of cords and nests of basaloid-appearing cells. These cells are associated with sebaceous cells in pagetoid nests in the parabasal areas and in larger clusters near the epithelial surface (Courtesy of R.J. Kurman, M.D., Baltimore, MD.)**

masses of pleomorphic basal cells. The connective tissue adjacent to the tumor frequently contains a chronic inflammatory cell infiltrate and occasionally shows a mucoid or myxomatous change.

Primary treatment is wide local excision [1]. Local recurrence occurs in approximately 9–20% of cases [119]. Metastasis to regional lymph nodes occurs but is rare [11]. The overall prognosis of patients with these tumors is excellent, with only a rare death reported [11].

Adenoid Basal Cell Carcinoma

Adenoid basal cell carcinoma is a variant of basal cell carcinoma in which tubular and glandlike differentiation is seen within a tumor that otherwise is a characteristic basal cell carcinoma.

Metatypical Basal Cell Carcinoma (Basosquamous Carcinoma)

Metatypical basal cell carcinoma, or basosquamous carcinoma, represents a mixture of both squamous and basal cell neoplastic elements. Unlike basal cell carcinomas, basosquamous carcinomas are locally aggressive and metastasize rarely, and should be managed like squamous cell carcinoma related to the stage of the tumor.

Sebaceous Cell Carcinoma

Sebaceous cell carcinoma is a rare tumor of the vulva that may be associated with vulvar intraepithelial neoplasia. The tumor has features of basosquamous cell carcinoma with sebaceous differentiation (*Fig. 2.32*) [21].

Glandular Tumors of the Vulva (Primary Adenocarcinomas of the Vulva)

Adenocarcinomas of the vulva are relatively rare. Many previous reports have been shown retrospectively to represent benign hidradenomas or foci of adnexal Paget disease. Adenocarcinoma in situ has been reported arising within vulvar papillary hidradenoma [143]. Most adenocarcinomas of the vulva arise as primary malignant tumors of the Bartholin gland; however, they also may arise from sweat glands or from other skin appendages, the urethra, the Skene gland, and from Paget disease [169]. Paget disease and Paget-like neoplastic lesions, including pagetoid urothelial intraepithelial neoplasia (PUIN), are described here.

Paget Disease

Clinical Features

Clinically, vulvar Paget disease can present as either an erythematous lesion, often involving the vestibule and adjacent areas, or an eczematous lesion that appears as a red to pink area with white islands of hyperkeratosis and usually involving hair-bearing skin (*Figs. 2.33* and *2.34*). The extent of involvement can be very focal, or extensive, extending about the anus, medial aspects of the upper thigh, or other contiguous sites [123].

Pruritus is present in more than half the patients, and was present for a median duration of 2 years before the diagnosis in a study of 100 patients [55]. Almost all patients are postmenopausal Caucasian women, with a median age of 70 years [55]. Paget disease may occur in younger women of reproductive age. Vulvar pruritus or pain may bring the patient to the attention of the physician. Because of its clinical resemblance to a dermatosis, these patients may be treated with various topical medications for some time before the diagnosis is made by biopsy.

Vulvar Paget disease and pagetoid urothelial intraepithelial neoplasia (PUIN) have recently been subclassified by Wilkinson and Brown into two distinct types, specifically cutaneous Paget disease and noncutaneous Paget disease based upon the origin of the neoplastic cells summarized as follows: [173]

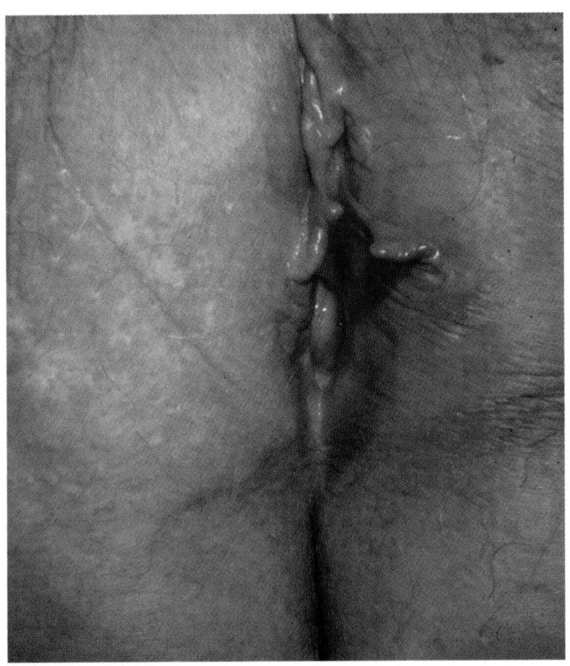

Fig. 2.33
Paget disease, primary type. **An eczematoid, slightly raised and white area is present on the medial anterior surface of the right labium majus, an eroded, red, ulcerated area is present on the left labia majus**

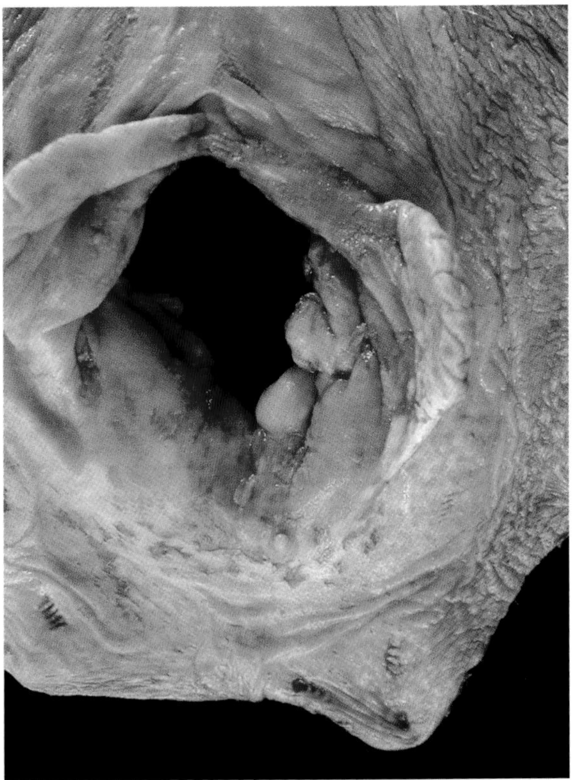

Fig. 2.34
Paget disease, primary type, partial deep vulvectomy. **The white and eczematoid epithelial changes reflect the Paget disease that involves the perineal body and left labia majus (photo courtesy R. Foss, PA, Gainesville, FL.)**

Primary Cutaneous Paget Disease

Primary vulvar cutaneous Paget disease is subdivided into three distinct groups (*Table 2.8*).

Primary cutaneous Paget disease can be an intraepithelial neoplasm or primary vulvar intraepithelial Paget disease. It characterized by an intraepithelial proliferation of atypical glandular-type cells and may be considered as an adenocarcinoma in situ (*Fig. 2.35*). Histopathologic features are characterized by relatively large cells, with prominent cytoplasm, that are within the squamous epithelium. These cells are generally larger than the adjacent keratinocytes and have large nuclei with prominent nucleoli. Their cytoplasm is finely granular and amphophilic to basophilic, and may be vacuolated, in contrast to the eosinophilic more homogeneous cytoplasm of keratinocytes. The neoplastic cells are typically clustered in groups or dispersed as single cells within the basal and

Table 2.8
Classification of primary and secondary vulvar Paget disease [169]

Primary Paget disease (primary cutaneous Paget disease)
Paget disease as an intraepithelial neoplasm/in situ Paget disease
Paget disease as an intraepithelial neoplasm with invasion/invasive primary Paget disease.
Paget disease as a manifestation of an underlying cutaneous neoplasm.
Secondary Paget disease: (Paget disease of noncutaneous origin)
Paget disease as a manifestation of anal-rectal adenocarcinoma
Paget disease related to other adenocarcinomas.
Paget disease as a manifestation of urothelial in situ or invasive carcinoma/pagetoid urothelial intraepithelial neoplasia (PUIN).

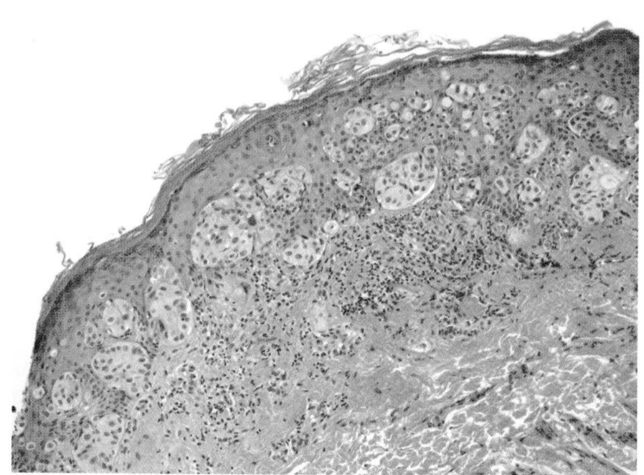

Fig. 2.35
Paget disease, primary type. **Large numbers of Paget cells within the basal and parabasal areas with Paget cells extending into the upper epithelium. Paget cells are present singly and in nests. Their pale cytoplasm differentiates them from surrounding keratinocytes. The nuclei of the Paget cells are larger, and their nuclear chromatin coarser, than in the adjacent keratinocytes**

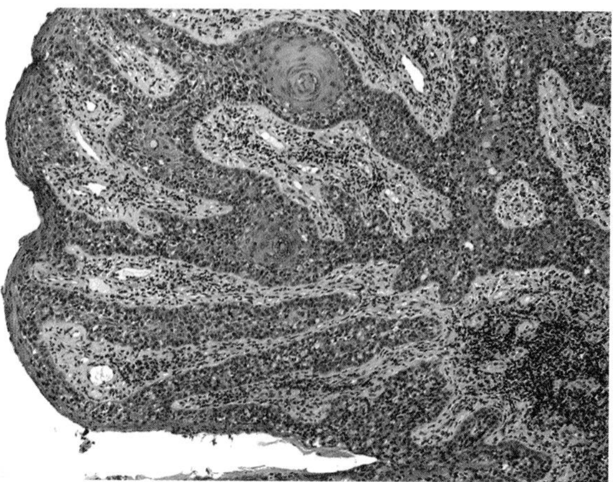

Fig. 2.36
Paget disease, primary type. **The tumor has a papillomatous, appearance and there is an associated superficial dermal chronic inflammatory cell infiltrate. Paget cells are present within the basal and parabasal epithelium (Case courtesy Dr. Michael J. Goldfischer, Hackensack University Medical center, Hackensack, NJ.)**

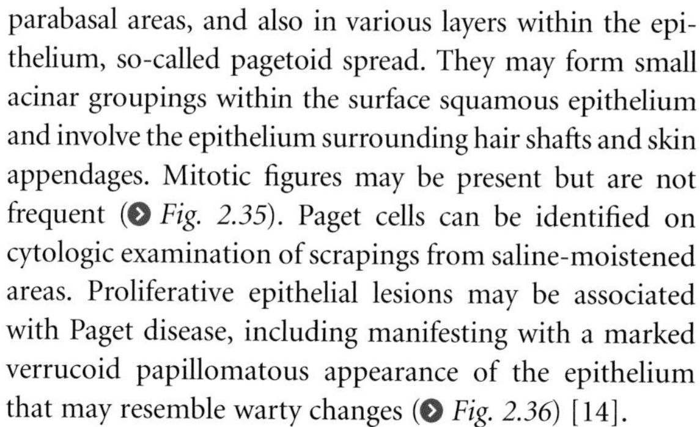

parabasal areas, and also in various layers within the epithelium, so-called pagetoid spread. They may form small acinar groupings within the surface squamous epithelium and involve the epithelium surrounding hair shafts and skin appendages. Mitotic figures may be present but are not frequent (*Fig. 2.35*). Paget cells can be identified on cytologic examination of scrapings from saline-moistened areas. Proliferative epithelial lesions may be associated with Paget disease, including manifesting with a marked verrucoid papillomatous appearance of the epithelium that may resemble warty changes (*Fig. 2.36*) [14].

Primary cutaneous Paget disease can present as a primary vulvar intraepithelial Paget disease with invasion. Dermal, or submucosal, invasion by intraepithelial Paget cells is well documented and has been reported in 12% in a series of 100 cases [55]. Vulvar Paget disease is therefore properly classified as a form of intraepithelial neoplasia that may become invasive.

Primary cutaneous Paget disease can present as a manifestation of a primary underlying adenocarcinoma of the vulva. Vulvar Paget disease associated with an underlying primary invasive adenocarcinoma of the vulva has been reported in 4% of vulvar Paget disease cases in one series [55]. Cases with associated adenocarcinoma of the Bartholin gland and squamous cell carcinoma of the vulva have been reported. Primary vulvar adenocarcinoma is identified beneath Paget disease in approximately 10–20% of the cases reported. Its origin may be from primary invasive Paget disease or adenocarcinoma of the Bartholin gland, specialized anogenital glands, or other vulvar glandular structures. Early investigators noted underlying adnexal adenocarcinoma beneath the skin in the vicinity of Paget disease in many extramammary cases. This finding led some to conclude that Paget cells in the epidermis represented an intradermal migration of neoplastic cells from an underlying cutaneous tumor, as occurs in the breast. This has been documented in a case of eccrine carcinoma of the vulva with pagetoid spread of the tumor cells within the vulvar skin, with resulting Paget disease of the involved skin [65]. This is a rare occurrence and is not the usual finding. The origin of such underlying adenocarcinomas associated with Paget disease does not appear to be usually associated with sweat gland tumors in that epidermal growth factor (EGF), which is typically present in approximately three fourths of eccrine or apocrine sweat gland tumors, was absent in vulvar Paget disease in a study of 17 cases [3]. Vulvar Paget disease may be of noncutaneous origin, and there are two major groups of such cases. One group is Paget disease as a manifestation of an associated adjacent primary anal, rectal, or other noncutaneous adenocarcinoma. The second group of noncutaneous Paget disease represents those cases that are a manifestation of bladder or other urothelial carcinoma. Wilkinson and Brown have proposed that this Paget-like neoplasm of the vulva be classified as pagetoid urothelial intraepithelial neoplasia (PUIN) to characterize this neoplasm as a manifestation of bladder (urothelial) neoplasia, and not of glandular origin [18,173].

Cases of Paget disease as a manifestation of an associated adjacent primary noncutaneous adenocarcinoma, include Paget disease associated with in situ or invasive rectal adenocarcinoma or colonic adenocarcinoma (➋ *Fig. 2.37*), or intraepithelial extension from an adjacent cervical adenocarcinoma. Perianal involvement by Paget disease is associated with a high frequency of adenocarcinoma or squamous carcinoma of the rectum and may present with perianal pruritus, pain and burning, or bleeding after defecation [99]. Primary perianal Paget disease may involve the vulva and should be distinguished from primary cutaneous vulvar Paget disease. Although cutaneous primary vulvar Paget disease involving the perianal area cannot be distinguished by routine histologic examination from primary anal Paget disease involving the vulva, the distinction can be made employing immunohistochemistry. Primary noncutaneous perianal Paget disease is immunoreactive for cytokeratin 20 and negative for gross cystic disease fluid protein-15 (GCDFP-15). It is also associated with rectal Paget disease and, in most reported cases, with rectal adenocarcinoma (➋ *Table 2.8*) [113]. Adenocarcinoma of the cervix manifesting as vulvar Paget disease has been reported [37]. In such cases, the immunohistochemistry would reflect a cervical adenocarcinoma, depending on cellular type, and would have a high probability of containing human papillomavirus, especially types 16 or 18. Paget cells typically are HPV negative.

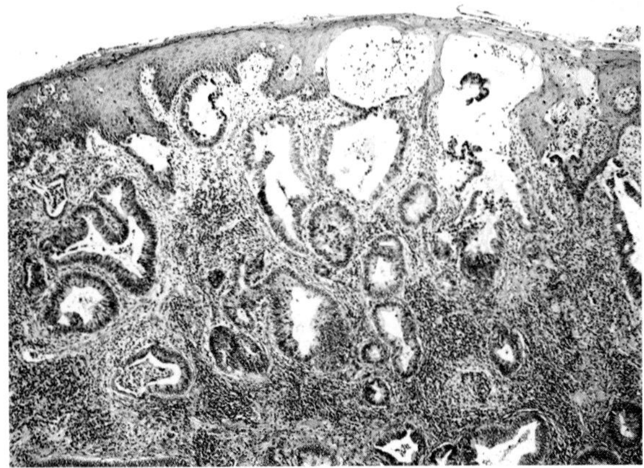

Fig. 2.37
Paget disease, secondary type, of anorectal adenocarcinoma origin. **The Paget lesion is focally contiguous with the invasive anal adenocarcinoma that invades the dermis and focally involves the overlying epithelium**

Paget disease of urothelial origin, pagetoid urothelial intraepithelial neoplasia (PUIN), is a cutaneous manifestation of bladder (urothelial) neoplasia: urinary tract malignancy has been reported with genital Paget disease, and the original report of extramammary Paget disease by Crocker in 1889 was of a man with penile and scrotal Paget disease associated with bladder carcinoma [113]. It has recently been recognized, however, that Paget-like vulvar mucosal and dermal changes associated with urothelial neoplasia can be recognized as a distinct entity [173]. In these cases, there is involvement of the vulvar vestibule, including the periurethral area, which is manifested as an erythematous lesion.

The cells of PUIN have the cytologic features of urothelial carcinoma in situ, with which PUIN is most commonly associated (➋ *Figs. 2.38* and ➋ *2.39*) [18,173]. Of key importance regarding the recognition of PUIN (Pagetoid intraepitheral neoplasia) is that this vulvar neoplasm is a manifestation of bladder urothelial neoplasia and is not associated with underlying adenocarcinoma.

Differential Diagnosis and Adjunctive Studies

The PUIN cells do not contain mucin, PAS-positive material, CEA, or GCDFP-15 as do the Paget cells of primary cutaneous Paget disease, or noncutaneous Paget disease related to adenocarcinoma anorectal area, or other nonvulvar primary site [172]. The cells of PUIN are immunoreactive for cytokeratin 7 and may be cytokeratin 20 positive and uroplakin III positive, as are one half of the primary urothelial carcinomas (➋ *Table 2.2*) [18,173].

Paget cells of primary cutaneous Paget disease, or noncutaneous Paget disease related to adenocarcinoma anorectal area, or other nonvulvar primary site are positive for PAS (diastase resistant), mucicarmine, aldehydefuschin, and Alcian blue. The cells stain pink against a background of greenish-blue with Movat stain. In addition, Paget cells of cutaneous type, as well as the cells and secretions of normal eccrine and apocrine glands, are rich in carcinoembryonic antigen (CEA) and gross cystic disease fluid protein-15 (GCDFP-15), and typically are negative for S-100 protein, HMB-45, and Melan-A [173]. Paget cells of cutaneous type are immunoreactive for cytokeratin 7 [37,172,173]. These reactions distinguish typical cutaneous Paget cells from PUIN, VIN, superficial spreading malignant melanoma, and pagetoid reticulosis. They may also be useful in evaluation of margins in permanent sections [61]. Melanoma is distinguished by being immunoreactive for S-100, HMB-45, and Melan-A, which are typically not identified in Paget cells [77,120]. Paget cells, however, may contain granules of melanin, demonstrable with Fontana–Mason stain, probably produced by neighboring melanocytes and engulfed secondarily by the Paget cell. Paget cells have not been demonstrated to be associated with common oncogenic or non-oncogenic genital human papillomaviruses [150]. Estrogen receptor expression, p53 immunoreactivity, and DNA ploidy do not appear predictive of clinical behavior or recurrence; however, DNA non-diploid Paget disease has been associated with an increased risk of recurrence, as compared to diploid Paget disease, in one study [138].

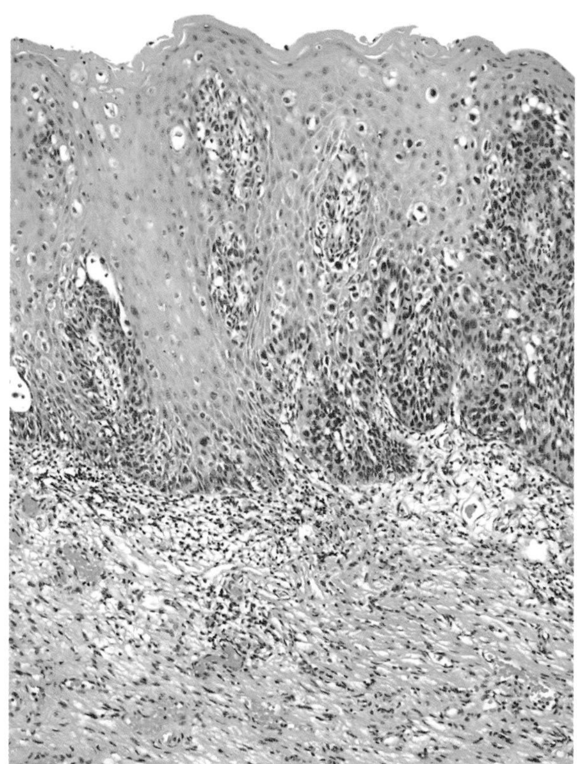

Fig. 2.38
Pagetoid urothelial intraepithelial neoplasia (PUIN); Paget disease, secondary type, of urothelial origin. **The epithelium has pagetoid urothelial cells throughout the full thickness, but most concentrated in the basal and parabasal areas. The "clefts" between the neoplastic urothelial cells and the adjacent epithelial keratinocytes are characteristic of PUIN**

Clinical Behavior and Treatment

The treatment and prognosis of Paget disease of the vulva depends on the type as described herein. For primary cutaneous Paget disease, prognosis depends on whether the lesion is intraepithelial only, or if there is an associated invasive Paget disease. For primary intraepithelial Paget disease, the lesion is usually a slowly progressive, indolent, superficial process. Accordingly, local excision of the visible lesion to the fascia, with 2 cm clinically visibly clear margins of excision, is sufficient. In cases associated with invasive Paget disease, or with underlying skin appendage or vulvar glandular adenocarcinoma, as determined by histopathologic evaluation, treatment includes ipsilateral inguinal–femoral lymphadenectomy. If the tumor extends to the margins of excision, or the excision is deemed inadequate in the face of invasive disease, more extended partial or total vulvectomy may be needed [9,37,55]. Recurrent vulvar Paget disease, occurring peripheral to an excised intraepithelial Paget lesion, does not appear to be associated with any significant risk of underlying adenocarcinoma and can be treated by a more conservative approach, such as superficial excision, or topical therapy, including imiquimod [54,72,99].

In the patient with vulvar primary cutaneous Paget disease, clinically normal-appearing skin may contain Paget cells. A careful topographic study [66] demonstrated

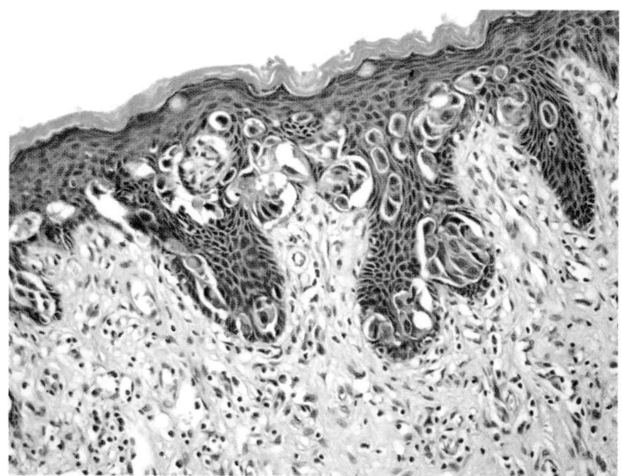

Fig. 2.39
Pagetoid urothelial intraepithelial neoplasia (PUIN); Paget disease, secondary type, of urothelial origin. **Large neoplastic intraepithelial urothelial cells are present throughout the epithelium**

that the outline of the histologically involved area was highly irregular and of much greater extent than the visible lesion. In addition, multicentric foci, some occurring in grossly normal-appearing skin, were noted; this accounts for the frequent "recurrences" of disease despite seemingly adequate excision. These clinically normal-appearing areas of skin, however, are not associated with underlying skin appendage adenocarcinoma or invasive primary cutaneous Paget disease. In the author's experience, when invasive primary cutaneous Paget disease or cutaneous Paget disease associated with an underlying skin appendage carcinoma (type 1c) is present, the adenocarcinoma is within the dermis of the skin or mucosa clinically involved with the Paget disease. In such cases, excision to the fascia of these clinically involved areas, to excise the Paget disease and the potential underlying adenocarcinoma, is necessary.

The depth of invasion influences prognosis in such cases. When the depth of dermal invasion was 1 mm or less, no nodal metastasis or death from tumor was observed in seven such patients, whereas all three patients with tumor invasion beyond 1 mm had inguinofemoral node metastasis [37]. Frozen section evaluation of clinically normal-appearing skin margins adjacent to primary cutaneous Paget disease has not been demonstrated either to improve survival or to reduce recurrence. In a study of 12 patients with involved margins following surgery, seven (58%) had recurrence, whereas recurrence was seen in one of four patients (25%) with negative margins [37]. Recurrences of primary cutaneous intraepithelial Paget disease after excision of the primary lesion have not demonstrated a significant risk of associated underlying adenocarcinoma. Recurrences at the site of the original tumor or remote from it can be treated by local superficial excision. Intraepithelial Paget disease has no significant risk of lymph node metastasis or death [37,55]. The issues regarding margin assessment specifically relate to primary cutaneous Paget disease. Margin assessment for Paget disease of noncutaneous origin, including PUIN, needs to be addressed. One study has reported reduced E-cadherin expression in primary vulvar Paget disease as correlating with disease progression [49].

In cases of perianal Paget disease, it is necessary to evaluate the rectum and the anus to determine if the lesion is a manifestation of underlying rectal Paget disease or rectal or anal adenocarcinoma. In such cases, therapy is directed toward treatment of the rectal or anal carcinoma, and the vulvar Paget disease can be treated as an intraepithelial neoplasm, with local superficial excision, or more conservatively.

In vulvar Paget disease associated with other adjacent adenocarcinomas, such as cervical adenocarcinoma, the treatment is focused on the primary adenocarcinoma and the associated Paget disease is treated as an intraepithelial neoplastic process, with superficial excision. The prognosis in such cases is dependent on the stage and behavior of the associated adenocarcinoma.

Therapy for vulvar PUIN is directed toward the bladder urothelial neoplasm, and the vulvar pagetoid intraepithelial urothelial neoplastic process is treated conservatively, as an intraepithelial neoplasm. Total vulvectomy and excision to the deep fascia is not indicated in this circumstance [173].

Adenocarcinoma of Cloacogenic Origin (Mucinous Adenocarcinoma Arising in the Surface Epithelium of the Vulva); Cloacogenic Carcinoma (Cloacogenic Adenocarcinoma)

All these rare tumors of the vulva have features of glandular tumors of the colon, and their origin is uncertain. They are usually solitary, but may involve more than one site. The tumor presents as a cutaneous mass and are polypoid, excoriated and/or inflamed [46,181]. They appear to be primary mucinous tumors of the vulvar epithelium and within the vulvar vestibule this may be a probable explanation. Benign-appearing mucinous glandular elements have been reported in the dermis deep to the tumor in one case [187]. It is also possible that they arise from some remnant of the early colaca within the vulva, as the term implies.

On microscopic examination the tumor may be entirely confined to the epithelium, with a verrucoid, or papillary appearance and with neoplastic colonic-type glandular epithelial cells on the surface of the tumor. They may resemble colonic villous adenoma when a predominant intraepithelial component is present. The neoplastic mucinous epithelium is in continuity with the overlying epithelium. If invasion is present, it is in continuity with the overlying neoplastic epithelium. The tumor is not associated with an underlying dermal glandular neoplasm as may be seen with Paget disease. The invasive adenocarcinoma resembles mucinous colonic carcinoma, with neoplastic colonic type epithelium with goblet cells and intracytoplasmic mucin. Apocrine differentiation is not observed [181,187].

On immunohistochemical study, these tumors are reported as being reactive with mucicarmine, Alcian blue pH 5, and immunoreactive for polyclonal CEA, cytokeratin 17, CAM 5.2, and p53 antigen. In addition, S-100 and chromogranin are also reported as immunoreactive in some neoplastic epithelial cells, evidence of the presence of endocrine cells. The tumors are not reactive for monoclonal CEA and estrogen receptor (ER) and progesterone receptor (PR). Electron microscopic studies have provided additional evidence of a colonic type epithelium within these tumors [46,181,187].

Although there is limited experience, treatment of tumors that are entirely intraepithelial would be more conservative than for invasive tumors. For these deeper tumors, risk of lymph node metastasis is limited although regional lymph node involvement is apparently rare. Treatment with partial deep vulvectomy (deep local excision) has reportedly been effective [181]. Gynecologic oncology consultation is recommended because of the very limited experience with these tumors.

Bartholin Gland Tumors

General Features

A wide variety of tumors may arise from the Bartholin gland. The criteria for the diagnosis of a tumor of Bartholin gland origin are that (1) the neoplasm must arise at the site of Bartholin gland, (2) be consistent histologically with a primary neoplasm of Bartholin gland, and (3) not be metastatic. Adenocarcinomas account for approximately 40% of Bartholin gland carcinomas, but others include squamous cell carcinoma (40%), adenoid cystic carcinoma (15%), transitional cell carcinoma (less than 5%), adenosquamous carcinoma (less than 5%), and poorly differentiated adenocarcinomas [40].

Clinical Features

Carcinoma of the Bartholin gland usually presents as an enlargement in the gland area and may present as an apparent Bartholin cyst. The average age of women with this tumor is 50 years, with most between 40 and 70 years.

Gross Findings

Bartholin gland tumors are typically solid, deeply infiltrative, and occupy the site of the gland, occasionally obscuring its presence. They range from 1 to 7 cm in diameter.

Microscopic Findings

Adenocarcinomas of the Bartholin gland usually are nonspecific in type, but mucinous and papillary types have been described. The tumors usually contain intracytoplasmic mucin and are immunoreactive for CEA. Fine-needle aspiration cytology may be of value in diagnosis.

Differential Diagnosis

The differential diagnosis of Bartholin gland adenocarcinoma includes adenocarcinoma of skin appendage origin and metastatic adenocarcinoma. These tumors typically do not involve the Bartholin gland, and the tumor type may not be consistent with a primary tumor of the Bartholin gland.

Other Primary Bartholin Gland Carcinomas

Squamous cell carcinomas arising in the Bartholin gland have the same microscopic appearance as those arising elsewhere in the vulva. These tumors are typically immunoreactive for CEA.

Adenoid cystic carcinomas arising in the Bartholin gland are similar to those occurring in salivary glands, the upper respiratory tract, and skin. They are composed of uniform, small cells arranged in cords and nests with a cribriform pattern [36]. Variable-sized cysts filled with amphophilic or eosinophilic acellular basement membrane-like material also may be encountered (➋ *Figs. 2.40* and ➋ *2.41*). Keratin and S-100 antigen are detectable by immunohistochemical techniques. The S-100 reactivity may demonstrate a myoepithelial cell element.

The differential diagnosis of adenoid cystic carcinoma includes adenocarcinoma, basal cell carcinoma, metastatic atypical carcinoid, and small cell carcinoma. Metastatic small cell carcinoma arising in the vagina has been reported as presenting as a Bartholin mass [104]. Adenocarcinomas lack the uniform acinar arrangement and intraluminal basement membrane material of adenoid cystic carcinoma. Basal cell carcinomas are more solid and lack the cystic spaces and the intracystic basement membrane-like material. Metastatic carcinoids and small cell carcinomas are more solid, have fewer lumens, contain argyrophil cells, and stain for neuron-specific enolase (NSE) in most cases. Carcinoid tumors almost always react with antibodies against chromogranin and other neuroendocrine markers.

Adenosquamous carcinoma of the Bartholin gland contains a mixture of squamous cells with intracellular bridges and glandular cells that typically contain mucin.

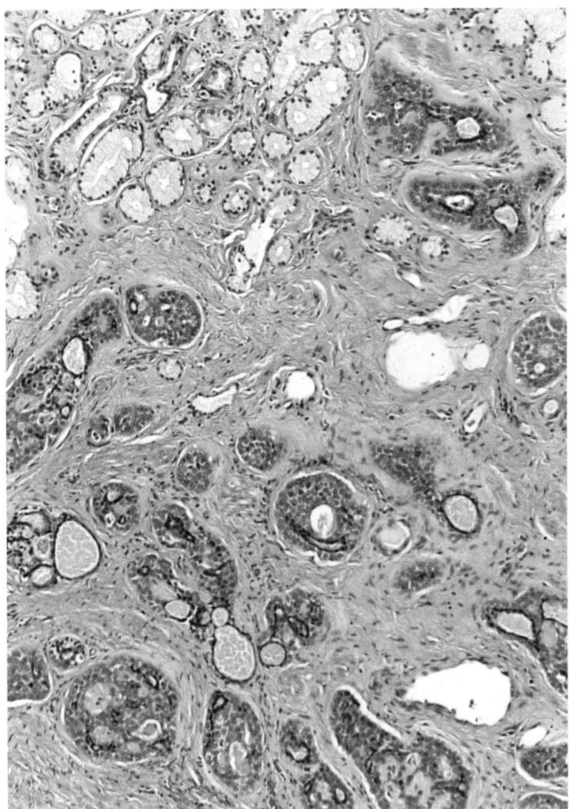

Fig. 2.40
Adenoid cystic carcinoma. **Relatively small cells surrounding sharply punched-out cystic spaces**

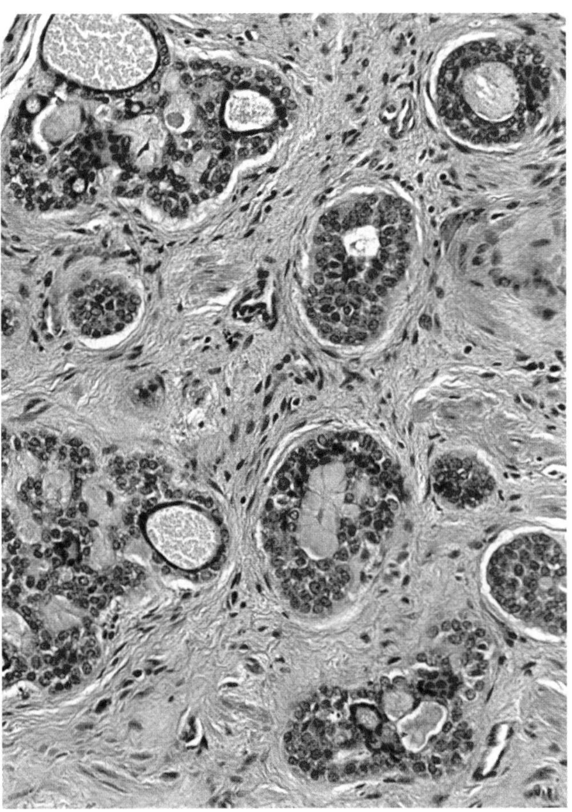

Fig. 2.41
Adenoid cystic carcinoma. **The tumor is composed of relatively small hyperchromatic cells arranged in well-circumscribed nests within the stroma. Well-defined cystic spaces are evident in this tumor. The surrounding stroma is desmoplastic (Courtesy of R.J. Kurman, M.D., Baltimore, MD.)**

Transitional cell carcinoma arising in the Bartholin gland is composed of uniform polyhedral or rounded epithelial cells often lining broad papillary fronds. Rare areas of glandular or squamous differentiation may be found. The differential diagnosis of primary transitional cell carcinoma of the Bartholin gland includes poorly differentiated squamous cell carcinoma and adenocarcinoma. If more than rare foci contain glands or show keratinization, the tumor is of mixed cell type and should be so designated, listing the different tumor types.

Clinical Behavior and Treatment

The primary treatment for Bartholin gland carcinoma is wide local excision to the fascia, hemivulvectomy, or total vulvectomy. Ipsilateral or bilateral inguinofemoral lymph node dissection is necessary, regardless of the type of primary excision [35,95,168]. Adjunctive radiation therapy to the vulva and regional lymph nodes also has been advocated [35].

Approximately 20% of carcinomas of the Bartholin gland are associated with metastases to the inguinofemoral lymph nodes. The overall 5-year survival of patients with Bartholin gland carcinomas is approximately 50% when the groin nodes are free of tumor, but decreases to 18% when two or more nodes are involved [168]. If the groin nodes are involved there is a 20% probability that pelvic lymph node metastasis also will be involved, but if the groin nodes are free of metastasis, there is essentially no risk of pelvic node metastasis.

Therapy for adenoid cystic carcinoma of the Bartholin gland is wide local excision with ipsilateral inguinofemoral lymphadenectomy [36]. Local recurrence is well documented and, when the tumor involves the margin, adjuvant radiotherapy may be beneficial. Survival is better with adenoid carcinoma than with other forms of carcinoma of the Bartholin gland.

The treatment of vulvar adenosquamous carcinoma is similar to that of squamous cell carcinoma. Adenosquamous carcinomas have a poorer prognosis than squamous cell carcinomas, partly because of the higher frequency of lymph node metastasis.

Mammary Gland-like Adenocarcinoma Arising in the Vulva

Specialized anogenital mammary-like glands, found typically in the interlabial sulcus, are thought to be the origin of vulvar mammary-like (breast-like) adenocarcinomas [162]. Other benign and malignant tumors, including papillary hidradenomas as well as fibrocystic-like disease, have been described within these specialized glands. The origin of these tumors had been previously thought to be ectopic breast tissue; however, current opinion is that these glands are not ectopic tissue, but rather normal anatomic elements composed of specialized anogenital mammary-like glands. The adenocarcinomas arising from these glands have histopathologic features very similar to those of primary mammary adenocarcinomas, and a few have been associated with breast adenocarcinoma. Most have a pattern of growth of infiltrating, well-differentiated adenocarcinoma. In some cases, an intraductal carcinoma component has been identified.

Metastases to inguinal lymph nodes from adenocarcinomas of vulvar mammary-like tumors have been observed. These adenocarcinomas contain secretory material similar to that of breast adenocarcinomas, including alpha-lactalbumin and milk fat globulin protein, and also may contain estrogen and progesterone receptors.

Metastatic adenocarcinoma to the vulva can be distinguished from primary adenocarcinomas if mammary-like glands or in situ adenocarcinoma is present. In the absence of mammary-like tissue, the distinction may not be possible. Treatment of primary adenocarcinoma arising within vulvar specialized anogenital glands is extended wide local excision and ipsilateral inguinofemoral lymphadenectomy.

Carcinomas of Sweat Gland Origin

Carcinomas of vulvar sweat gland origin, including Skene glands, are rare, comprising less than 1% of all vulvar carcinomas [169]. Patients typically present with a painless vulvar mass. In addition to undifferentiated sweat gland adenocarcinomas, ductal eccrine carcinoma, eccrine porocarcinoma, eccrine hidradenocarcinoma, clear cell hidradenocarcinoma, and apocrine carcinomas have been reported [169]. Adenosquamous carcinoma has been reported arising in a hidradenoma [10].

Sebaceous carcinoma of the vulva has also been reported, which may be associated with VIN [52,169]. Adenocarcinomas of the vulva may arise from the Skene glands [149].

Mucinous adenocarcinoma with focal squamous and neuroendocrine differentiation has been reported arising in the labium majus. This tumor expressed chromogranin A, protein gene product 9.5, serotonin, and vasoactive intestinal polypeptide [64].

Malignant Melanoma

General Features

Melanomas account for approximately 9% of all malignant tumors of the vulva, and vulvar melanoma accounts for approximately 3% of all melanomas in women and approximately 8–10% of all vulvar malignant neoplasms [25,41,82]. Melanomas occur predominantly in white women. The age-specific incidence in a comprehensive Swedish study is 75 years of age or older, occurring in 1.28 per 100,000. In women 60–74 years old, the incidence was 0.56; in those 45–59, 0.19. In those 30–44 it was 0.08, and 0.02 or less in women under 29 years of age [126]. Vulvar melanoma has been reported in children [19,47]. Vulvar bleeding was the most common symptom of 198 patients studied, being recorded in 35% of the patients. A vulvar mass was observed in 28%, an ulcer in 5%, and a mole in 5% [126]. Pruritus occurred in 15%, irritation and or burning in 14%, and discomfort with urination in 12%.

Vulvar melanomas may arise from a preexisting benign or atypical pigmented lesion [106,182]. Melanomas occur on the clitoris, labia minora, and labia majora with approximately equal frequency, although approximately one third of the cases arise at mucosal-cutaneous sites on the vulva. Of the cases available with data on site within the vulva, 90 melanomas occurred on glabrous skin, 69 on hairy–glabrous skin, and 23 on hairy skin. The mass usually is polypoid or nodular (40%) and, although generally pigmented, was nonpigmented in 27% in one series [126]. Satellite nodules may be present, and were observed in 20% of 198 cases [126].

Vulvar melanomas are of three distinct histopathologic types: superficial spreading melanoma (➲ *Figs. 2.42–2.44*), nodular melanoma (➲ *Figs. 2.45* and ➲ *2.46*), and mucosal–lentiginous (mucosal/acral lentiginous) melanoma (➲ *Figs. 2.48* and ➲ *2.49*) [127]. Some vulvar melanomas are mixed or otherwise unclassifiable. This group comprised approximately one quarter of the cases in one study [126]. Thin melanomas have also been reported [38]. The relative frequency of these types differs in various reports [41,165,167]. Mucosal/acral lentiginous melanoma was the most common type identified in the Karolinska series, observed in 52% of the cases, where as nodular melanoma accounted for 20% and superficial spreading melanoma 4% of the 198 cases reported [126].

Some of the variation in the type of vulvar melanoma reported may relate to differences in the criteria used to distinguish superficial spreading melanoma from nodular melanoma. Superficial spreading melanoma usually can be differentiated from nodular melanoma by evaluating the adjacent epithelium. If the radial growth of a melanoma or atypical melanocytes involves four or more adjacent rete ridges, the tumor should be classified as superficial spreading melanoma (see ➲ *Fig. 2.44*).

There is some variation in the frequency of melanoma type related to the vulvar anatomic site of the tumor. In one large series, mucosal/acral lentiginous melanomas were seen with similar frequency in glabrous, hairy–glabrous, and hairy skin, whereas nodular melanomas were seen primarily in glabrous and hairy–glabrous skin and less frequently in hairy skin. In contrast, superficial spreading melanomas were seen predominately in hairy skin [126].

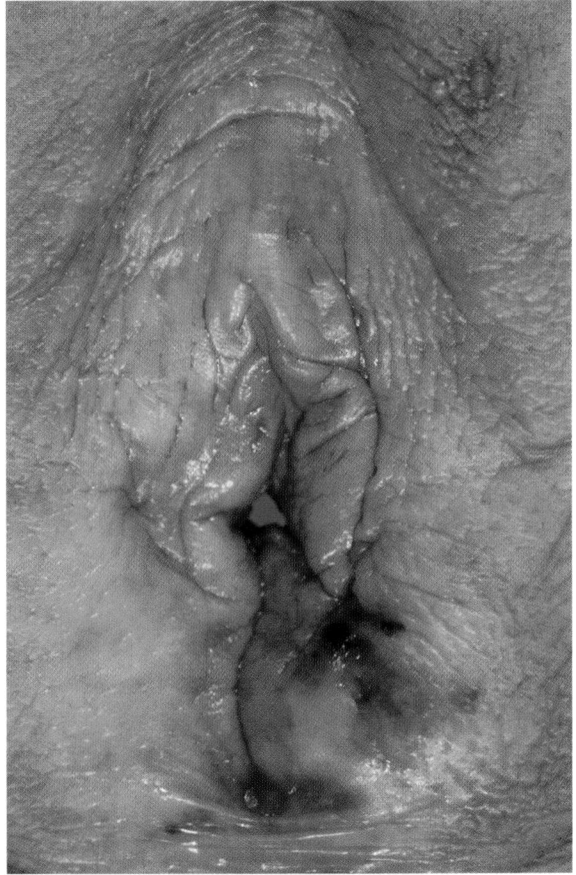

Fig. 2.42
Malignant melanoma. **A superficial spreading malignant melanoma with vertical growth within the field of a superficially spreading malignant melanoma (Courtesy of Linda S. Morgan, M.D., Gainesville, FL.)**

Microscopic Findings

Mucosal–lentiginous (mucosal/acral lentiginous) melanomas have both vertical growth, as is seen in nodular melanoma, and radial growth, as is seen in superficial spreading melanoma, and may be in situ or superficially invasive (➲ *Figs 2.48* and ➲ *2.49*). Atypical melanocytes usually can be identified within the epithelium adjacent to mucosal–lentiginous and superficial spreading melanomas. Malignant melanomas may consist predominantly of epithelioid, dendritic (nevoid), or spindle cell types, either pure or mixed, within a given tumor. The cells may contain no melanin, or variable amounts, ranging from minimal to very large quantities. The histopathologic features vary considerably, and certain features can be correlated with the subtype of the melanoma. In the invasive area of mucosal–lentiginous melanoma the cells may be dendritic and spindle like, with deeper and more central areas of invasion having more significant cytoatpyia (➲ *Fig. 2.49*). Within the invasive area of a superficial spreading melanoma, the malignant melanocytic cells usually are large and have relatively uniform nuclei with prominent nucleoli. Similar melanocytic cells can be found within the adjacent epithelium, representing the radial growth phase of the tumor. Junctional melanocytes are numerous and distributed within the epithelium in a pagetoid distribution.

In nodular melanomas, an intraepithelial component may be present in addition to an invasive component, but without an adjacent radial growth phase. The cells of nodular melanomas may be polygonal (epithelioid) or

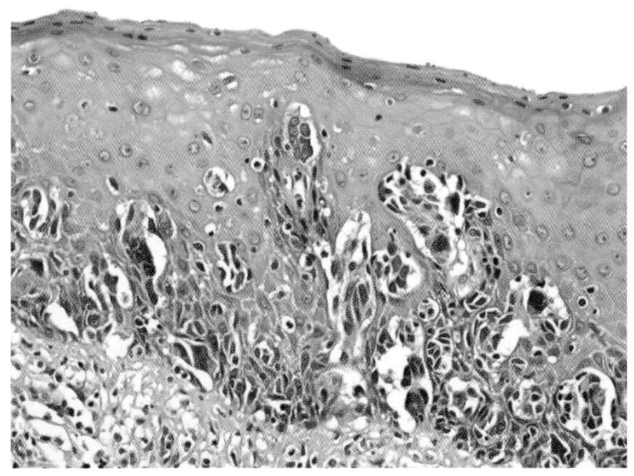

Fig. 2.43
Superficial spreading malignant melanoma. **Pagetoid spread of the melanoma cells into the upper third of the epidermis. Markedly atypical melanocytic cells are at the epithelial–dermal junction. No invasion is present**

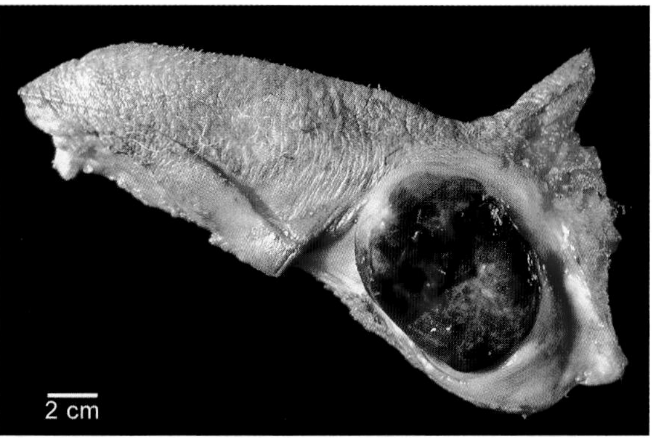

Fig. 2.45
Nodular melanoma, partial deep vulvectomy. **The tumor is deeply pigmented and clearly demarcated from the adjacent vulvar epithelium. The tumor is deeply invasive (Courtesy R. Foss, PA, Gainesville, FL.)**

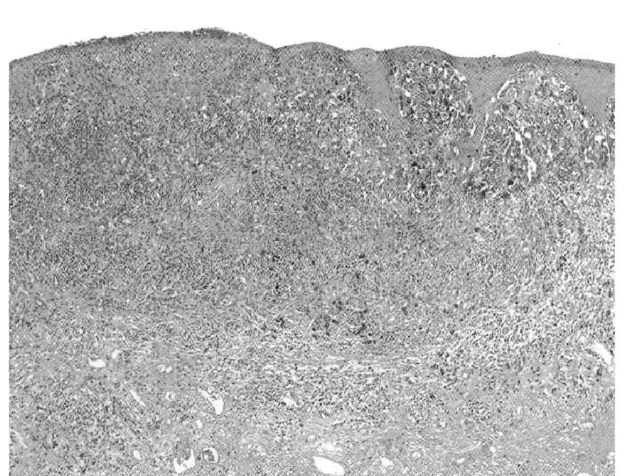

Fig. 2.44
Superficial spreading melanoma. **The tumor displays vertical, invasive, growth**

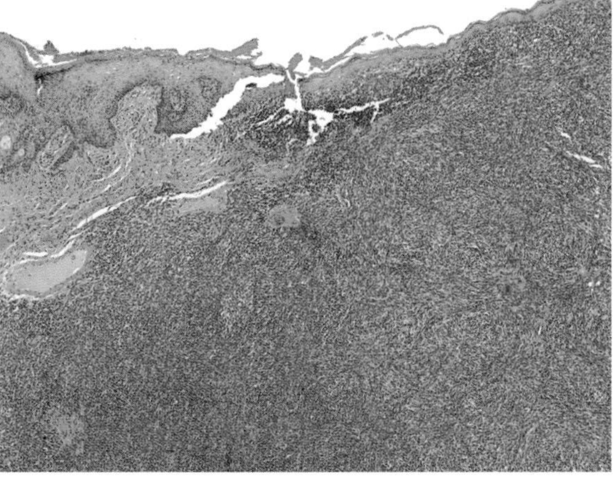

Fig. 2.46
Nodular melanoma. **The tumor is deep within the dermis, with overlying epithelium that does not have an intraepithelial melanocytic lesion**

spindle shaped (see *Fig. 2.46*). The polygonal cells contain abundant eosinophilic cytoplasm, large nuclei, and prominent nucleoli. The dendritic cells have tapering cytoplasmic extensions resembling nerve cells and show moderate nuclear pleomorphism. Spindle cells have smaller, oval nuclei and may be arranged in sheets or bundles (see *Fig. 2.47*). Mucosal/acral lentiginous melanomas of the vulva arise most commonly within the vestibule. They may show little or no pagetoid spread and are characterized by melanoma cells within the junctional zone. When there is extension into the adjacent dermis growth is in a diffuse pattern (see *Figs. 2.48* and *2.49*). The melanoma cells in the junctional area are relatively uniform with little nuclear pleomorphism, however with deeper invasion the cellular features may be more distinctive for melanoma. Within the subepithelial tissue, the tumor cells usually evoke a desmoplastic response.

Differential Diagnosis

Superficial spreading malignant melanoma must be distinguished from Paget disease, VIN, and dysplastic nevi. The cells of Paget disease usually are larger than superficial spreading melanoma, have more cytoplasm, and are clustered with occasional gland formation. Squamous cell carcinomas with tumor giant cells, or those predominantly composed of spindle cells, may resemble malignant melanoma. Typical squamous cell carcinoma may be identifiable adjacent to the giant cell or spindle cell component, which may establish the diagnosis. Spindle cell tumors of soft tissue origin, large cell lymphomas, pagetoid reticulosis, Kaposi sarcoma, and metastatic tumors, including choriocarcinoma, may be included in the differential diagnosis. In these cases, review of the clinical history and physical and radiologic findings, as well as thorough sectioning of the submitted tissue and appropriate immunohistochemical studies, as discussed next, usually will contribute evidence to establish the diagnosis. It should be emphasized that when faced with a poorly differentiated vulvar tumor that defies classification on initial microscopic examination, melanoma should be placed first on the list of the differential diagnosis.

Paget disease can be distinguished from melanoma with histochemical and immunohistochemical studies for mucin, CEA, S-100 protein, HMB-45 (or Melan-A), and cytokeratins. Paget cells, regardless of origin, are immunoreactive for cytokeratin and primary cutaneous Paget disease, and Paget disease of anorectal origin also typically contain cytoplasmic mucin, with mucicarmine stain, and are immunoreactive for CEA, whereas melanomas are not (see ➋ *Table 2.2*). Pagetoid reticulosis and Kaposi sarcoma will typically express CD 45 and related lymphoproliferative markers. Melanomas usually are immunoreactive for S-100 protein, HMB-45, and Melan-A, whereas the non-melanocytic tumors, including Paget, PUIN, VIN, squamous cell carcinoma, pagetoid/bowenoid reticulosis, and Kaposi sarcoma, are negative [173]. When the diagnosis of vulvar melanoma is difficult to resolve, the immunohistochemical studies should include epithelial markers, to identify squamous, glandular, and transitional cell neoplasms (e.g., AE1/3, cytokeratins 7 and 20, epithelial membrane antigen (EMA), CEA, GCDFP-15); hematopoietic markers, to identify lymphomas including Ki-1 lymphomas, pagetoid/bowenoid reticulosis, etc. (e.g., CD 45); muscle markers for leiomyosarcoma or rhabdomyosarcoma (e.g., desmin, smooth muscle actin); fibrohistiocytic markers (e.g., alpha-1-antitrypsin, alpha-1-antichymotrypsin); neural and neuroendocrine tumor markers (e.g., S-100,

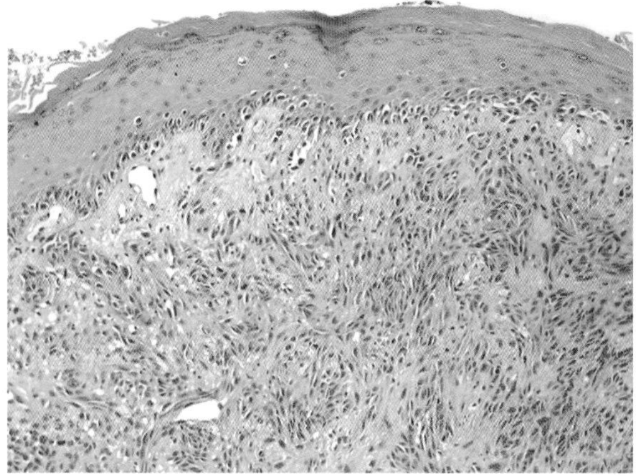

Fig. 2.47
Malignant melanoma, amelanotic, spindle cell type. **The overlying epithelium has in situ melanoma with neoplastic cells in the basal and parabasal epithelium. The invasive melanoma consists of spindle-shaped neoplastic cells. No melanin pigment is identified and the tumor is deeply invasive**

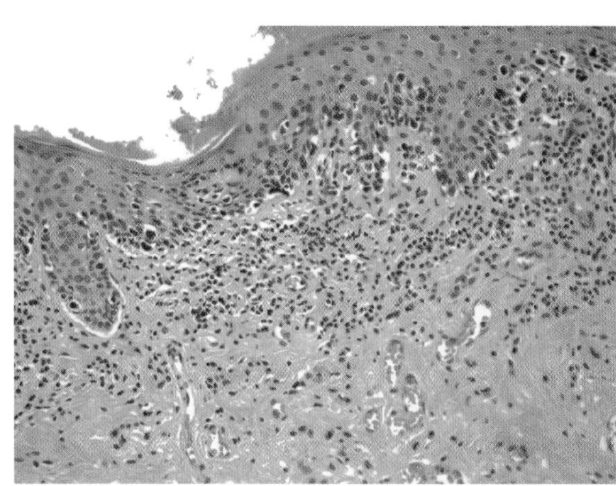

Fig. 2.48
Mucosal–lentiginous melanoma, in situ. **This variant of malignant melanoma is characterized by a radial component with a lentiginous pattern at the mucosal–submucosal interface. In this case, the basal epithelium of the vulvar vestibule is involved. The melanoma cells are relatively obscured by the associated inflammatory cells. Pagetoid spread is not evident. This type of malignant melanoma usually is found within the vulvar vestibule**

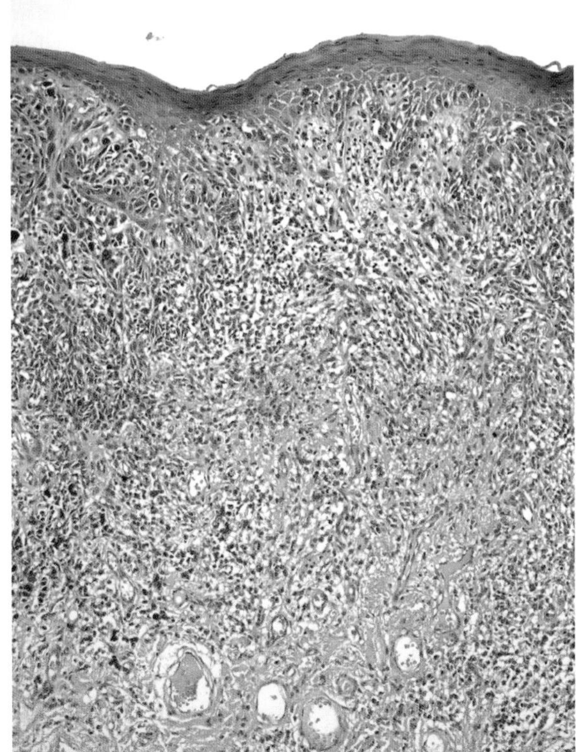

Fig. 2.49
Mucosal–lentiginous melanoma. **The melanoma involves the overlying mucosal epithelium predominately in the basal layer in a lentiginous pattern. No significant pagetoid growth is identified. Invasive melanoma is evident at the mucosal–submucosal interface with deep submucosal involvement**

chromogranin, synaptophysin, CD56); and melanoma markers (e.g., HMB-45, Melan-A, S-100).

Clinical Behavior and Treatment

Both the level of invasion of a malignant melanoma (Clark level) and its thickness have prognostic significance [127]. The Clark classification of cutaneous melanomas into five levels of invasion is well accepted and can be applied to melanomas of the vulva arising in keratinized skin, though they require some interpretation when arising within mucocutaneous areas such as the vulvar vestibule whereas the Breslow measurements for thickness are readily applicable in both sites [15]. A level I melanoma is a melanoma in situ; level II melanoma extends into the superficial papillary dermis; and level III melanoma fills and expands the papillary dermis; level IV melanoma invades the reticular dermis; and level V melanoma invades beyond the reticular dermis into fat or other deeper tissues.

Thickness measurements for cutaneous malignant melanomas as proposed by Breslow require measurement from the deep border of the granular layer of the overlying epithelium to the deepest point of tumor invasion [15]. If a lesion is less than 0.76 mm in thickness, it has little or no metastatic potential. This is also generally accepted for tumors with a thickness of 1 mm or less. Correlations between the thickness and the level of a vulvar melanoma can be made. Level I melanomas have no measurable thickness. In one study, level II melanomas had a thickness of 1 mm or less, level III melanomas had a thickness from 1 to 2 mm, and level IV melanomas had a thickness exceeding 2 mm, but did not involve subcutaneous fat or adjacent deeper structures.

Factors that adversely influence survival include a tumor thickness exceeding 2 mm, Clark level IV, a mitotic count exceeding 10 mm^2, surface ulceration, and a minimal or absent inflammatory reaction [182]. Vascular space invasion and tumor necrosis also are associated with a poorer prognosis and are seen more commonly with large melanomas. No recurrences of vulvar melanoma have been observed when the thickness was 0.75 mm or less [182]. An excellent prognosis has been associated with melanomas at Clark level II or less, and those with a thickness of 1.49 mm or less. A tumor volume of less than 100 mm^3 also correlates with an excellent prognosis. Other adverse prognostic factors reported include central location of the tumors, tumor ulceration, vascular space involvement, and a high mitotic rate [159].

Vulvar melanomas may recur locally, or in the cervix, urethra, vagina, or rectum. Distant metastasis may be the first sign of recurrence. Metastases to the lungs, brain, urinary bladder, bone marrow, and abdominal wall have all been observed. The prognosis after recurrence is guarded, with a 5-year survival of approximately 5%. The usual treatment for vulvar melanomas with a thickness of 0.75 mm or less is wide local excision with a 1 cm circumferential and 1–2 cm deep margins. This is also acceptable treatment for some melanomas with a thickness of 1 mm or less, although there is limited data available for vulvar melanomas with a thickness between 0.76 and 1.0 mm. Melanomas 1.1–4 mm thick require 2 cm surgical margins with deep margins of at least 1–2 cm. Melanomas with a thickness greater than 4 mm are usually treated by wide excision to the fascia or partial or total vulvectomy [159]. Depending on the size of the tumor, the surgical procedure may include bilateral inguinal lymphadenectomy [182]. Radical vulvectomy does not appear to improve survival when compared to radical local excision with bilateral groin lymphadenectomy. Regional lymph node metastasis, as well as the number of lymph nodes with metastatic tumor, significantly influence survival [120].

Other Malignant Tumors of the Vulva

Malignant Blue Nevus

Malignant blue nevus is a rare tumor but has been reported as a primary vulvar tumor, reported arising in the labium majus of a 28-year-old woman. This patient had an ovarian metastasis from this tumor 15 years after therapy. Malignant blue nevus typically has significant nuclear atypia, but a low mitotic rate [151].

Yolk Sac Tumor (Endodermal Sinus Tumor)

Yolk sac tumor is a germ cell tumor occurring in ovary and testis (see ➋ Chap. 16, Germ Cell Tumors of the Ovary). Its occurrence in extragonadal sites is rare. In the vulva, vagina, and pelvis, the tumor is reported primarily in children and young women [57]. The characteristic histopathological features are quite variable although Schiller–Duval bodies and eosinophilic hyaline droplets are classic features. These features may not be evident in cases with other patterns including reticular, micropapillary, microcystic, and hepatoid. The eosinophilic droplets are PAS positive, diastase resistant, and express alpha-fetoprotein (AFP) on immunohistochemical study. The histologic appearance does not appear to influence prognosis in tumors of the ovary, but there are insufficient cases within the vulva to evaluate this relationship. The variable patterns of growth may resemble adenocarcinoma, which is the primary differential diagnosis. Immunoperoxidase studies to demonstrate the presence of alpha-fetoprotein (AFP) and an elevated serum level of AFP support the diagnosis. Recommended therapy for vulvar yolk sac tumor is wide local excision and chemotherapy [57]. Platinum-based chemotherapy has markedly improved survival in patients with this tumor [57].

Primary Malignant Lymphoma

The vulva is the second most common site, after the cervix, for malignant lymphoma involving the genital tract (see ➋ Chap. 22, Soft Tissue Lesions Involving Female Reproductive Organs). These tumors predominately are found in women of reproductive age, and postmenopausal women, but may occur in children. The tumor may present as a Bartholin mass, clitoral enlargement, ulcerated or destructive neoplasm, or mimic other vulvar tumors [121,161,164]. Lymphomas involving the vulva are usually of the diffuse, B cell large cell type. Other tumor types have also been reported including diffuse mixed cell lymphoma, follicular large cell lymphoma, and peripheral T cell lymphoma. Kappa-positive lymphoplasmacytic lymphoma and angiocentric small and large mixed cell lymphoma, as well as plasmocytoma, have also been reported in the vulva [161,164]. Lymphoma involving the vulva may also represent metastatic involvement [164]. The diagnosis of lymphoma is confirmed by specific immunoperoxidase and/or flow cytometry studies including specific markers for lymphocytes, such as CD 45, and T and B cells, and studies for specific lymphocyte markers including specific molecular studies for gene rearrangements to identify the neoplastic cell population as lymphoma.

The differential diagnosis includes inflammatory conditions and dermatoses as well as lymphoepithelioma-like carcinoma [22]. Dermatoses and benign inflammatory processes, unlike lymphomas, contain mixed populations of lymphocytes and other inflammatory cells. Lymphoepithelioma-like carcinomas contain epithelial cells that express high molecular–weight cytokeratins and lack evidence of a monoclonal lymphocytic population [22]. Large cell lymphomas, including Ki-1 lymphomas, may mimic poorly differentiated carcinoma. Immunoperoxidase studies, including CD45 (LCA); and specific lymphocyte markers as well as epithelial markers are of value to distinguish these types. Appropriate aggressive chemotherapy is the treatment of choice for most lymphomas. Prognosis is dependent on the lymphoma type and stage of the tumor [161].

Merkel Cell Tumor

Merkel cell tumor of the vulva is rare, occurring predominately in older women [26,34,62,141]. These tumors typically present as an intradermal nodule or nodules with erythema of the overlying skin [34]. These tumors may be associated with VIN or squamous cell carcinoma. Both squamous differentiaition and glandular differentiation have been reported in one case. Three distinctive histopathologic types of Merkel cell tumor are recognized, namely the trabecular or carcinoid-like type, the intermediate cell type, and the small cell or oat cell-like type

(➋ *Figs. 2.50* and ➋ *2.51*). The distribution of these types among vulvar tumors has not been determined. The histopathologic features are that of a poorly differentiated neoplasm within the dermis and composed of a diffuse population of relatively small, uniform, hyperchromatic cells usually without prominent nucleoli (see ➋ *Figs. 2.50* and ➋ *2.51*). In some cases, the tumor may have pagetoid growth. Immunocytochemistry demonstrates a distinctive perinuclear cytoplasmic dot with low molecular–weight cytokeratin-specific antibodies such as AE1/3, Cam 5.2, and cytokeratin 20. The tumors are usually immunoreactive for neuron-specific enolase (NSE) [26,62]. Chromogranin may be negative. These tumors usually contain membrane bound neurosecretory granules that can be demonstrated by electron microscopy; ACTH production by a Merkle cell tumor with demonstrated neurosecretory granules has been reported.

The differential diagnosis includes other small cell tumors, of either primary or metastatic origin, including but not limited to neuroendocrine tumors, primitive neuroectodermal tumor (PNET), basal cell carcinoma, and basaloid squamous cell carcinoma. When pagetoid spread is present Paget disease, melanoma, or lymphoma must also be considered (see ➋ Paget Disease). Immunohistochemical findings will not distinguish Merkle cell tumor from a metastatic tumor of similar reactivity and morphology, but clinical history usually will. PNET expresses CD99 and lymphomas usually express CD 45; neither of these are expressed in Merkle cell tumor.

Merkel cell tumors are clinically very aggressive, with regional node metastasis and subsequent widespread metastasis often occurring within a year of diagnosis [26,62]. For local disease, therapy includes wide local excision (partial deep vulvectomy) with a 2 cm margin of excision with sentinel lymph node biopsy. If the sentinel node demonstrates metastatic tumor, regional lymphadenectomy and postoperative local radiation therapy to the primary and regional sites is recommended. If there is systemic disease, chemotherapy is recommended [26,29,62].

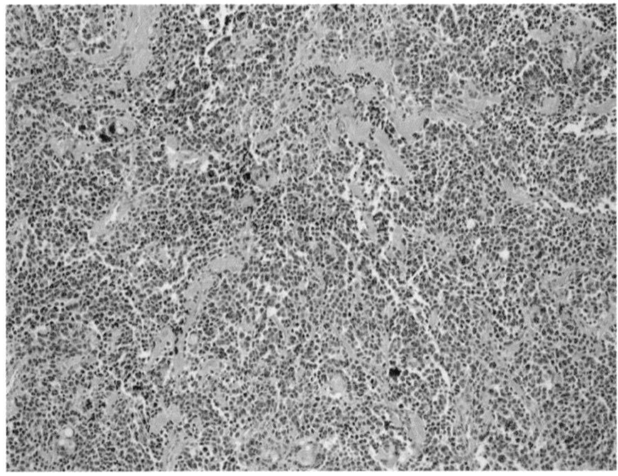

Fig. 2.50
Merkel cell carcinoma. **The tumor is within the dermis and composed of a diffuse population of relatively small, uniform cells with hyperchromatic nuclear chromatin. Prominent eosinophilic fibrovascular stroma is present between irregular- shaped groups of cells**

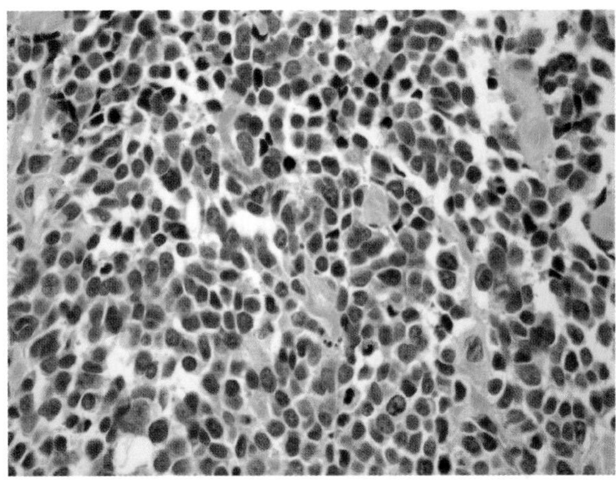

Fig. 2.51
Merkel cell carcinoma. **The tumor cells are relatively small and uniform with little cytoplasm and nuclei with dispersed chromatin. Nucleoli are not prominent**

Metastatic Tumors

Metastatic tumors comprise approximately 8% of all tumors of the vulva. Tumors from other sites of the genital tract are the most common tumors that metastasize to the vulva, with squamous carcinoma of the cervix being the most frequent, followed by carcinomas of the endometrium and ovary. Other common primary tumor sites include the bladder and urethra [102]. The vulva may be involved by direct extension of tumors arising in the vagina, urethra, bladder, or rectum. Other primary tumors that have metastasized to the vulva including malignancies of breast, kidney, lung, stomach and gestational choriocarcinoma, melanoma, and neuroblastoma [102,111,131,145].

Low-grade endometrial stromal sarcoma has been reported metastatic to the clitoris [7]. Malignant lymphomas also may metastasize to the vulva and the Bartholin gland [121,161,164]. Metastatic myeloid sarcoma presenting as a mass involving the labia majora has been reported as a presenting symptom of acute myeloid leukemia [51]. Eosinophilic granuloma has been reported involving the vulva [83]. Metastatic tumors typically involve the dermis and overlying epithelium and consequently are often associated with ulceration. Patients with metastatic carcinoma to the vulva have a poor prognosis. Treatment is primarily palliative; radical surgical approaches are not indicated.

Tumors of the Urethra

Urethral Carcinoma

Urethral carcinoma constitutes less than 1% of malignancies affecting the female genitalia and occurs almost exclusively in elderly women. Urethral bleeding, frequency, and dysuria are the most frequent presenting complaints. Tumors in the distal urethra usually give rise to symptoms early in their course (see *Table 2.9*). Most of these tumors arise in the distal urethra and are squamous cell carcinomas. Squamous cell carcinomas and transitional cell carcinomas may be papillary, forming papillomas or papillary carcinomas, or nonpapillary, presenting as carcinoma in situ of urothelial or squamous type or as solid high-grade urothelial carcinomas or squamous cell carcinomas. Urothelial (transitional cell) carcinomas may be seen in the distal as well as proximal urethra and have been described arising within a urethral diverticulum [6,108].

A pagetoid variant of urothelial carcinoma in situ has been described that primarily involves the bladder but is also described in the urethra [116]. Pagetoid urothelial intraepithelial neoplasia (PUIN) involving the urethral meatus and the vulvar vestibule, and clinically resembling vulvar Paget disease, has recently been described (see Paget Disease) [173]. Primary urothelial carcinomas express cytokeratin 7 and usually cytokeratin 20. In addition, uroplakin III is reported to be expressed in more than one half of primary urinary tract urothelial carcinoma cases studied and in approximately two thirds of the metastasis from urinary tract urothelial carcinomas [18].

Adenocarcinomas of the urethra are relatively rare, accounting for approximately 10% of all primary urethral carcinomas. They occur in the proximal urethra as well as within urethral diverticula [6]. Histopathologic types of adenocarcinoma include columnar/mucinous, clear cell, and colloid types [98,108,185]. Of these, clear cell adenocarcinoma of the urethra is of special interest in that this

Table 2.9
American Joint Committee on clinical staging of urethral carcinoma primary tumor (T), urethra

TX: Primary tumor cannot be assessed
T0: No evidence of primary tumor
Ta: Noninvasive papillary, polypoid, or verrucous carcinoma
Tis: Carcinoma in situ
T1: Tumor invades subepithelial connective tissue
T2: Tumor invades any of the following: periurethral muscle (in males includes corpus spongiosum and prostate)
T3: Tumor invades any of the following: anterior vagina, bladder neck
T4: Tumor invades other adjacent organs
Regional lymph nodes (N) related to urethral carcinoma are staged as follows:
NX: Regional lymph nodes cannot be assessed
NO: Ro regional lymph node metastasis
N1: Metastasis in a single lymph node, 2 cm or less in greatest dimension
N2: Metastasis in a single node more than 2 cm in greatest dimension, or in multiple nodes
Distant Metastasis (M)
MX: Distant metastasis cannot be assessed
M0: No distant metastasis
M1: Distant metastasis

Source: From [5].

tumor occurs in adults with a wide age range, has distinct immunohistochemical and morphologic features suggesting Müllerian differentiation, and appears to have a generally better prognosis, even with more advanced stages [45]. These tumors do not express prostate-specific antigen (PSA) or prostate acid phosphatase, and have tubulocystic, papillary, and diffuse patterns of growth similar to clear cell carcinomas of the female genital tract [45]. In one series, two thirds of the cases arose in a urethral diverticulum [115]. The differential diagnosis of these clear cell tumors includes metastatic tumor, mesonephric carcinoma, and nephrogenic metaplasia [108,185].

Primary adenocarcinomas arising in Skene glands and a periurethral cyst have also been reported [108,109]. Skene gland tumors are thought to arise from the luminal secretory cells of these glands and have been demonstrated to express PSA and prostate acid phosphatase, reflecting the homology between Skene periurethral glands and the prostate [149]. Both urethral squamous carcinomas and adenocarcinomas are usually immunoreactive for CEA.

The staging system for tumors of the urethra proposed by the AJCC is summarized in Table 2.9 [5].

The prognosis related to urethral carcinoma is relatively poor. Survival is better with tumors in the distal urethra, where 5-year survival may exceed 50%. Tumors in the proximal portions of the urethra have a poorer prognosis, and those patients with tumors involving the entire urethra have the poorest prognosis [108]. Survival in urethral carcinoma is influenced by the fact that up to one half of the women with urethral carcinoma have metastasis to superficial or deep pelvic nodes when first seen. Improved early detection, and individualized surgical and radiotherapy techniques, promise to substantially increase survival.

Other Malignant Tumors of the Urethra

Non-Hodgkin's lymphoma, [8,130], carcinosarcoma [90], and sarcomas have all been reported arising within the urethra. Urethral caruncles with atypical stromal cells, and a florid proliferation of reactive lymphoid cells, are the primary differential diagnosis in regard to lymphomas and sarcomas in this location [186]. Immunohistochemical studies to distinguish lymphocytic populations distinguish these benign processes from lymphoma. The atypical stromal cells in the urethral caruncles are immunoreactive for vimentin in approximately two thirds of the cases, and express alpha-smooth muscle actin in one half of cases [186].

A number of metastatic tumors may involve the urethra, either by direct mucosal growth or by lymphatic or vascular metastasis [108]. Metastatic involvement of the urethra from bladder carcinoma is observed in 8–16% of cases [27,101]. In these cases, direct mucosal-related metastasis and/or lymphatic metastasis may occur. Bladder neck involvement by the primary bladder carcinoma is the most significant risk factor for urethral involvement [27]. Metastatic tumors from vulvar, vaginal, cervical, or anal carcinomas, as well as endometrial and, rarely, ovarian carcinomas, may occur [70]. Metastatic ovarian carcinoma has been reported presenting as a urethral caruncle [70].

Gross Description, Processing and Reporting of Vulvar specimens

Vulvar Biopises

Vulvar biopsies may be diagnostic, where only a sampling of the lesion in question is made, or complete excisional, where the clinician attempts to excise the entire lesion. Diagnostic biopsies may be punch biopsies, such as performed with a Keyes punch biopsy, shave biopsies, or partial excisional biopsies, where a scalpel is used to excise a representative section of the lesion in question. Punch biopsies are usually preferred to evaluate inflammatory processes, such as lichen sclerosus, whereas excisional biopsies are preferred if the lesion is considered neoplastic and issues regarding possible invasive tumors are made. Shave biopsies are also useful for neoplastic lesions, provided issues such as depth of a tumor are not an issue. In general, vulvar biopsies should be handled like skin biopsies, and in all cases, effort should be made to keep the specimen well orientated so that on sectioning, right angle sections of the epithelial–dermal are made, to clearly identify the epithelial–dermal or mucosal stromal interface.

Several methods are in common use to assess both deep as well as lateral resection margins. Orientation is aided if the surgeon places a suture on one edge of the epithelium for orientation, or uses India ink, or tattoo dye to facilitate the recognition of the surface of the lesion. For lateral and deep margins one or more colored inks or dyes can be used to define the margins. Specimens should be sectioned into approximately 2 mm slices, with the plane of section at right angles to the surface of the specimen, and the entire specimen submitted for evaluation, unless it is very large in which case it is handled as any other partial vulvectomy. In most cases, several slices can be placed into a single cassette. Small punch biopsies are submitted totally and, when necessary, bisected perpendicular to the epithelial surface.

It is useful to request at the time of submission that the paraffin block(s) be cut at multiple levels. For example, cutting three sections from each block. This will usually give an excellent view of the lesion in question. This practice also shortens the turnaround time, since without it small biopsies frequently are sectioned inadequately the first time they are cut, often with only one section made. Remounting the block and cutting again to make additional slides takes more time than obtaining multiple levels at the onset, and may result in loss of valuable tissue.

Large Operative Specimens

Wide Local Excision (Partial Deep Vulvectomy) and Superficial Vulvectomy

Most specimens are highly variable in their composition, since these procedures are tailored to the extent of the lesion. Recently, wide local excision has been performed for Stage IA (<1 mm) invasive tumors, whereas laser techniques and/or topical medications are often used to treat vulvar intraepithelial neoplasia (VIN 3) or residual Paget disease once invasion has been excluded. The operative specimens may include all or part of the labia minora, labia majora, clitoris, perineal body, and perianal tissue without subcutaneous fat.

The gross description should specify the features and extent of the lesion as well as the anatomic structures involved. Since intraepithelial lesions are subtle, careful attention must be paid to coloration and surface texture. The lesions typically are red, brown, or white and often are roughened. They should be measured, and distances from the lesion to the resection margin should be recorded.

Because the disease process often is multifocal and difficult to discern with the naked eye, all surgical resection margins must be examined microscopically. This requires sections through all obvious lesions to rule out invasive carcinoma and sections from all the lateral resection margins. Sections parallel to the surgical margins (shave biopsies) often are taken to evaluate the excision lines, a method that uses fewer sections than those taken perpendicular to the line of resection. Multiple perpendicular sections, however, have the advantage that the central lesion, margin, and intervening areas can be included in one slide and tumor "close to" the margin is much easier to evaluate. To facilitate sectioning, pin the specimen on a corkboard or a block of paraffin and fix for 2–3 h before sectioning [31,171].

The surgical pathology report should include the microscopic diagnosis, extent of the involvement, and adequacy of the surgical resection margins (see: CAP synoptic reporting in this chapter) [31,171].

Total Vulvectomy: Superficial or Deep

The specimen includes the entire vulva. When superficial (skinning vulvectomy) is performed, the specimen consists of skin and minimal subcutaneous tissue. If deep, the excision includes the skin or mucosa, as well as the subcutaneous fat and skin adnexa, since the surgical dissection is carried down to the deep fascia. Superficial vulvectomy is used on occasion for extensive vulvar intraepithelial neoplasia. Total deep vulvectomy is performed primarily for larger invasive tumors, where deep partial vulvectomy is not considered adequate, or for extensive vulvar Paget disease where there may be serious concern for underlying or associated adenocarcinoma.

The gross description is similar to that outlined for the superficial vulvectomy. Although Paget disease of the vulva usually is an intraepithelial lesion, at times, it may be invasive or associated with an underlying sweat gland, Bartholin, or other carcinoma, and, therefore, the underlying subcutaneous tissue is removed. The specimen should be pinned, fixed, and then sectioned at approximately 0.5 cm intervals in order to evaluate adequately the underlying dermis for an invasive carcinoma. Microscopic involvement of Paget disease may exceed the visible extent of the lesion on gross examination. Occult foci of Paget disease also may be present within normal-appearing skin, and consequently the entire deep and lateral resection margins must be thoroughly evaluated in a similar manner as described for the superficial vulvectomy specimen. The surgical pathology report should include the microscopic diagnosis, extent of involvement, adequacy of the resection margins, and whether an underlying carcinoma is present (see: CAP synoptic reporting in this chapter) [31,171].

Total Deep Vulvectomy with En-Block Lymphadenectomy (Radical Vulvectomy, with Lymphadenectomy)

The specimen consists of the vulva, inguinal skin, subcutaneous tissue, femoral and inguinal lymph nodes, and portions of the saphenous veins. The procedure is performed for advanced invasive squamous carcinomas and has been somewhat superseded by total deep vulvectomy with separate incisions for inguinal–femoral lymphadenectomy.

The gross description should include the size, location, and depth of penetration of the primary lesion, and all resection margins, including the perirectal and vaginal margins. Examination often is aided if the specimen is first pinned out and fixed for a short period. Sections should include the tumor, showing the maximum depth of invasion, labia majora and minora, clitoris, resection margins including the vaginal margin, and all lymph nodes. Sections should evaluate the status of the skin immediately adjacent to the primary lesion, as preinvasive disease often is present. Separation of lymph nodes into superficial and deep groups requires communication with the gynecologic surgeon. Invasive vulvar neoplasms, in contrast to intraepithelial lesions, tend to be solitary and, consequently, evaluation of resection margins can be limited to the margins near the tumor. Because the specimen contains a considerable amount of fatty tissue, identification of lymph nodes may be difficult. In the fresh state, lymph nodes are recognized by palpation. The fatty tissue should be bread loafed at 1–2 cm intervals to allow adequate palpation and sectioning of node bearing tissue to identify as many nodes as possible. Location of lymph nodes is facilitated by an understanding of the lymphatic drainage of the vulva [31,171].

The surgical pathology report should include the microscopic diagnosis, tumor grade, dimensions, location and maximum depth of invasion, presence of lymphatic invasion, number and location of the involved lymph nodes, and status of resection margins [31,171] (see: CAP synoptic reporting in this chapter).

References

1. Abramova L, Parekh J, Irvin WP Jr, Rice LW, Taylor PT Jr, Anderson WA, Slingluff CL Jr (2002) Sentinel node biopsy in vulvar and vaginal melanoma: presentation of six cases and a literature review. Ann Surg Oncol 9(9):840–846
2. Al-Ghamdi A, Freedman D, Miller D, Poh C, Rosin M, Zhang L, Gilks CB (2002) Vulvar squamous cell carcinoma in young women: a clinicopathologic study of 21 cases. Gynecol Oncol 84(1):94–101
3. Al-Salameh A, Atawil A, Spiegal GW (2000) Absence of epithelial growth factor in anogenital Paget's disease argues against an origin from sweat glands. Mod Pathol 13:120A
4. American Cancer Society: Vulvar Cancer. State of Vulvar Cancer (2008) Cancer Facts & Figures 2008. American Cancer Society, Atlanta
5. American Joint Committee on Cancer. AJCC cancer staging handbook. In: AJCC cancer staging manual, 7th edn. (2010) Springer Science + Business, New York, NY, pp 463–467; pp 579–584
6. Amin MB, Young RH (1997) Primary carcinomas of the urethra. Semin Diagn Pathol 14:147–160
7. Androulaki A, Papathomas TG, Alexandrou P, Lazaris AC (2007) Metastatic low-grade endometrial stromal sarcoma of clitoris: report of a case. Int J Gynecol Cancer 17(1):290–293
8. Atalay AC, Karaman MI, Basak T et al (1998) Non-Hodgkin's lymphoma of the female urethra presenting as a caruncle. Int Urol Nephrol 30:609–610
9. Baehrendtz H, Einhorn N, Pettersson F, Silfversward C (1994) Paget's disease of the vulva: the radiumhemmet series 1975–1990. Int J Gynecol Cancer 4(1):1–6
10. Bannatyne P, Elliott P, Russell P (1989) Vulvar adenosquamous carcinoma arising in a hidradenoma papilliferum, with rapidly fatal outcome: case report. Gynecol Oncol 35(3):395–398
11. Benedet JL, Miller DM, Ehlen TG et al (1997) Basal cell carcinoma of the vulva: clinical features and treatment results in 28 patients. Obstet Gynecol 90:765–768
12. Benedet JL, Wilson PS, Matisic J (1991) Epidermal thickness and skin appendage involvement in vulvar intraepithelial neoplasia. J Reprod Med 36:608–612
13. Binder SW, Huang I, Fu YS et al (1990) Risk factors for the development of lymph node metastasis in vulvar squamous cell carcinoma. Gynecol Oncol 37:9–16
14. Brainard JA, Hart WR (2000) Proliferative epidermal lesions associated with anogenital Paget's disease. Am J Surg Pathol 24(4):543–552
15. Breslow A (1975) Tumor thickness, level of invasion and node dissection in stage I cutaneous melanoma. Ann Surg 182:572–575
16. Brinton LA, Nasca PC, Mallin K, Baptiste MS, Wilbanks GD, Richart RM (1990) Case-control study of cancer of the vulva. Obstet Gynecol 75:859–866
17. Brisigotti M, Moreno A, Murcia C et al (1989) Verrucous carcinoma of the vulva: a clinicopathologic and immunohistochemical study of five cases. Int J Gynecol Pathol 8:1–7
18. Brown HM, Wilkinson EJ (2002) Uroplakin-III to distinguish vulvar Paget disease secondary to urothelial carcinoma. Hum Pathol 33(5):545–548
19. Ca E, Bradley RR, Logsdon VK et al (1997) Vulvar melanoma in childhood. Arch Dermatol 133:345–348
20. Carlson JA, Ambros R, Malfetano J et al (1998) Vulvar lichen sclerosus and squamous cell carcinoma: a cohort, case control, and investigational study with historical perspective; implications for chronic inflammation and sclerosis in the development of neoplasia. Hum Pathol 29:932–948
21. Carlson JW, McGlennen RC, Gomez R et al (1996) Sebaceous carcinoma of the vulva: a case report and review of the literature. Gynecol Oncol 60:489–491
22. Carr KA, Bulengo S, Weiss LM et al (1992) Lymphoepithelioma-like carcinoma of the skin. Am J Surg Pathol 16:909–913
23. Caterson RJ, Furber J, Murray J et al (1984) Carcinoma of the vulva in two young renal allograft recipients. Transplant Proc 16:559
24. Chafe W, Richards A, Morgan L et al (1988) Unrecognized invasive carcinoma in vulvar intraepithelial neoplasia (VIN). Gynecol Oncol 31:154–162
25. Chang AE, Karnell LH, Menck HR (1998) The national cancer data base report on cutaneous and noncutaneous melanoma: a summary of 84, 836 cases from the past decade. The American College of surgeons Commission on Cancer and the American Cancer Society. Cancer 83:1664–1678
26. Chen KT (1994) Merkel's cell (neuroendocrine) carcinoma of the vulva. Cancer (Phila) 73:2186–2191
27. Chen ME, Pisters LL, Malpica A et al (1997) Risk of urethral, vaginal and cervical involvement in patients undergoing radical cystectomy for bladder cancer: results of a contemporary cystectomy series from M.D. Anderson Cancer Center. J Urol 157:2120–2123
28. Chiesa-Vottero A, Dvoretsky PM, Hart WR (2006) Histopathologic study of thin vulvar squamous cell carcinomas and associated cutaneous lesions: a correlative study of 48 tumors in 44 patients with analysis of adjacent vulvar intraepithelial neoplasia types and lichen sclerosus. Am J Surg Pathol 30(3):310–8
29. Cliby W, Soisson AP, Berchuck A et al (1991) Stage I small cell carcinoma of the vulva treated with vulvectomy, lymphadenectomy, and adjuvant chemo-therapy. Cancer (Phila) 67:2415–2417
30. Colgan TJ (1998) Vulvar intraepithelial neoplasia: a synopsis of recent developments. J Low Genital Tract Dis 2:31–36
31. College of American Pathologists: Surgical Pathology Cancer Case Summary (Checklist); Vulva: Excisional Biopsy, Resection. Author: Branton, PA., Protocol revision date: January 2005: www.CAP.org
32. Copas P, Dyer M, Comas FV et al (1982) Spindle cell carcinoma of the vulva. Diagn Gynecol Obstet 4:235–235
33. Cooper WA, Valmadre S, Russell P (2002) Sarcomatoid squamous cell carcinoma of the vulva. Pathology 34(2):197–199
34. Copeland LJ, Cleary K, Sneige N et al (1985) Neuroendocrine (Merkle cell) carcinoma of the vulva: a case report and review of the literature. Gynecol Oncol 22:367–378

35. Copeland LJ, Sneige N, Gershenson DM et al (1986) Bartholin gland carcinoma. Obstet Gynecol 67:794–801
36. Copeland LJ, Sneige N, Gershenson DM et al (1986) Adenoid cystic carcinoma of Bartholin's gland. Obstet Gynecol 67:115–120
37. Crawford D, Nimmo M, Clement PB et al (1999) Prognostic factors in Paget's disease of the Crum CP, Liskow A, Petras P, Keng WC, Frick HC II. Vulvar intraepithelial neoplasia (severe atypia and carcinoma in situ). A clinicopathologic analysis of 41 cases. Cancer 1984;54:1429–1434
38. de Giorgi V, Massi D, Salvini C, Mannone F, Cattaneo A, Carli P (2005) Thin melanoma of the vulva: a clinical, dermoscopic-pathologic case study. Arch Dermatol 141(8):1046–1047
39. DeHulla JA, Doting E, Piers DA et al (1998) Sentinel lymph node identification with technetium-99 m-labeled noncolloid in squamous cell cancer of the vulva. J Nucl Med 39:1381–1385
40. DePasquale SE, McGuinness TB, Mangan CE et al (1996) Adenoid cystic carcinoma of Bartholin's gland: a review of the literature and report of a patient. Gynecol Oncol 61:122–125
41. De Simone P, Silipo V, Buccini P, Mariani G, Marenda S, Eibenschutz L, Ferrari A, Catricalà C (2008) Vulvar melanoma: a report of 10 cases and review of the literature. Melanoma Res 18(2):127–133. Review
42. Dinh TV, Powell LC, Hanninan EV et al (1988) Simultaneously occurring condylomata acuminata, carcinoma in situ and verrucous carcinoma of the vulva and carcinoma in situ of the cervix in a young woman. J Reprod Med 33:510–513
43. Downey GO, Okagaki T, Ostrow RS et al (1988) Condylomatous carcinoma of the vulva with special reference to human papillomavirus DNA. Obstet Gynecol 72:68–72
44. Drew PA, Al-Abbadi MA, Orlando C et al (1996) Prognostic factors in carcinoma of the vulva: a clinicopathologic and DNA flow cytometric study. Int J Gynecol Pathol 15:235–241
45. Drew PA, Murphy WM, Civantos F et al (1996) The histogenesis of clear cell adenocarcinoma of the lower urinary tract. Case series and review of the literature. Hum Pathol 27:248–252
46. Dubé V, Veilleux C, Plante M, Têtu B (2004) Primary villoglandular adenocarcinoma of cloacogenic origin of the vulva. Hum Pathol 35(3):377–379
47. Egan CA, Bradley RR, Logsdon VK, Summers BK, Hunter GR, Vanderhooft SL (1997) Vulvar melanoma in childhood. Arch Dermatol 133(3):345–348
48. Ehrmann RL, Dwyer IM, Yavner BA, Hancock WW (1988) An immunoperoxidase study of laminin and type IV collagen distribution in carcinoma of the cervix and vulva. Obstet Gynecol 72:257–262
49. Ellis PE, Cano SD, Fear M, Kelsell DP, Ghali L, Crow JC, Perrett CW, MacLean AB (2008) Reduced E-cadherin expression correlates with disease progression in Paget's disease of the vulva but not Paget's disease of the breast. Mod Pathol 21(10):1192–1199. Epub 2008 May 9
50. Emanuels AG, Burger MP, Hollema H et al (1996) Quantitation of proliferation-associated markers Ag-NOR and Ki-67 does not contribute to the prediction of lymph node metastases in squamous cell carcinoma of the vulva. Hum Pathol 27:807–811
51. Erşahin C, Omeroglu G, Potkul RK, Salhadar A (2007) Myeloid sarcoma of the vulva as the presenting symptom in a patient with acute myeloid leukemia. Gynecol Oncol 106(1):259–261
52. Escalonilla P, Grilli R, Canamero M et al (1999) Sebaceous carcinoma of the vulva. Am J Dermatopathol 21:468–472
53. Esquius J, Brisigotti M, Matias-Guiu X et al (1991) Keratin expression in normal vulva, non-neoplastic epithelial disorders, vulvar intraepithelial neoplasia, and invasive squamous cell. Int J Gynecol Pathol 10:341–355
54. Ewing TL (1991) Paget's disease of the vulva treated by combined surgery and laser. Gynecol Oncol 43:137–140
55. Fanning J, Lambert HC, Hale TM et al (1999) Paget's disease of the vulva: prevalence of associated vulvar adenocarcinoma, invasive Paget's disease, and recurrence after surgical excision. Am J Obstet Gynecol 180:24–27
56. Feakins RM, Lowe DG (1997) Basal cell carcinoma of the vulva: a clinicopathologic study of 45 cases. Int J Gynecol Pathol 16:319–324
57. Flanagan CW, Parker JR, Mannel RS et al (1997) Primary endodermal sinus tumor of the vulva: a case report and review of the literature. Gynecol Oncol 66:515–518
58. Friedrich EG Jr, Wilkinson EJ, Fu YS (1980) Carcinoma in situ of the vulva: a continuing challenge. Am J Obstet Gynecol 136: 830–843
59. Fu YS, Reagan JW, Townsend DE et al (1981) Nuclear DNA study of vulvar intraepithelial and invasive squamous neoplasms. Obstet Gynecol 57:643–652
60. Fuste V, Alejo M, Clavero O et al (2009) HPV negative vuvar intraepithelial neoplasia (VIN) with basaloid features. An unrecognized variant of simplex (differentiated) VIN. Modern Pathol 22;1:214A
61. Ganjei P, Giraldo KA, Lampe B et al (1990) Vulvar Paget's disease. Is immunocytochemistry helpful in assessing the surgical margins? J Reprod Med 35:1002–1004
62. Gil-Moreno A, Garcia-Jimenez A, Gonzalez-Bosquet J et al (1997) Merkel cell carcinoma of the vulva. Gynecol Oncol 64:526–532
63. Gordon AN (1991) Current concepts in the treatment of invasive vulvar carcinoma. Clin Obstet Gynecol 34:587–598
64. Graf AH, Su HC, Tubbs RR et al (1998) Primary neuroendocrine differentiated mucinous adenocarcinoma of the vulva: case report and review of the literature. Anticancer Res 18:2041–2045
65. Grin A, Colgan T, Laframboise S, Shaw P, Ghazarian D (2008) "Pagetoid" eccrine carcinoma of the vulva: report of an unusual case with review of the literature. J Low Genit Tract Dis 12(2):134–139
66. Gunn RA, Gallager HS (1980) Vulvar Paget's disease: a topographic study. Cancer (Phila) 46:590–594
67. Hacker NF, Berek JS, Lagasse LD et al (1984) Individualization of treatment for stage I squamous cell vulvar carcinoma. Obstet Gynecol 63:155–162
68. Hacker NF, Nieberg RK, Berek JS et al (1983) Superficially invasive vulvar cancer with nodal metastases. Gynecol Oncol 15:65–77
69. Haefner HK, Tate JE, McLachlin CM et al (1995) Vulvar intraepithelial neoplasia: age, morphological phenotype, papillomavirus DNA, and coexisting invasive carcinoma. Hum Pathol 26:147–154
70. Hammadeh MY, Thomas K, Philp T (1996) Urethral caruncle: an unusual presentation of ovarian tumour. Gynecol Obstet Invest 42:279–280
71. Hart WR (2001) Vulvar intraepithelial neoplasia: historical aspects and current status. Int J Gynecol Pathol 20(1):16–30
72. Hatch KD, Davis JR (2008) Complete resolution of Paget disease of the vulva with imiquimod cream. J Low Genit Tract Dis 12(2):90–94
73. Heaps JM, Fu YS, Montz FJ et al (1990) Surgical-pathologic variables predictive of local recurrence in squamous cell carcinoma of the vulva. Gynecol Oncol 38:309–314
74. Heard I, Kazatchkine MD (1999) Regression of cervical lesions in HIV-infected women receiving HAART. AIDS Read 9:630–635

75. Hendricks JB, Wilkinson EJ, Kubilis P et al (1994) Ki-67 expression in vulvar carcinoma. Int J Gynecol Pathol 13:205–210
76. Herod JJ, Shafi MI, Rollason TP et al (1996) Vulvar intraepithelial neoplasia with superficially invasive carcinoma of the vulva. Br J Obstet Gynaecol 103:453–456
77. Hill SJ, Berkowitz R, Granter SR, Hirsch MS (2008) Pagetoid lesions of the vulva: a collision between malignant melanoma and extramammary Paget disease. Int J Gynecol Pathol 27(2):292–296
78. Homesley HD, Bundy BN, Sedlis A et al (1991) Assessment of current international federation of gynecology and obstetrics staging of vulvar carcinoma relative to prognostic factors for survival (a gynecologic oncology group study). Am J Obstet Gynecol 164:997–1004
79. Horn LC, Liebert UG, Edelmann J, Höckel M, Einenkel J (2008) Adenoid squamous carcinoma (pseudoangiosarcomatous carcinoma) of the vulva: a rare but highly aggressive variant of squamous cell carcinoma-report of a case and review of the literature. Int J Gynecol Pathol 27(2):288–291. Review
80. Husseinzadeh N, Recinto C (1999) Frequency of invasive cancer in surgically excised vulvar lesions with intraepithelial neoplasia (VIN 3). Gynecol Oncol 73:119–120
81. Husseinzadeh N, Zaino R, Nahhas WA, et al (1983) The significance of histologic findings in predicting nodal metastasis in invasive squamous cell carcinoma of the vulva. Gynecol Oncol 16:105–111
82. Irvin PW, Legallo RL, Stoler MH, Rice LW, Taylor PT Jr, Andersen WA (2001) Vulvar melanoma: a retrospective analysis and literature review. Gynecol Oncol 83:457–465
83. Issa PY, Salem PA, Brihi E et al (1980) Eosinophilic granuloma with involvement of the female genitalia. Am J Obstet Gynecol 137:608
84. Iversen T, Andreasson B, Bryson SCP et al (1990) Surgical-procedure terminology for the vulva and vagina: a report of an international society for the study of vulvar disease task force. J Reprod Med 35:1033–1034
85. Jones RW, Rowan DM (1994) Vulvar intraepithelial neoplasia. III: A clinical study of the outcome in 113 cases with relation to the later development of invasive vulvar carcinoma (see comments). Obstet Gynecol 84:741–745
86. Jones RW, Rowan DM, Stewart AW (2005) Vulvar intraepithelial neoplasia: aspects of the natural history and outcome in 405 women. Obstet Gynecol 106(6):1319–1326
87. Judson LJ, Habermann EB, Baxter NN, Durham SB, Virnig BA (2006). Trends in the incidence of invasive and in situ vulvar carcinoma. Obstet Gynecol 107:1018–1012
88. Kim YT, Thomas NF, Kessis TD, et al (1996) p53 mutations and clonality in vulvar carcinomas and squamous hyperplasias: evidence suggesting that squamous hyperplasias do not serve as direct precursors of human papillomavirus-negative vulvar carcinomas. Hum Pathol 27:389
89. Kneale BL (1984) Microinvasive cancer of the vulva: report of the international society for the study of vulvar disease task force, VIIth congress. J Reprod Med 29:454–456
90. Konno N, Mori M, Kurooka Y et al (1997) Carcinosarcoma in the region of the female urethra. Int J Urol 4:229–231
91. Kruse AJ, Bottenberg MJ, Tosserams J, Slangen B, van Marion AM, van Trappen PO (2008) The absence of high-risk HPV combined with specific p53 and p16INK4a expression patterns points to the HPV-independent pathway as the causative agent for vulvar squamous cell carcinoma and its precursor simplex VIN in a young patient. Int J Gynecol Pathol 27(4):591–595
92. Kurman RJ, Norris HJ, Wilkinson EJ (1992) Tumors of the cervix, vagina and vulva. In Atlas of Tumor Pathology, Fascicle 3. Armed Forces Institute of Pathology, Washington, DC (Fascicle 4: Kurman R, Ronette B, and Wilkinson EJ, in press, 2010)
93. Kurman RJ, Toki T, Schiffman MH (1993) Basaloid and warty carcinomas of the vulva. Distinctive types of squamous cell carcinoma frequently associated with human papillomaviruses. Am J Surg Pathol 17:133–145
94. Lerma E, Esteller M, Herman JG, Prat J (2002) Alterations of the p16^{INK4a}/Rb/Cyclin-D1 pathway in vulvar carcinoma, vulvar intraepithelial neoplasia, and lichen sclerosus. Hum Pathol 33(11): 1120–1125
95. Leuchter RS, Hacker NF, Voet RL et al (1982) Primary carcinoma of the Bartholin gland: a report of 14 cases and review of the literature. Obstet Gynecol 60:361–368
96. Logani S, Lu D, Quint WG, Ellenson LH, Pirog EC (2003) Low-grade vulvar and vaginal intraepithelial neoplasia: correlation of histologic features with human papillomavirus DNA detection and MIB-1 immunostaining. Mod Pathol 16(8):735–741
97. Lomo L, Crum CP (2004) Papillary carcinoma of the vulva. Mod Pathol 17:204a
98. Loo KT, Chan JKC (1992) Colloid adenocarcinoma of the urethra associated with mucosal in situ carcinoma. Arch Pathol Lab Med 116:976–977
99. MacLean AB, Makwana M, Ellis PE, Cunnington F (2004) The management of Paget's disease of the vulva. J Obstet Gynaecol 24(2):124–128
100. Magrina JF, Gonzalez-Bosquet J, Weaver AL et al (2000) Squamous cell carcinoma of the vulva stage IA: long-term results. Gynecol Oncol 76:24–27
101. Maralani S, Wood DP Jr, Grignon D et al (1997) Incidence of urethral involvement in female bladder cancer: an anatomic pathologic study. Urology 50:537–541
102. Mazur MT, Hsueh S, Gersell DJ (1984) Metastases to the female genital tract: analysis of 325 cases. Cancer (Phila) 53:1978–1984
103. McLachlin CM, Kozakewich H, Craighill M et al (1994) Histologic correlates of vulvar human papillomavirus infection in children and young adults. Am J Surg Pathol 18:728–735
104. Mirhashemi R, Kratz A, Weir MM et al (1998) Vaginal small cell carcinoma mimicking a Bartholin's gland abscess: a case report. Gynecol Oncol 68:297–300
105. Moore RG, DePasquale SE, Steinhoff MM, Gajewski W, Steller M, Noto R, Falkenberry S (2003) Sentinel node identification and the ability to detect metastatic tumor to inguinal lymph nodes in squamous cell cancer of the vulva. Gynecol Oncol 89(3):475–479
106. Morgan LS, Joslyn P, Chafe W et al (1988) A report on 18 cases of primary malignant melanoma of the vulva. Colp Las Sur 4:161–170
107. Mulayim N, Foster Silver D, Tolgay Ocal I, Babalola E (2002) Vulvar basal cell carcinoma: two unusual presentations and review of the literature. Gynecol Oncol 85(3):532–537
108. Murphy WM, Grignon DJ, Perlman EJ (2004) Tumors of the Kidney, Bladder, and Related Urinary Structures, vol 4, AFIP Atlas of Tumor Pathology. American Registry of Pathology, Washington DC, pp 263–273
109. Nagano M, Hasui Y, Ide H, Itoi T, Takehara T, Osada Y (2002) Primary adenocarcinoma arising from a paraurethral cyst in a female patient. Urol Int 69(3):244–246
110. Nascimento AF, Granter SR, Cviko A, Yuan L, Hecht JL, Crum CP (2004) Vulvar acanthosis with altered differentiation: a precursor to verrucous carcinoma. Am J Surg Pathol 28(5):638–643

111. Neto AG, Deavers MT, Silva EG, Malpica A (2003) Metastatic tumors of the vulva a clinicopathologic study of 66 cases. Am J Surg Pathol 27(6):799–804
112. Niebyl JR, Genadry R, Friedrich EG et al (1975) Vulvar carcinoma with hypercalcemia. Obstet Gynecol 45:343–348
113. Nowak MA, Guerriere-Kovach P, Pathan A et al (1998) Perianal Paget's disease: distinguishing primary and secondary lesions using immunohistochemical studies including gross cystic disease fluid protein-15 and cytokeratin 20 expression. Arch Pathol Lab Med 122:1077–1081
114. Obermair A, Koller S, Crandon AJ, Perrin L, Nicklin JL (2001) Primary Bartholin gland carcinoma: a report of seven cases. Aust NZ J Obstet Gynaecol 41(1):78–81
115. Oliva E, Young RH (1996) Clear cell adenocarcinoma of the urethra: a clinicopathologic analysis of 19 cases. Mod Pathol 9:513–520
116. Orozco RE, Vander ZR, Murphy WM (1993) The pagetoid variant of urothelial carcinoma in situ. Hum Pathol 24:1199–1202
117. Park JS, Jones RW, McLean MR et al (1991) Possible etiologic heterogeneity of vulvar intraepithelial neoplasia. A correlation of pathologic characteristics with human papillomavirus detection by in situ hybridization and polymerase chain reaction. Cancer (Phila) 67:1599–1607
118. Pinto AP, Signorello LB, Crum CP et al (1999) Squamous cell carcinoma of the vulva in Brazil: prognostic importance of host and viral variables. Gynecol Oncol 74:61–67
119. Piura B, Rabinovich A, Dgani R (1999) Basal cell carcinoma of the vulva. J Surg Oncol 70:172–176
120. Piura B, Rabinovich A, Dgani R (1999) Malignant melanoma of the vulva: report of six cases and review of the literature. Eur J Gynaecol Oncol 20:182–186
121. Plouffe L, Tulandi T, Rosenberg A et al (1984) Non-Hodgkin's lymphoma in Bartholin's gland: case report and review of literature. Am J Obstet Gynecol 148:608–609
122. Preti M, Micheletti L, Barbero M et al (1993) Histologic parameters of vulvar invasive carcinoma and lymph node metastases. J Reprod Med 38:28–32
123. Preti M, Micheletti L, Massobrio M, Ansai SI, Wilkinson EJ (2003) Vulvar paget disease: one century after first reported. J Low Genit Tract Dis 7(2):122–135
124. Rabah R, Farmer D (1999) Squamous cell carcinoma of the vulva in a child. J Low Genit Tract Dis 3:204–206
125. Raju RR, Goldblum JR, Hart WR (2003) Pagetoid squamous cell carcinoma in situ (Pagetoid Bowen's Disease) of the external genitalia. Int J Gynecol Pathol 22(2):127–135
126. Ragnarsson-Olding BK, Nilsson BR, Kanter-Lewensohn LR et al (1999) Malignant melanoma of the vulva in a nationwide, 25–year study of 219 Swedish females: predictors of survival. Cancer (Phila) 86:1285–1293
127. Raspagliesi F, Ditto A, Paladini D et al (2000) Prognostic indicators in melanoma of the vulva. Ann Surg Oncol 7(10):738–742
128. Redman R, Massoll NA, Wilkinson EJ (2005) Association between invasive squamous cell carcinoma of the vulva and ABO blood group. J Low Genit Tract Dis 9(2):89–92
129. Riethdorf S, Neffen EF, Cviko A, Löning T, Crum CP, Riethdorf L (2004) p16INK4A expression as biomarker for HPV 16-related vulvar neoplasias. Hum Pathol 35(12):1477–1483
130. Rikaniadis N, Konstadoulakis MM, Kymionis GD et al (1998) Long-term survival of a female patient with primary malignant melanoma of the urethra. Eur J Surg Oncol 24:607–608
131. Rocconi RP, Leath CA 3rd, Johnson WM 3rd, Barnes MN 3rd, Conner MG (2004) Primary lung large cell carcinoma metastatic to the vulva: a case report and review of the literature. Gynecol Oncol 94(3):829–831. Review
132. Rodke G, Friedrich EG Jr, Wilkinson EJ (1988) Malignant potential of mixed vulvar dystrophy (lichen sclerosis associated with squamous cell hyperplasia). J Reprod Med 33:545–550
133. Rufforny I, Wilkinson EJ, Liu C, Zhu H, Buteral M, Massoll NA (2005) Human papillomavirus infection and p16ink4a protein expression in vulvar intraepithelial neoplasia and invasive squamous cell carcinoma. J Low Genit Tract Dis 9 (2):108–113
134. Samama B, Lipsker D, Boehm N (2006) p16 expression in relation to human papillomavirus in anogenital lesions. Hum Pathol 37(5):513–519
135. Santeusanio G, Schiaroli S, Anemona L et al (1991) Carcinoma of the vulva with sarcomatoid features: a case report with immunohistochemical study. Gynecol Oncol 40:160–163
136. Santos LD, Krivanek MJ, Chan F, Killingsworth M (2006) Pseudoangiosarcomatous squamous cell carcinoma of the vulva. Pathology 38(6):581–584
137. Santos M, Montagut C, Mellado B et al (2004) Immunohistochemical Staining for p16 and p53 in Premalignant and Malignant Epithelial Lesions of the Vulva. Int J Gynecol Pathol 23:206–214
138. Scheistroen M, Trope C, Kaern J et al (1997) DNA ploidy and expression of p53 and C-erbB-2 in extrammammary Paget's disease of the vulva. Gynecol Oncol 64:88–92
139. Scully RE, BonfiglioTA KRJ, Silverberg SG, Wilkinson EJ (1994) Histological typing of female genital tract tumors, World Health Organization international histological classification of tumors, 2nd edn. Springer, New York
140. Scurry J, Beshay V, Cohen C et al (1998) Ki67 expression in lichen sclerosus of vulva in patients with and without associated squamous cell carcinoma. Histopathology (Oxf) 32:399–404
141. Scurry J, Brand A, Planner R et al (1996) Vulvar Merkel cell tumor with glandular and squamous differentiation. Gynecol Oncol 62:292–297
142. Sedlis A, Homesley H, Bundy BN et al (1987) Positive groin lymph nodes in superficial squamous cell vulvar cancer: a gynecologic oncology group study. Am J Obstet Gynecol 156:1159–1164
143. Shah SS, Adelson M, Mazur MT (2008) Adenocarcinoma in situ arising in vulvar papillary hidradenoma: report of 2 cases. Int J Gynecol Pathol 27(3):453–456
144. Shatz P, Bergeron C, Wilkinson EJ et al (1989) Vulvar intraepithelial neoplasia and skin appendage involvement. Obstet Gynecol 74:769–774
145. Sheen-Chen SM, Eng HL, Huang CC (2004) Breast cancer metastatic to the vulva. Gynecol Oncol 94(3):858–860
146. Short KA, Kalu G, Mortimer PS, Higgins EM (2005) Vulval squamous cell carcinoma arising in chronic hidradenitis suppurative. Clin Exp Dermatol 30(5):481–483
147. Sideri M, Jones RW, Wilkinson EJ, Preti M, Heller DS, Scurry J, Haefner H, Neill S (2005) Squamous vulvar intraepithelial neoplasia: 2004 modified terminology, ISSVD vulvar oncology subcommittee. J Reprod Med 50(11):807–810
148. Skapa P, Zamecnik J, Hamsikova E, Salakova M, Smahelova J, Jandova K, Robova H, Rob L, Tachezy R (2007) Human papillomavirus (HPV) profiles of vulvar lesions: possible implications for the classification of vulvar squamous cell carcinoma precursors and for the efficacy of prophylactic HPV vaccination. Am J Surg Pathol 31(12):1834–1843

149. Sloboda J, Zaviacic M, Jakubovsky J et al (1998) Metastasizing adenocarcinoma of the female prostate (Skene's paraurethral glands). Histological and immunohistochemical prostate markers studies and first ultrastructural observation. Pathol Res Pract 194:129–136
150. Snow SN, DeSouky S, Lo JS et al (1992) Failure to detect human papillomavirus DNA in extramammary Paget's disease. Cancer (Phila) 69:249–251
151. Spatz A, Zimmermann U, Bachollet B, Pautier P, Michel G, Duvillard P (1998) Malignant blue nevus of the vulva with late ovarian metastasis. Am J Dermatopathol 20(4):408–412
152. Srodon M, Stoler MH, Baber GB, Kurman RJ (2006) The distribution of low and high risk HPV types in vulvar and vaginal intraepithelial neoplasia (VIN and VaIN). Am J Surg Pathol 30(12):1513–1518
153. Steeper TA, Piscioli F, Rosai J (1983) Squamous cell carcinoma with sarcoma-like stroma of the female genital tract. Clinicopathologic study of four cases. Cancer (Phila) 52:890–898
154. Stehman FB, Bundy BN, Dvoretsky PM et al (1992) Early stage I carcinoma of the vulva treated with ipsilateral superficial inguinal lymphadenectomy and modified radical hemivulvectomy: a prospective study of the gynecologic oncology group. Obstet Gynecol 79:490–497
155. Sturgeon SR, Brinton LA, Devesa SS et al (1992) In situ and invasive vulvar cancer incidence trends (1973–1987). Am J Obstet Gynecol 166:1482
156. Todd RW, Etherington IJ, Luesley DM (2002) The effects of 5% imiquimod cream on high-grade vulval intraepithelial neoplasia. Gynecol Oncol 85(1):67–70
157. Toki T, Kurman RJ, Park JS et al (1991) Probable nonpapillomavirus etiology of squamous cell carcinoma of the vulva in older women: a clinicopathologic study using in situ. Int J Gynecol Pathol 10:107–125
158. Tran TA, Carlson JA (2008) Plasmacytoid squamous cell carcinoma of the vulva. Int J Gynecol Pathol 27(4):601–605
159. Trimble EL (1996) Melanomas of the vulva and vagina. Oncology (Basel) 10:1017–1023
160. Trimble CL, Diener-West M, Wilkinson EJ et al (1999) Reproducibility of the histopathological classification of vulvar squamous carcinoma and intraepithelial neoplasia. J Low Genit Tract Dis 3:98–103
161. Tuder RM (1992) Vulvar destruction by malignant lymphoma. Gynecol Oncol 45:52–57
162. Van der Putte SCJ (1994) Mammary-like glands of the vulva and their disorders. Int J Gynecol Pathol 13:150–160
163. van Seters M, van Beurden M, ten Kate FJ, Beckmann I, Ewing PC, Eijkemans MJ, Kagie MJ, Meijer CJ, Aaronson NK, Kleinjan A, Heijmans-Antonissen C, Zijlstra FJ, Burger MP, Helmerhorst TJ (2008) Treatment of vulvar intraepithelial neoplasia with topical imiquimod. New Engl J Med 358(14):1465–1473
164. Vang R, Medeiros LJ, Malpica A, Levenback C, Deavers M (2000) Non-Hodgkin's lymphoma involving the vulva. Int J Gynecol Pathol 19(3):236–242
165. Verschraegen CF, Benjapibal M, Supakarapongkul W, Levy LB, Ross M, Atkinson EN, Bodurka-Bevers D, Kavanagh JJ, Kudelka AP, Legha SS (2001) Vulvar melanoma at the M. D. Anderson Cancer Center: 25 years later. Int J Gynecol Cancer 11(5):359–364
166. Wade TR, Kopf AW, Ackerman AB (1979) Bowenoid papulosis of the genitalia. Arch Dermatol 115:306–308
167. Wechter ME, Reynolds RK, Haefner HK, Lowe L, Gruber SB, Schwartz JL, Johnston CM, Johnson TM (2004) Vulvar melanoma: review of diagnosis, staging, and therapy. J Low Genit Tract Dis 8(1):58–69
168. Wheelock JB, Goplerud DR, Dunn LJ et al (1984) Primary carcinoma of the Bartholin gland: a report of ten cases. Obstet Gynecol 63:820–824
169. Wick MR, Goellner JR, Wolfe JT et al (1985) Vulvar sweat gland carcinoma. Arch Pathol Lab Med 109:43–47
170. Wilkinson EJ (1991) Superficially invasive carcinoma of the vulva. Clin Obstet Gynecol 34:651–661
171. Wilkinson EJ (2000) Protocol for the examination of specimens from patients with carcinomas and malignant melanomas of the vulva: a basis for checklists. Cancer Committee of the College of American Pathologists. Arch Pathol Lab Med 124:51–56: Revised 2005
172. Wilkinson EJ, Brown H (2001) Vulvar pagetoid urothelial intraepithelial neoplasia (PUIN). Mod Pathol 13:134A
173. Wilkinson EJ, Brown HM (2002) Vulvar Paget disease of urothelial origin: a report of three cases and a proposed classification of vulvar Paget disease. Hum Pathol 33(5):549–554
174. Wilkinson EJ, Stone IK (2008) Atlas of vulvar disease, 2nd edn. Wolters Kluwer/Lippincott Williams and Wilkins Publishers, Philadelphia, PA
175. Wilkinson EJ, Teixeira MR (2003) The Vulva. In: Tavassoli FA, Deville T (eds) World health organization classification of tumours: pathology & genetics, tumours of the breast and female genital organs. IARC Press, Lyon, France, pp 316–326
176. Wilkinson EJ, Cook JC, Friedrich EG Jr et al (1988) Vulvar intraepithelial neoplasia: association with cigarette smoking. Colp Gynecol Las Sur 4:153–159
177. Wilkinson EJ, Croker BP, Friedrich EG Jr et al (1988) Two distinct pathologic types of giant cell tumor of the vulva: a report of two cases. J Reprod Med 33:519–522
178. Wilkinson EJ, Friedrich EG Jr, Fu YS (1981) Multicentric nature of vulvar carcinoma in situ. Obstet Gynecol 58:69–74
179. Wilkinson EJ, Morgan LS, Friedrich EG Jr (1984) Association of Franconi's anemia and squamous-cell carcinoma of the lower female genital tract with condyloma acuminatum. J Reprod Med 29:447–453
180. Wilkinson EJ, Kneale B, Lynch PJ (1986) Report of the ISSVD terminology committee. Proc VIII world congress, Stockholm, Sweden. J Reprod Med 31:973–974
181. Willen R, Bekassy Z, Carlen B, Bozoky B, Cajander S (1999) Cloacogenic adenocarinoma of the vulva. Gynecol Oncol 74(2): 298–301
182. Woolcott RJ, Henry RJ, Houghton CR (1988) Malignant melanoma of the vulva. J Reprod Med 33:699–702
183. Yang B, Hart WR (2000) Vulvar intraepithelial neoplasia of the simplex (differentiated) type: a clinicopathologic study including analysis of HPV and p53 expression. Am J Surg Pathol 24:429–441
184. Yoder BJ, Rufforny I, Massoll N, Wilkinson E (2008) Stage IA vulvar squamous cell carcinoma; an analysis of tumor invasive characteristics and risk. Am J Surg Pathol 32(5):765–772
185. Young RH, Scully RE (1985) Clear cell adenocarcinoma of the bladder and urethra. Am J Surg Pathol 9:816–826
186. Young RH, Oliva E, Garcia JA et al (1996) Urethral caruncle with atypical stromal cells simulating lymphoma or sarcoma – a distinctive pseudoneoplastic lesion of females. A report of six cases. Am J Surg Pathol 20:1190–1195
187. Zaidi SN, Conner MG (2001) Primary vulvar adenocarcinoma of cloacogenic origin. South Med J 94(7):744–746

3 Diseases of the Vagina

Richard J. Zaino · Marisa Nucci · Robert J. Kurman

R. J. Kurman, L. Hedrick Ellenson, B. M. Ronnett (eds.), *Blaustein's Pathology of the Female Genital Tract (6th ed.)*, DOI 10.1007/978-1-4419-0489-8_3,

The vagina, like other orifices that interface between the external environment and the interior milieu, acts as a barrier to many potentially invasive microorganisms. It is, thus, not surprising that the vagina is the site of a variety of infections, both sexually and nonsexually transmitted, and this, in fact, represents the predominant type of pathology of this organ. In contrast, neoplasms are relatively unusual in this site, which is somewhat unexpected in view of the relationship between infection (e.g., human papilloma virus infection) and the development of carcinoma of the vulva and cervix.

Because of its profound effects on the development of the vagina, the pathology of in utero diethylstilbestrol (DES) exposure has been integrated into the Developmental Disorders and Malignant Neoplasms sections of this chapter. This well-intended therapy for women with a history of early pregnancy loss had serious and wholly unexpected consequences that prompted research that elucidated many interrelationships among embryology, anatomy, physiology, and neoplasia of the vagina. The astute reader will note, however, that the failure to identify many aspects relating to the pathogenesis of numerous other diseases of the vagina reflects our current state of ignorance.

Development

The müllerian ducts first appear as funnel-shaped openings of the coelomic epithelium in the mesonephric ridge at about postconception day 37 [50]. They grow caudally as paired tubes, extending to meet the posterior wall of the urogenital sinus. At about day 54, the caudal portions of the müllerian ducts fuse, forming a straight uterovaginal canal that is lined by simple columnar epithelium. The uterovaginal canal continues to elongate caudally until about day 66. Shortly thereafter, the epithelium from the caudal tip of the canal to the external cervical os changes to a stratified squamous type; this results from a migration of squamous cells from the urogenital sinus, rather than from squamous metaplasia of the native müllerian columnar epithelium [242]. Continued stratification of the squamous epithelial lining progressively occludes the more caudal portion of the canal, leading to the development of a solid vaginal plate. In the 16th week, the squamous epithelium of the vagina and ectocervix begins to mature, becoming glycogenated and thickened. Desquamation subsequently results in the canalization of the vaginal plate. Vaginal development is essentially complete by the 18th–20th week. A band of subepithelial stroma extending from the endocervix to the vulva has been described, but the role of the vaginal stroma in induction of mucosal changes remains unclear [50, 247].

In the past, our knowledge of vaginal embryology was derived from classic dissections of the fetus. Several experiments of nature in humans (in utero exposure to DES, transverse vaginal septation, and partial vaginal agenesis) and in mice (testicular feminization syndrome and agenesis of the lower vagina [50]) as well as studies using human fetal grafts transplanted into the nude mouse [51] have provided the opportunity for elegant studies of altered development. Such studies reaffirm that the vagina is of dual origin, with a native lining of müllerian columnar cells that are retained unless there is a contribution of squamous cells from the urogenital sinus.

Anatomy

The vagina is a partially collapsed, midline, tubular structure that extends from the vestibule of the vulva to the uterine cervix. The vagina is posterior to the urinary bladder and anterior to the rectum, with an angle of more than 90° between the axis of the vagina and that of the uterus (➋ *Fig. 3.1*). In an adult, the vagina is about 9 cm in length. Its caliber and length are unrelated to sexual activity or symptoms of dyspareunia [309]. The anterior and posterior walls are in contact with each other, with the exception of the cranial (proximal) end where the vagina surrounds the ectocervix. Here, there are vaultlike recesses between the vaginal walls and the cervix, termed fornices, which are deepest posteriorly. In contrast to the slack anterior and posterior walls, the lateral walls are relatively rigid, resulting in a somewhat compressed lumen with an H shape in transverse sections.

The vagina is in contact anteriorly with the uterine cervix, the base of the bladder, and the urethra. The proximal third of the urethra is separated from the vagina by loose connective tissue; it enters into the vaginal wall distally, where their fasciae fuse into a single dense layer. Posteriorly, the upper fourth of the vaginal wall is bounded by peritoneum, and forms the anterior part of the cul-de-sac or pouch of Douglas. The rectovaginal septum connects the adventitia of the middle half of the vagina with the rectum, whereas the perineal body and anal and rectal sphincters separate the remaining more caudal portion from the anal canal. Laterally, each ureter, crossed by the uterine artery and vein, runs just above the lateral fornix. Caudally (distally), the levator ani and bulbocavernosus muscles partially surround the vagina, which ultimately opens into the vestibule (➋ *Fig. 3.2*).

Blood is supplied to the vagina primarily by branches of the internal iliac artery, including the uterine, vaginal, middle rectal, and internal pudendal arteries. Extensive

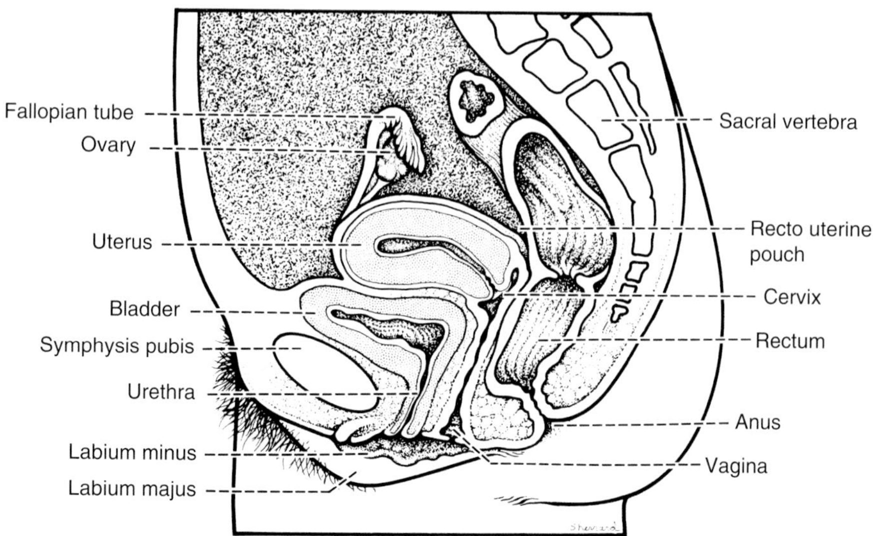

Fig. 3.1
Median sagittal section of the female pelvis

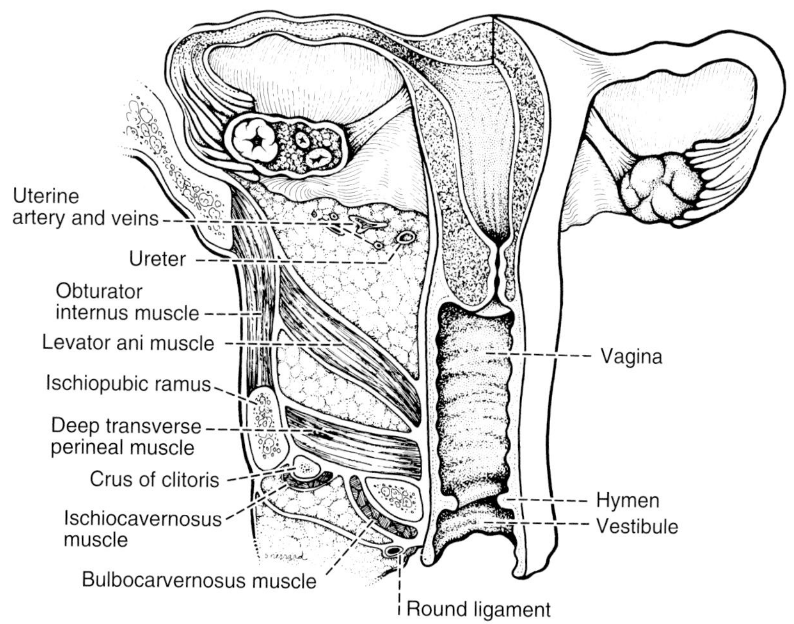

Fig. 3.2
Vagina, uterus, and supporting structures of the pelvis

anastomoses provide alternate routes of flow, which minimize the possibility of ischemic damage. A complex network of veins surrounds the vagina, forming a plexus with the uterine, pudendal, and rectal veins, which drain into the interior iliac vein.

The lymphatic drainage of the vagina is complex and variable. The lymphatics of the proximal anterior vagina and vaginal vault join those of the cervix and drain primarily into the external iliac lymph nodes. The posterior portion of the vagina drains into the inferior gluteal, sacral, and anorectal lymph nodes, whereas the distal part of the vagina, like the vulva, drains into the femoral lymph nodes. It is important to note that, as a consequence of extensive anastomotic channels, any pelvic, anorectal, or femoral node may be involved in the lymphatic drainage of any part of the vagina.

The innervation of the vagina is principally from the superior hypogastric plexus of the autonomic nervous system. This plexus bifurcates and is joined by branches of the second through fifth sacral nerves, forming the pelvic plexuses.

Histology and Physiology

The vaginal wall consists of three layers: mucosa, muscularis, and adventitia (➋ *Fig. 3.3a* and *b*). The vaginal mucosa is thrown into ill-defined laterally oriented folds or rugae of about 2–5 mm thickness (➋ *Fig. 3.4*). The thickness of the folds varies according to location and hormonal stimulation. The mucosal lining is a stratified squamous epithelium that is normally glycogenated and nonkeratinizing. Subdivision of the epithelium into layers is somewhat arbitrary but useful as it provides a basis for understanding the variable appearance of squamous cells in vaginal cytologic smears (➋ *Fig. 3.5*). The basal layer consists of a single layer of columnar cells, with the principal axis of the cells perpendicular to the basement membrane. The nuclei are oval and uniformly hyperchromatic, and are surrounded by relatively scant cytoplasm, resulting in a high nuclear/cytoplasmic ratio. The parabasal layer usually consists of two to five layers of cells of cuboidal shape, with a centrally located, round, and uniformly hyperchromatic nucleus. Mitoses usually are confined to the basal and parabasal layers. The intermediate layer is of variable thickness. The cells in this layer contain moderate quantities of slightly flattened cytoplasm and oval nuclei with finely dispersed chromatin. The long axis of both nucleus and cytoplasm is parallel to the basement membrane. The superficial layer also varies in thickness. The cells contain pyknotic nuclei, which are small, round, and hyperchromatic. The cytoplasm is abundant, with an orientation similar to intermediate cells. The three-dimensional configuration of these cells is that of a highly attenuated disk, resulting in a flattened appearance when viewed in cross section.

Variable quantities of glycogen may be present in the intermediate and superficial cell layers. The glycogen accumulates initially in a perinuclear location within

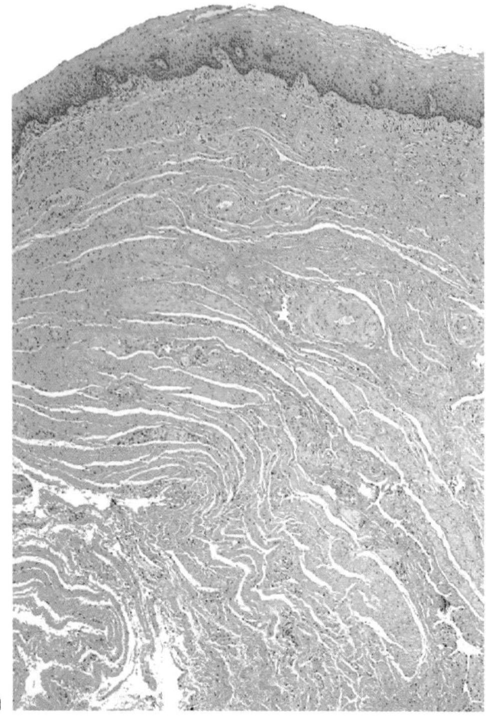

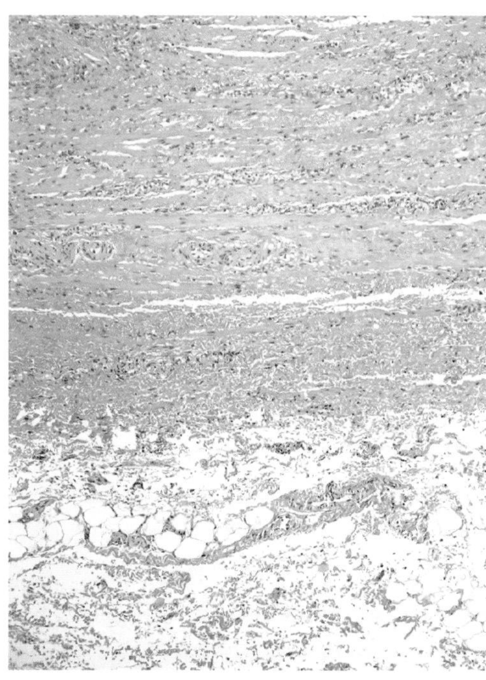

Fig. 3.3
Vaginal wall. **The vaginal muscularis is composed of ill-defined and variably sized smooth muscle bundles (a). The adventitia contains numerous blood vessels and nerves within adipose tissue (b)**

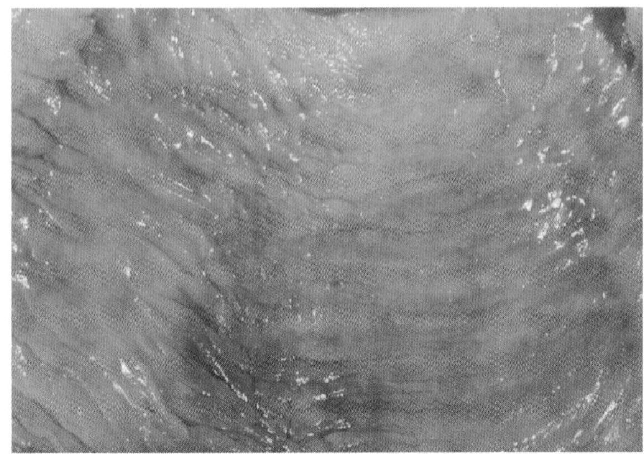

Fig. 3.4
Vaginal mucosa. **The mucosa is composed of ill-defined, laterally oriented folds or rugae**

intermediate cells, resulting in a clear zone around the nucleus. This appearance may cause confusion with the perinuclear clearing of koilocytes. However, the presence of nuclear membrane irregularity in koilocytes and the characteristic location of these normal cells in the middle rather than superficial third of the epithelium are helpful distinguishing features. Melanocytes have been identified as a normal constituent of the basal layer in about 3% of women.

The lamina propria, which lies beneath the squamous epithelium, consists of a loose fibrovascular stroma containing elastic fibers and nerves. A band of stroma extends from the endocervix to the vulva, which may contain atypical polygonal to stellate stromal cells with scant cytoplasm. Some of these cells are multinucleated or have multilobulated nuclei (*Figs. 3.6* and *3.7*). The muscularis consists of

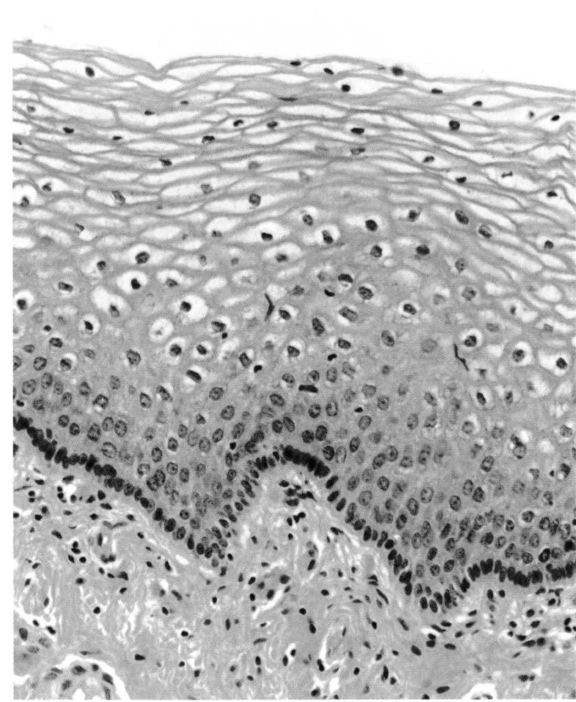

Fig. 3.5
Mature vaginal squamous epithelium. **The epithelium is composed of a basal layer, several layers of parabasal cells, and multiple layers of intermediate and superficial cells that progressively accumulate glycogen**

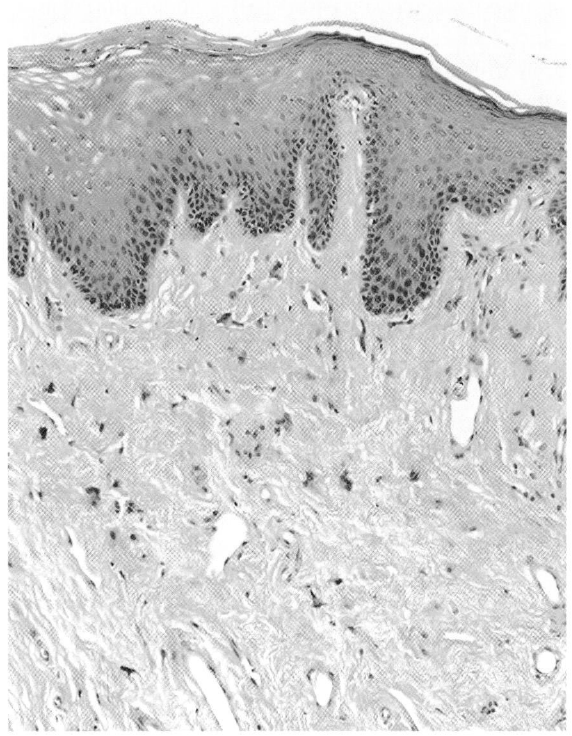

Fig. 3.6
Lamina propria of the vagina. **Beneath the squamous epithelium of the vagina is a poorly defined zone containing large, stellate, or spindle stromal cells. This zone extends in irregular fashion from the cervix to the vulva**

poorly delineated, inner circular, and outer longitudinal bundles of smooth muscle. Some of the outer longitudinal layers of muscle pass into the lateral pelvic wall to contribute to the inferior portion of the cardinal ligaments, whereas fibers of the bulbocavernosus form a sphincter around the distal vagina. The adventitia is a thin coat of dense connective tissue that merges with the loose connective tissue of the surrounding pelvis, which contains the lymphatic and venous plexuses and nerve bundles.

The squamous cells of the vagina contain intranuclear steroid receptors and represent a target tissue for sex steroids. The thickness and maturation of the epithelium varies throughout the menstrual cycle. Because the vagina is rarely biopsied but frequently sampled cytologically, the latter procedure has contributed greatly to our knowledge of normal and aberrant maturation. During the proliferative phase, the epithelium progressively proliferates and matures fully in response to estrogens. The addition of progesterone during the secretory phase is associated with an arrest of maturation at the intermediate cell level and a decrease in epithelial thickness. Although glycogen is found in the intermediate and superficial cells throughout the menstrual cycle, it is particularly abundant during pregnancy. Transient vaginal atrophy is found in some women postpartum, particularly in those who are lactating [313]. After menopause, a gradual reduction in the thickness of the epithelium occurs, first with a loss of superficial cells followed by intermediate cells, such that the mucosa of late menopausal women may be reduced to only six to eight layers of parabasal cells (➋ *Fig. 3.8*). As a consequence, a normal postmenopausal atrophic pattern may be confused with a high-grade intraepithelial lesion, unless care is taken to identify other nuclear abnormalities. Newborn infants, having been exposed to maternal steroids in utero, have a fully mature-appearing epithelium that rapidly regresses to atrophy within about 4 weeks. A gradual maturation of the epithelium follows the onset of menarche. Exposure of the postmenopausal vagina to estrogen leads to squamous maturation comparable to that observed in the proliferative phase of reproductive-age women. It is interesting to note that, in one study, the time required for

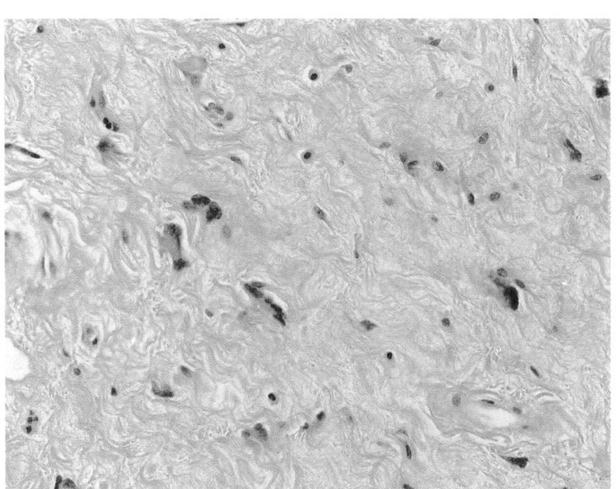

Fig. 3.7
Multinucleate stromal cells of the lamina propria. **Scattered bizarre, floret-type multinucleate cells are often admixed with other stellate or spindle cells in the superficial portion of the lamina propria. These may be the source of bizarre cells identified in some vaginal fibroepithelial (mesodermal) stromal polyps**

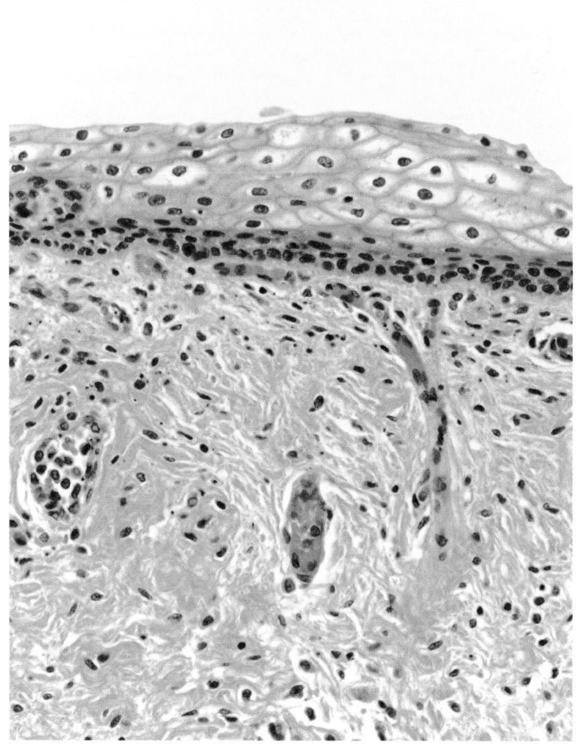

Fig. 3.8
Vaginal atrophy. **The epithelium is reduced to only a few layers of parabasal and basal cells**

a vaginal squamous cell to make the transition from progenitor cell through desquamation was about 5 days for both cycling and postmenopausal women [11].

There are few data concerning vaginal function during coitus or parturition [174]. Distension and lengthening of the proximal two thirds of the vagina occurs during the early phases of sexual response, followed by constriction of the distal third. The anterior portion of the levator ani, the pubococcygeus muscle, appears to be involved in orgasmic function, but the mechanism is speculative [174, 257]. Functional MRI has provided evidence that the vagus nerve may be either a primary or secondary pathway for nerve impulse conduction during vaginal orgasm [136]. Even the source of vaginal fluids that are present during arousal has been disputed. Glands are not normally present in the vagina, and candidate sources include secretions from sebaceous, sweat, Bartholin, and Skene glands or the endocervix. Fine droplets appear scattered throughout the rugal folds of the vaginal wall during arousal, followed by a rapid coalescence [174]. The fluid is believed to represent a transudate resulting from associated vasoconstriction within the venous plexus [174]. The fluid is usually acidic, with a pH around 4.6, but the pH rises during the sexual response. This fluid contains a variety of enzymes, enzyme inhibitors, and immunoglobulins, which may play a role in the liquefaction of coagulated semen and capacitation of spermatocytes or have antimicrobial activity. The immunoglobulin A levels are highest during the late proliferative phase [115], but the significance of this observation is unclear. During pregnancy and immediately postpartum, edema, vascular congestion, and loss of collagen have been noted in the lamina propria, which may serve to increase elasticity of vaginal tissues during delivery.

Developmental Disorders

Lesions Related to In Utero Exposure to DES

Diethylstilbestrol and the chemically related drugs hexestrol and dienestrol are synthetic, nonsteroidal estrogens that were administered frequently to gravid women who were thought to be at high risk for early pregnancy loss during the 1940s through the 1960s. An estimated five to ten million Americans received DES during pregnancy or were exposed to the drug in utero [95]. In 1971, the rare development of clear cell adenocarcinoma of the vagina in young women was linked to their in utero exposure to these drugs [113]. Subsequently, a number of nonneoplastic changes were identified in the genital tract of daughters of women exposed to DES, such as adenosis, cervical ectropion, various types of cervicovaginal ridges, and structural abnormalities of the uterine corpus and fallopian tube. DES was soon thereafter withdrawn from the market for use during pregnancy. Consequently, the population exposed in utero now averages about 55 years in age, with the youngest persons about 35 years old.

Gross Structural Changes of the Vagina and Cervix

Approximately one fifth of DES-exposed women demonstrate gross structural changes in the cervix or vagina [112]. Descriptive designations have included coxcomb (hood), collar (rim), pseudopolyp, and ridge. The pseudopolyp is caused by a peripheral concentric cervical band that gives the portio vaginalis central to it the appearance of a protruding cervical polyp; however, the presence of the external os at its center differentiates it from a true polyp. The cervix may be hypoplastic, the vaginal fornices may be obliterated, or the vagina may be traversed by a ridge (septum) consisting of fibrous connective tissue covered by squamous epithelium (➋ *Fig. 3.9*). The natural history of the structural abnormalities is not well understood, although some ridges have been observed to disappear as the cervix and vagina undergo remodeling with age.

Vaginal Epithelial Changes: Adenosis and Squamous Metaplasia

Vaginal adenosis and metaplastic squamous epithelium – vaginal epithelial changes (VECs) – are common in DES-exposed females. In the pre-DES era, vaginal adenosis was a clinical rarity, detected only occasionally in women, usually in their 30s or 40s, who often complained of an excessive mucous discharge from the vagina. The demographics are again changing. During the past decade, adenosis caused by DES exposure has become rare, although acquired adenosis in adult women with vaginal dysplasia treated with topical 5-fluorouracil occasionally have been reported [64, 98]. Clinically, adenosis should be suspected when the vaginal mucosa contains red granular spots or patches (➋ *Fig. 3.9*) and does not stain with an iodine solution. On colposcopy, adenosis appears as glandular or metaplastic epithelium replacing the native squamous epithelium of the vaginal mucosa.

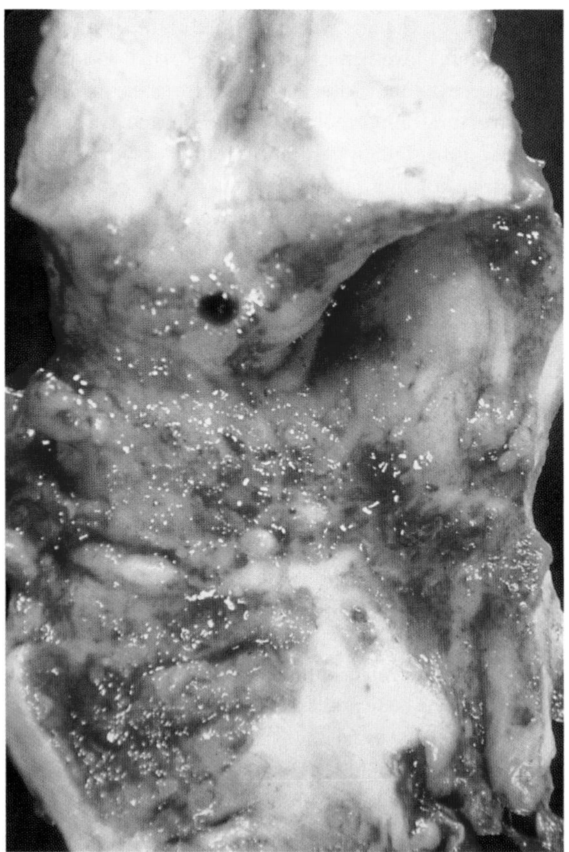

Fig. 3.9
Adenosis in a woman exposed to DES in utero. **There is a nodular deformity and ridge in the cervix visible in the upper portion of the photograph. The friable red granular epithelium that replaces much of the mucosa reflects regions of adenosis, most of which is of the tuboendometrioid type**

Adenosis involves the upper third of the vagina in 34% of DES-exposed women, the middle third in about 10%, and lower third in about 2% of exposed women. Mucinous columnar cells, which resemble those of the normal endocervical mucosa, comprise the glandular epithelium most frequently encountered as adenosis (62% of biopsy specimens with vaginal adenosis) (*Fig. 3.10*) [240]. Tuboendometrial adenosis with dark and light cells, often ciliated and resembling the lining cells of the fallopian tube and endometrium, is found in 21% of specimens with adenosis. These cells usually are found in glands in the lamina propria and not on the surface of the vagina. In most biopsy specimens, metaplastic squamous cells replace adenosis to some degree (*Fig. 3.11*), indicating the manner by which adenosis regresses. Reserve cell proliferation progresses through immature and mature stages of squamous metaplasia, with intercellular pools of mucin and droplets remaining as the final vestiges of adenosis. Eventual maturation of the metaplastic squamous epithelium with acquisition of glycogen makes it indistinguishable from the normal (native) squamous epithelium.

The Embryologic Basis of Vaginal Adenosis and Cervical Ectropion

The DES experience and the experimental studies it has fostered have provided insights into the development of the normal lower genital tract and the effects caused by prenatal DES exposure [239]. In brief, the embryonic squamous epithelium of the urogenital sinus normally extends up the vagina and exocervix, replacing the original columnar (müllerian) epithelium lining these organs. Recent experimental work has suggested that inhibition of p63 by DES may alter the urogenital sinus and müllerian duct epithelial differentiation and result in adenosis [143]. Further, the stroma of the vaginal wall (like the uterine corpus and fallopian tube) induces the growth of a tuboendometrial-type epithelium, while the stroma of the superficial endocervix favors mucinous columnar epithelium. In DES-exposed fetal organs, the stromal components of the uterine wall fail to segregate normally into an outer layer of smooth muscle and an inner layer of endometrial stroma [242].

Vaginal adenosis is not limited exclusively to women exposed to DES in utero, but has also been reported in 2–10% of non-exposed females who have no known risk factors [32, 229]. Adenosis may occur following topical treatment of squamous dysplasia with 5-fluorouracil [92], but the mechanism by which it induces glandular metaplasia remains unclear.

Imperforate Hymen

Imperforate hymen probably represents the most common significant congenital anomaly of the vagina. Its frequency is reported to be about 1 in 2,000 female patients. The presence of a thick mucoid secretion that distends the vagina may provide a clue to diagnosis in the neonate, but often an imperforate hymen is not recognized until puberty, when there is abdominal pain and retention of menstrual

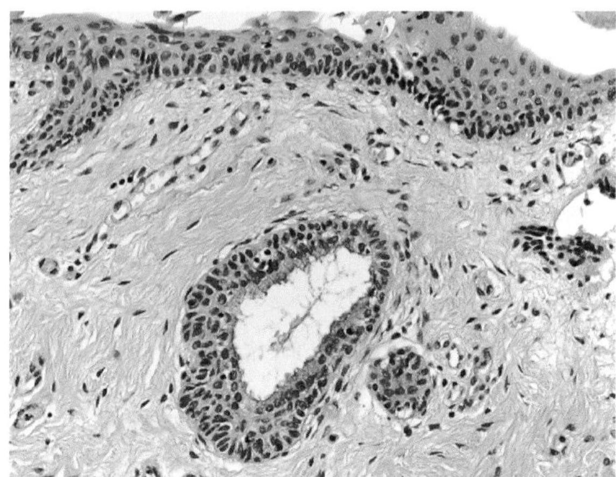

Fig. 3.10
Adenosis. **Glands within the lamina propria are lined by a mucin-secreting columnar epithelium**

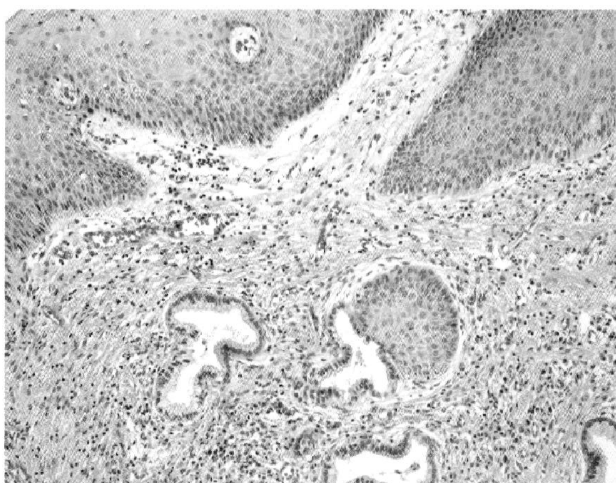

Fig. 3.11
Adenosis. **The mucinous glands display partial replacement by metaplastic squamous epithelium. With increasing age, mature squamous metaplasia obliterates all evidence of the adenosis**

detritus [220]. If it is not corrected promptly, infertility may result from endometriosis and pelvic adhesions associated with retrograde menstruation [311]. The treatment is surgical, with either a central incision or local excision [3]. No detailed pathologic description of this condition has been reported.

Vaginal Agenesis

Complete vaginal agenesis is relatively rare, occurring in about 1 in 5,000 female births [63, 82, 296]. As an isolated defect it results from incomplete caudal development and fusion of the lower part of the müllerian ducts (müllerian dysgenesis). The external genitalia usually appear normal, except for the introitus, where a short blind pouch may be present [311]. Therapy usually involves construction of an artificial vagina. Although this rarely results in a specimen for pathologic examination, the defect often is associated with the absence of the uterus and fallopian tubes (müllerian agenesis or Mayer–Rokitansky–Kuster–Hauser syndrome) [72] and with anomalies of the urinary tract [202]. The latter syndrome provides insight into embryologic development and demonstrates that an intact mesonephric duct is required for the growth and caudal lengthening of the müllerian duct during fetal life [163, 164]. Because the gonads are not of müllerian origin, they usually are normal. About 25% of women with vaginal agenesis have a uterus, and they may have complications from retrograde menstruation.

Transverse Vaginal Septum

A transverse vaginal septum is uncommon, with an estimated prevalence of about 1 in 50,000 women [220], and may occur anywhere within the vagina, but most frequently at the junction of the cranial and middle third. It presumably results from incomplete migration or excavation of the vaginal plate. A complete vaginal septum results in obstructive symptoms similar to an imperforate hymen, whereas a partial septum may allow passage of menstrual flow but cause dyspareunia or lacerate during childbirth. The microscopic appearance of the septum is typically that of a fibrovascular stroma covered on two surfaces by epithelium. Although the caudal surface is covered by a stratified nonkeratinizing squamous epithelium, the cranial aspect is covered typically by glandular epithelium, as might be predicted from the embryologic development.

Miscellaneous Congenital Disorders

Complete duplication of the vagina with a septum including muscularis extending to the introitus is rare, and typically is accompanied by cervical and uterine duplication [14]. Longitudinal septa that lack a muscular layer are more common; they often are clinically asymptomatic. Congenital rectovaginal fistulas often are associated with an imperforate anus. Typically, the anus opens into the posterior caudal portion of the vagina, near the fourchette.

Infectious Inflammatory Disorders

The normal vaginal flora is varied and changes from birth through menarche to menopause. Although it has long been evident that lactobacilli split glycogen to form lactic acid, thus reducing the pH of the vagina, this does not provide a complete explanation for the regulation of the vaginal flora. The ecosystem reflects a delicate balance that includes the interplay of steroid hormones, vascularity, vaginal acidity, and glycogen. It can be upset easily by mechanical, chemical, or hormonal manipulation. Approximately 10^9 obligate anaerobic and 10^8 facultative bacteria are present in a gram of vaginal secretion, of which lactobacilli probably are the most common [171]. Three hundred and forty-five organisms were represented in 52 specimens collected from healthy adults, including the following anaerobes: *Peptococcus*, *Bacteroides*, *Peptostreptococcus*, *Lactobacillus*, *Eubacterium* spp.; and aerobes: *Stapylococcus epidermidis*, *Corynebacterium* spp., and *Lactobacillus* sp [14]. The proportion of aerobic organisms decreases about 100-fold during the week before menses. During pregnancy, more lactobacilli and yeast, but fewer anaerobic bacteria, are present [157]. On the third day after parturition, there is a dramatic increase in the number of anaerobic bacteria. Postmenopausal women also have a relatively larger proportion of anaerobes, with more lactobacilli recovered from those treated with estrogen [149]. Organisms that at times are associated with vaginitis may colonize the vagina of healthy, asymptomatic women.

Table 3.1
Sexually transmitted pathogens

Sexually transmitted pathogens
Bacterial agents
Neisseria gonorrhoeae
Chlamydia trachomatis
Mycoplasma hominis
Ureaplasma urealyticum
Treponema pallidum
Gardnerella vaginalis
Haemophilus ducreyi
Shigella
Campylobacter
Group B streptococcus
Fungal agents
Candida albicans
Viral agents
Herpes simplex virus
Hepatitis B virus
Cytomegalovirus
Human papilloma virus
Molluscum contagiosum virus
Protozoan agents
Trichomonas vaginalis
Entamoeba histolytica
Giardia lamblia
Ectoparasites
Pediculus pubis
Sarcoptes scabiei

Vaginitis

Vaginitis is one of the most common reasons for a patient to visit her gynecologist, accounting for more than ten million office visits each year [132]. Abnormal colonization or invasive infection has been reported for practically all major types of organisms, including viruses, bacteria, fungi, and parasites. It is difficult to determine the most common organism responsible for vaginitis because frequency lists vary according to age, sexual activity, and method of microbial identification [265]. Currently, more than 20 bacterial, viral, and protozoan agents are considered to be responsible for sexually transmitted diseases (STDs) (*Table 3.1*). Because the notification that one has an STD frequently evokes a strong emotional response, it is important to remember that the distinction between sexually and nonsexually transmitted disease is at times arbitrary. Whereas many infectious agents make use of the opportunity afforded by close apposition of mucous membranes or secretions to spread, there is variability in the stringency of their demands.

The clinical diagnosis of vaginitis is frequently based on the presence of a vaginal discharge. Reliance on this finding alone may lead to overdiagnosis, as the production of vaginal fluid is a physiologic event caused by transudation of fluid through the vaginal wall, with additional contributions by cervical and uterine secretions, exfoliated epithelial cells, bacteria, and bacterial products. This event is particularly noticeable at mid-cycle when cervical mucus becomes watery and profuse and often is interpreted erroneously as a "discharge." Other relatively nonspecific criteria of vaginitis include subjective assessment of the color, odor, quantity, or quality of the discharge. In contrast to discharge caused by vaginitis, normal vaginal secretions are floccular rather than homogeneous, and neither malodorous nor associated with pruritis. Although accurate diagnosis of vaginitis does not require a biopsy, some infectious agents cause highly specific tissue reactions, with which the pathologist should be familiar.

Candida

Candida probably is the most common potential or active pathogen in the female genital tract. It can be isolated from the vagina of about 20% of asymptomatic healthy women, and about 70% of women will have a symptomatic candidal infection at some time during their lives [267]. *C. albicans* is found frequently in the colon of healthy individuals, and spread from the contaminated perineum probably is the usual method of introduction of the organism into the vagina [267]. Interestingly, fomites from bathtubs or toilet seats do not appear to be a common mechanism for transmission [9]. Sexual transmission plays a role in some patients, resulting from either oral–genital or less likely penile–genital transmission [30]. Factors associated with an increased risk of developing symptomatic infection include pregnancy, oral contraceptive use, antibiotic therapy, diabetes mellitus, and antibiotic use. Changes in the vaginal flora likely play a role in the development of candidiasis.

Vulvar pruritis is the typical presenting symptom, often accompanied by a white, granular vaginal discharge. The vagina appears reddened, and superficial erosion of the mucosa may be evident after the removal of a pseudomembrane of adherent granular debris.

Saline or potassium hydroxide suspensions of a discharge containing blastospores and pseudohyphae permit a presumptive microscopic diagnosis to be made immediately. Unfortunately, the sensitivity of the wet prep exam is only about 65% [180], and the morphologic appearance is not entirely specific. In one study, Papanicolaou-stained smears demonstrated the organism in 46% infected patients, compared with 85% for the wet prep and 94% for culture [179]. In daily practice, it is the experience of the examiner that seems to be the most critical determinant for accurate recognition of the organism. Definitive identification of the fungus is generally made by culture or polymerase chain reaction [173].

Biopsies, which are rarely obtained, contain relatively dense infiltrates of primarily mononuclear inflammatory cells and congested blood vessels in the stroma, with exocytosis of neutrophils into the overlying epithelium (*Fig. 3.12*) [130]. *Candida* are generally not identifiable unless the discharge remains adherent, where the organisms are visualized as yeast and pseudohyphae intertwined among the desquamated squamous cells (*Fig. 3.13*) [19]. First-line therapy of topical imidazole derivatives for 5–7 days has been used for the past 20 years, but the recent introduction of triazols permits equal efficacy with single-dose therapy [267]. However, recurrent infection remains common and may result from either failure to respond to medical therapy or endogenous reinfection by the identical strain of organism [300].

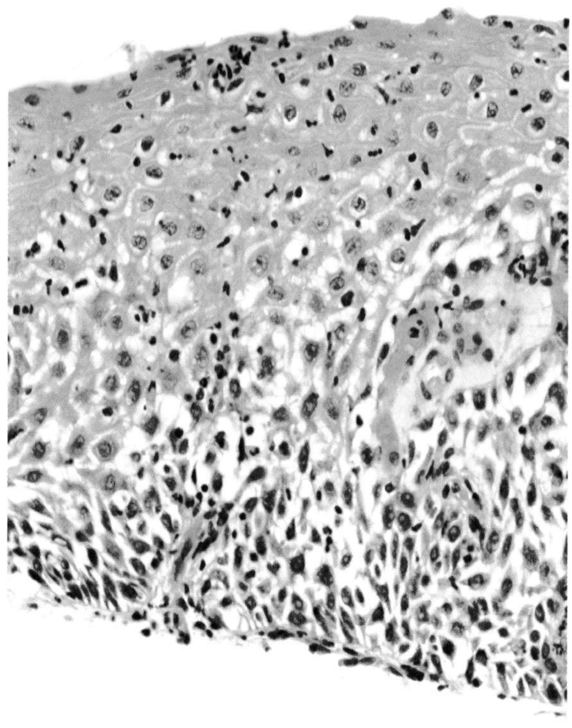

Fig. 3.12
Vaginitis caused by *Candida* or *Trichomonas*. **The histologic changes, including variably dense infiltrates of mononuclear inflammatory cells in the stroma and neutrophils in the epithelium, are similar for both organisms**

Candidal species other than *C. albicans* are responsible for about 10–20% of cases of fungal vaginitis [238, 267], and infection with *C. tropicalis* or *C. glabrata* is associated with a high rate of recurrence [238]. *C. glabrata* typically produces milder symptoms than *C. albicans* [21], but *C. glabrata* has been reported to cause a severe ulcerative vaginitis-simulating malignancy [37]. The microscopic appearances of most *Candida* species are similar, but *C. glabrata* produces only yeasts (blastospores), which are slightly smaller than those of *C. albicans* [21].

Bacterial Vaginosis

Organisms such as *Trichomonas* and *Candida* have long been known to produce vaginitis; however, until recently

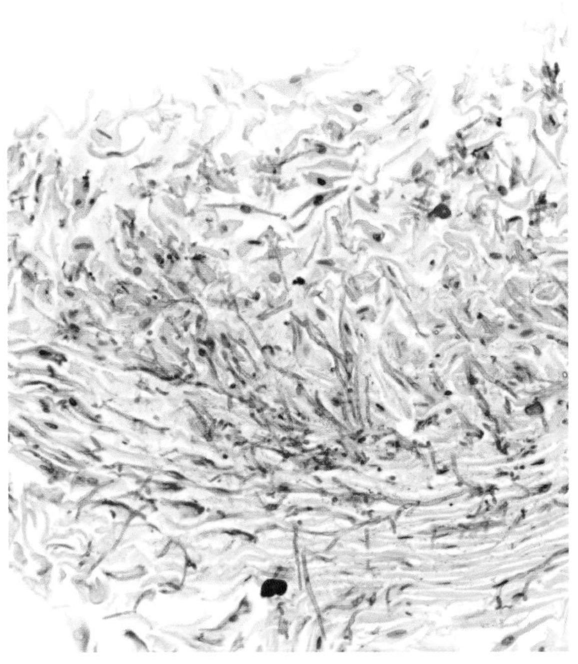

◘ Fig. 3.13
Candida vaginitis. **Yeast and pseudohyphae are present in a mat of exfoliated superficial squamous cells.** ***Candida*** **are usually not identified in biopsies of the vagina unless desquamated cells remain adherent to the intact mucosal surface (periodic acid–Schiff [PAS] stain)**

there have been a substantial number of women who have a copious vaginal discharge or pruritis in the absence of a readily identifiable pathogen. In the past, this condition was designated nonspecific vaginitis, but the term bacterial vaginosis currently is preferred because evidence of inflammation is typically absent [171]. *Gardnerella*, a gram-negative bacillus, has been isolated from women with vaginosis at a higher rate than asymptomatic women and thus was considered to be responsible for nonspecific vaginitis [87]. However, more recent studies cast doubt on this concept, because this organism and "clue" cells have been identified at times with similar frequency in healthy women without vaginal discharge [269]. Currently, it is believed that bacterial vaginosis is not an infection by a single organism, but rather an overgrowth of multiple colonizing bacteria including *Gardnerella* and a variety of anaerobes [216, 286, 303]. The flora typically found in affected women includes not only disproportionately large numbers of *Gardnerella vaginalis*, but also abundant *Prevotella bivia*, *Mycoplasma hominis*, *Mobiluncus mulieris*, and *Mobiluncus curtisii* [287]. In an animal model, the inoculation of *Gardnerella* and *Mobiluncus* together caused the clinical disease, although neither alone was capable of doing so [172]. The diagnosis of bacterial vaginosis is made if three of the following four criteria are present: (1) homogeneous, thin, malodorous discharge, (2) vaginal pH 4.5, (3) vaginal epithelial cells with numerous attached bacteria ("clue" cells) (➤ *Fig. 3.14*), and (4) fishy odor on alkalinization of vaginal secretions [7, 56, 255]. The diagnosis usually is confirmed by elimination of other pathogens, combined with identification of gram-negative to gram-variable bacilli and "clue" cells on wet mount or smears, or by culture [284]. The identification of squamous cells coated by large numbers of coccobacilli in a cervical vaginal cytology specimen represents a moderately sensitive and highly specific method for screening for bacterial vaginosis [56, 94]. No specific histopathologic features have been described.

Efforts to restore the local environment by topical administration of acetic acid, estrogen, or fermented milk products have been ineffective. In contrast, antimicrobial therapy with metronidazole or intravaginal clindamycin produces clinical cure in most women, further supporting the concept that anaerobes acting with *Gardnerella* produce bacterial vaginosis [269]. The initiating cause remains unknown, but sexual transmission occurs in many instances [150, 198]. Although bacterial vaginosis was previously thought to carry no appreciable morbidity, it recently has been associated with a 3- to 15-fold increased risk of upper genital tract infection, including salpingitis and endometritis [116, 138, 206, 276]. In addition, the anaerobic bacteria cultured from the endometrium and fallopian tubes of women with asymptomatic endometritis or symptomatic salpingitis were those associated with bacterial vaginosis [138, 268]. During pregnancy, bacterial vaginosis significantly increases the likelihood of premature onset of labor and chorioamnionitis [118, 176, 196, 268].

Trichomonas Vaginalis

Trichomoniasis is responsible for more than 2.5 million infections per year in the United States and about 180 million infections worldwide [285]. It is found in about 10% of asymptomatic women, and almost 50% of those attending STD clinics [275]. The organism is almost always sexually transmitted [320], although trichomonads reportedly may survive in tap water, soap water, and chlorinated swimming pools. The mechanism by which *Trichomonas* causes disease is unknown, but the organisms are found both in the vaginal lumen and adherent to squamous, but not columnar, epithelial cells [235]. Invasion of the squamous mucosa does not occur. *Trichomonas* is a strict anaerobe and there is frequently an alteration in the associated vaginal flora, with increased anaerobic bacteria [298]. Although the role of sex steroids is unclear, infection is generally lower in women taking oral contraceptives [24].

Symptoms of infection include vaginal discharge, intense pruritis, and dyspareunia, with exacerbations often temporally related to menses. However, in one study, only 17% of culture-positive women noted pruritis, and more than one third did not even complain of a vaginal discharge [178]. When present, the vaginal discharge usually is copious, homogeneous, yellow green to gray, and malodorous. Typically, the vaginal mucosa is erythematous and punctate hemorrhages may be present, particularly on the cervical mucosa, leading to what is unfortunately described as a "strawberry cervix."

The diagnosis usually is made by the microscopic identification of motile organisms accompanied by many neutrophils in a saline preparation. The protozoan is ovoid, about 10–20 mm in diameter, with polar flagella. Active motility, in the form of a jerky swaying motion, is provided by the flagella and undulating membrane. If the wet prep diagnosis is based on the presence of motile organisms, the specificity approaches 100%. Trichomonads also may be found in Papanicolaou-stained vaginal smears in about 70% of cases (➋ *Fig. 3.15*), a sensitivity similar to that of the wet prep [160]. Several recently introduced molecular amplification methods appear to provide both high sensitivity and specificity when applied to distal vaginal secretions [60, 106, 167, 314]. Culture methods are available, expensive, and generally unnecessary. The organism is not detectable in biopsy specimens from culture-positive women, although an inflammatory response of variable intensity may be seen, including dilated vessels in the stroma, accompanied by dense infiltrates of plasma cells and lymphocytes (➋ *Fig. 3.12*). The ectocervical as well as vagina mucosa is commonly spongiotic (➋ *Fig. 3.12*) [134]. Neutrophils frequently are present in large numbers among the squamous cells, sometimes forming intraepithelial abscesses. There may be irregular acanthosis of the epithelium, with pseuodepitheliomatous hyperplasia. A fibrinopurulent exudate composed of necrotic debris, neutrophils, and lymphocytes is found in the foci of ulceration. Metronidazole provides effective therapy, although recurrence is common if the typically asymptomatic male partner is not also treated. Unfortunately, the frequency of resistance to metronidazole is increasing [289].

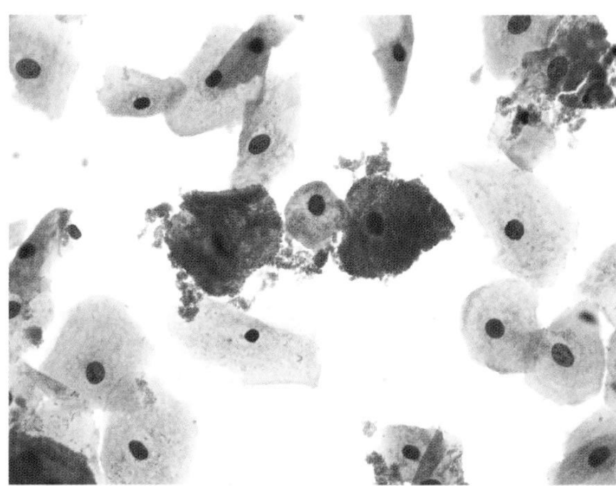

Fig. 3.14
Bacterial vaginosis. **Papanicolaou-stained cytologic preparation containing scattered intermediate squamous cells, two of which are covered by innumerable minute coccal bacteria (Clue cells). This represents one of the four criteria necessary for the diagnosis of bacterial vaginosis**

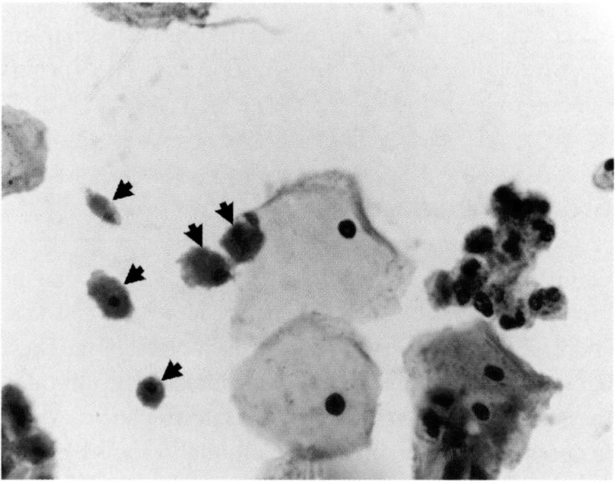

Fig. 3.15
Trichomonas vaginitis. **Papanicolaou-stained cytologic preparation of vaginal secretions containing several of the nucleated, ovoid protozoans, as well as three intermediate squamous cells and inflammatory cells**

Acquired Immunodeficiency Syndrome

Slightly more than one million persons in the US are living with human immunodeficiency virus (HIV)/acquired immunodeficiency virus syndrome (AIDS). Woman account for about one quarter of newly reported cases, and heterosexual contact represents the mode of transmission in about 28% of all cases in the United States. It is the fifth leading cause of death among American women 25–44 years of age. There are no gross or histopathologic changes of AIDS specific to the vagina.

Most HIV infections resulting from heterosexual contact have occurred in women who reported only vaginal intercourse [210]. The virus has been identified in both semen and cell-free seminal fluid [155]. Certain STDs are considered to be risk factors for sexual transmission of HIV, particularly those that cause ulceration of the vaginal mucosa, facilitating HIV exposure to vascular channels, as well as providing a large number of CD4 lymphocytes and macrophages that contain or could bind HIV at the site of injury [40]. It is estimated that a fivefold to tenfold increase in risk of heterosexual transmission of HIV is present in those with genital ulcers [302]. A twofold to fivefold increase in risk is associated with the presence of an inflammatory or exudative STD, presumably reflecting the presence of microscopic ulcerations or increased concentrations of CD4 lymphocytes in the discharge [153, 302]. Localization of simian immunodeficiency virus (SIV) in dendritic cells of the monkey vagina has been demonstrated in an experimental model, suggesting that heterosexual transmission of HIV may occur across an intact mucosa [183]. Nevertheless, the precise mechanism by which heterosexual transmission of HIV occurs remains to be defined.

Group B *Streptococcus*

Group B streptococci (*Streptococcus agalactiae*) can be found in 5–35% of normal females [119, 319] and thus are considered to be part of the normal vaginal flora. These bacteria frequently are sexually transmitted [115], although they also can ascend from the lower intestinal tract, which may serve as a reservoir [195]. Although group B streptococcal colonization of the vagina or urethra usually causes little morbidity to the adult female, a vaginitis at times may occur [115]. Histopathologic changes resulting from vaginal infection by group B streptococci have not been well described. More significantly, this organism is a frequent cause of abortion, chorioamnionitis, premature rupture of membranes, perinatal death, and intrapartum and postpartum bacteremia [233, 276]. For reasons that currently are unknown, only a small proportion of colonized mothers or infants develop symptomatic infection [276].

Actinomycetes

Actinomycetes have been implicated in upper genital tract infections in women with intrauterine contraceptive devices and also are found in the vagina of about one quarter of women without such devices. These organisms represent part of the normal oral and colonic flora, from which it may be introduced into the vagina. Vaginitis subsequently occurs when overgrowth is favored by the presence of a foreign body [53]. Actinomycetes are recognized in Papanicolaou-stained smears and tissue sections as a dense mass of fine, blue, filamentous bacteria, usually radiating from a central core (*Fig. 3.16*).

Malacoplakia and Xanthogranulomatous Pseudotumor

Malacoplakia and xanthogranulomatous pseudotumor of the vagina are closely related entities resulting from infection by gram-negative bacilli, usually *Escherichia coli* [156, 271]. Typically, yellow polypoid nodules arise from the vaginal mucosa, at times accompanied by a discharge.

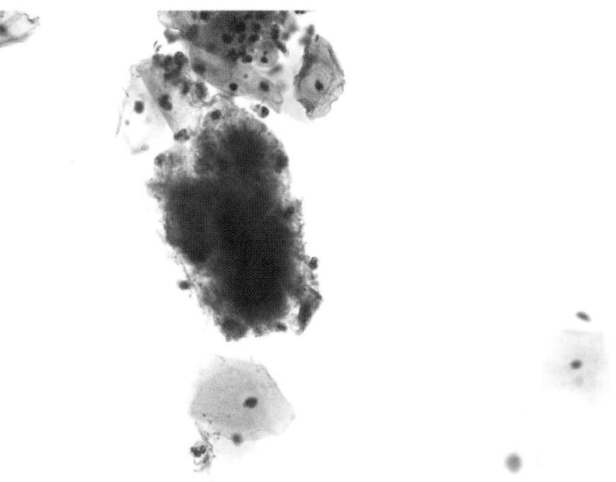

Fig. 3.16
Actinomycetes. **Papanicolaou-stained cytologic preparation with a dense collection of fine, blue, filamentous bacteria, which appear to radiate from a central core**

The microscopic findings are identical to those described in other body sites, and include the presence of large collections of histiocytes with abundant granular to pale foamy cytoplasms (von Hansemann cells), with interspersed plasma cells and lymphocytes. Both intracellular and extracellular, concentrically laminated basophilic masses (Michaelis–Gutmann bodies) are present in variable numbers. The clinical suspicion of tumor may lead the pathologist to the misdiagnosis of a rare neoplasm such as a granular cell tumor, unless care is taken to consider this lesion. The correct diagnosis may be confirmed by the finding of numerous gram-negative rodlike bacteria on tissue Gram stain, on silver stain, or by electron microscopy.

Tuberculosis

Genital tract tuberculosis is no longer frequent in the United States, but remains a significant problem in Third World nations. The vagina is involved in about only 1% of these women, and patients present with localized ulceration [199]. Characteristic microscopic features include necrotizing granulomata containing Langhans giant cells underlying an ulcerated epithelium [41].

Emphysematous Vaginitis

Emphysematous vaginitis is a rare entity (about 200 reported cases), characterized by multiple, discrete, gas-filled cystic cavities in the vaginal mucosa. Most patients present with symptoms of vaginal discharge, although some are aware of popping sounds associated with the rupture of the cysts during intercourse. The dramatic presentation and physical findings have prompted an interest disproportionate to the frequency or significance of the disease. There is evidence that it is an unusual manifestation of a common infection in an immunocompromised host [127, 288]. No single organism has been identified as the causative agent, although both *Trichomonas vaginalis* and *Gardnerella vaginalis* have been implicated [88]. Chemical analyses of the lesions have disclosed a wide variety of gases, including ammonia, hydrogen sulfide, nitrogen, oxygen, carbonic acid, and trimethylamine. The microscopic findings are variable, with cysts in the stroma lined by either multinucleated giant cells, squamous cells, or both. A scattering of chronic inflammatory cells accompanies the cysts [88, 140]. Bacterial or protozoan production of gas with transmucosal passage into the stroma has been suggested, but the pathogenesis remains obscure [88].

Unusual Types of Bacterial Vaginitis

Occasionally, vaginitis may be caused by bacteria that are commonly pathogenic in other sites. *Shigella vulvovaginitis* has been identified primarily as a cause of a chronic, sanguinous, and purulent vaginal discharge in children, unassociated with intestinal infection [54, 232]. Haemophilus influenzae, Coryne bacterium diphtheria, and *Neisseria meningitidis* also rarely cause vaginitis in children [31, 68, 69, 274], but the histologic changes have not been documented. Staphylococcal infection of the vagina after systemic antibiotic therapy was reported more than 30 years ago and thought to result from a disturbed indigenous flora [148] (see section ➋ Toxic Shock Syndrome).

Parasitic Vaginitis

Parasitic infection of the vagina, although currently rare in the United States, almost certainly will be encountered more commonly because of more frequent global travel.

Vaginal amebiasis caused by *Entamoeba histolytica* has been reported in Mexico, South Africa, and India, where the infection is endemic [107, 117, 188, 297]. Most patients present with a bloody vaginal discharge. The gross appearance mimics carcinoma, with one or more ulcerated, necrotic growths typically involving the vagina and cervix. Microscopically, the lesions are characterized by ulceration of the epithelium with replacement by a fibrinopurulent exudate containing trophozoites 15–60 micrometers in diameter. In cytologic preparations they appear somewhat larger than histiocytes, and approximate the size of parabasal cells. Positive staining with periodic acid–Schiff (PAS) stain or acid phosphatase provides further support for the diagnosis.

Eggs of *Enterobius vermicularis* or *Trichuris trichiura* usually are found after incidental contamination of the vagina associated with intestinal infestation by these worms [187]. Eggs and worms of *Schistosoma mansoni* and *hematobium* have been identified in pelvic tissues including the vagina, presumably reflecting anastomoses between hemorrhoidal and hypogastric veins [91]. They elicit a striking host inflammatory response, ultimately resulting in dense fibrosis.

Toxic Shock Syndrome

General Features

In 1978, Todd et al. described an acute, potentially life-threatening disease characterized by fever, hypotension, headache, confusion, rash, vomiting, diarrhea, and oliguria. The disease was termed toxic shock syndrome (TSS) because it was associated with infection with strains of *Staphylococcus* that produced a unique epidermal toxin [290]. By 1980, more than 98% of cases had been related to the use of tampons during menses [75]. The incidence is about 6 cases per 100,000 menstruating women per year. Although *S. aureus* rarely inhabits the vagina normally, it has been isolated from about 75% of women with TSS [55, 177]. More recently it has become evident that children or adults with any focal staphylococcal infection are also at risk for TSS, and about 11% of all reported cases are nonmenstrual [236].

Pathogenesis

There is a strong relationship between localized infection with *S. aureus* and the development of TSS. Studies of patients with TSS as well as experimental systems have revealed that some staphylococci elaborate a protein of about 22 kDa termed toxic shock syndrome toxin 1 (TSST-1), which produces essentially all the systemic biologic effects [20]. TSS can also occur in the absence of this toxin, and other staphylococcal enterotoxins (such as Staphylococcal exotoxin B), streptococcal exotoxins, and endotoxins from gram-negative bacteria have been implicated in some cases of TSS [230, 236]. The mechanism by which tampon use during menses predisposes to TSS remains somewhat unclear, but it is believed that microulcerations of the vaginal mucosa caused by tampons (see below, ➋ Tampon Ulcer) permit the growth of toxin-producing staphylococci. A diminished host immune response to the toxin, access of toxin through a denuded endometrial mucosa, and the normal menstrual phase decrease in lactobacilli that are inhibitory to the growth of staphylococci may facilitate the process [75, 252]. A multifactorial sequence is supported by the observation that about 10% of healthy women are colonized vaginally by *Staphylococcus aureus*, and 85% of women have antibodies to TSST-1 [205], whereas other women have recurrent episodes of the illness. A dramatic reduction in the incidence of TTS occurred when Rely superabsorbent tampons were withdrawn from the market in 1980 [142].

Clinical Features

The diagnosis of TSS is based on a constellation of clinical features, as follows: fever, hypotension, palmar or diffuse erythroderma followed by desquamation, hyperemia of conjunctivae or mucous membranes of vagina or pharynx, and multisystem dysfunction including vomiting; diarrhea; impaired renal, cerebral, or hepatic function; cardiopulmonary dysfunction; thrombocytopenia; elevated creatine phosphokinase; and decreased serum calcium and phosphate [55]. Vaginal erythema, erosions, or vaginitis, sometimes accompanied by a purulent exudate, typically are present [304]. Abdominal or bilateral adnexal tenderness is present in about half of cases [109].

Gross and Microscopic Findings

The disease is systemic, with pathologic abnormalities described in lung, liver, and kidney, as well as genital tract [1, 205]. Ulceration and discoloration of the vaginal and cervical mucosa are present focally. Microscopically, there is extensive desquamation of the epithelium, with underlying subacute vasculitis, perivascular inflammatory cell infiltrates, and platelet thrombi [1, 205]. Rare gram-positive cocci have been found in the fibrinopurulent exudate associated with ulcers. Deep tissue invasion by the organisms has not been described [205].

Clinical Behavior and Treatment

The spectrum of severity of TSS varies from a relatively mild to a rapidly fatal illness, with a mortality rate of about 4% [277]. The treatment includes beta-lactamase-resistant anti-staphylococcal antibiotics, and aggressive, supportive measures for systemic manifestations related to shock [236]. Intravenous immunoglobulin therapy also has been effective, supporting the concept that the symptoms of TSS result from a toxin that may be neutralized by infused antibodies [13].

Noninfectious Inflammatory Diseases

The vagina is occasionally the site of involvement by a systemic disease, a generalized disease of squamous mucosa, or by extension from a disease elsewhere in the pelvis. In one recent study of chronic vaginitis, the most common diagnoses were as follows: contact dermatitis (21%), recurrent vulvovaginal candidiasis (21%), atrophic vaginitis (15%), and vulvar vestibulitis syndrome (13%) [200].

Desquamative Inflammatory Vaginitis

Idiopathic desquamative inflammatory vaginitis is the term that has been applied to an unusual process in which bright red, well-delineated areas replace portions of the normal mucosa of the cranial half of the vagina. It must be distinguished from other disorders causing erosion such as pemphigus vulgaris, lichen planus, and pemphigoid [191]. A pseudomembrane at times replaces the ulcerated mucosa. A copious purulent to hemorrhagic vaginal discharge is present, smears of which display numerous neutrophils and a high proportion of parabasal cells. The women usually are premenopausal and have normal serum estrogen levels. In rare cases in which biopsies have been performed, a nonspecific mixed inflammatory cell infiltrate has been reported [192]. The etiology is unknown, and no single bacterial or viral agent has been identified by culture. Nevertheless, the replacement of long gram-positive bacilli by gram-positive cocci in the vaginal discharge of some affected women suggests an infectious etiology. Treatment with clindamycin and topical steroids results in clinical improvement in more than 95% of patients [266].

Ligneous Vaginitis

Ligneous vaginitis is one localized manifestation of a rare, inherited, and potentially life-threatening systemic disease in which afflicted individuals develop pseudomembranous lesions of mucosal surfaces in the acute phase [161]. Recent research indicates that it reflects a severe type 1 plaminogen (PLG) deficiency due to a variety of mutations in the PLG gene [283]. Clinical manifestations often include ligneous conjunctivitis, ligneous gingivitis, and occasional involvement of the respiratory or gastrointestinal tract. The chronic phase is characterized by asymptomatic sessile or pedunculated yellow-white to red firm masses. Histologically, these represent subepithelial accumulations of amorphic, eosinophilic material that represents fibrin and collagen [161], which may be accompanied by granulation tissue or chronic inflammatory cell infiltrates (➲ *Fig. 3.17*).

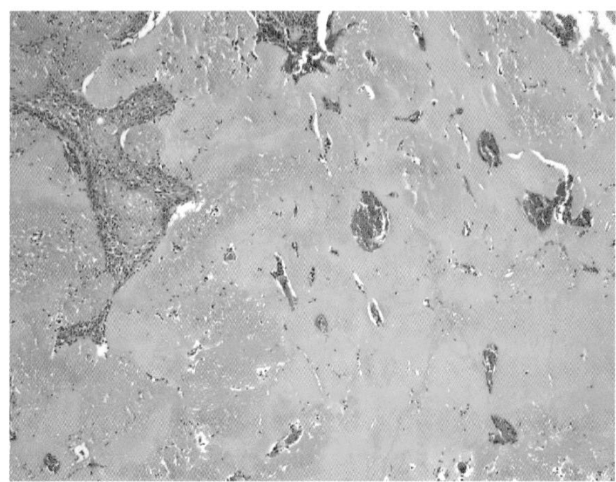

◘ Fig. 3.17
Ligneous vaginitis. **Extensive stromal deposition of amorphic, eosinophilic material is characteristic of a long-standing lesion and is frequently accompanied by overlying pseudoepitheliomatous hyperplasia**

Allergic Reactions to Seminal Fluid

A few women display allergic reactions after exposure to seminal fluid [152]. The severity of the response varies from localized vulvovaginal urticarial reactions to generalized urticaria and bronchospasm. The onset of symptoms immediately follows contact with seminal fluid, and the duration of the reaction is between 2 and 72 h.

Crohn Disease

About 20% of females with Crohn disease have vaginal symptoms [100]. Rectovaginal fistulas occur in some patients with Crohn disease [70], and they represent the site of about 9% of fistulas in women with this disease [5]. In situ squamous carcinoma of the vagina has been reported rarely [224].

Bullous Dermatoses

Vaginal stenosis may develop as a sequela of severe bullous erythema multiforme (Stevens–Johnson syndrome) in which extensive vulvar and vaginal ulceration occurred [101]. Acantholytic intraepithelial bullae may be found when there is vaginal involvement by familial benign chronic pemphigus (Hailey–Hailey disease) [295].

Giant Cell Arteritis and Polyarteritis

Giant cell arteritis is not always limited to the temporal arteries, and may be associated with either limited visceral, or much more rarely, generalized organ involvement [216]. A pan-arteritis, with fragmentation and destruction of the internal elastic lamella and phagocytosis of elastic material by multinucleated giant cells may be seen in the vagina as part of limited female genital tract involvement [16]. Arteritis limited to the genital tract is most commonly found in the cervix and endometrium and has a favorable prognosis in the absence of an elevated sedimentation rate [74]. The frequency of involvement of the vagina has not been determined, since vaginal tissues are infrequently sampled in the course of most surgical procedures.

Thrombotic Thrombocytopenic Purpura

Massive, acute hemorrhagic necrosis of the vagina has been reported as one of the initial manifestations of thrombotic thrombocytopenic purpura [85]. The disease usually is characterized by the pentad of fever, microangiopathic hemolytic anemia, thrombocytopenia, neurologic symptoms, and renal dysfunction. Numerous thrombi are found microscopically in the vaginal stroma, accompanied by superficial hemorrhage, necrosis, and sloughing of the epithelium.

Lesions That Follow Trauma, Surgery, and Radiation

Atrophic Vaginitis

Atrophy of the squamous epithelium of the vagina, accompanied by a loss of glycogen and an increase in the pH, are physiologic events in postmenopausal women that reflect estrogen deprivation. The response also includes a change in the vaginal flora, with a reduction in the lactobacilli that ordinarily inhibit other potential pathogens. The thin epithelium seems to offer little resistance to an altered flora, which may include *streptococci, staphylococci, E. coli,* and diphtheroids. As a result, minor trauma may facilitate a transition from simple atrophy to atrophic vaginitis. Many patients are asymptomatic, but there may be minor vaginal bleeding, pruritis, dysuria, or dyspareunia, accompanied at times by a watery discharge. Atrophy of the vagina produces a pale-appearing mucosa, with petechiae and loss of rugal folds. Microscopically, there is a variable reduction or a loss of the superficial and intermediate cell layers. Small ulcers with acute inflammation and granulation tissue may be interspersed among regions of intact epithelium. Elsewhere, the submucosa is infiltrated by lymphocytes and plasma cells (➲ *Fig. 3.18*). Although the histologic changes are relatively straightforward, occasionally there may be a confusion of atrophy with a high-grade squamous intraepithelial lesion (see below, ➲ Vaginal Intraepithelial Neoplasia). There usually is a good response to estrogen replacement, with epithelial cell maturation and a return to premenopausal flora and pH. Antibiotic therapy rarely is necessary.

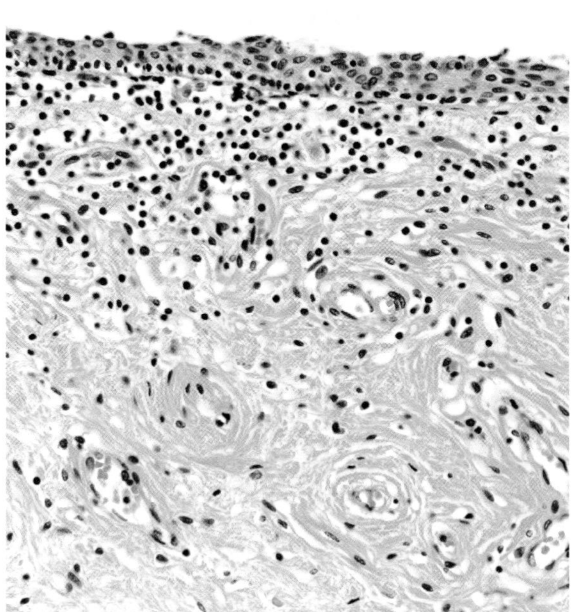

Fig. 3.18
Atrophic vaginitis. **In addition to profound atrophy of the epithelium, there is dense infiltration of the stroma by chronic inflammatory cells**

Tampon Ulcer

Although tampons have been in use for 60 years, there had been little interest in their effects on the vagina until about 1980, when mucosal ulceration and TSS were related to their use. In several series of cases, the women presented with abnormal vaginal discharge or intermenstrual bleeding. Typically, a single ulcer with an irregular border of granulation tissue was identified in one of the vaginal fornices. After neoplasms and infectious etiologies were excluded, a more detailed history revealed the frequent use of tampons. Microscopically, some of the ulcers contained fibrillar foreign bodies within the exudate [125].

The lesions healed spontaneously within 2–3 months after discontinuation of tampon usage [125]. Subsequently, Friedrich studied the vagina during tampon use, and characterized a sequence of clinically asymptomatic, colposcopic, and microscopic changes as follows: (1) mucosal dehydration, (2) layering or intraepithelial cleavage, and (3) microulceration [78]. Ultrastructural findings include a widening of the intercellular spaces separating squamous cells and a marked reduction in the number of desmosomes. He suggested that these changes resulted from a fluid shift across the vaginal epithelium due to the absorbent qualities of the tampon. This hypothesis explains the higher frequency of mucosal alteration with the use of superabsorbent tampons. However, this explanation may be incomplete because a colposcopic study demonstrated an inverse relationship between vaginal drying and the quantity of blood absorbed by different tampon types [255]. The great frequency with which tampons induce clinically inapparent vaginal microulcerations helps to explain their relationship to staphylococcal infections and the development of TSS. The observation that vaginal colonization by *Staphyloccous aureus* has increased from about 12% in 1980 to 23% in 2005 should be viewed with alarm [253].

Postoperative Spindle Cell Nodule

In 1984, Proppe et al. described a lesion of the lower genitourinary tract that closely simulated a sarcoma histologically but was benign [225]. The term postoperative spindle cell nodule was applied to the lesion because typically it arose within 1–3 months of surgery in the region, and usually presented as polypoid, poorly defined nodules. Lesions of similar histologic appearance have been reported in the urinary tract in the absence of a clinical history of surgery or instrumentation [318]. Similarly, these lesions may occur in the vagina in the absence of surgery. The microscopic appearance is characterized by intersecting fascicles of plump spindle cells with a delicate network of small blood vessels, sometimes accompanied by extravasated blood or hemosiderin (*Fig. 3.19*). Superficial ulceration may be present, and chronic inflammatory cells are scattered in the deeper portions of the lesions. The spindle cells have oval, elongated nuclei with evenly dispersed chromatin and abundant eosinophilic bipolar cytoplasmic processes. Because mitotic figures are numerous and the lesions are poorly circumscribed, they may easily be confused with sarcoma. Helpful distinguishing features include the lack of nuclear pleomorphism or nuclear hyperchromasia, an absence of abnormal mitotic figures, and the clinical history of a recent surgical procedure in the region of the lesion [225]. Local recurrence has not been reported, even after incomplete resection [225]. Recently, it has been suggested that this lesion should be included in the category of inflammatory myofibroblastic tumor (IMT), but most IMTs are not associated with prior surgery, and about 33% of them recur following local excision [185].

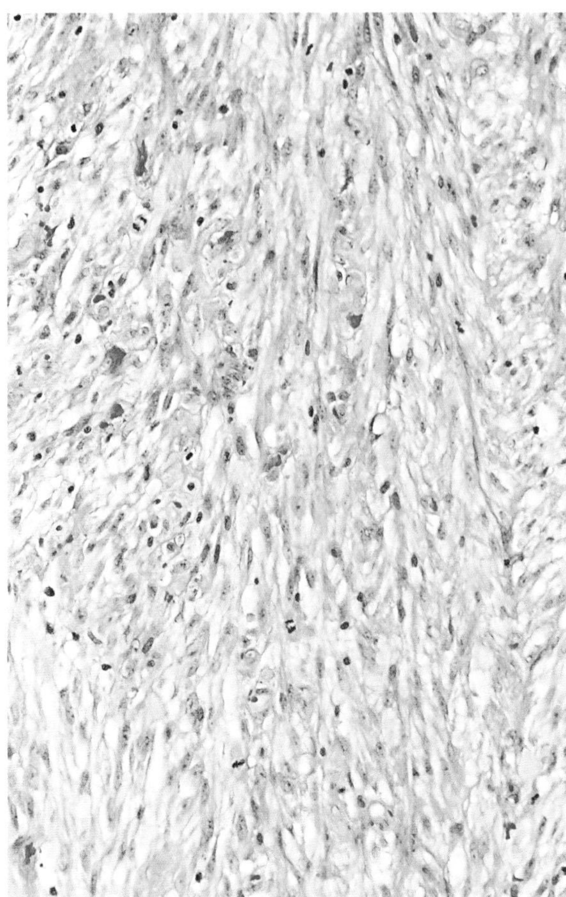

Fig. 3.19
Postoperative spindle cell nodule. **The spindle cells have oval, elongated nuclei with evenly dispersed chromatin and bipolar eosinophilic cytoplasmic processes. Extravasated red blood cells are a characteristic finding**

Vaginal Vault Granulation Tissue

Vaginal vault granulation tissue is a common finding after hysterectomy. One or more small, red, and soft granular to polypoid lesions may be seen grossly, which microscopically are composed of ulcerated, edematous, and granulation tissue containing numerous neutrophils superficially and lymphocytes and plasma cells in the deeper stroma. Occasionally, scattered bizarre stromal cells may cause confusion with a malignant neoplasm (➋ *Fig. 3.20*), particularly if the hysterectomy has been performed for a cervical or corpus tumor.

Fistula

Vesicovaginal and ureterovaginal fistulas may occur as a complication of hysterectomy, resulting from ischemic necrosis secondary to interruption of the vascular supply [280]. The surgical correction usually yields small fragments of tissue with variable amounts of granulation tissue, fibrosis, chronic inflammation, and little or no epithelium. Rarely, calculi are present. These are composed of urinary salts that develop in the vagina because of continuous leakage of urine from a vesicovaginal fistula. Vesicovaginal fistula and vaginal laceration also may be a consequence of coitus.

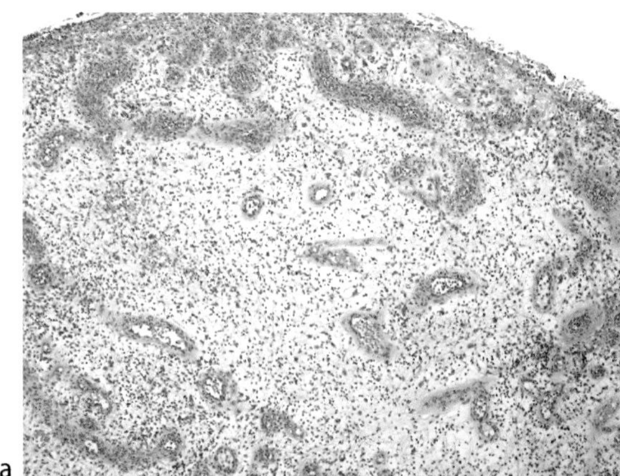

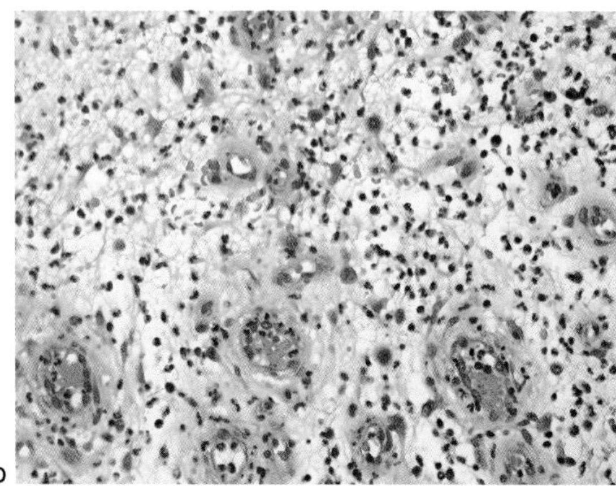

Fig. 3.20
Granulation tissue. **Polypoid, edematous, and vessel rich tissue (a) contains numerous inflammatory cells, scattered bizarre stromal cells and prominent endothelial cells, which may simulate malignancy (b)**

Radionecrosis

Radiation therapy to the vulva, vagina, or uterine cervix may cause necrosis, ulceration, or stenosis of the vagina [246]. The mechanism by which this injury develops reflects the sensitivity of endothelial cells to radiation, with thrombosis and subsequent stenosis or obliteration of small blood vessels, stromal fibrosis, and epithelial ulceration. The formation of granular to polypoid masses, particularly in the vaginal vault, may clinically simulate recurrent cervical carcinoma. In addition to the vascular changes, dense infiltrates of plasma cells, granulation tissue, and bizarre stromal cells with pleomorphic, hyperchromatic nuclei may be sprinkled through the stroma. Even in the absence of a gross lesion, one may anticipate extreme atrophy of the vaginal squamous mucosa as a consequence of radiation therapy combined with cessation of ovarian function (➋ *Fig. 3.21*). Careful examination of nuclear detail helps to distinguish radiation atrophy from intraepithelial carcinoma. Atrophic cells have high nuclear/cytoplasmic ratios such as those of intraepithelial carcinoma, but have a regular, round to oval nuclear shape with a uniform distribution of chromatin that may appear smudged, in contrast to the irregular nuclear contours and clumped chromatin of vaginal intraepithelial neoplasia. Occasionally, radiation may result in partially obliterated vascular channels lined by plump endothelial cells containing large nuclei with vesicular chromatin, which simulate cords of invasive carcinoma. The distinction may be assisted by immunohistochemistry. Although a positive immunostaining reaction is not always present, the localization of factor VIII antigen in the atypical cells coupled with the absence of staining for keratins provides evidence for reactive endothelial rather than epithelial cells.

Vaginal Prolapse

Cystocele, rectocele, and vaginal prolapse may occur after multiple vaginal deliveries. The surgical correction may include removal of elliptical fragments of vaginal mucosa in which variable degrees of acanthosis, hyperkeratosis, or parakeratosis are present (➋ *Fig. 3.22*).

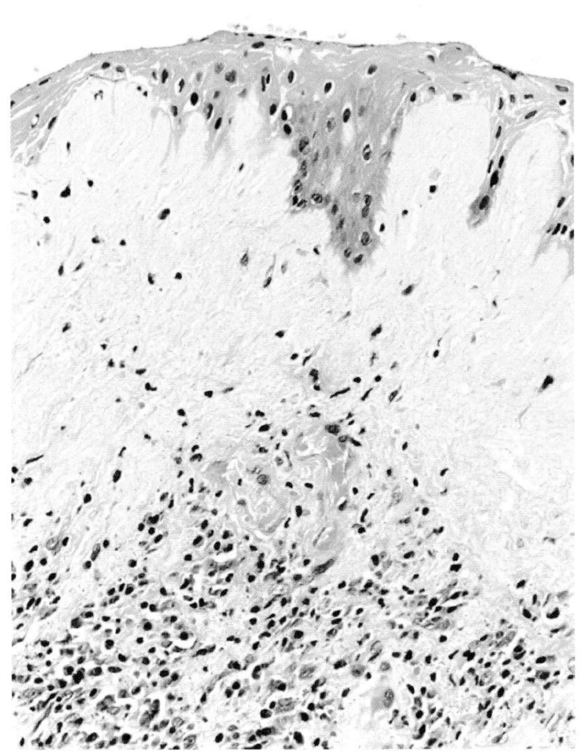

Fig. 3.21
Radiation change. **Long-term consequences of irradiation to the vagina include atrophy of the squamous epithelium, edema, fibrosis within the stroma, and obliteration of vascular channels**

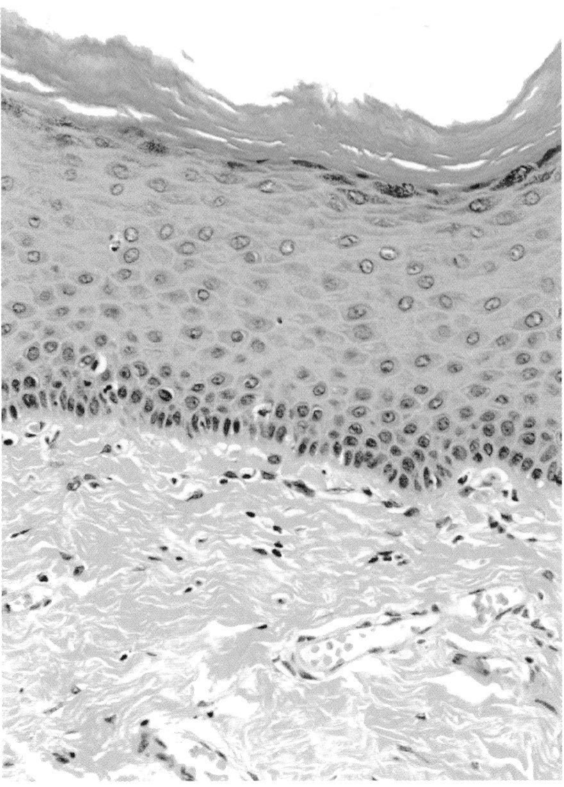

Fig. 3.22
Vaginal prolapse. **Acanthosis and hyperkeratosis of the squamous epithelium are present**

Fallopian Tube Prolapse

Prolapse of the fallopian tube into the vagina is a relatively uncommon complication of either vaginal or abdominal hysterectomy [29, 262]. Patients often present with abdominal pain, vaginal discharge, or vaginal bleeding. A red, granular mass or nodule usually is present at the vaginal apex, which grossly may be confused with granulation tissue or carcinoma. Manipulation of the prolapsed tube typically causes extreme pain. Microscopically, a complex pattern of tubular, glandular, and papillary structures may be present (*Fig. 3.23*). Nuclear crowding and stratification are common, and ciliated or secretory columnar cells of typical tubal type may be difficult to locate (*Fig. 3.24*) [262]. Fimbriae are rarely identifiable, and both a diligence and an awareness of the condition are required to avoid the misdiagnosis of adenocarcinoma. There is often associated inflammation and granulation tissue, and when prominent, this may

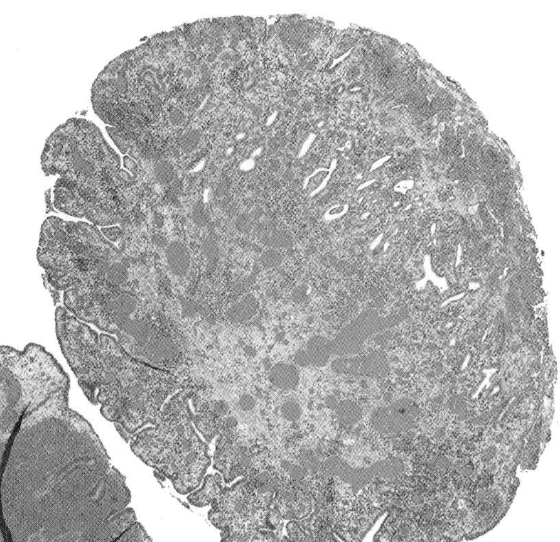

Fig. 3.23
Fallopian tube prolapse. **When the plicae are blunt, there may be confusion with adenocarcinoma**

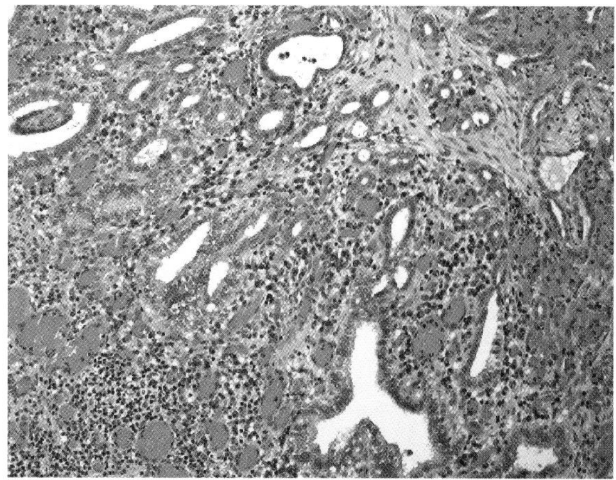

Fig. 3.24
Fallopian tube prolapse. **While the architectural complexity raises the possibility of malignancy, most cells are ciliated confirming that the structure is fallopian tube**

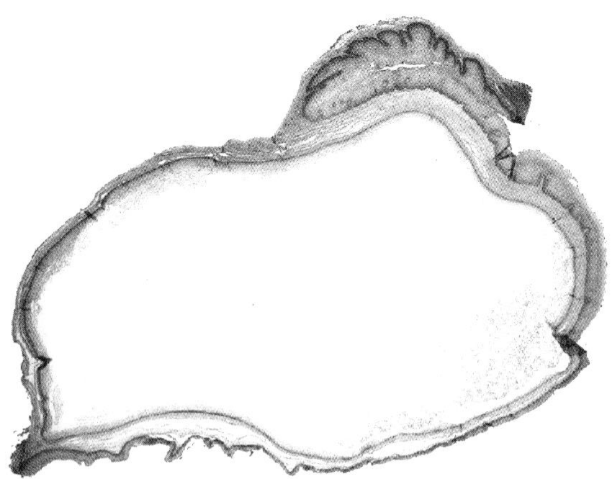

Fig. 3.25
Squamous inclusion cyst. **The cyst is lined by stratified squamous epithelium and contains keratinaceous debris**

be confused with either aggressive angiomyxoma or angiomyofibroblastoma [181, 299].

Cysts

Cysts of the vagina are relatively uncommon. Several classifications for cystic lesions have been proposed, reflecting a combination of good microscopic descriptions, an incomplete knowledge of embryology, and an assumption that histologic differentiation mirrors histogenesis [131, 139]. A functional classification scheme follows: squamous inclusion cysts, mesonephric cysts, müllerian cysts, and Bartholin gland cysts.

Squamous Inclusion Cyst

Squamous inclusion cysts are probably the most common of the vaginal cysts, resulting from the entrapment of fragments of mucosa during repair of a vaginal laceration or episiotomy and thus more commonly occur in the distal portion of the vagina [131]. These cysts are often asymptomatic and vary from a few millimeters to several centimeters in diameter. The microscopic appearance is that of a cyst wall formed by a stratified squamous epithelium, lacking rete ridges, with a central mass of keratin from desquamated cells (*Fig. 3.25*).

Mesonephric Cyst

Mesonephric cysts, also termed Gartners duct cysts, are most often located along the anterolateral wall of the vagina, following the route of the mesonephric duct. It is assumed that mesonephric cysts result from secretion by small isolated epithelial remnants after incomplete regression of the mesonephric duct. Mesonephric cysts are lined by low cuboidal, non-mucin-secreting cells, which are devoid of cytoplasmic mucicarmine or PAS-positive material (*Fig. 3.26*).

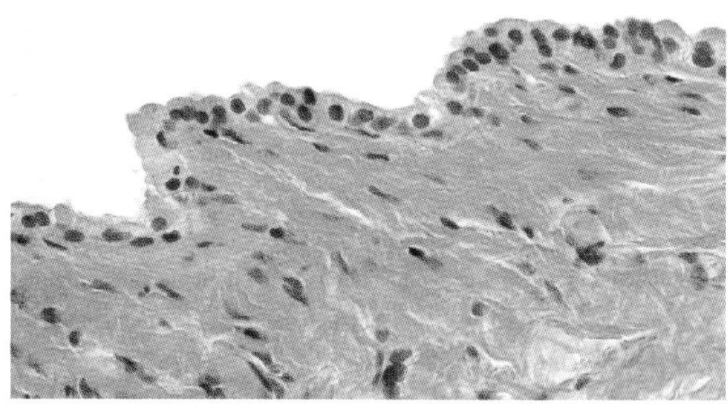

Fig. 3.26
Mesonephric cyst. **The cyst is typically small and lined by a simple cuboidal epithelium, lacking cilia or intracellular mucin**

Müllerian Cyst

The genesis of the müllerian cysts is poorly understood; perhaps some are derived from islands of adenosis [131]. They are located anywhere within the vagina are grossly indistinguishable from mesonephric duct cysts, and are usually less than 2 cm in diameter. The distinction is made on microscopic examination. Müllerian cysts may be lined by any of the epithelia of the müllerian duct, including mucinous endocervical, endometrial, and ciliated tubal types (➋ *Fig. 3.27*). Tall columnar mucin-secreting cells of endocervical type are most common, and squamous metaplasia may be observed.

Bartholin Gland Cyst

Bartholin gland cysts occur in the region of the ducts of Bartholin glands, near the opening of the primary duct into the vestibule. The pathogenesis is incompletely understood, but usually involves occlusion of the duct, associated with either a highly viscous thick mucoid secretion or infection of the gland [131]. The cyst may enlarge rapidly and cause dyspareunia. The cyst lining varies from mucin secreting to squamous or "transitional," reflecting the different types of epithelium lining the duct and gland (➋ *Fig. 3.28*). Histochemical and ultrastructural studies of the mucinous cells of normal Bartholin glands, as well as these cysts, reveal no differences from the cells of the endocervix [248]. The Bartholin gland is of urogenital sinus origin, whereas the cervix is of müllerian derivation; therefore, the weakness of a histogenetic classification of vaginal cysts based on histologic features is reinforced further by this observation. Cysts of identical histologic appearance may occur elsewhere in the vestibule, reflecting the presence of numerous minor vestibular glands of urogenital sinus origin. The treatment of vaginal cysts usually is excision, although marsupialization may be indicated for some Bartholin gland cysts.

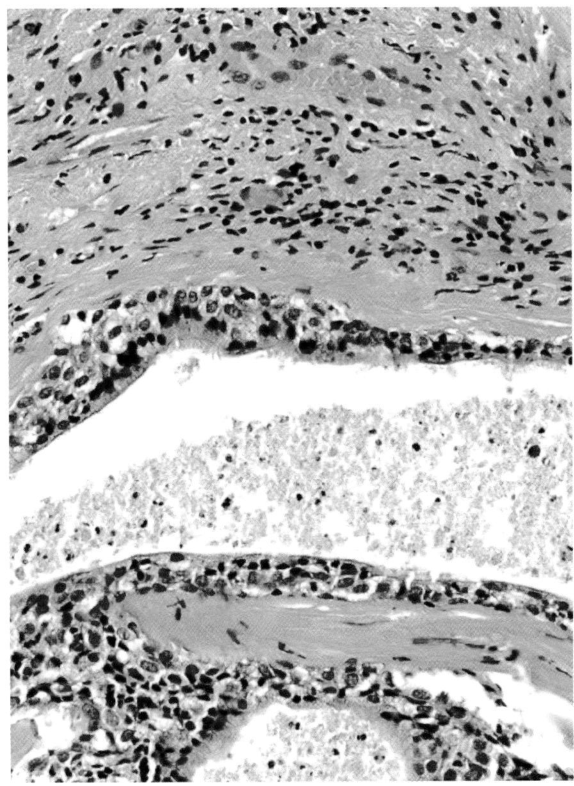

Fig. 3.27
Müllerian cyst. **The cyst is lined by cuboidal or columnar cells, which may be endocervical, tubal, or endometrial type. Note the cilia along the apical border of scattered cells**

Benign Neoplasms

Squamous Papilloma

Squamous papillomas may be single but are frequently multiple. These lesions usually are only a few millimeters in diameter, and most commonly occur in clusters near the hymenal ring, resulting in a condition referred to as squamous papillomatosis [144]. The lesions usually are asymptomatic, but may be associated with vulvar burning or dyspareunia. Squamous papillomas may be difficult to distinguish from condylomas by gross inspection. Colposcopic and microscopic examination reveal the squamous papilloma to be composed of a single papillary frond with a central fibrovascular core (➋ *Fig. 3.29*). It lacks the complex arborizing architecture, acanthosis, and cellular atypia (koilocytes) of the condyloma.

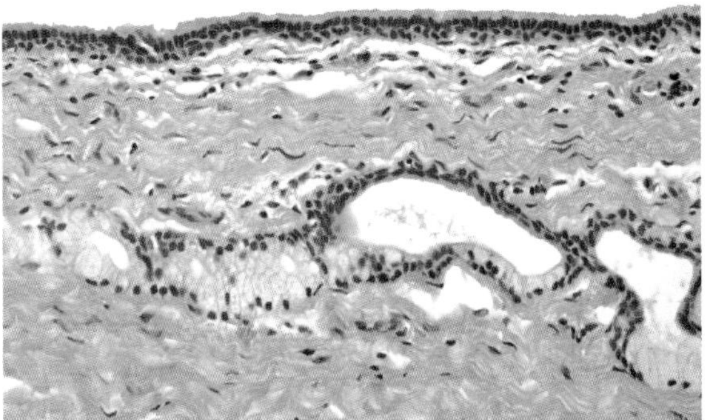

Fig. 3.28
Bartholin gland cyst. **The cyst is partially lined by mucin-containing cells similar to those seen in normal Bartholin's glands**

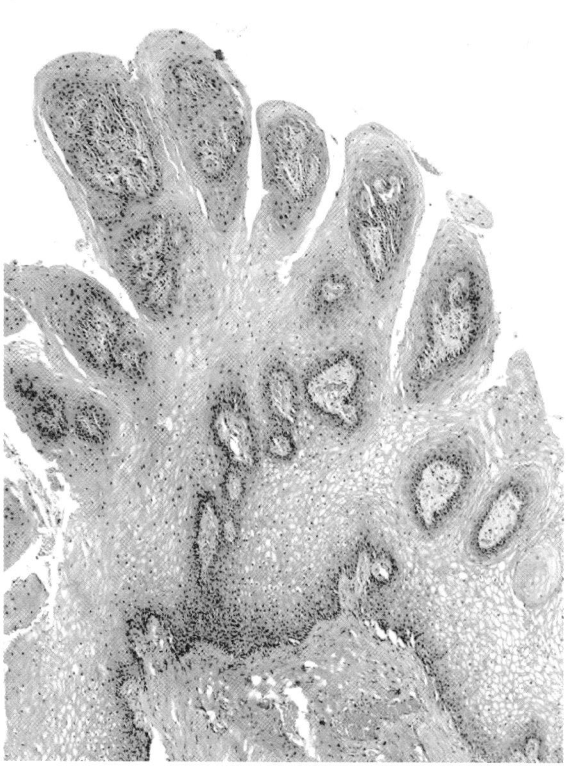

Fig. 3.29
Squamous papilloma. **In contrast to a condyloma, this lesion lacks koilocytes and complex branching papillae**

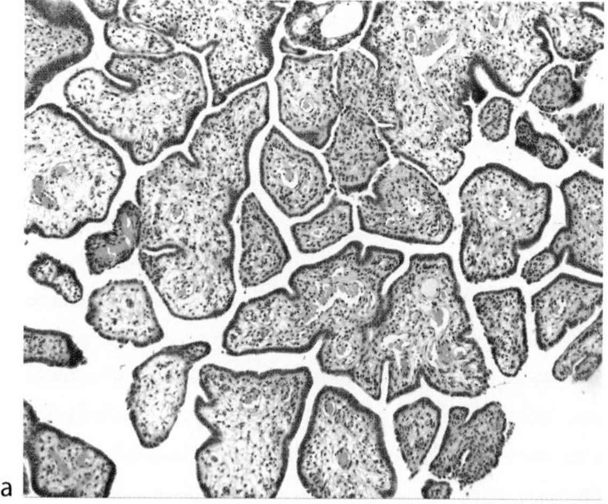

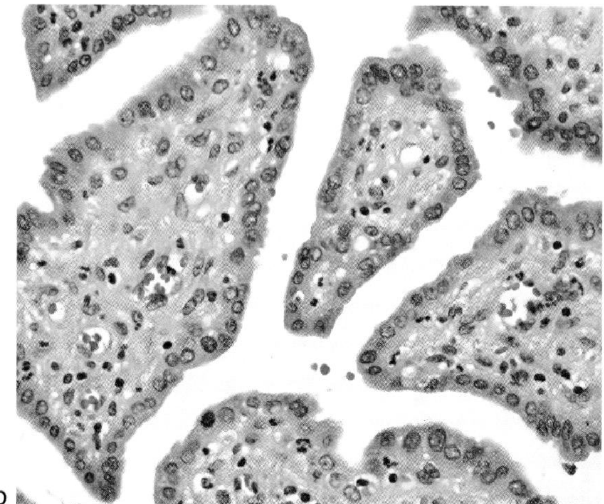

Fig. 3.30
Müllerian papilloma. **Complex, branching, thick fibrovascular cores (a) are covered by a bland low columnar epithelium (b)**

Condyloma Acuminatum

An extensive discussion of the features of condylomas is provided in Chap. 1, Benign Diseases of the Vulva, and Chap. 4, Benign Diseases of the Cervix. As the biologic and pathologic characteristics of vaginal condylomas are similar to those in the cervix and vulva, they are not described here.

Müllerian Papilloma

Müllerian papilloma is a rare benign neoplasm, first described by Ulbright et al., which typically occurs in the vagina (and cervix) of young girls, usually less than 5 years of age. As these lesions are typically exophytic papillary growths, patients most commonly present with vaginal bleeding. Microscopically, it is composed of a complex arborizing papillae with fibrovascular cores lined by bland-appearing epithelial cells, typically low columnar to cuboidal, which may sometimes form both solid masses and glandular lumina (*Fig. 3.30*) [294]. Although similar tumors displaying an exophytic growth pattern and covered by mucin-secreting, hobnail, or eosinophilic cells have been described in both the vagina and cervix of young girls as mesonephric müllerian papillomas [10, 44, 165, 175, 254, 279], the morphologic, immunophenotypic, and ultra-structural features, including microvilli, perinuclear arrays of microfilaments, tonofilaments, and complex cytoplasmic interdigitations, support a müllerian origin. These tumors are considered benign, although rare instances of recurrence and malignant transformation have been reported [2, 62].

Fibroepithelial Polyp (Mesodermal Stromal Polyp)

The fibroepithelial stromal polyp is a benign proliferation that most likely represents a reactive process that arises from the distinctive subepithelial myxoid stroma of the distal female genital tract rather than representing a neoplastic process; cells with a similar histologic appearance have been described in a band-like subepithelial stromal zone extending from the endocervix to the vulva of normal females and may represent the origin of these atypical cells. The fibroepithelial stromal polyp may occur at any age, with the age range extending from newborn to 77 years, but are most frequent during reproductive years with a mean age at diagnosis of about 40 years [34, 182, 186, 201, 203, 226]. The lesions usually are asymptomatic and are discovered incidentally, during pelvic examination, on the lateral wall of the lower third of the vagina. The size varies but they usually measure less than 5 cm, and the gross configuration may be that of a single edematous soft polyp resembling an acrochordon, a papillary lesion with fingerlike projections, or a cerebriform mass (➲ *Fig. 3.31*). Although usually single, multiple polyps may occur, particularly during pregnancy; about 25% of patients with fibroepithelial stromal polyps are pregnant at the time of diagnosis. Microscopically, these polypoid lesions have a fibroblastic stroma and a centrally located fibrovascular core, and are covered by a variably thickened stratified squamous epithelium. The most histologically distinctive component of these lesions is the stroma, which can vary from edematous and hypocellular with bland spindle-shaped cells with indistinct cytoplasm to lesions that are hypercellular and contain cells with markedly enlarged hyperchromatic nuclei. When the latter features are florid, which more commonly occur during pregnancy, these changes can mimic malignancy, particularly sarcoma botryoides; however, the fibroepithelial polyp lacks a "cambium layer," small undifferentiated stromal cells, rhabdomyoblasts, or invasion of the overlying squamous epithelium, which are typical features of sarcoma botryoides. Most fibroepithelial polyps occur in women over the age of 20, whereas sarcoma botryoides is confined almost always to children less than 5 years of age. Moreover, the presence of stellate and multinucleate cells, which are typically located near the epithelial stromal interface, as well as the lack of an interface between the lesional stromal cells and the overlying squamous epithelium are characteristic findings, even in floridly pseudosarcomatous lesions (➲ *Fig. 3.32*). However, the distinction from sarcoma is made primarily on the basis of superficial location, small size, lack of an identifiable lesional margin, extension of abnormal stromal tissue to the mucosal–stromal interface, and the presence of scattered multinucleate stromal cells [200]. The stromal cells are typically positive for desmin, vimentin, estrogen receptor, and progesterone receptor; actin is less commonly positive [104, 182, 186]. The immunolocalization of steroid receptors in these bizarre cells and frequent relationship to pregnancy, during which there may be multiple polyps (and following which they usually regress) supports the premise that fibroepithelial polyps are hormonally induced.

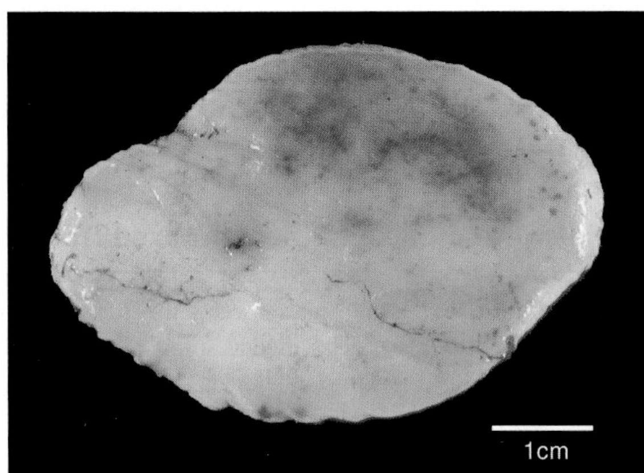

Fig. 3.31
Fibroepithelial stromal polyp. Cross section shows a homogeneous fibrous core

Leiomyoma

Benign smooth muscle tumors of the vagina are uncommon. The mean age at detection is about 40 years, with a reported range of 19–72 years [253]. The tumor may occur anywhere within the vagina, however, it more commonly involves the lateral aspect and is usually in a submucosal location. Vaginal leiomyomas vary from 0.5 to 15 cm in diameter, but are usually less than 5 cm [282]. Because most are relatively small, they often are asymptomatic. Larger tumors may produce pain, hemorrhage, dystocia, or dyspareunia.

The gross and microscopic appearances of vaginal leiomyomas resemble those of their uterine counterparts.

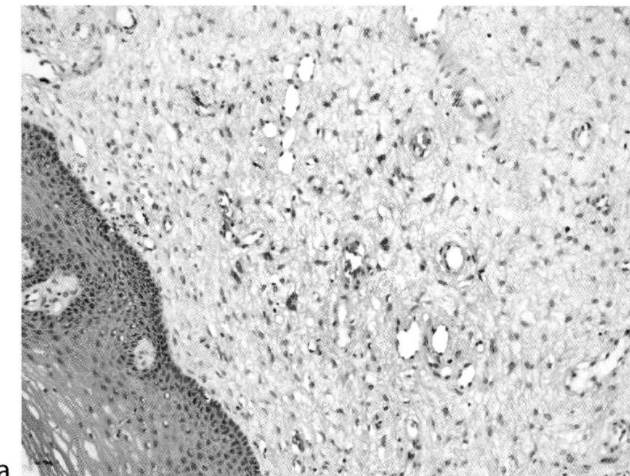

a

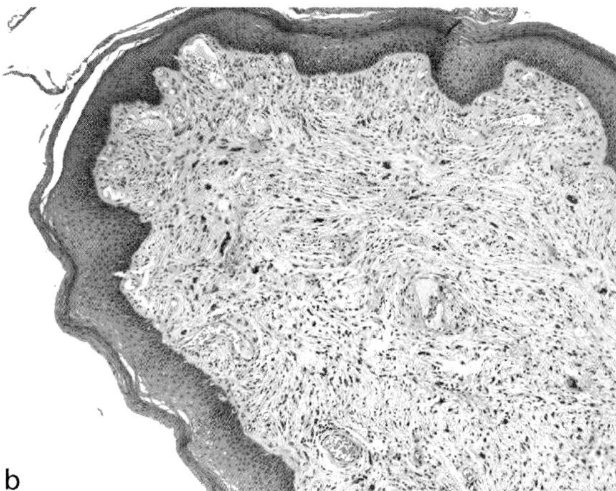

b

Fig. 3.32
Fibroepithelial stromal polyp. **The stroma varies in appearance from bland and hypocellular (a) to stroma with markedly atypical cells (b). Note the lack of an interface between the stromal cells and the overlying epithelium and the presence of multinucleate stromal cells near the epithelial–stromal interface**

They are well-circumscribed, firm masses that occasionally may contain foci of edema or hyalinization. Microscopically, they are well circumscribed without evidence of infiltration and are composed of interlacing fascicles of spindle-shaped cells, with elongated, oval nuclei with no mitotic activity or nuclear pleomorphism. Of the 60 cases of smooth muscle tumors of the vagina reviewed by Tavassoli and Norris, only 7 contained more than five mitoses per ten high-power fields (HPF). Five patients developed recurrence after local excision. All the recurrent tumors were in the subset with high mitotic activity and generally moderate to marked nuclear atypia [282]. Accordingly, it is recommended that the diagnosis of vaginal leiomyoma be reserved for those tumors that are histologically well circumscribed, are cytologically bland, and have fewer than five mitoses per ten HPF. However, it also should be noted that increased mitotic activity in the absence of aggressive behavior may be present in vaginal leiomyomas during pregnancy.

Rhabdomyoma

Rhabdomyoma is a rare benign tumor displaying well-formed skeletal muscle differentiation, about 20 cases of which have been reported arising within the vagina [96, 103, 123]. The average age at diagnosis is about 45 years, with a range extending from 34 to 57 years. Patients typically present with a solitary polypoid to nodular mass that varies from 1 to 11 cm in diameter. Symptoms are typically related to a mass lesion and include dyspareunia; bleeding is less common as the overlying mucosa is usually intact.

Microscopically, rhabdomyomas are located in the submucosa and are composed of a somewhat fascicular proliferation of benign-appearing fetal- or adult-type skeletal muscle cells surrounded by variable quantities of fibrous stroma (➲ *Fig. 3.33*). The cells are of spindle to oval shape, with plump oval nuclei and abundant granular, eosinophilic cytoplasm. Mitotic activity and nuclear pleomorphism are absent. The diagnosis is confirmed by identification of intracytoplasmic fibers with cross-striations (➲ *Fig. 3.34*), staining for which may be enhanced by phosphotungstic acid hematoxlin (PTAH) or trichrome preparations . Immunohistochemistry and electron microscopy usually are not needed to confirm the presence of skeletal muscle differentiation [96]. It is important not to confuse vaginal rhabdomyoma with embryonal rhabdomyosarcoma (see below), but this is generally not difficult because genital rhabdomyoma lacks nuclear atypia, mitotic activity, and a cambium layer; in addition it occurs in an older-age population. The behavior of rhabdomyoma is benign, and local excision provides adequate therapy.

Spindle Cell Epithelioma (Benign Mixed Tumor)

Tumors that histologically bear some resemblance to salivary gland neoplasms are classified as spindle cell epitheliomas or benign mixed tumors. These neoplasms are rare, and usually present as a slowly growing, painless, well-circumscribed, submucosal mass that may occur anywhere in the vagina, but most frequently near the hymenal ring [25, 263]. The mean age at diagnosis is 30 years. They range in size from 1.5 to 5 cm and often are diagnosed preoperatively as a polyp or cyst.

Microscopically, the neoplasm is a well-circumscribed, unencapsulated mass located near, but not connected to, the overlying epithelial surface and is characterized by a biphasic proliferation of spindle and epithelial cells (➋ *Figs. 3.35* and ➋ *3.36*). The spindle cell proliferation is variably cellular and loosely fascicular with paler hypocellular zones containing fibroblastic-type cells separating the cellular areas into interconnecting islands. The epithelial component, which may be only focally present, includes nests of bland-appearing glycogenated, stratified squamous cells and occasional glands lined by a mucin-secreting epithelium [83]. Eosinophilic hyaline globules, which likely represent condensation of the stromal matrix, are characteristic. The spindle cells are positive for keratin and smooth muscle actin [190], the combination of which led to the former designation of these lesions as mixed tumors. The behavior is benign and local excision is curative; one case of a recurrence has been reported 8 years following initial excision [316].

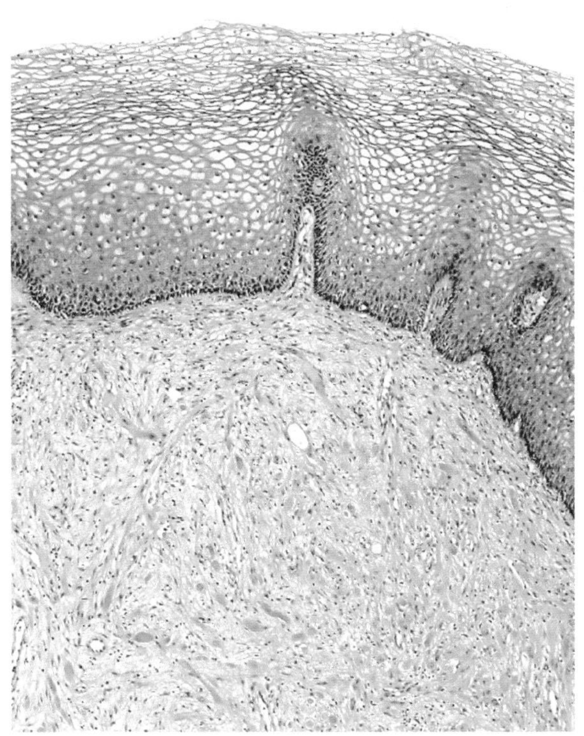

Fig. 3.33
Vaginal rhabdomyoma. **At low magnification, a nonencapsulated mass of plump, elongated cells is covered by a slightly thickened squamous epithelium**

Endometriosis

It is not uncommon for endometriosis to involve the vagina, either superficially implanted in the squamous mucosa or involving the deep stroma, particularly of the

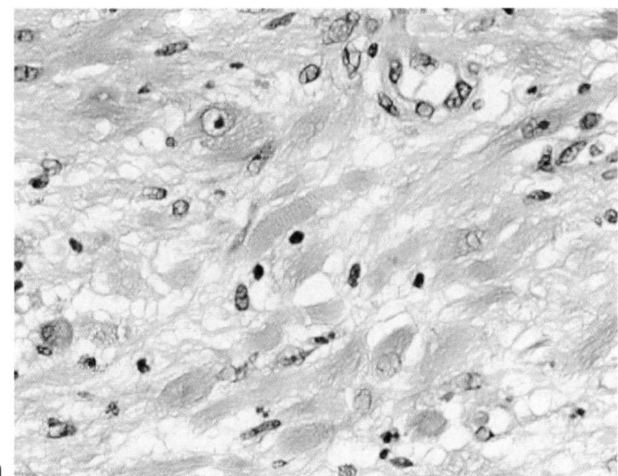

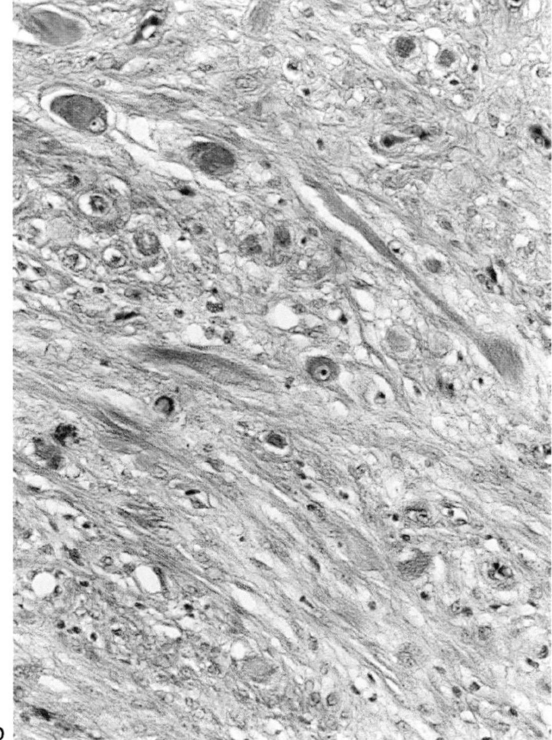

Fig. 3.34
Vaginal rhabdomyoma. **At higher magnification, cross striations can be seen in the eosinophilic cell cytoplasm (hematoxylin and eosin stain) (a); the cross striations are further enhanced with phosphotungstic acid–hematoxylin stain (b)**

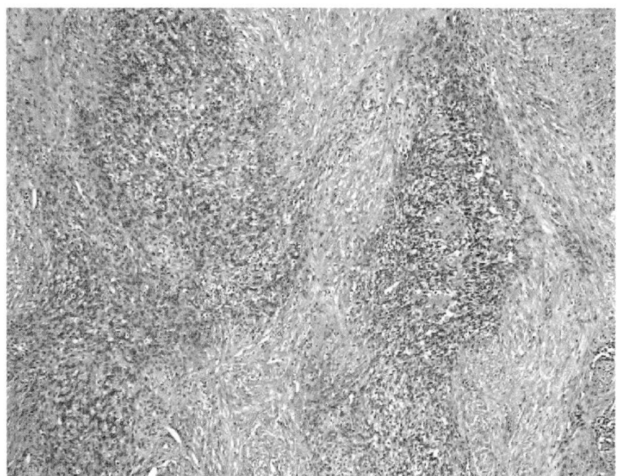

■ Fig. 3.35
Spindle cell epithelioma (benign mixed tumor of vagina). **The tumor often has a biphasic spindle cell population composed of hypo- and hypercellular zones**

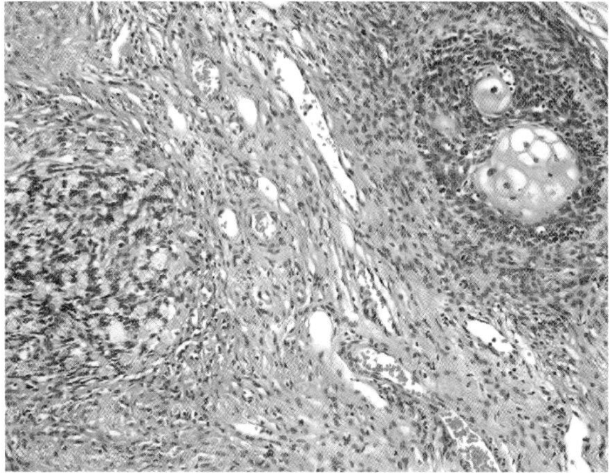

■ Fig. 3.36
Spindle cell epithelioma (benign mixed tumor of vagina). **A nest of stratified squamous epithelial cells is surrounded by irregular fascicles of spindled stromal cells**

rectovaginal septum [86, 133, 169, 301, 312]. A complete discussion of endometriosis is provided in Chap. 13, Diseases of the Peritoneum.

Miscellaneous Benign Tumors and Tumor-Like Lesions

In addition to those tumors that are highly characteristic for the vagina, sporadic cases of benign neoplasms and tumor-like processes have been reported, including adenomatoid tumor [159], villous adenoma (*Fig. 3.37*) [73], mature cystic teratoma [145], Brenner tumor

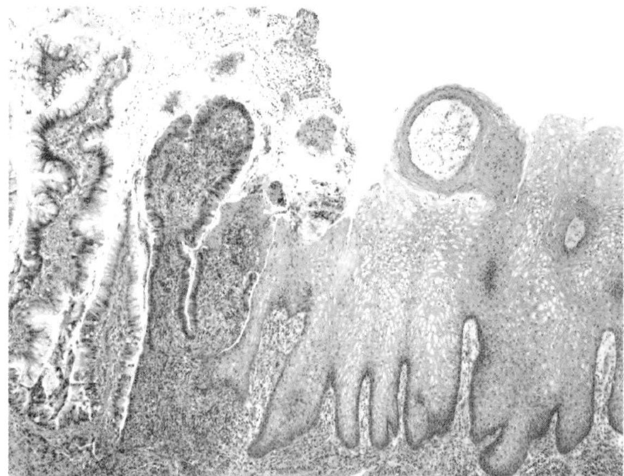

■ Fig. 3.37
Villous adenoma of the vagina. **The lesion presented as a polypoid mass. It is histologically identical to a villous adenoma in the colon**

[33], hemangioma [97], granular cell tumor [139], neurofibroma [58], paraganglioma [215], glomus tumor [270], blue nevus [289], and eosinophilic granuloma [320]. Thyroid and parathyroid glands have been described in the vaginal wall of a 3-year-old girl, but probably these represented monodermal differentiation within a benign vaginal teratoma [145].

Malignant Neoplasms

Vaginal Intraepithelial Neoplasia

In contrast to the high prevalence of intraepithelial lesions of the cervix and vulva, vaginal intraepithelial neoplasia (VAIN) is relatively rare. The reason for this discrepancy is unknown, but may be related to a lesser susceptibility of the vaginal mucosa to HPV infection than the cervical transformation zone. However, similar to the cervix, the range of HPV types that can affect this area is greater than those that occur in the vulva [270]. Understanding the reasons for this difference may prove pivotal to understanding carcinogenesis involving the squamous epithelium of the lower female genital tract. The terminology for intraepithelial neoplasia of the vagina continues to evolve, reflecting conceptual refinements, and parallels that for the cervix and vulva. *Squamous intraepithelial lesion* (SIL) and *dysplasia* represent alternative systems of nomenclature for *intraepithelial neoplasia*, reflecting differing social, political, and scientific efforts to best characterize the processes. Irrespective of terminology (VAIN), SIL displays nuclear atypia coupled with some loss of squamous maturation, disordered maturation, increased mitotic activity, sometimes accompanied by abnormal mitotic figures, acanthosis, and dyskeratosis.

General Features

The incidence of in situ carcinoma of the vagina is reported to be about 0.20 cases per 100,000 in Caucasian females and 0.31 cases per 100,000 in black females; this is less than 1% of the incidence for the same disease in the cervix [47, 110]. The highest incidence rates are observed in women over the age of 60, with the mean age at diagnosis of VAIN 3 about 53 years. These figures are 10 or more years greater than the age of detection of cervical intraepithelial neoplasia (CIN) 3 [121]. Risk factors for the development of VAIN paralleled that of the cervix and include immunosuppression, HPV infection, or squamous neoplasia elsewhere in the lower genital tract, irradiation, and in utero exposure to DES, although this latter factor is controversial [26]. During the mid-1970s, it was first suggested that DES-exposed offspring might be at risk for increased rates of dysplasia because of the extent of metaplastic tissue present in both the cervix and vagina. Multiple studies of prevalence rates subsequently conducted indicated that the frequency of dysplasia in both the exposed and unexposed populations was approximately the same. In 1984, the DESAD Project amplified its findings on the frequency of dysplasia. The incidence rates were slightly higher in exposed women. The new occurrence of squamous cell dysplasia in women under observation developed twice as frequently in DES-exposed women in contrast to those that were never exposed in utero [23, 241]. Some believe that the DESAD findings may not be valid, and that the increased rates of dysplasia, especially of mild form, may be caused by over- or misinterpretation of the HPV-infected tissue for dysplasia [238], especially as the DESAD study was conducted before many of the histologic intricacies of HPV infection were fully appreciated. Regardless of interpretation, DES itself is not believed to be the etiologic cause of dysplasia. Possibly, the metaplastic squamous epithelium, which is more extensive in the vagina in DES-exposed women, may be more susceptible to agents that give rise to dysplasia, but even this is speculative.

Almost 75% of women with VAIN have preceding or coexisting squamous carcinomas of the cervix or vulva [18, 128, 129, 151, 260]. These observations have generated the concept of a field effect, in which the squamous epithelium of the entire lower female genital tract is at risk for neoplastic transformation. This hypothesis is appealing, because the squamous epithelia of these sites do share a common embryonic derivation from the urogenital sinus, and all are susceptible to infection by various HPVs. Radiation therapy for cervical carcinoma results in exposure of the vagina to ionizing radiation, and women who have had pelvic radiation for benign as well as malignant diseases are at increased risk for development of VAIN [18, 89, 151].

Gross Findings

Women with VAIN are usually asymptomatic, and in most instances there is no grossly identifiable lesion in the vagina. Occasionally, the epithelium appears raised, roughened, and white or pink (*Fig. 3.38*). More often, the patient presents with an abnormal Papanicolaou smear and the diagnosis is confirmed by a colposcopically directed biopsy subsequent to an abnormal cytologic diagnosis in which sampling of the vagina as well as the cervix has been performed, or in vaginal samples after hysterectomy. The process is multifocal or diffuse in almost half of the cases, and usually is located in the upper third of the vagina [18, 151, 184, 251].

Microscopic Findings

The microscopic features of VAIN are analogous to those of CIN (see Chap. 5, Precancerous Lesions of the

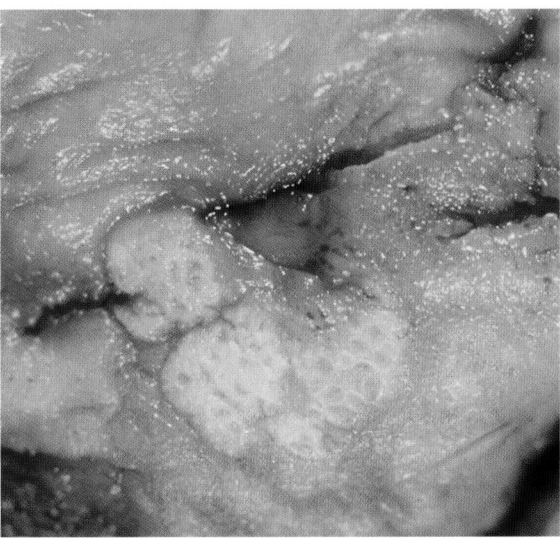

Fig. 3.38
Dysplasia of the vaginal vault. It appears as an irregular raised white plaque with a granular surface

Cervix), and similarly the term VAIN comprises lesions classified as condyloma (low-grade VAIN, VAIN I) and lesions classified as vaginal intraepithelial neoplasia (high-grade VAIN, VAIN II–III). Histologically, low-grade VAIN parallels CIN I and includes exophytic and flat condyloma. Exophytic condyloma is characterized by verucopapillary growth, acanthosis, and superficial koilocytotic atypia (*Fig. 3.39*); this lesion is highly associated with HPV types 6 and 11. Flat condyloma shares the superficial distribution of koilocytotic atypia but lacks exophytic growth (*Fig. 3.40*). High-grade VAIN is characterized histologically by the presence of nuclear abnormalities including enlargement with irregular shape, hyperchromasia, and irregular condensation of chromatin at all levels of the epithelium. Lesions that exhibit maturation at the surface are classified as VAIN II, whereas those with minimal maturation correspond to VAIN III (*Figs. 3.41* and *3.42*). SIL (VAIN) lesions nearly always display some loss of squamous maturation as well as disordered maturation, frequently including increased mitotic activity, abnormal mitotic figures, acanthosis, and dyskeratosis.

The differential diagnosis of SIL (VAIN) includes atrophy, radiation change, and immature squamous metaplasia in women with adenosis, all of which may display loss of glycogen and a relative increase in cellularity. The distinction rests primarily on the characteristic nuclear features of SIL (VAIN), which are absent in the other conditions. Radiation changes include nuclear enlargement, smudged chromatin, multinucleation, and vacuolization of cytoplasm, with lack of mitotic activity [80]. Occasionally, there may be significant nuclear atypia associated with inflammatory and reactive processes, but usually this is expressed as regular nuclear enlargement with vesicular chromatin and moderate-sized nucleoli. Such changes are referred to as reactive squamous atypia.

Clinical Behavior and Treatment

The natural history of SIL (VAIN) is uncertain. In one study, about 5% of SIL (VAIN) progressed to invasive carcinoma, with sequential changes documented by serial biopsies [251], but this figure probably significantly underestimates the biologic potential of VAIN because many lesions were treated [261]. Therapy generally is local excision, although topical 5-fluorouracil, laser vaporization, vaginectomy, and irradiation also have been successfully used [166, 272, 315]. In a study of 94 women with VAIN,

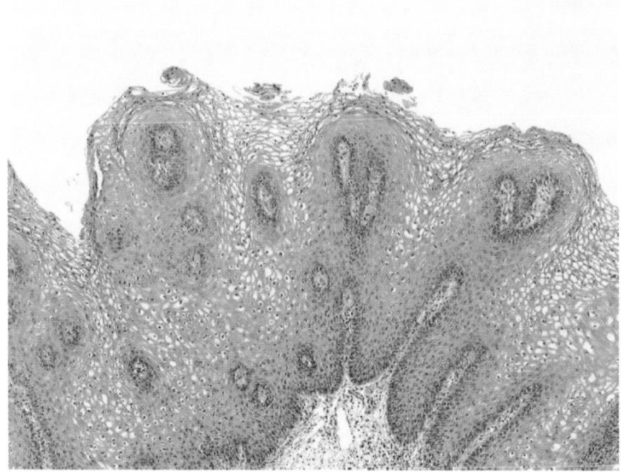

Fig. 3.39
VAIN I (low-grade SIL, exophytic condyloma). **There is papillomatosis and irregular acanthosis of this epithelium in addition to koilocytosis and nuclear features of intraepithelial neoplasia. The extensive cytoplasmic differentiation is diagnostic of VAIN I (low-grade SIL)**

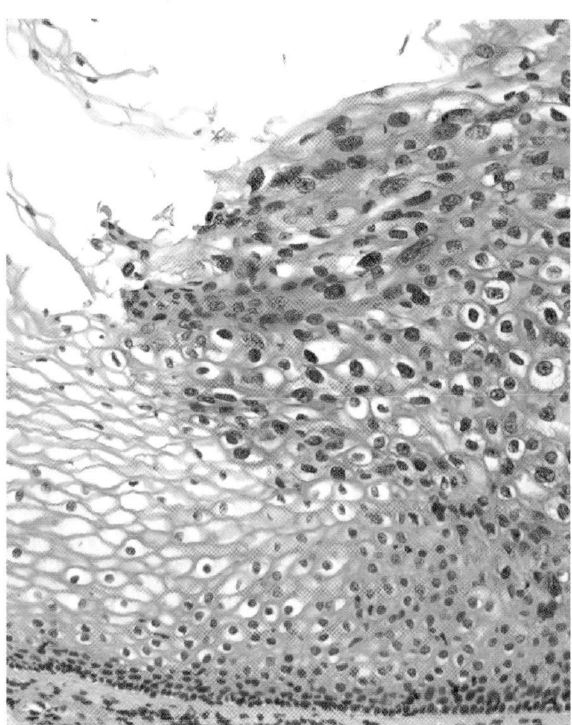

Fig. 3.40
VAIN 1 (low-grade SIL, flat condyloma). **This lesion shows striking superficial koilocytotic atypia but lacks exophytic growth. The nuclear features of intraepithelial neoplasia are evident, including nuclear enlargement, pleomorphism, coarse chromatin, and irregular nuclear contours. Koilocytosis is also present**

70% achieved remission after a single treatment of any type, but 24% required additional therapy with chemosurgery or upper vaginectomy; 5% progressed to invasive squamous carcinoma in spite of therapy and close follow-up [261].

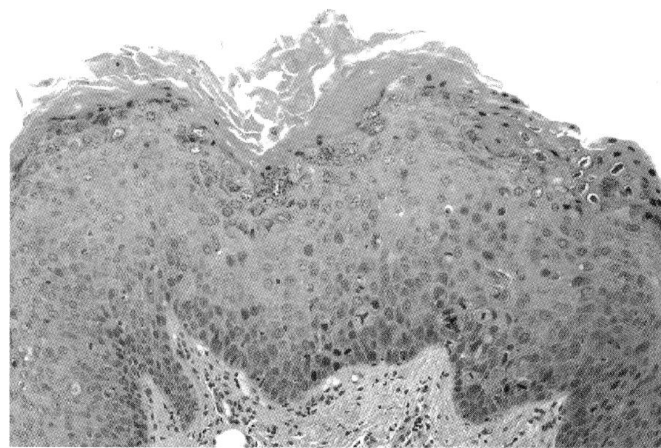

Fig. 3.41
VAIN 2 (high-grade SIL). **This intraepithelial process is characterized by enlargement and pleomorphism of nuclei, but preservation of some features of cytoplasmic differentiation is noted in cells of the intermediate and superficial layers**

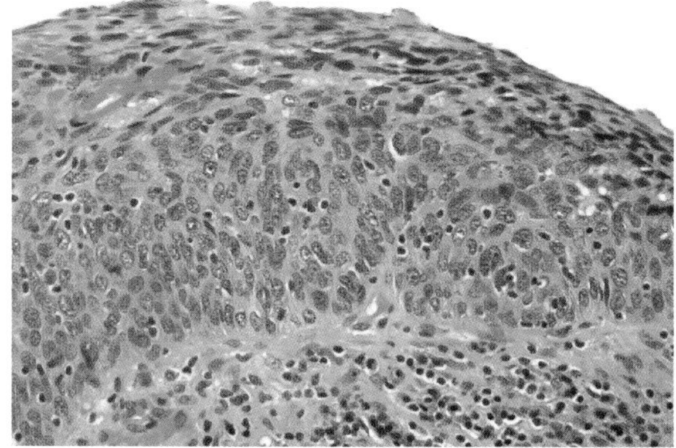

Fig. 3.42
VAIN 3 (high-grade SIL). **Cytoplasmic differentiation is limited to the uppermost layers of the squamous epithelium. The remaining cells have a high nuclear/cytoplasmic ratio, with a longitudinal nuclear axis perpendicular to the basement membrane**

Squamous Cell Carcinoma

General Features

Squamous cell carcinoma represents about 80% of malignant neoplasms primary to the vagina [48, 217]. The incidence in the United States is about 1,000 cases each year. The incidence is 0.42 cases per 100,000 in Caucasian women and 0.93 per 100,000 in black women [47, 217], which is about 1/50th the incidence of cervical squamous cell carcinoma [189]. Only 1% of malignant neoplasms of the female genital tract are classified as squamous cell carcinoma originating in the vagina [217]. The incidence reflects both the relative rarity of squamous cell carcinoma at this site and the extremely rigid criteria for diagnosis of vaginal as compared with cervical carcinoma, which results in underestimation of its true frequency. The International Federation of Gynecology and Obstetrics (FIGO) staging of vaginal cancer is analogous to that of cervical cancer and is based on clinical rather than pathologic examination (*Table 3.2*). To be considered a primary tumor of the vagina, the neoplasm must be located in the vagina, without clinical or histologic evidence of involvement of the cervix or vulva. Thus, bulky tumors located in the upper vagina that have extended onto the portio vaginalis of the cervix are classified as primary cervical carcinoma. Similarly, squamous cell carcinoma occurring in the vagina within 5 years of therapy for cervical carcinoma is considered to be recurrent cervical carcinoma rather than a new primary carcinoma of the vagina [212]. It is thus not surprising that only 10–20% of vaginal malignancies are classified as primary neoplasms of the vagina [80]. The risk factors for invasive squamous carcinoma of the vagina are the same as those for SIL (VAIN)

Table 3.2
FIGO staging of vaginal carcinoma (1978)

Stage	Clinical status
0	Intraepithelial
I	Limited to vaginal wall
II	Extends to subvaginal tissue but not to pelvic side wall
III	Extends to pelvic side wall
IV	Extends beyond the true pelvis or involves mucosa of the bladder or rectum (bullous edema does not consign the patient to stage IV)
IVa	Adjacent organs involved
IVb	Distant organs involved

[26, 251]. In a case control study of VAIN and invasive squamous carcinoma of the vagina, significant risk factors also included prior vaginal discharge, condyloma acuminata, or irritation, prior abnormal cervical vaginal cytology, and prior hysterectomy. Surprisingly, early age at first intercourse, multiple sexual partners, and a history of smoking were not associated with an elevated risk of neoplasia [26]. Occasionally, squamous cell carcinomas also have been reported in young women with congenital absence of the vagina 8 to 25 years after the creation of a neovagina [120, 250].

Clinical Features

The mean age at diagnosis of invasive vaginal squamous carcinoma is 64 years [144]. The presenting symptoms usually are painless vaginal bleeding or discharge, dysuria, or frequency [6]. There is a relationship between duration of symptoms and the size and spread of tumor. Unfortunately, about 20% of patients with vaginal cancer delay more than 7 months from onset of symptoms to initiation of therapy [219]. Most of the tumors arise in the upper third of the vagina [219], with 57% involving the posterior wall and 27% located on the anterior wall [218].

Gross Findings

Vaginal squamous carcinomas vary in size from clinically occult to larger than 10 cm. The gross configuration is similarly variable and includes polypoid, fungating, indurated, and ulcerated lesions (➋ *Fig. 3.43*).

Microscopic Findings

Squamous cell carcinomas of the vagina resemble those arising in the cervix (➋ *Fig. 3.44*). Histologic grade using either the method of Broders or Reagan and Wentz has not been related to prognosis [61, 207]. Microinvasive carcinoma is not currently a defined entity in the vagina; however, superficially invasive tumors, with less than 3 mm of stromal invasion and no vascular space invasion, appear to have a low likelihood of nodal metastasis [218]. The distinction of early invasive carcinoma from intraepithelial carcinoma is based on a constellation of findings, including the presence of angulated narrow cords of squamous cells at the stromal interface, frequently with acquisition of more abundant eosinophilic cytoplasm, and a desmosplastic or inflammatory host response. Unfortunately, these features are not present in every case of early invasive squamous carcinoma.

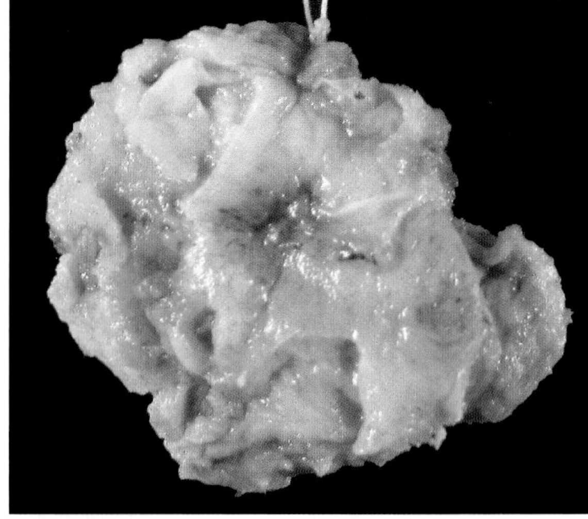

▪ Fig. 3.43
Squamous cell carcinoma. **The tumor has ulcerated the mucosa centrally within this specimen**

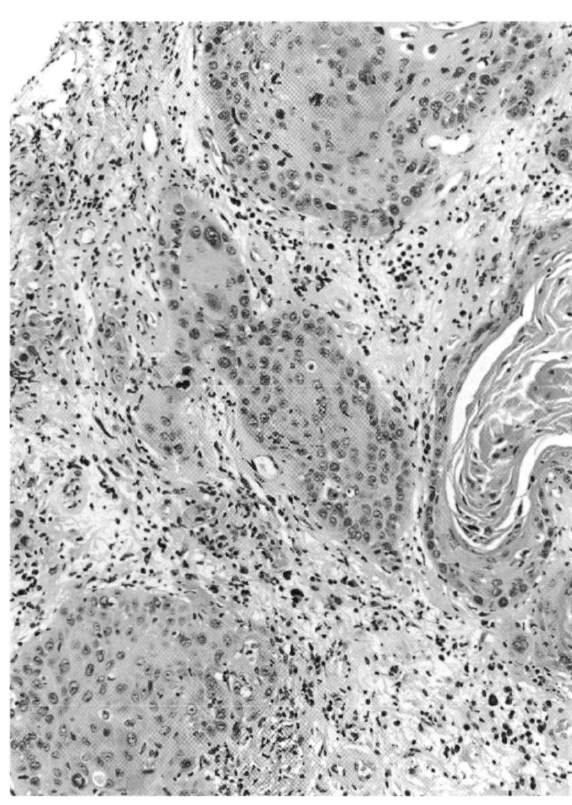

▪ Fig. 3.44
Squamous cell carcinoma of the vagina. **Irregular nests of neoplastic cells with highly pleomorphic nuclei infiltrate the stroma. Keratin pearl formation is evident**

Clinical Behavior and Treatment

Historically, the survival rates for women with squamous cell carcinoma of the vagina were low. However, recent studies indicate a considerably better prognosis, with rates comparable to those of cervical carcinoma when corrected for stage of disease [61, 208, 222]. In a review of 300 women with vaginal carcinoma treated over a 40-year interval at one institution, the overall 5- and 10-year survival rates were 60% and 49%, respectively [36]. The most important prognostic indicators included FIGO stage, tumor size, and location in the vagina (with better outcomes for those with lesions in the upper vagina). Results from the National Cancer Data Base between 1985 and 1994 and the FIGO 6th annual report of results of treatment in gynecologic cancer support the prognostic importance of stage [17, 48]. The relative 5-year survival rate for stage I disease was 73%, 53% for stage II tumors, and only 36% for stages III and IV [48]. Unfortunately, relatively few women are diagnosed with tumors confined to the vagina. Direct spread into the soft tissues of the pelvis or to the mucosa of the bladder or rectum occurs early because the wall of the vagina is thin and is separated from these organs by only a few millimeters of connective tissue. Consequently, at initial diagnosis, most tumors have invaded the soft tissues surrounding the vaginal wall and about 20% extend to the pelvic sidewall [36]. As discussed in the section on anatomy, the lymphatic drainage of the vagina is complex and variable, and any of the inguinal or pelvic lymph nodes may be the site of metastasis, although there is some relationship to the location of the tumor within the vagina [170].

Radiation therapy, including brachytherapy and external beam radiation, is the modality used primarily to treat vaginal squamous carcinoma, although radical vaginectomy may be indicated in selected instances. Although metastases may be discovered ultimately in the lungs or supraclavicular lymph nodes, recurrent disease is typically local and occurs within 2 years of diagnosis [144]. In one large study, local recurrences were identified at 5 years in 23% and distant metastases in 15% of patients [36]. Only 12% of the women who suffered a recurrence survived for 5 years.

Verrucous Carcinoma

The use of the term verrucous carcinoma should be reserved for those rare vaginal tumors that display the characteristic features described by Ackerman [4, 49]. Grossly, they are exophytic, fungating masses with a coarsely granular or undulating surface. Microscopically, the characteristic feature of verrucous carcinoma is the presence of squamous cells with bland cytologic features. At the deep margin of the tumor, the squamous cells invade in a pushing fashion as broad bulbous masses, creating a so-called baggy pants appearance. On the surface of the tumor, hyperkeratosis and acanthosis are common. The distinction of verrucous carcinoma from condyloma or pseudoepitheliomatous hyperplasia may be difficult and may not be possible in a superficial biopsy specimen. Some authors have indicated that verrucous carcinoma does not display the koilocytosis or surface papillae formed of fibrovascular cores covered by squamous cells, which are typical of condylomata or warty carcinomas [124, 144], but other investigators disagree [65, 162]. This issue, however, is not of primary importance because the diagnosis rests on the presence of bland cytologic features in the broad bulbous masses of squamous cells at the stromal interface. Verrucous carcinomas display a relatively indolent growth potential, with frequent local recurrence after incomplete excision. Lymph node metastasis occurs rarely, if ever. Because verrucous carcinomas not only are resistant to therapeutic irradiation but may actually transform to conventional squamous carcinoma after radiation therapy, the treatment is usually wide local or radical surgery [4, 141]. Tumors with a mixed pattern of both verrucous and conventional squamous carcinomas behave with the aggressiveness of typical squamous cancer and should be classified as such.

Warty Carcinoma

Squamous cell carcinomas in which many of the cells contain nuclear abnormalities and perinuclear cytoplasmic cavitation similar to the koilocytes in intraepithelial neoplasms have been designated warty carcinoma. These changes are not typically present in verrucous carcinoma. In addition, warty carcinomas have greater nuclear pleomorphism than verrucous carcinomas, as well as multinucleation, and an infiltrative pattern at the stromal interface. A detailed clinicopathologic analysis of warty carcinomas in the vagina has not been reported. Preliminary data from similar tumors in the vulva indicate that they behave in a low-grade malignant fashion, although metastases to regional lymph nodes occur occasionally (see ➋ Chap. 2, Premalignant and Malignant Tumors of the Vulva) [146].

Papillary Squamotransitional Cell Carcinoma

During the past decade, there has been increased recognition that lesions involving the lower genital tract may bear a close resemblance to those arising from urothelium. In addition to transitional cell metaplasia [311], malignant neoplasms have been reported, primarily in the cervix [135, 230], but with occasional cases originating in the vagina [15, 71, 249]. The diagnostic terminology has been varied, including papillary squamous carcinoma, transitional cell carcinoma, and mixed squamous and transitional (squamotransitional) cell carcinoma, reflecting the less than unambiguous histologic features that discriminate such epithelia [135]. Immunohistochemical studies have usually demonstrated the presence of cytokeratin CK-7 and the frequent absence of CK-20 in the papillary genital tract tumors, unlike the profile of transitional cell carcinomas of the urinary bladder, which typically react with both CK-7 and CK-20 [135].

The presenting symptom of papillary squamotransitional cell carcinoma is usually either abnormal bleeding or abnormal cervical–vaginal cytology. The gross tumor configuration is described as papillary, polypoid, or exophytic. The neoplasm is characterized microscopically by the presence of predominantly narrow fibrovascular cores covered by a multilayered epithelium that may resemble either transitional cells, squamous cells, or both (*Fig. 3.45*). Cytologic atypia is usually present in cells having oval nuclei, with frequent hyperchromasia and the occasional presence of longitudinal intranuclear grooves. Koilocytosis is rare, but mitoses are distributed throughout the epithelium. Often stromal invasion is not identifiable within the papillae of a superficial biopsy and must be sought at the deeper stromal interface. The invasive component may be identical to either conventional squamous or transitional cell carcinoma and usually elicits a desmoplastic host response.

The biologic behavior remains incompletely defined and has been described as either indolent or similar to that of conventional squamous carcinoma [135, 230]. Some of the cases have followed treatment of primary papillary transitional cell carcinomas of the urinary tract or have been associated with transitional cell metaplasia, suggesting the possibility of an extended urogenital field at risk for transitional cell neoplasia [71].

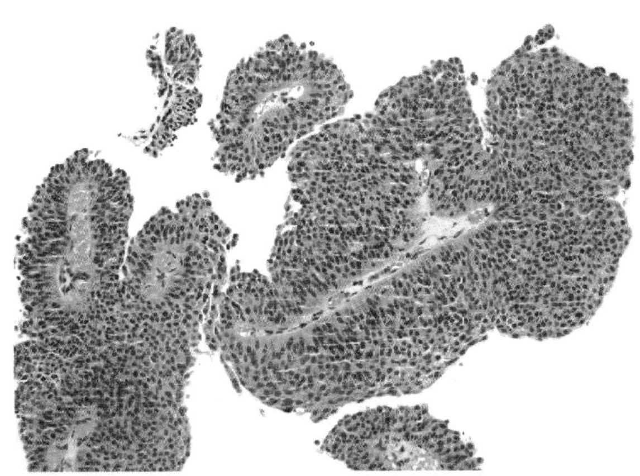

Fig. 3.45
Papillary squamotransitional cell carcinoma. **The tumor closely resembles a papillary urothelial cell carcinoma**

Clear Cell Adenocarcinoma

General Features

From the 1970s through the 1990s, most cases of vaginal clear cell adenocarcinoma occurred in young women with a documented history of DES exposure in utero. The median age at the time of diagnosis in the DES-exposed US population was 19 years, and the risk of tumor development was higher when the drug was started early in pregnancy. Fortunately, clear cell adenocarcinoma developed in only about 0.1% of exposed females up to the age of 24 years. As of 2008, 757 cases of clear cell adenocarcinoma of the cervix or vagina had been accessioned worldwide to the Registry for Research on Hormonal Transplacental Carcinogenesis. Consequent to the removal of DES from the market for the treatment of high-risk pregnancy in 1971, the exposed population has aged, and between 2003 and 2008, only 35 cases of clear cell carcinomas were reported to the Registry (personal communication). Our understanding of DES-mediated carcinogenesis remains incomplete. A high frequency of microsatellite instability and overexpression of wild-type p53 has been observed [306, 307]. Currently, many of the cases of clear cell adenocarcinoma of the vagina are diagnosed in older, non-DES-exposed women.

Clinical Features

Larger tumors almost always cause symptoms such as vaginal bleeding or discharge, while many small tumors are asymptomatic. Approximately 60% of lesions have been confined to the vagina. The remainder have been limited to the cervix or involved both the cervix and vagina.

Gross Findings

The tumor may involve any portion of the vagina and/or cervix. Most of the larger cancers are polypoid and nodular, but some are flat or ulcerated, having a granular or indurated surface. Small tumors may be invisible on colposcopic examination if confined to the lamina propria and covered by normal, or metaplastic squamous epithelium, and are detectable only by palpation (➲ *Fig. 3.46*).

Microscopic Findings

DES-associated clear cell adenocarcinoma is identical to the clear cell adenocarcinoma of the ovary and endometrium, which occur sporadically in older women. Several histologic patterns may be observed, either alone or in combination. A characteristic pattern, for which the tumor is named, consists of solid sheets of clear cells (➲ *Fig. 3.47*), the clear appearance of the cytoplasm being caused by the dissolution of glycogen when the specimen is processed for microscopic examination. A second (and the most frequent) pattern, the tubulocystic pattern (➲ *Fig. 3.48*), is characterized by tubules and cysts lined by hobnail cells, by flat cells, or by cells that resemble müllerian-type epithelium to varying degrees. The hobnail cell is characterized by a bulbous nucleus that protrudes into the lumen (➲ *Fig. 3.49*). Flat cells often appear cytologically bland. When only this type of epithelium is present in a small biopsy, it may be difficult to differentiate tumor from adenosis [256]. Less common patterns include a papillary and a tubular pattern resembling endometrial carcinoma. In any of these patterns, the lumen may contain mucin.

Atypical adenosis, characterized by glands with cellular stratification, nuclear pleomorphism, hyperchromasia, and prominent nucleoli, has been identified near the periphery of most clear cell carcinomas. The frequent finding of the tuboendometrial type of glandular cell and the rarity of the mucinous type of cell adjacent to the tumors suggest that the clear cell adenocarcinoma arises from the tuboendometrial cells [243, 244].

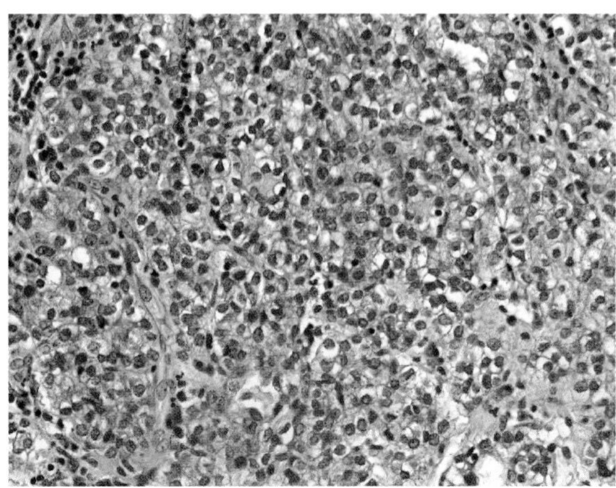

Fig. 3.47
Clear cell carcinoma. **Solid pattern of tumor, resembling clear cell carcinoma of ovary and endometrium**

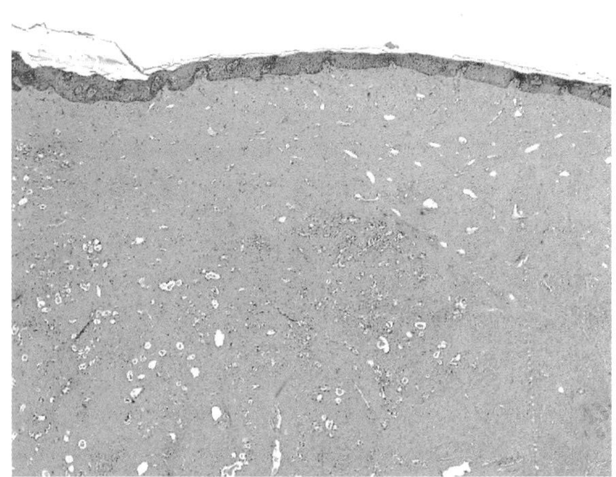

Fig. 3.46
Flat clear cell carcinoma of vagina. **This tumor was detectable only by palpation since the overlying mucosa underwent complete squamous metaplasia and the underlying neoplastic glands produced a small nodule**

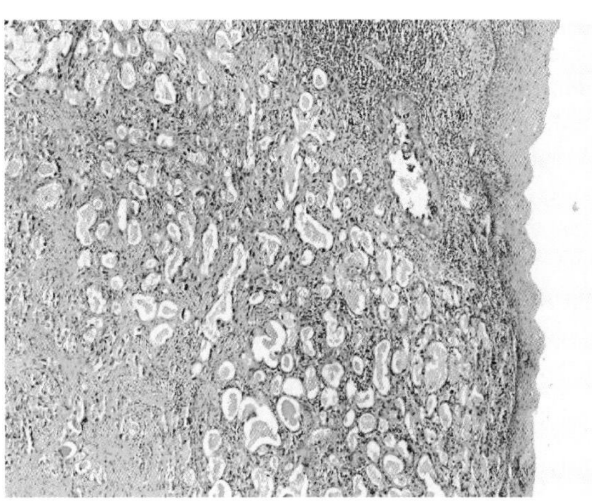

Fig. 3.48
Tubulocystic pattern of tumor in which small tubules are lined by neoplastic hobnail, cuboidal or flattened cells

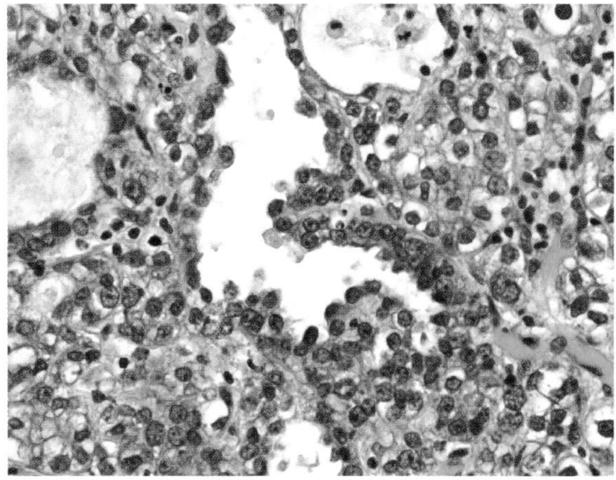

Fig. 3.49
Clear cell carcinoma. **Detail of solid and hobnail cells showing high nuclear/cytoplasmic ratio and apically located nuclei protruding into the cystic spaces**

Differential Diagnosis

Microglandular hyperplasia usually occurs in the cervix, but may arise in vaginal adenosis. It contains many small, closely packed glands devoid of intervening stroma (see Chap. 4, Benign Diseases of the Cervix). The presence of extensive nests of metaplastic squamous cells with pale eosinophilic cytoplasm may make the lesion difficult to distinguish from the solid pattern of clear cell carcinoma. A clue to the diagnosis is the presence of clefts lined by mucinous epithelium that course through the metaplastic squamous epithelium. The Arias–Stella reaction usually occurs in pregnant women. Although usually seen in the endometrium, the Arias–Stella reaction has been observed in the endocervix and occasionally in vaginal adenosis of the tuboendometrial type. Characteristically, hypersecretory glands are lined by cells with markedly enlarged nuclei resembling hobnail cells. However, in clear cell adenocarcinoma, the presence of sheets of clear cells or prominent papillae should enable the two lesions to be distinguished. In addition, the hobnail-like nuclei in the Arias–Stella reaction commonly contain smudged nuclear chromatin.

Clinical Behavior and Treatment

The tumor spreads locally and also metastasizes via lymphatics and blood vessels. Clear cell carcinoma extends outside the abdominal cavity more frequently than does squamous cell carcinoma of the vagina or cervix. Thirty-six percent of the initial recurrences of clear cell carcinomas are in the lung or a supraclavicular lymph node, in contrast to less than 10% for squamous cell carcinomas.

The 5-year actuarial survival rates for all patients with clear cell adenocarcinoma are high, about 93% at 5 years and 87% at 10 years when the tumor is at stage I [111]. Large size and/or deep invasion into the wall are associated with a poorer prognosis, but small or superficial tumors also may recur or metastasize. Recurrences develop most often within 3 years after primary therapy; however, recurrences as late as 19 years after treatment have been observed [28].

The prognosis for women with clear cell adenocarcinoma who have known exposure to DES in utero is significantly better than for those who have no history of DES exposure (5-year survival rates of 84% and 69%, respectively) [305]. Although some of this difference could reflect earlier detection in the intensively screened exposed population, the survival advantage persists even when the comparison is adjusted for stage of disease. Metastases to the lungs or supraclavicular lymph nodes are more frequent in the non-DES-exposed group.

Embryonal Rhabdomyosarcoma (Sarcoma Botryoides)

General Features

The most common malignant neoplasm of the vagina in infants and children is embryonal rhabdomyosarcoma, most of which is of the subtype designated sarcoma botyroides [46, 48, 197]. Nearly 90% of cases are diagnosed before 5 years of age [48, 76]. This is a rare tumor of unknown etiology and pathogenesis. Certainly the distribution of embryonal rhabdomyosarcomas does not correlate with the mass of skeletal muscle, as most of these neoplasms arise in or near the mucosa of either the head and orbit or the lower urogenital system.

Clinical Features

The mean age at diagnosis is 2 years, with a range extending from birth to 41 years [76]. Most children present with symptoms of a vaginal mass or bleeding. The tumors usually are located along the anterior wall of the vagina, and appear as papillae, small nodules, or pedunculated or sessile soft, polypoid masses with an intact overlying mucosa. Larger tumors may protrude through the introitus. The tumors usually are staged according to a modification of the Intergroup Rhabdomyosarcoma Study (IRS) classification, which is based on combined features of extent of disease, resectibility, and microscopic evaluation of margins of excision (➋ *Table 3.3*).

Gross Findings

Soft gray or tan, edematous, and nodular tumors are typical. The polypoid gross configuration is thought to result from relatively unrestricted growth into the lumen of a hollow organ (➋ *Fig. 3.50*).

Microscopic Findings

The distinction of sarcoma botryoides from the spindle or nonspecialized variants of embryonal rhabdomyosarcoma is based on the presence of a cambium tumor cell layer underlying an intact epithelium in at least one microscopic field [227]. The cambium layer is defined as the condensed subepithelial layer of rhabdomyoblasts that are scattered in a loose myxoid or dense collagenous stroma (➋ *Fig. 3.51*). The term cambium was chosen as an analogy to the peripheral, actively growing layer in tree trunks and branches, which it mimics at a microscopic level. The histologic criteria are more important in establishing the diagnosis than the gross demonstration of a polypoid or "grapelike" pattern of tumor growth. The cells in the cambium layer often are polyhedral, with little discernible cytoplasm, but extensive rhabdomyoblastic differentiation, with a spindled configuration of tumor cells, may predominate in this or other portions of the tumor. The tumor cells are of round to spindle shape, with oval nuclei, an open chromatin pattern, and inconspicuous nucleoli [293].

Focal evidence of rhabdomyogenesis may be evident in any of the patterns, with eosinophilic cytoplasm containing fibers in which cross-striations are present (➋ *Fig. 3.52*). However, in cases that lack such features immunohistochemical staining with antibodies directed against muscle-specific actin, desmin, myoglobin, or myogenin (myf 4) may be helpful in establishing the diagnosis [12, 27, 67, 144, 227]. Although the first two antibodies are more sensitive than myoglobin, they are not specific for skeletal muscle differentiation. It is important not to be misled to the erroneous diagnosis of melanoma by the presence of immunoreactivity for S-100 protein, which has been reported in about 20% of cases of rhabdomyosarcoma [227].

Table 3.3
IRSG surgical–pathologic grouping system

Group	Definition
I	Localized tumor, completely removed with pathologically clear margins and no regional lymph node involvement
II	Localized tumor, grossly removed with (a) microscopically involved margins, (b) involved, grossly resected regional lymph nodes, or (c) both
III	Localized tumor, with gross residual disease after grossly incomplete removal, or biopsy only
IV	Distant metastases present at diagnosis

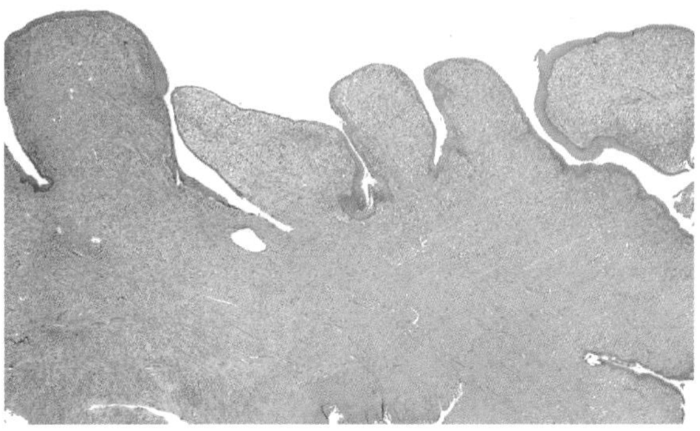

Fig. 3.50
Embryonal rhabdomyosarcoma, botryoid type. **Note the polypoid appearance of the tumor**

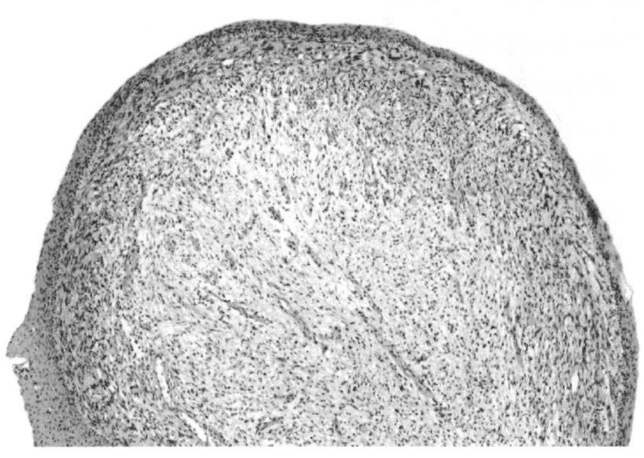

Fig. 3.51
Embryonal rhabdomyosarcoma, botryoid type. **The cambium layer is recognized as a condensed subepithelial layer of rhabdomyoblasts that are scattered in a loose myxoid or dense collagenous stroma**

The differential diagnosis includes fibroepithelial polyps, müllerian papillomas, and rhabdomyomas. The correct diagnosis can be made by considering the age at presentation and the microscopic features described above. After radiation or chemotherapy, occasionally there is difficulty in determining whether scattered mature-appearing skeletal muscle fibers represent residual tumor cells that are refractory to therapy or radiated benign muscle fibers of the pelvis. One study suggests that differentiation occurs more frequently with the botryoid variant of rhabdomyosarcoma following therapy and that it is associated with a favorable outcome [43].

Clinical Behavior and Treatment

The tumor initially grows into the vaginal wall and soft tissue of the pelvis, bladder, or rectum and subsequently metastasizes to lymph nodes, lungs, liver, and bone.

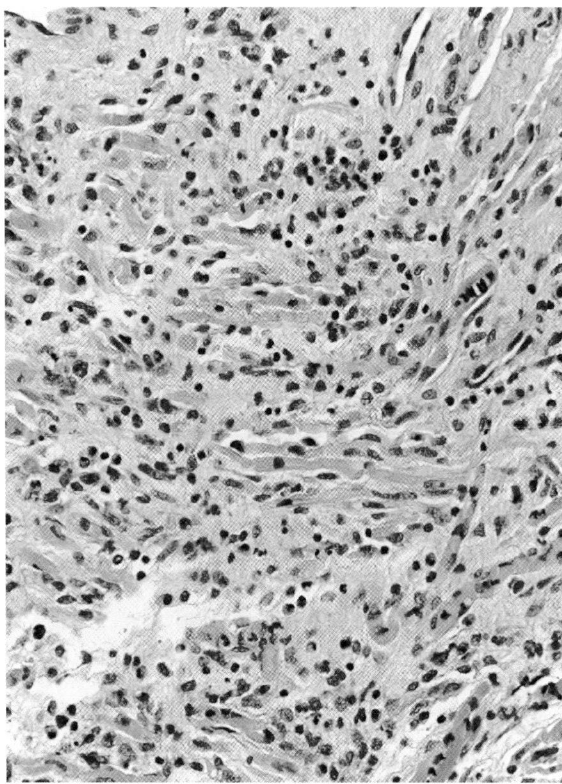

Fig. 3.52
Embryonal rhabdomyosarcoma, botryoid type. **In contrast to the vaginal rhabdomyoma, the embryonal rhabdomyosarcoma contains densely cellular regions composed of small primitive cells. Interspersed strap cells confirm the skeletal muscle differentiation**

Historically, the prognosis after radical surgery was poor, with survival rates of less than 20% [42]. The introduction of combined multiagent chemotherapy and in some cases radiotherapy, in addition to surgery, has dramatically improved the probability of survival [42, 93, 168, 197].

Based on five consecutive clinical trials conducted by the Intergroup Rhabdomyosarcoma Study Group (IRSG) [231], a number of prognostic factors have been identified that strongly correlate with patient outcome. These include clinical group (*Table 3.3*), stage of disease (*Table 3.4*), patient age, and histologic subtype. Fortunately, the botryoid type, the variant of embryonal rhabdomyosarcoma found most frequently in the vagina, has a superior prognosis, with a survival rate greater than 90% [108, 184, 227]; however, even the focal presence of an alveolar histology confers a worse prognosis [227]. In addition, a recent study suggests that the presence of cellular anaplasia may be of prognostic significance in patients with embryonal rhabdomyosarcoma [226]. Two examples of relapse approximately 10 years after initial diagnosis, a few months following menarche, have been reported, and a possible causal association with estrogen has been postulated [300].

Melanoma

General Features

More than 155 cases of vaginal melanoma have been reported, representing less than 5% of the malignant

Table 3.4
IRSG staging system

Stage	Sites of primary tumor	Tumor size (cm)	Regional lymph nodes	Distant metastases
1	Orbit, non-PM head, neck; GU non-bladder/ prostate; biliary tract	Any size	N0, N1	M0
2	All other sites	≤5	N0	M0
3	All other sites	≤5	N1	M0
		≤5	N0 or N1	
4		Any size	N0 or N1	M1

PM, parameningeal; GU, genitourinary; N0, regional bodes not clinically involved by tumor; N1, regional nodes clinically involved by tumor; M0, no distant metastases; M1, distant metastases at diagnosis.

neoplasms of the vagina and less than 1% of all melanomas [48, 59, 90, 102, 122, 214]. These tumors can occur at any age, with a range from 22 to 90 years; however, most patients are postmenopausal with a mean age of approximately 60 years [154, 214, 228]. Presenting symptoms include vaginal bleeding, discharge, and a mass. Although the tumors may arise anywhere within the vagina, there is a predilection for the distal third [35]. The etiology and pathogenesis are unknown, but a disproportionately large number of vaginal melanomas have occurred in Japanese women, followed in frequency by Caucasian and then black women [35, 48, 154]. In one autopsy study, melanocytes were identified in the basal layer of the vagina of 3 of 100 women. It has been suggested that such a condition, referred to as benign melanosis, is the setting from which melanoma occasionally may arise [105], and we have seen localized regions of melanosis in the vagina remote from melanomas. Unfortunately, the term melanosis also has been used to designate melanophages in the stroma and lentigo malignum-like lesions in mucosal tissues, further obscuring interpretation of the scant available literature.

Gross Findings

Melanomas may appear as nodular, polypoid, or fungating gray or black soft masses that vary from 0.5 to 8 cm in diameter (● *Fig. 3.53*) [35, 102, 264]. Frequently, there is ulceration of the overlying epithelium.

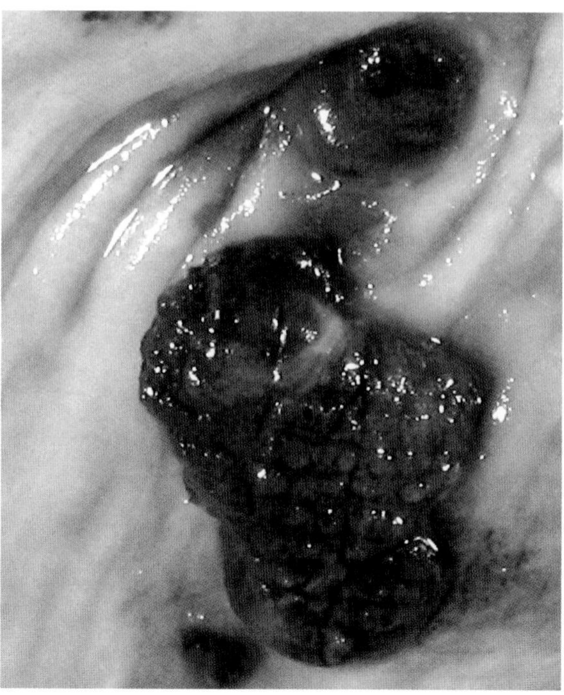

Fig. 3.53
Melanoma of the vagina. **Confluent nodular pigmented masses are present**

Microscopic Findings

Vaginal melanomas have no microscopic characteristics that are distinctive for this site. The diagnosis usually rests on a constellation of features. In addition to junctional activity, the presence of highly atypical melanocytes, either singly or in clusters, extending through the squamous epithelium is common (● *Fig. 3.54*). The infiltrating neoplastic cells may be epithelioid, spindled, or mixed (● *Fig. 3.55*). Melanin is common within both neoplastic melanocytes and benign melanophages. The lateral spread is typically of the lentiginous type, with single, spindled cells containing pleomorphic nuclei at the epithelial–stromal interface [35]. Rarely, a pagetoid junctional component consisting of epithelioid melanocytes in nests is present [35].

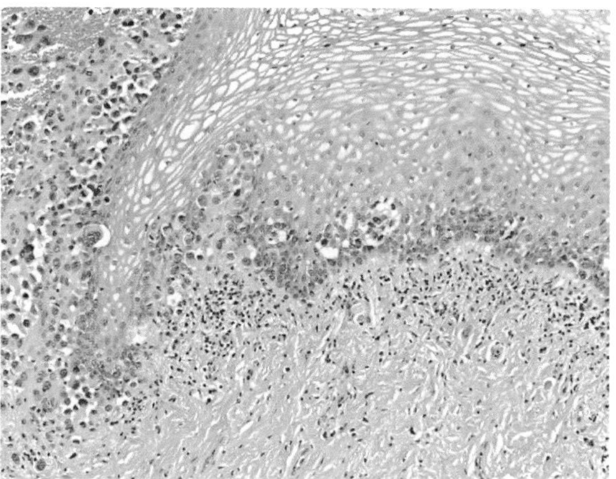

Fig. 3.54
Melanoma of the vagina. **Junctional involvement (right side of field) is frequently identified peripheral to ulcerated or intact central region of deep stromal invasion in primary vaginal melanomas**

Because Clark's levels are not appropriate for mucosal sites of melanoma, a system based entirely on tumor thickness has been proposed by Chung et al., as follows: level I, tumor confined to the surface epithelium; level II, invasion of 1 mm or less; level III, invasion of 1–2 mm; and level IV, invasion greater than 2 mm [35]. Unfortunately, most of the tumors are deeply invasive. In a group of 19 patients, only 1 was at level III; the remainder were at level IV [35].

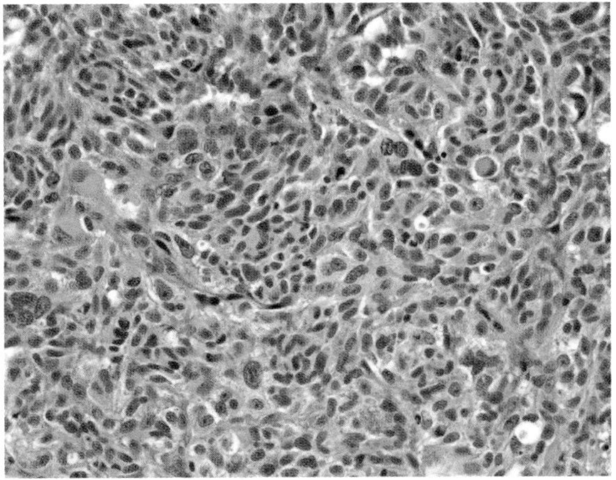

Fig. 3.55
Melanoma of the vagina. **The neoplastic cells may be of polyhedral or spindle configuration and may be confused in routinely stained sections with either squamous carcinoma or sarcoma, particularly if the overlying epithelium is ulcerated. Immunohistochemistry can help to resolve the diagnosis when melanin pigment is not apparent**

Differential Diagnosis

The diagnosis usually is straightforward as most vaginal melanomas are large, with gross and microscopic pigmentation. The differential diagnosis may include melanoma metastatic from other sites, poorly differentiated squamous carcinoma, sarcoma, and blue nevus. Because primary vaginal melanoma is rare, it is important to rule out metastasis from other sites. The presence of an extensive lateral junctional component is typical in melanomas arising in the vagina but relatively uncommon in metastases. A complete history is essential, and some cases can be confirmed only by postmortem examination. When large ulcerated lesions are devoid of pigment, immunohistochemistry and ultrastructural examination may permit discrimination of melanoma from other poorly differentiated neoplasms. Positive staining of malignant cells with antibodies directed against S-100 protein is a sensitive, but not specific, marker of melanocytic or neural differentiation. HMB-45 is a less sensitive (negative in 23% of cases in one study [102]) but more specific indicator of melanoma, and staining for keratin or desmin should be absent. Ultrastructural findings include premelanosomes and melanosomes, as well as abundant rough and smooth endoplasmic reticulum [105]. A high degree of nuclear atypia and numerous mitotic figures usually permit discrimination of melanoma from the rare benign vaginal nevus.

Clinical Behavior and Treatment

The prognosis for vaginal melanoma is poor, with 5-year survival rates of less than 10–20% [35, 48, 154, 228, 310]. Undoubtedly, this reflects the inherent aggressiveness of melanoma coupled with the typically deep invasion found at the time of diagnosis [35, 48, 59, 234]. In one study, survival was inversely related to the mitotic activity [22]. Both lymphatic and hematogenous metastases are common, with the vagina and groin being the most common initial sites of spread. Primary therapy usually includes radical local excision, although pelvic exenteration has been suggested as treatment for tumors greater than 3 mm in thickness. The value of groin node dissection, radiation, and chemotherapy remains unknown [154, 209].

Yolk Sac Tumor

Although the yolk sac tumor (endodermal sinus tumor [EST]) usually arises in the gonads, about 57 cases have been reported in the vagina [39]. It is appealing to consider that these tumors originate from germ cells that have failed to complete migration normally in the embryo from the hindgut to the gonad. However, this hypothesis does not provide an obvious explanation for the absence of other malignant germ cell tumors in the vagina, or the predilection of EST for the vagina.

Most vaginal ESTs have been diagnosed in children less than 4 years of age. The presenting symptom usually is a bloody vaginal discharge. The gross and microscopic features of vaginal EST closely resemble those of ovarian origin. Polypoid or sessile, soft, and tan or white vaginal masses 1–5 cm in diameter are typical [144]. A variety of histologic patterns may be present including the microcystic, reticular, papillary, and solid types of EST. Schiller–Duval bodies, composed of papillary arrangements of columnar cells separated from central vascular channels by an acellular zone of connective tissue, are characteristic findings. Extracellular hyaline droplets also are common. Although the histologic findings usually are typical, the diagnosis may not be considered initially because of the rarity of EST in the vagina. The differential diagnosis includes clear cell adenocarcinoma from which EST may be distinguished by the younger age and positive immunohistochemical reactions for alpha-fetoprotein and alpha-1-antitrypsin [317].

EST is an extremely aggressive tumor. In the past, the median survival was 11 months, and the survival rate at 5 years was less than 25% [45, 209]. Most patients developed recurrence and died within 2 years, even after radical surgery [45, 144]. The addition of multiagent chemotherapy, usually consisting of vincristine, actinomycin, and cyclophosphamide, since 1970 has resulted in a 95% disease-free survival at 2 years [8, 45, 317]. Preliminary data suggest that combination chemotherapy and conservative surgery may permit preservation of future sexual function and fertility as well as an excellent cure rate [209].

Leiomyosarcoma

About 65 leiomyosarcomas of the vagina have been reported [48, 52, 211]. The frequency and behavior have been difficult to establish because the pathologic criteria separating benign from malignant smooth muscle tumors have varied. Currently, it is recommended that smooth muscle tumors of greater than 3 cm diameter, with five or more mitotic figures per ten HPFs, moderate or marked cytologic atypia, and infiltrating margins be classified as leiomyosarcoma (➋ *Fig. 3.56*) [282]. The age range extends from 25 to 86 years with most patients being older than 40 years. Vaginal bleeding is the most common presenting symptom. The gross and microscopic features resemble those of uterine leiomyosarcoma, but the spread of tumor is by local invasion and hematogenous metastasis. The 5-year survival rate is about 35%, and the stage of the disease is the most important prognostic indicator [211]. The primary therapy is surgical, and exenteration may be required to provide an adequate margin around larger tumors.

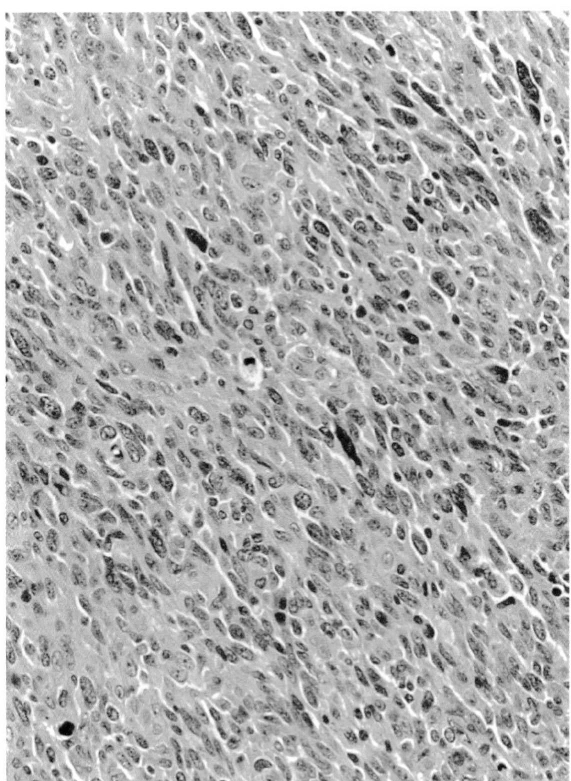

Fig. 3.56
Vaginal leiomyosarcoma. **The tumor resembles that of uterine origin, with fascicles of spindle cells having moderate or marked nuclear pleomorphism with increased mitotic activity**

Malignant Mixed Tumor

Probably unrelated to the benign vaginal mixed tumor is the reportedly malignant mixed tumor, which resembles either synovial sarcoma or a malignant tumor arising from mesonephric rests [201, 275, 278]. Two of these rare tumors occurred in women 24 and 33 years old, who presented with a polypoid nodule in the lateral vaginal fornix. The microscopic appearance is of an intact vaginal squamous mucosa with a subjacent mixture of solid nests of polyhedral-shaped cells and flattened epithelial cells in acinar or tubular arrays, bordered peripherally by smaller bundles of spindle cells resembling fibroblasts. Ultrastructural features resembling synovial sarcoma were noted in one case [201, 275]. The presence of mitotic activity as great as eight mitoses per ten HPFs coupled with nuclear pleomorphism and moderate-sized nucleoli suggested that the process was malignant. However, the biologic potential remains uncertain in the absence of long-term follow-up.

Secondary Neoplasms

Although primary neoplasms of the vagina are quite rare, secondary spread of malignant neoplasms to the vagina by

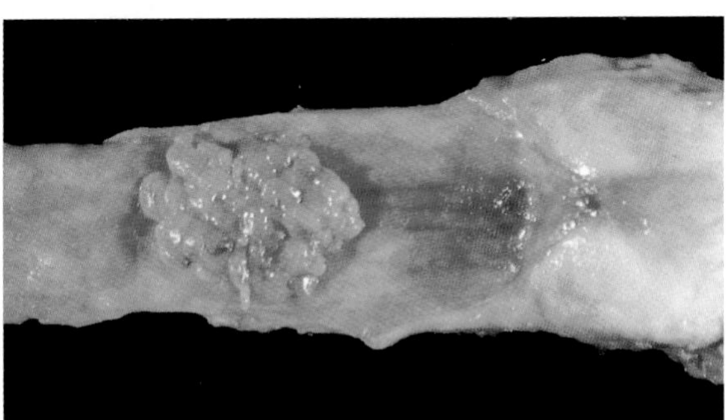

Fig. 3.57
Metastatic endometrial adenosarcoma to the vagina. **This tumor represents a recurrence of a uterine adenosarcoma initially resected 8 years earlier**

direct extension or lymphatic or hematogenous metastasis is quite common (➋ *Fig. 3.57*). Fu and Reagan found that only 58 (16%) of 355 invasive carcinomas involving the vagina represented primary neoplasms [81]. Spread from primary carcinoma of the cervix was most common (32%), followed by endometrium (18%), colon and rectum (9%), ovary (6%), vulva (6%), and urinary tract (4%) (➋ *Fig. 3.58*). Even among the squamous carcinomas found in the vagina, only a minority prove to be primary to this site. About 75% are secondary, arising in either the cervix (79%) or vulva (14%) [81].

About 70 cases of vaginal metastases from renal cell carcinoma have been reported (➋ *Fig. 3.59*) [281, 292, 315]. Metastases from clear cell carcinoma of the kidney may be very difficult to distinguish histologically from primary clear cell carcinoma of the vagina. This difficulty is complicated by the observation that in some instances the identification of the metastatic lesion has preceded the diagnosis of the renal tumor [292]. A young age, history of DES exposure in utero, prior or concurrent vaginal adenosis, and foci of neoplastic clear cells with a tubulocystic or papillary architecture are features that favor a vaginal primary, whereas older age and regions of granular, cytoplasm or sarcomatoid differentiation are more common in tumors that originate in the kidney. In rare cases, the histologic distinction of clear cell carcinoma of the vagina from a renal metastasis may be impossible.

Miscellaneous Malignant Neoplasms

Endometrioid adenocarcinomas, stromal sarcomas, and carcinosarcomas occasionally originate in the vagina, at times arising from a background of endometriosis (➋ *Fig. 3.60*) [99, 194, 211]. In addition, there are occasional reported cases of primary vaginal adenocarcinoma in situ [38], intestinal-type adenocarcinoma [79], adenosquamous

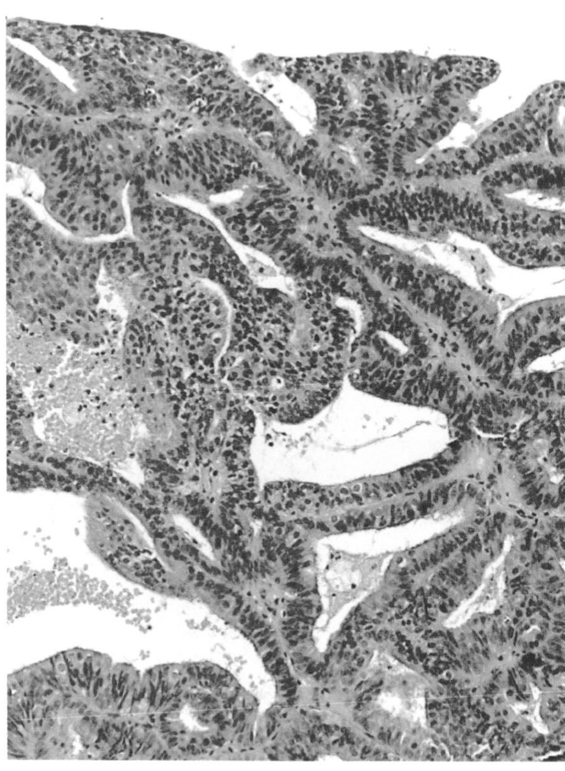

Fig. 3.58
Metastatic endometrial adenocarcinoma. **Vaginal recurrence of adenocarcinoma of the endometrium is common. There is great fidelity in most cases to the histologic appearance of the endometrial primary**

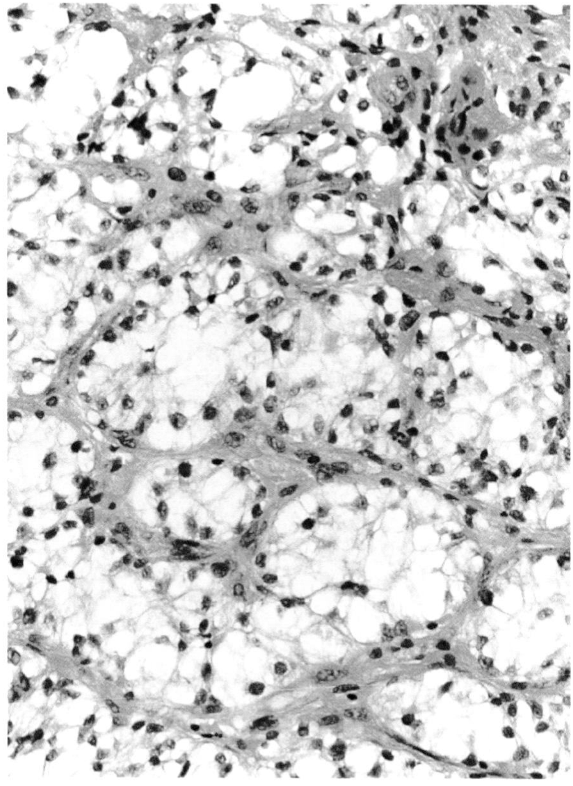

Fig. 3.59
Metastatic renal cell carcinoma. **Solid masses of polygonal cells with clear cytoplasm are separated from each other by delicate fibrovascular septa**

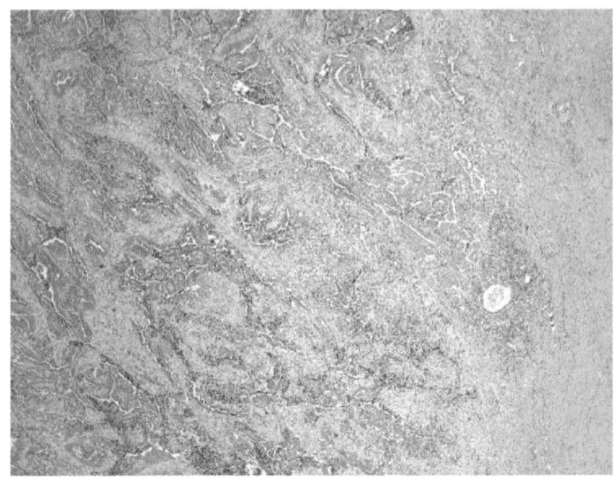

Fig. 3.60
Endometrioid adenocarcinoma of the vagina. **This primary endometrioid adenocarcinoma is arising in association with endometriosis (right side of illustration)**

carcinoma [237, 258, 273], adenocarcinoma arising in mesonephric duct remnants, adenoid basal cell carcinoma [193], adenoid cystic carcinoma [144], carcinoid tumor [84], small cell carcinoma [126, 236], malignant schwannoma [57], fibrosarcoma [204], malignant fibrous histiocytoma [308], angiosarcoma [223, 291], alveolar soft part sarcoma [30, 147].

References

1. Abdul-Karim FW, Lederman MM, Carter JR et al (1981) Toxic shock syndrome: clinicopathologic findings in a fatal case. Hum Pathol 12:16–22
2. Abu J, Nunns D, Ireland D, Brown L (2003) Malignant progression through borderline changes in recurrent Mullerian papilloma of the vagina. Histopathology 42:510–511
3. Acar A, Balci O, Karatayli R, Capar M, Colakoglu MC (2007) The treatment of 65 women with imperforate hymen by a central incision and application of Foley catheter. BJOG 114(11): p1376–p1379
4. Ackerman LV (1948) Verrucous carcinoma of the oral cavity. Surgery (St Louis) 23:670–678
5. Andreani SM, Dang HH, Grondona P, Khan AZ, Edwards DP (2007) Rectovaginal fistula in Crohn's disease. Dis Colon Rectum 50(12):2215–2222
6. Al-Durdi M, Monaghan JM (1977) Thirty-two years experience in management of primary tumors of the vagina. Br J Obstet Gynecol 127:513
7. Amsel R, Totten PA, Spiegel CA et al (1983) Nonspecific vaginitis: diagnostic criteria and micro-bial and epidemiologic associations. Am J Med 74:14–22
8. Anderson WA, Sabio H, Durso N et al (1985) Endodermal sinus tumor of the vagina. The role of primary chemotherapy. Cancer (Phila) 56:1025–1027
9. Andrew DE, Bumstead K, Kempton AG (1975) The role of fomites in the transmission of vaginitis. Can Med Assoc J 112:1181–1183
10. Arbo E, dos RR, Uchoa D et al (2004) Vaginal Mullerian papilloma in a 2-year-old child. Gynecol Obstet Invest 58:55–56
11. Averette HE, Weinstein GD, Frost P (1970) Autoradiographic analysis of cell proliferation kinetics in human genital tissues. I. Normal cervix and vagina. Am J Obstet Gynecol 108:8–17
12. Bale PM, Parsons RE, Stevens MM (1983) Diagnosis and behavior of juvenile rhabdomyosarcoma. Hum Pathol 14:596–611
13. Barry W, Hudgins L, Donta ST, Pesanti EL (1992) Intravenous immunoglobulin therapy for toxic shock syndrome. JAMA 267:3315–3316
14. Bartlett JG, Onderdonk AB, Drude E et al (1977) Quantitative bacteriology of the vaginal flora. J Infect Dis 136:271–277
15. Bass P, Birch B, Smart C, Theaker J, Wells M (1994) Low grade transitional cell carcinoma of the vagina – an unusual cause of vaginal bleeding. Histopathology (Oxf) 24:581–583
16. Bell DA, Mondschein M, Scully RE (1986) Giant cell arteritis of the female genital tract. A report of three cases. Am J Surg Pathol 10:696–701
17. Beller U, Benedet JL, Creasman WT, Ngan HY, Quinn MA, Maisonneuve P, Pecorelli S, Odicino F, Heintz AP (2006) Carcinoma of the vagina. FIGO 6th annual report on the results of treatment in gynecological cancer. Int J Gynaecol Obstet 95(Suppl 1):S29–S42
18. Benedet JL, Sanders BH (1984) Carcinoma in situ of the vagina. Am Obstet Gynecol 148:695–700
19. Bennett HG, Ehrlich HM (1941) Myoma of the vagina. Am J Obstet Gynecol 42:314
20. Bergdoll MS, Reiser RF, Crass BA et al (1981) A new staphylococcal enterotoxin, enterotoxin F, associated with toxic-shock-syndrome staphylococcus aureus isolates. Lancet 1:1017–1021
21. Boquet-Jiménez E, Alvarez San Cristóbal A (1978) Cytologic and microbiologic aspects of vaginal torulopsis. Acta Cytol 22:331–334
22. Borazjani G, Prem KA, Okagaki T et al (1990) Primary malignant melanoma of the vagina: a clinicopathological analysis of 10 cases. Gynecol Oncol 37:264–267
23. Bornstein J, Adam E, Adler-Storthz K, Kaufman RH (1988) Development of cervical and vaginal squamous cell neoplasia as a late consequence of in utero exposure to diethylstilbestrol. Obstet Gynecol Surv 43:15–21
24. Bramley M, Kinghorn G (1979) Do oral contraceptives inhibit Trichomonoas vaginalis? Sex Transm Dis 6:261–263
25. Branton PA, Tavassoli FA (1993) Spindle cell epithelioma, the so-called mixed tumor of the vagina. Am J Surg Path 17:509–515
26. Brinton LA, Nasca PC, Mallin K et al (1990) Case-control study of in situ and invasive carcinoma of the vagina. Gynecol Oncol 38:49
27. Brooks JJ (1982) Immunohistochemistry of soft tissue tumors. Myoglobin as a tumor marker for rhabdomyosarcoma. Cancer 50:1757
28. Burks RT, Schwarz AM, Wheeler JE, Antoniolli D (1990) Late recurrence of clear cell adenocarcinoma of the cervix: case report. Obstet Gynecol 76:525–527
29. Caceres A, McCarus SD (2008) Fallopian tube prolapse after total laparoscopic hysterectomy. Obstet Gynecol 112(2 Pt 2):494–495
30. Chapman GW, Benda JO, Williams T (1984) Alveolar soft part sarcoma of the vagina. Gynecol Oncol 18:125–129
31. Charles V, Charles SX (1978) A case of vulvo-vaginal diphtheria in a girl of seven years. Indian J Pediatr 15:257–258
32. Chattopadhyay I, Cruickshan DJ, Packer M (2001) Non diethylstilbesterol induced vaginal adenosis – a case series and review of literature. Eur J Gynaecol Oncol 22(4):p260–p262

33. Chen KTK (1981) Brenner tumor of the vagina. Diagn Gynecol Obstet 3:255
34. Chirayil SJ, Tobon H (1981) Polyps of the vagina: a clinicopathologic study of 18 cases. Cancer (Phila) 47:2904–2907
35. Chung AF, Casey MJ, Flannery JT et al (1980) Malignant melanoma of the vagina: report of 19 cases. Obstet Gynecol 55:720–727
36. Chyle V, Zagars GK, Wheeler JA, Wharton JT, Delclos L (1996) Definitive radiotherapy for carcinoma of the vagina: outcome and prognostic factors. Int J Radiat Oncol Biol Phys 35(5):891–905
37. Clark JFJ, Faggett T, Peters B, Sampson CC (1978) Ulcerative vaginitis due to torulopsis glabrata: a case report. J Natl Med Assoc 70:913–914
38. Clement PB, Benedet JL (1979) Adenocarcinoma in situ of the vagina. A case report. Cancer (Phila) 43:2479–2485
39. Clement PB, Young RH, Scully RE (1988) Extraovarian pelvic yolk sac tumors. Cancer (Phila) 62:620–626
40. Clemetson D, Moss G, Willerford D (1993) Detection of HIV DNA in cervical and vaginal secretions. JAMA 269:2860–2863
41. Coetzee LF (1972) Tuberculous vaginitis. South Afr Med J 46: 1225–1226
42. Coffin CM, Dehner LP (1992) The soft tissue. In: Stocker JT, Dehner LP (eds) Pediatric pathology, vol 2. Lippincott, Philadelphia, PA, pp 1091–1132
43. Coffin C, Rulon J, Smith L, Bruggers C, White F (1997) Pathologic features of rhabdomyosarcoma before and after treatment: a clinicopathologic and immunohistochemical analysis. Mod Pathol 10: 1175–1187
44. Cohen M, Pedemonte L, Drut R (2001) Pigmented mullerian papilloma of the vagina. Histopathology 39:541–543
45. Copeland LJ, Sneige N, Ordonez NG (1985) Endodermal sinus tumor of the vagina and cervix. Cancer (Phila) 55:2558–2565
46. Copeland LJ, Sneige N, Stringer CA et al (1985) Alveolar rhabdomyosarcoma of the female genitalia. Cancer (Phila) 56:849–855
47. Cramer DW, Cutler SJ (1974) Incidence and histopathology of malignancies of the female genital organs in the United States. Am J Obstet Gynecol 118:443–460
48. Creasman WT, Phillips JL, Menck HR (1998) The National Cancer Data Base report on cancer of the vagina. Cancer (Phila) 83(5): 1033–1040
49. Crowther ME, Lowe DG, Shepherd JH (1988) Verrucous carcinoma of the female genital tract: a review. Obstet Gynecol Surv 43:263–280
50. Cunha GR (1975) The dual origin of vaginal epithelium. Am J Anat 143:387–392
51. Cunha GR, Taguchi O, Namikawa R et al (1987) Teratogenic effects of clomiphene, tamoxifen, and diethylstilbestrol on the developing human female and genital tract. Hum Pathol 18:1132–1143
52. Curtin JP, Saigo P, Slucher B, Venkatraman ES, Mychalczak B, Hoskins WJ (1995) Soft-tissue sarcoma of the vagina and vulva: a clinicopathologic study. Obstet Gynecol 86(2):269–272
53. Curtis EM, Pine L (1981) Actinomyces in the vaginas of women with and without intrauterine contraceptive devices. Am J Obstet Gynecol 140:880–884
54. Davis TC (1975) Chronic vulvovaginitis in children due to Shigella flexneri. Pediatrics 56:41–44
55. Davis JP, Chesney PJ, Wand PJ, LaVenture M (1980) Toxic-shock syndrome. Epidemiologic features, recurrence, risk factors, and prevention. N Engl J Med 303:1429–1435
56. Davis JD, Connor EE, Clark P, Wilkinson EJ, Duff P (1997) Correlation between cervical cytologic results and Gram stain as diagnostic tests for bacterial vaginosis. Am J Obstet Gynecol 177(3):532–535
57. Davos I, Abell MR (1976) Sarcomas of the vagina. Obstet Gynecol 47(3):342–350
58. Dekel A, Avidan D, Bar-ziv J et al (1988) Neurofibroma of the vagina presenting with urinary retention. Review of the literature and report of a case. Obstet Gynecol Surv 43:325–327
59. De Matos P, Tyler D, Seigler HF (1998) Mucosal melanoma of the female genitalia: a clinicopathologic study of forty-three cases at Duke University Medical Center. Surgery (St Louis) 124(1):38–48
60. De Meo LR, Draper DL, McGregor JA et al (1996) Evaluation of a deoxyribonucleic acid probe for the detection of Trichomonas vaginalis in vaginal secretions. Am J Obstet Gynecol 174(4):1339–1342
61. Dixit S, Singhal S, Baboo HA (1993) Squamous cell carcinoma of the vagina: a review of 70 cases. Gynecol Oncol 48:80–87
62. Dobbs SP, Shaw PA, Brown LJ, Ireland D (1998) Borderline malignant change in recurrent mullerian papilloma of the vagina. J Clin Pathol 51:875–877
63. Droegemueller W, Herbst AL, Mishell DR Jr, Stenchever MA (1987) Comprehensive gynecology. Mosby, St. Louis, MO, p 974
64. Dungar C, Wilkinson E (1995) Vaginal columnar cell metaplasia. An acquired adenosis associated with topical 5-fluorouracil therapy. J Reprod Med 40(5):361–366
65. Dvoretsky PM, Bonfiglio TA (1986) The pathology of vulvar squamous cell carcinoma and verrucous carcinoma. In: Sommers SC, Rosen PP, Fechner RE (eds) Pathology annual, part 2, vol 21. Appleton-Century-Crofts, Norwalk, CT, pp 23–45
66. Elliott GB, Elliott JD (1973) Superficial stromal reactions of the lower genital tract. Arch Pathol 95:100–101
67. Eusebi V, Ceccarelli C, Gorza L et al (1986) Immunocytochemistry of rhabdomyosarcoma. The use of four different markers. Am J Surg Pathol 10:293
68. Fallon RJ, Robinson ET (1974) Meningococcal vulvovaginitis. Scand J Infect Dis 6:295–296
69. Farrand RJ (1971) Haemophilus influenzae infections of the genital tract. J Med Microbiol 4:357–358
70. Faulconer HT, Muldoon JP (1975) Rectovaginal fistula in patients with colitis: review and report of a case. Dis Colon Rectum 18:413–415
71. Fetissof F, Haillot O, Lanson Y, Arbeille B, Lansac J (1990) Papillary tumor of the vagina resembling transitional cell carcinoma. Pathol Res Pract 186:358–364
72. Fliegner JR (1987) Congenital atresia of the vagina. Surg Gynecol Obstet 165:387–391
73. Fox H, Wells M, Harris M et al (1988) Enteric tumors of the lower female genital tract: a report of three cases. Histopathology (Oxf) 12:167–176
74. Francke ML, Mihaescu A, Chaubert P (1998) Isolated necrotizing arteritis of the female genital tract: a clinicopathologic and immunohistochemical study of 11 cases. Int J Gynecol Pathol 17(3): 193–200
75. Friedell S, Mercer LJ (1986) Nonmenstrual toxic shock syndrome. Obstet Gynecol Surv 41:336–341
76. Friedman M, Peretz BA, Nissenbaum M, Paldi E (1986) Modern treatment of vaginal embryonal rhabdomyosarcoma. Obstet Gynecol Surv 41:614–618
77. Friedrich EG (1985) Vaginitis Am J Obstet Gyn 152:247–251
78. Friedrich EG, Siegesmund KA (1980) Tampon-associated vaginal ulcerations. Obstet Gynecol 55:149–156
79. Frick HC, Jacox HW, Taylor HC (1968) Primary carcinoma of the vagina. Am J Obstet Gynecol 101:695–703

80. Fu YS, Reagan JW (1989) Pathology of the uterine cervix, vagina, and vulva. Saunders, Philadelphia, PA, pp 193–224
81. Fu YS, Reagan JW (1989) Pathology of the uterine cervix, vagina, and vulva. Saunders, Philadelphia, PA, pp 336–379
82. Fujimoto V, Miller J, Klein N, Soules M (1997) Congenital cervical atresia: report of seven cases and review of the literature. Am J Obstet Gynecol 177(6):1419–1425
83. Fukunaga M, Endo Y, Ishikawa E, Ushigome S (1996) Mixed tumour of the vagina. Histopathology (Oxf) 28(5):457–461
84. Fukushima M, Twiggs LB, Okagaki T (1986) Mixed intestinal adenocarcinoma-argentaffin carcinoma of the vagina. Gynecol Oncol 23:387–394
85. Gallup DC, Nolan TE, Martin D et al (1991) Thrombotic thrombocytopenic purpura first seen as massive vaginal necrosis. Am J Obstet Gynecol 165:413–415
86. Gardner HL (1966) Cervical and vaginal endo-metriosis. Clin Obstet Gynecol 9:358–372
87. Gardner HL (1980) Haemophilus vaginalis vaginitis after twenty-five years. Am J Obstet Gynecol 137:385–391
88. Gardner HL, Fernet P (1964) Etiology of vaginitis emphysematosa. Report of ten cases and review of literature. Am J Obstet Gynecol 88:680–694
89. Geelhoed GW, Henson DE, Taylor PT et al (1976) Carcinoma in situ of the vagina following treatment for carcinoma of the cervix. A distinctive clinical entity. Am J Obstet Gynecol 124:510
90. Geisler JP, Look KY, Moore DA, Sutton GP (1995) Pelvic exenteration for malignant melanomas of the vagina or urethra with over 3 mm of invasion. Gynecol Oncol 59(3):338–341
91. Gelfand M, Ross MD, Blair DM, Weber MC (1972) Distribution and extent of schistosomiasis in female pelvic organs, with special reference to the genital tract, as determined at autopsy. Am J Trop Med Hyg 20:846–849
92. Georgiev D, Karag'ozov I, Velev M, Makaveeva V (2006) Three cases of vaginal adenosis after topical 5-fluorouracil therapy for vaginal HPV-associated lesions. Akusherstvo i Ginekologiia 45(3):59–61
93. Ghaemmaghami F, Karimi Zarchi M, Ghasemi M (2008) Lower genital tract rhabdomyosarcoma: case series and literature review. Arch Gynecol Obstet 278:65–69
94. Giacomini G, Calcinai A, Moretti D, Cristofani R (1998) Accuracy of cervical/vaginal cytology in the diagnosis of bacterial vaginosis. Sex Transm Dis 25(1):24–27
95. Giusti RM, Iwamoto K, Hatch EE (1995) Diethylstilbestrol revisited: a review of the long-term health effects. Ann Intern Med 122(10):778–788
96. Gold JH, Bossen EH (1976) Benign vaginal rhabdomyoma. A light and electron microscopic study. Cancer (Phila) 37:2283–2294
97. Gompel C, Silverberg SG (1977) Pathology in gynecology and obstetrics. Lippincott, Philadelphia, PA
98. Goodman A, Zukerberg LR, Nikrui N, Scully RE (1991) Vaginal adenosis and clear cell carcinoma after 5-fluorouracil treatment for condylomas. Cancer (Phila) 68(7):1628–1632
99. Goyert G, Budev H, Wright C et al (1987) Vaginal müllerian stromal sarcoma. A case report. J Reprod Med 32:129–130
100. Graham DB, Tishon JR, Borum ML (2008) An evaluation of vaginal symptoms in women with Crohn's disease. Digest Dis Sci 53(3):765–766
101. Graham-Brown RAC, Cochrane GW, Swinhoe JR et al (1981) Vaginal stenosis due to bullous erythema multiforme (Stevens-Johnson syndrome). Br J Obstet Gynaecol 88:1156–1157
102. Gupta D, Malpica A, Deavers MT, Silva EG (2002) Vaginal melanoma: a clinicopathologic and immunohistochemical study of 26 cases. Am J Surg Pathol 26:1450–1457
103. Hanski W, Hagel-Lewicka E, Daniszewski K (1991) Rhabdomyomas of female genital tract. Report on two cases. Zentralbl Pathol 137:439–442
104. Hartmann C-A, Sperling M, Stein H (1990) So-called fibroepithelial polyps of the vagina exhibiting an unusual but uniform antigen profile characterized by expression of desmin and steroid hormone receptors but no muscle-specific actin or macrophage markers. Am J Clin Pathol 93:604–608
105. Hasumi K, Sakamoto G, Sugano H et al (1978) Primary malignant melanoma of the vagina. Study of four autopsy cases with ultrastructural findings. Cancer (Phila) 42:2675–2686
106. Heine RP, Wiesenfeld HC, Sweet RL, Witkin SS (1997) Polymerase chain reaction analysis of distal vaginal specimens: a less invasive strategy for detection of Trichomonas vaginalis. Clin Infect Dis 24(5):985–987
107. Heinz KPW (1973) Amoebic infection of the female genital tract. A report of three cases. South Afr Med J 47:1795–1798
108. Hays DM, Shimada H et al (1985) Sarcomas of the vagina and the uterus: the Intergroup Rhabdomyosarcoma Study. J Pediatr Surg 20:718
109. Helms CM, Lengeling RW, Pinsky RL et al (1981) Toxic shock syndrome: a retrospective study of 25 cases from Iowa. Am J Med Sci 282:50–60
110. Henson D, Tarone R (1977) An epidemiologic study of cancer of the cervix, vagina, and vulva based on the Third National Cancer Survey in the United States. Am J Obstet Gynecol 129:525–532
111. Herbst AL (1992) Vaginal clear cell cancer: incidence, survival and screening. In: Long-term effects of exposure to diethylstilbestrol (DES) (NIH Workshop), April 23–24. Falls Church, VA, pp 19–20
112. Herbst AL, Poskanzer DC, Robboy SJ et al (1975) Prenatal exposure to stilbestrol: a prospective comparison of exposed female offspring with unexposed control. N Engl J Med 292:334
113. Herbst AL, Ulfelder H, Poskanzer DC (1971) Adenocarcinoma of the vagina: association of maternal stilbestrol therapy with tumor appearance in young women. N Engl J Med 284:878
114. Hilgers RD, Malkasian GD Jr, Soule EH (1970) Embryonal rhabdomyosarcoma (botryoid type) of the vagina: a clinicopathologic review. Am J Obstet Gynecol 107:484
115. Hill HR (1984) Group B streptococal infections. In: Holmes KK, Mårdh P-A, Sparling PF, Wiesner PJ (eds) Sexually transmitted diseases. McGraw-Hill, New York, pp 397–407
116. Hillier SL, Kiviat NB, Hawes SE et al (1996) Role of bacterial vaginosis-associated microorganisms in endometritis. Am J Obstet Gynecol 175(2):435–441
117. Hingorani V, Mahapatra LN (1964) Amebiasis of vagina and cervix. J Int Coll Surg 42:662–667
118. Holst E, Goffeng AR, Andersch B (1994) Bacterial vaginosis and vaginal microorganisms in idiopathic premature labor and association with pregnancy outcome. J Clin Microbiol 32(1):176–186
119. Hoogkamp-Korstanje JAA, Gerrards LJ, Cats BP (1982) Maternal carriage and neonatal acquisition of group B streptococci. J Infect Dis 145:800–803
120. Hopkins MP, Morley GW (1987) Squamous cell carcinoma of the neovagina. Obstet Gynecol 69:525–527
121. Hummer WK, Mussey E, Decker DG, Dockerty MB (1970) Carcinoma in situ of the vagina. Am J Obstet Gynecol 108:1109–1116

122. Irvin WP Jr, Bliss SA, Rice LW, Taylor PT Jr, Andersen WA (1998) Malignant melanoma of the vagina and locoregional control: radical surgery revisited. Gynecol Oncol 71(3):476–480
123. Iversen UM (1996) Two cases of benign vaginal rhabdomyoma. Case reports. APMIS 104(7–8):575–578
124. Japaze H, Dinh TV, Woodruff JD (1982) Verrucous carcinoma of the vulva: study of 24 cases. Obstet Gynecol 60:462–466
125. Jimerson SD, Becker JD (1980) Vaginal ulcers associated with tampon usage. Obstet Gynecol 56:97–99
126. Joseph RE, Enghardt MH, Doering DL et al (1992) Small cell neuroendocrine carcinoma of the vagina. Cancer (Phila) 70:784–789
127. Josey WE, Campbell WG (1990) Vaginitis emphysematosa. J Reprod Med 35:974–977
128. Kalogirou D, Antoniou G, Karakitsos P, Botsis D, Papadimitriou A, Giannikos L (1997) Vaginal intraepithelial neoplasia (VAIN) following hysterectomy in patients treated for carcinoma in situ of the cervix. Eur J Gynaecol Oncol 18(3):188–191
129. Kanbour AI, Klionski B, Murphy AI (1974) Carcinoma of the vagina following cervical cancer. Cancer (Phila) 34:1838–1841
130. Kaufman RH (1980) The origin and diagnosis of "nonspecific vaginitis. N Engl J Med 303:637–638
131. Kaufman RH, Friedrich EG, Gardner HL (1989) Cystic tumors. In: Benign diseases of the vulva and vagina, 3rd ed. Year Book, Chicago, pp 237–285
132. Kent HL (1991) Epidemiology of vaginitis. Am J Obstet Gynecol 165:1168
133. Keyzer C, Lilford R, Gordon W, Bloch B (1982) Pyoderma gangrenosum, vesicovaginal fistula and endometriosis. A case report. South Afr Med J 61:843–845
134. Kiviat NB, Paavonen JA, Wølner-Hanssen P et al (1990) Histopathology of endocervical infection caused by Chlamydia trachomatis, herpes simplex virus, Trichomonas vaginalis, and Neisseria gonorrhoeae. Hum Pathol 21:831–837
135. Koenig C, Turnicky R, Kankam C, Tavassoli F (1997) Papillary squamotransitional cell carcinoma of the cervix: a report of 32 cases. Am J Surg Pathol 21:915–921
136. Komisaruk BR, Whipple B, Komisaruk BR, Whipple B (2005) Functional MRI of the brain during orgasm in women. Ann Rev Sex Res 16:62–86
137. Kondi-Pafiti A, Grapsa D, Papakonstantinou K, Kairi-Vassilatou E, Xasiakos D (2008) Vaginal cysts: a common pathologic entity revisited. Clin Exper Obstet Gynecol 35(1):41–44
138. Korn AP, Bolan G, Padian N, Ohm-Smith M, Schachter J, Landers DV (1995) Plasma cell endometritis in women with symptomatic bacterial vaginosis. Obstet Gynecol 85(3):387–390
139. Koskela O (1964) Granular cell myoblastoma of the vagina. Ann Chir Gynaecol Fenn 53:270–273
140. Kramer K, Tobin H (1987) Vaginitis emphysematosa. Arch Pathol Lab Med 111:746–749
141. Kraus FT, Perez-Mesa C (1966) Verrucous carcinoma. Clinical and pathologic study of 105 cases involving oral cavity, larynx and genitalia. Cancer (Phila) 19:26–38
142. Krause RM (1992) The origin of plagues: old and new. Science 257:1073–1078
143. Kurita T, Cunha GR, Robboy SJ, Mills AA, Medina RT (2005) Differential expression of p63 isoforms in female reproductive organs. Mech Dev 122(9):1043–1055
144. Kurman RJ, Norris HJ, Wilkinson E (1992) Tumors of the vagina. In: Atlas of tumor pathology, 3rd series, fasc 4. Tumors of the cervix, vagina, and vulva. Armed Forces Institute of Pathology, Washington DC, pp 141–178
145. Kurman RJ, Prabha AC (1973) Thyroid and parathyroid glands in the vaginal wall: report of a case. Am J Clin Pathol 59:503–507
146. Kurman RJ, Toki T, Schiffman MH (1993) Basaloid and warty carcinomas of the vulva. Distinctive types of squamous cell carcinoma frequently associated with human papillomaviruses. Am J Surg Pathol 17(2):133–145
147. Lakshminarasimhan S, Doval DC, Rajashekhar U et al (1996) Preleukemic granulocytic sarcoma of vagina. A case report with review of literature. Indian J Cancer 33(3):145–148
148. Lang WR, Israel SL, Fritz MA (1958) Staphylococcal vulvovaginitis. A report of two cases following antibiotic therapy. Obstet Gynecol 11:352–354
149. Larsen B, Galask RP (1980) Vaginal microbial flora: practical and theoretic relevance. Obstet Gynecol 55:100S–113S
150. Larsson P-G, Platz-Christensen J-J, Sundström E (1991) Is bacterial vaginosis a sexually transmitted disease? Int J STD AIDS 2:362–364
151. Lenehan PM, Meffe F, Lickrish GM (1986) Vaginal intraepithelial neoplasia: biologic aspects and management. Obstet Gynecol 68:333–337
152. Levine BB, Sriaganian RP, Schenkein I (1973) Allergy to human seminal plasma. N Engl J Med 288:894
153. Levine WC, Pope V, Bhoomkar A et al (1998) Increase in endocervical CD4 lymphocytes among women with nonulcerative sexually transmitted diseases. J Infect Dis 177(1):167–174
154. Levitan Z, Gordon AN, Kaplan AL, Kaufman RH (1989) Primary malignant melanoma of the vagina: report of four cases and review of the literature. Gynecol Oncol 33:85–90
155. Lifson AR (1992) Transmission of the human immunodeficiency virus. In: DeVita VT, Hellman S, Rosenberg SA (eds) AIDS: Etiology, diagnosis, treatment, and prevention. Lippincott, Philadelphia, PA, pp 111–117
156. Lin JI, Caracta PF, Chang CH et al (1979) Malacoplakia of the vagina. South Med J 72:326–328
157. Lindner JGEM, Plantema FHF, Hoogkamp-Korstanje JAA (1978) Quantitative studies of the vaginal flora of healthy women and of obstetric and gynaecologic patients. J Med Microbiol 11:233
158. Liu L-Y, Hou Y-J, Li J-Z (1987) Primary malignant melanoma of the vagina: a report of seven cases. Obstet Gynecol 70:569–572
159. Lorenz G (1978) Adenomatoid tumor of the ovary and vagina. Zentbl Gynakkol 100:1412–1416
160. Lossick JG, Kent HL (1991) Trichomoniasis: trends in diagnosis and management. Am J Obstet Gynecol 165:1217–1222
161. Lotan TL, Tefs K, Schuster V, Miller J, Manaligod J, Filstead A, Yamada SD, Krausz T (2007) Inherited plasminogen deficiency presenting as ligneous vaginitis: a case report with molecular correlation and review of the literature. Hum Pathol 38(10):1569–1575
162. Lucas WE, Benirschke K, Lebherz TB (1974) Verrucous carcinoma of the female genital tract. Am J Obstet Gynecol 119:435–440
163. Ludwig K (1998) The Mayer-Rokitansky-Kuster syndrome. An analysis of its morphology and embryology. Part I: Morphology. Arch Gynecol Obstet 262(1–2):1–26
164. Ludwig K (1998) The Mayer-Rokitansky-Kuster syndrome. An analysis of its morphology and embryology. Part II: Embryology. Arch Gynecol Obstet 262(1–2):27–42
165. Luttges JE, Lubke M (1994) Recurrent benign müllerian papilloma of the vagina. Immunohistological findings and histogenesis. Arch Gynecol Obstet 255(3):157–160

166. MacLeod C, Fowler A, Dalrymple C, Atkinson K, Elliott P, Carter J (1997) High-dose-rate brachy-therapy in the management of high-grade intraepithelial neoplasia of the vagina. Gynecol Oncol 65(1):74–77
167. Madico G, Quinn TC, Rompalo A, McKee KT Jr, Gaydos CA (1998) Diagnosis of Trichomonas vaginalis infection by PCR using vaginal swab samples. J Clin Microbiol 36(11):3205–3210
168. Maharaj NR, Nimako D, Hadley GP (2008) Multimodal therapy for the initial management of genital rhabdomyosarcoma in childhood. Int J Gynecol Cancer 18:190–192
169. March CM, Israel R (1976) Rectovaginal endometriosis: an isolated engima. Am J Obstet Gynecol 125:274–275
170. Marcus SL (1960) Primary carcinoma of the vagina. Obstet Gynecol 15:673
171. Mårdh P-A (1991) The vaginal ecosystem. Am J Obstet Gynecol 165:1163–1168
172. Mårdh P-A, Holst E, Moller BR (1984) The Grivet monkey as a model for study of vaginitis. In: Mårdh P-A, Taylor-Robinson D (eds) Bacterial vaginosis. Almquist and Wiksell International, Stockholm, p 201
173. Mardh PA, Novikova N, Witkin SS, Korneeva I, Rodriques AR (2003) Detection of candida by polymerase chain reaction vs microscopy and culture in women diagnosed as recurrent vulvovaginal cases. Int J STD AIDS 14(11):753–756
174. Masters WH (1960) The sexual response cycle of the human female. I. Gross anatomic considerations. West J Surg Obstet Gynecol 68:57–72
175. McCluggage WG, Nirmala V, Radhakumari K (1999) Intramural mullerian papilloma of the vagina. Int J Gynecol Pathol 18:94–95
176. McGregor JA, French JI, Jones W et al (1994) Bacterial vaginosis is associated with prematurity and vaginal fluid mucinase and sialidase: results of a controlled trial of topical clindamycin cream. Am J Obstet Gynecol 170(4):1048–1059; discussion 1059–1060
177. McKenna UG, Meadows JA, Brewer NS et al (1980) Toxic shock syndrome, a newly recognized disease entity. Report of 11 cases. Mayo Clin Proc 55:663–672
178. McLellan R, Spence MR, Brockman M et al (1982) The clinical diagnosis of trichomoniasis. Obstet Gynecol 60:30
179. McLennan MT, Smith JM, McLennan CE (1972) Diagnosis of vaginal mycosis and trichomoniasis: reliability of cytologic smear, wet smear and culture. Obstet Gynecol 40:231–234
180. Merkus JMWM, Bisschop MPJM, Stolte LAM (1985) The proper nature of vaginal candidosis and the problem of recurrence. Obstet Gynecol Surv 40:493–504
181. Michal M, Rokyta Z, Mejchar B, Pelikan K, Kummel M, Mukensnabl P (2000) Prolapse of the fallopian tube after hysterectomy associated with exuberant angiomyofibroblastic stroma response: a diagnostic pitfall. Virchows Arch 437(4):436–439
182. Miettinen M, Wahlström T, Vesterinen E, Saksela E (1983) Vaginal polyps with pseudosarcomatous features. A clinicopathologic study of seven cases. Cancer (Phila) 51:1148–1151
183. Miller CJ, Vogel P, Alexander NJ (1992) Localization of SIV in the genital tract of chronically infected female rhesus macaques. Am J Pathol 141:655–660
184. Minucci D, Cinel A, Insacco E, Oselladore M (1995) Epidemiological aspects of vaginal intraepithelial neoplasia (VAIN). Clin Exp Obstet Gynecol 22(1):36–42
185. Montgomery EA, Shuster DD, Burkart AL, Esteban JM, Sgrignoli A, Elwood L, Vaughn DJ, Griffin CA, Epstein JI (2006) Inflammatory myofibroblastic tumors of the urinary tract: a clinicopathologic study of 46 cases, including a malignant example inflammatory fibrosarcoma and a subset associated with high-grade urothelial carcinoma. Am J Surg Pathol 30(12):1502–1512
186. Mucitelli DR, Charles EZ, Kraus FT (1990) Vulvovaginal polyps. Histologic appearance, ultrastructure, immunocytochemical characteristics and clinicopathologic correlations. Int J Gynecol Pathol 9:20–40
187. de Mundi ZA, del Alamo CM, de Blas LL, San Cristobal AA (1978) Egg of Trichuris trichiura in a vaginal smear. Acta Cytol 22:119–120
188. Munguia H, Franco E, Valenzuela P (1966) Diagnosis of genital amebiasis in women by the standard Papanicolaou technique. Am J Obstet Gynecol 94:181–188
189. Murad TM, Durant JR, Maddox WA, Dowling EA (1975) The pathologic behavior of primary vaginal carcinoma and its relationship to cervical cancer. Cancer (Phila) 35:787–794
190. Murdoch F, Sharma R, Al Nafussi A (2003) Benign mixed tumor of the vagina: case report with expanded immunohistochemical profile. Int J Gynecol Cancer 13:543–547
191. Murphy R (2004) Desquamative inflammatory vaginitis. Dermatol Therapy 17(1):47–49
192. Murphy R, Edwards L (2008) Desquamative inflammatory vaginitis: what is it? J Reprod Med 53(2):124–128
193. Naves AE, Monti JA, Chichoni E (1980) Basal cell-like carcinoma of the upper third of the vagina. Am J Obstet Gynecol 137:136–137
194. Neesham D, Kerdemelidis P, Scurry J (1998) Primary malignant mixed müllerian tumor of the vagina. Gynecol Oncol 70(2):303–307
195. Newton ER, Butler MC, Shain RN (1996) Sexual behavior and vaginal colonization by group B streptococcus among minority women. Obstet Gynecol 88(4 pt 1):577–582
196. Newton ER, Piper J, Peairs W (1997) Bacterial vaginosis and intraamniotic infection. Am J Obstet Gynecol 176(3):672–677
197. Newton WA, Soule EH, Hamoudi AB et al (1988) Histopathology of childhood sarcomas, intergroup rhabdomyosarcoma studies I and II: clinicopathologic correlation. J Clin Oncol 6:67–75
198. Nilsson U, Hellberg D, Shoubnikova M, Nilsson S, Mardh PA (1997) Sexual behavior risk factors associated with bacterial vaginosis and Chlamydia trachomatis infection. Sex Transm Dis 24(5):241–246
199. Nogales-Ortiz F, Tarancón I, Nogales F (1979) The pathology of female genital tuberculosis. Obstet Gynecol 53:422–428
200. Nucci MR, Young R, Fletcher C (2000) Cellular pseudosarcomatous fibroepithelial stromal polyps of the lower female genital tract: an underrecognized lesion often misdiagnosed as sarcoma. Am J Surg Pathol 24:231–240
201. Okagaki T, Ishida T, Hilgers RD (1976) A malignant tumor of the vagina resembling synovial sarcoma. A light and electron microscopic study. Cancer (Phila) 37:2306–2320
202. Opitz JM (1987) Editorial comment: Vaginal atresia (von Mayer-Rokitansky-Küster or MRK anomaly) in hereditary renal adysplasia (HRA). Am J Med Genet 26:873–876
203. Östör AG, Fortune DW, Riley CB (1988) Fibroepithelial polyps with atypical stromal cells (pseudosarcoma botryoides) of vulva and vagina. A report of 13 cases. Int J Gynecol Pathol 7:351–360
204. Palmer JP, Biback SM (1954) Primary cancer of the vagina. Am J Obstet Gynecol 67:377–397
205. Paris AL, Herwaldt LA, Blum D et al (1982) Pathologic findings in twelve fatal cases of toxic shock syndrome. Ann Intern Med 96:852–857
206. Peipert JF, Montagno AB, Cooper AS, Sung CJ (1997) Bacterial vaginosis as a risk factor for upper genital tract infection. Am J Obstet Gynecol 177(5):1184–1187

207. Perez CA, Arneson AN, Dehner LP et al (1974) Radiation therapy in carcinoma of vagina. Obstet Gynecol 44:862
208. Perez CA, Camel HM, Galakatos AE et al (1988) Definitive irradiation in carcinoma of the vagina: long-term evaluation of results. Int J Radiat Oncol Biol Phys 15:1283
209. Perez CA, Gersell DJ, Hoskins WJ, McGuire WP III (1992) Vagina. In: Hoskins WJ, Perez CA, Young RC (eds) Principles and practice of gynecologic oncology. Lippincott, Philadelphia, PA, pp 567–590
210. Peterman TA, Stoneburner RL, Allen JR et al (1988) Risk of human immunodeficiency virus transmission from heterosexual adults with transfusion-associated infections. JAMA 259:55
211. Peters WA, Kumar NB, Anderson WA, Morley GW (1985) Primary sarcoma of the adult vagina: a clinicopathologic study. Obstet Gynecol 65:699–704
212. Peters WA, Kumar NB, Morley GW (1985) Carcinoma of the vagina: factors influencing treatment outcome. Cancer (Phila) 55:892
213. Peters WA, Kumar NB, Morley GW (1985) Microinvasive carcinoma of the vagina: a distinct clinical entity? Am J Obstet Gynecol 153:505–507
214. Petru E, Nagele F, Czerwenka K et al (1998) Primary malignant melanoma of the vagina: long-term remission following radiation therapy. Gynecol Oncol 70(1):23–26
215. Pezeshkpour G (1981) Solitary paraganglioma of the vagina. Report of a case. Am J Obstet Gynecol 139:219–221
216. Pheifer TA, Forsyth PS, Durfee MA et al (1978) Nonspecific vaginitis. Role of Haemophilus vaginalis and treatment with metronidazole. N Engl J Med 298:1429–1434
217. Platz C, Benda J (1995) Female genital tract cancer. Cancer (Phila) 75:270–294
218. Plentl AA, Friedman EA (1971) Lymphatic system of the female genitalia. The morphologic basis of oncologic diagnosis and therapy. Saunders, Philadelphia, PA, pp 51–74
219. Podczaski E, Herbst AL (1986) Cancer of the vagina and fallopian tube. In: Knapp RC, Berkowitz RS (eds) Gynecologic oncology. Macmillan, New York, pp 399–424
220. Polasek P, Erickson L, Stanhope C (1995) Transverse vaginal septum associated with tubal atresia. Mayo Clin Proc 70(10):965–968
221. Prasad CJ, Ray JA, Kessler S (1992) Primary small cell carcinoma of the vagina arising in a background of atypical adenosis. Cancer (Phila) 70:2484–2487
222. Premptee T, Amornmarn R (1985) Radiation treatment of primary carcinoma of the vagina: patterns of failure after definitive therapy. Acta Radiol Oncol 24:51
223. Premptee T, Tang C-K, Hatef A et al (1983) Angiosarcoma of the vagina: a clinicopathologic report. Cancer (Phila) 51:618–622
224. Prezyna AP, Kalyanaraman U (1977) Bowen's carcinoma in vulvovaginal Crohn's disease (regional enterocolitis). Report of first case. Am J Obstet Gynecol 128:914–916
225. Proppe KH, Scully RE, Rosai J (1984) Postoperative spindle cell nodules of genitourinary tract resembling sarcomas. A report of eight cases. Am J Surg Pathol 8:101–108
226. Pul M, Yilmaz N, Gürses N, Ozoran Y (1990) Vaginal polyp in a newborn – a case report and review of the literature. Clin Pediatr 29:346
227. Qualman S, Coffin C, Newton W et al (1998) Intergroup rhabdomyosarcoma study: update for pathologists. Pediatr Dev Pathol 1:550–561
228. Raghavaiah NV, Devi AI (1980) Primary vaginal stones. J Urol 123:771–772
229. Ragnarsson-Olding B, Johansson H, Rutqvist LE, Ringborg U (1993) Malignant melanoma of the vulva and vagina. Trends in incidence, age distribution, and long-term survival among 245 consecutive cases in Sweden 1960–1984. Cancer 71:1893–1897
230. Randall M, Andersen W, Mills S, Kim J-A (1986) Papillary squamous cell carcinoma of the uterine cervix. Int J Gynecol Pathol 5:1–10
231. Rajagopalan G, Smart MK, Murali N, Patel R, David CS (2007) Acute systemic immune activation following vaginal exposure to staphylococcal enterotoxin B – implications for menstrual shock. J Reprod Immunol 73(1):51–59
232. Rajkumar S, Narayanaswamy G, Laude TA (1979) Shigella vulvovaginitis in childhood: a case report. J Natl Med Assoc 71:1005–1006
233. Regan JA, Klebanoff MA, Nugent RP et al (1996) Colonization with group B streptococci in pregnancy and adverse outcome. VIP Study Group. Am J Obstet Gynecol 174(4):1354–1360
234. Reid GC, Schmidt RW, Roberts JA et al (1989) Primary melanoma of the vagina: a clinicopathologic analysis. Obstet Gynecol 74: 190–199
235. Rein MF, Müller M (1990) Trichomonas vaginalis. In: Holmes KK, Mårdh P-A, Sparling PF, Wiesner PJ (eds) Sexually transmitted diseases, 2nd edn. McGraw-Hill, New York
236. Resnick SD (1990) Toxic shock syndrome: recent developments in pathogenesis. J Pediatr 116:321–328
237. Rhatigan RM, Mojadidi Q (1973) Adenosquamous carcinomas of the vulva and vagina. Am J Clin Pathol 59:208–217
238. Richart RM (1986) The incidence of cervical and vaginal dysplasia after exposure to DES. JAMA 255:36–37
239. Robboy SJ (1983) A hypothetic mechanism of diethylstilbestrol (DES)-induced anomalies in prenatally exposed women. Hum Pathol 14:831
240. Robboy SJ, Kaufman RH, Prat J et al (1979) Pathologic findings in young women enrolled in national cooperative diethylstilbestrol adenosis (DESAD) project. Obstet Gynecol 53:309
241. Robboy SJ, Noller KL, O'Brien P et al (1984) Increased incidence of cervical and vaginal dysplasia in 3, 980 diethylstilbestrol (DES)-exposed young women: Experience of the National Collaborative DES-Adenosis (DESAD) Project. JAMA 252:2979
242. Robboy SJ, Taguchi O, Cunha GR (1982) Normal development of the human female reproductive tract and alterations resulting from experimental exposure to diethylstilbestrol. Hum Pathol 13:190–198
243. Robboy SJ, Welch WR, Young RH et al (1982) Topographic relation of adenosis, clear cell adenocarcinoma and other related lesions of the vagina and cervix in DES-exposed progeny. Obstet Gynecol 60:546
244. Robboy SJ, Young RH, Welch WR et al (1984) Atypical (dysplastic) adenosis: forerunner and transitional state to clear cell adenocarcinoma in young women exposed in utero to diethylstilbestrol. Cancer (Phila) 54:869
245. Robboy SJ, Prade M, Cunha G (1992) Vagina. In: Sternberg SS (ed) Histology for pathologists. Raven Press, New York, pp 881–892.
246. Roberts WS, Hoffman MS, LaPolla JP et al (1991) Management of radionecrosis of the vulva and distal vagina. Am J Obstet Gynecol 164:1235–1238
247. Roberts DK, Walker NJ, Parmley TH, Horbelt DV (1988) Interaction of epithelial and stromal cells in vaginal adenosis. Hum Pathol 19:855–861

248. Rorat E, Ferenczy A, Richart RM (1975) Human Bartholin gland, duct, and duct cyst. Histochemical and ultrastructural study. Arch Pathol 99:367–374
249. Rose P, Stoler M, Abdul-Karim F (1998) Papillary squamotransitional cell carcinoma of the vagina. Int J Gynecol Pathol 17:372–375
250. Rotmensch J, Rosenshein N, Dillon M et al (1983) Carcinoma arising in the neovagina: case report and review of the literature. Obstet Gynecol 61:534
251. Rutledge F (1967) Cancer of the vagina. Am J Obstet Gynecol 97:635–655
252. Sanders CC, Sanders WE, Fagnant JE (1982) Toxic shock syndrome: an ecologic imbalance within the genital microflora of women? Am J Obstet Gynecol 142:977–982
253. Sangwan K, Khosla AH, Hazra PC (1996) Leiomyoma of the vagina. Aust N Z J Obstet Gynaecol 36(4):494–495
254. Schmedding A, Zense M, Fuchs J, Gluer S (1997) Benign papilloma of the cervix in childhood: immunohistochemical findings and review of the literature. Eur J Pediatr 156(4):320–322
255. Schwebke JR, Hillier SL, Sobel JD, McGregor JA, Sweet RL (1996) Validity of the vaginal Gram stain for the diagnosis of bacterial vaginosis. Obstet Gynecol 88(4 pt 1):573–576
256. Scurry J, Planner R, Grant P (1991) Unusual variants of vaginal adenosis: a challenge for diagnosis and treatment. Gynecol Oncol 41(2):172–177
257. Senekjian EK, Hubby M, Bell DA et al (1986) Clear cell adenocarcinoma (CCA) of the vagina and cervix in association with pregnancy. Gynecol Oncol 24:207–219
258. Sheets JL, Dockerty MD, Decker DG, Welch JS (1964) Primary epithelial malignancy in the vagina. Am J Obstet Gynecol 89:121–128
259. Shevchuk MM, Fenoglio CM, Lattes R (1978) Malignant mixed tumor of the vagina probably arising in mesonephric rests. Cancer (Phila) 42:214–223
260. Sillman FH, Sedlis A, Boyce JG (1985) A review of lower genital intraepithelial neoplasia and the use of topical 5-fluorouracil. Obstet Gynecol Surv 40:190–220
261. Sillman FH, Fruchter RG, Chen YS, Camilien L, Sedlis A, McTigue E (1997) Vaginal intraepithelial neoplasia: risk factors for persistence, recurrence, and invasion and its management. Am J Obstet Gynecol 176(1 pt 1):93–99
262. Silverberg SG, Frabler WJ (1974) Prolapse of fallopian tube into vaginal vault after hysterectomy. Histopathology, cytopathology, and differential diagnosis. Arch Pathol 97:100–103
263. Sirota RL, Dickerson GR, Scully RE (1981) Mixed tumors of the vagina: a clinicopathologic analysis of eight cases. Am J Surg Pathol 5:413–422
264. Smith YR, Quint EH, Hinton EL (1998) Recurrent benign mullerian papilloma of the cervix. J Pediatr Adolesc Gynecol 11(1):29–31
265. Sobel JD (1990) Vaginal infections in adult women. Med Clin North Am 74:1573–1602
266. Sobel JD (1994) Desquamative inflammatory vaginitis: a new subgroup of purulent vaginitis responsive to topical 2% clindamycin therapy. Am J Obstet Gynecol 171(5):1215–1220
267. Sobel JD, Brooker D, Stein GE et al (1995) Single oral dose fluconazole compared with conventional clotrimazole topical therapy of Candida vaginitis. Fluconazole Vaginitis Study Group. Am J Obstet Gynecol 172(4 pt 1):1263–1268
268. Soper DE, Brockwell NJ, Dalton HP, Johnson D (1994) Observations concerning the microbial etiology of acute salpingitis. Am J Obstet Gynecol 170(4):1008–1014; discussion 1014–1017
269. Spiegel CA, Amsel R, Eschenbach D et al (1980) Anaerobic bacteria in nonspecific vaginitis. N Engl J Med 303:601–607
270. Spitzer M, Molho L, Seltzer VL et al (1985) Vaginal glomus tumor: case presentation and ultrastructural findings. Obstet Gynecol 66:86S–88S
271. Strate SM, Taylor WE, Forney JP, Silva FG (1983) Xanthogranulomatous pseudotumor of the vagina: evidence of a local response to an unusual bacterium (mucoid Escherichia coli). Am J Clin Pathol 79:637–643
272. Stuart GCE, Flagler EA, Nation JG et al (1988) Laser vaporization of vaginal intraepithelial neoplasia. Am J Obstet Gynecol 158:240–243
273. Sulak P, Barnhill D, Heller P et al (1988) Nonsquamous cancer of the vagina. Gynecol Oncol 29:309–320
274. Sunderland WA, Harris HH, Spence DA, Lawson HW (1972) Meningococcemia in a newborn infant whose mother had meningococcal vaginitis (Letter to the Editor). J Pediatr 81(856):310
275. Sweet RL, Gibbs RS (1985) Infectious vulvovaginitis. In: Infectious diseases of the female genital tract. Williams & Wilkins, Baltimore, MD, pp 89–96
276. Sweet RL (1995) Role of bacterial vaginosis in pelvic inflammatory disease. Clin Infect Dis 20(2):S271–S275
277. Sweet RL, Gibbs RS (1985) Perinatal infections. Infectious diseases of the female genital tract. Williams & Wilkins, Baltimore, MD, pp 206–214
278. Sweet RL, Gibbs RS (1985) Toxic shock syndrome. Infectious diseases of the female genital tract. Williams & Wilkins, Baltimore, MD, pp 78–88
279. Takehara M, Hayakawa O, Itoh E, Sagae S, Suzuki T, Kudo R (1998) A case of a malignant mixed tumor in the vagina. J Obstet Gynaecol Res 24(1):7–11
280. Tancer ML (1980) The post-total hysterectomy (vault) vesicovaginal fistula. J Urol 123:839–840
281. Tarraza HM Jr, Meltzer SE, De Cain M, Jones MA (1998) Vaginal metastases from renal cell carcinoma: report of four cases and review of the literature. Eur J Gynaecol Oncol 19(1):14–18
282. Tazvassoli FA, Norris HJ (1979) Smooth muscle tumors of the vagina. Obstet Gynecol 53:689–693
283. The Working Group on Severe Streptococcal Infections (1993) Defining the Group A streptococcal toxic shock syndrome. Rationale and consensus definition. JAMA 269:390–391
284. Thomason JL, Anderson RJ, Gelbart SM et al (1992) Simplified Gram stain interpretive method for diagnosis of bacterial vaginosis. Am J Obstet Gynecol 167:16–19
285. Thomason JL, Gelbart SM (1989) Trichomonas vaginalis. Obstet Gynecol 74:536–541
286. Thomason JL, Gelbart SM, Anderson RJ et al (1990) Statistical evaluation of diagnostic criteria for bacterial vaginosis. Am J Obstet Gynecol 162:155–160
287. Thorsen P, Jensen IP, Jeune B et al (1998) Few microorganisms associated with bacterial vaginosis may constitute the pathologic core: a population-based microbiologic study among 3596 pregnant women. Am J Obstet Gynecol 178(3):580–587
288. Tjugum J, Jonassen F, Olsson JH (1986) Vaginitis emphysematosa in a renal transplant patient. Acta Obstet Gynecol Scand 65(377):378
289. Tobon H, Murphy AI (1977) Benign blue nevus of the vagina. Cancer (Phila) 40:3174
290. Todd J, Fishaut M, Kapral F, Welch T (1978) Toxic-shock syndrome associated with phage-group-I staphylococci. Lancet 2:1116–1118

291. Tohya T, Katabuchi H, Fukuma K et al (1991) Angiosarcoma of the vagina. A light and electronmicroscopy study. Acta Obstet Gynecol Scand 70:169–172
292. Torne A, Pahisa J, Castelo-Branco C, Fabregues F, Mallofre C, Iglesias X (1994) Solitary vaginal metastasis as a presenting form of unsuspected renal adenocarcinoma. Gynecol Oncol 52(2):260–263
293. Tsokos M, Webber BL, Parham DM et al (1992) Rhabdomyosarcoma. A new classification scheme related to prognosis. Arch Pathol Lab Med 116:847–855
294. Ulbright TM, Alexander RW, Kraus FT (1981) Intramural papilloma of the vagina: evidence of müllerian histogenesis. Cancer 48:2260–2266
295. Václavínková V, Neumann E (1981) Vaginal involvement in familial benign chronic pemphigus (morbus Hailey-Hailey). Acta Dermatovenerал (Stockh) 62:80–81
296. Van Lingen B, Reindollar R, Davis A, Gray M (1998) Further evidence that the WT1 gene does not have a role in the development of the derivatives of the mullerian duct. Am J Obstet Gynecol 179(3 pt 1):597–603
297. van den Broek N, Emmerson C, Dunlop W (1996) Benign mixed tumour of the vagina: an unusual cause for postmenopausal bleeding. Eur J Obstet Gynecol Reprod Biol 69(2):143–144
298. van der Meijden WI, Duivenvoorden HJ, Both-Patoir HC et al (1988) Clinical and laboratory findings in women with bacterial vaginosis and trichomoniasis versus controls. Eur J Obstet Gynecol Reprod Biol 28:39–52
299. Vasquez R, Collini P, Meazza C, Favini F, Casanova M (2008) Ferrari A. Late relapse of embryonal rhabdomyosarcoma, botyroid variant, of the vagina Cancer 51:140–141
300. Vazquez JA, Sobel JD, Demitriou R, Vaishampayan J, Lynch M, Zervos MJ (1994) Karyotyping of Candida albicans isolates obtained longitudinally in women with recurrent vulvovaginal candidiasis. J Infect Dis 170(6):1566–1569
301. Venter PF, Anderson JD, Van Velden DJJ (1979) Postmenopausal endometriosis. A case report. South Afr Med J 56:1136–1138
302. de Virgiliis G, Sideri M, Rossi A et al (1985) "DES-Like" anomalies. I. Biological and clinical problems. A study on 12, 285 cases. Cervix Low Female Genital Tract 3:297–312
303. Vontver LA, Eschenbach DA (1981) The role of gardnerella vaginalis in nonspecific vaginitis. Clin Obstet Gynecol 24:439–460
304. Wager GP (1983) Toxic shock syndrome: a review. Am J Obstet Gynecol 146:93–102
305. Waggoner SE, Mittendorf R, Biney N, Anderson D, Herbst AL (1994) Influence of in utero diethylstilbestrol exposure on the prognosis and biologic behavior of vaginal clear-cell adenocarcinoma. Gynecol Oncol 55(2):238–244
306. Waggoner SE, Anderson SM, Luce MC, Takahashi H, Boyd J (1996) p53 protein expression and gene analysis in clear cell adenocarcinoma of the vagina and cervix. Gynecol Oncol 60(3):339–344
307. Ways SC, Mortola JF, Zvaifler NJ et al (1987) Alterations in immune responsiveness in women exposed to diethylstilbestrol in utero. Fertil Steril 48:193–197
308. Webb MJ, Symmonds RE, Weiland LH (1974) Malignant fibrous histiocytoma of vagina. Am J Obstet Gynecol 119:190–192
309. Weber A, Walters M, Schover L, Mitchinson A (1995) Vaginal anatomy and sexual function. Obstet Gynecol 86(6):946–949
310. Weinstock MA (1994) Malignant melanoma of the vulva and vagina in the United States: patterns of incidence and population-based estimates of survival. Am J Obstet Gynecol 171(5):1225–1230
311. Wheelock JB, Schneider V, Goplerud DR (1985) Prolapsed fallopian tube masquerading as adenocarcinoma of the vagina in a postmenopausal woman. Gynecol Oncol 21:369–375
312. Williams GA (1965) Postsurgical and post-traumatic tumors. Clin Obstet Gynecol 8:1020–1034
313. Wisniewski PM, Wilkinson EJ (1991) Postpartum vaginal atrophy. Am J Obstet Gynecol 165:1249–1254
314. Witkin SS, Inglis SR, Polaneczky M (1996) Detection of Chlamydia trachomatis and Trichomonas vaginalis by polymerase chain reaction in introital specimens from pregnant women. Am J Obstet Gynecol 175(1):165–167
315. Wooduff JD, Parmley TH, Julian CG (1975) Topical 5-fluorouracil in the treatment of vaginal carcinoma in situ. Gynecol Oncol 3:124–125
316. Yokoyama Y, Sato S, Kawaguchi T, Saito Y (1998) A case of concurrent uterine cervical adenocarcinoma and renal-cell carcinoma, and subsequent vaginal metastasis from the renal-cell carcinoma. J Obstet Gynaecol Res 24(1):37–43
317. Young RH, Scully RE (1984) Endodermal sinus tumor of the vagina: a report of nine cases and review of the literature. Gynecol Oncol 18:380–392
318. Yousem HL (1961) Adenocarcinoma of Gartner's duct cyst presenting as a vaginal lesion. A case report. Sinai Hosp J 10:112–114
319. Yow MD, Leeds LJ, Thompson PK et al (1980) The natural history of group B streptococcal colonization in the pregnant woman and her offspring. I. Colonization studies. Am J Obstet Gynecol 137:34–38
320. Zhang ZF (1996) Epidemiology of trichomonas vaginalis. A prospective study in China. Sex Transm Dis 23(5):415–424

4 Benign Diseases of the Cervix

Thomas C. Wright · Brigitte M. Ronnett · Alex Ferenczy

R. J. Kurman, L. Hedrick Ellenson, B. M. Ronnett (eds.), *Blaustein's Pathology of the Female Genital Tract (6th ed.)*, DOI 10.1007/978-1-4419-0489-8_4,

Gross Anatomy

The uterus is divided into the corpus, isthmus, and cervix [63]. The cervix (term taken from the Latin, meaning *neck*) is the most inferior portion of the uterus, protruding into the upper vagina. The transition between the endocervix and the lower portion of the uterine corpus is termed the *isthmus* or *lower uterine segment*. The latter is used for descriptive purposes during gestation and labor and is an important landmark for the pathologist when describing cancers of the uterine corpus. The muscular layer in the region of the isthmus is less well developed than in the corpus, a feature that facilitates effacement and dilation during labor. The vagina is fused circumferentially and obliquely to the distal part of the cervix and is divided into an upper, supervaginal, and lower vaginal portion. The cervix measures 2.5–3 cm in length in the adult nulligravida, and when normally positioned, is angled slightly downward and backward. The vaginal portion (portio vaginalis) of the cervix, also referred to as the *exocervix*, is delimited by the anterior and posterior vaginal fornices; it has a convex elliptical surface. The portio may be divided into anterior and posterior lips, of which the anterior is shorter and projects lower than the posterior lip. In the center of the exocervix is the external os. The external os is circular in the nulligravida and slit-like in the parous woman (➋ *Fig. 4.1a, b*). The external os is connected to the isthmus of the cervical canal (endocervix). The canal is an elliptical cavity, measuring 8 mm in its greatest diameter and contains longitudinal mucosal ridges, the plicae palmatae.

The blood supply of the cervix is provided by the descending branches of the uterine arteries, reaching the lateral walls along the upper margin of the paracervical ligaments (cardinal ligaments of Mackenrodt) (➋ *Fig. 4.2*). These ligaments and the uterosacral ligaments, which attach the supervaginal portion of the cervix to the second through fourth sacral vertebrae, are the main sources of fixation, support, and suspension of the organ. The venous drainage parallels the arterial system, with communication between the cervical plexus and neck of the urinary bladder. The lymphatics of the cervix have a dual origin: coursing beneath the mucosa and deep in the fibrous stroma. Both systems collect into two lateral plexuses in the region of the isthmus and give origin to four efferent channels running toward the external iliac and obturator nodes, the hypogastric and common iliac nodes, the sacral nodes, and the nodes of the posterior wall of the urinary bladder (➋ *Fig. 4.2*). The innervation of the cervix is chiefly limited to the endocervix and peripheral deep portion of the exocervix. This distribution is responsible for the relative insensitivity to pain of the inner two-thirds of the portio vaginalis. The cervical nerves are derived from the pelvic autonomic system, the superior, middle, and inferior hypogastric plexuses.

a

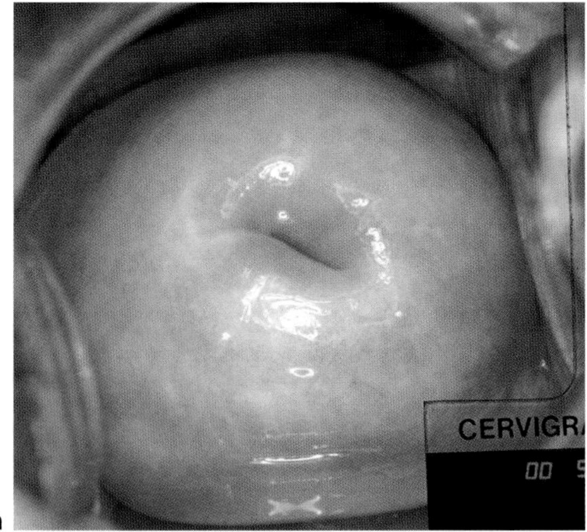

b

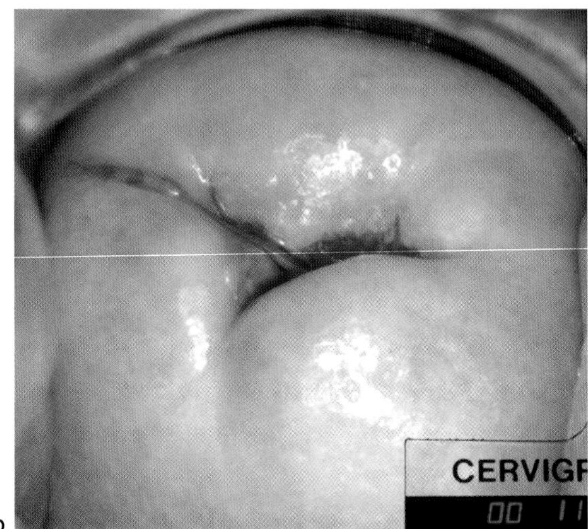

Fig. 4.1
Normal cervix uteri. **(a)** Nulliparous cervix **(b)** Parous cervix

Histology and Physiology

The cervix is composed of an admixture of fibrous, muscular, and elastic tissue and is lined by columnar and squamous epithelium. Fibrous connective tissue is the predominant component. Smooth muscle comprises 15% of

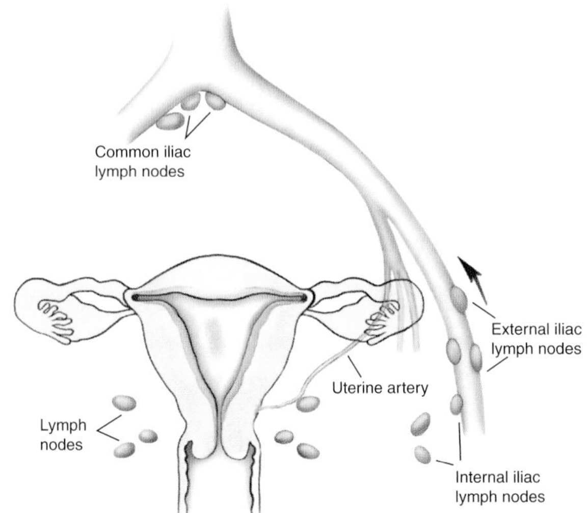

Fig. 4.2
Anatomy of the cervix. **The blood supply and lymphatic drainage of the cervix are demonstrated**

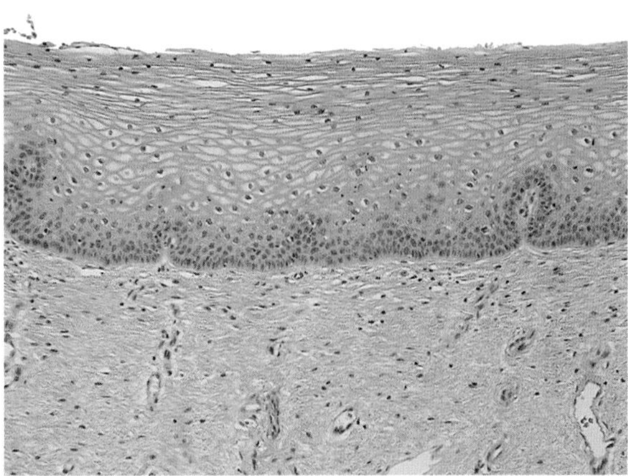

Fig. 4.3
Normal squamous epithelium. **The mature squamous epithelium of the portio of the cervix shows a gradual ascending maturation, vacuolization of midzone cells, and a single layer of basal cells in which the nuclei are perpendicularly oriented to the basal lamina. The stromal–epithelial junction contains finger-like, fibrovascular stromal papilla penetrating the lower portion of the epithelium**

the substance and is located mainly in the endocervix, the portio vaginalis being nearly devoid of smooth muscle fibers. In contrast, at the isthmus, 50–60% of the supportive tissue consists of concentrically arranged smooth muscle, which acts as a sphincter.

Squamous Epithelium

Histology

The mature nonkeratinized squamous epithelium of the exocervix is similar to the vaginal epithelium but under normal circumstances lacks the rete pegs seen in the vagina. It is divided into three zones: the basal/parabasal or germinal cell layer, which is responsible for continuous epithelial renewal, the midzone or stratum spinosum, the dominant portion of the epithelium, and the superficial zone, containing the most mature cell population (➲ *Fig. 4.3*).

The basal/parabasal or germinal layer contains two types of cells. One type is the true *basal cell*, which is about 10 μm in diameter, with scant cytoplasm and oval nuclei oriented perpendicularly to the underlying basal lamina (➲ *Fig. 4.4*). The other type of cell is termed the *parabasal cell* because of its geographic placement. Parabasal cells are larger than basal cells and have more cytoplasm. Parabasal cells typically form a layer that is one-to-two-cells thick over the basal layer.

Epithelial regeneration is the major function of the basal and parabasal layers. Accordingly, epidermal growth factor receptors including HER-2/neu, and receptors for estrogen and progesterone are found predominantly in the basal and parabasal cells [8, 54]. The number of growth factor receptors becomes reduced as the squamous epithelial cells differentiate into the intermediate cell layer. Basal cells appear to act as stem cells, whereas parabasal cells comprise the actively replicating compartment. Indeed, mitotic figures are usually found in parabasal but not basal cells, and other markers for actively proliferating cells such as Ki-67 antigen, PCN, and other cyclins are localized to parabasal cells (➲ *Table 4.1*) [12, 60, 80].

The midzone is occupied by cells that are undergoing maturation, characterized by a gradual increase in the volume of the cytoplasm. Nuclear size, however, remains stable up to the most superficial cell level. These cells are referred to as *intermediate cells* when they exfoliate. They do not divide. Intermediate cells have abundant periodic-acid Schiff (PAS)-positive, diatase-labile intracellular glycogen, which is responsible for the clear, vacuolated appearance of their cytoplasm.

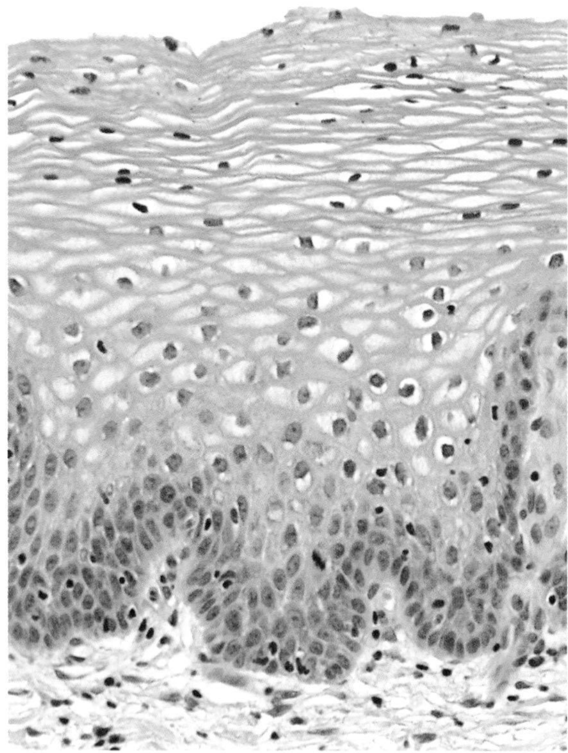

Fig. 4.4
Normal squamous epithelium. **Under normal conditions the basal layer acts as a reserve cell layer, and mitoses are only identified in parabasal cells**

The superficial zone forms the most differentiated compartment of the squamous epithelium. These cells are flattened and have a larger area of cytoplasm (50 µm in diameter) and smaller pyknotic nuclei than the underlying intermediate cells. The pink, eosinophilic cytoplasm has abundant intermediate filaments, which provide rigidity membrane-bound keratinosomes by electron microscopy (*Fig. 4.5*).

The squamous epithelium of the portio is supported by fibrous connective tissue, devoid of endocervical glands. It has occasional finger-like extensions into the epithelium, the stromal papillae (*Fig. 4.3*). The penetrating vessels within the papillae supply the epithelial cells with nutrients and oxygen. Occasional free nerve endings are seen entering the stromal papilla.

In postmenopausal women, who no longer produce ovarian hormones, the squamous epithelium is atrophic with little or no intracytoplasmic glycogen (*Fig. 4.6*). Surface epithelial maturation and stromal papillae are absent. These cellular alterations should not be confused with cervical intraepithelial neoplasia (Chap. 5, Precancerous Lesions of the Cervix). The atrophic epithelial covering does not adequately protect the subepithelial vasculature against trauma, a situation that frequently leads to bleeding and inflammation.

Effect of Estrogen and Progesterone

The epithelium of the exocervix is remodeled by proliferation, maturation, and desquamation during the reproductive period. The epithelium is completely replaced by a new population of cells every 4–5 days; the process of squamous epithelial maturation can be accelerated to 3 days by the administration of estrogenic compounds [61]. Estrogen receptors have been localized to nuclei in the basal, parabasal, and intermediate cell layers [54, 60]. Compared to the endometrium in the cervix, only a small increase of estrogen receptor levels occurs during the follicular phase as compared to the luteal phase. In atrophic and highly inflamed exocervical epithelium, the amount of estrogen receptor is reduced. No, or only low levels, of progesterone receptors are detected immunohistochemically in the exocervical epithelium during the follicular phase of the menstrual cycle, whereas during the luteal phase and during pregnancy, progesterone receptors appear in the parabasal cell layer [60]. Both estrogen and progesterone receptors can be detected in stromal fibroblasts of the exocervix throughout the menstrual cycle.

In general, estradiol-17β stimulates epithelial proliferation, maturation, and desquamation, whereas progesterone inhibits maturation at the upper midzone level of the epithelium. Accordingly, the portio epithelium during the postnatal period is fully mature and contains large amounts of glycogen as a result of maternal estrogen stimulation. Maturation ceases and glycogen rapidly disappears as the serum hormone levels fall. The epithelium remains atrophic during childhood until menarche when, under the stimulatory effect of ovarian hormones, maturation occurs again and glycogen reappears. During pregnancy, when progesterone levels are elevated, superficial cell maturation is absent.

Columnar Epithelium

Histology

A single layer of mucin-secreting, columnar epithelium lines both the surface of the endocervical canal and the

Table 4.1

Immunohistochemical staining patterns of normal cervical tissues

Antibody	Cells of stratified squamous epithelium				Reserve cells/squamous metaplasia	Endocervical columnar cells
	Basal	Parabasal	Intermediate	Superficial		
Growth factors/receptors						
Her 2/neu [8]	+	+	–	–	+	+
EGF receptor [8]	+	+	–	–	+	–
Estrogen receptor [31, 54, 84]	±	+	+	–	+	+
Progesterone receptor [31, 54, 84]	–	+[a]	–	–	+	+
Cell cycle proteins						
PCN [6, 55, 80, 90]	–	+	–	–	NA	+
MIB-1 (Ki-67) [70, 97]	–	±	–	–	–	–
bcl-2 [84, 97]	+		–	–	+	±
Cyclin B1 [54]	–	+	–	–	unknown	unknown
Cyclin D1 [12]	+	+	–	–	+	+
Other proteins						
CD44 [45]	+	+	–	–	+	–
CEA	–	–	–	–	–	+

[a]Expressed during luteal phase of menstrual cycle and during pregnancy

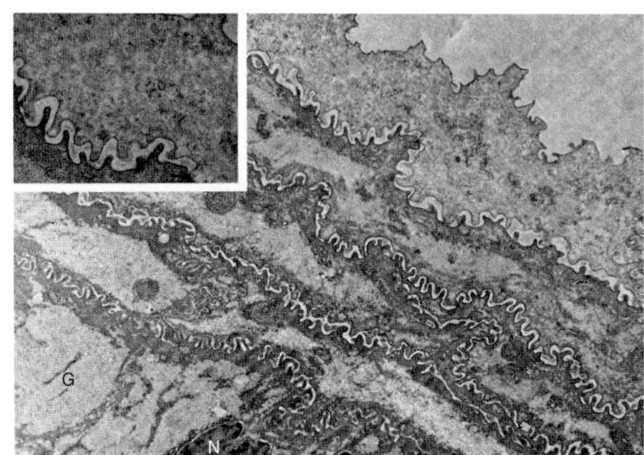

Fig. 4.5
Normal squamous epithelium. **Electron microscopy of the superficial cells. These cells have pyknotic nuclei (N) and flattened cytoplasm packed with glycogen (G). The most superficial cells are rich in microfilaments and contain irregular surface membrane projections. Note the lack of desmosomal attachments between the most superficial cells, a feature facilitating desquamation. X4795. *Inset*: Higher magnification of intracytoplasmic microfilaments in the most superficial cells. X11,370**

underlying glandular structures. The latter are traditionally called *compound, tubular racemose, endocervical glands.* Three-dimensional plastic reconstructions from serial histological sections demonstrate that the endocervical glands actually represent deep, cleft-like infoldings of the surface epithelium with numerous blind, tunnel-like collaterals (*Fig. 4.7*) [28]. Because of the complex architecture of these clefts, or grooves, including oblique, transverse, and longitudinal arrangements, they appear as isolated glands in histological sections. The epithelium lining the clefts is identical with that lining the surface, and consequently the endocervical mucin-producing apparatus is not considered glandular but a complex infolding mucinous membrane. True glands, in contrast, have different epithelial lining in their secretory apparatus compared to their ductal and surface epithelial portions.

The columnar epithelial cells characteristically have basally placed nuclei and tall, uniform, finely granular cytoplasm filled with mucinous droplets (*Fig. 4.8*). The droplets have great affinity for Alcian blue stains, reflecting their sulfated, sialic acid, mucopolysacchride content [23]. Cells lining the luminal surface have been termed *picket cells* because of their resemblance to a picket

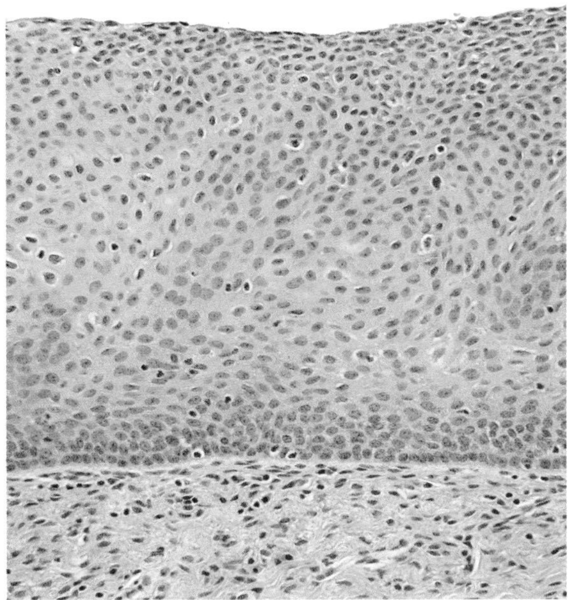

Fig. 4.6
Atrophic squamous epithelium. **The epithelium is devoid of glycogen-rich vacuolated cells. The normal cellular orientation is disrupted, but cellular cohesion is normal and cytologic atypia is absent**

fence. Occasionally, nonsecretory cells with cilia are observed (*Fig. 4.9*), the main function of which is to distribute and mobilize the endocervical mucus [35]. Isolated neuroendocrine, argyrophil and argentaffin cell types also are identified within the endocervical epithelium by histochemical stains [26]. The argentaffin-positive cells often contain serotonin. The physiologic purpose of these rare endocrine endocervical cells is obscure. Biochemically and immunohistochemically, the columnar cells of the endocervix have features of simple epithelia, characterized by the presence of only low molecular weight cytokeratins, including cytokeratins 7, 8, 18, and 19 [29].

Mitoses in the normal columnar epithelium are very rarely observed. It is not known whether regeneration occurs from the underlying subcolumnar reserve cells, which under normal circumstances are seldom seen even at the ultrastructural level, or from the persisting mature endocervical cells [35]. Unlike the attenuated vascular stromal papillae of the original squamous portio epithelium, the subepithelial capillary network in the endocervical mucosa is well developed.

The stroma of the endocervix is comparatively better innervated than that of the exocervix. Fibers run parallel to muscle bundles, but sensory free endings have not been clearly demonstrated. True lymphoid follicles, with or without germinal centers, are encountered in the subepithelial stroma of both the exocervix and the endocervix.

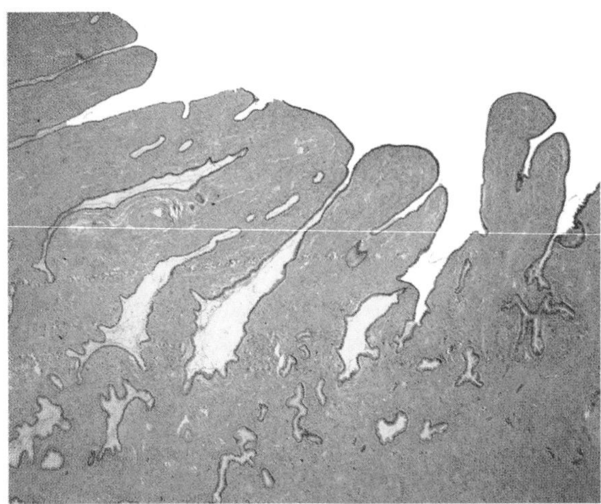

Fig. 4.7
Endocervical mucosa. **There are cleft-like infoldings and tunnel-like collaterals. The neighboring gland-like structures represent tangentially sectioned cleft-tunnel complexes**

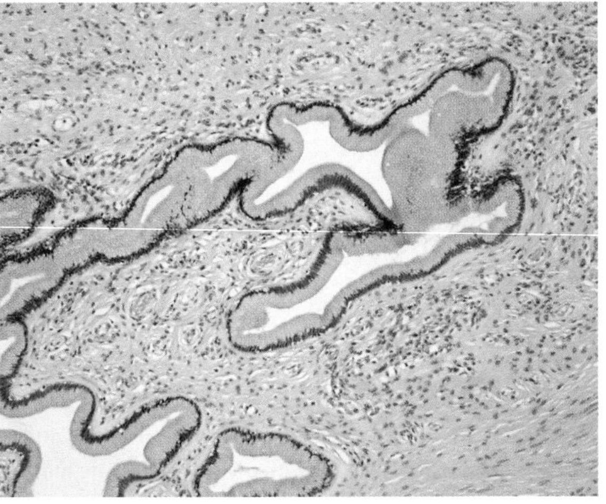

Fig. 4.8
Endocervical mucosa. **Tall columnar mucin-filled endocervical cells with basal nuclei**

Effects of Estrogen and Progesterone

The cervical mucus is subject to profound cyclic changes. Under estrogenic stimulation, the endocervical secretions are profuse, watery, and alkaline, facilitating sperm penetration. During the postovulatory phase, secretions are scant, thick, and acid, containing numerous leukocytes and act as a barrier to sperm penetration. Endocervical secretory activity operates by both the apocrine and the merocrine type of expulsion of secretory products [24]. In the former, a portion of apical cytoplasm packed with secretory granules is detached whereas, in the latter, secretory products are released from apical granules through pore-like openings of the surface cytoplasmic membrane.

Langerhans Cells and Lymphoid-Derived Cells

Mucosal immunity is an important component of the host's defense mechanism against viral and bacterial pathogens. Components of the secretory (IgA antibody mediated), humoral (IgG antibody mediated) as well as the cellular immune systems are present in the cervix. A variety of lymphocyte and dendritic macrophage subsets are present in both the epithelium of the exo- and endocervix as well as the subepithelial stroma [68]. Dendritic cells include both mature and immature forms. They are primarily responsible for antigen recognition and the earliest stage of cellular immune response.

Large numbers of T lymphocytes are also present in the cervix under normalConditions [47]. CD3+ T lymphocytes are concentrated in a band directly beneath both the squamous epithelium of the exocervix and the columnar epithelium of the endocervix [47, 72]. These cells are predominately cytotoxic T-lymphocytes (e.g., CD8+), although helper T lymphocytes (e.g., CD4+) are also present. Variable numbers of B lymphocytes and plasma cells are also found in the lamina propria of the cervix [47]. Because the presence of lymphocytes as well as lymphoid follicles (➲ *Fig. 4.10*) is a normal finding in the cervix, the diagnosis of chronic cervicitis should be reserved for specimens showing a marked infiltration of lymphocytes.

The Transformation Zone

The squamocolumnar junction of the cervix is defined as the border between the stratified squamous epithelium and the mucin-secreting columnar epithelium of the

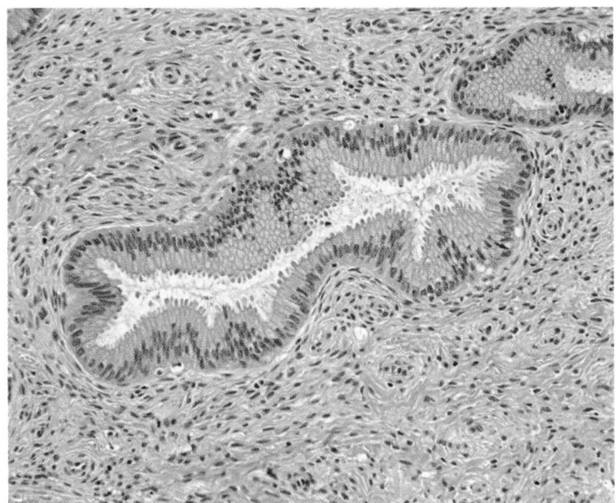

Fig. 4.9
Endocervical mucosa. **When endocervical cells engage in apocrine secretion, portions of atypical cytoplasm are expelled**

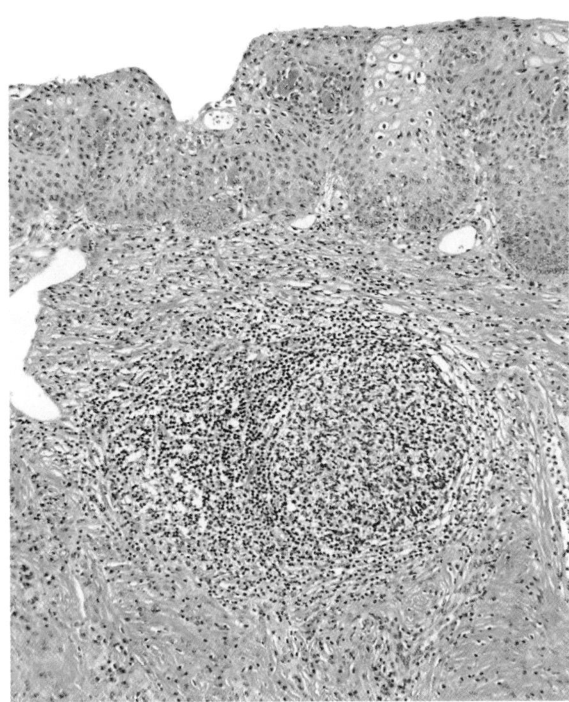

Fig. 4.10
Lymphoid follicles. **Occasional lymphoid follicles can be seen in the cervical stroma in the absence of cervicitis**

endocervix. Morphogenetically, there are two different squamocolumnar junctions (➋ *Fig. 4.11*). One is termed the *original* squamocolumnar junction and is the site at which the native squamous epithelium of the exocervix abuts the endocervical columnar epithelium at the time of birth. At birth, most newborns have some mucin-secreting columnar endocervical epithelium present on the exocervix, which forms an *ectropion* or cervical *ectopy*. The exact location of the original squamocolumnar junction and, therefore, the amount of endocervical ectopy present at birth depends on the extent of inward migration of squamous epithelium from the lower third of the vagina.

At about the age of 1 year, the cervix begins to elongate. This results in the migration of the squamocolumnar junction toward the external os. This migration is frequently incomplete. Hormonal and other physical factors influence the size and distribution of the cervical ectopy by altering the shape and volume of the cervical lips. At the time of menarche or during pregnancy both the uterus and the cervix enlarge. Enlargement of the cervix is accompanied by alterations in its shape, which result in more of an "eversion" or rolling outward of endocervical columnar epithelium onto the portio (➋ *Fig. 4.11*). As a result, in most women during the reproductive period, cervical ectopy is present, and the size of the ectopy is most

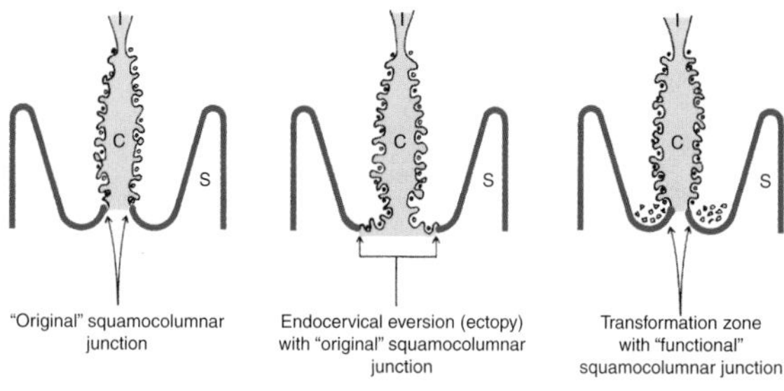

Fig. 4.11
The transformation zone. **Schematic representation of original and functional squamocolumnar junctions and three basic types of portios. *Left*: Diagram of a portio completely covered with native squamous epithelium. The squamocolumnar junction is at the external os. *Middle*: Denotes cervical ectopy, with the squamocolumnar junction being located on the exocervix below the external os. *Right*: Indicates areas of cervical ectopy that have become covered with squamous epithelium. This area is the cervical transformation zone. The new, or functional, squamocolumnar junction of the transformation zone is at the external os. S, squamous epithelium; C, endocervical columnar epithelium; I, uterine isthmus**

extensive in women under 20 years of age and following the first pregnancy. When viewed with the naked eye, the endocervical mucosa appears as a red, velvety zone, sharply contrasting with the neighboring pink, translucent squamous portio epithelium (➋ *Fig. 4.12a*).

Over time, the columnar epithelium that composes the cervical ectopy is remodeled and replaced by metaplastic squamous epithelium. As this occurs, the histological squamocolumnar junction moves toward the exocervical os. This newly formed squamocolumnar junction is called the *physiologic*, *functional*, or *new* squamocolumnar junction. While the original squamocolumnar junction is usually quite abrupt, the junction between the columnar and squamous epithelium at the physiologic or functional squamocolumnar junction can be either abrupt or gradual (➋ *Fig. 4.12b*). The region between the original squamocolumnar junction and the postpubertal functional squamocolumnar junction is termed the *transformation zone*. The transformation zone is histologically characterized by the presence of metaplastic epithelium (see section ➋ Squamous Metaplasia).

The concept of the transformation zone is extremely important for understanding the pathogenesis of squamous cell carcinomas of the cervix and its precursors, since virtually all cervical squamous neoplasia begins at the new squamocolumnar junction and because the extension and limits of cervical cancer precursors coincide with the distribution of the transformation zone. It is also important to remember that during the childbearing years and during pregnancy, the transformation zone is located, in almost all instances, on the exposed portion of the cervix. Consequently, the vast majority of cervical neoplasias can be removed for histologic diagnosis by punch biopsy. Movement of the functional squamocolumnar junction continues throughout the reproductive years. Therefore, in older and postmenopausal women, the functional squamocolumnar junction is nearly always located within the external os (➋ *Fig. 4.12c*).

Pregnancy and Puerperium

The morphologic alterations that occur in the antepartum or postpartum cervix are not pathognomonic of pregnancy or parturition but are seen more commonly at these times than in the nonpregnant postpartum state. They are related to the stimulatory effects of elevated steroid hormones. The spongy enlargement of the pregnant cervix is caused by increased vascularity and edema of the stroma accompanied by acute inflammation. The massive destruction of collagen fibers and accumulation

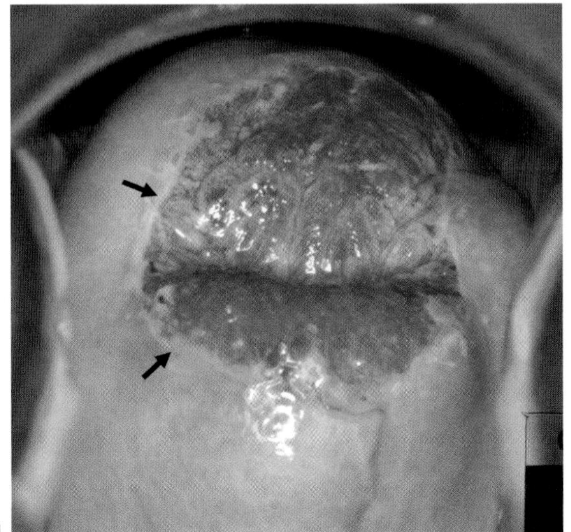

a

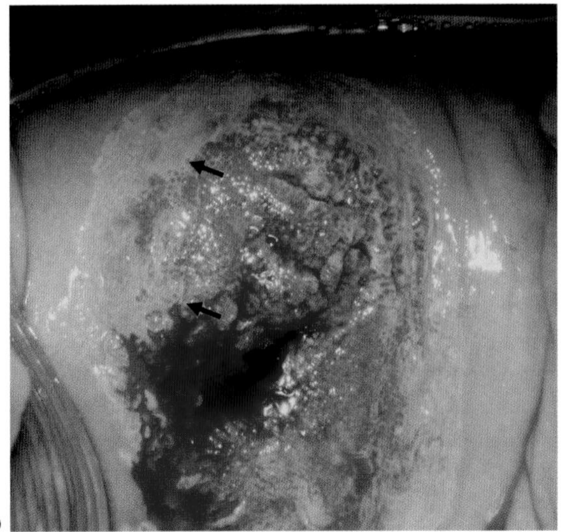

b

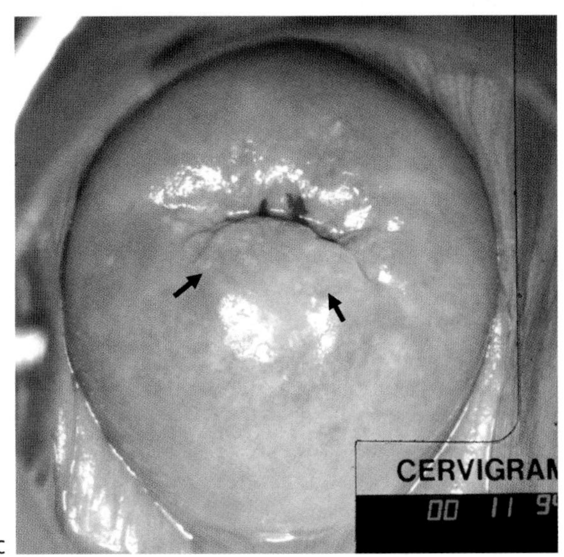

c

Fig. 4.12
The transformation zone. **Colpophotographs of endocervical eversion of the transformation zone. (a) Endocervical mucosa is everted on both the anterior and the posterior lip and surrounds the anatomic external os. The original squamocolumnar junction (SCJ) is on the portio of the cervix (*arrows*). (b) Squamous metaplasia is occurring and the new SCJ (*arrows*) is now internal to the original SCJ. The area between the original and new SCJ is the transformation zone. (c) The transformation zone is completely mature and the SCJ is inside the endocervical canal. Residual endocervical gland mouths are present (*arrows*)**

of extracellular glycoprotein ground substance before labor result in cervical softening and effacement, facilitating dilation of the cervix to about 10 cm during labor. Gestational cervical mucus is thick, tenacious, rich in leukocytes, and forms a mucous plug that obliterates the cervical canal, sealing the endometrial cavity from the vagina and thus preventing bacterial invasion. Squamous metaplasia and lobules of tightly packed small endocervical glandular units, forming polypoid protrusions into the canal are often seen.

Pseudodecidual Reaction

Pseudodecidualization of the stroma, either patchy or diffuse, occurs in about one-third of the cervices examined histologically and disappears by 2 months postpartum [49]. It is presumably mediated by the high levels of progesterone during pregnancy. The appearance of pseudodecidualized cervical is identical to decidualized stroma at other sites. The cells develop abundant pink cytoplasm, with well-defined cellular borders (➋ *Fig. 4.13a, b*).

Arias-Stella Reaction

During pregnancy, the gestational Arias-Stella reaction can develop in both endocervical glands and in ectopic endometrial glands within the cervix. In one study of 191 gravid hysterectomy specimens, an Arias-Stella reaction of endocervical glands was seen, at least focally, in 9% of the cases [85]. The Arias-Stella reaction of the endocervix is usually focal and is more commonly present in the proximal portion of the endocervix involving superficial as opposed to deeply situated glands. Microscopically, the Arias-Stella reaction that occurs in the endocervical glands during pregnancy is identical to that which occurs in the endometrium. The cells within the affected glands are markedly enlarged with irregular, frequently hyperchromatic nuclei that can project into the glandular lumen in a hobnail pattern. The cells are pseudostratified and have hypersecretory cytoplasmic features with abundant vacuolated cytoplasm (➋ *Fig. 4.14*). Papillary processes with fibrovascular cores, lined by enlarged epithelial cells can project into the endocervical gland lumen.

The Arias-Stella reaction can occasionally be mistaken for clear cell carcinoma or adenocarcinoma in situ of the cervix. Differentiation from clear cell carcinoma is made by the lack of a mass lesion and clear-cut stromal invasion as well as by the absence of the classic tubular and papillary areas typical of clear cell carcinoma. The cells in adenocarcinoma in situ have more uniform nuclei and less cytoplasmic vacuolization. The Arias-Stella reaction lacks mitotic activity, whereas both clear cell carcinoma and adenocarcinoma in situ are mitotically active. Because of the possibility of confusing Arias-Stella reaction with clear cell carcinoma or adenocarcinoma in situ, the diagnosis of the later two entities should be made with caution in the pregnant patient.

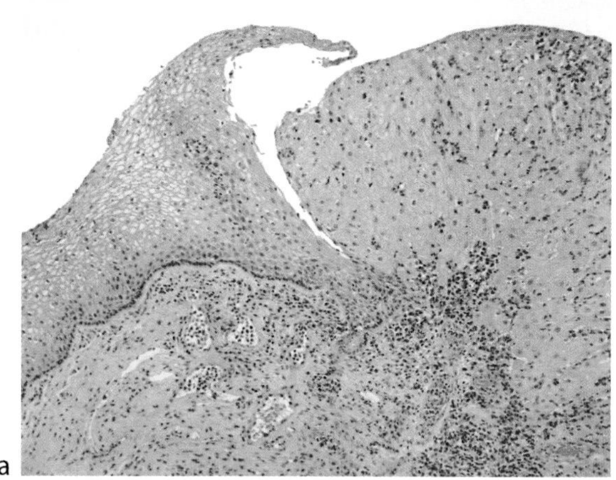

a

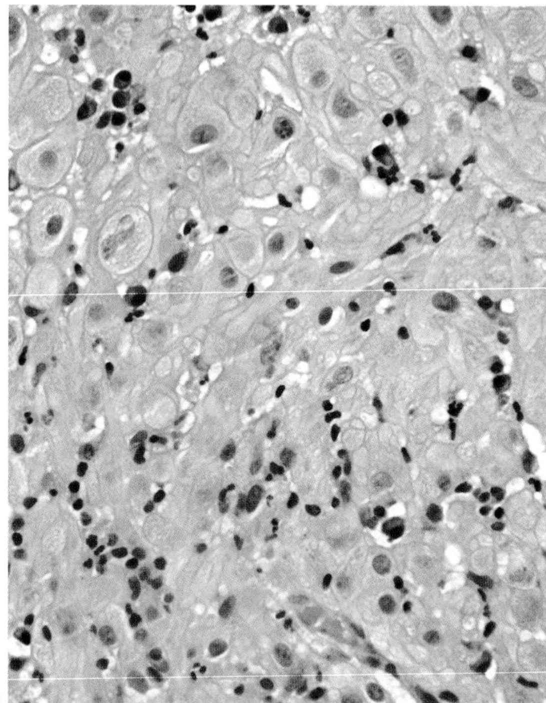

b

Fig. 4.13
Pseudodecidual reaction. **A pseudodecidual reaction of cervical stromal cells can occur during pregnancy. (a) In this case, the pseudodecidual reaction forms a discrete nodule. (b) The decidualized stromal cells are identical with gestational decidual cells of the endometrium**

Metaplasia

Squamous Metaplasia

Metaplasia is defined as the replacement of one type of mature tissue by another equally mature type of tissue. In the cervix, squamous metaplasia is the replacement of the mucin-producing columnar epithelium by stratified squamous epithelium and appears to occur by two different mechanisms (➋ *Fig. 4.15*). One mechanism consists of direct ingrowth from the native portio epithelium

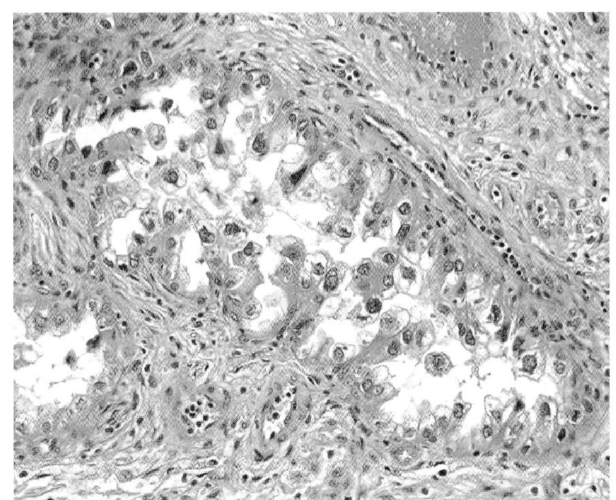

■ Fig. 4.14
Arias-Stella reaction. **The Arias-Stella reaction should not be confused with clear cell adenocarcinoma of the cervix**

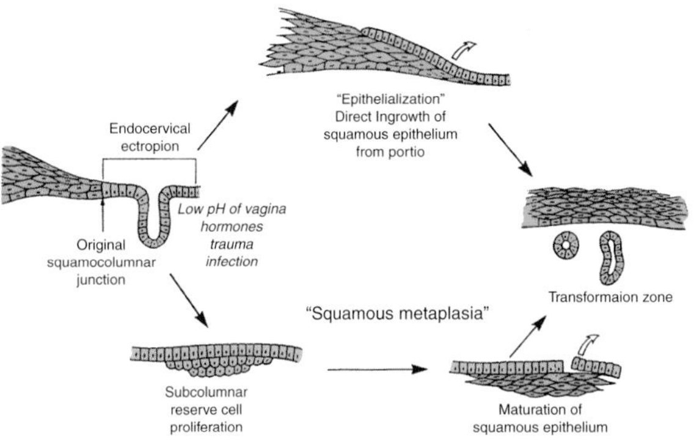

■ Fig. 4.15
Squamous metaplasia. **There are two histogenic mechanisms by which the endocervical mucosa is replaced by squamous epithelium. The first is the direct ingrowth of squamous epithelium from the portio, which is referred to as squamous epithelialization (*top*). The other is through proliferation of subcolumnar reserve cells and their subsequent maturation into a squamous epithelium, which is called squamous metaplasia (*bottom*). Both result in a mature squamous epithelium overlying endocervical mucus-producing glands (*right*)**

bordering the columnar epithelium, a process frequently referred to as "squamous epithelialization." The second mechanism involves a proliferation of undifferentiated subcolumnar reserve cells of the endocervical epithelium, which differentiate into squamous epithelium. This process has been termed *squamous metaplasia.*

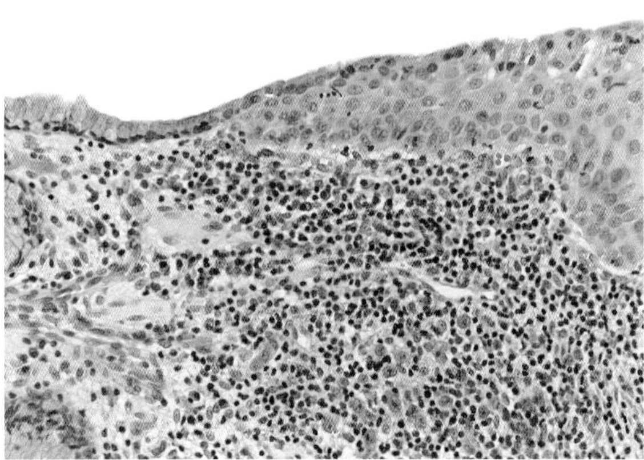

■ Fig. 4.16
Squamous epithelialization. **During squamous epithelialization a narrow tongue of squamous epithelium from the portio grows under the everted endocervical mucosa and lifts it off the basement membrane. The endocervical cells then degenerate and are sloughed**

During squamous epithelialization, tongues of native squamous epithelium of the portio grow beneath the adjacent columnar epithelium and expand between the mucinous epithelium and its basement membrane. As the squamous cells expand and mature, the endocervical cells are gradually displaced upward, degenerate, and eventually are sloughed (➋ *Fig. 4.16*). The progression of squamous transformation of the endocervical ectropion has been hypothesized to be primarily dependent on local (vaginal) environmental factors initiated by the low (acid) pH of the vagina after puberty [16]. Trauma, chronic irritation, or cervical infection also play a role in development and maturation of the transformation zone by stimulating repair and remodeling; eventually the ectocervix is covered by a protective surface of mature squamous epithelium (➋ *Fig. 4.17*). The process of squamous epithelialization is thought to be responsible for the obliteration of the outer two-thirds of endocervical ectopy. Rapid squamous re-epithelialization of the columnar epithelium of the transformation zone may also be produced iatrogenically by electrocautery, cryosurgery or laser surgery.

The second mechanism involved in replacement of columnar epithelium by a squamous epithelium and the function of the transformation zone is squamous metaplasia. The first stage of squamous metaplasia is the appearance of small cuboidal cells beneath the columnar mucinous epithelium, the so-called subcolumnar reserve

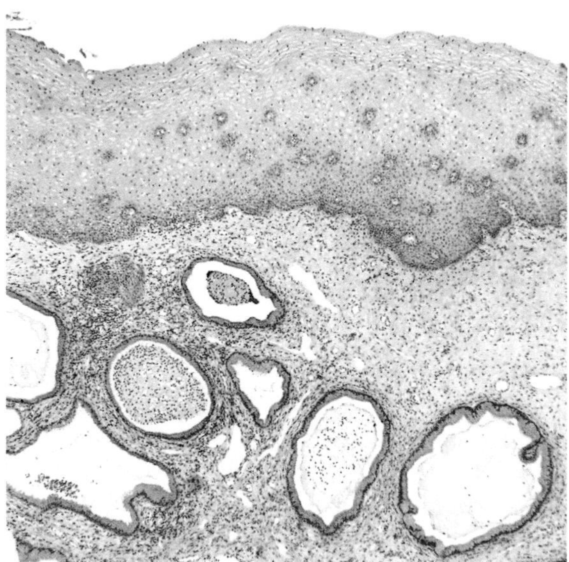

Fig. 4.17
Mature transformation zone. **Mature squamous epithelium covers the underlying endocervical glands that are distended with mucin**

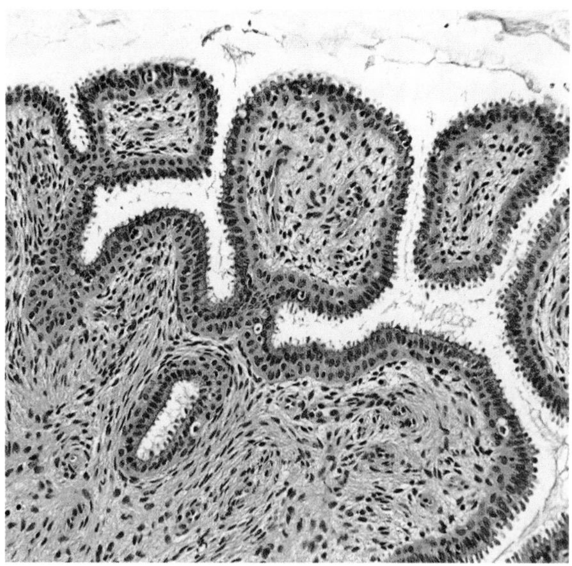

Fig. 4.18
Reserve cell hyperplasia. **Reserve cells are seen under the columnar epithelium**

cells (*Fig. 4.18*). *Reserve cells* have large, uniformly shaped, round nuclei with faintly granular chromatin and occasional aggregates of chromatin (i.e., chromocenters of reserve cells). The cell borders are poorly defined and the cells have only scant amounts of cytoplasm. The origin of subcolumnar reserve cells is controversial. Some investigators suggest a direct derivation from columnar mucinous secretory cells, whereas others favor an origin from the basal cells of the squamous portio epithelium, embryonal rests of urogenital origin, or stromal cells as possible sources.

Progressive growth and stratification of reserve cells (subcolumnar reserve cell hyperplasia), followed by the differentiation into immature squamous metaplasia followed by an additional maturation, result in the formation of a fully mature squamous epithelium indistinguishable from the native portio epithelium (*Figs. 4.19a–c* and *4.20*). Immature squamous metaplastic epithelium is distinguished from its mature counterpart by a lack of surface maturation and inconspicuous intracytoplasmic glycogen. It is, characteristically, sharply demarcated from the native portio epithelium by a perpendicular or oblique line to the surface. As a result, the uninitiated observer may mistake immature squamous metaplasia for a squamous intraepithelial lesion (SIL), particularly when the process also involves the underlying glands. In contrast to neoplastic epithelium, the immature squamous metaplastic epithelium maintains cell organization and cohesion, nuclear atypia is absent and, frequently, a single row of endocervical cells overlies the squamous cells. Biochemically and immunohistochemically, immature squamous metaplasia shares features of both the mature squamous epithelium and the columnar mucinous epithelium.

Tubal Metaplasia

Tubal metaplasia refers to endocervical glands that are lined by a Mullerian-type epithelium that closely resembles that of the fallopian tube. In pure tubal metaplasia, the endocervical glands are lined by an epithelium that more closely resembles that of the fallopian tube and contains many more ciliated cells than are normally present in the endocervical epithelium as well as tubal type secretory cells and reserve or intercalary cells (*Fig. 4.21a, b*) [50, 74, 96]. Tubal metaplasia can be found in up to 31% of patients and does not appear to be related to the phase of menstrual cycle, the presence of inflammatory changes, or low-grade SIL (CIN 1) [50].

Tubal metaplasia can be quite extensive and can occasionally be mistaken for endocervical glandular neoplasia. However, the bland cytological features, lack of mitotic activity, and prominent cilia seen at the apical surfaces of tubal metaplasia usually allow it to be differentiated

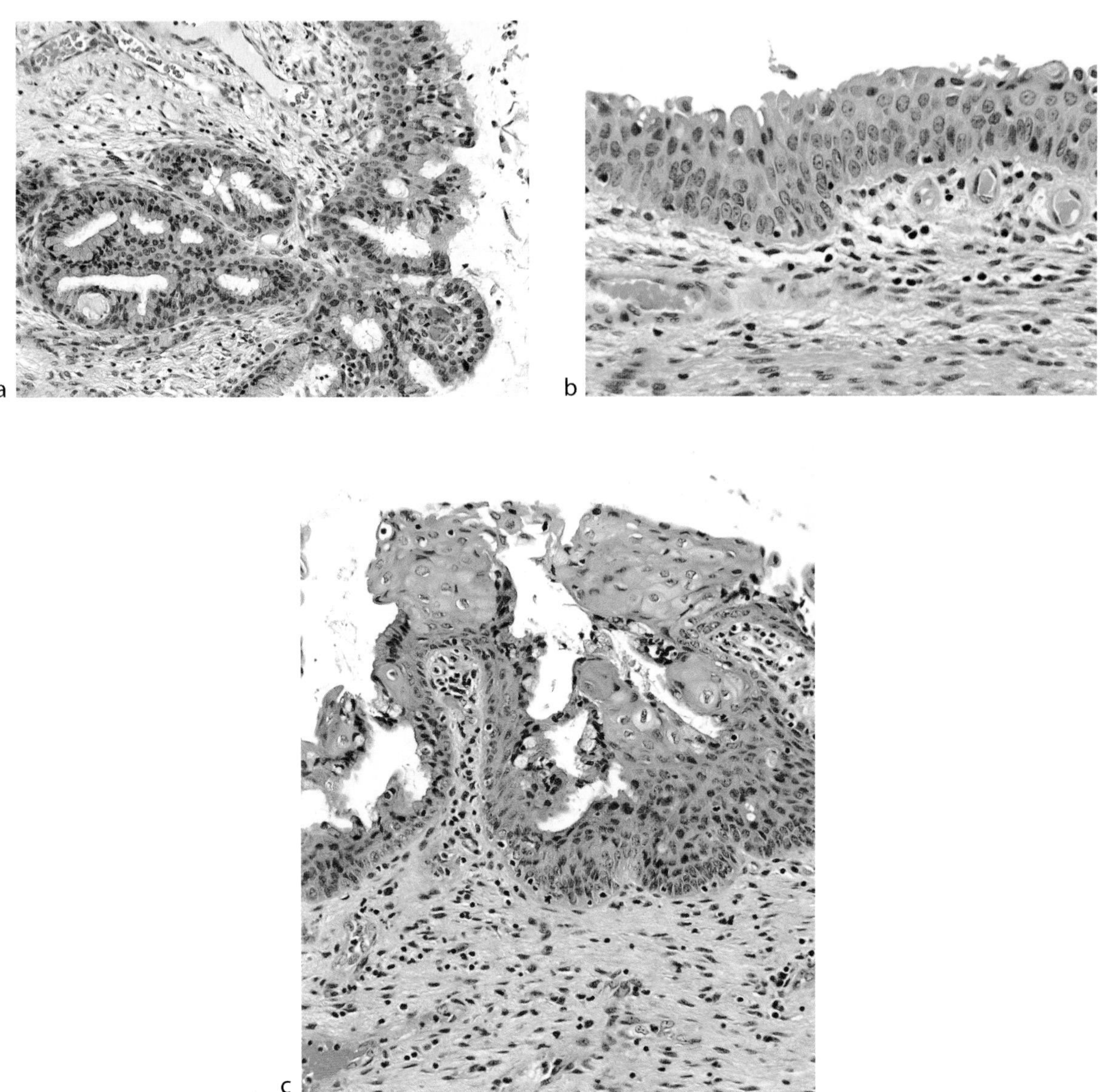

■ Fig. 4.19
Squamous metaplasia. **(a)** Reserve cells proliferate and are stratified under the columnar epithelium. **(b)** Columnar differentiation is lost, resulting in a multilayered squamous epithelium composed of immature metaplastic cells. Note occasional mucinous endocervical cells at the surface. **(c)** The immature metaplastic epithelium begins to differentiate

from a neoplastic lesion. Other features that can aid in distinguishing between tubal metaplasia and glandular neoplasia are the location and shape of the glands and the surrounding stroma. Glands demonstrating tubal metaplasia are typically confined to the superficial third of the cervical wall (i.e., they extend less than 7 mm into the cervical stroma) and typically show only slight variation in size and shape. Moreover, the stroma-surrounding glands involved by tubal metaplasia is usually normal appearing and is neither desmoplastic nor edematous appearing. Cases of tubal metaplasia demonstrating glandular architectural abnormalities or hypercellularity of the adjacent stroma can present diagnostic difficulties [76].

Atypical tubal metaplasia is a form of tubal metaplasia in which the glands are lined by ciliated and nonciliated cells that are crowded and have larger, more hyperchromatic nuclei than that observed in typical tubal metaplasia (*Fig. 4.22*). The cells of atypical tubal metaplasia are frequently pseudostratified. Atypical tubal metaplasia frequently presents a diagnostic problem since it histologically can be confused with adenocarcinoma in situ. Differentiation from adenocarcinoma in situ is based on a lack of significant mitotic activity, the absence of architectural abnormalities such as cribiforming and papillary projections, and the failure of cells to stain for p16^{ink}. However, one should be cautioned that atypical tubal metaplasia can occur in association with adenocarcinoma in situ of the cervix, including both tubal and non-tubal types (Chap. 5, Precancerous Lesions of the Cervix).

Tubo-Endometrioid Metaplasia

Tubo-endometrioid metaplasia of the cervix is a type of metaplasia that is histologically similar to the tubal metaplasia that can develop in the endometrium in patients with unopposed estrogenic stimulation. Endocervical glands demonstrating tubo-endometrioid metaplasia are lined by a pseudostratified epithelium composed of columnar cells with a high nuclear:cytoplasmic ratio (*Fig. 4.23*). Many of these cells are ciliated or have secretory features with apical snouts, but the glands lack an associated endometrial stroma. Tubo-endometrioid metaplasia occurs commonly after cervical conization and has been interpreted as a form of aberrant differentiation following cervical injury [46]. Because of the pseudostratification and high nuclear:cytoplasmic ratio, these glands can be misinterpreted as representing adenocarcinoma in situ. As with tubal metaplasia, the features that indicate a metaplastic, as opposed to a neoplastic, process are the location and shape of the glands and lack of a desmoplastic or edematous stromal response.

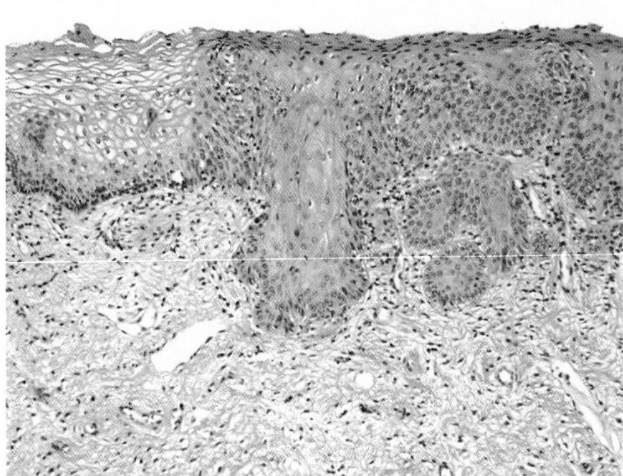

Fig. 4.20
Transformation zone epithelium. **On the *left*, the native portio epithelium is present with full maturation. On the *right*, metaplastic squamous epithelium is present. Note the sharp boundary. Metaplasia has extended into the endocervical crypts and completely replaced the columnar epithelium**

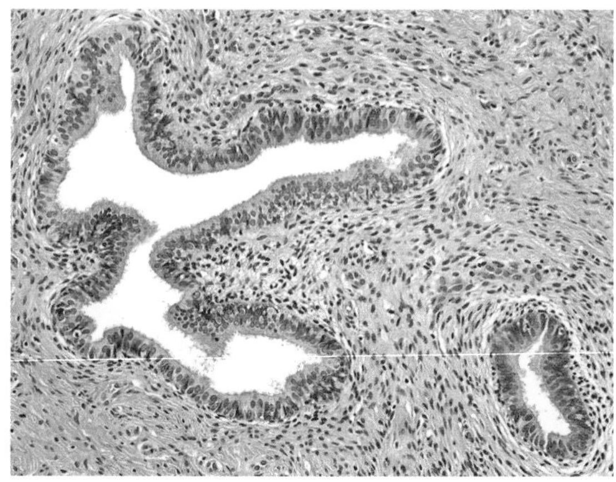

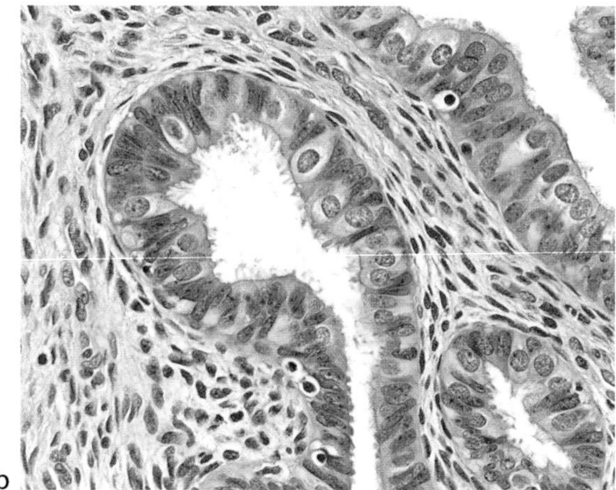

Fig. 4.21
Tubal metaplasia. **(a) The columnar, mucus-producing epithelium has been replaced by a tubal type epithelium with ciliated, secretory and intercalated cells. (b) At higher magnification the resemblance to the epithelium of the fallopian tube is obvious**

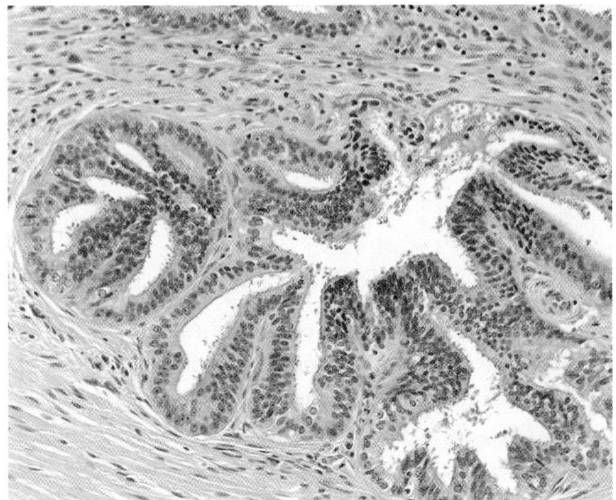

Fig. 4.22
Atypical tubal metaplasia. **The epithelium is more crowded and pseudostratified than in typical tubal metaplasia. The cells have larger, hyperchromatic nuclei. Ciliated cells are present, but mitotic figures are uncommonly seen**

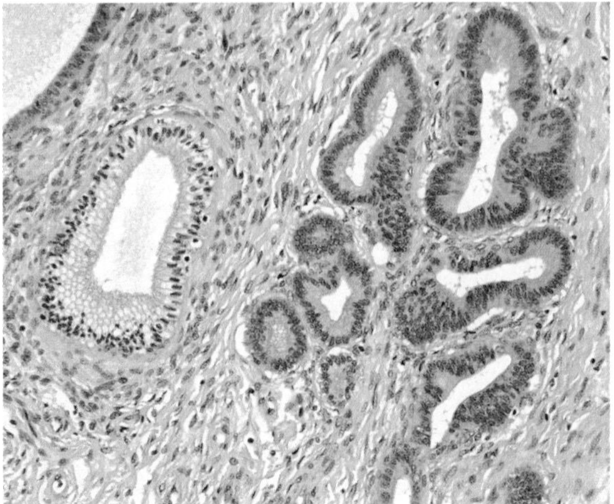

Fig. 4.23
Tubo-endometrioid metaplasia. **Typical endocervical epithelium on the *left*. On the *right* columnar, mucus-producing epithelium has been replaced by pseudostratified epithelium with high nuclear: cytoplasmic ratios**

Transitional Cell Metaplasia

Transitional cell metaplasia refers to a controversial type of metaplasia in which the surface of the cervix and endocervical crypts is lined by an epithelium that is interpreted by some to resemble a hyperplastic urothelium [19, 20, 51, 98]. By definition, the epithelium has a "disordered" appearance that is comprised of over ten layers of cells that have oval- to spindle-shaped nuclei and are oriented vertically in the deeper layers (*Fig. 4.24*). The cells of the superficial layer often resemble the umbrella cells of the normal urothelium and have horizontally oriented nuclei.

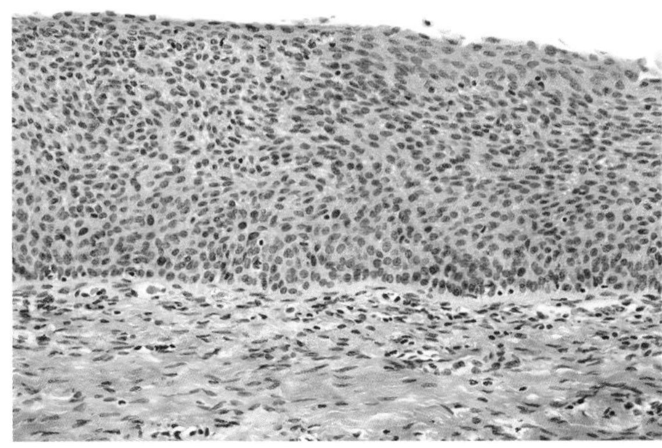

Fig. 4.24
Transitional cell metaplasia. **The squamous epithelium in this postmenopausal patient is more than ten layers thick and is disorganized. This type of change is referred to by some as "transitional cell metaplasia"**

The controversy surrounding transitional cell metaplasia revolves around whether it represents a unique histopathological entity that has a specific biology or whether it simply represents a biologically insignificant histological variation of other well-described histological entities. Almost all of the reported examples of transitional cell metaplasia have been identified in postmenopausal women. In the two largest series, the mean ages of women with the lesion were 60 and 67.8 years [20, 98]. Some of these women have had previous abnormal Papanicolaou smears, and it has been suggested that some of the cases may represent atrophic high-grade SIL [62]. In addition to arising in the transformation zone, transitional cell metaplasia can also be identified in the exocervix and the vagina [98]. This suggests that in some cases, transitional cell metaplasia may simply represent a histological variant of atrophy, either of the original squamous epithelium or of a fully mature metaplastic squamous epithelium, in which the number of cell layers is not reduced. Immunohistochemical studies using cytokeratin antibodies have shown that foci of transitional cell metaplasia express cytokeratins 13, 17, and 18, which are expressed in normal urothelium but do not express cytokeratin 20 and the asymmetric unit membrane that are related to urothelial differentiation [39].

Inflammatory Diseases

Cervicitis can be divided into two categories, based on whether the etiology of the disorder is noninfectious or infectious. Whatever the etiology, the tissue response of the cervix to injury is limited and reflects the basic mechanisms of inflammation and repair. Two types of morphologic changes, however, that are often encountered in association with a variety of inflammatory diseases deserve specific attention. These are atypia of repair and hyperkeratosis and parakeratosis.

Atypia of Repair

In cases of severe, acute, long-standing chronic inflammation or infection with epithelial injury of any kind – true erosion, biopsy, or conization – the squamous and endocervical epithelia undergo reactive changes characterized by epithelial disorganization and nuclear atypia. These changes are often confused, histologically and cytologically, with high-grade squamous intraepithelial lesions (HSIL). In reactive squamous atypia, the cytoplasmic membrane is well defined, the nuclei are uniform in shape and size, and the chromatin is aggregated in prominent aggregates or clumps (➋ *Fig. 4.25a, b*). The epithelium is often infiltrated with migrating inflammatory cells. Mitotic figures are normal and are confined to the proliferative basal and parabasal cell populations. Characteristically, the cells in the upper half of the epithelium are normal, and maturation occurs in an orderly fashion.

When reparative changes affect endocervical columnar cells, the morphological alterations include nuclear enlargement and hyperchromasia with irregularity of nuclear size and shape and smudgy chromatin. There can also be cytoplasmic eosinophilia and loss of mucinous droplets (➋ *Fig. 4.26a, b*). The combination of endocervical cell

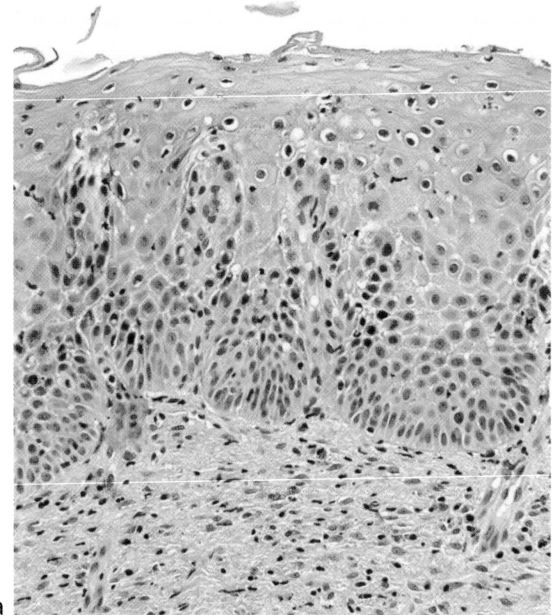

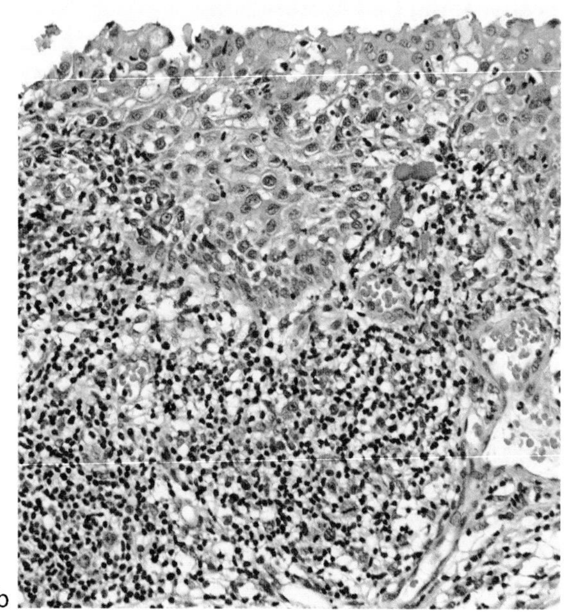

Fig. 4.25
Squamous reparative atypia. **(a) When reparative changes develop in mature squamous epithelium, there is usually basal cell hyperplasia that involves the lower one-third of the epithelium. The nuclei contain prominent chromocenters but lack nuclear abnormalities associated with neoplasia. Intermediate and superficial epithelial cells continue to show maturation but often develop perinuclear halos and some degree of nuclear enlargement. However, the superficial cells lack the nuclear atypia characteristic of HPV-infected cells. (b) When reparative changes develop in immature metaplastic squamous epithelium, the epithelium exhibits intercellular edema, and acute and chronic inflammatory cells often infiltrate both the epithelium and stroma. The nuclei of the metaplastic cells become hyperchromatic and enlarged and typically have prominent chromocenters. Microabsesses are frequently seen**

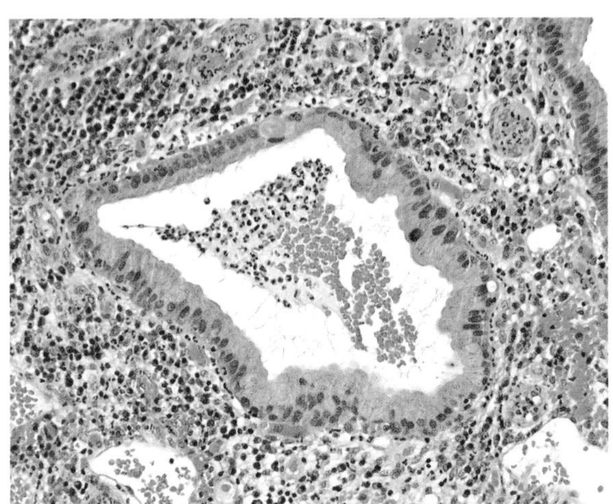

Fig. 4.26
Endocervical reparative atypia. **The endocervical epithelium develops nuclear enlargement, mitosis, microabscesses, and inconspicuous intracellular mucus. Note the diffuse distribution of nuclear chromatin, the cytoplasmic eosinophilia, and the absence of abnormal mitoses, features distinguishing endocervical atypia of inflammation from in situ adenocarcinoma of the cervix**

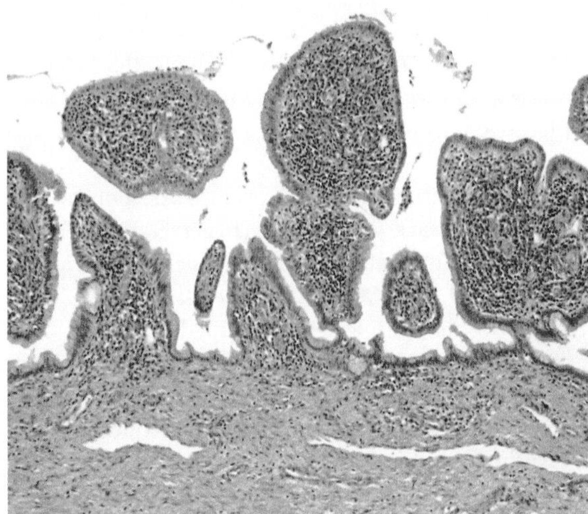

Fig. 4.27
Papillary endocervical reparative change. **The marked inflammation of the stroma results in the endocervical epithelium being raised into papillary projections**

enlargement with dense, eosinophilic, focally vacuolated cytoplasm and varying degrees of nuclear atypia has been referred to as "atypical oxyphilic metaplasia." Although this type of glandular epithelium appears atypical, the changes are focal, alternating with normal mucinous columnar cells, and are confined to areas with inflammation or mucosal injury. In addition, the deep cytoplasmic eosinophilia, when it is present, and the absence of abnormal mitoses are features that distinguish the inflammatory lesions from an in situ adenocarcinoma of the endocervix (AIS). In both squamous and endocervical cell atypia of repair, immunostaining for p16^{ink} is uniformly negative. The use of the antibody is of great help for distinguishing HSIL and AIS from their mimic, for example, epithelial atypia of repair (Chap. 5, Precancerous Lesions of the Cervix). Occasionally, when there is an endocervical inflammation, the stroma becomes filled with chronic inflammatory cells and this results in the endocervix taking on a papillary configuration (*Fig. 4.27*).

Radiation-Induced Atypia

Treatment of the cervix with therapeutic levels of radiation can cause morphological changes in both the squamous and glandular epithelium. The atypical squamous cells that develop post radiation have nuclear enlargement and can be multinucleated. The cells can have abundant amounts of vacuolated cytoplasm and are usually detected in cervical cytological preparations. Radiation-induced changes in the endocervical glandular epithelium include cellular enlargement, a loss of polarity of nuclei, dense eosinophilic, enlarged nucleoli that can be multiple [66]. The stroma in women who have received therapeutic radiation is frequently fibrotic, often with hyalinization. Blood vessels often have an intimal hyaline thickening and can be totally occluded. "Radiation fibroblasts" are usually not present [66]. These morphological changes can exist up to 17 years after the radiation therapy.

Hyperkeratosis and Parakeratosis

Hyperkeratosis and parakeratosis can be detected cytologically in up to 8% of all women undergoing routine Pap smear screening [48]. Both hyperkeratosis and parakeratosis have the gross appearance of a thickened, white epithelium and can be either focal or diffuse. When diffuse, the entire portio is covered by a thickened, white, and wrinkled epithelial membrane. When focal, a slightly raised white plaque is present. The etiology of cervical hyperkeratosis is poorly understood, but in some cases it appears to be related to chronic irritation. For example, most patients with diffuse hyperkeratosis have prolapsed uteri. Focal areas of hyperkeratosis can be associated with a local chronic irritation, such as that seen in women who wear a diaphragm or pessary and in women with cervical neoplasia. However, in most cases there is no known cause.

Microscopically, the whitish plaque corresponds to the presence of a thick keratin layer (hyperkeratosis), which may or may not contain pyknotic nuclei (parakeratosis) (*Figs. 4.28* and *4.29*). The epithelium is often acanthotic and has a well-developed granular layer, prominent intercellular bridges and elongated rete pegs. Characteristically, the epithelial cells contain sparse glycogen, but cytological atypia is absent. Frequently, there is epithelial hyperplasia and chronic inflammation. Mature squamous metaplasia is often associated with parakeratosis.

Although there is neither morphological nor clinical evidence that parakeratosis represents precursor lesions to cervical neoplasia, both hyperkeratosis and parakeratosis can occur in association with HSIL and invasive cervical cancer. Because of this association, some experts have suggested that all women with otherwise negative Pap smears but demonstrating these findings need colposcopy. However, several studies have reported that less than 4% of women with hyperkeratosis or parakeratosis without nuclear atypia on an otherwise negative Pap smear had SIL and that in all instances the SIL was low grade. This suggests that the routine colposcopic evaluation is unnecessary in such women [48]. It should be emphasized, however, that since hyperkeratosis may occasionally overlie HSIL and invasive carcinomas, all grossly visible white plaques on the portio vaginalis or vaginal epithelium should be biopsied.

Noninfectious Cervicitis

Noninfectious cervicitis is, for the most part, chemical or mechanical in nature, and the inflammatory response is nonspecific. Common causes include chemical irritation secondary to douching or local trauma produced by foreign bodies, including tampons, diaphragms, pessaries, and intrauterine contraceptive devices. Surgical instrumentation and therapeutic intervention are common iatrogenic causes of cervical tissue injury and inflammation. Stromal edema, vascular congestion, and neutrophilic infiltration of the stroma and epithelium characterize

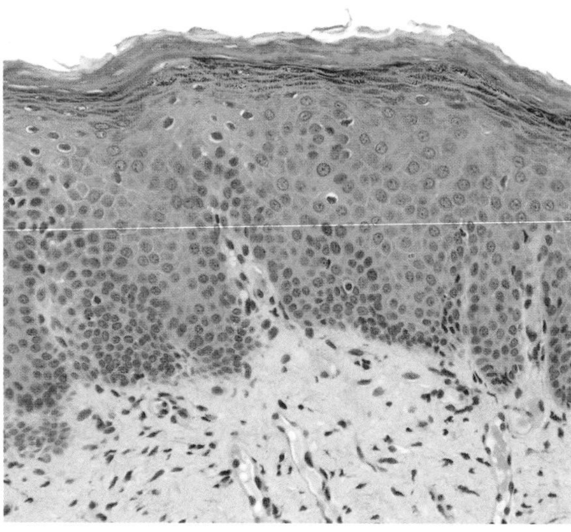

Fig. 4.28
Hyperkeratosis of the cervix. **A superficial layer of anucleated, keratinized squamous cells, which is frequently accompanied by a thickened granular layer is present**

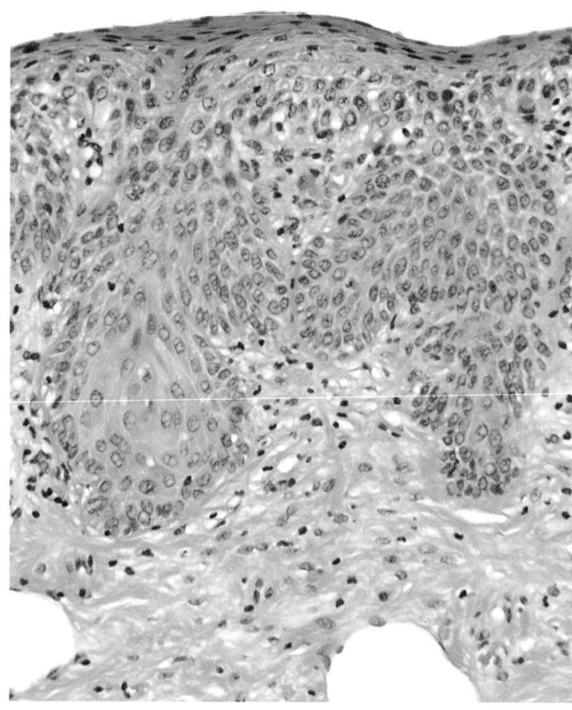

Fig. 4.29
Parakeratosis of the cervix. **Pyknotic nuclei are retained in the superficial cell layer. Parakeratosis is frequently accompanied by hyperkeratosis**

acute cervicitis. Clinically, the cervix appears swollen, erythematous and friable, and there may be an associated purulent endocervical discharge. Prolonged or severe acute inflammation eventually leads to degenerative changes in the epithelial surface, loss of endocervical secretory activity, and ulceration.

In chronic cervicitis, round cells, including lymphocytes, plasma cells, and histiocytes, predominate in the inflammatory infiltrate and are associated with varying amounts of granulation tissue and stromal fibrosis. The diagnosis of chronic cervicitis should be reserved for cases where there is definite clinical and histological evidence of a significant chronic inflammatory process. Otherwise, a histological diagnosis based on the presence of scattered lymphocytes has no clinical significance and is meaningless. Occasionally, lymphoid follicles with germinal centers are found beneath the epithelium in noninfectious cervicitis (*Fig. 4.30*). The presence of lymphoid follicles beneath the cervical epithelium is frequently referred to as *follicular cervicitis*. In some instances, the lymphoid inflammatory reactions may produce lymphoma-like lesions, raising the question of lymphoma (see below).

Infectious Cervicitis

Table 4.2 summarizes some of the important or pathologically significant etiologic organisms of infectious cervicitis. It is apparent from this listing that infectious cervicitis is important because of its epidemic proportions and because of its central role in the pathogenesis of pelvic inflammatory disease and endometrial infections. According to the understanding of the pathogenesis of pelvic inflammatory disease, infectious cervicitis is the initial event of the pelvic inflammatory disease. It is also the primary infectious focus in related syndromes such as postpartum and postabortal endometritis. Spontaneous abortion, premature delivery, chorioamnionitis, stillbirth, and neonatal pneumonia and septicemia have been directly related to concurrent bacterial infection of the cervix. Even when asymptomatic, infectious cervicitis

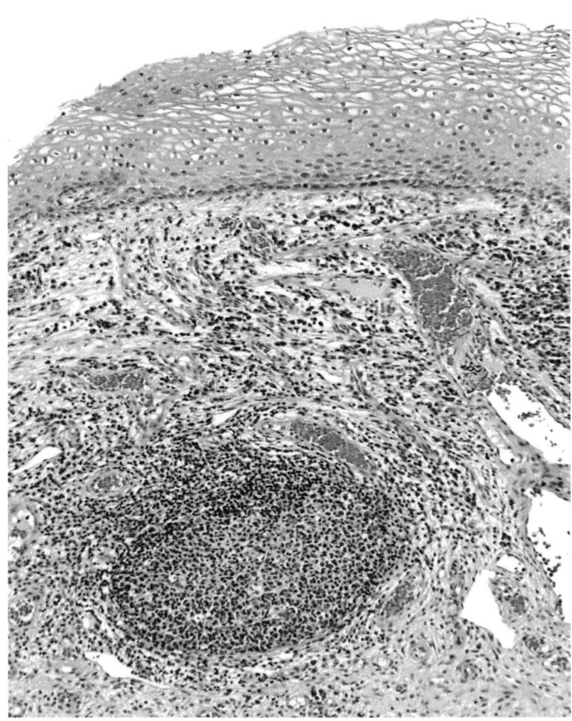

Fig. 4.30
Chronic cervicitis. **A subepithelial lymphoid follicle with a prominent germinal center is present. When lymphoid follicles are numerous, the condition is referred to as *follicular cervicitis***

Table 4.2
Microorganisms causing infectious cervicitis

Bacteria, chlamydia, mycobacteria, polymicrobial, endogenous vaginal aerobes and anaerobes
Chlamydia trachomatis
Neisseria gonorrhoeae
Mycoplasma hominis
Group B Streptococcus
Ureaplasma ureolyticum
Gardnerella vaginalis
Actinomyces israelii
Mycobacterium tuberculosis
Treponema pallidum
Viruses
Herpes simplex virus
Human papillomavirus
Fungi
Candida
Aspergillus
Protozoa and parasites
Trichomonas vaginalis
Ameba
Schistosomes

can be clinically important since it can act as a source of sexual transmission to male partners, as well as ascending infection in the female, and vertical transmission during pregnancy.

Infectious cervicitis can affect either the endocervical-type columnar epithelium producing *endocervicitis* (mucopurulent cervicitis) or affect the stratified squamous epithelium of the exocervix producing *exocervicitis* [42]. The infectious agents that cause endo- and exocervicitis tend to differ, although some agents can cause both.

Bacterial and Chlamydial Cervicitis

Bacterial and chlamydial infections of the cervix are the most common cause of infectious cervicitis and are associated with a nonspecific inflammatory response. The columnar epithelium of the endocervix is much more susceptible to bacterial and chlamydial infections than is the surrounding squamous epithelium, and endocervicitis is characteristic. The infectious agents that most commonly cause clinically significant endocervicitis are *Chlamydia trachomatis* and *Neisseria gonorrhoea.* Infection with either of these two agents requires no predisposing factors and is primarily dependent on exposure and size of the inoculum.

Histologically, follicular cervicitis is frequently found in patients with *chlamydia trachomatis* infection, and *chlamydia trachomatis* is now presumed to be a major cause of this condition in younger women. *Chlamydia trachomatis* cervicitis has also been associated with a dense, diffuse inflammatory exudate as well as reactive squamous and endocervical atypia [17].

Actinomycosis

Actinomyces israelii is a frequent commensual organism found in the female lower genital tract. Culture and immunofluorescence studies of cervical and vaginal secretions indicate that 3–27% of asymptomatic women without obvious risk factors are infected with *Actinomyces israelii* [67]. Aggregates of bacteria with the morphological appearance of actinomyces have been reported to occur in approximately 0.13% of all Papanicolaou smears [78]. The organism is more commonly identified in women wearing intrauterine devices (IUDs) than in women in the general population, and detection is related to the length of time that the IUD has been in place [18, 67, 78]. Structures resembling the "sulfur granules" observed in *Actinomyces israelii* infections are sometimes identified in endocervical curettings of asymptomatic women. In the majority of cases these are "pseudoactinomycotic radiate granules," which are nonspecific collections of bacteria or foreign material (e.g., fragments from nylon strings of IUD), glycoproteins, and lipids rather than actual collections of *Actinomyces israelii* [9].

The identification of *Actinomyces israelii* in asymptomatic women has little clinical significance and does not warrant antibiotic therapy [67]. Rarely *Actinomyces israelii* can be associated with pelvic abscesses.

Tuberculosis

Tuberculosis of the cervix is almost invariably secondary to tuberculous salpingitis and endometritis and is typically associated with pulmonary tuberculosis (➔ Chap. 7, Benign Diseases of the Endometrium, ➔ Chap. 11, Diseases of the Fallopian Tube and Paratubal Region). The prevalence of cervical tuberculosis in a population with genital tuberculosis varies between 2% and 82% [4]. Macroscopically, the cervix may appear normal, inflamed, or may simulate invasive carcinoma. Histologically, tuberculous infection of the cervix is recognized by the presence of multiple granulomas or tubercles, characterized by central caseous necrosis, epithelioid histiocytes, and multinucleated Langhans giant cells. Granulomas typically disappear after successful anti-tubercular therapy [4]. Tuberculous cervicitis may appear as a noncaseating, granulomatous lesion. Since caseating, nontuberculous granulomas due to lymphogranuloma venereum or sarcoidosis may be encountered in the cervix, the unequivocal diagnosis of tuberculous cervicitis requires demonstration of acid-fast *Mycobacterium tuberculosis,* a straight, rod-shaped bacillus, by Ziehl–Neelsen-stained sections, or by culture [22]. Because culture yields far better results than staining of tissue sections, unfixed biopsy material should be obtained for microbiologic testing whenever tuberculosis is suspected. The most common granulomatous lesions to be distinguished from tuberculous cervicitis include foreign body giant cell granulomas secondary to sutures, crystals, or cotton, lymphogranuloma venereum, schistosomiasis, and sarcoidosis. Cervical granuloma may occasionally develop after a biopsy or operation as a reaction to local tissue necrosis [22].

Other Granulomatous Infections

Certain venereally transmitted diseases commonly encountered in the vulva may also involve the cervix

(➊ Chap. 1, Benign Diseases of the Vulva). These include syphilis, either as the primary chancre, secondary mucous patches, or tertiary gumma, lymphogranuloma venereum, granuloma inguinale, and chancroid. All these conditions may resemble carcinoma clinically. This is particularly a problem with granuloma inguinale that is endemic in areas of Africa that have high prevalence of invasive cervical cancer. Up to 50% of women with granuloma inguinale may be initially misdiagnosed as having carcinoma of the cervix. Many of these women are thought to have high stage tumors because of the spread of the infection to the parametrial tissue [43]. In addition to the characteristic morphologic features, specific bacteriologic and immunologic techniques are available for identifying each of these diseases.

Viral Diseases

In contrast to bacterial infections of the cervix, the most common cervical viral infections – human papillomavirus (HPV) and herpes simplex virus (HSV) – have a predilection for the squamous epithelium and produce characteristic morphologic changes. Cytomegalovirus, although often isolated from cervical secretions, is not typically associated with cervicitis, and its role in cervical infection is poorly understood.

Herpesvirus Infection (HSV)

Although the precise prevalence of cervical HSV infection (herpes genitalis) is not known, it is far greater than generally recognized. At least 50 million individuals in the USA have genital HSV infection [100]. Up to 70% of HSV-2 infections appear to be asymptomatic. Both HSV-1 and HSV-2 can cause genital herpes and in some populations, HSV-1 is more common or the cause of initial herpes infection than is HSV-2 [100]. However, HSV-2 is responsible for the majority of cases of recurrent HSV. Cervical involvement can be detected in 70–90% of women with primary genital HSV-2 infections. Occasionally, in women with cervical involvement, the ulceronecrotic process is so extensive that a fungating, necrotic mass appears on the cervical portio, which can be mistaken for carcinoma. During the vesicular phase of a cervical lesion, a biopsy may reveal the presence of suprabasal intraepidermal vesicles filled with serum, degenerated epidermal cells, and multinucleated giant cells, some containing eosinophilic, intranuclear inclusions surrounded by a clear halo (➊ *Fig. 4.31*).

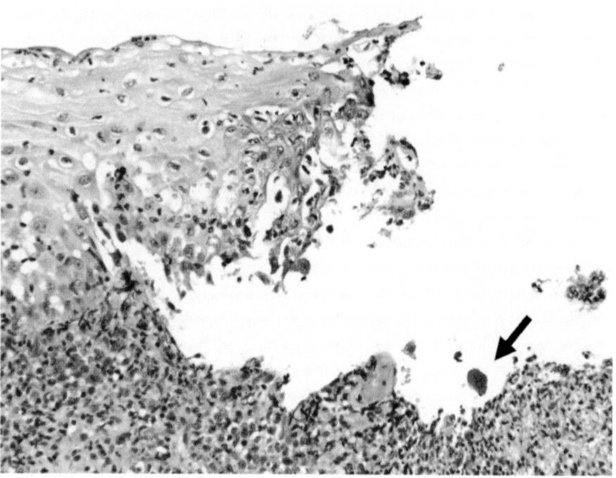

Fig. 4.31
Herpetic cervicitis. **Suprabasal vesicle in squamous epithelium of the portio. A multinucleated squamous cell with a ground-glass intranuclear viral inclusion is present in the *lower right***

Herpes-Like Lesions

Vesicular and bullous lesions of the cervical squamous mucous membrane, other than herpetic cervicitis, have been reported [11]. Pemphigus vulgaris of the cervix is a common finding in women with generalized disease [56]. Microscopically, there are multiple intraepithelial bullae in a suprabasal location containing the characteristic acantholytic Tzanck cells.

Human Papillomavirus (HPV)

Exophytic condyloma acuminata are one of the common manifestations of human papillomavirus type infection of the lower anogenital tract and are usually caused by HPV type 6 and less frequently type 11 [95]. When florid condylomas of the vulva are identified, multicentric disease can occur and internal vaginal or cervical exophytic condylomas can be occasionally identified. Exophytic condylomas of the cervix without vulvovaginal involvement are rare. They are commonly multifocal and may involve the mature squamous epithelium of the native cervical portio as well as the immature squamous epithelium of the transformation zone, including metaplastic squamous epithelium, replacing endocervical glands. Extension into the endocervical canal may occur. Grossly and colposcopically, condyloma accuminata appear white, and the degree of whiteness depends largely on the thickness of the associated surface hyperkeratosis (➊ *Fig. 4.32*). Other configurations of cervical exophytic

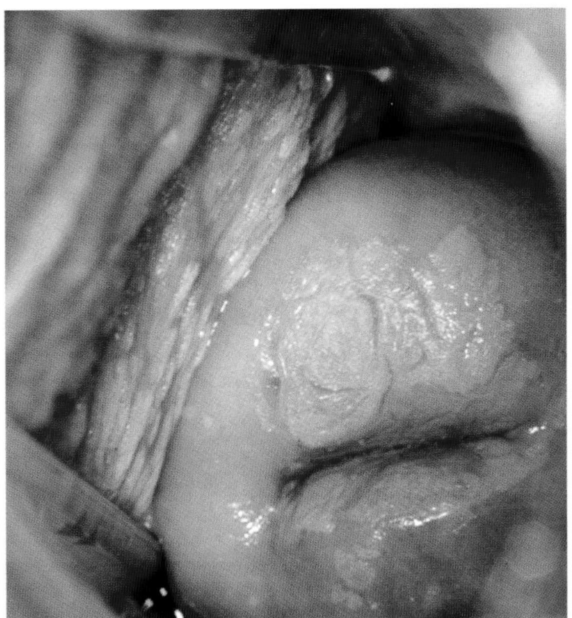

Fig. 4.32
Exophytic condyloma acuminata. **The lesions are multifocal and form raised white projections on both the vagina and cervix**

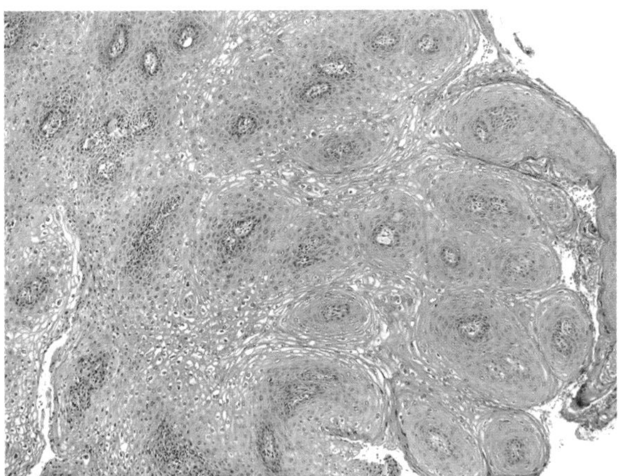

Fig. 4.33
Exophytic condyloma acuminata. **The classic histological features are papillomatosis with acanthosis, parakeratosis, hyperkeratosis, as well as cytological alterations including multinucleation, koilocytosis and nuclear atypia**

condylomas include myriad of minute, maculopapular, only slightly raised, condylomas involving the vagina and the cervix.

Microscopically, the histological features of exophytic cervical condyloma acuminata include architectural alterations such as papillomatosis, acanthosis, parakeratosis, and hyperkeratosis as well as cytologic alterations including koilocytosis (manifested by perinuclear cytoplasmic cavitation), nuclear enlargement and atypia. Multinucleation is also frequently observed (*Fig. 4.33*) (Chap. 1, Benign Diseases of the Vulva, Chap. 5, Precancerous Lesions of the Cervix).

The natural history of exophytic cervical condyloma accuminata is one of the spontaneous regressions, good response to conservative therapy, unpredictable recurrence, and sometimes persistence. Lesion regression or apparent cure following biopsy is fairly common. The natural history of genital condylomata in general may be modified by host factors, notably immunosuppression and steroid hormone levels.

Fungal Diseases

Cervical fungal infection by *Candida albicans* usually occurs as part of a generalized lower genital tract infection involving the vagina and vulva. Antibiotic therapy, poorly controlled diabetes mellitus, and immunosuppression all favor fungal overgrowth [93]. Cervical candidal infections can be associated with increased numbers of polymorpholeukocytes present in the upper layers of the epithelium and fungal hyphae that can be identified by periodic acid-Schiff (PAS) stains, both at the surface of the epithelium and within the superficial layers of the epithelium.

Protozoal and Parasitic Diseases

Cervical infestation by *Trichomonas vaginalis* is quite frequent and most often associated with concurrent trichomonal vaginitis. Acute trichomonal cervicitis may provoke an intense inflammatory response with prominent reparative atypia in exfoliated squamous and endocervical cells, with corresponding gross and colposcopic abnormalities.

Rare instances of parasitic infestations such as echinococcosis or hydatid cysts, Chagas' disease, and ulceronecrotic amebiasis have been encountered in the cervix [15]. In contrast, schistosomiasis (bilharziasis) of the cervix, generally caused by *Schistosoma mansoni*, is very common in Africa (Egypt), South America, Puerto Rico, and several Asian countries [81]. A large number of cases of cervical schistosomiasis are associated with urinary schistosomiasis and sterility. Microscopically, noncaseating granulomas (pseudotubercles) with ova surrounded by multinucleated giant cells are seen and the ova are often calcified (➋ *Fig. 4.34*). *S. mansoni* has a long lateral spine, whereas *S. haematobium* has a short spine extending from one of its poles. Cervical schistosomiasis may be associated with extensive pseudoepitheliomatous hyperplasia of the cervical squamous epithelium, masquerading both clinically and histologically as carcinoma. Although it was previously thought that chronic, untreated cervical schistosomiasis plays a role in the genesis of cervical carcinoma in populations where schistosomiasis is prevalent, there is now evidence indicating no association between schistosomiasis and cervical cancer [82].

Cervicovaginitis Emphysematosa

Multiple, blue-gray, subepithelial cysts of the portio vaginalis and vagina characterize this unusual disease [33]. In rare cases, the cysts have been misdiagnosed as an invasive cervical cancer [5]. The cause of this condition is unknown, but it is often associated with trichomoniasis [33]. Gas-forming bacteria have never been identified within the cysts. The cysts are dilated connective tissue spaces without lining epithelium that contain air and carbon dioxide. Multinucleated foreign body giant cells surround some of the cysts, and often the subepithelial veins and lymphatics are dilated.

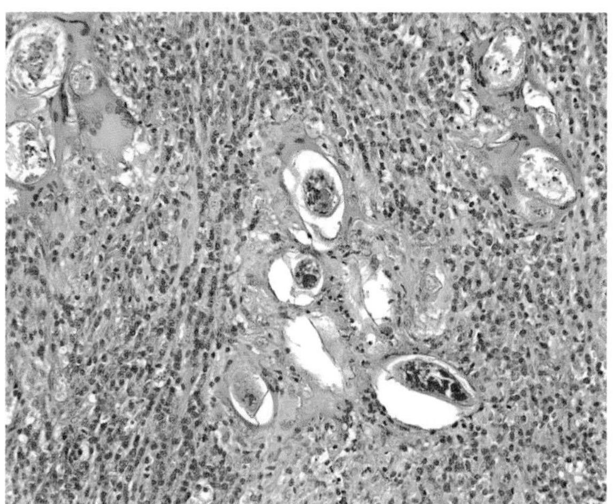

Fig. 4.34
Cervical schistosomiasis. Note calcified *Schistosoma haematobiium* ova

Cervical Vasculitis

Isolated arteritis of the cervix, histologically identical but clinically unrelated to polyarteritis nodosa, may rarely be encountered [65]. It may be asymptomatic or may be associated with bleeding and may clinically resemble cancer. Gynecologic vasculitides are encountered in 0.04% and 0.1% of surgically removed gynecologic specimens. Most are isolated, single organ disease and the cervix is the most frequently involved organ [40]. In most cases, medium-sized arteries contain non-granulomatous vasculitis and is usually an incidental finding in surgical specimens. The pathogenesis of single organ gynecologic vasculitis is unknown and if no systemic disease is identified, no further therapy is indicated.

Pseudoneoplastic Glandular Conditions (Hyperplasias) and Endometriosis

Microglandular Endocervical Hyperplasia

Microglandular endocervical hyperplasia is a benign proliferation of endocervical glands. Microglandular hyperplasia is frequently detected as an incidental finding on a cervical biopsy, cone biopsy or a hysterectomy specimen. If clinically apparent, it most often resembles a cervical polyp, measuring 1–2 cm in size. These patients may complain of postcoital bleeding or spotting. Microglandular hyperplasia is most common in women of reproductive ages and has been detected in up to 27% of cone biopsies or hysterectomy specimens [10]. Early studies reported that the microglandular hyperplasia typically occurs in patients with a history of recent progesterone exposure, either as a result of oral contraceptive use or pregnancy, and concluded that it represents a progestin-induced lesion. However, a number of cases have been reported in which there is no associated hormonal history, and a recent comprehensive study did not find a relationship between microglandular hyperplasia and progestin exposure [36]. Therefore, the role of progestin exposure in the pathogenesis of this lesion is currently unclear.

Histologically, microglandular hyperplasia may present in a single focus or be distributed in multiple foci. It may involve the surface and/or deeper portions of endocervical clefts. The most common form consists of tightly packed varying-sized glandular or tubular units, lined by flattened to cuboidal cells with eosinophilic granular cytoplasm containing small quantities of mucin (➋ *Fig. 4.35a, b*). The glands vary in size and shape from

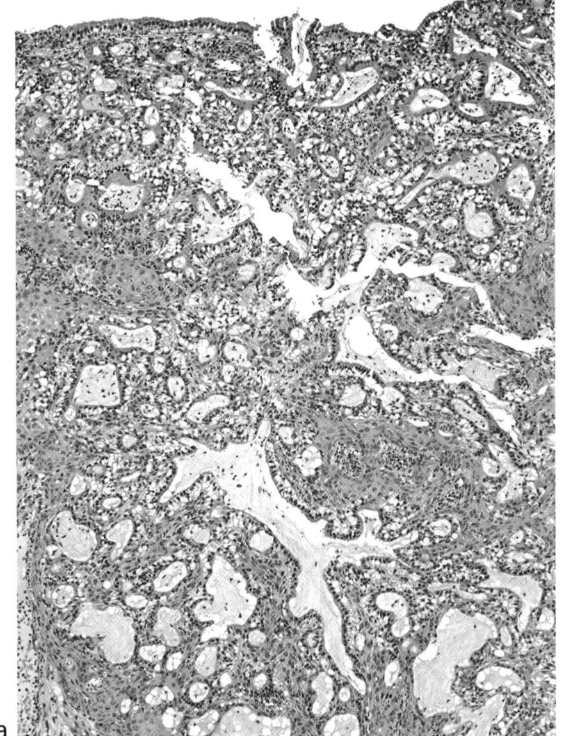

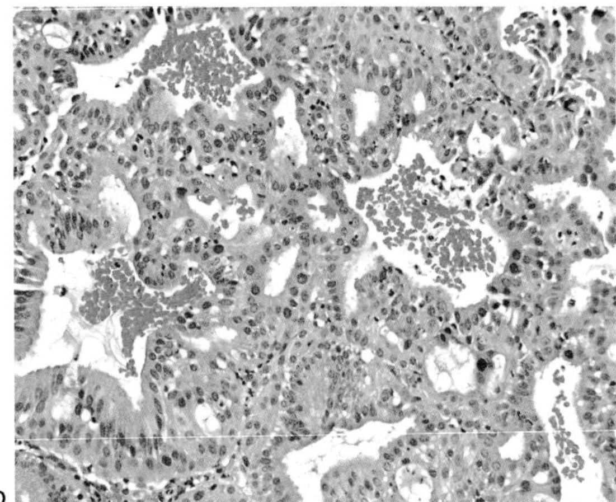

Fig. 4.35
Microglandular hyperplasia. **(a) There is an adenomatous pattern with cuboidal lining cells and focal squamous metaplasia. (b) At higher magnification the cells appear uniform and form a reticular pattern. Note the extensive vacuolization of the lesion that is caused by cystic dilation of intercellular spaces. There is a paucity of intracellular mucin**

round and small to large irregularly dilated cystic structures. The stroma separating the glands is usually infiltrated with acute and chronic inflammatory cells. The nuclei of the endocervical cells are uniform, with occasional pleomorphism and hyperchromasia, but mitotic activity is quite low with only 1 mitotic figure per 10 high-power fields [105]. Associated squamous metaplasia and subcolumnar reserve cell hyperplasia are seen in a large number of cases. Foci with a solid proliferation of cells, including signet ring cells, can also be present. In more florid forms of microglandular hyperplasia, the glandular elements are arranged in a reticulated or solid pattern with areas of nuclear hyperchromasia and pleomorphism. The significance of the florid forms of microglandular hyperplasia is that the irregularly arranged glands can impart an infiltrative appearance and they can be mistaken for adenocarcinoma, in particular, clear cell adenocarcinoma. Microglandular hyperplasia with solid areas, especially when the solid component predominates or when signet ring cells are present, can also be difficult to distinguish from adenocarcinomas [105]. The benign nature of these florid lesions is usually demonstrable by a lack of clear-cut stromal invasion and the low mitotic activity of microglandular hyperplasia as compared to endocervical adenocarcinoma. In addition, florid forms of microglandular hyperplasia almost always contain areas with the more typical histological features of microglandular hyperplasia.

Mesonephric Hyperplasia and Remnants

The vestigial elements of the distal ends of the mesonephric ducts are found in 1–22% of adult cervices and in up to 40% of the cervices of newborns and children [44, 92]. The wide variation in the reported prevalence of these remnants appears to be a function of how extensively the cervix is sampled and the site of sampling [25]. Mesonephric remnants are most commonly present in the lateral aspects of the cervix, a region that is usually not sampled on routine hysterectomy specimens. They consist of small tubules or cysts that are usually located deep in the lateral cervical wall. Characteristically, the tubules are arranged in small clusters or have an orderly distribution reminiscent of the ampullary portion of the fetal mesonephric duct. The tubules are lined by nonciliated, low columnar, or cuboidal epithelium. The lining cells contain no glycogen or mucin, features that distinguish mesonephric from endocervical epithelium (*Fig. 4.36*). The tubular lumen, however, is often filled with pink, homogeneous, PAS-positive secretions.

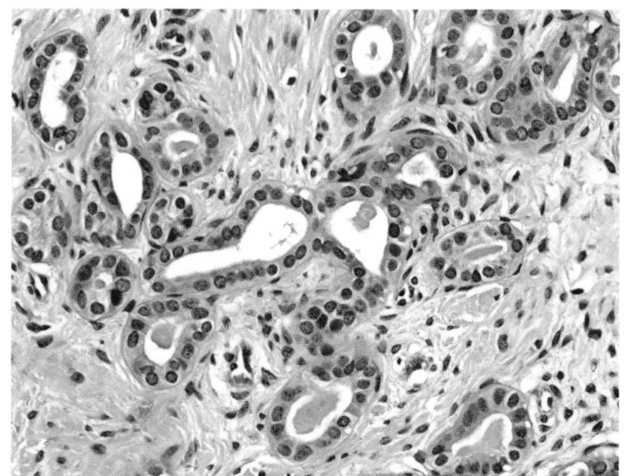

Fig. 4.36
Mesonephric remnants. **The mesonephric tubules are lined by cuboidal epithelium with bland nuclei. Occasional tubules contain pink, homogenoeous intraluminal secretions**

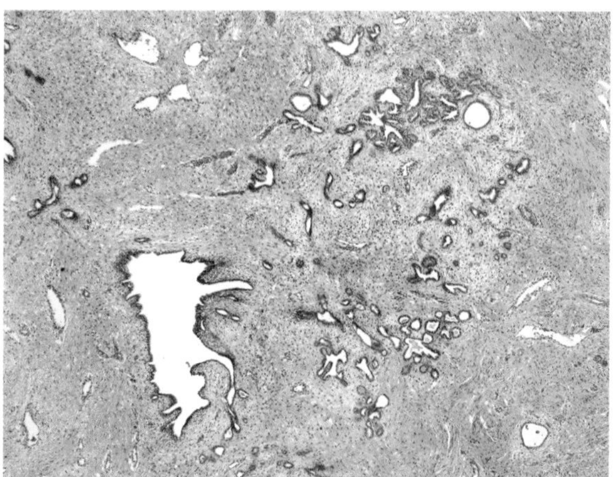

Fig. 4.37
Florid mesonephric hyperplasia. **Extensive mesonephric tubular-ductal proliferation in the deeper portion of the cervix, resembling an invasive adenocarcinoma. Unlike the latter, the lobular architecture is maintained in hyperplasia. Note the mesonephric duct in the lower left surrounded by a proliferation of small tubules**

Mesonephric remnants may become hyperplastic, resulting in a florid, tubuloglandular proliferation with transmural involvement of the cervix (*Fig. 4.37*). Based on the architecture of the glandular structures, mesonephric hyperplasia has been classified by some authors into different histological types [25, 87]. The most common type is called the lobular type and is characterized by clustered mesonephric tubules, with or without a centrally placed duct. The lobular form tends to occur at a younger age, is less extensive, and tends to arise deeper in the cervical stroma. The less common type is called the diffuse type and is characterized by a nonclustered diffuse pattern or proliferation of mesonephric tubules. The histological subdivision of mesonephric hyperplasia into different forms does not have a clinical significance.

Mesonephric hyperplasia is almost always asymptomatic and is detected on either cervical biopsy, cone biopsy or hysterectomy specimens. Histological differentiation between mesonephric hyperplasia and mesonephric remnants is quite arbitrary, and of little clinical importance. Mesonephric hyperplasia is a benign condition that is of pathological significance, because it can be misinterpreted as a minimal deviation adenocarcinoma of the endocervix (Chap. 6, Carcinoma and Other Tumors of the Cervix). Mesonephric hyperplasia is distinguished from carcinoma by lack of a complex glandular pattern, mitosis, intracellular mucin, and periglandular stromal edema. In contrast to most cervical adenocarcinomas, carcinoembryonic antigen (i.e., CEA) is absent in mesonephric hyperplasia, and these lesions have low Ki-67 staining indices [69]. In addition, normal mesonephric remnants are usually admixed with the hyperplastic tubules.

Lobular Endocervical Glandular Hyperplasia (LEGH)

Endocervical hyperplasia can sometimes be encountered and can take several different forms. Lobular endocervical glandular hyperplasia (LEGH) is a rare form, first described by Nucci et al. [75]. Later studies have shown that it has a distinctive gastric phenotype (pyloric gland metaplasia) by demonstrating immunohistochemical positivity for H1K1083, an antibody specific for gastric pyloric mucin [71]. Most cases are incidental findings in hysterectomy specimens; some patients, however, complain of abundant mucoid or watery discharge. Microscopically, there is a proliferation of tightly packed, small-sized endocervical glands displaying a well-demarcated, multilobular pattern. Several of the lobules are centered by a larger glandular structure (*Fig. 4.38a, b*). Typically, LEGH is confined to the inner one-half of the cervical wall, and the gland-lining cells are devoid of "malignant" atypia, and mitoses do not exceed 2 per 10 high-power fields. LEGH may be mistaken for adenoma malignum (Chap. 6, Minimal Deviation Endocervical Adenocarcinoma). The orderly,

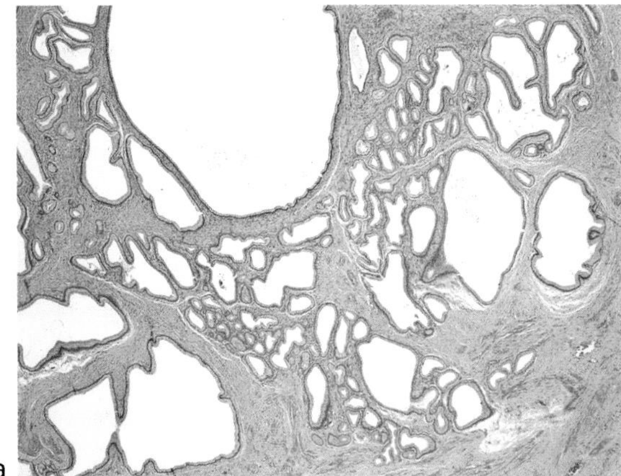

a

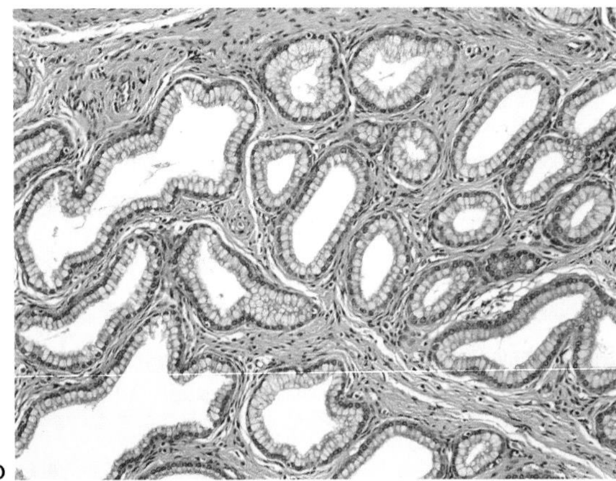

b

Fig. 4.38
Lobular endocervical glandular hyperplasia (LEGH).
(a) There is a proliferation of highly packed, small-sized endocervical glands in a lobular pattern. (b) The cells lack cellular atypia and have a gastric phenotype with a large number of goblet type cells

lobular architecture of glandular units, absence of irregular, deep stromal infiltration and desmoplasia, and immunonegativity for CEA are features distinguishing the former from the latter. Occasionally, LEGH is associated with in situ and invasive adenocarcinoma, particularly adenoma malignum of endocervix, as well as benign, borderline, and invasive endocervical-type mucinous lesions of the endometrium, tubes, and ovaries [74]. The possibility of LEGH being a precursor of malignant endocervical neoplasms has been raised, however, not via the high-risk HPV-related carcinogenesis pathway, for it is uniformly HPV DNA negative by PCR and in situ hybridization [57]. Its association with malignancy may be a reflection of chromosomal inbalances common to adenoma malignum [57]. It has been suggested, furthermore, that the association may be predominantly limited to those cases in which both LEGH and cervical adenocarcinoma display gastro-pyloric glandular metaplasia [71].

Diffuse Laminar Endocervical Glandular Hyperplasia (DLEGH)

Diffuse laminar endocervical glandular hyperplasia (DLEGH) is another rare form of hyperplasia described by Jones et al. [53] in which tightly packed, small to medium-sized endocervical glands are typically confined to the upper one-third of the cervical wall (*Fig. 4.39a, b*). Unlike LEGH, its laminar counterpart is devoid of lobulation and is clearly demarcated from the underlying stroma exhibiting a straight line at its base. The lining epithelium of glandular structures is cytologically normal without mitoses, and stromal desmoplasia is not seen. These features and its superficial position distinguish DLEGH from adenoma malignum.

Occasionally, cases of endocervical hyperplasia are encountered which do not fit the published descriptions of either LEGH or DLEGH. We utilize the descriptive term *endocervical hyperplasia – NOS* to describe such cases. *Figure 4.40a, b* illustrates such as case which lacks both a lobular architecture as well as a well-demarcated laminar architecture. Follow-up studies of such lesions are not published, but most cases are diagnosed on hysterectomy specimens and appear to be incidental findings.

Endocervicosis

Endocervicosis is a very rare condition described by Zaino [106] and Young et al. [102] in which the outer aspect of the cervical wall is enlarged, rubbery and may be grossly cystic. Histologically, glands varying in shape and size, often cystically dilated, are lined by mucinous-type endocervical cells and typically occupy the outer one-third of the cervical wall with extension to the paracervical tissues (*Fig. 4.41*). The lining epithelium is normal to flattened with very occasional mitotic figures, and occasional glands can be surrounded by endometrial-like stroma. Overall, the lesion resembles endocervicosis of urinary bladder and its distinctive feature from adenoma malignum is that it is located in the outer wall of the cervix with clear demarcation from the upper, normal endocervical glands of the endocervical mucosal layer [102].

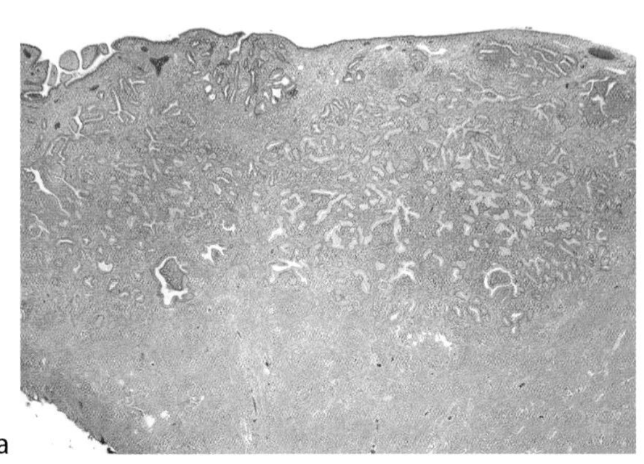

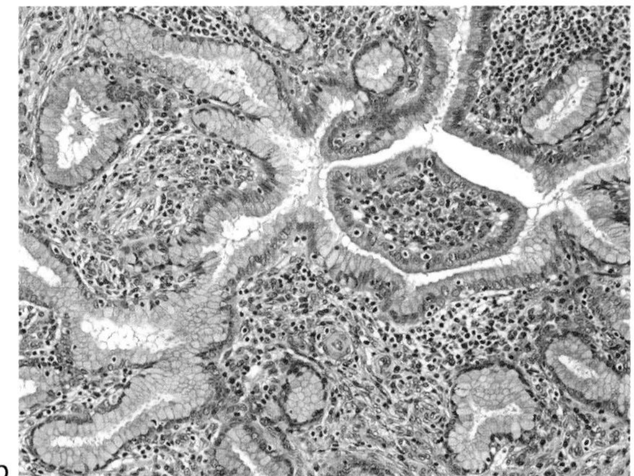

Fig. 4.39
Diffuse laminar endocervical glandular hyperplasia (DLEGH). **(a) There is a proliferation of highly packed, small-sized endocervical glands that is clearly demarcated from the underlying cervical stroma. (b) The cells lack cellular atypia and have a normal endocervical appearance**

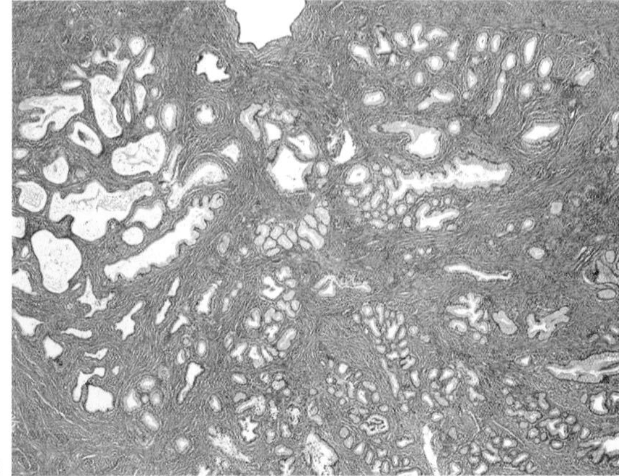

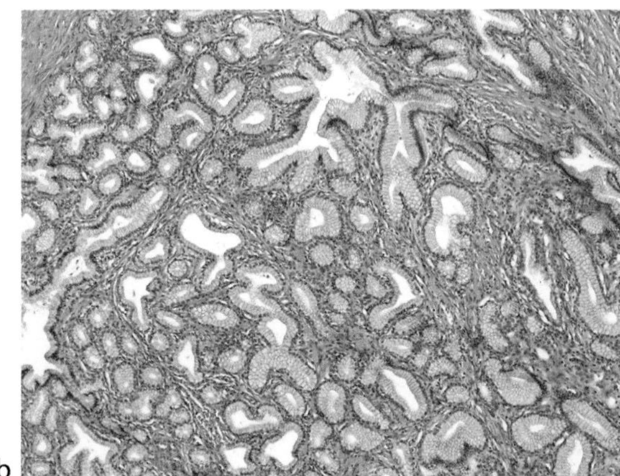

Fig. 4.40
Endocervical glandular hyperplasia – NOS. **(a) There is a proliferation of loosely packed endocervical glands. (b) The cells lack cellular atypia or mitotic activity and there is no stromal reaction to the proliferation**

Endometriosis

Endometriosis refers to lesions that are composed of ectopic endometrial glands and stroma (Chap. 9, Endometrial Carcinoma), whereas *tubo-endometrioid metaplasia* refers to endocervical glands that are lined by ciliated cells or secretory-type cells with apical snouts that resemble those that can be seen in the endometrium but which lack endometrial stroma. Endometriosis of the cervix may occur on the portio or in the endocervical canal. The process is usually confined to the superficial third of the cervical wall [7]. Most areas of endometriosis of the exocervix appear as one or more, small, blue or red nodules, measuring a few millimeters in diameter. Occasionally, however, the lesion may be larger or cystic and may produce abnormal vaginal bleeding. Histologically, the glands and stroma resemble proliferative endometrium (*Fig. 4.42*). Rarely, the glands are secretory. Decidua may be seen in pregnancy or with progestin therapy.

The mechanism responsible for the development of endometriosis is unknown, but it is clear that cervical endometriosis frequently develops following cervical trauma. Cervical endometriosis is encountered in 5–43% of patients undergoing cervical cautery or cold-knife cone biopsy or loop excisional procedures [32]. This association has been interpreted by some investigators as evidence supporting the implantation theory of endometriosis. According to this theory, endometrial tissue is implanted into the cervical mucosa or submucosa, following postmenstrual cauterization or during delivery. However, the frequent occurrence of posttraumatic endometriosis could also be interpreted as supporting the view that cervical endometriosis represents a reparative/metaplastic process. Support for the concept that the cervical endometriosis develops as a metaplastic process, as opposed to direct implantation, also comes from the frequent demonstration of glands with either *tubo-endometrioid* or pure *tubal metaplasia* in posttraumatic cervices.

Benign Tumors

Endocervical Polyps

Endocervical polyps constitute the most common new growths of the uterine cervix. Cervical polyps are focal, hyperplastic protrusions of endocervical folds, including the epithelium and substantia propria. Cervical polyps are most often found during the fourth to sixth decades and in multigravidas. They may present with profuse leukorrhea due to hypersecretion of mucus from inflamed endocervical epithelium or abnormal bleeding from ulceration of the surface epithelium. Clinically, cervical polyps are rounded or elongated with a smooth or lobulated surface that is often reddened because of increased vascularity. Most polyps are single and measure from a few millimeters to 2–3 cm. In rare instances, they may reach gigantic dimensions, protruding beyond the introitus and resembling carcinoma. Various cervical lesions with a polypoid gross appearance are presented in *Table 4.3*. Microscopically, cervical polyps display a variety of patterns that vary according to the preponderance of one or another of the tissue components. The most common type is the endocervical mucosal polyp. It is composed of mucinous epithelium that lines crypts, with or without cystic changes (*Fig. 4.43*). Occasionally, they may be mainly fibrous, representing an overgrowth of the connective tissue stroma of the portio. In other cases, blood

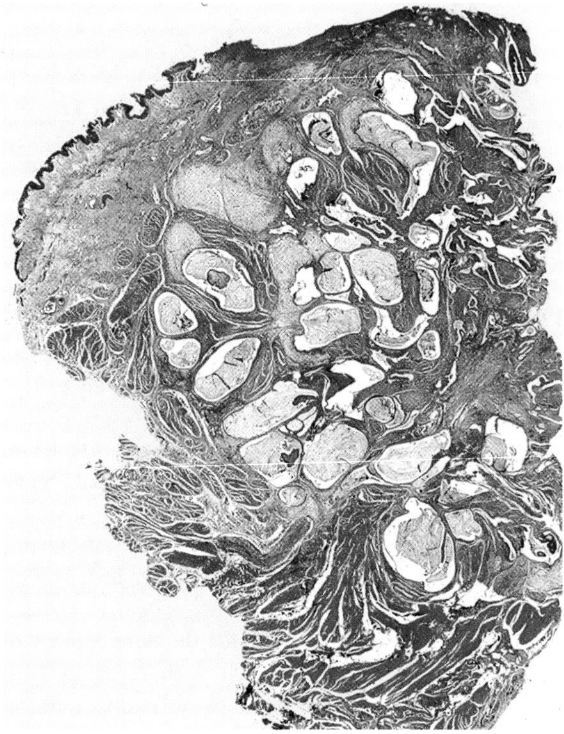

Fig. 4.41
Endocervicosis of the cervix. **Cystically dilated endocervical glands extend into the outer third of the wall of the cervix (Photograph courtesy of Dr. Phillip Clement of Vancouver, Canada)**

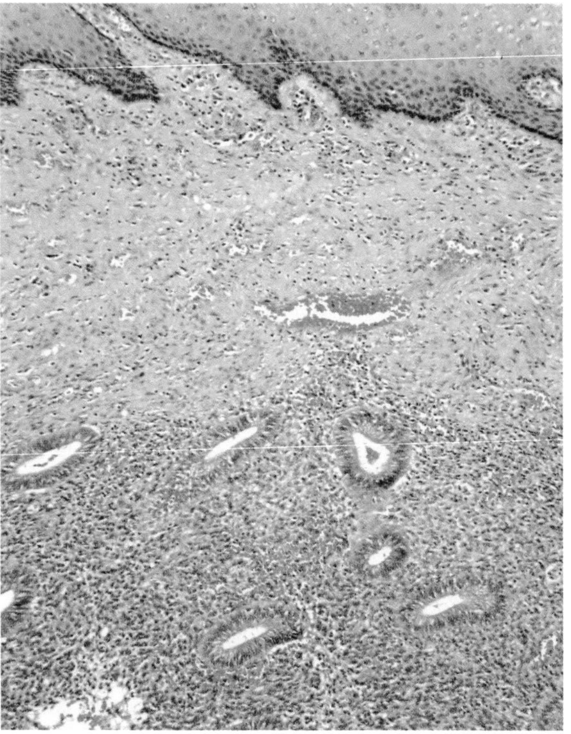

Fig. 4.42
Endometriosis of the cervix. **Both typical endometrial glands and stroma are present beneath the squamous portio epithelium**

vessels predominate and the lesion is called a *vascular polyp*. Squamous metaplasia involving the surface or glandular epithelium of polyps is frequently observed. The supporting connective tissue of polyps is generally loose, with centrally placed feeding vessels and is almost always infiltrated by a chronic inflammatory infiltrate. Occasionally, such infiltration may be so extensive as to be the principal tissue constituent of the polyp. In these cases, polypoid granulation tissue devoid of surface epithelium is observed (➲ *Fig. 4.44*). Polyps originating in the isthmus often have an admixture of endocervical- and endometrial-type epithelial components and are referred to as *mixed polyps*.

Table 4.3
Differential clinical diagnosis of polypoid lesions of the cervix

Polyp	Squamous papilloma
Microglandular endocervical hyperplasia	Condyloma acuminatum
	Papillary adenofibroma
Decidua	Squamous cell carcinoma
Granulation tissue	Adenocarcinoma
Leiomyoma Adenomyoma	Sarcoma, primary Sarcoma, secondary
Fibroadenoma	

High-grade SIL, carcinoma, either in situ or invasive (adeno- or squamous), arising in cervical polyps is extremely rare. Endocervical polyps with adenocarcinomatous changes must be differentiated from polypoid adenocarcinoma of the endocervix and from endocervical polyps that are secondarily involved by an adjacent adenocarcinoma. The most useful criterion for differentiating between the two is to determine whether or not the base of the pedicle of the polyp is involved by carcinoma. The base of a polyp that harbors a primary tumor is free of disease, and the carcinoma usually has a focal distribution within an otherwise benign polyp. In a polypoid carcinoma, the entire mass is malignant, including its base and neighboring areas. A focus of carcinoma in a cervical polyp without involvement of its base but associated with similar carcinoma in the adjacent regions should be regarded as a secondary rather than a primary focus. Adenocarcinoma confined to a polyp has an excellent prognosis [2].

Mesodermal Stromal Polyp

Mesodermal stromal polyps are benign, exophytic proliferations of stroma and epithelium that can occur in the vagina and cervix of women of reproductive ages. These lesions are seen most frequently in pregnant patients and arise more commonly from the vagina than from the cervix [73]. Histologically, these polyps are composed of an edematous stroma that is covered by a benign

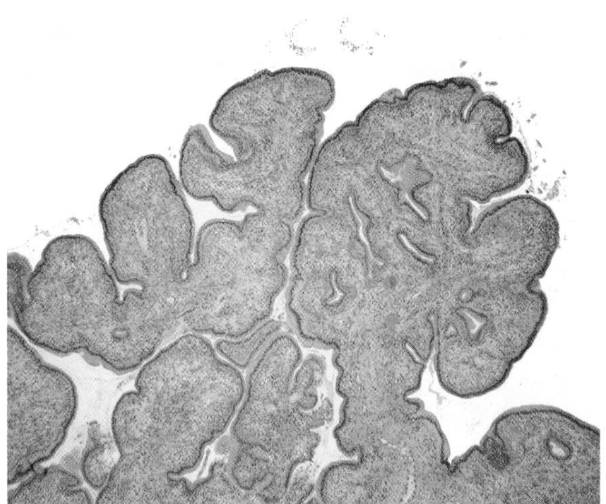

Fig. 4.43
Endocervical polyp. **This is the most common type of endocervical polyp. Endocervical-type, tall columnar, mucinous epithelium covers the surface and crypts**

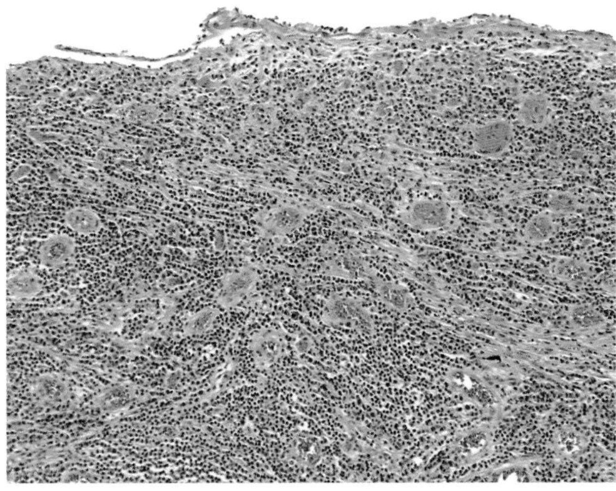

Fig. 4.44
Granulation tissue. **Polypoid nodules of granulation tissue can grossly resemble an endocervical polyp. This type of lesion often leads to bleeding**

appearing stratified squamous epithelium (➲ *Fig. 4.45a*). The stromal component is usually comprised of bland appearing plump stromal fibroblasts. However in some cases, there can be focal areas of bizarre fibroblasts with irregular, occasionally multinucleated hyperchromatic nuclei that resemble the fibroblasts in radiation reactions (➲ *Fig. 4.45b*) [13]. Occasional multinucleated stromal giant cells can be identified in approximately 25% of cone biopsy or hysterectomy specimens when carefully searched for [38]. These cells stain negatively for cytokeratin, desmin, factor VIII, and S100 protein but stain positively for vimentin and alpha1-antichymotrypsin. When stromal polyps contain large number of these cells, they can appear quite alarming and simulate the appearance of sarcoma botryoides [21]. However, careful inspection will allow these lesions to be differentiated from sarcoma botryoides by the absence of mitotic figures, lack of rhabdomyoblasts, and lack of a cambium layer.

Placental Site Trophoblastic Nodule

Placental site trophoblastic nodules can be found in the endocervix, immediately beneath the epithelium. They are sometimes detected in endocervical curettages. These lesions are histologically identical to early implantation sites that can be detected in the endometrium of women of reproductive ages [105]. Microscopically, placental site trophoblastic nodules are well-defined lesions that have a hyalinized appearance and contain intermediate trophoblasts and inflammatory cells (➲ *Fig. 4.46*). The intermediate trophoblast cells are frequently degenerated and have an

a

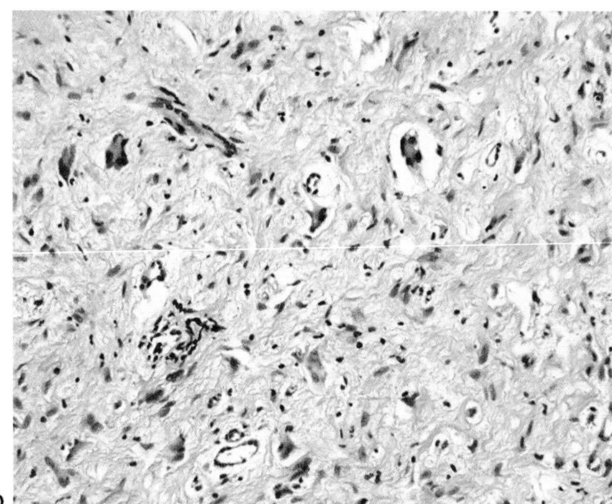

b

Fig. 4.45
Mesodermal stromal polyp. **(a) Spindle-shaped and stellate fibroblasts are embedded in a loose myxoid stroma that has a stratified squamous surface epithelium. (b) At higher magnification, stellate atypical fibroblasts can be seen in the stroma**

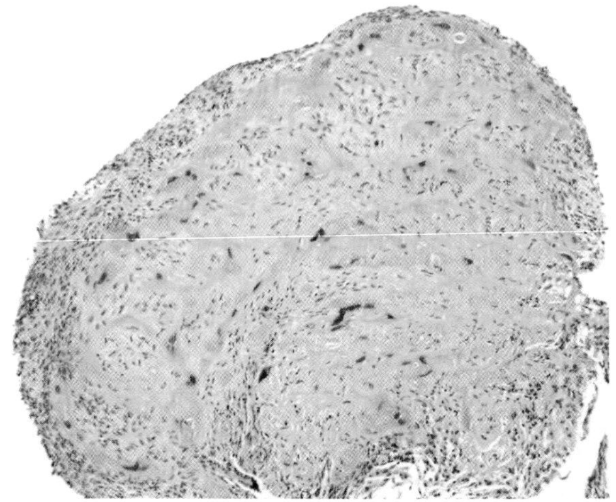

Fig. 4.46
Placental site nodule. **A hyalinized nodule containing intermediate trophoblast is identified in an endocervical curettage obtained several months postpartum**

extensive cytoplasmic vacuolization but lack significant nuclear atypia, lack mitotic activity, and have very low Ki-67 labeling indices [89]. Intermediate trophoblast stains positively with antibodies against cytokeratins, human placental lactogen, and Mel-CAM, a cell adhesion molecule of the immunoglobulin gene superfamily [89]. The lack of significant nuclear atypia and mitotic activity, as well as staining with antibodies against human placental lactogen, allow these lesions to be microscopically differentiated from invasive nonkeratinizing squamous cell carcinomas.

Leiomyoma

Cervical leiomyomas are much less common than uterine myomata. They usually occur singly and produce unilateral enlargement of the cervical portio. At times, the lesion may protrude from the canal, resembling an endocervical polyp, and in pregnancy may produce dystocia. Cervical leiomyomas are grossly similar to those observed in the myometrium; microscopically they tend to be more vascularized than those of the uterus; a variety of histological patterns may be encountered, including atypical leiomyoma, which contains cells with bizarre nuclei (Chap. 10, Mesenchymal Tumors of the Uterus).

Adenomyoma and Papillary Adenofibroma

These neoplasms are rare and are composed of an admixture of fibroconnective tissue and smooth muscle elements, intermingling with glands lined by a predominately endocervical-type epithelium. The tumors typically measure 1.3–8 cm in diameter and usually present as asymptomatic cervical polyps [34]. The epithelial component is typically composed of irregular, large glands that may be accompanied by smaller glands in a lobular arrangement. These tumors can be distinguished from endocervical adenocarcinomas by the lack of invasion of the stromal component by the epithelial component, lack of nuclear atypia, and minimal mitotic activity. Adenomyomas can persist or recur, but there are no reported instances of extracervical spread or metastasis [34].

Papillary adenofibromas are rare benign neoplasm with histological characteristics similar to the ovarian adenofibroma. Only several cases have been reported in the literature. They consist of an admixture of fibroconnective tissue and glands lined by either endocervical-type epithelium or a tubal type epithelium. The fibroconnective tissue usually forms papillary projections (*Fig. 4.47*) [1, 30].

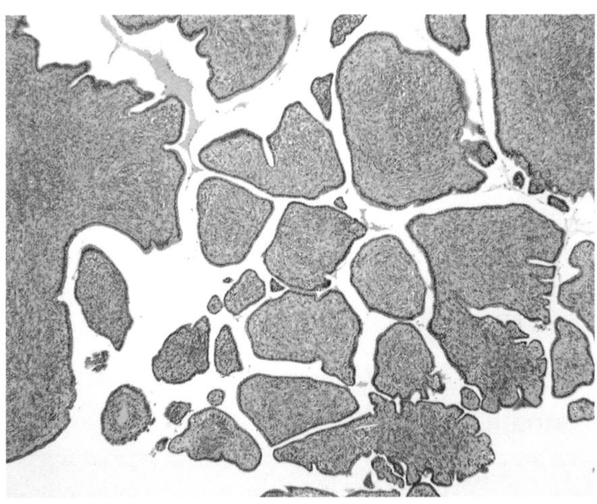

Fig. 4.47
Papillary adenofibroma of the endocervix. **Fibroepithelial papillae project from the cervix. The papillae are covered with an endocervical-type epithelium**

Miscellaneous Tumors

Hemangiomas are rarely found in the cervix. They may be of capillary or cavernous type [37]. A single instance of cervical lymphangioma was reported by Stout and several cases of lipoma of the cervix are on record [94]. Neoplasms of neurogenic derivation arising in the cervix are extremely rare and include neurofibroma and ganglioneuroma. Benign blue nevi of the endocervix, indistinguishable from those arising in the dermis, are seen occasionally [77]. They are composed of melanin-containing fusiform cells with dendritic cytoplasmic processes, located in the stroma of the endocervix. Cervical melanosis is an uncommon finding characterized by the hyperpigmentation of the cervical basal epithelium. It is reported to occur either with or without accompanying basal melanocytes [101].

Cysts

Nabothian Cyst

Nabothian cysts are the most common type of cyst of the cervix and develop within the transformation zone secondary to squamous metaplasia, covering over and obstructing endocervical glands. Grossly, these lesions appear as yellow white cysts that are frequently multiple and can measure up to 1.5 cm in diameter.

Microscopically, they are lined by a somewhat flattened, single layer of mucin-producing endocervical epithelium (➋ *Fig. 4.48*). In some cases, squamous metaplasia of the lining epithelium occurs. The lining epithelium is almost always at least focally positive with mucicarimine stains, allowing these lesions to be distinguished from traumatic inclusion cysts and mesonephric duct cysts. Although nabothian cysts are usually confined to the superficial portion of the cervix, they may extend through the wall of the cervix [14].

Tunnel Clusters

Endocervical tunnel clusters are benign collections of endocervical glands that are usually located close to the surface epithelium of the cervix. Tunnel clusters are quite common and become more prevalent with increasing age. In the Fluhmann's original description of this condition, they were detected in 8% of all adult women and 13% of the postmenopausal women [27]. They appear to be more common in pregnant women. These lesions are asymptomatic and are detected as incidental findings in either hysterectomy specimens or cone biopsies obtained for unrelated reasons [86].

Two types of tunnel clusters were originally described. One type represents a cluster of closely packed glands that are noncystic and are lined by tall columnar epithelium. The other type is grossly cystic and lined by a cuboidal or flattened epithelium (➋ *Fig. 4.49*). These collections of glands have a clustered appearance with a rounded margin and do not invade into the deep cervical stroma. The importance of tunnel clusters is that they are occasionally misinterpreted as minimal deviation adenocarcinomas of the cervix [52, 86]. However, tunnel clusters do not have nuclear atypia, mitotic activity, and most importantly do not invade into the deep cervical stroma.

Inclusion Cyst

Traumatic inclusion cysts are a form of epidermal inclusion cysts that commonly occur in the vagina at sites of surgical repair of episiotomies or vaginal intrapartum lacerations (➋ Chap. 3, Diseases of the Vagina). They are thought to develop from viable fragments of epithelium, which

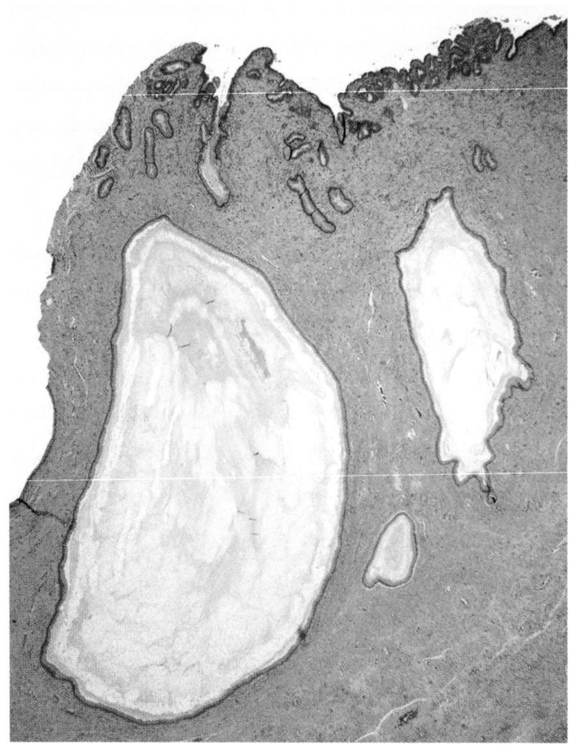

Fig. 4.48
Nabothian cysts. **Nabothian cysts are lined by a flattened layer of mucin-producing epithelium**

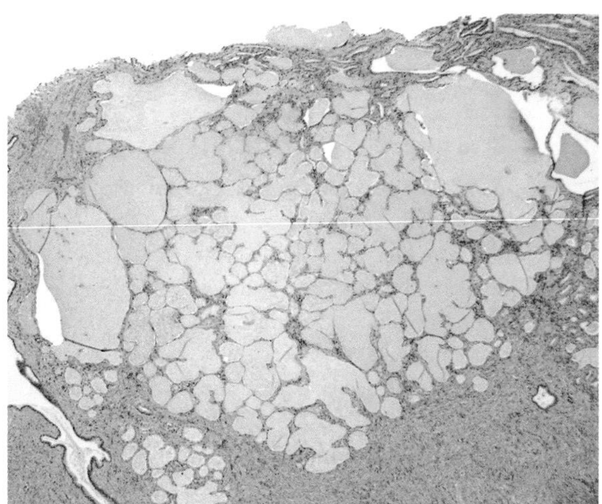

Fig. 4.49
Endocervical tunnel cluster. **Closely packed cystically dilated glands lined by a flattened epithelium. The condition is well demarcated and does not extend beyond the depth of the normal endocervical glands**

become entrapped within the stroma at the time of obstetrical trauma or subsequent surgical repair. Inclusion cysts are uncommonly found on the cervix. Grossly, they present as unilocular cystic structures measuring 1–2 cm in diameter beneath the native portio epithelium [28]. Microscopically, traumatic inclusion cysts are lined by a stratified squamous epithelium similar to that of the vaginal mucosa but usually somewhat thinner. The epithelium shows normal maturation with the basal cells, oriented away from the cyst cavity that is filled with desquamated epithelial cells. The cyst contents are identical to those of epidermal inclusion cysts at other sites and are thick, white, and cheesy.

Tumor-Like Lesions

Decidual Pseudopolyp

The gross appearance of the pseudodecidual change that can occur during pregnancy depends on the site. If the change occurs on the exocervix, it frequently presents as a raised plaque or pseudopolyp that can be mistaken for invasive carcinoma both colposcopically and microscopically. During gestation, cervical polyps may also contain focal stromal pseudodecidual changes, and rarely massive decidualization of endocervical stroma occurs, producing a polypoid protrusion from the endocervix. Clinically, decidualized polyps need to be differentiated from extruded fragments of decidua that may indicate an impeding miscarriage. Distinction is made by identifying a stalk for the decidualized polyp, whereas expulsed fragments of decidua lack a stalk. Areas of pseudodecidualization are microscopically differentiated from invasive nonkeratinizing squamous cell carcinoma by the lack of significant nuclear atypia, as well as lack of mitotic figures, a coexisting squamous intraepithelial lesion (SIL) and continuity with the surface epithelium. In difficult cases, immunohistochemistry using antibodies against cytokeratin proteins can be used to differentiate cytokeratin-negative decidual reactions from cytokeratin-positive nonkeratinizing squamous cell carcinoma.

Mullerian Papilloma

Rare instances of a benign, papillary growth of the cervix that occur primarily in children have been described [41, 64, 88]. They are composed of complex papillary projections, lined by flat cuboidal epithelium with cores

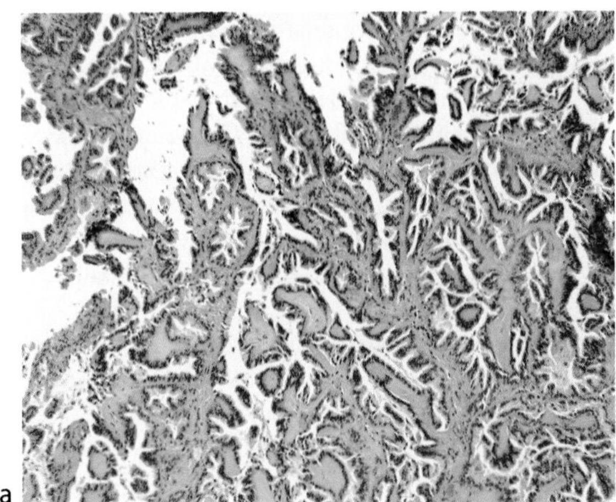
a

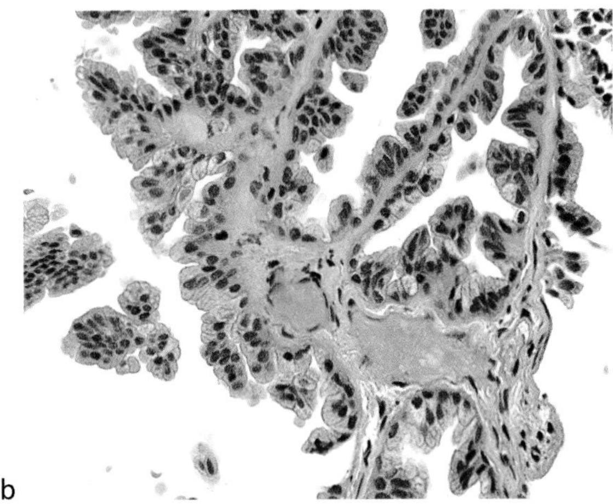
b

Fig. 4.50
Mullerian papilloma. **(a) Papillary projections; (b) papillary projections covered with cuboidal to columnar epithelium**

of loose fibrovascular tissue (*Fig. 4.50a, b*). Cytologic atypia and mitoses are absent. In the past, the lesions were thought to be of mesonephric duct origin, although they have not been encountered in association with mesonephric remnants. Although the histogenesis of these lesions remains uncertain, recent studies favor a Mullerian origin.

Postoperative Spindle Cell Nodule and Inflammatory Pseudotumor

Postoperative spindle cell nodules of the cervix are clinically and histologically identical to their more common counterparts of the vulva and vagina [58, 79]. These lesions may develop after either a cervical biopsy or some other form of trauma. They resemble nodular fasciitis and are composed of actively proliferative spindle cells with oval nuclei arranged in interlacing bundles (➋ Chap. 3, Diseases of the Vagina). The cells may vary slightly in size and mitotic figures are often present. A characteristic feature is the presence of neutrophils and erythrocytes in the lesion, giving it the appearance of granulation tissue.

Inflammatory pseudotumor refers to a lesion closely related to postoperative spindle cell nodule that occurs in the absence of a known history of trauma [3]. Inflammatory pseudotumor is a proliferative process of an unknown etiology with a polymorphic morphology. The lesions contain two cellular components: a fibrohistiocytic component consisting of fibroblasts, myofibroblasts and histiocytes and a polymorphous inflammatory component consisting of lymphocytes and plasma cells. The lesion can be differentiated from other neoplastic processes by the lack of atypia, mitoses, and the presence of a polymorphous inflammatory infiltrate.

Lymphoma-Like Lesions

Lymphoma-like lesions (pseudolymphomas) are marked inflammatory lesions of the cervix, extensive enough to cause confusion with a lymphoproliferative lesion [105]. Lymphoma-like lesions are composed of a superficial band of large lymphoid cells admixed with mature lymphocytes and plasma cells. The lymphoid infiltrates commonly include macrophages and germinal centers, which help to distinguish them from lymphomas. Another feature, which helps to distinguish lymphoma-like lesions from lymphomas, is the superficial localization of the infiltrate. Lymphoma-like lesions rarely infiltrate deeper than 3 mm from the surface epithelium, whereas lymphomas of the cervix usually extend beyond the depth of the endocervical glands (➋ Chap. 6, Carcinoma and Other Tumors of the Cervix).

Heterologous Tissue

Glia

There are 15 recorded cases of neuroglial tissue in the cervix or the endometrium (➋ Chap. 7, Benign Diseases of the Endometrium) [91]. Although the term glioma is used for this condition, the high degree of differentiation of the glial tissue, the absence of mitoses, and the absence of recurrence are against its being neoplastic. The lesion should not be confused with a pure heterologous sarcoma or a teratoma. The neural tissue is believed to represent either implantation of fetal cerebral glia at the time of instrumentation of the gravid uterus or heterotopic maldevelopment during embryogenesis. When the cervix is involved, the lesion usually appears as a polyp that bleeds readily.

Skin

Among the pathologic curiosities of the cervix are cases of true epidermidization of the cervical mucosa. In these instances, sebaceous glands, hair, sweat glands, and occasionally mantle structure are found. The presence of these ectodermal structures, which are normally appendages of the epidermis, on a mucous membrane of mesodermal derivation is difficult to explain. It is conceivable, however, that stratified squamous epithelium under certain circumstances, such as long-standing chronic inflammation or congenital misplacement, can form the appendages of its epidermal analogue [59].

Cartilage

Four cases of heterotopic mature cartilage in the cervix are on record [83]. The finding of these structures alone has no clinical significance. They should not be confused with a malignant mixed mesodermal tumor.

References

1. Abell MR (1971) Papillary adenofibroma of the uterine cervix. Am J Obstet Gynecol 110(7):990–993
2. Abell MR, Gosling JRG (1962) Gland cell carcinoma (adenocarcinoma) of the uterine cervix. Am J Obstet Gynecol 83:729
3. Abenoza P, Shek YH, Perrone T (1994) Inflammatory pseudotumor of the cervix. Int J Gynecol Pathol 13:80–86
4. Agarwal J, Gupta JK (1993) Female genital tuberculosis – a retrospective clinico-pathologic study of 501 cases. Indian J Pathol Microbiol 36(4):389–397
5. Akang EE, Matiluko AA, Omigbodun AO et al (1997) Cervicovaginitis emphysematosa mimicking carcinoma of the cervix: a case report. Afr J Med Med Sci 26(1–2):99–100
6. Al-Nafussi AI, Klys HS, Rebello G et al (1993) The assessment of proliferating cell nuclear antigen (PCNA) immunostaining in the uterine cervix and cervical squamous neoplasia. Int J Gynecol Cancer 3:154–158
7. Baker PM, Clement PB, Bell DA et al (1999) Superficial endometriosis of the uterine cervix: a report of 20 cases of a process that may be

confused with endocervical glandular dysplasia or adenocarcinoma in situ. Int J Gynecol Pathol 18:198–205

8. Berchuck A, Rodriguez G, Kamel A et al (1990) Expression of epidermal growth factor receptor and HER-2/Neu in normal and neoplastic cervix, vulva and vagina. Obstet Gynecol 76:381–387
9. Bhagavan BS, Ruffier J, Shinn B (1982) Pseudoactinomycotic radiate granules in the lower female genital tract: relationship to the Splendore-Hoeppli phenomenon. Hum Pathol 13(10):898–904
10. Brown LJR, Wells M (1986) Cervical glandular atypia associated with squamous intraepithelial neoplasia: a premalignant lesion? J Clin Pathol 39:22–28
11. Burd LI, Easterly JR (1971) Vesicular lesions of the uterine cervix. Am J Obstet Gynecol 110:887–888
12. Cho NH, Kim YT, Kim JW (1997) Correlation between G1 cyclins and HPV in the uterine cervix. Int J Gynecol Pathol 16:339–347
13. Clement PB (1985) Multinucleated stromal giant cells of the uterine cervix. Arch Pathol Lab Med 109:200–202
14. Clement PB, Young RH (1989) Deep Nabothian cysts of the uterine cervix. A possible source of confusion with minimal-deviation adenocarcinoma (adenoma malignum). Int J Gynecol Pathol 8:340–348
15. Concetti H, Retegui M, Perez G et al (2000) Chagas' disease of the cervix uteri in a patient with acquired immunodeficiency syndrome. Hum Pathol 31(1):120–122
16. Coppleson M, Pixley E, Reid B (1971) Colposcopy: a scientific and practical approach to the cervix in health and disease. Charles C. Thomas, Springfield, IL
17. Crum CP, Mitao M, Winkler B et al (1984) Localizing chlamydial infection in cervical biopsies with the immunoperoxidase technique. Int J Gynecol Pathol 3(2):191–197
18. Curtis EM, Pine L (1981) Actinomyces in the vaginas of women with and without intrauterine contraceptive devices. Am J Obstet Gynecol 140(8):880–884
19. Duggan MA (2000) Cytologic and histologic diagnosis and significance of controversial squamous lesions of the uterine cervix. Mod Pathol 13(3):252–60
20. Egan AJ, Russell P (1997) Transitional (urothelial) cell metaplasia of the uterine cervix: morphological assessment of 31 cases. Int J Gynecol Pathol 16(2):89–98
21. Elliott GB, Elliott JDA (1973) Superficial stromal reactions of the lower genital tract. Arch Pathol 95:100–101
22. Evans CS, Goldman RL, Klein HZ et al (1984) Necrobiotic granulomas of the uterine cervix: a probable postoperative reaction. Am J Surg Pathol 8(11):841–844
23. Fand SB (1973) The histochemistry of human cervical epithelium. In: Blandau RJ, Moghissi K (eds) The biology of the cervix. University of Chicago Press, Chicago, IL, pp 103–124
24. Ferenczy A, Richard RM (1974) Female reproductive system: dynamics of scan and transmission electron microscopy. Wiley, New York
25. Ferry JA, Scully RE (1990) Mesonephric remnants, hyperplasia, and neoplasia in the uterine cervix – a study of 49 cases. Am J Surg Pathol 14(12):1100–1111
26. Fetissof F, Serres G, Arbeille B et al (1991) Argyrophilic cells and ectocervical epithelium. Int J Gynecol Pathol 10(2):177–190
27. Fluhmann CF (1961) Focal hyperplasia (tunnel clusters) of the cervix uteri. Obstet Gynecol 17:206–214
28. Fluhmann FC (1961) The cervix uteri and its diseases. W.B. Saunders, Philadelphia, PA
29. Franke WW, Moll R, Achtstaetter T et al (1986) Cell typing of epithelial and carcinomas of the female genital tract using cytoskeletal proteins as markers. In: Peto R, zur Hausen H (eds) Banbury report 21: Viral etiology of cervical cancer. Cold Spring Harbor Laboratory, Cold Spring Harbor, NY
30. Fratini D, Cavaliere A (1996) Papillary adenofibroma of the uterine cervix: a case report. Pathologica 88(2):135–136
31. Fujiwara H, Tortolero-Luna G, Mitchell MF et al (1997) Adenocarcinoma of the cervix: expression and clinical significance of estrogen and progesterone receptors. Cancer 79(3):505–512
32. Gardner HL (1966) Cervical and vaginal endometriosis. Clin Obstet Gynecol 9:358
33. Gardner HL, Fernet P (1964) Etiology of vaginitis emphysematosa. Am J Obstet Gynecol 88:680
34. Gilks CB, Young RH, Clement PB et al (1996) Adenomyomas of the uterine cervix of endocervical type: a report of ten cases of a benign cervical tumor that may be confused with adenoma malignum. Mod Pathol 9(3):220–224
35. Gould PR, Barter RA, Papadimitriou JM (1979) An ultrastructural, cytochemical and autoradiographic study of the mucous membrane of the human cervical canal with reference to subcolumnar cells. Am J Pathol 95:1–16
36. Greeley C, Schroeder S, Silverberg SG (1995) Microglandular hyperplasia of the cervix: a true "pill" lesion? Int J Gynecol Pathol 14(1):50–54
37. Gudson JT (1965) Hemangioma of the cervix. Am J Obstet Gynecol 91:204
38. Hariri J, Ingemanssen JL (1993) Multinucleated stromal giant cells of the uterine cervix. Int J Gynecol Pathol 12:228–234
39. Harnden P, Kennedy W, Andrew AC et al (1999) Immunophenotype of transitional metaplasia of the uterine cervix. Int J Gynecol Pathol 18(2):125–129
40. Hernandez-Rodriguez J, Tan CD, Rodriguez ER et al (2009) Gynecologic vasculitis: an analysis of 163 patients. Medicine (Baltimore) 88(3):169–181
41. Hollowell ML, Goulart RA, Gang DL et al (2007) Cytologic features of mullerian papilloma of the cervix: mimic of malignancy. Diagn Cytopathol 35(9):607–611
42. Holmes KK, Stamm WE (1999) Lower genital tract infections in women. In: Holmes KK, Sparling PF, Mardhet P-A (eds) Sexually transmitted diseases. McGraw-Hill, New York, pp 761–782
43. Hoosen AA, Draper G, Moodley J et al (1990) Granuloma inguinale of the cervix: a carcinoma look-alike. Genitourin Med 66(5):380–382
44. Huffman JW (1948) Mesonephric remnants in the cervix. Am J Obstet Gynecol 56:23–40
45. Ibrahim EM, Blackett AD, Tidy JA et al (1999) CD44 is a marker of endocervical neoplasia. Int J Gynecol Pathol 18:101–108
46. Ismail SM (1991) Cone biopsy causes cervical endometriosis and tubo-endometrioid metaplasia. Histopathol 18(2):107–114
47. Johansson EL, Rudin A, Wassen L et al (1999) Distribution of lymphocytes and adhesion molecules in human cervix and vagina. Immunology 96(2):272–277
48. Johnson CA, Lorenzetti LA, Liese BS et al (1991) Clinical significance of hyperkeratosis on otherwise normal Papanicolaou smears. J Fam Pract 33(4):354–358
49. Johnson LD (1973) Dysplasia and carcinoma in-situ in pregnancy. In: Norris HJ, Hertig AT, Abell MR (eds) The Uterus International Academy of Pathology monographs. Williams & Wilkins, Baltimore, MD, pp 382–412
50. Jonasson JG, Wang HH, Antonioli DA et al (1992) Tubal metaplasia of the uterine cervix: a prevalence study in patients with gynecologic pathologic findings. Int J Gynecol Pathol 11(2):89–95
51. Jones MA (1998) Transitional cell metaplasia and neoplasia in the female genital tract: an update. Adv Anat Pathol 5(2):106–113

52. Jones MA, Young RH (1996) Endocervical type A (noncystic) tunnel clusters with cytologic atypia. A report of 14 cases. Am J Surg Pathol 20:1312–1318
53. Jones MA, Young RH, Scully RE (1991) Diffuse laminar endocervical glandular hyperplasia: a benign lesion often confused with adenoma malignum. Am J Surg Pathol 15:1123–1129
54. Kanai M, Shiozawa T, Xin L et al (1998) Immunohistochemical detection of sex steroid receptors, cyclins, and cyclin-dependent kinases in the normal and neoplastic squamous epithelia of the uterine cervix. Cancer 82(9):1709–1719
55. Karakitsos P, Kyroudes A, Apostolaki C et al (1994) The evaluation of PCNA/cyclin expression in cervical intraepithelial lesions. Gynecol Oncol 55:101–107
56. Kaufman RH, Watts JM, Gardner HL (1969) Pemphigus vulgaris: genital involvement. Report of two cases. Obstet Gynecol 33(2):264–266
57. Kawauchi S, Kusuda T, Liu XP et al (2008) Is lobular endocervical glandular hyperplasia a cancerous precursor of minimal deviation adenocarcinoma?: a comparative molecular-genetic and immunohistochemical study. Am J Surg Pathol 32(12):1807–1815
58. Kay S, Schneider V (1985) Reactive spindle cell nodule of the endocervix simulating uterine sarcoma. Int J Gynecol Pathol 4:255–257
59. Kazakov DV, Mukensnabl P, Kacerovska D et al (2009) Mantle structures in the uterine cervix. Int J Gynecol Pathol 28(6):568–569
60. Konishi I, Fujii S, Nonogaki H et al (1991) Immunohistochemical analysis of estrogen receptors, Ki-67 antigen, and human papillomavirus DNA in normal and neoplastic epithelium of the uterine cervix. Cancer 68:1340–1350
61. Koss LG (1992) Diagnostic cytology and its histopathologic basis. J.B. Lippincott, New York
62. Koss LG (1998) Transitional cell metaplasia. Adv Anat Pathol 5(3):202–203
63. Krantz KE (1973) The anatomy of the human cervix, gross and microscopic. In: Blandau RJ, Moghissi K (eds) The biology of the cervix. University of Chicago Press, Chicago, IL
64. Lane BR, Ross JH, Hart WR et al (2005) Mullerian papilloma of the cervix in a child with multiple renal cysts. Urology 65(2):388
65. Laurtizen AF, Meinecke G (1987) Isolated arteritis of the uterine cervix. Acta Obstet Gynecol Scand 66:659–660
66. Lesack D, Wahab I, Bilks CB (1996) Radiation-induced atypia of endocervical epithelium: a histological, immunohistochemical and cytometric study. Int J Gynecol Pathol 15:242–247
67. Lippes J (1999) Pelvic actinomycosis: a review and preliminary look at prevalence. Am J Obstet Gynecol 180(2 Pt 1):265–269
68. Manickam A, Sivanandham M, Tourkova IL (2007) Immunological role of dendritic cells in cervical cancer. Adv Exp Med Biol 601:155–162
69. McCluggage WG (2007) Immunohistochemistry as a diagnostic aid in cervical pathology. Pathology 39(1):97–111
70. McCluggage WG, Buhidma M, Tang L et al (1996) Monoclonal antibody MIB1 in the assessment of cervical squamous intraepithelial lesions. Int J Gynecol Pathol 15:131–136
71. Mikami Y, Kiyokawa T, Sasajima Y et al (2009) Reappraisal of synchronous and multifocal mucinous lesions of the female genital tract: a close association with gastric metaplasia. Histopathol 54(2): 184–191
72. Miller CJ, McChesney M, Moore PF (1992) Langerhans cells, macrophages and lymphocyte subsets in the cervix and vagina of rhesus macaques. Lab Invest 67(5):628–634
73. Norris HJ, Taylor HB (1966) Polyps of the vagina: a benigh lesion resembling sarcoma botryoides. Cancer 19:226
74. Novotny DB, Maygarden SJ, Johnson DE et al (1992) Tubal metaplasia: a frequent potential pitfall in the cytologic diagnosis of endocervical glandular dysplasia on cervical smears. Acta Cytol 36(1):1–10
75. Nucci MR, Clement PB, Young RH (1999) Lobular endocervical glandular hyperplasia, not otherwise specified: a clinicopathologic analysis of thirteen cases of a distinctive pseudoneoplastic lesion and comparison with fourteen cases of adenoma malignum. Am J Surg Pathol 23(8):886–891
76. Oliva E, Clement PB, Young RH (1995) Tubal and tubo-endometrioid metaplasia of the uterine cervix: unemphasized features that may cause problems in differential diagnosis: a report of 25 cases. Am J Clin Pathol 103(5):618–623
77. Patel DS, Bhagavan BS (1985) Blue nevus of the uterine cervix. Hum Pathol 16:79–86
78. Petitti DB, Yamamoto D, Morgenstern N (1983) Factors associated with actinomyces-like organisms on Papanicolaou smear in users of intrauterine contraceptive devices. Am J Obstet Gynecol 145(3):338–341
79. Proppe KH, Scully RE, Rosai J (1984) Postoperative spindle cell nodules of geniturinary tract resembling sarcomas: a report of eight cases. Am J Surg Pathol 8:101–108
80. Raju GC (1994) Expression of the proliferating cell nuclear antigen in cervical neoplasia. Int J Gynecol Pathol 13(4):337–341
81. Rand RJ, Lowe JW (1998) Schistosomiasis of the uterine cervix. Br J Obstet Gynaecol 105(12):1329–1331
82. Riffenburgh RH, Olson PE, Johnstone PA (1997) Association of schistosomiasis with cervical cancer: detecting bias in clinical studies. East Afr Med J 74(1):14–16
83. Roth E, Taylor HB (1966) Heterotopic cartilage in the uterus. Obstet Gynecol 27:838
84. Saegusa M, Takano Y, Hashimura M et al (1995) The possible role of bcl-2 expression in the progression of tumors of the uterine cervix. Cancer 76(11):2297–2303
85. Schneider V (1981) Arias-stella reaction of the endocervix: frequency and location. Acta Cytol 25(3):224–228
86. Segal GH, Hart WR (1990) Cystic endocervical tunnel clusters: a clinicopathologic study of 29 cases of so-called adenomatous hyperplasia. Am J Surg Pathol 14:895–903
87. Seidman JD, Tavassoli FA (1995) Mesonephric hyperplasia of the uterine cervix: a clinicopathologic study of 51 cases. Int J Gynecol Pathol 14(4):293–299
88. Seltzer V, Sall S, Castadot MJ et al (1979) Glassy cell cervical carcinoma. Gynecol Oncol 8:141–151
89. Shih IM, Kurman RJ (1998) Ki-67 labeling index in the differential diagnosis of exaggerated placental site, placental site trophoblastic tumor, and choriocarcinoma: a double immunohistochemical staining technique using Ki-67 and Mel-CAM antibodies. Hum Pathol 29(1):27–33
90. Shurbaji MS, Brooks SK, Thurmond TS (1993) Proliferating cell nuclear antigen immunoreactivity in cervical intraepithelial neoplasia and benign cervical epithelium. Am J Clin Pathol 100(1):22–26
91. Slavutin L (1979) Uterine gliosis and ossificiation. Am J Diag Gynecol Obstet 1:351
92. Sneeden VD (1958) Mesonephric lesions of the cervix. A practical means of demonstration and a suggestion of incidence. Cancer 11:334–336
93. Sobel JD (1997) Vaginitis. N Engl J Med 337(26):1896–1903
94. Stout AP (1943) Hemangioendothelioma: a tumor of blood vessels featuring vascular endothelial cells. Ann Surg 118:445

95. Sugase M, Moriyama S, Matsukura T (1991) Human papillomavirus in exophytic condylomatous lesions on different female genital regions. J Med Virol 34(1):1–6
96. Suh KS, Silverberg SG (1990) Tubal metaplasia of the uterine cervix. Int J Gynecol Pathol 9(2):122–128
97. ter Harmsel B, Kuijpers J, Smedts F et al (1997) Progressing imbalance between proliferation and apoptosis with increasing severity of cervical intraepithelial neoplasia. Int J Gynecol Pathol 16:205–211
98. Weir MM, Bell DA, Young RH (1997) Transitional cell metaplasia of the uterine cervix and vagina: an underrecognized lesion that may be confused with high-grade dysplasia. A report of 59 cases [see comments]. Am J Surg Pathol 21(5):510–517
99. Witkiewicz AK, Hecht JL, Cviko A et al (2005) Microglandular hyperplasia: a model for the de novo emergence and evolution of endocervical reserve cells. Hum Pathol 36(2):154–161
100. Workowski KA, Berman SM (2006) Sexually transmitted diseases treatment guidelines, 2006. MMWR Recomm Rep; 55(RR-11):1–94
101. Yilmaz AG, Chandler P, Hahm GK et al (1999) Melanosis of the uterine cervix: a report of two cases and discussion pigmented cervical lesions. Int J Gynecol Pathol 18:73–76
102. Young RH, Clement PB (2000) Endocervicosis involving the uterine cervix: a report of four cases of a benign process that may be confused with deeply invasive endocervical adenocarcinoma. Int J Gynecol Pathol 19(4):322–328
103. Young RH, Scully RE (1989) Atypical forms of microglandular hyperplasia of the cervix simulating carcinoma. Am J Surg Pathol 13:50–56
104. Young RH, Harris NL, Scully RE (1985) Lymphoma-like lesions of the lower female genital tract: a report of 16 cases. Int J Gynecol Pathol 4(4):289–299
105. Young RH, Kurman RJ, Scully RE (1988) Proliferations and tumors of intermediate trophoblast of the placental site. Semin Diagn Pathol 5:223–237
106. Zaino RJ (2000) Glandular lesions of the uterine cervix. Mod Pathol 13(3):261–274

5 Precancerous Lesions of the Cervix

Thomas C. Wright · Brigitte M. Ronnett · Robert J. Kurman · Alex Ferenczy

R. J. Kurman, L. Hedrick Ellenson, B. M. Ronnett (eds.), *Blaustein's Pathology of the Female Genital Tract (6th ed.)*, DOI 10.1007/978-1-4419-0489-8_5,

Precursors of Squamous Cell Carcinoma

Terminology and Historical Perspective

The histopathological classification of a disease should reflect both current concepts of its pathogenesis as well as its clinical behavior. Over the last 50 years, our understanding of the pathobiology and behavior of cervical cancer precursors has evolved considerably. As a result, the terminology used to classify preinvasive lesions of the cervix has frequently changed. Although these changes in nomenclature and the resulting lack of a uniform terminology have been an ongoing source of confusion to both gynecologists and pathologists, each change has actually reduced the number of specific pathological categories and has made clinical decision making more straightforward.

The existence of precursor lesions for invasive cervical cancer has been recognized for over a century. As early as 1886, Sir John Williams commented on the presence of noninvasive epithelial abnormalities adjacent to the invasive squamous cell carcinomas of the cervix [198]. The spatial relationships and the histological appearance of these noninvasive epithelial lesions were better described by Cullen in 1900 who recognized that these intraepithelial lesions histologically resembled the adjacent invasive cancers [44]. In the 1930s, Broders reintroduced the term *carcinoma in situ* that was first used by Schottlander and Kermauner to refer to these intraepithelial cervical lesions [24]. A temporal relationship between carcinoma in situ and invasive cancer was subsequently reported by Smith and Pemberton, as well as by Galvin, Jones, and Telinde who diagnosed carcinoma in situ in several patients months to years before the development of invasive cervical cancer [148]. The recognition that there were both a spatial and temporal relationship between carcinoma in situ and invasive squamous cell carcinoma led to the hypothesis that invasive squamous cell carcinoma develops from a histologically well-defined precursor lesion [24]. This hypothesis was subsequently substantiated by long-term follow-up studies, which clearly demonstrated that a significant proportion of untreated patients with carcinoma in situ subsequently develop invasive squamous cell carcinoma [102, 104].

Once it was accepted that carcinoma in situ was a precursor to invasive squamous cell carcinoma, population-based cytological screening programs were begun to detect and treat precursor lesions prior to the actual development of cancer. As large numbers of women began to be screened for cervical disease, it became apparent that many women had cervical epithelial abnormalities that were cytologically/histologically less severe than carcinoma in situ. These lesions formed a histological spectrum that ranged from lesions in which the majority of the cells had the cytological features of carcinoma in situ to those in which the degree of atypicality was much less. The term *dysplasia* was used to refer to this spectrum of cervical abnormalities with features intermediate between those of carcinoma in situ and normal cervical epithelium [157].

The key distinguishing feature of dysplasia was that the atypical cells did not extend through the full thickness of the epithelium or invade the basement membrane. In the cytological nomenclature, dysplasia was considered to be a benign to possibly malignant squamous epithelial atypia, whereas carcinoma in situ was designated as positive for malignant cells.

The separation of noninvasive cervical lesions into two groups, dysplasia and carcinoma in situ, implied that there was a biologic distinction between these two entities and that the two could be reproducibly distinguished from each other. In most centers, dysplasia was considered to be a potentially reversible process and therefore was either ignored, followed, or treated depending on a variety of clinical factors, whereas carcinoma in situ was considered to be a highly significant lesion and patients with this diagnosis were usually treated with hysterectomy. This classification of noninvasive precursor lesions into dysplastic and carcinoma in situ lesions was based solely on arbitrary histological differences that were often quite subtle [28, 103]. In the 1960s, several studies of inter- and intraobserver variability of histological diagnosis demonstrated that pathologists could not reproducibly distinguish between severe dysplasia and carcinoma in situ [41, 100].

A number of studies in the late 1960s suggested that the cellular changes of dysplasia and carcinoma in situ were qualitatively similar and remained constant throughout the histological spectrum. Both dysplasia and carcinoma in situ were found to be monoclonal proliferations of abnormal squamous epithelial cells with an aneuploid nuclear DNA content [65]. On the basis of these descriptive biologic studies, Richart introduced the concept that all types of precursor lesions to squamous cell carcinoma of cervix represented a single disease process that he termed *cervical intraepithelial neoplasia* (CIN) [159].

The CIN terminology divided cervical cancer precursors into three groups: CIN 1 corresponds to lesions previously diagnosed as mild dysplasia, CIN 2 corresponds to moderate dysplasia, and CIN 3 to both severe dysplasia and carcinoma in situ, since pathologists could not reproducibly distinguish between the two. At the time of its introduction, CIN was thought to define a spectrum of histological changes that shared a common etiology, biology, and natural history. Furthermore, the diagnostic term CIN implied that such lesions, if untreated, had a significant, albeit individually unknown risk of developing into invasive carcinoma in the future. As a corollary, it was presumed that when the histological changes of CIN were diagnosed and the lesion adequately treated, the development of invasive cancer could be prevented. The CIN terminology became the most widely used histological terminology for cervical cancer precursors in the 1970s and the 1980s. However, over the last 2 decades, there has been an explosion of information about the etiology of cervical cancer and its precursor lesions. It is now widely accepted that both invasive squamous cell carcinomas and adenocarcinomas of the cervix, as well as their respective precursor lesions, are caused by specific types of high-risk human papillomavirus (HPV) that infect the anogenital tract [213, 214]. Since infection with specific high-risk types of HPV plays a critical role in the development of cervical cancer, a new model of cervical carcinogenesis has been developed (➋ *Fig. 5.1*). This model has three discrete steps: (1) initial infection with a high-risk type of HPV, (2) progression to a histologically defined precursor lesion that requires persistence of the HPV infection, and (3) invasion [167, 176, 209]. Based on this biological model, it is highly unlikely that cervical cancer develops according to a stepwise progression that envisions CIN 1, progressing to CIN 2, to CIN 3, and on to cancer. Moreover, it now appears that the basic premise underlying the CIN terminology is incorrect; the spectrum of histological changes that are referred to as CIN do not represent a single disease process at different stages in its development but instead two distinct biological entities, one a productive viral infection and the other a true neoplastic process confined to the epithelium [202].

Productive HPV infections of the cervical squamous epithelium are self-limited in the majority of patients and commonly result in flat cervical lesions (➋ *Fig. 5.2*) and less frequently in exophytic ones (condylomata acuminata). Flat HPV-associated lesions in which productive viral infection is occurring display cytoplasmic cavitation and nuclear abnormalities. Traditionally, flat and exophytic condylomas were not classified as CIN 1 since they do not have the degree of nuclear atypia usually present in CIN. However, in the 1980s, it was found that the HPV types found in the cervical flat and exophytic condylomas are the same types that can be found in CIN 1 lesions [43]. Moreover, flat condylomas and CIN 1 lesions are similar with respect to their ploidy status [63]. Therefore, both exophytic and flat condylomatous lesions of the cervix were combined into the CIN 1 category. These lesions have been designated in the past as *koilocytotic atypia*, *koilocytosis*, or *flat condyloma*.

The other entity subsumed within the morphologic CIN spectrum is histologically "high grade." High-grade

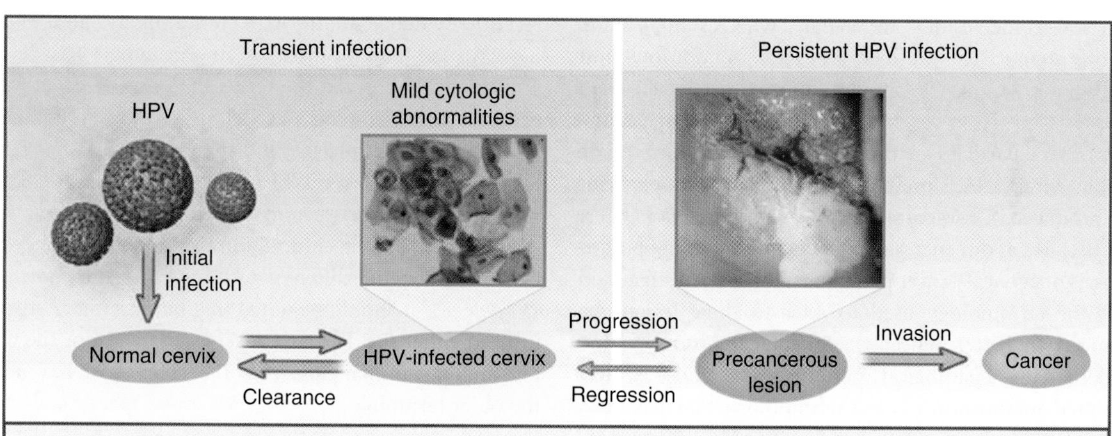

The three steps of cervical carcinogenesis.

The steps can be conceptualized as infection with specific high-risk types of human papillomavirus (HPV), progression to a precancerous lesion, and invasion, HPV infections are usually transient and are often associated with mild cytologic abnormalities. Persistent infection with high-risk types of HPV is uncommon and is required for progression.

Fig. 5.1
Steps in the development of cervical cancer. **Three steps in cervical carcinogenesis (Used with permission from [209])**

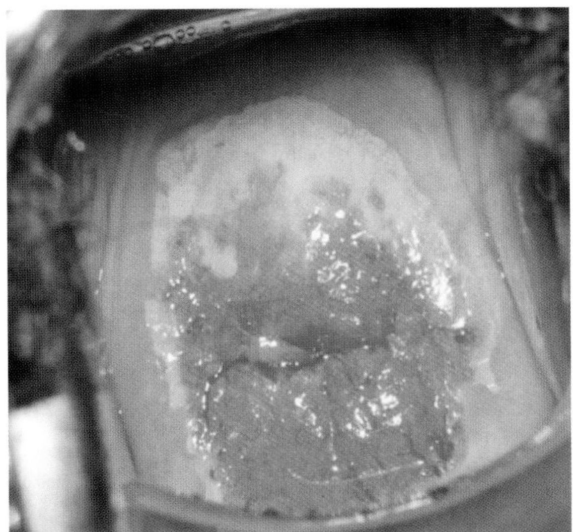

Fig. 5.2
Flat HPV-associated cervical lesion. **This flat white lesion seen after the application of a weak solution of acetic acid represents productive HPV infection of the cervix**

lesions are frequently aneuploid and represent true intraepithelial neoplasia with a potential to progress to invasive squamous cell carcinoma if left untreated. They are composed of proliferating basal-type atypical cells with a high nuclear : cytoplasmic ratio and have been designated *moderate dysplasia, severe dysplasia, carcinoma in situ*, or *CIN 2* or *3*. There is a common misconception that low-grade lesions are "viral," whereas high-grade lesions are not. The prevalence of HPV in both low- and high-grade lesions is similar, approximately 80–90% [36, 37, 175]. However, in low-grade lesions, large numbers of viral particles are produced, whereas in high-grade lesions, viral DNA is present, but infectious viral particles are produced in comparatively lower amounts, *Fig. 5.3*.

Because of our increased understanding of the pathogenesis of cervical cancer precursors, it has been suggested that the terminology used to refer to these lesions be changed to better reflect the biological processes that underlie the histological patterns. The most widely accepted modification is the terminology that has been incorporated into the Bethesda System (TBS) of cytological diagnosis. This terminology uses the term *low-grade squamous intraepithelial lesion* (LSIL) for lesions previously classified as koilocytotic atypia and CIN 1 and *high-grade squamous intraepithelial lesion* (HSIL) for lesions previously called CIN 2 and CIN 3 [116, 177]. For histopathological reporting, it has been suggested that the terms LSIL and HSIL also be used [205]. Therefore, in this chapter, we have adopted the use of the Bethesda Terminology for reporting cytopathology and the terms LSIL (CIN 1) and HSIL (CIN 2, 3) for histopathology. The rationale for adapting the two-tiered terminology for histopathology is the same as for using a two-tiered terminology for cytology. First, LSIL (previously referred to as CIN 1) represents a biologically distinct group compared to HSIL (previously referred to as CIN 2 and CIN 3). HSIL are heterogeneous with respect to associated HPV types, clonality, ploidy, and loss of heterozygosity (LOH) at specific chromosomal loci, whereas HSIL are homogeneous with respect to these parameters. Moreover, the natural history of LSIL is characterized by higher rates of spontaneous regression and lower rates of progression than compared to HSIL. In our opinion, using the term "lesion" rather than "neoplasia" better reflects the natural history of these histopathological entities, since the majority of CIN are histologically low grade and represent self-limited HPV infections that will spontaneously resolve in the absence of therapy. "Intraepithelial lesion" better describes these low-grade viral infections than does the term "intraepithelial neoplasia." It must be emphasized that different terminologies are currently in use by different pathology laboratories. Although many laboratories in the USA have switched to the two-tiered or modified CIN terminology, some continue to utilize the original three-tiered CIN terminology and some even utilize the terms dysplasia and carcinoma in situ. This is expected to change over the next several years since the World Health Organization (WHO) recently switched to the CIN terminology, and in the new Armed Forces Institute of Pathology Fasicle on Tumors of the Cervix, the terms LSIL and HSIL are utilized for histopathology, as well as cytology [107, 196]. However, some clinicians find the use of LSIL and HSIL for both cytology and histology somewhat confusing since distinction between cytologically and histologically diagnosed lesions is clinically important [202]. Correlations between the different terminologies are shown in *Table 5.1*. It should be noted that because older studies utilized either the dysplasia/carcinoma in situ or the CIN terminology, in many places in this chapter we have used the older terminology.

General Features

Prevalence

SIL is predominantly a disease of women in their reproductive years, with a large population impact and risk

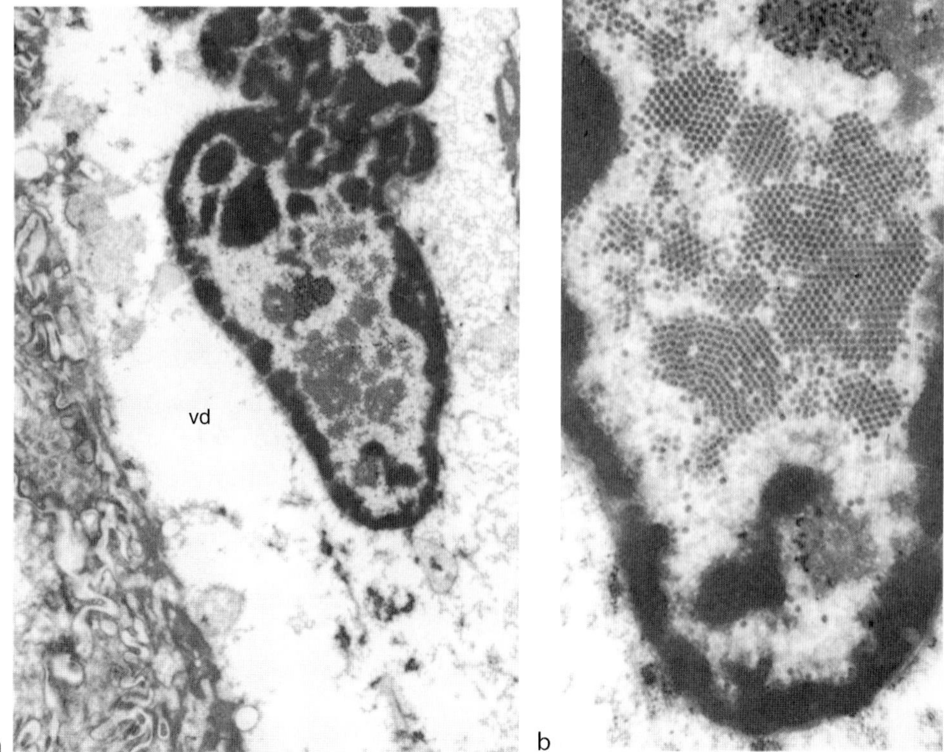

Fig. 5.3
HPV-infected cells. **Electron microscopy of cells productively infected with HPV. (a) There are intranuclear aggregates of HPV in a koilocytotic, superficial cell of an HSIL. The marginated nuclear chromatin is agglutinated, and the cytoplasmic substance displays vacuolar degeneration (vd). The latter corresponds to koilocytotic ballooning on light microscopy. (b) Higher magnification of HPV particles in the nucleus**

Table 5.1
Terminologies for cervical cancer precursor lesions

Older classification	WHO[a] classification	Bethesda system terminology
Mild dysplasia	CIN 1	Low-grade squamous intraepithelial lesion (LSIL)
Moderate dysplasia	CIN 2	High-grade squamous intraepithelial lesion (HSIL)
Severe dysplasia/ Carcinoma in situ	CIN 3	HSIL

[a]World Health Organization.
CIN, cervical intraepithelial lesion

factors characteristic of a sexually transmitted disease (STD). The prevalence of SIL in different countries and populations within a country varies widely depending on the underlying risk factors in the population and the extent of cytological screening. Although SIL is not a reportable disease, good estimates of the prevalence of cytologic abnormalities in women undergoing screening in the USA are available from a number of sources. One of the most comprehensive surveys is the College of American Pathologists (CAP) "Q-Probes" study that compiles rates of cytological abnormalities diagnosis from over 300 U.S. cytology laboratories. According to this survey, in 2003 the mean reporting rate of LSIL was 2.6% and it was 0.7% for HSIL [47]. Age has a profound impact on both the rate of detection of cytological abnormalities as well as the histologically confirmed SIL lesions. In the Kaiser Permanente health plan, the highest rate of LSIL is in adolescents between 15 and 19 years of age [84]. Almost 4% of Papanicolaou tests (Pap tests) obtained from adolescents enrolled in the Kaiser Permanente health plan were diagnosed as LSIL. The LSIL rate drops with an increasing age and was only approximately 1% in women 25–40 years of age and was much lower in women over the age of 40 years. In contrast, the rate of HSIL increases up until 25–29 years and then decreases, ➋ *Fig. 5.4*. In the recent quadrivalent HPV vaccine trial, the prevalence of LSIL on enrollment cytology in the North American participants 16–26 years of age (mean age 20 years) was 6.2% and the prevalence of HSIL was 0.5% (Barr 2008). The same impact of age as is seen with cytological abnormalities is also found for histologically diagnosed LSIL and HSIL lesions in Kaiser, ➋ *Fig. 5.5* [84]. The peak age for the diagnosis of HSIL is 25–29 years of age. Another large national program that compiles statistics of cytological abnormalities among women in the USA is the National Breast and Cervical Cancer Early Detection Program (NBCCEDP). The overall rate of cytological abnormalities in this program between 1995 and 1998 was 2.3% and 0.8% for LSIL and HSIL, respectively [12]. In this program, the rates of histologically identified LSIL and HSIL are highest in women under the age of 30 years. Rates tend to increase up until the age of 30 years and then begin to decrease, with lowest rates in women 60 years and older [12, 166]. In contrast, the rate of histologically confirmed invasive cervical cancer reported in the U.S. Surveillance Epidemiology and End Results (SEER) cancer registry increases until 40 years of age and then shows only minimal changes through 65 years of age, ➋ *Fig. 5.6* [192]. After the age of 65 years, there is a minimal decline. It is also important to note that during the 1970s–1990s that the rates of HSIL appear to have increased both in Western Europe and the USA. In Iceland, for example, the rate of detection of HSIL in women 20–24 years of age increased almost fourfold from 1979–1983 to 1994–1998 and then leveled out, ➋ *Fig. 5.7* [173]. In women 25–29 years of age, it almost doubled during this time period and then appears to have begun to decrease.

Etiology

Epidemiologic studies have documented that the major risk factors for cervical cancer are infection with specific

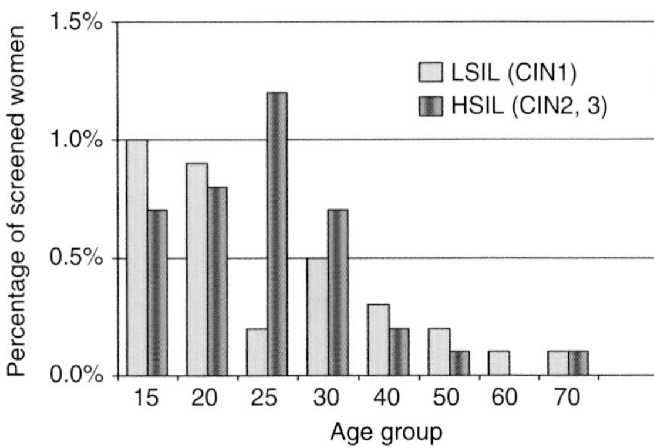

Fig. 5.5
Impact of age on histologically confirmed SIL. **The data come from Kaiser Northern California (Modified from [84])**

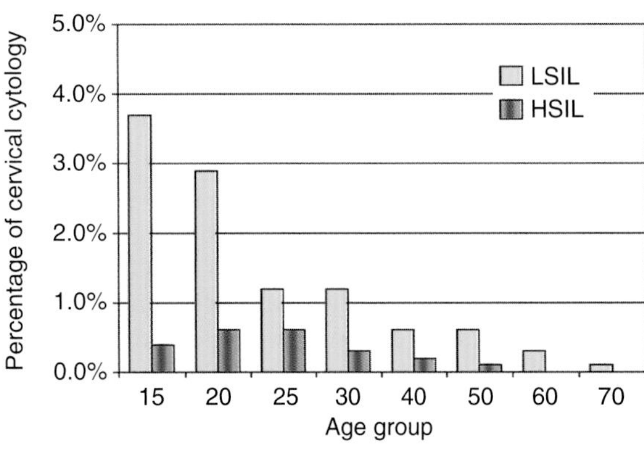

Fig. 5.4
Impact of age on cytological abnormalities. **The data come from Kaiser Northern California (Modified from [84])**

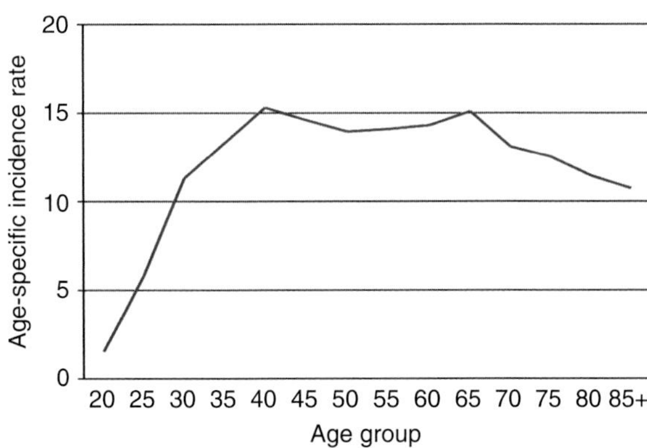

Fig. 5.6
Incidence of cervical cancer in the USA. **The impact of age on the incidence of cervical cancer is derived from surveillance data from the National Cancer Institutes' Surveillance Epidemiology and End Results (SEER) cancer registry (Modified from [192])**

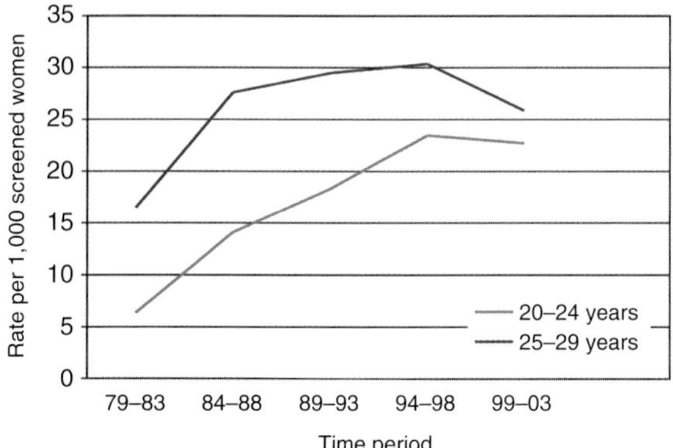

Fig. 5.7
Changes in detection of HSIL in Iceland between 1979 and 1998 (Modified from [173])

Table 5.2
Risk factors associated with SIL in various epidemiological studies

Risk factors
Sexual activity
Number of sexual partners
Early sexual activity (especially less than 16 years of age)
Sexually transmitted diseases
Human papillomavirus
Herpes simplex virus
Chlamydia trachomatis
Early age of first pregnancy
Parity
Low socioeconomic class
Cigarette smoking
Human immunodeficiency virus
Immunosuppression from any cause
Vitamin deficiencies
Interval since last Pap smear
Oral contraceptive use

SIL, squamous intraepithelial lesion

high-risk types of HPV and a lack of cervical cancer screening, *Table 5.2*. Other risk factors that have classically been associated with cervical cancer play a much less important role. Among women infected with high-risk types of HPV, other factors such as smoking, immunosuppression, and long-term use of oral contraceptives can result in a doubling or tripling of risk for HSIL and invasive cancer [167]. The mechanisms of action of any of the risk factors other than infection with high-risk types of HPV and lack of cervical cancer screening are not understood.

Human Papillomaviruses

In the late 1970s, based on theoretical considerations, Dr. Harald zur Hausen suggested that there might be an association between HPV and cervical cancer, an achievement for which he received the Nobel Prize in Medicine in 2008 [212, 214]. A large number of epidemiological, clinicopathological, and molecular studies subsequently linked the presence of specific types of HPV to the development of anogenital cancers and their precursors and it is now accepted that high-risk HPVs play a critical role in the pathogenesis of most cervical cancers and their precursor lesions [83].

Classification of HPV and Association with Specific Types of Anogenital Lesions

Papillomaviruses are classified as members of the family Papillomaviridae [83]. They are double-standard DNA tumor viruses that have a double-stranded DNA genome of approximately 8,000 base pairs in length, a non-enveloped virion that measures 45 to 55 nm in diameter, and an icosahedral capsid composed of 72 capsomers. They are widely distributed throughout nature. There are bovine, canine, avian, rabbit, deer, and human papillomaviruses. They are all highly species-specific viruses that infect only one species. Within a given species, many types and subtypes of papillomaviruses may exist. Unlike many other viruses in which specific viral isolates have capsid proteins with different antigenic structures, the capsid proteins of papillomavirus are highly conserved and antibodies directed against BPV capsid proteins cross-react with human papillomaviruses [90]. Therefore, DNA sequence is used to classify different viral types (genotypes). The classification of papillomaviruses is based on phylogenetic algorithms that compare either the whole viral genomic sequence or specific subgenomic segments. To date, the phylogenetic classification of papillomaviruses includes 118 distinct types, *Fig. 5.8* [50]. The human papillomaviruses are included in the genus alpha-papillomavirus and consists of a number of closely related groupings referred to as species or clades. The most important of these are the A9 clade that has HPV 16 as the prototypic virus and the A7 clade that includes HPV 18 and 45. The genetic sequence of papillomaviruses is quite stable and changes in molecular sequence through either mutation or recombination appears to be quite uncommon [191]. For example, there are three distinct lineages

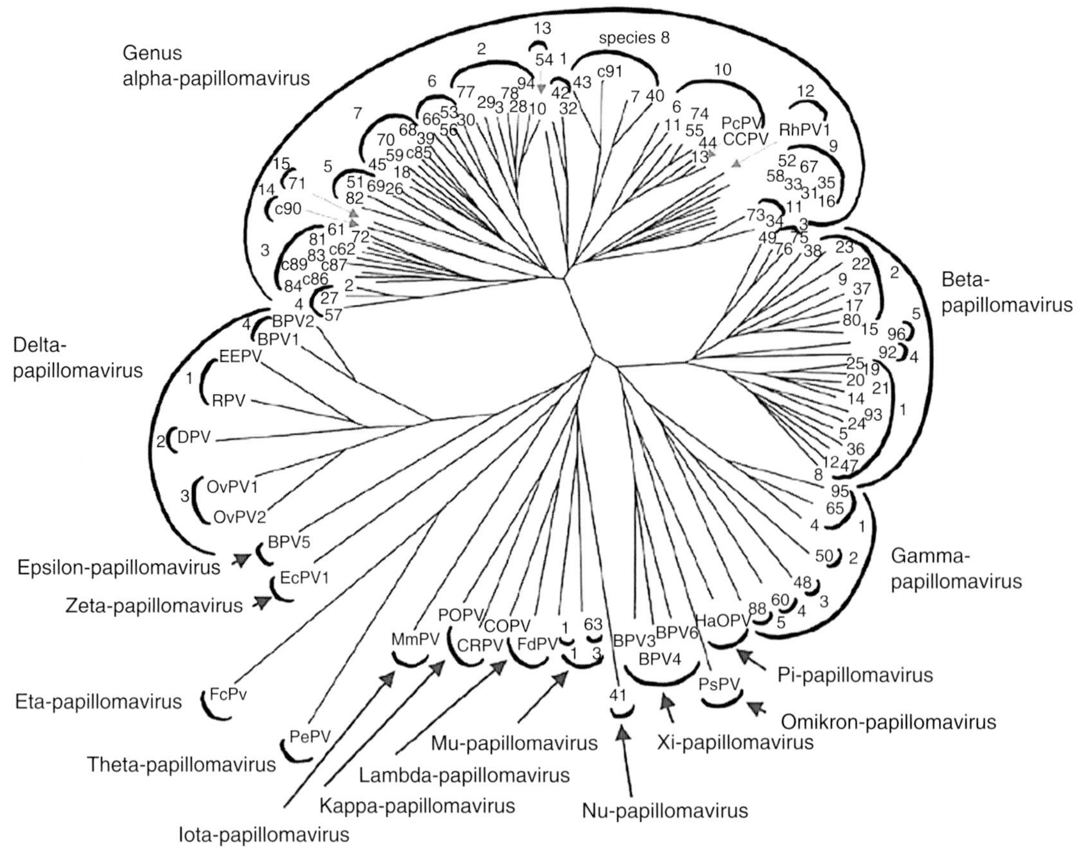

Fig. 5.8

Phylogenetic classification of papillomaviruses. **Based on their DNA sequence, papillomaviruses can be group in closely related clusters or clades (Used with permission from [50])**

of HPV 18 variants and these appear to have diverged about the time *Homo sapiens* began establishing residence in difference continents [14]. Over 118 types of papillomaviruses have been molecularly cloned and sequenced and more than 120 putative novel types have been partially characterized [83]. Although the different types of HPV are quite similar structurally, they have significant specificity with regard to the anatomic location of the epithelia that they infect and the type of lesions that they produce at the site of infection. In addition to types, there also are subtypes or variants of specific types, such as HPV 16. In order to be considered a subtype or variant, a virus must differ by 2–5% from the original isolate. Different subtypes of HPV 16 have been shown to have different biological potential and specific variants appear more likely to be associated with invasive cervical cancers than others [48].

Papillomaviruses are epitheliotropic viruses that predominantly infect skin and mucous membranes and produce characteristic epithelial proliferations at the sites of infection. These benign epithelial proliferations or papillomas have the capacity to undergo malignant transformation under certain circumstances. Examples of this in animals include the papillomas induced in domestic rabbits by the cottontailed rabbit papillomavirus (CRPV) that can progress to invasive squamous cell carcinomas when treated with topical applications of methylcholanthrene and alimentary tract papillomas induced in cattle by bovine papillomavirus (BPV), which undergo malignant transformation when the animals eat radiomimetic bracken ferns. In humans, HPV infections occur on the skin and mucous membranes, on the conjunctiva, oral cavity, larynx, tracheobronchial tree, esophagus, bladder, anus, and genital tract of both sexes. HPVs appear to be

Table 5.3

Oncogenic risk of common types of anogenital human papillomavirus

Low oncogenic risk[a]	6, 11, 42, 43, 44, 53
High oncogenic risk	16, 18, 31, 33, 35, 39, 45, 51, 52, 56, 58, 59, 66
Unclear oncogenic risk	26, 68, 73, 82

[a]For cervical cancer

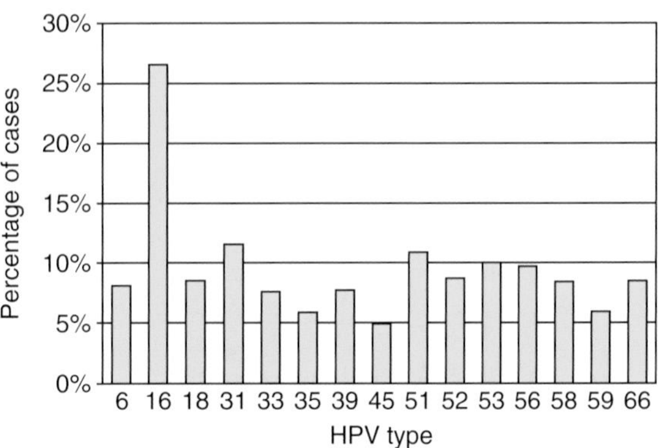

Fig. 5.9

Prevalence of anogenital HPV types in LSIL (Modified from [36])

fastidious in their growth requirements and replicate only in the nucleus of infected cells. In addition to being species specific, papillomaviruses are also relatively tissue- and site specific.

More than 40 types of HPV can infect the anogenital tract. The most commonly encountered ones are shown in *Table 5.3*. Based on their associations with cervical and anogenital cancers, 13 anogenital HPVs have been classified by the International Agency for Research on Cancer (IARC) as oncogenic. These are HPV 16, 18, 31, 33, 35, 39, 45, 51, 52, 56, 58, 59, and 66 [83]. Others also consider HPV types 68 and 82 to be oncogenic [135]. HPV types 6 and 11, which are the two types most commonly found in association with condyloma acuminata, are not implicated in the development of cervical cancer, but are associated with squamous cell carcinomas of the larynx and various carcinomas of the vulva, penis, and anus [83].

More than 80% of SIL lesions are found to be associated with HPV when sensitive molecular methods are used to detect HPV DNA. LSIL can be associated with any of the anogenital types identified in women in the general population. A meta-analysis of HPV types identified in women with either cytologically identified LSIL or histologically diagnosed LSIL lesions found that HPV was detected in 80% of LSIL from North America and approximately 70% for LSIL from other regions of the world [36, 37]. This difference most likely is due to regional differences in how lesions are diagnosed. HPV 16 was the most common genotype, being found in 26% of HPV positive cases, *Fig. 5.9*. HPV types 31, 51, and 53 were the next most commonly identified types, each being identified in approximately 10–12% of lesions. HPV 16 was less likely to be found in lesions from Africa and HPV 18 was more common in lesions from North America than in lesions from Europe or Latin America. All of the associations are complicated by the fact that multiple types of HPV are frequently found in association with low-grade lesions.

In contrast to LSIL, most studies have found that almost half of HSIL are associated with HPV 16. The prevalence of HPV 16 in cytologically identified HSIL and histologically diagnosed HSIL in studies from different areas of the globe range from 30% to 70% [36, 175]. A recent meta-analyses of the distribution of HPV in HSIL has concluded that HPV 16 is identified in 45.3% of the lesions, HPV 18 in 6.9% and HPV 31 in 8.6%, *Fig. 5.10a* [175]. HPV 16 and 18 were found in 52% of the HSIL lesions. HPV types 31, 33, 58, and 52 are the next most common types found in HSIL. Multiple types of HPV are less commonly found in HSIL than in LSIL.

The distribution of HPV types in invasive cervical cancers shows an even stronger enrichment for HPV 16 and 18 that is observed in women with HSIL, *Fig. 5.10b*. HPV 16 and 18 are found in approximately 70% of invasive cervical cancers worldwide [175]. HPV 31, 33, 35, and 45 are each found in 3–4% of cervical cancers [175]. None of the other high-risk types are found in association with more than 2.5% of cervical cancers and most are found in less than 1%. As with HSIL, multiple HPV types are rarely found in association with invasive cervical cancers.

Genomic Organization of HPV

The genomic organization of the different types of HPV appears to be similar, *Fig. 5.11*. The viral genome can be divided into three regions: an upstream regulatory region (also referred to as the long control region or LCR), the early region, and the late region. The LCR is a noncoding region of the viral genome that is important in regulating viral replication and transcription of downstream sequences in the early region. The early region is

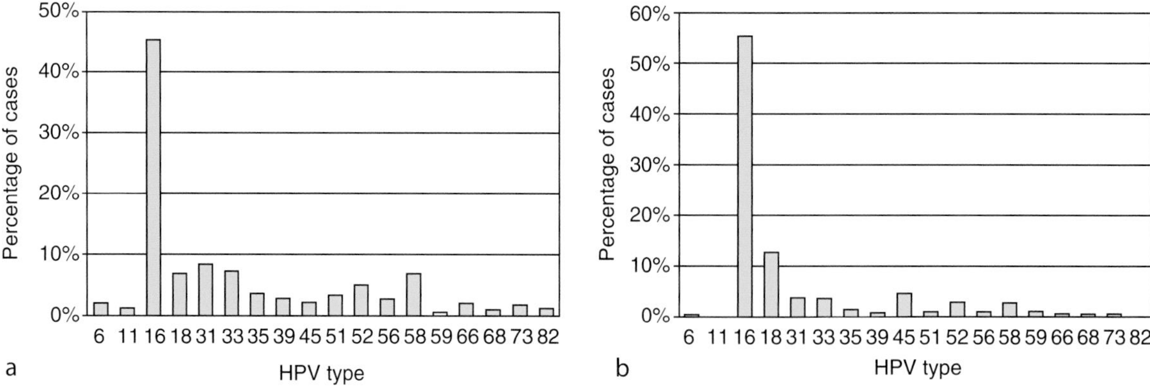

Fig. 5.10
Prevalence of anogenital HPV types. **(a) HSIL. (b) Invasive cervical cancer (Modified from [175])**

transcribed early in the viral life cycle (hence its name) and encodes predominately for proteins that are important in viral replication, whereas the late region encodes for viral structural proteins that are produced late in the viral life cycle.

The early region open reading frames (ORFs) encode for proteins required for viral replication and maintenance of a high viral copy number in infected cells [52]. The early region also includes the transforming regions of the HPV genome: E5, E6, and E7. The E6 and E7 ORFs encode the major transforming genes of HPV [213]. The E5 ORF encodes a protein with weak transforming capacity. Both, the E6 and E7 proteins are small zinc-binding proteins that lack endogenous enzymatic activity and exert their transforming activity through binding to cell regulatory proteins. E6 can bind to p53 and results in rapid proteolytic degradation of p53 through an ubiquitin-dependent pathway, thus blocking apoptosis. E7 binds to the retinoblastoma (Rb) gene product, as well as other "Rb-like proteins." Binding of E7 to Rb blocks the cell proliferation inhibiting function of these endogenous tumor suppressors. E7 can also activate cyclins A and E as well as block the cell proliferation inhibiting functions of WAF-1 and p27, two cyclin-dependent kinase inhibitors. The end result of overexpression of E6 and E7 within cells is unrestricted cell proliferation and a blockage of apoptosis.

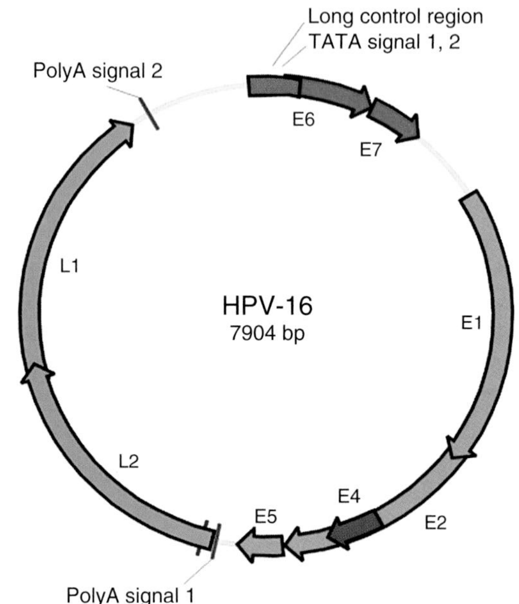

Fig. 5.11
Genomic organization of HPV. **HPV is a double-stranded, circular, DNA tumor virus whose genome can be divided into three regions: the upstream regulatory region (URR), the early region, and the late region**

The late region of HPV is downstream of the early region and contains two ORFs termed L1 and L2 that encode capsid proteins. The L1-encoded protein is the major capsid protein and is highly conserved among papillomaviruses from all species. The L2-encoded protein is a minor capsid protein that is much more variable among viral types. Transcription from the L1 and L2 ORFs occurs as a late event in the viral life cycle at a time when infectious virus is being produced. L1 capsid proteins produced in in vitro culture systems are capable of associating and forming viral-like particles (VLPs) that are similar to native virions, but lack the viral genome. VLPs composed of L1 capsid proteins have recently been introduced as prophylactic HPV vaccines.

Life Cycle of HPV

Although the HPV life cycle is not completely characterized, the rough outlines of the process are known, ➋ *Fig. 5.12* [167, 176]. The initial site of infection is thought to be either basal cells or primitive "basal-like" cells of the immature squamous epithelium that HPV reaches presumably through defects in the epithelium. Localization in the basal layer may be due to the presence of specific receptors for HPV on the basal cells. Once HPV enters into the basal cells, it can exist within the cells in two distinct biological states. One is as a nonproductive infection in which HPV DNA continues to reside in the basal cells, but infectious virions are not produced. In the literature, nonproductive HPV infections have frequently been referred to as *latent infections.* Usually in nonproductive latent infections a small number of copies of the HPV genome remain in the nucleus in a free circular form called an *episome.* Replication of the episomal DNA in latent infections is tightly coupled to the replication of the epithelial cells and only occurs in concert with replication of the host cell's chromosomal DNA. Since complete viral particles are presumably not produced in latent infections, the characteristic cellular effects of a HPV infection are not present and HPV can only be identified using molecular methods. Latently infected epithelium displays no morphologic abnormality. Thus, latent infection is used to characterize HPV infections in which there is no gross or microscopic evidence of a HPV-induced epithelial lesion, and the virus is present at such low copy number in the epithelium that it cannot be detected with routine molecular detection methods.

The other form of HPV infection is *a productive viral infection.* In productive viral infections, viral DNA replication occurs independently of host chromosomal DNA synthesis. This independent viral DNA replication produces large amounts of viral DNA and results in infectious virions. Viral DNA replication takes place predominantly

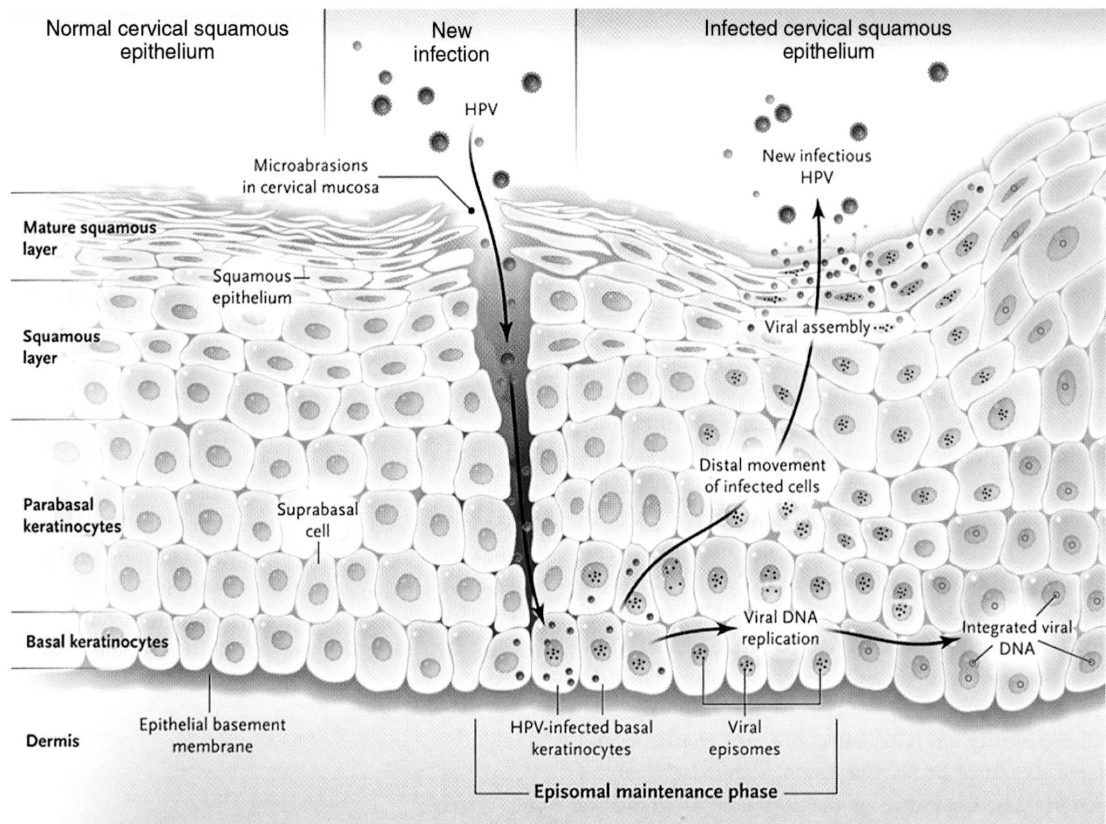

■ Fig. 5.12

HPV life cycle (Source: Kahn JA (2009) HPV vaccination for the prevention of cervical intraepithelial neoplasia (CIN). N Engl J Med 361:273)

in the intermediate and superficial cell layers of the stratified squamous epithelium. As the virally infected epithelial cells mature and move toward the epithelial surface, cell-derived, differentiation-specific transcriptional factors produced by the epithelium stimulate the production of viral capsid proteins. This allows large amounts of intact virions to be formed and produces the characteristic virally associated effects of HPV that can be detected both cytologically and histologically, ➋ *Fig. 5.13a, b*. These viral-associated effects include acanthosis, cytoplasmic vacuolization, koilocytosis, multinucleation, and nuclear atypia.

Epidemiology of HPV Infections

Anogenital HPV infections are primarily transmitted by direct skin-to-skin or mucosa-to-mucosa contact. Based on prevalence studies among both men and women in the population, it appears that although sexual intercourse is the most common route of infection, intercourse is not required for transmission [27]. The efficiency of transmission during sexual intercourse is unknown, but clearly quite high with some estimates indicating a 40% transmission risk per act of intercourse [27]. Infection with multiple types of HPV is seen in 20–30% of infected young men and women. Condom use reduces but does not eliminate the risk of transmission to women. It also appears that male circumcision reduces transmission and carriage of HPV [199].

Most women become infected with HPV within several years of initiating sexual activity [25, 200]. Cumulative exposure is difficult to measure because most infections are transient and relatively short-lived, and serology is an insensitive indicator of exposure since many infected women do not produce measurable levels of antibody [78]. However, prospective follow-up studies of female college students report that after 5 years of follow-up 80% have been infected at some point with HPV [200]. Follow-up studies indicate that a frequent pattern of infection in sexually active young women is multiple serial infections with different types of HPV with each infectious episode being of relatively short duration [25].

The majority of HPV infections are transient and undergo clearance or become latent within 1–2 years of detection [27]. Clearance or development of latency is presumed to be mediated by cell-mediated immunity. High oncogenic risk HPV infections tend to clear more slowly than those caused by low oncogenic HPV types. After an infection has been persistent for 36 months, the potential for future clearance diminishes considerably [167]. Moreover, the longer an infection persists, the greater the likelihood that a high-grade precursor lesion will develop [167]. Therefore, infections caused by high

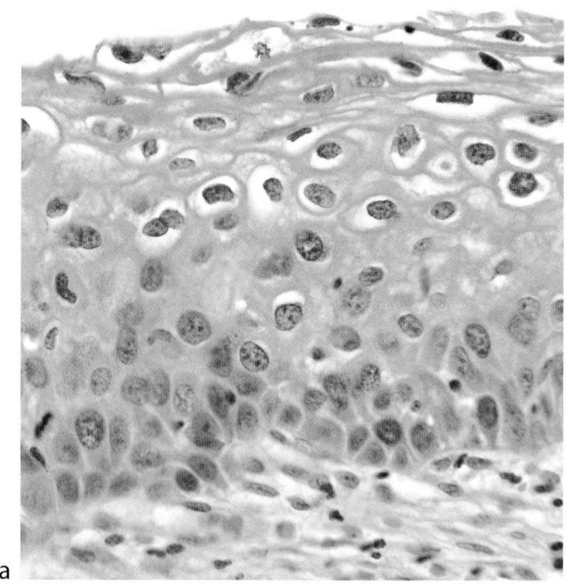

a

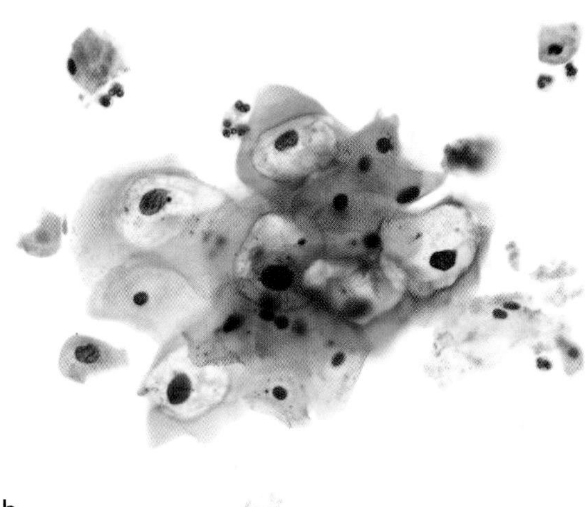

b

Fig. 5.13
Cytopathic effects of HPV. **The cytopathic effects of HPV include nuclear enlargement, nuclear pyknosis or hyperchromaticity, anisocytosis, multinucleation, and perinuclear cytoplasmic vacuolization. (a) Histological features of a lesion is classified LSIL. (b) Cytological features of LSIL**

oncogenic risk HPV infections that persist for two or more years pose the greatest risk to women since these are the infections that may progress to a high-grade cervical cancer precursor or even an invasive cervical cancer. Approximately 10% of HPV infections will persist for two or more years. Long-term prospective cohort studies have demonstrated that in some women, HPV infections that have appeared to have cleared can reappear. Moreover, follow-up studies of HIV-infected women show a strong relationship between increasing levels of immune suppression and detection of HPV [204]. This suggests that in many instances women who appear to have cleared HPV infections actually harbor latent HPV infections in which the virus remains in the epithelium at a low copy number. The combination of multiple anogenital types of HPV, all of which appear to be highly transmissible in sexually active populations, combined with the transient nature of most infections explains the prevalence of HPV in the population. Prevalence of high-risk HPV DNA positivity is high in women with normal cytology in their late teens and 20s and drops with increasing age, ➲ *Fig. 5.14* [46]. Reactivity of latent infections could explain the slight increase in HPV prevalence seen in postmenopausal women [49]. Developmental status of the country of residence also appears to be important [49]. The reasons for the increased HPV prevalence in less-developed countries are unknown, but many relate to sexual practices and poor hygienic conditions, as well as an increase in burden of comorbid disease in the population.

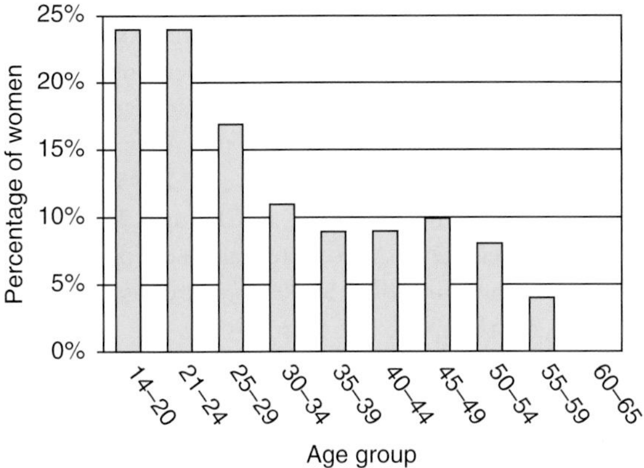

◻ Fig. 5.14
Prevalence of high-risk HPV DNA in women with normal cytology in the USA. This data come from a large, CDC surveillance survey (Modified from [46])

Development of Cervical Disease After HPV Infection

About one-third of the HPV DNA positive women will have a cytological abnormality [167]. The cumulative incidence of minor cytological abnormalities in HPV-infected women with initial normal cytology is 25–50% within 1–2 years. The risk of a cytological abnormality declines to baseline level in the population by 4 years [34, 131]. Risk factors for HPV persistence and the subsequent development of HSIL are not yet well characterized; however, HPV type is clearly important. HPV 16 infections are especially oncogenic and the cumulative risk for HSIL approaches 40% in women with persistent HPV infections for 3–5 years. Risk for HSIL is increased in women who are infected with multiple types of HPV, but this may simply reflect the sum of the risks for each individual type [197]. Risks of persistence and subsequent development of HSIL are also increased for HIV-infected and other immunosuppressed women [204].

In light of our current understanding of the pathogenesis of SIL, it would be expected that LSIL would be frequently multicellular in origin, since it develops within a field of latently infected cervical epithelium and frequently is associated with multiple types of HPV. In contrast, HSIL is typically associated with only a single type of HPV, is frequently aneuploid, and may contain integrated HPV DNA. Therefore, HSIL would be expected to be unicellular in origin. Studies that have utilized PCR-based detection methods to identify X-chromosome linked genetic markers have shown that SIL can be either monoclonal or polyclonal. Park et al. analyzed clonality by evaluating inactivation of the human androgen receptor gene that is located in the X-chromosome [144]. They found that LSIL associated with low-risk HPV types are typically polyclonal, whereas LSIL associated with high-risk HPV types are typically monoclonal, as are almost all HSIL. This indicates that LSIL associated with low risk or novel types of HPV are biologically different at their inception from lesions that are histologically low grade, but associated with high-risk HPV types. This conclusion is supported by studies that have determined the rates of regression, persistence, and progression of CIN 1 and CIN 2 lesions have found that 83% of monoclonal lesions progress or persist, whereas 64% of polyclonal lesions regress [189]. Other studies that have looked at LOH at specific chromosomal loci have found that a relatively small proportion of LSIL have LOH, but frequent LOH in HSIL [35, 108].

There is no unanimous opinion on the cellular origin of SIL. Three cellular sites of origin have been proposed: basal cells of the squamous epithelium of the portio, basal cells of the transformation zone epithelium, and reserve cells of the endocervix [91]. Most SIL begins at the squamocolumnar junction of the transformation zone, with one edge of the lesion bordering the endocervical columnar epithelium. Only about 10% of SIL will involve the endocervical canal without involving the squamocolumnar junction [1]. In general, the portion of SIL on the exocervical portio surface is low grade, whereas the portion of SIL that extends into the endocervical canal is high grade, *Fig. 5.15*. From these observations, it is now thought that most SIL arises in the basal cells of the transformation zone epithelium that is formed by the coalescence of squamous metaplastic epithelium with native squamous epithelium.

The subsequent development of invasive cervical cancer in persistently infected women appears to take a decade or more since the peak prevalence of HPV infection in the population is in the late teens/early 20s, whereas cervical cancer incidence in the unscreened populations plateaus from around 35–55 years of age. High-grade cervical cancer precursors are consistently more common than are invasive cervical cancers in the unscreened populations, suggesting that only a minority of high-grade precursors develop the capacity to become invasive cancers [80]. Long-term follow-up studies of untreated or partially treated HSIL have found that 30–50% progress to invasive cancer over a 30-year follow-up period [125].

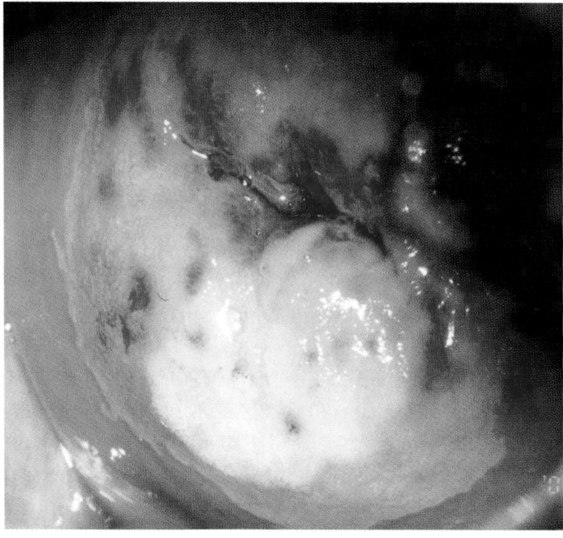

Fig. 5.15
Distribution of SIL on the cervix. **When both HSIL and LSIL are present on the cervix, the HSIL generally develops internally to the LSIL. It is much more likely that HSIL will extend into the endocervical canal**

Other Risk Factors

It should be stressed that although infection with specific high-risk types of HPV is necessary for the development of invasive cervical cancer, it is not sufficient for the development of cervical cancer. The long latency between the initial exposure to HPV and the development of cervical cancer, as well as the fact that only a small fraction of women exposed to HPV develop cervical disease suggest that additional steps and perhaps other cofactors are necessary in the pathogenesis of cervical neoplasia.

Smoking, Diet, Oral Contraceptives

Cigarette smoking has also been associated with the development of cervical cancer [22]. In a comprehensive review of the literature, Szarewski concluded that a positive association between cigarette smoking and the development of cervical cancer had been reported by the majority of studies designed to address this question [182]. There are a number of possible mechanisms that could account for an association between cervical cancer and cigarette smoking. One is the secretion of cigarette smoke by-products, including nicotine and cotinine, in cervical mucous of tobacco users and women passively exposed to cigarette smoke [122]. Another possible mechanism that could account for the association is the effect of cervical smoke by-products on the number and distribution immune effector and regulatory cells such as Langerhan's cells in the cervix [183].

The use of combined oral contraceptives is now recognized as a significant risk factor for the development of both cervical cancer precursors and invasive cervical cancers. A meta-analysis of 28 studies evaluating the risk of cervical cancer in women on oral contraceptives demonstrated that the relative risk of invasive cervical cancer increased with increasing duration of contraceptive use. After 10 years of use, the summary relative risks for were 2.2 (95% CI. 1.9–2.2) for all women and 2.5 (95% CI. 1.6–3.9) for HPV positive women [174]. A recent reanalysis of epidemiological studies involving over 50,000 women has confirmed that oral contraceptive use increases the risk of cervical cancer [6]. The impact of exogenous hormone use and cervical disease could be explained by a number of mechanisms including direct interactions between the hormones and the HPV genome, as well as by indirect effects such as a reduction in blood folate levels that is occasionally observed in women on oral contraceptives. It is unclear whether there is an association between endogenous hormone levels and invasive cervical cancer. No association has been found between age at menarche or age of menopause and cervical squamous cell carcinoma.

Only a few studies have focused on relationships between cervical cancer and diet, but some studies of the association between micronutrients and cervical neoplasia have shown a probable protective effect for folate, retinol, and vitamin E and possibly for vegetable and several other micronutrients [67, 180]. However, there has been no confirmation of the role of any micronutrients in supplementation trials. A review of the cervical disease and antioxidant nutrients concluded that there are only six studies that have properly controlled for HPV [31]. In these six well-controlled studies, an inverse relationship was observed between serum carotene and cervical carcinogenesis. Other studies have found an inverse association between cervical neoplasia and serum lycopene and beta-carotene [31]. Folate deficiency may also be a risk factor and a case-control study recently reported that higher folate levels are associated with significantly lower risk of SIL [29, 151]. Other factors that may be important include coinfection with *Chlamydia trachomatis* and low socioeconomic status (even after accounting for screening) [167].

Immunosuppression

Although cellular immune response against HPV are rather poorly characterized, they clearly play an important role in determining whether HPV infections are ultimately cleared or whether they persist and can develop into cervical neoplasia [179]. The human leukocyte antigen DRB1*1301 appears to confirm a protective effect in epidemiological studies from diverse populations [194]. Immunosuppression is a well-established risk factor for the development of both SIL and cervical cancer. Renal transplant recipients have a relative risk of 13.6 for the development of cervical carcinoma in situ compared to women in the general population [204]. There is also an association between cervical disease and infection with the human immunodeficiency virus (HIV) [204]. HPV infections are more prevalent, and tend to be more persistent in HIV-infected women. Numerous studies have documented a higher prevalence of cervical neoplasia among HIV-infected women compared to various control groups of HIV-uninfected women [204]. There also appears to be an increase in invasive cervical cancer, and cervical cancer is classified as an AIDS-defining condition. Among women in New York City, the standardized incidence ratio for cervical cancer is 9.2 times higher in HIV infected compared to noninfected women [59]. It is clear that the invasive cervical cancers that do develop in HIV-infected women act aggressively and respond poorly to standard forms of therapy [117].

Clinical Features

SIL appears to be somewhat more frequently detected on the posterior lip of the cervix compared to the anterior lip of the cervix and is rarely seen at the lateral cervical angles [73, 153]. SIL may expand horizontally and involve the entire transformation zone, but it usually does not extend onto the native portio epithelium. The endocervical extension of SIL is not restricted and extension along the entire endocervical canal and into the uterus can rarely occur. The size and endocervical distribution of SIL tend to vary directly with increasing severity of lesion grade. HSIL usually has the largest surface area and more frequently involves the endocervical canal.

Pathologic Findings

SIL is characterized by abnormal cellular proliferation, abnormal maturation, and cytologic atypia. The cytologic abnormalities include hyperchromatic nuclei, abnormal chromatin distribution, nuclear pleomorphism, and increased nuclear : cytoplasmic ratio. Nuclear atypia is the hallmark of SIL. The nuclear borders are irregular, and the chromatin is coarse, granular (salt and pepper), or filamentous throughout the nuclear mass [134, 149].

Ultrastructurally, both the nuclear and cytoplasmic alterations of SIL are consistent with a progressive lack of normal differentiation [172]. There is a decrease in glycogen, tonofilaments, desmosomes, and specialized junctional units with increasing histologic dedifferentiation. These alterations are correlated with a progressive decrease in cellular adhesion, basal pseudopodia, and cell contact inhibition demonstrated by time-lapse cinematography in cells grown in vitro [161]. The surface ultrastructure of SIL also differs from the normal architecture. The most outstanding feature is the absence of surface microridges and the presence of abundant microvilli.

The traditional grading of SIL was based on the proportion of the epithelium occupied by basaloid, undifferentiated cells, reflecting a progressive loss of epithelial maturation, and decreasing glycogenization with increasing lesion severity. The spectrum of epithelial alterations that comprises SIL was therefore semiquantitatively classified into three categories: CIN grade 1 – neoplastic, basaloid cells occupying the lower third of the epithelium; CIN grade 2 – basaloid cells occupying the lower third to two-thirds of the epithelium; and CIN grade 3 – basaloid cells occupying two-thirds to full thickness of the epithelium, ➋ *Fig. 5.16*. Adoption of TBS nomenclature to histologic classification results in a two-tier rather than a three-tier grading system.

LSIL

HPV-induced cytologic and histologic changes are considered the most characteristic features of LSIL (CIN 1). The most important of these changes is significant nuclear atypia. Nuclear atypia is characterized by variation in nuclear size with nuclear enlargement, hyperchromasia, and irregularity, and wrinkling of the nuclear membrane. Nuclei often vary up to threefold in size and have quite variable staining patterns, ➋ *Fig. 5.17*. However, in LSIL there is usually minimal nuclear atypia in the epithelial cells residing in the lower third of the epithelium, ➋ *Fig. 5.18*. Cells in the superficial layers of the epithelium may have nuclei that are somewhat smaller and pyknotic. Squamous cells with productive HPV infections also frequently show perinuclear cytoplasmic cavitation or halos that are accompanied by thickening of the cytoplasmic membrane, ➋ *Fig. 5.19a*. These halos are best appreciated in cytology specimens, ➋ *Fig. 5.19b*. They develop because productive HPV infections induce cytoskeletal abnormalities that may lead to cytoplasmic cavitation. The combination of significant nuclear atypia and cytoplasmic halos has been termed *koilocytosis* or *koilocytotic atypia* and is pathognomonic of a productive HPV infected. Mitotic spindle abnormalities also occur in productive HPV infections and these appear to interfere with mitosis and cytokinesis. This leads to the polyploidy and bi- or multinucleated cells that are usually present in productive HPV infections, ➋ *Figs. 5.13* and ➋ *5.19* [62]. Polyploid cells are cytologically atypical and are readily recognized as being "abnormal" on either cytology or histology. Taken together, the histological and cytological features of koilocytosis, nuclear atypia, architectural abnormalities, and multinucleation are pathognomonic of an HPV-infected epithelium at any site in the lower genital tract and are especially prominent in LSIL.

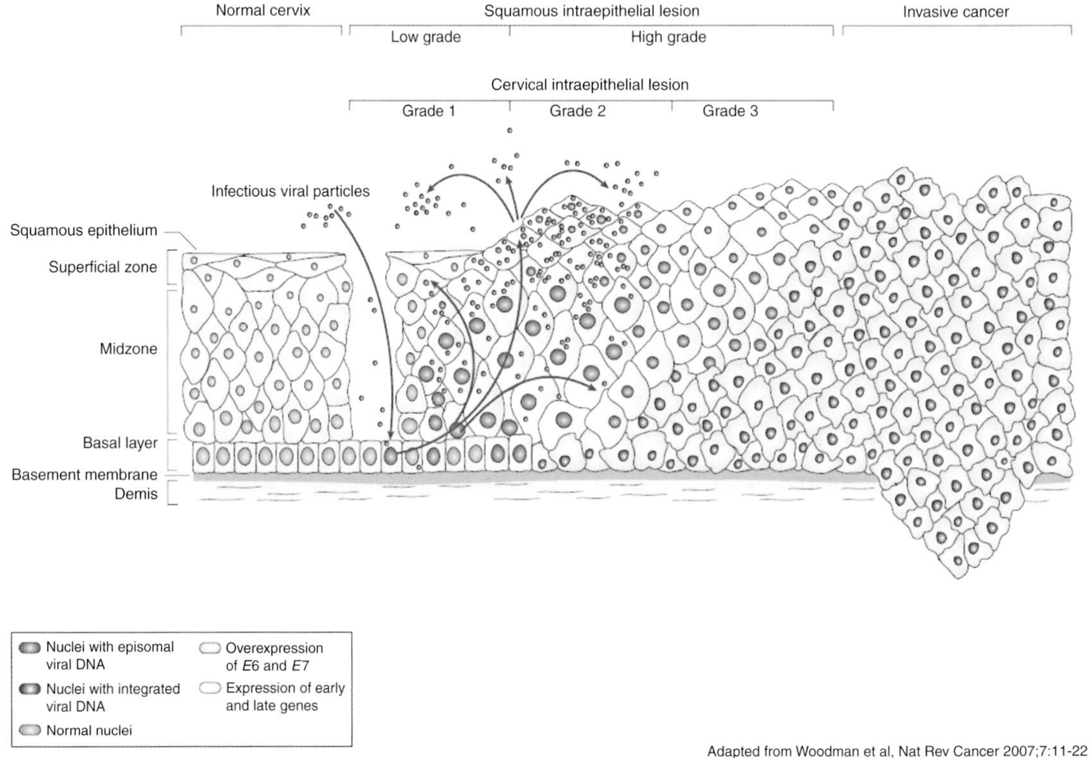

Fig. 5.16

Cervical squamous carcinoma precursors. **Schematic representation of cervical cancer precursors and the different terminologies that have been used to refer to them. The risk of developing microinvasion from different states of SIL is arbitrarily represented and is not necessarily proportional to that illustrated in this scheme**

The architectural abnormalities associated with low-grade SIL are due to a proliferation of basal and parabasal cells in the infected epithelium. The architectural abnormalities associated with LSIL causes the lesional tissue to appear quite different from the adjacent epithelium. Therefore, LSIL can usually be identified at lower magnifications based on the increased thickness of the epithelium accompanied by cells with prominent hyperchromatic nuclei in the upper levels of the epithelium, ● *Fig. 5.20.* HPV-induced hyperplasia can be highly variable and takes many forms, but is most commonly characterized by papillomatosis and acanthosis, ● *Fig. 5.21.* One of the more common patterns of the acanthosis is that of moderate epithelial thickening and an undulating, slightly raised surface. In the older literature, cervical lesions with HPV-associated cytopathic effects and only a moderate degree of epithelial thickening were referred to as *condyloma planum* or *flat condyloma.* Other types of epithelial hyperplasia that can occur in productive HPV infection are multiple papillary fronds containing fibrovascular cores and pointed epithelial spikes, ● *Fig. 5.22.* Colposcopically, these can present as an

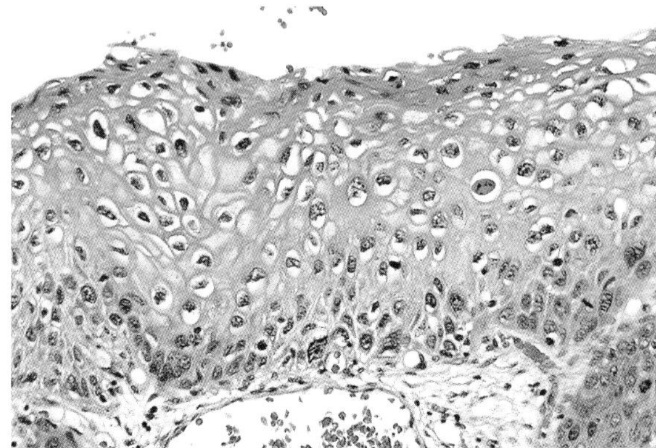

■ Fig. 5.17
Nuclear atypia in LSIL. **The most significant feature of LSIL is nuclear atypia. This is characterized by nuclear enlargement, hyperchromasia, nuclear irregularity, and variation in nuclear size**

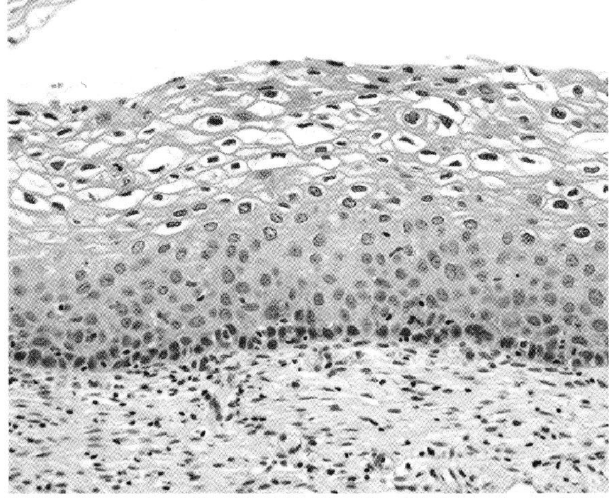

■ Fig. 5.18
LSIL with minimal cytological atypia in lower third of the epithelium. **Typically, the cells in lower third of the epithelium show minimal atypia in LSIL**

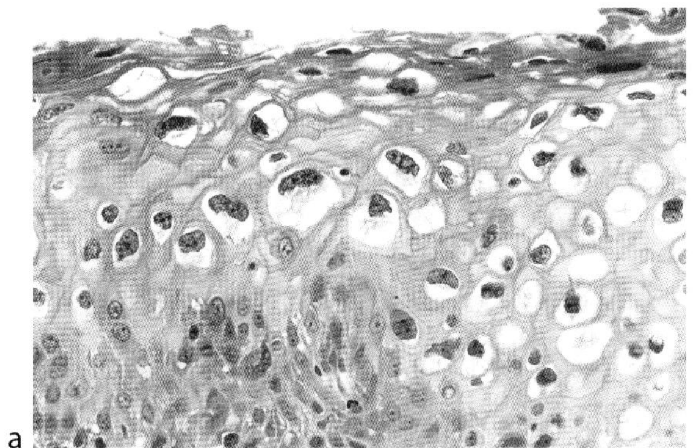

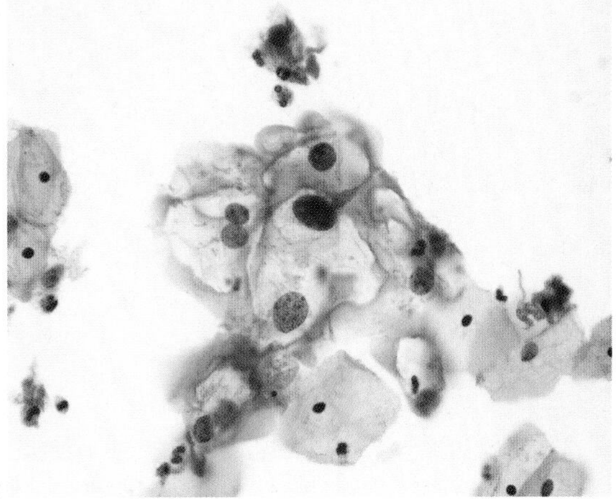

■ Fig. 5.19
Koilocytosis in LSIL. **The cytological features of a productive HPV infection include multinucleation and perinuclear cytoplasmic cavitation or halos. The combination of nuclear atypia and cytoplasmic halos is referred to as *koilocytosis*. (a) Koilocytosis on histology, (b) Koilocytosis on cytology**

exophytic condyloma acuminatum similar to those that occur on the vulva or vagina or as a less-exophytic lesion with prominent, fine surface spikes. The latter are frequently referred to in the colposcopic literature as *spiked condyloma*. A third type of papillary low-grade CIN is referred to as immature condyloma (e.g., papillary immature metaplasia). These represent infections of the transformation zone epithelium by HPV 6 or 11. These lesions typically have a filiform papillary architecture, ➋ *Fig. 5.23a*. Immature condylomas can be viewed as part of a histologic spectrum that ranges from squamous papillomas at the benign end to papillary carcinomas at the malignant end. Because HPV 6- and 11-infected transformation zone epithelial cells do not mature, koilocytotic features are minimized and these lesions retain an immature metaplastic phenotype, ➋ *Fig. 5.23b*. Cells in immature condylomas demonstrate only a mild degree of nuclear atypia and typically have a relatively low mitotic index.

The surface of LSIL frequently has a layer of parakeratosis and somewhat less commonly hyperkeratosis with an associated granular layer, ➋ *Fig. 5.24*. When gland involvement by the HPV-infected epithelium and acanthosis predominate, the histological pattern appears endophytic and superficially resembles that of an inverted nasal papilloma.

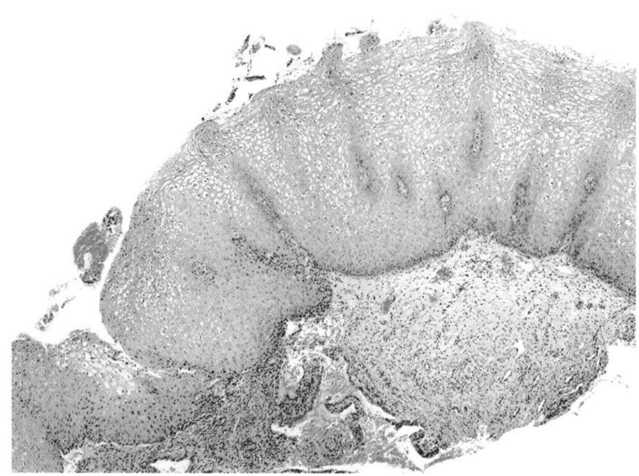

Fig. 5.20
LSIL recognized at low magnification. **LSIL can usually be recognized at relatively low magnification based on the increased thickness of the epithelium accompanied by prominent hyperchromatic nuclei in upper level of the epithelium**

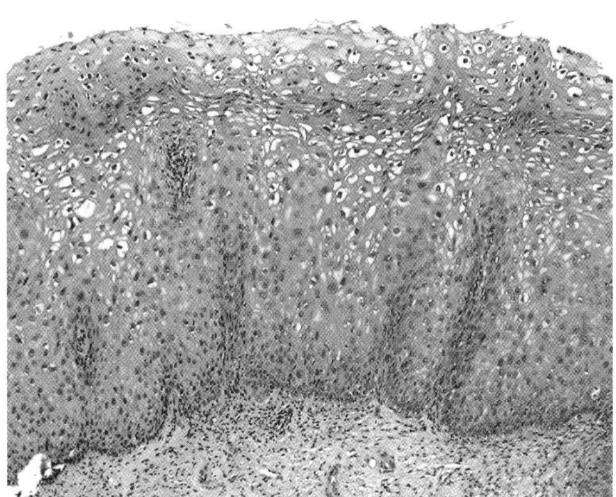

Fig. 5.21
LSIL. **Papillomatosis, acanthosis, parakeratosis, and hyperkeratosis are frequently present**

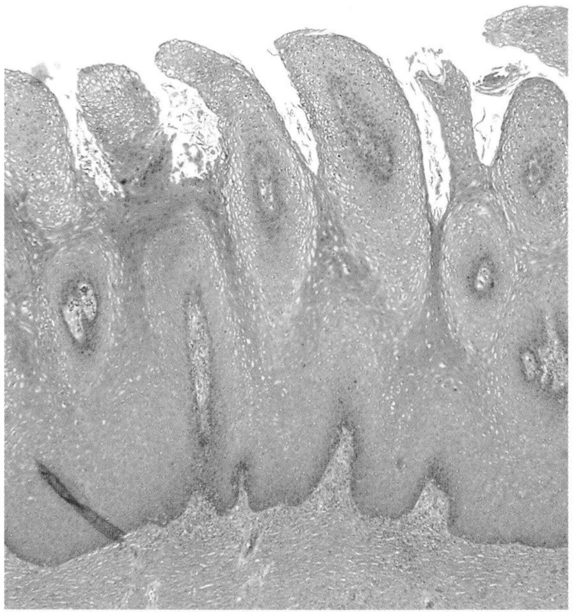

Fig. 5.22
LSIL of type referred to as *spiked condyloma*. **This lesion shows exaggerated epithelial thickening with multiple papillary fronds, each of which contains a fibrovascular core. The individual cells in these lesions are similar to the cells seen in flat lesions. Such lesions are referred to as "spiked condyloma" on colposcopy**

Differential Diagnosis

Studies measuring interobserver variability of histological diagnosis of cervical lesions demonstrate that although agreement between pathologists is excellent for invasive lesions, and moderately good for HSIL, it is poor for LSIL [87, 163, 171, 181]. In the NCI-sponsored ALTS (ASCUS-LSIL Traige Study) multicenter study, 2,237 colposcopically directed biopsies that had been initially diagnosed at the clinical performance sites were reviewed by a quality control panel of pathologists. Only 43% of the biopsies initially diagnosed as LSIL were classified as LSIL after review, ➋ *Table 5.4.* Most of the discrepancies were due to the inability of the pathologists to distinguish LSIL from reactive squamous proliferations. This suggests that the morphologic criteria routinely used to distinguish these two lesions have serious shortcomings.

Prospective follow-up studies indicate that the majority of LSIL lesions spontaneously regress over a several year period of time [126]. Therefore, it is not surprising that lesions are frequently encountered that have some, but not all of the features of LSIL. Such lesions may represent regressing LSIL and are classified as *borderline condyloma* by some authors [64]. Such lesions as described as having mild acanthosis and mild cellular proliferation in the parabasal layers remain quite organized. They show rare, mildly atypical squamous cells in the intermediate and superficial layers that are characterized by minor nuclear enlargement, hyperchromasia, and sometimes binucleation, ➋ *Fig. 5.25a, b.* It is important to recognize that there are no good molecular : histopathological correlation studies of these lesions and therefore the clinical significance of *borderline condylomas* is unknown and we do not recommend the use of this term.

Two biomarkers, $p16^{ink}$ and Ki-67, appear to be useful for differentiating SIL from other conditions. $p16^{ink}$ is a cyclin-dependent protein kinase inhibitor that is overexpressed in almost all HSIL and invasive cervical cancers [96, 101, 188]. $p16^{ink}$ is particularly attractive as a biomarker for HPV-associated SIL since overexpression within cervical neoplasia has been directly linked to the continued expression of the HPV oncogene E7. Moreover, $p16^{ink}$ overexpression appears to be independent of

a

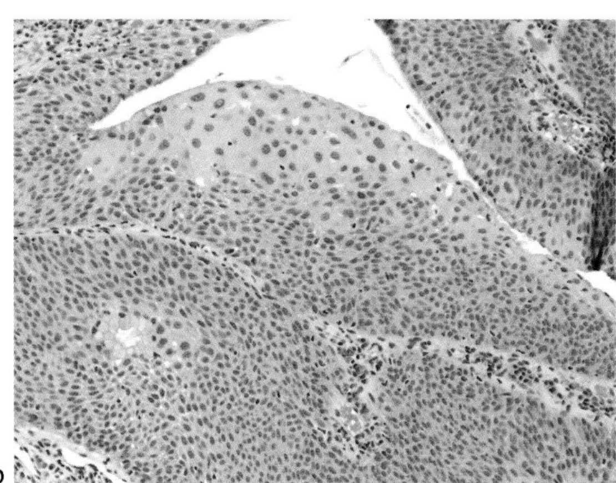

b

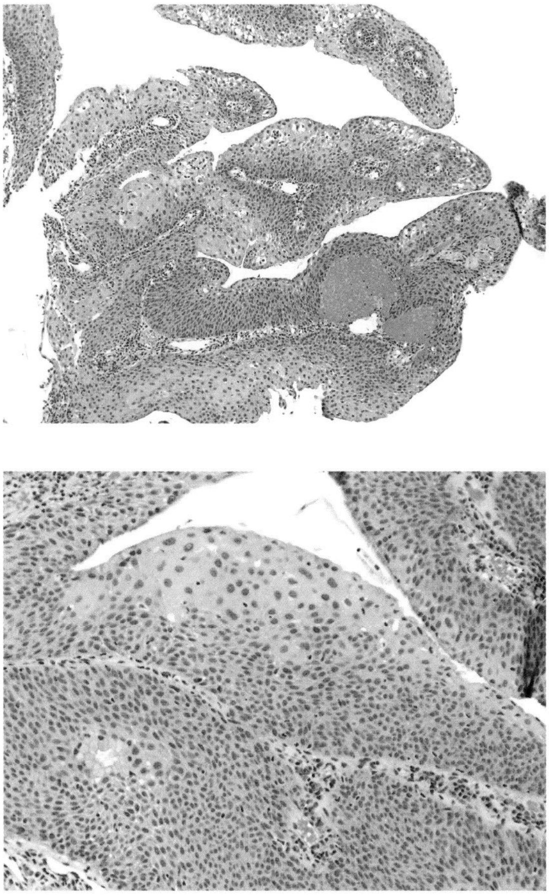

■ Fig. 5.23
LSIL of type referred to as *immature condyloma*. **These lesions occur in the transformation zone and are associated with HPV 6 or 11. (a) They typically form thin, papillary projections. (b) Typically, the cells have a metaplastic phenotype with minimal koilocytosis**

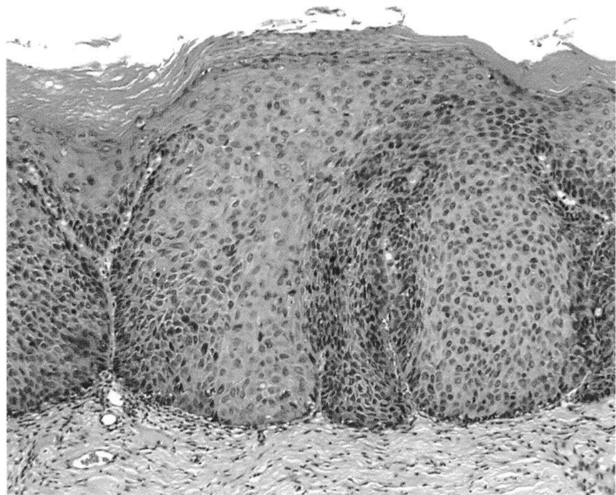

■ Fig. 5.24
LSIL with both hyperkeratosis and parakeratosis. **Both hyperkeratosis and parakeratosis are frequently associated with LSIL**

Table 5.4
Variability in histopathological diagnoses in ALTS

Initial Dx	Quality control panel review diagnosis				
	WNL (%)	ASCUS (%)	LSIL (%)	HSIL (%)	Total
WNL	91	22	4	3	685
ASCUS	77	10	9	4	184
LSIL	44	4	43	13	887
HSIL	7	2	14	77	481

Modified from [181].

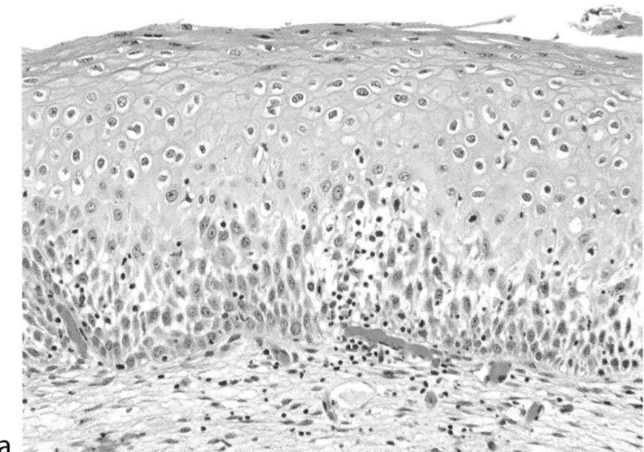

a

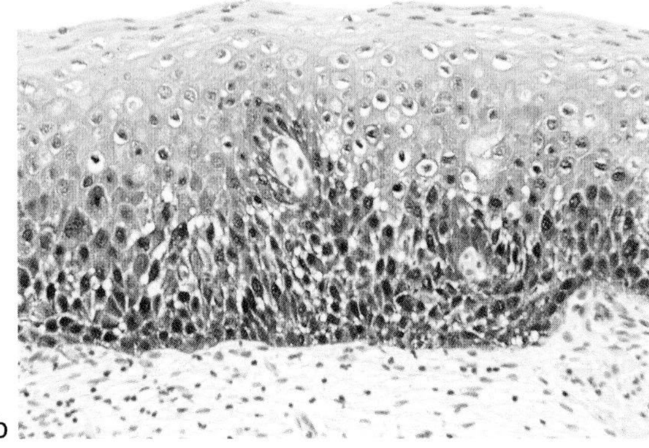

b

Fig. 5.25
LSIL of the type referred to as *borderline condyloma*.
(a) Lesions of this type have less nuclear atypia and acanthosis than usually seen in LSIL. This lesion contains considerable numbers of multinucleated cells. (b) It stains positively with p16^{ink} and we would classify it as LSIL

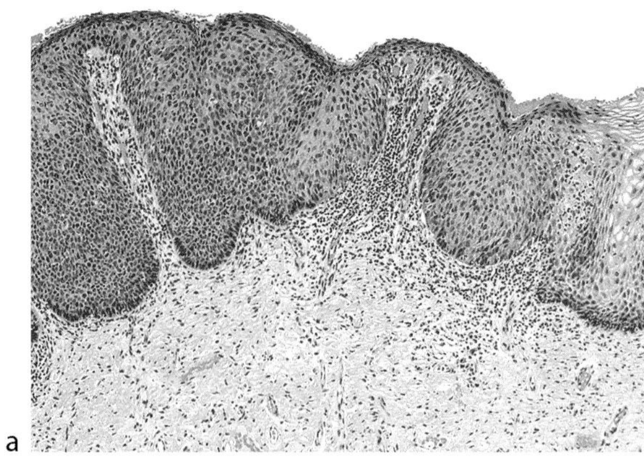

a

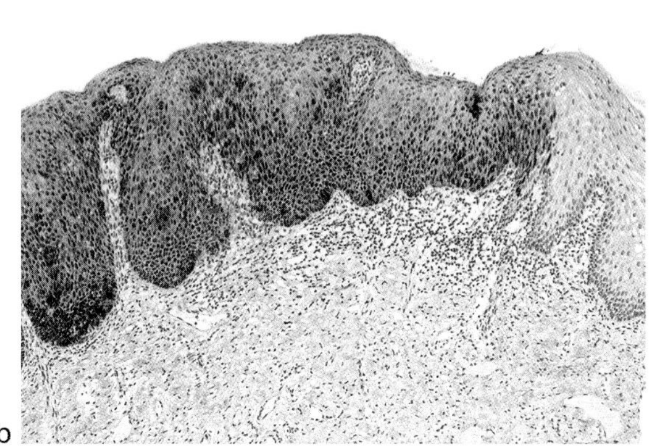

b

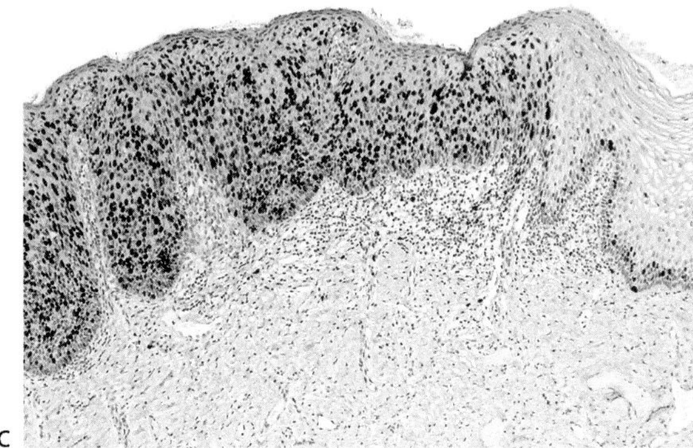

c

Fig. 5.26
Junction between HSIL and normal squamous epithelium.
(a) This section shows the junction between a HSIL and normal squamous epithelium. Both (b) p16^{ink} and (c) Ki-67 staining demonstrates how sharp the demarcation usually is between lesional and non-lesional tissue

the particular type of high-risk HPV-associated with the lesion. Studies have uniformly shown p16^{ink} staining to be absent in normal squamous epithelium and benign inflammatory/reparative conditions, ➋ *Fig. 5.26b* [155, 188, 193, 211]. Therefore, it has been suggested that p16^{ink} immunostaining could improve the ability of pathologists to differentiate between immature squamous metaplasia or reaction/reparative conditions and SIL associated with high-risk types of HPV. Since approximately two-thirds of LSIL is associated with a high-risk type of HPV, it is not surprising that approximately one-third to half of LSIL will show strong diffuse staining of the basal layer with p16^{ink}, ➋ *Fig. 5.27a, b*, and another one-third show focal p16^{ink} staining [75, 193, 211]. Therefore, although absence of p16^{ink} staining does not mean that a lesion is not LSIL, the presence of strong diffuse staining of the lower half of the epithelium is a fairly good indicator that a lesion is a SIL. Ki-67 is a marker of cellular proliferation that is also useful for the identification of SIL that show staining in the upper two-thirds of the epithelium whereas normal squamous epithelium typically shows only limited staining in the parabasal cell layer, ➋ *Figs. 5.26c* and ➋ *5.27c* [86, 154]. However, unlike p16^{ink}, Ki-67 staining may be positive in HPV-negative squamous metaplasia and reactive/reparative conditions that reduces its usefulness in differentiating these conditions from SIL.

Overdiagnosis of LSIL can be reduced if it is remembered that significant nuclear atypia is the hallmark of SIL. Correlation of HPV DNA with specific cytologic/histologic findings has uniformly found that perinuclear halos in the absence of significant nuclear atypia are nonspecific features [60, 130, 195]. Therefore, the diagnosis of LSIL should be made only when significant nuclear atypia accompanies perinuclear halos and the indiscriminate use of the term "koilocytosis" whenever the cervical squamous epithelium demonstrates the slightest hint of "cytoplasmic vacuolization" should be discouraged. Cytoplasmic vacuolization in the absence of nuclear atypia is a nonspecific change that may occur as a reflection of atrophy-related vacuolar degeneration or with prominent glycogen vacuolization of the normal squamous epithelium, ➋ *Fig. 5.28a, b*. Although LSIL does occur in postmenopausal women, it is uncommon. "Pseudokoilocytes" can also be seen in non-HPV-related infections, such as trichomoniasis, *Gardnerella vaginalis*, and candidiasis, ➋ *Fig. 5.29*. In contrast to the focal distribution of koilocytes in LSIL, cells of normal squamous epithelium that have perinuclear clearing are not sharply demarcated, the nuclei are not enlarged or atypical, and multinucleated cells are infrequent. In addition to the

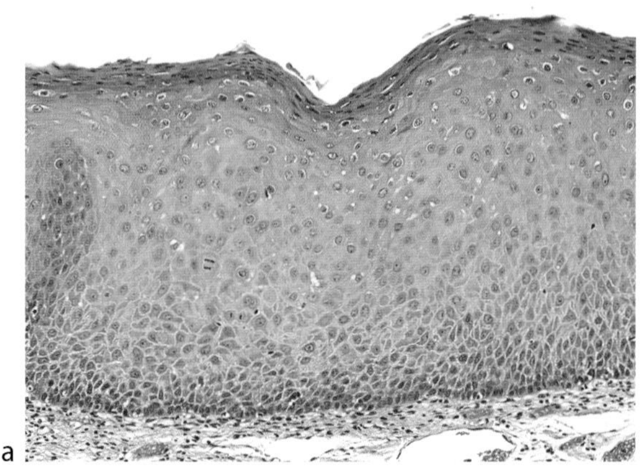

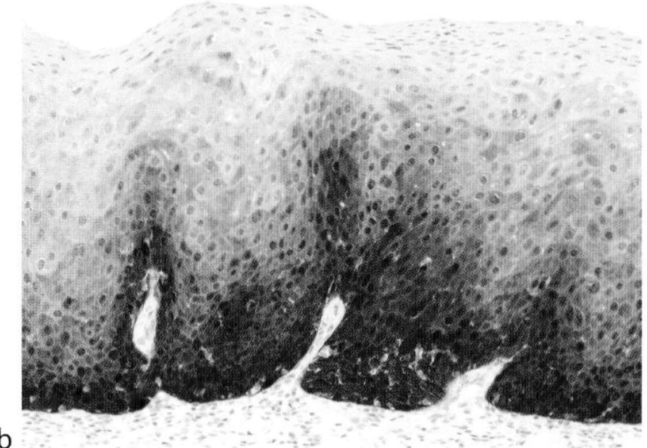

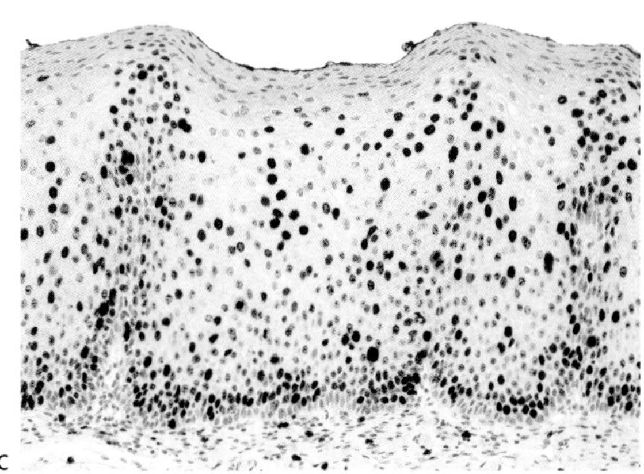

▪ Fig. 5.27
p16^{ink} and Ki-67 staining of LSIL. **Approximately one-third of LSIL will show strong diffuse staining of the lower portion of the epithelium with p16^{ink}. Most LSIL will have an increased Ki-67 labeling index. (a) H&E, (b) p16^{ink}, and (c) Ki-67 staining**

absence of nuclear atypia, normal stratification and maturation are maintained in such conditions, whereas in HPV-associated lesions, there is some degree of cellular disorganization, particularly near the surface, and there is disturbance in the normal pattern of maturation.

Misdiagnosis of LSIL as HSIL can be avoided by recognizing that LSIL generally does not have a high mitotic index, loss of cell polarity, and abnormal mitotic figures (AMFs). Although a diagnosis of LSIL requires significant atypia, the atypia does not usually involve the basal or parabasal cell layers. The classification of lesions that have the characteristic histologic features of LSIL, but also have

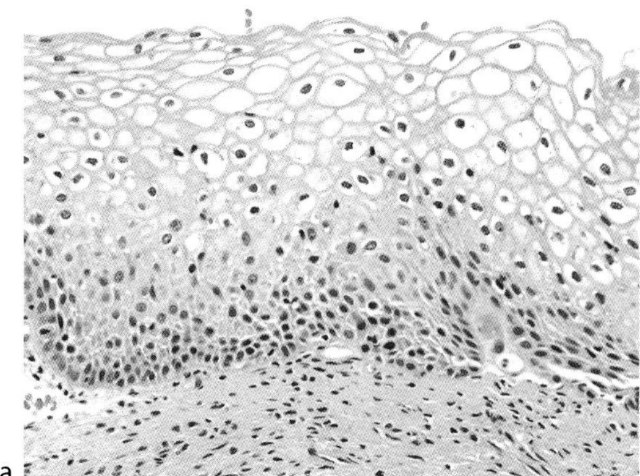

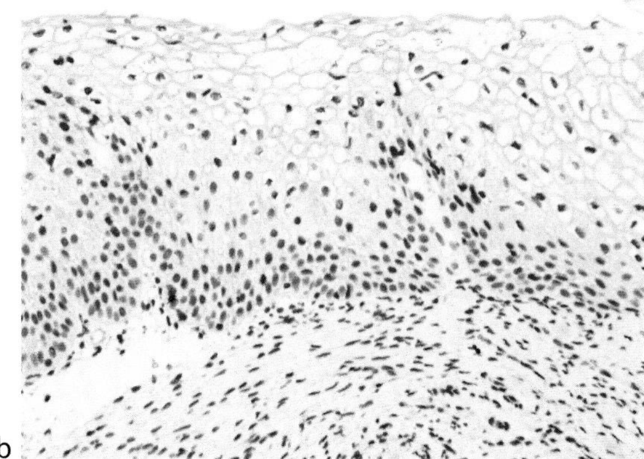

Fig. 5.28
Atrophy-related perinuclear halos. **(a)** Biopsy from a postmenopausal patient. The squamous epithelial cells show prominent perinuclear halos, but do not have significant nuclear atypia. **(b)** This lesion does not stain for $p16^{ink}$

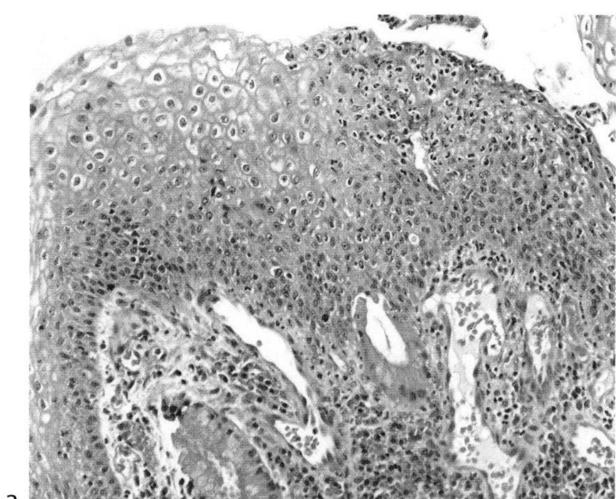

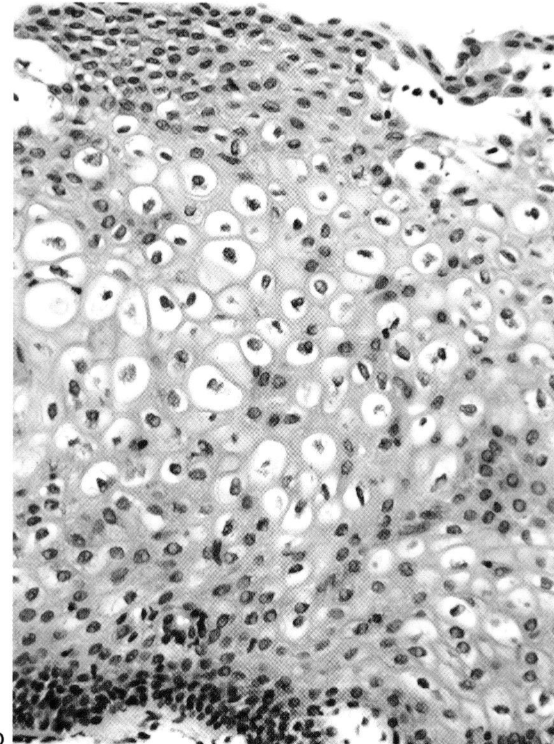

Fig. 5.29
Pseudokoilocytosis secondary to infection. **(a)** Infection-related perinuclear halos are frequently observed in women with non-HPV-related infections. Generally in infection considerable numbers of inflammatory cells are present. **(b)** At higher magnification, the nuclei are not as enlarged or atypical as usually seen in LSIL and multinucleated cells are infrequent

AMFs is controversial. AMFs generally indicate that a lesion is aneuploid, ➋ *Fig. 5.30.* Therefore, an argument could be made that lesions with AMFs should be classified as HSIL, although in the absence of significant basal or parabasal atypia many pathologists would classify low-grade-appearing lesions with only one or two AMFs as LSIL. It is also important to note that many HSIL have significant koilocytotic change in the upper layers of the epithelium, so simply having koilocytosis and differentiation in the upper half of the epithelium should not result in a lesion being classified as LSIL if it has significant basal–parabasal nuclear atypia, ➋ *Fig. 5.31.* ➋ *Figure 5.32* is a lesion that might be classified as LSIL by some pathologists. However, the lesion has significant basal and parabasal nuclear atypia, as well as a mitosis in the midportion of the epithelium and an AMF. Therefore, we would classify this lesion as a HSIL.

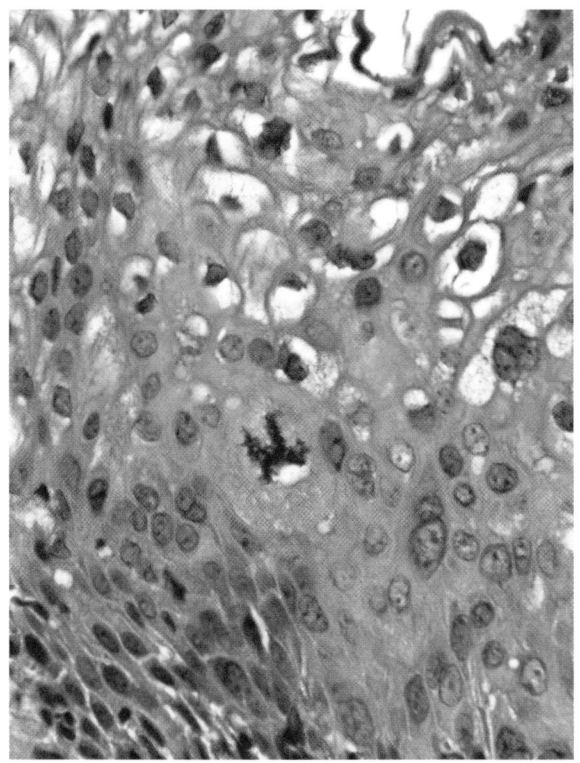

Fig. 5.30
Abnormal mitotic figures (AMFs) in SIL. **AMFs indicate that a lesion is aneuploid and are typically found in HSIL**

HSIL

In HSIL (CIN 2, 3), atypia should be present in all layers of the squamous epithelium, but to an extent and degree that exceeds what is seen in LSIL. There is significant basal-parabasal nuclear atypia and AMFs. Immature basal-type cells typically occupy more than the lower third of the

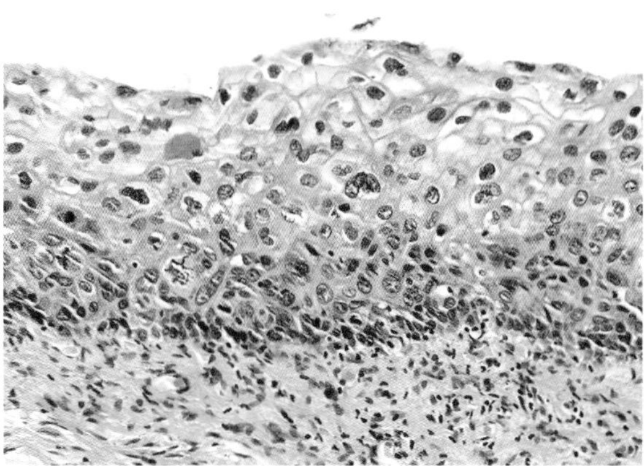

Fig. 5.31
HSIL mimicking an LSIL. **This lesion has marked koilocytosis in the upper half of the epithelium, but has significant atypia of the basal, parabasal layers and abnormal mitotic figures (AMFs). Because of the atypia in the basal and parabasal layers, this should be classified as HSIL**

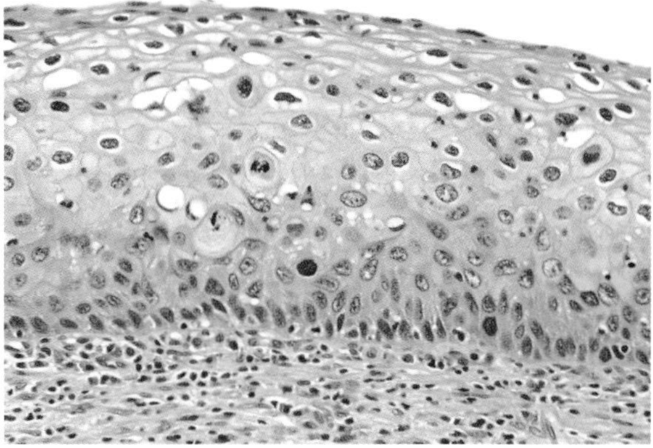

Fig. 5.32
LSIL versus HSIL. **Sometimes it is difficult to differentiate between LSIL and HSIL. This lesion has many features of LSIL, but also has a mitosis in the middle of the epithelium and an abnormal mitotic figure (AMF) and based on this it should be classified as HSIL**

epithelium, ➲ *Fig. 5.33*. In addition, there is nuclear crowding, pleomorphism, and loss of the normal cell polarity. The nuclei of the immature basal-type cells are enlarged when compared to the nuclei of cells at comparable levels of the normal epithelium. This nuclear enlargement is frequently most pronounced in the lower half of the epithelium although in all cases the superficial cells demonstrate some degree of nuclear enlargement. As in LSIL, the nuclei are hyperchromatic and the chromatin is finely to coarsely granular, ➲ *Fig. 5.34*. Prominent nuclei or chromocenters are uncommon. Normal and abnormal mitotic figures are present and mitoses are usually present in the upper half of the epithelium. Cytoplasm is usually scant resulting in an increase in the nuclear : cytoplasmic ratio. Cell borders between the primitive cells are usually indistinct. The cells overlying the basal-type cells also have atypical nuclei but have more cytoplasm and therefore lower nuclear : cytoplasmic ratios, more distinct cell boundaries, and can have prominent HPV cytopathic effects, including perinuclear halos and bi- or multinucleation. In the superficial layers of the epithelium, individual dyskeratotic cells may be seen, ➲ *Fig. 5.35*. These cells are small with pyknotic hyperchromatic nuclei and dense acidophilic cytoplasm. Another characteristic feature of HSIL is the variability in nuclear size (anisonucleosis), ➲ *Fig. 5.36*. It should be stressed, however, that this is a variable histological feature. In some HSIL lesions, particularly those that were previously termed carcinoma in situ, the nuclei at first glance appear relatively uniform in size, although careful scrutiny will reveal some variation in nuclear size and shape, ➲ *Fig. 5.37*. Many HSIL lesions also have koilocytotic features in the upper layers of the epithelium similar to what is seen in LSIL, ➲ *Fig. 5.38*. However, these koilocytotic features are often associated with bizarre nuclei and abnormal keratinization. These lesions were previously classified as CIN 2.

The original CIN terminology subdivides HSIL into two categories: CIN 2 and CIN 3. This distinction is made based on the proportion of the epithelial thickness occupied by undifferentiated neoplastic cells. In CIN 2, the immature basaloid-type cells occupy up to two-thirds of the epithelial thickness, but do not extend into the upper third of the epithelium, ➲ *Fig. 5.38*. Similarly, mitoses are found in the lower two-thirds of the epithelium, but not in the upper third. In CIN 3 lesions, immature basaloid-type cells occupy the upper third of the epithelium and mitoses can be present at any level, ➲ *Fig. 5.39*. Studies of the reproducibility of the histopathological diagnosis of different grades of cervical cancer precursors have shown that diagnosis of CIN 2 is not reproducible [33, 87, 163]. The lack of reproducibility of the diagnosis of CIN 2 is due to

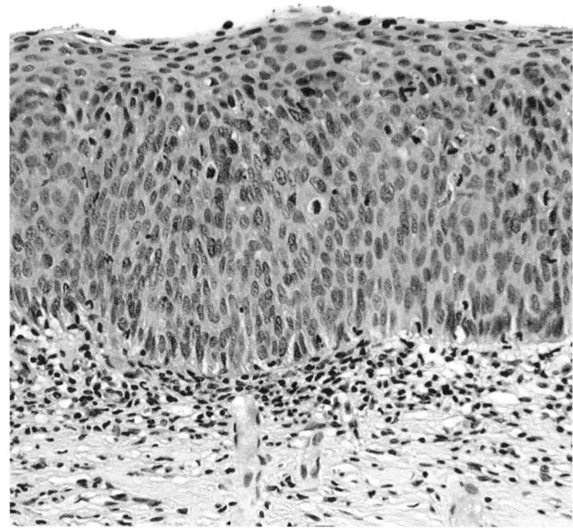

Fig. 5.33
HSIL. Undifferentiated neoplastic cells replace 50–70% of the epithelium. The nuclear : cytoplasmic ratio is high, and the cytoplasmic membranes and the basal layer are indistinct

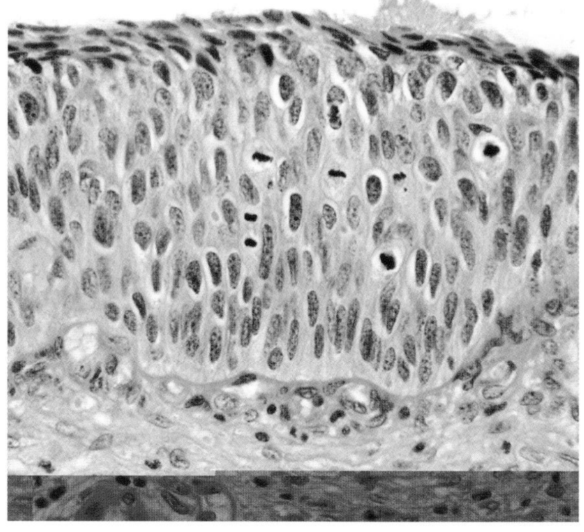

Fig. 5.34
HSIL. This is a typical HSIL with numerous mitoses in the middle portion of the epithelium and immature basaloid cells extending almost to the surface

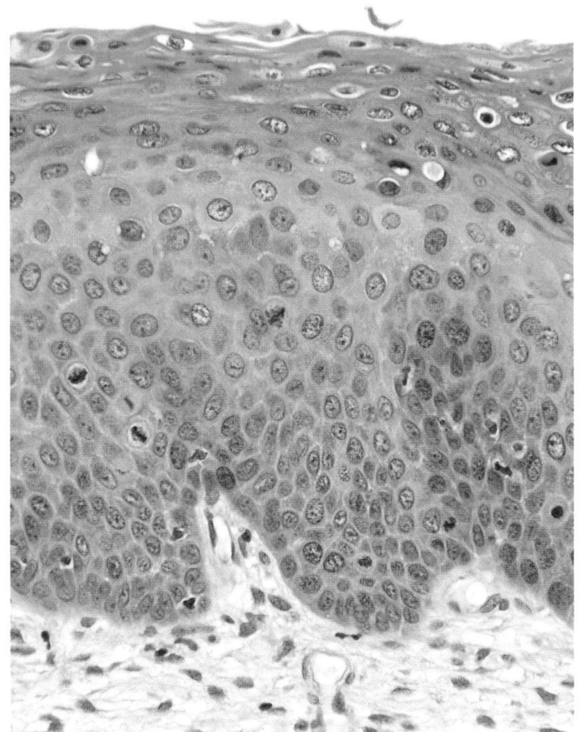

■ Fig. 5.35
HSIL with dyskeratotic cells. **This HSIL shows both parakeratosis and dyskeratotic cells (small dark cells with pyknotic nuclei and eosinophilic cytoplasm) in the upper half of the epithelium**

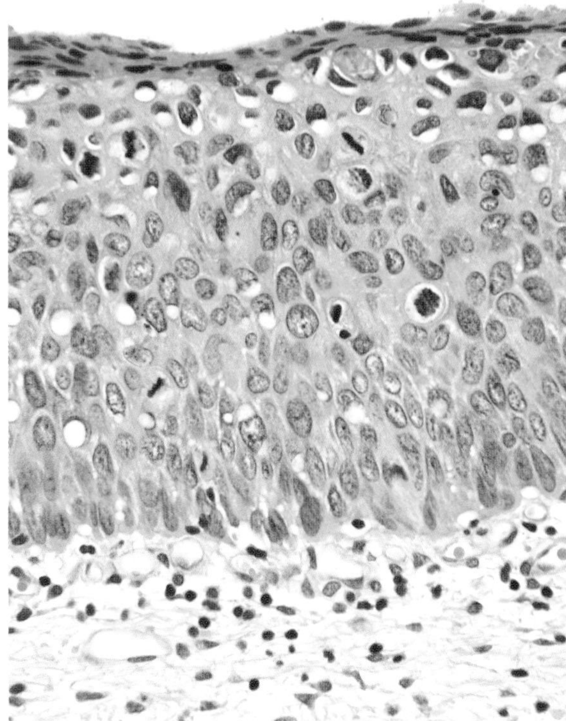

■ Fig. 5.36
HSIL with marked variability in nuclear size (anisonucleosis). **Anisonucleosis is a variable feature of HSIL**

the subjective criteria used to separate the different grades of CIN and the fact that the thickness of the epithelium occupied by immature basaloid-type cells varies considerably, even in cervical biopsy specimens.

In most tissues, aneuploidy is a marker of malignant potential and multiple studies have shown that the majority of HSIL lesions are aneuploid [17, 19, 20]. A number of studies have compared histologic features with ploidy levels and found that cervical lesions with diploid or polyploid DNA contents generally retain polarity of the basal cell layer and lack AMFs, whereas aneuploid lesions have more marked nuclear atypia and more cellular disorganization. The best histologic correlate of aneuploid is AMFs [13, 63]. Therefore, some authors have suggested that AMFs other than multipolar and dispersed metaphases are an accurate histologic surrogate of aneuploidy and can be used as a histological determinate for discriminating between LSIL and HSIL [160]. Although AMFs are commonly seen in HSIL, ➲ *Fig. 5.39*, they should not be used as the sole criterion for discriminating between LSIL and HSIL for several reasons: (1) they can be difficult to distinguish from karyorrhexis, (2) detection of AMFs is influenced by variables that are independent of ploidy level, including size of biopsy, quality of fixation, quality of the microscopic section, and number of levels examined, and (3) some HSIL lesions, and even some invasive cancers, lack AMFs and are not aneuploid [74, 134]. Therefore, although a lesion showing the above features with unequivocal AMFs should be classified as HSIL, the converse is not true. Lesions with the other histological features of a HSIL should be classified as such even in the absence of AMFs. It is also important to point out that using these criteria, some high-grade lesions will have cells with prominent HPV cytopathic effects similar to those seen in LSIL, ➲ *Figs. 5.31* and ➲ *5.32*. The presence of such cells should not be taken as evidence that the lesion is low grade if other features of a high-grade lesion are present. Therefore, the criteria that are used for distinguishing LSIL from HSIL include other features such as the distribution of immature, basal-type cells, the level at which mitotic figures in the epithelium are identified, the extent

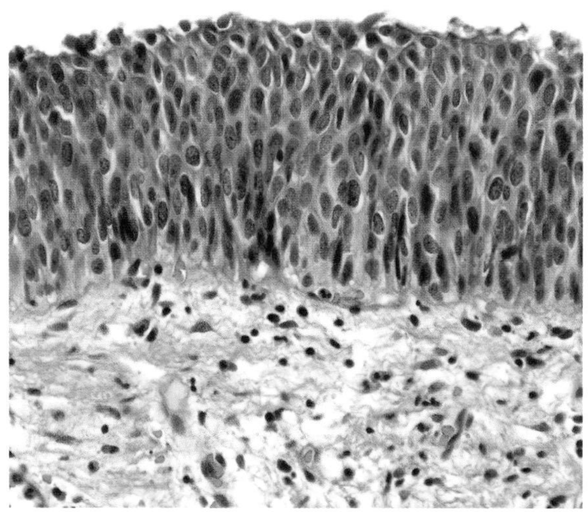

Fig. 5.37
HSIL. **The full thickness of the epithelium is composed of small, undifferentiated neoplastic cells. This is the classic *small cell carcinoma in situ*. Note numerous mitotic figures, loss of cellular maturation and organization, and lack of koilocytes**

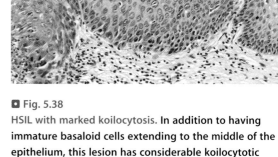

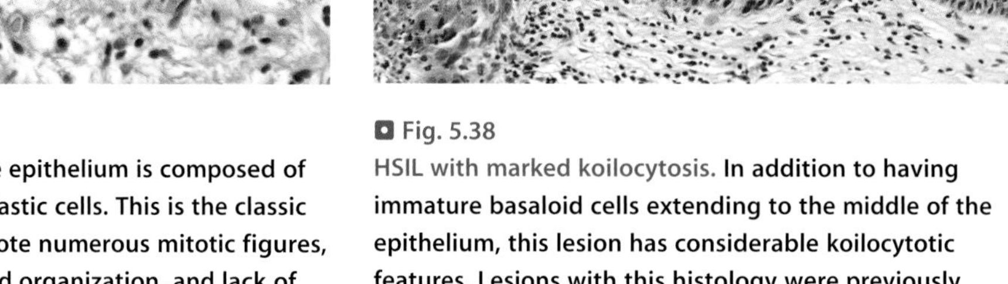

Fig. 5.38
HSIL with marked koilocytosis. **In addition to having immature basaloid cells extending to the middle of the epithelium, this lesion has considerable koilocytotic features. Lesions with this histology were previously classified as CIN 2**

of abnormalities of differentiation and polarity, and the degree of nuclear atypia, *Table 5.5*.

It is important to recognize that HSIL has quite a variable histological presentation, especially with respect to size of the cells, extent of koilocytosis, degree of atypia, and degree of keratinization. The most common different presentations include a mature or koilocytotic form that is characterized by prominent HPV features (i.e., koilocytosis) accompanied by atypia of the basal and parabasal cell layers together with mitotic figures, including abnormal forms, in the upper two-thirds of the epithelium. Another commonly encountered presentation is keratinizing HSIL that has quite prominent superficial keratinization accompanied by cells with the typical histological and cytological features of HSIL, *Fig. 5.40*. Other HSILs show less keratinization but have a prominent layer of parakeratotic cells, *Fig. 5.41*. Perhaps the most difficult forms of HSIL to recognize are those that have an immature metaplastic phenotype. These lesions resemble immature squamous metaplasia and are sometimes encountered underneath an intact columnar epithelium, *Fig. 5.42*. Compared to immature squamous metaplasia, HSIL with an immature metaplastic phenotype shows a greater degree of hyperchromasia and anisonucleosis. Nuclear density does not decrease in the superficial cell layers and a syncytium of nuclei can

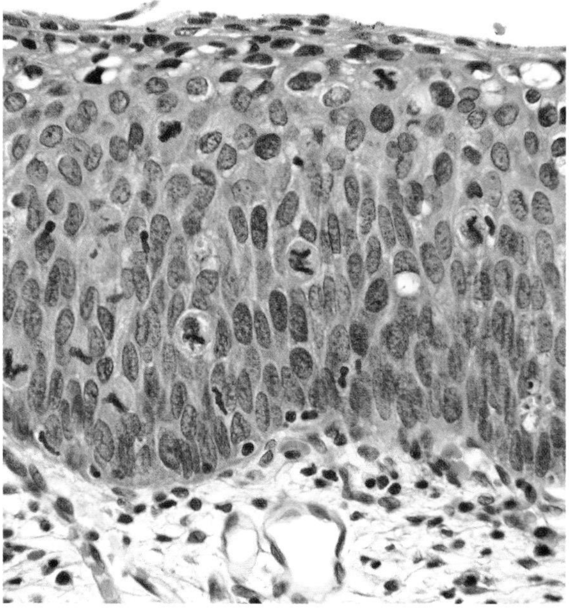

Fig. 5.39
HSIL. **This form of HSIL has immature basaloid cells and mitoses extending almost to the surface. Lesions with this histology were previously classified as CIN 3**

Table 5.5
Distinguishing features of LSIL and HSIL

Feature	LSIL	HSIL
HPV types	Any anogenital HPV	High-risk types[a]
Koilocytosis	Frequently present	Occasionally present
Ploidy	Mostly diploid or polyploid	Usually aneuploid
Abnormal mitotic figures (AMFs)	Absent	Frequent
Location of undifferentiated cells and mitotic figures	Lower third	Upper two-thirds

[a]High risk types of HPV include 16, 18, 31, 33, 35, 39, 45, 51, 52, 56, 58, 59, 66.

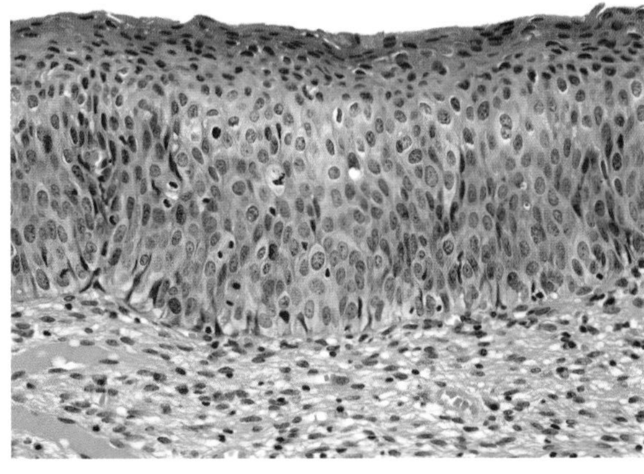

Fig. 5.41
HSIL with prominent abnormal parakeratosis. **This HSIL has a superficial layer of compacted parakeratotic cells that appear abnormally keratinized**

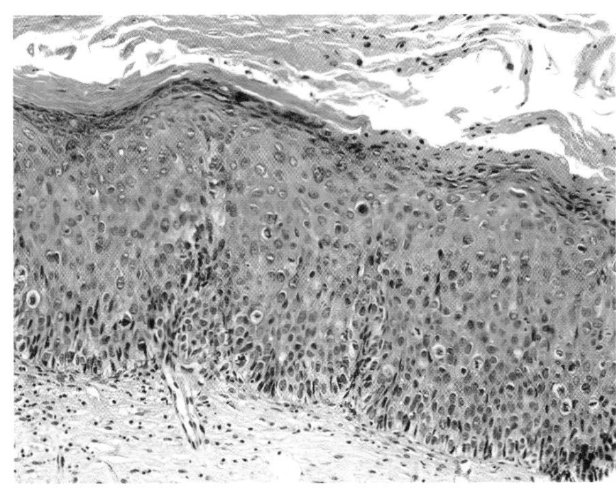

Fig. 5.40
HSIL with hyperkeratosis and parakeratosis. **Prominent keratinization is frequently seen in HSIL. This HSIL has a thick plaque of keratin on the surface that can often be seen at the time of a gynecological examination. Clinicians call plaques of keratin on the surface of the cervix leukoplakia. Parakeratosis is also present**

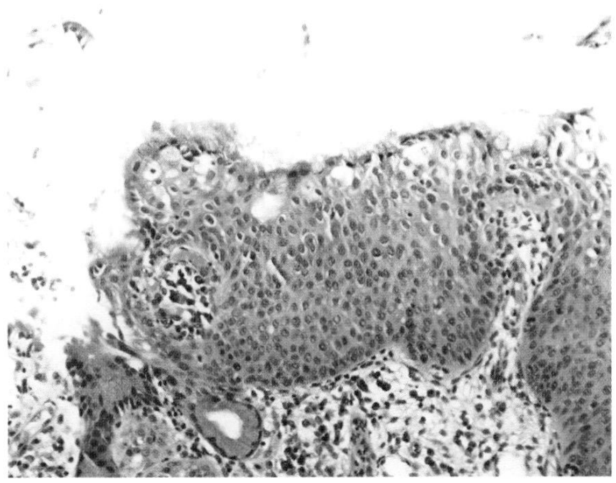

Fig. 5.42
HSIL with metaplastic features. **This HSIL has a metaplastic appearance and is covered by columnar epithelium. The degree of nuclear atypia is too great for this to be metaplasia**

sometimes be seen in the superficial layers. p16[Ink] is very useful in diagnosing these lesions, *Fig. 5.43a, b.* In addition, some HSIL have both squamous and mucinous differentiation, *Fig. 5.44a.* This reflects the multipotential nature of the cells in the transformation zone. These lesions with both squamous and mucinous differentiation have been referred to as *stratified mucin-producing intraepithelial lesion* (SMILE) and contain cells with prominent mucin droplets [145]. SMILE usually shows a high Ki-67 labeling index and strong diffuse staining with p16[Ink], *Fig. 5.44b, c.* These lesions are often found in association with both HSIL and adenocarcinoma in situ (AIS) [145].

In the past, some investigators have proposed formally subtyping high-grade precursors into small cell anaplastic, large cell keratinizing, and large cell non-keratinizing dysplasia [147, 157]. Because accurate studies concerning the invasive potential of each of these subtypes are lacking, prediction of the likelihood of progression to invasive carcinoma should not be based on the above subclassification.

Differential Diagnosis

Immature metaplasia, reactive/reparative processes, and atrophy are the most common lesions mistaken for HSIL. This is because cells of these lesions can show immaturity of the squamous epithelium, nuclear atypia, and inflammatory cellular changes. In immature

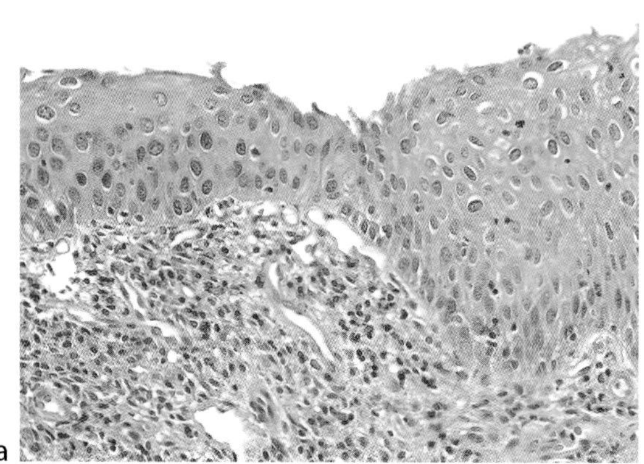

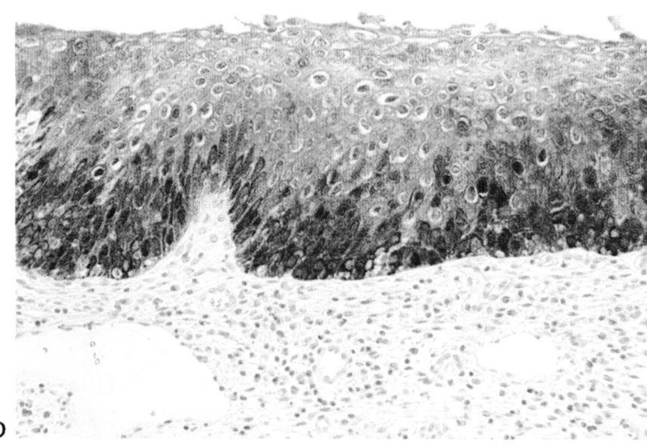

Fig. 5.43
HSIL with metaplastic features. **(a)** This lesion is relatively bland appearing, but has considerable numbers of mitotic figures. **(b)** $P16^{ink}$ staining demonstrates strong diffuse positivity

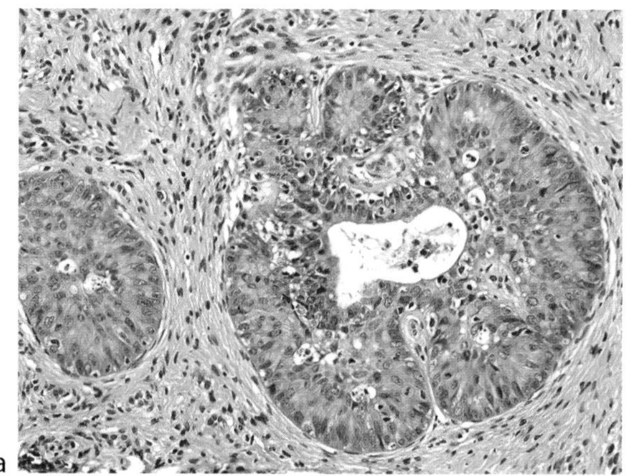

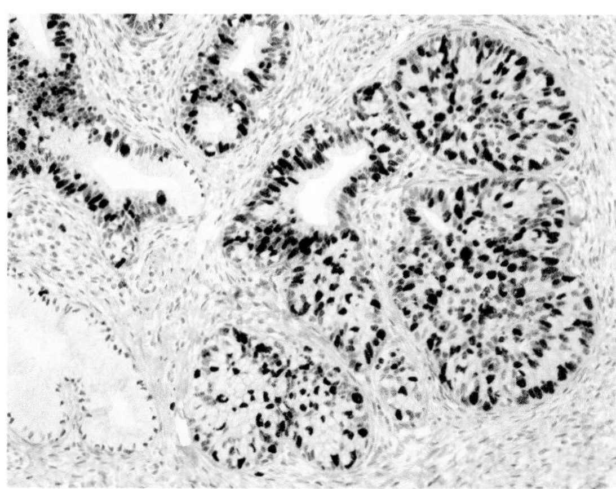

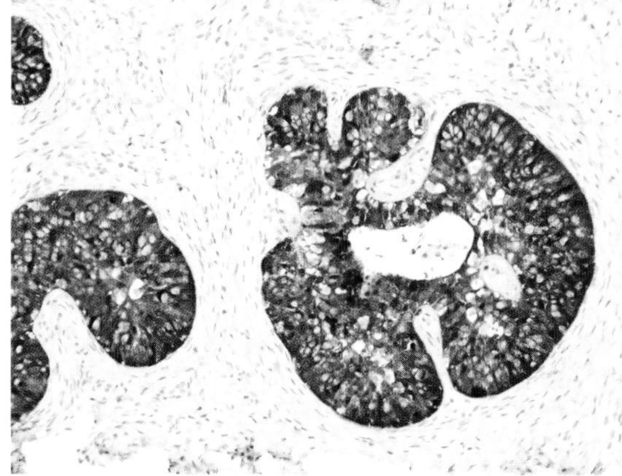

Fig. 5.44
Stratified mucin-producing intraepithelial lesion (SMILE). **(a)** These HSIL show both mucinous and squamous differentiation. **(b)** It has a high Ki-67 labeling index and **(c)** stains positively for $p16^{ink}$

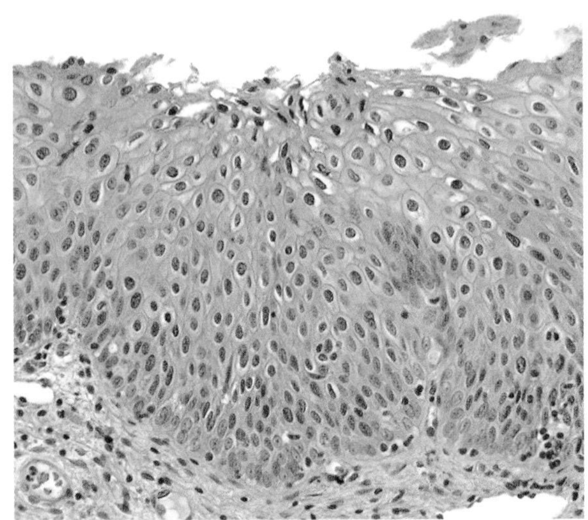

Fig. 5.45
Immature squamous metaplasia. **Metaplastic squamous cells are regularly oriented with uniformly disposed nuclear chromatin and cellular borders. Intracellular bridges are present**

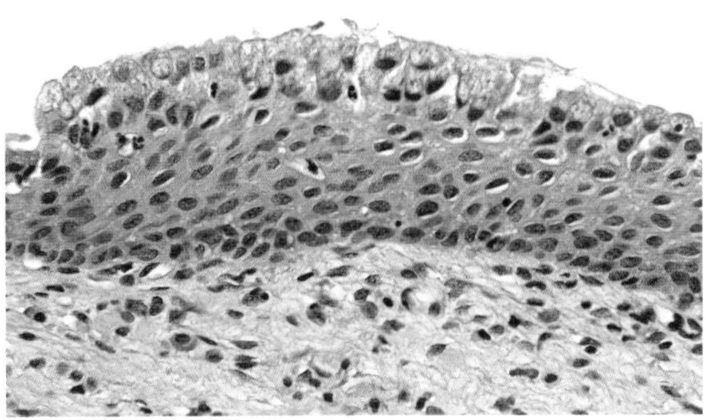

Fig. 5.46
Immature squamous metaplasia. **This lesion has a relatively uniform metaplastic appearance, but the nuclei are hyperchromatic and irregular. Some mitoses are present. However, the lesion is found underlying columnar epithelium and the degree of nuclear atypia is insufficient to warrant a diagnosis of HSIL**

metaplasia, the full thickness of the epithelium is composed of immature parabasal cells with a high nuclear : cytoplasmic ratio, *Fig. 5.45*. The cells usually are vertical and the nuclei are only slightly hyperchromatic. The most helpful feature in distinguishing HSIL with an immature metaplastic phenotype from immature metaplasia is the absence of nuclear pleomorphism in the latter. The chromatin in metaplastic squamous epithelium is finer and more evenly distributed than in HSIL. In addition, cellular polarity is retained, cell membranes are clearly defined, and cellular crowding is not marked. Immature metaplasia typically shows a regularity of nuclear spacing and the lesions lack significant variation in nuclear size and staining pattern. Atypical cells are rarely seen in the superficial layers of the epithelium and the superficial layers of the epithelium often appear more normal than the lower half. Mucinous epithelium is often present on the surface of immature metaplastic squamous epithelium but only occasionally overlies HSIL, *Fig. 5.46*. Immature metaplasia may have mitotic activity, but AMFs are not present. When significant numbers of mitoses are present it is more likely that the lesion represents a HSIL, *Fig. 5.47*. Sometimes, there may be more pronounced nuclear atypia within immature metaplasia, *Fig. 5.48a, b*. Such lesions are designated by some as *atypical immature metaplasia* (AIM) [42]. Histologically, AIM lesions have a monomorphic population of squamous cells that retain

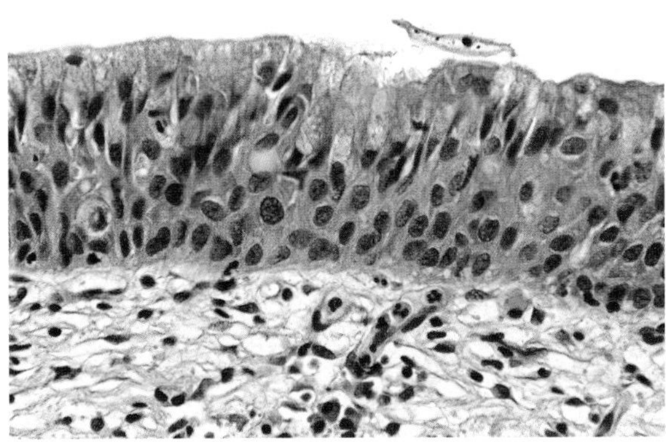

Fig. 5.47
HSIL. **This lesion has a relatively uniform metaplastic appearance, but has considerable numbers of mitoses and exhibits loss of polarity. It is somewhat similar to the lesion shown in *Fig. 5.46*. However, this lesion showed strong diffuse p16^{ink} staining throughout its full thickness (not shown) and was associated with classic HSIL in other sections. Immunohistochemical staining for p16^{ink} is helpful in classifying lesions of this type**

their cellular polarity. They are more cellular than the usual immature squamous metaplasia but show a low mitotic activity, usually less than one mitoses per ten high-powered fields and very few cells are Ki-67 positive [64]. The use of the term AIM is not generally recommended unless clarified with a note because it is not widely accepted and may be confusing to clinicians. Moreover, an AIM diagnosis is poorly reproducible and many of the lesions diagnosed as AIM will be accompanied by a concurrent or subsequent diagnosis of HSIL [143]. In one study, 80% of high-risk HPV positive patients with AIM lesions had a follow-up or concurrent diagnosis of HSIL [70] suggesting that the lesions classified as AIM were very likely subtle forms of HSIL.

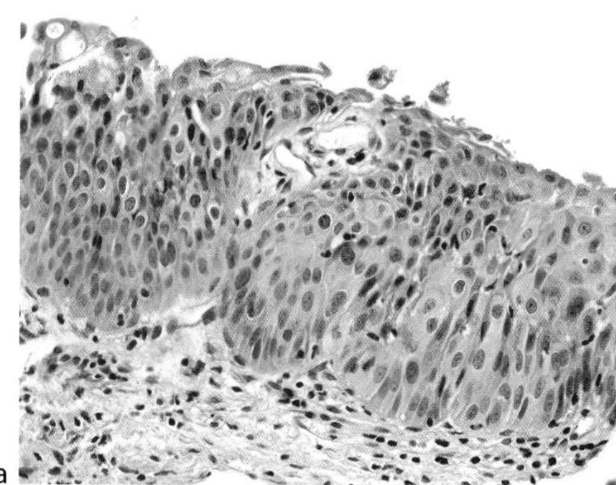

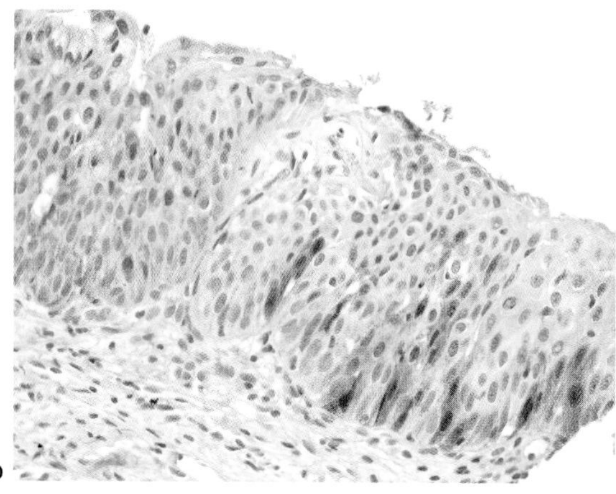

Fig. 5.48
Atypical immature metaplasia (AIM). **(a) This immature squamous metaplastic lesion has more pronounced nuclear atypia than usually seen in metaplasia. Lesions with this histology are referred to by some as AIM lesions. (b) This particular lesion has negative/patchy p16^{ink} staining**

Reparative processes are also sometimes very difficult to differentiate from HSIL, *Fig. 5.49*. In reparative processes atypical basal cells occupy the lower half of the epithelium but the cells have a regular nuclear outline, prominent nucleoli, and usually have distinct cell membranes. In addition, dense acute and chronic inflammatory infiltrates are usually present. In reactive/reparative processes there is usually intracellular edema which leads to spongiosis of the epithelium. Multinucleated cells are generally not observed and the superficial epithelial cells lack the marked variability in nuclear size, shape, and density that characterize HSIL.

Atrophy can have a variety of histological appearances and is occasionally difficult to distinguish from HSIL because it is composed of basal and parabasal cells showing no differentiation. In most instances the atrophic cells are immature but they are quite bland appearing. Although there is a high nuclear : cytoplasmic ratio, atrophic epithelium is thin and shows no nuclear pleomorphism, mitotic activity, atypia, or lack of polarity.

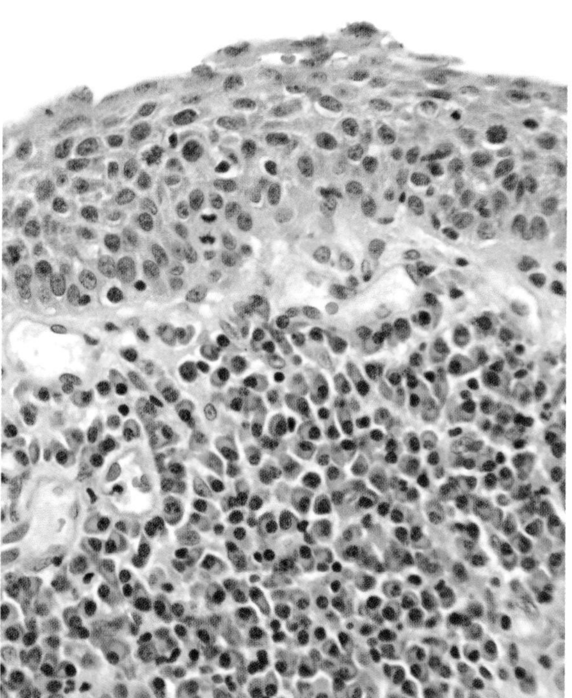

Fig. 5.49
Reparative process mimicking HSIL. **This reparative process shows more nuclear variability than usually seen in repair. However, there is considerable inflammation present**

These cases rarely are mistaken for HSIL, provided the patient's age is known. However, in other instances atrophy results in disturbances in cellular maturation with pseudokoilocytotic cells and cells with nuclear enlargement and nuclear hyperchromasia, ➋ *Fig. 5.50.* Finally, HSIL, particularly with extensive gland involvement, may be confused with microinvasive carcinoma (see ➋ Chap. 6, Carcinoma and Other Tumors of the Cervix), ➋ *Fig. 5.51.*

In our experience it is sometimes simply impossible to distinguish immature metaplasia, AIM, reactive/reparative changes, or atrophy from HSIL based on histopathology alone. In these cases, immunohistochemical staining is essential in differentiating HSIL from the other conditions. P16^{ink} is overexpressed in almost all HSIL and invasive cervical cancers and almost all HSILs show strong, diffuse staining of the epithelium, ➋ *Fig. 5.52* [96, 101, 188]. Both reparative/metaplastic processes and atrophic epithelium do not stain with p16^{ink}, ➋ *Figs. 5.48b* and ➋ *5.50c.* Atrophic epithelium shows either absent or

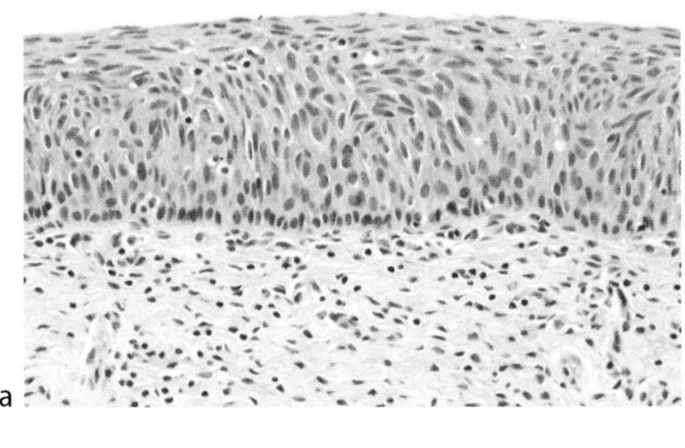

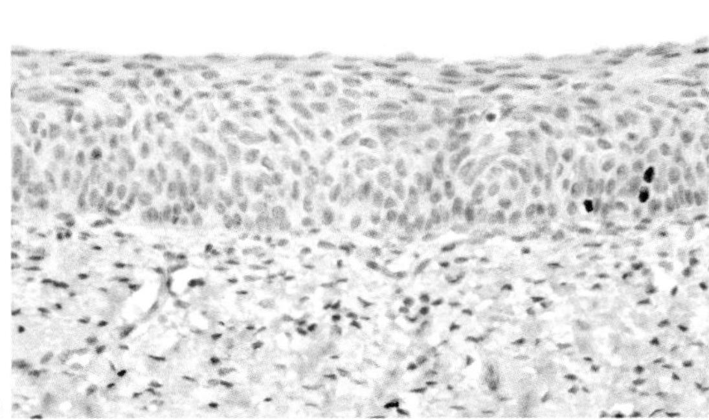

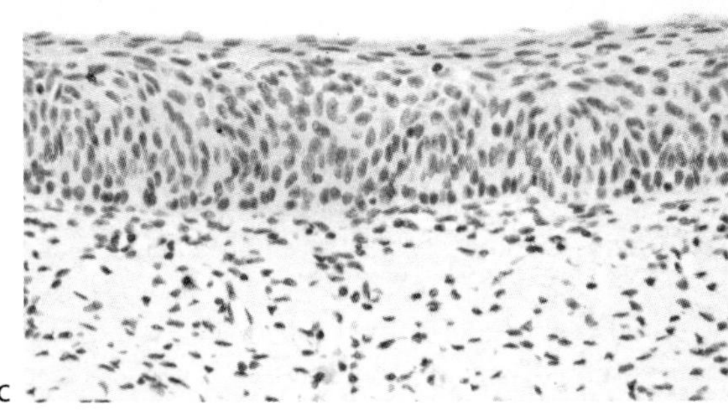

Fig. 5.50
Atrophy mimicking HSIL. **(a) In severe atrophy, there can be considerable variation in nuclear size and irregularly oriented cells mimicing HSIL. (b) Atrophy has a very low Ki-67 staining index and (c) does not stain with p16^{ink}**

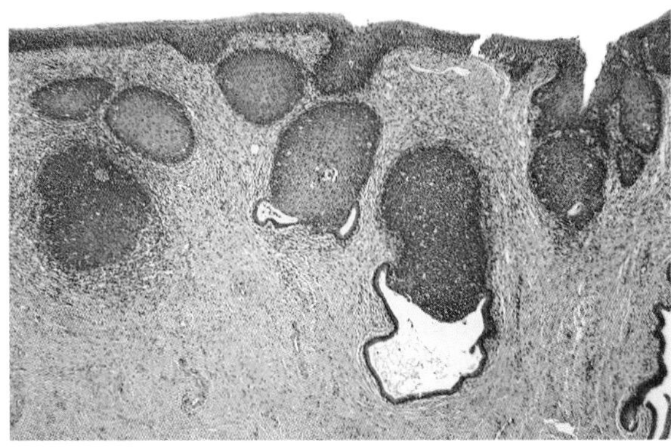

Fig. 5.51
HSIL extending into endocervical glands. **When HSIL extends into endocervical crypts or glands, it can sometimes be misinterpreted as an invasive lesion**

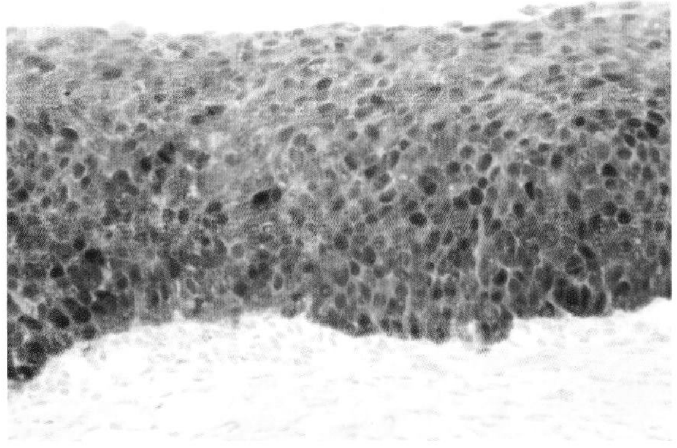

Fig. 5.52
p16^{ink} immunostaining of HSIL. **HSIL typically shows strong, diffuse staining with p16^{ink}**

minimal staining with Ki-67, whereas HSIL shows considerable numbers of labeled cells in all layers of the epithelium.

Behavior of SIL

Before discussing the behavior of SIL, it is important to emphasize that most natural history studies were conducted in the 1970s and 1980s prior to our enhanced understanding of the role of HPV in the pathogenesis of cervical cancer and the realization that LSIL is simply a cytological and histological marker for a productive HPV infection. Moreover, over the last decade, we have come to realize that not only is the interpretation of cervical biopsies and cytology subjective and prone to considerable error, but also that colposcopy is much less accurate than previously thought [66, 120, 181]. Nevertheless, the older natural history studies remain important because they provide insight into both the likelihood that a woman with SIL will spontaneously clear her lesion and the likelihood that she will develop an invasive cervical cancer. Since these studies used the dysplasia/CIS or CIN terminology, in this section those terms will be retained in order to accurately describe the findings from these studies. Two approaches have been used to determine the natural history of SIL. These are prospective, clinical follow-up studies of individual women with cervical lesions and epidemiological studies linking cytology records with cancer registries. Prospective clinical follow-up studies of the "natural history" or behavior of SIL have provided widely varying estimates of the rate of progression and regression in the different lesions. This is not surprising since various studies have used different entry criteria, different diagnostic criteria for categorizing lesions as SIL, and different study designs. For example, some studies have used punch biopsy and endocervical curettage (ECC) to establish the diagnosis. These diagnostic methods may remove (treat) lesions and therefore may interfere with long-term analysis by increasing the frequency of spontaneous regression and decreasing the frequency of progression [137].

➲ *Table 5.6* provides a summary of a meta-analysis of clinical follow-up studies of biopsy-confirmed CIN published through the mid-1990s [129]. The higher the grade of a lesion, the more likely it is to persist and the less likely it is to regress. Overall, it appears that approximately 57% of CIN 1 lesions spontaneously regress in the absence of therapy, and 11% progress to carcinoma in situ. The rates of persistence and progression are greater for high-grade CIN. Forty-three percent of CIN 2 lesions regress and 22% progress to carcinoma in situ. The equivalent rates for CIN 3 lesions were 32% regression and 12% progression to carcinoma in situ. Overall, the progression of all grades of CIN to invasive cancer in the published observational studies is 1.7%. More recently, Castle et al. published estimates of the rate of spontaneous regression of biopsy-confirmed CIN 2 and found that after 24 months of follow-up 43% of the lesions had regressed, which is almost identical to what was found by the meta-analysis of older studies [32].

Table 5.6

Natural history of CIN is dependent of lesional grade

	% Regression	% Persist	Progress to CIS
CIN 1	57	32	11
CIN 2	43	35	22
CIN 3	32	56	12

From [129]

In 1998, Melnikow et al. performed a meta-analysis of studies in which women with a cytologic result of SIL were followed [126]. The analysis included 13,226 women with a cytologic result of LSIL who were followed for at least 6 months and had a median-weighted follow-up of 29 months. There were 10,026 women with HSIL who had a median-weighted follow-up of 25 months. The pooled estimates for regression to normal were 47% for LSIL and 35% for HSIL, ➲ *Fig. 5.53*. No evidence of a relationship between the proportion of subjects regressing to normal and the length of follow-up was observed. Rates of progression of LSIL were 7% at 6 months and 21% at 24 months. For HSIL, the 6- and 24-month pooled progression rates were 7 and 24%. The pooled progression rates for invasive cancer at 6 and 24 months for LSIL were 0.04 and 0.15%, respectively. For HSIL, they were 0.15% at 6 months and 1.44% at 24 months. A much higher rate of regression of cytologically diagnosed LSIL has been reported by Moscicki et al. who prospectively followed a cohort of young women with LSIL. After 12 months of follow-up, 61% had regressed and by 36 months of follow-up 91% had regressed [133].

Another very informative study evaluated the records of the largest cytology laboratory serving the Toronto (Canada) region and linked these records with the Ontario Tumor Registry for the years of 1962–1980 [80]. During this period of time, most women with dysplasia who were evaluated by this laboratory were managed conservatively and did not undergo treatment. This study provides a unique insight into the long-term natural history of

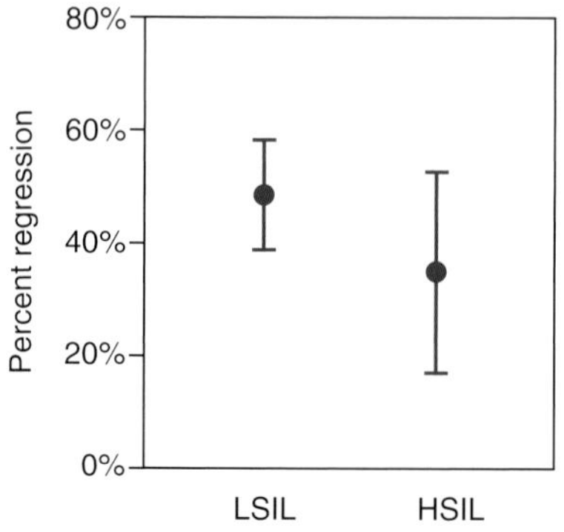

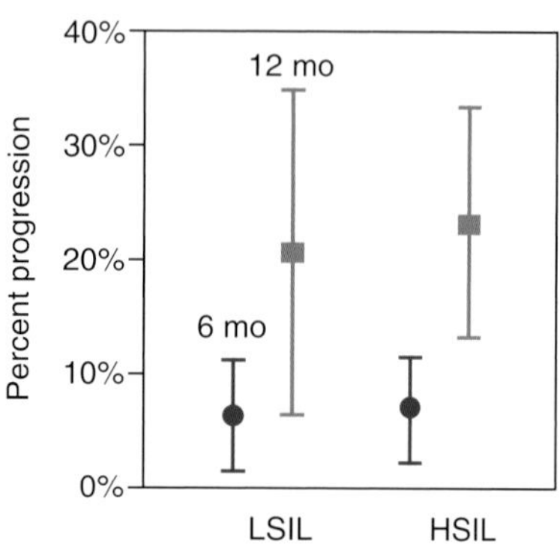

Fig. 5.53

Pooled estimates of the rates of spontaneous regression (*left panel*) of a cytologic diagnosis of LSIL and HSIL. Pooled estimates of the rates of spontaneous progression (*right panel*) of LSIL and HSIL after 6 months (*circles*) and 12 months (*squares*). Progression of HSIL is from CIN 2 to CIN 3 or carcinoma in situ. Bars represent 95% confidence intervals (Modified from reference [126])

Table 5.7

Toronto long-term follow-up of abnormal cervical cytology

Grade of lesion	2 years	10 years
Regression rates[a]		
Mild dysplasia	44%	88%
Moderate dysplasia	33%	83%
Progression rates[b]		
Mild dysplasia	0.6%	12%
Moderate dysplasia	1.5%	17%
Severe dysplasia	2.8%	21%

[a]Regression to within normal limits.
[b]Progression to carcinoma in situ or worse.
Modified from [80].

untreated SIL, *Table 5.7*. The key findings of this study were that after 10 years of follow-up only 12% of untreated mild dysplasia and 17% of untreated moderate dysplasia were diagnosed with carcinoma in situ. At 10 years, 88% of the mild dysplasia and 83% of cases of moderate dysplasia had regressed [80].

What these studies show is that the vast majority of LSIL spontaneously regress in the absence of treatment and the risk that a woman with a LSIL will be subsequently diagnosed with either carcinoma in situ or invasive cervical cancer is relatively low. They also demonstrate that the likelihood that HSIL will regress in the absence of treatment is higher than many clinicians realize and that it generally takes many years for a HSIL to progress to an invasive carcinoma.

Management

Colposcopy combined with colposcopically directed cervical biopsies are the primary modality by which women with abnormal Pap smears are evaluated. Colposcopic examination consists of viewing the cervix with a long-focal-length, dissecting-type microscope at a magnification of about 16× after a solution of dilute (4%) acetic acid has been applied to the cervix. The acetic acid solution acts to remove and dissolve the cervical mucus and causes SIL to become whiter than the surrounding epithelium (acetowhite), *Fig. 5.54*. This coloration allows the colposcopist to identify and biopsy epithelial lesions. In addition to allowing the detection of acetowhite areas, colposcopy also allows for the detection of blood vessel patterns that can indicate HSIL and the detection of invasive cancers. Colposcopy and appropriately directed biopsy have greatly facilitated the management of patients with preinvasive lesions of the cervix because it allows the clinician to rule out invasive cancer and determine the limits of preinvasive disease. Conservative ablative treatment modalities such as cryosurgery, laser ablation, and loop electrosurgical excision procedure (LEEP) can then be used to treat preinvasive disease, with success rates similar to those obtained with cone biopsies.

Precursors of Cervical Adenocarcinoma

Terminology and Historical Perspective

The first indication that precursor lesions for invasive endocervical adenocarcinomas exist came in 1952 when

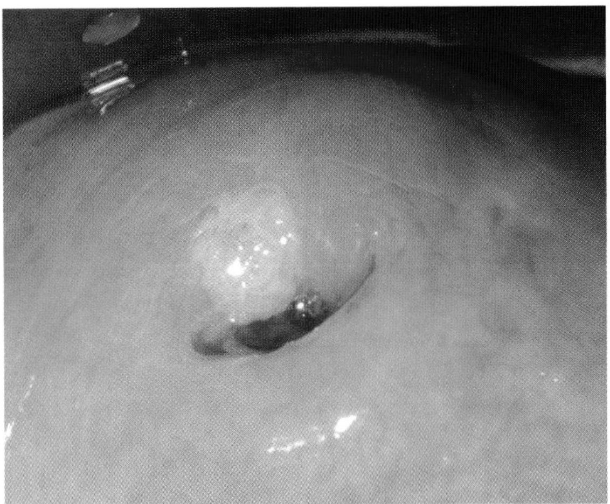

Fig. 5.54
Colposcopic appearance of SIL. **An acetowhite, well-circumscribed lesion is present at the external os**

Helper described highly atypical neoplastic cells lining architecturally normal endocervical glands adjacent to frankly invasive endocervical adenocarcinomas [76]. Shortly thereafter, Friedell and McKay described two patients with atypical glandular lesions of the cervix and designated these lesions AIS because of their histological resemblance to invasive endocervical adenocarcinoma [61]. One of these patients had a coexistent invasive adenocarcinoma of the cervix and one, squamous "carcinoma in situ."

By analogy to squamous cell cervical cancer precursors, some authors have proposed parallel classification schemata for endocervical adenocarcinoma precursors that include lesions with a lesser degree of abnormality than AIS [23, 26, 69, 115]. Such low-grade putative glandular precursor lesions were originally termed *endocervical dysplasia* by Bousfield et al. but other terms such as *atypical hyperplasia* are also used to refer to lesions that resemble AIS, but have a somewhat lesser degree of nuclear atypia and mitotic activity [23, 81]. Gloor and associates suggested that the term *cervical intraepithelial glandular neoplasia* (*CIGN*) be used to refer to both endocervical glandular dysplasia and AIS and that endocervical glandular dysplasia be classified as either CIGN grade 1 or 2 and AIS be classified as CIGN grade 3 [71]. The World Health Organization utilizes the term *glandular dysplasia* to describe a "glandular lesion characterized by significant nuclear abnormalities that are more striking than those in glandular atypia, but fall short of the criteria for adenocarcinoma in situ" [186]. Because of the relative rarity of endocervical glandular dysplasia, the subjective nature of the morphologic criteria used to distinguish it from AIS, and the infrequent coexistence of endocervical glandular dysplasia with AIS, the significance of endocervical glandular dysplasia is not known [110]. A number of studies have utilized objective biomarkers including HPV DNA positivity, proliferation markers such as Ki-67/MIB-1, p16^{INK}, and selective mucin staining to determine whether endocervical glandular dysplasia acts as a precursor to AIS or invasive endocervical adenocarcinoma [3, 10, 71, 77, 109, 111, 136, 162, 185]. Although some of these studies have shown a similar pattern of biomarker expression in both endocervical glandular dysplasia and AIS, most recent studies have not [85, 110, 162]. Investigators who advocate the use of the term "glandular dysplasia" do so under the misguided notion that there is a similar relationship of glandular precursors to HPV infection as there is for squamous precursor lesions. As previously discussed, the histologic manifestation of productive viral infection is LSIL (mild dysplasia). Productive HPV infection is tightly linked to squamous differentiation. Glandular epithelium does not support productive infection. Accordingly, there is no comparable low-grade lesion in glandular epithelium. Since the term glandular dysplasia implies a relationship to AIS and invasive carcinoma that does not exist, the use of this term should be discontinued. Instead, atypical glandular proliferations that fall short of AIS should be evaluated using biomarkers such as p16^{INK} and Ki-67 and classified as reparative changes if they are p16^{INK} negative and show a low Ki-67 labeling index. In contrast, if they express p16^{INK} strongly and diffusely and show a high Ki-67 proliferation index they are classified as AIS.

Epidemiology and Etiology

Over the last 3 decades, endocervical glandular lesions have received increasing attention. This is attributable to a variety of factors. One is a perception that the prevalence of adenocarcinomas of the cervix and its precursor lesions is increasing. There has been a documented absolute increase in the prevalence of invasive adenocarcinomas in specific groups of women in both the USA and Europe. This may be due, in part, to the increased routine use of cytobrushes in screening and the widespread adoption of excisional methods for treating SIL such as the LEEP that permit pathological examination of the entire transformation zone. In addition, there is an increased awareness of these lesions by pathologists, and an awareness by colposcopists that certain types of glandular lesions are difficult to recogniz colposcopically.

The prevalence of AIS is not known but it is considerably less common than SIL. In most series, the ratio between AIS and HSIL has ranged from 1:26 to 1:237. Estimates for the USA as a whole are available in the SEER public database that contains data from patients entered into the database between 1976 and 1995, which is the last year that in situ carcinomas were reported to the database [5, 192]. In the SEER registry, there are a total of 149,178 women with either in situ or invasive cervical cancer. Of these, 96% had squamous lesions and 4% had glandular lesions. 121,793 (82%) of all cervical lesions were classified as in situ and of these, 120,317 (99%) were squamous cell carcinoma in situ and only 1,476 (1%) were AIS. For comparison, of the 27,385 women with invasive cervical cancer, 4,369 (16%) had invasive adenocarcinoma. In 1991–1995, the age-adjusted incidence rate in the SEER database for squamous carcinoma in situ in White women was 27.93 cases per 100,000, whereas the age-adjusted incidence rate for AIS was only 1.25 per 100,000 [152, 192]. Although the overall incidence of AIS remains quite low, the incidence increased approximately sixfold from the 1970s to the 1990s [192]. Because AIS is no longer reported, we do not know if the incidence has continued to increase over the last 2 decades. AIS rates peak at age 35–44 years in both White and Black women [192].

The age relationship between AIS and invasive adenocarcinoma is similar to that of HSIL and invasive squamous cell carcinoma, suggesting that AIS is a precursor lesion [152]. However, unlike squamous lesions of the cervix in which high-grade precursors occur more frequently than invasive cancer, exactly the opposite relationship exists for AIS and invasive adenocarcinoma of the cervix. The incidence of invasive glandular lesions is higher than that of noninvasive glandular lesions in all age groups [152]. A number of reasons have been proposed for this apparent discrepancy, including the fact that AIS is more difficult to detect both cytologically and colposcopically than is SIL and, therefore, might not be detected prior to the development of invasive adenocarcinoma. The experience reported for both Finland and Australia indicates that few women with endocervical adenocarcinoma are identified through screening [128, 140]. Additional support implicating AIS as a precursor of invasive adenocarcinoma comes from several anecdotal case reports and two small series of patients who had cytological or histological evidence of AIS several years prior to the detection of invasive adenocarcinoma [18, 21, 95]. Although these studies have been interpreted as indicating that AIS is a precursor lesion, it is conceivable that an unrecognized invasive cancer was present at the time of the original Pap test or cervical biopsy.

The proportion of AIS that occurs in association with SIL ranges from 24% to 75% [4, 38, 51]. This suggests that the two types of lesions may share a common etiology. Moreover, many of the risk factors are similar between glandular and squamous lesions. These include multiple sex partners, use of oral contraceptives, early onset of sexual activity, and low socioeconomic class [190]. Both squamous and glandular lesions also appear to be associated with high-risk types of HPV. Using in situ hybridization, Tase and coworkers examined eight cases of AIS for the presence of HPV DNA and found that five of the cases contained HPV but that, unlike SIL lesions analyzed with the same method, the majority of AIS was associated with HPV 18 as opposed to HPV 16 in SIL [184]. Since this initial report, other groups have analyzed AIS for the presence of HPV DNA, and it appears clear that most AIS is associated with HPV DNA and that HPV 16 and 18 are the most commonly encountered types. Duggan analyzed a series of 37 cases of AIS using PCR with dot blot enhancement and identified HPV 18 in 43% of cases and HPV 16 in 23% [55]. HPV DNA positivity was not correlated with any clinical variable in that series. Recently, Quint et al. analyzed 31 cases of AIS using a highly sensitive PCR method and identified HPV DNA in all of the cases. HPV 18 was found in 26% and HPV 16 in 70% [156].

Clinical Features

Most women with AIS are asymptomatic and the lesions are detected either during screening or fortuitously on an ECC, cervical punch biopsy, cone or loop excisional biopsy performed during the workup for SIL. In women who are symptomatic, the most common complaint is abnormal vaginal bleeding, either postcoital, postmenopausal, or out of phase. Rarely, symptomatic patients present with an abnormal discharge.

AIS is difficult to detect both cytologically and colposcopically [57, 158]. The detection of AIS on ECC can also be difficult [4]. In one histological study of 42 women with AIS, only 45% of the women had atypical glandular cells (AGC) detected cytologically on the prediagnosis cervical cytology [51]. The other cases were detected fortuitously on biopsies taken to evaluate SIL. In another study of 36 women with AIS, glandular abnormalities were detected on the prediagnosis cytology in only one-half of the women [4]. However, a large case-control study of AIS from Australia using data from a statewide registry found that the screening histories of 307 women with AIS were similar to that of healthy, control women which was interpreted as indicating that AIS is usually detected through screening [127].

The distribution of AIS in the cervix is important for determining the most appropriate clinical management of these patients. AIS involves both the surface and glands in almost all cases. In 65% of cases, it involves the transformation zone [4, 15] and in the vast majority of cases it is unifocal. It can extend for a distance of up to 3 cm into the endocervical canal [15, 45].

Pathologic Findings

AIS is characterized by the presence of endocervical glands lined by atypical columnar epithelial cells that cytologically resemble the cells of invasive adenocarcinoma but which occur in the absence of invasion, ➲ *Fig. 5.55*. These cells have elongated, cigar-shaped, hyperchromatic nuclei with coarse granular chromatin, ➲ *Fig. 5.56*. The amount of cytoplasm is greatly reduced and there is only minimal intracellular mucin. This produces an increased nuclear : cytoplasmic ratio. The cells are crowded and pseudostratified, forming two or more rows. AIS may involve glands either focally, multifocally, or diffusely. Typically, some glands show an abrupt transition between normal epithelium and AIS, ➲ *Fig. 5.57*. Mitotic figures including AMFs are common and apoptotic bodies are also commonly seen in the epithelium, usually subadjacent to the nucleus, ➲ *Fig. 5.58*. Architecturally, the glands of AIS can have numerous outpouchings and complex papillary infoldings and may display a cribriform pattern focally, ➲ *Fig. 5.57*.

Ostor et al. have described two histological types of AIS [142]. One is the typical endocervical type of AIS described above. The other has features of an intestinal, as opposed to endocervical, mucosa with goblet cells and sometimes Paneth cells, ➲ *Fig. 5.59*. The colonic type is uncommon and usually occurs in association with typical endocervical AIS. The goblet cells in colonic AIS contain

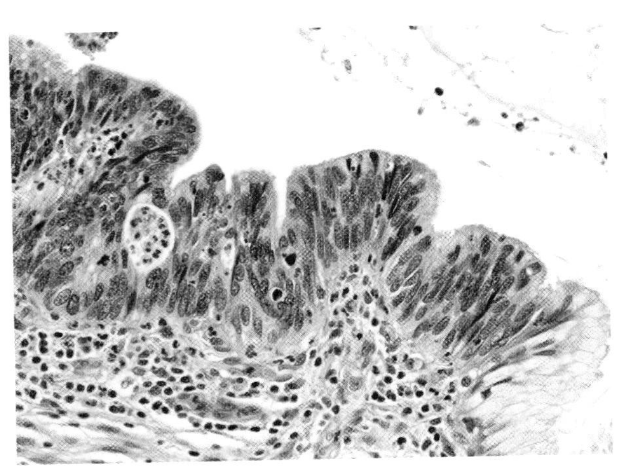

Fig. 5.56
Adenocarcinoma in situ (AIS). **The cells of AIS are pseudostratified and have elongated, hyperchromatic nuclei**

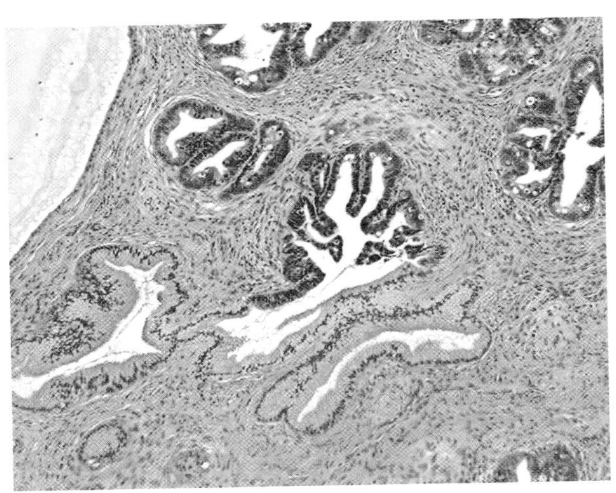

Fig. 5.55
Adenocarcinoma in situ (AIS). **AIS is characterized by endocervical glands lined by atypical columnar cells resembling the cells of adenocarcinoma**

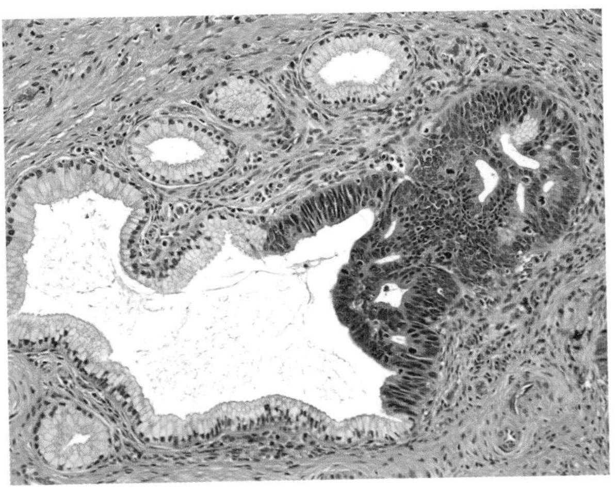

Fig. 5.57
Adenocarcinoma in situ (AIS). **Frequently there is a sharp transition between the normal columnar epithelium and the neoplastic glandular epithelium**

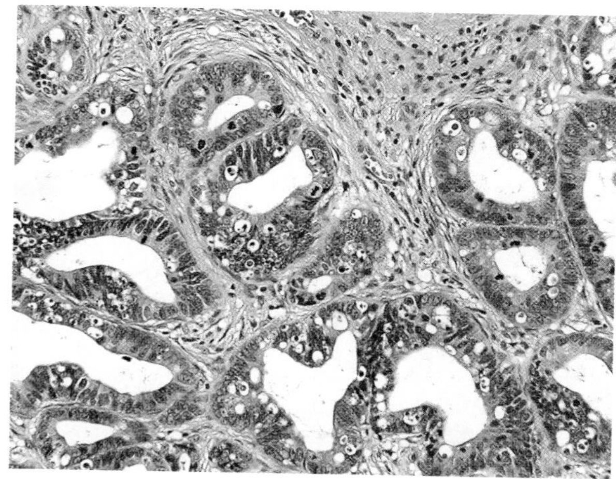

Fig. 5.58
Adenocarcinoma in situ (AIS). **Mitotic figures and apoptotic bodies are usually present**

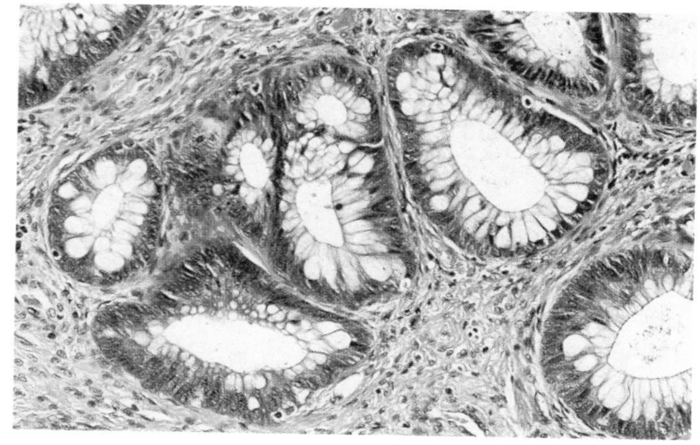

Fig. 5.59
Adenocarcinoma in situ (AIS) of the intestinal type. **The intestinal type of AIS shows goblet cells and sometimes even Paneth cells**

O-acetylated sialomucin, which is a marker of intestinal differentiation. Some intestinal types of AIS also contain argentaffin and Paneth cells [88, 187]. Endometrioid types of AIS and more rarely, adenosquamous, and clear cell AIS also occur [71, 89].

Invasion should be suspected if the involved glands extend beyond the glandular field or beyond the deepest uninvolved endocervical crypt. In addition, in AIS there should be no desmoplasia or stromal reaction around the involved glands. Other worrisome features that can be associated with invasion are exuberant glandular budding, an extensive cribiform pattern, foci in which the glands become confluent or back to back and the formation of papillary projections from the endocervical surface [105, 141].

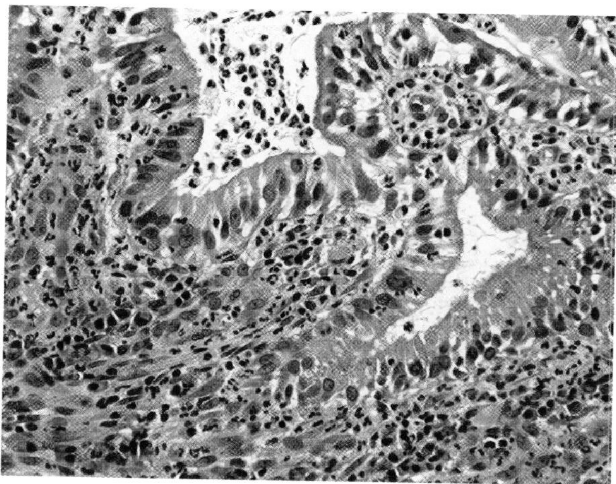

Fig. 5.60
Reparative changes of endocervical epithelium. **When reactive processes involve the endocervical epithelium the nuclei become enlarged and have prominent nucleoli, but they lack hyperchromasia, nuclear clearing, and have few mitotic figures**

Differential Diagnosis

The differential diagnosis of AIS includes reparative/reactive glandular atypia secondary to inflammation, radiation or viral infections, Arias-Stella reaction, microglandular hyperplasia, endometriosis, tubal metaplasia, mesonephric remnants, and invasive adenocarcinoma. Endocervical glands may display a wide range of cytological and architectural changes in response to inflammation and radiation. In reactive/reparative atypia, the nuclei become enlarged and have prominent nucleoli, but have nuclear clearing and lack hyperchromasia, ➲ *Fig. 5.60*. Nuclei may be pleomorphic but the chromatin is usually smudged and degenerative in appearance. Mitotic activity is usually absent or minimal, as is pseudostratification. Care must be taken to distinguish between true pseudostratification and tangential sectioning through glands that can appear as pseudostratification. Inflamed endocervical glands with reserve cell hyperplasia can also appear as pseudostratification, ➲ *Fig. 5.61*. Although intraglandular papillary projections

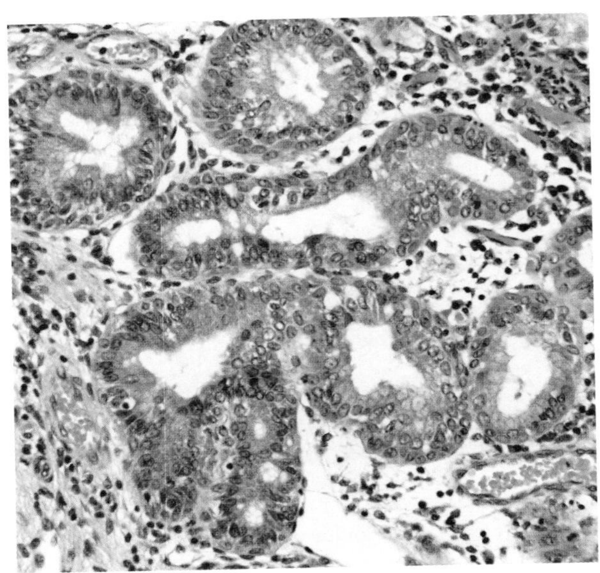

Fig. 5.61
Inflamed endocervical epithelium with reserve cell hyperplasia. **When endocervical glands are inflamed and also have reserve cell hyperplasia, they can appear to be pseudostratified and occasionally be mistaken for AIS**

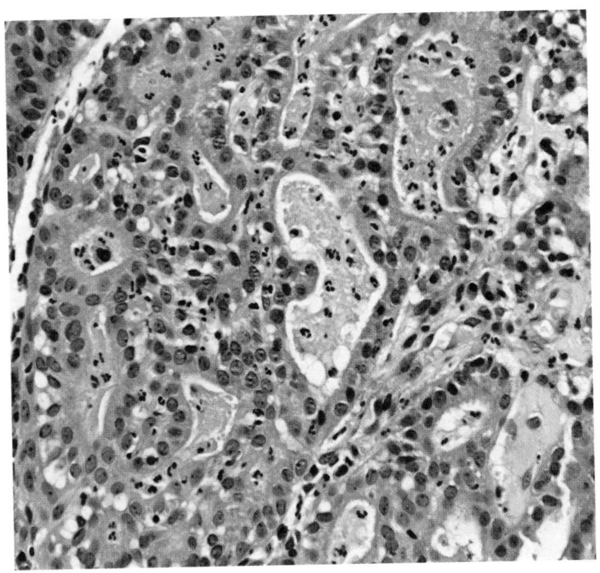

Fig. 5.62
Microglandular hyperplasia with reparative changes. **When significant inflammation is present microglandular hyperplasia can become somewhat atypical and mistaken for AIS. Even when inflamed, mitotic figures are uncommon in microglandular hyperplasia and there is a lack of pseudostratification and minimal nuclear atypia**

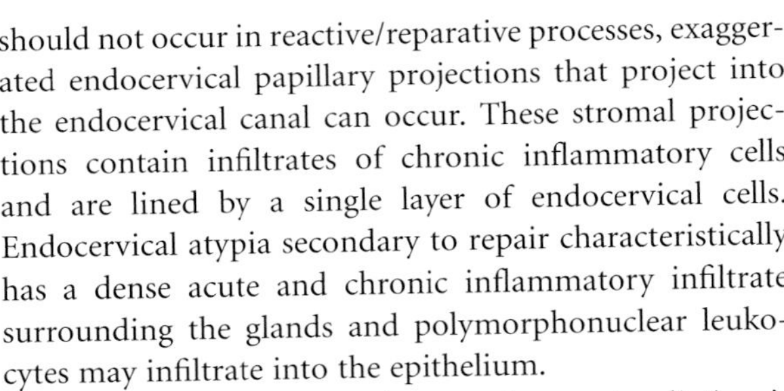

should not occur in reactive/reparative processes, exaggerated endocervical papillary projections that project into the endocervical canal can occur. These stromal projections contain infiltrates of chronic inflammatory cells and are lined by a single layer of endocervical cells. Endocervical atypia secondary to repair characteristically has a dense acute and chronic inflammatory infiltrate surrounding the glands and polymorphonuclear leukocytes may infiltrate into the epithelium.

Reactive glandular atypia secondary to irradiation is characterized by nuclear enlargement and pleomorphism, but the cytoplasm is frequently vacuolated or granular. Pseudostratification and mitotic figures are absent. Atypia due to irradiation has greater cell-to-cell variation in size and shape than AIS or endocervical glandular atypia. Glands with the Arias-Stella reaction have a single layer of hyperchromatic, enlarged nuclei that frequently protrude into the gland lumen (i.e., hobnail cells). Typically, Arias-Stella reaction involves only a portion of a gland and mitotic activity is absent. Although microglandular hyperplasia, especially when inflamed, can occasionally be confused with AIS, microglandular hyperplasia lacks significant nuclear atypia, lacks pseudostratification, and has few mitotic figures, ➲ *Fig. 5.62*. Moreover, microglandular hyperplasia has a characteristic pattern of closely packed, small, uniform glands. Atypical forms of microglandular hyperplasia have been described that form solid masses of epithelium and have significant degrees of cytological atypia [210]. These lesions almost always contain areas of typical microglandular hyperplasia that allow them to be identified as atypical forms of microglandular hyperplasia (see ➲ Chap. 6, Carcinoma and Other Tumors of the Cervix). Similarly, endometriosis of the cervix is usually readily recognizable and easily distinguished from AIS. Typical endometriosis consists of glands and endometrial-type stroma. The cells lining the glands are basally located endometrial-type cells that can be pseudostratified and mitotically inactive. Both tubal metaplasia and mesonephric remnants should not be mistaken for AIS since they have bland, non-mitotically active nuclei and typical histological features that allow them to be recognized (see ➲ Chap. 6, Carcinoma and Other Tumors of the Cervix). However, tubal metaplasia can occasionally have more enlarged nuclei with coarse chromatin that can make it difficult to distinguish from AIS, ➲ *Fig. 5.63*.

Immunohistochemical staining can be quite useful in distinguishing AIS from other glandular lesions. Most, but not all, AIS lesions demonstrate diffuse nuclear and/or cytoplasmic immunoreactivity for p16^{INK}, ➲ *Fig. 5.64* [30, 138, 162]. Reactive/reparative lesions and microglandular hyperplasia are usually p16^{INK} negative. Tubal metaplasia is not infrequently p16^{INK} positive, but the staining pattern is different than that seen with AIS. In tubal metaplasia the staining with p16^{INK} is usually focal and weak, as opposed to diffuse and strong as seen in AIS, ➲ *Fig. 5.65* [123]. Another useful marker is Ki-67 (MIB1). The Ki-67 proliferation index in tubal metaplasia and endometriosis is usually quite low, less than 10% of the cells will stain positively, whereas the Ki-67 proliferation index in AIS is much higher [30, 124, 150]. Over 30% of the cells in AIS lesions usually show nuclear staining with Ki-67 and in most instances the majority of AIS cells will stain positively, ➲ *Fig. 5.64b*. Bcl-2 has also been used to help differentiate AIS from endometriosis and tubal metaplasia. Bcl-2 appears to have anti-apoptotic properties and both tubal metaplasia and endometriosis stain positively for bcl-2, whereas AIS lesions that show significant degrees of apoptosis stain either negatively or only focally positive with bcl-2 [30]. Carcinoembryonic antigen (CEA) is expressed cytoplasmically in 67% of AIS, whereas the normal columnar epithelium of the endocervix is either negative or demonstrates only luminal, as opposed to cytoplasmic staining [82, 119]. Immunohistochemical staining for vimentin typically is negative in AIS lesions but shows cytoplasmic positivity in tubal metaplasia and endometriosis [119]. Similarly, both tubal metaplasia

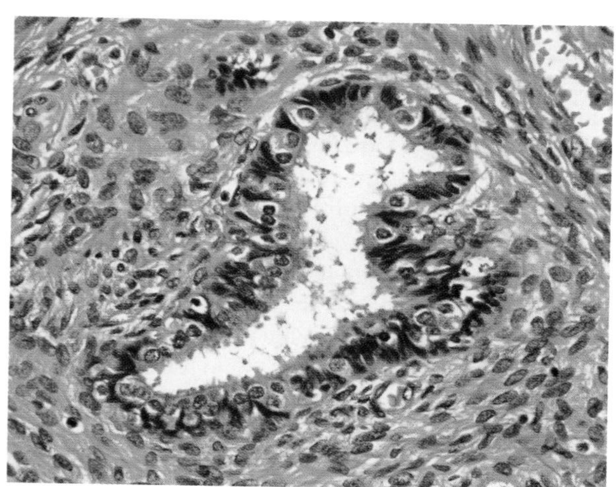

Fig. 5.63
Atypical tubal metaplasia. **Occasionally, tubal metaplasia becomes more hyperchromatic and has enlarged nuclei with coarse chromatin. When this occurs it can be misinterpreted as AIS. However, such lesions typically lack mitotic activity and pseudostratification**

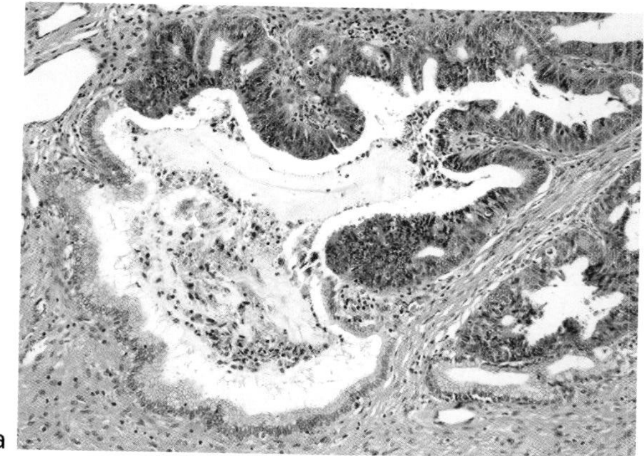

a

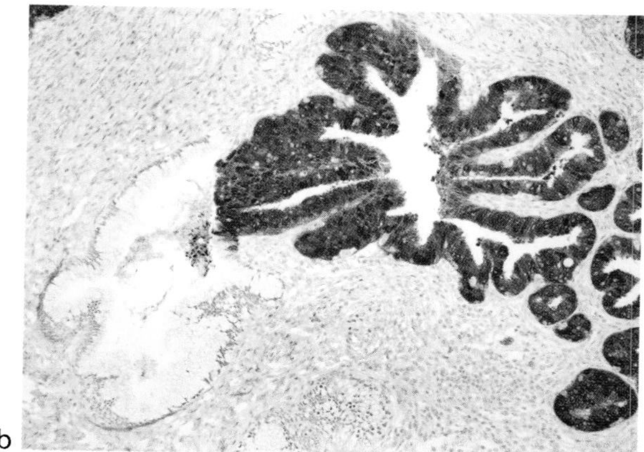

b

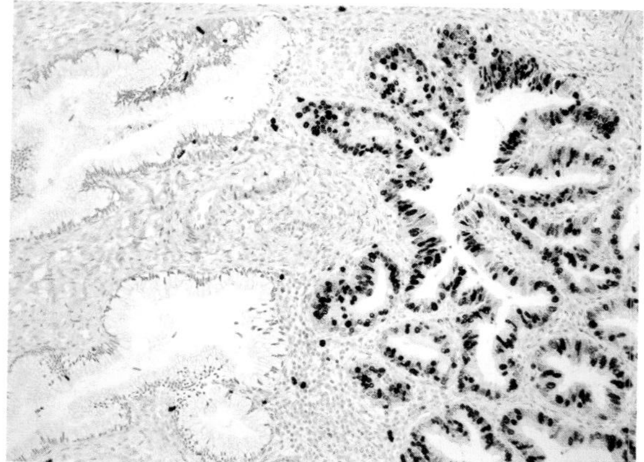

c

Fig. 5.64
p16^{ink} staining of adenocarcinoma in situ (AIS). **(a) Classic AIS showing sharp demarcation between normal and neoplastic tissue. (b) The neoplastic tissue stains strongly with p16^{ink}. (c) It has a high Ki-67 labeling index**

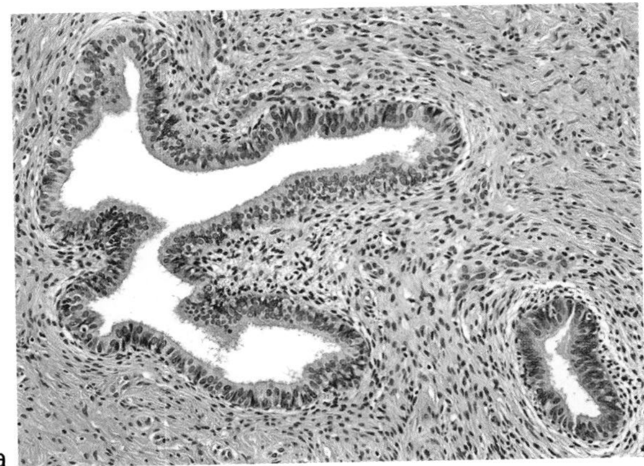
a

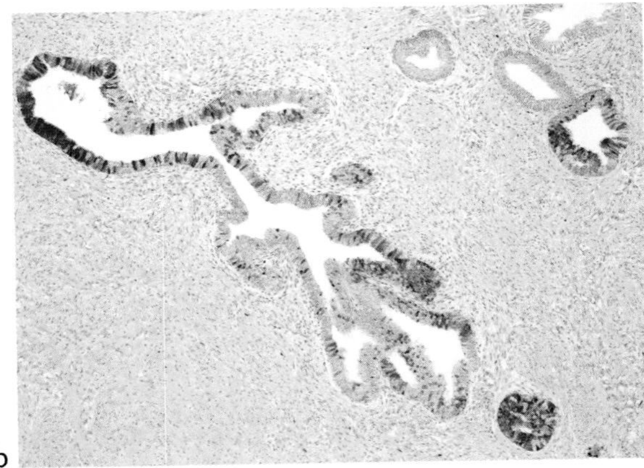
b

Fig. 5.65
Typical tubal metaplasia. **Tubal metaplasia shows focal weak staining with p16^{ink}, as opposed to the strong diffuse staining seen in AIS. (a) H&E, (b) p16^{ink} immunostaining**

and endometriosis usually stain positively for estrogen receptors, whereas AIS does not. Some authors have recommended that a panel of antibodies be utilized when trying to identify difficult cases of AIS. This panel includes Ki-67, p16^{ink}, bcl-2, monoclonal CEA, vimentin, and estrogen receptor antibodies [123]. In our experience, a panel of p16, Ki-67, estrogen and progesterone receptors suffices.

Clinical Behavior and Treatment

Due to the relative rarity of AIS, no natural history studies have been published and therefore the evidence that these lesions are precursors for invasive endocervical adenocarcinoma remains circumstantial. Despite this, until recently the treatment of choice was simple hysterectomy. Recently, however, there have been several series of patients with AIS who have been followed after cone biopsy. These studies have generally shown relatively low rates of invasive adenocarcinoma and recurrent AIS among women treated by means of a cone biopsy, provided the endocervical margin is negative. A recent meta-analysis found that of 671 patients who had been treated by cone biopsy and followed, 26% with negative margins developed recurrent disease, and 0.1% developed invasive adenocarcinoma [165]. Women with positive endocervical margins are at significantly greater risk for having an undiagnosed invasive cervical adenocarcinoma or for developing recurrent AIS. Invasive adenocarcinoma was found in 5.2% of such patients in the above meta-analysis. Based on these studies, conservative management by cone biopsy alone is now considered to be an option in women with AIS desirous of maintaining their fertility, if the cone biopsy margins are negative.

Cervical Cytology

Strengths and Limitations of Cervical Cytology

Although it was introduced over a half century ago, cervical cytologic screening continues to be the most effective cancer prevention test available. The cytologic screening has never been tested in a prospective double-blind study; however, over the half century since it was introduced, so much epidemiological and modeling data have accumulated demonstrating the effectiveness of cytology that it has become the index by which all other cancer screening tests are compared. Cytologic screening performed only twice in a woman's lifetime can reduce her risk for invasive cervical cancer by up to 43% and yearly screening is estimated to reduce a woman's risk by over 90% [72, 146]. However, despite the effectiveness of cytologic screening, it is important to remember that no screening, diagnostic, or therapeutic technique used in medicine is perfect, and cervical cytology is no exception. Some women will develop invasive cervical cancer, despite annual cytologic screening.

Over the last decade, numerous advances have been made in cervical cytology collection techniques, how cytological preparations are evaluated, and the classification systems used for reporting cytologic diagnosis. One of the most important advances has been the recent introduction of liquid-based cytology. With liquid-based cytology, the cells collected from the cervix are transferred directly to a liquid fixation solution that is shipped to the cytology laboratory where the slide is prepared. One of the primary advantages of liquid-based cytology is that HPV DNA testing can be performed directly from liquid-based specimens when a diagnosis of ASCUS is made (i.e., "reflex" HPV DNA testing).

TBS Terminology

In 1988, TBS for reporting cervical/vaginal cytological diagnoses was developed to provide uniform guidelines for reviewing and reporting gynecological Pap tests. TBS classification was subsequently modified in 1991 and 2001 [201]. This is now the most widely used classification for cervical cytology in the USA. There are two distinct parts to the report: a statement of specimen adequacy and a general categorization, Table 5.8. In addition, in many instances a descriptive diagnosis is provided. This is designed to assist clinicians by answering three basic questions: (1) Was the sample adequate? (2) Was the Pap test normal? (3) If the test was not completely normal, what specifically was wrong?

Cytological Appearance of Cervical Cancer Precursors

TBS classification categorizes precursors to cervical cancer as "epithelial cell abnormalities." The category "epithelial cell abnormalities" is subdivided into abnormalities of squamous cells and abnormalities involving glandular cells, either endocervical or endometrial. Cytological changes previously classified as mild squamous cytological atypia and atypical endocervical cells are also included in this category.

Squamous Cell Abnormalities

ASC The ASC category is used to designate cytological changes suggestive of a squamous intraepithelial lesion that are quantitatively or qualitatively insufficient for a definitive diagnosis of SIL. There are several points that need to be made with respect to ASC. First, a diagnosis of ASC is one of exclusion; the cells are abnormal, but they do not warrant a diagnosis of SIL. Second, a diagnosis of ASC should not be used when the underlying process is inflammatory or reactive, such slides should be classified as "negative for intraepithelial lesion or malignancy" rather than ASC. Third, although the ASC category is sometimes disparagingly referred to as a "cytological wastebasket," there are specific criteria that should be used for making this diagnosis. If these criteria are adhered to, the rate of ASC in a routine cytology laboratory should be no greater than about 5% of all cytology specimens and the ASC rate should be approximately twice the SIL rate.

The 2001 Bethesda System subdivides the ASC category into two subdivisions. Atypical squamous cells of

Table 5.8
The Bethesda system (TBS) 2001 classification.

Adequacy of the specimen
Satisfactory for evaluation
Unsatisfactory for evaluation
General categorization
Negative for intraepithelial lesion or malignancy
Epithelial cell abnormalities
Squamous Cell
Atypical squamous cells (ASC)
Atypical squamous cells – undetermined significance (ASCUS)
Atypical squamous cells – cannot exclude HSIL (ASC-H)
Low-grade squamous intraepithelial lesion (LSIL) encompassing human papillomavirus[a] and mild dysplasia/CIN 1
High-grade squamous intraepithelial lesion (HSIL) encompassing moderate and severe dysplasia, CIS/CIN 2 and CIN 3
Squamous cell carcinoma
Glandular cell
Atypical glandular cells
Atypical glandular cells (unqualified)
Atypical endocervical cells (unqualified)
Atypical endometrial cells (unqualified)
Atypical glandular cells, favor neoplastic
Atypical endocervical cells, favor neoplastic
Adenocarcinoma in situ (AIS)
Endocervical adenocarcinoma
Endometrial adenocarcinoma
Adenocarcinoma, nonspecific
Other
Hormonal evaluation (applies to vaginal smears only)
Hormonal pattern compatible with age and history
Hormonal pattern incompatible with age and history (specify)
Hormonal evaluation not possible because of. . .(specify)

[a]Cellular changes of human papillomavirus, previously termed koilocytosis koilocytotic atypia, and condylomatous atypia are included in the category of LSIL.
CIN, cervical intraepithelial neoplasia; CIS, carcinoma in situ.

Table 5.9
Criteria used to diagnose atypical squamous cells (ASC)

Atypical squamous cells of undetermined significance (ASCUS)
Cells resemble superficial or intermediate squamous cells in size and configuration
Nuclei are 2–3 times the size of a normal intermediate cell
Nuclei are round to oval with minimal irregularities
Nuclei are normochromatic to slightly hyperchromatic
Atypical squamous cells – cannot exclude HSIL (ASC-H)
Cells resemble parabasal or basal cells in size and configuration
Nuclei often have uneven chromatin and are hyperchromatic
Nuclear contour is often irregular

undetermined significance (*ASCUS*) refers to samples in which the cytological changes are suggestive of LSIL, but lack sufficient cytological abnormalities to allow a definitive diagnosis. Atypical squamous cells – cannot exclude HSIL (*ASC-H*) refers to samples in which the cytological changes are suggestive of HSIL but the cytological abnormalities are insufficient to allow a definitive interpretation [170].

The specific criteria used to diagnose ASC are given in *Table 5.9*. One of the major criteria used to distinguish ASCUS from benign cellular changes is nuclear size. In ASCUS, the nuclei are typically 2–3 times the size of a normal intermediate cell. In addition, to changes in nuclear size, the nuclei in ASCUS are somewhat irregular and frequently hyperchromatic, *Fig. 5.66*. However, the degree of nuclear changes considered sufficient to warrant a diagnosis of ASCUS is highly subjective and varies between cytologists. This introduces a degree of uncertainty with respect to a diagnosis of ASCUS, and studies have shown that a diagnosis of ASCUS is the least reproducible of all cytological diagnoses [39, 40, 68, 181]. In the recent NCI-sponsored ALTS trial, only 55% of the referral Pap tests originally classified as ASCUS were classified as ASCUS by the pathology quality control panel [181]. It should also be noted that a diagnosis of ASCUS is sometimes made when there are cells with some, but not all of the criteria necessary for a diagnosis of LSIL, *Fig. 5.67*.

In the USA, the median reporting rate of ASCUS is 4.7% according to a 2003 College of American Pathology survey [47]. Approximately, 7–12% of women with a diagnosis of ASC will have HSIL when colposcopy is performed [2, 9, 113, 118, 206].

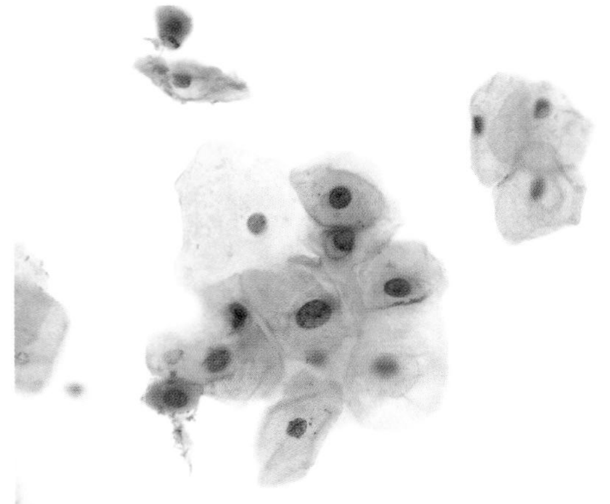

Fig. 5.66
Atypical squamous cells of undetermined significance (ASCUS). **Intermediate squamous epithelial cells demonstrate nuclear enlargement and hyperchromasia. No organisms or inflammatory changes were identified on the smear**

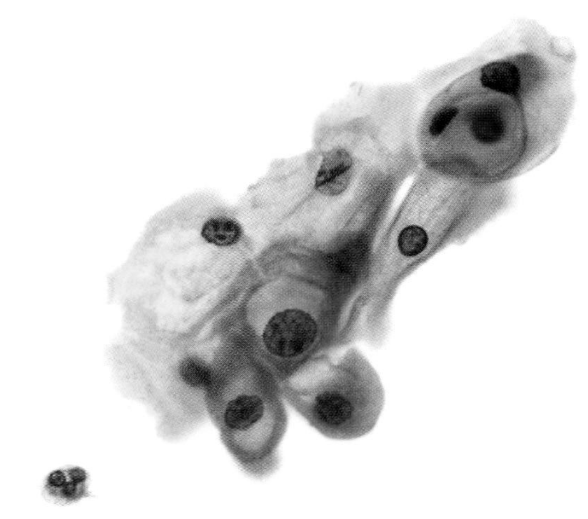

Fig. 5.67
Atypical squamous cells of undetermined significance (ASCUS). **These cells are suggestive, but not diagnostic of a LSIL since they have a considerable degree of nuclear enlargement and perinuclear halos. However, the findings are not sufficient to allow a diagnosis of LSIL and there were only a limited number of such cells present so a diagnosis of ASCUS was rendered**

In ASC-H, the cells resemble parabasal or basal cells in size and configuration. These cells frequently have irregular nuclear contours and uneven chromatin, *Fig. 5.68.* There are varying degrees of hyperchromasia. The differential diagnosis in such cases is between atypical immature squamous metaplasia and HSIL. The median reporting rate of ASC-H in the USA in 2003 was 0.4% according to the CAP survey [47]. The majority of women with ASC-H are high-risk HPV DNA positive and HSIL (CIN 2, 3) lesions are identified at the time of colposcopy in 12–68% of women with ASC-H [11, 112, 170]. Because of the high prevalence of HSIL (CIN 2, 3) lesions in women with ASC-H, it has been suggested that ASC-H would be more appropriately referred to as "equivocal HSIL" [207].

LSILs The LSIL category in TBS includes both HPV effects and mild dysplasia (CIN 1). The cells of LSIL are of the superficial or intermediate cell type. They have enlarged nuclei that are 4–6 times the size of a normal intermediate cell nucleus (*Fig. 5.69*), but many vary in size and in LSIL with marked HPV cytopathic effects, the nuclei are often only two times the size of a normal intermediate cell nucleus, *Fig. 5.70.* In LSIL, the nuclei are

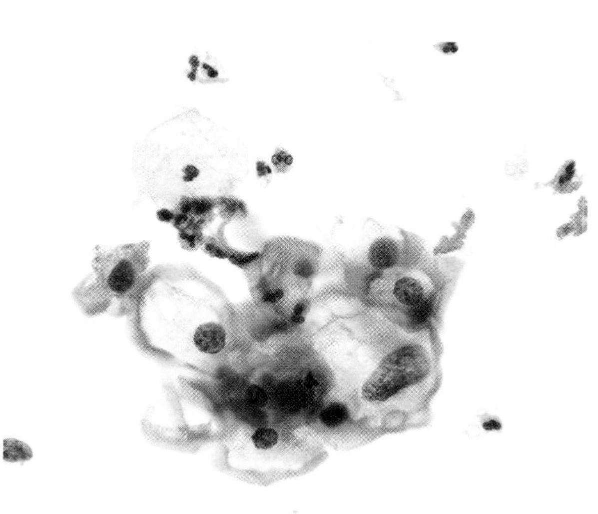

Fig. 5.69
LSIL. **The cells are of the intermediate type with nuclear enlargement and prominent koilocytosis. One of the nuclei is more than 10 times the size of a normal intermediate cell**

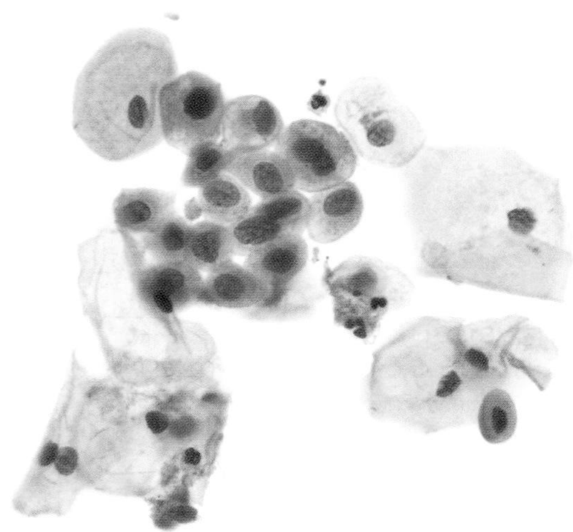

Fig. 5.68
Atypical squamous cells of undetermined significance cannot exclude HSIL (ASC-H). **A cluster of atypical immature metaplastic type cells is present. The cells have an increased nuclear : cytoplasmic ratio, hyperchromasia, and slightly irregular nuclei. However, the cells have more cytoplasm than usually associated with HSIL and only a few clusters were present**

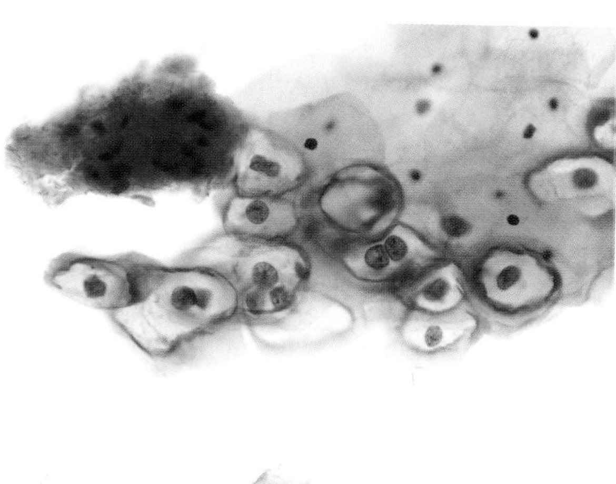

Fig. 5.70
LSIL. **Cells from this lesion demonstrate considerable koilocytosis with multinucleation and prominent halos**

◘ Table 5.10
Criteria used to diagnosed squamous epithelial cell abnormalities

Bethesda system	LSIL	HSIL		
CIN terminology	CIN 1	CIN 2	CIN 3	
WHO terminology	Mild dysplasia	Moderate dysplasia	Severe dysplasia	CIS
Cell type	Superficial or intermediate	Parabasal	Basal	Basal, spindle, pleomorphic
Cell arrangement	Singly or sheets	Singly or sheets	Singly or sheets	Singly or sheets or syncitia
Number abnormal cells	+	++	+++	++++
Koilocytosis	+++	+	+/–	+/–
Nuclear size	+++	++	+	+
Hyperchromasia	+	++	+++	++++
Nuclear:cytoplasmic ratio	+	++	+++	++++

usually hyperchromatic, and multinucleation is common. The chromatin is finely granular and uniformly distributed. The cells typically occur as individual cells or as sheets of cells with well-defined cell borders. With cytology methods such as liquid-based cytology and computerized imaging systems, the rate of LSIL appears to be increasing in the USA. In surveys taken in the 1990s, the median reporting rate of LSIL in U.S. laboratories was 1.6% but by 2004 this has increased to 2.4% [47, 92]. A recent report of the impact of implementing a computerized cytology imaging system in a tertiary military medical center reported that after implementation the rate of LSIL increased from 2.6% to 3.9% [54].

HSILs Because TBS combines moderate and severe dysplasia together with carcinoma in situ in the HSIL category, there is a wide variation in the cytological appearance of HSIL. As the severity of the lesion increases, the degree of differentiation and the amount of cytoplasm decreases, the nuclear : cytoplasmic ratio increases, and the degree of nuclear atypia increases, ➋ *Table 5.10*. HSIL of the type previously classified as moderate dysplasia typically contains cells similar to those seen in LSIL, as well as atypical immature cells of the parabasal type, ➋ *Fig. 5.71*. The nuclei of these cells are more hyperchromatic and irregular than typically seen in LSIL. In HSIL of the type previously classified as severe dysplasia, the overall size of the cells is reduced compared to HSIL previously classified as moderate dysplasia, but because the cells demonstrate minimal differentiation, the nuclear : cytoplasmic ratio is greatly increased, ➋ *Fig. 5.72*. In these cases, there are usually greater numbers of neoplastic cells and individual dysplastic cells are frequently found. According to the CAP 2003 survey, the mean reporting rate of HSIL in the USA is 0.7% [47]. The rate of HSIL varies with age. In one U.S. center, the rate of HSIL in women 20–29 years old was 0.6% compared with 0.2% and 0.1% in women 40–49 years old and 50–59 years old, respectively [84]. A diagnosis of HSIL connotes a high risk for significant cervical disease. Recent studies have found that HSIL (CIN 2, 3) is found in 84–97% of women evaluated using a loop electrosurgical excision [56, 121].

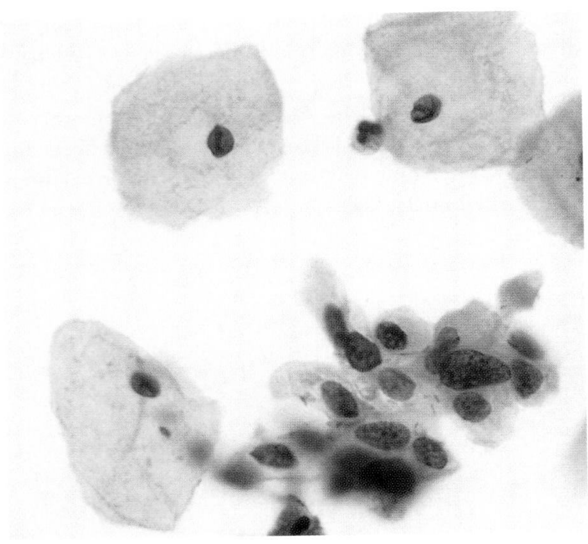

◘ Fig. 5.71
HSIL. **HSIL of the type previously referred to as moderate dysplasia. Many of the cells have a considerable amount of cytoplasm, but the nuclear : cytoplasmic ratio is higher than usually seen in LSIL**

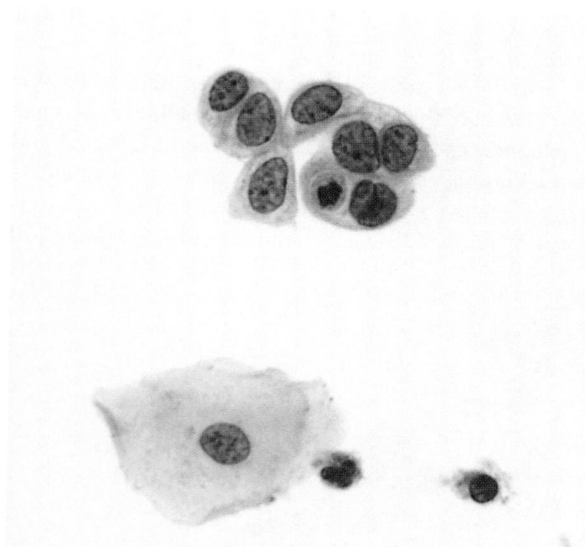

◘ Fig. 5.72
HSIL. **HSIL of the type previously referred to as severe dysplasia. The atypical parabasal type cells have hyperchromatic nuclei and a high nuclear : cytoplasmic ratio**

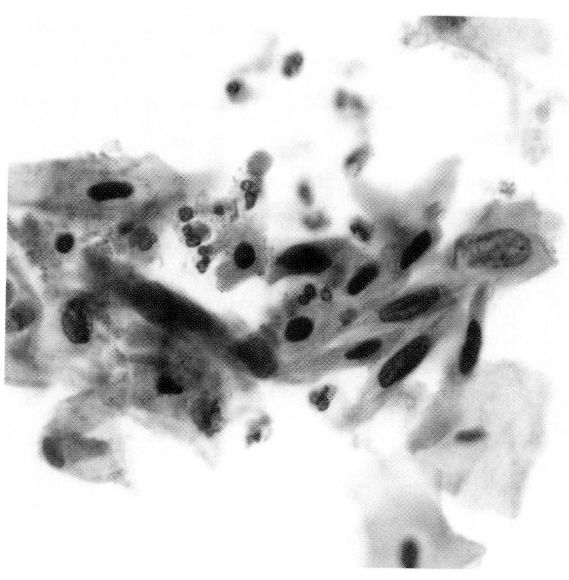

◘ Fig. 5.73
High-grade SIL. **High-grade SIL of the type previously referred to as keratinizing large cell type carcinoma in situ. Many of the cells are keratinized and have quite hyperchromatic nuclei. It is often difficult to distinguish between HSIL of this type and keratinizing invasive squamous cell carcinoma**

HSIL that was previously classified as carcinoma in situ can be of the small cell type, of the large cell non-keratinizing type, or of the large cell keratinizing (pleomorphic) type. Although separation of carcinoma in situ into these three different cytological types has no clinical significance, they do differ in cytological appearance. Small cell lesions consist of small basal-type cells similar to those seen in severe dysplasia but which demonstrate even less cytoplasm and higher nuclear : cytoplasmic ratios. Because of their small size, these cells can be easily overlooked during routine screening and these cases account for a disproportionate percentage of false negative Pap tests. The cells of large cell nonkeratinizing lesions typically form syncytial-like cell sheets in which individual cell membranes are difficult to identify. These cells have enlarged, hyperchromatic nuclei and minimal amounts of cytoplasm. The keratinizing large cell type of carcinoma in situ is composed of pleomorphic, highly atypical cells many of which have thick orangophilic, keratinized, cytoplasm, ➲ *Fig. 5.73*. These cells are often spindled or "tadpole" shaped and have extremely dense nuclear chromatin.

Invasive Squamous Cell Carcinoma Squamous cell carcinomas of the cervix are subdivided into keratinizing and non-keratinizing types. Non-keratinizing carcinomas typically have large numbers of malignant cells that form loose cell sheets and syncytial arrangements. The cells have enlarged nuclei that are 2–3 times the size of a normal intermediate cell nucleus, coarsely clumped chromatin, prominent macronucleoli, and focal chromatin clearing, ➲ *Fig. 5.74*. These cells are often smaller than those seen in SIL. Using conventional cytology, squamous cell carcinomas often have a "dirty" background containing blood, cellular debris, fibrin, and necrotic material. This is often referred to as a tumor diathesis. This characteristic background is less prominent in liquid-based cytology specimens. However, in liquid-based cytology, there is often a distinctive necrotic background that is easy to recognize since it surrounds the cellular material in a "clumped" appearance and large, necrotic tissue fragments are sometimes present, ➲ *Fig. 5.75*.

Pap tests from women with keratinizing carcinomas contain malignant cells, demonstrating a variety of cell shapes and sizes, ➲ *Fig. 5.76*. Some of the cells are pleomorphic or tadpole shaped. These cells have abundant orangophilic cytoplasm. There is frequently abundant hyperkeratosis and parakeratosis. The nuclei are irregular in shape and quite hyperchromatic. Sometimes the nuclei are degenerated, appearing as opaque masses or "inkblots." Unlike nonkeratinizing squamous cell carcinoma, keratinizing squamous cell carcinomas usually do not have "dirty" background or evidence of tumor diathesis.

Glandular Cell Abnormalities

In the 2001 Bethesda System, all types of glandular cell abnormalities, including both atypical endocervical and endometrial cells are combined together in a single entity referred to as glandular cell abnormalities. Benign appearing endometrial cells occurring in postmenopausal women are now classified as "Other." Glandular cell abnormalities are divided into three categories: AGC, either unqualified or favor neoplastic; AIS; and invasive adenocarcinoma.

AGC All AGC lacking the diagnostic features of adenocarcinoma, irrespective of whether they are of endometrial or endocervical origin, are classified by the 2001 Bethesda System as AGC with a specification as to whether they are endocervical, endometrial, or of uncertain origin. There are two categories of AGC. The first is AGC (either endocervical, endometrial, or unclassified), not qualified and the second is AGC, favor neoplastic.

Glandular cytological abnormalities are considerably less common than squamous abnormalities and most cytologists tend to be less comfortable recognizing and diagnosing them. In addition, the criteria used to differentiate reactive endocervical changes, endocervical dysplasia, endocervical AIS, and invasive endocervical

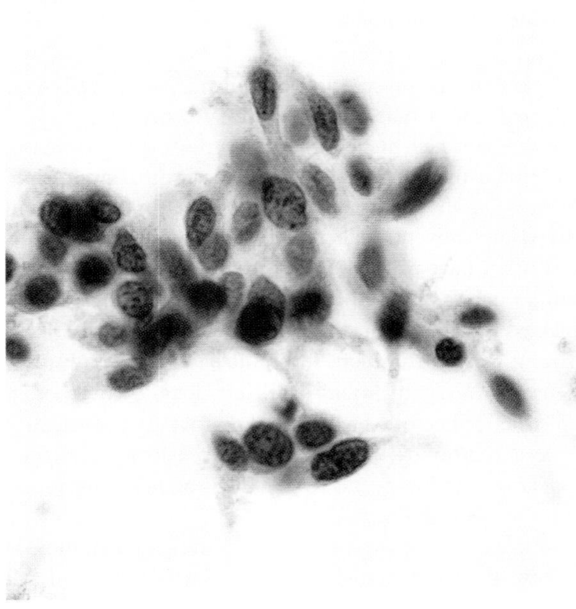

Fig. 5.74
Invasive squamous cell carcinoma. **The cells of this nonkeratinizing squamous cell carcinoma are polygonal and arranged in syncytial sheets. They are highly atypical, but smaller than the cells of many intraepithelial lesions**

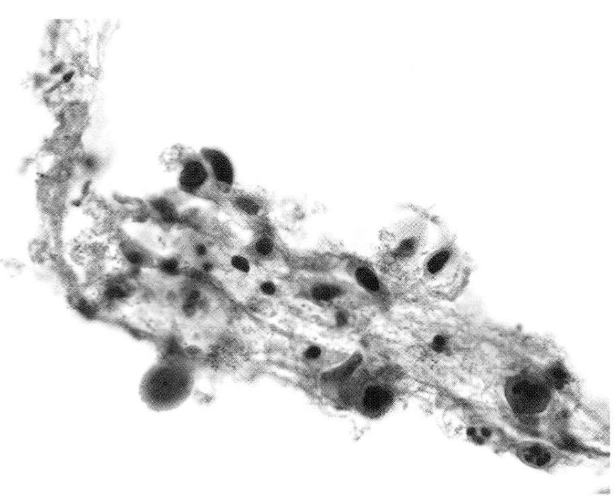

Fig. 5.75
Tumor diathesis. **This liquid-based cytology preparation from a woman with squamous cell carcinoma shows necrotic material surrounding malignant cells giving it a "clumped" appearance**

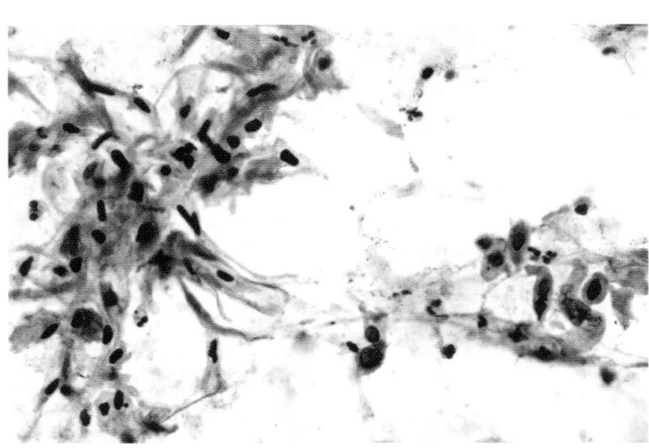

Fig. 5.76
Invasive squamous cell carcinoma. **The cells of this keratinizing squamous cell carcinoma are quite pleomorphic and include spindle-shaped, elongate, and caudate forms. The nuclei of some cells are extremely hyperchromatic**

adenocarcinoma are less well established than those used for squamous lesions. Cytologists even have difficulty in differentiating atypical endocervical cells from cases of HSIL that have extended into endocervical crypts. This accounts for the high prevalence of squamous abnormalities (approximately 30%) detected in women referred to colposcopy for AGC [97, 164].

The cytological features of atypical endocervical cells vary depending on the degree of the underlying histopathologic abnormality. Cases of the type designated by cytopathologists as atypical endocervical cells – unqualified have minor degrees of variability in nuclear size and shape, ➋ *Fig. 5.77*. Endocervical cells form dense two- or three-dimensional aggregates that have minor degrees of nuclear overlapping. In some cases, the chromatin is somewhat granular and nuclear feathering can be seen at the periphery of the cellular aggregates. Atypical endocervical cells favor neoplasia includes those cases where the cytological features are suggestive of AIS, but are insufficient to allow a definitive diagnosis. These cases typically have more nuclear hyperchromasia, variability in nuclear size, and granularity of the cytoplasm than is observed in cases of atypical endocervical cells, unqualified, ➋ *Fig. 5.78*.

AIS In cases of AIS, there are usually a larger number of AGC that form crowded cellular clusters. The sheets are usually three-dimensional and sometimes retain the architecture of the underlying glands, ➋ *Fig. 5.79*. The cells

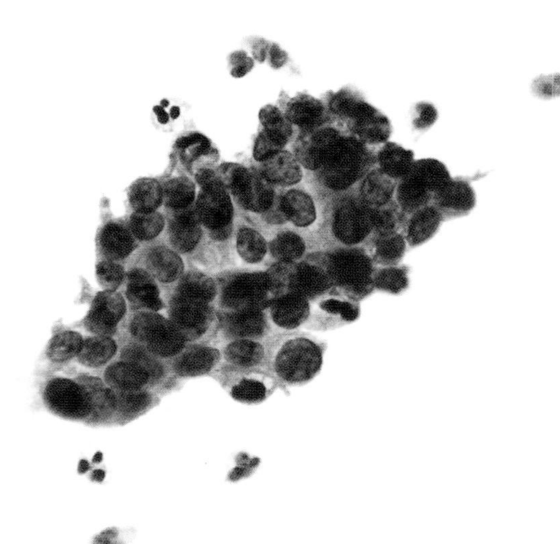

▣ Fig. 5.78
Atypical glandular cells (AGC) – favor neoplasia. **These endocervical cells are somewhat suggestive of adenocarcinoma in situ (AIS). The nuclei are hyperchromatic and the chromatin is coarsely clumped. There is variation in nuclear size and the cells form a three-dimensional aggregate**

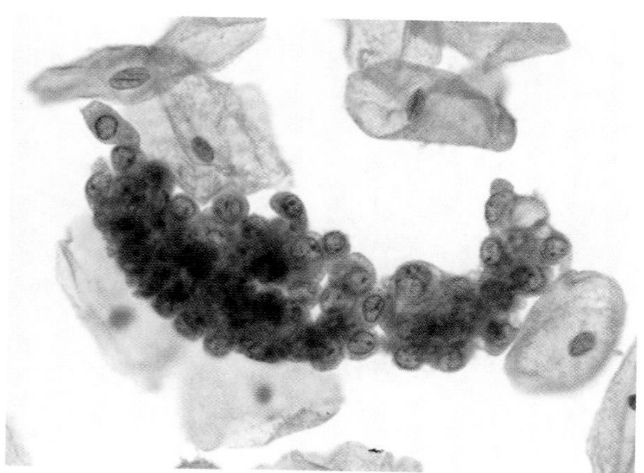

▣ Fig. 5.77
Atypical glandular cells – endocervical type (AGC-EC). **These endocervical cells have enlarged nuclei, prominent nucleoli, and vary somewhat in size and shape. The smear was obtained 6 weeks postpartum and follow-up examination was completely negative**

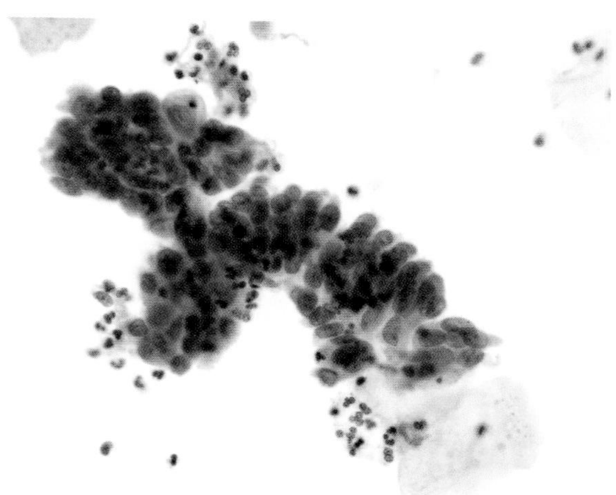

▣ Fig. 5.79
Adenocarcinoma in situ (AIS). **These endocervical cells form a tight three-dimensional structure that is similar to the outline of an endocervical gland. Large numbers of these formations are often present in specimens from AIS**

within these sheets occasionally form rosettes and have extensive feathering of the cells at the periphery. Individual endocervical cells are highly atypical with enlarged round, oval, or elongated nuclei that vary in size from cell to cell. In most cases, the chromatin is coarsely clumped and multiple mitoses are seen, *Fig. 5.80*. Sometimes, it is difficult for the cytologist to determine whether the atypical cells represent AGC or HSIL cells that have extended into an endocervical crypt or "gland." In these cases, highly atypical nuclei are identified in the center of a cell aggregate and some of the cells at the periphery of the aggregate appear to be endocervical cells.

Adenocarcinoma TBS subclassifies invasive adenocarcinomas into "adenocarcinoma-endocervical type," "adenocarcinoma-endometrial type," and "adenocarcinoma-not otherwise specified." The cytological diagnosis of invasive adenocarcinoma is relatively straightforward. Adenocarcinoma cells from either an endocervical or an endometrial primary have enlarged nuclei, high nuclear : cytoplasmic ratios, coarsely clumped chromatin, and prominent nucleoli, *Fig. 5.81*. They can occur singly or in clusters. Cytologists should try to distinguish between endometrial and endocervical primary adenocarcinomas whenever possible. Key features that allow discrimination between endometrial and endocervical origin in cytology include number of abnormal cells, size of the cells, retention of columnar configuration, appearance of cytoplasm, and unclear structure [139]. Typically, adenocarcinoma of the cervix shows considerably larger numbers of cells than does endometrial adenocarcinoma. Cells derived from endocervical adenocarcinoma typically retain a columnar configuration that is lost in most endometrial carcinomas. The cytoplasm of cells exfoliated from endocervical adenocarcinoma is typically eosinophilic and glandular, whereas the cytoplasm from cells of endometrial adenocarcinoma is typically finely vacuolated cytoplasm and cyanophilic. The nuclei of cells of endometrial adenocarcinoma have less glandular chromatin, are less hyperchromatic, are smaller, and less frequently have multiple nucleoli than do the nuclei of cells of endocervical adenocarcinoma.

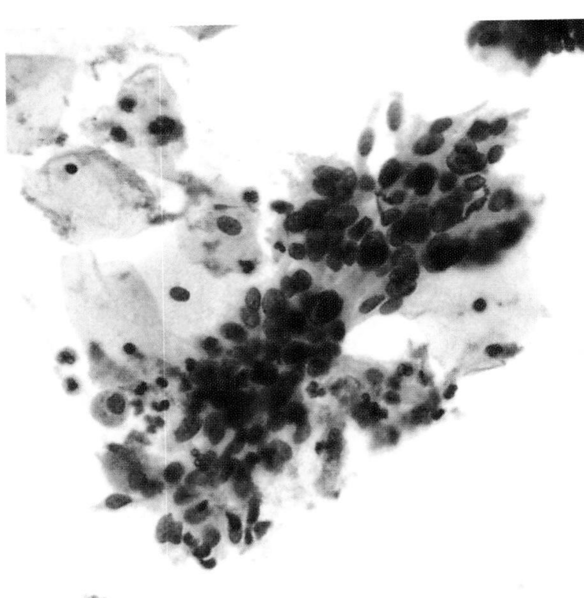

Fig. 5.80
Adenocarcinoma in situ (AIS). **The individual atypical endocervical cells are hyperchromatic with coarsely clumped chromatin. They show the characteristic feathering of the nuclei at the edge of the cluster that is typical of AIS**

Management of Cytologic Abnormalities and Cervical Cancer Precursors

In 2006, the American Society for Colposcopy and Cervical Pathology sponsored a consensus workshop to update the 2001 Consensus Guidelines for the Management of

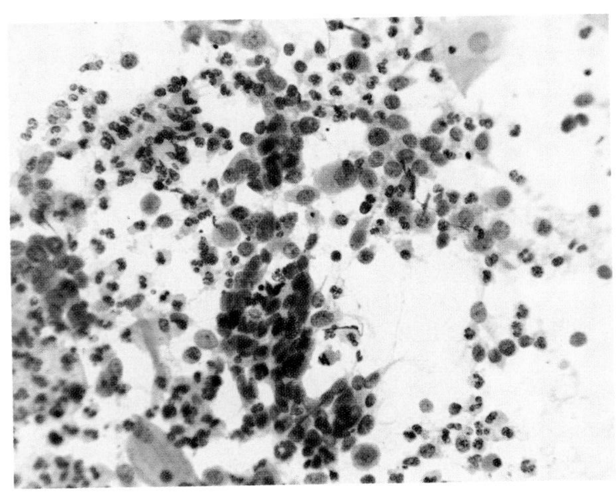

Fig. 5.81
Endocervical adenocarcinoma. **These endocervical cells have the features of frank adenocarcinoma. The nuclei are quite enlarged, the chromatin is coarsely clumped and marginated, and there are prominent nucleoli. The background shows inflammation and necrosis indicating tumor diathesis is present**

Women with Cytological Abnormalities and Cervical Cancer Precursors [206, 208]. These guidelines are widely used in the USA and are evidence based with each recommendation accompanied by a grading of both the strength of the recommendation and the strength of the data supporting the recommendation. What follows is a brief synopsis of the guidelines. The complete recommendations and management algorithms are available at www.asccp.org.

ASC

The prevalence of biopsy-confirmed HSIL among women undergoing colposcopy for an ASC cytology varies from 5% to 17% [206]. The prevalence of HSIL in women with ASC depends on the number of factors including the patient's age, history, and the subclassification of the result. Overall, it appears that approximately half of women with histologically confirmed HSIL have ASC as their initial abnormal cervical cytology result [99, 114]. However, it should be noted that the risk that a woman with ASC has invasive cervical cancer is quite low (about one per thousand).

Atypical Squamous Cells of Undetermined Significance (ASCUS)

Three methods are considered acceptable for managing women in the general population with ASC; immediate colposcopy, high-risk HPV DNA testing, and repeating the cervical cytology twice at 6-month intervals, ➋ *Fig. 5.82.* HPV DNA testing identifies more cases of HSIL than does a single repeat cervical cytology, but refers approximately equivalent numbers of women for colposcopy [7]. Moreover, cost-effectiveness modeling has demonstrated that HPV DNA testing for women with ASCUS is highly attractive when the initial ASCUS cytology was obtained from a liquid-based sample [98, 106]. Thus,

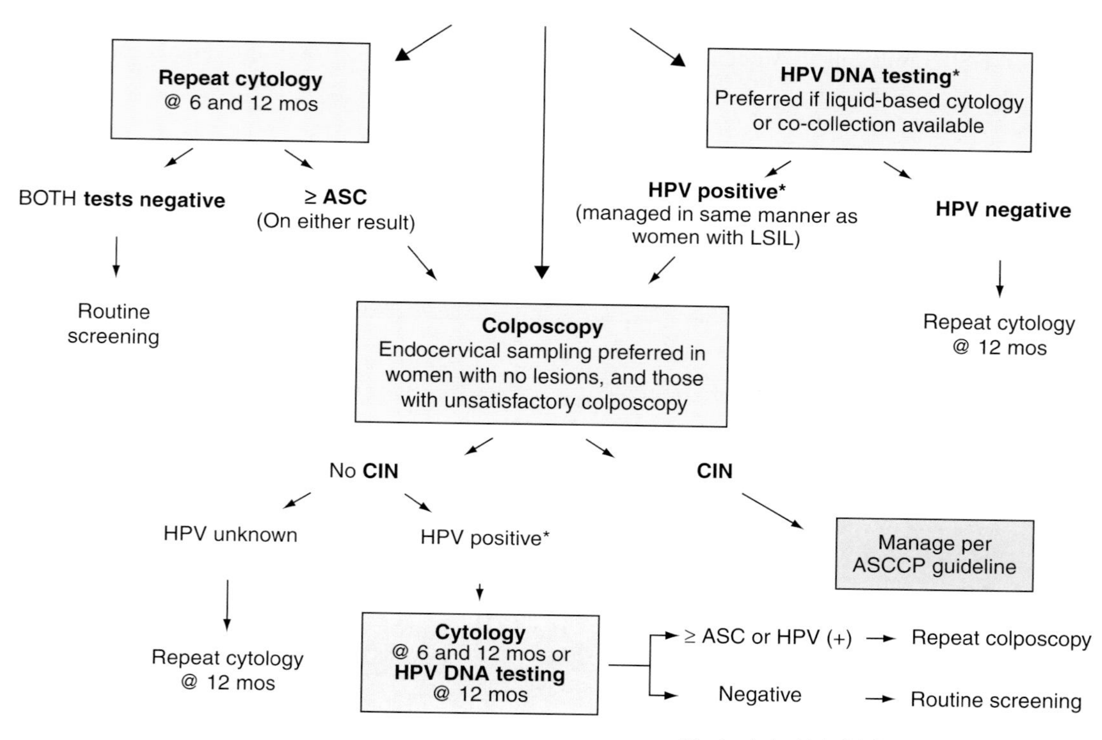

Fig. 5.82
ASCCP Consensus Conference algorithm for managing women with ASCUS

high-risk HPV DNA testing is the preferred approach to managing women with ASCUS whenever liquid-based cytology is used for screening [206]. Women found to be high-risk HPV DNA positive should be referred to colposcopy, whereas HPV DNA negative women should be rescreened in 12 months.

Since the prevalence of HPV DNA positivity is much higher in young women with ASCUS than in older women and is extremely high in adolescents with ASCUS, HPV DNA testing is not recommended for adolescents with ASCUS [16, 169, 206]. Instead, adolescents should be managed using annual repeat cytological examinations and only referred to colposcopy if the repeat Pap tests are diagnosed as HSIL or are persistently abnormal for a period of 2 years, ❯ *Fig. 5.83* [206]. Management options for pregnant patients with ASCUS are identical to those for nonpregnant patients with the exception that it is acceptable to defer the colposcopic examination until the patient is 6–8 weeks postpartum [206].

ASC-H

ASC-H is a much more concerning cytology result than ASCUS since biopsy-confirmed HSIL is identified in 24–94% of women with ASC-H [203]. Thus, for the purposes of management, ASC-H should be considered to be an equivocal HSIL result and all women with ASC-H should be referred for a colposcopic evaluation [206]. If SIL is not identified, followed-up utilizing either repeat cytology at 6 and 12 months or high-risk HPV DNA testing at 12 months is acceptable.

LSIL

Biopsy-confirmed HSIL is found in 15–30% of women with LSIL on cervical cytology [8, 94, 114]. Therefore, all women in the general population with a cytological result of LSIL should be referred to colposcopy, ❯ *Fig. 5.84* [206]. A diagnostic excisional procedure is not necessary when a woman with LSIL cytology is found to have an unsatisfactory colposcopic examination. Since invasive cervical cancer is very uncommon in adolescents and prospective studies have shown that over 90% of LSIL will spontaneously clear in adolescents, adolescents with LSIL should not be referred to colposcopy, but should be followed using yearly Pap tests for a period of 2 years [131, 132, 206]. Another "special population" is postmenopausal women with LSIL. Both the prevalence of HPV DNA and the prevalence of HSIL are lower in postmenopausal women than in women in the general population with LSIL. Therefore, postmenopausal women with LSIL can be managed in the same manner as women with

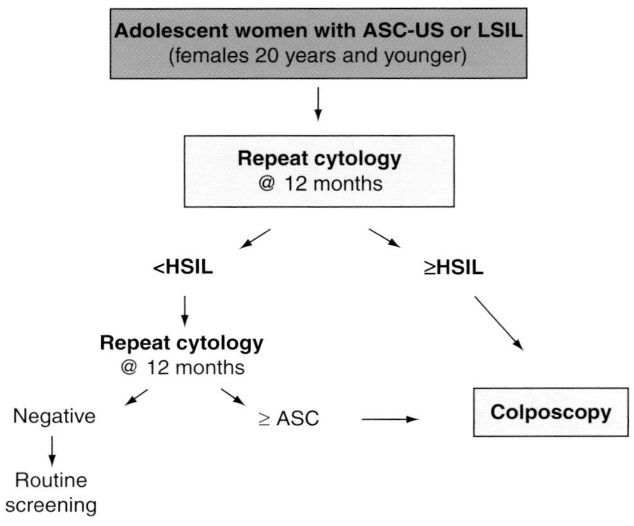

Fig. 5.83
ASCCP Consensus Conference algorithm for managing adolescents with either ASCUS or LSIL

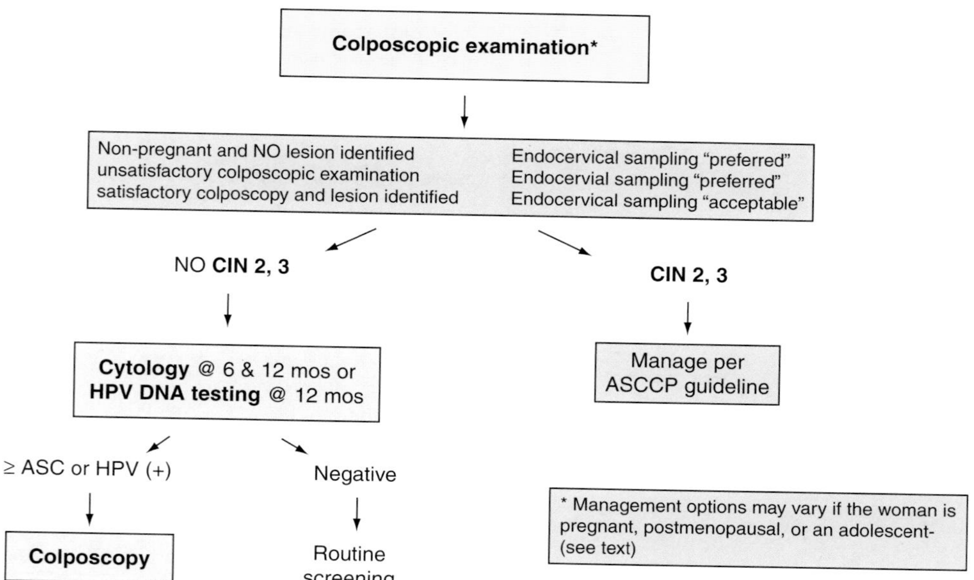

Fig. 5.84
ASCCP Consensus Conference algorithm for managing women with LSIL

ASCUS. This includes using reflex HPV DNA testing to determine who should undergo colposcopy [58, 169].

HSIL

Histologically confirmed HSIL is identified in 53–97% of women with a cytological result of HSIL and invasive cervical cancer is found in approximately 2% [47, 92, 93, 206]. Therefore, women with a cytological result of HSIL should be referred for either a colposcopic evaluation or an immediate LEEP, *Fig. 5.85* [206]. If histologically confirmed HSIL is not identified after colposcopy and the colposcopic examination is satisfactory and endocervical sampling is negative, either a diagnostic excisional procedure or follow-up using colposcopy and cytology at 6-month intervals is acceptable for 1 year. Nonpregnant women with HSIL who have an unsatisfactory colposcopic examination require a diagnostic excisional procedure.

AGC

AGC is a relatively uncommon cytological diagnosis with a mean reporting rate of 0.4% in the USA in 2003 according to a survey of the CAP [47]. Most clinicians consider a diagnosis of AGC to much more concerning than a diagnosis of ASCUS. This is because women with AGC are much more likely to have a significant underlying condition of the cervix or endometrium. Either HSIL, AIS, or invasive cancer is found in 9–38% of women with AGC and invasive cancer of either the cervix or endometrium is found in 3–17% [206]. Therefore, the initial work-up of women with AGC generally includes both evaluation of the cervix using colposcopy and endocervical curettage to exclude HSIL, AIS, and cervical cancer, as well as endometrial sampling to rule out endometrial hyperplasia and cancer, *Fig. 5.86*. Endometrial sampling is not necessary in women under the age of 35 years who do not have other risk factors for endometrial disease such as abnormal bleeding or polycystic ovarian syndrome since these women are at low risk for having endometrial pathology. Similarly, colposcopy can be deferred until after the results of endometrial and endocervical sampling are available in women who have atypical endometrial cells since these women are much more likely to have endometrial as opposed to cervical disease. Subsequent management of women with AGC depends not only on the findings at the time of colposcopy and endometrial sampling, but also on the patient's HPV DNA status and on the subclassification of the referral AGC cytology result, *Fig. 5.87*. If the referral cytology was classified as atypical endocervical,

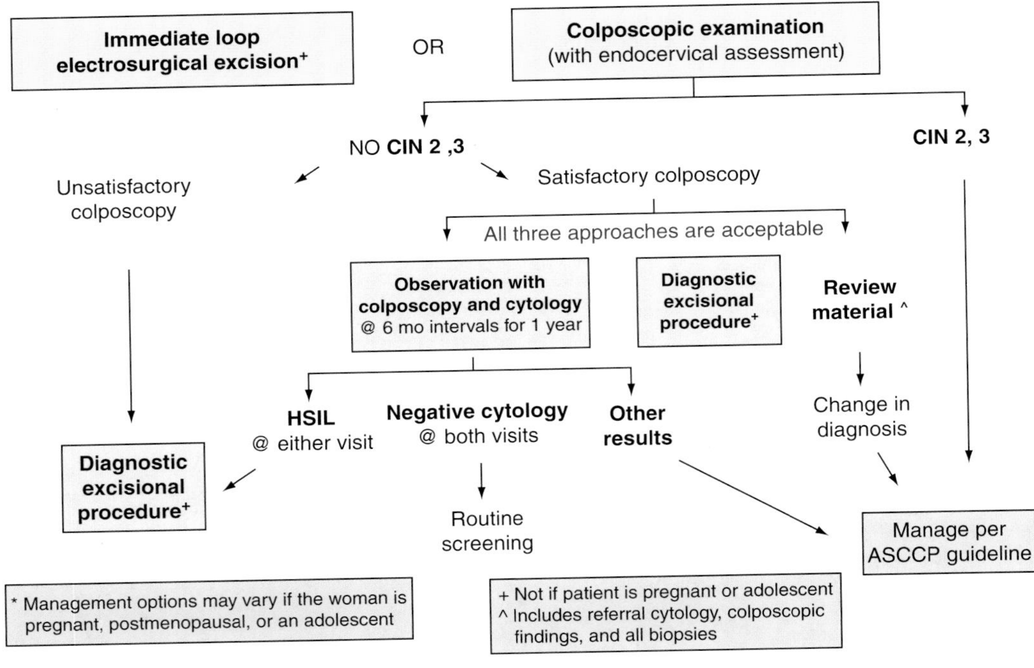

Fig. 5.85
ASCCP Consensus Conference algorithm for managing women with HSIL

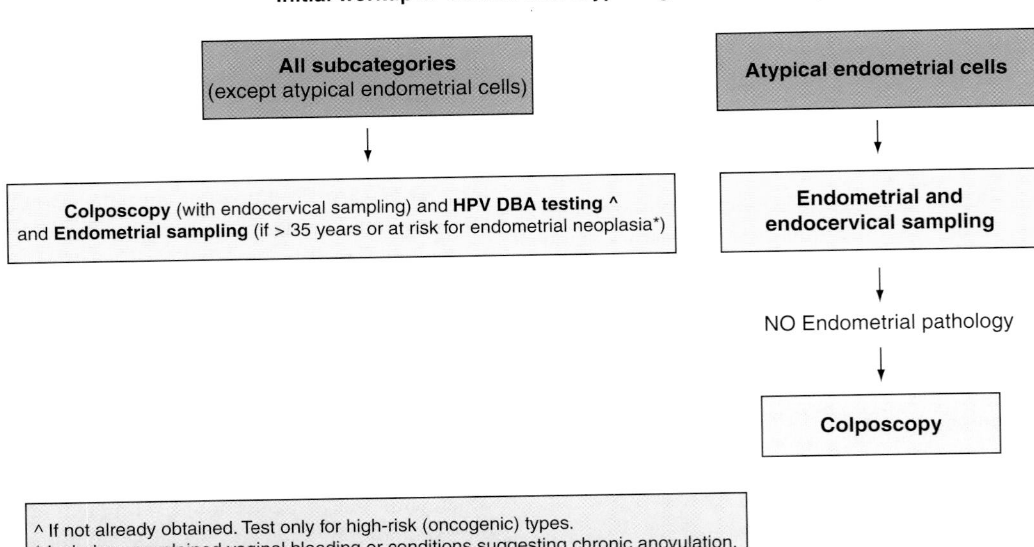

Fig. 5.86
ASCCP Consensus Conference algorithm for the initial management of women with AGC cytology results

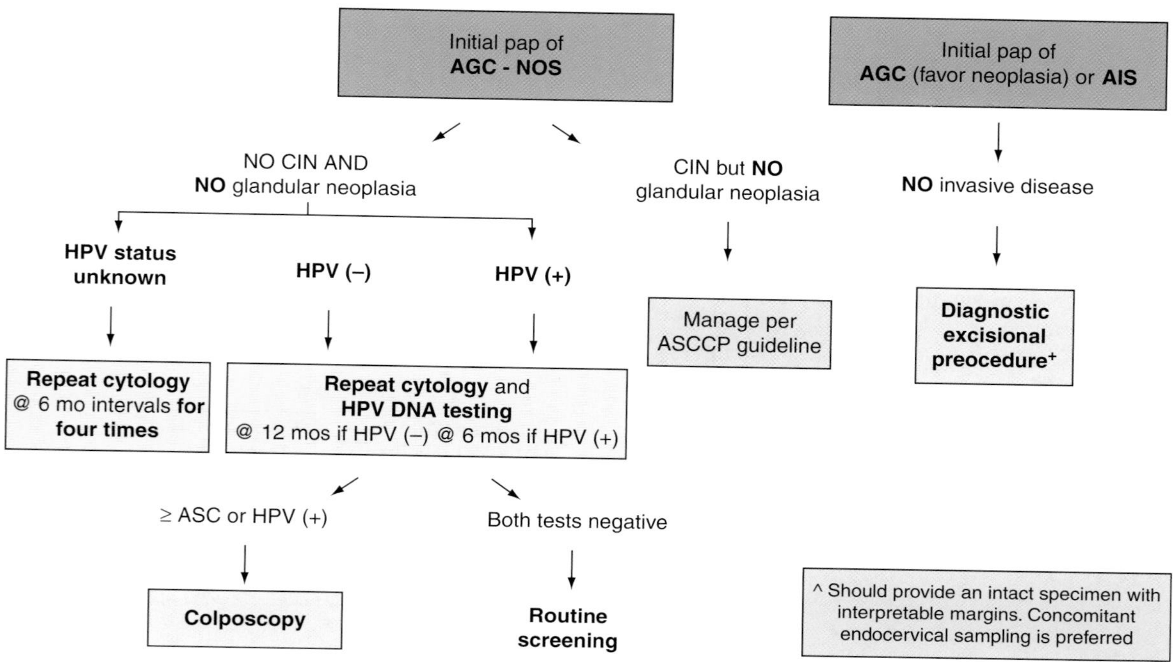

Fig. 5.87
ASCCP Consensus Conference algorithm for the subsequent management of women with AGC cytology results

endometrial, or glandular cells not otherwise specified (NOS) and significant disease is not identified during initial workup, the patient can be followed up with repeat cytologic testing combined with HPV DNA testing. However, if the referral AGC cytology was atypical glandular cells "favor neoplasia" or AIS, the patient should undergo a diagnostic excisional procedure which can be either a cold-knife or loop excisional conization [206].

Histologically confirmed LSIL

There is a considerable degree of overdiagnosis of reactive reparative conditions as LSIL and the majority of histologically confirmed LSIL will spontaneously regress in the absence of therapy. Therefore, it is recommended that histologically confirmed LSIL preceded by ASCUS, ASC-H, or LSIL cytology undergo conservative follow-up consisting of either HPV DNA testing every 12 months or repeat cervical cytology every 6–12 months, Fig. 5.88. If histologically confirmed LSIL persists for at least 2 years, either continued follow-up or treatment is acceptable. Since the risk of an undetected HSIL or glandular lesion is expected to be higher in women referred for the evaluation of a HSIL or AGC on cytology, women with histologically confirmed LSIL preceded by HSIL or AGC cervical cytology can undergo either a diagnostic excisional procedure or be followed using both colposcopy and cytology at 6-month intervals for 1 year, provided the colposcopic examination is satisfactory and endocervical sampling is negative [208].

Histologically confirmed HSIL

Women with histologically confirmed HSIL are at significantly high risk of progressing to invasive cervical cancer and therefore treatment is recommended. Provided the colposcopic examination is satisfactory and there is no suggestion of invasive disease (e.g., either by colposcopy, cytology, or histology), both ablative and excisional treatment modalities are considered acceptable forms of treatment [208]. A diagnostic excisional procedure is recommended for all women with histologically confirmed HSIL and an unsatisfactory colposcopic examination or with recurrent disease.

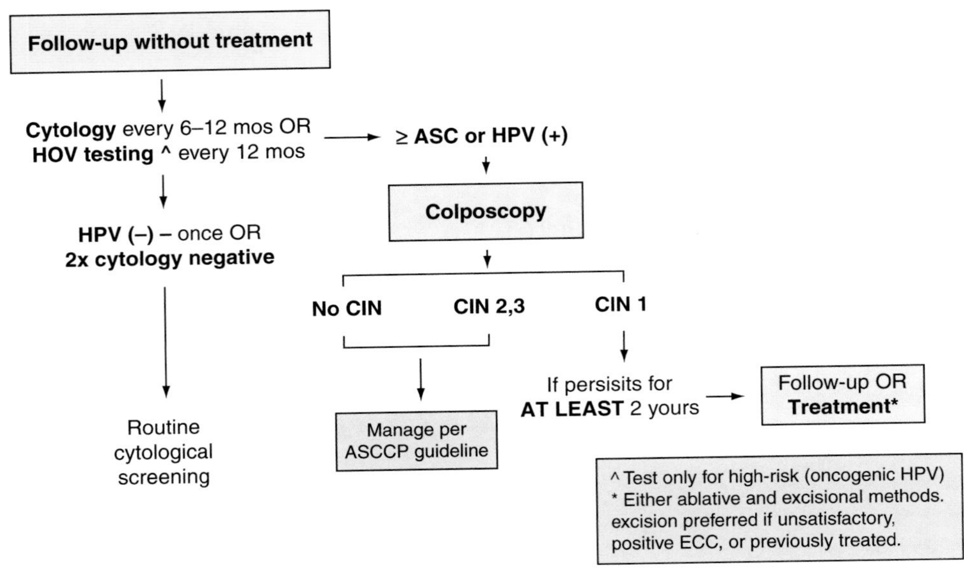

Fig. 5.88
ASCCP Consensus Conference algorithm for managing women with histologically confirmed LSIL

ECC

ECC is performed to evaluate lesion distribution and morphology within the endocervical canal and to exclude the presence of invasive carcinoma, and unsuspected cervical AIS and invasive adenocarcinoma. Recently, the utility of ECC has become the subject of considerable debate [53]. In ALTS, the ECC provided only a minimal 2.2% increase in the detection of HSIL when performed in women under the age of 40 years, but provided a 13% increased detection of high-grade CIN when performed in women 40 years and older [178]. Nevertheless, many clinicians perform an ECC during colposcopic evaluation of the cervix.

The ECC specimen consists of endocervical tissue fragments, blood, mucus, and, when positive, strips of atypical epithelium, ➋ *Fig. 5.89*. To avoid the loss of tiny tissue fragments during processing, the clinician should collect and concentrate the sample, including mucus and blood, on a small square of lens paper or using a cytobrush and immediately place it in the fixative [79]. By this method, even the smallest tissue fragments can be recovered easily in the laboratory, embedded, and sectioned entirely.

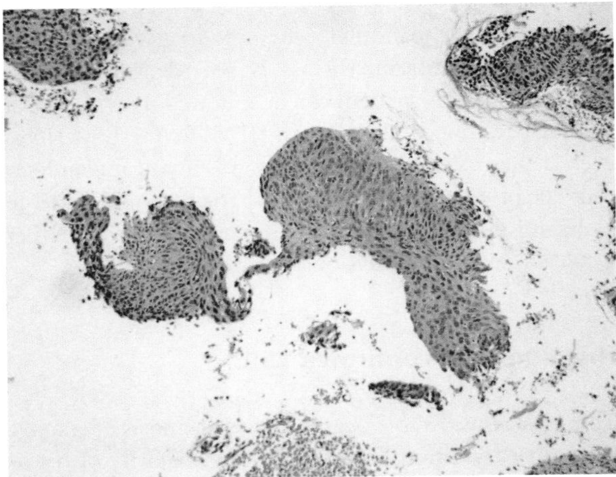

Fig. 5.89
HSIL present in an endocervical curetting

In most instances, when atypical epithelium is detected in the ECC it lacks underlying stroma and orientation is not possible. As a result, the pathologist can neither rule out underlying invasion nor grade an intraepithelial lesion. In other cases, where the atypical epithelium is well oriented, the pathologist is able to grade the lesion and can, if desired. It is also helpful if the pathologist conveys an estimate of the amount of atypical epithelium that is present in the ECC. If only a few small fragments of atypical epithelium are present in the ECC, these may represent "pickups" from a lesion that is actually confined to the portio and does not extend into the endocervical canal. In such cases, it may be preferable to reexamine the patient with the colposcope rather than proceeding directly with a diagnostic excisional procedure. Frequently the second carefully performed curettage yields no atypical epithelium and the patient may be managed on a conservative, outpatient basis. Conversely, the pathologist should be careful not to discount or overlook a few or even a single fragment of atypical epithelium in an ECC. In a review of 21 women who developed invasive cancer after cryotherapy, 7 out of 18 ECCs taken before cryotherapy were found on review to contain SIL that had been missed at the time of original diagnosis [168].

References

1. Abdul-Karim FW, Fu YS, Reagan JW et al (1982) Morphometric study of intraepithelial neoplasia of the uterine cervix. Obstet Gynecol 60:210–214
2. Alvarez RD, Wright TC (2007) Effective cervical neoplasia detection with a novel optical detection system: a randomized trial. Gynecol Oncol 104(2):281–289
3. Anciaux D, Lawrence WD, Gregoire L (1997) Glandular lesions of the uterine cervix: prognostic implications of human papillomavirus status. Int J Gynecol Pathol 16:103–110
4. Andersen ES, Arffmann E (1989) Adenocarcinoma in situ of the uterine cervix: a clinico-pathologic study of 36 cases. Gynecol Oncol 35:1–7
5. Anonymous (2001) SEER Program – National Cancer Institute, USA. http://www-seer.ims.nci.nih.gov/ScientificSystems/. Retrieved 20 Mar, 2003, 2009
6. Appleby P, Beral V, Berrington de Gonzalez A et al (2007) Cervical cancer and hormonal contraceptives: collaborative reanalysis of individual data for 16,573 women with cervical cancer and 35,509 women without cervical cancer from 24 epidemiological studies. Lancet 370(9599):1609–1621
7. Arbyn M, Sasieni P, Meijer CJ et al (2006) Chapter 9: Clinical applications of HPV testing: a summary of meta-analyses. Vaccine 24(Suppl 3):S78–S89
8. ASCUS-LSIL Traige Study (ALTS) Group (2003) A randomized trial on the management of low-grade squamous intraepithelial lesion cytology interpretations. Am J Obstet Gynecol 188(6):1393–1400
9. ASCUS-LSIL Traige Study (ALTS) Group (2003) Results of a randomized trial on the management of cytology interpretations of atypical squamous cells of undetermined significance. Am J Obstet Gynecol 188(6):1383–1392
10. Baker AC, Eltoum I, Curry RO et al (2006) Mucinous expression in benign and neoplastic glandular lesions of the uterine cervix. Arch Pathol Lab Med 130(10):1510–1515
11. Bandyopadhyay S, Austin RM, Dabbs D et al (2008) Adjunctive human papillomavirus DNA testing is a useful option in some clinical settings for disease risk assessment and triage of females with ASC-H Papanicolaou test results. Arch Pathol Lab Med 132(12):1874–1881
12. Benard VB, Lee NC, Piper M et al (2001) Race-specific results of Papanicolaou testing and the rate of cervical neoplasia in the National Breast and Cervical Cancer Early Detection Program, 1991–1998 (United States). Cancer Causes Control 12(1):61–68
13. Bergeron C, Ferenczy A, Shah K et al (1987) Multicentric human papillomavirus infections of the female genital tract. Correlation of viral types with abnormal mitotic figures, colposcopic presentation, and location. Obstet Gynecol 69:736–742
14. Bernard H-U, Chan S-Y, Delius H (1994) Evolution of papillomaviruses. Curr Top Microbiol Immunol 186:33–54
15. Bertrand M, Lickrish GM, Colgan TJ (1987) The anatomic distribution of cervical adenocarcinoma in situ: implications for treatment. Am J Obstet Gynecol 157:21–25
16. Boardman LA, Stanko C, Weitzen S et al (2005) Atypical squamous cells of undetermined significance: human papillomavirus testing in adolescents. Obstet Gynecol 105(4):741–746
17. Bocking A, Nguyen VQ (2004) Diagnostic and prognostic use of DNA image cytometry in cervical squamous intraepithelial lesions and invasive carcinoma. Cancer 102(1):41–54
18. Boddington MM, Spriggs AI, Cowdell RH (1976) Adenocarcinoma of the uterine cervix: cytological evidence of a long preclinical evolution. Br J Obstet Gynecol 83:900–903
19. Bollmann R, Mehes G, Speich N et al (2005) Aberrant, highly hyperdiploid cells in human papillomavirus-positive, abnormal cytologic samples are associated with progressive lesions of the uterine cervix. Cancer 105(2):96–100
20. Bollmann R, Mehes G, Torka R et al (2003) Human papillomavirus typing and DNA ploidy determination of squamous intraepithelial lesions in liquid-based cytologic samples. Cancer 99(1):57–62
21. Boon ME, Baak JPA, Kurver PJH et al (1981) Adenocarcinoma in situ of the cervix: an underdiagnosed lesion. Cancer 48:768–773
22. Bosch FX, de Sanjose S (2007) The epidemiology of human papillomavirus infection and cervical cancer. Dis Markers 23(4):213–227
23. Bousfield L, Pacey F, Young Q et al (1980) Expanded cytologic criteria for the diagnosis of adenocarcinoma in situ of the cervix and related lesions. Acta Cytol 24(4):283–296
24. Broders AC (1932) Carcinoma in situ contrasted with benign penetrating epithelium. JAMA 99:1670–1674
25. Brown DR, Shew ML, Qadadri B et al (2005) A longitudinal study of genital human papillomavirus infection in a cohort of closely followed adolescent women. J Infect Dis 191(2):182–192
26. Brown LJR, Wells M (1986) Cervical glandular atypia associated with squamous intraepithelial neoplasia: a premalignant lesion? J Clin Pathol 39:22–28
27. Burchell AN, Winer RL, de Sanjose S et al (2006) Chapter 6: Epidemiology and transmission dynamics of genital HPV infection. Vaccine 24(Suppl 3):S52–S61
28. Burghardt E (1991) Colposcopy-cervical pathology. Thieme Medical, New York
29. Butterworth CEJ, Hatch KD, Macaluso M et al (1992) Folate deficiency and cervical dysplasia. JAMA 267:528–533
30. Cameron RI, Maxwell P, Jenkins D et al (2002) Immunohistochemical staining with MIB1, bcl2 and p16 assists in the distinction of

cervical glandular intraepithelial neoplasia from tubo-endometrial metaplasia, endometriosis and microglandular hyperplasia. Histopathology 41(4):313–321
31. Castle PE, Giuliano AR (2003) Chapter 4: Genital tract infections, cervical inflammation, and antioxidant nutrients – assessing their roles as human papillomavirus cofactors. J Natl Cancer Inst Monogr (31):29–34
32. Castle PE, Schiffman M, Wheeler CM et al (2009) Evidence for frequent regression of cervical intraepithelial neoplasia-grade 2. Obstet Gynecol 113(1):18–25
33. Castle PE, Stoler MH, Solomon D et al (2007) The relationship of community biopsy-diagnosed cervical intraepithelial neoplasia grade 2 to the quality control pathology-reviewed diagnoses: an ALTS report. Am J Clin Pathol 127(5):805–815
34. Castle PE, Wacholder S, Sherman ME et al (2002) Absolute risk of a subsequent abnormal pap among oncogenic human papillomavirus DNA-positive, cytologically negative women. Cancer 95(10): 2145–2151
35. Chung TK, Cheung TH, Lo WK et al (2000) Loss of heterozygosity at the short arm of chromosome 3 in microdissected cervical intraepithelial neoplasia. Cancer Lett 154(2):189–194
36. Clifford G, Franceschi S, Diaz M et al (2006) Chapter 3: HPV type-distribution in women with and without cervical neoplastic diseases. Vaccine 24(Suppl 3):S26–S34
37. Clifford GM, Rana RK, Franceschi S et al (2005) Human papillomavirus genotype distribution in low-grade cervical lesions: comparison by geographic region and with cervical cancer. Cancer Epidemiol Biomarkers Prev 14(5):1157–1164
38. Colgan TJ, Lickrish GM (1990) The topography and invasive potential of cervical adenocarcinoma in situ, with and without associated squamous dysplasia. Gynecol Oncol 36:246–249
39. Confortini M, Bondi A, Cariaggi MP et al (2007) Interlaboratory reproducibility of liquid-based equivocal cervical cytology within a randomized controlled trial framework. Diagn Cytopathol 35(9):541–544
40. Confortini M, Carozzi F, Dalla Palma P et al (2003) Interlaboratory reproducibility of atypical squamous cells of undetermined significance report: a national survey. Cytopathology 14(5):263–268
41. Crocker J, Fox H, Langley FA (1968) Consistency in the histological diagnosis of epithelial abnormalities of the cervix uteri. J Clin Pathol 21:67–70
42. Crum CP, Egawa K, Fu YS et al (1983) Atypical immature metaplasia (AIM): a subset of human papillomavirus infection of the cervix. Cancer 51:2214–2219
43. Crum CP, Egawa K, Levine RU et al (1983) Human papillomavirus infection (condyloma) of the cervix and cervical intraepithelial neoplasia: a histological and statistical analysis. Gynecol Oncol 15:88
44. Cullen TS (1900) Cancer of the uterus. Appleton, New York
45. Cullimore JE, Luesley DM, Rollason TP et al (1992) A prospective study of conization of the cervix in the management of cervical intraepithelial glandular neoplasia (CIGN) – a preliminary report. Br J Obstet Gynecol 99:314–318
46. Datta SD, Koutsky LA, Ratelle S et al (2008) Human papillomavirus infection and cervical cytology in women screened for cervical cancer in the United States, 2003–2005. Ann Intern Med 148(7): 493–500
47. Davey DD, Neal MH, Wilbur DC et al (2004) Bethesda 2001 implementation and reporting rates: 2003 practices of participants in the College of American Pathologists Interlaboratory Comparison Program in Cervicovaginal Cytology. Arch Pathol Lab Med 128(11):1224–1229
48. de Araujo Souza PS, Maciag PC, Ribeiro KB et al (2008) Interaction between polymorphisms of the human leukocyte antigen and HPV-16 variants on the risk of invasive cervical cancer. BMC Cancer 8:246
49. de Sanjose S, Diaz M, Castellsague X et al (2007) Worldwide prevalence and genotype distribution of cervical human papillomavirus DNA in women with normal cytology: a meta-analysis. Lancet Infect Dis 7(7):453–459
50. de Villiers EM, Fauquet C, Broker TR et al (2004) Classification of papillomaviruses. Virology 324(1):17–27
51. Denehy TR, Gregori CA, Breen JL (1997) Endocervical curettage, cone margins, and residual adenocarcinoma in situ of the cervix. Obstet Gynecol 90(1):1–6
52. Doorbar J (2006) Molecular biology of human papillomavirus infection and cervical cancer. Clin Sci (Lond) 110(5):525–541
53. Driggers RW, Zahn CM (2008) To ECC or not to ECC: the question remains. Obstet Gynecol Clin North Am 35(4):583–597; viii
54. Duby JM, DiFurio MJ (2009) Implementation of the ThinPrep Imaging System in a tertiary military medical center. Cancer Cytopathol 117(4):264–270
55. Duggan MA, Benoit JL, McGregor SE et al (1994) Adenocarcinoma in situ of the endocervix: Human papillomavirus determination by dot blot hybridization and polymerase chain reaction amplification. Int J Gynecol Pathol 13(2):143–149
56. Dunn TS, Burke M, Shwayder J (2003) A "see and treat" management for high-grade squamous intraepithelial lesion pap smears. J Low Genit Tract Dis 7(2):104–106
57. Duska LR (2009) Can we improve the detection of glandular cervical lesions: the role and limitations of the Pap smear diagnosis atypical glandular cells (AGC). Gynecol Oncol 114(3):381–382
58. Evans MF, Adamson CS, Papillo JL et al (2006) Distribution of human papillomavirus types in ThinPrep Papanicolaou tests classified according to the Bethesda 2001 terminology and correlations with patient age and biopsy outcomes. Cancer 106(5):1054–1064
59. Fordyce EJ, Wang Z, Kahn AR et al (2000) Risk of cancer among women with AIDS in New York City. AIDS Public Policy J 15(3–4):95–104
60. Franquemont DW, Ward BE, Anderson WA et al (1989) Prediction of "high-risk" cervical papillomavirus infection by biopsy morphology. Am J Clin Pathol 92(5):577–582
61. Friedell GH, McKay DG (1953) Adenocarcinoma in situ of endocervix. Cancer 6:887–897
62. Fu YS, Braun L, Shah KV et al (1983) Histologic, nuclear DNA, and human papillomavirus studies of cervical condylomas. Cancer 52:1705–1711
63. Fu YS, Huang I, Beaudenon S et al (1988) Correlative study of human papillomavirus DNA, histopathology and morphometry in cervical condyloma and intraepithelial neoplasia. Int J Gynecol Pathol 7: 297–307
64. Fu YS, Reagan JW (2002) Pathology of the uterine cervix, vagina, and vulva. WB Saunders, Philadelphia
65. Fu YS, Reagan JW, Richart RM (1983) Precursors of cervical cancer. Cancer Surv 2:359–382
66. Gage JC, Hanson VW, Abbey K et al (2006) Number of cervical biopsies and sensitivity of colposcopy. Obstet Gynecol 108(2): 264–272
67. Garcia-Closas R, Castellsague X, Bosch X et al (2005) The role of diet and nutrition in cervical carcinogenesis: a review of recent evidence. Int J Cancer 117(4):629–637
68. Gatscha RM, Abadi M, Babore S et al (2001) Smears diagnosed as ASCUS: interobserver variation and follow-up. Diagn Cytopathol 25(2):138–140

69. Genest DR, Stein L, Cibas E et al (1993) A binary (Bethesda) system for classifying cervical cancer precursors: criteria, reproducibility, and viral correlates. Hum Pathol 24(7):730–736
70. Geng L, Connolly DC, Isacson C et al (1999) Atypical immature metaplasia (AIM) of the cervix: is it related to high-grade squamous intraepithelial lesion (HSIL)? Hum Pathol 30(3):345–351
71. Gloor E, Hurlimann J (1986) Cervical intraepithelial glandular neoplasia (adenocarcinoma in situ and glandular dysplasia). A correlative study of 23 cases with histologic grading, histochemical analysis of mucins and immunohistochemical determination of the affinity for four lectins. Cancer 58:1272–1280
72. Goldie SJ, Kim JJ, Wright TC (2004) Cost-effectiveness of human papillomavirus DNA testing for cervical cancer screening in women aged 30 years or more. Obstet Gynecol 103(4):619–631
73. Guido RS, Jeronimo J, Schiffman M et al (2005) The distribution of neoplasia arising on the cervix: results from the ALTS trial. Am J Obstet Gynecol 193(4):1331–1337
74. Hanselaar AG, Vooijs GP, Oud PS et al (1988) DNA ploidy patterns in cervical intraepithelial neoplasia grade III, with and without synchronous invasive squamous cell carcinoma: Measurements in nuclei isolated from paraffin-embedded tissue. Cancer 62: 2537–2545
75. Hariri J, Oster A (2007) The negative predictive value of p16INK4a to assess the outcome of cervical intraepithelial neoplasia 1 in the uterine cervix. Int J Gynecol Pathol 26(3):223–228
76. Helper TK, Dockerty MB, Randall LM (1952) Primary adenocarcinoma of the cervix. Am J Obstet Gynecol 63:800–808
77. Higgins GD, Phillips GE, Smith LA et al (1992) High prevalence of human papillomavirus transcripts in all grades of cervical intraepithelial glandular neoplasia. Cancer 70:136–146
78. Ho GY, Studentsov YY, Bierman R et al (2004) Natural history of human papillomavirus type 16 virus-like particle antibodies in young women. Cancer Epidemiol Biomarkers Prev 13(1):110–116
79. Hoffman MS, Sterghos S Jr, Gordy LW et al (1993) Evaluation of the cervical canal with the endocervical brush. Obstet Gynecol 82(4 Pt 1):573–577
80. Holowaty P, Miller AB, Rohan T et al (1999) Natural history of dysplasia of the uterine cervix. J Natl Cancer Inst 91(3):252–258
81. Hopkins MP, Roberts JA, Schmidt RW (1988) Cervical adenocarcinoma in situ. Obstet Gynecol 71:842–844
82. Hurlimann J, Gloor E (1984) Adenocarcinoma in situ and invasive adenocarcinoma of the uterine cervix. An immunohistologic study with antibodies specific for several epithelial markers. Cancer 54(1):103–109
83. IARC (2007) Human Papillomaviruses. IARC, Lyon
84. Insinga RP, Glass AG, Rush BB (2004) Diagnoses and outcomes in cervical cancer screening: a population-based study. Am J Obstet Gynecol 191(1):105–113
85. Ioffe OB, Sagae S, Moritani S et al (2003) Symposium part 3: Should pathologists diagnose endocervical preneoplastic lesions "less than" adenocarcinoma in situ?: point. Int J Gynecol Pathol 22(1):18–21
86. Isacson C, Kessis TD, Hedrick L et al (1996) Both cell proliferation and apoptosis increase with lesion grade in cervical neoplasia but do not correlate with human papillomavirus type. Cancer Res 56(4):669–674
87. Ismail SM, Colelough AB, Dinnen JS et al (1989) Observer variation in histopathological diagnosis and grading of cervical intraepithelial neoplasia. BMJ 298:707–710
88. Jakobsen A, Kristensen PB, Poulsen HK (1983) Flow cytometric classification of biopsy specimens from cervical intraepithelial neoplasia. Cytometry 4:166–169
89. Jaworski RC, Pacey NR, Greenberg ML et al (1988) The histologic diagnosis of adenocarcinoma in situ and related lesions of the cervix uteri. Adenocarcinoma in situ. Cancer 61:1171–1181
90. Jenson AB, Rosenthal JD, Olson C et al (1980) Immunologic relatedness of papillomavirus from different species. J Natl Cancer Instit 64:495–500
91. Johnson LD (1969) The histopathological approach to early cervical neoplasia. Obstet Gynecol Surv 24:735–767
92. Jones BA, Davey DD (2000) Quality management in gynecologic cytology using interlaboratory comparison. Arch Pathol Lab Med 124(5):672–681
93. Jones BA, Novis DA (1996) Cervical biopsy-cytology correlation. A College of American Pathologists Q-Probes study of 22,439 correlations in 348 laboratories. Arch Pathol Lab Med 120(6): 523–531
94. Jones BA, Novis DA (2000) Follow-up of abnormal gynecologic cytology: a college of American pathologists Q-probes study of 16132 cases from 306 laboratories. Arch Pathol Lab Med 124(5):665–671
95. Kashimura M, Shinohara M, Oikawa K et al (1990) An adenocarcinoma in situ of the uterine cervix that developed into invasive adenocarcinoma after 5 years. Gynecol Oncol 36:128–133
96. Keating JT, Cviko A, Riethdorf S et al (2001) Ki-67, cyclin E, and p16INK4 are complimentary surrogate biomarkers for human papilloma virus-related cervical neoplasia. Am J Surg Pathol 25(7):884–891
97. Kim TJ, Kim HS, Park CT et al (1999) Clinical evaluation of follow-up methods and results of atypical glandular cells of undetermined significance (AGUS) detected on cervicovaginal Pap smears. Gynecol Oncol 73(2):292–298
98. Kim JJ, Wright TC, Goldie SJ (2002) Cost-effectiveness of alternative triage strategies for atypical squamous cells of undetermined significance. JAMA 287(18):2382–2390
99. Kinney WK, Manos MM, Hurley LB et al (1998) Where's the high-grade cervical neoplasia? The importance of minimally abnormal Papanicolaou diagnoses. Obstet Gynecol 91(6):973–976
100. Kirkland JA (1963) Atypical epithelial changes in the uterine cervix. J Clin Pathol 16:150–154
101. Klaes R, Friedrich T, Spitkovsky D et al (2001) Overexpression of p16(INK4A) as a specific marker for dysplastic and neoplastic epithelial cells of the cervix uteri. Int J Cancer 92(2):276–284
102. Kolstad P, Klem V (1976) Long-term followup of 1121 cases of carcinoma in situ. Obstet Gynecol 48(2):125–129
103. Koss LG (1978) Dysplasia. A real concept or a misnomer? Obstet Gynecol 51:374
104. Koss LG, Stewart FW, Foote FW et al (1963) Some histological aspects of behavior of epidermoid carcinoma in situ and related lesions of the uterine cervix. Cancer 16(9):1160–1211
105. Kudo R, Sagai S, Hayakawa O et al (1991) Morphology of adenocarcinoma in situ and microinvasive adenocarcinoma of the uterine cervix. Acta Cytol 35:109–116
106. Kulasingam SL, Kim JJ, Lawrence WF et al (2006) Cost-effectiveness analysis based on the atypical squamous cells of undetermined significance/low-grade squamous intraepithelial lesion Triage Study (ALTS). J Natl Cancer Inst 98(2):92–100
107. Kurman RJ, Ronnett BM, Sherman ME et al (2009) Tumors of the cervix, vagina and vulva. American Registry of Pathology in conjunction with Armed Forces Institute of Pathology, Washington, DC
108. Larson AA, Kern S, Curtiss S et al (1997) High resolution analysis of chromosome 3p alterations in cervical carcinoma. Cancer Res 57:4082–4090

109. Leary J, Jaworski R, Houghton R (1991) In-situ hybridization using biotinylated DNA probes to human papillomavirus in adenocarcinoma in-situ and endocervical glandular dysplasia of the uterine cervix. Pathology 23:85–89
110. Lee KR (2003) Symposium part 4: Should pathologists diagnose endocervical preneoplastic lesions "less than" adenocarcinoma in situ?: counterpoint. Int J Gynecol Pathol 22(1):22–24
111. Lee KR, Sun D, Crum CP (2000) Endocervical intraepithelial glandular atypia (dysplasia): a histopathologic, human papillomavirus, and MIB-1 analysis of 25 cases. Hum Pathol 31(6):656–664
112. Liman AK, Giampoli EJ, Bonfiglio TA (2005) Should women with atypical squamous cells, cannot exclude high-grade squamous intraepithelial lesion, receive reflex human papillomavirus-DNA testing? Cancer 105(6):457–460
113. Lonky NM, Felix JC, Naidu YM et al (2003) Triage of atypical squamous cells of undetermined significance with hybrid capture II: colposcopy and histologic human papillomavirus correlation. Obstet Gynecol 101(3):481–489
114. Lonky NM, Sadeghi M, Tsadik GW et al (1999) The clinical significance of the poor correlation of cervical dysplasia and cervical malignancy with referral cytologic results. Am J Obstet Gynecol 181(3):560–566
115. Luesley DM, Jordan JA, Woodman CBJ et al (1987) A retrospective review of adenocarcinoma-in-situ and glandular atypia of the uterine cervix. Br J Obstet Gynaecol 94:699–703
116. Luff RD (1992) The Bethesda System for reporting cervical/vaginal cytologic diagnoses: report of the 1991 Bethesda workshop. The Bethesda System Editorial Committee. Hum Pathol 23(7):719–721
117. Maiman M (1998) Management of cervical neoplasia in human immunodeficiency virus-infected women. J Natl Cancer Instit 23:43–49
118. Manos MM, Kinney WK, Hurley LB et al (1999) Identifying women with cervical neoplasia: using human papillomavirus DNA testing for equivocal Papanicolaou results. JAMA 281(17):1605–1610
119. Marques T, Andrade LA, Vassallo J (1996) Endocervical tubal metaplasia and adenocarcinoma in situ: role of immunohistochemistry for carcinoembryonic antigen and vimentin in differential diagnosis. Histopathology 28(6):549–550
120. Massad LS (2006) More is more: improving the sensitivity of colposcopy. Obstet Gynecol 108(2):246–247
121. Massad LS, Collins YC, Meyer PM (2001) Biopsy correlates of abnormal cervical cytology classified using the Bethesda system. Gynecol Oncol 82(3):516–522
122. McCann MF, Irwin DE, Walton LA et al (1992) Nicotine and cotinine in the cervical mucus of smokers, passive smokers, and nonsmokers. Cancer Epidemiol Biomarkers Prev 1:125–129
123. McCluggage WG (2007) Immunohistochemistry as a diagnostic aid in cervical pathology. Pathology 39(1):97–111
124. McCluggage WG, Maxwell P, McBride HA et al (1995) Monoclonal antibodies Ki-67 and MIB1 in the distinction of tuboendometrial metaplasia from endocervical adenocarcinoma and adenocarcinoma in situ in formalin-fixed material. Int J Gynecol Pathol 14(3):209–216
125. McCredie MR, Sharples KJ, Paul C et al (2008) Natural history of cervical neoplasia and risk of invasive cancer in women with cervical intraepithelial neoplasia 3: a retrospective cohort study. Lancet Oncol 9(5):425–434
126. Melnikow J, Nuovo J, Willan AR et al (1998) Natural history of cervical squamous intraepithelial lesions: a meta-analysis. Obstet Gynecol 92(4 Pt 2):727–735
127. Mitchell H, Hocking J, Saville M (2004) Cervical cytology screening history of women diagnosed with adenocarcinoma in situ of the cervix: a case-control study. Acta Cytol 48(5):595–600
128. Mitchell H, Medley G, Gordon I et al (1995) Cervical cytology reported as negative and risk of adenocarcinoma of the cervix: no strong evidence of benefit. Br J Cancer 71(4):894–897
129. Mitchell MF, Tortolero-Luna G, Wright T et al (1996) Cervical human papillomavirus infection and intraepithelial neoplasia: a review. J Natl Cancer Inst Monogr 21:17–25
130. Mittal KR, Chan W, Demopoulos RL (1990) Sensitivity and specificity of various morphological features of cervical condylomas. Arch Pathol Lab Med 114:1038–1041
131. Moscicki AB, Hills N, Shiboski S et al (2001) Risks for incident human papillomavirus infection and low-grade squamous intraepithelial lesion development in young females. JAMA 285:2995–3002
132. Moscicki AB, Schiffman M, Kjaer S et al (2006) Chapter 5: Updating the natural history of HPV and anogenital cancer. Vaccine 24 (Suppl 3):S42–S51
133. Moscicki AB, Shiboski S, Hills NK et al (2004) Regression of low-grade squamous intra-epithelial lesions in young women. Lancet 364(9446):1678–1683
134. Mourits MJE, Pieters WJ, Hollema H et al (1992) Three-group metaphase as a morphologic criterion of progressive cervical intraepithelial neoplasia. Am J Obstet Gynecol 167(3):591–595
135. Muñoz N, Castellsagué X, De González AB et al (2006) Chapter 1: HPV in the etiology of human cancer. Vaccine 24(Suppl 3):S1–S10. Epub 2006 Jun 23
136. Murphy N, Heffron CC, King B et al (2004) p16INK4A positivity in benign, premalignant and malignant cervical glandular lesions: a potential diagnostic problem. Virchows Arch 445(6):610–615
137. Nasiell K, Nasiell M, Vaclavinkova V (1983) Behavior of moderate cervical dysplasia during long-term follow-up. Obstet Gynecol 61:609–614
138. Negri G, Egarter-Vigl E, Kasal A et al (2003) p16INK4a is a useful marker for the diagnosis of adenocarcinoma of the cervix uteri and its precursors: an immunohistochemical study with immunocytochemical correlations. Am J Surg Pathol 27(2):187–193
139. Ng A (1993) Glandular diseases of the uterus. In: Keebler CM, Somrak TM (eds) The manual of cytotechnology. American Society of Clinical Pathologists, Chicago
140. Nieminen P, Kallio M, Hakama M (1995) The effect of mass screening on incidence and mortality of squamous and adenocarcinoma of cervix uteri. Obstet Gynecol 85(6):1017–1021
141. Ostor AG, Duncan A, Quinn M et al (2000) Adenocarcinoma in situ of the uterine cervix: an experience with 100 cases. Gynecol Oncol 79(2):207–210
142. Ostor AG, Pagano R, Davoren RAM et al (1984) Adenocarcinoma in situ of the cervix. Int J Gynecol Pathol 3:179–190
143. Park JJ, Genest DR, Sun D et al (1999) Atypical immature metaplastic-like proliferations of the cervix: diagnostic reproducibility and viral (HPV) correlates. Hum Pathol 30(10):1161–1165
144. Park TJ, Richart RM, Sun X-W et al (1996) Association between HPV type and clonal status of cervical squamous intraepithelial lesions (SIL). J Natl Cancer Instit 88(66):355–358
145. Park JJ, Sun D, Quade BJ et al (2000) Stratified mucin-producing intraepithelial lesions of the cervix: adenosquamous or columnar cell neoplasia? Am J Surg Pathol 24(10):1414–1419
146. Parkin DM (1991) Screening for cervix cancer in developing countries. In: Miller AB, Chamberlain J, Day NE, Hakama M, Prorok PC

(eds) Cancer screening. Cambridge University Press, Cambridge, pp 184–198

147. Patten SF (1978) Diagnostic cytopathology of the uterine cervix. Karger, Basal
148. Pemberton FA, Smith GV (1929) The early diagnosis and prevention of carcinoma of the cervix: a clinical pathologic study of borderline cases treated at the Free Hospital for women. Am J Obstet Gynecol 17:165
149. Pieters WJ, Koudstaal J, Ploem-Zaajer JJ et al (1992) The three group metaphase as morphologic indicator of high ploidy cells in cervical intraepithelial neoplasia. Anal Quant Cytol Histol 14:227–232
150. Pirog EC, Isacson C, Szabolcs MJ et al (2002) Proliferative activity of benign and neoplastic endocervical epithelium and correlation with HPV DNA detection. Int J Gynecol Pathol 21(1):22–26
151. Piyathilake CJ, Macaluso M, Alvarez RD et al (2009) Lower risk of cervical intraepithelial neoplasia in women with high plasma folate and sufficient vitamin B12 in the post-folic acid fortification era. Cancer Prev Res 2(7):658–664
152. Plaxe SC, Saltzstein SL (1999) Estimation of the duration of the preclinical phase of cervical adenocarcinoma suggests that there is ample opportunity for screening. Gynecol Oncol 75(1):55–61
153. Pretorius RG, Zhang X, Belinson JL et al (2006) Distribution of cervical intraepithelial neoplasia 2, 3 and cancer on the uterine cervix. J Low Genit Tract Dis 10(1):45–50
154. Queiroz C, Silva TC, Alves VA et al (2006) Comparative study of the expression of cellular cycle proteins in cervical intraepithelial lesions. Pathol Res Pract 202(10):731–737
155. Queiroz C, Silva TC, Alves VA et al (2006) P16(INK4a) expression as a potential prognostic marker in cervical pre-neoplastic and neoplastic lesions. Pathol Res Pract 202(2):77–83
156. Quint KD, de Koning MN, Geraets DT et al (2009) Comprehensive analysis of Human Papillomavirus and *Chlamydia trachomatis* in in-situ and invasive cervical adenocarcinoma. Gynecol Oncol 114(3):390–394
157. Ratnam S, Franco EL, Ferenczy A (2000) Human papillomavirus testing for primary screening of cervical cancer precursors. Cancer Epidemiol Biomarkers Prev 9(9):945–951
158. Renshaw AA, Mody DR, Lozano RL et al (2004) Detection of adenocarcinoma in situ of the cervix in Papanicolaou tests: comparison of diagnostic accuracy with other high-grade lesions. Arch Pathol Lab Med 128(2):153–157
159. Richart RM (1973) Cervical intraepithelial neoplasia: a review. Pathol Ann 8:301–328
160. Richart RM (1990) A modified terminology for cervical intraepithelial neoplasia. Obstet Gynecol 75(1):131–133
161. Richart RM, Lerch V, Baron B (1967) A time-lapse cinematographic study in vitro of mitosis in normal human cervical epithelium, dysplasia and carcinoma in situ. J Natl Cancer Instit 39:571
162. Riethdorf L, Riethdorf S, Lee KR et al (2002) Human papillomaviruses, expression of p16, and early endocervical glandular neoplasia. Hum Pathol 33(9):899–904
163. Robertson AJ, Anderson JM, Beck JS et al (1989) Observer variability in histopathological reporting of cervical biopsy specimens. J Clin Pathol 42(3):231–238
164. Ronnett BM, Manos MM, Ransley JE et al (1999) Atypical glandular cells of undetermined significance (AGUS): cytopathologic features, histopathologic results, and human papillomavirus DNA detection. Hum Pathol 30(7):816–825
165. Salani R, Puri I, Bristow RE (2009) Adenocarcinoma in situ of the uterine cervix: a metaanalysis of 1278 patients evaluating the predictive value of conization margin status. Am J Obstet Gynecol 200(2):182e1–182e5
166. Sawaya GF, McConnell KJ, Kulasingam SL et al (2003) Risk of cervical cancer associated with extending the interval between cervical-cancer screenings. N Engl J Med 349(16):1501–1509
167. Schiffman M, Castle PE, Jeronimo J et al (2007) Human papillomavirus and cervical cancer. Lancet 370(9590):890–907
168. Schmidt C, Pretorius RG, Bonin M et al (1992) Invasive cervical cancer following cryotherapy for cervical intraepithelial neoplasia or human papillomavirus infection. Obstet Gynecol 80(5):797–800
169. Sherman ME, Schiffman M, Cox JT et al (2002) Effects of age and HPV load on colposcopic triage: data from the ASCUS LSIL Triage Study (ALTS). J Natl Cancer Instit 94:102–107
170. Sherman ME, Tabbara SO, Scott DR et al (1999) "ASCUS, rule out HSIL": cytologic features, histologic correlates, and human papillomavirus detection. Mod Pathol 12(4):335–342
171. Shin CH, Schorge JO, Lee KR et al (2000) Conservative management of adenocarcinoma in situ of the cervix. Gynecol Oncol 79(1):6–10
172. Shingleton HM, Richart RM, Wiener J et al (1968) Human cervical intraepithelial neoplasia. Fine structure of dysplasia and carcinoma in situ. Cancer Res 28:695–706
173. Sigurdsson K, Sigvaldason H (2007) Is it rational to start population-based cervical cancer screening at or soon after age 20? Analysis of time trends in preinvasive and invasive diseases. Eur J Cancer 43(4):769–774
174. Smith JS, Green J, Berrington de Gonzalez A et al (2003) Cervical cancer and use of hormonal contraceptives: a systematic review. Lancet 361(9364):1159–1167
175. Smith JS, Lindsay L, Hoots B et al (2007) Human papillomavirus type distribution in invasive cervical cancer and high-grade cervical lesions: a meta-analysis update. Int J Cancer 121(3):621–632
176. Snijders PJ, Steenbergen RD, Heideman DA et al (2006) HPV-mediated cervical carcinogenesis: concepts and clinical implications. J Pathol 208(2):152–164
177. Solomon D, Davey D, Kurman R et al (2002) The 2001 Bethesda System: terminology for reporting results of cervical cytology. JAMA 287(16):2114–2119
178. Solomon D, Stoler M, Jeronimo J et al (2007) Diagnostic utility of endocervical curettage in women undergoing colposcopy for equivocal or low-grade cytologic abnormalities. Obstet Gynecol 110(2):288–295
179. Stanley M (2003) Chapter 17: Genital human papillomavirus infections – current and prospective therapies. J Natl Cancer Inst Monogr (31):117–124
180. Steben M, Duarte-Franco E (2007) Human papillomavirus infection: epidemiology and pathophysiology. Gynecol Oncol 107(2 Suppl 1):S2–S5
181. Stoler MH, Schiffman M (2001) Interobserver reproducibility of cervical cytologic and histologic interpretations: realistic estimates from the ASCUS-LSIL Triage Study. JAMA 285(11):1500–1505
182. Szarewski A, Cuzick J (1998) Smoking and cervical neoplasia; a review of the evidence. J Epidemiol Biostat 3:229
183. Szarewski A, Maddox P, Royston P et al (2001) The effect of stopping smoking on cervical Langerhans' cells and lymphocytes. BJOG 108(3):295–303
184. Tase T, Okagaki T, Clark BA et al (1989) Human papillomavirus DNA in adenocarcinoma in situ, microinvasive adenocarcinoma of the uterine cervix and coexisting cervical squamous intraepithelial neoplasia. Int J Gynecol Pathol 8(1):8–17

185. Tase T, Okagaki T, Clark BA et al (1989) Human papillomavirus DNA in glandular dysplasia and microglandular hyperplasia: presumed precursors of adenocarcinoma of the uterine cervix. Obstet Gynecol 73(6):1005–1008
186. Tavassoli FA, Devilee P (eds) (2003) Pathology and genetics of tumours of the breast and female genital organs. World Health Organization Classification of Tumors. IARC, Lyon
187. Trowell JE (1985) Intestinal metaplasia with argentaffin cells in the uterine cervix. Histopathology 9:561–569
188. Tsoumpou I, Arbyn M, Kyrgiou M et al (2009) p16(INK4a) immunostaining in cytological and histological specimens from the uterine cervix: a systematic review and meta-analysis. Cancer Treat Rev 35(3):210–220
189. Ueda Y, Enomoto T, Miyatake T et al (2003) Monoclonal expansion with integration of high-risk type human papillomaviruses is an initial step for cervical carcinogenesis: association of clonal status and human papillomavirus infection with clinical outcome in cervical intraepithelial neoplasia. Lab Invest 83(10):1517–1527
190. Ursin G, Pike MC, Preston-Martin S et al (1996) Sexual, reproductive, and other risk factors for adenocarcinoma of the cervix: results from a population-based case-control study (California, United States) [see comments]. Cancer Causes Control 7(3):391–401
191. Van Ranst MS, Tachezy R, Delius H et al (1993) Taxonomy of the human papillomaviruses. Papillomavirus Rep 4:61–65
192. Wang SS, Sherman ME, Hildesheim A et al (2004) Cervical adenocarcinoma and squamous cell carcinoma incidence trends among white women and black women in the United States for 1976–2000. Cancer 100(5):1035–1044
193. Wang SS, Trunk M, Schiffman M et al (2004) Validation of p16INK4a as a marker of oncogenic human papillomavirus infection in cervical biopsies from a population-based cohort in Costa Rica. Cancer Epidemiol Biomarkers Prev 13(8): 1355–1360
194. Wang SS, Wheeler CM, Hildesheim A et al (2001) Human leukocyte antigen class I and II alleles and risk of cervical neoplasia: results from a population-based study in Costa Rica. J Infect Dis 184(10):1310–1314
195. Ward BE, Burkett BA, Peterson C et al (1990) Cytological correlates of cervical papillomavirus infection. Int J Gynecol Pathol 9:297–305
196. Wells M, Ostor AG, Franceschi S et al (2003) Epithelial tumors of the uterine cervix. In: Tavassoli FA, Devilee P (eds) Tumors of the breast and female genital organs. IARC, Lyon, pp 221–232
197. Wheeler CM, Hunt WC, Schiffman M et al (2006) Human papillomavirus genotypes and the cumulative 2-year risk of cervical precancer. J Infect Dis 194(9):1291–1299
198. Williams J (1888) Cancer of the uterus: Harveian lectures for 1886. Lewis, London
199. Winer RL, Hughes JP, Feng Q et al (2006) Condom use and the risk of genital human papillomavirus infection in young women. N Engl J Med 354(25):2645–2654
200. Winer RL, Lee SK, Hughes JP et al (2003) Genital human papillomavirus infection: incidence and risk factors in a cohort of female university students. Am J Epidemiol 157(3):218–226
201. Workshop NCI (1991) The revised Bethesda System for reporting cervical/vaginal cytologic diagnoses. Report of the 1991 Bethesda Workshop. JAMA 267:1892
202. Wright TC Jr (2006) Chapter 3: Pathology of HPV infection at the cytologic and histologic levels: basis for a 2-tiered morphologic classification system. Int J Gynaecol Obstet 94(Suppl 1):S22–S31
203. Wright TC Jr, Cox JT, Massad LS et al (2002) 2001 consensus guidelines for the management of women with cervical cytological abnormalities. JAMA 287(16):2120–2129
204. Wright TC, Kuhn L (2006) Immunosuppression and the cervix: human immunodeficiency virus (HIV). In: Jordan JA, Singer A (eds) The cervix. Blackwell, Malden, pp 450–517
205. Wright TC, Kurman RJ (1994) A critical review of the morphologic classification systems of preinvasive lesions of the cervix: the scientific basis of the paradigm. Papillomavirus Rep 5:175–181
206. Wright TC Jr, Massad LS, Dunton CJ et al (2007) 2006 consensus guidelines for the management of women with abnormal cervical cancer screening tests. Am J Obstet Gynecol 197(4):346–355
207. Wright TC Jr, Massad LS, Dunton CJ et al (2007) 2006 consensus guidelines for the management of women with abnormal cervical screening tests. J Low Genit Tract Dis 11(4):201–222
208. Wright TC Jr, Massad LS, Dunton CJ et al (2007) 2006 consensus guidelines for the management of women with cervical intraepithelial neoplasia or adenocarcinoma in situ. Am J Obstet Gynecol 197(4):340–345
209. Wright TC, Schiffman M (2003) Adding a test for human papillomavirus DNA to cervical-cancer screening. New Eng J Med 348(6):489–490
210. Young RH, Scully RE (1989) Atypical forms of microglandular hyperplasia of the cervix simulating carcinoma. Am J Surg Pathol 13:50–56
211. Zhang Q, Kuhn L, Denny LA et al (2007) Impact of utilizing p16INK4A immunohistochemistry on estimated performance of three cervical cancer screening tests. Int J Cancer 120(2):351–356
212. zur Hausen H (1977) Human papillomaviruses and their possible role in squamous cell carcinomas. Curr Top Microbiol Immunol 78:1–30
213. zur Hausen H (2002) Papillomaviruses and cancer: from basic studies to clinical application. Nat Rev Cancer 2(5):342–350
214. zur Hausen H (2009) The search for infectious causes of human cancers: where and why (Nobel lecture). Angewandte Chemie 48(32):5798–5808

6 Carcinoma and Other Tumors of the Cervix

Agnieszka K. Witkiewicz · Thomas C. Wright · Alex Ferenczy · Brigitte M. Ronnett · Robert J. Kurman

R. J. Kurman, L. Hedrick Ellenson, B. M. Ronnett (eds.), *Blaustein's Pathology of the Female Genital Tract (6th ed.)*, DOI 10.1007/978-1-4419-0489-8_6,

Invasive Carcinoma

The World Health Organization (WHO) recognizes three general categories of invasive carcinoma of the cervix: squamous cell carcinoma, adenocarcinoma, and "other epithelial tumors" (➋ *Table 6.1*) [278]. The "other epithelial tumors" include adenosquamous carcinoma, adenoid basal cell carcinoma, adenoid cystic carcinomas, as well as neuroendocrine tumors and undifferentiated carcinoma (➋ *Table 6.1*) [278]. The relative frequency of these different tumor types varies between studies; in general, squamous cell carcinoma is the most common histologic subtype accounting for 70–80% of invasive carcinomas. Adenocarcinoma and adenosquamous carcinoma comprise 10–15% of all cases, and all others 10–15% [45, 245, 271].

The most widely accepted staging system for tumors of the cervix is the four-stage system of the International Federation of Gynecologists and Obstetricians (FIGO) (➋ *Table 6.2*) [205]. Stage I includes all tumors confined to the cervix and is divided into two subcategories: those that invade 5 mm or less into the stroma and are macroscopically not visible, and those that either invade more than 5 mm or are macroscopically visible. As such, staging of cervical cancer is based on clinical, not surgical, examination of the cervix. Stage II tumors extend beyond the cervix, but not to the pelvic sidewall, and do not invade the lower third of the vagina. Stage III tumors include those that extend to the pelvic sidewall, cause hydronephrosis, or invade the lower third of the vagina. Stage IV tumors extend beyond the true pelvis or clinically involve the mucosa of the bladder or rectum.

Table 6.1
Modified World Health Organization histological classification of invasive carcinomas of the uterine cervix

Squamous cell carcinoma
Microinvasive (early invasive) squamous cell carcinoma
Invasive squamous cell carcinoma
Keratinizing
Nonkeratinizing
Basaloid
Verrucous
Warty
Papillary
Squamotransitional
Lymphoepithelioma-like carcinoma
Adenocarcinoma
Usual type adenocarcinoma
Mucinous adenocarcinoma
Endocervical type
Intestinal type
Signet-ring type
Minimal deviation
Villoglandular
Endometrioid adenocarcinoma
Clear cell adenocarcinoma
Serous adenocarcinoma
Mesonephric adenocarcinoma
Other epithelial tumors
Adenosquamous carcinoma
Glassy cell variant
Adenoid cystic carcinoma
Adenoid basal carcinoma
Neuroendocrine tumors
Carcinoid
Atypical carcinoid
Small cell carcinoma
Large cell neuroendocrine carcinoma
Undifferentiated carcinoma

Squamous Cell Carcinoma

Microinvasive Squamous Cell Carcinoma

The concept of prognostically favorable, microinvasive carcinoma (MICA) of the cervix was first introduced in 1847 by Mestwerdt. Microinvasive carcinoma is considered a preclinical stage in the spectrum of squamous intraepithelial lesions (SIL), and frank clinical invasive carcinoma of the cervix. Most patients who die of disseminated squamous cell carcinoma have either lymphatic involvement, tumors that invade beyond 5 mm into the cervical stroma, or tumors more than 2.5 cm^3 in volume. Therefore, microscopic tumors that invade <5 mm beyond the base of the epithelium, either surface or glandular, and with horizontal spread not exceeding 7 mm (stage IA) are defined by FIGO as MICA (see ➋ *Table 6.2*). Tumors that qualify as stage IA are further subdivided into those that invade no more than 3 mm (stage IA1) and those that invade more than 3 mm, but <5 mm, into the cervical stroma (stage IA2). The presence of lymphvascular invasion does not exclude a tumor from FIGO Stage IA. Proponents who believe that classification systems should guide clinical treatment consider only FIGO stage IA1 as MICA.

The Society of Gynecological Oncologists (SGO) in the United States has proposed a more restricted definition for MICA. According to that definition, histologically detected lesions with <3 mm stromal invasion and no vascular invasion are considered MICA [52]. Lesions that

Table 6.2
2009 modification of FIGO staging of carcinoma of the cervix uteri [205]

Stage	Definition
I	Cervical carcinoma confined to uterus (extension to the corpus should be disregarded)
IA	Invasive carcinoma diagnosed only by microscopy; all macroscopically visible lesions, even with superficial invasion, are stage IB
IA1	Stromal invasion no greater than 3.0 mm in depth and 7.0 mm or less in horizontal spread
IA2	Stromal invasion more than 3.0 mm and not more than 5.0 mm with a horizontal spread of 7.0 mm or less
IB	Clinically visible lesion confined to the cervix or microscopic lesion greater than IA2[a]
IB1	Clinically visible lesion 4.0 cm or less in greatest dimension
IB2	Clinically visible lesion more than 4.0 cm in greatest dimension
II	Tumor invades beyond the uterus but not to pelvic wall or to lower third of the vagina
IIA	Without parametrial invasion
IIA1	Clinically visible lesion ≤4.0 cm in greatest dimension
IIA2	Clinically visible lesion >4 cm in greatest dimension
IIB	With parametrial invasion
III	Tumor extends to the pelvic wall and/or involves lower third of vagina and/or causes hydronephrosis or nonfunctioning kidney[b]
IIIA	Tumor involves lower third of vagina with no extension to pelvic wall
IIIB	Tumor extends to pelvic wall and/or causes hydronephrosis or nonfunctioning kidney
IV	The carcinoma has extended beyond the true pelvis or has involved (biopsy proven) the mucosa of the bladder or rectum. A bullous edema, as such, does not permit a case to be allotted to stage IV
IVA	Spread of the growth to adjacent organs
IVB	Spread to distant organs

[a]The depth of invasion should not be more than 5 mm taken from the base of the epithelium, either surface or glandular, from which it originates. The depth of invasion is defined as the measurement of the tumor from the epithelial–stromal junction of the adjacent most superficial epithelial papilla to the deepest point of invasion. Vascular space involvement, venous or lymphatic, does not affect classification.
[b]On rectal examination, there is no cancer-free space between the tumor and the pelvic wall. All cases with hydronephrosis or non-functioning kidney are included, unless they are known to be due to another cause.

fulfill the SGO definition of MICA have virtually no potential for metastases or recurrence. Therefore, this definition appears to be the most appropriate one for guiding clinical management. Patients with MICA by SGO criteria are sometimes treated conservatively, usually with conization, while those that have tumors measuring >3 mm in depth or with lymphatic invasion are often considered for more radical therapy [55]. It is important to stress that because the lesion cannot be visualized on gross inspection, the diagnosis of MICA is always based on histologic examination of a cone biopsy specimen that includes the entire lesion.

General Features

The majority of MICA occurs in women 35–46 years of age. In screened populations, MICA accounts for approximately 20% of all cervical cancers [36, 177]. The reported frequency of MICA in patients with a squamous intraepithelial lesion (SIL) varies from <1% to >50%. This wide variation in prevalence reflects differences in the definition of MICA, methods of sampling of cervical specimens, and the criteria used for diagnosing invasion. A 4% prevalence of MICA has been demonstrated in serial step sections of specimens with a squamous intraepithelial lesion (SIL) [28, 136]. However, it should be noted that such studies typically identify only microscopic foci of a few epithelial cells invading the stroma. Estimates of the prevalence of MICA in the general population can be obtained from population-based cervical cancer registries. A population-based registry from British Columbia, Canada, estimates the prevalence of MICA to be 4.8 per 100,000 women screened, whereas the prevalence of carcinoma in situ is 316 per 100,000 women screened [23]. With the widespread adoption of shallow laser excisional conization and loop electrosurgical excision procedure (LEEP) as diagnostic and therapeutic methods for SIL, better estimates for the prevalence of MICA in patients with all grades of SIL have been obtained. Larger studies of specimens obtained by LEEP have reported colposcopically undetected MICA in 0.4–3% of all patients with biopsy-confirmed SIL [251]. In an audit of the National Health Service (NHS) Cervical Cancer Screening Program in the United Kingdom During the 1991–1993 period, the incidence of MICA was 3.6 per 100,00 total female population [100]. In assessing the probability of MICA developing in women with SIL, the size as well as grade of the lesion is important. Microinvasive squamous cell carcinoma appears to be most commonly associated with extensive high-grade

SIL involving the endocervical crypts [8]. Two additional histologic features predicting microinvasion include presence of luminal necrosis and intraepithelial squamous maturation [8].

Clinical Features

Most patients with MICA are asymptomatic with a grossly normal cervix or nonspecific findings such as chronic cervicitis or erosion. Cytologic studies do not accurately predict the presence of microinvasion [200]. In a study of 536 women undergoing laser conization, cytology predicted the presence of invasion in only 27.3% of women with MICA [10]. In another study, cytology predicted invasion only in 12.5% of women with MICA [36]. A definitive diagnosis of microinvasion is made by histologic evaluation of cervical tissue removed by conization or at hysterectomy. Colposcopically, areas of MICA usually show acetowhitening consistent with high-grade SIL, and may contain one or more foci of bizarre surface branching vessels [159]. However, microinvasion frequently cannot be accurately detected using colposcopy. In a study that correlated colposcopic appearances with histologic findings from a large number of LEEP specimens, Murdoch et al. demonstrated that accurate colposcopic detection of MICA requires invasion of more than 1 mm into the cervical stroma [187]. Because it is difficult to colposcopically identify MICA, most colposcopists routinely treat all large biopsy-confirmed, high-grade SIL using excisional methods such as LEEP.

Pathologic Features

The diagnosis of MICA is based on the presence of one or more tongues of malignant cells penetrating the basement membrane of the squamous epithelium (➋ *Figs. 6.1–6.4*). The squamous epithelium invariably demonstrates varying grades of SIL, and in most instances the underlying endocervical glands are extensively replaced by the intraepithelial disease. Within the microinvasion foci, the cells are better differentiated with abundant eosinophilic cytoplasm and prominent nucleoli as compared to the associated SIL. Occasionally, small foci of keratinization are seen within the microinvasive foci. Because of focal disruption of the basement membrane, the margin of the invading nests is ragged, flanked by intact basement membrane on either side. This irregular contour is probably the most reliable criterion for the diagnosis of MICA. It is easily distinguished from the smooth and regular contour

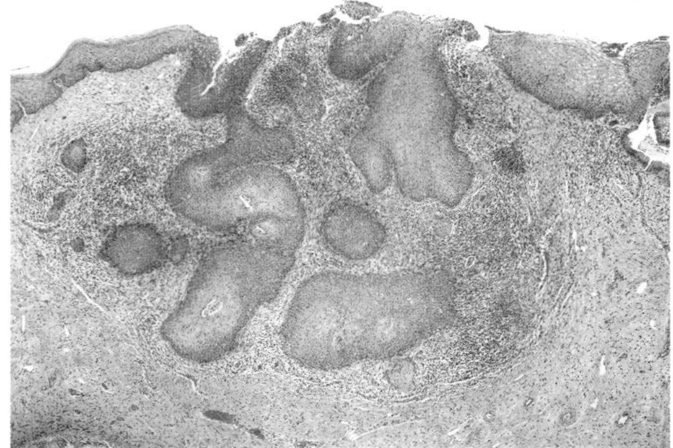

Fig. 6.1
Microinvasive squamous carcinoma. **Irregular islands of squamous cell carcinoma invade superficial cervical stroma but do not exceed 5 mm in depth or 7 mm in horizontal extent**

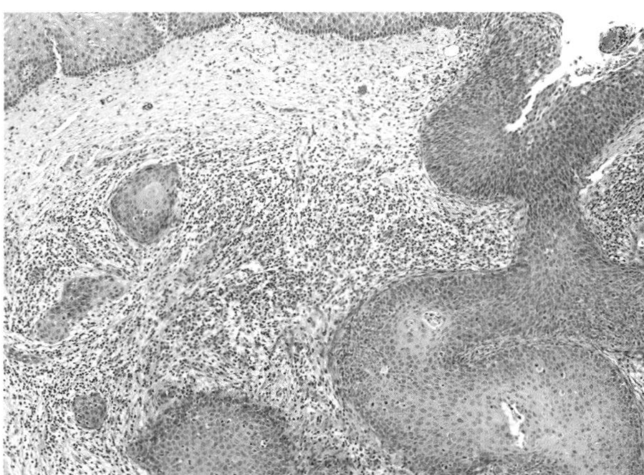

Fig. 6.2
Microinvasive squamous carcinoma. **Some small nests of squamous cell carcinoma are isolated in superficial stroma, whereas one larger island remains attached to the overlying high-grade squamous intraepithelial lesion**

of endocervical gland involved by high-grade SIL. There is often a conspicuous lymphoplasmacytic infiltrate surrounding the tips of the invasive epithelial tongues, and frequently there is a desmoplastic response in the adjacent stroma. Two additional histologic features that are reported to be helpful for diagnosing MICA, particularly when there is a marked inflammatory infiltrate, are apparent duplication or folding of the neoplastic epithelium

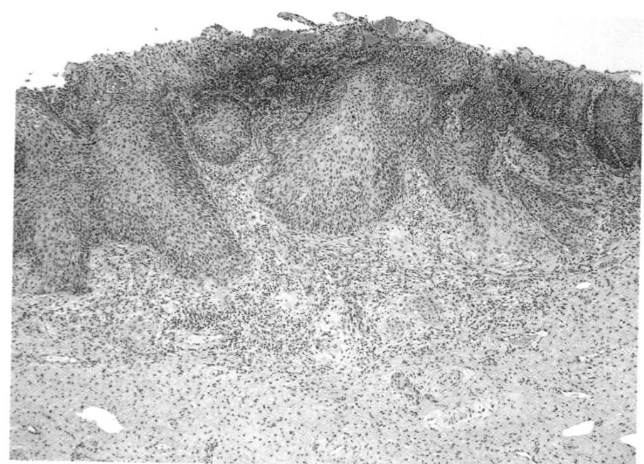

Fig. 6.3
Microinvasive squamous cell carcinoma. **Small foci of squamous cell carcinoma present in superficial stroma not exceeding 5 mm in depth from the basement membrane of the overlying high-grade squamous intraepithelial lesion and not exceeding 7 mm in horizontal extent**

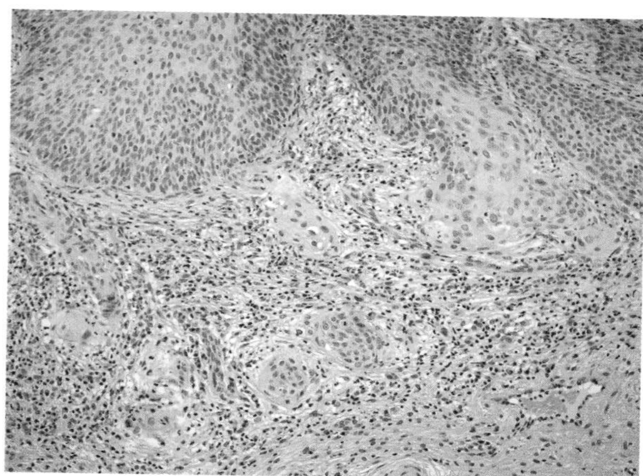

Fig. 6.4
Microinvasive squamous cell carcinoma. **Small detached nests and one attached elongated tongue of squamous cell carcinoma are present in superficial stroma beneath the overlying high-grade squamous intraepithelial lesion**

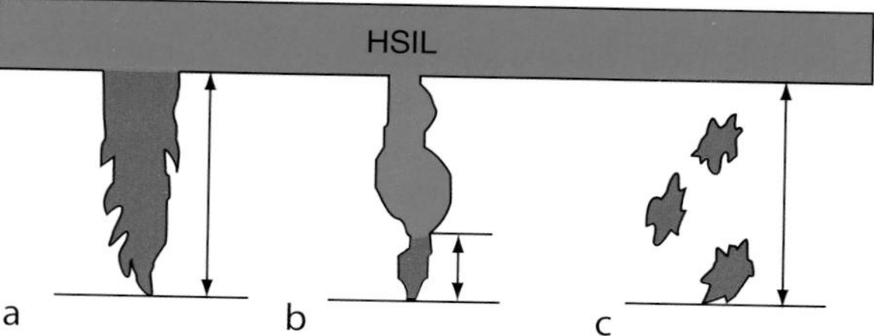

Fig. 6.5
Methods of measuring depth of invasion of microinvasive squamous cell carcinoma of the cervix. **The pattern of stromal invasion determines the stromal depth measurement that is most appropriate. (a) Origin of invasion at surface HSIL: depth of stromal invasion is measured from point of origin of invasion downward to the last cell of the invasive focus. (b) Origin of invasion at HSIL with gland involvement: depth of stromal invasion is measured from site of origin downward to the last cell of the invasive focus. (c) Origin of invasion not seen: depth of stromal invasion is measured from basal lamina of surface HSIL downward to the last cell of the invasive focus**

and scalloping of the margins of the epithelium at the dermal–epidermal interface [57].

After establishing a diagnosis of MICA, the pathologist evaluates the surgical margins, depth of stromal invasion, greatest lateral extent of the lesion, and whether lymphvascular invasion is present. For consistency in the measurement of the depth of stromal invasion, the following guidelines are recommended. The depth of neoplastic projections should be measured from the initial site of invasion, either from the basal lamina of the surface epithelium or from endocervical glands replaced by intraepithelial neoplasia (*Fig. 6.5*). There are cases, however, in which direct continuity between invasive foci and SIL cannot be demonstrated, even in deeper cuts of the paraffin block. In such instances, it is assumed that the invasion originated from basal cells of the overlying SIL. Therefore, the depth of invasion is arbitrarily measured from the basal lamina of the surface SIL. The most accurate method to measure the depth of stromal penetration is with a calibrated slide or ocular micrometer. A more convenient, but perhaps less accurate, method of establishing the size and depth of penetrating foci consists of direct microscopic visualization with a transparent metric ruler. The depth of invasion also depends on the angle at which sections are prepared, and therefore efforts should be made to secure vertically sectioned tissue samples. The lateral extent of MICA is measured as described for the depth of stromal invasion. Measurements are made between the two farthest lateral points where invasion is identified.

At the site of initial stromal invasion, disruption of the basement membrane has been historically identified using electron microscopy. Therefore, a number of studies have attempted to use immunohistochemistry and antibodies directed against basement membrane constituents such as laminin or type IV collagen as a way of enhancing the recognition of early stromal invasion in cervical lesions. However, small basement membrane disruptions (as defined by laminin and type IV collagen staining) frequently occur both in the normal cervical epithelium and in squamous intraepithelial lesions that lack microinvasion, especially in areas with severe stromal inflammatory infiltrates [159, 187]. In addition, foci of basement membrane staining frequently occur in areas of invasion, and the amount of staining tends to increase as the degree of differentiation of the invading tumor advances [66]. Furthermore, metastatic foci of squamous cell carcinoma in the lymph nodes were found to be surrounded by basement membrane [96]. Therefore, immunohistochemistry appears to be of limited value in assessing questionable early stromal invasion.

Differential Diagnosis

The detection of microscopic foci of invasion in SIL can be difficult by light microscopy. The problem is often compounded by the presence of dense, obscuring inflammatory infiltrates, the small size of the biopsy specimens, and artifacts associated with shallow cervical excisions. Therefore, MICA is frequently misdiagnosed. Of 265 purported cases of MICA submitted to a group of reference pathologists of the Gynecologic Oncology Group (GOG), 132 cases (approximately 50%) were rejected [232]. Another study from the United Kingdom that reviewed 286 cases initially diagnosed as MICA found that 41% were incorrectly diagnosed [180]. Special attention should be paid to the interpretation of recently biopsied conization specimens as these may harbor nests of neoplastic epithelium buried within the cervical stroma at the site of a previous punch biopsy. Both SIL and immature squamous metaplasia with extensive gland involvement should also be distinguished from MICA. A prominent stromal desmoplastic response, abundant eosinophilic cytoplasm, and an irregular margin or scalloping of the epithelial nest are associated with invasive foci.

Risk Factors

Factors that have been reported to increase an individual's risk for nodal metastases, recurrence, and death are (1) depth of stromal invasion, (2) presence of lymphvascular invasion, (3) tumor volume, and (4) involvement of the resection margin. However, the lack of a uniform definition of MICA and methodology for measuring the depth of invasion together with different follow-up time and treatment methods make interpretation of the published data difficult. For example, the maximal depth of stromal invasion in studies of MICA varies from 1 to 5 mm. Some studies characterize microinvasion by the absence of confluency of invasive foci or the absence of lymphvascular invasion, whereas in others these features do not exclude the diagnosis of MICA. As a result, the frequency of pelvic node metastasis associated with MICA in the published literature varies from 0% to 9% [56, 232].

Depth and Pattern of Invasion

Depth of stromal invasion is a major factor in determining the outcome of patients with MICA. Early studies reported that no residual carcinoma was detected in the subsequent hysterectomy specimen when MICA invaded 1 mm or less in the cone biopsy. In contrast, residual carcinoma was detected in a significant proportion of cases when MICA in the cone biopsy invaded 3 mm or more. Histologic analysis of lymph nodes removed at the time of radical surgery has shown a clear relationship between the depth of stromal invasion and the presence of lymph node metastases (➲ *Table 6.3*). Lymph node metastases are very uncommon in patients with stromal invasion of 3 mm or less. In contrast, the prevalence of lymph node metastases is 7.6% in women with 3.1–5 mm of invasion [17, 51, 56, 61, 98, 152, 163, 232, 234, 242, 263, 267].

The development of recurrent disease or death from cervical cancer in women with <1 mm of stromal invasion who have been managed with either a cone biopsy or a simple hysterectomy is infrequent [53, 56, 142, 190]. In three long-term follow-up studies involving 403 women, not a single patient with <1 mm of stromal invasion treated with a cone biopsy or simple hysterectomy died of their tumor (➲ *Table 6.4*) [34, 53, 142].

Table 6.3

Pelvic node metastasis with early invasive carcinoma according to depth of stromal penetration

Depth of invasion (mm)[a]	No. of patients	Percent (%) of patients with lymph node metastasis
<1	367	0.2
1.0–3.0	941	1.9
3.1–5.0	243	7.6

[a]Depth of stromal invasion regardless of presence or absence of vascular invasion and confluency.
Modified from [17].

Table 6.4

Outcome of women with microinvasive squamous cell carcinoma with 1 mm or less invasion managed by cone biopsy or simple hysterectomy

Author	No. of patients	No. of deaths from tumor
Burghardt et al.	259	0
Coppleson et al.	54	0
Koldstad	90	0
Total	403	0

Modified from [34, 53, 142].

Similarly, recurrent disease occurs in approximately 0.4% of patients when tumors invade <3 mm (➋ *Table 6.5*) [56, 66, 96, 180, 233, 285]. Recurrence occurs in approximately 5% of patients when there is 3.1–5 mm of invasion (➋ *Table 6.5*).

Confluency of neoplastic epithelium in MICA has not been associated with pelvic node metastases, vaginal recurrence, or cancer death in most series [142, 263]. A reproducible definition of what constitutes a confluent pattern of invasion has been difficult to achieve, particularly for smaller lesions [22]. Therefore, clinical outcome is strongly influenced by the depth but not the pattern of invasion.

Lymphvascular Space Invasion (LVSI)

Roche and Norris defined lymphatic space invasion as endothelial-lined (capillary-like) spaces containing tumor cells that are contiguous with the stroma [219]. In view of the difficulties in distinguishing small blood

Table 6.5

Percent (%) of patients with recurrent invasive cancer after therapy for early invasive squamous cell carcinoma of the cervix with differing depths of invasion

Author	No of Patients	<3.0 mm of invasion[a]	3.1–5.0 mm of invasion[a]
Sedlis et al.	132	0.9	4.8
Sevin et al.	110	0	11.1
Copeland et al.	673	1.4	2.5
Maiman et al.	95	0	0
Simon et al.	69	0	0
van Nagell et al.	177	0	9.4
Total	1,256	0.4	4.6

[a]Irrespective of presence or absence of lymphvascular space involvement or horizontal extent of tumor.
Modified from [51, 163, 232, 234, 242, 267].

Table 6.6

Relationship between depth of invasion and presence of lymphvascular space involvement

Depth of invasion (mm)	No. of patients	Percentage of specimens showing lymphvascular space involvement	
		Mean (%)	Range (%)
<1.0	548	4.4	0–10
1.0–3.0	596	16.4	3–30
3.1–5.0	350	19.7	2–36

Adopted from [27, 66, 98, 180, 217, 242, 267, 271].

vessels and capillaries from small lymphatic channels, the term lymphvascular space(s) invasion (LVSI) is used in this chapter. Identification of early LVSI, particularly in the cervical stroma adjacent to the overlying epithelium, may be difficult and is often hampered by technical processing artifacts. A recently developed monoclonal antibody D2-40, specific for lymphatic endothelium, is helpful in distinguishing between true LVSI and processing artifacts [88]. The relationship between LVSI and clinical outcome in women with early invasive squamous cell carcinoma is less clear-cut than the relationship between the depth of invasion and lymph node metastases. LVSI is reported to occur in 0–10% of MICA that invade <1 mm and in 3–30% of MICA invading 1–3 mm (➋ *Table 6.6*) [27, 66, 98, 180, 217, 242, 267, 271].

The large variation between the different reports results from several factors, including the number of pathologic sections evaluated and interobserver variability in determining LVSI. Shrinkage of stroma surrounding invasive nests can result in the formation of artifactual spaces that can be erroneously interpreted as LVSI. One study of early invasive squamous cell carcinoma reported that the frequency of LVSI detection increased from 30% to 57% when step sections were cut through the site of invasion [219]. Despite the problems with recognizing LVSI, most studies have found a relationship between the increasing depth of invasion and the increased frequency of LVSI (➒ *Table 6.6*). Most studies indicate that the presence of LVSI is an adverse prognostic factor [34, 51, 56, 163, 232, 267]. Three of 96 patients (3.1%) with <3 mm invasion and LVSI developed recurrence compared to 3 of 486 patients (0.6%) who did not have LVSI. In patients with 3–5 mm invasion and LVSI, 8 of 51 (15.7%) had recurrent disease. This was in contrast to only 2 of 115 patients (1.7%) who developed recurrence with similar depth of invasion but absence of LVSI. LVSI also appears to be a predictor of the presence of invasive carcinoma in subsequent hysterectomy specimens and lymph node metastasis [22, 61]. Therefore, although FIGO does not take LVSI into account in staging, the prevailing opinion in the United States is that LVSI should be assessed in women with early invasive squamous cell carcinoma; its presence excludes a diagnosis of MICA.

Tumor Volume and Horizontal Extent

Burghardt and Holzer have introduced the concept of tumor volume as applied to MICA and have reported no pelvic node metastases in patients with 420 mm^3 of cancer or less, with the exception of one case in which vascular invasion was noted [35]. In recent years, the concept of MICA tumor volume has been emphasized by some authors. However, MICA tumor volume estimation by serially sectioning cone specimens is both cumbersome and time-consuming, and is unlikely to become a routine laboratory method. Other investigators and FIGO have used lateral extent of spread as a surrogate for measuring tumor volume. The lateral extent of spread of early invasive squamous cell carcinoma has been correlated with the frequency of residual neoplasia in postcone hysterectomy specimens (➒ *Table 6.7*) [232]. In a study of 402 patients with stromal invasion of 5 mm or less, Takeshima et al. found that 18% had >7 mm of horizontal spread [253]. As the depth of invasion increased, there was an increase in horizontal spread. Only 6.3% of lesions with 3 mm of invasion or less had >7 mm horizontal spread, whereas 61% of those with 3–5 mm of invasion had more than 7 mm lateral spread [253].

Table 6.7

Residual invasive tumor in postconization hysterectomy specimens according to lateral extent of carcinoma with as much as 5 mm stromal invasion

Lateral extent of invasion (mm)	No. of patients	Percent (%) with residual disease in postconization hysterectomy specimen
4	55	2
4–8	26	27
8	23	35

Adapted from [232], #Thomas C. Wright, Alex Ferenczy, and Robert J. Kurman

Surgical Margins

Perhaps one of the most important contributions of the pathologist to the appropriate management of early invasive squamous cell carcinoma is evaluating surgical margins of conization specimens [56, 94, 119, 152, 232]. In fact, the status of cone margins may well be the most important single parameter in deciding the therapeutic approach to patients with early invasive squamous cell carcinoma. In most studies, women with cone margins positive for either SIL or invasive disease are much more likely to have residual invasive disease in the hysterectomy specimens than are women with a negative margin. Furthermore, the residual invasion may actually be deeper than that found in the cone biopsy specimen (➒ *Table 6.8*).

Treatment

The therapy for IA1 MICA is more conservative than that for stage IA2, and treatment is often individualized based on (1) the definition of the lesion (FIGO vs. SGO), (2) lateral extent, and (3) involvement of cone margins. The data on risk factors for nodal metastases, recurrence, and death suggest that lesions with 3 mm or less stromal invasion without LVSI have virtually no potential for metastasis or recurrence. Those invading 3 mm or less but with LVSI may potentially metastasize,

Table 6.8

Relationship between status of cone biopsy margin in patients with early invasive squamous cell carcinoma of the cervix and residual disease in the postcone hysterectomy specimen

Author	Negative margins: No. of patients (% with residual cancer)	Positive margins[a]: No. of patients (% with residual cancer)
Creasman et al.	45 (4.4)	13 (77)
Greer et al.	17 (24)	33 (82)
Jones et al.	25 (4)	46 (35)
Leman et al.	24 (0)	23 (39)
Sedlis et al.	85 (4)	15 (80)
Total	196 (5.1)	130 (57)

[a]Positive margin includes either microinvasive carcinoma or high-grade SIL at the margin.
Adapted from [56, 94, 119, 152, 232].

although the risk is small, about 3.5%. Therefore, most authorities believe that women with <3 mm of stromal invasion who lack LVSI can be managed with procedures less radical than those required for higher-stage invasive squamous cell carcinomas [24, 151, 181]. Patients who are managed with less radical procedures should have had a diagnostic conization that removed the entire lesion with negative resection margins and a negative endocervical curettage obtained at the time of conization.

At most centers the recommended therapy for MICA, by the SGO definition, is a simple hysterectomy. Most authorities now agree that women with MICA who desire to remain fertile can be managed safely with conization, provided they clearly understand that there is a low risk of developing pelvic lymph node metastases or recurrent disease. Such patients have to return for regular follow-up examinations including cytology, colposcopy, and HPV testing [25, 151, 181]. In one series with medium follow up of 45 months, 10% of patients developed cervical intraepithelial neoplasis 3 [81]. At present, radical hysterectomy with pelvic lymphadenectomy is considered the most appropriate therapeutic approach for most stage IA2 early squamous cell carcinomas of the cervix and stage IA1 tumors with LVSI. In women desiring to preserve fertility, radical trachelectomy (amputation of cervix) and laparoscopic bilateral pelvic lymphadenectomy can be performed [63].

Invasive Squamous Cell Carcinoma

General Features

Worldwide, cervical cancer is second only to breast cancer in incidence and is the third leading cause of cancer mortality (after lung and breast cancers) [77]. Over the past 3 decades the incidence of cervical carcinoma in the United States has declined by almost one third, mostly due to a decrease in squamous cell carcinoma (SCC) [270]. In 2008, there were 11,270 new cases and 4,070 deaths due to cervical cancer [116]. Despite the decrease in incidence, cervical cancer is the second leading cause of mortality in women aged 21–39 in the United States [116]. Regardless of the advances in detection and management in developed countries, cervical cancer continues to be a significant health problem worldwide. Cervical cancer is the most frequent type of cancer in women in some developing countries, whereas it is the seventh most frequent type in much of the developed world [211]. The regions of the world where the incidence is greatest include eastern and southern Africa, Central and South America, and south-central Asia. The highest incidence rate is in eastern Africa, where there is an age-standardized rate of 42.7. The lowest reported incidence rates are from China and western Asia, with age-standardized incidence rates of 6.8 and 5.8, respectively [203]; however, cervical cancer incidence has been increasing in China among women under age 50 [286].

The majority of women with invasive SCC are diagnosed in their mid-40s or 50; however, cervical carcinoma can occur at almost any age between 17 and 90 years [209]. Patients with invasive SCC are 15–23 years older than patients with high-grade SIL and 8 years older than patients with microinvasive carcinoma. In recent years there has been increased recognition that cervical cancer can occur in women under 35 years. Women under 35 years account for 22.1% of all patients with invasive cervical cancer in the United States [192].

There is little doubt that cytologic screening plays a major role in reducing both the incidence and mortality of invasive cervical cancer. According to the American Cancer Society, in 1961 only 30% of all US women had ever had a Pap smear, but this number increased to 87% by 1987 [214]. In 1940, the incidence of invasive cervical cancer in the United States was 32.6 per 100,000 women, which is similar to that currently seen in the developing world, whereas by 2008 the incidence was 8.3 per 100,000 women [192]. The reduction in incidence was paralleled by a reduction in mortality. Despite the low incidence of invasive cervical cancer in the United States, cervical cancer continues to be a problem among selected groups of women. The incidence among African-American women is almost 50% higher than the incidence of white women in the United States, and the incidence among Hispanic women is twice that of Caucasian women. The incidence of cervical cancer deaths is highest for black women (5.3 per 100,000), followed by Hispanic women (3.5 per 100,000), and Caucasian women (2.5 per 100,000) [115]. A significant proportion of the remaining cases of invasive cervical carcinoma in the United States could be prevented if all women at risk underwent routine cytologic screening and colposcopic evaluation of significant cytologic abnormalities. In the United States, 56% of the women who developed invasive cervical cancer had not had a Pap smear in the preceding 3 years [286].

Pathogenesis and Etiology

Molecular, clinical, and epidemiological studies have implicated HPV infection in the pathogenesis of cervical carcinoma. More than 90% of cervical carcinoma contains DNA sequences of specific HPV types, especially HPV 16 and HPV 18 [48]. The distribution of HPV types in invasive cervical cancers shows only minor geographic variations. Globally, HPV 16 is most frequently detected in invasive cervical cancer, followed by HPV 18. HPV types 31, 33, 35, 45, 52, and 58 are the next most common types found in cancers globally with minor variations seen in their relative importance by region [185]. The failure to detect HPV DNA in a small subset of invasive squamous cell carcinomas appears to be caused by a number of factors including failure to adequately sample the lesion, presence of a HPV type other than those assayed for, and loss of, part of the HPV genome from the malignant cells. A study that investigated supposedly HPV DNA-negative tumors using multiple molecular techniques detected HPV DNA in most of the cases and concluded that the worldwide prevalence of HPV in cervical carcinomas is 99.7% [272]. In patients with metastatic cervical carcinoma, HPV DNA can also be identified in distant metastases, with viral DNA hybridization patterns frequently matching those of the primary cervical tumor [298]. Based on the strength of the molecular and epidemiologic evidence linking HPV to invasive squamous cell carcinoma of the cervix, 13 high-risk types of HPV (16, 18, 31, 33, 35, 39, 45, 51, 52, 56, 58, 59, and 66) have been classified as carcinogenic to humans by the WHO.

There is a considerable body of evidence indicating that invasive squamous cell carcinoma develops from SIL and women with invasive squamous cell carcinoma have similar epidemiologic characteristics to those with preinvasive precursor lesions (see Chap. 5, Precancerous Lesions of the Cervix). Like women with SIL, the majority of women with invasive cancer of the cervix are from lower socioeconomic groups, began heterosexual activity early in life, married early, are multiparous, and have many sexual partners or have partners who have been sexually promiscuous even if they have not been [113, 201, 228].

There is also considerable epidemiologic evidence indicating that factors other than HPV are important in the development of invasive squamous cell carcinoma of the cervix. Two studies found that even after controlling for HPV, there continued to be a significant associations between cervical cancer and number of sexual partners, smoking, and histories of venereal disease [15, 42]. In women infected with high-risk carcinogenic HPV, long-term use of oral contraceptive can significantly increase the risk of developing high-grade SIL and carcinoma [243]. Genetic and immunologic host factors and viral factors such as viral load and viral integration are probably important but their precise roles have not yet been clarified [186].

It has been estimated that approximately 1–5% of untreated low-grade SIL eventually progress to invasive cancer [280]. In the Ontario Cancer Registry study of more than 17,000 women with a history of abnormal Pap smears, the actual rate of untreated low-grade SIL progressing to carcinoma in situ or invasive cervical cancer was 2.8% for women followed more than 10 years [105]. The percentage of carcinoma in situ that progressed to invasive squamous cell carcinoma has been between 6% and 74% in various follow-up series (see Chap. 5, Precancerous Lesions of the Cervix).

The presenting symptoms of patients with invasive carcinoma of the cervix of all histologic types appear to be dependent on the size and stage of the lesion [214]. Early series from the 1950s through the 1970s were composed predominantly of patients with bulky, late-stage disease. Nearly all these patients had clinically visible cancers and nearly all complained of abnormal vaginal bleeding. The most significant and common feature was bleeding following intercourse or douching. Intermittent spotting, serosanguinous discharge, and frank hemorrhage were also frequently encountered. Around 10–20% of the patients complained of bloody malodorous discharge and pain, often radiating to the sacral region. Weakness, pallor, weight loss, edema of the lower extremities, rectal pain, and hematuria are symptoms and signs of either locally advanced or metastatic disease.

More recent studies include a much higher percentage of patients with stage I disease. Patients with stage I disease are frequently asymptomatic, particularly those with endophytic cancers. In these cases, cytology is often negative, i.e., contains no abnormal cells. About two thirds of exophytic lesions are detected on the basis of an abnormal Pap smear [100, 214]. Primary presentation correlates well with disease severity and survival. Patients who present with an abnormal Pap smear have a disease free survival of 96% as compared to 51% for those with vaginal bleeding and 21% for those presenting with pain [214]. Accurate detection and diagnosis of frank invasive carcinoma is based on cytology, colposcopy, and colposcopically directed punch biopsy [24]. Cervical cancers are clinically staged based on biopsy, physical examination, and chest x-ray results. If the stage is >IB1, CT or MRI of the abdomen and pelvis is typically done to identify metastases, estimate tumor volume, and determine parametrial involvement. If MRI and CT are not available, cystoscopy, sigmoidoscopy, and IV urography, when clinically indicated, may be used, but are not required, for staging [24, 205].

Invasive carcinoma of either the squamous or glandular type can develop in the cervical stump that remains following subtotal hysterectomy in 0.1–3% of patients [235, 283]. In a study of 173 women with carcinoma of the cervical stump, Wolff et al. divided patients into those that developed carcinoma less than and more than 2 years from the operation [283]. The 5-year survival of patients in the first group was worse (30%) than those in the second group (49%) or those with cancer of the cervix in general. Based on these observations, it has been suggested that cervical stump cancers occurring within the first 2 years following surgery represent residual malignancy, whereas those discovered after 2 years are "new" cancers arising from the cervical stump.

Cervical cancer is the most common gynecologic cancer in pregnancy, but the incidence is low (1.5–12 per 100,000 pregnancies) [109, 120]. Routine cervical cytology is a part of the initial prenatal examination. The mean age of pregnant women with invasive cervical cancer is 32 years, which is considerably lower than that of women in the general population with invasive cervical cancer. Women who are pregnant usually present with early-stage tumors; in one series 83% were stage I [120]. The treatment of pregnant patients with invasive cervical cancer depends on the clinical stage and gestational age. In general, prognosis is not altered by pregnancy.

Gross Findings

The gross appearance of invasive squamous cell carcinoma varies widely. Early lesions may be focally indurated, ulcerated, or present as a slightly elevated, granular area that bleeds readily. Colposcopic examination usually reveals atypical, tortuous vessels varying widely in size and configuration. Approximately 98% of early carcinomas are localized within the transformation zone, with variable degrees of encroachment onto the neighboring native portio. Most advanced tumors are endophytic or exophytic. Endophytic carcinomas are ulcerated or nodular; they tend to develop within the endocervical canal and frequently invade deeply into the cervical stroma to produce an enlarged, hard, barrel-shaped cervix. In some patients with endophytic carcinomas, the cervix appears grossly normal. The exophytic varieties of cervical carcinoma have a polypoid or papillary appearance.

Microscopic Findings

Microscopically, invasive squamous cell carcinoma is characterized by anastomosing tongues or cords of neoplastic epithelium infiltrating the stroma (➲ *Fig. 6.6*). Characteristically, the contour of the infiltrating nests and clusters is irregular and ragged. In other cases, the tumor invades either as individual cells or almost completely replaces the stroma with large masses of neoplastic squamous cells. Cells in the center of the invading nests frequently become necrotic or undergo extensive keratinization. Individual

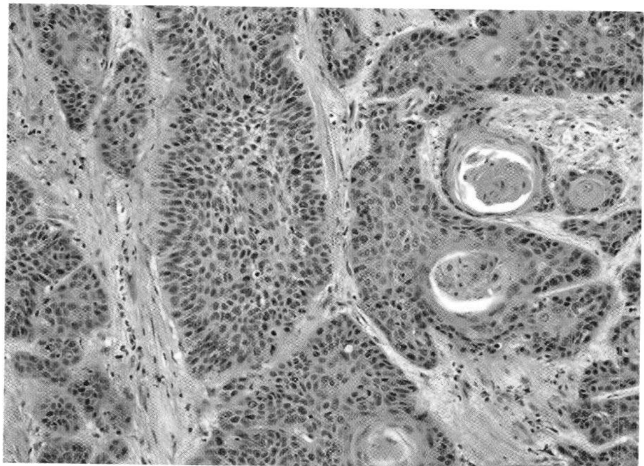

■ Fig. 6.6
Invasive squamous carcinoma. **Well to moderately differentiated carcinoma is composed of islands and nests of neoplastic squamous epithelium with keratinization invading stroma**

cells are generally polygonal or oval with eosinophilic cytoplasm and prominent cellular membranes. Intracellular bridges may or may not be visible. In some cases, the nuclei are relatively uniform, whereas in others they are quite pleomorphic. In most cases, the chromatin is coarse and clumped, and mitotic figures, including abnormal forms, commonly are encountered.

Histological Typing

One of the earliest approaches to classifying cervical squamous cell carcinomas was based on the predominant cell type. The classification separated squamous cell carcinomas into large cell keratinizing, large cell nonkeratinizing, and small cell nonkeratinizing. In the experience of Wentz and Reagan, the best 5-year survival rate after radiation therapy was associated with large cell nonkeratinizing carcinomas (68.3%), followed by the large cell keratinizing type (41.7%), and small cell carcinomas (20%) [279]. Because there has been frequent confusion between the small cell nonkeratinizing squamous cell carcinomas described by Wentz and Reagan and small cell carcinomas with neuroendocrine features similar to those described in the lung, the current WHO classification of invasive cervical cancers places small cell undifferentiated carcinoma with neuroendocrine features in a separate category and divides invasive squamous cell carcinomas into two groups, keratinizing and nonkeratinizing [278].

Keratinizing carcinomas are characterized by the presence of well-differentiated squamous cells that are arranged in nests or cords that vary greatly in size and configuration. The defining feature of keratinizing carcinomas is the presence of keratin pearls within the epithelium, and the presence of a single keratin pearl is sufficient to classify a tumor as a keratinizing carcinoma. Keratin pearls are composed of clusters of squamous cells that have undergone keratinization and are arranged in a concentric nest. The neoplastic squamous cells not forming keratin pearls frequently have abundant eosinophilic cytoplasm and prominent intracellular bridges. The nuclei are often enlarged, but mitotic figures are not numerous.

Nonkeratinizing squamous cell carcinoma is characterized by nests of neoplastic squamous cells that frequently undergo individual cell keratinization but, by definition, do not form keratin pearls. The cells have relatively indistinct cell borders. The nuclei tend to be round to oval with coarsely clumped chromatin. Mitotic figures are numerous. In some cases SCC is composed of solid sheets of cells with clear cytoplasm (➲ *Fig. 6.7*). Other nonkeratinizing squamous cell carcinomas are composed of masses and nests of small basaloid cells with scant cytoplasm and hyperchromatic uniform nuclei with numerous mitotic figures (➲ *Fig. 6.8*). These tumors are similar to the basaloid carcinomas of the vulva and vagina.

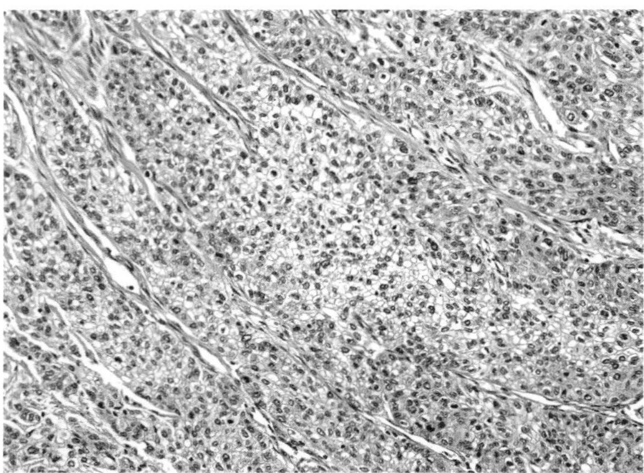

Fig. 6.7
Squamous cell carcinoma. **Solid sheets of carcinoma contain cells with clear cytoplasm; this variant lacks the characteristic cytologic and architectural features of clear cell carcinoma and should not be misclassified as such**

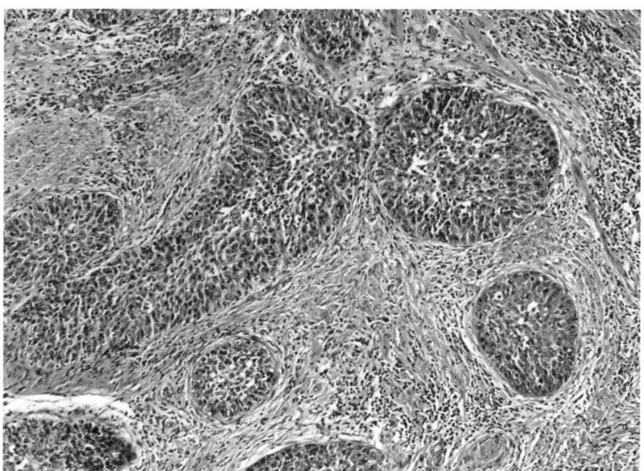

Fig. 6.8
Squamous cell carcinoma. **Basaloid variant resembles high-grade squamous intraepithelial lesion within endocervical glands but nests within desmoplastic cervical stroma are indicative of invasive tumor**

Some investigators have reported that this classification has prognostic significance in patients treated with radiotherapy [279]. Others authors have reported no significant difference in prognosis between patients with large cell nonkeratinizing and large cell keratinizing squamous carcinomas when treated with radical surgery [297].

Microscopic Grading

The most commonly used grading system for squamous cell carcinoma is a modification of the original system proposed by Broders in 1920 [32]. This method was based on the proportion of the tumor undergoing keratinization with the formation of squamous pearls and a number of mitoses. Currently histologic grading divides squamous cell carcinomas into three groups, well differentiated (grade 1), moderately differentiated (grade 2), and poorly differentiated (grade 3). Most squamous cell carcinomas are moderately differentiated (grade 2), followed by poorly differentiated (grade 3) and well differentiated (grade 1).

In well-differentiated (grade 1) tumors, the most striking feature is abundant keratin, which is deposited as keratin pearls in the center of neoplastic epithelial nests. The cells appear mature, with abundant eosinophilic cytoplasm. Individual cell keratinization (dyskeratosis) characterized by intense cytoplasmic eosinophilia may also be present. The cells are tightly packed and have well-developed intercellular bridges. The nuclei are large, irregular, and hyperchromatic. Mitotic figures are present most notably at the periphery of the advancing epithelial nests. The stroma is often infiltrated by chronic inflammatory cells, and occasionally a foreign body giant cell reaction is observed.

In moderately differentiated (grade 2) squamous cell carcinomas, the neoplastic cells are more pleomorphic than in grade 1 tumors, have large irregular nuclei, and have less abundant cytoplasm. The cellular borders and intercellular bridge appear indistinct. Keratin pearl formation is rare, but individual cell keratinization is seen in the center of nests of tumor cells. Mitotic figures are more numerous than in grade 1 carcinomas (see *Fig. 6.6*).

Poorly differentiated (grade 3) squamous cell carcinomas are generally composed of cells with hyperchromatic oval nuclei and scant indistinct cytoplasm, resembling the malignant cells of high-grade SIL (*Fig. 6.9*). Clear-cut squamous differentiation manifested by keratinization may be difficult to find. Mitoses and areas of necrosis are abundant. Poorly differentiated lesions are occasionally composed of large, pleomorphic cells with giant, bizarre nuclei and abnormal mitotic figures. In rare instances, the neoplastic cells assume a spindle-shaped configuration resembling a sarcoma (*Fig. 6.10*). Immunohistochemical staining for epithelial membrane antigen and cytokeratins demonstrates the epithelial nature of the spindle cells in these cases. Although in some studies tumor grade was associated with patients survival [18], most studies have failed to confirm that histopathologic grade influences clinical outcome [103, 252]. A study from the Gynecologic Oncology Group (GOG) evaluated a number of different tumor-grading systems including

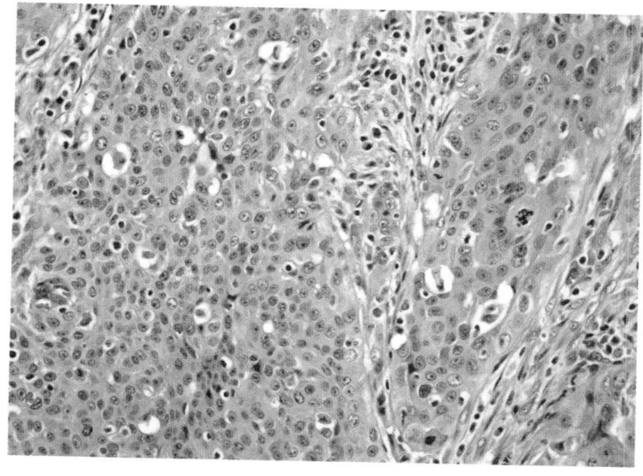

Fig. 6.9
Squamous cell carcinoma. **Poorly differentiated carcinoma is composed of sheets of atypical cells**

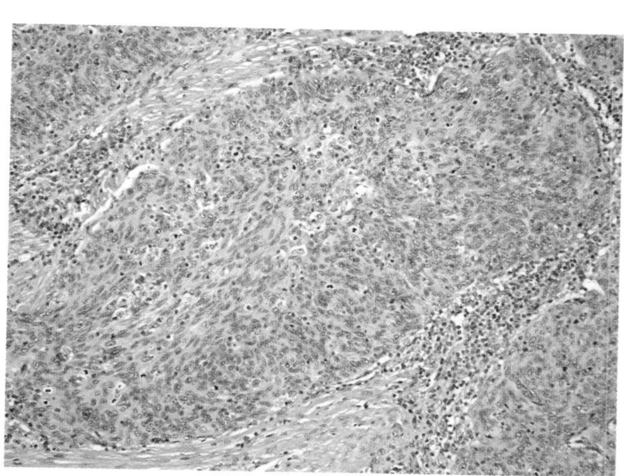

Fig. 6.10
Squamous cell carcinoma. **Poorly differentiated carcinoma has some cells with spindled morphology**

those proposed by Warren, Reagan, and Broder in surgically treated stage IB cervical cancers. Although there was good reproducibility between observers (76–92%), none of the grading systems had prognostic significance. Nuclear grade, degree of keratinization, mitotic activity, pattern of infiltration, and degree of lymphoid response all lacked prognostic significance [297]. Because histopathologic grade has failed to predict clinical outcome in many studies, systems taking into account growth pattern at the invasive tumor front have been developed. Three patterns of invasion have been described: pushing, finger-like, and spray-like [106]. The pushing pattern of invasion is characterized by a well-delinated tumor border. The finger-like pattern of invasion shows a trabecular tumor growth in solid cords. The spray-like pattern is defined by the presence of small groups and/or single cells at the invasive tumor front. In several studies spray-like growth pattern has been associated with a reduced 5-year survival in cervical cancer patients with primary surgical treatment [106, 239], but this finding was not confirmed by other authors [225, 297].

Prognostic Biomarkers

Several studies have investigated the immunohistochemical detection of prognostic biomarkers in squamous cell carcinomas of the cervix. In a study of 129 women with squamous cell carcinoma, a high number of CD4 positive tumor infiltrating lymphocytes were associated with good prognosis, while a high Ki-67 index among the tumor cells predicted poor prognosis in patients with late-stage cervical cancer. In the same study, expression of the transmembrane protein, leucine-rich repeats, and immunoglobulin-like domains 1 (LRIG1) were associated with a favorable prognosis in early-stage cervical cancer [99]. LRIG1 has been shown to restrict growth factor signaling by enhancing ubiquitylation and degradation of epidermal growth factor receptor (EGFR) and inhibiting the function of cellular oncogenes Met and Ret [95, 149, 236]. High cyclooxygenase 2 (COX-2) expression in cervical cancer cells has been associated with poor survival in several studies [70, 158]. COX-2 is the key enzyme in the conversion of arachidonic acid to prostaglandins and its overexpression increases metastatic potential and angiogenesis, while decreasing host immune response and apoptosis. In addition, a recent study has demonstrated that COX-2 transcription is regulated by HPV 16 oncoproteins E6 and E7 through EGFR signaling [248]. Synchronous co-expression of EGFR and COX-2 has been reported in 32% of cervical cancers and also correlates with poor outcome [137]. Ferrandina et al. have reported that in celecoxib-treated patients, tumor biopsies showed decreased expression of COX-2, Ki-67 (a cellular proliferation marker), and CD31 (an angiogenesis marker), as well as a decrease in microvessel density [71]. These data were used as the background for two clinical trials of celecoxib in advanced cervical cancer. Despite biologic promise, two phase II trials testing specific COX-2 inhibitors as radio-sensitizers in locally advanced cervical cancer demonstrated increased toxicity with no change in therapeutic effect [83, 101].

The presence of EGFR and human EGFR 2 (HER2) has been associated with accelerated tumor progression and therapeutic resistance in several malignancies including cervical cancer. Previous studies have shown that EGFR is expressed in up to 76% of cervical cancers and correlates with poor prognosis [134]. EGFR inhibitors are currently undergoing testing in clinical trials. In a recent phase II trial, EGFR expression levels, evaluated by immunohistochemistry, did not correlate with tumor response and disease control in patients treated with gefitinib (EGFR inhibitor) [89]. Using the standardized HercepTest scoring criteria, HER2 expression is considered a rare event in cervical cancer [138].

High peritumoral lymphatic vessel density evaluated by counting D2-40-positive (a selective marker for lymphatic endothelium) vessels has shown significant correlation with higher tumor stage, lymph node metastases, and poor survival in 111 cervical squamous cell carcinomas FIGO stage 1A–IIA [88]. Another recent study using an antibody against lymphatic vessel endothelial hyaluronan receptor-1 has also shown that increased lymphatic vessel density was associated with lymph node metastasis and lymphatic vessel invasion in early-stage cervical carcinoma [300].

The dependence of tumor growth and metastasis on blood vessels makes angiogenesis one of the fundamental hallmarks of cancer and a target for therapy. One of the major pathways involved in angiogenesis is the vascular endothelial growth factor (VEGF) family of proteins and receptors. Overexpression of VEGF has been associated with tumor progression and poor prognosis in several tumors, including cervical cancer. Intratumoral protein levels of VEGF are increased in cervical cancer compared to normal cervical tissue and higher VEGF levels correlate with higher stage and increased risk of lymph nodes metastasis [41]. It has also been demonstrated that higher VEGF expression and increased tumor vascularization are independent predictors of shorter disease-free interval and overall poor survival [160]. There is also data suggesting that HPV may directly stimulate VEGF production through upregulation of the E6 oncoprotein [260]. In phase II clinical trials, bevacizumab (a recombinant humanized anti-VEGF monoclonal antibody) was well tolerated and active as second- and third-line treatment of patients with recurrent cervical cancer [178].

P53 and RAS mutations are rare in cervical squamous cell carcinoma and in recent studies have not been associated with tumor stage, tumor grade, or survival [199, 256]. Amplification and overexpression of cellular oncogene c-myc have been demonstrated in approximately 20% of cervical squamous cell carcinomas and shown to be associated with the presence of HPV16. Overexpression of c-myc has also been associated with worse prognosis in some studies [14, 99].

Differential Diagnosis

Histologically, the lesions most commonly confused with invasive squamous cell carcinomas are squamous metaplasia, high-grade SIL with extensive endocervical gland involvement, gestational decidual reaction with degenerative features, trophoblastic lesions such as placental site nodules and epithelioid trophobastic tumors, condylomata acuminata, and reparative changes associated with chronic granulomatous diseases such as lymphogranuloma venereum and granuloma inguinale. Both squamous metaplasia and high-grade SIL are frequently extensive and extend into endocervical glands. Even though a low level of mitotic activity can be present in squamous metaplasia, careful evaluation of the cytologic appearance of the metaplastic cells reveals their benign nature because the cells are relatively uniform in size and shape and lack significant nuclear atypia. Moreover, the borders of endocervical glands involved with either squamous metaplasia or high-grade SIL are rounded and distinct and lack the irregular margins, scalloping, and desmoplasia in the stroma adjacent to the glands. A decidual reaction with degenerative features lacks mitotic activity and in difficult cases can be differentiated from invasive squamous cell carcinomas by the use of immunohistochemical staining because decidual cells do not contain cytokeratin. Placental site nodules appear as well-circumscribed nodules or plaques containing intermediate trophoblastic cells. These cells lack mitotic activity and are arranged in nests surrounded by hyaline material. Epithelioid trophoblastic tumors in contrast to squamous lesions have a more nested appearance and typically display a characteristic pattern of geographic necrosis. In difficult cases immunohistochemistry can be used to discriminate cervical neoplastic lesions from trophoblastic lesions as the latter express inhibin and CK 18 but are negative for p16, while the converse expression patterns occur in cervical neoplasia.

It can also be difficult to distinguish between poorly differentiated squamous cell carcinomas composed of small, basaloid cells and small (oat) cell carcinomas of the neuroendocrine type, lymphoma, and malignant melanoma. Small cell carcinomas of the neuroendocrine type typically invade the stroma diffusely as individual cells or as small discohesive nests and show extensive crush artifact; they frequently form rosettes or trabeculae and the cells characteristically have smudged, intensely hyperchromatic nuclei and lack nucleoli. In contrast, poorly differentiated squamous cell carcinomas invade as cohesive nests, and the cells have oval nuclei with granular chromatin. In difficult cases immmunohistochemical stain for p63 can be used to confirm squamous differentiation. In a study of 250 invasive carcinomas, a strong, diffuse p63 expression was present in 97% of squamous cell carcinomas, including 91% of small cell nonkeratinizing squamous cell carcinomas. All neuroendocrine carcinomas did not show p63 staining or only focal expression (<30% of tumor cells) [274]. Malignant melanoma and lymphoma are p63 and cytokeratin negative.

Squamous cell carcinomas that contain large amounts of cytoplasmic glycogen can sometimes be confused with clear cell carcinomas (➋ *Fig. 6.7*). Like clear cell carcinomas, cells in these tumors have clear cytoplasm and distinct cell membranes. However, squamous cell carcinoma with clear cytoplasm lacks the characteristic hobnail cells and the papillary or tubulocystic areas that are typical of clear cell carcinomas. In squamous cell carcinoma, a careful search of multiple sections will usually detect areas with unambiguous squamous differentiation. Expression of p63 confirms squamous differentiation.

In rare cases, primitive neuroendocrine tumors occur in the cervix [164]. Membranous staining for CD99, nuclear staining for FLI-1, and negative p63 staining help to differentiate these tumors from poorly differentiated squamous cell carcinomas [76]. In addition, primitive neuroendocrine tumors have t(11;12)(q24;q12) chromosomal translocation, which can be demonstrated by reverse transcription polymerase chain reaction and fluorescence in situ hybridization.

Although diffuse p16 expression is a surrogate marker for the presence of high-risk HPV in cervical neoplasia, it is important to remember that positive immohistochemical p16 staining may occur in non-HPV-related neoplasms (➋ *Fig. 6.11*) [139]. Therefore, molecular testing for HPV using sensitive methods such as PCR or HPV in situ hybridization can be used to determine origin of

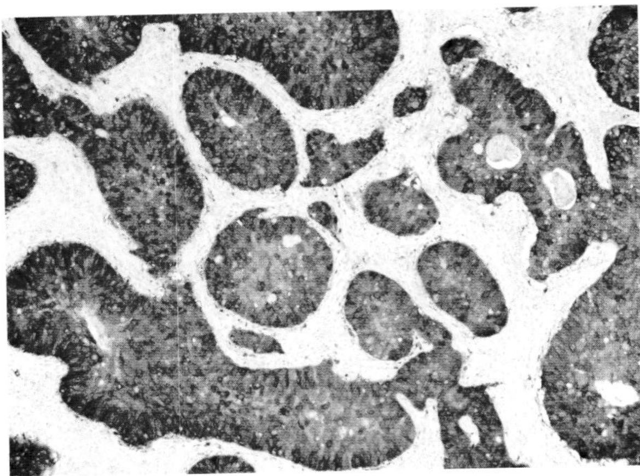

Fig. 6.11
Squamous cell carcinoma. **Tumor exhibits characteristic diffuse/strong p16 expression of a high-risk HPV-related carcinoma**

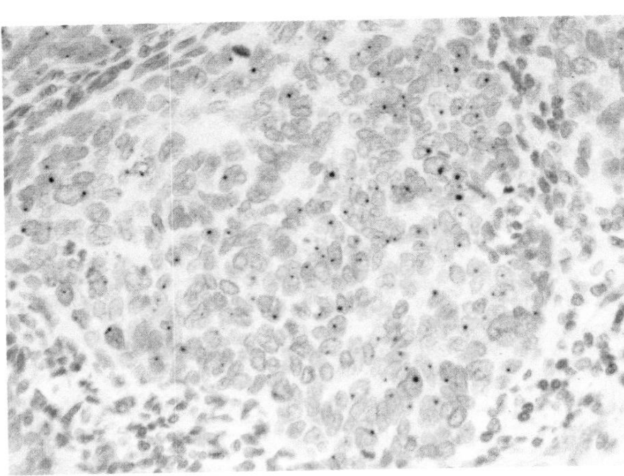

Fig. 6.12
Squamous cell carcinoma. **In situ hybridization demonstrates punctate nuclear signals in tumor nuclei indicating the presence of HPV 16 DNA**

metastatic squamous cell carcinoma when cervical origin is suspected (*Fig. 6.12*). However, when paraffin-embedded material is utilized for testing many of the broad spectrum primer sets used for PCR-based HPV testing have a relatively low sensitivity for HPV and therefore absence of HPV DNA does not definitively rule out a cervical primary.

Histopathologic Prognostic Features

Stage is the most important prognostic factor in cervical carcinoma. Histologic typing and grading have little direct influence on survival within any stage (see "Microscopic grading"). The most significant pathologic prognostic factors in women with surgically treated stage IB and IIA squamous cell carcinoma are tumor size, depth of invasion, parametrial involvement, and nodal status [62, 144, 297]. A study of 188 women undergoing radical hysterectomy with bilateral pelvic lymphadenectomy for stage IB squamous cell carcinoma found that patients with tumors measuring <2 cm in diameter or larger tumors that only invaded <10 mm into the cervical stroma had a 5-year disease-free survival of 95%. In contrast, all other patients had a 5-year disease-free survival of 52% [61]. In the GOG series of patients with stage IB squamous cell carcinoma treated surgically, women whose tumors invaded the inner third of the cervical stroma had a 98% 5-year progression-free survival, whereas for those whose tumors invaded the outer third progression-free survival was only 63% [297]. In the same GOG series, the 5-year progression-free interval was 70% in tumors with lymphvascular invasion (LVSI) compared to 83% in cases without LVSI [297]. In most series of surgically treated stage IB cancers, LVSI has proven to be somewhat less important than tumor size and depth of invasion. Accordingly, in reporting squamous cell carcinomas, the depth of invasion (in millimeters or the proportion of the wall invaded), the presence or absence of LVSI, and the size of the tumor (greatest tumor dimension) should be reported.

Among stage IB patients, presence of LVSI has been associated with four to five times increased risk of pelvic lymph node metastases. In a GOG study of 732 IB patients, Delgado et al. reported 3-year disease-free survival of 74% and 86% for those with and without lymph node metastases [62]. In a series of 978 Stage IB–IIA patients, the median survival was 5.3 years for those with negative nodes and decreased to 3.2 and 1.3 years for those with positive pelvic and paraaortic lymph nodes, respectively [18].

Parametrial extension correlates with LVSI, lymph node metastases, tumor recurrence, and poor survival [61]. In 69 radical hysterectomy specimens performed for stage IB and IIA carcinomas, evaluation of the entire parametria by a giant section technique revealed parametrial involvement in 31% of IB tumors, 63% of IB2, and 58% of IIA tumors. Survival was significantly higher for the patients with negative parametrial findings compared with those with positive parametrial findings (100% vs. 78%) [25].

Another factor that may influence prognosis is patient age. In 1952, Lindell, and subsequently others, demonstrated that survival was improved for older women [157]. However, other large studies, including one that analyzed more than 10,000 women with invasive cervical cancer, reported that younger women had a better prognosis than older women [172]. When stratified by stage it appears that there is little difference in prognosis between younger and older women with early-stage disease, however, with high-stage disease younger women have poorer survival [222].

HPV DNA Status

Several studies have assessed the effect of HPV type on prognosis and most show a significant correlation between HPV 18 and poor prognosis. In a study of 296 Stage IB-IV cancers, detection of HPV 18 DNA was associated with an approximately threefold increase in the risk of death in stage IB disease. This association was independent of established cervical carcinoma prognostic factors, such as FIGO stage and tumor size [231]. A recent study evaluated prognostic significance of HPV type in 1,067 patients with Stage IA–IIA disease. HPV 18 was detected in 16.5% of the samples, a typical prevalence for this genotype in most series. In a multivariant analysis of FIGO stage II tumors, deep stromal invasion, parametrial extension, and HPV 18 positivity were significant predictors for death [147]. Recent studies have suggested that patients infected with multiple HPV types had a significantly shorter cancer-specific survival and do not respond as well to radiation treatment as patients with a single HPV type [19, 184].

Spread and Metastases

Squamous cell carcinoma of the cervix spreads principally by direct local invasion of adjacent tissues and lymphatics and less commonly through blood vessels. Initially, the tumor grows by extending along tissue planes, such as the perineural and perivascular tissues, into the para-cervical and parametrial areas, and into the cardinal and uterosacral ligaments. Ultimately, lateral spread may reach the bony pelvis, encompassing and obstructing one or both ureters. Direct extension may also involve the uterine cavity and vagina, with extension into the urinary bladder and rectum, resulting in vesicovaginal and rectovaginal fistulas.

The spread of cervical cancer via lymphatics occurs relatively early and is present in 25–50% of patients with stage IB and II carcinomas. The most common sites of lymph node metastases are the internal iliac, obturator, external iliac, and common iliac lymph nodes. Later in the course of the disease, extension to the lateral sacral, paraaortic, and inguinal nodes can occur. Isolated invasion of the sacral, external iliac, and hypogastric nodes is occasionally observed. Distant lymph node metastases above the diaphragm including the supraclavicular lymph nodes are uncommon and are a feature of widespread disease. In these cases, cancer cells are transported from the paraaortic nodes into the mediastinum and then into the thoracic duct. Hematogenous dissemination is the least common metastatic pathway of cervical carcinoma. Blood-borne metastases to the lung, liver, bone, heart, skin, and brain are generally seen in stage IV tumors or when the local growth has previously been irradiated.

Ureteral obstruction caused by tumor invasion of the ureteral wall or by compression due to tumor in periureteral lymphatics leads to hydroureter, hydronephrosis, hydronephrotic renal atrophy, pyelonephritis, and loss of renal function. Obstruction of both ureters results in uremia and is a leading cause of death. Although the frequency of ureteral involvement was unchanged between 1930 and 1960, advances in radiation therapy during the 1970s reduced the number of patients dying of ureteral obstruction and uremia from 28% to 6.7% [131]. Peritonitis caused by obstruction and bowel perforation, respiratory failure associated with pulmonary metastasis, massive edema, hemorrhage, cardiac failure, massive venous thrombosis, pulmonary embolism, and complications of radiation therapy represent the major causes of death in order of frequency.

Behavior and Treatment

The three basic therapeutic modalities for squamous cell carcinoma are surgery, radiation, and combinations of radiation and surgery or radiation with concurrent chemotherapy. Recently targeted therapies have shown some promise. In stage IB and early stage II patients, virtually identical results are seen with radical hysterectomy with bilateral pelvic lymphadenectomy and radiation therapy. In young women with Stage IA1/2 and IB1 lesions, particularly those measuring <2 cm in diameter and desire to preserve their fertility, radical trachelectomy combined with laparoscopic pelvic lymphadenectomy has been widely accepted [63]. The 5-year disease-free survival in these women has been 96%. The pregnancy rate ranges between 41% and 79%, and 44% to 64% of pregnancies resulted in live births. A large randomized GOG trial compared radiation therapy followed by adjunctive extrafascial hysterectomy for bulky-stage IB cervical cancers with radiation therapy combined with concurrent cisplatin chemotherapy and adjunctive extrafascial hysterectomy. The concurrent use of cisplatin and radiation significantly improved survival [135]. Other recent trials that have incorporated combinations of combined external and intracavitary radiotherapy with concurrent platinum-based chemotherapy for stage II and stage III cancers have also shown significant improvements in survival with the addition of chemotherapy compared to radiation alone [179]. A recent Cochrane Review of the treatment of early-stage cervical cancer concluded that the addition of platinum-based chemotherapy to radiotherapy may offer clinical benefit in early-stage cervical cancer with risk factors for recurrence [221].

Morphologic changes in cervical squamous carcinoma cells that are considered evidence of response to ionizing radiation are cellular differentiation with keratinization, cell degeneration with cytoplasmic vacuolization, pyknosis, and nucleomegaly. Radiation-induced changes in adenocarcinoma of cervix include nuclear shrinkage and pyknosis, cytoplasmic vacuolization, and decrease in mucin synthesis.

Chemotherapy using a variety of regimens, most of which use cisplatin either alone or in combination with other drugs, has been recommended by the National Cancer Institute and GOG for concurrent therapy in women with stage IB2 and locally advanced (stage II–IVA) cervical cancer undergoing radiation therapy. A subsequent meta-analysis of 19 randomized controlled trials totaling 4,580 patients verified that the addition of chemotherapy to radiation therapy improved progression-free and overall survival [145]. Although 40–70% of such patients being treated for the first time will respond to cisplatin-containing regimens, the proportion of patients with prolonged responses is considerably less [161]. In addition, chemotherapy is used for patients with metastatic or recurrent cancer previously treated with surgery or radiation therapy. Response rates for cisplatin-based therapy in these recurrent or late-stage patients ranges 20–30% and overall survival is less than 10 months. Since effective treatment options are limited for advanced cervical cancer, therapies targeting cervical cancer signaling pathways are currently being investigated.

The 5-year survival for treated stage I patients is 90–95%, for stage II 50–70%, for stage III 30%, and <20% for patients with stage IV disease [24]. The survival rates are reduced even in patients with low-stage disease when metastases to lymph nodes are present; survival rates appear to correlate with the number of positive nodes [111]. Metastatic node involvement occurs in 8–25% of stage I, 21–38% of stage II, and 32–46% of stage III lesions [194]. Typically, the majority of recurrences appear within 2 years after initial therapy.

Verrucous Carcinoma

Verrucous carcinoma is a rare variant of squamous cell carcinoma. In the female genital tract, the region most commonly involved is the vulva, but well-documented cases have been described in the cervix [129, 299]. In the past, this tumor has been reported as giant condyloma acuminatum of Buschke and Lowenstein, but the implication that this tumor is a type of condyloma is erroneous and the term is no longer used. More recently some studies have implicated HPV as an etiologic agent since low- and high-risk HPV types were identified in verrucous carcinoma [37, 78].

Clinically, verrucous carcinoma appears as a large, sessile tumor that grossly resembles a condyloma. Verrucous carcinoma is a slow-growing, locally invasive malignant tumor. Because it is frequently diagnosed incorrectly, it may become quite advanced and lead to death. Five of eight patients in one series died shortly after the diagnosis was made [162]. Histologically, cervical verrucous carcinomas are identical to the more common vulvar tumors and are predominately exophytic and characterized by frondlike papillae with or without surface keratinization (*Fig. 6.13*). The epithelium lacks significant cytologic

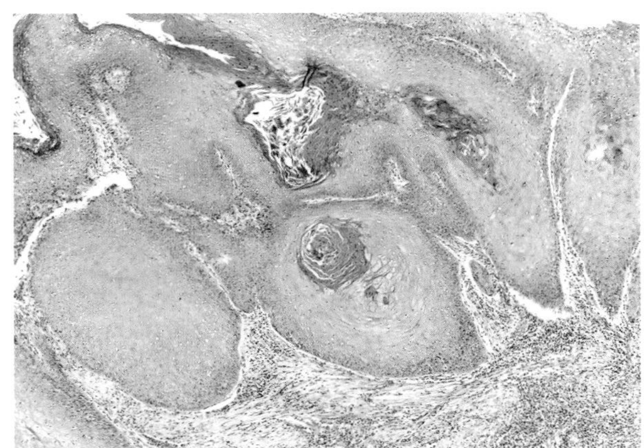

Fig. 6.13
Verrucous carcinoma. **Broad, bulbous nests of very well-differentiated neoplastic squamous epithelium invade superficial stroma with a pushing border**

atypia and mitotic activity, although in some cases mitoses may be found in the deep layers. The base of the tumor is composed of invasive nests of epithelium that are broad and expansile with a well-circumscribed pushing margin. There is a conspicuous inflammatory reaction at the epithelial stromal junction. For accurate diagnosis the biopsy should be large to include the rete ridge pattern at the base of the tumor as well as more superficial areas. If only superficial keratotic areas are examined the correct diagnosis is impossible.

Verrucous carcinoma should be distinguished from warty carcinoma (see section Warty (Condylomatous) Carcinoma) and condylomata acuminatum. Unlike condyloma acuminatum, verrucous carcinoma lacks the central fibroconnective tissue cores in the epithelial papillae that are characteristic of condylomata. Typically, these tumors recur locally but do not metastasize unless they are inadequately radiated, in which case accelerated growth and metastasis may occur [129]. The most appropriate therapy is wide local excision if possible. However, these lesions can frequently be deeply invasive, even extending into the endometrium or adjacent pelvic tissue [162, 250]. Regional lymph nodes are rarely involved, and distant metastases are exceedingly rare [162].

Warty (Condylomatous) Carcinoma

Warty (condylomatous) carcinoma is a variant of squamous cell carcinoma of the cervix that has marked condylomatous changes. Unlike verrucous carcinoma, warty carcinomas demonstrate features of a typical squamous cell carcinoma at the deep margin. In addition, many of the malignant cells have cytoplasmic vacuolization and nuclear changes closely resembling koilocytotic atypia. Although clinical experience with these tumors is very limited, they appear to behave less aggressively than typical well-differentiated squamous cell carcinomas of the cervix. In one study, multiple types of HPV including low-risk types were identified in two thirds of these tumors [43].

Papillary Squamous Cell (Transitional) Carcinoma

Papillary squamous cell carcinoma is a rare variant of squamous cell carcinoma of the cervix. These tumors were initially described by Randall et al., who reported that they had a histologic resemblance to transitional cell carcinoma of the bladder [215]. A comprehensive study from the Armed Forces Institute of Pathology of 32 cases of papillary cervical carcinomas reported that these papillary tumors of the cervix can be subdivided into three groups based on their histologic appearance: predominately squamous, predominantly transitional, and mixed squamous and transitional [141]. However, all three histologic subdivisions demonstrated similar immunohistochemical staining patterns for cytokeratin 7 and 20. The tumors were typically positive for cytokeratin 7 and negative for cytokeratin 20, which is a pattern more typical of cervical squamous lesions than of transitional cell tumors of the urinary tract. Follow-up was available for 12 patients, and 3 were reported to have died of their disease [141]. However, no apparent differences were observed in the clinical behavior of the three subtypes. Therefore, it appears that papillary squamous cell carcinomas of the cervix present a spectrum of histologic appearances with some tumors appearing more squamous and others more transitional. Because they demonstrate a spectrum of histologic appearances, these tumors have been referred to as papillary squamotransitional carcinomas. HPV 16 has been identified in three cases of papillary squamous cell carcinoma of the cervix [31].

Histologically, papillary squamous cell carcinomas are composed of papillary projections that are covered by several layers of atypical epithelial cells (*Fig. 6.14*). In cases that appear more transitional, the cells are oval with their long axis oriented perpendicular to the surface and there is minimal flattening of the cells as they reach the surface. In cases with more squamous differentiation, the

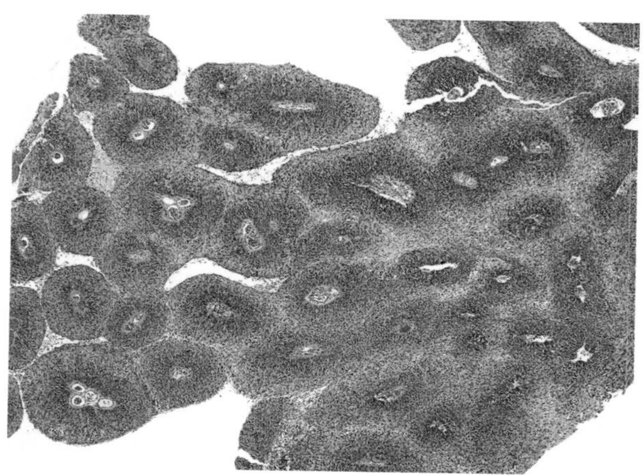

Fig. 6.14
Papillary squamous cell carcinoma. **Papillary fronds are lined by atypical squamous epithelium**

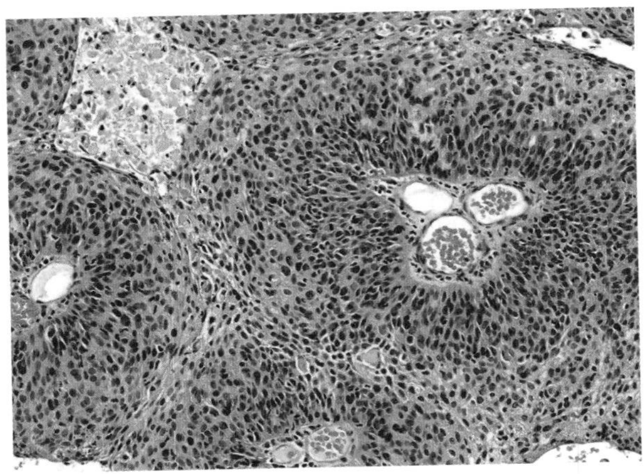

Fig. 6.15
Papillary squamous cell carcinoma. **Atypical squamous epithelium displaying loss of maturation and nuclear hyperchromasia with pleomorphism**

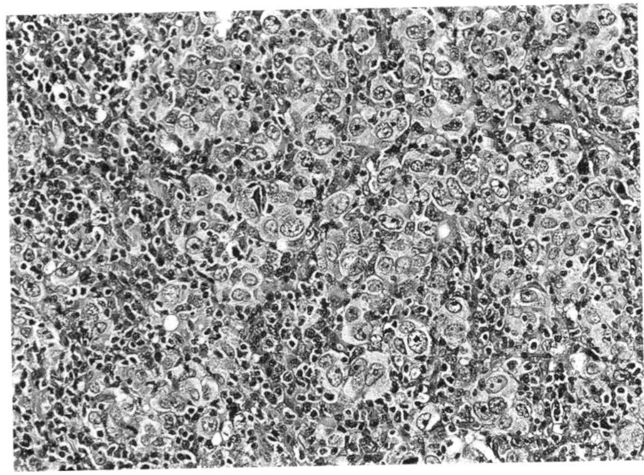

Fig. 6.16
Lymphoepithelioma-like carcinoma. **Large, atypical, discohesive cells simulating lymphoma are intimately associated with a mixed chronic inflammatory cell infiltrate**

cells are more basaloid and resemble those of a high-grade SIL (*Fig. 6.15*). The cells have hyperchromatic, oval nuclei, and minimal amounts of cytoplasm. Mitoses are frequent. Focally, there are usually areas of squamous differentiation. Typical invasive squamous cell carcinoma can often be identified at the base of the tumor, appearing as well-circumscribed nests of epithelium in continuity with papillae that extend deeply into the stroma. Focal invasion of the papillae themselves also sometimes occurs. The behavior of papillary squamous cell carcinoma is similar to that of invasive squamous cell carcinoma with the exception that late recurrences have been reported in the larger series [215].

Papillary squamous cell carcinoma can be mistaken for a papillary squamous cell carcinoma in situ on a superficial biopsy. Because papillary squamous cell carcinoma is capable of acting aggressively and metastasizing, it is important that a cone biopsy performed to rule out invasion whenever a papillary squamous cell carcinoma in situ is diagnosed. These tumors can also be mistakenly diagnosed as verrucous carcinoma or as condyloma accuminatum with atypia. Papillary squamous cell carcinomas lack the condylomatous changes and degree of cytoplasmic differentiation present in the other lesions.

Lymphoepithelioma-like Carcinoma

Lymphoepithelioma-like carcinomas (LELC) are a distinctive subset of squamous cell carcinomas of the cervix that are typically well circumscribed and composed of undifferentiated cells surrounded by a dense stromal inflammatory infiltrate [167]. These tumors are reported to have a better prognosis than typical squamous cell carcinoma. LELC represent only 0.7% of all primary cervical malignancies in Western countries but up to 5.5% of cervical cancers in some series from Asia [262]. The pathogenesis of cervical LELC is still unclear. The Epstein-Barr virus (EBV) has been suggested as a potential causative agent and has been detected in 75% of cervical LELC cases in Asian women [166, 262]. In contrast, a role for EBV in LELC pathogenesis in women in Western countries seems less likely since EBV has not been detected in cervical LELC in Caucasian women so far. A possible role for the human papillomavirus (HPV) in the pathogenesis of cervical LELC has also been suggested [20, 193]. The cells composing LELC are relatively undifferentiated but have abundant cytoplasm and uniform vesicular nuclei (*Fig. 6.16*). The cell borders tend to be indistinct and form what has been described as a syncytium. The nests of undifferentiated cells are surrounded by a marked chronic inflammatory infiltrate composed of lymphocytes, plasma cells, and eosinophils.

LELC can be mistaken for either glassy cell carcinoma or true lymphoproliferative disorders. Glassy cell carcinomas have a very poor prognosis and are characterized by prominent cell borders, ground glass cytoplasm, and prominent nucleoli. Lymphoproliferative disorders can be easily differentiated from LELC by immunohistochemical staining with antibodies against leukocyte common antigen, cytokeratin, and epithelial membrane antigen.

Adenocarcinoma

Adenocarcinomas of the cervix comprise a heterogeneous group of neoplasms that displays a variety of histologic patterns (see ➋ *Table 6.1*). Because these cell types and patterns are frequently admixed, the histologic classification of these tumors is based on the predominant cell type. If additional histologic components comprise at least 10% of the tumor, some authors recommend classifying the tumor according to the predominant pattern and listing the individual components as part of the diagnosis.

The most common cervical adenocarcinoma type is the usual type, also referred to as "mucinous type," followed by endometroid adenocarcinoma [6, 290]. Although some studies have found endometrioid adenocarcinomas to be more prevalent than usual type adenocarcinomas, in most series endometrioid adenocarcinomas account for 7–30% of cervical adenocarcinomas [223, 277, 290].

Prevalence

The relative proportion and absolute incidence of squamous cell carcinoma and adenocarcinoma of the cervix has been changing in the United States and Western Europe since the introduction of widespread cytologic screening programs. The incidence of all invasive cervical cancer and of cervical squamous cell carcinoma has been decreasing, however the incidence of cervical adenocarcinoma (i.e., adenosquamous carcinoma and adenocarcinoma) among young women has increased in developed countries, even those with widespread screening programs and histology-specific cancer registration [33, 271]. In the 1950s and 1960s, approximately 95% of all invasive cervical carcinomas were classified as squamous cell carcinomas and only 5% as adenocarcinomas [175]. However, invasive cervical cancer series published since the early 1970s have found that squamous cell carcinomas account for 75–80% of the cases, while the remaining 20–25% include various types of adenocarcinomas, adenosquamous carcinomas, and other epithelial tumors [33, 271]. Between 1973 and 1996, the overall age-adjusted incidence of invasive cervical cancer in the United States decreased by 36.9%. At the same time, the age-adjusted incidence of adenocarcinoma increased by 29.1% and the proportion of adenocarcinoma relative to squamous cell carcinoma increased by 95% [245]. In contrast to squamous cell carcinoma, rates of adenocarcinoma were significantly lower among African-American women than in Caucasian women. Rates of adenocarcinoma were significantly higher in Hispanic women than among non-Hispanics [226]. Most studies have noted increasing rates of adenocarcinoma among younger women, particularly under the age of 40 [245, 275, 301]. An international study monitoring trends in adenocarcinoma incidence from 1973 to 1991 reported increasing risk in cohorts born after 1935 in England, Scotland, Denmark, Sweden, Slovenia, and Slovakia [271]. A recent review from 13 European countries confirmed this report, and with data spanning the 1990s also showed increased adenocarcinoma incidence in Estonia, Spain, Finland, and Italy, countries previously reported to have either stable or decreasing trends [30].

Pathogenesis and Risk Factors

The cell of origin for invasive cervical adenocarcinoma is thought to be the pluripotential subcolumnar reserve cell of the columnar endocervical epithelium, and adenocarcinoma in situ is regarded as the immediate precursor to invasive endocervical adenocarcinoma. Many of the epidemiologic risk factors for the development of adenocarcinoma of the cervix are similar to those described for invasive squamous cell carcinomas [39]. Both are frequently associated with SIL, multiple sexual partners (more than 10 partners has a relative risk of 10.9 and 2.9 for adenocarcinoma and squamous cell carcinoma, respectively), and young age at first intercourse (intercourse before the age of 15 has a relative risk of 2.0 for both adenocarcinoma and squamous cell carcinoma) [140]. Tobacco smoking is associated with increased risk of squamous cell but not adenocarcinoma of the cervix [113]. Epidemiologic studies have shown a strong association between HPV and cervical adenocarcinoma, suggesting a causal relationship, as is the case for the squamous cell carcinoma. HPV 16 and 18 are the most common types of HPV found in association with both squamous cell carcinomas and adenocarcinomas of the cervix. However, HPV 18 is more commonly found in association with adenocarcinomas than with squamous cell carcinomas [11, 39, 210]. Use of oral contraceptives for more than 10 years, particularly those with a large progestational component, has been shown to be a risk factor for invasive cervical adenocarcinoma [39, 277]. Some studies comparing the risk factors for invasive adenocarcinomas with those of squamous cell carcinomas have revealed no significant differences in oral contraceptive usage between the two groups of women after controlling for HPV and sexual factors [93, 113]. It should also be noted that one study has reported a significant association between the use of hormone replacement therapy in older women and invasive adenocarcinomas of the cervix [146].

A genetic predisposition to invasive cervical adenocarcinoma has been documented in women with Peutz–Jeghers syndrome in whom minimal deviation adenocarcinoma of the cervix occurs more frequently than in the general population [50]. It also appears that a generalized predisposition to the development of adenocarcinoma of the ovary and cervix can occur because dual primary cervical and ovarian adenocarcinomas develop in some women [174, 291]. Mucinous tumors of the ovary appear to be particularly prevalent in women with minimal deviation mucinous adenocarcinomas of the cervix [291].

Clinical Features

The most common presenting symptom is abnormal vaginal bleeding, occurring in about 75% of patients [153]. Occasionally women present with vaginal discharge or with pelvic pain. The majority of invasive cervical adenocarcinomas arise in the transformation zone, and on gross examination 50% of patients have a fungating, polypoid, or papillary mass [110]. In approximately 15% of patients, the cervix is either diffusely enlarged or nodular. In another 15%, no gross lesions are visible. Although the majority of patients with grossly inapparent tumors have early-stage tumors, some have deep invasion because the carcinoma arose deep within the endocervical canal [223]. Adenocarcinoma of the cervix is confined to the cervix (stage I) or the parametrium/vagina (stage II) in 80% of women at the time of diagnosis. The diagnostic accuracy of cytopathology in the detection of cervical adenocarcinoma varies according to the expertise of the pathologist and the sampling techniques used. In most large series the majority of patients with cervical adenocarcinomas have cytologic abnormalities [183, 195].

Microinvasive Adenocarcinoma

Definition

The current definition FIGO definition for microinvasive (stage IA) cervical cancer applies to both squamous cell carcinoma and adenocarcinoma. However it is important to emphasize that recognizing microinvasive adenocarcinoma is often problematic and less is known about behavior of microinvasive adenocarcinoma compared to microinvasive squamous cell carcinoma [195, 295]. The irregular distribution and architecture of the normal endocervical crypts in the cervical stroma makes it difficult to differentiate between early stromal invasion and adenocarcinoma in situ [195]. In cases with admixed adenocarcinoma in situ and superficially invasive adenocarcinoma the actual depth of the invasion may be very difficult to measure (see below).

Microscopic Findings

Several growth patterns can be present in microinvasive carcinoma. Presence of a finger-like extension of epithelium with abundant pink cytoplasm into the stroma from a gland demonstrating the histologic features of adenocarcinoma in situ is often the first histologic sign of invasion [195]. More advanced areas of invasion show glands that lack the lobular architecture of crypts involved by adenocarcinoma in situ (*Fig. 6.17*). These glands are often separated by stroma and may be within the zone of normal endocervical mucosa. There may or may not be a stromal response with edema, inflammation, and desmoplasia. However, in some cases of early invasive adenocarcinoma these features are not present and invasion is indicated by the gland pattern and haphazard distribution on low power examinations. Confluent glandular pattern and complex gland architecture are more

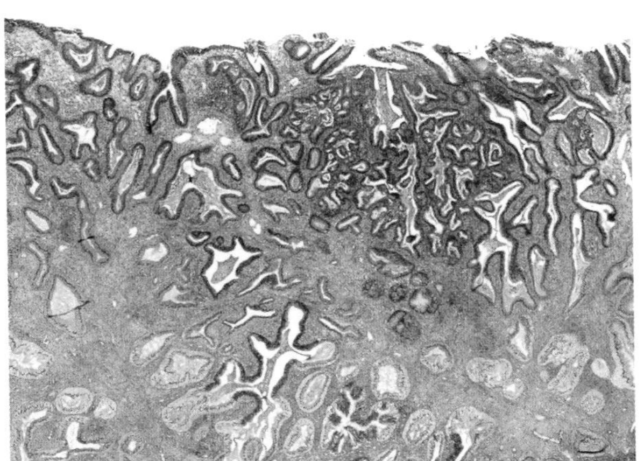

Fig. 6.17
Superficially invasive endocervical adenocarcinoma associated with adenocarcinoma in situ. **A region of confluent glandular growth within extensive adenocarcinoma in situ indicates superficial stromal invasion**

subtle patterns of invasion [195]. Smooth-contoured, dilated glands with complex intraglandular cribriform or papillary growth patterns also indicate invasion as well as presence of glands below the deep margin of normal endocervical glands [150]. Finally, if the distance between neoplastic glands and thick-walled blood vessels is less than the thickness of the vessel wall, invasion should be strongly suspected [281]. Most patients have coexisting adenocarcinoma in situ and some also have HSIL. After establishing invasion, the depth of invasion and horizontal extent of the invasive component should be measured. Measurements with a calibrated optic are recommended. The depth of invasion is measured from the surface (when the in situ component is not present on a section with the deepest invasion) or from overlying the in situ carcinoma. Similar to microinvasive SCC a definitive diagnosis of microinvasive adenocarcinoma requires examination of the entire lesion in a cold knife cone biopsy or hysterectomy specimen.

Clinical Behavior and Treatment

Microinvasive adenocarcinoma accounts for 12% of adenocarcinomas [195]. The average age at presentation is 39 years, approximately 7 years younger than the peak age for frankly invasive adenocarcinoma. The natural history of microinvasive cervical adenocarcinoma is not well understood since a cone biopsy is necessary to confirm the diagnosis and is often curative. There are rare documented cases of in situ adenocarcinoma progressing to invasive carcinoma after conservative treatment with cone excision [104, 132]. In a recent review of microinvasive adenocarcinomas 2 of 228 (0.8%) stage IA1 and 3 of 179 (1.6%) stage IA2 had lymph node metastasis [212]. In a literature review of 26 reports of microinvasive adenocarcinomas, totaling 436 cases of invasive adenocarcinoma defined as 5 mm or less of invasion, only 5 (2%) of 219 patients undergoing lymphadenectomy had metastases [195]. Review of 531 cases from the SEER (Surveillance, Epidemiology, and End Results) database confirmed low incidence (1.28%) of lymph node metastasis in Stage IA1 and IA2 tumors [244]. Data on lymphvascular space involvement are difficult to extract since most series do not comment on the presence or absence of this feature.

Kaspar et al. analyzed 25 cases with stage IA adenocarcinoma and found tumor volume to be a better predictor of lymph node metastasis and recurrence. None of the patients with tumor volume $<500\ mm^3$ had lymph node metastases or recurrence whereas two of two patients with tumor volume more than $500\ mm^3$ had recurrence and one of two developed lymph node metastases [130]. Other studies confirmed this observation [54, 124]. There is also very little information on margin status at conization and residual disease in a subsequent hysterectomy specimen. In two studies, patients who underwent conization with negative margins did not have residual disease in the subsequent hysterectomy specimen. Half of the patients with positive margins had tumor in the uterus [195, 212]. The overall prognosis for microinvasive adenocarcinoma (stage IA1 and IA2) is excellent. Based on SEER data the risk for stage IA1 versus IA2 for lymph node metastases (1.45 vs. 1.73%), recurrence (1.54 vs. 1.96%), and death (0.85% vs. 1.12%) was not statistically different [244]. In the same study there was no difference in recurrence and death of disease between patients treated conservatively (with conization or simply hysterectomy) and those undergoing radical hysterectomy. However, 10% of the patients in the study received adjuvant radiotherapy or underwent a pelvic lymphadenectomy. Therefore, a conization alone for patients with stage IA1 adenocarcinoma was not recommended. In a recent report none of four patients with stage IA1 adenocarcinoma treated with conization developed recurrence after 2–13 years of follow-up [284]. All the patients had a term delivery. No residual invasive adenocarcinoma was present in three of four patients who underwent radical hysterectomy with pelvic lymph node dissection. Prospective, long-term follow-up studies for patients with microinvasive adenocarcinoma treated with conization are lacking.

Endocervical Adenocarcinoma

Cervical adenocarcinoma displays a wide variety of morphologic patterns but over 75% of the tumors display a relatively similar pattern. The WHO classification adopted the traditional approach of referring to these tumors as "mucinous carcinomas" but since they have little, if any, intracytoplasmic mucin evident on H&E and mucin stains, we prefer the designation "endocervical adenocarcinoma of usual type" [6]. True endometrioid-type endocervical adenocarcinoma is relatively uncommon, accounting for approximately 10% of cervical adenocarcinomas. The remainder of cervical adenocarcinomas comprises a diverse group that includes mucinous adenocarcinoma, of which there are three variants (endocervical type, intestinal type, and signet ring type), minimal deviation adenocarcinoma, villoglandular adenocarcinoma, clear cell carcinoma, serous carcinoma, mesonephric carcinoma, and a number of uncommon variants.

Adenocarcinoma, Usual Type

Gross Findings

Most adenocarcinomas are papillary or polypoid, whereas some are nodular and may ulcerate the cervix. Some are high in the endocervical canal and are therefore very difficult to visualize on clinical examination. Others diffusely infiltrate and enlarge the cervix resulting in a "barrel" configuration.

Microscopic Findings

This is far and away the most common histologic type of cervical adenocarcinoma and although it has a somewhat similar appearance to endometrioid carcinoma, the glands exhibit a hybrid of endocervical and endometrioid differentiation (➋ *Figs. 6.18–6.21*). The cells are columnar with elongated, hyperchromatic nuclei that may show marked atypia with nuclear pleomorphism and coarse chromatin. The cells are often stratified and contain amphophilic or eosinophilic apical cytoplasm. Mitotic figures, which typically appear to be "floating" in the cytoplasm, are frequent as are apoptotic bodies. The glands may be widely spaced or densely arranged in a complex racemose pattern. A cribriform pattern is very common and papillae commonly project into gland lumens.

The usual-type adenocarcinomas of the cervix are graded on the basis of architectural features, in a manner similar to that used for endometrial adenocarcinomas. Well-differentiated tumors are defined as those in which <10% of the tumor volume is composed of solid sheets of cells, the remainder of the tumor being glandular; in moderately differentiated tumors, 11–50% of the tumor is composed of solid sheets of cells; and in poorly differentiated tumors, >50% of the tumor is solid.

Measurement of the depth of invasion is more difficult than for squamous cell carcinomas because of the difficulty in determining the point of origin. Measurement

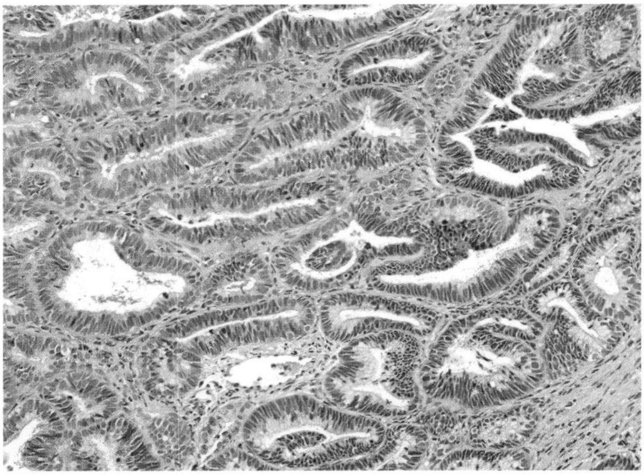

Fig. 6.18
Endocervical adenocarcinoma, usual type. **Crowded glands within desmoplastic stroma exhibit a hybrid of endometrioid and mucinous features**

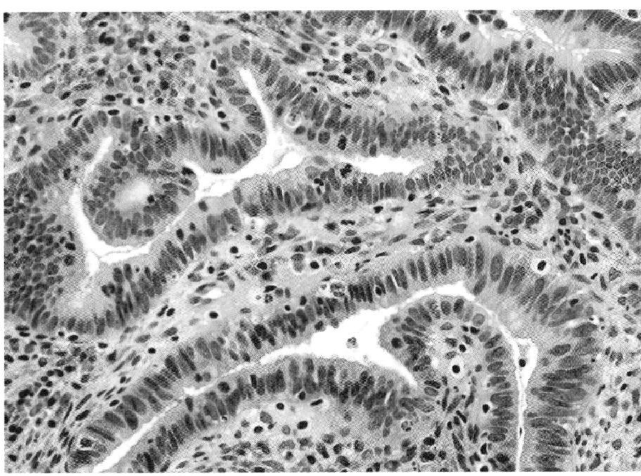

Fig. 6.19
Endocervical adenocarcinoma, usual type. **Glandular epithelium exhibits a hybrid of endometrioid and mucinous features and numerous mitotic figures and apoptotic bodies are characteristic**

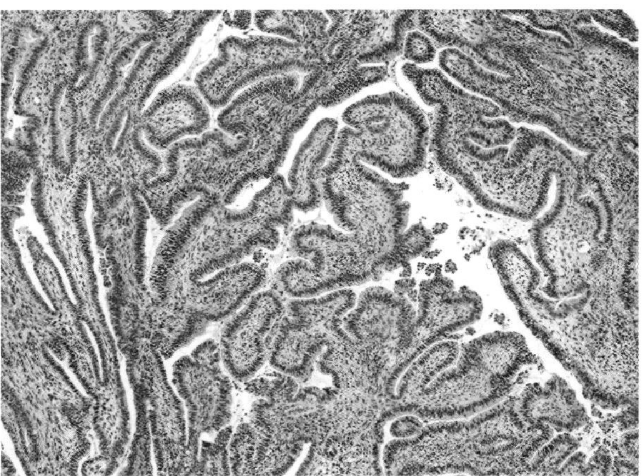

Fig. 6.20
Endocervical adenocarcinoma, usual type. **Complex labyrinthine glandular pattern indicates an invasive adenocarcinoma**

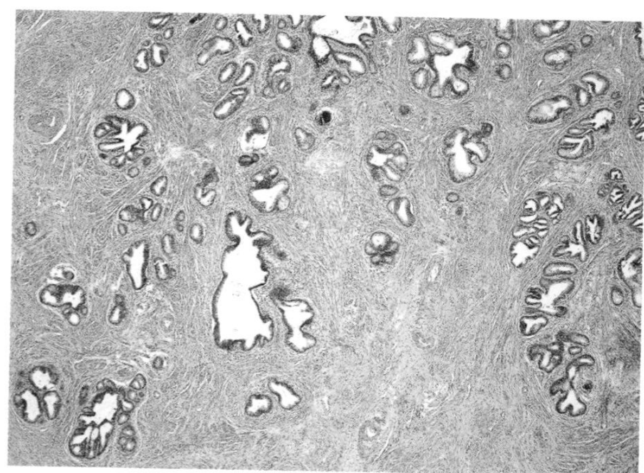

Fig. 6.21
Invasive endocervical adenocarcinoma. **Glands resemble adenocarcinoma in situ and are surrounded by nonreactive stroma but the deep extent and diffuse pattern indicate an invasive adenocarcinoma**

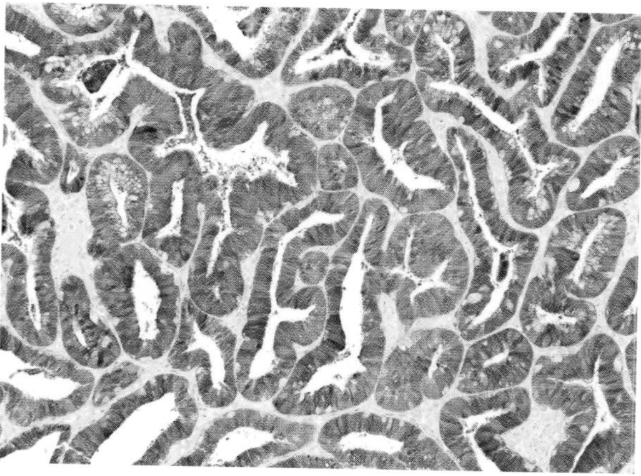

Fig. 6.22
Endocervical adenocarcinoma, usual type. **Tumor exhibits diffuse/strong p16 expression**

can be expressed either in millimeters or centimeters or as the percentage of involvement of the wall. Measurements with a calibrated eyepiece or microscopic fields are recommended. The presence of vascular invasion should be noted.

Immunohistochemical Findings

Distinction of endometrial endometrioid carcinomas from endocervical adenocarcinomas is important because surgical management of these tumors often differs. The vast majority of endocervical adenocarcinomas (~90%) are HPV-related and exhibit diffuse/moderate-strong p16 expression due to complex molecular mechanisms by which high-risk HPV-transforming proteins (E6, E7) interact with cell cycle regulatory proteins (p53, pRb) to generate a futile feedback loop resulting in p16 overexpression (*Fig. 6.22*). Interestingly, these HPV-related endocervical adenocarcinomas also often lack hormone receptor expression (estrogen [ER] and progesterone [PR] receptors) [171, 220, 247, 288] (*Fig. 6.23*). In contrast, endometrial endometrioid carcinomas are considered etiologically unrelated to HPV. They have been shown to exhibit generally patchy p16 expression of variable intensity, with mean/median extent of expression in 30–40% of tumor cells across all FIGO grades, and only rare tumors exhibiting diffuse/strong expression [289]. This patchy pattern is distinct from the diffuse/strong

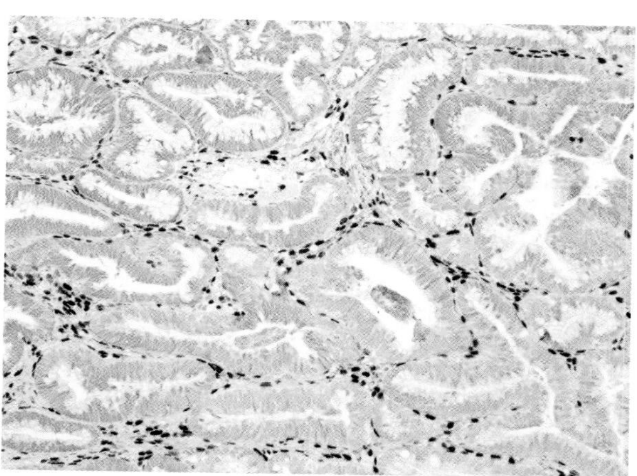

Fig. 6.23
Endocervical adenocarcinoma, usual type. **Tumor has loss of progesterone receptor expression (estrogen receptor expression is usually also lost). Positive intervening stromal cells serve as an internal control**

expression characteristic of HPV-related endocervical adenocarcinomas. In addition, most endometrial endometrioid carcinomas, particularly FIGO grade 1 and 2 tumors but also many FIGO grade 3 tumors, express hormone receptors [148, 171, 247]. Thus, a panel of immunohistochemical markers comprised of ER, PR, and p16 has been shown to be useful for distinguishing endometrial endometrioid carcinomas from endocervical adenocarcinomas [12, 170, 176, 247, 288]. Typical endometrial endometrioid carcinomas are p16 focal+/ER+/PR+, whereas typical endocervical adenocarcinomas are p16 diffuse+/ER−/PR−, with some of the latter retaining focal/limited expression of hormone receptors. We specifically recommend the use of PR in conjunction with ER based on our published [220, 247, 288] and unpublished experiences indicating that the subset of endocervical carcinomas that retains some expression of hormone receptors most often retains ER expression to some degree (often focal/weak-moderate) but entirely loses PR expression; thus, PR is the more discriminatory marker of the two when trying to distinguish endocervical adenocarcinomas from endometrial endometrioid carcinomas.

A number of studies have suggested that using a combination of inhibin, ER, and CEA staining can distinguish between endocervical and endometrial adenocarcinomas [59, 171, 296]. However others have found that this combination of stains is influenced not only by the site of origin of the adenocarcinoma, but also by the pattern of differentiation of the tumor [128]. The state of differentiation of the tumor (mucinous vs. endometriod) had a strong impact on whether or not a tumor stained positively with either vimentin or CEA. Furthermore, in our experience with numerous consultation cases, immunostains for CEA and vimentin are often difficult to interpret due to problems in discerning the localization of staining in tumor epithelium versus intimately associated stroma (for vimentin) or apical/luminal secretions (for CEA), and not infrequently, focality of staining for both markers can be observed in tumors of both sites. For these reasons, a panel comprised of p16, ER, and PR is recommended as most useful because differential expression patterns are based on biologic differences between endocervical and endometrial adenocarcinomas. Expression of p16 is also useful for identifying metastatic endocervical adenocarcinoma in the ovary. These ovarian metastases have a propensity to simulate primary ovarian endometrioid and mucinous tumors (atypical proliferative (borderline) tumors and carcinomas). Ovarian endometrioid and mucinous tumors, with few exceptions, are characterized by generally patchy p16 expression (or lack of expression) whereas metastatic HPV-related endocervical adenocarcinomas are diffusely/strongly positive [220, 268]. In the absence of a known primary endocervical adenocarcinoma, demonstrating high-risk HPV by in situ hybridization can be used for arriving at a definitive diagnosis [220] (➋ *Fig. 6.24*). Although it should be recognized that in most laboratories in situ hybridization has a relatively low sensitivity for detecting HPV in carcinomas, it should also be noted that p16 has no utility for identifying minimal-deviation-type endocervical adenocarcinomas since these tumors are unrelated to high-risk HPV and thus do not exhibit diffuse/strong p16 expression.

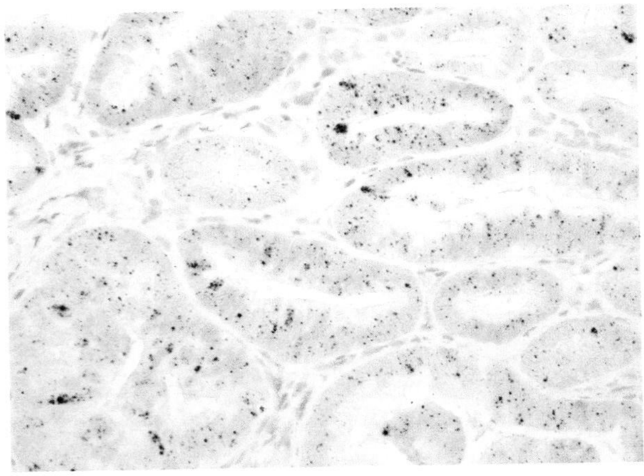

Fig. 6.24
Endocervical adenocarcinoma, usual type. **In situ hybridization demonstrates punctate nuclear signals indicating the presence of HPV 16 DNA**

A recent study reviewed expression of CDX2 in cervical adenocarcinomas [249]. CDX2 is a member of the caudal-related homeobox gene family that is expressed during the normal development of the intestinal tract. CDX2 is highly sensitive for the identification of colorectal adenocarcinomas; however its expression has been described in other tumors showing intestinal-type differentiation. Sullivan at al. have demonstrated that nuclear CDX2 expression in cervical adenocarcinomas is not restricted to intestinal type tumors but may be seen in 30% of the more common subtypes (endocervical and endometrioid) [249]. Therefore, CDX2 has limited value in determining origin of metastatic carcinoma when colorectal, pancreaticobiliary, mucinous ovarian, and endocervical adenocarcinomas are possible primary sites.

Differential Diagnosis

Invasive adenocarcinoma must be distinguished from adenocarcinoma in situ (AIS), primary endometrial adenocarcinoma with extension into the endocervical canal, and metastatic adenocarcinoma. Features favoring a benign glandular process include lack of an infiltrative pattern, lobular arrangement of glands, superficial location and a well-demarcated margin as well as lack of a desmoplastic stromal response and cytologic atypia. It is important to note that occasionally normal cervical glands may extend deep into the cervical wall. Absence of cytologic atypia, stromal reaction, and usually a widely scattered distribution allow exclusion of a malignant process [60]. It is important to make sure that the stromal reaction elicited by an infiltrating adenocarcinoma does not represent reaction to extravasated mucin from a ruptured benign gland. Cytologic atypia can be seen in the Arias-Stella reaction, atypical oxyphilic metaplasia, radiation changes, and rarely, viral infection. An Arias-Stella reaction involving endocervical glands is detected in 10–50% of gravid uteri [229]. Occasionally glandular changes similar to the Arias-Stella occur in nonpregnant women, usually in patients taking exogenous hormones. Whereas the distinctive cyto- and nucleomegaly raises concern for malignancy, lack of mitoses and partial gland involvement help to establish the correct diagnosis. The degenerative nature of atypia with enlarged, hyperchromatic nuclei containing smudged chromatin, cytoplasmic vacuolation, and preservation of the nuclear to cytoplasmic ratio are features of atypical oxyphilic metaplasia and radiation induced atypia [122, 156]. Distinctive cytopathic features associated with cytomegalovirus (CMV) and herpes simplex virus (HSV) infections and immunohistochemistry for detection of the specific pathogen assist in diagnosis.

One of the common benign mimics, tunnel clusters, has to be distinguished from cervical adenocarcinoma with a microcystic pattern [254]. Tambouret et al. described a small series of microcystic endocervical adenocarcinomas resembling type B tunnel clusters. In addition to architecture simulating a benign process, some of the cases had largely denuded atypical epithelium. High power examination of the lesion is recommended to look for the presence of cytologic atypia, which indicates that the lesion is microcystic endocervical adenocarcinoma. Other benign lesions that must be distinguished from invasive adenocarcinoma of the cervix are microglandular hyperplasia and hyperplastic mesonephric remnants. Microglandular hyperplasia tends to occur in young women and is frequently polypoid. Like endocervical adenocarcinoma, microglandular hyperplasia is CEA positive. In contrast to cervical adenocarcinoma, microglandular hyperplasia is composed of relatively uniform, small glands lined by a single layer of bland epithelium with few mitoses. Mesonephric remnants are tubular, retain a clustered arrangement associated with a mesonephric duct, and are usually deep in the cervical stroma. The epithelium lining the tubules is usually cuboidal and not stratified. Cytologic atypia is minimal [74].

Adenocarcinoma in situ of the cervix is distinguished from invasive cervical adenocarcinoma by the lack of extension beyond the depth to which normal endocervical glands extend, lack of desmoplasia surrounding the glands, and lack of foci of closely packed glands. The normal endocervical glandular architecture is maintained in adenocarcinoma in situ. Morphologically, endocervical adenocarcinoma can be distinguished from endometrial adenocarcinoma extending to the cervix by the presence of squamous metaplasia and foamy histiocytes in the latter. Immunohistochemical stains (as discussed earlier) may be useful in difficult cases. Metastatic adenocarcinoma of the cervix usually occurs in the setting of a patient with a known, widely metastatic primary lesion and is histologically characterized by a lack of surface involvement and widespread lymphvascular involvement. In assessing whether a carcinoma is of primary endocervical origin or is metastatic in the cervix, the pathologist should evaluate the following morphologic features: (1) neoplastic growth pattern, (2) coexistent in situ changes, (3) cell type, and (4) immunohistochemical characteristics. Transition between in situ and invasive carcinoma provides the strongest evidence for a primary origin and is found in approximately 50% of primary cervical adenocarcinomas.

Risk Factors

Major prognostic indicators for cervical adenocarcinoma include tumor size, depth of invasion, involvement of lymphvascular spaces, parametrial involvement, stage, age, and presence or absence of lymph node metastases [16, 26, 68]. Poor prognostic features include size >3 cm, uterine enlargement and high histologic grade. Women with poorly differentiated stage I tumors have a 5-year survival of 41–62% compared to 80–90% for those with well-differentiated adenocarcinomas [68]. Young age at presentation has been associated with a good prognosis in several series [16, 238]. Infection with HPV 18 has been associated with poor survival [191].

Clinical Behavior and Treatment

Adenocarcinoma of the cervix spreads in a fashion similar to squamous cell carcinoma and, in general, both squamous and adenocarcinomas are treated similarly. The most commonly used therapeutic modalities for stage I and II adenocarcinoma are radiation alone, radiation with concurrent chemotherapy, radiation followed by simple hysterectomy, or radical surgery [208]. Only a few studies have directly compared the therapeutic results achieved with invasive squamous cell and adenocarcinomas over the same time period and from the same institution, and these studies have produced conflicting data. Some studies have found that that the overall 5-year survival rates are lower for adenocarcinoma (48–65%) than for squamous cell carcinoma patients (68%) [26, 68]. In a study of 1,538 stage IB squamous cell carcinomas of the cervix and 229 adenocarcinomas initially treated with radiation therapy, Eifel et al. observed a worse outcome in women with adenocarcinoma [68]. A large retrospective analysis of 3,678 cases of cervical cancer from Taiwan found that the difference in survival between adenocarcinomas and squamous cell carcinomas appeared to be predominantly the result of a poorer outcome in early-stage lesions [40]. In data from the United States, reported survival is lower for adenocarcinoma versus squamous cell carcinoma for stage II disease but not for stage I or stage III or IV disease [238, 245]. Other comparison studies, as well as several population-based studies, have failed to confirm that prognosis, and survival are affected by histologic type [13, 114, 153]. Therefore, the prognosis of cervical adenocarcinoma relative to squamous carcinoma remains a controversial issue.

Mucinous Adenocarcinoma

Endocervical-Type Mucinous Carcinoma

Endocervical-type adenocarcinomas are composed of cells that have basal nuclei and abundant pale granular cytoplasm, which stains positively with mucicarmine stains. The cells resemble those in the normal endocervical glands but nuclear atypia is significant and mitotic figures are present. The majority of the endocervical-type adenocarcinomas are well-to-moderately differentiated, and the glandular elements are arranged in a pattern simulating the cleft–tunnel configuration of the normal endocervical mucosa (*Fig. 6.25*). In less-differentiated tumors, the cells contain less cytoplasm but usually still form recognizable glandular structures. Cells are typically stratified, and there may be considerable nuclear atypia with variation in nuclear size, coarsely clumped chromatin, and prominent nucleoli. Mitoses are usually numerous. Large amounts of mucin may be found in the stroma, forming mucin lakes or pools.

Intestinal-Type Mucinous Carcinoma

The intestinal-type mucinous carcinoma is composed of cells similar to those present in adenocarcinomas of the

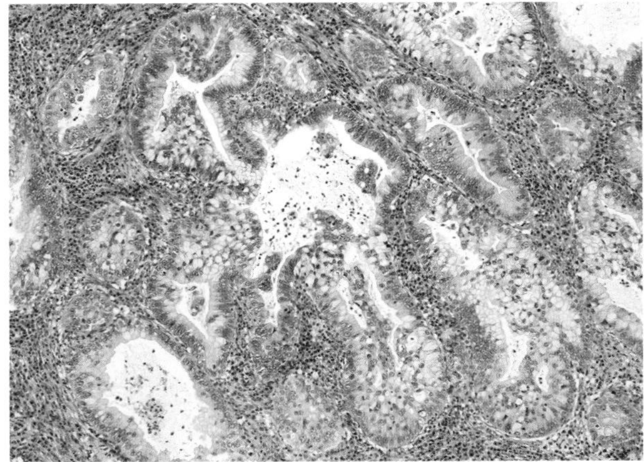

Fig. 6.25
Endocervical adenocarcinoma, mucinous type. **Invasive glands have prominent apical mucinous cytoplasm**

large intestine. These tumors frequently contain goblet cells and more rarely argentaffin cells and Paneth cells. In the intestinal type, the tumor cells tend to be pseudostratified, and contain only small amounts of intracellular mucin. They can either form glands with papillae or infiltrate throughout the stroma in a pattern similar to that of colonic adenocarcinoma.

Signet-Ring Cell-Type Mucinous Carcinoma

Signet-ring cell carcinomas rarely occur in a pure form and are usually admixed with intestinal or endocervical adenocarcinomas.

Minimal Deviation Adenocarcinoma

Minimal deviation adenocarcinoma is an extremely well-differentiated variant of cervical adenocarcinoma in which most of the cells lack the cytologic features of malignancy. These tumors were originally referred to as adenoma malignum. Because of their close cytologic resemblance to normal endocervical glands, in 1975 Silverberg and Hurt introduced the term "minimal deviation adenocarcinoma" (MDA) for these lesions [241]. Although all the tumors in the original description were extremely well-differentiated mucin-producing adenocarcinomas, MDA has been expanded to include endometrioid and clear cell variants [257, 293].

Minimal deviation adenocarcinomas are uncommon tumors and account for only 1–3% of all cervical adenocarcinomas [102, 127]. In a study of 389 primary adenocarcinomas of the cervix on file at the Armed Forces Institute of Pathology, only 1.3 % of cases represented MDA [127]. Patients with MDA range in age from 25 to 72 years (average 42 years). When sensitive PCR techniques are utilized, MDA are usually found to be negative for HPV [210]. MDA is more likely to either precede or develop coincidentally with an ovarian carcinoma than other types of cervical adenocarcinomas. The ovarian neoplasms with which MDA is most likely to be associated include mucinous adenocarcinomas and sex cord tumors with annular tubules. Both MDA of the cervix and ovarian sex cord tumors with annular tubules have been strongly associated with Peutz–Jeghers syndrome [294]. In one series, 4 of 27 women with Peutz–Jeghers syndrome developed MDA [294]. Therefore, close surveillance of women with Peutz–Jeghers syndrome is recommended, including careful endocervical cytologic examination and periodic endocervical curettage.

The characteristic microscopic features of MDA are the presence of cytologically low-grade but architecturally atypical glands that vary in size, shape, and location (➲ *Figs. 6.26–6.28*). In the mucin-producing forms, the glands are lined by a single layer of tall columnar epithelium that usually has minimal, if any, nuclear atypia but careful scrutiny will almost always disclose cells with clear-cut atypia. The nuclei are bland, may have conspicuous nucleoli, and are located at the base of the epithelium (➲ *Figs. 6.29–6.30*). In the endometrioid type, the cells lining the glands resemble either normal proliferative or hyperplastic endometrium. Although the glands may exhibit a branching arrangement similar to that of the normal endocervical glands, characteristically glands with bizarre angular outpouchings, which vary greatly in size, are present [86]. Desmoplasia is frequently present surrounding the angular outpouchings of MDA or in the deep portion of the tumor. Large areas of invasive tumor may be devoid of any stromal reaction. In such areas, the presence of glands adjacent to thick-walled blood vessels is a helpful finding in determining that stromal invasion is present. The most reliable criterion to assess the malignant

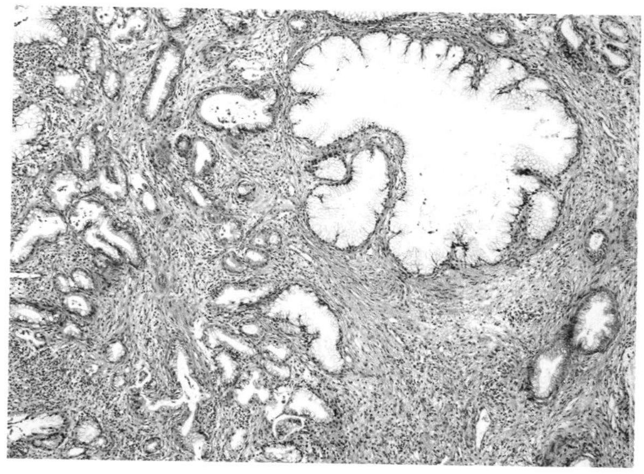

Fig. 6.27
Minimal deviation adenocarcinoma. **Smaller invasive well-differentiated mucinous glands within desmoplastic stroma are present adjacent to a larger hyperplastic gland**

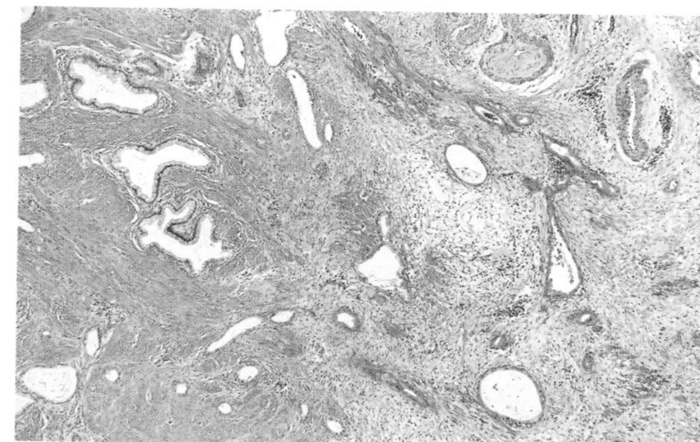

Fig. 6.26
Minimal deviation adenocarcinoma. **Highly differentiated mucinous glands in fibrous stroma are present along with irregular infiltrative glands in deeper edematous stroma**

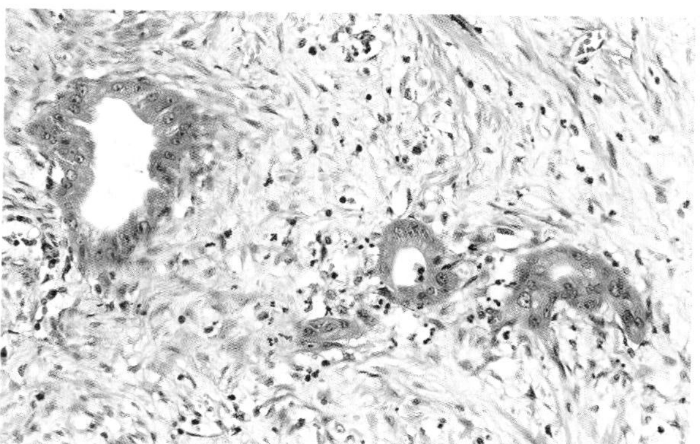

Fig. 6.28
Minimal deviation adenocarcinoma. **Smaller invasive well-differentiated mucinous glands within desmoplastic stroma are present adjacent to a larger hyperplastic gland**

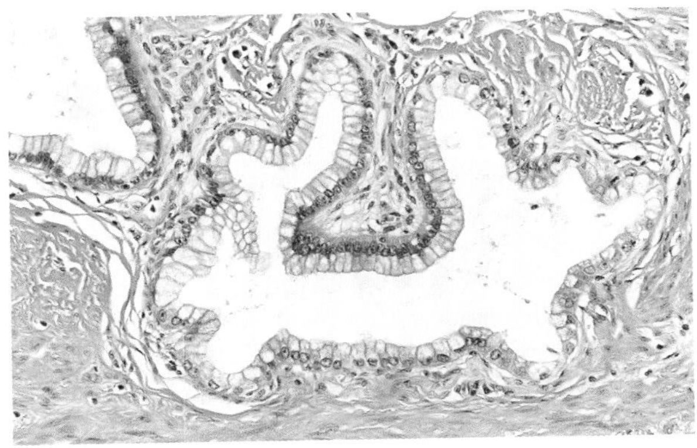

Fig. 6.29
Minimal deviation adenocarcinoma. **Very well-differentiated mucinous gland has vesicular nuclei with conspicuous nucleoli, the characteristic cytologic features of this adenocarcinoma**

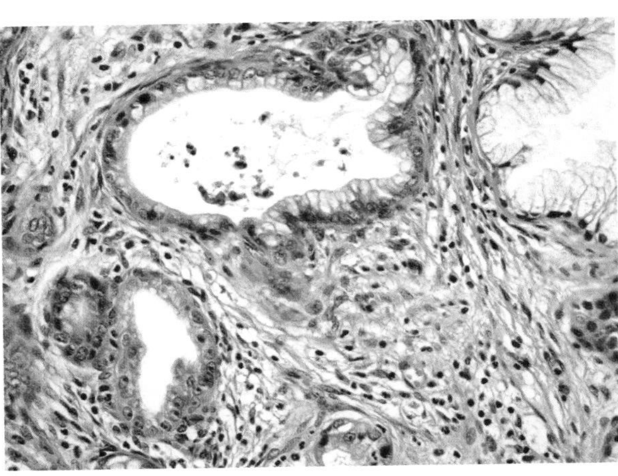

Fig. 6.30
Minimal deviation adenocarcinoma. **Invasive glands have atypical vesicular nuclei with nucleoli whereas hyperplastic gland has small uniformly hyperchromatic basally situated nuclei**

nature of MDA is the haphazard arrangement of glands that extend beyond the level of normal endocervical glands and the presence of occasional mitoses in glandular cells. Mitoses are quite uncommon in the normal, nonneoplastic, endocervical epithelium, and the presence of mitoses should alert the pathologist to the possible presence of MDA. However, occasional mitotic figures in otherwise normal-appearing glands should not be taken as sufficient for a diagnosis of MDA. Minimal deviation adenocarcinoma often involves more than two thirds of the thickness of the cervical stroma and should be regarded as invasive because the normal endocervical crypts and tunnels do not extend beyond 7 mm [86, 127]. Because the depth of penetration of the glands is an essential histologic feature of MDA, in most cases, the diagnosis cannot be made on a superficial cervical biopsy, but instead requires either a cone biopsy or hysterectomy specimen. Immunohistochemical studies using CEA have found highly variable staining of MDA with only focal areas of positivity, and CA 125 staining is significantly reduced compared to normal endocervical glands [86, 259]. Immunohistochemical staining for estrogen and progesterone receptors is uniformly negative in MDA, and this criterion can be used to help differentiate these tumors from variants of normal endocervical glands [259]. Stains for p16 are negative or only focally positive since MDA is not associated with high-risk HPV infection and Ki-67 proliferation index is often low. Immunoreactivity for a monoclonal antibody to gastric gland mucous cell mucin (HIK1083) has been reported; however it is also positive in gastric metaplasia associated with lobular endocervical glandular hyperplasia [173]. Some authors believe that MDA can be derived from lobular endocervical glandular hyperplasia and morphologically usual-type AIS showing gastric phenotype [173].

The differential diagnosis of MDA includes several conditions in which nonneoplastic glands extend beyond 7 mm from the surface. These conditions include endocervical tunnel clusters, deeply situated nabothian cysts, endocervicosis of the cervical wall, and mesonephric hyperplasia [290]. The glands of endocervical tunnel clusters, mesonephric hyperplasia, and deep nabothian cysts are usually much more uniform in size than are the glands of MDA and lack the bizarre branching and irregular outpouchings that are characteristic of the glands of MDA. The benign processes also lack a desmoplastic response.

Villoglandular Adenocarcinoma

Villoglandular adenocarcinoma is a well-differentiated form of cervical adenocarcinoma that occurs predominantly in young women and has an excellent prognosis [121, 292]. The characteristic features of this tumor are a surface component that is composed of papillae lined by epithelium that has only mild cytologic atypia (*Fig. 6.31*). The epithelial cells lining the papillae can display endocervical, endometrioid, or intestinal features (*Figs. 6.32–6.34*). Because of the large number of surface

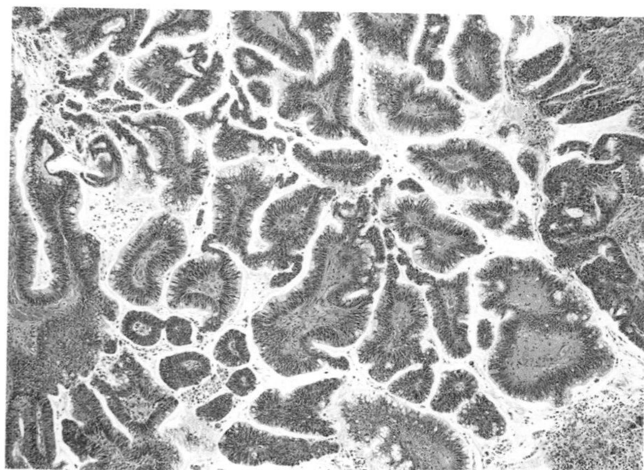

Fig. 6.31
Endocervical adenocarcinoma, villoglandular type. **Tumor is composed of papillary structures with central fibrous cores**

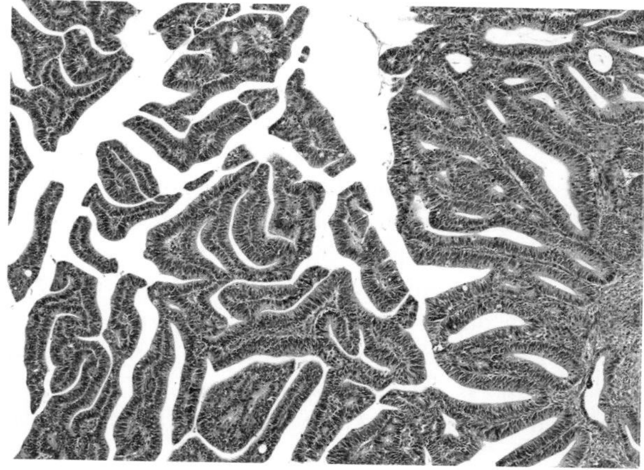

Fig. 6.33
Endocervical adenocarcinoma, villoglandular type. **Elongated villous papillary structures have an endometrioid appearance at lower magnification**

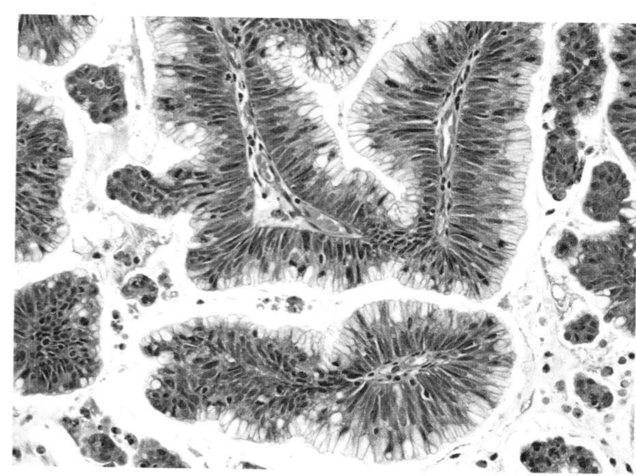

Fig. 6.32
Endocervical adenocarcinoma, villoglandular type. **Epithelium lining papillae exhibits mucinous differentiation**

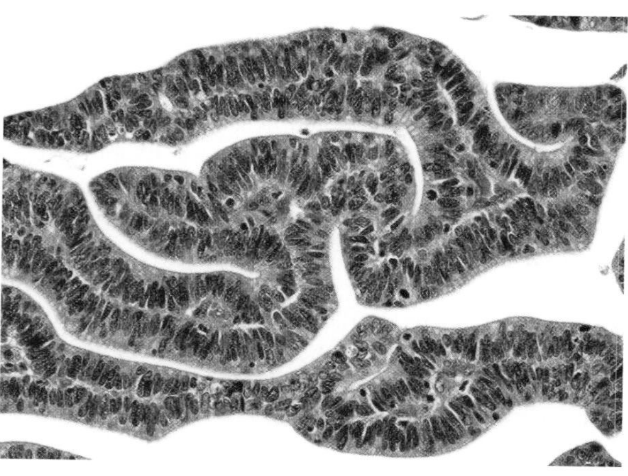

Fig. 6.34
Endocervical adenocarcinoma, villoglandular type. **Villous structures have thin fibrovascular cores and are lined by epithelium with a hybrid of endometrioid and mucinous features ("usual type" differentiation)**

papillae, these tumors frequently form an exophytic, friable tumor mass. Most of the papillae have central cores containing spindle-shaped stromal cells resembling those of the normal cervical stroma and a variable number of inflammatory cells. The papillae can be either long and thin or thick and short. Small papillary tufts composed entirely of epithelial cells of the type characteristic of serous carcinomas of the ovary are absent. Beneath the papillary surface, the infiltrating portion of the tumor is composed of irregular branching glands that are typically surrounded by only a minimal desmoplastic response.

The differential diagnosis of these tumors includes papillary endocervicitis, papillary adenofibromas of the cervix, and müllerian papillomas. All three of these lesions lack the degree of cellular atypia that is present in villoglandular adenocarcinomas. The müllerian papilloma is a lesion of children, whereas the age of patients with villoglandular adenocarcinomas ranges from 27 to 54 years, with a mean of 37 in one series [121]. In contrast to villoglandular adenocarcinoma, adenofibroma of the cervix and müllerian papilloma have a more prominent stromal component. Villoglandular adenocarcinoma must also be distinguished from serous papillary carcinomas of the cervix. Serous papillary carcinomas have more irregular papillae that are lined by cells with marked nuclear atypia and high mitotic counts, which frequently form cellular tufts.

Villoglandular adenocarcinomas have been associated with the use of oral contraceptives and are frequently associated with high-risk types of HPV [117]. In the majority of cases, the tumor is superficially invasive, although deep invasion with extension into the uterine corpus may occur. In most of the cases published to date, the clinical outcome of patients with villoglandular adenocarcinomas has been excellent. In the two largest series, all patients, including those who were treated by simple excisional biopsy or cone biopsy, were alive and well with no evidence of recurrent disease after 7–77 months of follow-up [121]. There are also reports of villoglandular adenocarcinomas treated successfully with conization in young patients who wished to preserve fertility [143]. Conservative treatment should be considered only if the tumor is superficial, does not involve lymphvascular spaces, and there is no residual disease in the cone margins. In a series of seven cases from Japan the presence of lymphvascular space involvement was associated with lymph node metastases in two cases and resulted in death in one patient [125]. Rarely, villoglandular carcinomas may be mixed with other types of carcinomas. The authors are aware of two such cases in which lymph node metastasis has occurred (unpublished observations).

Endometrioid Adenocarcinoma

Endometrioid adenocarcinomas of the cervix are defined as tumors composed of cells that resemble those of primary adenocarcinomas of the uterine corpus. In different series endometrioid carcinomas accounted for 7–50% of endocervical adenocarcinomas [230, 296]. This wide range is due to the fact that at times it can be difficult to differentiate endometrioid adenocarcinoma from the more common, usual type of cervical adenocarcinoma as the latter frequently has endometrioid features. Many tumors classified as endometrioid adenocarcinomas may actually represent poorly differentiated mucinous tumors that have lost their capacity to produce mucin [290].

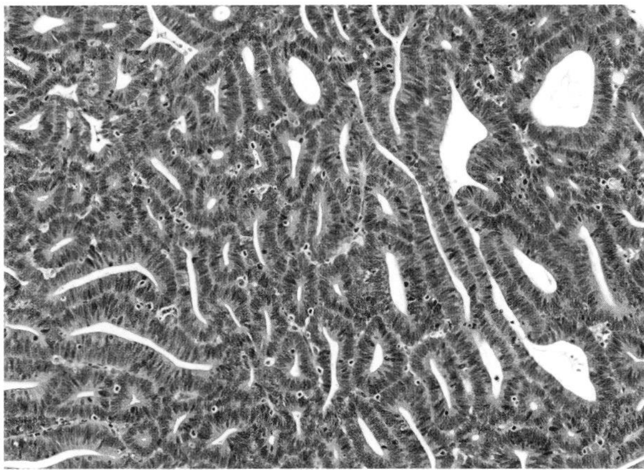

Fig. 6.35
Endocervical adenocarcinoma, endometrioid type.
Crowded glands have columnar cells with elongated nuclei and little apical cytoplasm, analogous to primary endometrial endometrioid carcinoma

The cells of endometrioid adenocarcinomas tend to be stratified and have oval nuclei that are arranged with their long axis perpendicular to the basement membrane of the gland (*Fig. 6.35*). The cells do not contain mucin and have less cytoplasm than the cells of the usual type of endocervical adenocarcinomas. Endometrioid adenocarcinomas frequently contain small foci of squamous epithelium. It can also be difficult to differentiate between an endometrioid carcinoma primary in the cervix and a primary endometrial adenocarcinoma extending to cervix. Primary uterine corpus tumors are usually bulky tumors that have invaded the myometrium by the time they extend to the cervix and therefore cause uterine enlargement. In contrast, primary cervical adenocarcinomas often cause cervical enlargement in the absence of uterine enlargement. Even with large, destructive primary cervical adenocarcinomas, differentiation from primary endometrial adenocarcinomas can be made if normal endometrium is present either on a fractional dilation and curettage or on an endometrial biopsy. Contamination, however, of the endometrial sample can occur while passing the curette or biopsy instrument through the involved endocervical canal. In these cases, a careful search through multiple sections may reveal atypical endometrial hyperplasia in primary endometrial tumors and either AIS, SIL, or foci with features of a typical endocervical carcinoma in primary endocervical tumors. Immunohistochemistry can also assist (see above).

Clear Cell Adenocarcinoma

Clear cell carcinomas account for approximately 4% of adenocarcinomas of the cervix. Most of the cases of clear cell adenocarcinoma diagnosed during the 1970s, 1980s, and 1990s have been linked to prenatal exposure to diethylstilbestrol (DES) [218]. Cases diagnosed more recently have developed in the absence of exposure to DES [169]. Tumors that develop in the absence of DES exposure occur more commonly in postmenopausal women, whereas those in women exposed to DES occur in younger women [97]. The sporadically developing tumors arise in either the exocervix or endocervix, whereas the tumors developing in DES-exposed women develop predominately on the exocervix. The microscopic features of clear cell carcinoma, developing in women with or without DES exposure, are the same. There are three basic microscopic patterns: solid, tubulocystic, and papillary. The cells comprising the tumor have abundant clear cytoplasm due to the accumulation of glycogen or granular eosinophilic cytoplasm, with prominent nuclei that can be quite hyperchromatic and pleomorphic and project into the lumen of the cysts and tubules to form "hobnail cells" (➋ *Fig. 6.36*). The papillae often have hyalinized cores.

The differential diagnosis of clear cell carcinomas includes other types of cervical adenocarcinomas as well as benign processes such as the Arias-Stella reaction and microglandular and mesonephric remnant hyperplasia. Distinguishing between these entities can be difficult, especially on small biopsy samples. Microglandular hyperplasia usually lacks the degree of nuclear atypica of clear cell carcinoma and it usually contains mucin.

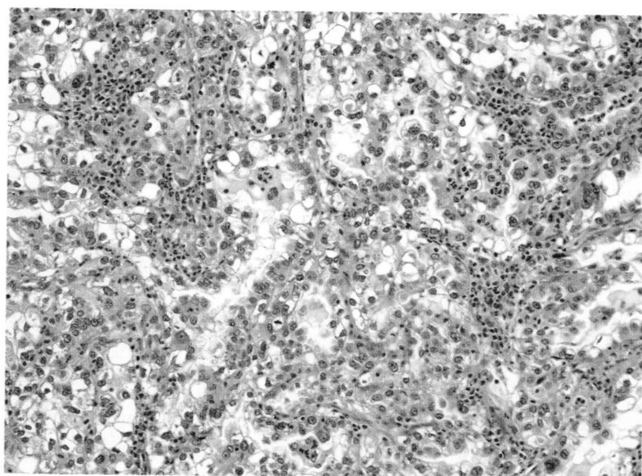

■ Fig. 6.36
Clear cell carcinoma of the cervix. **Glands are lined by markedly atypical cells with clear cytoplasm**

Microglandular hyperplasia develops in women of reproductive age, whereas most clear cell carcinomas currently occur in older women. The Arias-Stella reaction can be differentiated on the basis of lack of mitotic activity, lack of the classic patterns of clear cell carcinoma, and the clinical history of pregnancy. Rarely on low-power magnification, mesonephric remnant hyperplasia can mimic the tubulocystic pattern of clear cell carcinomas; however, examination at high power does not reveal clear or hobnail cells.

The prognosis of surgically treated patients with stage IB–IIB clear cell carcinomas without exposure to DES is similar to patients with non-clear cell adenocarcinomas [216]. The overall survival of DES exposed women with clear cell adenocarcinoma has been higher than non-DES exposed women likely due to early detection [126].

Serous Adenocarcinoma

Serous adenocarcinoma of the cervix is an uncommon form of cervical adenocarcinoma that histologically is identical to serous adenocarcinomas arising in the endometrium. The diagnosis of primary serous cervical adenocarcinoma should be made only if spread from other gynecologic sites has been excluded. These tumors are composed of papillary tufts and complex papillae lined by cells with pleomorphic, high-grade nuclei [302]. In the largest reported series this histological variant has been associated with a poor prognosis when diagnosed at an advanced stage, but the outcome for patients with stage I tumors is similar to that of patients with cervical adenocarcinomas of the usual type [302].

Mesonephric Carcinoma

Mesonephric duct remnants are detected in up to 20% of cervices removed during routine hysterectomy, and adenocarcinomas can rarely develop in these remnants [108]. Mesonephric carcinomas are very rare, and in the past were confused with clear cell carcinomas of the cervix. Patients range in age from 34 to 72 years and most present with abnormal vaginal bleeding [46, 74, 240]. In most cases, gross inspection of the cervix reveals a mass that can be exophytic or endophytic. In contrast to the superficial location of cervical clear cell adenocarcinomas, true mesonephric adenocarcinomas develop deep in the lateral wall of the cervix, in a site corresponding to the location of mesonephric duct remnants. Therefore, they often extend into the outer third of the cervical wall. The tumors can be either pure adenocarcinomas or adenocarcinomas that are mixed with a spindle cell component. In one series, 50% of the mesonephric carcinomas contained a spindle cell component [46]. The most common appearance has been termed the ductal pattern and consists of tubular glands that vary in size and are lined by one to several layers of columnar cells (➲ *Figs. 6.37* and ➲ *6.38*). Some of the gland lumens contain PAS-positive, diastase-resistant eosinophilic secretions. Other patterns that have been described include a retiform pattern, a tubular pattern, and a sex cord pattern [46]. Mesonephric hyperplasia,

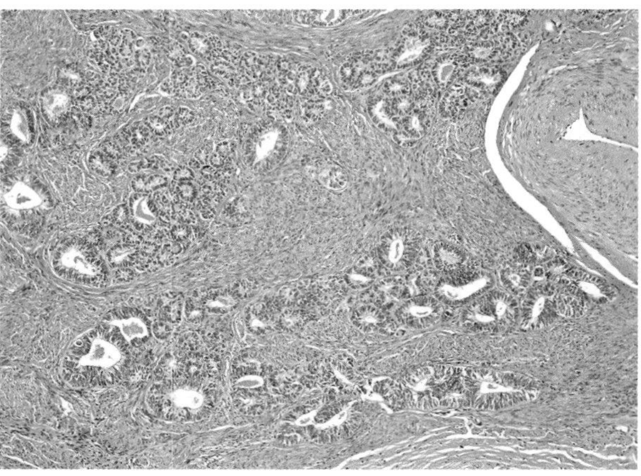

Fig. 6.37
Mesonephric carcinoma. **Tubular glands with eosinophilic secretions invade deep cervical stroma in a haphazard fashion**

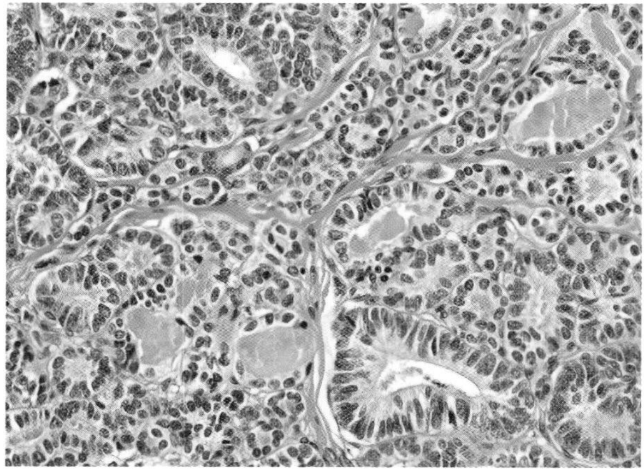

Fig. 6.38
Mesonephric carcinoma. **Densely packed small tubular glands are lined by atypical cells and contain eosinophilic secretions**

often with atypical architectural and nuclear features, is often found at the periphery of the tumor or admixed with it. The immunohistochemical profile of mesonephric carcinomas is similar to that of normal mesonephric duct remnants. Epithelial markers (including CK7 and EMA) are positive and vimentin expression is present in 70% of cases. Calretinin is found in 88%, and androgen receptor in 33% cases, whereas monoclonal CEA, estrogen receptor protein, progesterone receptor protein, and CK20 are absent [240].

Distinguishing mesonephric carcinoma from florid mesonephric hyperplasia can be difficult because the majority of carcinomas develop in the setting of diffuse mesonephric hyperplasia [74]. In contrast to mesonephric hyperplasia, the carcinoma does not have a lobular architecture and the nuclei appear cytologically malignant. Mesonephric carcinomas with a prominent spindle cell component have to be distinguished from cervical carcinosarcoma. The carcinomatous component in the latter entity is often squamous or basaloid in contrast to tubules and glands present in mesonephric carcinomas with a prominent spindle cell component. Since there are morphologic similarities between mesonephric carcinoma and clear cell carcinoma, a diagnosis of mesonephric carcinoma should only be made if the tumor is located deep in the wall of the cervix, the endocervical mucosa is uninvolved, and there is no evidence that the patient was exposed to DES.

Stage I mesonephric carcinomas seem to have a more indolent behavior than other types of cervical adenocarcinoma [46]. However, several high-stage tumors have had an aggressive course and several tumors with a sarcomatoid component have metastasized [240].

Other Epithelial Tumors

Adenosquamous Carcinoma

Adenosquamous carcinomas are defined as tumors that contain an admixture of histologically malignant squamous and glandular cells. Adenosquamous carcinomas account for between 3.6% and 25% of all cervical cancers [69, 238, 269, 287]. They occur in both young and old women and can occur during pregnancy. The squamous component generally includes areas that are well differentiated and contain either keratin "pearls" or sheets of cells with individual cell keratinization. To make the diagnosis of adenosquamous carcinoma, there must be sufficient differentiation of the adenocarcinomatous component so that glands are histologically recognizable (➲ *Fig. 6.39*).

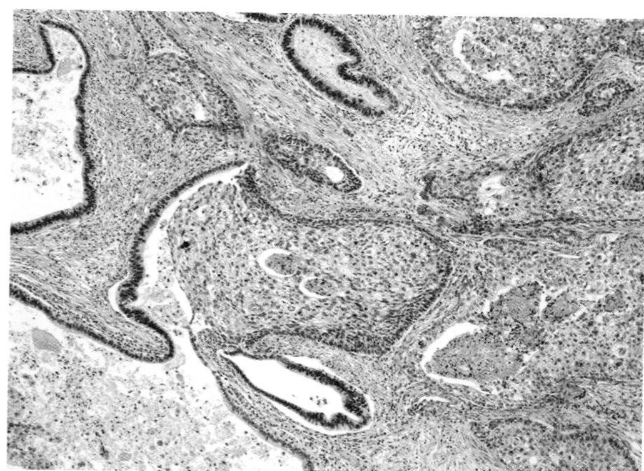

Fig. 6.39
Adenosquamous cell carcinoma. **Invasive nests of carcinoma display both squamous and glandular differentiation**

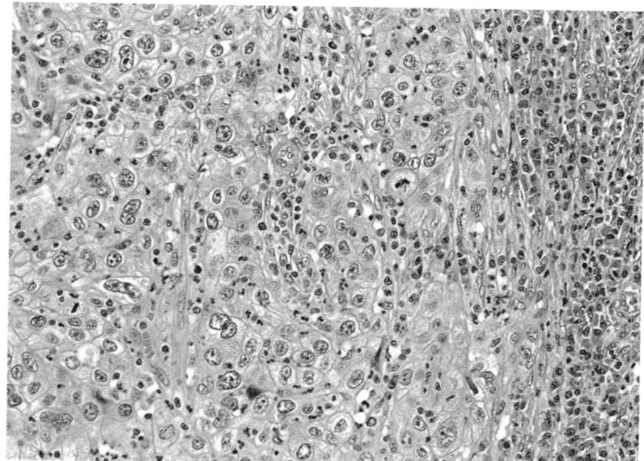

Fig. 6.40
Glassy cell carcinoma. **This poorly differentiated variant of adenosquamous carcinoma is characterized by notably atypical cells with abundant eosinophilic to amphophilic, "ground glass" cytoplasm, distinct cell membranes, and a prominent inflammatory infiltrate**

Although the well-differentiated forms are usually easily recognized, when the adenocarcinomatous component is less well differentiated and is present in relatively small amounts, it can easily be overlooked. The term adenosquamous carcinoma is not used for adenocarcinomas that have bland (nonmalignant)-appearing squamous differentiation. Instead, such tumors are classified as endometrioid adenocarcinomas of the cervix with squamous metaplasia. Lesions with mixed patterns of epithelial differentiation are thought to arise from the pluripotential subcolumnar reserve cells of the endocervical mucous epithelium and represent biphasic differentiation. In a recent study, squamous and glandular components were shown to be monoclonal in origin and had identical types of HPV supporting origin from a common precursor cell [264]. The prevalence of adenosquamous carcinomas may be increased in young women, and these tumors metastasize to pelvic lymph nodes twice as frequently as squamous cell carcinomas or adenocarcinomas [223, 269]. Despite the increase in pelvic lymph node metastases, the prognosis in patients with adenosquamous carcinomas has not been significantly worse than that of patients with squamous cell carcinomas in some studies, although other series have reported a poorer prognosis associated with these tumors [69, 238, 269, 287].

Glassy Cell Carcinoma

Glassy cell carcinoma is a poorly differentiated adenosquamous carcinoma with distinct microscopic features. It comprises <1% of cervical cancers. On gross examination glassy cell carcinomas are generally large and produce a barrel-shaped cervix (➋ *Fig. 6.40*). The distinctive microscopic features include: (1) uniform large polygonal cells with finely granular ground glass-type cytoplasm (hence the name glassy cell), (2) distinct cell membranes, and (3) prominent nucleoli (Fig. 6.43). The glassy cell appearance is due to abundant filaments and dilated rough endocytoplasmic reticulum [266]. In addition, the cells lack intercellular bridges, dyskeratosis, and intracellular glycogen. Mitotic figures are abundant. Lymphoplasmacytic and eosinophilic inflammatory cells characteristically heavily infiltrate the stroma. Occasionally, areas of keratin pearl and abortive lumen formation are seen together with signet-ring cells and intracellular mucin. Glassy cell carcinoma has to be distinguished from adenosquamous carcinoma treated with neoadjuvant chemoradiation therapy.

Glassy cell carcinoma has an extremely aggressive clinical course, with a poor response to radiation and surgery [197, 255]. More recently patients treated with neoadjuvant chemotherapy have been reported to have longer survival [189].

Clear Cell Adenosquamous Carcinoma

Adenosquamous carcinoma in which at least 70% of tumor cells have vacuolated, clear cytoplasm containing large amounts of glycogen has been referred to as clear cell adenosquamous carcinoma [80]. The cohesive sheets of tumor cells are frequently subdivided by connective tissue septa, which can have a prominent lymphocytic infiltrate that produces a lobulated appearance. The tumors demonstrate focal gland formation and stain positively with a mucin stain such as mucicarmine. In some clear cell adenosquamous carcinomas there are spindle-shaped cells suggesting squamous differentiation. Clear cell adenosquamous carcinomas need to be distinguished from clear cell carcinomas and glassy cell carcinoma of the cervix. Unlike clear cell carcinomas, clear cell adenosquamous carcinomas lack papillary or tubulocystic areas and hobnail cells. Clear cell adenosquamous carcinoma is associated with HPV 18 and has an aggressive clinical course. In one series, 7 of the 11 patients died of their disease, including 3 of 5 patients with stage IB disease [80].

Mucoepidermoid Carcinoma

Mucoepidermoid carcinoma (MEC) is not recognized as separate entity in the recent WHO classification of cervical tumors but is included within the category of adenosquamous carcinoma. Rearrangements of CRTC1 and MAML2 genes (translocation involving these two genes is common in minor salivary gland MEC) have been recently described [155]. None of the analyzed cervical adenosquamous carcinomas harbored rearrangements of either locus suggesting that cervical MEC is distinct from conventional cervical adenosquamous carcinoma. Morphologic criteria for diagnosing cervical MEC are identical to those of salivary gland MEC and include the presence of three cell types (epidermoid, intermediate, and mucin-producing) and lack of recognizable glands [64, 258]. In mucoepidermoid carcinoma, the squamous component is usually large cell nonkeratinizing or focally keratinizing, and the mucin-producing cells are frequently localized in the center of nests of squamous cell carcinoma. The mucinous component includes goblet or signet-ring-type cells that contain mucinocarminophilic, periodic acid-Schiff (PAS)-positive, diastase-resistant mucopolysaccharides. The mucin from these cells is extruded into the intercellular spaces or fibrous stroma, where it may collect in small or large lakes.

In some studies, MEC is more common in younger patients and has been associated with an increased risk of lymph node metastases [224, 258]. This association has led some authors to propose that MEC has a distinctive clinical presentation and contributes to a subset of highly aggressive cervical cancers occurring in young women. However, most studies have failed to detect a significant clinical difference between patients with MEC and those with pure squamous cell carcinomas of the cervix [224, 269].

Adenoid Cystic Carcinoma

Adenoid cystic carcinoma of the cervix is a relatively uncommon tumor accounting for <1% of all cervical adenocarcinomas. The tumor is most often seen in patients between the sixth and seventh decades (mean age of 71 years in the largest series) and is more common in blacks than whites [91].

Clinically, these tumors generally present as hard palpable masses that can be ulcerated or friable. The histologic features are similar to those seen in salivary gland adenoid cystic carcinomas. The tumor is characterized by nests of small basaloid cells of varying size with high nuclear-to-cytoplasmic ratios that have a cribriform appearance due to cylindrical hyaline bodies or small acini or cysts [91, 188]. In cross section, the hyaline cylinders appear round or ovoid, giving the neoplasm a sieve-like appearance (Fig. 6.41). These tumors frequently display peripheral palisading of the cells. The nuclei of the cells are small, only mildly pleomorphic, and there are occasional mitotic figures. Focal squamous differentiation and necrosis may be present. Lymphvascular invasion is common. At the electron microscopic level, the hyaline

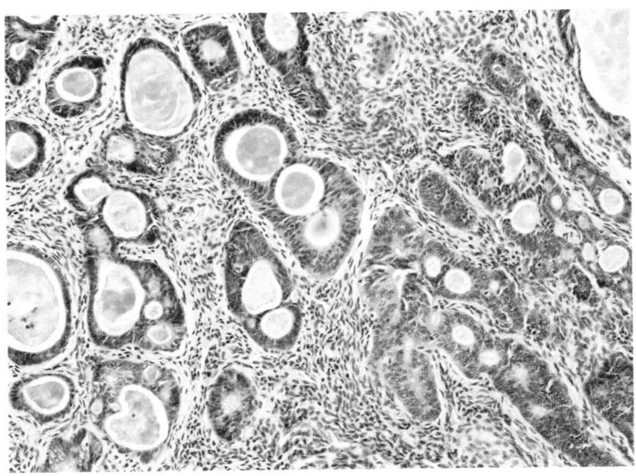

Fig. 6.41
Adenoid cystic carcinoma. **Glands demonstrate focal cribriform growth and contain central eosinophilic material**

material is partly composed of coalesced masses of basal lamina produced by the epithelial tumor cells and partly of fine precollagen and collagen fibers of fibroblastic origin. This material stains positively on immunohistochemistry for laminin and type IV collagen [91]. Unlike adenoid cystic carcinomas of other sites, cervical adenoid cystic carcinomas contain few myoepithelial cells as detected by electron microscopy or S-100 and actin immunohistochemical stains. The basaloid cells stain positively on immunohistochemistry with MNF 116 and CAM 5.2 (low molecular weight cytokeratin) [91]. A predominance of solid foci is seen in up to 20% of cases (so-called solid variant of adenoid cystic carcinoma) [5].

Integration of high-risk HPV DNA, including 16, has been implicated in the pathogenesis of adenoid cystic carcinoma [204]. Grayson has proposed the "reserve cell origin" for the tumor claiming that adenoid cystic carcinoma and the basaloid cystic carcinoma of the cervix derive from a common progenitor cell [91].

Adenoid cystic carcinoma behaves aggressively with frequent local recurrences or metastatic spread. In a review of 43 cases, overall survival for patients with stage I disease was 56% at 3–5 years [213]. While some studies have reported a higher survival rate, it appears to be considerably lower than other types of stage I cervical cancer. Adenoid cystic carcinoma of the cervix should be differentiated from adenoid basal carcinoma of the cervix.

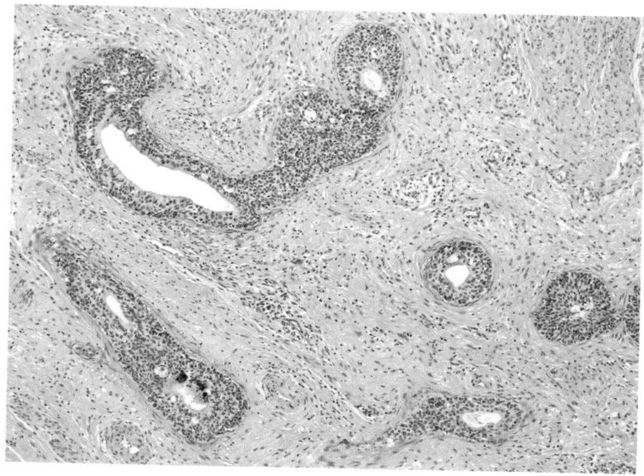

◘ Fig. 6.42
Adenoid basal carcinoma. **Nests and islands of carcinoma deep in cervical stroma exhibit basaloid features with central glandular differentiation**

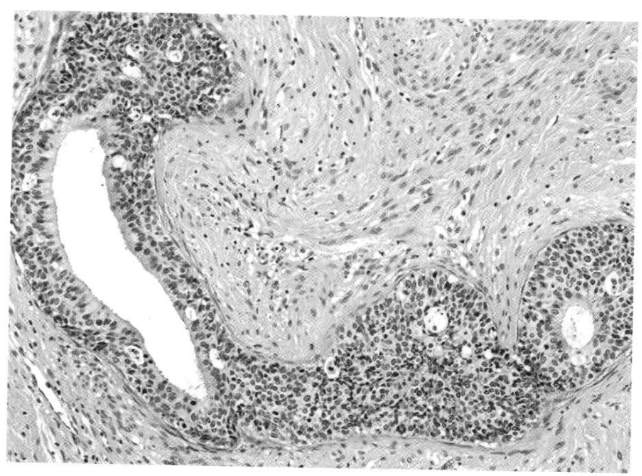

◘ Fig. 6.43
Adenoid basal carcinoma. **Island of carcinoma demonstrates both basaloid and central glandular differentiation; nuclei are hyperchromatic and several mitotic figures are evident**

Adenoid Basal Carcinoma

Adenoid basal carcinoma shares histologic features with adenoid cystic carcinoma and the two entities are often confused. Adenoid basal carcinomas are uncommon neoplasms that account for less than 1% of cervical adenocarcinomas and usually are found in postmenopausal, especially black, women [29, 73]. The mean age of patients with adenoid basal carcinoma is approximately 64 years.

Patients with adenoid basal carcinoma are usually asymptomatic without grossly detectable masses. Adenoid basal carcinomas are usually detected as unexpected findings in patients undergoing hysterectomy or cone biopsy for a coexistent SIL or another reason. Tumors are composed of small, uniform basaloid cells resembling basal cell carcinomas of the skin. The cells are arranged in small nests and cords with a rounded or lobulated appearance (➲ *Figs. 6.42* and ➲ *6.43*). At the periphery of the nests palisading of the nuclei is seen, and some of the nests have central cystic spaces that can be filled with necrotic debris. In the center of the nests there also can be squamous or glandular differentiation. Adenoid basal carcinoma shares some histologic features with adenoid cystic carcinoma and the two entities are often confused. Adenoid basal carcinomas can usually be distinguished from adenoid cystic carcinomas by the lack of the characteristic intraluminal hyaline material frequently present in adenoid cystic carcinomas; the presence of smaller, less pleomorphic nuclei; and less mitotic activity than is characteristic of adenoid cystic carcinomas [29]. Both adenoid basal and adenoid cystic carcinomas are frequently associated with SIL. Therefore, these features should not be used to distinguish between the two types of tumors. It should be noted that adenoid basal carcinomas can be found in association with adenoid cystic carcinomas, adenosquamous cell carcinomas, and squamous cell carcinomas of the cervix and are associated with high-risk types of HPV [72, 204].

Adenoid basal carcinomas of the type reported in the older literature (which is dominated by tumors having features of "adenoid basal epithelioma" – see below) almost uniformly pursue a benign clinical course. Although tumors can penetrate into the wall of the cervix and almost half the reported cases are classified as stage IB, tumors with typical histologic features of adenoid basal carcinoma do not metastasize or show any evidence of aggressive clinical behavior. There are rare reported cases that acted aggressively. Aggressive tumors typically have irregularly shaped nests of basaloid cells that infiltrate into the stroma and elicit a stromal reaction analogous to morpheaform basal cell carcinoma of the skin [72, 91].

Recently, in view of overwhelmingly benign behavior of tumors traditionally referred to as adenoid basal carcinomas, it has been proposed that adenoid basal tumors be divided into benign and malignant types based on morphologic features. The term "adenoid basal epithelioma" has been suggested for the low-grade variety; these tumors resemble basal cell carcinoma of the skin with squamous differentiation [29] (➲ *Figs. 6.44* and ➲ *6.45*). The high-grade variety, which is often associated with adenoid basal epithelioma, has an infiltrative component with architectural and cytologic features of carcinoma and is classified as "adenoid basal carcinoma." Additional diagnostic terms can be applied to describe any other accompanying specific components of carcinoma, which can include basaloid, squamous, and adenoid cystic carcinoma components [29, 204].

Neuroendocrine Tumors

Neuroendocrine tumors of the cervix are relatively rare. The terminology that has been used to describe these tumors has varied over the last 25 years resulting in difficulties in interpreting clinicopathologic studies. Because the morphologic features of cervical neuroendocrine tumors are similar to those in the lung, the current WHO classification for cervical tumors is the same as the one used for the lung. The four categories of neuroendocrine tumors of the cervix include: (1) typical carcinoid tumor, (2) atypical carcinoid tumor, (3) large cell neuroendocrine carcinoma, and (4) small cell carcinoma.

The exact cellular origin of neuroendocrine tumors of the cervix is unknown. Small numbers of argyrophil cells, a potential precursor for neuroendocrine tumors, are present in the exocervical epithelium of ~40% of women and in the endocervical epithelium in about 20% of women [75]. However argyrophil cells are also detected in about 60% of minimal deviation adenocarcinomas of the cervix

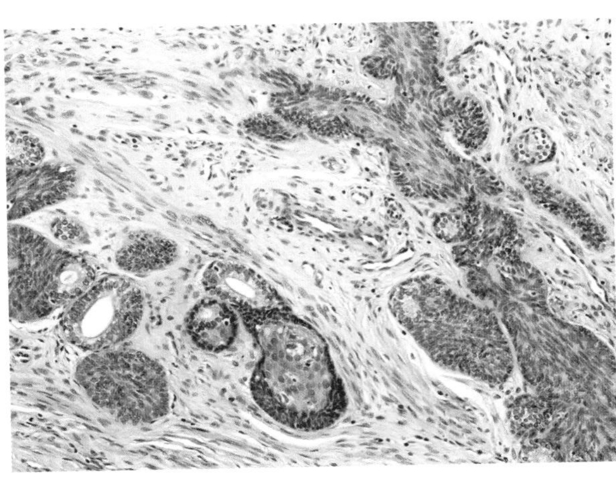

Fig. 6.44
Adenoid basal epithelioma. **Small nests of bland tumor with basaloid, squamous, and focal central glandular differentiation are situated within cervical stroma**

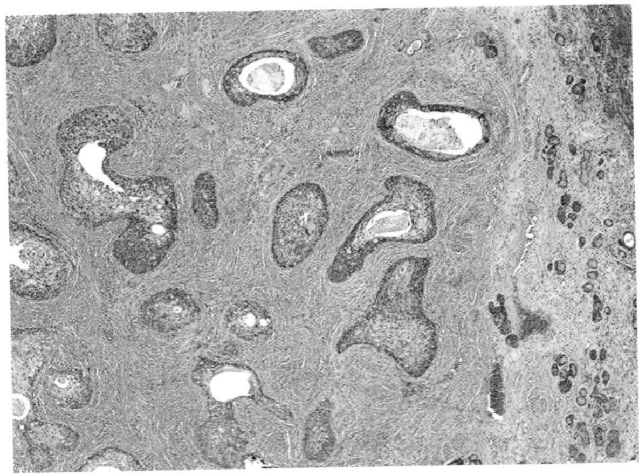

Fig. 6.45
Adenoid basal epithelioma associated with invasive squamous cell carcinoma. **Larger islands of squamous cell carcinoma invade cervical stroma, with smaller adjacent nests of adenoid basal epithelioma**

and in 14% of other types of cervical adenocarcinomas or adenosquamous carcinomas [67].

Typical and Atypical Carcinoid Tumor

Tumors that have been categorized as well-differentiated carcinoid tumors of the cervix were originally described by Albores-Saavedra et al., and were classified as carcinoid tumors because they contained neuroendocrine granules and were histologically similar to intestinal carcinoid tumors [4]. Microscopically these well-differentiated tumors grow in trabecular, nodular, or cord-like patterns. Rosette-like structures are common, but follicles with eosinophilic material are uncommon. The neoplastic cells have round to oval spindle-shaped nuclei and finely granular cytoplasm. Mitoses are rare. Atypical carcinoids share the same architectural patterns of growth as typical carcinoids, but are much more cellular than typical carcinoids and have increased mitotic activity (5–10 mitoses/10 high-power fields), moderate cytologic atypia, and focal areas of necrosis (*Table 6.9*) [3]. These tumors stain positively for synaptophysin, chromogranin A, and neuron-specific enolase. Neurosecretory granules can be identified in these tumors by electron microscopy.

Typical and atypical carcinoid tumors are uncommon [282]. Some of the tumors that have been previously described as well-differentiated cervical carcinoid tumors appear to be adenocarcinomas of the cervix that focally resemble carcinoid tumors of the intestinal tract and have neuroendocrine differentiation. It should be noted that neurosecretory granules can be identified in many carcinomas of the cervix if a diligent search is made. Although early reports suggested that these tumors had a relatively good prognosis, more recent reports demonstrate that these tumors can act in a malignant fashion with local and distant metastasis. To date, none of the published cases has been associated with the carcinoid syndrome.

Large Cell Neuroendocrine Carcinoma

Large cell neuroendocrine carcinomas are poorly differentiated tumors that typically grow in organoid, trabecular, or cord-like patterns, although some cases only grow in sheets (*Fig. 6.46*). Peripheral palisading of the cells and

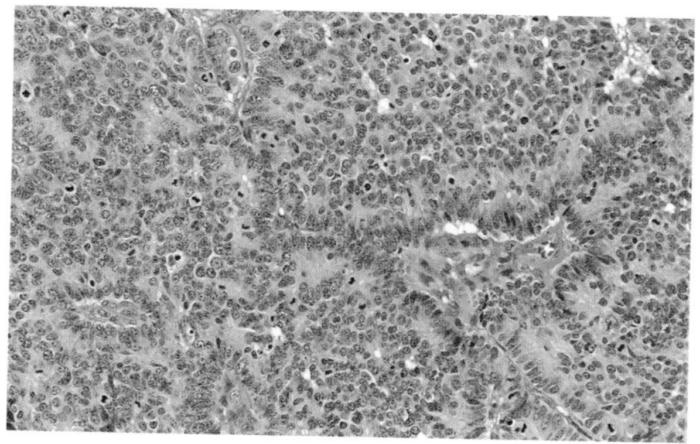

Fig. 6.46
Neuroendocrine carcinoma. **Solid islands of carcinoma exhibit some cords and palisading typical of neuroendocrine differentiation; nuclei are atypical and numerous mitotic figures are evident**

Table 6.9
Histologic features used for distinguishing neuroendocrine tumors of the cervix

Tumor	Patterns	Mitoses	Nuclear atypia	Neurosecretory granules[a]	Necrosis
Typical carcinoid tumor	Trabecular, insular, sheetlike	Rare	No	Yes	No
Atypical carcinoid tumor	Trabecular, insular, sheetlike	5–10/10 HPF	Moderate	Yes	Focal
Large cell neuroendocrine carcinoma	Sheets, organoid trabecular, cordlike	10/10 HPF	Marked	Yes	Moderate
Small cell carcinoma	Sheets, nests, trabecular, cordlike	10/10 HPF	Moderate	Sometimes	Extensive

[a]By electron microscopy or immunohistochemistry.
HPF, high-power fields.
Adapted from [3, 87]

geographic patterns of necrosis are frequently present. The cells of large cell neuroendocrine carcinomas are large with abundant eosinophilic cytoplasm, and small eosinophilic cytoplasmic granules can sometimes be identified on hematoxylin- and eosin-stained sections. The cells have vesicular high-grade nuclei with prominent nucleoli. Mitotic figures are numerous (>10 mitoses/10 high-power fields). The tumor cells usually stain for neuron-specific enolase, chromogranin A, and synaptophysin. Cytokeratin stains are often positive and CEA is expressed in 70% of cases [87]. Large cell neuroendocrine carcinomas are often associated with glandular lesions. In the series of Gilks et al., 66% of large cell neuroendocrine carcinomas had a coexisting adenocarcinoma in situ and 25% had a coexisting cervical adenocarcinoma [87].

Atypical carcinoids and large cell neuroendocrine carcinomas can be distinguished based on mitotic activity, nuclear atypia, and degree of necrosis (*Table 6.9*) [3]. It is more difficult to differentiate between large cell neuroendocrine carcinoma and poorly differentiated cervical adenocarcinomas or squamous cell carcinomas. It is important that trabecular and insular growth patterns be looked for in poorly differentiated cervical tumors and that stains for neuroendocrine markers be used whenever there is an indication of neuroendocrine differentiation. It should be cautioned, however, that occasional typical cervical adenocarcinomas and adenosquamous carcinomas can stain focally with neuroendocrine markers or contain occasional argyrophilic cells [227]. In contrast, large cell neuroendocrine carcinoma have evidence of neuroendocrine differentiation by routine light microscopy and show more diffuse expression of neuroendocrine markers. Finally large cell neuroendocrine carcinoma has to be distinguished from malignant melanoma. Presence of melanin pigment and immunoreactivity for S-100 and HMB-45 facilitate the distinction between these tumors.

Several studies have explored the role of HPV in large cell neuroendocrine carcinomas. In the largest series, HPV 16 was detected by in situ hybridization or polymerase chain reaction in 58% and HPV 18 in 16% cases [90]. Large cell neuroendocrine carcinomas are highly aggressive neoplasms. In the review of 31 published cases, 65% patients died of disease within 3 years of diagnosis [87].

Small Cell Carcinoma

Small cell carcinomas of the cervix are histologically identical to their counterparts at other sites such as the lung. In most series these tumors account for 1–2% (range 0.5–5%) of all cervical tumors [1, 85]. The age of the patients ranges from 21 to 87 years with mean and median ages in the fifth decade in most series [1, 85]. In a study comparing small cell carcinoma to nonkeratinizing squamous carcinoma composed of small cells, the mean age of women with small cell carcinoma was 36 years compared to 50 years for squamous carcinoma [9]. Most patients present with abnormal vaginal bleeding and have an obvious mass on pelvic examination. In rare cases, patients present with abdominal symptoms related to ovarian metastases [293]. The number of patients presenting with abnormal cytologic examination is smaller than in patients with squamous cell carcinoma. This results from lack of an in situ component and rapid growth of the tumor [273].

Pathologic Findings

Grossly, small cell carcinomas range in size from small, clinically inapparent lesions to large ulcerated lesions measuring more than 6 cm in greatest dimension [85]. Microscopically tumors are composed of sheets and cords of closely packed, small, scant cells with inconspicuous cytoplasm, closely resembling the cells of "oat cell" carcinoma of the lung. The cells have hyperchromatic nuclei with finely stippled chromatin, inconspicuous nucleoli, and high nuclear to cytoplasmic ratios. Mitotic rate is high with three or more mitoses present in most high-power fields (*Fig. 6.47*). The nuclear shape varies from

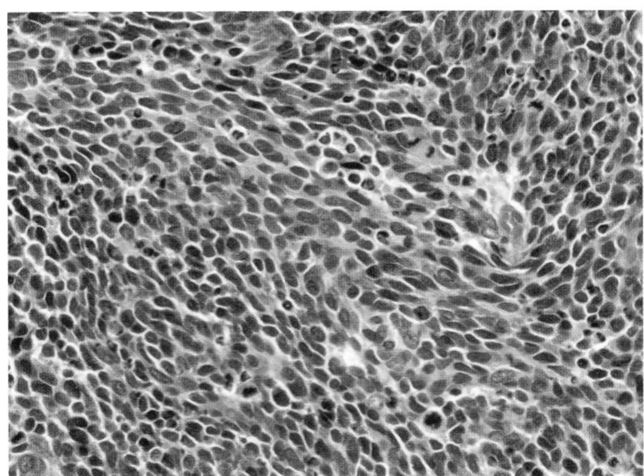

Fig. 6.47
Small cell carcinoma. **Tumor is composed of cells with enlarged, atypical hyperchromatic nuclei, numerous mitotic figures, scanty cytoplasm. Cellular molding also is present**

round to spindled, and nuclear molding is a characteristic feature. Smudging of the nucleus and extensive crush artifact frequently obscures nuclear detail and nucleoli. Small areas of either squamous or glandular differentiation can be present but should account for less than 5% of the total tumor volume [85].

Immunohistochemical and Molecular Genetic Findings

Neuroendocrine dense-core granules can be detected using Grimelius stains or electron microscopy in most cases. Although small cell carcinomas have been associated with ectopic ACTH, insulin, and gastrin production, clinical symptoms related to ectopic hormone production are uncommon [85, 293]. This suggests that hormones are produced in an inactive form, in insufficient amount, or are rapidly inactivated. By immunohistochemistry, neuroendocrine markers such as neuron-specific enolase, chromogranin, or synaptophysin are present in many cases; however, staining might be very focal [85]. Small cell carcinomas show variable expression of cytokeratins, epithelial membrane antigen, as well as variety of hormones and polypeptides including ACTH, calcitonin, serotonin, gastrin, substance P, VIP and somatostatin [1, 9, 112, 265].

In recent studies virtually all cervical small cell carcinomas have been associated with high-risk HPV types 18 and 16, with type 18 being the most prevalent, detected in 82% of the cases [107, 275]. Data on *TP53* mutation in small cell carcinomas are conflicting. Wistuba et al. has reported *TP53* gene mutations and loss of heterozygosity at the 17p/p53 locus in six of eight cervical small cell carcinomas, among which four cases were positive for HPV 18 or 16 [282]. However, no mutations or loss of heterozygosity at the 17p/p53 locus were found in other studies [165, 198, 276].

Differential Diagnosis

Differentiation between small cell carcinoma and nonkeratinizing squamous carcinoma with small cells can be difficult. The diagnosis of small cell carcinoma should be reserved for tumors composed of small cells in which squamous or glandular differentiation is absent or minor. Women with small cell carcinoma tend to be younger than women with nonkeratinizing squamous carcinoma with small cells. Histologically, cells of nonkeratinizing squamous carcinoma with small cells resemble those of high-grade SIL and lack the nuclear molding and extensive crush artifact present in most small cell carcinomas. Small cell carcinomas invade the stroma diffusely in trabeculae and poorly defined nests. In contrast, nonkeratinizing squamous carcinomas with small cells invade the stroma in discrete nests. In an individual case, immunohistochemistry for neuroendocrine markers may not be helpful because 40% of nonkeratinizing squamous carcinomas with small cells are positive for neuroendocrine markers and 40% of small cell carcinomas are positive for cytokeratins [9]. Nuclear staining for p63 confirms squamous differentiation in nonkeratinizing small cell carcinomas, while neuroendocrine type small cell carcinomas are negative for this marker [274]. Due to the presence of high-risk HPV in nonkeratinizing small cell carcinomas, they are positive for p16. Expression of thyroid transcription factor 1 (TTF1) has been reported in cervical small cell carcinomas and can cause diagnostic problems in tumors that metastasize to the lungs [2]. Immunohistochemical staining with antibodies against leukocyte common antigen and neuroendocrine markers can be useful for differentiating between small cell carcinoma from lymphoproliferative disorders.

Clinical Behavior and Treatment

Small cell carcinoma of the cervix is a highly aggressive tumor [1, 303]. Lymphvascular invasion is present in 90% of cases and is often extensive [1]. The prognosis of small cell carcinoma of the cervix is worse than that of stage-comparable, poorly differentiated squamous carcinoma [9]. Most patients have advanced disease at the time of hysterectomy even if they present clinically with stage I disease. In one study, 57% of clinical stage IB or IIA patients had lymph node metastases [237]. In another series, 9 of 12 patients died as a direct result of their tumor, and the median duration of survival of those dying of disease was only 12.5 months [273]. Similarly, in the series of Gersell et al., 10 of 15 patients died as a direct result of their tumor [85].

Combined modality treatments with chemotherapy and radiotherapy are currently used in management of small cell carcinoma. In a recent series, patients with early stage disease treated with platinum-based chemotherapy in addition to radiation had significantly better overall and disease-free survival when compared to patients who did not receive chemotherapy as part of their initial treatment [303].

Mixed Epithelial and Mesenchymal Tumors

Malignant mesenchymal tumors that can arise in the cervix include leiomyosarcoma, endocervical stromal sarcoma, embryonal rhabdomyosarcoma (botryoid type), alveolar soft part sarcoma, malignant schwannomas, and osteosarcomas (see Chap. 10, Mesenchymal Tumors of the Uterus) (*Figs. 6.48* and *6.49*). Primary cervical sarcomas are rare, of which the most common is leiomyosarcoma.

Primary cervical mixed epithelial and mesenchymal tumors include müllerian adenosarcomas and malignant müllerian mixed tumors (MMMT) of the cervix. Cervical MMMT are less common than their much more common uterine counterparts [47]. Both usually occur in postmenopausal women and both typically form polypoid or pedunculated masses. The mean age of patients was 65 years in the largest published series [47]. However, cervical MMMTs differ in their histologic appearance from MMMTs arising in the uterus. The carcinomatous component in cervical MMMT is in the form of cervical carcinoma type rather than endometrial carcinoma as seen in uterine MMMT. The most common carcinomatous pattern in cervical tumors is a basaloid pattern that consists of anastomosing densely cellular trabeculae composed of small cells with scant cytoplasm and peripheral palisading. Other epithelial patterns include typical squamous cell carcinoma and endometrioid adenocarcinoma. Adenoid basal and adenoid cystic components have also been reported in several cases [168]. The sarcomatous element is typically homologous and frequently has the appearance of a fibrosarcoma or endometrial stromal sarcoma. The sarcomatous element is frequently high grade and may have myxoid change.

Extension of uterine MMMT to the cervix is in the differential diagnosis of cervical MMMT. The correct diagnosis is based on the dominant location of the tumor, the appearance of the carcinomatous component and detection of HPV. In a study of eight patients with cervical MMMT, HPV-DNA was detected by polymerase chain reaction in all cases. Interestingly, using in-situ hybridization HPV-16 DNA was detected in both epithelial and sarcomatous components in three cases [92]. Although the number of reported cases is small, cervical MMMTs may have a better prognosis than their uterine counterparts.

Only a small number of müllerian adenosarcomas of the cervix have been reported. They may occur more frequently than reported because they are frequently misdiagnosed [84, 118, 133]. Adenosarcomas occur in women between the ages of 14 and 67 years, with a mean age of 38 years [118, 133]. Women typically present with vaginal bleeding or recurrent cervical polyps. Microscopically, tumors usually demonstrate thick papillae covered with a typical endocervical-type endothelium. The appearance of the sarcomatous component can vary considerably. In some tumors, it consists of mitotically active, plump spindle cells that form periglandular cuffs and

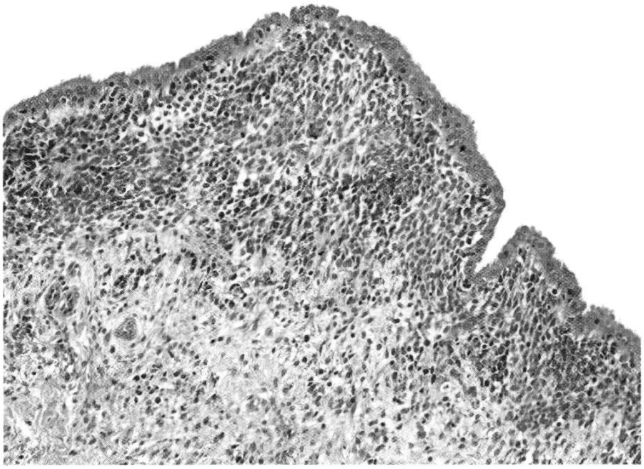

Fig. 6.48
Embryonal rhabdomyosarcoma. **Polypoid tumor has a cambium layer of hypercellular stroma immediately beneath the benign endocervical epithelium**

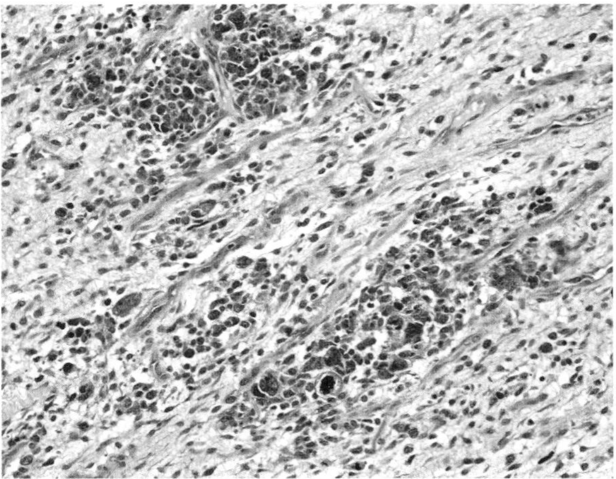

Fig. 6.49
Embryonal rhabdomyosarcoma. **Hypercellular foci within background edematous hypocellular stroma are composed of immature atypical cells with scant cytoplasm; mitotic figures and apoptotic bodies are usually evident**

a cambium layer under the surface epithelium. At least two mitotic figures per 10 high power fields are required to make a diagnosis of adenosarcoma, but in most cases the mitotic index exceeds 4 per 10 high power fields. In other tumors, the stromal component contains foci that are more embryonic in appearance, with small, undifferentiated round cells that are mitotically active. Heterologous sarcomatous elements including strap cells, lipoblasts, cartilage, and osteoid can be present.

The differential diagnosis includes adenofibroma, atypical endocervical polyp, adenomyoma of the cervix, and MMMT. Adenofibroma is also a biphasic lesion, but both the epithelium and stroma are benign. Atypical endocervical polyps show increased stromal cellularity and reactive nuclear atypia but these changes are often focal and mitotic activity is absent. Adenomyomas can be distinguished from adenosarcoma by the presence of well-defined myomatous component. The prognosis of cervical adenosarcoma is usually good after surgical therapy, although several patients have died of disease or developed recurrent tumor [84, 118, 133].

Miscellaneous Tumors

Primary malignant melanoma is among the least common of the malignant tumors that arise in the cervix; 27 patients have been reported [38, 44]. Common presenting signs include vaginal bleeding, frequently of short duration. In most instances, the lesion is pigmented and dark brown. The diagnosis of primary melanoma of the cervix is based on the histologic demonstration of junctional changes in the squamous epithelium and the absence of similar lesions elsewhere in the body. Morphologically, it is identical to melanoma arising in the skin and extragenital mucous membranes; it frequently contains intracytoplasmic melanin pigment granules. Some tumors are amelanotic and have to be distinguished from undifferentiated carcinoma. Rarely cervical malignant melanoma can be composed of clear cells. Immunohistochemical staining for HMB 45, Melan-A (MART-1), S-100 protein and absence of epithelial markers are helpful to rule out clear cell carcinoma. Spindle cell malignant melanoma has to be distinguished from leiomyosarcoma or malignant peripheral nerve sheet tumor. In contrast to malignant melanoma, leiomyocarcoma expresses smooth muscle markers and is negative for melanocytic markers. The cell pigmentation, nesting, and the presence of an atypical epidermal or junctional component, together with diffuse, strong reactivity for S100 protein and positivity for other melanocytic markers help to differentiate melanoma from malignant peripheral nerve sheet tumor [58]. The prognosis of primary malignant melanoma is poor, with only 25% survival rate for patients with stage I disease [44].

Primary choriocarcinoma and epithelioid trophoblastic tumors in the cervix are rare [123]. The gross and microscopic appearance, as well as the clinical course, is identical with those found in the uterine corpus.

Primary cervical germ cell tumors have been described: these include both the mature teratomas and yolk sac tumors [21, 52]. There are also case reports of primitive neuroectodermal tumors (PNET) of the cervix [246]. These tumors appear to be identical to PNETs occurring at other sites, and in some cases have stained positive on immunohistochemistry for the restricted surface antigen MIC-2 and contained the EWS/FLI-1 chimeric mRNA transcript characteristic of PNET/Ewing's sarcoma family.

Secondary Tumors

Direct extension from a pelvic tumor is the most common source of cervical involvement by secondary carcinoma, often originating in the endometrium, rectum, or bladder. Intrapelvic and intragenital, lymphatic, or vascular metastases to the cervix occur less frequently. These lesions are usually associated with ovarian carcinoma, endometrial adenocarcinoma, and less commonly with transitional cell carcinoma of the bladder [154, 182]. Another lesion that has a relatively high rate of cervical metastasis is choriocarcinoma. Sarcomas of the uterine corpus may also involve the cervix. Metastases to the cervix from distant primary sites are rare, the most common being the gastrointestinal tract (colon and stomach), ovary, and breast. Instances of metastatic carcinoma from the kidney, gallbladder, pancreas, lung, thyroid, and malignant melanoma have also been described. On occasion, metastases may occur primarily as cervical involvement and pose a differential diagnostic problem. Unusual gross appearance or histologic patterns, e.g., signet-ring cell carcinoma or clear cell carcinoma, provide a clue to the possibility of origin from a distant primary site.

References

1. Abeler VM, Holm R et al (1994) Small cell carcinoma of the cervix. A clinicopathologic study of 26 patients. Cancer 73(3):672–677
2. Agoff SN, Lamps LW et al (2000) Thyroid transcription factor-1 is expressed in extrapulmonary small cell carcinomas but not in other extrapulmonary neuroendocrine tumors. Mod Pathol 13(3):238–242

3. Albores-Saavedra J, Gersell D et al (1997) Terminology of endocrine tumors of the uterine cervix: results of a workshop sponsored by the College of American Pathologists and the National Cancer Institute. Arch Pathol Lab Med 121(1):34–39
4. Albores-Saavedra J, Larraza O et al (1976) Carcinoid of the uterine cervix: additional observations on a new tumor entity. Cancer 38(6):2328–2342
5. Albores-Saavedra J, Manivel C et al (1992) The solid variant of adenoid cystic carcinoma of the cervix. Int J Gynecol Pathol 11(1):2–10
6. Alfsen GC, Kristensen GB et al (2001) Histologic subtype has minor importance for overall survival in patients with adenocarcinoma of the uterine cervix: a population-based study of prognostic factors in 505 patients with nonsquamous cell carcinomas of the cervix. Cancer 92(9):2471–2483
7. Alfsen GC, Thoresen SO et al (2000) Histopathologic subtyping of cervical adenocarcinoma reveals increasing incidence rates of endometrioid tumors in all age groups: a population based study with review of all nonsquamous cervical carcinomas in Norway from 1966 to 1970, 1976 to 1980, and 1986 to 1990. Cancer 89(6): 1291–1299
8. al-Nafussi AI, Hughes DE (1994) Histological features of CIN3 and their value in predicting invasive microinvasive squamous carcinoma. J Clin Pathol 47(9):799–804
9. Ambros RA, Park JS et al (1991) Evaluation of histologic, morphometric, and immunohistochemical criteria in the differential diagnosis of small cell carcinomas of the cervix with particular reference to human papillomavirus types 16 and 18. Mod Pathol 4(5):586–593
10. Andersen ES, Nielsen K et al (1995) The reliability of preconization diagnostic evaluation in patients with cervical intraepithelial neoplasia and microinvasive carcinoma. Gynecol Oncol 59(1):143–147
11. Andersson S, Rylander E et al (2001) The role of human papillomavirus in cervical adenocarcinoma carcinogenesis. Eur J Cancer 37(2):246–250
12. Ansari-Lari MA, Staebler A et al (2004) Distinction of endocervical and endometrial adenocarcinomas: immunohistochemical p16 expression correlated with human papillomavirus (HPV) DNA detection. Am J Surg Pathol 28(2):160–167
13. Anton-Culver H, Bloss JD et al (1992) Comparison of adenocarcinoma and squamous cell carcinoma of the uterine cervix: a population-based epidemiologic study. Am J Obstet Gynecol 166(5):1507–1514
14. Aoyama C, Peters J et al (1998) Uterine cervical dysplasia and cancer: identification of c-myc status by quantitative polymerase chain reaction. Diagn Mol Pathol 7(6):324–330
15. Appleby P, Beral V et al (2006) Carcinoma of the cervix and tobacco smoking: collaborative reanalysis of individual data on 13,541 women with carcinoma of the cervix and 23,017 women without carcinoma of the cervix from 23 epidemiological studies. Int J Cancer 118(6):1481–1495
16. Attanoos R, Nahar K et al (1995) Primary adenocarcinoma of the cervix. A clinicopathologic study of prognostic variables in 55 cases. Int J Gynecol Cancer 5(3):179–186
17. Averette HE, Nelson JH Jr et al (1976) Diagnosis and management of microinvasive (stage IA) carcinoma of the uterine cervix. Cancer 38(1 SUPPL):414–425
18 Averette HE, Nguyen HN et al (1993) Radical hysterectomy for invasive cervical cancer. A 25-year prospective experience with the Miami technique. Cancer 71(4 Suppl):1422–1437
19. Bachtiary B, Obermair A et al (2002) Impact of multiple HPV infection on response to treatment and survival in patients receiving radical radiotherapy for cervical cancer. Int J Cancer 102(3):237–243
20. Bais AG, Kooi S et al (2005) Lymphoepithelioma-like carcinoma of the uterine cervix: absence of Epstein-Barr virus, but presence of a multiple human papillomavirus infection. Gynecol Oncol 97(2): 716–718
21. Bell MC, Schmidt-Grimminger DC et al (1996) A cervical teratoma with invasive squamous cell carcinoma in an HIV-infected patient: a case report. Gynecol Oncol 60(3):475–479
22. Benedet JL, Anderson GH (1996) Stage IA carcinoma of the cervix revisited. Obstet Gynecol 87(6):1052–1059
23. Benedet JL, Anderson GH et al (1985) Colposcopic accuracy in the diagnosis of microinvasive and occult invasive carcinoma of the cervix. Obstet Gynecol 65(4):557–562
24. Benedet JL, Bender H et al (2000) FIGO staging classifications and clinical practice guidelines in the management of gynecologic cancers. FIGO Committee on Gynecologic Oncology. Int J Gynaecol Obstet 70(2):209–262
25. Benedetti-Panici P, Maneschi F et al (2000) Early cervical carcinoma: the natural history of lymph node involvement redefined on the basis of thorough parametrectomy and giant section study. Cancer 88(10): 2267–2274
26. Berek JS, Hacker NF et al (1985) Adenocarcinoma of the uterine cervix: histologic variables associated with lymph node metastasis and survival. Obstet Gynecol 65(1):46–52
27. Bohm JW, Krupp PJ et al (1976) Lymph node metastasis in microinvasive epidermoid cancer of the cervix. Obstet Gynecol 48(1):65–67
28. Boyes DA, Worth AJ et al (1970) The results of treatment of 4389 cases of preclinical cervical squamous carcinoma. J Obstet Gynaecol Br Commonw 77(9):769–780
29. Brainard JA, Hart WR (1998) Adenoid basal epitheliomas of the uterine cervix: a reevaluation of distinctive cervical basaloid lesions currently classified as adenoid basal carcinoma and adenoid basal hyperplasia. Am J Surg Pathol 22(8):965–975
30. Bray F, Carstensen B et al (2005) Incidence trends of adenocarcinoma of the cervix in 13 European countries. Cancer Epidemiol Biomarkers Prev 14(9):2191–2199
31. Brinck U, Jakob C et al (2000) Papillary squamous cell carcinoma of the uterine cervix: report of three cases and a review of its classification. Int J Gynecol Pathol 19(3):231–235
32. Broders AC (1920) Squamous-cell epithelioma of the lip: a study of five hundred and thirty-seven cases. JAMA 74:656–664
33. Bulk S, Visser O et al (2005) Cervical cancer in the Netherlands 1989-1998: Decrease of squamous cell carcinoma in older women, increase of adenocarcinoma in younger women. Int J Cancer 113(6): 1005–1009
34. Burghardt E, Girardi F et al (1991) Microinvasive carcinoma of the uterine cervix (International Federation of Gynecology and Obstetrics Stage IA). Cancer 67(4):1037–1045
35. Burghardt E, Holzer E (1977) Diagnosis and treatment of microinvasive carcinoma of the cervix uteri. Obstet Gynecol 49(6):641–653
36. Cairns M, Cruickshank M (2007) A review of women with microinvasive cervical cancer in the Grampian region. J Low Genit Tract Dis 11(4):290–293
37. Cantu de Leon D, Perez Montiel D et al (2009) Serous adenocarcinoma of the fallopian tube, associated with verrucous carcinoma of the uterine cervix: a case report of synchronic rare gynecological tumors. World J Surg Oncol 7:20

38. Cantuaria G, Angioli R et al (1999) Primary malignant melanoma of the uterine cervix: case report and review of the literature. Gynecol Oncol 75(1):170–174
39. Castellsague X, Diaz M et al (2006) Worldwide human papillomavirus etiology of cervical adenocarcinoma and its cofactors: implications for screening and prevention. J Natl Cancer Inst 98(5):303–315
40. Chen RJ, Lin YH et al (1999) Influence of histologic type and age on survival rates for invasive cervical carcinoma in Taiwan. Gynecol Oncol 73(2):184–190
41. Cheng WF, Chen CA et al (2000) Vascular endothelial growth factor and prognosis of cervical carcinoma. Obstet Gynecol 96(5 Pt 1): 721–726
42. Chichareon S, Herrero R et al (1998) Risk factors for cervical cancer in Thailand: a case-control study. J Natl Cancer Inst 90(1):50–57
43. Cho NH, Joo HJ et al (1998) Detection of human papillomavirus in warty carcinoma of the uterine cervix: comparison of immunohistochemistry, in situ hybridization and in situ polymerase chain reaction methods. Pathol Res Pract 194(10):713–720
44. Clark KC, Butz WR et al (1999) Primary malignant melanoma of the uterine cervix: case report with world literature review. Int J Gynecol Pathol 18(3):265–273
45. Clement PB, Scully RE (1982) Carcinoma of the cervix: histologic types. Semin Oncol 9(3):251–264
46. Clement PB, Young RH et al (1995) Malignant mesonephric neoplasms of the uterine cervix. A report of eight cases, including four with a malignant spindle cell component. Am J Surg Pathol 19(10):1158–1171
47. Clement PB, Zubovits JT et al (1998) Malignant mullerian mixed tumors of the uterine cervix: a report of nine cases of a neoplasm with morphology often different from its counterpart in the corpus. Int J Gynecol Pathol 17(3):211–222
48. Clifford G, Franceschi S et al (2006) Chapter 3: HPV type-distribution in women with and without cervical neoplastic diseases. Vaccine 24(S3):26–34
49. Clifford GM, Smith JS et al (2003) Human papillomavirus types in invasive cervical cancer worldwide: a meta-analysis. Br J Cancer 88(1):63–73
50. Connolly DC, Katabuchi H et al (2000) Somatic mutations in the STK11/LKB1 gene are uncommon in rare gynecological tumor types associated with Peutz-Jegher's syndrome. Am J Pathol 156(1): 339–345
51. Copeland LJ, Silva EG et al (1992) Superficially invasive squamous cell carcinoma of the cervix. Gynecol Oncol 45(3):307–312
52. Copeland LJ, Sneige N et al (1985) Endodermal sinus tumor of the vagina and cervix. Cancer 55(11):2558–2565
53. Coppleson M (1992) Early invasive squamous and adnocarcinoma of the cervix (FIGO stage Ia): clinical features and management. In: Gynecological oncology. Churchill Livingstone, Edinburgh, pp 631–634
54. Covens A, Kirby J et al (1999) Prognostic factors for relapse and pelvic lymph node metastases in early stage I adenocarcinoma of the cervix. Gynecol Oncol 74(3):423–427
55. Creasman WT (1995) New gynecologic cancer staging. Gynecol Oncol 58(2):157–158
56. Creasman WT, Fetter BF et al (1985) Management of stage IA carcinoma of the cervix. Am J Obstet Gynecol 153(2):164–172
57. Crum CP (1993) Papillomavirus-related changes and premalignant and malignant squamous lesions of the uterine cervix. In: Clement PB, Young RH (eds) Tumors and tumorlike lesions of the uterine corpus and cervix. Churchill Livingstone, New York, pp 51–83
58. Cruz J, Reis-Filho JS et al (2004) Malignant peripheral nerve sheath tumour-like primary cutaneous malignant melanoma. J Clin Pathol 57(2):218–220
59. Dabbs DJ, Sturtz K et al (1996) The immunohistochemical discrimination of endometrioid adenocarcinomas. Hum Pathol 27(2):172–177
60. Daya D, Young RH (1995) Florid deep glands of the uterine cervix. Another mimic of adenoma malignum. Am J Clin Pathol 103(5):614–617
61. Delgado G, Bundy BN et al (1989) A prospective surgical pathological study of stage I squamous carcinoma of the cervix: a Gynecologic Oncology Group Study. Gynecol Oncol 35(3):314–320
62. Delgado G, Bundy B et al (1990) Prospective surgical-pathological study of disease-free interval in patients with stage IB squamous cell carcinoma of the cervix: a Gynecologic Oncology Group study. Gynecol Oncol 38(3):352–357
63. Diaz JP, Sonoda Y et al (2008) Oncologic outcome of fertility-sparing radical trachelectomy versus radical hysterectomy for stage IB1 cervical carcinoma. Gynecol Oncol 111(2):255–260
64. Dinges HP, Werner R et al (1977) Mucoepidermoid carcinoma of the cervix uteri. Zentralbl Gynakol 99(7):396–403
65. Edwards BK, Brown ML et al (2005) Annual report to the nation on the status of cancer, 1975-2002, featuring population-based trends in cancer treatment. J Natl Cancer Inst 97(19):1407–1427
66. Ehrmann RL, Dwyer IM et al (1988) An immunoperoxidase study of laminin and type IV collagen distribution in carcinoma of the cervix and vulva. Obstet Gynecol 72(2):257–262
67. Eichhorn JH, Young RH (2001) Neuroendocrine tumors of the genital tract. Am J Clin Pathol 115(Suppl):S94–S112
68. Eifel PJ, Morris M et al (1990) Adenocarcinoma of the uterine cervix. Prognosis and patterns of failure in 367 cases. Cancer 65(11):2507–2514
69. Farley JH, Hickey KW et al (2003) Adenosquamous histology predicts a poor outcome for patients with advanced-stage, but not early-stage, cervical carcinoma. Cancer 97(9):2196–2202
70. Ferrandina G, Lauriola L et al (2002) Increased cyclooxygenase-2 expression is associated with chemotherapy resistance and poor survival in cervical cancer patients. J Clin Oncol 20(4):973–981
71. Ferrandina G, Ranelletti FO et al (2003) Celecoxib modulates the expression of cyclooxygenase-2, ki67, apoptosis-related marker, and microvessel density in human cervical cancer: a pilot study. Clin Cancer Res 9(12):4324–4331
72. Ferry JA (1997) Adenoid basal carcinoma of the uterine cervix: evolution of a distinctive clinicopathologic entity. Int J Gynecol Pathol 16(4):299–300
73. Ferry JA, Scully RE (1988) "Adenoid cystic" carcinoma and adenoid basal carcinoma of the uterine cervix. A study of 28 cases. Am J Surg Pathol 12(2):134–144
74. Ferry JA, Scully RE (1990) Mesonephric remnants, hyperplasia, and neoplasia in the uterine cervix. A study of 49 cases. Am J Surg Pathol 14(12):1100–1111
75. Fetissof F, Berger G et al (1985) Endocrine cells in the female genital tract. Histopathology 9(2):133–145
76. Folpe AL, Goldblum JR et al (2005) Morphologic and immunophenotypic diversity in Ewing family tumors: a study of 66 genetically confirmed cases. Am J Surg Pathol 29(8): 1025–1033
77. Franco EL, Schlecht NF et al (2003) The epidemiology of cervical cancer. Cancer J 9(5):348–359

78. Frega A, Lukic A et al (2007) Verrucous carcinoma of the cervix: detection of carcinogenetic human papillomavirus types and their role during follow-up. Anticancer Res 27(6C):4491–4494
79. Fuchs I, Vorsteher N et al (2007) The prognostic significance of human epidermal growth factor receptor correlations in squamous cell cervical carcinoma. Anticancer Res 27(2):959–963
80. Fujiwara H, Mitchell MF et al (1995) Clear cell adenosquamous carcinoma of the cervix. An aggressive tumor associated with human papillomavirus-18. Cancer 76(9):1591–1600
81. Gadducci A, Sartori E et al (2003) The clinical outcome of patients with stage Ia1 and Ia2 squamous cell carcinoma of the uterine cervix: a Cooperation Task Force (CTF) study. Eur J Gynaecol Oncol 24(6):513–516
82. Gaffney DK, Holden J et al (2001) Elevated cyclooxygenase-2 expression correlates with diminished survival in carcinoma of the cervix treated with radiotherapy. Int J Radiat Oncol Biol Phys 49(5):1213–1217
83. Gaffney DK, Winter K et al (2007) A Phase II study of acute toxicity for Celebrex (celecoxib) and chemoradiation in patients with locally advanced cervical cancer: primary endpoint analysis of RTOG 0128. Int J Radiat Oncol Biol Phys 67(1):104–109
84. Gallardo A, Prat J (2009) Mullerian adenosarcoma: a clinicopathologic and immunohistochemical study of 55 cases challenging the existence of adenofibroma. Am J Surg Pathol 33(2):278–288
85. Gersell DJ, Mazoujian G et al (1988) Small-cell undifferentiated carcinoma of the cervix. A clinicopathologic, ultrastructural, and immunocytochemical study of 15 cases. Am J Surg Pathol 12(9): 684–698
86. Gilks CB, Young RH et al (1989) Adenoma malignum (minimal deviation adenocarcinoma) of the uterine cervix. A clinicopathological and immunohistochemical analysis of 26 cases. Am J Surg Pathol 13(9):717–729
87. Gilks CB, Young RH et al (1997) Large cell neuroendocrine [corrected] carcinoma of the uterine cervix: a clinicopathologic study of 12 cases. Am J Surg Pathol 21(8):905–914
88. Gombos Z, Xu X et al (2005) Peritumoral lymphatic vessel density and vascular endothelial growth factor C expression in early-stage squamous cell carcinoma of the uterine cervix. Clin Cancer Res 11(23):8364–8371
89. Goncalves A, Fabbro M et al (2008) A phase II trial to evaluate gefitinib as second- or third-line treatment in patients with recurring locoregionally advanced or metastatic cervical cancer. Gynecol Oncol 108(1):42–46
90. Grayson W, Rhemtula HA et al (2002) Detection of human papillomavirus in large cell neuroendocrine carcinoma of the uterine cervix: a study of 12 cases. J Clin Pathol 55(2):108–114
91. Grayson W, Taylor LF et al (1999) Adenoid cystic and adenoid basal carcinoma of the uterine cervix: comparative morphologic, mucin, and immunohistochemical profile of two rare neoplasms of putative "reserve cell" origin. Am J Surg Pathol 23(4):448–458
92. Grayson W, Taylor LF et al (2001) Carcinosarcoma of the uterine cervix: a report of eight cases with immunohistochemical analysis and evaluation of human papillomavirus status. Am J Surg Pathol 25(3):338–347
93. Green J, Berrington de Gonzalez A et al (2003) Risk factors for adenocarcinoma and squamous cell carcinoma of the cervix in women aged 20-44 years: the UK National Case-Control Study of Cervical Cancer. Br J Cancer 89(11):2078–2086
94. Greer BE, Figge DC et al (1990) Stage IA2 squamous carcinoma of the cervix: difficult diagnosis and therapeutic dilemma. Am J Obstet Gynecol 162(6):1406–1409, discussion 1409-1411
95. Gur G, Rubin C et al (2004) LRIG1 restricts growth factor signaling by enhancing receptor ubiquitylation and degradation. Embo J 23(16):3270–3281
96. Gusterson BA, Clinton S et al (1986) Studies of early invasive and intraepithelial squamous cell carcinomas using an antibody to type IV collagen. Histopathology 10(2):161–169
97. Hanselaar A, van Loosbroek M et al (1997) Clear cell adenocarcinoma of the vagina and cervix. An update of the central Netherlands registry showing twin age incidence peaks. Cancer 79(11):2229–2236
98. Hasumi K, Sakamoto A et al (1980) Microinvasive carcinoma of the uterine cervix. Cancer 45(5):928–931
99. Hellberg D, Tot T et al (2009) Pitfalls in immunohistochemical validation of tumor marker expression–exemplified in invasive cancer of the uterine cervix. Gynecol Oncol 112(1):235–240
100. Herbert A, Anshu et al (2009) Screen-detected invasive cervical carcinoma and its clinical significance during the introduction of organized screening. BJOG 116(6):854–859
101. Herrera FG, Chan P et al (2007) A prospective phase I-II trial of the cyclooxygenase-2 inhibitor celecoxib in patients with carcinoma of the cervix with biomarker assessment of the tumor microenvironment. Int J Radiat Oncol Biol Phys 67(1):97–103
102. Hirai Y, Takeshima N et al (1998) A clinicocytopathologic study of adenoma malignum of the uterine cervix. Gynecol Oncol 70(2): 219–223
103. Ho CM, Chien TY et al (2004) Multivariate analysis of the prognostic factors and outcomes in early cervical cancer patients undergoing radical hysterectomy. Gynecol Oncol 93(2):458–464
104. Hocking GR, Hayman JA et al (1996) Adenocarcinoma in situ of the uterine cervix progressing to invasive adenocarcinoma. Aust NZ J Obstet Gynaecol 36(2):218–220
105. Holowaty P, Miller AB et al (1999) Natural history of dysplasia of the uterine cervix. J Natl Cancer Inst 91(3):252–258
106. Horn LC, Fischer U et al (2006) Pattern of invasion is of prognostic value in surgically treated cervical cancer patients. Gynecol Oncol 103(3):906–911
107. Horn LC, Lindner K et al (2006) p16, p14, p53, and cyclin D1 expression and HPV analysis in small cell carcinomas of the uterine cervix. Int J Gynecol Pathol 25(2):182–186
108. Huffman JW (1948) Mesonephric remnants in the cervix. Am J Obstet Gynecol 56(1):23–40
109. Hunter MI, Monk BJ et al (2008) Cervical neoplasia in pregnancy. Part 1: screening and management of preinvasive disease. Am J Obstet Gynecol 199(1):3–9
110. Hurt WG, Silverberg SG et al (1977) Adenocarcinoma of the cervix: histopathologic and clinical features. Am J Obstet Gynecol 129(3):304–315
111. Inoue T, Morita K (1990) The prognostic significance of number of positive nodes in cervical carcinoma stages IB, IIA, and IIB. Cancer 65(9):1923–1927
112. Inoue T, Yamaguchi K et al (1984) Production of immunoreactive-polypeptide hormones in cervical carcinoma. Cancer 53(7): 1509–1514
113. International Collaboration of Epidemiological Studies of Cervical Cancer (2007) Comparison of risk factors for invasive squamous cell carcinoma and adenocarcinoma of the cervix: collaborative reanalysis of individual data on 8, 097 women with squamous cell carcinoma and 1,374 women with adenocarcinoma from 12 epidemiological studies. Int J Cancer 120(4): 885–891

114. Ishikawa H, Nakanishi T et al (1999) Prognostic factors of adenocarcinoma of the uterine cervix. Gynecol Oncol 73(1):42–46
115. Jemal A, Siegel R et al (2006) Cancer statistics, 2006. CA Cancer J Clin 56(2):106–130
116. Jemal A, Siegel R et al (2008) Cancer statistics, 2008. CA Cancer J Clin 58(2):71–96
117. Jones MW, Kounelis S et al (2000) Well-differentiated villoglandular adenocarcinoma of the uterine cervix: oncogene/tumor suppressor gene alterations and human papillomavirus genotyping. Int J Gynecol Pathol 19(2):110–117
118. Jones MW, Lefkowitz M (1995) Adenosarcoma of the uterine cervix: a clinicopathological study of 12 cases. Int J Gynecol Pathol 14(3):223–229
119. Jones WB, Mercer GO et al (1993) Early invasive carcinoma of the cervix. Gynecol Oncol 51(1):26–32
120. Jones WB, Shingleton HM et al (1996) Cervical carcinoma and pregnancy. A national patterns of care study of the American College of Surgeons. Cancer 77(8):1479–1488
121. Jones MW, Silverberg SG et al (1993) Well-differentiated villoglandular adenocarcinoma of the uterine cervix: a clinicopathological study of 24 cases. Int J Gynecol Pathol 12(1):1–7
122. Jones MA, Young RH (1997) Atypical oxyphilic metaplasia of the endocervical epithelium: a report of six cases. Int J Gynecol Pathol 16(2):99–102
123. Kairi-Vassilatou E, Papakonstantinou K et al (2007) Primary gestational choriocarcinoma of the uterine cervix. Report of a case and review of the literature. Int J Gynecol Cancer 17(4): 921–925
124. Kaku T, Kamura T et al (1997) Early adenocarcinoma of the uterine cervix. Gynecol Oncol 65(2):281–285
125. Kaku T, Kamura T et al (1997) Adenocarcinoma of the uterine cervix with predominantly villogladular papillary growth pattern. Gynecol Oncol 64(1):147–152
126. Kaminski PF, Maier RC (1983) Clear cell adenocarcinoma of the cervix unrelated to diethylstilbestrol exposure. Obstet Gynecol 62(6):720–727
127. Kaminski PF, Norris HJ (1983) Minimal deviation carcinoma (adenoma malignum) of the cervix. Int J Gynecol Pathol 2(2):141–152
128. Kamoi S, AlJuboury MI et al (2002) Immunohistochemical staining in the distinction between primary endometrial and endocervical adenocarcinomas: another viewpoint. Int J Gynecol Pathol 21(3):217–223
129. Kashimura M, Tsukamoto N et al (1984) Verrucous carcinoma of the uterine cervix: report of a case with follow-up of 6 1/2 years. Gynecol Oncol 19(2):204–215
130. Kaspar HG, Dinh TV et al (1993) Clinical implications of tumor volume measurement in stage I adenocarcinoma of the cervix. Obstet Gynecol 81(2):296–300
131. Katz HJ, Davies JN (1980) Death from cervix uteri carcinoma: the changing pattern. Gynecol Oncol 9(1):86–89
132. Kennedy AW, elTabbakh GH et al (1995) Invasive adenocarcinoma of the cervix following LLETZ (large loop excision of the transformation zone) for adenocarcinoma in situ. Gynecol Oncol 58(2):274–277
133. Kerner H, Lichtig C (1993) Mullerian adenosarcoma presenting as cervical polyps: a report of seven cases and review of the literature. Obstet Gynecol 81(5 Pt 1):655–659
134. Kersemaekers AM, Fleuren GJ et al (1999) Oncogene alterations in carcinomas of the uterine cervix: overexpression of the epidermal growth factor receptor is associated with poor prognosis. Clin Cancer Res 5(3):577–586
135. Keys HM, Bundy BN et al (1999) Cisplatin, radiation, and adjuvant hysterectomy compared with radiation and adjuvant hysterectomy for bulky stage IB cervical carcinoma. N Engl J Med 340(15): 1154–1161
136. Killackey MA, Jones WB et al (1986) Diagnostic conization of the cervix: review of 460 consecutive cases. Obstet Gynecol 67(6): 766–770
137. Kim GE, Kim YB et al (2004) Synchronous coexpression of epidermal growth factor receptor and cyclooxygenase-2 in carcinomas of the uterine cervix: a potential predictor of poor survival. Clin Cancer Res 10(4):1366–1374
138. Kim JY, Lim SJ et al (2005) Cyclooxygenase-2 and c-erbB-2 expression in uterine cervical neoplasm assessed using tissue microarrays. Gynecol Oncol 97(2):337–341
139. Kim WY, Sharpless NE (2006) The regulation of INK4/ARF in cancer and aging. Cell 127(2):265–275
140. Kjaer SK, Brinton LA (1993) Adenocarcinomas of the uterine cervix: the epidemiology of an increasing problem. Epidemiol Rev 15(2):486–498
141. Koenig C, Turnicky RP et al (1997) Papillary squamotransitional cell carcinoma of the cervix: a report of 32 cases. Am J Surg Pathol 21(8):915–921
142. Kolstad P (1989) Follow-up study of 232 patients with stage Ia1 and 411 patients with stage Ia2 squamous cell carcinoma of the cervix (microinvasive carcinoma). Gynecol Oncol 33(3): 265–272
143. Korach J, Machtinger R et al (2009) Villoglandular papillary adenocarcinoma of the uterine cervix: a diagnostic challenge. Acta Obstet Gynecol Scand 88(3):355–358
144. Kristensen GB, Abeler VM et al (1999) Tumor size, depth of invasion, and grading of the invasive tumor front are the main prognostic factors in early squamous cell cervical carcinoma. Gynecol Oncol 74(2):245–251
145. Kuzuya K (2004) Chemoradiotherapy for uterine cancer: current status and perspectives. Int J Clin Oncol 9(6):458–470
146. Lacey JV Jr, Brinton LA et al (2000) Use of hormone replacement therapy and adenocarcinomas and squamous cell carcinomas of the uterine cervix. Gynecol Oncol 77(1):149–154
147. Lai CH, Chang CJ et al (2007) Role of human papillomavirus genotype in prognosis of early-stage cervical cancer undergoing primary surgery. J Clin Oncol 25(24):3628–3634
148. Lax SF, Pizer ES et al (1998) Clear cell carcinoma of the endometrium is characterized by a distinctive profile of p53, Ki-67, estrogen, and progesterone receptor expression. Hum Pathol 29(6): 551–558
149. Ledda F, Bieraugel O et al (2008) Lrig1 is an endogenous inhibitor of Ret receptor tyrosine kinase activation, downstream signaling, and biological responses to GDNF. J Neurosci 28(1):39–49
150. Lee KR, Flynn CE (2000) Early invasive adenocarcinoma of the cervix. Cancer 89(5):1048–1055
151. Lee SW, Kim YM et al (2009) The efficacy of conservative management after conization in patients with stage IA1 microinvasive cervical carcinoma. Acta Obstet Gynecol Scand 88(2):209–215
152. Leman MH Jr, Benson WL et al (1976) Microinvasive carcinoma of the cervix. Obstet Gynecol 48(5):571–578
153. Leminen A, Paavonen J et al (1990) Adenocarcinoma of the uterine cervix. Cancer 65(1):53–59
154. Lemoine NR, Hall PA (1986) Epithelial tumors metastatic to the uterine cervix. A study of 33 cases and review of the literature. Cancer 57(10):2002–2005

155. Lennerz JK, Perry A et al (2009) Mucoepidermoid carcinoma of the cervix: another tumor with the t(11;19)-associated CRTC1-MAML2 gene fusion. Am J Surg Pathol 33(6):835–843
156. Lesack D, Wahab I et al (1996) Radiation-induced atypia of endocervical epithelium: a histological, immunohistochemical and cytometric study. Int J Gynecol Pathol 15(3):242–247
157. Lindell A (1952) Carcinoma of the uterine cervix; incidence and influence of age; a statistical study. Acta Radiol Suppl 92:1–102
158. Lindstrom AK, Stendahl U et al (2007) Predicting the outcome of squamous cell carcinoma of the uterine cervix using combinations of individual tumor marker expressions. Anticancer Res 27(3B): 1609–1615
159. Liu WM, Chao KC et al (1989) Colposcopic assessment in microinvasive carcinoma of the cervix. Zhonghua Yi Xue Za Zhi (Taipei) 43(3):171–176
160. Loncaster JA, Cooper RA et al (2000) Vascular endothelial growth factor (VEGF) expression is a prognostic factor for radiotherapy outcome in advanced carcinoma of the cervix. Br J Cancer 83(5):620–625
161. Long HJ 3rd, Bundy BN et al (2005) Randomized phase III trial of cisplatin with or without topotecan in carcinoma of the uterine cervix: a Gynecologic Oncology Group Study. J Clin Oncol 23(21):4626–4633
162. Lucas WE, Benirschke K et al (1974) Verrucous carcinoma of the female genital tract. Am J Obstet Gynecol 119(4):435–440
163. Maiman MA, Fruchter RG et al (1988) Superficially invasive squamous cell carcinoma of the cervix. Obstet Gynecol 72(3 Pt 1): 399–403
164. Malpica A, Moran CA (2002) Primitive neuroectodermal tumor of the cervix: a clinicopathologic and immunohistochemical study of two cases. Ann Diagn Pathol 6(5):281–287
165. Mannion C, Park WS et al (1998) Endocrine tumors of the cervix: morphologic assessment, expression of human papillomavirus, and evaluation for loss of heterozygosity on 1p, 3p, 11q, and 17p. Cancer 83(7):1391–1400
166. Martinez-Leandro EP, Martorell M et al (1994) Lymphoepithelial-like carcinoma of the uterine cervix. Study of a case with in situ hybridization of the Epstein-Barr virus genome and the human papillomavirus genome. Acta Obstet Gynecol Scand 73(7):589–592
167. Martorell MA, Julian JM et al (2002) Lymphoepithelioma-like carcinoma of the uterine cervix. Arch Pathol Lab Med 126(12): 1501–1505
168. Mathoulin-Portier MP, Penault-Llorca F et al (1998) Malignant mullerian mixed tumor of the uterine cervix with adenoid cystic component. Int J Gynecol Pathol 17(1):91–92
169. Matias-Guiu X, Lerma E et al (1997) Clear cell tumors of the female genital tract. Semin Diagn Pathol 14(4):233–239
170. McCluggage WG, Jenkins D (2003) p16 immunoreactivity may assist in the distinction between endometrial and endocervical adenocarcinoma. Int J Gynecol Pathol 22(3):231–235
171. McCluggage WG, Sumathi VP et al (2002) A panel of immunohistochemical stains, including carcinoembryonic antigen, vimentin, and estrogen receptor, aids the distinction between primary endometrial and endocervical adenocarcinomas. Int J Gynecol Pathol 21(1):11–15
172. Meanwell CA, Kelly KA et al (1988) Young age as a prognostic factor in cervical cancer: analysis of population based data from 10,022 cases. Br Med J (Clin Res Ed) 296(6619):386–391
173. Mikami Y, Kiyokawa T et al (2004) Gastrointestinal immunophenotype in adenocarcinomas of the uterine cervix and related glandular lesions: a possible link between lobular endocervical glandular hyperplasia/pyloric gland metaplasia and "adenoma malignum". Mod Pathol 17(8):962–972
174. Mikami Y, Kiyokawa T et al (2009) Reappraisal of synchronous and multifocal mucinous lesions of the female genital tract: a close association with gastric metaplasia. Histopathology 54(2):184–191
175. Mikuta JJ, Celebre JA (1969) Adenocarcinoma of the cervix. Obstet Gynecol 33(6):753–756
176. Missaoui N, Hmissa S et al (2006) p16INK4A overexpression and HPV infection in uterine cervix adenocarcinoma. Virchows Arch 448(5):597–603
177. Mobius G (1993) Cytological early detection of cervical carcinoma: possibilities and limitations. Analysis of failures. J Cancer Res Clin Oncol 119(9):513–521
178. Monk BJ, Sill MW et al (2009) Phase II trial of bevacizumab in the treatment of persistent or recurrent squamous cell carcinoma of the cervix: a gynecologic oncology group study. J Clin Oncol 27(7):1069–1074
179. Monk BJ, Tewari KS et al (2007) Multimodality therapy for locally advanced cervical carcinoma: state of the art and future directions. J Clin Oncol 25(20):2952–2965
180. Morgan PR, Anderson MC et al (1993) The Royal College of Obstetricians and Gynaecologists micro-invasive carcinoma of the cervix study: preliminary results. Br J Obstet Gynaecol 100(7): 664–668
181. Mota F (2003) Microinvasive squamous carcinoma of the cervix: treatment modalities. Acta Obstet Gynecol Scand 82(6):505–509
182. Mulvany NJ, Nirenberg A et al (1996) Non-primary cervical adenocarcinomas. Pathology 28(4):293–297
183. Mulvany N, Ostor A (1997) Microinvasive adenocarcinoma of the cervix: a cytohistopathologic study of 40 cases. Diagn Cytopathol 16(5):430–436
184. Munagala R, Dona MG et al (2009) Significance of multiple HPV infection in cervical cancer patients and its impact on treatment response. Int J Oncol 34(1):263–271
185. Munoz N, Bosch FX et al (2003) Epidemiologic classification of human papillomavirus types associated with cervical cancer. N Engl J Med 348(6):518–527
186. Munoz N, Castellsague X et al (2006) Chapter 1: HPV in the etiology of human cancer. Vaccine 24(S3):1–10
187. Murdoch JB, Grimshaw RN et al (1992) The impact of loop diathermy on management of early invasive cervical cancer. Int J Gynecol Cancer 2(3):129–133
188. Musa AG, Hughes RR et al (1985) Adenoid cystic carcinoma of the cervix: a report of 17 cases. Gynecol Oncol 22(2):167–173
189. Nagai T, Okubo T et al (2008) Glassy cell carcinoma of the uterine cervix responsive to neoadjuvant intraarterial chemotherapy. Int J Clin Oncol 13(6):541–544
190. Nair SA, Nair MB et al (1997) The basement membrane and tumor progression in the uterine cervix. Gen Diagn Pathol 142(5–6):297–303
191. Nakagawa S, Yoshikawa H et al (1996) Type of human papillomavirus is related to clinical features of cervical carcinoma. Cancer 78(9):1935–1941
192. National Cancer Institute (2006) SEER Fact Sheet Cervical Cancer. http://seer.cancer.gov/statfacts/html/cervix.html. Accessed 4 October 2010
193. Noel J, Lespagnard L et al (2001) Evidence of human papilloma virus infection but lack of Epstein-Barr virus in lymphoepithelioma-like carcinoma of uterine cervix: report of two cases and review of the literature. Hum Pathol 32(1):135–138

194. Nogales F, Botella Llusia J (1965) The frequency of invasion of the lymph nodes in cancer of the uterine cervix. A study of the degree of extension in relation to the histological type of tumor. Am J Obstet Gynecol 93:91–94
195. Ostor AG (2000) Early invasive adenocarcinoma of the uterine cervix. Int J Gynecol Pathol 19(1):29–38
196. Ostor A, Rome R et al (1997) Microinvasive adenocarcinoma of the cervix: a clinicopathologic study of 77 women. Obstet Gynecol 89(1):88–93
197. Pak HY, Yokota SB et al (1983) Glassy cell carcinoma of the cervix. Cytologic and clinicopathologic analysis. Cancer 52(2):307–312
198. Pao CC, Kao SM et al (1994) State of mutational alterations of p53 and retinoblastoma susceptibility genes in papillomavirus-negative small cell cervical carcinomas. J Surg Oncol 57(2):87–93
199. Pappa KI, Choleza M et al (2006) Consistent absence of BRAF mutations in cervical and endometrial cancer despite KRAS mutation status. Gynecol Oncol 100(3):596–600
200. Paraskevaidis E, Kitchener HC et al (1992) A population-based study of microinvasive disease of the cervix–a colposcopic and cytologic analysis. Gynecol Oncol 45(1):9–12
201. Parazzini F, Chatenoud L et al (1998) Determinants of risk of invasive cervical cancer in young women. Br J Cancer 77(5): 838–841
202. Park JY, Kim DY et al (2009) Human papillomavirus test after conization in predicting residual disease in subsequent hysterectomy specimens. Obstet Gynecol 114(1):87–92
203. Parkin DM, Bray F et al (2005) Global cancer statistics, 2002. CA Cancer J Clin 55(2):74–108
204. Parwani AV, Smith Sehdev AE et al (2005) Cervical adenoid basal tumors comprised of adenoid basal epithelioma associated with various types of invasive carcinoma: clinicopathologic features, human papillomavirus DNA detection, and P16 expression. Hum Pathol 36(1):82–90
205. Pecorelli S (2009) Revised FIGO staging for carcinoma of the vulva, cervix, and endometrium. Int J Gynaecol Obstet 105(2): 103–104
206. Pecorelli S, Zigliani L et al (2009) Revised FIGO staging for carcinoma of the cervix. Int J Gynaecol Obstet 105(2):107–108
207. Perez-Regadera J, Sanchez-Munoz A et al (2009) Negative prognostic impact of the coexpression of epidermal growth factor receptor and c-erbB-2 in locally advanced cervical cancer. Oncology 76(2):133–141
208. Peters WA 3rd, Liu PY et al (2000) Concurrent chemotherapy and pelvic radiation therapy compared with pelvic radiation therapy alone as adjuvant therapy after radical surgery in high-risk early-stage cancer of the cervix. J Clin Oncol 18(8): 1606–1613
209. Pinto AP, Crum CP (2000) Natural history of cervical neoplasia: defining progression and its consequence. Clin Obstet Gynecol 43(2):352–362
210. Pirog EC, Kleter B et al (2000) Prevalence of human papillomavirus DNA in different histological subtypes of cervical adenocarcinoma. Am J Pathol 157(4):1055–1062
211. Pisani P, Bray F et al (2002) Estimates of the world-wide prevalence of cancer for 25 sites in the adult population. Int J Cancer 97(1): 72–81
212. Poynor EA, Marshall D et al (2006) Clinicopathologic features of early adenocarcinoma of the cervix initially managed with cervical conization. Gynecol Oncol 103(3):960–965
213. Prempree T, Villasanta U et al (1980) Management of adenoid cystic carcinoma of the uterine cervix (cylindroma): report of six cases and reappraisal of all cases reported in the medical literature. Cancer 46(7):1631–1635
214. Pretorius R, Semrad N et al (1991) Presentation of cervical cancer. Gynecol Oncol 42(1):48–53
215. Randall ME, Andersen WA et al (1986) Papillary squamous cell carcinoma of the uterine cervix: a clinicopathologic study of nine cases. Int J Gynecol Pathol 5(1):1–10
216. Reich O, Tamussino K et al (2000) Clear cell carcinoma of the uterine cervix: pathology and prognosis in surgically treated stage IB-IIB disease in women not exposed in utero to diethylstilbestrol. Gynecol Oncol 76(3):331–335
217. Richards CJ, Furness PN (1990) Basement membrane continuity in benign, premalignant and malignant epithelial conditions of the uterine cervix. Histopathology 16(1):47–52
218. Robboy SJ, Young RH et al (1984) Atypical vaginal adenosis and cervical ectropion. Association with clear cell adenocarcinoma in diethylstilbestrol-exposed offspring. Cancer 54(5):869–875
219. Roche WD, Norris HJ (1975) Microinvasive carcinoma of the cervix. The significance of lymphatic invasion and confluent patterns of stromal growth. Cancer 36(1):180–186
220. Ronnett BM, Yemelyanova AV et al (2008) Endocervical adenocarcinomas with ovarian metastases: analysis of 29 cases with emphasis on minimally invasive cervical tumors and the ability of the metastases to simulate primary ovarian neoplasms. Am J Surg Pathol 32(12):1835–1853
221. Rosa DD, Medeiros LR et al (2009) Adjuvant platinum-based chemotherapy for early stage cervical cancer. Cochrane Database Syst Rev 3:CD005342
222. Rutledge FN, Mitchell MF et al (1992) Youth as a prognostic factor in carcinoma of the cervix: a matched analysis. Gynecol Oncol 44(2):123–130
223. Saigo PE, Cain JM et al (1986) Prognostic factors in adenocarcinoma of the uterine cervix. Cancer 57(8):1584–1593
224. Samlal RA, Ten Kate FJ et al (1998) Do mucin-secreting squamous cell carcinomas of the uterine cervix metastasize more frequently to pelvic lymph nodes? A case-control study? Int J Gynecol Pathol 17(3):201–204
225. Samlal RA, van der Velden J et al (1997) Identification of high-risk groups among node-positive patients with stage IB and IIA cervical carcinoma. Gynecol Oncol 64(3):463–467
226. Saraiya M, Ahmed F et al (2007) Cervical cancer incidence in a prevaccine era in the United States, 1998–2002. Obstet Gynecol 109(2 Pt 1):360–370
227. Savargaonkar PR, Hale RJ et al (1996) Neuroendocrine differentiation in cervical carcinoma. J Clin Pathol 49(2):139–141
228. Schiffman M, Castle PE et al (2007) Human papillomavirus and cervical cancer. Lancet 370(9590):890–907
229. Schneider V (1981) Arias-stella reaction of the endocervix: frequency and location. Acta Cytol 25(3):224–228
230. Schorge JO, Lee KR et al (1999) Early cervical adenocarcinoma: selection criteria for radical surgery. Obstet Gynecol 94(3): 386–390
231. Schwartz SM, Daling JR et al (2001) Human papillomavirus and prognosis of invasive cervical cancer: a population-based study. J Clin Oncol 19(7):1906–1915
232. Sedlis A, Sall S et al (1979) Microinvasive carcinoma of the uterine cervix: a clinical-pathologic study. Am J Obstet Gynecol 133(1): 64–74
233. Seski JC, Abell MR et al (1977) Microinvasive squamous carcinoma of the cervix: definition, histologic analysis, late results of treatment. Obstet Gynecol 50(4):410–414

234. Sevin BU, Nadji M et al (1992) Microinvasive carcinoma of the cervix. Cancer 70(8):2121–2128
235. Shah AN, Olah KS (2002) Cervical stump carcinoma following subtotal hysterectomy. J Obstet Gynaecol 22(6):701
236. Shattuck DL, Miller JK et al (2007) LRIG1 is a novel negative regulator of the Met receptor and opposes Met and Her2 synergy. Mol Cell Biol 27(5):1934–1946
237. Sheets EE, Berman ML et al (1988) Surgically treated, early-stage neuroendocrine small-cell cervical carcinoma. Obstet Gynecol 71(1):10–14
238. Shingleton HM, Bell MC et al (1995) Is there really a difference in survival of women with squamous cell carcinoma, adenocarcinoma, and adenosquamous cell carcinoma of the cervix? Cancer 76(10 Suppl):1948–1955
239. Shinohara S, Ochi T et al (2004) Histopathological prognostic factors in patients with cervical cancer treated with radical hysterectomy and postoperative radiotherapy. Int J Clin Oncol 9(6): 503–509
240. Silver SA, Devouassoux-Shisheboran M et al (2001) Mesonephric adenocarcinomas of the uterine cervix: a study of 11 cases with immunohistochemical findings. Am J Surg Pathol 25(3): 379–387
241. Silverberg SG, Hurt WG (1975) Minimal deviation adenocarcinoma ("adenoma malignum") of the cervix: a reappraisal. Am J Obstet Gynecol 121(7):971–975
242. Simon NL, Gore H et al (1986) Study of superficially invasive carcinoma of the cervix. Obstet Gynecol 68(1):19–24
243. Smith JS, Green J et al (2003) Cervical cancer and use of hormonal contraceptives: a systematic review. Lancet 361(9364): 1159–1167
244. Smith HO, Qualls CR et al (2002) Is there a difference in survival for IA1 and IA2 adenocarcinoma of the uterine cervix? Gynecol Oncol 85(2):229–241
245. Smith HO, Tiffany MF et al (2000) The rising incidence of adenocarcinoma relative to squamous cell carcinoma of the uterine cervix in the United States–a 24-year population-based study. Gynecol Oncol 78(2):97–105
246. Snijders-Keilholz A, Ewing P et al (2005) Primitive neuroectodermal tumor of the cervix uteri: a case report – changing concepts in therapy. Gynecol Oncol 98(3):516–519
247. Staebler A, Sherman ME et al (2002) Hormone receptor immunohistochemistry and human papillomavirus in situ hybridization are useful for distinguishing endocervical and endometrial adenocarcinomas. Am J Surg Pathol 26(8):998–1006
248. Subbaramaiah K, Dannenberg AJ (2007) Cyclooxygenase-2 transcription is regulated by human papillomavirus 16 E6 and E7 oncoproteins: evidence of a corepressor/coactivator exchange. Cancer Res 67(8):3976–3985
249. Sullivan LM, Smolkin ME et al (2008) Comprehensive evaluation of CDX2 in invasive cervical adenocarcinomas: immunopositivity in the absence of overt colorectal morphology. Am J Surg Pathol 32(11):1608–1612
250. Szczepulska E, Nasierowska-Guttmejer A et al (1999) Cervical verrucous carcinoma involving endometrium. Case report. Eur J Gynaecol Oncol 20(1):35–37
251. Szurkus DC, Harrison TA (2003) Loop excision for high-grade squamous intraepithelial lesion on cytology: correlation with colposcopic and histologic findings. Am J Obstet Gynecol 188(5):1180–1182
252. Takeda N, Sakuragi N et al (2002) Multivariate analysis of histopathologic prognostic factors for invasive cervical cancer treated with radical hysterectomy and systematic retroperitoneal lymphadenectomy. Acta Obstet Gynecol Scand 81(12):1144–1151
253. Takeshima N, Yanoh K et al (1999) Assessment of the revised International Federation of Gynecology and obstetrics staging for early invasive squamous cervical cancer. Gynecol Oncol 74(2): 165–169
254. Tambouret R, Bell DA et al (2000) Microcystic endocervical adenocarcinomas: a report of eight cases. Am J Surg Pathol 24(3):369–374
255. Tamimi HK, Ek M et al (1988) Glassy cell carcinoma of the cervix redefined. Obstet Gynecol 71(6 Pt 1):837–841
256. Tenti P, Pavanello S et al (1998) Analysis and clinical implications of p53 gene mutations and human papillomavirus type 16 and 18 infection in primary adenocarcinoma of the uterine cervix. Am J Pathol 152(4):1057–1063
257. Teshima S, Shimosato Y et al (1985) Early stage adenocarcinoma of the uterine cervix. Histopathologic analysis with consideration of histogenesis. Cancer 56(1):167–172
258. Thelmo WL, Nicastri AD et al (1990) Mucoepidermoid carcinoma of uterine cervix stage IB. Long-term follow-up, histochemical and immunohistochemical study. Int J Gynecol Pathol 9(4):316–324
259. Toki T, Shiozawa T et al (1997) Minimal deviation adenocarcinoma of the uterine cervix has abnormal expression of sex steroid receptors, CA125, and gastric mucin. Int J Gynecol Pathol 16(2):111–116
260. Toussaint-Smith E, Donner DB et al (2004) Expression of human papillomavirus type 16 E6 and E7 oncoproteins in primary foreskin keratinocytes is sufficient to alter the expression of angiogenic factors. Oncogene 23(17):2988–2995
261. Trottier H, Mahmud S et al (2006) Human papillomavirus infections with multiple types and risk of cervical neoplasia. Cancer Epidemiol Biomarkers Prev 15(7):1274–1280
262. Tseng CJ, Pao CC et al (1997) Lymphoepithelioma-like carcinoma of the uterine cervix: association with Epstein-Barr virus and human papillomavirus. Cancer 80(1):91–97
263. Tsukamoto N, Kaku T et al (1989) The problem of stage Ia (FIGO, 1985) carcinoma of the uterine cervix. Gynecol Oncol 34(1):1–6
264. Ueda Y, Miyatake T et al (2008) Clonality and HPV infection analysis of concurrent glandular and squamous lesions and adenosquamous carcinomas of the uterine cervix. Am J Clin Pathol 130(3):389–400
265. Ueda G, Shimizu C et al (1989) An immunohistochemical study of small-cell and poorly differentiated carcinomas of the cervix using neuroendocrine markers. Gynecol Oncol 34(2):164–169
266. Ulbright TM, Gersell DJ (1983) Glassy cell carcinoma of the uterine cervix. A light and electron microscopic study of five cases. Cancer 51(12):2255–2263
267. Van Nagell JR Jr, Greenwell N et al (1983) Microinvasive carcinoma of the cervix. Am J Obstet Gynecol 145(8):981–991
268. Vang R, Gown AM et al (2007) p16 expression in primary ovarian mucinous and endometrioid tumors and metastatic adenocarcinomas in the ovary: utility for identification of metastatic HPV-related endocervical adenocarcinomas. Am J Surg Pathol 31(5):653–663
269. Vesterinen E, Forss M et al (1989) Increase of cervical adenocarcinoma: a report of 520 cases of cervical carcinoma including 112 tumors with glandular elements. Gynecol Oncol 33(1):49–53
270. Vinh-Hung V, Bourgain C et al (2007) Prognostic value of histopathology and trends in cervical cancer: a SEER population study. BMC Cancer 7:164

271. Vizcaino AP, Moreno V et al (1998) International trends in the incidence of cervical cancer: I. Adenocarcinoma and adenosquamous cell carcinomas. Int J Cancer 75(4):536–545
272. Walboomers JM, Jacobs MV et al (1999) Human papillomavirus is a necessary cause of invasive cervical cancer worldwide. J Pathol 189(1):12–19
273. Walker AN, Mills SE et al (1988) Cervical neuroendocrine carcinoma: a clinical and light microscopic study of 14 cases. Int J Gynecol Pathol 7(1):64–74
274. Wang TY, Chen BF et al (2001) Histologic and immunophenotypic classification of cervical carcinomas by expression of the p53 homologue p63: a study of 250 cases. Hum Pathol 32(5):479–486
275. Wang HL, Lu DW (2004) Detection of human papillomavirus DNA and expression of p16, Rb, and p53 proteins in small cell carcinomas of the uterine cervix. Am J Surg Pathol 28(7):901–908
276. Wang SS, Sherman ME et al (2004) Cervical adenocarcinoma and squamous cell carcinoma incidence trends among white women and black women in the United States for 1976–2000. Cancer 100(5):1035–1044
277. Wang SS, Sherman ME et al (2006) Pathological characteristics of cervical adenocarcinoma in a multi-center US-based study. Gynecol Oncol 103(2):541–546
278. Wells M, Ostor AG et al (2002) Tumours of the uterine cervix. In: Tavassoli FA, Devilee P (eds) Tumors of the breast and female genital organs. IARC, Lyon, pp 260–286
279. Wentz WB, Reagan JW (1959) Survival in cervical cancer with respect to cell type. Cancer 12(2):384–388
280. Wheeler CM (2008) Natural history of human papillomavirus infections, cytologic and histologic abnormalities, and cancer. Obstet Gynecol Clin North Am 35(4):519-36; vii
281. Wheeler DT, Kurman RJ (2005) The relationship of glands to thick-wall blood vessels as a marker of invasion in endocervical adenocarcinoma. Int J Gynecol Pathol 24(2):125–130
282. Wistuba II, Thomas B et al (1999) Molecular abnormalities associated with endocrine tumors of the uterine cervix. Gynecol Oncol 72(1):3–9
283. Wolff JP, Lacour J et al (1972) Cancer of the cervical stump. Study of 173 patients. Obstet Gynecol 39(1):10–16
284. Yahata T, Numata M et al (2008) Conservative treatment of stage IA1 adenocarcinoma of the cervix during pregnancy. Gynecol Oncol 109(1):49–52
285. Yajima A, Noda K (1979) The results of treatment of microinvasive carcinoma (stage iA) of the uterine cervix by means of simple and extended hysterectomy. Am J Obstet Gynecol 135(5):685–688
286. Yang L, Parkin DM et al (2004) Estimation and projection of the national profile of cancer mortality in China: 1991–2005. Br J Cancer 90(11):2157–2166
287. Yazigi R, Sandstad J et al (1990) Adenosquamous carcinoma of the cervix: prognosis in stage IB. Obstet Gynecol 75(6):1012–1015
288. Yemelyanova A, Ji H et al (2009) Utility of p16 expression for distinction of uterine serous carcinomas from endometrial endometrioid and endocervical adenocarcinomas: immunohistochemical analysis of 201 cases. Am J Surg Pathol 33(10):1504–1514
289. Yemelyanova A, Vang R et al (2009) Endocervical adenocarcinomas with prominent endometrial or endomyometrial involvement simulating primary endometrial carcinomas: utility of HPV DNA detection and immunohistochemical expression of p16 and hormone receptors to confirm the cervical origin of the corpus tumor. Am J Surg Pathol 33(6):914–924
290. Young RH, Clement PB (2002) Endocervical adenocarcinoma and its variants: their morphology and differential diagnosis. Histopathology 41(3):185–207
291. Young RH, Scully RE (1988) Mucinous ovarian tumors associated with mucinous adenocarcinomas of the cervix. A clinicopathological analysis of 16 cases. Int J Gynecol Pathol 7(2):99–111
292. Young RH, Scully RE (1989) Atypical forms of microglandular hyperplasia of the cervix simulating carcinoma. A report of five cases and review of the literature. Am J Surg Pathol 13(1):50–56
293. Young RH, Scully RE (1993) Minimal-deviation endometrioid adenocarcinoma of the uterine cervix. A report of five cases of a distinctive neoplasm that may be misinterpreted as benign. Am J Surg Pathol 17(7):660–665
294. Young RH, Welch WR et al (1982) Ovarian sex cord tumor with annular tubules: review of 74 cases including 27 with Peutz-Jeghers syndrome and four with adenoma malignum of the cervix. Cancer 50(7):1384–1402
295. Zaino RJ (2002) The fruits of our labors: distinguishing endometrial from endocervical adenocarcinoma. Int J Gynecol Pathol 21(1):1–3
296. Zaino RJ (2002) Symposium part I: adenocarcinoma in situ, glandular dysplasia, and early invasive adenocarcinoma of the uterine cervix. Int J Gynecol Pathol 21(4):314–326
297. Zaino RJ, Ward S et al (1992) Histopathologic predictors of the behavior of surgically treated stage IB squamous cell carcinoma of the cervix. A Gynecologic Oncology Group study. Cancer 69(7):1750–1758
298. Zannoni GF, Sioletic S et al (2008) The role of HPV detection and typing in diagnosis of pulmonary metastatic squamous cell carcinoma of the uterine cervix. Histopathology 53(5):604–606
299. Zbroch T, Grzegorz Knapp P et al (2005) Verrucous carcinoma of the cervix–diagnostic and therapeutic difficulties with regards to HPV status. Case report. Eur J Gynaecol Oncol 26(2):227–230
300. Zhang SQ, Yu H et al (2009) Clinical implications of increased lymph vessel density in the lymphatic metastasis of early-stage invasive cervical carcinoma: a clinical immunohistochemical method study. BMC Cancer 9:64
301. Zheng T, Holford TR et al (1996) The continuing increase in adenocarcinoma of the uterine cervix: a birth cohort phenomenon. Int J Epidemiol 25(2):252–258
302. Zhou C, Gilks CB et al (1998) Papillary serous carcinoma of the uterine cervix: a clinicopathologic study of 17 cases. Am J Surg Pathol 22(1):113–120
303. Zivanovic O, Leitao MM Jr et al (2009) Small cell neuroendocrine carcinoma of the cervix: Analysis of outcome, recurrence pattern and the impact of platinum-based combination chemotherapy. Gynecol Oncol 112(3):590–593

7 Benign Diseases of the Endometrium

W. Glenn McCluggage

R. J. Kurman, L. Hedrick Ellenson, B. M. Ronnett (eds.), *Blaustein's Pathology of the Female Genital Tract (6th ed.)*, DOI 10.1007/978-1-4419-0489-8_7,

Embryology and Anatomy

The endometrium and the myometrium are of mesodermal origin and are formed secondary to fusion of the müllerian (paramesonephric) ducts between the 8th and 9th postovulatory weeks. The cervix is generally considered to be of müllerian origin, although it has been claimed that its mucous membrane is derived from the urogenital sinus; however, the exact contribution of müllerian and sinus tissue to the cervix remains uncertain [47]. Until the 20th week of gestation, the endometrium consists of a single layer of columnar epithelium supported by a thick layer of fibroblastic stroma. After the 20th gestational week, the surface epithelium invaginates into the underlying stroma, forming glandular structures that extend toward the underlying myometrium. At birth, the uterus, which is made up of the uterine corpus and uterine cervix, measures approximately 4 cm in length, the majority of which is made up of the cervix. The endometrium measures less than 0.5 mm in thickness, and the surface and glands are lined by a low columnar to cuboidal epithelium devoid of either proliferative or secretory activity, which resembles the inactive endometrium of postmenopausal women.

During the prepubertal years, the endometrium remains inactive, and the cervix continues to comprise the major part of the uterus. In the reproductive years, the dimensions and weight of a normal uterus varies widely according to parity. In nulliparous women, the uterus measures approximately 8 cm in length, 5 cm in width at the level of the fundus, and 2.5 cm in thickness; most weigh between 40 and 100 g. Multigravid uteri are larger with increasing length and weight with increasing parity. The internal os, a fibromuscular junction, separates the muscular uterine corpus from the fibrous uterine cervix. The uterine corpus is divided into the fundus, body, and isthmus. The fundus is that part of the uterus above the orifices of the fallopian tubes, and the isthmus represents the lower uterine segment. The uterus is located between the rectum (posteriorly) and the urinary bladder (anteriorly); it is supported by the round ligaments and the utero-ovarian ligaments and covered by the pelvic peritoneum. The endometrium during the reproductive period undergoes cyclical morphologic changes (described in detail below), which are particularly evident in the superficial two thirds, the so-called functionalis layer. Morphologic alterations are minimal in the deeper one third, the so-called basalis layer. In postmenopausal women, the endometrial morphology is similar to that in the prepubertal years (see section ❯ Postmenopausal Endometrium).

Vascular Anatomy

The endometrium has an abundant vascular supply that originates from the radial arteries of the underlying myometrium. These arteries penetrate the endometrium at regular intervals and give rise to the basal arteries, which in turn divide into horizontal and vertical branches, the former providing the blood supply to the endometrial basalis and the latter to the overlying functionalis layer. The endometrial vessels in the functionalis layer are referred to as spiral arteries. Their development and arborization near the endometrial surface and their connections with the subsurface epithelial precapillary system, as well as extreme coiling during the menstrual cycle, are influenced by ovarian steroid hormones and prostaglandins.

A differentiating feature between the endometrial and myometrial arteries is the absence of subendothelial elastic tissue in the endometrial arteries, except for those in the basal layer, and its presence in the myometrial arteries. Veins and lymphatics are closely associated with the endometrial arteries and glands, respectively. Uterine lymphatics drain from subserosal uterine plexuses to the pelvic and para-aortic lymph nodes.

Congenital Defects

Congenital abnormalities of the uterus are uncommon. They may be secondary to the effects of exogenous hormones, such as diethylstilbestrol (DES), in utero [70], or imbalances in endogenous hormones associated with abnormal gonads and chromosomal defects. In utero exposure to DES is, of course, nowadays rare. Genotypically normal females with normal gonads may also have müllerian duct abnormalities. These developmental aberrations, such as defects in the fusion of the müllerian ducts, are caused by errors in embryogenesis. The etiology of these developmental errors is mostly unknown, but hormonal imbalances or genetic abnormalities may be implicated. These disorders are frequently associated with malformations in the urinary system and the distal gastrointestinal tract. For practical purposes, müllerian duct abnormalities can be divided into two categories, namely abnormalities of fusion and abnormalities caused by atresia.

Fusion Defects of the Müllerian Ducts

Normally, the upper one third of the vagina and the uterus are formed by fusion of the paired müllerian ducts.

After fusion, the intervening wall degenerates, forming the endometrial cavity and the upper vaginal canal. Nonfusion of the müllerian ducts results in a bicornuate uterus. If the ducts fuse but the wall between the two lumens persists, an abnormal septate uterus results. Occasionally a carcinoma develops in one cavity, and only the other normal cavity is sampled during the investigation of abnormal uterine bleeding. If the defect is minor or confined to the fundus, the uterus is referred to as arcuatus. If the full length of the uterus and the upper vagina is divided by a septum, the condition results in uterus didelphys with a partially double vagina. These congenital anomalies may result in infertility or spontaneous abortion and in some cases require surgical correction.

Atresia of the Müllerian Ducts and Vagina

Atresia of the müllerian ducts and the vagina may be partial or complete. The etiology of these conditions is obscure, although a genetic cause is suggested in families with multiple affected siblings. The pattern of inheritance may be autosomal recessive or dominant. If only one of the müllerian ducts is involved, only the tubal fimbria and a small muscular mass at the pelvic sidewall will form. With bilateral atresia, the upper genital tract may consist of bilateral noncanalized muscular tissue located on the lateral pelvic walls. In Rokitansky–Kuster–Hauser syndrome, a severe defect characterized by müllerian and vaginal aplasia, patients may have urinary tract anomalies such as a pelvic kidney or anephria. Vertebral and other skeletal abnormalities may also be present, suggesting a more generalized morphogenetic abnormality. Patients with these conditions are endocrinologically normal with normal gonads. It has been postulated that activating mutations affecting the gene coding for antimüllerian hormone or its receptor may be related to the development of these syndromes [78]. If the anomaly is associated with obstruction of the vagina and functional endometrial tissue is present, hydrocolpos may be present at birth, or patients may present with primary amenorrhea. A uterus bicornis unicollis may develop in women with one affected müllerian duct, resulting in a pelvic mass and cyclic pelvic pain associated with menses. A number of multiple malformation syndromes have been associated with müllerian or vaginal agenesis. Winter syndrome, a genetically inherited autosomal recessive disorder, is characterized by vaginal agenesis, renal agenesis, and middle ear anomalies [156]. Management of patients with complete vaginal atresia requires surgery to create a neovagina. If the anomaly is isolated vaginal atresia, as most commonly occurs, the patient will usually be fertile if a normal uterus and fallopian tubes are present.

Normal Cyclical Endometrium

In the reproductive years, the endometrium is characterized by cyclical growth, shedding, and regrowth in response to estrogen and progesterone secretion by the ovaries. Endometrial morphology, as a consequence, is continually altering depending on the levels of estrogen and progesterone [33, 107]. During the proliferative phase of the menstrual cycle, the endometrium has a relatively constant morphology, which does not differ significantly from day to day; as such, accurate dating is not possible in the proliferative phase. Following ovulation, the morphological appearances in the secretory phase have been considered relatively specific from day to day such that it is possible to accurately date secretory phase endometrium to within 1 or 2 days. However, this view has been challenged with one study finding that traditional endometrial histologic dating criteria are much less temporally distinct and discriminating than originally described [102]. Nowadays, most endometrial biopsies are performed during the investigation of abnormal uterine bleeding, and it is relatively uncommon to be asked to date the endometrium, although formerly this was often requested in the investigation of infertility. The typical endometrial cycle is 28 days, although the length varies between women and even in the same woman. In general, the differences in cycle length are due to variation in the duration of the proliferative phase, the secretory phase usually being constant and lasting 14 days from the time of ovulation to the onset of menstruation. In the reproductive years, the endometrium is divided into two regions, namely the superficial functionalis (stratum spongiosum) and the basalis (stratum basale). The former exhibits the greatest degree of hormonal responsiveness, while the latter is much more unresponsive, the morphology not varying greatly during the menstrual cycle; as such, a biopsy consisting entirely of basalis is not adequate for dating of the menstrual cycle. Usually, the endometrial glands are regularly spaced and have a perpendicular arrangement from the basalis to the surface. The basalis abuts the myometrium and regenerates the functionalis following its shedding during menstruation. The basalis is composed of inactive appearing glands, cellular stroma, and spiral arteries that have thicker muscular walls than those in the functionalis. Accurate typing of the endometrium is, in general, not possible when polyps, endometritis, or other pathological lesions are present.

Proliferative Phase

The onset of menstruation is the first day of the menstrual cycle. Following menstruation, the uterus is lined by shallow basal endometrium and the deeper part of the functionalis. The endometrium begins to proliferate on the third or fourth day of the cycle, and during the proliferative phase, it increases in thickness up to 4 or 5 mm. Between the 5th and 14th days of a typical 28-day cycle, there is glandular, stromal, and vascular growth, the endometrium progressively increasing in depth until ovulation. The endometrial glands are uniform, widely and regularly spaced, and on cross section are tubular (➋ *Fig. 7.1*). An occasional mildly dilated gland is a normal feature and of no significance. Mitotic figures are easily identified within the glands, and the presence of mitotic activity should be confirmed before labeling an endometrium as proliferative in type. The glandular epithelium is composed of pseudostratified cuboidal or low columnar cells with a moderate amount of basophilic cytoplasm. The nuclei are oval or rounded and may contain small nucleoli; they remain orientated to the basement membrane. Proliferative activity is maximal between the 8th and 10th days of the cycle, and, at this stage, the glandular epithelium becomes more stratified and mitoses more frequently seen. In the late-proliferative phase, the glands become progressively more convoluted and tortuous and appear more variable in size and shape. Occasional subnuclear vacuoles may be seen. During the proliferative phase, the endometrial stroma is usually densely cellular, and the stromal cells are small and oval with hyperchromatic nuclei and indistinct cytoplasm and cell borders. Mitotic figures are present within the stroma, although less numerous than within the glands. Scanty thin-walled stromal blood vessels are present. The degree of mitotic activity within both the glands and stroma decreases in the late-proliferative phase, and early stromal edema develops. Estrogenic activity during the proliferative phase often results in focal ciliation of the surface epithelial cells; thus, surface ciliated cells are a feature of normal proliferative endometrium, and this does not indicate ciliated or tubal metaplasia (discussed below).

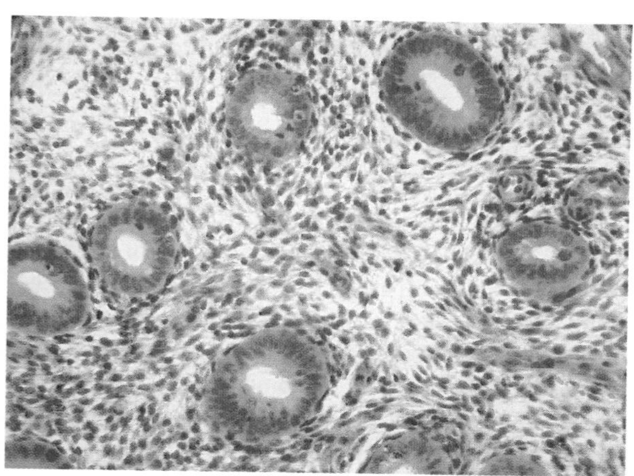

Fig. 7.1
Proliferative endometrium. **Widely spaced tubular glands exhibit mitotic activity**

Secretory Phase

Secretory endometrium is characterized by glandular secretion, stromal maturation, and vascular differentiation occurring in response to progesterone produced by the postovulatory corpus luteum. The endometrium increases in thickness up to 7 or 8 mm. The secretory phase may be divided into three stages, namely the early secretory phase (from the 2nd to 4th postovulatory day; days 16–18 of a normal 28-day cycle), the mid-secretory phase (from the 5th to 9th postovulatory day; days 19–23 of a normal 28-day cycle), and the late-secretory phase (from the 10th to 14th postovulatory day; days 24–28 of a normal 28-day cycle). These phases are continuous and not sharply demarcated, and some areas of endometrium may appear at a slightly more advanced stage than others.

There is an interval of 36 to 48 h between ovulation and the first morphologically recognizable signs of early secretory activity. In the early secretory phase, the endometrial glands still have a tubular appearance and mitotic activity may be identified. The initial morphological feature of ovulation is the appearance within the glandular epithelium of subnuclear vacuoles. These typically appear on the 16th day of the typical 28-day cycle, that is, the 2nd postovulatory day. Initially, subnuclear vacuoles are identified only within occasional cells and are irregularly distributed but usually most obvious in the mid-zone of the functionalis. There is a progressive increase in the number of and distribution of subnuclear vacuoles until they involve almost all cells within most glands in the functionalis (➋ *Fig. 7.2*). Subnuclear vacuoles are maximal between the 17th and 18th day of the cycle (3rd and 4th postovulatory days). As stated, some areas of endometrium may appear at a slightly more advanced stage than others, and in the early secretory phase, there may be an admixture of glands exhibiting proliferative and secretory activity; in fact, an individual gland may exhibit both mitotic activity and subnuclear vacuolation. It is generally

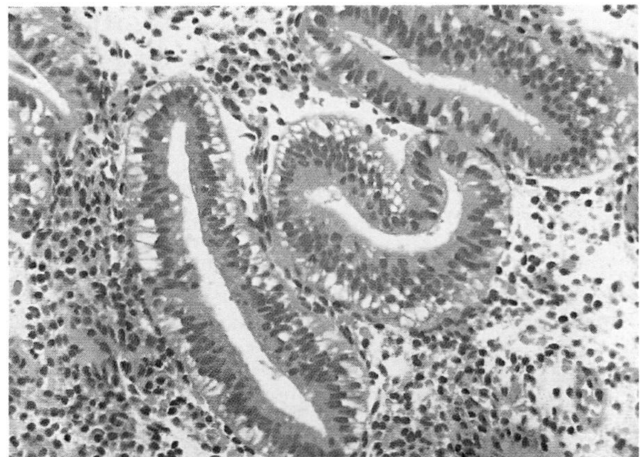

Fig. 7.2
Early secretory phase endometrium. **Tubular glands exhibit subnuclear vacuolation**

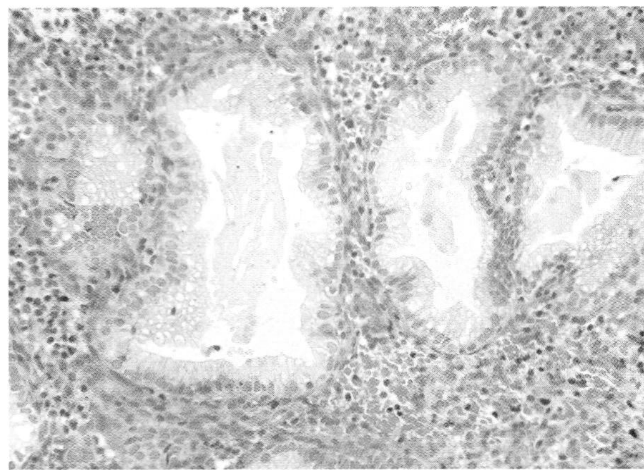

Fig. 7.3
Mid-secretory endometrium. **The glands contain supranuclear vacuoles with secretions within glandular lumina**

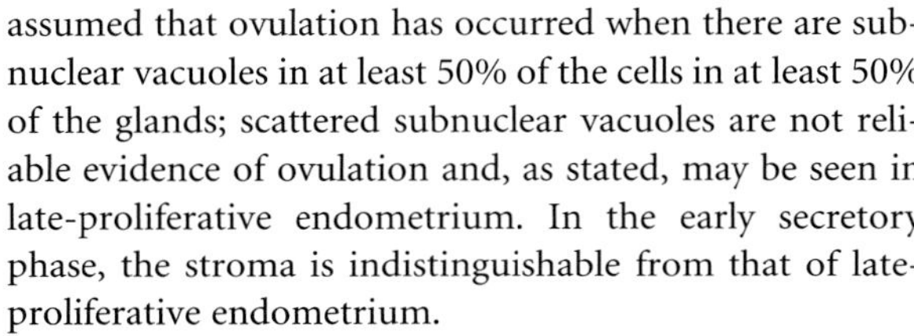

assumed that ovulation has occurred when there are subnuclear vacuoles in at least 50% of the cells in at least 50% of the glands; scattered subnuclear vacuoles are not reliable evidence of ovulation and, as stated, may be seen in late-proliferative endometrium. In the early secretory phase, the stroma is indistinguishable from that of late-proliferative endometrium.

Between the 19th and 23rd day of a typical 28-day cycle (the mid-secretory phase), the degree of glandular secretion increases. Cytoplasmic vacuoles become supranuclear and secretions are seen within glandular lumina (➲ *Fig. 7.3*); it is important to realize that secretory material within glandular lumina is not specific to secretory endometrium but may also be seen in proliferative, hyperplastic, and malignant endometria. Mid-secretory glands are usually angular in shape, and mitotic activity is no longer apparent. The glands in the superficial layers of the functionalis tend to exhibit less secretory activity, and, as a result, superficial biopsies may produce a false impression of poorly developed secretory activity. Stromal edema progressively increases, is most obvious in days 22 and 23, and is most prominent in the mid-zone (➲ *Fig. 7.4*). Spiral arteries become apparent. At this stage, the stromal cells have more conspicuous eosinophilic cytoplasm; these cells are referred to as predecidual cells.

In the late-secretory phase (days 24 to 28 of a typical 28-day cycle or 10th to 14th postovulatory days), there is typically diminution of glandular secretory activity (secretory exhaustion), and the glands become serrated. Predecidual stromal change increases, initially being most apparent in the cells surrounding the spiral arteries

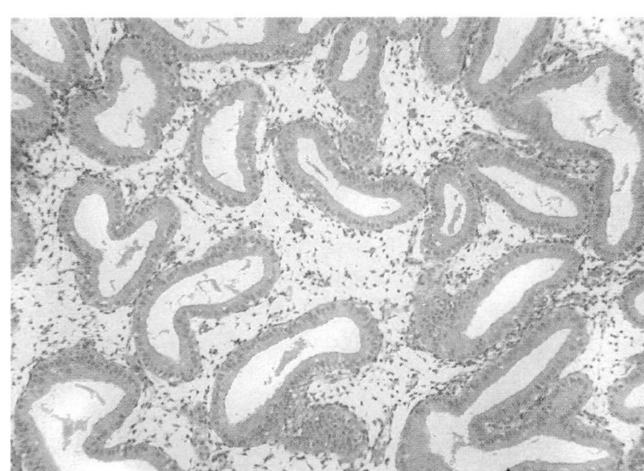

Fig. 7.4
Mid-secretory endometrium. **There is marked stromal edema**

(➲ *Fig. 7.5*). The predecidual change results in formation of the so-called compact layer (stratum compactum) beneath the surface epithelium, the deeper layers of stroma exhibiting less predecidual change. Sometimes, the predecidual cells may have a spindle cell or even signet-ring morphology and may not be readily appreciated as predecidual cells. Occasional mitoses may reappear in the predecidual stromal cells on day 26 or 27. A stromal infiltrate of granulated lymphocytes (described in detail later) is now obvious, and occasional neutrophils may appear in the premenstrual phase; the presence of granulated

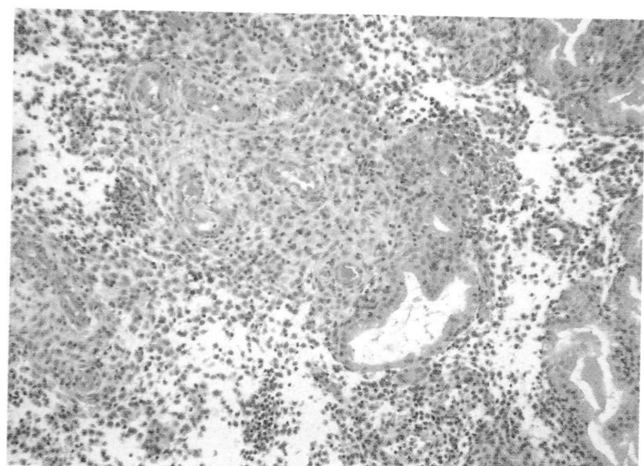

Fig. 7.5
Late-secretory endometrium. **There is predecidual change surrounding the spiral arteries**

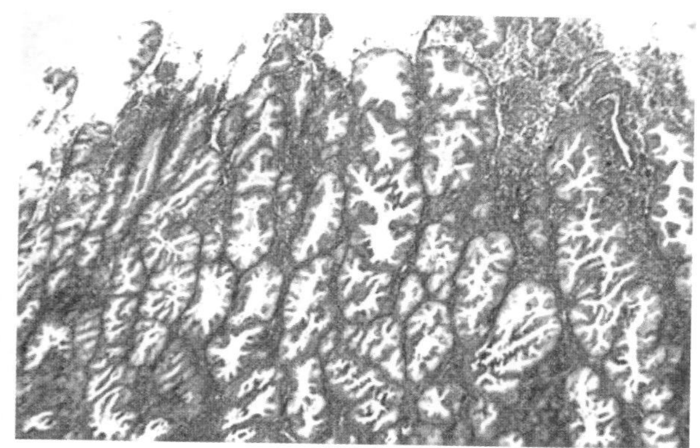

Fig. 7.6
Late-secretory endometrium. **The glands may be closely packed superficially resembling a hyperplastic endometrium**

lymphocytes and neutrophils should not be misinterpreted as evidence of an endometritis. In late-secretory endometrium, the glands may be closely packed (this impression can be exacerbated by tangential sectioning), and this can superficially resemble hyperplastic endometrium (*Fig. 7.6*); however, other features of a hyperplastic endometrium, such as mitotic activity, are absent. In some late-secretory endometria, the glands have a "hypersecretory" appearance, resembling Arias-Stella effect endometrium (*Fig. 7.7*); this should not, in itself, be interpreted as evidence of early pregnancy. In the immediate premenstrual days, apoptotic activity is seen within glands, fibrin thrombi appear in small blood

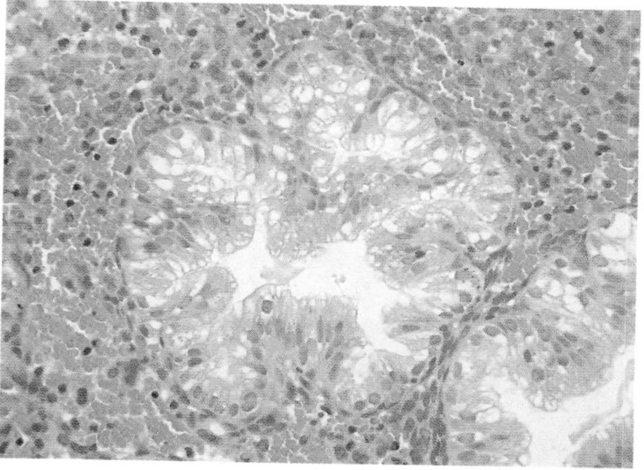

Fig. 7.7
Late-secretory endometrium. **The glands exhibit the Arias-Stella reaction**

vessels, and there is extravasation of red blood cells into the stroma.

Menstrual Phase

Menstruation occurs after the 28th day of the normal cycle (the onset of menstruation is the first day of the menstrual cycle) and is characterized by glandular and stromal breakdown. Menstruation usually lasts for about 4 days. The endometrial glands are serrated and collapsed. Some of the glands remain vacuolated and of secretory appearance. The stroma is condensed and collapsed, and the stromal cells aggregate into tightly packed balls (stromal blue balls) and separate from the glands (*Fig. 7.8*); the presence of tightly aggregated balls of stromal cells with hyperchromatic nuclei may be worrisome to the unwary. The predecidual appearance of the stromal cells is lost. Other features include the presence of necrotic debris, neutrophil infiltration, interstitial hemorrhage, and fibrin deposition. Apoptotic bodies are identified within both the glands and the stroma (*Fig. 7.9*). When menstrual activity is well developed, little or no stromal tissue may remain, and the glands become closely packed, sometimes with a back to back appearance; to the unwary, this may result in consideration of a hyperplasia or carcinoma. Following breakdown, the endometrial glands assume a surface micropapillary architecture (*Fig. 7.10*). The term papillary syncytial metaplasia (discussed later) is used for this appearance, but this is an inaccurate term since this is not strictly speaking a metaplasia but rather a regenerative or degenerative process secondary to tissue

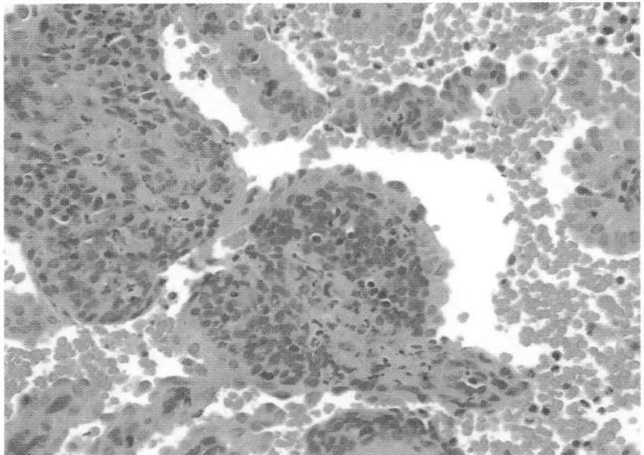

Fig. 7.8
Menstrual phase endometrium. **The stromal cells aggregate into "blue balls"**

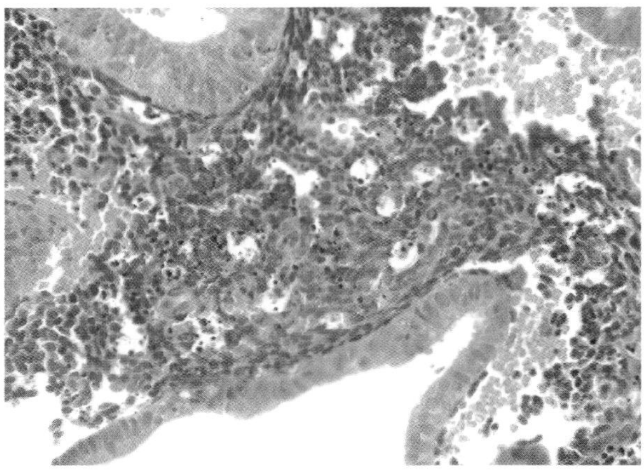

Fig. 7.9
Menstrual phase endometrium. **Apoptotic bodies are present within endometrial glands and stroma**

breakdown. Mitotic figures may be present within the papillary proliferations. Papillary syncytial metaplasia is also seen following surface breakdown associated with non-menstrual conditions. On occasions, the micropapillary architecture is particularly striking, and, if associated with mitotic activity, this raises the possibility of a serous carcinoma; appreciation of the accompanying features of breakdown and immunohistochemical staining with p53 may be of value. Most serous carcinomas exhibit diffuse intense nuclear immunoreactivity with p53, while papillary syncytial metaplasia is negative, or there may be a pattern of staining, which has been described as weak and heterogeneous [123].

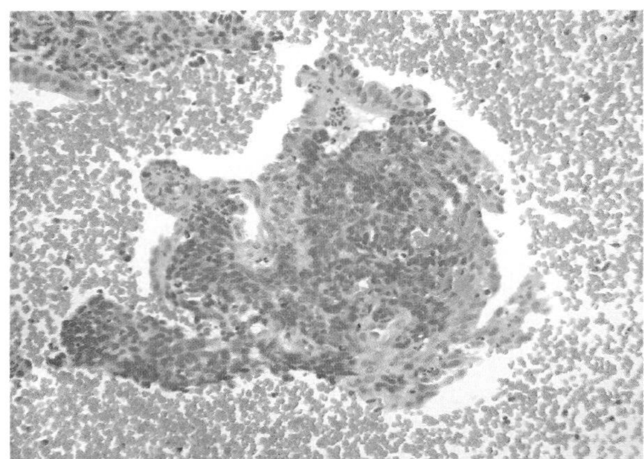

Fig 7.10
Papillary syncytial metaplasia. **Following breakdown, the endometrial glands regenerate with a surface micropapillary architecture**

Lower Uterine Segment Endometrium

Lower uterine segment or isthmic endometrium is poorly responsive to steroid hormones, and the morphology does not alter significantly during the menstrual cycle; as is the case with the endometrial basalis, lower uterine segment endometrium is not useful for dating the menstrual cycle. Lower uterine segment endometrium is composed of inactive poorly developed glands that are often ciliated (*Fig. 7.11*). They are irregularly distributed, and some may be dilated. The stroma typically has a fibrous appearance, and the stromal cells are more elongate and "fibroblast-like" than in the corpus. Given these features, lower uterine segment endometrium may be mistaken for a polyp in a biopsy specimen. In the inferior part of the lower uterine segment, the glands merge with mucinous type glands from the upper endocervix, and the stroma becomes even more fibrous.

Steroid Hormone, Steroid Hormone Receptor, and Immunopeptide Interactions in the Endometrial Cycle

As detailed, the menstrual cycle in postmenarchal, premenopausal women follows a regular series of morphological and physiological events characterized by proliferation, secretory differentiation, shedding, and regeneration of the uterine lining. These alterations are controlled by the cyclical release of the steroid sex hormones estradiol (E2) and progesterone (P) from the

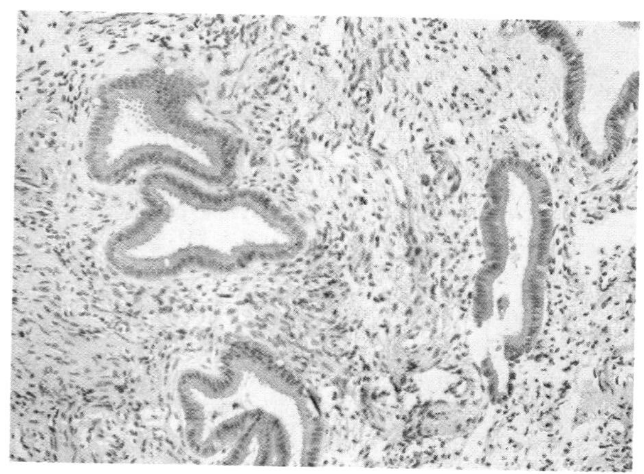

Fig. 7.11
Lower uterine segment endometrium. **This is composed of a mixture of ciliated and mucinous glands within a fibrous stroma**

ovaries; the endometrium is thus a highly sensitive indicator of the hypothalamic–pituitary–ovarian axis. Steroid hormone control of endometrial epithelial and stromal cells is mediated by estrogen receptors (ER) and progesterone receptors (PR). These steroid receptors are proteins concentrated in the nuclei of endometrial epithelial and stromal cells that have high affinity to bind E2 and P. Because they are sex steroid hormone (ligand) specific, a particular receptor may display high affinity for a closely related class of hormones, and these classes may compete for available binding sites. For example, ER effectively binds not only E2 but also estrone (E1), as well as synthetic estrogens, such as diethylstilbestrol (DES).

Although E2 plays a crucial role in the proliferation of endometrial cells in vivo, E2 alone is not able to induce proliferation of endometrial cells in primary culture. It has been suggested that the mitogenic action of E2 is mediated indirectly via a paracrine effect by the polypeptide growth factor, epidermal growth factor (EGF). EGF promotes the transition of cells from the G_0 to G_1 phase of the cell cycle [144]. Human endometrial cells possess EGF receptors and mRNA for EGF. EGF-like immunoreactivity is seen in both the endometrial epithelial and stromal cells, with higher concentrations in the epithelium than the stroma, and parallels the fluctuation of cyclic sex steroid hormones during the menstrual cycle. It appears that the regulation of EGF receptor content is regulated by ovarian E2 and P secretion (autocrine control). Indeed, EGF alone fails to influence cell proliferation, but in combination with E2, it increases the mean glandular but not stromal cell counts by more than 50% in vitro. The immunolocalization of EGF in normal human endometrium and the stimulation of epithelial cell proliferation in culture by EGF and E2 provide support for a role of EGF in endometrial growth.

The continuous dynamic remodeling of the endometrium results from a delicate balance of cellular proliferation and programmed cell death within specific subpopulations of stromal and epithelial cells, a process that is modulated by steroid hormones. A ladder pattern of DNA cleavage characteristic of apoptosis is seen in the late-secretory, menstrual, and early-proliferative phases. Localization of apoptotic subpopulations using in situ assays for DNA breakage has shown that the majority of apoptotic cells represent glandular cells within the basalis and these cells increase in number throughout the secretory phase and peak during menses [141]. The apoptotic effects of steroid hormones are likely mediated through a complex network of inhibitors and initiators. Progestins have been shown to decrease endometrial secretion of the apoptosis inhibitor bcl-2 [51], a process that is reversed upon administration of antiprogestogenic agents [32]. Progestins may also positively promote apoptosis by increasing levels of the apoptosis inducer gene BAK. The concentrations of ER and PR in the normal endometrium vary during the normal menstrual cycle according to fluctuating plasma levels of E2 and P. The highest values of ER (approximately 400 fmol/mg protein) and PR (approximately 1,000 fmol/mg protein) occur during the mid-proliferative phase (8th–10th day of the cycle) and correspond to rising plasma levels of E2. E2 promotes the synthesis of both ER and PR, whereas P inhibits the synthesis of ER. Monoclonal antibodies to ER allow the precise intracellular localization of ER by means of immunohistochemistry. Most ER is localized in the nuclei rather than the cytoplasm of endometrial epithelial and stromal cells. Endothelial cells fail to stain with ER antibodies. The concept of the mechanisms of sex steroid hormone–receptor action in target cells includes the following major steps: (1) circulating and unbound steroid hormone molecules are taken up from the cytoplasmic membrane, presumably by cytoplasmic receptors; (2) the hormone molecules enter the nucleus, which contains most (90–95%) of the cellular receptors; (3) the intranuclear hormone molecules induce conversion of the inactive (nonfunctional) 4S form of receptor to the active (functional) 5S form of the receptor; (4) the hormonally activated 5S receptor binds to acceptor genes in the nucleus and influences gene expression by stimulating RNA polymerase and thus mRNA transcription; and (5) the newly formed mRNA is transported to the cytoplasm, where it is translated into proteins, including anabolic and catabolic enzymes, as well as new receptors (receptor replenishment). According to this concept, the most significant effect of sex hormones is intranuclear activation of receptors that in turn initiate a sequence of events, which results in alterations in the physiologic functions of target cells.

Immunohistochemistry of Normal Endometrium

The normal endometrial glands and stroma are estrogen receptor (ER) and progesterone receptor (PR) positive (➋ *Fig. 7.12*). Endometrial glands are diffusely positive with the anti-apoptotic protein bcl-2 during the proliferative phase of the menstrual cycle. There is marked diminution in staining during the early and mid-secretory phases with reappearance during the late-secretory phase [13, 51, 101]. A minor population of endometrial epithelial cells exhibit nuclear immunoreactivity with p63; it has been speculated that these are reserve cells or basal cells and the origin of metaplastic endometrial epithelial cells [111]. Endometrial glands are cytokeratin 7 positive and cytokeratin 20 negative. The normal endometrial stroma is CD10 (➋ *Fig. 7.13*) and bcl-2 positive [86] and CD34 negative, in contrast to cervical stroma, which is largely CD10 and bcl-2 negative and CD34 positive [9], although there may be immunoreactivity with CD10 of stromal cells surrounding endocervical glands [89]. This differing immunophenotype may be useful in assessing whether the stroma accompanying a neoplasm is endometrial or cervical in type and in assessing tumor origin when this is problematic. The immunophenotype of lower uterine segment stroma overlaps with that of the endometrial and the cervical stroma. Normal endometrial stroma may be smooth muscle actin positive but is desmin negative. The immunohistochemistry of endometrial hematopoietic cells is discussed in the next section.

Hematopoietic Cells Within the Endometrium

The normal endometrium contains a variety of hematopoietic cells, the composition of which varies depending on the stage of the menstrual cycle and the menopausal status. Lymphocytes, including lymphoid aggregates and occasionally lymphoid follicles with germinal centers, are found at all stages of the menstrual cycle and in the postmenopausal endometrium. In the normal menstrual cycle, lymphoid aggregates are most common in the proliferative phase. They are more commonly seen postmenopausally within the basal endometrium; it is not clear whether this is due to lymphoid aggregates being more numerous postmenopausally or whether they are more obvious secondary to the glandular atrophy. Immunohistochemical studies have demonstrated that B lymphoid cells (CD20 and CD79a positive) constitute approximately 1% of the normal lymphoid population of the endometrium and are present mainly in aggregates in the basalis and rarely as individual cells in the functionalis. T lymphocytes (CD3 positive) are more common and are present throughout the endometrial stroma, usually as individual cells [37]. The distribution of B and T lymphoid cells is altered in endometritis; this is discussed below. Granulated lymphocytes (CD56 positive)

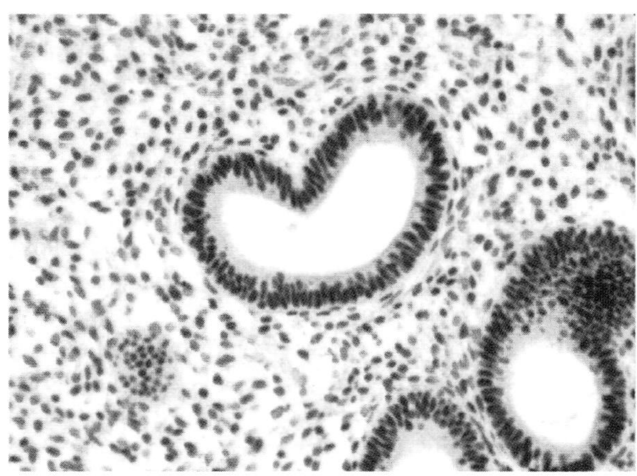

◘ Fig. 7.12
Estrogen receptor in endometrium. **The normal endometrial glands and stroma are positive with estrogen receptor**

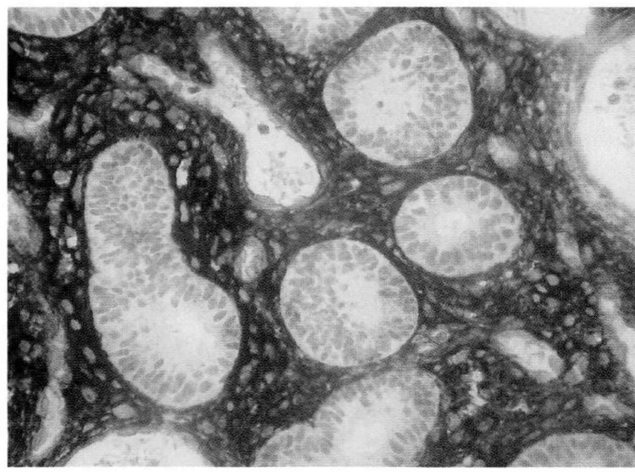

◘ Fig. 7.13
CD10 in endometrium. **The normal endometrial stroma is CD10 positive**

are present in large numbers in predecidualized endometrial stroma in the mid- and late-secretory phases [16, 17] (➲ *Fig. 7.14*); these were formerly designated endometrial stromal granulocytes and have a mononuclear or bilobed nucleus and abundant eosinophilic cytoplasm containing a variable number of granules. The function of granulated lymphocytes is not entirely clear but they have the characteristics of natural killer cells and, as well as being positive with CD56, are immunoreactive with T cell markers. Neutrophils are present in small numbers throughout the menstrual cycle but only become morphologically evident in large numbers in association with the tissue breakdown and necrosis associated with menses. In contrast to lymphocytes and neutrophils, plasma cells are not considered to be a component of the normal endometrium, although the presence of an occasional plasma cell is allowable in an otherwise morphologically normal endometrium. Plasma cells are, of course, a feature of endometritis (discussed below). Rare mast cells, demonstrable with toluidine blue or Giemsa staining, may be found in the endometrium, primarily within the basalis. Mast cells are also found normally in the myometrium, in endometrial polyps and in leiomyomas, often in large numbers in the latter. The number of mast cells in the endometrium and myometrium tends to decrease with advancing age. Histiocytes are also seen in the normal endometrium (discussed later – section ➲ Contaminants and Other Elements in Endometrial Biopsies). Eosinophils are not a component of the normal endometrium. Rarely, foci of extramedullary hematopoiesis are present in the endometrium, usually in association with an underlying hematopoietic disorder or occasionally representing remnants of fetal tissue [31].

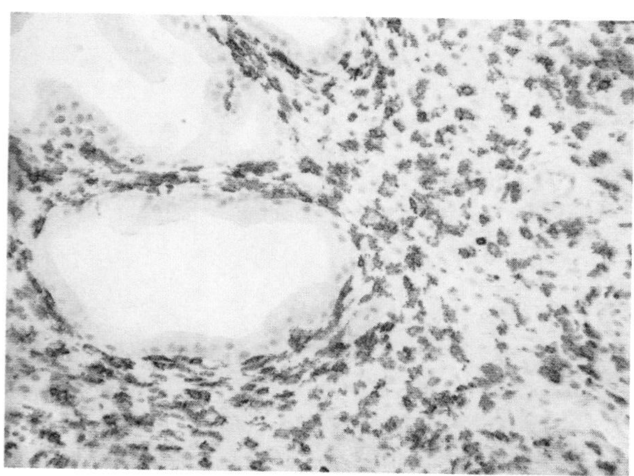

Fig. 7.14
CD56 in endometrium. **CD56 positive granulated lymphocytes are present in large numbers in predecidualized endometrial stroma in the mid-and late-secretory phases**

Gestational Endometrium

Pregnancy is characterized by morphological changes involving the endometrial glands and stroma. The trophoblastic populations in an intrauterine gestation are covered in ➲ Chap. 20, Gestational Trophoblastic Tumors and Related Tumor-Like Lesions. Early in pregnancy, the endometrium displays hypertrophic and hypersecretory features that have been referred to as "gestational hyperplasia." The endometrium is characterized by (1) glandular ferning with epithelial and intraluminal secretions, (2) stromal edema and vascular congestion, and (3) decidual reaction of the stromal cells. The changes are similar to but quantitatively exaggerated compared to those of nongestational endometrium at days 22 to 26 of the menstrual cycle. In the normal cycle, each of these alterations is prominent on a given day of the secretory phase, whereas during early pregnancy they occur simultaneously. The features described are not pathognomonic of early pregnancy but may occasionally be seen in other situations (see section ➲ Arias-Stella Reaction).

Immediately after implantation of the blastocyst on the endometrial surface, changes begin to occur in the endometrial glands and the stroma, although the overall morphology of late-secretory endometrium is maintained for several days. The early changes include glandular serration and distension, increase in glandular secretions, stromal edema, and a stromal predecidual reaction. The morphological features during the first 2 weeks of gestation are subtle, but after approximately 15 days, they become more characteristic with the formation of decidual cells. Compared to predecidual cells, decidual cells are larger with prominent cell membranes and more abundant eosinophilic cytoplasm that may contain small vacuoles (➲ *Fig. 7.15*). The nuclei of decidual cells are round to ovoid with finely dispersed chromatin and indistinct nucleoli. Stromal granulated lymphocytes are present during early pregnancy and spiral arteries become more apparent; they have thicker walls than in nongestational secretory endometrium. Some of the spiral arteries display acute atherosis with concentric intimal proliferation of myofibroblasts and accumulation of foamy cells. As the pregnancy progresses, decidual cells become widespread with better defined cell borders and develop an epithelioid appearance. Small numbers of granulated lymphocytes remain throughout the gestation. Some of the glands become atrophic while others have a hypersecretory appearance. Four to eight weeks after implantation, the glands often exhibit, at least focally, the Arias-Stella reaction, which is a response to the presence of trophoblastic tissue in the uterus or at an ectopic site. Histologically, the Arias-Stella reaction is characterized by cellular stratification, secretory activity, vacuolated cytoplasm, and enlargement of the epithelial cell nuclei and cytoplasm (➔ *Fig. 7.16*). The nuclei may be enlarged up to three times normal and can exhibit considerable atypia and a hobnail appearance with bulging into the glandular lumina. Mitotic figures may be present, although these are rarely prominent and there is a low MIB1 proliferation index. Atypical mitoses have rarely been described [3]. The Arias-Stella reaction may be extensive, involving many glands, or focal with involvement of only a few glands or even part of a gland. The changes persist for at least 8 weeks following delivery. Several histological variants have been described, namely atypical, early secretory pattern, hypersecretory pattern, regenerative pattern, and monstrous cell pattern [4]. However, there is considerable overlap between these patterns, and there is no value in attempting to subclassify Arias-Stella effect endometrium. The Arias-Stella reaction may also be seen in the glandular epithelium of the cervix and fallopian tube and involving endometriosis or vaginal adenosis [109].

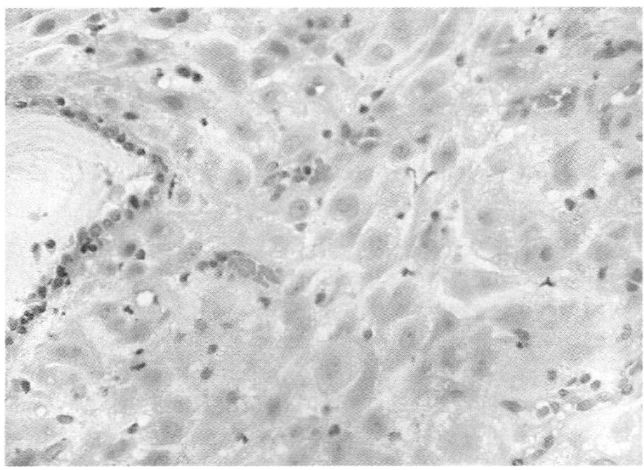

Fig. 7.15
Gestational endometrium. **The stroma is expanded and composed of decidualized cells with abundant eosinophilic cytoplasm**

Apart from the Arias-Stella reaction, the endometrial glands may undergo other changes in the presence of trophoblastic tissue. These include abundant clear glycogen-rich cytoplasm; this overlaps with the Arias-Stella reaction, but the nuclear enlargement of the latter is not present. Another pregnancy-related change is the presence of optically clear nuclei within the endometrial epithelium [98] (➔ *Fig. 7.17*). This may occur in association with the Arias-Stella reaction or independently. This appearance is due to the intranuclear accumulation of biotin and may simulate the ground glass nuclei of herpes simplex virus infection [157]. However, the nuclei lack the Cowdry type A eosinophilic intranuclear inclusions and nuclear

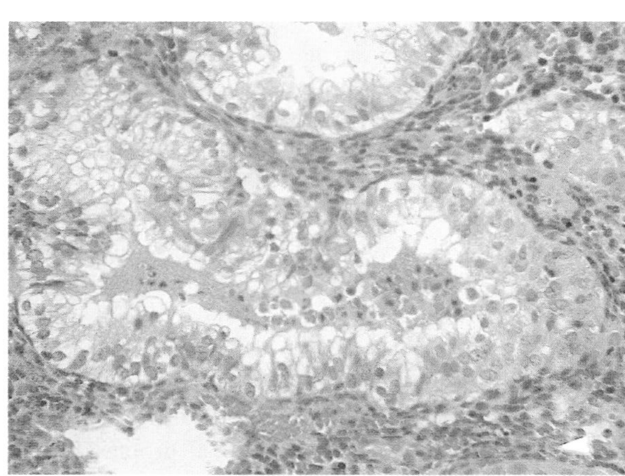

Fig. 7.16
Arias-Stella reaction in pregnancy. **There is cellular stratification, vacuolated cytoplasm, and enlargement of the epithelial cell nuclei**

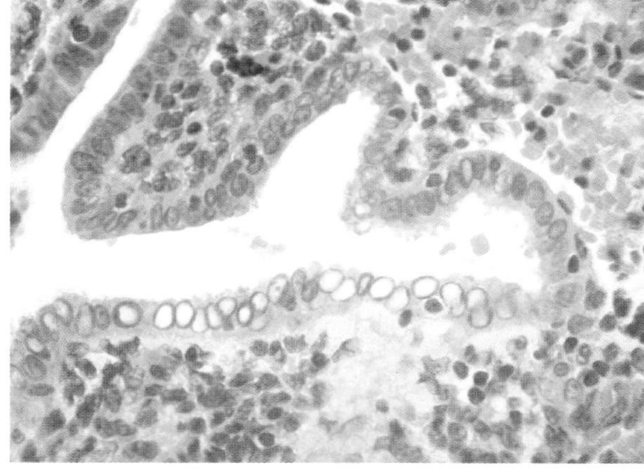

Fig. 7.17
Optically clear nuclei in pregnancy. **Endometrial glands in pregnancy may contain cells with optically clear nuclei**

molding characteristic of herpes simplex virus infection. Localized endometrial glandular proliferations have also been described during pregnancy, usually in first trimester gestations of women in their 4th or 5th decades. These rare focal lesions are characterized by glandular expansion, nuclear stratification, a cribriform architecture, and intraluminal calcifications [49] (*Fig. 7.18*). There is mitotic activity, but the cytology is bland. These appear to be benign lesions based on uneventful follow-up and an unusual response to pregnancy.

In early pregnancy, endometrial glands become strongly S100 positive [106]. This immunoreactivity disappears after the 12th week of gestation. The reason for this S100 positivity is not clear.

It is emphasized that the endometrial morphological changes of pregnancy described may be seen with both an intrauterine gestation and an ectopic pregnancy. Confirmation of an intrauterine gestation requires the presence of trophoblast, either in the form of chorionic villi or a placental site reaction (described in Chap. 20, Gestational Trophoblastic Tumors and Related Tumor-Like Lesions). In the placental site, intermediate trophoblast infiltrates the decidua. On occasions, it may be difficult to distinguish between decidual cells and implantation site intermediate trophoblast, although intermediate trophoblastic cells are larger and more variable in size and shape, ranging from polygonal to spindle shaped. The nuclei are lobated and hyperchromatic and binucleate or multinucleate cells may be present. There may be prominent nucleoli and sharply defined cytoplasmic vacuoles. In contrast, the nuclei of decidualized stromal cells are uniform and round to oval with finely dispersed chromatin and inconspicuous nucleoli. In problematic cases, immunohistochemical staining may assist in distinguishing between intermediate trophoblastic cells at the placental site and decidualized stromal cells. Markers of value are discussed in Chap. 20, Gestational Trophoblastic Tumors and Related Tumor-Like Lesions but trophoblastic cells are immunoreactive with broad-spectrum cytokeratins, cytokeratin 7, human placental lactogen, HLA-G, inhibin and mel-CAM (CD146), while decidua is negative [75, 82, 112].

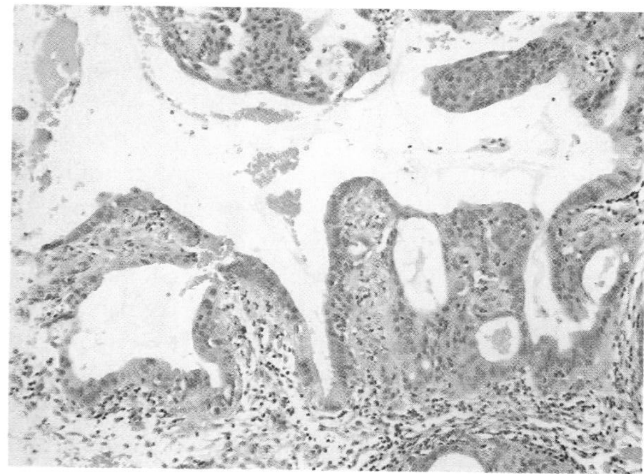

Fig. 7.18
Endometrial glandular proliferation of pregnancy. In rare cases, the endometrial glands in pregnancy exhibit proliferation with papillary and cribriform arrangements

Endometrium Associated with Ectopic Pregnancy

The morphology of gestational endometrium is discussed in the previous section. Endometrial changes also occur with an ectopic pregnancy. The features are variable but by day 22 to 28 of the ectopic gestation, the endometrial glands usually exhibit secretory or hypersecretory features, sometimes with Arias-Stella reaction, at least focally. Occasionally, the endometrial glands are atrophic. If the ectopic trophoblast regresses, the endometrial glands have a variable appearance, ranging from proliferative to secretory to a picture identical to that seen in disordered proliferation or progestogen effect. The endometrial stroma in association with an ectopic gestation is usually decidualized and devoid of inflammation. Thick-walled spiral arteries are present. Trophoblastic tissue, in the form of chorionic villi or a placental site reaction, is absent.

Postmenopausal Endometrium

The age of the menopause with cessation of ovulation and resultant diminution of hormone production by the ovaries is variable but is usually around age 50. Postmenopausally, the endometrium becomes thin and atrophic, unless there is continuing estrogenic drive, either in the form of endogenous production or exogenous hormone use. When there is no estrogenic drive, the functionalis is absent and the endometrium is composed only of a basalis, similar to the basalis of the reproductive years and of the premenarchal endometrium.

The histological appearance of the postmenopausal endometrium is variable. The endometrium is usually thin and this is appreciated in hysterectomy or endometrial resection specimens. The glands do not exhibit proliferative activity and vary from consisting entirely of small widely spaced atrophic tubules (*Fig. 7.19*) to cystically dilated glands throughout (so-called cystic atrophy or senile cystic atrophy) (*Fig. 7.20*); a mixture of small

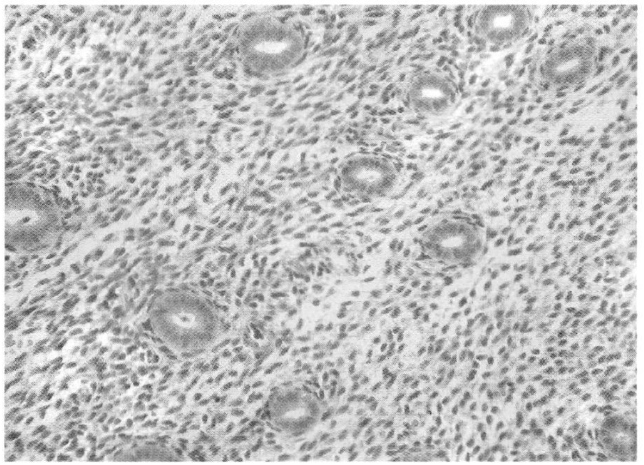

Fig. 7.19
Atrophic endometrium. **There are widely spaced small atrophic tubules**

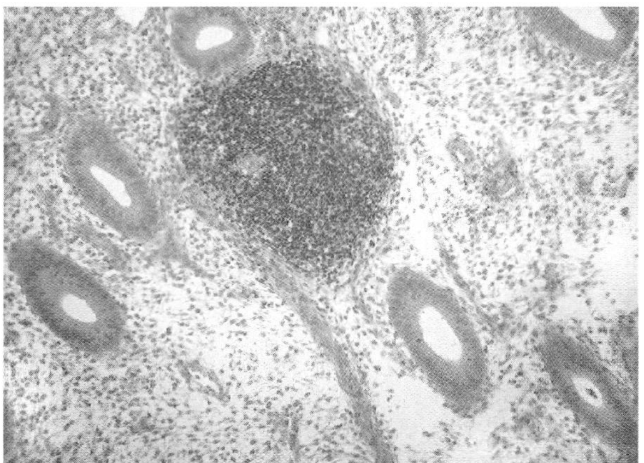

Fig. 7.21
Lymphoid aggregates in endometrium. **Lymphoid aggregates are a normal phenomenon within the endometrial stroma**

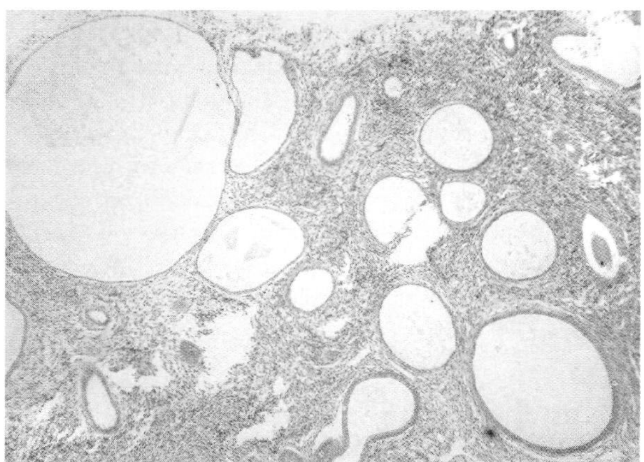

Fig. 7.20
Cystic atrophy. **Cystically dilated glands are present within a fibrous stroma**

tubules and cystically dilated glands may occur. The cystic glands seen in atrophic endometria in hysterectomy or resection specimens may not be observed in endometrial biopsies because tissue fragmentation during the procedure disrupts the glands. Usually, tubular glands are more prominent in the years immediately following the menopause while cystic atrophy is more common in older women but this is variable. The glandular cells have small dark regular nuclei that may be round, ovoid, or low columnar; in cystic glands, the nuclei are often compressed and attenuated. Sometimes, there is a degree of nuclear pseudostratification, which may result in a false impression of proliferative activity. The cytoplasm is usually scanty. High-power examination is required to confirm an absence of mitotic activity, and this is especially so in the distinction between proliferative endometrium and atrophy with small tubular glands and between cystic forms of atrophy and simple hyperplasia. The stroma in postmenopausal endometria may be densely cellular and composed of ovoid to spindle-shaped cells with scant cytoplasm or have a more fibrous appearance than in the premenopausal endometrium; the stroma tends to become more hypocellular and fibrous with advancing age. This may be the direct cause of the cystic change because of blockage of the glands. Lymphoid aggregates are often prominent (*Fig. 7.21*), more so than in premenopausal endometria; it is not clear whether this is due to an actual increase in the number of aggregates or due to them being more obvious because of the glandular atrophy. Sometimes, occasional mitotic figures are seen in the glands of postmenopausal endometria with no proven source of estrogenic stimulation. This may occur in women in whom the menopause appears gradually and also with uterine prolapse. The postmenopausal endometrium is hormone receptor positive, like that of premenopausal endometria, and retains the capacity to respond to estrogenic stimulation.

The morphological features of postmenopausal endometria are similar to those of atrophic endometrium due to other causes, for example, exogenous hormones, although there is often also stromal decidualization in those patients taking progestogen-only compounds or combined preparations containing a progestogen. Atrophic endometrium may also occur in young patients with premature ovarian failure, either idiopathic or due to surgical removal, chemotherapy, or radiotherapy.

Endometrial Sampling

Most endometrial samples are taken during the investigation of abnormal uterine bleeding in pre-, peri-, or postmenopausal women. Traditionally, most endometrial samples were obtained by cervical dilatation and curettage (D and C). It was believed that this had a therapeutic effect in some cases of abnormal uterine bleeding, as well as producing a sample for histological examination. Nowadays, most endometrial samples are outpatient biopsies performed by pipelle or other methods of endometrial sampling. In contrast to the traditional D and C sample, pipelle biopsies do not require an anesthetic and are often performed in conjunction with ultrasound examination and/or hysteroscopy, both of which may identify focal lesions that could be missed by pipelle biopsy. The disadvantages of a pipelle biopsy are that often only very scant tissue is obtained, especially in a postmenopausal woman with an atrophic endometrium, and focal lesions may be missed. Issues relating to adequacy of endometrial samples are discussed below. On occasions, a pipelle biopsy is followed by a D and C, for example, when there is a suspicion of malignancy and pipelle biopsy produces only a scant amount of tissue, which is nondiagnostic or when there are worrying features on the pipelle sample that are not diagnostic of malignancy. As stated earlier, endometrial sampling is nowadays not widely undertaken in the investigation of infertility, but when this is the case, the timing of the biopsy is important; ideally, the biopsy should be taken in the mid-secretory phase between the 7th and 11th postovulatory days. Endometrial polypectomy may be undertaken, and in such instances, sampling of the non-polypoid endometrium should also be undertaken. Transcervical resection of the endometrium (TCRE) may be performed under a variety of circumstances, such as in the management of menorrhagia or multiple polyps or occasionally when conservative nonsurgical management of an endometrial hyperplasia or a low-grade endometrioid adenocarcinoma is undertaken. This procedure produces a specimen consisting of multiple chippings, similar to prostatic chips. Chips should be weighed (this should also be done when biopsy or D and C yields a significant amount of tissue but may be impractical with very scant specimens). All endometrial specimens should be submitted in their entirety for histological examination. The exception is large endometrial polyps where representative sampling may be undertaken; it should be remembered that endometrial polyps may be involved by small carcinomas or by serous endometrial intraepithelial carcinoma (serous EIC), and, as a rule of thumb, at least one block per cm should be taken of large endometrial polyps. Endometrial chips should be orientated if possible since poorly orientated specimens, especially if tangentially sectioned, may result in a histological suspicion of adenomyosis; it is doubtful whether adenomyosis can be reliably diagnosed on a TCRE sample, although this can be suspected on well-orientated specimens, especially when there is smooth muscle hypertrophy surrounding the islands of endometrial tissue within the myometrium. A related, although uncommon, problem with endometrial resection specimens is the potential for overdiagnosis of myometrial invasion in cases of endometrial hyperplasia or adenocarcinoma; again, this is due to poor orientation and tangential sectioning.

In evaluating any endometrial specimen, an adequate clinical history is important, including the age of the patient and the reason for biopsy. Knowledge of the menopausal status as well as the date of onset of the last menstrual period (LMP) and the length of the menstrual cycle in premenopausal women should be provided. In some cases of "postmenopausal bleeding," the patient is not actually postmenopausal but rather perimenopausal with a prolonged interval between periods, resulting in the clinician and the patient assuming that the woman is postmenopausal. Many women with abnormal uterine bleeding have been prescribed exogenous hormones, especially progestins, before biopsy to control the bleeding and this information is not always conveyed to the pathologist. Other women may be taking hormone replacement therapy (HRT) or contraceptive agents. These hormonal compounds may alter the morphological appearance of the endometrium and a knowledge that these, and relevant medications such as tamoxifen, are being taken is paramount to the pathologist.

Criteria for Adequacy of Endometrial Sample

With the increasing trend to perform outpatient endometrial pipelle biopsies rather than formal curettage, pathologists are dealing with increasing numbers of endometrial specimens in which there is scant, or even no, endometrial tissue, especially when the endometrium is atrophic. These specimens may consist entirely of superficial strips or wisps of atrophic glands (➋ *Fig. 7.22*), with little or no stroma, admixed with cervical mucus, ectocervical or endocervical tissue, and tissue from the

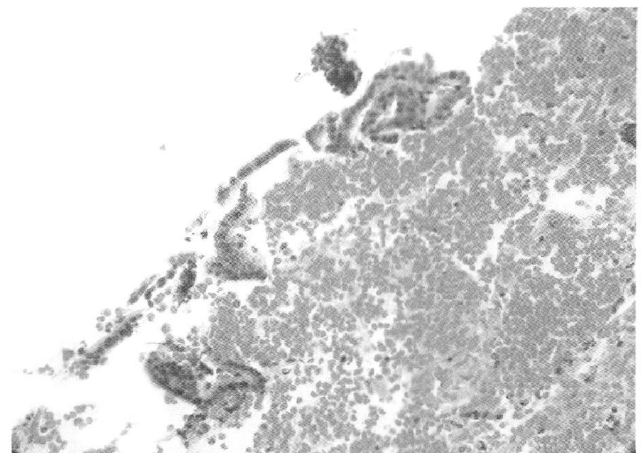

Fig. 7.22
Scanty endometrial biopsy. **Endometrial pipelle biopsy in postmenopausal woman where the specimen consists entirely of superficial strips of atrophic endometrial glands without accompanying endometrial stroma**

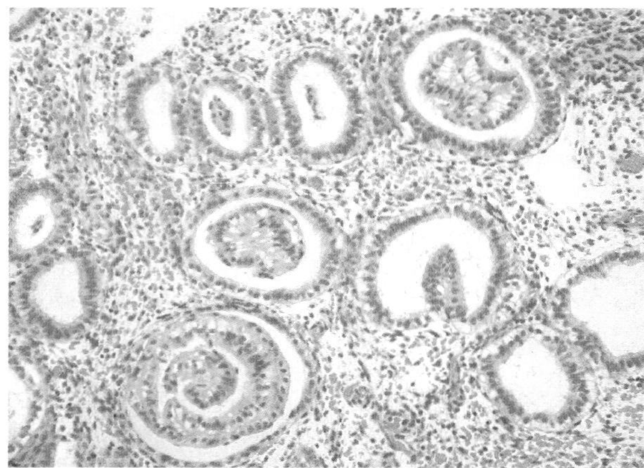

Fig. 7.23
Telescoping (glands within glands). **This is a common artifact in endometrial biopsy specimens**

lower uterine segment. Paradoxically, it often takes the pathologist longer to examine such specimens since no underlying architecture is present, and the tissue must be examined carefully under high power to look for mitotic activity, which is abnormal in a postmenopausal endometrium. In specimens such as this, it is controversial as to what constitutes an adequate or inadequate specimen. Designation of a biopsy as inadequate may be of importance since this can have management and medicolegal implications. For example, some clinicians routinely perform a repeat biopsy when an earlier sample has been reported as inadequate while others do not. A biopsy reported as inadequate may suggest to some that the clinician is at fault or has not undertaken the biopsy procedure correctly. While this may be the case in some instances, in most it is not. In published studies, inadequate rates of outpatient endometrial biopsies range from 4.8 to 33% [1, 2, 22, 52, 94], but in most of these studies, the criteria for adequacy are not clear. It is also worth noting that studies have shown that with an atrophic endometrium and no focal lesion, minimal tissue is the norm with a pipelle biopsy, and there is little chance of missing significant pathology [7]. Although it is difficult to recommend precise criteria for adequacy, caution should be exercised before categorizing an endometrial biopsy as inadequate or insufficient. In the majority of cases, the presence of only scant tissue in an endometrial specimen is not a reason for a repeat biopsy, provided the endometrial cavity has been entered, and at least some endometrial tissue is present in the biopsy specimen to confirm this, although theoretically endometrial type glands with or without stroma could be derived from tuboendometrial metaplasia or endometriosis within the cervix.

It has been suggested that with an endometrial biopsy containing scant tissue that cannot be typed, the term unassessable is more appropriate than inadequate or insufficient [120]. In such cases, the gynecologist should correlate the biopsy results with the ultrasonic and/or hysteroscopic findings. If there is a clinical suspicion of hyperplasia or malignancy, for example, if there is recurrent postmenopausal bleeding, or if the ultrasonic and/or hysteroscopic findings are worrying, then D and C should be performed. If the above investigations suggest an atrophic endometrium, rebiopsy is probably unnecessary.

Artifacts in Endometrial Biopsy Specimens

There are several common artifacts in endometrial biopsy specimens that have received scant attention in the literature [91]. Occasionally, these may be misinterpreted as an endometrial hyperplasia or even a carcinoma if not appreciated to be artifactual. Telescoping is common and refers to the presence of glands within glands (*Fig. 7.23*). This artifact seems to be a result of mechanical disruption and "snap back" of the glands during biopsy, resulting in a form of intussusception. Artifactual crowding and compression of glands are also common and may result in consideration of a complex endometrial hyperplasia. With this artifact, the glands often become "molded" together, and there is commonly tearing of the tissue around the glands, which is a clue to the artifactual nature (➋ *Fig. 7.24*). An artifact that is especially common with, but not exclusive to, outpatient biopsies is the presence of superficial strips of endometrial epithelium, sometimes accompanied by a little stroma, with a pseudopapillary architecture (➋ *Fig. 7.25*). This may result in consideration of a wide range of papillary lesions, benign and malignant, which occur in the endometrium. Such superficial strips of pseudopapillary epithelium, which are generally atrophic, should be examined carefully under high power to look for proliferative activity and nuclear atypia. Crushed endometrial glands and stroma may be extremely cellular and can cause concern. Extensive crush artifact is more likely to occur in biopsies from atrophic endometrium in postmenopausal patients. As with the examination of other tissues, crushed elements should not be viewed in isolation. Problems associated with poorly orientated endometrial resection specimens have already been described. Another artifact that may be seen in endometrial resection specimens and which is secondary to cautery is vacuolation of the endometrial stromal cells, resulting in a signet-ring appearance (➋ *Fig. 7.26*); this is a similar phenomenon to the vacuolation of cervical stromal cells, which may occur secondary to cautery [93].

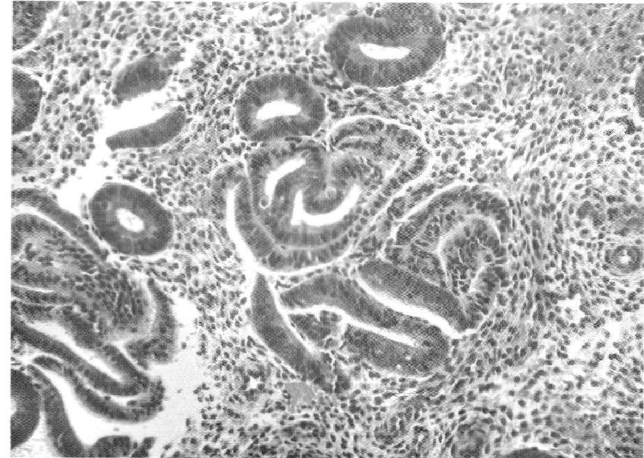

Fig. 7.24
Glandular molding. **A common artifact in endometrial biopsies is glandular "molding." There is tearing of the tissue around the glands, which is a clue to the artifactual nature**

Contaminants and Other Elements in Endometrial Biopsies

Not uncommonly, fragments of tissue other than from the endometrium are present in endometrial biopsy or curettage specimens. Superficial myometrium is commonly seen, especially in vigorous curettage specimens and in postmenopausal women with an atrophic endometrial lining. It is very common to see cervical mucus, often admixed with neutrophils, histiocytes and giant cells (➋ *Fig. 7.27*), and cervical tissue in endometrial biopsy specimens. The cervical tissue usually takes the form of strips of

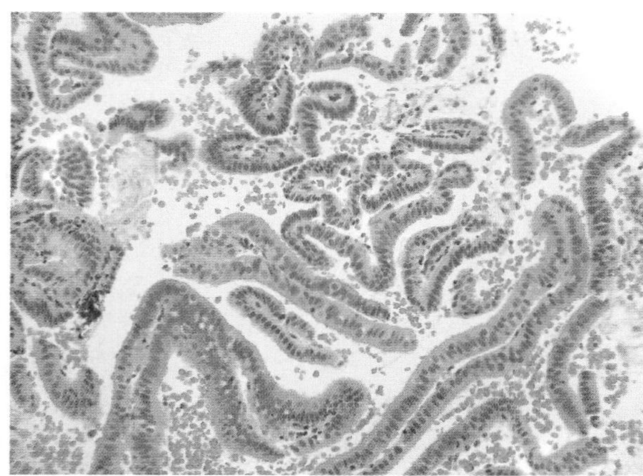

Fig. 7.25
Pseudopapillary endometrium. **Endometrial biopsy composed of superficial strips of endometrial epithelium with a pseudopapillary architecture**

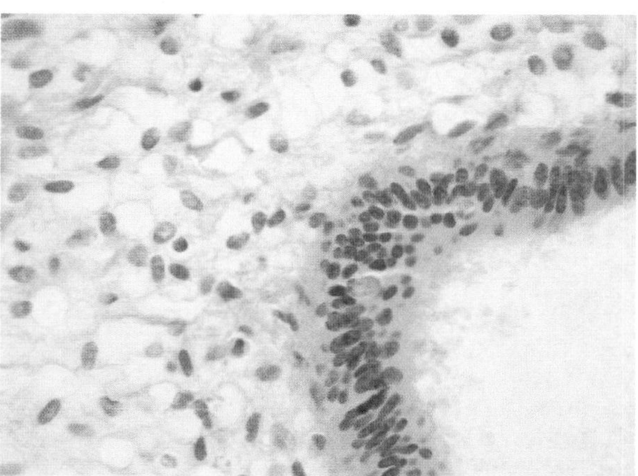

Fig. 7.26
Vacuolation of endometrial stromal cells. **Vacuolation, resulting in a signet-ring appearance, may occur secondary to thermal artifact**

endocervical glandular or squamous epithelium, sometimes with accompanying stroma. The squamous epithelium may be immature metaplastic in type. Usually the cervical origin is obvious but occasionally this is not the case and diagnostic confusion may ensue. For example, if cervical glandular elements exhibiting microglandular hyperplasia are identified within an endometrial biopsy specimen, this may result in consideration of an endometrial hyperplasia or carcinoma. The confusion may be heightened by artifactual apposition such that it can appear that the endometrial and cervical tissue is in continuity; assessment of whether the accompanying stroma is endometrial or cervical in type may assist in interpretation. Sometimes, dysplastic cervical squamous or glandular epithelium or tissue derived from a cervical neoplasm is present in an endometrial biopsy specimen. Fragments of fallopian tube epithelium may also be seen occasionally.

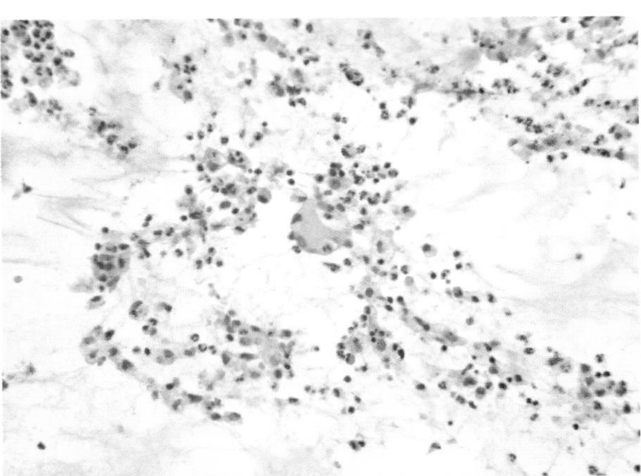

Fig. 7.27
Cervical mucus in endometrial biopsy specimen. **In many endometrial biopsies, mucus derived from the cervix is present, often admixed with neutrophils, histiocytes, and giant cells**

On occasions, aggregates or sheets of histiocytes may be seen in an endometrial biopsy specimen, either free floating or within the endometrial stroma. Small numbers of histiocytes are not uncommon and are usually inconspicuous but when present in large aggregates this may result in consideration of an epithelial or stromal neoplasm (*Fig. 7.28*). Recognition of the characteristic lobated, reniform, or coffee-bean nucleus of histiocytes assists and immunohistochemical staining for histiocytic markers, such as CD68 or lysozyme, may be of value. The histiocytes are probably a reaction to debris within the endometrial cavity and, when present in large numbers, this has been referred to as nodular histiocytic hyperplasia [74]. Occasionally, mitotic figures may be identified within the aggregates of histiocytes, and there may be prominent cell membranes. Rarely, the histiocytes have intracytoplasmic vacuoles and a signet-ring appearance [66] (*Fig. 7.29*) raising the possibility of a signet-ring carcinoma; staining for epithelial and histiocytic markers facilitates the diagnosis. Decidualized and predecidualized endometrial stromal cells may also contain intracytoplasmic vacuoles and simulate signet-ring cell

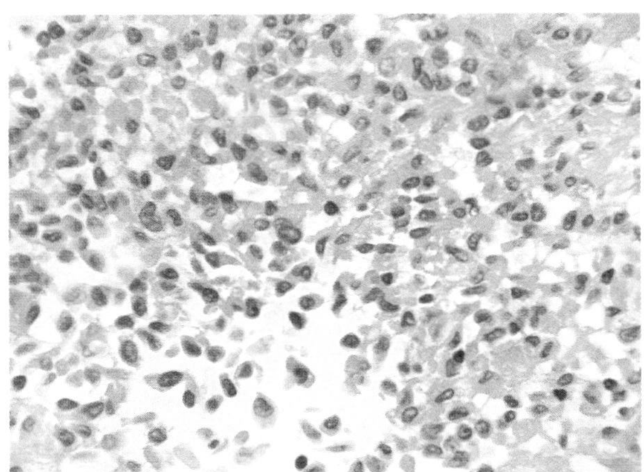

Fig. 7.28
Histiocytes in endometrial biopsy. **Aggregate of histiocytes in an endometrial biopsy composed of cells with a coffee-bean nucleus and abundant eosinophilic cytoplasm**

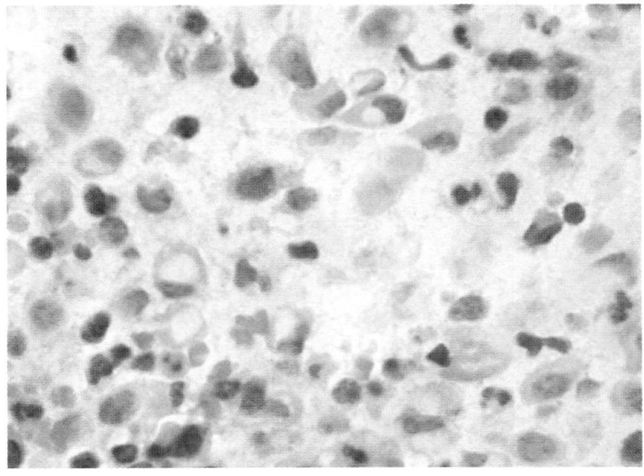

Fig. 7.29
Histiocytes in endometrial biopsy. **Sometimes histiocytes contain intracytoplasmic vacuoles imparting a signet-ring appearance**

carcinoma. Foamy histiocytes with abundant cytoplasm may also occur within the endometrium, either in association with an endometrial hyperplasia, carcinoma, or pyometra, or as a manifestation of xanthogranulomatous endometritis.

Extrauterine Tissues in Endometrial Biopsy Specimens

Rarely, extrauterine tissues are present in an endometrial biopsy specimen and this raises the possibility that uterine perforation has occurred during the current biopsy procedure or some time previously and that a fistulous tract is present. The most common extrauterine tissue is adipose tissue. Although this may potentially be derived from a uterine lipoleiomyoma, lipoma, hamartomatous lesion [83], other pathological lesion containing adipose tissue or represent metaplastic adipose tissue within the endometrial stroma, in most instances the adipose tissue is derived from the pelvic soft tissues or omentum and indicates perforation. Occasionally, the adipose tissue is accompanied by fibrinous material and mesothelial cells; this is a reflection of underlying pelvic pathology with resultant mesothelial proliferation, which results in fixation of the uterus within the pelvis and makes perforation more likely. In some cases, the patient comes to no harm because of the perforation, presumably due to contraction of myometrial smooth muscle sealing off the defect, but in other instances, a pelvic and/or abdominal inflammatory process ensues and the patient becomes symptomatic. For this reason, the identification of adipose tissue in an endometrial biopsy specimen should prompt a phone call to the clinician. Rarely, other extrauterine tissues, such as intestinal mucosa, may be present in an endometrial biopsy specimen secondary to perforation.

Endometritis

Endometritis is a histological diagnosis based upon the identification within the endometrium of an abnormal pattern of inflammatory infiltrate; as such, it must be distinguished from the normal hematopoietic component of the endometrium (see above). Most cases of endometritis occur in the reproductive years but sometimes postmenopausal women are affected. Presentation is typically with abnormal vaginal bleeding, most commonly intermenstrual bleeding or menorrhagia. Endometritis may have both an infective and noninfective etiology. The endometrium is relatively resistant to ascending infection from the lower female genital tract because of the barrier created by the cervix and the cervical mucus. However, on occasions, an endometritis occurs secondary to ascending infection, and this is often a component of pelvic inflammatory disease with inflammation elsewhere in the genital tract. Predisposing factors to endometritis include a recent pregnancy, the presence of an intrauterine device (IUD), cervical stenosis, and prior instrumentation. Endometritis may also accompany a pathological lesion within the uterus, such as an endometrial polyp, hyperplasia, carcinoma, or a leiomyoma. Usually, the morphological appearances are nonspecific, and, in the absence of an associated pathological lesion, an underlying cause cannot be determined, although occasionally the histological features suggest a particular etiology. Specific forms of endometritis are discussed later. Endometritis has traditionally been divided into acute and chronic forms, but these constitute a continuum, and often there is an admixture of acute and chronic inflammatory cells.

Endometritis may be focal or diffuse and can range from a subtle finding to a pronounced inflammatory reaction. Usually, the endometrial glands exhibit proliferative activity, and there may be mild glandular architectural distortion, in the form of occasional dilated glands. There is often associated surface breakdown with features identical to those seen in menstrual breakdown and breakdown due to non-menstrual causes. In some cases, an initial low-power clue to the diagnosis of endometritis is spindle cell alteration of the stroma (➲ *Fig. 7.30*), although this feature is not specific and is not always present. In other cases, the stroma may be edematous. In acute endometritis, the predominant inflammatory cells are neutrophils and collections of these may be seen within glandular

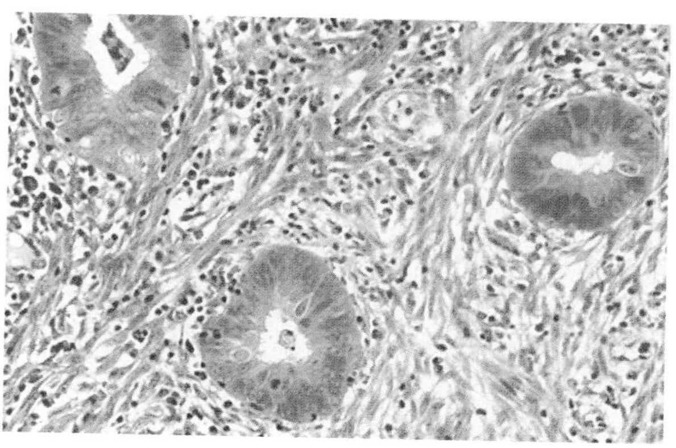

Fig. 7.30
Endometritis. **In some cases of endometritis, the endometrial stroma has a spindle cell appearance**

lumina, forming microabscesses (Fig. 7.31), or surrounding glands; neutrophils are often most easily seen just deep to the surface endometrium. In some cases, there is surface erosion with fibrinous debris and numerous acute inflammatory cells. By tradition, an unequivocal diagnosis of endometritis requires the presence of plasma cells (Fig. 7.32) since neutrophils are found normally in the endometrium just prior to and in association with menstruation and lymphocytes, including lymphoid aggregates, are a normal component of the endometrial stroma. However, in acute forms of endometritis, plasma cells may be absent or few in number. Plasma cells are usually most numerous surrounding endometrial glands and just deep to the surface epithelium. A form of endometritis without plasma cells has been described and termed focal necrotizing endometritis [12]. The histological features of this are of focal, patchy inflammation comprising lymphocytes and neutrophils and centered on individual glands. Due to the focal nature, this form of endometritis can be easily overlooked.

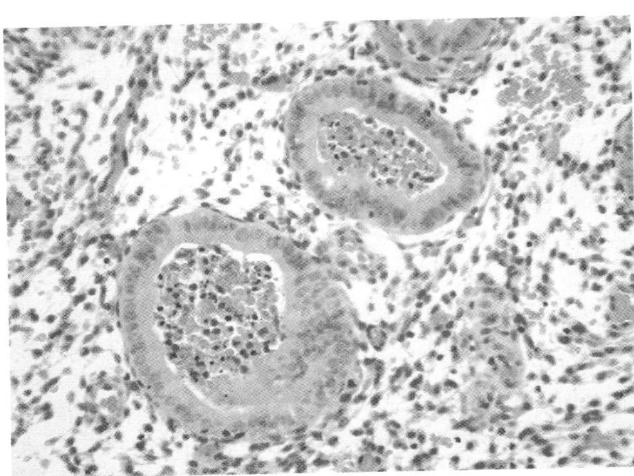

Fig. 7.31
Acute endometritis. **In acute endometritis, neutrophils are present, sometimes forming microabscesses within glandular lumina**

Besides plasma cells, there are also increased numbers of lymphocytes in chronic endometritis, sometimes with prominent and unusually large lymphoid aggregates and occasionally with the formation of lymphoid follicles. Other inflammatory cells, which may be a component of endometritis, include eosinophils and histiocytes. Usually, histiocytes are inconspicuous since they are admixed with other inflammatory cells but occasionally large numbers of histiocytes, sometimes with abundant foamy cytoplasm, are present. When these are abundant, this is referred to as xanthogranulomatous endometritis (Fig. 7.33). Xanthogranulomatous endometritis may occur in association with an endometrial hyperplasia or carcinoma and secondary to cervical stenosis and obstruction.

In endometritis, reactive and metaplastic changes may involve the endometrial surface and glandular epithelium. Squamous, ciliated, eosinophilic, and other forms of epithelial metaplasia can occur, and there may be mild nuclear atypia with nuclear enlargement and prominent

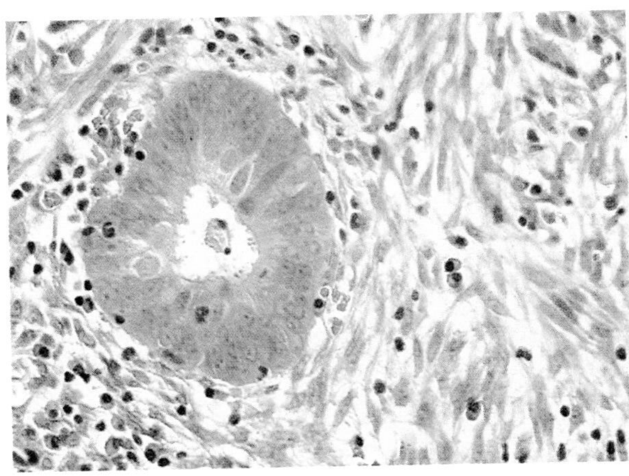

Fig. 7.32
Chronic endometritis. **In cases of chronic endometritis, plasma cells are present within the endometrial stroma**

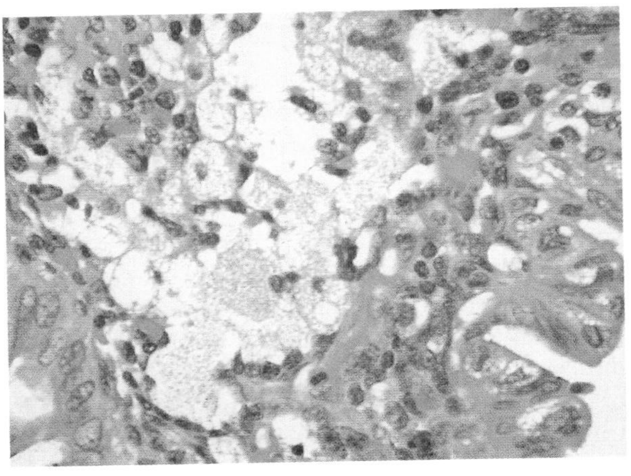

Fig. 7.33
Xanthogranulomatous endometritis. **Large numbers of foamy histiocytes are present within the endometrial stroma**

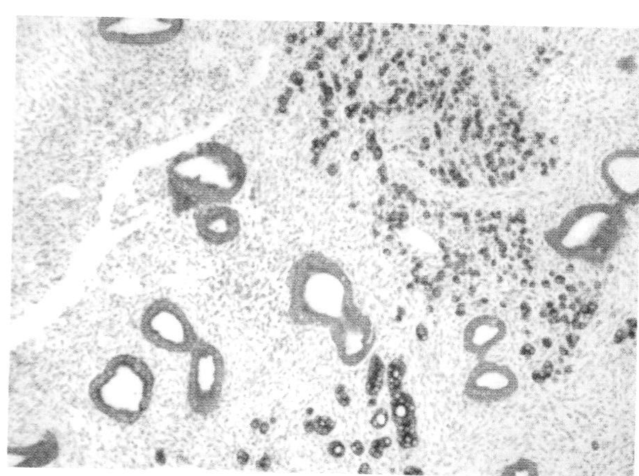

Fig. 7.34
Syndecan immunohistochemical stain in endometritis. **Syndecan (CD138) immunohistochemical staining may be useful in identifying plasma cells. The endometrial glands are also positive**

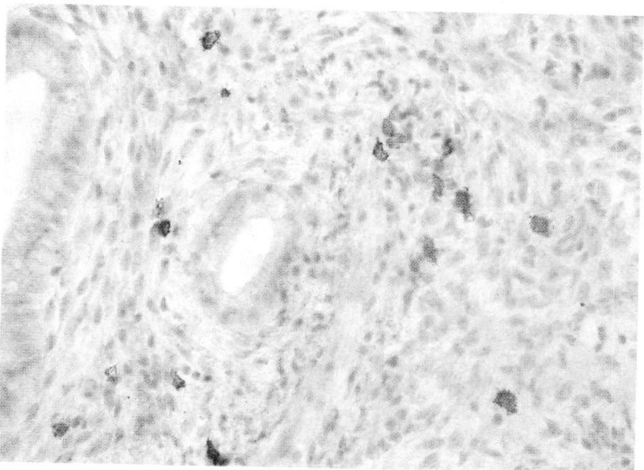

Fig. 7.35
CD20 in chronic endometritis. **Chronic endometritis in which increased numbers of B lymphoid cells (CD20 positive) are present within the endometrial stroma**

nucleoli. As stated, sometimes there are mild architectural changes with occasional dilated glands, but significant glandular crowding is not a feature of endometritis.

As stated, there may be problems in identifying plasma cells when they are few in number, especially in suboptimally stained sections. Endometrial stromal cells may have a plasmacytoid appearance, especially pre-decidualized cells in the mid-and late-secretory phase, and unequivocal plasma cells with eccentric nuclei and a perinuclear hof should be present. Occasional plasma cells may be seen in an otherwise normal endometrium and, in the absence of at least some of the other features of endometritis described, a rigorous search for plasma cells is not justified. Plasma cells may be present in the stroma of an endometrial polyp and this is not classified as an endometritis unless these are also seen in the non-polypoid endometrium. In problematic cases, histochemical or immunohistochemical stains may be of value in identifying plasma cells. Histochemical stains include methyl green pyronin and immunohistochemistry may be performed using plasma cell markers such as VS38 or syndecan (CD138) [10, 11, 77]. However, endometrial glandular epithelium commonly reacts with both VS38 and syndecan (➋ *Fig. 7.34*) and endometrial stromal cells may be VS38 positive; therefore, syndecan is more useful than VS38, in that although endometrial glandular epithelium is commonly positive, stromal cells are negative. Immunohistochemistry or in situ hybridization for kappa and lambda immunoglobulin light chains may also help demonstrate plasma cells but this is not routinely performed [41]. Immunohistochemical staining with B lymphoid markers (CD20 and CD79a) may also assist in distinguishing between the physiological endometrial lymphocytic infiltrate and the inflammatory infiltrate of endometritis. Normally, the vast majority of lymphoid cells within the endometrial stroma are T cells (CD3 positive) with B lymphocytes accounting for about 1% of all endometrial leucocytes [96]. B lymphoid cells are largely confined to lymphoid aggregates within the endometrial basalis with occasional individual cells in the functionalis. In most cases of chronic endometritis, there are increased numbers of B lymphoid cells, and these also have an abnormal location being found outside lymphoid aggregates within the stroma and sometimes intraepithelially and within glandular lumina (➋ *Fig. 7.35*) [37]. The number of T lymphocytes, histiocytes, and granulated lymphocytes in endometritis does not differ significantly from controls. It is emphasized that plasma cells do not usually stain with CD20 but are positive with CD79a.

Specific Forms of Endometritis

Chlamydia Trachomatis

Chlamydia trachomatis has been isolated from cases of both acute and chronic endometritis. However, it is unclear whether the organism is causative in such cases or an accompanying pathogen. Chlamydia trachomatis is a relatively common infection in both the upper and lower female genital tract and may be associated with pelvic inflammatory disease and infertility. Endometritis secondary to Chlamydia trachomatis has no specific histological features, although the inflammatory infiltrate may be intense and lymphoid follicles and large numbers of blasts may be seen [115]. Stromal necrosis and reactive atypia of the endometrial epithelium may be present. Definitive diagnosis in most cases requires culture. However, Chlamydia trachomatis inclusion bodies have been identified within endometrial epithelial cells; these are extremely difficult to detect on hematoxylin-and eosin-stained sections but can occasionally be recognized on Giemsa stain. Immunohistochemical staining may also be of value [155], positivity being localized to the epithelial cells in the form of stippling within supranuclear intracytoplasmic vacuoles. Molecular investigations may also be of value in demonstrating Chlamydia trachomatis infection.

Cytomegalovirus

Cytomegalovirus (CMV) endometritis is rare. It is most common in immunosuppressed patients but occasionally occurs in women with no underlying immune disorder. Typical intranuclear and cytoplasmic CMV inclusions are seen, mainly in epithelial cells but occasionally in stromal or endothelial cells. The other histological features are nonspecific; granulomas have been described in occasional cases [48].

Herpes Simplex Virus

Herpes simplex virus type II rarely results in an endometritis, usually secondary to ascending infection from the cervix and sometimes in women who are immunosuppressed. Typical herpes simplex virus inclusions are present within the glandular epithelium and there are multinucleate cells with molded ground glass nuclei. The other histological features are nonspecific, but patchy necrosis of the endometrial glands and stroma with an associated inflammatory infiltrate may occur [38]. Optically clear nuclei, due to the accumulation of biotin, associated with the presence of trophoblast may superficially resemble herpes simplex virus inclusions; immunohistochemical staining may be of value in such instances.

Mycoplasma

Rarely mycoplasma organisms, usually ureaplasma urealyticum, result in an endometritis. The inflammatory infiltrate is typically focal and has been termed "subacute focal endometritis" [73]. The inflammatory cells comprise mainly lymphocytes and histiocytes with few neutrophils and plasma cells and they tend to be concentrated beneath the surface epithelium, adjacent to glands, or around spiral arteries. Granulomas have rarely been described.

Actinomyces

The gram-positive anaerobic bacterium actinomyces may result in an endometritis, often in association with a long-term IUD. The bacterial colonies form the so-called actinomycotic granules (AMGs), referred to as sulfur granules because of their tan to yellow color on gross examination. It is important to recognize actinomyces since the organism may result in ascending infection with resultant tubo-ovarian abscess formation and pelvic inflammatory disease. Histologically, AMGs are usually seen on the endometrial surface or within the superficial stroma as non-refractile granules with thin basophilic radiating filaments and sometimes a dense more eosinophilic granular core (*Fig. 7.36*). They are Gram positive on Brown and Brenn stain and are highlighted with Gomori methenamine silver stain [122]. Although the diagnosis can be strongly suspected on morphological examination, culture is recommended for confirmation since other gram-positive filamentous bacteria may be found in the gynecological tract. Because of the potential complications, actinomyces must be distinguished from pseudoactinomycotic radiate granules (pseudo-sulfur granules).

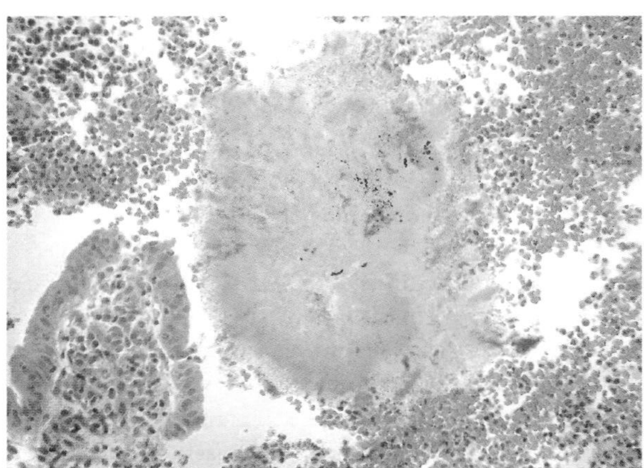

Fig. 7.36
Actinomycotic granules. **Actinomycotic granules (AMGs) composed of thin basophilic radiating filaments with a dense more eosinophilic granular core**

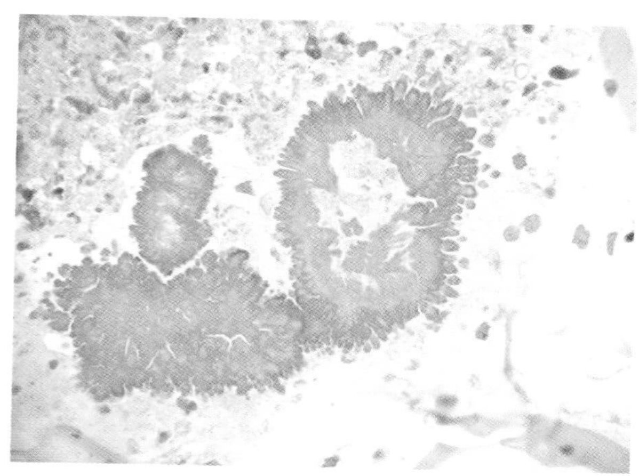

Fig. 7.37
Pseudoactinomycotic radiate granules.
Pseudoactinomycotic radiate granules with thick irregular club-like peripheral projections without a central dense core

These are noninfectious lesions, most commonly seen in association with an IUD, but sometimes in non-IUD users. They consist of thick irregular club-like peripheral projections without a dense central core (*Fig. 7.37*). An associated inflammatory response may be present. With Brown and Brenn stains, there is diffuse, intense nonspecific staining, while silver stains are negative. Pseudoactinomycotic radiate granules are probably more common than actinomyces [110] and occasionally the two coexist. The former may also be seen in association with pelvic inflammatory disease. The noninfectious nature of pseudoactinomycotic radiate granules is supported by microbiological and histochemical studies and ultrastructural analysis. Their exact composition and nature is unknown but they may represent an unusual response to foreign bodies (Splendore-Hoeppli phenomenon). Their main significance is that they may be mistaken for AMGs.

Fungi and Parasites

Fungi and parasites may rarely result in an endometritis, more commonly in underdeveloped countries. Blastomycosis (*Blastomyces dermatitidis*) and coccidioidomycosis (*Coccidioides immitis*) may result in an endometritis as part of a disseminated infection. Granulomas may be a component of the inflammatory infiltrate. There have been occasional reports of candidal and cryptococcal endometritis. Gomori methenamine silver and periodic acid-Schiff (PAS) stains are helpful in identifying these organisms.

Schistosoma, *Enterobius vermicularis*, and *Echinococcus granulosus* are rare causes of endometritis in developed countries but schistosomiasis is endemic in some parts of the world. Schistosomal endometritis may be mild or severe and is characterized by granulomatous inflammation with lymphocytes, plasma cells, eosinophils, and histiocytes, sometimes closely simulating a tubercle. The endometrial surface may be ulcerated and replaced by granulation tissue. Diagnosis is made by identifying the ova in tissue sections or in smears of vaginal secretions. Toxoplasmosis (*Toxoplasma gondii*) evokes a nonspecific inflammatory reaction in the endometrium. The microorganism can be identified by immunofluorescence.

Malakoplakia

Malakoplakia may involve several organs, most commonly the urinary bladder, and is characterized by the presence of sheets of foamy histiocytes (von Hansemann's histiocytes) containing Michaelis–Gutmann bodies. These are small, round, laminated calcospherites, which are present in the cytoplasm of the histiocytes and in an extracellular location. They contain calcium and can be demonstrated by von Kossa stain. The histiocytes are often admixed with other inflammatory cells, including plasma cells and neutrophils. Occasional examples have been reported in the endometrium [145]. Malakoplakia is a result of an abnormal immune response to bacteria, most commonly Escherichia coli, which are retained within the phagolysosomes of the histiocytes but are not digested; the Michaelis–Gutmann bodies are the result of mineral encrustation of incompletely digested bacteria.

Lymphoma-like Lesion

The so-called lymphoma-like lesions are more common within the cervix but have rarely been described in the endometrium [158] (see Chap. 21, Hematologic Neoplasms and Selected Tumor-Like Lesions Involving the Female Reproductive Organs). Histologically, they are characterized by dense aggregates of lymphoid cells, often with large numbers of blasts and a starry-sky appearance, forming a superficial band-like infiltrate, this only being appreciated on a hysterectomy or endometrial resection specimen. Lymphoid follicles with germinal centers, which may be large and ill defined, are typically present. Along with germinal centers and large numbers of blasts, a mixed inflammatory infiltrate is present with small lymphocytes, plasma cells, neutrophils, and histiocytes. Lymphoma-like lesions represent an exaggerated form of chronic endometritis. The polymorphic nature of the infiltrate together with the presence of germinal centers and the superficial location of the inflammation (as stated, only appreciated on hysterectomy or endometrial resection specimens) help to distinguish lymphoma-like lesion from malignant lymphoma, as does the absence of a mass lesion grossly. Immunohistochemistry for kappa and lambda light chains or molecular investigations to demonstrate a polyclonal population may also be of value. Occasional cervical cases have been associated with Epstein–Barr virus infection [158].

Endometrial Granulomas

Granulomas within the endometrium are rare. Worldwide, the most common cause is tuberculosis and, although rare in developed countries, granulomatous endometritis should be considered as tuberculous in origin until proven otherwise. Tuberculosis of the endometrium usually occurs in premenopausal women and is rare after the menopause. Caseous necrosis is characteristic of tuberculous granulomas but due to the constant shedding associated with menstruation, endometrial granulomas in patients with tuberculosis are often noncaseating. Tubercle bacilli are seldom identified on Ziehl–Neelson stained sections, and culture should be undertaken in all cases in which histological examination raises the possibility of tuberculosis. Other infectious causes of granulomatous endometritis include various fungi, schistosomiasis, *Enterobius vermicularis*, and *Toxoplasma gondii* (see section ➋ Fungi and Parasites). As already discussed, granulomas are occasionally a feature of cytomegalovirus and mycoplasma endometritis.

Endometrial granulomas, especially when well circumscribed, also raise the possibility of sarcoidosis and there have been rare reports of sarcoidosis involving the endometrium [117]. A granulomatous reaction to keratin may be seen in association with an endometrioid adenocarcinoma or atypical polypoid adenomyoma exhibiting squamous differentiation. Occasionally, such keratin granulomas may also be found on the surface of the ovaries, the fallopian tubes, or on the omentum or peritoneum; this is secondary to spread of keratin through the fallopian tubes and in the absence of associated neoplastic cells does not represent tumor spread. Foreign body granulomas in the endometrium may be secondary to talc or other substances and in association with an IUD. A palisading granuloma with fibrinoid material and a surrounding histiocytic and giant cell reaction, the features resembling a rheumatoid nodule, may occur secondary to endometrial ablation; usually, the entire endometrium or much of the endometrium is affected, and well-circumscribed granulomas are not generally found. A similar picture may be seen secondary to endometrial resection. In rare instances, there is no obvious cause for endometrial granulomatous inflammation, so-called idiopathic granulomatous endometritis (➋ *Fig. 7.38*).

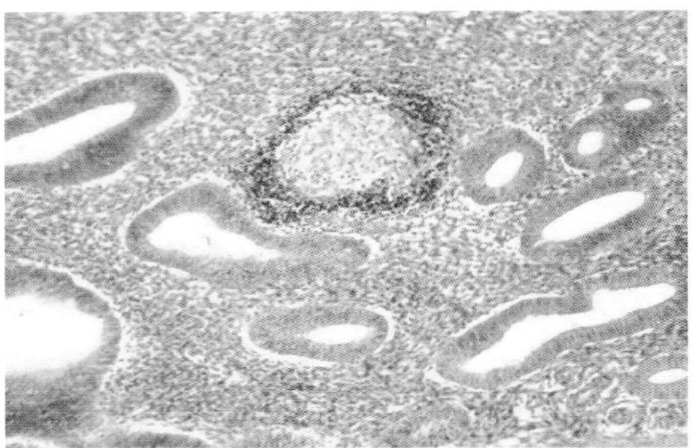

Fig. 7.38
Granulomatous endometritis. **A single granuloma is present within the endometrial stroma**

Ligneous (Pseudomembranous) Endometritis

Ligneous (pseudomembranous) endometritis is discussed here, although the term endometritis is not strictly appropriate since there is often little or no inflammatory infiltrate. Ligneous disease is an inherited autosomal recessive condition. The histological features in the endometrium are identical to those when other sites are affected, most commonly the conjunctiva. Ligneous disease is rare in the female genital tract and most commonly affects the cervix, vulva, or vagina. Rare endometrial cases have been described [129]. When the endometrium is affected, this may result in dysmenorrhea and infertility. Histology shows amorphous eosinophilic material, somewhat similar to amyloid, but Congo red negative, which represents fibrin. There may be associated mild inflammation, including occasional multinucleate giant cells. The inflammatory infiltrate may be more severe if there is surface ulceration. The underlying etiology is due to absent or low plasminogen levels, which results in accumulation of fibrin.

Dysfunctional Uterine Bleeding

Dysfunctional uterine bleeding (DUB) is abnormal uterine bleeding in a premenopausal woman resulting from alterations in the normal cyclical changes of the endometrium and without an underlying specific pathological cause such as endometritis, polyps, exogenous hormones, hyperplasia, or carcinoma. In many cases, DUB is probably secondary to endogenous hormone imbalance. There are several morphological alterations of the endometrium that are characteristic of DUB, the most common being those associated with anovulatory cycles or luteal phase defects. These can be regarded as estrogen-related and progesterone-related, respectively, and are discussed in the next sections. Often DUB is managed by hormonal therapy and a biopsy only performed when symptoms persist; the hormone therapy may result in modification of the morphology. It is stressed that DUB is not a pathological diagnosis but rather a clinical term. A common, but not invariable, feature of biopsies from patients with DUB is the presence of glandular and stromal breakdown. The features associated with this are not unique to DUB and are seen in menstrual endometrium and in bleeding associated with a variety of organic disorders. It is important to recognize the features of breakdown and to distinguish them from other pathological lesions. It is also important to realize that glandular and stromal breakdown is a nonspecific feature and that the intact endometrium must be assessed to evaluate the underlying abnormality. Glandular and stromal breakdown may also occur in an atrophic endometrium. The changes associated with glandular and stromal breakdown are described in the next paragraphs. In menstrual endometrium, the features of breakdown are diffuse and occur on a background of secretory endometrium. In contrast, in DUB, the background endometrium is typically nonsecretory in type and breakdown is usually a focal phenomenon, resulting in a heterogeneous pattern with intact fragments of endometrium admixed with fragments exhibiting the features of breakdown. Furthermore, in menstrual endometrium the changes are acute and there are no features of chronic bleeding, such as hemosiderin deposition and accumulation of foam cells.

The morphological features associated with glandular and stromal breakdown are summarized in ➋ *Table 7.1*. An early feature is the accumulation of nuclear (apoptotic) debris in the basal cytoplasm of the glandular cells (➋ *Fig. 7.39*) [139]. The stromal cells collapse and aggregate into tight clusters, which are separated by lakes of blood. These clusters of stromal cells, sometime called "stromal blue balls," may form small polypoid extrusions or become detached from the surrounding tissue (➋ *Fig. 7.40*). They are characterized by tightly packed cells with hyperchromatic nuclei and scanty cytoplasm admixed with apoptotic debris. They can exhibit nuclear molding and to the unwary may raise the possibility of small cell carcinoma. However, they are often covered by an epithelial lining, which may be flat or may exhibit the features of papillary syncytial metaplasia (see below) and are associated with other features of breakdown. Because of the stromal collapse, the endometrial glands become disrupted and crowded (➋ *Fig. 7.41*). This glandular crowding may mimic hyperplasia or even

Table 7.1
Features of endometrial breakdown

Glandular changes
Nuclear (apoptotic) debris in basal cytoplasm of glandular cells
Papillary syncytial metaplasia
Glandular crowding
Stromal changes
Stromal collapse
Aggregates of stromal cells
Nuclear (apoptotic) debris in stroma
Fibrin thrombi
Hemosiderin pigment deposition
Foam cell accumulation
Fibrosis and hyalinization

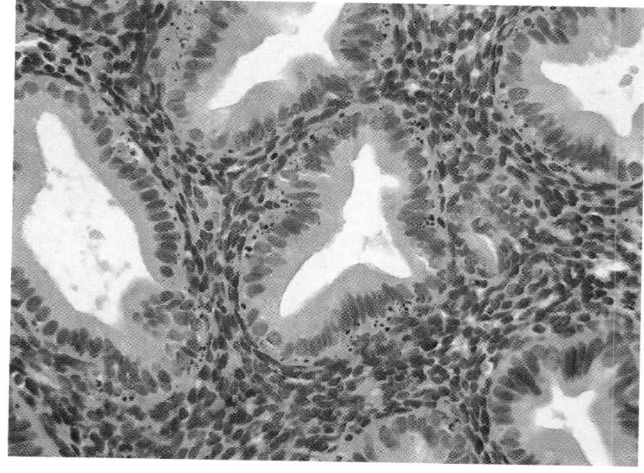

Fig. 7.39
Glandular and stromal breakdown. **An early feature is the accumulation of apoptotic debris in the cytoplasm of the glandular epithelial cells**

adenocarcinoma but recognition of the other features of breakdown facilitates the diagnosis. Fibrin thrombi are usually seen in small blood vessels, either in the spiral arteries or in superficial ectatic stromal vessels (➋ *Fig. 7.42*). Another consistent feature of breakdown is papillary syncytial metaplasia (➋ *Fig. 7.10*). Synonymous terms include eosinophilic syncytial change and surface syncytial change. The term papillary syncytial metaplasia is a misnomer since this is not a true metaplasia but has rather been variously considered a regenerative reaction to surface breakdown or a degenerative or regressive process [131]. Papillary syncytial metaplasia is characterized histologically by syncytial sheets of epithelial cells with indistinct cell borders that form micropapillary structures, sometimes with small glandular lumina. The syncytia are devoid of stromal support, lacking fibrovascular stromal cores. The cells usually have eosinophilic cytoplasm and there is often a neutrophilic infiltrate. There may be mild nuclear atypia and sometimes mitoses are identified.

Other features of breakdown, which are not present in all cases, include hemosiderin deposition, free either within the stroma or within histiocytes (➋ *Fig. 7.43*) and

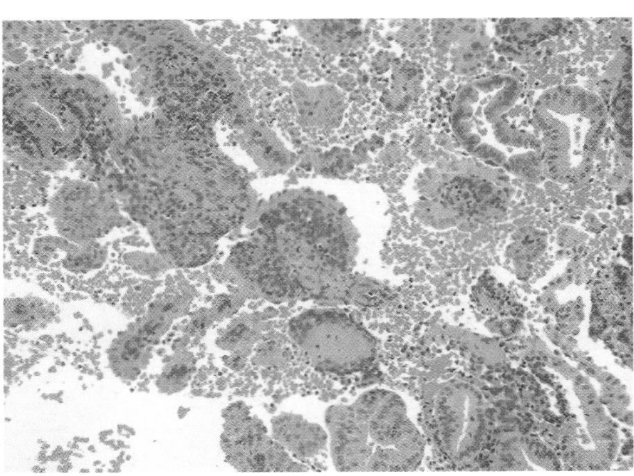

■ Fig. 7.40
Breaking down endometrium. **With breakdown, the stromal cells aggregate into stromal "blue balls"**

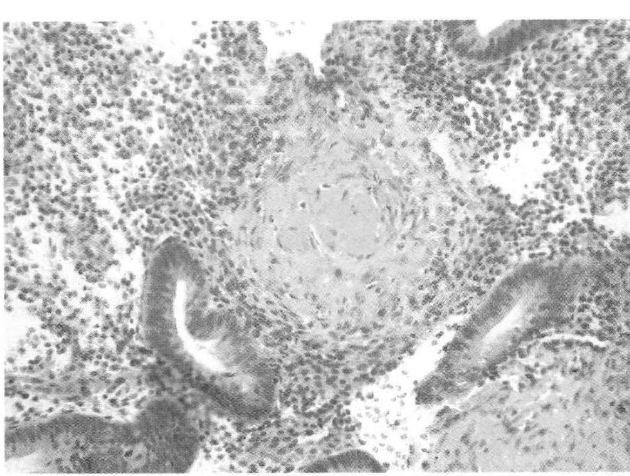

■ Fig. 7.42
Breaking down endometrium. **With breakdown, fibrin thrombi are typically seen within blood vessels**

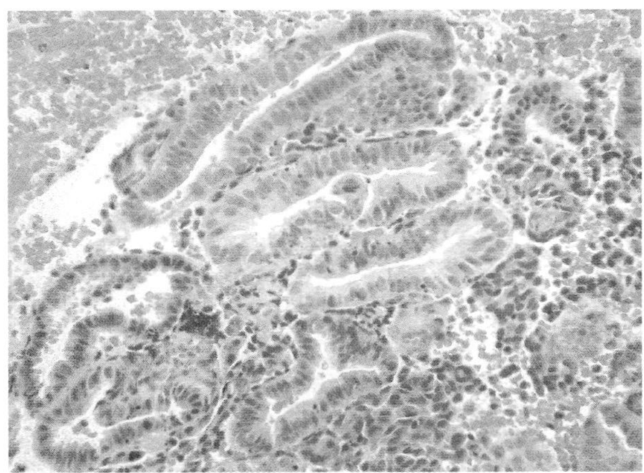

■ Fig. 7.41
Breaking down endometrium. **With breakdown, the endometrial glands become disrupted and crowded because of stromal collapse**

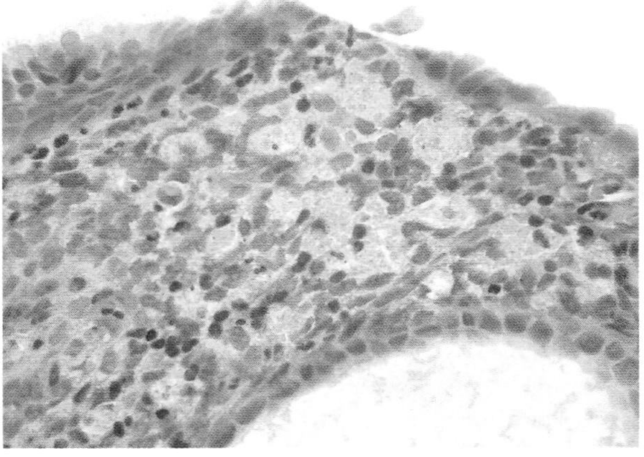

■ Fig. 7.43
Chronic breakdown. **With chronic breakdown, hemosiderin pigment may accumulate within histiocytes within the endometrial stroma**

accumulation of foam cells, neither of which occurs in normal cyclical endometrium during the reproductive years. These features usually indicate chronic bleeding. The foam cells were initially thought to represent histiocytes, but it has been suggested that they may represent endometrial stromal cells, which become distended with lipid following erythrocyte breakdown [42]. Chronic bleeding may also occasionally result in focal stromal fibrosis and hyalinization.

Estrogen Related Dysfunctional Uterine Bleeding, Including Endometrium Associated with Anovulatory Cycles

This endometrial morphology is most common in the perimenopausal years where it is usually secondary to anovulatory cycles with resultant absence of development of the corpus luteum and decrease in progesterone secretion; in fact, this is sometimes referred to as anovulatory endometrium. The term persistent proliferative endometrium has also been used. The underlying causes are complex but many cases may be a result of hypothalamic dysfunction. The developing follicles persist for a variable period of time and produce estradiol before undergoing atresia at which time estrogen withdrawal bleeding occurs. In other cases, estrogen breakthrough bleeding occurs when the persisting follicles produce estradiol resulting in the proliferating endometrium becoming thicker and outgrowing its blood supply. The usual presentation is with perimenopausal bleeding, but younger women may also be affected, for example, perimenarchal adolescents in whom regular ovulatory cycles are not established, those with polycystic ovarian syndrome (Stein–Leventhal syndrome), or older women taking unopposed estrogens or with an increase in endogenous estrogens, for example, secondary to obesity. Anovulatory cycles may also occur sporadically throughout the reproductive years. The histological features involve the entire endometrial compartment and are those of proliferative endometrium but with superimposed breakdown, as described above [103]. The extent of breakdown is highly variable and ranges from minute focal changes to a widespread phenomenon involving most of the specimen. There are often foci of ciliated (tubal) or other types of epithelial metaplasia that are randomly dispersed.

With chronic anovulatory cycles, there is abundant proliferative endometrium and mild degrees of disorganization with dilated glands may occur. This results in a picture, which is neither normal proliferative nor hyperplastic and which is referred to as disordered proliferative endometrium (*Fig. 7.44*). Occasional dilated glands within an otherwise normal proliferative endometrium does not warrant a diagnosis of disordered proliferation; in other words, there should be significant numbers of dilated glands and these should have a widespread distribution, although they are admixed with normal proliferative glands. In disordered proliferative endometrium, the normal gland to stroma ratio is largely maintained although there may be focal mild glandular crowding and branching. In cases with significant numbers of dilated glands, the morphological appearances merge with and overlap with those of simple hyperplasia; in fact, disordered proliferative endometrium and simple hyperplasia almost certainly constitute a continuum, and it is likely that both represent a response to unopposed estrogens and not a true premalignant lesion, although there is a small increased risk of the development of an endometrioid adenocarcinoma. In simple hyperplasia, there is usually more glandular dilatation, with a paucity of normal proliferative glands, and the glands exhibit more budding and branching. However, there is significant interobserver variability in the distinction between disordered proliferative endometrium and simple hyperplasia, and, as stated, these form part of a continuum without sharply defined borders. Disordered proliferative endometrium may occasionally be confused with a polyp because of the glandular architectural distortion and dilatation; however, the fibrous stroma and thick-walled stromal blood vessels characteristic of a polyp are absent and disordered proliferation involves the entire endometrium.

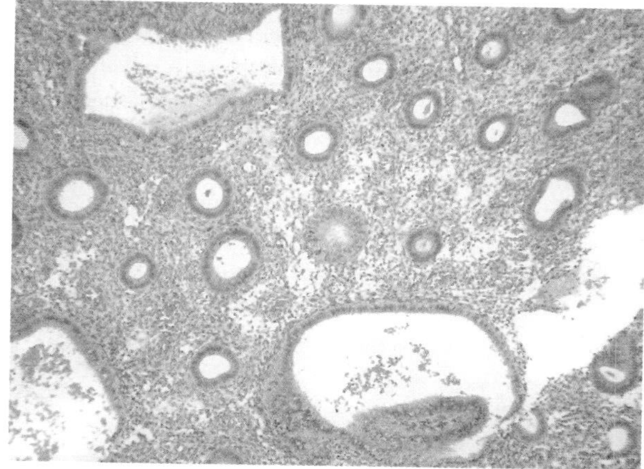

Fig. 7.44
Disordered proliferative endometrium. **Occasional cystically dilated glands are present within an otherwise typical proliferative endometrium**

Cystic atrophy may also enter into the differential diagnosis but in this there is an absence of mitotic activity and the cells lining the glands are attenuated. Menstrual shedding following ovulation often results in disordered proliferative endometrium reverting to normal.

Progesterone-Related Dysfunctional Uterine Bleeding-Luteal Phase Defects

Luteal phase defects (also known as inadequate luteal phase, secretory insufficiency, or inadequate secretory phase) are a relatively common cause of DUB and also of ovulatory infertility. Although ovulation occurs, there is a relative or absolute insufficiency of progesterone secretion by the corpus luteum, which may either regress prematurely or fail to produce an adequate amount of progesterone. As a consequence, the luteal (secretory) phase does not develop appropriately, the secretory features in the endometrium being poorly developed. The underlying cause is unknown but is thought to be a result of hypothalamic or pituitary dysfunction, which results in decreased levels of follicle stimulating hormone (FSH) and abnormal luteinizing hormone (LH) secretion. Because of inadequate progesterone secretion, there may be a lag in the histological date of the endometrium of at least two days compared to the actual postovulatory date. Other morphological features in some cases include discordance in development of the glands and stroma and different areas of the endometrium exhibiting marked variation in development; for example, some areas may exhibit early secretory activity while others show predecidual change. Alternatively, the glands may exhibit hypersecretory features while the stroma lacks predecidual change. Although the endometrium exhibits a secretory pattern, often this cannot be assigned to any day of the normal cycle. In addition to the features described, there is surface breakdown. The diagnosis can be made by a combination of repeated biopsies over several cycles and serial hormone measurements. In other cases, irregular shedding may be a result of a persistent corpus luteum with prolonged progesterone production. This is a poorly understood form of DUB and, as such, the histological features are not well described.

Effects of Exogenous Hormonal Agents and Drugs

There are a plethora of exogenous hormonal agents in widespread use for a variety of indications including contraception, alleviation of menopausal symptoms, management of organic lesions or DUB, treatment of infertility, management of endometrial hyperplasia or carcinoma, and endometrial prophylaxis in patients with hyperestrogenic states or taking medications such as tamoxifen. The effects of the various hormonal agents on the endometrium is varied, although in many instances predictable, and depends on a number of factors, including the menopausal status of the patient, the exact composition of the hormonal preparation, and the dose and duration of administration. Not uncommonly, the endometrium is biopsied in patients taking exogenous hormones, for example, when abnormal bleeding occurs, when hormones do not correct suspected DUB, or when the effect of hormonal agents on the endometrium is assessed. Hysterectomy or endometrial resection may also be performed in patients taking exogenous hormones. Some nonhormonal agents may also result in endometrial morphological changes, although much less commonly than with hormonal compounds. In the following sections, the effects on the endometrium of the most common hormonal agents and of some nonhormonal medications are described. Full details regarding the preparations being taken are obviously of paramount importance to the pathologist in assessing the endometrium but often the details are incomplete or not relayed to the pathologist at all. As such, the pathologist should always suspect the possibility of exogenous hormone use, especially when the endometrial morphology does not correspond to a normal cyclical or postmenopausal appearance.

Estrogen-Only Hormone Replacement Therapy (HRT)

There are various synthetic preparations of estrogens that are largely given to perimenopausal or postmenopausal women to treat menopausal symptoms. In women with a uterus, estrogen-only HRT (unopposed estrogen) is contraindicated due to the risk of endometrial proliferative lesions, including hyperplasia and endometrioid adenocarcinoma, and, as such, the use of estrogen-only preparations is unusual in a woman with a uterus. The morphological features in the endometrium vary, but there may be proliferative activity, a picture identical to disordered proliferation, any type of endometrial hyperplasia, or an endometrioid adenocarcinoma [40]. There may be associated surface breakdown and epithelial cytoplasmic change, including squamous and ciliated metaplasia. The risk of malignancy increases with the dose and duration of therapy; those adenocarcinomas that develop are usually, but not always, low grade and early stage. Unopposed estrogens result in endometrial hyperplasia in approximately 20% of women following 1 year of treatment. The "postmenopausal estrogen/progestin intervention (PEPI) trial" concluded that women taking estrogens alone had a high incidence of simple (27.7%), complex (22.7%), and atypical (11.7%) hyperplasia; this was significantly higher than in those taking placebos. The reported risk ratio for endometrial carcinoma in women taking unopposed estrogens has ranged from 2.3 to 10 [53, 116]; the risk persists for many years after estrogen treatment is discontinued [15, 132]. Estrogen-only preparations may also result in proliferative changes and the development of premalignant and malignant lesions in endometriosis; as such, caution should be exercised before prescribing unopposed estrogens following hysterectomy in a woman with known endometriosis.

Combined Estrogen and Progestin Hormone Replacement Therapy

Because of the potential adverse effects of unopposed estrogens, in most women with a uterus an estrogen is combined with a progestin for HRT. Estrogen and progestin combinations may be given sequentially or continuously. Sequential (cyclic) regimes are variable but usually employ daily estrogens for the first 21 to 25 days or the whole of the month with daily progestins added for the last 10 to 13 days; these regimes result in a withdrawal bleed. Continuous combined regimes use both estrogen and progestin daily. With continuous regimes, breakthrough bleeding may occur during the first 6 months, but this bleeding then usually stops. Patients receiving sequential or continuous regimes may undergo biopsy as part of routine surveillance or when unexpected bleeding occurs; there is no correlation between bleeding patterns and endometrial histology. With sequential regimes, the endometrium may exhibit atrophy, secretory, or weak proliferative activity, the latter especially if the biopsy is taken during the period of estrogen therapy. If the endometrium is biopsied during the period of progestin therapy, there may be poorly developed secretory activity in the glands with cytoplasmic vacuoles and scant luminal secretions. Focal glandular and stromal breakdown may also be seen. Sequential regimes do not completely eliminate the risk of carcinoma associated with unopposed estrogen therapy; the prevalence of endometrial hyperplasia associated with sequential HRT is 5.4% and that of atypical hyperplasia 0.7% [140]. It should be remembered that HRT is most commonly taken by postmenopausal women, and in this

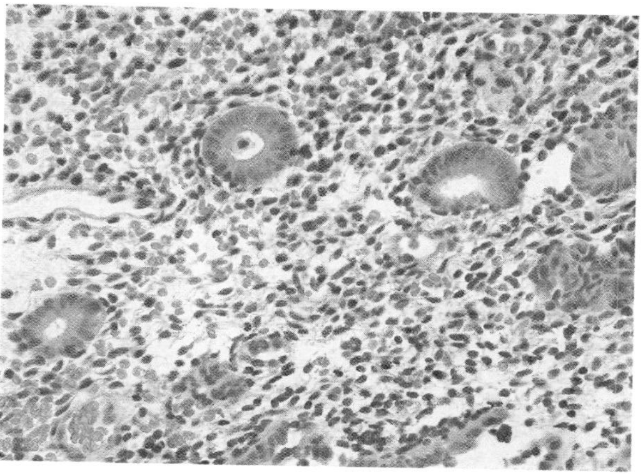

Fig. 7.45
Endometrium associated with continuous combined hormone regimes. **With continuous combined hormone regimes, the endometrium is usually atrophic**

age group, there is a background incidence of endometrial hyperplasia and carcinoma. With the continuous combined regimes, the endometrium is usually atrophic or exhibits weak secretory activity (*Fig. 7.45*) and, in many instances, biopsies yield scanty material. There is no increased risk of endometrial proliferative lesions with continuous combined HRT [105], and, in fact, these regimes may protect against the development of endometrial hyperplasia and carcinoma and normalize endometria that have exhibited complex hyperplasia [40, 43, 136]. This suggests that continuous combined HRT is suitable for long-term use in perimenopausal and postmenopausal women. Endometrial polyps are relatively common in women taking combined HRT and appear more common with sequential than continuous regimes [43].

Progestin-Only Compounds

Various forms of synthetic analogues of progesterone, termed progestins, are in widespread use, either alone or in combination with an estrogen. Progestin-only hormonal compounds, taken either orally or systemically, are usually prescribed for abnormal uterine bleeding and result in suppression of ovulation and inhibition of endometrial growth. Progestins may also be given for the management of conditions such as endometriosis, for contraception, or for endometrial protection in patients taking tamoxifen. The effects of progestins on the endometrium are variable and depend on the degree of estrogen priming as well as the type of progestin and the dose

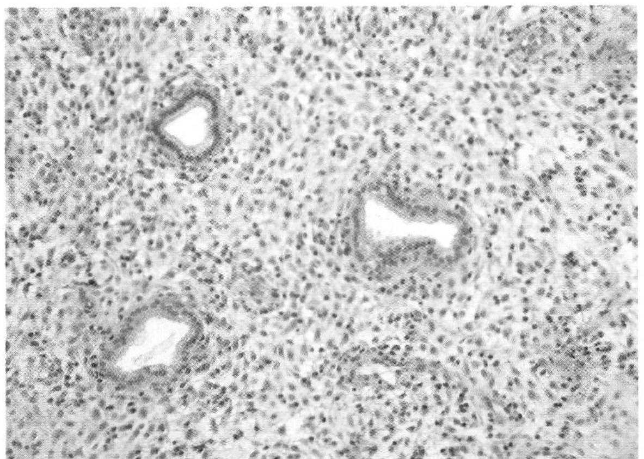

Fig. 7.46
Endometrium associated with progestin-only compound. **With progestin-only compounds, the stroma is typically expanded and composed of decidualized cells**

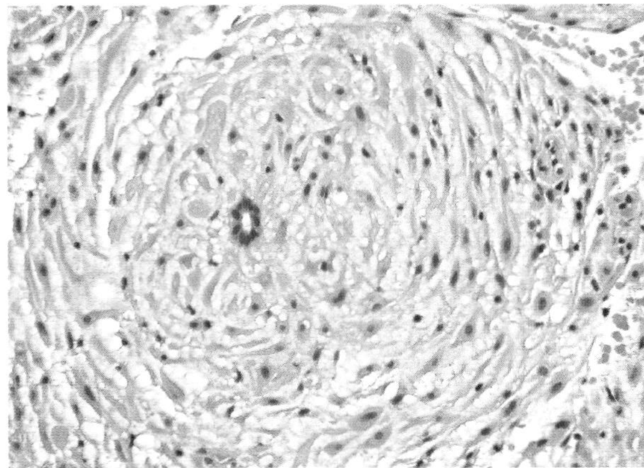

Fig. 7.47
Decidualized endometrial stroma. **Occasionally decidualized stroma contains cells with enlarged nuclei with cytoplasmic vacuolation and stromal myxoid change**

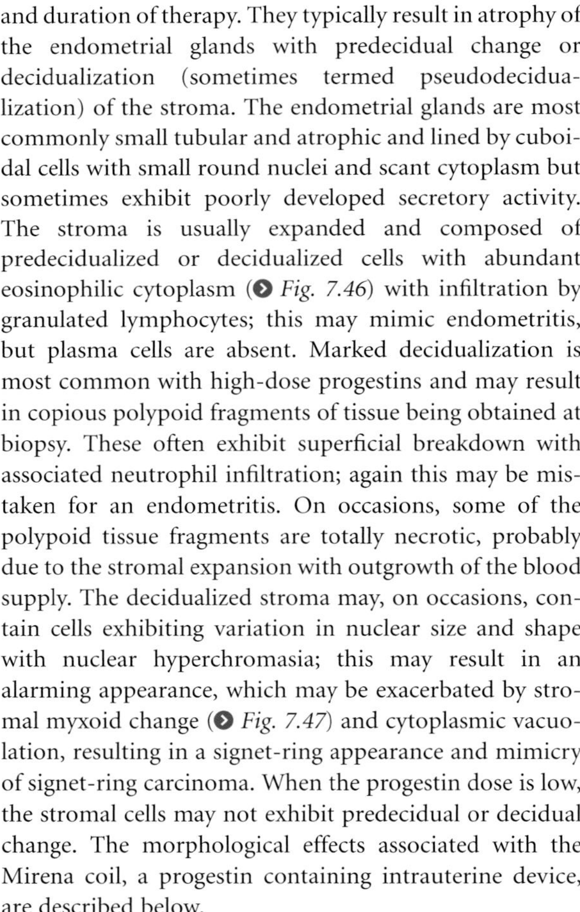

and duration of therapy. They typically result in atrophy of the endometrial glands with predecidual change or decidualization (sometimes termed pseudodecidualization) of the stroma. The endometrial glands are most commonly small tubular and atrophic and lined by cuboidal cells with small round nuclei and scant cytoplasm but sometimes exhibit poorly developed secretory activity. The stroma is usually expanded and composed of predecidualized or decidualized cells with abundant eosinophilic cytoplasm (➋ *Fig. 7.46*) with infiltration by granulated lymphocytes; this may mimic endometritis, but plasma cells are absent. Marked decidualization is most common with high-dose progestins and may result in copious polypoid fragments of tissue being obtained at biopsy. These often exhibit superficial breakdown with associated neutrophil infiltration; again this may be mistaken for an endometritis. On occasions, some of the polypoid tissue fragments are totally necrotic, probably due to the stromal expansion with outgrowth of the blood supply. The decidualized stroma may, on occasions, contain cells exhibiting variation in nuclear size and shape with nuclear hyperchromasia; this may result in an alarming appearance, which may be exacerbated by stromal myxoid change (➋ *Fig. 7.47*) and cytoplasmic vacuolation, resulting in a signet-ring appearance and mimicry of signet-ring carcinoma. When the progestin dose is low, the stromal cells may not exhibit predecidual or decidual change. The morphological effects associated with the Mirena coil, a progestin containing intrauterine device, are described below.

Progestin-like Effect Without Exogenous Hormone Use

Occasionally the endometrium exhibits identical changes to those occurring with progestins, namely atrophic glands and stromal decidualization, in a patient not taking exogenous hormones. This may occur in both premenopausal and postmenopausal women and the etiology is, in most cases, poorly understood. In very rare cases, the changes will be secondary to a progesterone secreting neoplasm in an ovary or elsewhere. Most other cases are probably secondary to a persistent functioning corpus luteum or a luteinized unruptured follicle where a follicle develops without ovulation and persists with luteinization of the granulosa and theca cells that produce progesterone. There have also been occasional reports of changes identical to those of progestin effect in postmenopausal women not taking exogenous hormones [24]. The changes may be a result of local mechanical factors rather than a response to progesterone-like hormones. Mechanical stimulation, including biopsy or the presence of an intrauterine device, may rarely result in predecidual or decidual change in the endometrium.

Gonadotropin-Releasing Hormone Agonists

Gonadotropin-releasing hormone agonists (GnRH agonists), including buserelin acetate, goserelin acetate, and leuprolide acetate, are commonly used in the management of uterine leiomyomas and endometriosis. After initial stimulation of the pituitary gland with increased production of luteinizing hormone (LH) and follicle stimulating hormone (FSH), further administration results in desensitization of the pituitary to GnRH and a subsequent decreased production of LH and FSH. This results in decreased estrogen production by the ovaries and a hypo-estrogenic state. As a consequence, there is shrinkage of uterine leiomyomas, thus alleviating symptoms and potentially allowing myomectomy rather than hysterectomy or vaginal hysterectomy rather than abdominal hysterectomy. The endometrium in patients taking GnRH agonists is typically atrophic with small tubular glands or sometimes the glands exhibit weak proliferative activity. When GnRH agonists are used in conjunction with a progestogen, the endometrium may exhibit decidualization of the stroma.

Androgens

Several androgens are in widespread use, for example, danazol and livial. The main indications for these preparations are the treatment of endometriosis but androgens may also be used in the management of menorrhagia or endometrial hyperplasia or as HRT. In the early stages of androgen therapy, the glands may exhibit weak secretory activity, but with prolonged therapy, the endometrium becomes atrophic [95].

Progesterone Receptor Modulators

Progesterone receptor modulators (PRMs) are synthetic compounds that interact with the progesterone receptor to inhibit or stimulate a downstream hormonal response. Compounds with progesterone receptor antagonist activity are used in contraception and in the management of uterine leiomyomata or endometriosis. The endometrial effects of PRMs have been described [104]. While in some cases, the endometrium is inactive or has a normal cyclical appearance, in a subset of cases, there is asymmetry of stromal and epithelial growth, resulting in prominent cystically dilated glands with admixed estrogenic (mitotic) and progestogenic (secretory) activity. Vascular changes described include a chicken wire vasculature and the presence of thick-walled and ectatic vessels. These novel changes are termed PRM-associated endometrial changes.

Tamoxifen

Tamoxifen is a nonsteroidal triphenylethyl compound that is widely used as adjuvant therapy in the treatment of breast cancer. It is a selective estrogen receptor modulator (SERM) and prolongs overall and disease-free survival in breast cancer, reduces the likelihood of disease in the contralateral breast, and may reduce the risk of development of breast cancer in asymptomatic women with a strong family history. Results from the National Surgical Adjuvant Breast and Bowel Project Breast Cancer Prevention study demonstrated that 5 years of tamoxifen use at a dose of 20 mg/day reduced breast cancer risk in high-risk women by 49% [45]. The efficacy of tamoxifen in breast cancer is due to its antiestrogenic properties that are mediated by competitive binding to the estrogen receptor. However, tamoxifen may also exert a weak estrogenic effect and act on the human endometrium [68, 69, 130]. Transvaginal ultrasonography has shown that the endometrium of tamoxifen-treated postmenopausal patients is significantly thicker than that of age-matched controls of women not taking tamoxifen [19]. Benign postmenopausal endometria of patients treated with tamoxifen exhibit a higher Ki-67 proliferation index than controls of patients not taking tamoxifen [54]. Tamoxifen therapy may result in a spectrum of endometrial proliferative lesions, including polyps, simple, complex, and atypical hyperplasia, and adenocarcinomas. Various other malignancies have also been described in association with tamoxifen. Since the majority of women taking tamoxifen are postmenopausal, most of the information regarding the endometrial side effects is related to this age group. The effects of tamoxifen on the endometrium appear to depend on the menopausal status, as well as on the dose and duration of tamoxifen usage.

Non-neoplastic endometrium in postmenopausal patients taking tamoxifen is most commonly atrophic while in other cases there is proliferative activity. The stroma is often fibrous and, as a result, endometrial biopsies in patients taking tamoxifen are often very scanty. There may be glandular dilatation secondary to obstruction of the glands by stromal fibrosis. Stromal decidualization is usually secondary to simultaneous progestin administration [28]. One of the most characteristic and common endometrial lesions in women taking tamoxifen is polyps, which may be single or multiple and may occur on a background of hyperplasia, such that there is merging of polypoid and non-polypoid endometrium. There are no pathognomonic features of tamoxifen-associated endometrial polyps but they tend to be larger than sporadic polyps. Periglandular stromal condensation, staghorn-shaped glands polarized along the long axis of the polyp, stromal edema and myxoid change, and epithelial metaplasias are all more common in tamoxifen-associated than sporadic polyps [72, 127], although all these features may be seen in sporadic polyps. Polyp cancers may develop in tamoxifen-associated polyps and can be of endometrioid or serous type. The presumed precursor lesion of serous carcinoma, serous endometrial intraepithelial carcinoma (serous EIC), may also involve tamoxifen-associated polyps [90, 134]. Rarely, a metastatic breast carcinoma, usually of lobular type, is identified within a tamoxifen-associated endometrial polyp [60].

As stated earlier, endometrial carcinomas may develop in association with tamoxifen. It is generally accepted that the risk of developing endometrial carcinoma in patients taking tamoxifen is two to three times higher than in an age-matched population of women not taking tamoxifen. It is probable that it is women who have been taking tamoxifen for a prolonged period of time and with a high cumulative dose who are at greatest risk. Most carcinomas are endometrioid in type but type 2 endometrial carcinomas, especially serous, are possibly proportionally more common than in the general population, although it is impossible to draw firm conclusions. Since most endometrial cancers that develop in association with estrogenic stimulation are low-grade endometrioid in type, it might be expected that carcinomas associated with tamoxifen would have a similar profile. However, although some studies support this [147], it has also been suggested that high-grade endometrial cancers, including serous carcinomas and carcinosarcomas (in reality metaplastic carcinomas or carcinomas with sarcomatous metaplasia) [87], are more common in patients taking tamoxifen and that the development of these cancers is not secondary to estrogenic stimulation but due to other mechanisms such as the formation of DNA adducts [84, 133]. Occasional uterine leiomyosarcomas, endometrial stromal sarcomas, adenofibromas, and adenosarcomas have been described in patients taking tamoxifen [27, 63, 81]; it is possible that these complications arise simply by chance since tamoxifen is widely used. Adenomyosis has been shown to be more common in postmenopausal patients taking tamoxifen [29], and this may exhibit unusual morphological features, such as stromal fibrosis, glandular dilatation, and epithelial metaplasias [85]. A rapid increase in size of uterine leiomyomas has been observed with tamoxifen therapy.

Other SERMs, such as raloxifene, have a similar efficacy to tamoxifen in the management of breast cancer. In contrast to tamoxifen, these seem to be pure estrogen antagonists, lacking the weak estrogen agonist effects of tamoxifen and do not result in endometrial proliferative lesions [35].

Taxanes

Taxanes, such as paclitaxel, are commonly used chemotherapeutic agents as first-line treatment in ovarian, breast, and lung cancer. Taxanes act by the simultaneous promotion of tubulin assembly into microtubules and inhibition of microtubule disassembly. The morphological features in the endometrium have been rarely reported but numerous mitoses in metaphase arrest with the formation of ring mitoses have been described [67]. Similar morphological changes are seen in other organs, such as the gastrointestinal tract, in association with taxanes.

Endometrial Epithelial Metaplasia (Epithelial Cytoplasmic Change)

Endometrial epithelial metaplasias are non-neoplastic alterations (metaplasias may coexist with endometrial hyperplasia or carcinoma but, in themselves, are non-neoplastic) in which the normal endometrial epithelium is replaced, focally or diffusely, by another type of differentiated epithelium. The variety of epithelial metaplasias encountered within the endometrium reflects the capacity of epithelium derived from the müllerian ducts to undergo differentiation into any other form of epithelium found in the müllerian system. The various epithelial metaplasias commonly coexist. It has been suggested that metaplasia is an inappropriate term for some of the alterations as strictly speaking the term metaplasia refers to the replacement of one type of epithelium by another that is not normally found in that organ [57]. For this reason, some authors use the term "epithelial cytoplasmic change" rather than metaplasia.

Metaplasia usually involves nonsecretory endometrium and is often associated with hyperestrogenism. Metaplasias are common within endometrial polyps. Other associations include exogenous hormone therapy, especially but not exclusively unopposed estrogens, the presence of an intrauterine device, chronic endometritis, and pyometra; the latter two conditions are particularly associated with squamous metaplasia. In some cases, there is no obvious underlying cause. It has been suggested that progestin therapy given for endometrial hyperplasia or endometrioid adenocarcinoma may result in various epithelial metaplasias within the malignant or premalignant lesion [154]. Metaplasia by itself is not associated with clinical symptoms but if there is an associated endometrial hyperplasia or carcinoma, there may be abnormal bleeding related to this [88].

A particular problem with epithelial metaplasias is their tendency to be associated with endometrial hyperplasias [18] or endometrioid adenocarcinoma. Squamous metaplasia and mucinous metaplasia are particularly common in endometrioid adenocarcinomas. In such instances, it may be difficult, at the lower end of the spectrum, to distinguish between a metaplasia with mild glandular complexity and a hyperplasia with coexistent metaplasia. It is important to make this distinction, since metaplasia by itself has no premalignant potential, and it is recommended that similar criteria are employed to those that are used in the diagnosis of endometrial hyperplasia without metaplasia (➲ Chap. 8, Precursor Lesions of Endometrial Carcinoma).

With some epithelial metaplasias, such as clear cell metaplasia and papillary syncytial metaplasia, the differential diagnosis may be between a metaplasia and a type 2 endometrial cancer or serous endometrial intraepithelial carcinoma (serous EIC). In such instances, immunohistochemistry may be of value in that serous EIC and type 2 cancers often exhibit diffuse intense nuclear p53 immunoreactivity while ER is generally negative or weakly positive. In contrast, most epithelial metaplasias are ER positive and exhibit a pattern of p53 immunoreactivity, which has been described as weak and heterogenous [123]. A minor population of endometrial epithelial cells exhibit nuclear immunoreactivity with p63; it has been speculated that these are reserve cells or basal cells and the origin of the various epithelial metaplasias [111].

Squamous Metaplasia

Squamous metaplasia is one of the commonest forms of endometrial epithelial metaplasia. Although usually a focal finding, on occasions there may be widespread squamous metaplasia with obliteration of the glandular lumina such that it is difficult to assess the underlying glandular component. This is especially common when the squamous metaplasia is of morular type (see below). Squamous metaplasia is common in endometrioid adenocarcinoma and in endometrial hyperplasias; these should be excluded by careful examination of the glandular elements. Squamous metaplasia may also be seen in endometrial polyps. There are two types of squamous metaplasia, namely typical squamous metaplasia and morular metaplasia, although these sometimes coexist. Typical squamous elements are characterized by sheets of cells exhibiting obvious squamous differentiation in the form of intercellular bridges, prominent cell membranes, or keratinization (➲ *Fig. 7.48*). Sometimes there is a histiocytic and giant cell reaction to keratin. Typical squamous metaplasia rarely involves much of or the entire endometrial surface such that the endometrial cavity is extensively lined by squamous epithelium, the condition known as ichthyosis uteri. This condition most commonly develops secondary to longstanding cervical obstruction or chronic inflammation. Usually, in ichthyosis uteri, the squamous epithelium is of normal appearance, but rarely, it may have the features of a condyloma acuminatum [137] or intraepithelial neoplasia [121]. It may rarely extend to involve the fallopian tubes and ovaries. Rarely an invasive squamous carcinoma develops in this manner.

Squamous morules are morphologically distinct structures, which were named so because of their three-dimensional resemblance to mulberries [39]. They are composed of rounded aggregates or syncytial sheets of cells that often fill glandular lumina (➲ *Fig. 7.49*). The constituent cells have central bland round, ovoid, or spindle shaped, evenly spaced nuclei, sometimes with small nucleoli. Some of these nuclei may contain optically clear biotin-rich inclusions. The cell borders are indistinct. Mitoses are rare or absent. There may be central necrosis. It is controversial whether morules actually exhibit squamous differentiation. Morphological features of overt squamous differentiation, such as keratinization, intercellular bridges, and prominent cell membranes, are typically absent in morules. Immunohistochemically,

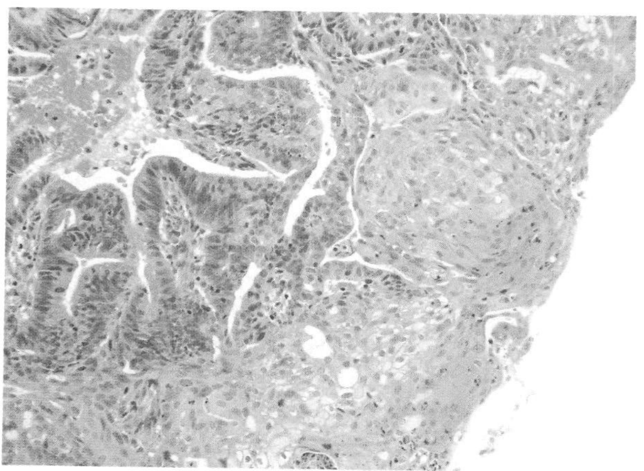

◘ Fig. 7.48
Squamous metaplasia in endometrium. **Typical squamous metaplasia with obvious squamous differentiation in the form of prominent cell membranes**

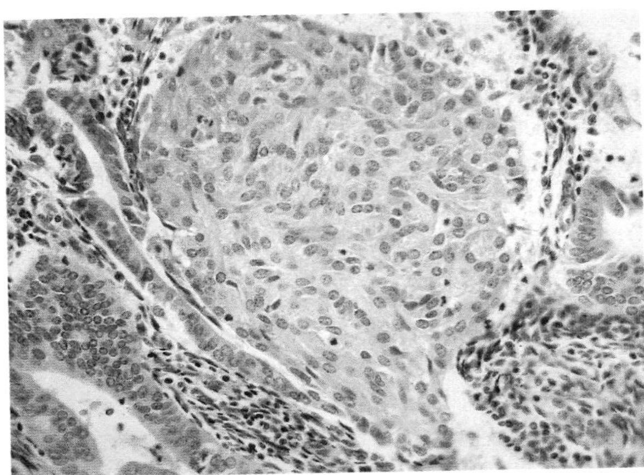

Fig. 7.49
Squamous morules in endometrium. **Squamous morules are composed of rounded aggregates or syncytial sheets of cells filling glandular lumina**

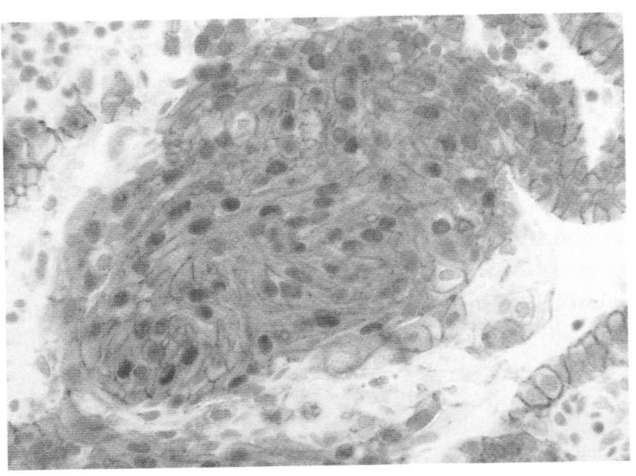

Fig. 7.50
Beta-catenin immunohistochemistry in squamous morules. **Morules exhibit nuclear and cytoplasmic immunoreactivity with beta-catenin**

morules exhibit a somewhat different immunophenotype to that of typical squamous elements. Morules exhibit nuclear and cytoplasmic positivity with beta-catenin (*Fig. 7.50*) [14, 124] while in typical squamous elements the "normal" membranous pattern of immunoreactivity is maintained [62]. Endometrial proliferative lesions with morules often exhibit beta-catenin gene mutation, and this results in the cytoplasmic and nuclear immunoreactivity. Morules are usually estrogen receptor (ER) and p63 negative [21], diffusely positive with CD10 [20], and

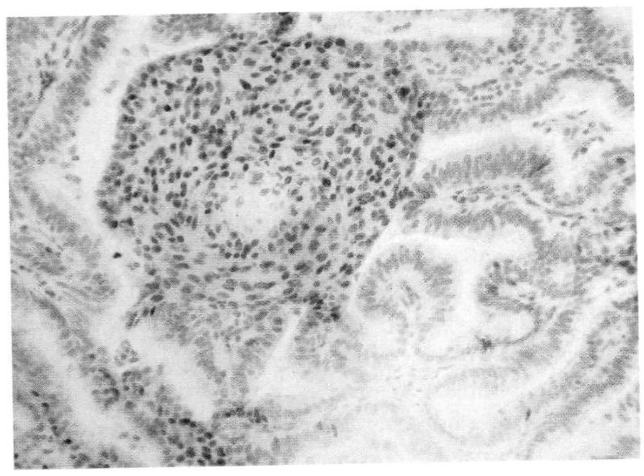

Fig. 7.51
CDX2 immunohistochemistry in squamous morules. **Morules exhibit nuclear immunoreactivity with the intestinal transcription factor CDX2**

exhibit nuclear immunoreactivity with the intestinal transcription factor CDX2 (*Fig. 7.51*) [62, 152]; it has been suggested that this is secondary to beta-catenin gene mutation. In contrast, typical squamous elements are usually positive with ER, p63, and CD10, and negative with CDX2. On the basis of the immunophenotype, it has been concluded that morules exhibit no firm immunohistochemical evidence of squamous differentiation, although immature squamous features cannot be excluded [62]. It has been suggested that the term morular metaplasia is used instead of squamous morules.

Mucinous Metaplasia

Mucinous metaplasia is a relatively uncommon form of endometrial epithelial metaplasia and is most commonly seen in association with a premalignant or malignant lesion. It may also be seen in endometrial polyps. A diagnosis of mucinous metaplasia should be reserved for cases in which the endometrial epithelial cells are replaced by cells with abundant intracytoplasmic mucin, the cells resembling endocervical cells (*Fig. 7.52*). Normal endometrial epithelial cells contain a little intracytoplasmic mucin, especially with a luminal distribution, and so abundant intracytoplasmic mucin is required to diagnose mucinous metaplasia. Rarely, intestinal metaplasia has been described in the endometrium where the mucinous epithelium contains goblet cells [153]. Enteric type mucins may be demonstrable with mucin stains in cases without morphological evidence of

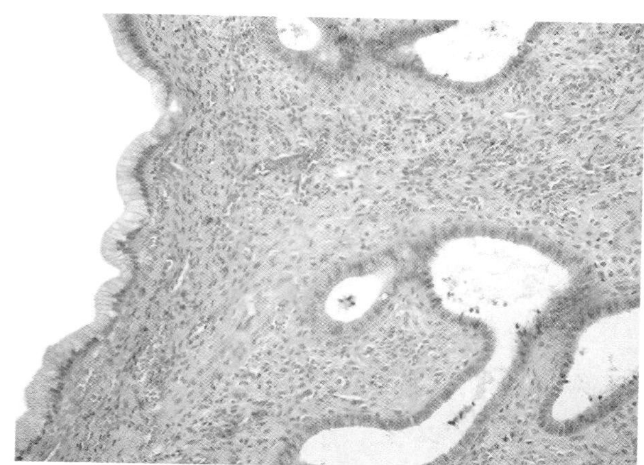

Fig. 7.52
Mucinous metaplasia in endometrium. **Focally the cells have abundant mucinous cytoplasm**

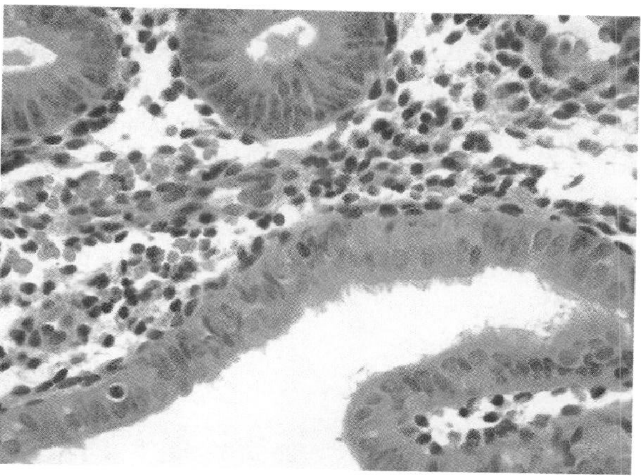

Fig. 7.53
Ciliated metaplasia in endometrium. **The endometrial glands are lined by ciliated cells with abundant eosinophilic cytoplasm**

intestinal metaplasia [80]. In mucinous metaplasia without an associated premalignant or malignant glandular proliferation, there are often small micropapillary projections. The nuclei are small and uniform and mitoses are rare or absent. An important point with a florid mucinous proliferation of the endometrium is that mucinous adenocarcinomas, even those exhibiting myometrial invasion, can be cytologically bland with little in the way of mitotic activity. As such, complex mucinous proliferations of the endometrium present a particular diagnostic problem, especially, but not exclusively, in biopsy material [150]. Mucinous proliferations of the endometrium have been divided into three categories depending on the degree of architectural complexity and association with underlying adenocarcinoma [108]. With any architecturally complex mucinous proliferation in an endometrial biopsy, a diagnosis of well-differentiated mucinous adenocarcinoma should be considered, and the term "complex endometrial mucinous proliferation" may be applied with a comment that there is a significant risk of a well-differentiated mucinous adenocarcinoma in the uterus. Rarely, mucinous metaplasia in the endometrium is accompanied by mucinous lesions elsewhere in the female genital tract, for example in the cervix and the ovary, perhaps as a manifestation of a field-change effect [6].

Ciliated (Tubal) Metaplasia

Ciliated epithelial cells are normal on the endometrial surface, especially in the proliferative phase of the menstrual cycle. A diagnosis of ciliated metaplasia should be made only when one or more endometrial glands contain ciliated cells, which may be interspersed among non-ciliated cells or be extensive and line most of the gland (*Fig. 7.53*). The nuclei may be rounded, mildly stratified, and contain small nucleoli but are cytologically bland. Ciliated cells often have abundant eosinophilic cytoplasm. Ciliated metaplasia is particularly associated with estrogenic stimulation. As with other types of epithelial metaplasia, ciliated cells may be found in non-neoplastic, hyperplastic, and malignant endometria. The presence or absence of hyperplasia or adenocarcinoma is evaluated by the usual parameters.

Clear Cell Metaplasia

Clear cell metaplasia is rare and is characterized by replacement of endometrial epithelial cells by cells with abundant clear cytoplasm (*Fig. 7.54*). This may be a feature of pregnancy when the features overlap with Arias-Stella reaction. Clear cell metaplasia may be misdiagnosed as clear cell carcinoma, especially on a biopsy specimen. Distinction is based on the bland nuclear features and the fact that in clear cell metaplasia the endometrial glands maintain a normal architecture and distribution. Other features favoring clear cell metaplasia over clear cell carcinoma include the focal nature of the lesion, absence of a grossly visible tumor, absence of stromal invasion, and strong estrogen receptor positivity. Some, but not all, endometrial clear cell carcinomas are estrogen receptor negative.

Hobnail Cell Metaplasia

Hobnail cell metaplasia or change is rare and is characterized by the presence of cells with rounded apical blebs, which may involve the endometrial surface or protrude into glandular lumina (➋ *Fig. 7.55*). Hobnail cell metaplasia may be a reparative phenomenon following endometrial curettage or may be seen on the surface of a polyp. It may also occur in pregnancy. Hobnail cells are also a feature of some clear cell carcinomas and this may enter into the differential diagnosis. Criteria useful in the distinction of hobnail cell metaplasia from clear cell carcinoma are similar to those used in distinction of the latter from clear cell metaplasia.

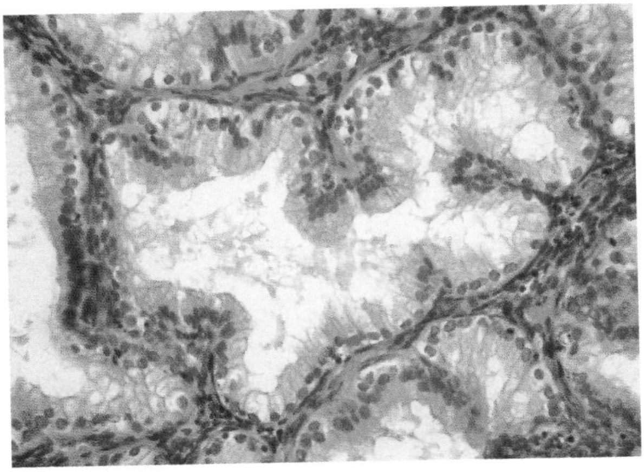

Fig. 7.54
Clear cell metaplasia in endometrium. **The endometrial glands are replaced by cells with abundant clear cytoplasm**

Eosinophilic (Oxyphilic, Oncocytic) Metaplasia

Eosinophilic or oxyphilic metaplasia is relatively common and is characterized by the presence of epithelial cells with abundant eosinophilic cytoplasm (➋ *Fig. 7.56*). The cytoplasm may be granular, in which case the term oncocytic metaplasia has been used. Ultrastructurally, abundant cytoplasmic mitochondria may be present, as is characteristic of oncocytes in other organs. The term pink cell metaplasia has also been used. Ciliated metaplasia is often characterized by abundant eosinophilic cytoplasm and overlaps with eosinophilic metaplasia. The epithelial cells in eosinophilic metaplasia can exhibit a significant degree of nuclear atypia (➋ *Fig. 7.57*); this is analogous to the degenerative nuclear atypia that is common in oncocytic cells in other organs. The main differential diagnosis is the eosinophilic or oxyphilic variant of endometrioid adenocarcinoma. Distinction from adenocarcinoma is based on the absence of a grossly visible lesion and maintenance of the normal glandular architecture.

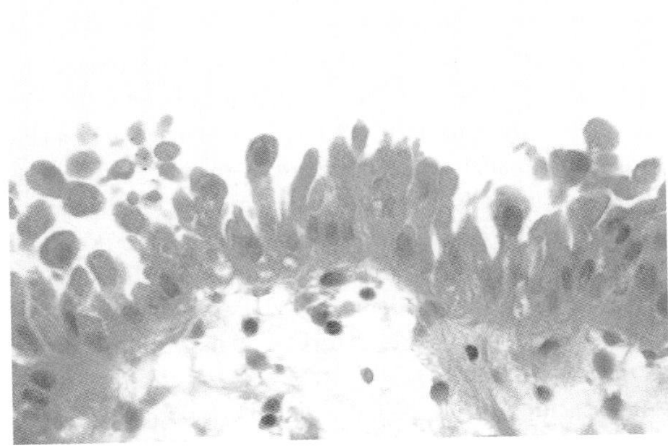

Fig. 7.55
Hobnail cell metaplasia in endometrium. **Hobnail cells are present on the surface of an endometrial polyp**

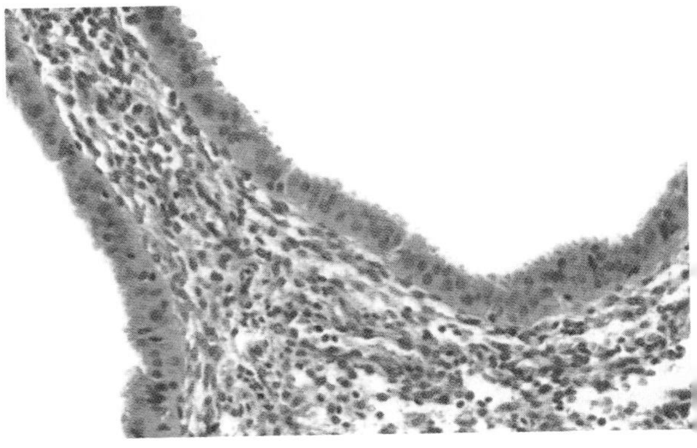

Fig. 7.56
Eosinophilic metaplasia in endometrium. **The epithelial cells contain abundant eosinophilic cytoplasm**

Papillary Syncytial Metaplasia

The term papillary syncytial metaplasia is a misnomer since this does not actually represent a metaplasia but rather a degenerative or reparative phenomenon associated with surface breakdown, either menstrual or nonmenstrual in type. However, since the term papillary syncytial metaplasia is in widespread use, it is discussed here. Synonymous terms include eosinophilic syncytial change and surface syncytial change. It has been suggested that papillary syncytial metaplasia is a degenerative or regressive phenomenon based on a low proliferation and mitotic index [131]. Papillary syncytial metaplasia is common and is characterized by small syncytia or micropapillary proliferations of endometrial epithelial cells, which may contain small glandular lumina and which are devoid of stromal support, lacking fibrovascular stromal cores (*Fig. 7.10*). The cells usually have eosinophilic cytoplasm and there is often a neutrophilic infiltrate. There may be mild nuclear atypia and in a minority of cases, mitoses are present. The distinction between papillary syncytial metaplasia and serous adenocarcinoma or serous EIC has been discussed earlier. Another important consideration is that foci similar to papillary syncytial metaplasia may occur on the surface of some endometrioid adenocarcinomas. The distinction between papillary syncytial metaplasia and papillary adenocarcinomas of endometrioid or serous type is facilitated by recognition that papillary syncytial metaplasia is limited to the endometrial surface and is associated with other morphological features of breakdown such as apoptotic debris, neutrophils, and adjacent glandular and stromal breakdown.

Arias-Stella Reaction

Arias-Stella reaction (Arias-Stella effect or change) has been discussed earlier and is almost always associated with pregnancy, either intrauterine or ectopic, or with trophoblastic disease. It rarely occurs secondary to hormone therapy, especially progestins; occasionally there is no obvious cause [64]. The most important differential diagnosis is clear cell carcinoma, but the diagnosis of Arias-Stella reaction is usually straightforward if the patient is known to be pregnant and if other morphological features of pregnancy are present, such as decidualization of the stroma. Arias-Stella reaction involves preexisting endometrial glands without evidence of stromal infiltration and there is no mass lesion. Although there is nuclear enlargement and atypia, a low nuclear to cytoplasmic ratio is maintained.

Papillary Proliferation of Endometrium

The term hyperplastic papillary proliferation of the endometrium has been used for a lesion, usually occurring in postmenopausal women, characterized by the presence of papillae with fibrovascular stromal cores and variable degrees of branching and cellular tufting (*Fig. 7.58*). The papillae are lined by epithelial cells with bland nuclei [76]. Although not strictly a metaplasia, the lesion is discussed here since epithelial metaplasias, most commonly mucinous, eosinophilic, or ciliated, are often also

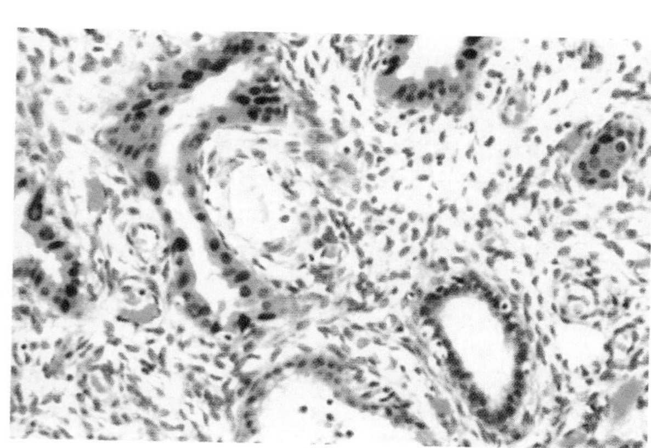

Fig. 7.57
Eosinophilic metaplasia in endometrium. **In eosinophilic metaplasia, a significant degree of nuclear atypia may be present**

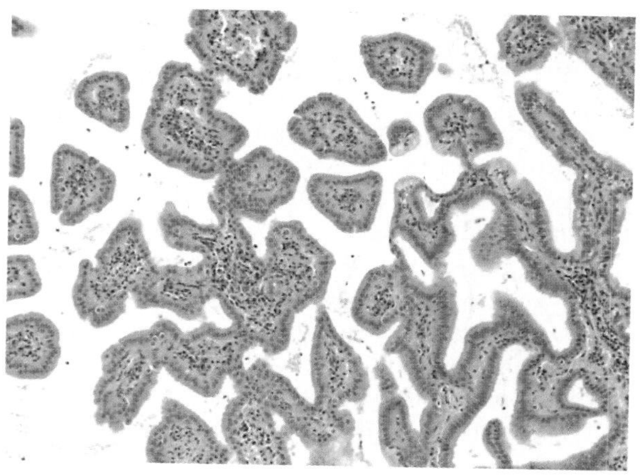

Fig. 7.58
Papillary proliferation of endometrium. **Papillary projections lined by bland epithelial cells on the surface of an endometrial polyp**

present. Sometimes the papillae are entirely intracystic (projecting into cystically dilated endometrial glands) while in other instances they involve the endometrial surface. Papillary proliferation is most commonly seen on the surface of an endometrial polyp and, in some instances, the features are florid. There may be an association with hormonal preparations. A misdiagnosis of an adenocarcinoma of endometrioid or serous type is possible, especially if an underlying polyp is not present or not obvious. Awareness of this phenomenon and the realization that it often occurs in a polyp are clues to the diagnosis, although both endometrioid and serous adenocarcinomas may arise in and be confined to a polyp. An absence of nuclear atypia helps to exclude an adenocarcinoma. It has been considered that these papillary proliferations are a form of hyperplasia that is closely associated with epithelial metaplasia. However, given the uneventful outcome in those cases with follow-up, the term hyperplasia may not be appropriate.

Endometrial Mesenchymal Metaplasia

Various forms of mesenchymal metaplasia, all of which are rare, may involve the endometrial stroma. There are two theories regarding the pathogenesis of the various mesenchymal metaplasias. They may result from metaplasia of the endometrial stroma or represent remnants of fetal tissue following abortion or instrumentation. They should be distinguished from heterologous mesenchymal components within a carcinosarcoma or another uterine neoplasm.

Smooth Muscle Metaplasia

This is the most common mesenchymal metaplasia in the endometrium. Given the common embryonic origin of endometrial stromal and smooth muscle cells, it is thought that a multipotential cell exists in the uterus, which has the capacity to differentiate into endometrial stroma and smooth muscle. This is in keeping with the observation that hybrid endometrial stromal and smooth muscle neoplasms exist. It is not uncommon to find small foci of smooth muscle within the endometrial stroma, and these foci have sometimes been referred to as intraendometrial leiomyomas. It is probable that some intraendometrial smooth muscle nodules are a result of the irregular nature of the normal endometrial–myometrial junction, but others reflect the capacity of endometrial stroma to differentiate into smooth muscle.

Cartilaginous and Osseous Metaplasia

Rarely, foci of benign cartilage or bone are found within endometrial biopsies, either within the endometrial stroma or free floating [5]. In most cases, it is likely that this is of fetal origin, and this is especially likely if these tissues are found in the endometrium of a young woman with a past history of abortion. In other cases, the cartilage or bone is truly metaplastic. These tissues may also rarely be found within the stroma of an endometrial carcinoma. Benign cartilaginous or osseous metaplasia in an endometrial carcinoma should not be mistaken for the heterologous sarcomatous component of a carcinosarcoma. Rarely, endometrial ossification is associated with Asherman's syndrome.

Glial Metaplasia

The presence of glial tissue in the endometrium is extremely rare. In most cases, glial tissue (confirmed if necessary by positive immunohistochemical staining with glial fibrillary acidic protein (GFAP)) is a consequence of a previous abortion. Support for this may come from the identification of other elements such as cartilage or bone.

Adipose Metaplasia

Metaplastic adipose tissue is rarely found within endometrial stroma or within the stroma of an endometrial polyp. If identified in an endometrial biopsy or curettage specimen, the possibility of uterine perforation must be raised. Other explanations for the presence of adipose tissue in an endometrial biopsy specimen include derivation from a lipoma, a lipoleiomyoma, a uterine hamartomatous-like lesion containing adipose tissue [83], or a carcinosarcoma.

Extramedullary Hematopoiesis

Rarely, foci of extramedullary hematopoiesis are present in the endometrium, usually in association with an underlying hematopoietic disorder or occasionally representing remnants of fetal tissue [31].

Endometrial Polyps

Endometrial polyps are common and have been identified in between 2 and 23% of patients undergoing endometrial biopsy because of abnormal uterine bleeding [126]. Polyps occur in pre- and postmenopausal women and are thought to be related in some way to hyperestrogenism, possibly originating as a localized hyperplasia of the endometrial basalis secondary to hormonal influences. There is an increased incidence of endometrial polyps with HRT usage, either estrogen-only HRT or combined preparations. Tamoxifen is also associated with an increased risk of the development of endometrial polyps. Molecular studies have demonstrated that many endometrial polyps represent monoclonal endometrial stromal overgrowths with secondary induction of polyclonal benign glands through undefined stromal–epithelial interactions [46]. They may contain abnormalities of chromosome 6 [34].

Polyps may be single or multiple, sessile or broad based, pedunculated or attached to the endometrium by a slender stalk. They usually have a smooth surface and small cysts may be seen on sectioning. They can arise anywhere in the endometrium, including the lower uterine segment, but are most common in the fundus. When large, they may fill the endometrial cavity and extend into the endocervical canal.

The pathological diagnosis is generally straightforward if the gynecologist is aware of the presence of a polyp, has conveyed this information to the pathologist, and has removed the polyp intact. On occasions, the gynecologist believes that a polyp is present but histological examination shows a cyclical endometrium, often secretory in type, reflecting the fact that an abundant secretory endometrium may have a polypoid appearance. In many cases, the gynecologist is not aware of the presence of a polyp, which is removed piecemeal with the result that in biopsy material, fragments derived from the polyp are admixed with fragments of non-polypoid endometrium, making the diagnosis difficult. In biopsies performed because of abnormal uterine bleeding, the pathologist should always consider the possibility of a polyp. Under low-power examination, the initial clue to the diagnosis is often the admixture of fragments of normal cyclical or atrophic endometrium and fragments that are morphologically different. The histological features of a polyp, not all of which are present in every case, include the following:

1 Polypoid pieces of tissue lined by epithelium on three sides,
2 Glands set in a stroma that is qualitatively different than the endometrial stroma in the non-polypoid fragments. The stroma is often, but not always, more fibrous than that in the non-polypoid fragments and is sometimes markedly hyalinized (➲ *Fig. 7.59*),
3 Glandular architectural abnormality with dilated glands and sometimes mild glandular crowding (➲ *Fig. 7.60*),

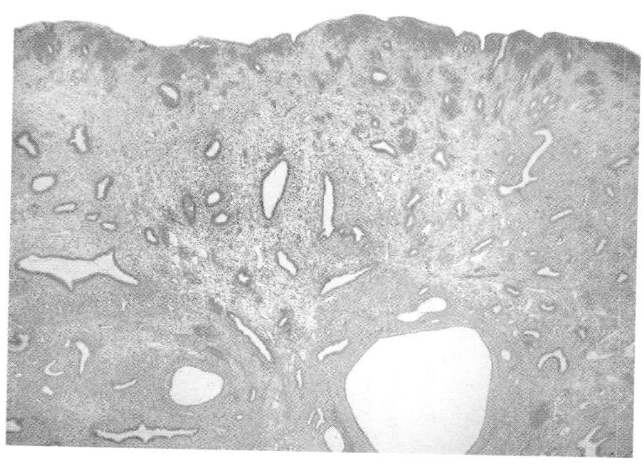

Fig. 7.59
Endometrial polyp. **Dilated glands are set in a fibrous stroma**

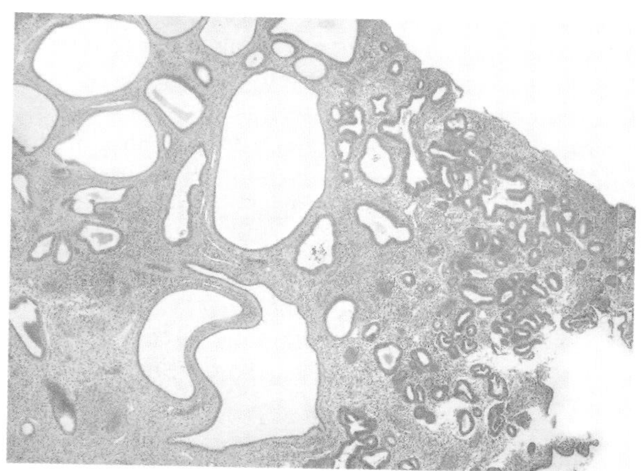

Fig. 7.60
Endometrial polyp. **There may be a mild degree of glandular crowding within some endometrial polyps**

4 Glands that appear different to those in the surrounding endometrium; for example, the glands of the non-polypoid endometrium may be secretory in type while the glands within the polyp are atrophic or exhibit poorly developed secretory or proliferative activity,
5 Collections of thick-walled stromal blood vessels (➲ *Fig. 7.61*).

The glands within a polyp are usually endometrioid in type but not uncommonly exhibit metaplastic change, including ciliated, eosinophilic, mucinous, and squamous metaplasia. The epithelium may be atrophic but often exhibits proliferative activity, even when the patient is postmenopausal and the surrounding endometrium is atrophic. The presence of proliferative activity in a polyp in a postmenopausal woman is of no clinical importance, although it is useful to comment in the pathology report on whether non-polypoid endometrium is also present and whether this exhibits proliferative activity. The stroma of a polyp is often more fibrous than that of the non-polypoid endometrium but this is not invariable and, in some polyps, the stroma is dense and cellular and resembles that of normal proliferative endometrium. As stated, collections of thick-walled stromal blood vessels are a characteristic feature of endometrial polyps, and ectatic thin-walled vessels are also sometimes seen. Some authors have divided endometrial polyps into different types, such as proliferative/hyperplastic (proliferative, sometimes crowded, glands), atrophic (atrophic glands), and functional (glands resembling those in the surrounding cyclical endometrium). However, these patterns often overlap and assignment to a specific type may be difficult; moreover, there is no clinical significance attached to the different types. Some polyps originate at the junction of the upper endocervix and lower uterine segment and contain both endocervical and ciliated lower uterine segment type glands.

A variety of morphological appearances affecting the epithelium or stroma may be seen in endometrial polyps and can result in diagnostic difficulty. Papillary proliferations with fibrovascular cores (see section Papillary Proliferation of Endometrium) occasionally occur on the surface of an endometrial polyp or within cystically dilated glands. The epithelium on the surface of a polyp may exhibit a degree of atypia, often with degenerate appearing nuclei (*Fig. 7.62*), and sometimes hobnail cell change. There may be focal surface glandular and stromal breakdown and, on occasions, polyps are extensively necrotic secondary to torsion or if they outgrow their blood supply; vascular thrombosis may be seen in such cases. In some instances, this may result in the formation of a necrotic polypoid mass with only the surface epithelium or the ghost outlines of glands remaining (*Fig. 7.63*). Variable amounts of stromal edema and occasionally myxoid change may be present as well as

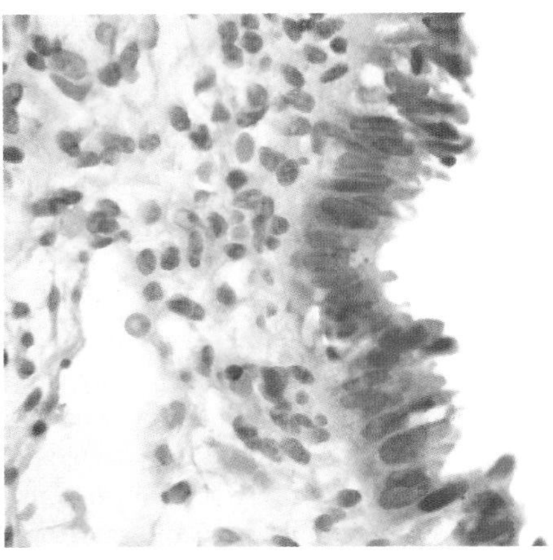

Fig. 7.62
Endometrial polyp. **The epithelium on the surface of a polyp may exhibit a degree of nuclear atypia with a degenerate appearance**

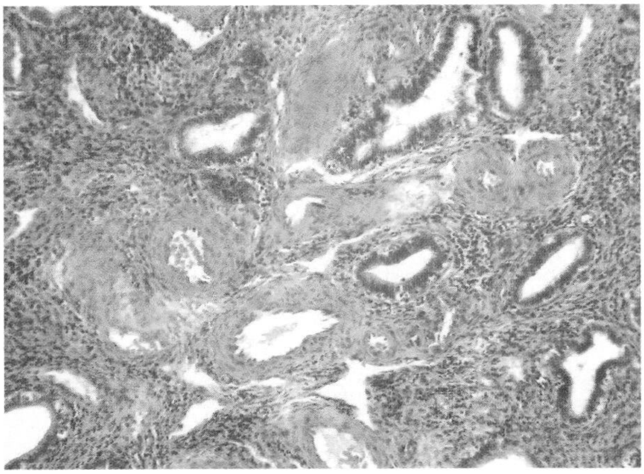

Fig. 7.61
Endometrial polyp. **Collections of thick-walled stromal blood vessels are a characteristic feature of endometrial polyps**

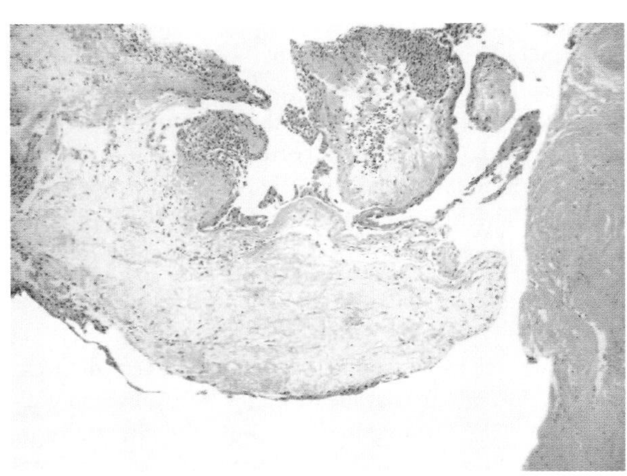

Fig. 7.63
Necrotic endometrial polyp. **Necrosis has occurred secondary to torsion**

hemosiderin pigment and foamy histiocytes. Sex cord-like areas have rarely been described in the stroma of an endometrial polyp [36]. Some endometrial polyps contain bundles of smooth muscle within the stroma, often in close proximity to thick-walled blood vessels. This is usually a minor feature and of no significance. However, when the smooth muscle is prominent, the term adenomyomatous polyp has been used (see section ➲ Adenomyomatous Polyp). Stromal inflammatory cells, including plasma cells, may be present in endometrial polyps; this should not be interpreted as an endometritis unless plasma cells are also present in the non-polypoid endometrium. Stromal decidualization or pseudodecidualization may occur secondary to progestational compounds but the degree of decidualization is typically less than in the surrounding endometrium.

As discussed previously, there is an increased frequency of endometrial polyps in patients taking tamoxifen. The polyps may be single or multiple and may be large. There are no pathognomonic histological features of tamoxifen-associated endometrial polyps, but an increased incidence of epithelial metaplasias, periglandular stromal condensation, stromal edema, and myxoid change and staghorn-shaped glands polarized along the long axis of the polyp have been reported [72].

As stated, diagnosing an endometrial polyp is generally straightforward when the polyp is large and removed intact. However, when small and fragmented, the diagnosis is more difficult. Lower uterine segment endometrium may be mistaken for a polyp because of the irregular glandular architecture and fibrous stroma. The spindle cell alteration of the stroma seen in some cases of endometritis may resemble the fibrous stroma of a polyp. However, other morphological features of a polyp are absent and there is a plasma cell infiltrate within the stroma; it should be remembered, however, that plasma cells may occur within the stroma of an endometrial polyp. Especially in large polyps with a degree of stromal condensation and increased cellularity around the glands, the differential diagnosis may include an adenosarcoma. Adenosarcoma typically has a leaf-like or club-like architecture, with broad papillae lined by surface epithelium, and intraglandular stromal projections, the overall architecture resembling a phyllodes tumor of the breast. In contrast, endometrial polyps usually have a smooth outline. The stroma in adenosarcoma is usually more cellular than in a benign polyp with increased mitotic activity and a degree of nuclear atypia, especially immediately surrounding the glands. With multiple recurrent endometrial polyps, a diagnosis of adenosarcoma should be suspected since the morphological features may be subtle. Adenofibroma may also be considered but this is rare and exhibits a similar low-power architecture to adenosarcoma. In polyps with a stromal smooth muscle component, an atypical polypoid adenomyoma may be considered. However, the stroma of atypical polypoid adenomyoma exhibits more extensive smooth muscle differentiation, the glandular architecture is more complicated, and there is often extensive squamous morule formation. Polyps in which the glands are mildly crowded and exhibit proliferative activity may be confused with an endometrial hyperplasia. In such cases, the identification of normal background endometrium facilitates the diagnosis since hyperplasia is usually a diffuse process.

Endometrial Polyp with Atypical Stromal Cells

Rare endometrial polyps contain stromal cells with markedly atypical symplastic-like nuclei (➲ *Fig. 7.64*), resembling those seen in polypoid lesions elsewhere in the female genital tract, such as in fibroepithelial stromal polyps of the vulva and vagina [143]. These atypical stromal cells are of no significance.

Adenomyomatous Polyp

As discussed, some endometrial polyps contain a minor component of stromal smooth muscle bundles, often in close proximity to thick-walled blood vessels. When the

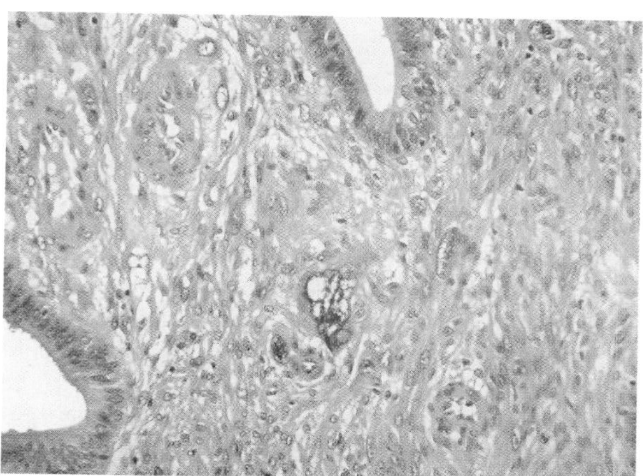

Fig. 7.64
Endometrial polyp with atypical stromal cells. Rare endometrial polyps contain stromal cells with markedly atypical nuclei

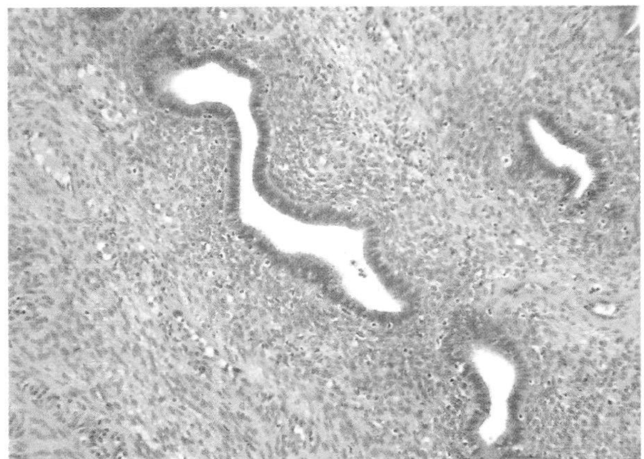

Fig. 7.65
Adenomyomatous polyp (adenomyoma). **Endometrioid type glands are surrounded by endometrial type stroma, which is in turn surrounded by smooth muscle**

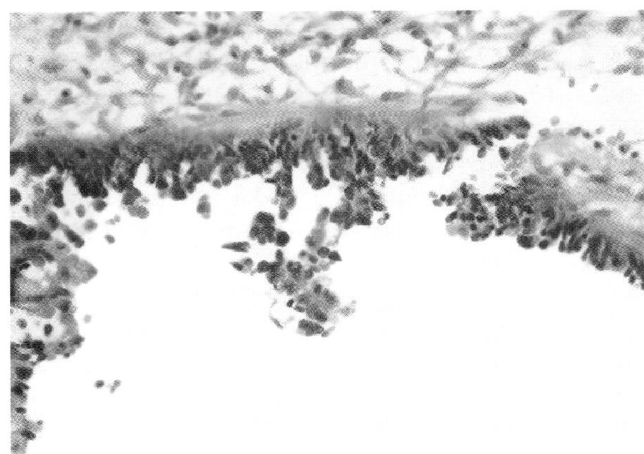

Fig. 7.66
Endometrial polyp with serous endometrial intraepithelial carcinoma (serous EIC). **Serous endometrial intraepithelial carcinoma rarely arises on the surface of an endometrial polyp**

smooth muscle is prominent, the term adenomyomatous polyp has been used. This term and the term adenomyoma have also been used for a lesion in which endometrioid type glands, sometimes with minor foci of ciliated, mucinous, or squamous metaplasia, are surrounded by endometrial stroma, which is in turn surrounded by smooth muscle [50, 142] (*Fig. 7.65*). These lesions, which may also be non-polypoid and located entirely within the myometrium can be associated with underlying adenomyosis. They should not be confused with atypical polypoid adenomyoma. In adenomyomas, the glands are usually surrounded by endometrioid type stroma, which is in turn surrounded by smooth muscle [50, 142].

Hyperplasia and Carcinoma Arising in Endometrial Polyp

Occasionally a hyperplasia or carcinoma arises within or involves a benign endometrial polyp [18]. A diagnosis of simple hyperplasia should not be made in a polyp since proliferative activity with glandular dilatation is a feature of many endometrial polyps. Complex and atypical hyperplasia is diagnosed in the same way as in non-polypoid endometrium. The hyperplasia may be confined to the polyp but also involves the non-polypoid endometrium in approximately 50% of cases [71, 100]. Both endometrioid and serous carcinomas (and occasionally other morphological types of malignancy) may arise within or involve an endometrial polyp and sometimes be confined to this. Serous carcinomas have a particular tendency to arise in or involve endometrial polyps as does

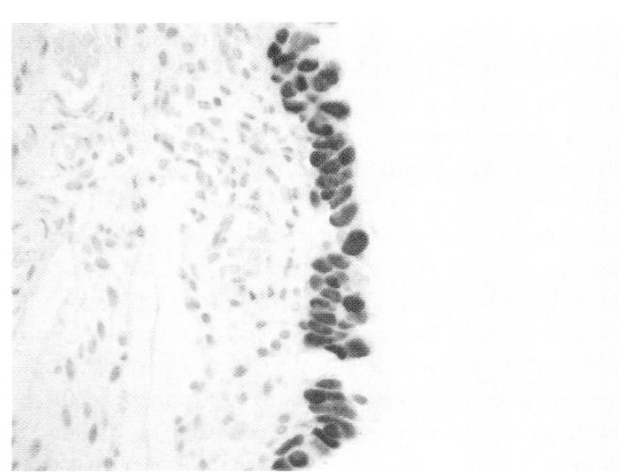

Fig. 7.67
p53 immunohistochemistry in serous endometrial intraepithelial carcinoma. **Diffuse intense nuclear p53 immunoreactivity of serous endometrial intraepithelial carcinoma on surface of an endometrial polyp**

the presumed precursor lesion serous endometrial intraepithelial carcinoma (serous EIC) [65, 134]. When serous EIC involves an endometrial polyp, there is partial replacement of the surface epithelium or sometimes the epithelium of the glands by cells with markedly atypical hyperchromatic nuclei, sometimes with prominent nucleoli, and prominent mitotic activity (*Fig. 7.66*). Immunohistochemical staining may assist in highlighting the serous proliferation since the cells of EIC typically exhibit diffuse intense nuclear immunoreactivity with p53 (➔ *Fig. 7.67*) and there is a high MIB1 proliferation index. ER is usually negative. In contrast, the benign epithelium within the polyp exhibits a low MIB1 proliferation index, is ER positive and is negative or only scattered nuclei are positive with p53. p53 staining may reveal that the EIC is more extensive than is appreciated on initial morphological examination. Rarely a carcinosarcoma arises in and is confined to an endometrial polyp. Occasional cases of metastatic carcinoma, especially breast lobular carcinoma, have been reported in endometrial polyps [60].

Atypical Polypoid Adenomyoma

Atypical polypoid adenomyoma is a biphasic polypoid lesion composed of endometrioid type glands in a myomatous or fibromyomatous stroma [97, 159]. Since the stroma may be fibromyomatous rather than overtly myomatous, some prefer the designation atypical polypoid adenomyofibroma [79]. Most patients are premenopausal or perimenopausal (average age 40 years) and present with abnormal uterine bleeding, usually in the form of menorrhagia. In some cases, the diagnosis is made during investigations for infertility. Occasional cases occur in postmenopausal women, and rare examples have been described in patients with Turner's syndrome who have been prescribed unopposed estrogens [23]. A single study has investigated molecular events in atypical polypoid adenomyoma and found MLH-1 promotor hypermethylation in some cases, a molecular alteration characteristic of some atypical hyperplasias and endometrioid adenocarcinomas [114].

Atypical polypoid adenomyoma is most commonly located in the lower uterine segment, although some cases involve the fundus, uterine body, or endocervix. In most cases, the lesion has an obvious polypoid gross appearance, in the form of either a sessile or broad-based polyp, but sometimes the polypoid nature is not grossly obvious, especially in smaller lesions.

The diagnosis may be made on endometrial biopsy, or polypectomy, or at hysterectomy. Histology shows architecturally irregular endometrioid type glands that may be widely separated and haphazardly arranged or somewhat crowded and arranged in groups, sometimes with a vaguely lobular pattern (➔ *Fig. 7.68*). The endometrioid epithelium varies in appearance from cuboidal to low columnar to pseudostratified. The nuclei are usually round, sometimes with prominent nucleoli, and exhibit

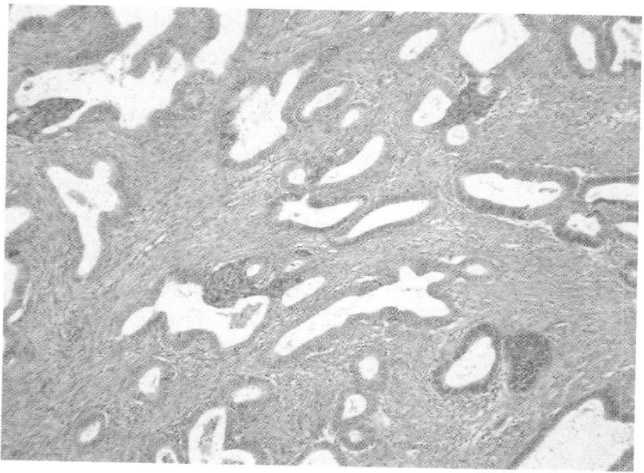

Fig. 7.68
Atypical polypoid adenomyoma. **Endometrioid type glands are embedded within a myomatous stroma**

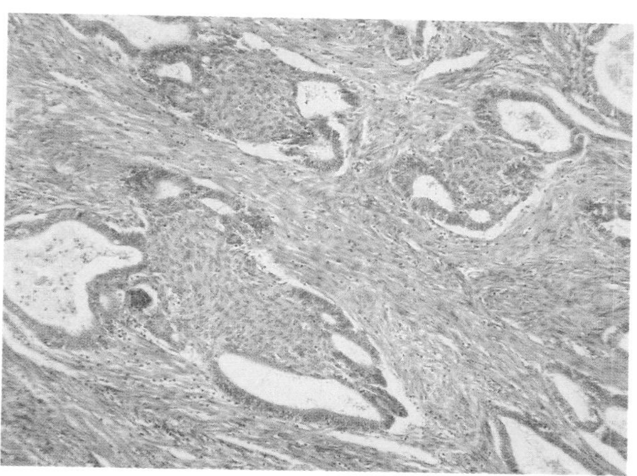

Fig. 7.69
Atypical polypoid adenomyoma. **There is abundant squamous morule formation**

mild or, at the most, moderate cytological atypia. Occasional foci of ciliated or mucinous epithelium may be present. A characteristic histological feature that is present in most, but not all, cases is abundant squamous morule formation (➔ *Fig. 7.69*); sometimes, the morules exhibit central necrosis. The glands are set in an abundant stroma, which varies from obviously smooth muscle in nature to fibromyomatous. Endometrial stroma is not present. The stromal cells are often arranged in short interlacing fascicles. Occasional mitotic figures may be identified within the stroma. The margin between the lesion and the underlying myometrium is usually rounded and well delineated but occasionally there is merging with underlying adenomyosis.

In some cases, there is significant glandular crowding with a back-to-back architecture and stromal exclusion, such that there are foci, which are virtually indistinguishable from, and which are best regarded as, grade I endometrioid adenocarcinoma. The term atypical polypoid adenomyoma of low malignant potential has been used for lesions with marked architectural complexity [79], but this term is not recommended. Very rarely, there is underlying myometrial invasion, and/or an endometrioid adenocarcinoma is present in the surrounding endometrium.

Atypical polypoid adenomyoma is generally a benign lesion, but there is a risk of recurrence if curettage or polypectomy is undertaken. In one series, 45% of cases treated by curettage or polypectomy recurred [79]. Given this risk of recurrence and the small, but definite, risk of transition to endometrioid adenocarcinoma, which was estimated at 8.8% in one meta-analysis [55], hysterectomy is the treatment of choice if the diagnosis is made on biopsy or polypectomy. In a woman who wishes to retain her uterus and in whom a confident diagnosis of atypical polypoid adenomyoma has been made on biopsy or polypectomy, complete removal by curettage or polypectomy may be undertaken with close follow-up and imaging. Successful pregnancies have ensued in patients managed in this way. It has been suggested that recurrence is more likely in cases with marked architectural complexity.

The most important differential diagnosis is an endometrioid adenocarcinoma exhibiting myometrial invasion or with a prominent desmoplastic stroma, an obviously important distinction since most atypical polypoid adenomyomas exhibit a benign behavior with a potential for conservative management. Recognition of the polypoid nature of the lesion assists in establishing the diagnosis. Marked cytological atypia favors a myoinvasive adenocarcinoma since in atypical polypoid adenomyoma, there is usually no more than mild to moderate cytological atypia. The stromal component of atypical polypoid adenomyoma grows in short interlacing fascicles, in contrast to the elongated fibers of the normal myometrium. In curettings or biopsy from an atypical polypoid adenomyoma, there are usually also fragments of normal background endometrium, and with an endometrioid adenocarcinoma, it would be unusual on biopsy to obtain only myoinvasive neoplasm without free tumor fragments. Immunohistochemistry is of little value in distinguishing between atypical polypoid adenomyoma and a myoinvasive endometrioid adenocarcinoma since the stromal component of atypical polypoid adenomyoma and myometrium infiltrated by carcinoma are both desmin and smooth muscle actin positive [135]. It has been suggested that CD10 may be of value since this is negative in the stromal component of atypical polypoid adenomyoma while the myoinvasive glands of endometrioid adenocarcinoma are typically surrounded by CD10 positive stromal cells [113]. The differential diagnosis can also include a benign endometrial polyp in which there may be a minor component of smooth muscle within the stroma. So-called typical adenomyomatous polyps or adenomyomas also occur (discussed earlier) and are composed of benign endometrioid type glands in a myomatous stroma [50, 142]. Often, endometrioid stroma surrounds the glands and this in turn is surrounded by smooth muscle. Rarely a carcinosarcoma enters into the differential diagnosis because of the admixture of epithelial and stromal elements. However, both the epithelial and mesenchymal components of a carcinosarcoma are obviously malignant and typically high grade.

Adenofibroma

Adenofibroma is a mixed tumor of the endometrium (and rarely also of the cervix) consisting of a benign epithelial and a benign mesenchymal component, both of which are integral components of the neoplasm. Adenofibromas most commonly occur in postmenopausal women but the age range is wide. The most common presenting symptom is abnormal vaginal bleeding. Occasional cases have arisen in patients taking tamoxifen [63]. Adenofibroma is rare and must be distinguished from the more common adenosarcoma with a subtle malignant stromal component [160] (discussed in ➋ Chap. 10, Mesenchymal Tumors of the Uterus). Grossly, adenofibroma occupies the uterine cavity, typically arising as a broad-based polypoid mass. The cut surface may be spongy or overtly cystic. Bland epithelium that is usually of endometrioid type but which may be mucinous, ciliated, or even squamous covers broad or fine papillary stromal fronds (➋ *Fig. 7.70*). Cells of fibroblastic type and more rarely endometrial stroma or smooth muscle make up the mesenchymal element. The stroma may be cellular or fibrous and the constituent cells are cytologically bland without nuclear pleomorphism. Mitotic figures are usually absent and should not exceed 1 per 10 high power fields; greater mitotic activity than this warrants a diagnosis of adenosarcoma, which is more common.

Periglandular cuffing by stromal cells should also result in consideration of adenosarcoma. Occasionally, an adenocarcinoma arises within an adenofibroma but this is probably a coincidental association [151].

While the adenofibroma is benign, hysterectomy is the most appropriate treatment. This is because adenosarcoma cannot be excluded in curettings or biopsy and also because recurrence of an adenofibroma treated by curettage or local excision may occur. It is for these reasons that some consider that adenofibroma does not exist, but rather is a well-differentiated form of adenosarcoma. At the heart of the controversy whether or not adenofibroma exists as an entity is the ability to distinguish it from adenosarcoma. The important features are the degree of mitotic activity in the stroma, the morphology of the stromal cells, and the presence of periglandular cuffing by stromal cells. A mitotic count greater than 1 per 10 high power fields warrants a diagnosis of adenosarcoma, a diagnosis that should also be made if there is more than mild nuclear atypia or significant periglandular stromal cuffing. It is difficult to make a confident diagnosis of adenofibroma on curetted or avulsed material because theoretically adenosarcoma cannot be excluded unless the whole tumor is available for examination. Thus, a hysterectomy is required to ensure that the tissue examined was not just the most benign area of an adenosarcoma. Using these strict criteria, the diagnosis of adenofibroma is made only rarely. Cases have been reported in which repeated curettages have been carried out because the lesion was wrongly thought to be benign before a diagnosis of adenosarcoma has eventually been made [26]. It is also important to differentiate between adenofibroma and a benign endometrial polyp since the latter does not require further treatment. While the distinction can be difficult, adenofibroma should be considered if the lesion has a papillary surface and a stroma that is cellular. The stroma of endometrial polyps tends to be more hyaline than that of adenofibroma, although there is considerable overlap.

Effects of Intrauterine Device (IUD)

Intrauterine devices (IUDs) are in widespread use, mainly for contraceptive purposes. Older devices were usually composed entirely of plastic while more modern devices are often composed of plastic with a copper coating. The effects of the Mirena coil, a progestin containing IUD, are discussed in the next section. The histological features in the endometrium in association with an IUD are largely due to local mechanical effects. The surface endometrium may take on the configuration of the IUD due to a direct pressure effect. There may be surface micropapillary formations and focal reactive changes with nuclear enlargement, mild nuclear atypia, small nucleoli, and cytoplasmic vacuolation (*Fig. 7.71*). When micropapillary fragments of epithelium exhibiting these features are present in an endometrial biopsy, this may result in diagnostic difficulty. The glandular epithelium may also exhibit epithelial cytoplasmic change, including squamous metaplasia, and there may be surface ulceration. The endometrial glands at the site of contact, and immediately surrounding this, may

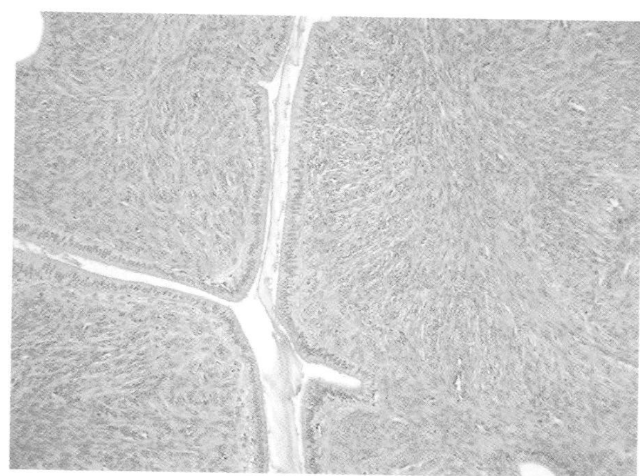

Fig. 7.70
Adenofibroma of endometrium. **Adenofibroma containing benign glands with underlying bland fibrous stroma**

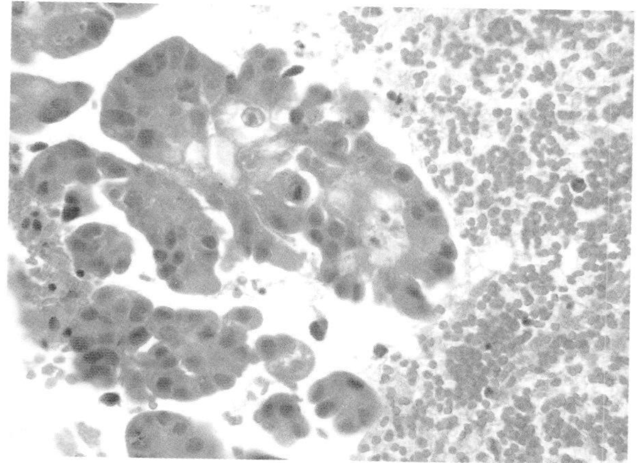

Fig. 7.71
Reaction to intrauterine device (IUD). **Micropapillary formations are present, in keeping with a reaction to an intrauterine device**

exhibit a different pattern of maturation from the rest of the endometrium. With long-term usage, the endometrium adjacent to the IUD may on occasions be fibrosed or simplified and composed of a monolayer. Rarely there is stromal microcalcification. Although the features may be subtle, a focal inflammatory infiltrate is commonly present consisting of polymorphs, lymphocytes, histiocytes, and plasma cells. Foreign body type giant cells and granulomas may be a component of the inflammatory infiltrate, the severity of which may be related to the type of IUD and the duration of use. In most cases, the inflammation is superficial and largely confined to the site of contact but in other instances it is more widespread. When confined to the IUD site, the inflammation is probably a consequence of irritation rather than infection but when more widespread it may be secondary to infection; in such cases, the inflammatory infiltrate, as well as being more widespread, is typically more intense. Infection appears more common with plastic devices than with copper-coated devices. Usually, a mixture of organisms is present. Long-term IUD use is associated with infection by the gram-positive anaerobic bacterium actinomyces (discussed earlier).

A rare but serious complication of IUD use is uterine perforation or laceration, most commonly occurring at the time of insertion. The risk of perforation is greatest in the postpartum period when the tissues are soft and expanded. Displacement of the IUD into the pelvis with an associated inflammatory reaction may ensue secondary to perforation and spontaneous expulsion may also occur.

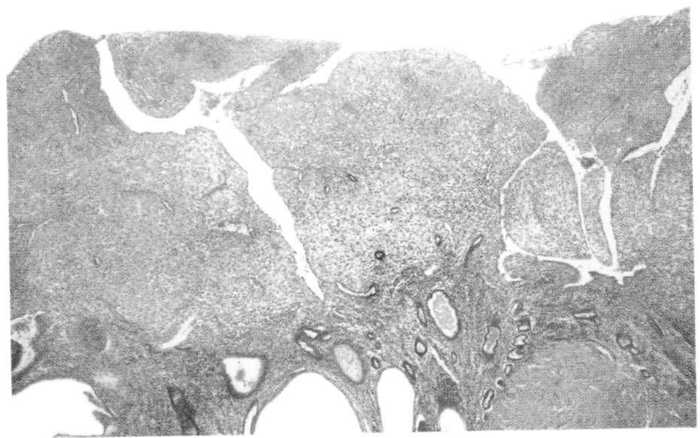

Fig. 7.72
Mirena coil–associated endometrium. **There is a low-power polypoid architecture**

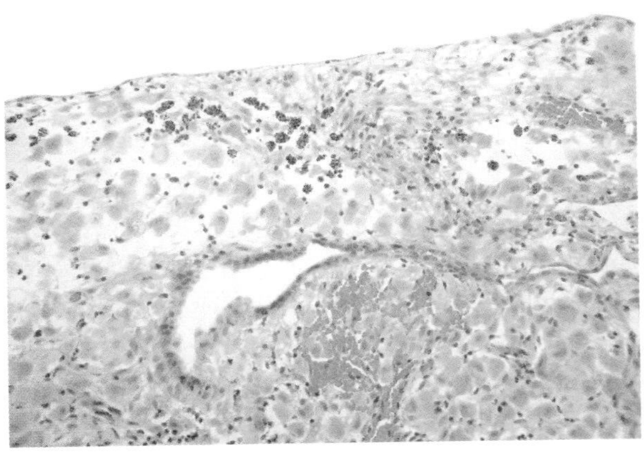

Fig. 7.73
Mirena coil–associated endometrium. **There is stromal expansion and decidualization. Hemosiderin pigment is present within the stroma**

Effects of Mirena Coil

The Mirena coil is a levonorgestrel (a progestin)-releasing IUD that is in widespread use as a highly effective contraceptive. The Mirena coil is also licensed for the management of idiopathic menorrhagia and has been used to deliver progestin for endometrial protection in postmenopausal hormone replacement regimes. It has also been suggested that the Mirena coil can be used to prevent endometrial hyperplastic changes in patients taking tamoxifen or estrogen-only HRT.

The histological features of the endometrium in association with the Mirena coil include a low-power polypoid architecture (*Fig. 7.72*), probably secondary to a direct mechanical effect. Ulceration, surface micropapillary proliferations, and reactive atypia of the surface endometrium may also be present. The endometrial glands are usually small tubular and atrophic but occasionally exhibit weak secretory activity. There is stromal expansion and decidualization or pseudodecidualization with infiltration by granulated lymphocytes (*Fig. 7.73*) [119]. Other histological features found in some cases include stromal myxoid or mucinous change, hemosiderin pigment and glandular metaplastic changes. Stromal necrosis, infarction, and microcalcifications are found in a small percentage of cases. In some cases, plasma cells are present within the stroma, indicating a coexistent chronic endometritis, secondary to the presence of the IUD. Stromal hyaline

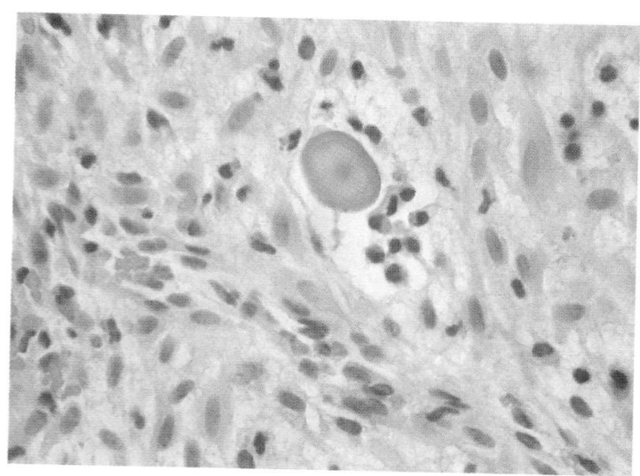

Fig. 7.74
Mirena coil–associated endometrium. **Stromal hyaline nodules may be seen in Mirena coil–associated endometrium**

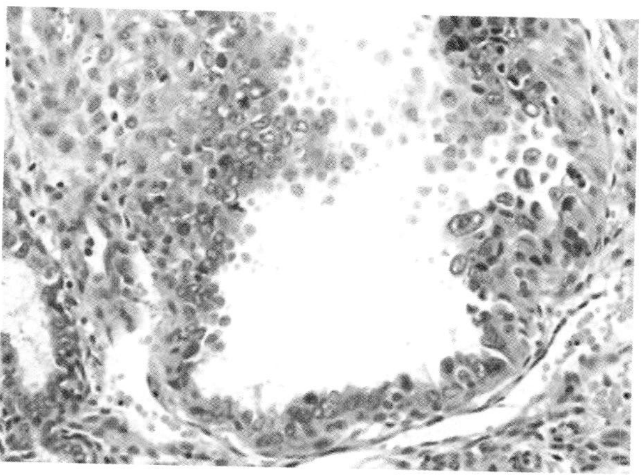

Fig. 7.75
Radiation effect endometrium. **Glands are lined by cells with enlarged atypical nuclei**

nodules have also been described (*Fig. 7.74*) [56]. There may be associated progestational effects in the cervix, including microglandular hyperplasia and stromal decidualization.

Radiation Effects on the Endometrium

The endometrial morphology can be altered by the effects of radiation, which may have been administered many years earlier. Radiation effect endometrium is characterized by surface endometrium or glands lined by cells with enlarged atypical, sometimes bizarre, hyperchromatic nuclei (*Fig. 7.75*). The nuclear chromatin may be smudged and indistinct or there may be prominent nucleoli. Hobnail cells may be present. There is usually abundant cytoplasm that can be eosinophilic, clear, or vacuolated. The normal glandular architecture is typically maintained or there may be glandular loss. The stroma can be fibrotic with associated vascular changes characteristic of radiation. The presence of cells with enlarged atypical nuclei can raise the possibility of serous EIC. Knowledge of the history of prior radiation is obviously paramount in establishing the diagnosis; a lack of mitotic activity and a low nuclear to cytoplasmic ratio are other diagnostic clues. p53 immunohistochemistry may assist since serous EIC usually exhibits diffuse intense nuclear immunoreactivity while in radiation effect the nuclei are negative or exhibit weak heterogeneous staining. Prior radiation is associated with an increased risk of the subsequent development of uterine malignancies. These may be of any morphological type but carcinosarcomas are proportionally overrepresented.

Effects of Endometrial Ablation or Resection

Endometrial ablation is commonly undertaken as a nonsurgical procedure in the management of abnormal uterine bleeding, especially in premenopausal women where the suspicion of malignancy is low and preservation of fertility is not an issue. The object of endometrial ablation is destruction of the entire endometrium and superficial myometrium using thermal coagulation (electrosurgical rollerball), laser vaporization, or resection. Most patients become amenorrheic or hypomenorrheic following the ablation but some have continuous bleeding and/or pain and repeat endometrial biopsy or sometimes hysterectomy is undertaken either soon after the procedure or some time later. The histological features depend on the time interval between the ablation and the subsequent biopsy or hysterectomy. In the early stages (up to 3 months), there may be complete or almost complete necrosis of the endometrium and superficial myometrium with replacement of this by a coagulum of necrotic fibrinoid material with a surrounding histiocytic and giant cell reaction (*Fig. 7.76*), the morphological features resembling that of a rheumatoid nodule or a necrotizing granulomatous process [30, 44]. Spicules of thermally damaged tissue may be identified and there is a variable

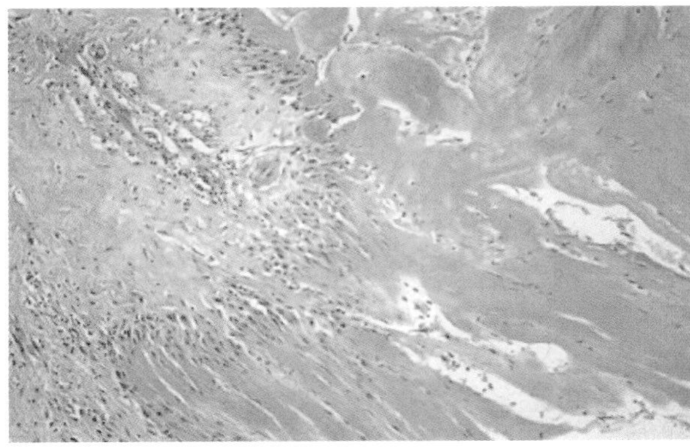

Fig. 7.76
Reaction to previous endometrial ablation. **Endometrium is replaced by fibrinoid material with a surrounding histiocytic and giant cell reaction**

degree of inflammation. Later, necrotic tissue is no longer present but a giant cell and granulomatous reaction may persist, sometimes with pigment within giant cells. There is usually striking fibrosis and there may be regeneration of the endometrium with the formation of a monolayer of simple cuboidal epithelium directly abutting the myometrium. In other cases, the endometrium is histologically relatively normal. Scarring may result in obstruction and the subsequent development of hematometra or pyometra. The histological features following endometrial resection are similar [92].

Usually, an endometrial biopsy is taken just prior to ablation being performed. Rarely this contains an unsuspected carcinoma and hysterectomy is performed soon after the ablation. In such instances, the endometrial carcinoma may have undergone total or extensive necrosis, secondary to the ablation procedure.

Effects of Curettage

Morphological changes may be seen in the endometrium secondary to recent curettage, especially if this has been vigorous. The changes are transient and will only be seen if repeat endometrial sampling or hysterectomy is undertaken a short time after curettage. There may be focal surface erosion with an associated mixed inflammatory infiltrate; in some cases, eosinophils are conspicuous [99]. Following this, there is usually epithelial regeneration, sometimes with a micropapillary architecture, hobnail cell change, and mild reactive nuclear atypia. Usually, the changes are minor, result in no particular diagnostic difficulties, and return to normal within 10 to 14 days. A similar phenomenon has been described in the endocervix secondary to recent endometrial sampling and termed atypical reactive proliferation of the endocervix ([128].)

Asherman's Syndrome

Asherman's syndrome is characterized by focal or diffuse endometrial fibrosis and loss of distinction between the functionalis and basalis. The endometrium may be composed of a monolayer of epithelium with underlying fibrous tissue and adhesions may form across the cavity. The endometrial stroma is fibrosed, may be calcified and, on rare occasions, even ossified. The endometrial glands are typically sparse, inactive, and may be cystically dilated. Asherman's syndrome can result in infertility, amenorrhea, or hypomenorrhea. Pregnancies may be complicated by premature labor, placenta previa, or placenta accreta. In some, but not all, cases, there is a known cause for the Asherman's syndrome, which may be secondary to previous surgery, curettage or ablation, infection, miscarriage, or retained products of conception. Hysteroscopic lysis of adhesions can result in successful pregnancies.

Postoperative Spindle Cell Nodule

Postoperative spindle cell nodule represents an exaggerated reparative response at the site of previous surgery or biopsy and, in the female genital tract, is most common in the vagina. It has rarely been described in the endometrium [25]. Postoperative spindle cell nodule occurs within weeks or months of the inciting procedure and consists of a cellular proliferation of spindle-shaped cells with admixed vascular channels and inflammatory cells. There may be abundant mitotic activity, raising the possibility of a sarcoma, usually a leiomyosarcoma. However, the high mitotic activity contrasts with the bland nuclear features and lack of cytological atypia. The history of a recent procedure is obviously paramount in establishing the diagnosis. The constituent cells may be positive with smooth muscle actin, desmin and, on rare occasions, cytokeratins.

Psammoma Bodies in the Endometrium

Calcified psammoma bodies may be seen in the endometrium in association with benign and malignant lesions and rarely in normal endometrium. They are present in up to one third of uterine serous carcinomas, a lower frequency than in ovarian serous carcinomas [58]. More uncommonly, they are seen in other morphological types of endometrial malignancy, such as endometrioid carcinoma. Psammoma bodies are occasionally seen in normal endometria (usually atrophic or proliferative in type), sometimes in association with hormonal preparations, and in benign lesions, most commonly endometrial polyps [59, 146]. They are often located within glandular lumina (➲ *Fig. 7.77*), in which case it is likely that they represent calcification of inspissated secretions. In other cases, they are situated within the stroma where they may be secondary to prior inflammation or the presence of an IUD. In the absence of a malignant lesion, the occurrence of psammoma bodies within glandular lumina or endometrial stroma is not an indication for evaluation of the upper female genital tract to exclude malignancy. However, free-floating psammoma bodies without attachment to tissue may be an indication of an extrauterine serous carcinoma.

Emphysematous Endometritis

There have been occasional reports of emphysematous (pneumopolycystic) endometritis characterized by the presence of gas-filled cysts in the endometrial stroma [118, 149]. There may be simultaneous involvement of the cervix or the condition may be confined to the endometrium. Histology shows empty cystic spaces of variable size and contour within the endometrial stroma lined by flattened stromal cells with occasional histiocytes and/or giant cells. Spontaneous resolution usually occurs. Emphysematous endometritis should be distinguished from sectioning artifact, dilated vascular spaces, and gas gangrene of the uterus, which is life threatening and associated with tissue necrosis.

Benign Endometrial Stromal Proliferations

Endometrial stromal neoplasms are discussed in ➲ Chap. 10, Mesenchymal Tumors of the Uterus, as is the differential diagnosis of fragments of tissue composed entirely of endometrial stroma in an endometrial biopsy. Occasional cases of multifocal microscopic benign endometrial stromal proliferations confined to the endometrium without invasive growth have been reported [138]. These have been termed focal endometrial stromal hyperplasia and may mimic an endometrial stromal nodule or endometrial stromal sarcoma in biopsy samples. Rarely, markedly atypical stromal cells with a symplastic appearance are present within an otherwise normal endometrium [148] (➲ *Fig. 7.78*).

Benign Trophoblastic Lesions

Benign lesions of intermediate trophoblast, namely placental site nodule or plaque (PSNP) and exaggerated placental site, are discussed in ➲ Chap. 20, Gestational Trophoblastic Tumors and Related Tumor-Like Lesions.

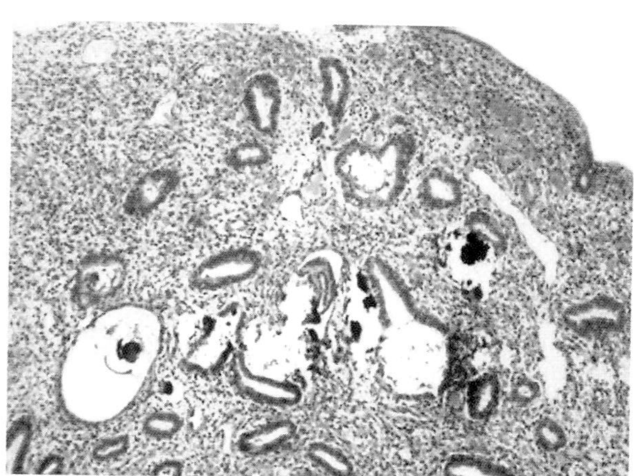

Fig. 7.77
Psammoma bodies in endometrium. **Psammoma bodies within glandular lumina within an endometrial polyp**

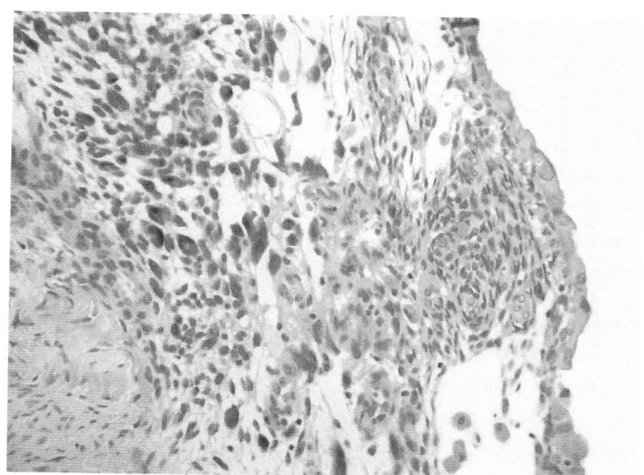

Fig. 7.78
Atypical endometrial stromal cells. **Rarely endometrial stromal cells with atypical symplastic-like nuclei are present in the normal endometrium**

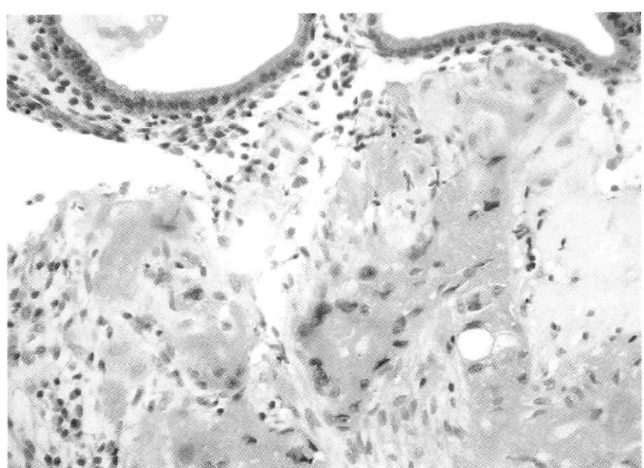

Fig. 7.79
Placental site nodule or plaque. **A well-circumscribed lesion is composed of epithelioid cells with abundant cytoplasm**

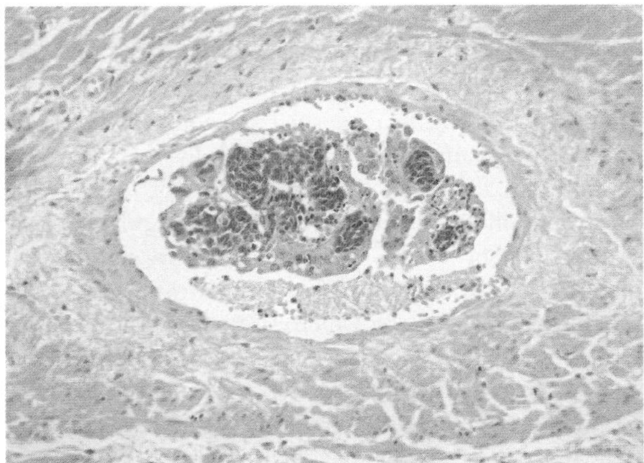

Fig. 7.80
Intravascular menstrual endometrium. **Menstrual endometrium within myometrial blood vessels is occasionally seen and is of no significance**

An endometrial PSNP may be identified in a biopsy, resection, or hysterectomy specimen many years following a pregnancy or abortion and rarely even in a postmenopausal woman. PSNP is characterized histologically by a well-circumscribed lesion composed of cells with large degenerate, often atypical nuclei and abundant eosinophilic cytoplasm (*Fig. 7.79*). The immunophenotype is discussed in detail later in Chap. 20, Gestational Trophoblastic Tumors and Related Tumor-Like Lesions.

Intravascular Endometrium

Occasionally in a hysterectomy specimen, menstrual endometrium is present within myometrial vascular channels (*Fig. 7.80*) [8]. Rarely there is extensive vascular involvement and even invasion of parametrial vessels. Intravascular menstrual endometrium is of no significance other than that it may be mistaken for neoplastic involvement of vascular channels. It should also be distinguished from intravascular foci of adenomyosis [125].

Endometrial Autolysis

Hysterectomies are performed for a wide variety of benign and malignant conditions. Especially with large uteri, the formalin does not penetrate into the endometrial cavity and, as a consequence, fixation is often not adequate and the endometrium may be markedly autolyzed. This not uncommonly results in problems in morphological assessment of the endometrium, which in some cases is so autolyzed that interpretation is impossible. This is important in all uteri but particularly so with endometrial neoplasms where autolysis may result in problems in assessing tumor type and grade. Bisection of the uterus soon after surgery may improve fixation, but this often results in distortion of the specimen making assessment of parameters such as the depth of myometrial invasion by tumor problematic. Packing the cavity with absorbable tissue paper following bisection and ensuring that the two halves of the uterus remain apposed minimizes the distortion. Uteri may also be injected with formalin using a needle and syringe directed alongside a probe, which is inserted through the external cervical os into the endometrial cavity [61]. This initiation results in significantly less endometrial autolysis.

References

1. Antoni J, Folch E, Costa J et al (1997) Comparison of cystopat and pipelle endometrial biopsy instruments. Eur J Obstet Gynecol Reprod Biol 72:57–61
2. Archer DF, McIntyre-Seltman K, Wilborn WW Jr et al (1991) Endometrial morphology in asymptomatic postmenopausal women. Am J Obstet Gynecol 165:317–320
3. Arias-Stella J Jr, Arias-Velasquez A, Arias-Stella J (1994) Normal and abnormal mitoses in the atypical endometrial change associated with chorionic tissue effect. Am J Surg Pathol 18:694–701
4. Arias-Stella J (2002) The Arias-Stella reaction: facts and fancies four decades after. Adv Anat Pathol 9:12–23
5. Bahceci M, Demirel LC (1996) Osseous metaplasia of the endometrium: a rare cause of infertility and its hysteroscopic management. Hum Reprod 11:2537–2539

6. Baird DB, Reddick RL (1991) Extraovarian mucinous metaplasia in a patient with bilateral mucinous borderline ovarian tumors: a case report. Int J Gynecol Pathol 10:96–103
7. Bakour SH, Khan KS, Gupta JK (2000) Controlled analysis of factors associated with insufficient sample on outpatient endometrial biopsy. Br J Obstet Gynaecol 107:1312–1314
8. Banks ER, Mills SE, Frierson HF Jr (1991) Uterine intravascular menstrual endometrium simulating malignancy. Am J Surg Pathol 15:407–412
9. Barroeta JE, Pasha TL, Acs G et al (2007) Immunoprofile of endometrial and endocervical stromal cells and its potential application in localization of tumour involvement. Int J Gynecol Pathol 26:76–82
10. Bayer-Garner IB, Korourian S (2001) Plasma cells in chronic endometritis are easily identified when stained with syndecan-1. Mod Pathol 14:877–879
11. Bayer-Garner IB, Nickell JA (2004) Routine syndecan-1 immunohistochemistry aids in the diagnosis of chronic endometritis. Arch Pathol Lab Med 128:1000–1003
12. Bennett AE, Rathmore S, Rhatigan RM (1999) Focal necrotizing endometritis: a clinicopathologic study of 15 cases. Int J Gynecol Pathol 18:220–225
13. Bozdogan O, Atasoy P, Erekul S et al (2002) Apoptosis-related proteins and steroid hormone receptors in normal, hyperplastic and neoplastic endometrium. Int J Gynecol Pathol 21:375–382
14. Brachtel EF, Sánchez-Estevez C, Moreno-Bueno G et al (2005) Distinct molecular alterations in complex endometrial hyperplasia (CEH) with and without immature squamous metaplasia (squamous morules). Am J Surg Pathol 29:1322–1329
15. Brinton LA, Hoover RN, Endometrial Cancer Collaborative Group (1993) Estrogen replacement therapy and endometrial cancer risk: a meta-analysis. Obstet Gynecol 81:265–271
16. Bulmer JN, Hollings D, Ritson A (1987) Immunocytochemical evidence that endometrial stromal granulocytes are granulated lymphocytes. J Pathol 155:281–287
17. Bulmer JN, Lunny DP, Hagin SV (1988) Immunohistochemical characterization of stromal leucocytes in non-pregnant human endometrium. Am J Reprod Immunol Microbiol 17:83–90
18. Carlson JW, Mutter GL (2008) Endometrial intraepithelial neoplasia is associated with polyps and frequently has metaplastic change. Histopathology 53:325–332
19. Cheng WF, Lin HH, Torng PL, Huang SC (1997) Comparison of endometrial changes among symptomatic tamoxifen-treated and non-treated premenopausal and postmenopausal breast cancer patients. Gynecol Oncol 66:233–237
20. Chiarelli S, Buriticá C, Litta P et al (2006) An immunohistochemical study of morules in endometrioid lesions of the female genital tract: CD10 is a characteristic marker of morular metaplasia. Clin Cancer Res 12:4251–4256
21. Chinen K, Kamiyama K, Kinjo T et al (2004) Morules in endometrial carcinoma and benign endometrial lesions differ from squamous differentiation tissue and are not infected with human papillomavirus. J Clin Pathol 57:918–926
22. Clark TJ, Mann CH, Shah N et al (2001) Accuracy of outpatient endometrial biopsy in the diagnosis of endometrial hyperplasia. Acta Obstet Gynecol Scand 80:784–793
23. Clement PB, Young RH (1987) Atypical polypoid adenomyoma of the uterus associated with Turner's syndrome. Int J Gynecol Pathol 6:104–113
24. Clement PB, Scully RE (1988) Idiopathic postmenopausal decidual reaction of the endometrium. Int J Gynecol Pathol 7:152–161
25. Clement PB (1988) Postoperative spindle-cell nodule of the endometrium. Arch Pathol Lab Med 112:566–568
26. Clement PB, Scully RE (1990) Mullerian adenosarcoma of the uterus: a clinicopathologic analysis of 100 cases and review of the literature. Hum Pathol 21:363–381
27. Clement PB, Oliva E, Young RH (1996) Mullerian adenosarcoma of the uterine corpus associated with tamoxifen therapy: a report of six cases and a review of tamoxifen – associated endometrial lesions. Int J Gynecol Pathol 15:222–229
28. Cohen I, Figer A, Altaras MM et al (1996) Common endometrial decidual reaction in postmenopausal breast cancer patients treated with tamoxifen and progestogens. Int J Gynecol Pathol 15:17–22
29. Cohen I, Beyth Y, Shapira J et al (1997) High frequency of adenomyosis in postmenopausal breast cancer patients treated with tamoxifen. Gynecol Obstet Invest 44:200–205
30. Colgan TJ, Shah R, Leyland N (1999) Post-hysteroscopic ablation reaction: A histopathologic study of electrosurgical ablation. Int J Gynecol Pathol 18:325–331
31. Creagh TM, Bain BJ, Evans DJ et al (1995) Endometrial extramedullary haematopoiesis. J Pathol 176:99–104
32. Critchley HO, Tong S, Cameron ST et al (1999) Regulation of bcl-2 gene family members in human endometrium by antiprogestin administration in vivo. J Reprod Fertil 115:389–395
33. Crum CP, Hornstein MD, Nucci MR (2003) Hertig and beyond: a systematic and practical approach to the endometrial biopsy. Adv Anat Pathol 10:301–318
34. Dal Cin P, De Wolf F, Klerckx P et al (1992) The 6p21 chromosome region is nonrandomly involved in endometrial polyps. Gynecol Oncol 46:393–396
35. Delmas PD, Bjarnson NH, Mitlak BH et al (1997) Effects of raloxifene on bone mineral density, serum cholesterol concentrations, and uterine endometrium in postmenopausal women. N Eng J Med 337:1641–1647
36. De Quintall MM, De Angelo Andrade LA (2006) Endometrial polyp with sex cord-like pattern. Int J Gynecol Pathol 25:170–172
37. Disep B, Innes BA, Cochrane HR et al (2004) Immunohistochemical characterization of endometrial leucocytes in endometritis. Histopathology 45:625–632
38. Duncan DA, Varner RE, Mazur MT (1989) Uterine herpes virus infection with multifocal necrotizing endometritis. Hum Pathol 20:1021–1024
39. Dutra F (1959) Intraglandular morules of the endometrium. Am J Clin Pathol 31:60–65
40. The Writing Group for the PEPI Trial (1996) Effects of hormone replacement therapy on endometrial histology in postmenopausal women. The Postmenopausal Estrogen/Progestin Interventions (PEPI) Trial. JAMA 275:370–375
41. Euscher E, Nuovo GJ (2002) Detection of kappa-and lamda-expressing cells in the endometrium by in-situ hybridisation. Int J Gynecol Pathol 21:383–390
42. Fechner RE, Bossart MI, Spjut HJ (1979) Ultrastructure of endometrial stromal foam cells. Am J Clin Pathol 72:628–633
43. Feeley KM, Wells M (2001) Hormone replacement therapy and the endometrium. J Clin Pathol 54:435–440
44. Ferryman SR, Stephens M, Gough D (1992) Necrotising granulomatous endometritis following endometrial ablation therapy. Br J Obstet Gynaecol 99:928–930
45. Fisher B, Consantino JP, Wickerham DL et al (1998) Tamoxifen for prevention of breast cancer: report of the National Surgical Adjuvant Breast and Bowel Project P-1 Study. J Natl Cancer Inst 90:1371–1388

46. Fletcher JA, Pinkus GS, Donovan K et al (1992) Clonal rearrangement of chromosome band 6p21 in the mesenchymal component of pulmonary chondroid hamartoma. Cancer Res 52:6224–6228
47. Fluhmann CF (1960) The developmental anatomy of the cervix uteri. Obstet Gynaecol 15:62–69
48. Frank TS, Himebaugh KS, Wilson MD (1992) Granulomatous endometritis associated with histologically occult cytomegalovirus in a healthy patient. Am J Surg Pathol 16:716–720
49. Genest DR, Brodsky G, Lage JA (1995) Localized endometrial proliferations associated with pregnancy: Clinical and histopathologic features of 11 cases. Hum Pathol 26:1233–1240
50. Gilks CB, Clement PB, Hart WR et al (2000) Uterine adenomyomas excluding atypical polypoid adenomyomas and adenomyomas of endocervical type: a clinicopathologic study of 30 cases of an underemphasized lesion that may cause diagnostic problems with brief consideration of adenomyomas of other female genital tract sites. Int J Gynecol Pathol 19:195–205
51. Gompel A, Sabourin JC, Martin A et al (1994) Bcl-2 expression in normal endometrium during the menstrual cycle. Am J Pathol 144:1195–1202
52. Gordon SJ, Westgate J (1999) The incidence and management of failed pipelle sampling in a general outpatient clinic. Aust N Z J Obstet Gynaecol 39:115–118
53. Grady D, Gebrestsadik T, Kerlikowske K et al (1995) Hormone replacement therapy and endometrial cancer risk: a meta-analysis. Obstet Gynaecol 85:304–313
54. Hachisuga T, Hideshima T, Kawarabayashi T et al (1999) Expression of steroid receptors, Ki-67 and epidermal growth factor receptor in tamoxifen-treated endometrium. Int J Gynecol Pathol 18:297–303
55. Heatley MK (2006) Atypical polypoid adenomyoma: a systematic review of the English literature. Histopathology 48:609–610
56. Hejmadi RK, Chaudhri S, Ganesan R, Rollason TP (2007) Morphologic changes in the endometrium associated with the use of the mirena coli: a retrospective study of 106 cases. Int J Surg Pathol 15:148–154
57. Hendrickson MR, Kempson RL (1980) Endometrial epithelial metaplasias: proliferations frequently misdiagnosed as adenocarcinoma. Report of 89 cases and proposed classification. Am J Surg Pathol 4:525–542
58. Hendrickson M, Ross J, Eifel P et al (1982) Uterine papillary serous carcinoma: a highly malignant form of endometrial adenocarcinoma. Am J Surg Pathol 6:93–108
59. Herbold DR, Magrane DM (1986) Calcifications of the benign endometrium. Arch Pathol Lab Med 110:666–669
60. Houghton J, Ioffe O, Silverberg SG et al (2003) Metastatic breast lobular carcinoma involving tamoxifen-associated endometrial polyps: report of two cases and review of tamoxifen-associated polypoid uterine lesions. Mod Pathol 16:395–398
61. Houghton JP, Roddy S, Carroll S, McCluggage WG (2004) A simple method for the prevention of endometrial autolysis in hysterectomy specimens. J Clin Pathol 57:332–333
62. Houghton O, Connolly LE, McCluggage WG (2008) Morules in endometrioid proliferations of the uterus and ovary consistently express the intestinal transcription factor CDX2. Histopathology 53:156–165
63. Huang KT, Chen CA, Cheng WF et al (1996) Sonographic characteristics of adenofibroma of the endometrium following tamoxifen therapy for breast cancer: two case reports. Ultrasound Obstet Gynecol 7:363–366
64. Huettner PC, Gersell DJ (1994) Arias-Stella reaction in nonpregnant women: a clinicopathologic study of nine cases. Int J Gynecol Pathol 13:241–247
65. Hui P, Kelly M, O'Malley DM et al (2005) Minimal uterine serous carcinoma: a clinicopathological study of 40 cases. Mod Pathol 18:75–82
66. Iezzoni JC, Mills SE (2001) Nonneoplastic endometrial signet-ring cells. Vacuolated decidual cells and stromal histiocytes mimicking adenocarcinoma. Am J Clin Pathol 115:249–255
67. Irving JA, McFarland D, Stuart DS et al (2000) Mitotic arrest of endometrial epithelium after paclitaxel therapy for breast cancer. Int J Gynecol Pathol 19:395–397
68. Ismail SM (1994) Pathology of endometrium treated with tamoxifen. J Clin Pathol 47:827–833
69. Ismail SM (1999) Gynaecological effects of tamoxifen. J Clin Pathol 52:83–88
70. Kaufman RH, Binder GL, Gray PN et al (1977) Upper genital tract changes associated with exposure in utero to diethylstilbestrol. Am J Obstet Gynecol 128:51
71. Kelly P, Dobbs SP, McCluggage WG (2007) Endometrial hyperplasia involving endometrial polyps: report of a series and discussion of the significance in an endometrial biopsy specimen. Br J Obstet Gynaecol 114:944–950
72. Kennedy MM, Baigrie CF, Manek S (1999) Tamoxifen and the endometrium: review of 102 cases and comparison with HRT-related and non-HRT-related endometrial pathology. Int J Gynecol Pathol 18:130–137
73. Khatamee MA, Sommers SC (1989) Clinicopathologic diagnosis of mycoplasma endometritis. Int J Fertil 34:52–59
74. Kim KR, Lee YH, Ro JY (2002) Nodular histiocytic hyperplasia of the endometrium. Int J Gynecol Pathol 21:141–146
75. Kurman RJ, Young RH, Norris HJ et al (1984) Immunocytochemical localization of placental lactogen and chorionic gonadotropin in the normal placenta and trophoblastic tumors, with emphasis on intermediate trophoblast and the placental site trophoblastic tissue. Int J Gynecol Pathol 3:101
76. Lehman MB, Hart WR (2002) Simple and complex hyperplastic papillary proliferations of the endometrium: a clinicopathologic study of nine cases of apparently localized papillary lesions with fibrovascular stromal cores and epithelial metaplasia. Am J Surg Pathol 25:1347–1354
77. Leung ASY, Vinyuvat S, Leong FJWM et al (1997) Anti-CD38 and VS38 antibodies for detection of plasma cells in the diagnosis of chronic endometritis. Appl Immunohistochem Mol Morphol 5:189–193
78. Lindenman E, Shepard MK, Pescovitz OH (1997) Clinical commentary. Müllerian agenesis: an update Obstet Gynecol 90:307–312
79. Longacre TA, Chung MH, Rouse RV et al (1996) Atypical polypoid adenomyofibromas (atypical polypoid adenomyomas) of the uterus. A clinicopathologic study of 55 cases. Am J Surg Pathol 20:1–20
80. McCluggage WG, Roberts N, Bharucha H (1995) Enteric differentiation in endometrial adenocarcinomas: a mucin histochemical study. Int J Gynecol Pathol 14:250–254
81. McCluggage WG, Varma V, Weir P, Bharucha H (1996) Uterine leiomyosarcoma in patient receiving tamoxifen therapy. Acta Obstet Gynecol Scand 75:593–595
82. McCluggage WG, Ashe P, McBride H et al (1998) Localization of the cellular expression of inhibin in trophoblastic tissue. Histopathology 32:252–256
83. McCluggage WG, Hamal P, Traub AI, Walsh MY (2000) Uterine adenolipoleiomyoma: a rare hamartomatous lesion. Int J Gynecol Pathol 19:183–185
84. McCluggage WG, Abdulkader M, Price JH et al (2000) Uterine carcinosarcomas in patients receiving tamoxifen: a report of 19 cases. Int J Gynecol Cancer 10:280–284

85. McCluggage WG, Desai V, Manek S (2000) Tamoxifen-associated postmenopausal adenomyosis exhibits stromal fibrosis, glandular dilatation and epithelial metaplasias. Histopathology 37:340–346
86. McCluggage WG, Sumathi VP, Maxwell P (2001) CD10 is a sensitive and diagnostically useful immunohistochemical marker of normal endometrial stroma and of endometrial stromal neoplasms. Histopathology 39:273–278
87. McCluggage WG (2002) Malignant biphasic uterine tumours: carcinosarcomas or metaplastic carcinomas? J Clin Pathol 55:321–325
88. McCluggage WG (2003) Metaplasias in the female genital tract. In: Lowe D, Underwood J (eds) Recent Advances in Histopathology, vol 20. Royal Society of Medicine Press Ltd, London
89. McCluggage WG, Oliva E, Herrington CS et al (2003) CD10 and calretinin staining of endocervical glandular lesions, endocervical stroma and endometrioid adenocarcinomas of the uterine corpus: CD10 positivity is characteristic of, but not specific for, mesonephric lesions and is not specific for endometrial stroma. Histopathology 43:144–150
90. McCluggage WG, Sumathi VP, McManus DT (2003) Uterine serous carcinoma and endometrial intraepithelial carcinoma arising in endometrial polyps: report of 5 cases, including 2 associated with tamoxifen therapy. Hum Pathol 34:939–943
91. McCluggage WG (2006) My approach to the interpretation of endometrial biopsies and curettings. J Clin Pathol 59:801–812
92. McCullough TA, Wagner B, Duffy S et al (1995) The pathology of hysterectomy specimens following transcervical resection of the endometrium. Histopathology 27:541–547
93. McKenna M, McCluggage WG (2008) Signet ring cells of stromal derivation in the uterine cervix secondary to cauterization: report of a previously undescribed phenomenon. J Clin Pathol 61:648–651
94. Machado F, Moreno J, Carazo M et al (2003) Accuracy of endometrial biopsy with the Cornier pipelle for diagnosis of endometrial cancer and atypical hyperplasia. Eur J Gynecol Oncol 24:279–281
95. Marchini M, Fedele L, Bianchi S et al (1992) Endometrial patterns during therapy with danazol or gestrinone for endometriosis- structural and ultrastructural study. Hum Pathol 23:51–56
96. Marshall RJ, Jones DB (1988) An immunohistochemical study of lymphoid ADD in human endometrium. Int J Gynecol Pathol 7:225–235
97. Mazur MT (1981) Atypical polypoid adenomyomas of the endometrium. Am J Surg Pathol 5:473–482
98. Mazur MT, Hendrickson MR, Kempson RL (1983) Optically clear nuclei. An alteration of endometrial epithelium in the presence of trophoblast Am J Surg Pathol 7:415–423
99. Miko TL, Lampe LG, Thomazy VA et al (1988) Eosinophilic endomyometritis associated with diagnostic curettage. Int J Gynecol Pathol 7:162–172
100. Mittal K, Da Costa M (2008) Endometrial hyperplasia and carcinoma in endometrial polyps: clinicopathologic and follow-up findings. Int J Gynecol Pathol 27:45–48
101. Morsi HM, Leers MP, Jager W et al (2000) The patterns of expression of an apoptosis-related CK18 neoepitope, the bcl-2 proto-oncogene, and the Ki67 proliferation marker in normal, hyperplastic, and malignant endometrium. Int J Gynecol Pathol 19:118–126
102. Murray MJ, Meyer WR, Zaino RJ et al (2004) A critical analysis of the accuracy, reproducibility, and clinical utility of histologic endometrial dating in fertile women. Fertil Steril 81:1333–1343
103. Mutter GL, Zaino RJ, Baak JPA et al (2007) Benign endometrial hyperplasia sequence and endometrial intraepithelial neoplasia. Int J Gynecol Pathol 26:103–114
104. Mutter GL, Bergeron C, Deligdish L et al (2008) The spectrum of endometrial pathology induced by progesterone receptor modulators. Mod Pathol 21:591–598
105. Nand SL, Webster MA, Baber R et al (1998) Bleeding pattern and endometrial changes during continuous combined hormone replacement therapy. Obstet Gynecol 91:678–684
106. Nakamura Y, Moritsuka Y, Ohta Y et al (1989) S-100 protein in glands within decidua and cervical glands during early pregnancy. Hum Pathol 20:1204–1209
107. Noyes FW, Hertig AT, Rock J (1950) Dating the endometrial biopsy. Fertil Steril 1:3–25
108. Nucci MR, Prasad CJ, Crum CP, Mutter GL (1999) Mucinous endometrial epithelial proliferations: A morphologic spectrum of changes with diverse clinical significance. Mod Pathol 12:1137–1142
109. Nucci MR, Young RH (2004) Arias-Stella reaction of the endocervix: a report of 18 cases with emphasis on its varied histology and differential diagnosis. Am J Surg Pathol 2004(28):608–612
110. O'Brien PK, Roth-Moyo LA, Davis BA (1981) Pseudo-sulfur granules associated with intrauterine contraceptive devices. Am J Clin Pathol 75:822–825
111. O'Connell JT, Mutter GL, Cviko A et al (2001) Identification of a basal/reserve cell immunophenotype in benign and neoplastic endometrium: a study with the p53 homologue p63. Gynecol Oncol 80:30–36
112. O'Connor DM, Kurman RJ (1988) Intermediate trophoblast in uterine curettings in the diagnosis of ectopic pregnancy. Obstet Gynecol 72:665–670
113. Ohishi Y, Kaku T, Kobayashi H et al (2008) CD10 immunostaining distinguishes atypical polypoid adenomyofibroma (atypical polypoid adenomyoma) from endometrial carcinoma invading the myometrium. Hum Pathol 39:1446–1453
114. Ota S, Catasus L, Matias-Guiu X et al (2003) Molecular pathology of atypical polypoid adenomyoma of the uterus. Hum Pathol 34:784–788
115. Paavonen J, Aine R, Teisala K et al (1985) Chlamydial endometritis. J Clin Pathol 38:726–732
116. Paganini-Hill A, Ross RK, Henderson BE (1989) Endometrial cancer and patterns of oestrogen replacement therapy. Cancer 59:445–447
117. Pearce KF, Nolan TA (1996) Endometrial sarcoidosis as a cause of postmenopausal bleeding. J Reprod Med 41:878–888
118. Perkins MB (1960) Pneumopolycystic endometritis. Am J Obstet Gynecol 80:332–336
119. Phillips V, Graham CT, Manek S, McCluggage WG (2003) The effects of the levonorgestrel intrauterine system (Mirena coil) on endometrial morphology. J Clin Pathol 56:305–307
120. Phillips VP, McCluggage WG (2005) Results of a questionnaire regarding criteria for adequacy of endometrial biopsies. J Clin Pathol 58:417–419
121. Pins MR, Young RH, Crum CP et al (1997) Cervical squamous cell carcinoma in situ with intraepithelial extension to the upper genital tract and invasion of tubes and ovaries: report of a case with human papillomavirus analysis. Int J Gynecol Pathol 16:272–278
122. Pritt B, Mount SL, Cooper K, Blaszyk H (2006) Pseudoactinomycotic radiate granules of the gynaecological tract: review of a diagnostic pitfall. J Clin Pathol 59:17–20
123. Quddus MR, Sung CJ, Zheng W, Lauchlan SC (1999) p53 immunoreactivity in endometrial metaplasia with dysfunctional uterine bleeding. Histopathology 35:44–49
124. Saegusa M, Okayasu I (2001) Frequent nuclear beta-catenin accumulation and associated mutations in endometrioid-type

endometrial and ovarian carcinomas with squamous differentiation. J Pathol 194:59–67
125. Sahin AA, Silva EG, Landon G et al (1989) Endometrial tissue in myometrial vessels not associated with menstruation. Int J Gynecol Pathol 8:139–146
126. Schindler AE, Schmidt G (1980) Postmenopausal bleeding: A study of more than 1000 cases. Maturitas 2:269–274
127. Schlesinger C, Kamoi S, Ascher SM et al (1998) Endometrial polyps: a comparison study of patients receiving tamoxifen with two control groups. Int J Gynecol Pathol 17:302–311
128. Scott M, Lyness RW, McCluggage WG (2006) Atypical reactive proliferation of endocervix: a common lesion associated with endometrial carcinoma and likely related to prior endometrial sampling. Mod Pathol 19:470–474
129. Scurry J, Planner R, Fortune DW, Lee CS, Rode J (1993) Ligneous (pseudomembranous) inflammation of the female genital tract: a report of two cases. J Reprod Med 38:407–412
130. Seidman JD, Kurman RJ (1999) Tamoxifen and the endometrium. Int J Gynecol Pathol 18:293–296
131. Shah SS, Mazur MT (2008) Endometrial eosinophilic syncytial change related to breakdown: immunohistochemical evidence suggests a regressive process. Int J Gynecol Pathol 27:534–538
132. Shapiro S, Kelly JP, Rosenberg L et al (1985) Risk of localized and widespread endometrial cancer in relation to recent and discontinued use of conjugated estrogens. New Eng J Med 313:969–972
133. Shibutani S, Ravindernath A, Suzuki N et al (2000) Identification of tamoxifen-DNA adducts in the endometrium of women treated with tamoxifen. Carcinogenesis 21:1461–1467
134. Silva EG, Jenkins R (1990) Serous carcinoma in endometrial polyps. Mod Pathol 3:120–128
135. Soslow RA, Chung MH, Rouse RV et al (1996) Atypical polypoid adenomyofibroma (APA) versus well-differentiated endometrial carcinoma with prominent stromal matrix: an immunohistochemical study. Int J Gynecol Pathol 15:209–216
136. Staland B (1981) Continuous treatment with natural oestrogens and progestagens. A method to avoid endometrial stimulation. Maturitas 3:145–156
137. Stasny JF, Ben-Ezra J, Stewart JA et al (1995) Condyloma and cervical intraepithelial neoplasia of the endometrium. Gynecol Obstet Invest 39:277–280
138. Stewart CJR, Michie BA, Kennedy JH (1998) Focal endometrial stromal hyperplasia. Histopathology 33:75–79
139. Stewart CJ, Campbell-Brown M, Critchley HO, Farqharson MA (1999) Endometrial apoptosis in patients with dysfunctional uterine bleeding. Histopathology 34:99–105
140. Sturdee DW, Ulrich LG, Barlow DH et al (2000) The endometrial response to sequential and continuous combined oestrogen-progestogen replacement therapy. Br J Obstet Gynaecol 107:1392–1400
141. Tabibzadeh S, Kong Q, Satyaswaroop P et al (1994) Distinct regional and menstrual cycle dependent distribution of apoptosis in human endometrium. Potential regulatory role of T cells and TNF-alpha. Endocrinol J 2:87–95
142. Tahlan A, Nanda A, Mohan H (2006) Uterine adenomyoma: a clinicopathologic review of 26 cases and a review of the literature. Int J Gynecol Pathol 25:361–365
143. Tai LH, Tavassoli FA (2002) Endometrial polyps with atypical (bizarre) stromal cells. Am J Surg Pathol 26:505–509
144. Taketani Y, Masahiko M (1991) Evidence for direct regulation of epidermal growth factor receptors by steroid hormones in human endometrial cells. Human Reprod 6:1365–1369
145. Thomas W Jr, Sadeghieh B, Fresco R et al (1978) Malacoplakia of the endometrium, a probable cause of postmenopausal bleeding. Am J Clin Pathol 69:637–641
146. Truskinovsky AM, Gerscoich EO, Duffield CR, Vogt PJ (2008) Endometrial microcalcifications detected by ultrasonography: clinical associations, histopathology and potential etiology. Int J Gynecol Pathol 27:61–67
147. Turbiner J, Moreno-Bueno G, Dahiya S et al (2008) Clinicopathological and molecular analysis of endometrial carcinoma associated with tamoxifen. Mod Pathol 21:925–936
148. Usubutun A, Karamn N, Ayhan A et al (2005) Atypical endometrial stromal cells related with a polypoid leiomyoma with bizarre nuclei: a case report. Int J Gynecol Pathol 24:352–354
149. Val-Bernal JF, Villoria F, Cagigal ML et al (2006) Pneumopolycstic endometritis. Am J Surg Pathol 30:258–261
150. Vang R, Tavassoli FA (2003) Proliferative mucinous lesions of the endometrium: Analysis of existing criteria for diagnosing carcinoma in biopsies and curettings. Int J Surg Pathol 11:261–270
151. Venkatraman L, Elliott H, Steele EK et al (2003) Serous adenocarcinoma arising in an adenofibroma of the endometrium. Int J Gynecol Pathol 22:194–197
152. Wani Y, Notohara K, Saegusa M et al (2008) Aberrant Cdx2 expression in endometrial lesions with squamous differentiation: important role of Cdx2 in squamous morula formation. Mod Pathol 39:1072–1079
153. Wells M, Tiltman A (1989) Intestinal metaplasia of the endometrium. Histopathology 15:431–433
154. Wheeler DT, Bristow RE, Kurman RJ (2007) Histologic alterations in endometrial hyperplasia and well-differentiated carcinoma treated with progestins. Am J Surg Pathol 31:988–998
155. Winkler B, Reumann W, Mitao M et al (1984) Chlamydia endometritis: a histological and immunohistochemical analysis. Am J Surg Pathol 8:771–778
156. Winter JD, Kohn G, Mellinin WJ et al (1968) A familial syndrome of renal, genital, and middle ear anomalies. J Pediatr 72:88
157. Yokomyama S, Kashima K, Inoue S et al (1993) Biotin-containing intranuclear inclusions in endometrial glands during gestation and puerperium. Am J Clin Pathol 99:13–17
158. Young RH, Harris NL, Scully RE (1985) Lymphoma-like lesions of the lower female genital tract: a report of 16 cases. Int J Gynecol Pathol 4:289–299
159. Young RH, Treger T, Scully RE (1986) Atypical polypoid adenomyoma of the uterus: a report of 27 cases. Am J Clin Pathol 86:139–145
160. Zaloudek CJ, Norris HJ (1991) Adenofibroma and adenosarcoma of the uterus: a clinicopathologic study of 35 cases. Cancer 48:354–366

8 Precursor Lesions of Endometrial Carcinoma

Lora Hedrick Ellenson · Brigitte M. Ronnett · Robert J. Kurman

R. J. Kurman, L. Hedrick Ellenson, B. M. Ronnett (eds.), *Blaustein's Pathology of the Female Genital Tract (6th ed.)*, DOI 10.1007/978-1-4419-0489-8_8,

Endometrial hyperplasia often precedes the development of endometrioid carcinoma, the most common type of endometrial carcinoma. More recently, studies have found that the risk of endometrial hyperplasia is associated with increasing body mass index and nulliparity [24]. In addition, obesity, anovulatory cycles, and exogenous hormones are associated with both endometrioid carcinoma and hyperplasia. All of these factors are thought to result in unopposed estrogen stimulation of the endometrium. The role of unopposed estrogen stimulation in the development of endometrial hyperplasia and carcinoma is further supported by studies demonstrating elevated serum estrogen levels in patients with endometrioid carcinoma [14, 72]. However, other histologic types of endometrial carcinoma appear to be unrelated to hormonal factors and hyperplasia [81]. Serous carcinoma is the prototypic endometrial carcinoma that is not related to estrogenic stimulation or hyperplasia. It usually arises in atrophic endometrium through a precursor lesion called endometrial intraepithelial carcinoma (EIC). Over the past 3 decades, clinicopathologic, immunohistochemical, and molecular genetic studies have provided data to support the development of a dualistic model of endometrial carcinogenesis. In this model, two types of precursor lesions precede the two most common types of endometrial carcinoma. Atypical hyperplasia (AH) is recognized as the precursor for endometrioid carcinoma and endometrial intraepithelial carcinoma (EIC) is recognized as the precursor for serous carcinoma. The following discussion summarizes current knowledge about these precursor lesions including their differential diagnosis, treatment, and relationship to endometrial carcinoma.

Endometrial Hyperplasia

Definition and Classification

In the past, the terms "adenomatous hyperplasia" and "atypical hyperplasia" were used to denote proliferative lesions of the endometrium with varying degrees of architectural complexity and cytologic atypia [15, 32, 37, 70, 93]. In addition, the term "carcinoma in situ" was proposed to describe small lesions, with or without glandular crowding, having the cytologic features of carcinoma but lacking invasion [37, 89, 93]. Carcinoma in situ was never clearly defined and therefore the term was abandoned. In retrospect, many of these lesions would be classified today as hyperplasia with eosinophilic change. Recently, the term has been applied to an entirely different lesion (see below), adding further confusion [64]. In this chapter, we will utilize the World Health Organization (WHO) classification [77], which does not recognize carcinoma in situ as a diagnostic term.

In summary, pathologists have recognized for decades that endometrial cancer precursors are morphologically and biologically heterogeneous. However, early studies designed to clarify the significance of these lesions were limited by the lack of standardized diagnostic criteria, failure to consider cytologic and architectural features separately, and inclusion of irradiated patients, which may have altered the natural history of the lesions studied [12, 17, 32, 37, 93]. Many of these limitations have been addressed in more recent studies (see "Behavior of Hyperplasia"). However, as will be discussed below, there remain significant issues in diagnostic reproducibility.

Endometrial hyperplasia is defined as a proliferation of glands of irregular size and shape with an associated increase in the gland/stroma ratio compared with proliferative endometrium. Although the process is often diffuse, it may also be focal. The World Health Organization (WHO) classification, presently the most widely used, is a four-tier classification system that takes into account both cytologic and architectural abnormalities [77]. Over the years, studies have raised doubts about the clinical significance of the architectural categories in this classification system and have suggested that endometrial hyperplasia could be simply subdivided into two broad categories: hyperplasia without cytologic atypia and hyperplasia with cytologic atypia (atypical hyperplasia) (Table 8.1). The rationale for this classification is based on the natural history of the disease as shown in long-term follow-up studies [8, 26, 49]. In one natural history study, fewer than 2% of hyperplasias without cytologic atypia progressed to carcinoma, whereas 23% of hyperplasias with cytologic atypia (atypical hyperplasia) progressed to carcinoma. In addition, a more recent epidemiologic study added further support for this simplified classification by showing that the only lesion that significantly increased the relative risk of carcinoma was atypical hyperplasia [53]. In that study, non-atypical hyperplasia (both

Table 8.1
Classification of endometrial hyperplasia

Hyperplasia without atypia
Simple hyperplasia without atypia
Complex hyperplasia without atypia
Atypical hyperplasia
Simple atypical hyperplasia (very rare)
Complex atypical hyperplasia

simple and complex) had a 10% chance of progression whereas atypical hyperplasia (both simple and complex) had a 40% chance of progression to carcinoma. Thus, the presence of cytologic atypia appears to be the main characteristic of hyperplasia that determines the risk of progression. Although increasing degrees of glandular complexity and crowding (architectural abnormalities) show a trend in increasing the likelihood of progression to carcinoma, these features are not statistically significant. Thus for practical purposes, it is reasonable to classify noninvasive proliferative lesions of the endometrium as either hyperplasia without atypia or atypical hyperplasia.

Clinical Features

Patients with endometrial hyperplasia typically have abnormal bleeding. Occasionally, the lesion is detected fortuitously by endometrial biopsy performed during the course of an infertility workup or before the start of hormone replacement therapy in postmenopausal women. Hyperplasia develops as a result of unopposed estrogenic stimulation, and consequently most patients with hyperplasia have a history of either persistent anovulation or exogenous unopposed estrogen usage. Although anovulation occurs at menarche and in perimenopausal women, hyperplasia is not usually encountered in young women. This may be because bleeding in menarchial women is seldom evaluated by an endometrial biopsy, although hyperplasia has been reported in a patient at 16 years of age [55]. During the reproductive years, hyperplasia is relatively uncommon, typically occurring in women with polycystic ovarian disease (Stein–Leventhal syndrome). In the original description of this syndrome, these women were reported to be anovulatory, obese, infertile, and exhibit hirsutism, but many women with this disorder lack these features. Conversely, women who are obese but who do not have polycystic ovarian disease may have hyperplasia, presumably as a result of peripheral conversion of androstenedione to estrogen in adipose tissue.

Diabetes mellitus and hypertension may occur in women with hyperplasia, but often these disorders are not present. Although hyperplasia or carcinoma should always be suspected in a postmenopausal woman with abnormal uterine bleeding, atrophy is the most common cause of bleeding in this age group. In one study of postmenopausal women with bleeding, 7% had endometrial cancer, 15% had various types of hyperplasia, and 56% had atrophy [58]. Typically, women with hyperplasia or carcinoma have moderate or heavy vaginal bleeding compared with women with atrophic endometria who present with spotting.

Pathologic Findings

Hyperplastic endometrium is not distinctive grossly. In hysterectomy specimens, hyperplasia may have a velvety, knobby surface of pale, spongy tissue with vague borders. Although diffuse thickening of the endometrium is common, hyperplasia can be focal and may simulate a polyp. The volume of tissue obtained in curettings is usually increased, but it may be quite variable and less than that obtained during the secretory phase of the normal cycle. A diagnosis of hyperplasia, therefore, depends on the histologic pattern and not on the volume of tissue.

Hyperplasia Without Cytologic Atypia

Hyperplasia is characterized by an increased gland/stroma ratio and a variety of abnormal architectural patterns. Glands typically vary in size and shape. Dilatation and outpouching of glandular epithelium characterize the lesser degrees of architectural abnormalities. In simple hyperplasia, the glands are cystically dilated, with occasional outpouchings surrounded by abundant cellular stroma (➲ *Fig. 8.1*). In other instances, the glands are only minimally dilated but focally crowded (➲ *Fig. 8.2*). Admixtures of the various patterns frequently occur (➲ *Fig. 8.3*). The cells lining the glands are stratified and

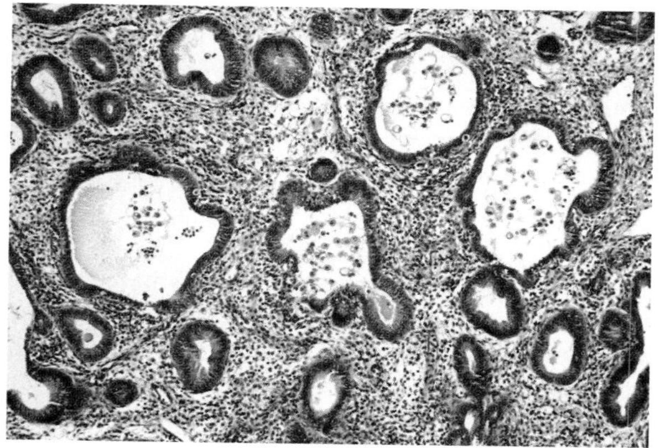

Fig. 8.1
Simple hyperplasia (without atypia). **Glands are only minimally crowded but are dilated and have outpouchings**

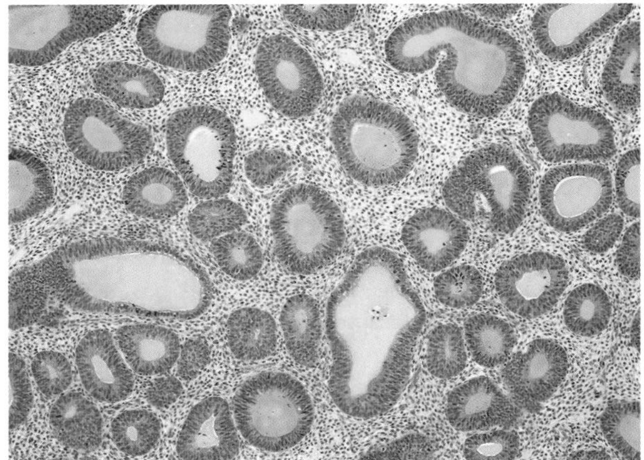

◘ Fig. 8.2
Simple hyperplasia (without atypia). **Glands are mildly crowded and some are cystically dilated**

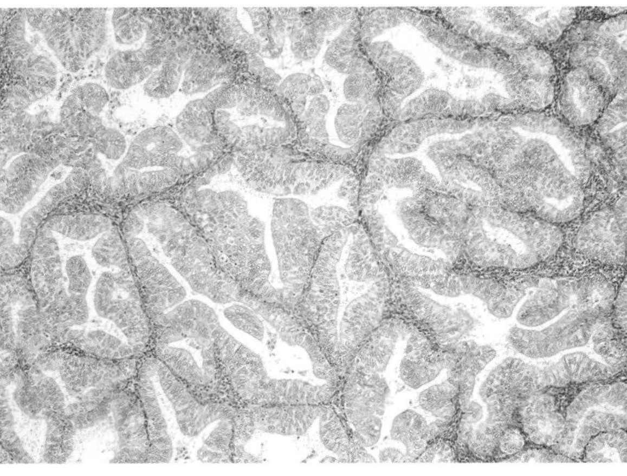

◘ Fig. 8.4
Complex atypical hyperplasia (AH). **Glands with complex profiles and papillary infoldings are crowded in a back-to-back fashion, compressing intervening normal endometrial stroma**

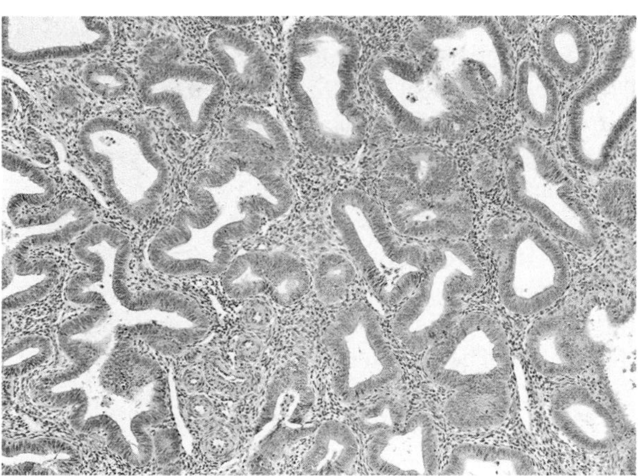

◘ Fig. 8.3
Simple hyperplasia (without atypia). **Glands are mildly crowded and dilated, with some exhibiting outpouchings and simple branching**

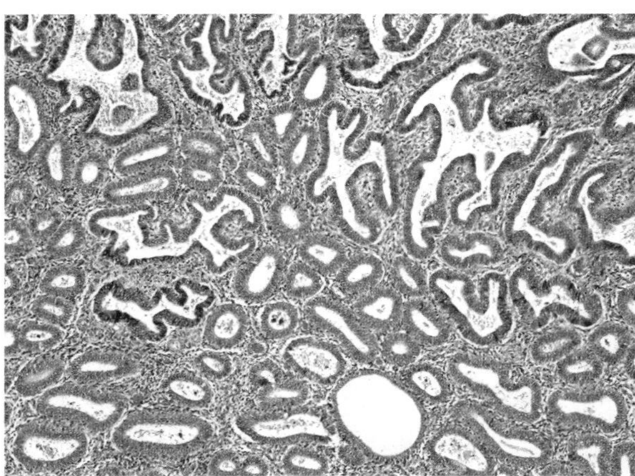

◘ Fig. 8.5
Complex hyperplasia (without atypia). **Branching and tubular glands are sufficiently crowded for classification as complex hyperplasia, despite the presence of some glands with simple tubular profiles**

columnar with amphophilic cytoplasm. Mitotic activity is variable. With increasing degrees of architectural abnormality, glands become complex and branched with irregular outlines and papillary infoldings into the lumens. In addition, with increased proliferation glands become crowded, compressing the intervening stroma, resulting in "back-to-back" glandular crowding. Thus, complex hyperplasia is composed of crowded glands with little intervening stroma [49] (➲ *Figs. 8.4–8.7*). Usually the glandular outlines are highly complex (➲ *Fig. 8.4*) but at times are tubular, with or without dilatation (➲ *Figs. 8.6* and ➲ *8.7*). Epithelial stratification can range from two to four layers, but some glands may exhibit little or no stratification. Mitotic activity is variable and is usually less than five mitotic figures per 10 high-power fields. Even in highly complex hyperplasia with marked stratification, mitotic figures may be

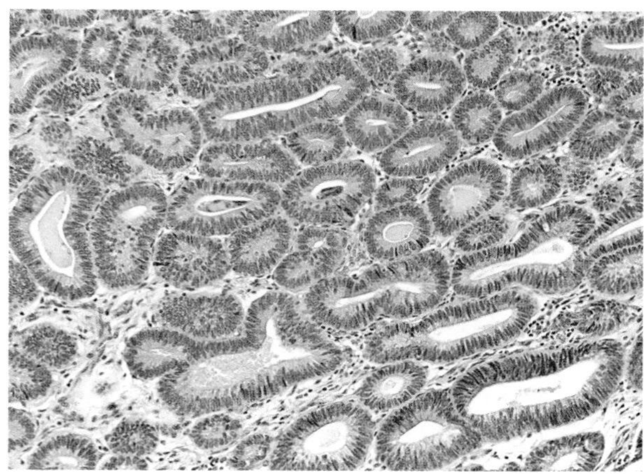

Fig. 8.6
Complex hyperplasia (without atypia). **Glands are sufficiently crowded for classification as complex hyperplasia, despite the presence of glands having only simple tubular profiles**

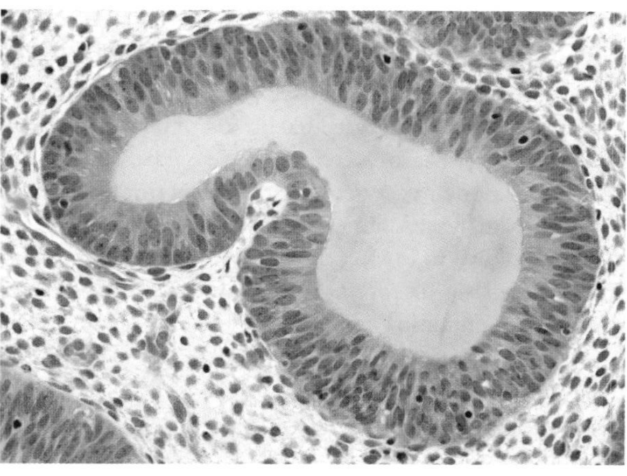

Fig. 8.8
Simple hyperplasia (without atypia). **Nuclei are elongated, oriented perpendicular to the basement membrane, and have even chromatin**

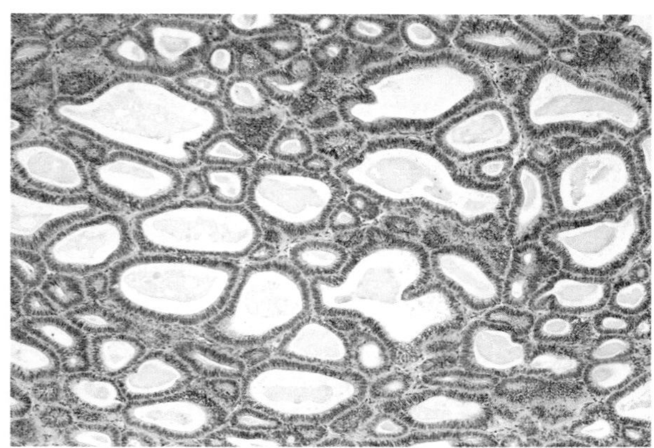

Fig. 8.7
Complex hyperplasia (without atypia). **Dilated glands resemble those seen in simple hyperplasia but are sufficiently crowded for classification as complex hyperplasia**

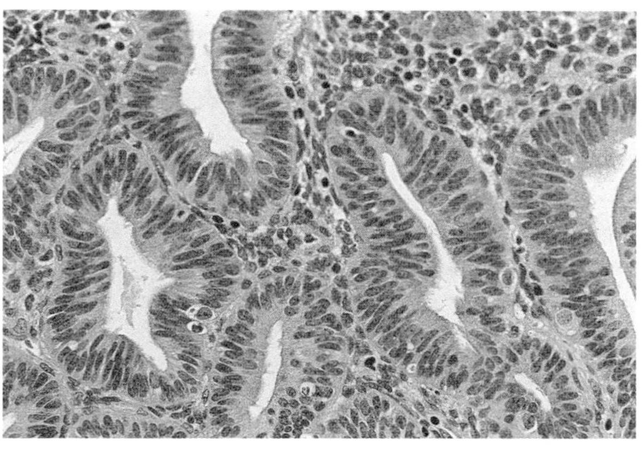

Fig. 8.9
Complex hyperplasia (without atypia). **Nuclei are elongated, oriented perpendicular to the basement membrane, and have even chromatin**

inconspicuous. In hyperplasia lacking atypia the epithelial cells contain oval, basally oriented bland nuclei with smooth, uniform contours resembling those in normal proliferative glands (*Figs. 8.8–8.11*). In simple hyperplasia, the stromal cells are more densely packed than in proliferative endometrium. The cells retain their spindle shape but are plump, with enlarged nuclei and indistinct cytoplasm. Mitotic activity in endometrial stromal cells is variable but may be increased. In complex hyperplasia, the stromal cells are spindle shaped and compressed by the glandular proliferation. In addition to densely packed stromal cells, clusters of foamy, lipid-laden cells may be present in the stroma of simple and complex hyperplasias, atypical hyperplasias, and well-differentiated adenocarcinomas [19, 83]. Foam cells have small pyknotic nuclei and cytoplasm that contain lipid droplets but no mucin. The foam cells have been shown to be histiocytes by immunohistochemistry [83]. These histiocytic cells may also be observed in atrophic and nonneoplastic endometria. The isolated finding of histiocytes in cervicovaginal smears of asymptomatic postmenopausal women has not been associated with an increased likelihood of detecting endometrial hyperplasia or carcinoma [33]. The presence of histiocytes alone in cervicovaginal smears from postmenopausal women with abnormal uterine bleeding also has not been shown to predict the presence of either endometrial hyperplasia or carcinoma. However, the finding of histiocytes containing phagocytosed acute inflammatory cells or normal endometrial cells in postmenopausal women with abnormal uterine bleeding has been associated with a three- to fourfold greater likelihood of coexistent endometrial carcinoma or hyperplasia [68].

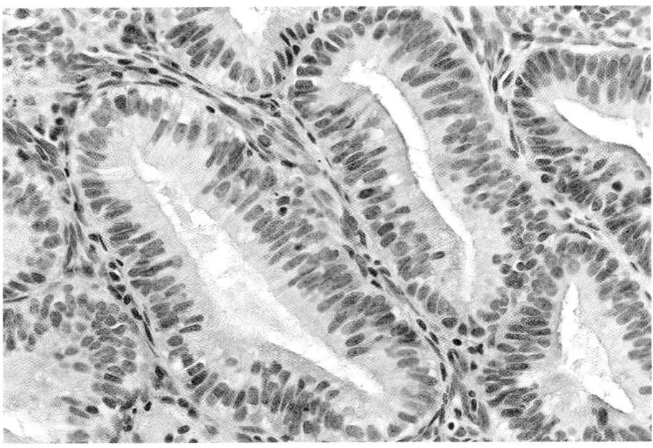

Fig. 8.10
Complex hyperplasia (without atypia). **Nuclei are elongated, oriented perpendicular to the basement membrane, and are evenly hyperchromatic**

Atypical Hyperplasia

The most important feature in the evaluation of endometrial hyperplasia is the presence or absence of nuclear atypia. Cells with nuclear atypia are stratified and show loss of polarity and an increase in the nuclear/cytoplasmic ratio (*Figs. 8.12–8.16*). The nuclei are enlarged, irregular in size and shape, with coarse chromatin clumping, a thickened irregular nuclear membrane, and prominent nucleoli. Nuclei tend to be round as compared with the oval nuclei of proliferative endometrium and hyperplasia without atypia. As a result, the nuclei often have a cleared or vesicular appearance with condensation of the chromatin around the nuclear membrane. Nuclear atypia is variable, both qualitatively and quantitatively. Not all glands contain atypical cells, and in an individual gland some cells are atypical and others are not. Rare atypical cells should be ignored, but if cellular atypia is evident without a diligent search, the diagnosis of atypical hyperplasia should be made. One of the main issues facing diagnostic surgical pathologists is the intra- and interobserver variability in the identification of atypia. Thus, grading atypia as mild, moderate, or severe is not recommended, as it is subjective and not reproducible. Furthermore, assessment of atypia is often problematic

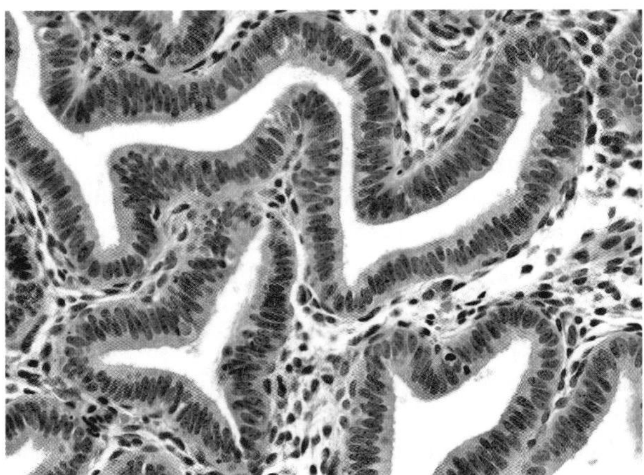

Fig. 8.11
Complex hyperplasia (without atypia). **Nuclei are elongated, oriented perpendicular to the basement membrane, and are evenly hyperchromatic**

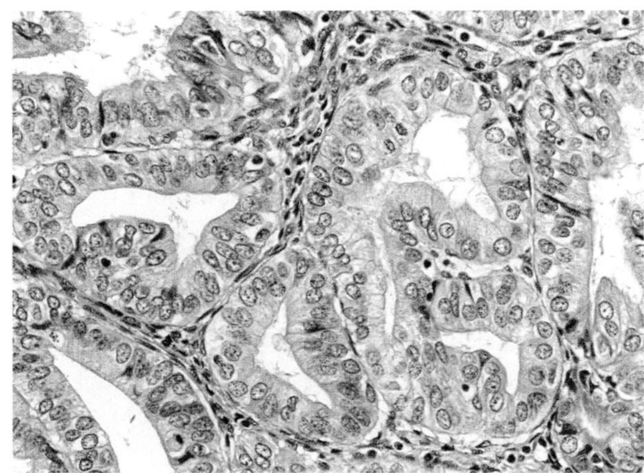

Fig. 8.12
Complex atypical hyperplasia. **Nuclei are rounded and have vesicular chromatin**

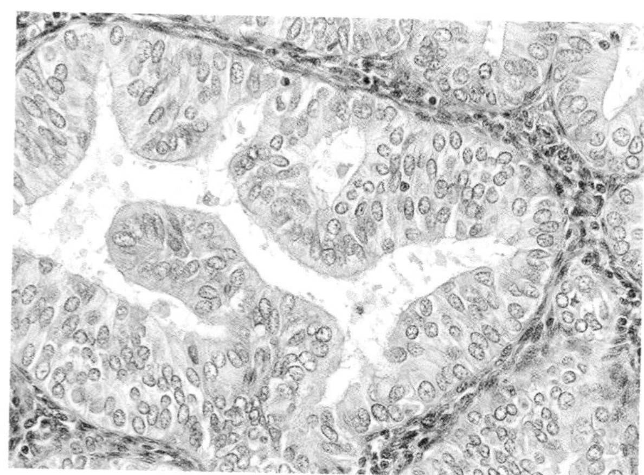

■ Fig. 8.13
Complex atypical hyperplasia. **Nuclei are rounded, have vesicular chromatin, and display stratification and loss of polarity**

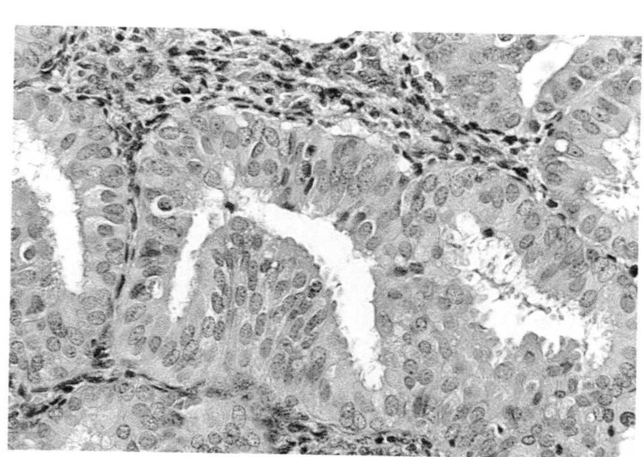

■ Fig. 8.14
Complex atypical hyperplasia. **Nuclei are enlarged and rounded, have vesicular chromatin with fine granularity, and display stratification and loss of polarity**

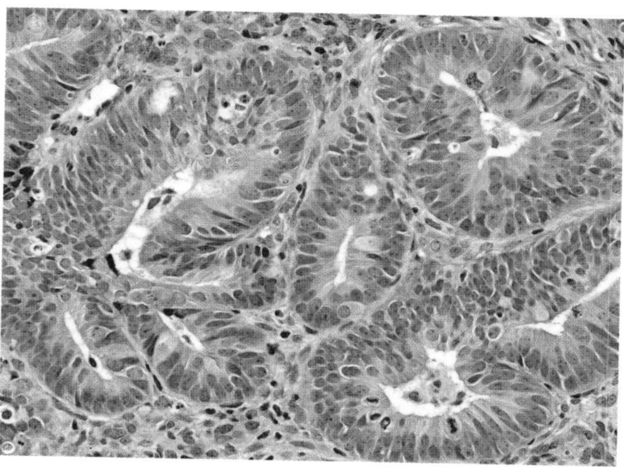

■ Fig. 8.15
Complex atypical hyperplasia. **Nuclei vary from ovoid to rounded, have even chromatin with evident nucleoli and mitotic figures, and display some stratification and loss of polarity**

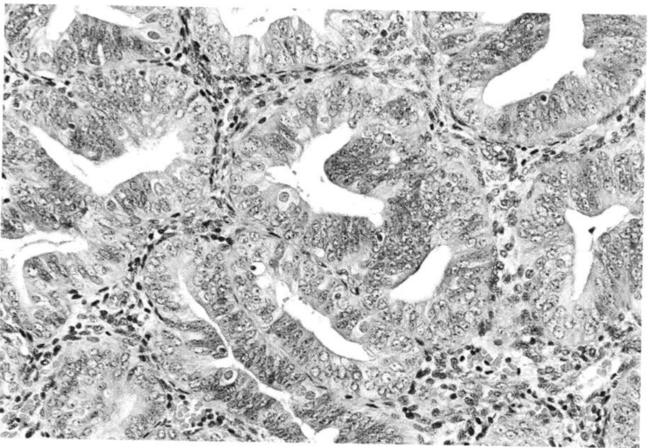

■ Fig. 8.16
Complex atypical hyperplasia. **Nuclei are enlarged and rounded, have vesicular chromatin with fine granularity and evident nucleoli, and display stratification and loss of polarity**

in the setting of metaplasias (see below). The nuclear enlargement, rounding and vesicular change seen in tubal metaplasia, for example, can suggest cytologic atypia, but this metaplastic change is not interpreted as true atypia as it has not been shown to affect clinical outcome [35]. Moreover, metaplasia and atypia can occur together in the same glands, so if the nuclear changes are present in cells that are not metaplastic a diagnosis of atypical hyperplasia can be made even in the setting of metaplasia (➔ *Fig. 8.17*).

The architectural features of simple atypical and complex atypical hyperplasia are similar to their counterparts without cytologic atypia. The glandular outlines in simple atypical hyperplasia may show minimal complexity or they may be more irregular with intraglandular tufting. The glands are separated by abundant stroma; back-to-back crowding is absent. In complex atypical hyperplasia, the glands almost invariably demonstrate marked structural complexity with irregular outlines and back-to-back

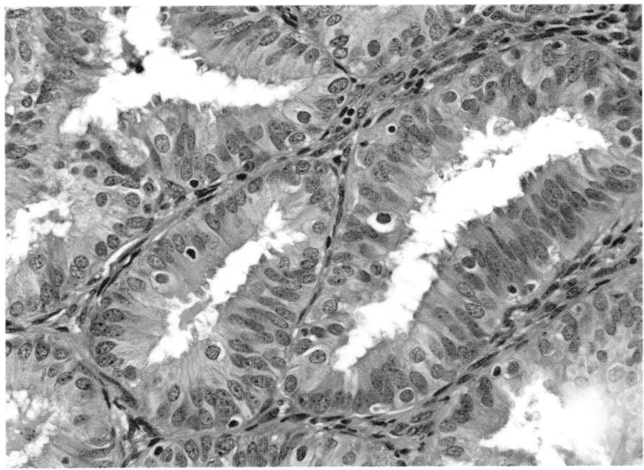

Fig. 8.17
Complex hyperplasia with tubal metaplasia and atypia. **Nuclei vary from ovoid to rounded, have finely granular chromatin, and display some stratification and loss of polarity. Ciliated cells are present, indicating tubal metaplasia. Some nuclear changes are related to the tubal metaplasia but the loss of polarity and stratification are beyond those attributable to metaplasia (compare with *Figs. 8.39* and *8.40*)**

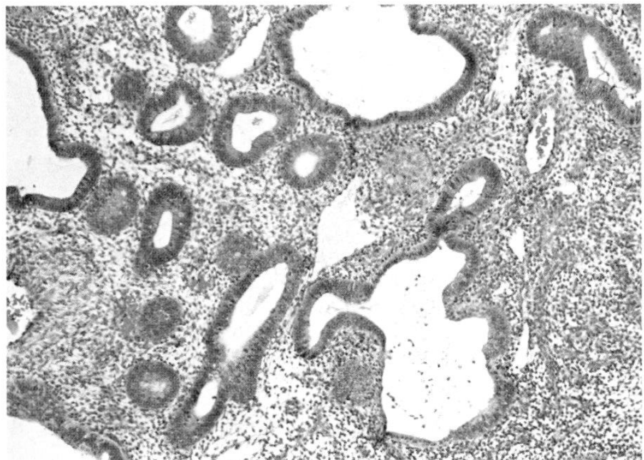

Fig. 8.18
Disordered proliferative endometrium. **Cystically dilated glands with outpouchings are admixed with small tubular proliferative glands**

crowding (*Fig. 8.4*). Epithelial stratification and mitotic activity are variable. Papillary infoldings also are seen. Some atypical hyperplasias have little stratification, and mitotic activity may be inconspicuous. Since simple atypical hyperplasia is exceedingly rare, recent studies have included it in the category with complex atypical hyperplasia.

Differential Diagnosis

Simple and complex hyperplasia should be distinguished from disordered proliferative phase, polyps, ciliated cell change (tubal metaplasia), cystic atrophy, and endometrial glandular and stromal breakdown. Disordered proliferative phase is similar qualitatively to simple hyperplasia but is a focal lesion characterized by irregularly shaped and enlarged glands that are interspersed among normal proliferative glands (*Fig. 8.18*). The latter may be focally crowded. The key feature that distinguishes disordered proliferative phase from simple hyperplasia is the focal nature of the glandular abnormality in disordered proliferative phase. The fragments of endometrium containing the disordered glands should not have the appearance of a polyp. Hyperplastic endometrial polyps often contain areas of simple and complex hyperplasia that are confined to one or just a few fragments of polypoid tissue. The polyp usually stands out as a large rounded tissue fragment in sharp contrast to the remainder of the uninvolved endometrium. Polyps typically have dense fibrous stroma and contain clusters of thick-walled blood vessels near the center of the fragment. The fragments usually are covered on three sides by surface endometrium (see Chap. 7, Benign Diseases of the Endometrium).

Endometrial glands with ciliated cell change are often found in association with simple and complex hyperplasia. When found with hyperplasia, the presence of ciliated cell change does not need to be specified. Ciliated glands are usually slightly dilated. When a few isolated glands show ciliated cell change in the absence of hyperplasia, a diagnosis of ciliated cell change (tubal metaplasia) is justified (see following). Ciliated cell change often contains scattered vesicular nuclei with occasional nucleoli that should not be mistaken as cytologic atypia when found in association with hyperplasia.

Distinction of cystic atrophy from simple hyperplasia is seldom a problem in curettings because atrophic glands collapse as a result of the procedure. In hysterectomy specimens, glands are dilated and lined by a single layer of cells that are often flattened. Mitotic activity is not present. In contrast, in simple hyperplasia there is pseudo-stratification of columnar epithelial cells. Mitotic activity is variable but present.

In endometrial glandular and stromal breakdown caused by estrogen withdrawal, proliferative-type glands appear back-to-back because of loss of intervening endometrial stroma. Glands are often fragmented, and apoptotic bodies are present. Clusters of stromal cells and fragmented glands surrounded by blood are consistent features (see ➑ Chap. 7, Benign Diseases of the Endometrium). In contrast, in complex hyperplasia the glandular outlines are more irregular and complex than the tubular, proliferative-type glands in breakdown. Furthermore, glandular fragmentation, apoptotic bodies, and rounded clusters of stromal cells, so-called stromal blue balls, are usually absent in hyperplasia. In addition, the tissue fragmentation and artifactual apposition of segments of surface epithelium encountered in biopsy and curettage specimens can complicate interpretation and should be considered prior to rendering a diagnosis of hyperplasia (➑ *Fig. 8.19*).

Atypical hyperplasia must be distinguished from an atypical polypoid adenomyoma and from well-differentiated adenocarcinoma. The atypical polypoid adenomyoma is composed of glands that show variable architectural complexity and some cytologic atypia (➑ *Fig. 8.20*). Squamous differentiation in the form of squamous morules is an almost constant feature of the atypical polypoid adenomyoma. Characteristically, the glands in the atypical polypoid adenomyoma are surrounded by smooth muscle, in contrast with the dense proliferative stroma found in hyperplasia and the altered or desmoplastic stroma found in association with well-differentiated carcinoma.

Most endometrial carcinomas are readily identified. However, several recent studies highlight the difficulty in distinguishing some cases of well-differentiated carcinoma from atypical hyperplasia on preoperative endometrial sampling by either biopsy or curettage. Specific histologic features can often be used to separate hyperplasia from well-differentiated carcinoma that reduce the subjectivity of the evaluation. In the presence of invasion the endometrial stroma interacts directly with malignant cells, and the morphologic changes it undergoes can serve as a means of identifying carcinoma. The stromal and epithelial alterations associated with invasive carcinoma are referred to collectively as endometrial stromal invasion. There are three useful criteria, any of which identifies stromal invasion: (1) an irregular infiltration of glands associated with an altered fibroblastic stroma (desmoplastic response); (2) a confluent glandular pattern in which individual glands, uninterrupted by stroma merge, at times creating a cribriform pattern; and (3) an extensive papillary pattern. It should be noted that on occasion complex hyperplasias can display a papillary architecture, including the presence of fibrovascular cores, but in contrast to the papillary pattern of carcinoma, complex hyperplasia is characterized by bland cytology, absence of epithelial stratification, and a low level of mitotic activity [56]. It has been reported that a process manifesting the features of invasion must be sufficiently extensive to involve half (2.1 mm) of a low-power field 4.2 mm in diameter to have value in predicting the

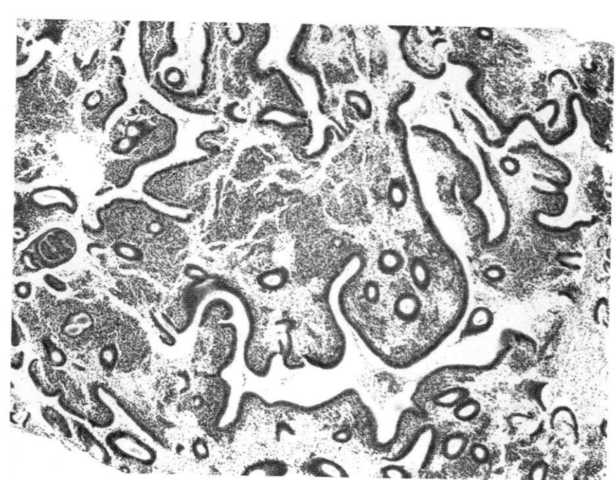

Fig. 8.19
Artifactual glandular crowding. **Apposition of surface epithelium of fragments of proliferative endometrium simulates the cystically dilated glands of simple hyperplasia but is an artifact**

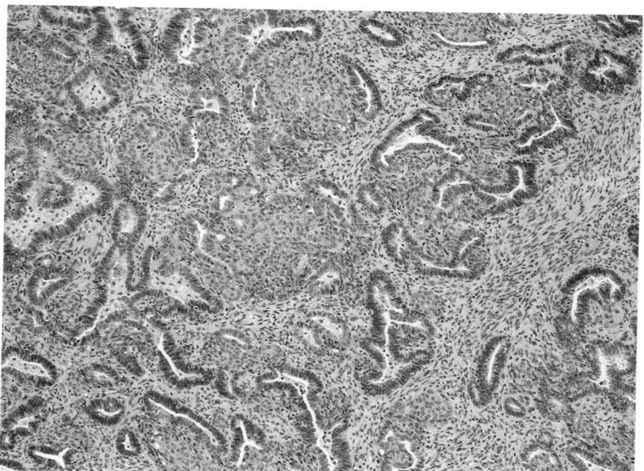

Fig. 8.20
Atypical polypoid adenomyoma. **Crowded complex glands with squamous morules are surrounded by a fibromuscular stroma**

presence of a biologically significant carcinoma in the uterus [50, 69]. This criterion, however, should not be applied too rigidly in view of the potential of missing a carcinoma in small samples. If unequivocal evidence of stromal invasion is present in an area measuring less than one half of a low-power field, a diagnosis of well-differentiated carcinoma should be made (➲ *Figs. 8.21* and ➲ *8.22*). The quantification criterion does not apply to moderately or poorly differentiated carcinomas. The three criteria for the identification of stromal invasion are described in greater detail below.

1. The altered stroma that reflects invasion contains parallel, densely arranged fibroblasts with more fibrosis than normal endometrial stroma, that disrupts the usual glandular pattern (➲ *Fig. 8.23*). The stromal cells are more spindle shaped than are the stromal cells of proliferative endometrium, with more elongated nuclei. Collagen compresses the stromal cells so that they have an eosinophilic and wavy appearance (➲ *Fig. 8.24*), compared with the basophilic naked-nucleus appearance of stromal cells found in proliferative endometrium and hyperplasia. In specimens containing fragments of polyps with fibrous stroma, or specimens from the lower uterine segment, these features cannot be applied. The distinction of hyperplasia from carcinoma in these cases is based on the identification of a confluent pattern (see below). Atypical polypoid adenomyomas (see ➲ Chap. 7, Benign Diseases of the Endometrium) contain smooth muscle and may simulate myometrial invasion (see ➲ *Fig. 8.20*) [62]. In contrast with the atypical polypoid adenomyoma, smooth muscle is rarely identified in curettings of well-differentiated carcinoma even

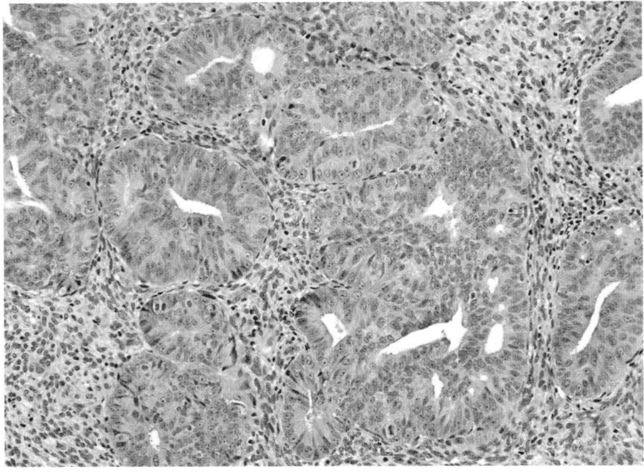

Fig. 8.22
Complex atypical hyperplasia with foci of well-differentiated endometrioid carcinoma. **Small aggregates of glands demonstrate gland fusion and early cribriform growth**

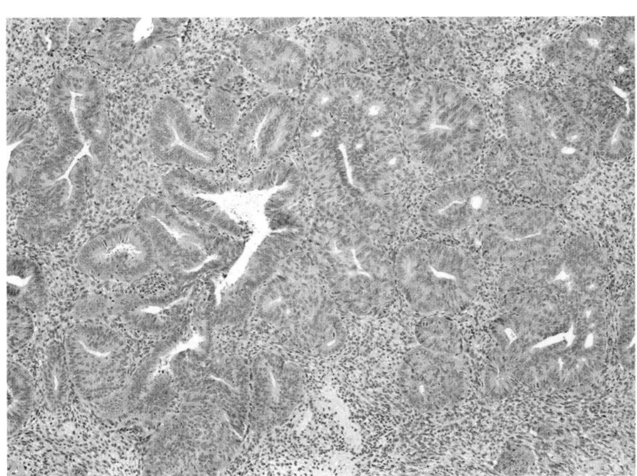

Fig. 8.21
Complex atypical hyperplasia with foci of well-differentiated endometrioid carcinoma. **Small aggregates of fused glands consistent with early endometrioid carcinoma are architecturally distinct from the individual larger glands of associated complex atypical hyperplasia**

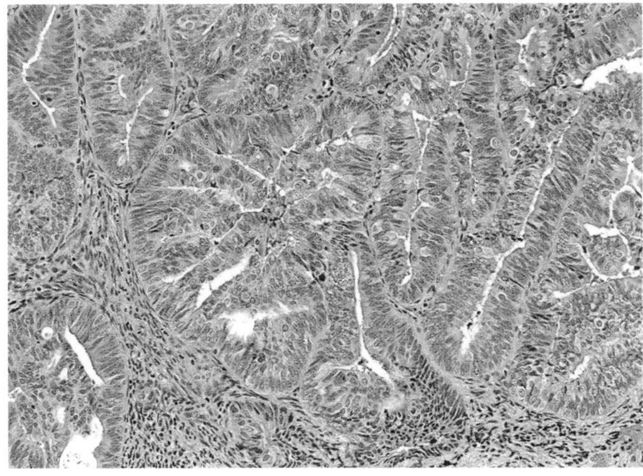

Fig. 8.23
Well-differentiated endometrioid carcinoma. **Crowded atypical glands with early glandular confluence are surrounded by eosinophilic spindled stromal cells, which constitute a desmoplastic stromal reaction, indicating stromal invasion by carcinoma**

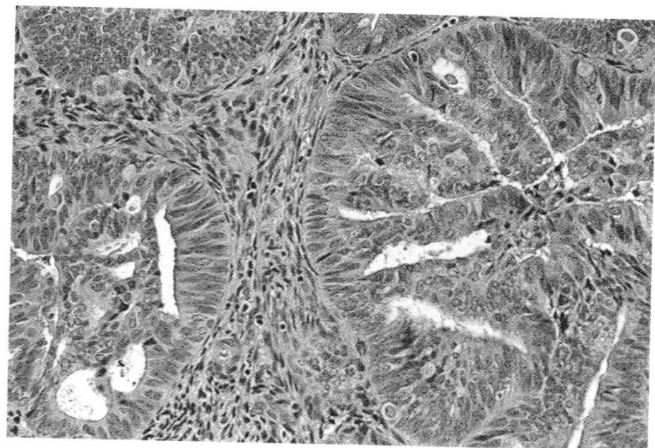

Fig. 8.24
Well-differentiated endometrioid carcinoma. **Stromal desmoplasia, a manifestation of endometrial stromal invasion by endometrioid carcinoma, is characterized by spindled cells with a fibroblastic appearance**

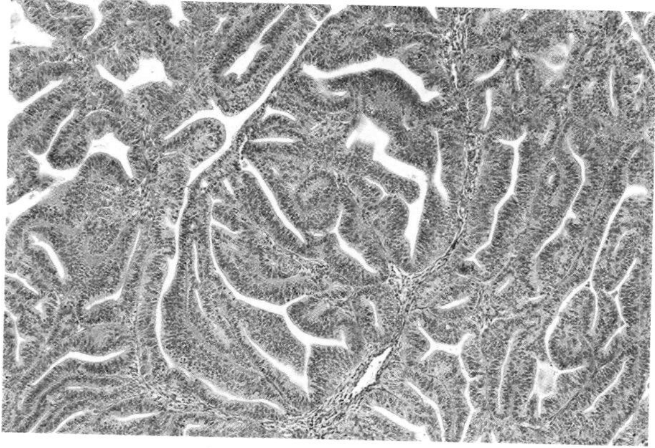

Fig. 8.26
Well-differentiated endometrioid carcinoma. **Complex branching glands creating a confluent glandular/labyrinthine pattern and altered (desmoplastic) stroma indicate endometrial stromal invasion by carcinoma**

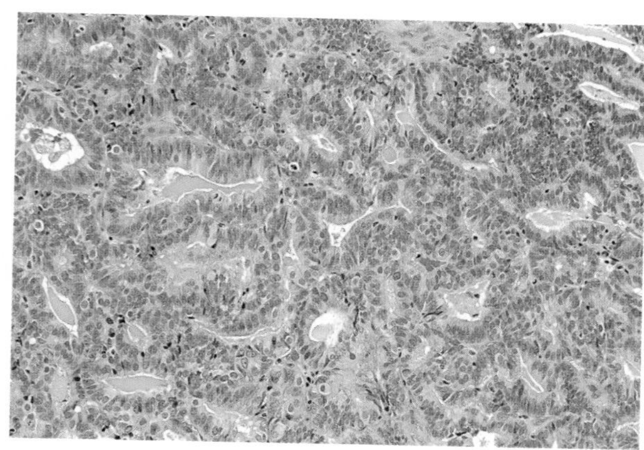

Fig. 8.25
Well-differentiated endometrioid carcinoma. **Glands are fused and interconnected in a confluent glandular pattern, without intervening stroma, indicating endometrial stromal invasion by carcinoma**

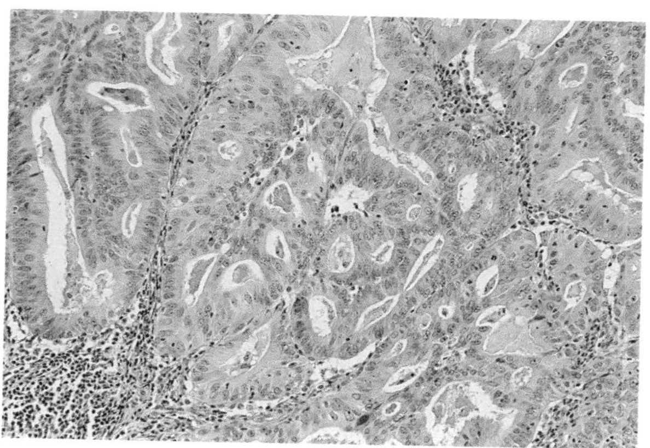

Fig. 8.27
Well-differentiated endometrioid carcinoma. **Fused glands creating a cribriform pattern indicate endometrial stromal invasion by carcinoma**

when there is deep myometrial invasion because only the exophytic portion of the tumor is removed in biopsies and curettings.

2. Confluent glandular aggregates without intervening stroma reflect stromal invasion (*Figs. 8.25* and *8.26*). Confluent patterns are characterized by glandular configurations in which individual glands are not surrounded by stroma. Instead, glands appear to merge into one another to form a complex labyrinth. Some proliferations are cribriform, resulting from proliferation and bridging of epithelium (*Fig. 8.27*).
3. Complex papillary patterns represent stromal invasion if multiple, branching, fibrous processes lined by epithelium are present (*Figs. 8.28* and *8.29*). Often, these papillary structures create a villoglandular pattern. Intraglandular epithelial papillations lacking a fibrovascular core do not qualify as a feature of invasion; such proliferation is often encountered in eosinophilic metaplasia within complex hyperplasia

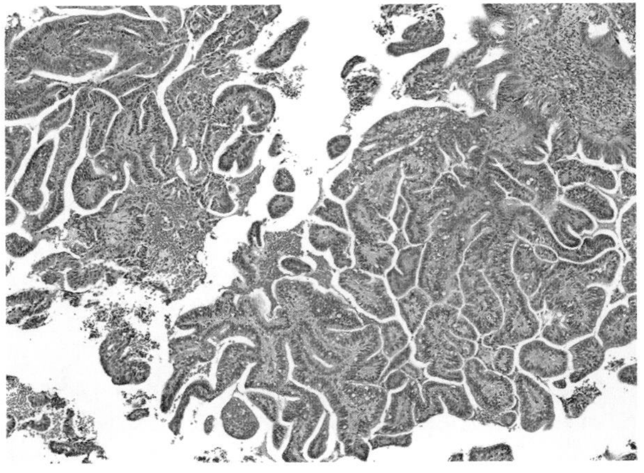

◘ Fig. 8.28
Well-differentiated endometrioid carcinoma. **A papillary/villoglandular proliferation indicates carcinoma when the papillary/villous structures have an exophytic growth pattern and are not merely intraglandular epithelial papillae**

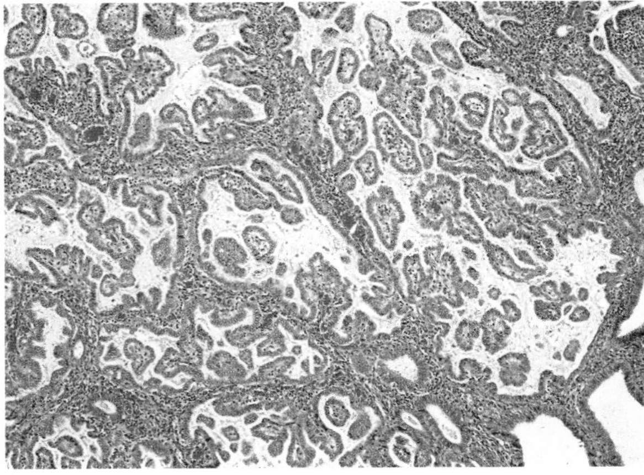

◘ Fig. 8.30
Complex papillary hyperplasia. **Intraglandular papillae reflect a papillary variant of hyperplasia rather than carcinoma (compare with ➲ *Fig. 8.28*)**

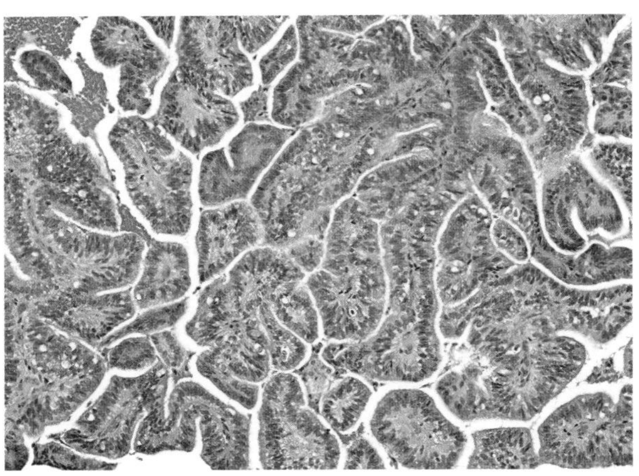

◘ Fig. 8.29
Well-differentiated endometrioid carcinoma. **A papillary/villoglandular pattern indicates carcinoma when the papillary/villous structures are lined by atypical endometrioid epithelium along the external aspect and have a central fibrovascular core**

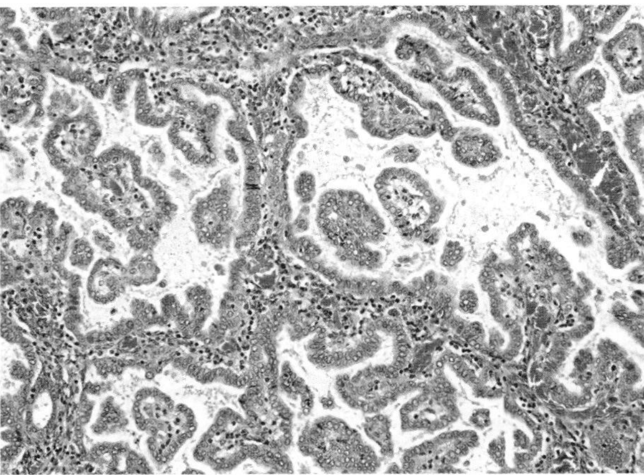

◘ Fig. 8.31
Complex papillary hyperplasia. **Papillae can lack or contain fibrovascular cores; their intraglandular location and absence of atypia indicates a hyperplasia rather than a papillary pattern of carcinoma**

(see below). Delicate papillary structures (with or without fibrovascular cores), often accompanied by metaplastic changes (mucinous, eosinophilic cell) and often occurring in polyps, are a feature of simple and complex papillary hyperplasias (➲ *Figs. 8.30* and ➲ *8.31*) [56]. In these lesions, the cytology is bland and the epithelium overlying the fibrovascular cores is not stratified. The mitotic index and the Ki-67 proliferation index are very low.

In the past, the presence of masses of squamous epithelium replacing the endometrial stroma was considered a feature of invasion [50]. Masses of squamous epithelium with minimal nuclear atypia that extensively replace the

Table 8.2

Hysterectomy findings when atypical hyperplasia[a] is present in curettings (89 patients)

Finding	No. (%)
Carcinoma	15 (17)
Grade	
Well differentiated	15 (100)
Moderately differentiated	0
Poorly differentiated	0
Myometrial invasion	
None	8 (53)[b]
Inner one third	7 (47)[b]
1 mm or less	5
2–4 mm	2

[a]A diagnosis of atypical hyperplasia based on cytological atypia in the absence of endometrial stromal invasion.
[b]The percentages refer to the proportion of carcinomas in the hysterectomy specimen.
Adapted with permission from [50].

Table 8.3

Hysterectomy findings when well-differentiated carcinoma[a] is present in curettings (115 patients)

Finding	No. (%)
Carcinoma	58 (50)
Grade	
Well differentiated	38 (66)[b]
Moderately differentiated	14 (24)[b]
Poorly differentiated	6 (10)[b]
Myometrial invasion	42 (72)[b]
Inner one third	28 (48)[b]
Middle and outer third	14 (24)[b]

[a]A diagnosis of well-differentiated carcinoma based on identification of endometrial stromal invasion.
[b]The percentages refer to the proportion of carcinomas in the hysterectomy specimen.
Adapted with permission from [50].

endometrium (over a 2-mm^2 area) reflect stromal invasion only if they are associated with a desmoplastic response or a confluent glandular pattern.

Increasing degrees of nuclear atypia, mitotic activity, and stratification of cells in curettings are associated with a higher frequency of carcinoma in the uterus but are of limited value because even a mild degree of these changes is associated with carcinoma in nearly one third of cases [56]. Even with mild atypia, low mitotic activity, and lesser degrees of stratification in curettings, 20% of residual carcinomas in the resected uterus are moderately or poorly differentiated, and 10% deeply invade the myometrium. These other features in curettings, although useful, therefore are not sufficiently accurate to predict whether a biologically significant lesion is present in the uterus. Unfortunately, assessing varying degrees of nuclear atypia in this borderline group of lesions is subjective and not easily reproduced. In contrast, when stromal invasion is absent in curettings, carcinoma is found in the uterus in only 17% of cases, and the carcinomas are well differentiated and either confined to the endometrium or only superficially invasive (*Table 8.2*).

If stromal invasion is present in curettings, residual carcinoma is found in the uterus in half; more than one third of the carcinomas are moderately or poorly differentiated, and a fourth of them invade deeply into the myometrium (*Table 8.3*). A small proportion (7%) of patients with invasion in curettings will have extrauterine metastases at hysterectomy, and half with metastasis will die of tumor [50]. Thus, the absence of stromal invasion provides the basis for distinguishing atypical hyperplasia from a biologically significant, well-differentiated carcinoma [46, 50]. A number of more recent studies have found higher frequencies of endometrial carcinoma (43–52%) in hysterectomy specimens following a diagnosis of atypical hyperplasia [39, 92, 96]. Of the carcinomas detected in two of these studies, 43% were stage IC or greater. In the most recent study, only 10.6% were stage IC while 30.9% were stage IB and the remaining were stage IA. These studies included patients who had been diagnosed by either curettage or biopsy, but there were no significant differences in the frequencies with which carcinoma was detected at hysterectomy in those patients who received a curettage compared to those who had been biopsied. However, in one of these studies, the biopsy and curettage specimens were not reviewed to confirm the absence of features of stromal invasion in these specimens [39]. More recently, additional studies have demonstrated that clinically significant endometrial proliferations, that is, those that have a high likelihood of myometrial invasion, can be recognized when either sufficient architectural complexity or nuclear atypia, including prominence of nucleoli, is present [60, 63]. In addition, the strong association of a desmoplastic stromal response with a myoinvasive lesion was confirmed.

The identification of stromal invasion is important because it is semiquantitative, therefore less subjective than other criteria, and it delineates a biologically significant lesion that has a much greater likelihood of metastasis than one in which invasion is absent. Experimental studies of neoplasms from the breast, colon, pancreas, and lung lend support to the division of endometrial proliferations into noninvasive and invasive forms based on the histologic alterations observed in the endometrial stroma. These studies demonstrate profound molecular and structural alterations in the stroma adjacent to invasive as compared with noninvasive tumors. Invasive tumors can induce a conversion of stromal fibroblasts into myofibroblasts, which elaborate extracellular matrix components, such as type V collagen and proteoglycans, which are increased in desmoplasia and are readily observed by light microscopy using the criteria for stromal invasion as outlined. It has been shown that tumor cells produce growth factors such as platelet-derived growth factor, epidermal-derived growth factor, and insulin-like growth factor, which may play a role in stimulating the growth of stromal cells surrounding tumors.

Reproducibility Studies and Adjunctive Techniques in the Classification of Endometrial Hyperplasias

A number of studies have addressed the reproducibility of the diagnosis of endometrial hyperplasia and its distinction from well-differentiated carcinoma [11, 44, 97]. One study of 100 endometrial biopsy and curettage specimens ranging from proliferative endometrium to well-differentiated carcinoma found substantial interobserver agreement for diagnoses of hyperplasia without atypia and well-differentiated carcinoma but only moderate agreement for the diagnosis of atypical hyperplasia [44]. Several histologic features, including nuclear enlargement, vesicular change, nuclear pleomorphism, chromatic irregularities, loss of polarity, nuclear rounding, and presence of nucleoli, were associated with a diagnosis of atypical hyperplasia by univariable logistic regression analysis. However, of the histologic features evaluated, the only feature that was associated with the distinction of atypical hyperplasia from hyperplasia without atypia in multivariable logistic regression analysis was the presence of nucleoli.

The features that were associated with the distinction of carcinoma from atypical hyperplasia in both univariable and multivariable analysis included stromal alteration (stromal desmoplasia) and glandular confluence. A more recent study found similar values for intraobserver agreement and slightly lower values for interobserver agreement [11]. In addition, the study confirmed that the category of atypical hyperplasia has the lowest diagnostic reproducibility of the various categories. Similar histologic features were found to be useful for distinguishing the various diagnostic categories, although the utility of the presence of nucleoli for diagnosing atypical hyperplasia and of stromal alteration for diagnosing well-differentiated carcinoma were somewhat less, as evidenced by lower mean interobserver agreement values for these features. Thus, interobserver agreement is lowest for the diagnostic category of atypical hyperplasia, indicating that further refinement of the histologic criteria, enhanced endometrial sampling techniques, and novel objective analyses are required to improve the reproducibility of the diagnosis of atypical hyperplasia.

Some investigators have attempted to use computerized morphometric analyses of endometrial hyperplasias to predict coexistent carcinoma in hysterectomy specimens [2, 4, 6, 7, 22]. Nuclear morphometry alone has been shown to be insufficiently sensitive and specific to properly distinguish hyperplasias that are associated with carcinoma from those that are not [2, 4]. Although, the combination of architectural and nuclear morphometric features has been shown to be useful for predicting risk of endometrial carcinoma in patients with hyperplasia it has not become widely used because it is labor intensive and too costly to be practical for most laboratories [5–8, 22].

More recently, investigators have proposed that endometrial proliferations be broadly divided into two categories based on the molecular genetic analysis of clonality [65–67]. Proliferations that are polyclonal are regarded as a response to an abnormal hormonal environment – either unopposed estrogenic stimulation associated with anovulatory cycles or exogenous estrogenic stimulation – and are designated "hyperplasia." Monoclonal lesions, on the other hand, are associated with an increased risk of progression to carcinoma and are designated "endometrial intraepithelial neoplasia" (EIN). The rationale cited for this approach is that therapy for hyperplasia should be aimed at treating the suspected cause and symptoms, whereas EIN should be removed or ablated. Since progestin treatment can frequently suppress atypical hyperplasia and well-differentiated endometrioid carcinoma this is not a good reason for adopting the EIN classification. Because clonality cannot routinely be performed on diagnostic specimens in most laboratories, it has been proposed that the diagnosis of EIN be made when glandular crowding results in a volume percentage of stroma less than 55%. Ideally, this parameter would be assessed by morphometric analysis, which has been shown to separate hyperplasias, particularly those classified as non-atypical by light microscopic assessment, into monoclonal and polyclonal lesions [67]. For practicality, routine light microscopic assessment aided by an ocular graticule and a web-based tutorial that correlates patterns of endometrial proliferations with clonality data has been proposed as an alternative to morphometry. However, in a recent nested case-control study the risk of progression to carcinoma was similar after either a diagnosis of EIN or atypical hyperplasia [54]. In addition, the diagnostic reproducibility of the light microscopic assessment of volume percentage stroma has not been adequately determined. Finally, cytologic atypia that allegedly differs from atypia as shown in the WHO classification is required for the diagnosis of EIN and is defined as cytology that differs from normal endometrial glands present in the same sample. Thus, when compared to a simplified version of the WHO classification system that collapses the four categories into two (hyperplasia and atypical hyperplasia) there are no apparent advantages to the use of the EIN system. In the future, molecular genetic data will undoubtedly play a role in the classification of these lesions, but at present since the WHO system is well understood and in widespread use, the proposed hyperplasia–EIN classification system is not recommended for clinical practice.

Molecular Genetics and Immunohistochemistry

Molecular genetic studies are mentioned only briefly here with a more detailed discussion in the chapter on "Endometrial Carcinoma" (see ➲ Chap. 9, Endometrial Carcinoma). There have been a number of molecular genetic alterations identified in atypical endometrial hyperplasia, including microsatellite instability and mutations in the *PTEN* tumor suppressor gene and the *KRAS* oncogene [57]. Of note, these are the most common molecular genetic alterations in endometrioid carcinoma. These findings support clinicopathologic and epidemiologic data indicating that atypical endometrial hyperplasia is the immediate precursor for endometrioid carcinoma. *PTEN* mutations are found at approximately the same frequency in complex atypical hyperplasia and carcinoma and have rarely been described in hyperplasia without atypia [34]. In addition, *KRAS* mutations and microsatellite instability have been reported in complex atypical hyperplasia [23, 25, 57]. Only a relatively small number of hyperplasias without atypia have been analyzed for mutations in *PTEN*, *KRAS*, and for microsatellite instability. Studies suggest that all of these alterations occur before the development of invasion but it is not clear when in the progression of the disease they occur.

Currently, immunohistochemistry does not play a role in the diagnosis of endometrial hyperplasia. Although a number of studies have been done with a wide variety of antibodies, none have been found to have diagnostic utility.

Behavior

Many of the past studies designed to determine the outcome of women with endometrial hyperplasia did not consider cytologic and architectural features separately. This issue was addressed in a retrospective analysis of 170 patients with endometrial hyperplasia on curettings with a mean follow-up of 13.4 years in which hysterectomy was not performed before 1 year after the initial diagnosis. Various histologic features were evaluated, and cytologic and architectural abnormalities were analyzed independently in an effort to delineate the histologic features associated with an increased risk of progression to carcinoma. A third of the patients with both non-atypical and atypical hyperplasia were asymptomatic after the diagnostic curettage and required no further treatment. Only 2 (2%) of 122 patients with hyperplasia lacking cytologic atypia, one with simple and one with complex hyperplasia, progressed to carcinoma. The two cases of simple hyperplasia that progressed to carcinoma first developed atypical hyperplasia. In contrast, 11 (23%) of the 48 women with atypical hyperplasia progressed to carcinoma (➲ *Table 8.4*); 8% of patients with simple atypical hyperplasia and 29% of patients with complex atypical hyperplasia progressed to carcinoma (➲ *Table 8.5*). The presence of glandular complexity and crowding superimposed on atypia, therefore, appears to place the patient at greater risk than does cytologic atypia alone. The differences in progression to carcinoma among the four subgroups, however, were not statistically significant. Similar findings were subsequently reported by other

Table 8.4
Follow-up of hyperplasia and atypical hyperplasia in 170 patients

Type of hyperplasia	No. of patients	Regressed		Persisted		Progressed to carcinoma	
		No.	(%)	No.	(%)	No.	(%)
Hyperplasia	122	97	(80)	23	(19)	2	(2)
Atypical hyperplasia	48	29	(60)	8	(17)	11	(23)

Adapted with permission from [49].

investigators [8, 26]. More recently a nested case-control study of 138 cases diagnosed with endometrial hyperplasia followed by carcinoma at least 1 year later with 241 controls (matched for age, date and follow-up duration, and counter-matched for endometrial hyperplasia diagnosis) showed that women with both simple and complex endometrial hyperplasia without atypia, had a 10% probability of developing carcinoma in contrast to a 40% probability for women with atypical hyperplasia, both simple and complex [53]. These studies show that cytologic atypia is the most useful feature in identifying a lesion that might progress to carcinoma.

The carcinomas that develop in patients with hyperplasia are relatively innocuous [32, 49]. In one study, the mean duration of progression of hyperplasia without atypia to carcinoma is nearly 10 years, and it takes a mean of 4 years to progress from atypical hyperplasia to clinically evident carcinoma [49]. In another study the median interval from atypical hyperplasia to carcinoma was 6.7 years. A comparison of the clinicopathologic features and behavior of the carcinomas developing after a diagnosis of atypical hyperplasia in women at the age of 40 years or younger compared with women over the age of 40 years is shown in Table 8.6. Although all but one of the carcinomas that developed from atypical hyperplasia were well differentiated and minimally invasive, one well-differentiated tumor that extended into the endocervix metastasized to the pelvic peritoneum and a paraaortic lymph node. After abdominal radiation the patient was disease free 19 years later. These findings and others suggest [10] that carcinomas associated with hyperplasia are relatively innocuous compared with carcinomas without associated hyperplasia.

It has been shown that 17–43% of women with atypical hyperplasia in curettings will have a well-differentiated carcinoma in the uterus if a hysterectomy is performed within 1 month of the curettage [46, 89]. Increasing degrees of nuclear atypia, mitotic activity, and stratification of cells in curettings are associated with a higher frequency of carcinoma in the uterus. With long-term follow-up, however, only 11–40% of women with atypical hyperplasia develop carcinoma if a hysterectomy is not done [32, 49]. Thus, the lesion designated as well-differentiated carcinoma usually remains stable for a long period of time. Reasons that may account for the relatively low rate of progression to carcinoma in

Table 8.5

Follow-up of simple and complex hyperplasia and atypical hyperplasia in 170 patients

Type of hyperplasia	No. of patients	Regressed		Persisted		Progressed to carcinoma	
		No.	(%)	No.	(%)	No.	(%)
Simple	93	74	(80)	18	(19)	1	(1)
Complex	29	23	(80)	5	(17)	1	(3)
Simple atypical	13	9	(69)	3	(23)	1	(8)
Complex atypical	35	20	(57)	5	(14)	10	(29)

Adapted with permission from [49].

Table 8.6

Clinical and pathological findings from 11 "untreated" women with progression of atypical hyperplasia to carcinoma

	40 years and younger (8 patients)	Over 40 years (3 patients)
Age range	23–40 years	43–50 years
Polycystic ovarian disease	4 (50%)	0
Obese	4 (50%)	1
Mean time of progression	3.3 years	7.8 years
Grade 1 adenocarcinoma	8 (100%)	2 (66%)
Grade 2 adenocarcinoma	0	1 (33%)
Carcinoma confined to endometrium or superficially invasive	8 (100%)	3 (100%)
Metastatic carcinoma	1[a]	0

[a]Grade 1 adenocarcinoma with squamous differentiation that extended to the endocervix subsequently metastasized to pelvic peritoneum and a paraaortic lymph node. Patient was treated with abdominal radiation and is alive and well 19 years later.
Adapted with permission from [49].

untreated patients with atypical hyperplasia include a general tendency for the highest grade of atypical hyperplasia to be selected for hysterectomy, leaving the lesser degree of atypia for conservative management, and atypical hyperplasia may not be the precursor of all forms of endometrial cancer, but only of a type that is slowly progressive.

A more recent study of the behavior of endometrial hyperplasia found that most cases of endometrial hyperplasia without atypia regressed spontaneously whereas those with complex atypical hyperplasia were much more likely to persist [90]. Another recent study confirmed the significance of cytologic atypia in predicting increased risk of associated endometrial carcinoma in hysterectomy specimens [38]. Because most atypical hyperplasias have complex architecture, it is complex atypical hyperplasia that is associated with a significant risk of persistence and progression to carcinoma. Hence, this lesion is regarded as a direct precursor of well-differentiated endometrioid carcinoma of the endometrium. However, hyperplasia is identified in a prior endometrial specimen or in the hysterectomy specimen in only 35–75% of women with endometrial carcinoma [3, 10, 13, 20, 31, 42]. In those reports that specified the number of hyperplasias that were classified as atypical, 14–36% of women with endometrial carcinoma had associated atypical hyperplasia [31, 42]. It is unclear whether failure to identify an associated atypical hyperplasia in all cases of endometrioid carcinoma reflects overgrowth of a preexisting hyperplasia by carcinoma or the development of carcinoma through a different pathway.

Management

Management of patients with endometrial hyperplasia is based on clinical factors, which include the desire to preserve fertility in young women and associated medical conditions that render older women at high risk for a surgical procedure, and microscopic findings [47].

Premenopausal Women (Less Than 40 Years of Age)

Most premenopausal women who present with abnormal bleeding have nonspecific hormonal disorders that are self-limited. These women are at low risk of having carcinoma (Table 8.7). In a study of 460 women 40 years of age and younger, 6 (1.3%) had "mild" hyperplasia (simple hyperplasia) but none had atypical hyperplasia or carcinoma [43]. Therefore, most women in this age group with abnormal bleeding do not require an endometrial biopsy. Women with risk factors for endometrial cancer, such as polycystic ovarian disease or obesity, and women with persistent bleeding should have an endometrial biopsy performed. Traditionally, evaluation of such patients has been by curettage in the operating room but it

Table 8.7
Pertinent findings in endometrium in women with abnormal bleeding according to age

	Age					
	Premenopausal [43] 40 years (*n* = 5,460)		Perimenopausal [43] 40–55 years (*n* = 5,748)		Postmenopausal [58] 55 years (*n* = 5,226)	
Finding in endometrial specimen[a]	No.	(%)	No.	(%)	No.	(%)
Carcinoma	0	(—)	3	(0.4)	15	(7)
Atypical hyperplasia	0	(—)	5	(0.7)	NK[b]	
Hyperplasia	6	(1)	41	(6).0	34	(15)
Atrophy	7	(2)	51	(7).0	127	(56)
Polyp	6	(1)	13	(2).0	19	(8)
Proliferative	139	(29)	273	(36)	31	(14)
Secretory	241	(50)	287	(38)	0	(—)

[a]Not all the endometrial findings in the study by Kaminski and Stevens are listed and therefore percentages do not total 100%.
[b]A category of atypical hyperplasia was not specified in this study.
NK, not known.

has been shown by some studies that office-based endometrial sampling devices such as the Pipelle device are comparable and are substantially less expensive, with 96% agreement between the biopsy and hysterectomy findings [30, 82, 87].

If a diagnosis of simple or complex hyperplasia is made, the patient can be treated conservatively because these lesions have an extremely low risk (1–2%) of progression to carcinoma. Because the transit time to carcinoma is approximately 10 years and hyperplasia without cytologic atypia first progresses through atypical hyperplasia before becoming carcinoma, follow-up and periodic endometrial biopsies suffice [49]. Conservative management of young women with simple hyperplasia and complex hyperplasia resulted in subsequent pregnancies in 29% and 20% of these women, respectively, in one study (➋ *Table 8.8*) [49].

Women with atypical hyperplasia on an endometrial biopsy who wish to preserve their fertility should be treated with progestin suppression. In view of the very similar accuracy of endometrial biopsy and curettage and the low risk of an associated endometrial carcinoma in women younger than 40 years of age, a curettage need not be performed to exclude carcinoma but close follow-up and periodic endometrial biopsies are necessary. A conservative plan of management is justified because the risk of progression to carcinoma in young women is low and the carcinomas that do develop tend to be innocuous (➋ *Table 8.9*); 20% of those women less than 40 years of age can subsequently become pregnant and have normal deliveries [74]. A recent study of complex hyperplasia with and without atypia found that progestin therapy resulted in regression of complex atypical hyperplasia (➋ *Table 8.10*) but that the majority of complex hyperplasias without atypia regressed with or without progestin therapy [75]. This study also found that higher doses and longer duration of progestin therapy increase the likelihood of regression of complex atypical hyperplasia (➋ *Table 8.11*).

Conservative management also can be considered for women diagnosed with well-differentiated carcinoma. One study of progestin treatment of atypical hyperplasia and well-differentiated carcinoma in women under age 40 found that 75% of women with carcinoma and 95% with atypical hyperplasia had regression of their lesions [74]. In addition, all patients were alive without evidence of progressive disease during the follow-up period. The median duration of progestin treatment necessary to effect regression was 9 months. In another study, 62% of women under the age of 40 years treated with progestins alone for endometrial carcinoma responded to the hormonal therapy, although 23% of these later developed recurrent disease [45]. Ninety percent of the patients were alive without evidence of disease during the follow-up period. The lower frequency of responders in this study may have been a result of the relatively short duration of the hormonal therapy. Thus, in premenopausal women, atypical hyperplasia and well-differentiated carcinoma can be

Table 8.8

Subsequent pregnancies in "untreated" women with hyperplasia and atypical hyperplasia

Diagnosis	No. of patients,40	No. of patients who became pregnant	No. of full-term pregnancies
Simple hyperplasia	35	10 (29%)	19
Complex hyperplasia	15	3 (20%)	4
Atypical hyperplasia (simple and complex)	24	3 (13%)	4

Adapted from [49].

Table 8.9

Hysterectomy findings according to the presence of atypical hyperplasia or well-differentiated adenocarcinoma in curettings in women under 40 years of age

	Curettings	
	Atypical hyperplasia (*n* = 517)	Well-differentiated carcinoma (*n* = 535)
Hysterectomy findings	No.	No.
Carcinoma	2 (12%)	13 (37%)
Grade 1	2	10
Grade 2	0	3
Myometrial invasion		
Endometrium only	2	3
Inner one third	0	9
Middle one third	0	1

Adapted from [50].

Table 8.10

Risk of persistence/progression of complex hyperplasia with and without atypia in relation to progestin therapy

Treatment	Complex hyperplasia without atypia (n = 115)		Complex atypical hyperplasia (n = 70)	
	Regression (n = 82)	Persist/progress (n = 33)	Regression (n = 44)	Persist/progress (n = 26)
No progestin (n = 20)	14 (70%)	6 (30%)	6 (33%)	12 (67%)
Progestin (n = 95)	68 (72%)	27 (28%)	38 (73%)	14 (27%)

Table 8.11

Risk of persistence/progression of complex hyperplasia with and without atypia in relation to duration of progestin therapy

Duration of Rx	Complex hyperplasia without atypia (n = 115)		Complex atypical hyperplasia (n = 70)	
	Regression (n = 82)	Persist/progress (n = 33)	Regression (n = 44)	Persist/progress (n = 26)
<3 months	71%	30%	62%	38%
>3 months	73%	28%	87%	13%

regarded as a single clinicopathologic entity for management purposes. Nonetheless, pathologists should distinguish atypical hyperplasia from well-differentiated carcinoma since atypical hyperplasia is more likely to respond to progestin treatment. If conservative management is elected, magnetic resonance imaging (MRI) must be performed to exclude deep myometrial invasion or the presence of a coexisting ovarian neoplasm.

Perimenopausal Women (40 to 55 Years of Age)

Abnormal bleeding in the perimenopausal age group can be managed in a similar fashion as in younger women because perimenopausal women also are at low risk of having carcinoma (see *Table 8.7*). Most simple and complex hyperplasias in the 40- to 55-year-old age group are related to anovulation and are self-limited. Nonetheless, a biopsy is usually performed to exclude carcinoma. Patients with a diagnosis of atypical hyperplasia can be treated with progestins or a hysterectomy.

Nearly 60% of atypical hyperplasias regress, but the likelihood of residual carcinoma in the uterus after a curettage increases with age. For patients in the 40- to 55-year age range, treatment should be individualized. Regression occurs frequently, and the risk of residual carcinoma is lower than in older women. Therefore, observation or suppression with progestins monitored by endometrial biopsies every 3 months suffices. If the lesion persists, a hysterectomy may have to be performed.

Postmenopausal Women (Over 55 Years of Age)

Women in the postmenopausal age group who have abnormal bleeding have a significant risk of having either carcinoma or atypical hyperplasia (see *Table 8.7*). Accordingly, abnormal bleeding requires immediate evaluation with an endometrial biopsy. A diagnosis of hyperplasia or atypical hyperplasia should be evaluated with a fractional curettage. If the curettings demonstrate hyperplasia without atypia, conservative management is an option because these types of hyperplasia are related to unopposed estrogenic stimulation, either from exogenous hormone treatment or because of peripheral conversion of androgens to estrogen in adipose tissue. Most (80%) hyperplasias treated with cyclic medroxyprogesterone acetate at 10 mg/day for 14 days regress; none progressed to carcinoma in a prospective study of 65 postmenopausal women [26]. Conservative management, which makes use of either observation only or treatment with medroxyprogesterone to produce a medical curettage, therefore, is adequate. Repeated episodes of irregular bleeding that are not responsive to hormone treatment require a hysterectomy. Hysterectomy is the treatment of choice for a diagnosis of atypical hyperplasia based on a curettage. In postmenopausal women with surgical risk factors that preclude a hysterectomy, continuous treatment with 20–40 mg/day megestrol acetate can be used effectively to avoid surgery. In a study of 70 women treated with complex hyperplasia (38 women) and atypical hyperplasia (32 women), surgery was avoided in 93% of patients. The hyperplasias (atypical and non-atypical) completely regressed in 85% after a mean follow-up of more than 5 years. None of the lesions progressed to carcinoma [28].

For postmenopausal women with hyperplasia or atypical hyperplasia who are receiving exogenous estrogen, termination of the estrogen usually suffices even for atypical hyperplasia, because these proliferations regress after the stimulus for their growth has been removed. Alternatively, the addition of cyclically or continuous administered medroxyprogesterone in women being treated with estrogen can be considered because the use of even low doses of progestins substantially reduces the risk of development of endometrial hyperplasia and carcinoma [91]. Using a 7- to 14-day regimen of orally administered 10 mg medroxy-progesterone to postmenopausal women receiving estrogen, 5 endometrial carcinomas were detected in 5,402 woman-years of continuous estrogen therapy [29]. This incidence is not greater than that of untreated postmenopausal women, in whom the expected incidence of endometrial cancer is 1–2 per 1,000 woman-years, that is, 5.4–9.8 cases. The addition of continuous low doses of norethindrone acetate to estradiol therapy also reduces the incidence of endometrial hyperplasia in postmenopausal women. Hyperplasia developed in 15% of women receiving unopposed estradiol therapy compared to less than 1% of those receiving continuous low doses of norethindrone combined with estradiol [52].

Morphologic Changes Associated with Progestin Treatment

Treatment with progestins for women with complex atypical hyperplasia and well-differentiated carcinoma has become an accepted alternative to hysterectomy. Correct interpretation of the morphologic changes that result from the treatment is required for the appropriate management of women who chose this therapeutic approach. Unfortunately, there have been few studies to describe these changes. One recent study, described a number of histologic changes including decreased gland-to-stroma ratio, decreased glandular cellularity, reduced to absent mitotic activity, loss of cytologic atypia, and a variety of metaplastic changes (➲ *Figs. 8.32* and ➲ *8.33*) [94]. In addition, cribriform and papillary architectural changes may be induced by treatment and confused with disease progression. Importantly, the persistence of architectural abnormalities and/or cytologic atypia after 6 months of treatment were the only histologic features found to be associated with treatment failure. Based on these findings, a classification of progestin-treated lesions was proposed (➲ *Table 8.12*). It is important that the pretreatment specimen be available for review in order for the pathologist to evaluate the response to progestin treatment, and therefore provide information to the gynecologist that will assist in modifying or discontinuing therapy.

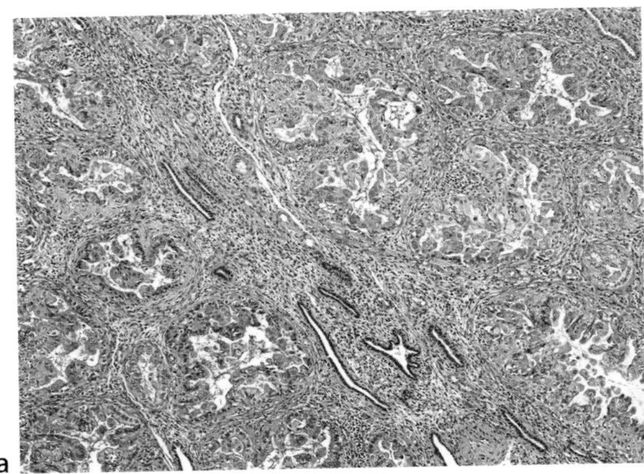
a

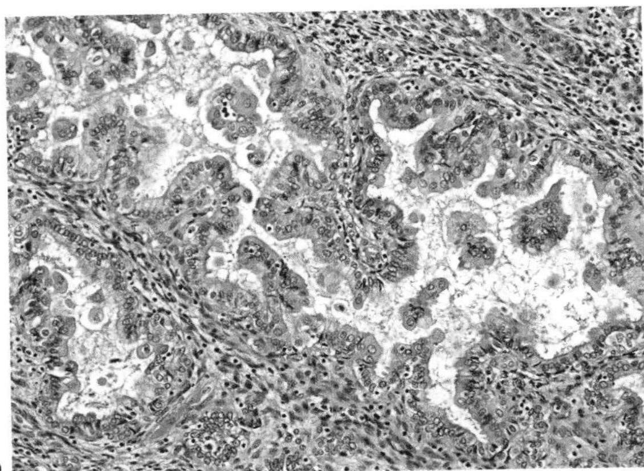
b

■ Fig. 8.32
Complex hyperplasia with treatment (progestin) effect.
Individual glands with complex profiles are interspersed with inactive glands within endometrial stroma (a). The confluent glandular pattern of the prior endometrioid carcinoma is absent. Glands exhibit mucinous change (b)

Endometrial Cellular Changes: Metaplasia, Cellular Differentiation

In contrast to hyperplasia, which is a proliferative response to estrogenic stimulation, metaplasia represents cytoplasmic differentiation. The cytoplasmic alterations (metaplasia) are manifested by eosinophilic, ciliated cell (tubal), squamous, secretory/clear, and mucinous differentiation. Metaplasias develop most commonly in response to estrogenic and progestational stimulation, although these changes may develop in response to various other stimuli as well. Thus, the morphologic response of the endometrium to hormonal stimulation is complex and is reflected by a combination of architectural, nuclear, and cytoplasmic alterations. Although classifications separate hyperplasia and the various metaplasias, both are usually intimately associated and cannot always be separately classified.

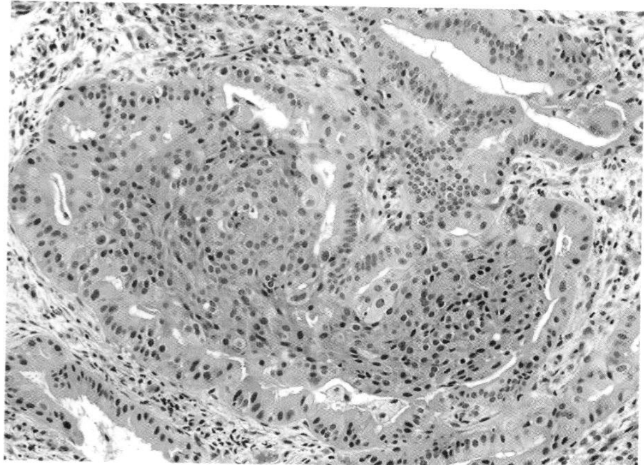

Fig. 8.33
Complex hyperplasia with treatment (progestin) effect.
Complex glands exhibit prominent metaplastic changes (eosinophilic, mucinous, tubal), which are commonly seen, along with reduction of nuclear atypia, as a result of progestin therapy

Table 8.12
Classification of progestin-treated lesions of the endometrium

Diagnosis	Histologic features
Progestin-treated complex hyperplasia	No cytologic atypia with crowded, back-to-back glands and/or a confluent glandular pattern (cribriform and/or papillary)
Progestin-treated CAH	Cytologic atypia with crowded, back-to-back glands that lack a confluent glandular pattern
Progestin-treated well-differentiated carcinoma	Cytologic atypia with confluent glandular pattern (cribriform and/or papillary pattern)

Adapted with permission from [94].

Definitions and Classification

Metaplasia is defined as replacement of one type of adult tissue by another type that is not normally found in that location. In the endometrium, most of the changes that are designated as metaplasia represent a variety of cytoplasmic alterations or forms of differentiation that are not encountered in normal proliferative endometrium but do not qualify as true metaplasia. Accordingly, it has been suggested that a more appropriate term is change [84]. Use of the term change also has the advantage of providing a descriptive designation without employing a specific mechanism of development. In this chapter, the terms metaplasia, change, and differentiation are used interchangeably. The various forms of cellular differentiation are typically focal when unaccompanied by hyperplasia but can be diffuse when hyperplasia is present. The WHO classification subdivides endometrial metaplasia as follows: squamous, mucinous, ciliary, hobnail, clear cell, eosinophilic, surface syncytial, papillary proliferation, and Arias–Stella effect [77]. This classification combines both cytologic and architectural alterations, some of which have different etiologies. As previously noted, the endometrial epithelium can undergo a variety of cytoplasmic changes in response to different stimuli that can be observed in both benign and malignant conditions. A simplified classification of these cytoplasmic changes is shown in *Table 8.13*. It is important to recognize the various cytoplasmic changes because they are benign and can be confused with hyperplasia. When hyperplasia and the cytoplasmic alterations coexist, as they often do, the hyperplasia should be classified, but it is not necessary to describe the cytoplasmic changes because they do not influence prognosis (see section Behavior).

Clinical Features

The frequent association of the various endometrial cytoplasmic changes with hyperplasia probably results from a hyperestrogenic state. More than 70% of perimenopausal

Table 8.13
Classification of endometrial cellular (cytoplasmic) changes

Eosinophilic (including syncytial change)
Squamous (squamous metaplasia)
Ciliated cell (tubal metaplasia)
Secretory and clear cell
Mucinous

and postmenopausal women with metaplasia had received exogenous estrogen in one study [35]. In addition, most young women with metaplasia have clinical manifestations of persistent anovulation and primary infertility, features of polycystic ovarian disease [18, 35]. Metaplasia also may occur in various benign conditions, including polyps, endometritis, trauma, and vitamin A deficiency [18, 27, 35, 36].

Pathologic Findings

The various types of endometrial cytoplasmic changes have no distinctive gross features.

Eosinophilic Change

Eosinophilic change is the most common cytoplasmic alteration (➋ *Figs. 8.34* and ➋ *8.35*). Several types of eosinophilic cytoplasmic transformation occur, all of them innocuous. Ciliated cells, squamous cells, oncocytes, and papillary and surface syncytial change all may have eosinophilic cytoplasm. However, eosinophilic cells also occur in association with hyperplasia, particularly atypical hyperplasia. Glands may be partially or completely lined by eosinophilic cells. Eosinophilic cells that line glands can show considerable variation in shape. They may be columnar when associated with atypical hyperplasia, rounded when associated with ciliated cells, or polygonal, forming pavement-like aggregates, when they merge with cells that show squamous differentiation. In hyperplastic lesions, aggregates of eosinophilic cells often form intraglandular papillary tufts and bridges, thus simulating carcinoma. Eosinophilic cells contain variable amounts of cytoplasm that at times can be partially vacuolated. The nuclei tend to be round and somewhat stratified. In most instances, the nuclei are smaller, more uniform, and lack the irregular nuclear membrane, coarse chromatin, and nucleoli that characterize cells with true cytologic atypia. Occasionally, the nuclei can be enlarged and contain a single prominent nucleolus. Mitotic figures are rarely present. On the endometrial surface, cells with eosinophilic cytoplasm typically merge into a syncytium that either can be flat or more commonly form papillary processes [76]. Typically, the papillary processes lack connective tissue support and contain small cystic spaces filled with polymorphonuclear leukocytes. This lesion has been referred to as surface syncytial change, papillary syncytial change, or papillary metaplasia [36, 84]. We prefer the term eosinophilic

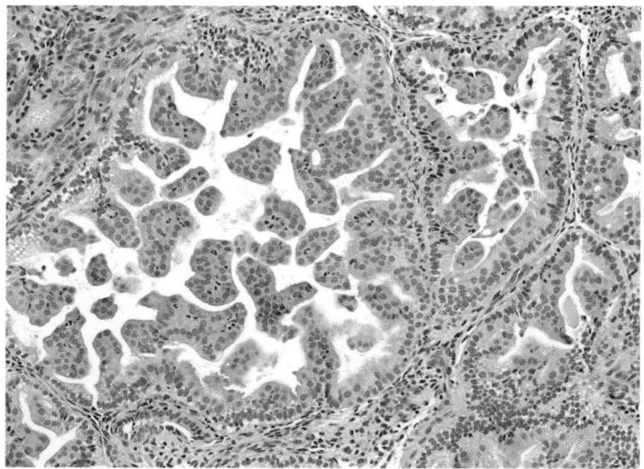

Fig. 8.34
Complex hyperplasia (without atypia) with eosinophilic metaplasia. **Intraglandular epithelial tufts composed of bland cells with abundant eosinophilic cytoplasm are present within a non-atypical hyperplasia**

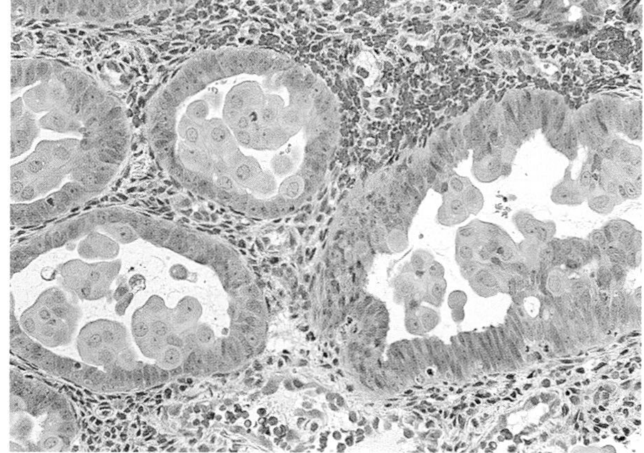

Fig. 8.35
Complex atypical hyperplasia with eosinophilic metaplasia. **Intraglandular epithelial clusters composed of rounded cells with abundant eosinophilic cytoplasm are present within an atypical hyperplasia; assessment of atypia is based on the appearance of the glandular epithelium, which displays vesicular nuclei with prominent nucleoli and loss of polarity**

syncytial change because the lesion is characteristically composed of eosinophilic cells forming a syncytium and can involve glands as well as the surface. Eosinophilic syncytial change is commonly associated with endometrial stromal breakdown or inflammation, suggesting that it is a degenerative or a reparative process [98]. A recent study using immunohistochemical stains for proliferation further support the regressive nature of this type of epithelial change [78]. The nuclei within the syncytium are arranged haphazardly and piled up; they generally are small and bland but at times may be round and vesicular and display alterations in shape and chromatin texture. Mitotic figures are rare. Hyperchromatic nuclei with smudged chromatin and irregular nuclear membranes appear degenerated whereas enlarged, vesicular nuclei with a prominent nucleolus and smooth nuclear membranes appear reactive. These degenerative and reparative changes should not be interpreted as nuclear atypia. Eosinophilic change can be seen in combination with hobnail secretory change on occasion. In fact, typically the various types of metaplasia occur concomitantly.

Squamous Differentiation (Squamous Metaplasia)

Squamous differentiation may occur in all forms of hyperplasia (*Figs. 8.36–8.38*) as well as in carcinoma. It is especially common in the more atypical endometrial proliferations and is rare in normally cycling endometrium or in simple and complex hyperplasias. The squamous cells are usually cytologically bland. The degree of nuclear atypia, when present, generally parallels that of the glandular cells. Typically, the squamous cells have a moderate amount of eosinophilic cytoplasm and are surrounded by a well-defined cell membrane. Often they merge with eosinophilic cells that qualify as eosinophilic change. The squamous cells tend to be rounded or polygonal but may be spindle shaped, forming a circumscribed nest (squamous morule) within the gland lumen (*Fig. 8.37*). Morules reflect immature or incomplete squamous differentiation. The cells are smaller and the cytoplasm is less prominent than in more completely differentiated squamous cells. Central keratinization and necrosis rarely occur. Eventually, proliferation results in protrusion of the squamous cells into the lumen, leading to replacement of the lumen by nests of squamous cells and coalescence with neighboring glands undergoing the same process. Mitotic activity is rare. A recent study found that squamous morules in hyperplastic proliferations lack expression of the estrogen and progesterone receptors and demonstrate rare to undetectable Ki-67 proliferative activity when compared to the associated hyperplastic epithelium. However, the glandular and squamous components had identical *PTEN* mutations indicating that the squamous component is clonally related to the glandular

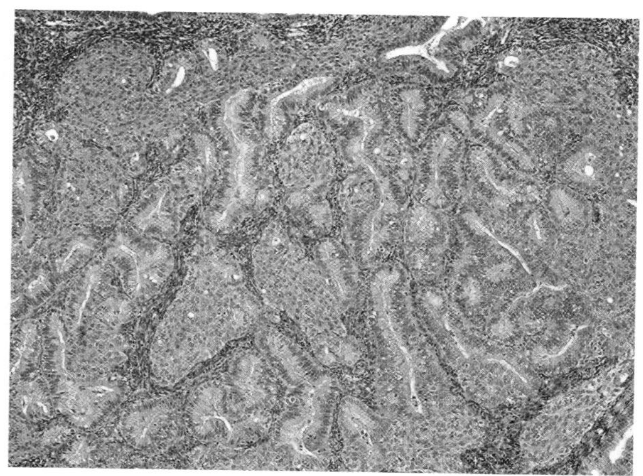

Fig. 8.36
Complex hyperplasia (without atypia) with squamous metaplasia. **Islands of squamous metaplastic epithelium are intimately admixed with non-atypical hyperplastic glands**

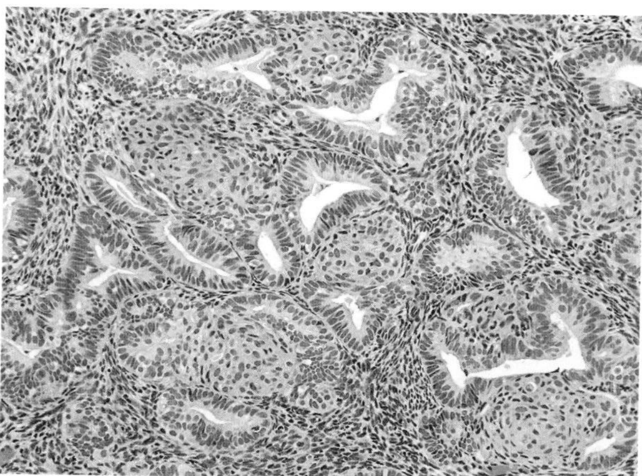

Fig. 8.37
Complex hyperplasia (without atypia) with squamous metaplasia. **Squamous morules are intimately admixed with non-atypical hyperplastic glands exhibiting tubal metaplasia as well**

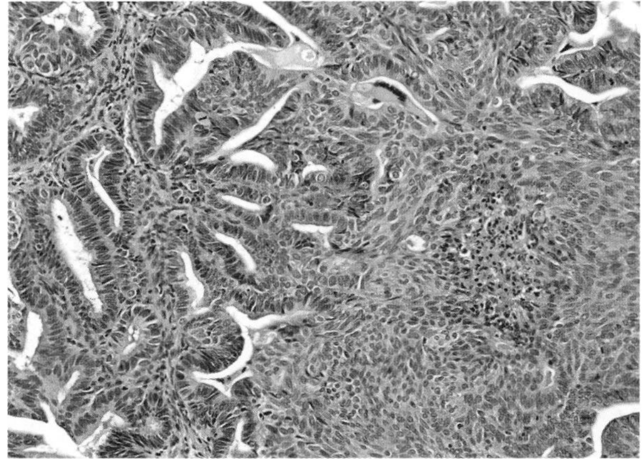

■ Fig. 8.38
Complex hyperplasia (without atypia) with squamous metaplasia. **Squamous metaplastic epithelium with central necrosis forms a confluent mass intimately admixed with non-atypical hyperplastic glands but should not be interpreted as an indicator of stromal invasion when the glandular component does not manifest confluence or induce desmoplasia**

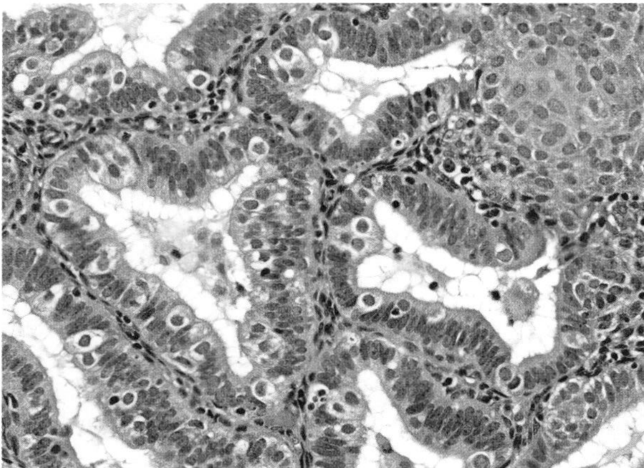

■ Fig. 8.39
Complex hyperplasia (without atypia) with tubal metaplasia. **Crowded glands have multiple cell types, including ciliated cells and those with rounded nuclei and cytoplasmic clearing (halos), similar to those seen in fallopian tube epithelium**

component. The authors concluded that the squamous morules are inert elements of the proliferative lesions. Importantly, since they are often associated with complex atypical hyperplasia and endometrioid carcinoma their presence on endometrial sampling, in the absence of an identifiable proliferative process, should result in close follow-up of the patient for the possibility of an under sampled or occult glandular lesion [59].

Ciliated Cell Change (Tubal Metaplasia)

Cilia are not usually evident microscopically in proliferative endometrial glandular cells, although they may be observed on the endometrial surface [61]. Ciliated cells occasionally are observed in isolated glands in atrophic or inactive endometria or in polyps in the absence of hyperplasia. The presence of a significant number of ciliated glandular cells is referred to as ciliated cell change or tubal metaplasia because of the resemblance to the epithelium of the fallopian tube. The ciliated cells are often round and slightly enlarged, but the nuclear membranes are smooth and uniform and the chromatin is fine and evenly dispersed. There is no nuclear atypia. The ciliated cells may be interspersed singly or in small groups among non-ciliated cells, or they may line a larger segment of a gland. Mitotic activity is limited to the adjacent non-ciliated cells. Ciliated cell change may occur in glands in the absence of hyperplasia. Dilated venous sinusoids are also frequently present. All these changes reflect a mild degree of estrogenic stimulation. Ciliated cell change frequently accompanies simple, complex, or atypical hyperplasia (➲ *Figs. 8.39–8.41*).

Secretory and Hobnail Change

Secretory change is characterized by columnar cells with sub- or supranuclear vacuoles containing clear glycogenated cytoplasm resembling the glandular cells of early secretory endometrium. These cells also can be observed in nonneoplastic proliferative endometria but are seen more often in association with hyperplasia or carcinoma (➲ *Fig. 8.42*) [48, 51]. Rarely, the cells in secretory change can display hobnail morphology reminiscent of the Arias–Stella reaction (➲ *Fig. 8.43*); such hobnail change, with or without the cytoplasmic vacuolization of secretory change (➲ *Fig. 8.44*), should not be misinterpreted as endometrial intraepithelial carcinoma (see below). At times secretory change can result from progestational stimulation, but often there is no such association. Columnar cells with secretory change may merge with polygonal-shaped clear cells and with squamous cells containing clear glycogenated cytoplasm. The accumulation of glycogen can occur in the cytoplasm of a variety of cell types.

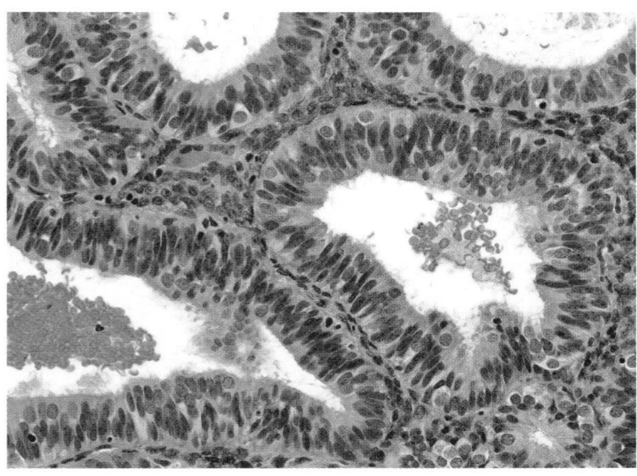

Fig. 8.40
Complex hyperplasia (without atypia) with tubal metaplasia. **Crowded glands have some ciliated cells and cells with nuclear rounding and cytoplasmic clearing**

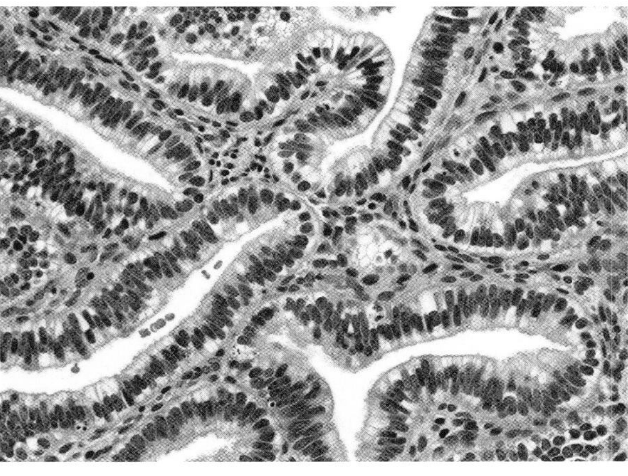

Fig. 8.42
Complex hyperplasia (without atypia) with secretory change. **Crowded glands have elongated nuclei and discrete sub- and supranuclear vacuoles, reminiscent of day 18 secretory endometrium**

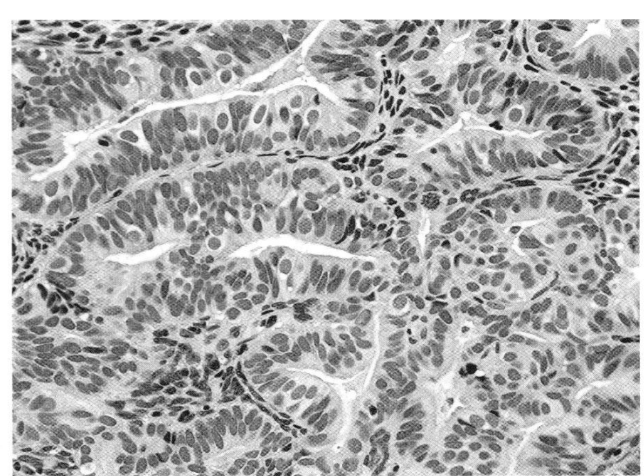

Fig. 8.41
Complex atypical hyperplasia with tubal metaplasia. **Markedly crowded glands have some cells with rounded nuclei and cytoplasmic clearing indicating underlying tubal metaplasia but the nuclear enlargement and loss of polarity are beyond that attributable to metaplasia and indicate atypia**

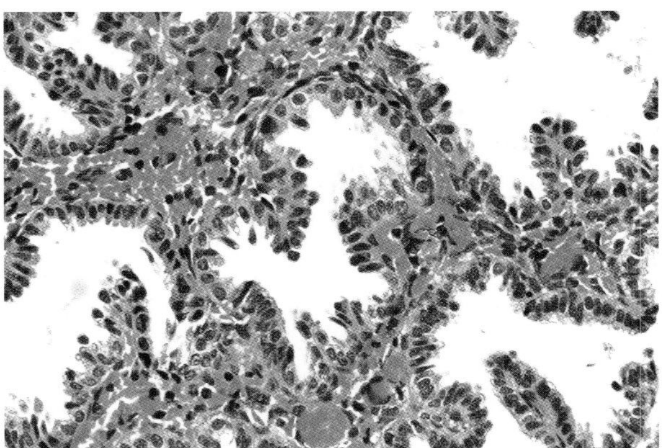

Fig. 8.43
Complex hyperplasia (without atypia) with hobnail change. **Crowded glands with cells containing hyperchromatic rounded nuclei that bulge into the gland lumen and some cytoplasmic clearing with vacuolization are reminiscent of the Arias–Stella reaction**

Mucinous Change

Mucinous change is characterized by mucinous epithelium resembling that of the endocervix cytologically, histochemically, and ultrastructurally [21]. Although it is one of the least commonly encountered cytoplasmic alterations, it occurs more frequently than generally described. The mucinous epithelium tends to be distributed focally and is composed of tall columnar cells with bland, basally oriented nuclei and clear, slightly granular cytoplasm (*Figs. 8.45* and *8.46*). At times mucinous change is accompanied by a papillary proliferation. The papillary processes contain normal but compressed stromal cells and are lined by nonstratified

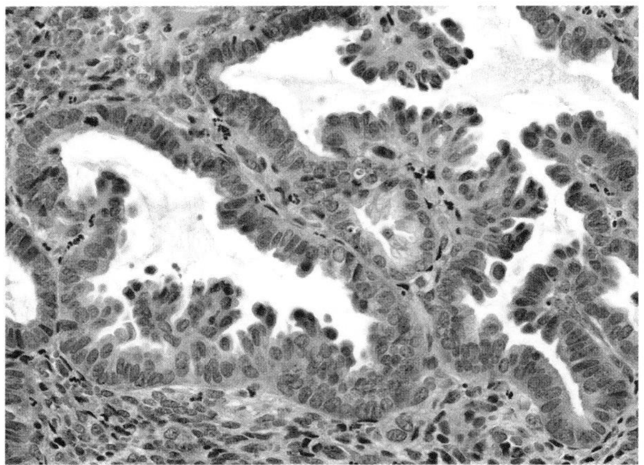

Fig. 8.44
Complex hyperplasia (without atypia) with hobnail change. **Crowded glands are partially lined by epithelial tufts containing cells with hyperchromatic rounded nuclei that bulge into the gland lumen. These tufts also share features with eosinophilic cell change**

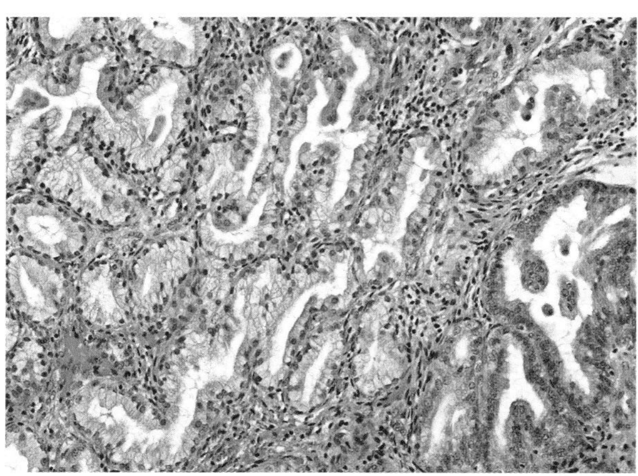

Fig. 8.45
Complex hyperplasia (without atypia) with mucinous change. **Crowded glands have abundant pale mucinous cytoplasm and basally situated small nuclei**

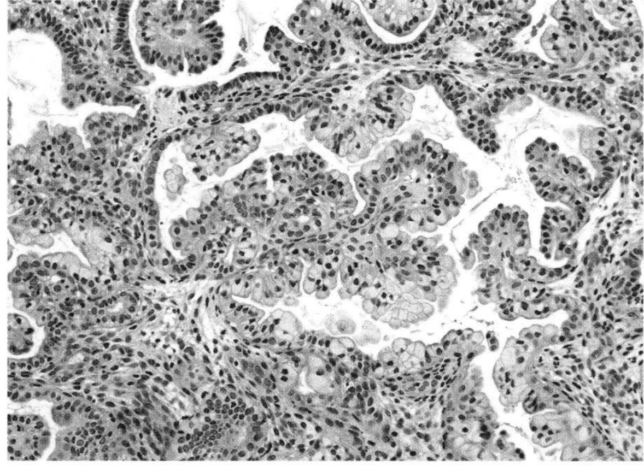

Fig. 8.46
Complex hyperplasia (without atypia) with mucinous change. **Crowded glands are lined by cells with pale mucinous cytoplasm and small round nuclei, with some forming papillary tufts**

columnar epithelium, which may have mucinous areas. Mitotic figures are rare. The cytoplasm is clear in hematoxylin and eosin (H&E) stains because it contains mucin, which is periodic acid–Schiff (PAS) positive and diastase resistant and stains with mucicarmine, toluidine blue, and alcian blue. In contrast to mucinous epithelium, the vacuolated cytoplasm of secretory endometrium contains glycogen. On rare occasion, the mucinous epithelium may contain goblet cells and is referred to as intestinal metaplasia.

Mucinous differentiation can be seen in a spectrum of epithelial proliferations ranging from benign to malignant. In one study, the likelihood of finding carcinoma associated with mucinous proliferations of the endometrium varies according to the degrees of architectural complexity and cytologic atypia of the lesions [71]. Architecturally simple lesions with papillary projections into luminal spaces and no cytologic atypia were found to have carcinoma on follow-up only when the initial specimen also contained atypical hyperplasia; otherwise, none of these simple mucinous proliferations were associated with carcinoma on follow-up. More complex proliferations with microglandular or cribriform patterns and minimal cytologic atypia, often presenting as endometrial surface lesions without coexistent atypical hyperplasia, were found to have well-differentiated noninvasive or minimally invasive carcinoma on follow-up in 65% of cases. Highly complex proliferations with glandular budding, cribriform growth, and branching of villous structures that also displayed moderate to severe cytologic atypia were invariably associated with carcinoma on follow-up (*Fig. 8.47*). Importantly, 80% of the study patients were over age 50. Thus, in perimenopausal and postmenopausal women with complex mucinous proliferations, including those with and without cytologic atypia, the risk of finding coexistent carcinoma is high.

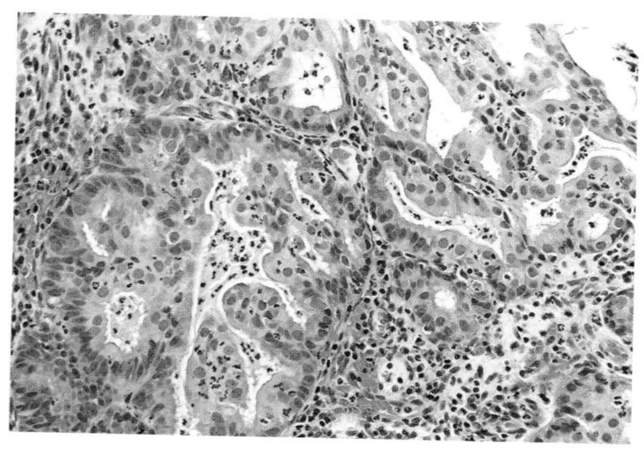

Fig. 8.47
Complex atypical mucinous proliferation. **This term is used for limited specimens in which crowded, fused, or cribriform glands with mucinous cytoplasmic change and atypical nuclei are concerning for at least complex atypical hyperplasia but there is little or no associated stroma to diagnose stromal invasion. Such lesions are often associated with FIGO gradel endometrioid carcinoma on follow-up, as occurred in this case**

Mixed Cellular Changes

Mixtures of different types of cellular changes are common. Most are closely related and represent different morphologic responses to a variety of stimuli, including estrogenic stimulation [35]. For example, eosinophilic change, especially eosinophilic syncytial change, may resemble squamous epithelium and often is associated with squamous metaplasia. Likewise, eosinophilic and ciliated cell change share many morphologic features and commonly occur together.

Differential Diagnosis

The most important aspect of the evaluation of the various metaplasias and cellular changes is not to confuse them with hyperplasia or carcinoma, which is best accomplished by evaluating the glandular architecture and cytological features. In hyperplasia, the glandular outlines are irregular and complex and there is stratification of the epithelium reflecting a proliferative process. In contrast, in the various cytoplasmic changes the glandular outlines are regular and have a tubular configuration, although cystic dilatation and slight glandular irregularity occasionally can occur.

Although the various cellular changes may be accompanied by slight nuclear enlargement, the cells lack the abnormal chromatin patterns that characterize the nuclei in atypical hyperplasia. At times the various cellular changes may look ominous and suggest carcinoma, but evidence of stromal invasion is lacking and therefore a diagnosis of carcinoma is not justified. For example, extensive squamous metaplasia may suggest a diagnosis of carcinoma but without a desmoplastic response or a confluent glandular pattern, a diagnosis of carcinoma should not be made. Squamous and eosinophilic change associated with hyperplasia can fill and bridge gland lumens but lack a true confluent or cribriform pattern. Mucinous change at times can form complex papillary processes, but the stroma of the papillae is composed of normal endometrial stroma and the epithelium lacks cytologic atypia.

Behavior

Cytoplasmic changes, other than eosinophilic syncytial change, rarely occur in the absence of hyperplasia or carcinoma [41]. In the absence of hyperplasia, these changes (metaplasia) had no clinical significance in one study of 89 patients [35]. In a long-term follow-up study of endometrial hyperplasia, 5 of 11 patients with atypical hyperplasia and associated squamous metaplasia eventually developed carcinoma, indicating that atypical hyperplasia with squamous metaplasia has malignant potential [49]. Inasmuch as the cytoplasmic changes by themselves have no prognostic significance, the importance of recognizing them lies in not confusing these benign processes with hyperplasia or carcinoma.

Management

The management of endometrial cytoplasmic changes depends entirely on the nature of the associated proliferative process. If hyperplasia is present it should be managed accordingly. Endometrial cytoplasmic changes without hyperplasia do not require treatment.

Endometrial Intraepithelial Carcinoma

Definition and Pathologic Findings

Serous carcinoma is the prototypic endometrial carcinoma that is not related to estrogenic stimulation and typically occurs in the setting of endometrial atrophy. Serous carcinoma is frequently associated with a putative precursor lesion, termed "endometrial intraepithelial carcinoma" (EIC). The lesion also has been referred to as "carcinoma in situ" [86] and "uterine surface carcinoma" [100], but we prefer the term EIC to CIS because EIC can be associated with metastatic disease (see following), whereas the term CIS implies a lesion that does not have metastatic potential. In view of the association of EIC with serous as opposed to endometrioid carcinoma it is reasonable to use the term serous EIC as has been proposed in the WHO classification. EIC is characterized by markedly atypical nuclei, identical to those of invasive serous carcinomas, lining the surfaces, and glands of the atrophic endometrium The lesion can be very small and focal and is often present on the surface of a polyp (*Figs. 8.48–8.54*) [1, 80]. EIC often has

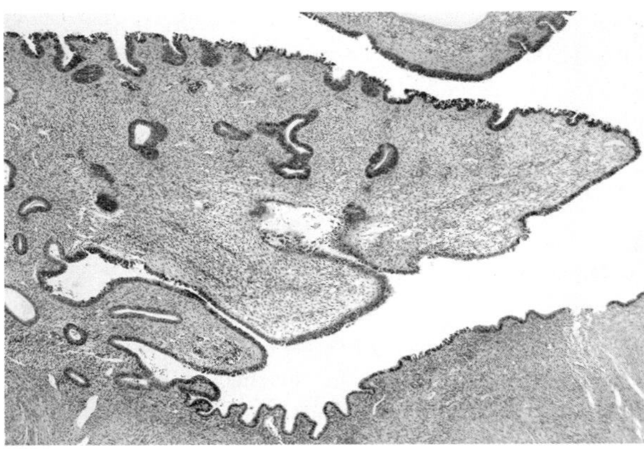

Fig. 8.48
Endometrial intraepithelial carcinoma (EIC) involving a polyp. **The surface epithelium of the polyp (best seen in blunt papillary structures along upper left and middle surface) is lined by markedly atypical cells of EIC (see *Fig. 8.49*)**

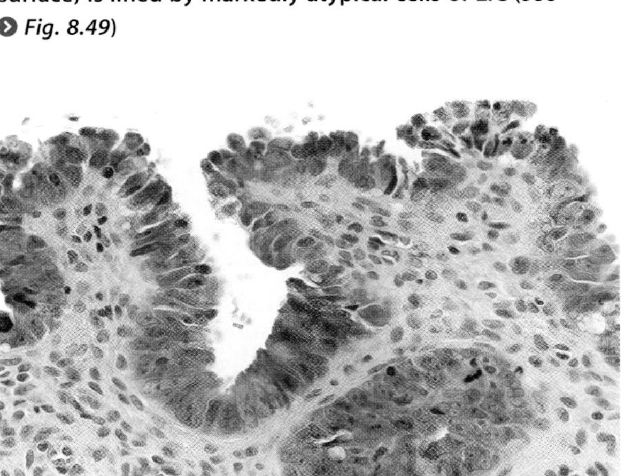

Fig. 8.49
Endometrial intraepithelial carcinoma (EIC) involving a polyp. **Higher magnification of an area of the polyp in *Fig. 8.48* shows markedly atypical cells containing enlarged vesicular nuclei with prominent nucleoli, hobnail cells, and apoptotic bodies lining the surface and involving an underlying gland**

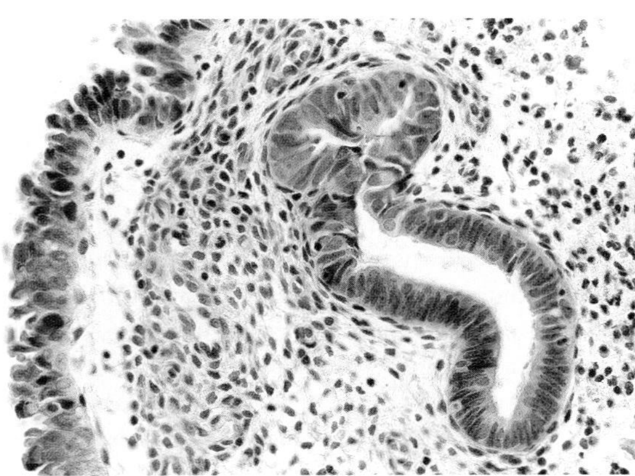

Fig. 8.50
Endometrial intraepithelial carcinoma (EIC). **Markedly atypical cells containing enlarged vesicular nuclei with prominent nucleoli, hobnail cells, and apoptotic bodies are lining the surface epithelium and partially involving an underlying gland**

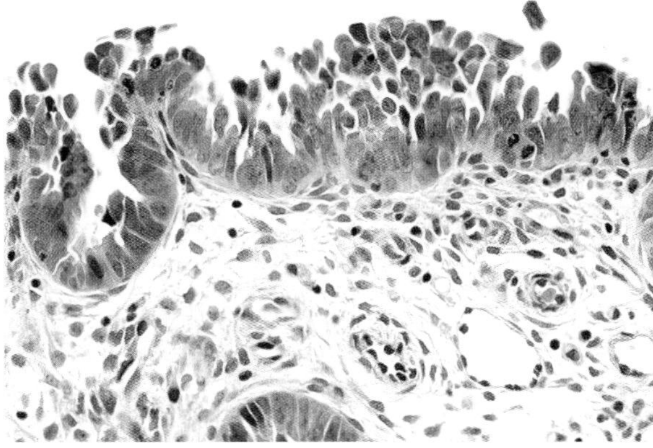

Fig. 8.51
Endometrial intraepithelial carcinoma (EIC). **Markedly atypical cells lining the surface epithelium have enlarged vesicular nuclei with prominent nucleoli and prominent hobnail morphology**

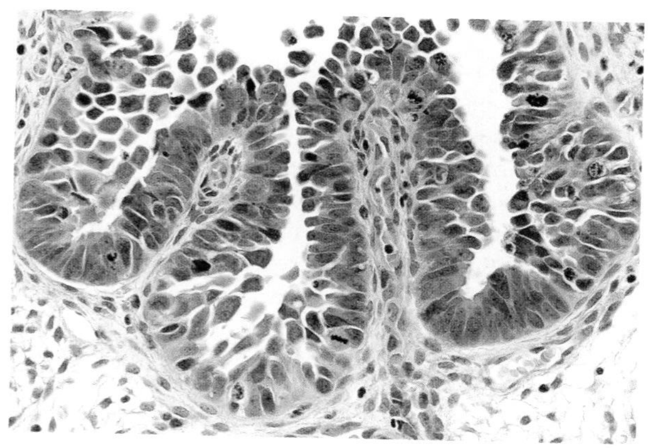

■ Fig. 8.52
Endometrial intraepithelial carcinoma (EIC). **Markedly atypical cells lining endometrial glands have enlarged vesicular nuclei with prominent nucleoli, numerous mitotic figures and apoptotic bodies, and prominent hobnail morphology**

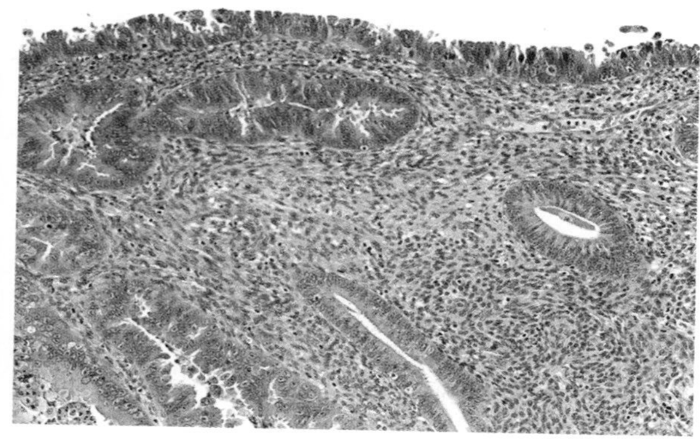

■ Fig. 8.53
Endometrial intraepithelial carcinoma (EIC). **Markedly atypical cells lining endometrial surface and underlying glands (*upper, middle,* and *lower left*) have enlarged vesicular nuclei with prominent nucleoli, distinct from the elongated nuclei in the normal glands (*lower middle* and *middle right*)**

a slightly papillary contour and some cells display hobnail morphology and smudged, hyperchromatic nuclei. The nuclei are enlarged, and frequently display enlarged eosinophilic nucleoli. Numerous mitotic figures, including atypical ones, are present. On occasion, the abnormal proliferation involves only a portion of an endometrial

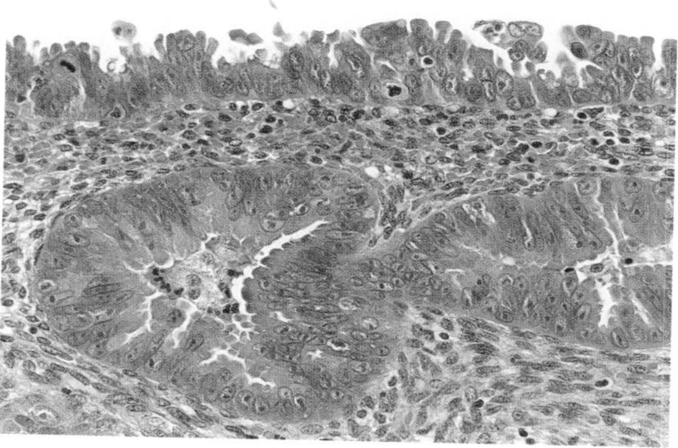

■ Fig. 8.54
Endometrial intraepithelial carcinoma (EIC). **Markedly atypical cells lining endometrial glands have enlarged vesicular nuclei with prominent red nucleoli**

gland (➋ *Fig. 8.50*). More recently a lesion has been described, termed endometrial glandular dysplasia, which also exhibits cytologic atypia with serous features but lacks the marked atypia associated with EIC [101]. It has been proposed that this lesion represents the precursor of EIC and serous carcinoma.

Molecular Biology and Immunohistochemistry

Molecular genetic evidence supports the concept that EIC is a precursor lesion of serous carcinoma. Studies have demonstrated immunohistochemical overexpression of p53 protein, loss of heterozygosity of chromosome 17p, and corresponding p53 gene mutations in a high proportion of serous carcinomas and EIC (➋ *Fig. 8.55*) [79, 88]. The finding of diffuse, intense staining for p53 is highly correlated with identification of p53 mutation in these cases. Lack of immunoreactivity for p53, however, does not exclude the presence of a mutation in p53 because mutations have been detected in a small number of serous carcinomas that were nonreactive for p53 due to the formation of a truncated or unstable protein [88]. Identical p53 gene mutations have been found in the EIC and adjacent serous carcinoma in several cases. Examples of pure EIC unassociated with serous carcinoma also have been shown to contain p53 mutations. In addition, a case of pure EIC has been shown to contain p53 mutation in the absence of loss of heterozygosity of chromosome 17p, suggesting that p53 mutation occurs early in the evolution of serous carcinoma [88]. The finding of EIC unassociated with invasive carcinoma and the presence of identical p53 mutations in both lesions support the view that EIC is the precursor lesion of serous carcinoma. As mentioned above, endometrial glandular dysplasia has been suggested as a precursor to EIC, in part based on a study that has shown that these lesions show intense staining for p53, as well as p53 mutations. Additional preliminary studies have suggested that endometrial glandular dysplasia is preceded by histologically normal lesions that demonstrate increased expression of p53 and p53 mutations. These histologically normal appearing glands have been called "p53 signatures" because of the expression of p53 [40, 99]. Presently, their relationship to serous carcinoma has not been definitely determined, but future studies will likely be done to further our understanding of their biologic significance in the pathogenesis of serous carcinoma.

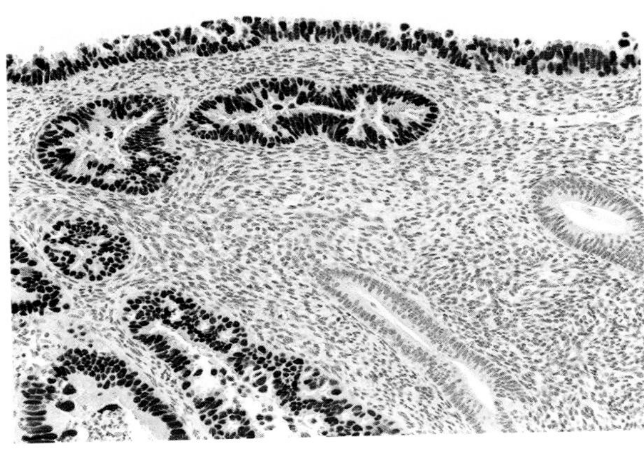

Fig. 8.55
Endometrial intraepithelial carcinoma (EIC). **Surface epithelium and underlying glands involved by EIC are highlighted by diffuse/strong nuclear expression of p53; normal glands are negative**

Differential Diagnosis

The distinction of extensive EIC from early serous carcinoma has not been well defined. Crowded glands involved by EIC within a polyp or within the endometrium should be classified as extensive EIC when the proliferation lacks a confluent glandular pattern, demonstrates no evidence of stromal desmoplasia (stromal invasion), and is less than 1 cm in greatest dimension. When either glandular confluence or stromal invasion is present and the proliferation exceeds 1 cm in greatest dimension, the lesion qualifies as serous carcinoma. Lesions with glandular confluence or stromal invasion but measuring less than 1 cm can be subclassified as minimal uterine serous carcinoma (*Figs. 8.56* and *8.57*; see following). It is important to note, however, that metastatic serous carcinoma can be

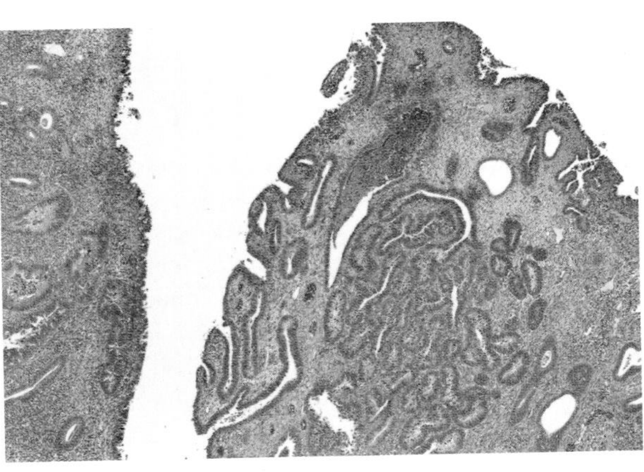

Fig. 8.56
Extensive endometrial intraepithelial carcinoma (EIC)/ minimal uterine serous carcinoma. **An endometrial polyp involved by EIC on its surface, as well as in the adjacent endometrium (*left*), contains crowded glands measuring less than 1 cm but verging on being confluent, suggesting early stromal invasion**

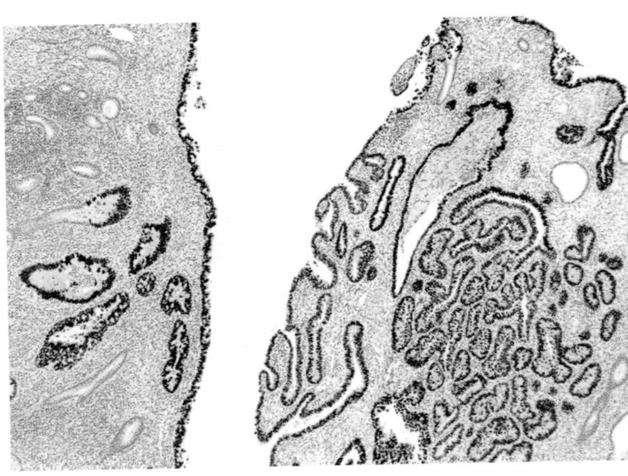

Fig. 8.57
Extensive endometrial intraepithelial carcinoma (EIC)/ minimal uterine serous carcinoma. **Immunohistochemical stain for p53 highlights the extent of the lesion in *Fig. 8.56***

found in other sites in the genital tract and in the abdomen in the absence of demonstrable invasion in uteri with EIC, indicating that EIC is capable of metastasizing without first invading the stroma of the endometrium [9, 85].

EIC must be distinguished from benign metaplastic endometrial lesions that can mimic the nuclear changes seen in EIC, which include eosinophilic cell change, hobnail change, and tubal metaplasia. At times, eosinophilic cell change and hobnail change can display enlarged, smudged, hyperchromatic nuclei, but these nuclei usually have a degenerative appearance and typically lack the prominent nucleoli seen in EIC. On occasion, however, the nuclei can appear more overtly atypical, with prominent nucleoli, suggesting EIC (see *Figs. 8.43* and *8.44*). Tubal metaplasia typically displays enlarged, hyperchromatic nuclei, but these are admixed with other cell types, including ciliated cells and intercalated cells, and nucleoli are usually not prominent. Immunohistochemistry for Ki-67, a proliferation marker, is very useful for distinguishing EIC from eosinophilic cell change and tubal metaplasia in that EIC typically displays a very high proliferation index (virtually all the nuclei express Ki-67), whereas the metaplasias have very low proliferation indices. In addition, EIC is usually diffusely and strongly positive for p53, whereas eosinophilic metaplasia is typically negative or occasionally displays weak or scattered moderate nuclear staining. Preliminary data based on a small number of cases indicate that tubal metaplasia and eosinophilic metaplasia do not strongly overexpress p53 [73]. Thus, the combination of Ki67 and p53 immunohistochemical stains is useful to distinguish EIC from metaplasia when the distinction is difficult by morphologic assessment alone.

Behavior and Treatment

There are limited data on the behavior of pure EIC. A recent study found that patients with pure EIC, and those with minimal uterine serous carcinoma (less than 1 cm of carcinoma in the endometrium) lacking myometrial or vascular invasion and no evidence of extrauterine disease, had an overall survival of 100% after a mean follow-up of 27 months [95]. The majority of these patients received no treatment after hysterectomy. In addition, the few patients with involvement of endocervical glands by EIC (stage IIA disease) were also alive without evidence of disease at intervals ranging from 12 to 54 months. Similarly, in another study of stage IA serous carcinoma, 11 of 13 patients were alive without evidence of disease after a median follow-up of 38 months [16]. In contrast, patients with either EIC or minimal serous carcinoma and evidence of extrauterine disease (even microscopic disease) all died of disease despite intensive chemotherapy [95]. Accordingly, patients with a diagnosis of EIC in an endometrial biopsy or curettage specimen should undergo careful surgical staging at the time of hysterectomy.

References

1. Ambros RA et al (1995) Endometrial intraepithelial carcinoma: a distinctive lesion specifically associated with tumors displaying serous differentiation. Hum Pathol 26:1260–1267
2. Ausems EW, van der Kamp JK, Baak JP (1985) Nuclear morphometry in the determination of the prognosis of marked atypical endometrial hyperplasia. Int J Gynecol Pathol 4:180–185
3. Ayhan A, Yarali H, Ayhan A (1991) Endometrial carcinoma: a pathologic evaluation of 142 cases with and without associated endometrial hyperplasia. J Surg Oncol 46:182–184
4. Baak JP (1986) Further evaluation of the practical applicability of nuclear morphometry for the prediction of the outcome of atypical endometrial hyperplasia. Anal Quant Cytol Histol 8:46–48
5. Baak JP, Kuik DJ, Bezemer PD (1994) The additional prognostic value of morphometric nuclear arrangement and DNA-ploidy to other morphometric and stereologic features in endometrial hyperplasias. Int J Gynecol Cancer 4:289–297
6. Baak JP et al (1988) Architectural and nuclear morphometrical features together are more important prognosticators in endometrial hyperplasias than nuclear morphometrical features alone. J Pathol 154:335–341
7. Baak JP et al (1992) Assessment of the risk on endometrial cancer in hyperplasia, by means of morphological and morphometrical features. Pathol Res Pract 188:856–859
8. Baak JP et al (2001) Prospective multicenter evaluation of the morphometric D-score for prediction of the outcome of endometrial hyperplasias. Am J Surg Pathol 25:930–935
9. Baergen RN et al (2001) Early uterine serous carcinoma: clonal origin of extrauterine disease. Int J Gynecol Pathol 20:214–219
10. Beckner ME, Mori T, Silverberg SG (1985) Endometrial carcinoma: nontumor factors in prognosis. Int J Gynecol Pathol 4:131–145
11. Bergeron C et al (1999) A multicentric European study testing the reproducibility of the WHO classification of endometrial hyperplasia with a proposal of a simplified working classification for biopsy and curettage specimens. Am J Surg Pathol 23:1102–1108
12. Beutler HK, Dockerty MB, Randall LM (1963) Precancerous lesions of the endometrium. Am J Obstet Gynecol 86:433–443
13. Bokhman JV (1983) Two pathogenetic types of endometrial carcinoma. Gynecol Oncol 15:10–17
14. Brinton LA et al (1992) Reproductive, menstrual, and medical risk factors for endometrial cancer: results from a case-control study. Am J Obstet Gynecol 167:1317–1325
15. Campbell PE, Barter RA (1961) The significance of atypical endometrial hyperplasia. J Obstet Gynaecol Br Commonw 68:668–672
16. Carcangiu ML, Tan LK, Chambers JT (1997) Stage IA uterine serous carcinoma: a study of 13 cases. Am J Surg Pathol 21:1507–1514
17. Chamlian DL, Taylor HB (1970) Endometrial hyperplasia in young women. Obstet Gynecol 36:659–666

18. Crum CP, Richart RM, Fenoglio CM (1981) Adenoacanthosis of endometrium: a clinicopathologic study in premenopausal women. Am J Surg Pathol 5:15–20
19. Dawagne MP, Silverberg SG (1982) Foam cells in endometrial carcinoma–a clinicopathologic study. Gynecol Oncol 13:67–75
20. Deligdisch L, Cohen CJ (1985) Histologic correlates and virulence implications of endometrial carcinoma associated with adenomatous hyperplasia. Cancer 56:1452–1455
21. Demopoulos RI, Greco MA (1983) Mucinous metaplasia of the endometrium: ultrastructural and histochemical characteristics. Int J Gynecol Pathol 1:383–390
22. Dunton CJ et al (1996) Use of computerized morphometric analyses of endometrial hyperplasias in the prediction of coexistent cancer. Am J Obstet Gynecol 174:1518–1521
23. Enomoto T et al (1993) Alterations of the p53 tumor suppressor gene and its association with activation of the c-K-ras-2 protooncogene in premalignant and malignant lesions of the human uterine endometrium. Cancer Res 53:1883–1888
24. Epplein M et al (2008) Risk of complex and atypical endometrial hyperplasia in relation to anthropometric measures and reproductive history. Am J Epidemiol 168:563–570; discussion 571–576
25. Esteller M et al (1999) hMLH1 promoter hypermethylation is an early event in human endometrial tumorigenesis. Am J Pathol 155:1767–1772
26. Ferenczy A, Gelfand M (1989) The biologic significance of cytologic atypia in progestogen-treated endometrial hyperplasia. Am J Obstet Gynecol 160:126–131
27. Fluhmann CF (1954) Comparative studies of squamous metaplasia of the cervix uteri and endometrium. Am J Obstet Gynecol 68:1447–1463
28. Gal D (1986) Hormonal therapy for lesions of the endometrium. Semin Oncol 13:33–36
29. Greenblatt RB, Gambrell RD Jr, Stoddard LD (1982) The protective role of progesterone in the prevention of endometrial cancer. Pathol Res Pract 174:297–318
30. Grimes DA (1982) Diagnostic dilation and curettage: a reappraisal. Am J Obstet Gynecol 142:1–6
31. Gucer F et al (1998) Concomitant endometrial hyperplasia in patients with endometrial carcinoma. Gynecol Oncol 69:64–68
32. Gusberg SB, Kaplan AL (1963) Precursors of Corpus Cancer. IV. Adenomatous Hyperplasia as Stage O Carcinoma of the Endometrium. Am J Obstet Gynecol 87:662–678
33. Hall TE, Stapleton JJ, McCance JM (1982) The isolated finding of histiocytes in Papanicolaou smears from postmenopausal women. J Reprod Med 27:647–650
34. Hayes MP et al (2006) PIK3CA and PTEN mutations in uterine endometrioid carcinoma and complex atypical hyperplasia. Clin Cancer Res 12:5932–5935
35. Hendrickson MR, Kempson RL (1980) Endometrial epithelial metaplasias: proliferations frequently misdiagnosed as adenocarcinoma. Report of 89 cases and proposed classification. Am J Surg Pathol 4:525–542
36. Hendrickson MR, Kempson RL (1980) Surgical pathology of the uterine corpus, vol 12. Saunders, Philadelphia
37. Hertig AT, Sommers SC (1949) Genesis of endometrial carcinoma: study of prior biopsies. Cancer 2:946–956, illust
38. Hunter JE et al (1994) The prognostic and therapeutic implications of cytologic atypia in patients with endometrial hyperplasia. Gynecol Oncol 55:66–71
39. Janicek MF, Rosenshein NB (1994) Invasive endometrial cancer in uteri resected for atypical endometrial hyperplasia. Gynecol Oncol 52:373–378
40. Jarboe EA et al (2009) Evidence for a latent precursor (p53 signature) that may precede serous endometrial intraepithelial carcinoma. Mod Pathol 22:345–350
41. Kaku T et al (1992) Endometrial metaplasia associated with endometrial carcinoma. Obstet Gynecol 80:812–816
42. Kaku T et al (1996) Endometrial carcinoma associated with hyperplasia. Gynecol Oncol 60:22–25
43. Kaminski PF, Stevens CW (1985) The value of endometrial sampling in abnormal uterine bleeding. Am J Gynecol Health II:33–36
44. Kendall BS et al (1998) Reproducibility of the diagnosis of endometrial hyperplasia, atypical hyperplasia, and well-differentiated carcinoma. Am J Surg Pathol 22:1012–1019
45. Kim YB et al (1997) Progestin alone as primary treatment of endometrial carcinoma in premenopausal women. Report of seven cases and review of the literature. Cancer 79:320–327
46. King A, Seraj IM, Wagner RJ (1984) Stromal invasion in endometrial adenocarcinoma. Am J Obstet Gynecol 149:10–14
47. Kraus FT (1985) High-risk and premalignant lesions of the endometrium. Am J Surg Pathol 9:31–40
48. Kumar NB, Hart WR (1982) Metastases to the uterine corpus from extragenital cancers. A clinicopathologic study of 63 cases. Cancer 50:2163–2169
49. Kurman RJ, Kaminski PF, Norris HJ (1985) The behavior of endometrial hyperplasia. A long-term study of "untreated" hyperplasia in 170 patients. Cancer 56:403–412
50. Kurman RJ, Norris HJ (1982) Evaluation of criteria for distinguishing atypical endometrial hyperplasia from well-differentiated carcinoma. Cancer 49:2547–2559
51. Kurman RJ, Scully RE (1976) Clear cell carcinoma of the endometrium: an analysis of 21 cases. Cancer 37:872–882
52. Kurman RJ et al (2000) Norethindrone acetate and estradiol-induced endometrial hyperplasia. Obstet Gynecol 96:373–379
53. Lacey JV Jr et al (2008) Endometrial carcinoma risk among women diagnosed with endometrial hyperplasia: the 34-year experience in a large health plan. Br J Cancer 98:45–53
54. Lacey JV Jr et al (2008) Risk of subsequent endometrial carcinoma associated with endometrial intraepithelial neoplasia classification of endometrial biopsies. Cancer 113:2073–2081
55. Lee KR, Scully RE (1989) Complex endometrial hyperplasia and carcinoma in adolescents and young women 15 to 20 years of age. A report of 10 cases. Int J Gynecol Pathol 8:201–213
56. Lehman MB, Hart WR (2001) Simple and complex hyperplastic papillary proliferations of the endometrium: a clinicopathologic study of nine cases of apparently localized papillary lesions with fibrovascular stromal cores and epithelial metaplasia. Am J Surg Pathol 25:1347–1354
57. Levine RL et al (1998) PTEN mutations and microsatellite instability in complex atypical hyperplasia, a precursor lesion to uterine endometrioid carcinoma. Cancer Res 58:3254–3258
58. Lidor A et al (1986) Histopathological findings in 226 women with post-menopausal uterine bleeding. Acta Obstet Gynecol Scand 65:41–43
59. Lin MC et al (2009) Squamous morules are functionally inert elements of premalignant endometrial neoplasia. Mod Pathol 22:167–174
60. Longacre TA et al (1995) Proposed criteria for the diagnosis of well-differentiated endometrial carcinoma. A diagnostic test for myoinvasion. Am J Surg Pathol 19:371–406
61. Masterton R, Armstrong EM, More IA (1975) The cyclical variation in the percentage of ciliated cells in the normal human endometrium. J Reprod Fertil 42:537–540

62. Mazur MT (1981) Atypical polypoid adenomyomas of the endometrium. Am J Surg Pathol 5:473–482
63. McKenney JK, Longacre TA (2009) Low-grade endometrial adenocarcinoma: a diagnostic algorithm for distinguishing atypical endometrial hyperplasia and other benign (and malignant) mimics. Adv Anat Pathol 16:1–22
64. Mittal K et al (2009) Presence of endometrial adenocarcinoma in situ in complex atypical endometrial hyperplasia is associated with increased incidence of endometrial carcinoma in subsequent hysterectomy. Mod Pathol 22:37–42
65. Mutter GL (2000) Endometrial intraepithelial neoplasia (EIN): will it bring order to chaos? The Endometrial Collaborative Group. Gynecol Oncol 76:287–290
66. Mutter GL, Chaponot ML, Fletcher JA (1995) A polymerase chain reaction assay for non-random X chromosome inactivation identifies monoclonal endometrial cancers and precancers. Am J Pathol 146:501–508
67. Mutter GL et al (2000) Endometrial precancer diagnosis by histopathology, clonal analysis, and computerized morphometry. J Pathol 190:462–469
68. Nguyen TN et al (1998) Clinical significance of histiocytes in the detection of endometrial adenocarcinoma and hyperplasia. Diagn Cytopathol 19:89–93
69. Norris HJ, Tavassoli FA, Kurman RJ (1983) Endometrial hyperplasia and carcinoma. Diagnostic considerations. Am J Surg Pathol 7:839–847
70. Novak E, Rutledge F (1948) Atypical endometrial hyperplasia simulating adenocarcinoma. Am J Obstet Gynecol 55:46–63
71. Nucci MR et al (1999) Mucinous endometrial epithelial proliferations: a morphologic spectrum of changes with diverse clinical significance. Mod Pathol 12:1137–1142
72. Potischman N et al (1996) Case-control study of endogenous steroid hormones and endometrial cancer. J Natl Cancer Inst 88:1127–1135
73. Quddus MR et al (1999) p53 immunoreactivity in endometrial metaplasia with dysfunctional uterine bleeding. Histopathology 35:44–49
74. Randall TC, Kurman RJ (1997) Progestin treatment of atypical hyperplasia and well-differentiated carcinoma of the endometrium in women under age 40. Obstet Gynecol 90:434–440
75. Reed SD et al (2009) Progestin therapy of complex endometrial hyperplasia with and without atypia. Obstet Gynecol 113:655–662
76. Rorat E, Wallach RC (1984) Papillary metaplasia of the endometrium: clinical and histopathologic considerations. Obstet Gynecol 64:90S–92S
77. Scully RE, Bonfiglio TA, Kurman RJ, Silverberg SG, Wilkinson EJ (1994) Histologic typing of female genital tract tumors (international histological classification of tumors), 2nd edn. Springer, New York, pp 1–189
78. Shah SS, Mazur MT (2008) Endometrial eosinophilic syncytial change related to breakdown: immunohistochemical evidence suggests a regressive process. Int J Gynecol Pathol 27:534–538
79. Sherman ME, Bur ME, Kurman RJ (1995) p53 in endometrial cancer and its putative precursors: evidence for diverse pathways of tumorigenesis. Hum Pathol 26:1268–1274
80. Sherman ME et al (1992) Uterine serous carcinoma. A morphologically diverse neoplasm with unifying clinicopathologic features. Am J Surg Pathol 16:600–610
81. Sherman ME et al (1997) Risk factors and hormone levels in patients with serous and endometrioid uterine carcinomas. Mod Pathol 10:963–968
82. Silver MM, Miles P, Rosa C (1991) Comparison of Novak and Pipelle endometrial biopsy instruments. Obstet Gynecol 78: 828–830
83. Silver SA, Sherman ME (1998) Morphologic and immunophenotypic characterization of foam cells in endometrial lesions. Int J Gynecol Pathol 17:140–145
84. Silverberg SG, Kurman RJ (1992) Atlas of tumor pathology. Tumors of the uterine corpus and gestational trophoblastic disease, third series, fascicle 3. Armed Forces Institute of Pathology, Washington, D.C
85. Soslow RA, Pirog E, Isacson C (2000) Endometrial intraepithelial carcinoma with associated peritoneal carcinomatosis. Am J Surg Pathol 24:726–732
86. Spiegel GW (1995) Endometrial carcinoma in situ in postmenopausal women. Am J Surg Pathol 19:417–432
87. Stovall TG, Ling FW, Morgan PL (1991) A prospective, randomized comparison of the Pipelle endometrial sampling device with the Novak curette. Am J Obstet Gynecol 165:1287–1290
88. Tashiro H et al (1997) p53 gene mutations are common in uterine serous carcinoma and occur early in their pathogenesis. Am J Pathol 150:177–185
89. Tavassoli F, Kraus FT (1978) Endometrial lesions in uteri resected for atypical endometrial hyperplasia. Am J Clin Pathol 70:770–779
90. Terakawa N et al (1997) The behavior of endometrial hyperplasia: a prospective study. Endometrial Hyperplasia Study Group. J Obstet Gynaecol Res 23:223–230
91. The Postmenopausal Estrogen/Progestin Interventions (PEPI) Trial (1996) Effects of hormone replacement therapy on endometrial histology in postmenopausal women. JAMA 275:370–375
92. Trimble CL et al (2006) Concurrent endometrial carcinoma in women with a biopsy diagnosis of atypical endometrial hyperplasia: a Gynecologic Oncology Group study. Cancer 106:812–819
93. Welch WR, Scully RE (1977) Precancerous lesions of the endometrium. Hum Pathol 8:503–512
94. Wheeler DT, Bristow RE, Kurman RJ (2007) Histologic alterations in endometrial hyperplasia and well-differentiated carcinoma treated with progestins. Am J Surg Pathol 31:988–998
95. Wheeler DT et al (2000) Minimal uterine serous carcinoma: diagnosis and clinicopathologic correlation. Am J Surg Pathol 24: 797–806
96. Widra EA et al (1995) Endometrial hyperplasia and the risk of carcinoma. Int J Gynecol Cancer 5:233–235
97. Zaino RJ et al (2006) Reproducibility of the diagnosis of atypical endometrial hyperplasia: a Gynecologic Oncology Group study. Cancer 106:804–811
98. Zaman SS, Mazur MT (1993) Endometrial papillary syncytial change. A nonspecific alteration associated with active breakdown. Am J Clin Pathol 99:741–745
99. Zhang X et al (2009) Molecular identification of "latent precancers" for endometrial serous carcinoma in benign-appearing endometrium. Am J Pathol 174:2000–2006
100. Zheng W et al (1998) p53 immunostaining as a significant adjunct diagnostic method for uterine surface carcinoma: precursor of uterine papillary serous carcinoma. Am J Surg Pathol 22: 1463–1473
101. Zheng W et al (2004) Endometrial glandular dysplasia: a newly defined precursor lesion of uterine papillary serous carcinoma. Part I: morphologic features. Int J Surg Pathol 12:207–223

9 Endometrial Carcinoma

Lora Hedrick Ellenson · Brigitte M. Ronnett · Robert A. Soslow · Richard J. Zaino · Robert J. Kurman

R. J. Kurman, L. Hedrick Ellenson, B. M. Ronnett (eds.), *Blaustein's Pathology of the Female Genital Tract (6th ed.)*, DOI 10.1007/978-1-4419-0489-8_9,

Epidemiology

Endometrial carcinoma is the most common invasive neoplasm of the female genital tract and the fourth most frequently diagnosed cancer in women in the USA. In 2008, it is estimated there will have been 40,100 new cases and 7,470 deaths resulting from this neoplasm. These figures represent an estimated 6% of the new cancer cases and 3% of the cancer deaths in women [377]. Worldwide, approximately 150,000 cases are diagnosed each year, making endometrial carcinoma the fifth most common cancer in women [304, 305]. The incidence of endometrial cancer varies widely throughout the world. The highest rates occur in North America and Europe, whereas rates in developing countries and Japan are four to five times lower. The incidence is also about twice as high in whites compared to blacks. However, the proportion of endometrial cancer related deaths is higher in blacks due to a relative increase in the incidence of high-risk endometrial carcinoma in the black population. The reason for this is not well understood but access to and quality of health care as well as genetics are considered possible factors [17].

Classification

Based on clinicopathologic and molecular genetic features, endometrial carcinoma can be broadly divided into two major categories, referred to as type I and type II. As discussed, factors associated with unopposed estrogenic stimulation, such as obesity and exogenous hormone use, as well as the presence of endometrial hyperplasia, are related to the development of the most common form of endometrial carcinoma, the endometrioid subtype, which is the prototype of type I carcinoma [44]. More recent studies have confirmed this association by demonstrating elevated serum estrogen levels in patients with endometrioid carcinoma [50, 323]. It also has been recognized that some forms of endometrial carcinoma appear to be unrelated to hormonal factors and hyperplasia [363]. Serous carcinoma is the most common form of endometrial carcinoma that is not related to estrogenic stimulation and represents type II carcinoma. Molecular genetic studies, as discussed below, have provided further support for the dualistic categorization by identifying significant molecular genetic differences between the two types (Table 9.1). Most of the other histologic subtypes of endometrial carcinoma can be classified as variants of either type I or II on the basis of clinicopathologic, immunohistochemical, and molecular features. Thus, other low-grade carcinomas, which are associated with endometrial hyperplasia and estrogenic stimulation, such as mucinous or low-grade endometrioid with squamous differentiation, are type I carcinomas. In contrast, some clear cell carcinomas share features with serous carcinoma and are considered a type II carcinoma. However, recent data suggests that clear cell carcinomas are a heterogenous group of tumors and that some may fit in the type I category (see below in Clear Cell Carcinoma).

Table 9.1
Pathogenetic forms of endometrial carcinoma

Feature	Type I	Type II
Unopposed estrogen	Present	Absent
Menopausal status	Pre- and perimenopausal	Postmenopausal
Precursor lesion	Atypical hyperplasia	Endometrial intraepithelial carcinoma
Tumor grade	Low	High
Myometrial invasion	Variable, often minimal	Variable, often deep
Histologic subtypes	Endometrioid	Serous and clear cell
Behavior	Indolent	Aggressive
Genetic alterations	PTEN mutation	P53 mutation
	Microsatellite instability	
	K-ras mutation	

A modified version of the recent World Health Organization (WHO) and International Society of Gynecological Pathologists (ISGYP) classification of endometrial carcinoma is shown in Table 9.2 [356]. This classification has certain limitations. The WHO classification uses the term papillary in the designation of serous carcinoma. Although uterine serous carcinomas often demonstrate papillary growth, a papillary pattern can be seen in other carcinomas, including villoglandular, mucinous, and clear cell carcinomas. Thus, papillary growth is not specifically associated with serous differentiation. Hence, its use in designating subtypes of endometrial carcinoma should be avoided. Malignant Mesodermal (Müllerian) mixed tumors (MMMTs, carcinosarcomas) are classified as mixed epithelial and nonepithelial tumors in the WHO classification of uterine tumors but as epithelial tumors in

Table 9.2
Classification of endometrial carcinoma[a]

Endometrioid adenocarcinoma
Villoglandular
Secretory
Ciliated cell
Endometrioid adenocarcinoma with squamous differentiation
Serous carcinoma
Clear cell carcinoma
Mucinous carcinoma
Squamous carcinoma
Mixed types of carcinoma
Undifferentiated carcinoma

[a]Modified World Health Organization and International Society of Gynecological Pathologists Histologic Classification of Endometrial Carcinoma.

the ovarian tumor classification. This inconsistency reflects the confusion over the histogenesis and classification of carcinosarcomas in different anatomic sites. Recent molecular genetic data support the concept that both components in these biphasic tumors are clonally derived from a transformed epithelial cell. Accordingly, many investigators now consider these neoplasms as poorly differentiated carcinomas that display sarcomatous differentiation (see the following).

Etiology

Hormonal Stimulation

The strong association between replacement estrogen therapy and the development of endometrial cancer was demonstrated in a number of case-control studies in the late 1970s [155, 157, 253, 264, 360, 376, 449]. More recent reviews summarize the data generated by numerous studies of hormonal therapy and risk of endometrial cancer and confirm the increased risk of unopposed estrogen therapy [39, 315]. A study of endogenous hormones and endometrial cancer demonstrated that the risk associated with elevated levels of unopposed estrogen varies according to menopausal status [323]. In particular, high estrone and albumin-bound estradiol levels were associated with increased risk in postmenopausal women, but high levels of total, free, and albumin-bound estradiol were unrelated to increased risk in premenopausal women. In addition, high circulating levels of androstenedione were identified as a risk factor in both pre- and postmenopausal women. In both age groups, the risk associated with obesity was not affected by adjustment for hormones. Factors that lower the exposure of the endometrium to unopposed estrogen reduce the risk of endometrial cancer; these include the addition of progestin to hormone replacement regimens, the use of oral contraceptives, and smoking [1, 32, 39, 131, 139, 156, 211, 243, 306, 315, 422]. It has been shown that women using unopposed estrogen for more than 2 years have a two- to threefold increase in the risk of endometrial cancer, whereas women receiving progestins in conjunction with estrogen have no increased risk [309]. One large case-control study demonstrated that the use of oral contraceptives for at least 1 year reduces the risk of endometrial carcinoma by 50% and that protection persists at least 15 years after discontinuation [1]. The risk of endometrial carcinoma may also be effected by polymorphisms in the estrogen receptor genes; however, the mechanism responsible is not currently understood [31].

The data on the risk of endometrial cancer in patients on tamoxifen are conflicting [358]. Tamoxifen is a nonsteroidal compound that acts by competing with estrogen for estrogen receptors. In reproductive age women it therefore has an antiestrogenic effect, but in postmenopausal (hypoestrogenic) women it has weak estrogenic effects. Some large studies have reported that there is a significantly increased risk of endometrial cancer, apparently related to dose and duration of use, whereas others have not shown a significant risk [25, 42, 86, 127, 128, 130, 210, 330, 338, 339, 390, 411]. In addition, some studies have reported a higher proportion of high-risk types of carcinomas in tamoxifen-treated women whereas others have found predominantly low-grade carcinomas [36, 128, 255, 370]. Thus, some investigators are convinced that tamoxifen confers an increased risk of endometrial cancer while others believe the evidence is inconclusive [90, 185, 189, 199, 223, 254].

Constitutional Factors

Obesity, like estrogen replacement therapy, is a well-defined risk factor for endometrial cancer [415], with reported relative risks ranging from 2 to 10 [304, 305]. The risk can be explained by the increased availability of peripheral estrogens as a result of aromatization of androgens to estrogens in adipose tissue and lower concentrations of sex hormone-binding globulins in obese women [114].

Diabetes has been repeatedly associated with an increased risk of endometrial cancer, ranging from 1.2 to 2.1, and this risk appears to be independent of other frequently associated variables such as obesity [50, 304, 305]. Other factors that have been associated with an increased risk of endometrial cancer include early age of menarche, later age of menopause, and nulliparity. The association with nulliparity appears to be primarily on the basis of infertility due to chronic anovulation in which unopposed estrogenic stimulation occurs [50, 305]. The protective effect of pregnancy appears to be related and restricted to the first full-term pregnancy because abortions and increasing numbers of births do not influence the risk.

Diet

Endometrial cancer risk is correlated with total caloric intake, total protein intake, and frequency of consumption of meat, eggs, milk, fats, and oils. These dietary factors, as well as decreased energy expenditure and physical exercise associated with a sedentary lifestyle, are major determinants of obesity, which is an established risk factor. The independent contribution of specific dietary factors to endometrial cancer risk has not been clearly established [245, 305]. A recent study suggests that activity decreases the risk of endometrial cancer independent of body weight [415].

Molecular Genetics

Since the initial proposal that endometrial carcinoma could be divided into two broad disease entities, it has been recognized by pathologists that there is a general correlation of the clinical type with the morphologic features of the endometrial tumor. For the most part, type I tumors are associated with endometrioid features and arise in the setting of hyperplasia, whereas type II tumors are often of serous histology and present in a background of endometrial atrophy. Although somewhat oversimplified given the diversity of histologic subtypes of endometrial carcinoma, this histologic distinction is important to the understanding of endometrial carcinoma at the molecular level. For conceptual and practical reasons, this section does not attempt to provide an exhaustive list of the cancer-causing genes that have been studied but rather is intended to provide the reader with an overview of the current understanding of the molecular genetics of endometrial carcinoma. For this reason, the two tumor types are discussed separately, recognizing that many of the early molecular studies did not clearly classify the tumors by morphologic type.

Endometrioid Carcinoma

Over the past 3 decades, a number of cancer-causing genes have been analyzed in endometrial carcinoma. Recently, a number of studies have shown that the most frequently altered gene in endometrioid carcinoma is the *PTEN* tumor suppressor gene, which is mutated in 30–54% of cases [333, 395]. *PTEN* is located on chromosome 10q23.3 and encodes a dual-specificity phosphatase [247]. The primary target is the lipid molecule phosphatidylinositol-3,4,5-triphosphate (PIP3) that is involved in a signal transduction pathway that regulates cell growth and apoptosis. The dephosphorylation of PIP3 counteracts the activity of a protein complex called PI3K (phosphoinositol 3 kinase) that leads to the conversion of PIP2 (phosphatidylinositol-4,5-diphosphate) to PIP3. Consequently, the inactivating mutations in *PTEN* result in increased levels of PIP3, which activates downstream molecules including phosphorylation of AKT. AKT is a central regulator of numerous pathways involved in cell proliferation, cell growth, and apoptosis that are altered in cancer development. Although the specific consequences of *PTEN* mutation have not been completely elucidated in endometrial carcinoma development it has been noted that the frequency of *PTEN* mutation is similar in all three grades of endometrioid carcinoma. In addition, it is mutated in approximately 20–48% of atypical and nonatypical hyperplasias [246, 259]. These findings suggest that inactivation of this gene is important early in the pathogenesis of endometrioid carcinoma. Genetic mouse models with germline heterozygous deletion of *PTEN* spontaneously develop endometrial hyperplasia in 100% of female mice with 20% of female mice showing progression to carcinoma supporting an early role of *Pten* in endometrial tumorigenesis [320]. Furthermore, a recent epidemiologic study found that the presence of *PTEN* mutations in complex atypical hyperplasia did not predict progression to carcinoma [230]. In sum, these findings suggest that *PTEN* mutations may be central to the development of hyperplasia, but may not play a role in the transition to carcinoma.

Of further interest, recent publications have identified mutations in the *PIK3CA* oncogene, the catalytic subunit of PI3K, in endometrioid carcinoma [170, 301]. The mutations are found in endometrioid carcinoma with and without *PTEN* mutations but are more common in tumors with *PTEN* mutations. An additional study showed that while *PTEN* mutations occur in a similar frequency in complex atypical hyperplasia and carcinoma, *PIK3CA* mutations are rare in complex atypical hyperplasia and occur in approximately 39% of carcinoma and are present in all three tumor grades [170]. These studies suggest that the inactivation of *PTEN* and the activation of *PIK3CA* have different roles in the development of endometrioid carcinoma. While *PTEN* is important in the development of hyperplasia, mutations in *PIK3CA* may play a role in the transition of complex atypical hyperplasia to carcinoma. Although the biologic basis of this has not yet been elucidated, understanding *PTEN* and *PIK3CA* mutations and their roles in the development of endometrial hyperplasia and carcinoma may provide targets for therapeutic intervention before the development of malignant disease.

The *p53* tumor suppressor gene has been extensively studied in endometrial cancer, as in other tumors. *p53* encodes a DNA-binding phosphoprotein that is involved in cell cycle control and apoptosis. Mutations in *p53* are found in approximately 10% of all endometrioid carcinomas, with most occurring in grade 3, and occasionally in grade 2, tumors. Overall, *p53* mutations occur in approximately 50% of grade 3 tumors, and they have not been identified in grade 1 tumors or endometrial hyperplasia [234]. This finding is consistent with a role for p53 in the progression, but not the initiation, of endometrioid carcinoma.

Another molecular alteration in endometrioid carcinomas that has received substantial attention is the molecular phenotype called microsatellite instability. Microsatellite instability is defined as alterations in the length of short, repetitive DNA sequences, called microsatellites, in tumors when compared to DNA prepared from the same patient's normal tissue. This molecular phenotype is detected in tumors that lack an intact DNA mismatch repair system, a fundamental cellular mechanism for preventing DNA alterations that are created largely during DNA replication. In tumors that display microsatellite instability, the DNA mismatch repair system has been inactivated either through mutation or "silencing" by promoter hypermethylation of one of the DNA mismatch repair genes [118]. The consequence of inactivating the DNA mismatch repair system is an increase in the rate at which mutations occur, a factor that clearly contributes to tumorigenesis. Microsatellite instability is found in tumors from patients affected by hereditary nonpolyposis colorectal carcinoma (HNPCC), a syndrome in which endometrial carcinoma is the most common noncolorectal malignancy [115]. Microsatellite instability also is present in approximately 20% of sporadic endometrial cancers and can be found in complex atypical hyperplasias that are associated with cancers that demonstrate instability [107, 246, 280]. Recent reports have suggested that like colorectal carcinoma, endometrial carcinomas with microsatellite instability may demonstrate specific histologic features (see below in discussion of ➲ Hereditary Nonpolyposis Colorectal Carcinoma) [52]. Unlike the familial cases, which are due to germline mutations in one of the DNA mismatch repair genes (*MSH2*, *MLH1*, *MSH6*, or *PMS2*), microsatellite instability in the sporadic cases is most commonly due to inactivation of the *MLH1* gene by promoter hypermethylation. This epigenetic alteration results in lack of expression of MLH1, which can be detected by immunohistochemistry. Interestingly, the hypermethylation of *MLH1* can be found in complex atypical hyperplasia that does not demonstrate microsatellite instability [116]. Thus, it remains unclear exactly when in the development of endometrial neoplasia the DNA mismatch repair system becomes inactivated. Further studies of endometrial hyperplasia are warranted to address this important biologic and potentially clinically relevant question.

A number of oncogenes have been studied in endometrial carcinomas, but only a few are altered in a significant number of cases. Mutations in the *KRAS* proto-oncogene have been identified consistently in 10–30% of endometrial cancers in several studies [48, 113, 234]. The mutations have been found in all grades of endometrioid carcinoma and have been reported in complex atypical hyperplasia, suggesting a relatively early role for *KRAS* mutations in this tumor type. *KRAS* encodes a guanine nucleotide-binding protein of 21 kDa that plays a role in the regulation of cell growth and differentiation by transducing signals from activated transmembrane receptors. In the mutant form, *KRAS* is constitutively "on" even in the absence of an activated receptor. Recently, mutations in *FGFR2* (fibroblast growth factor receptor 2) have been identified in 16% of endometrioid carcinomas and that *KRAS* and *FGFR2* mutations are mutually exclusive [55, 321]. In addition, mutations in the *CTNNB1* gene, which encodes the β-catenin protein, have been found in approximately 15–20% of endometrioid carcinomas, occurring primarily in tumors with squamous differentiation [133, 220, 353]. Other oncogenes that have been found to be overexpressed or amplified are *EGFR*, *CMYC*, *HER-2/neu*, *BCL2*, and *CFMS* [47, 177, 242, 397]. Additional studies on these genes are needed to more definitively determine their role in endometrial cancer.

Serous Carcinoma

Compared to endometrioid carcinoma, relatively little is known about serous carcinoma at the molecular level, partly because of its relative infrequency and because this tumor type is not analyzed separately in many molecular studies. Although a number of candidate cancer genes have been analyzed in serous carcinoma, only the *p53* tumor suppressor gene has been shown to be altered in a significant number, with mutations identified in almost 90% of cases [273, 396]. In fact, there are few other solid tumors that demonstrate a mutation frequency in a single gene as high as that of *p53* in serous endometrial carcinoma. Furthermore, approximately 75% of endometrial intraepithelial carcinomas, the putative precursor of serous carcinoma, have mutations in *p53* [396]. In this setting, it has been shown that intense, diffuse immunohistochemical staining for *p53* correlates well with *p53* mutation. These findings suggest that in serous carcinoma *p53* mutations occur relatively early and are central to the development of this tumor type; this is in contrast to endometrioid carcinoma, in which *p53* mutations are relatively uncommon and, when they do occur, they are largely confined to grade 3 tumors. Thus, it is possible that the mutation of *p53* early in the pathogenesis of serous carcinoma is an important factor that accounts for its aggressive behavior. In addition, the fact that *p53* mutations occur most commonly in grade 3 endometrioid and serous carcinomas most likely explains the finding that it is an indicator of tumors that behave aggressively [16].

In contrast to endometrioid carcinoma, mutations in *KRAS* and *PTEN* appear to be very uncommon in serous carcinoma, and microsatellite instability has not definitively been detected in this tumor type [234]. A recent study has described mutations in *PIK3CA* in 15% of serous carcinoma suggesting that the PI3K/PTEN/AKT pathway may be involved in the pathogenesis of a subset of this tumor type [169]. The same study found that 56% of serous carcinoma demonstrated staining for EGFR although they lacked intragenic mutations in the commonly mutated exons and failed to show significant amplification by flourescent in situ hybridization (FISH) analysis. Studies have suggested that there is amplification and overexpression of *CMYC* and *HER-2/neu*; however, it is not clear from the literature what percentage of serous carcinomas demonstrates these alterations.

As is apparent from this discussion, relatively little is known about the molecular pathogenesis of the two major types of endometrial carcinoma and almost nothing is known about the more uncommon histologic types of endometrial carcinoma. However, it is evident from the studies just described that endometrioid and serous carcinoma of the endometrium are distinct biologic entities. As in other tumor systems, the molecular studies of endometrial cancer support the notion that epithelial-derived tumors often develop from preinvasive precursors that accumulate a combination of genetic alterations, thus providing the cell with the attributes necessary for unregulated growth. In endometrioid carcinoma it appears that *PTEN* alterations may be central to the initiation of proliferative lesions that then acquire mutations in other cancer-causing genes (e.g., *PIK3CA*, DNA mismatch repair genes, *KRAS*, and *p53*) in the progression to malignancy. On the other hand, *p53* mutations appear to be important in the conversion of relatively quiescent, atrophic endometrium to an intraepithelial form of serous carcinoma that then sets the stage for the accumulation of alterations in yet unidentified cancer-causing genes.

The genes that have been described to play a role in endometrial cancer to date have been genes discovered in other tumor systems that have subsequently been found to have alterations in endometrial cancer. It is likely, with the technologic advances occurring in human genetics and the information being provided by the human genome project, novel genes that are involved in endometrial carcinogenesis will be identified.

Hereditary Syndromes

Hereditary Nonpolyposis Colorectal Carcinoma (Lynch Syndrome)

Lynch syndrome is the most common cause of familial endometrial carcinoma. It is due to germline transmission of defective DNA mismatch repair genes (*MSH2*, *MLH1*, *MSH6*, and *PMS2*) resulting in an autosomal-dominant inheritance pattern. As described above, mutations in DNA mismatch repair genes result in the molecular phenotype of microsatellite instability (MSI), which is thought to result in an increased rate of mutations in cancer-causing genes, thus predisposing affected individuals to the development of various cancers. Endometrial carcinoma is an integral part of HNPCC and women with early onset endometrial carcinoma may be probands for affected families (discussed below).

Up to one-third of endometrioid carcinomas demonstrate abnormal DNA MMR protein expression [101, 272, 308, 414]. This results from *MLH1* promoter hypermethylation in most cases or mutation of *MLH1*, *MSH2*, *MSH6*, or *PMS2* in the rest. Mutation, but not loss of expression alone, of one of these genes indicates that the affected patient may be part of HNPCC kindred. Therefore, DNA MMR protein immunohistochemistry serves as a screen for HNPCC; it is not a diagnostic test. For practical purposes, loss of expression of MSH2 and/or

MSH6 is considered a surrogate for the presence of a mutation involving one of the corresponding genes, whereas loss of expression of *MLH1* and/or *PMS2* is more likely associated with an epigenetic etiology unassociated with HNPCC.

In an effort to define a target endometrial cancer population in which the DNA MMR stains might be informative, several institutions have now begun testing for DNA MMR abnormalities in endometrial carcinomas that occur in women younger than 50 years and in older women whose tumors exhibit morphologic features that have been reported to covary with high levels of microsatellite instability (MSI-H). Such morphologic features, although not specific and currently considered of debatable significance, include dense peritumoral lymphocytes and [140] tumor infiltrating lymphocytes (greater than 40 TILs per ten high power fields), and tumors with undifferentiated components [365]. Most HNPCC tumors are endometrioid, but a proportion of clear cell and undifferentiated carcinomas, and perhaps even serous carcinomas and MMMTs, may also belong to this group [52]. It is increasingly recognized that clear cell carcinoma of the endometrium might represent a manifestation of HNPCC [60]; as such, there are rare clear cell carcinomas with loss of *MSH2* and *MSH6*, related to mutations in the corresponding genes. The preliminary data from a study investigating the feasibility and utility of testing such patients' tumors for DNA MMR expression indicate disproportionate representation of tumors lacking *MSH2* and *MSH6* expression, indirectly indicating mutation in either of the corresponding genes and possible membership in an HNPCC kindred [140]. Any patient with an abnormal immunohistochemical result should be referred for a comprehensive genetics evaluation that might include MSI testing and, when indicated, methylation and mutational analysis of the candidate genes.

Loss of expression tends to occur in couplets (*MLH1* with *PMS2* and *MSH2* with *MSH6*), although examples of isolated *PMS2* loss (without *MLH1*) or *MSH6* loss (without *MSH2*) are certainly on record. Only complete expression loss in the setting of a valid positive internal control is considered interpretable. Valid internal controls include nonneoplastic endometrial stroma and glands with reproducibly stained nuclei see below in ➋ Endometrioid Carcinoma Immunohistochemical Findings. Care should be taken to ensure that the lesion being assessed is carcinoma, not hyperplasia. It is also extremely important that the immunohistochemical methodology and interpretation of stains be performed with the strictest guidelines in mind, as performing and interpreting the *MLH1* stain, in particular, can be very problematic. Interpreting an *MLH1* stain as negative in the absence of a valid positive internal control is a rather common occurrence. Common pitfalls interpreting these stains are discussed in a recent review [364]. In one series, IHC with *MLH1* and *MSH2* antibodies had a sensitivity of 69% and a specificity of 100% in detecting MSI-H [272]. The addition of *PMS2* and *MSH6* antibodies improved the sensitivity to 91%, but decreased the specificity to 83%. The decreased specificity was primarily due to loss of *MSH6*, likely due to mutation of *MSH6*, which has been found in endometrial carcinomas that are MSI-low or MS-stable [166]. It has been proposed that a simple immunohistochemical panel including only *MSH6* and *PMS2* could allow recognition of all colorectal carcinoma mutation carriers but this has not yet been tested in endometrial carcinoma patients [366].

Cowden Syndrome

Cowden syndrome is an autosomal-dominant disorder caused by mutations in the *PTEN* tumor suppressor gene and is defined by a number of benign conditions and an increase in the risk of malignancies of the breast, thyroid, and endometrium. The risk of endometrial carcinoma in women with Cowden syndrome is estimated to be between 5% and 10% lifetime risk versus a 2.6% in the general population. The syndrome is recognized in approximately one in 200,000 individuals and the histologic type of endometrial carcinoma has not been described [283]. As discussed above, given the increase in lifetime risk, it is currently recommended that women with Cowden syndrome be screened for endometrial carcinoma with blind biopsies annually starting at 35–40 years of age or 5 years prior to the earliest diagnosis of endometrial carcinoma in the family and with annual endometrial ultrasound in postmenopausal women.

Clinical and Pathologic Features of Specific Types of Carcinomas

Endometrioid Carcinoma

Endometrioid carcinoma is the most common form of endometrial carcinoma, accounting for more than three-fourths of all cases. These tumors are referred to as endometrioid because they resemble proliferative-phase endometrium and to maintain consistency with the terminology used for describing tumors with the same histologic appearance in the cervix, ovary, or fallopian tube. The tumors in this category, by definition, do not contain areas showing more than 10% of serous, mucinous, or clear cell differentiation. Such foci are common in endometrioid carcinoma and are designated as mixed (see Mixed Types of Carcinoma).

Clinical Features

Patients with endometrioid carcinoma range in age from the second to the eighth decade, with a mean age of 59 years. Most women are postmenopausal, as the disease is relatively uncommon in young women. Only 1–8% of endometrial carcinomas occur in women under 40 years [96, 105, 151, 312, 336]. A small number of cases have been reported in women under the age of 30 years, the youngest being 15 years [121, 239]. In young women, the tumor is generally low grade and minimally invasive. In most series, the majority of patients have had clinical evidence of polycystic ovary disease (irregular menses, infertility, obesity, or hirsutism) but in some reports the patients lacked these features. Rarely, endometrioid carcinoma occurs during pregnancy [179]. In pregnant women, endometrial carcinomas are nearly always low grade, superficially invasive or noninvasive, and have an excellent prognosis.

The initial manifestation of endometrial carcinoma usually is abnormal vaginal bleeding, although rarely the patient is asymptomatic and the diagnosis is made fortuitously. In one study, 24 asymptomatic women with unsuspected endometrial carcinoma were detected among 8,998 women dying of unrelated causes who were autopsied at the Yale–New Haven and Massachusetts General Hospitals [183]. The estimated rates of undetected endometrial carcinoma were 22 and 31 per 10,000, respectively. These rates were four to five times higher than the diagnosis of endometrial carcinoma recorded by the Connecticut State Tumor Registry, indicating that a number of endometrial carcinomas may be asymptomatic and are undetected during life.

A number of studies have evaluated cytologic screening of endometrial cancer. Both direct endometrial sampling and examination of cervical cytologic smears for the presence of endometrial carcinoma have been performed. In a study of 2,586 asymptomatic women the prevalence of occult carcinoma using endometrial cytological sampling was 6.96 per 1,000; however, four cases were missed [226]. In addition, the investigators emphasized that endometrial smears were difficult to interpret and that the detection methods were only moderately reliable. About a third of the cases would have been detected using a vaginal pool specimen. In a population-based study from Australia, it was found that when a cervical smear was reported as showing endometrial carcinoma, the lesion was confirmed histologically in only 64% of cases [270]. Conversely, among women with endometrial carcinoma a cervical smear performed in the 2 years preceding the diagnosis predicted the presence of endometrial carcinoma in only 28% of cases. Because the sensitivity and specificity of cytologic examination for the detection of endometrial carcinoma is low in asymptomatic women, it is not a cost-effective screening tool for endometrial cancer. In an attempt to use cytologic screening in specific high-risk populations, it was reported that among 597 asymptomatic women over the age of 45 with diabetes and/or hypertension the diabetic women had a significantly higher rate of atypical hyperplasia compared with women with hypertension, suggesting that screening might be useful in diabetic patients [160]. In another study of endometrial cytology in 541 women, all 16 carcinomas were detected by cytologic examination; however, because all but one patient were symptomatic, the ability to detect cancers in asymptomatic women could not be assessed [405]. Similarly, endometrial brush sampling detected all but one of 13 cancers in 1,042 symptomatic patients in another study [219]. Cytologic detection methods in symptomatic women are thus of little value as women with abnormal vaginal bleeding are evaluated by either endometrial biopsy or curettage, which yields a more easily interpreted specimen.

Gross Findings

The gross appearance of endometrioid carcinoma is similar to the various other types of endometrial carcinoma with the possible exception of serous carcinoma or malignant mesodermal mixed tumors (see Serous Carcinoma and Malignant Mesodermal Mixed Tumors). The endometrial surface is shaggy, glistening, and tan and may be focally hemorrhagic. Endometrioid carcinoma is almost uniformly exophytic even when deeply invasive. The neoplasm may be focal or diffuse. At times the tumor may appear to be composed of separate polypoid masses. Necrosis usually is not evident macroscopically in well-differentiated carcinomas but may be seen in poorly differentiated tumors, sometimes in association with ulcerated or firm areas. Myometrial invasion by carcinoma may result in the enlargement of the uterus, but a small atrophic uterus may harbor carcinoma diffusely invading the myometrium. Myometrial invasion usually appears as well-demarcated, firm, gray-white tissue with linear extensions beneath an exophytic mass or as multiple, white nodules with yellow areas of necrosis within the uterine wall. However, uncommon cases of well-differentiated carcinoma may show extensive myometrial invasion in the absence of a grossly identifiable invasive component.

Extension into the lower uterine segment is common, whereas the involvement of the cervix occurs in approximately 20% of cases.

Microscopic Findings: Grading

The grade of endometrioid carcinoma is determined by the microscopic appearance of the tumor. It is based on the architectural pattern, nuclear features, or both (➲ *Figs. 9.1–9.16*). The architectural grade is determined by the extent to which the tumor is composed of solid masses of cells as compared with well-defined glands (➲ *Table 9.3*) (➲ *Figs. 9.1*, ➲ *9.3–9.7*, ➲ *9.10*, ➲ *9.12*, ➲ *9.13*, ➲ *9.15*). In endometrioid carcinomas with squamous differentiation, it is important to exclude masses of squamous epithelium in determining the amount of solid growth (see the following). The nuclear grade is determined by the variation in nuclear size and shape, chromatin distribution, and size of the nucleoli. Grade 1 nuclei are oval, mildly enlarged, and have evenly dispersed chromatin (➲ *Figs. 9.2* and ➲ *9.8*). Grade 3 nuclei are markedly enlarged and pleomorphic, with irregular coarse chromatin, and prominent eosinophilic nucleoli (➲ *Fig. 9.14*). Grade 2 nuclei have features intermediate to grades 1 and 3 (➲ *Figs. 9.9* and ➲ *9.16*). Mitotic activity is an independent histologic variable, but it is generally increased with increasing nuclear grade, as are abnormal mitotic figures.

The most recent revision of the FIGO (International Federation of Gynecology and Obstetrics) Staging System (➲ *Table 9.4*) and the WHO Histopathologic Classification of uterine carcinoma recommend that tumors be graded using both architectural and nuclear criteria [89, 356]. The grade of tumors that are architecturally grade 1 or 2 should be increased by one grade in the presence of "notable" nuclear atypia, defined as grade 3 nuclei [438]. For example, a tumor that is grade 2 by

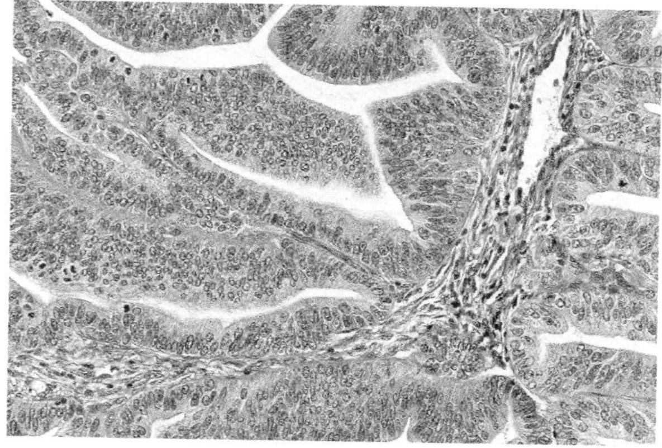

◘ Fig. 9.2
Endometrioid carcinoma, FIGO grade 1 (architectural grade 1, nuclear grade 1). **Well-formed glands have small, round to oval nuclei with uniform chromatin**

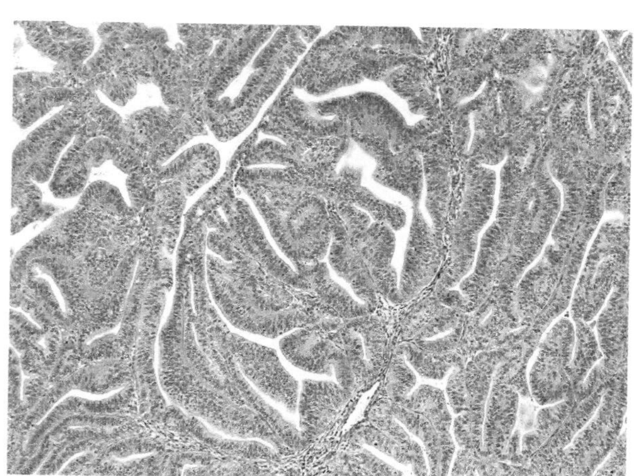

◘ Fig. 9.1
Endometrioid carcinoma, FIGO grade 1 (architectural grade 1, nuclear grade 1). **Well-differentiated glands display a confluent glandular pattern with surrounding desmoplastic stroma; these features indicate endometrial stromal invasion by carcinoma** (Courtesy of EC Pirog and K Loukeris)

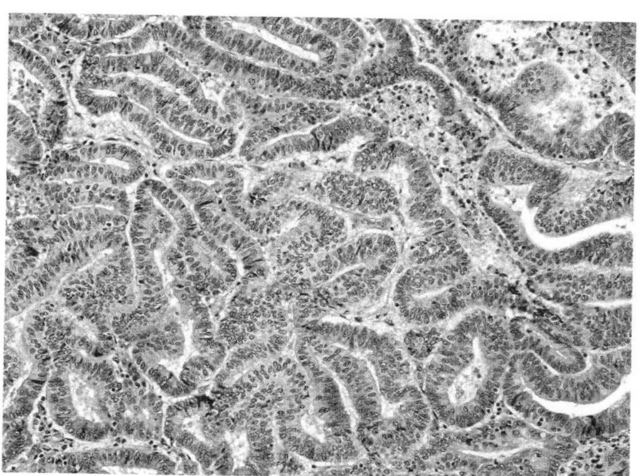

◘ Fig. 9.3
Endometrioid carcinoma, FIGO grade 1 (architectural grade 1, nuclear grade 1). **Glandular epithelium displays a confluent pattern indicating endometrial stromal invasion by carcinoma**

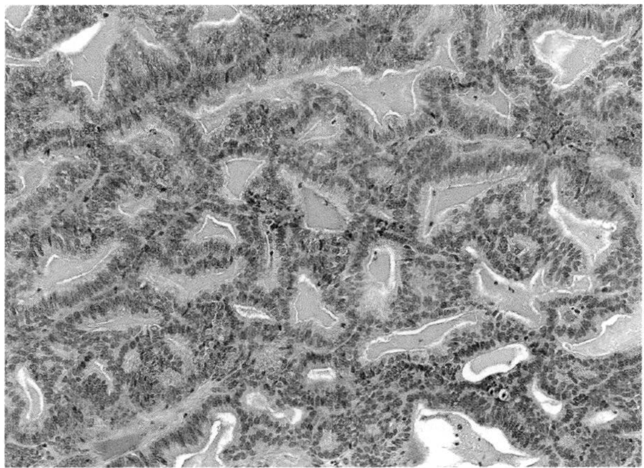

◘ Fig. 9.4
Endometrioid carcinoma, FIGO grade 1 (architectural grade 1, nuclear grade 1). **Well-differentiated glands are back-to-back with foci of fusion. The latter is indicative of carcinoma**

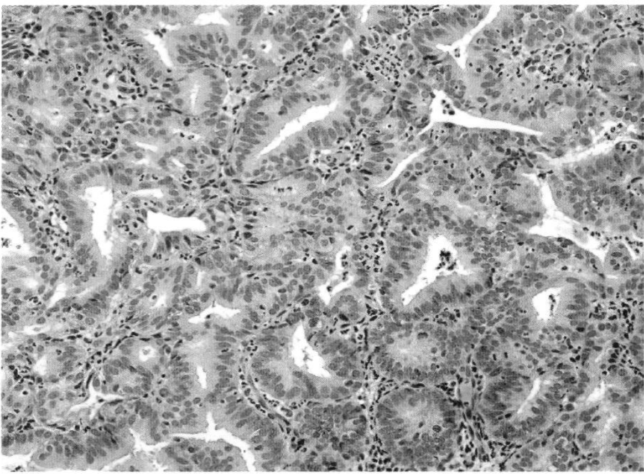

◘ Fig. 9.6
Endometrioid carcinoma, FIGO grade 1 (architectural grade 1, nuclear grade 1). **Fused glands are consistent with carcinoma**

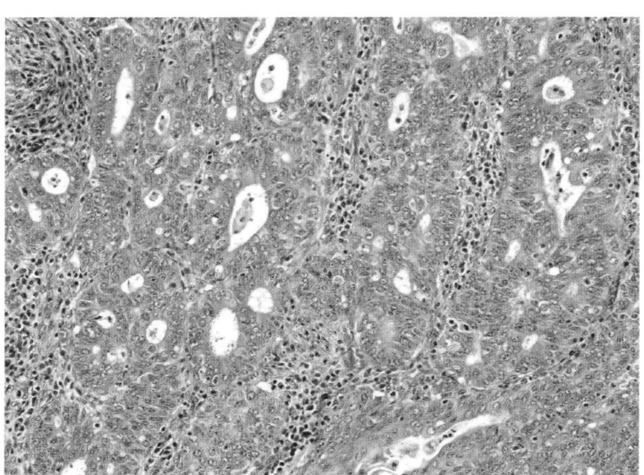

◘ Fig. 9.5
Endometrioid carcinoma, FIGO grade 1 (architectural grade 1, nuclear grade 2). **Well-differentiated glands exhibit cribriform growth, a pattern indicating endometrial stromal invasion by carcinoma**

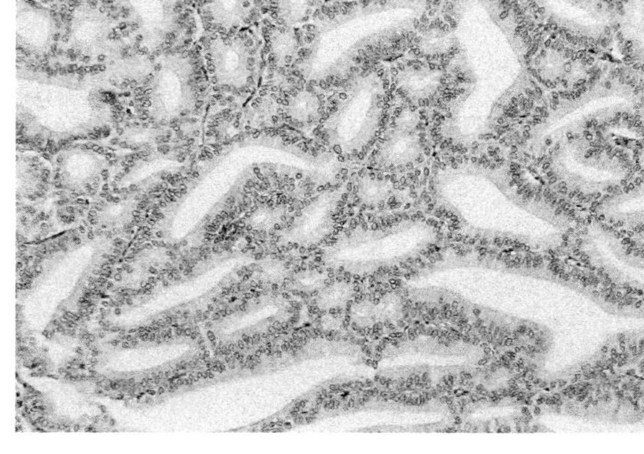

◘ Fig. 9.7
Endometrioid carcinoma, FIGO grade 1 (architectural grade 1, nuclear grade 1). **Back-to-back and fused well-differentiated glands have mucinous features**

architecture but in which there is marked nuclear atypia (nuclear grade 3) should be upgraded to grade 3. Thus, tumors are graded primarily by their architecture, with the overall grade modified by the nuclear grade when there is discordance. Marked discordance between nuclear and architectural grade is unusual in endometrioid carcinoma and should raise suspicion that the tumor is a serous carcinoma (see ➋ Serous Carcinoma). For a further discussion of grading, see ➋ Histologic Grade.

Marked differences in architectural grade can be seen within a tumor. It is not unusual to see well-formed glandular elements immediately adjacent to solid masses of cells. When a tumor displays this type of heterogeneity, the architectural grade should be based on the overall appearance. The heterogeneity in differentiation accounts for the differences in grade that can be observed between the endometrial curettings and the hysterectomy specimen. Discordance between the curettage and hysterectomy specimens occurs in 15–25% of cases [99, 232, 299].

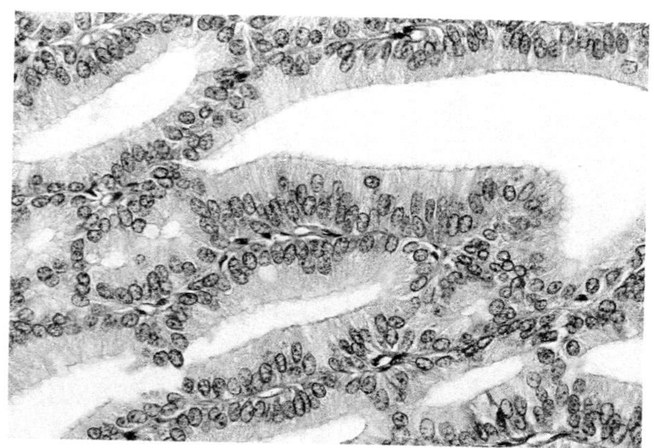

Fig. 9.8
Endometrioid carcinoma, FIGO grade 1 (architectural grade 1, nuclear grade 1). **Nuclei are round to oval with uniform chromatin**

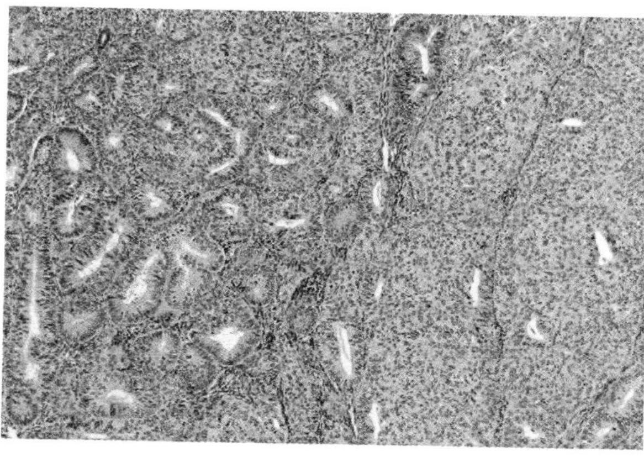

Fig. 9.10
Endometrioid carcinoma, FIGO grade 2 (architectural grade 2, nuclear grade 1). **Well-formed glands are admixed with solid nonsquamous nests of tumor, with the latter comprising more than 5% but less than 50% of the overall tumor**

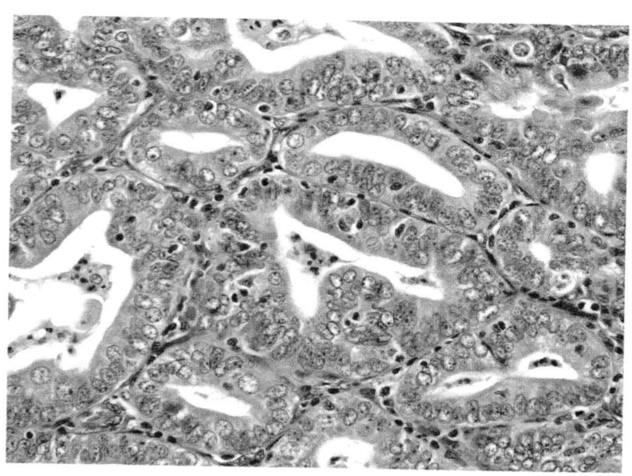

Fig. 9.9
Endometrioid carcinoma, FIGO grade 1 (architectural grade 1, nuclear grade 2). **Nuclei are somewhat enlarged, rounded, and have granular to vesicular chromatin with occasional small nucleoli**

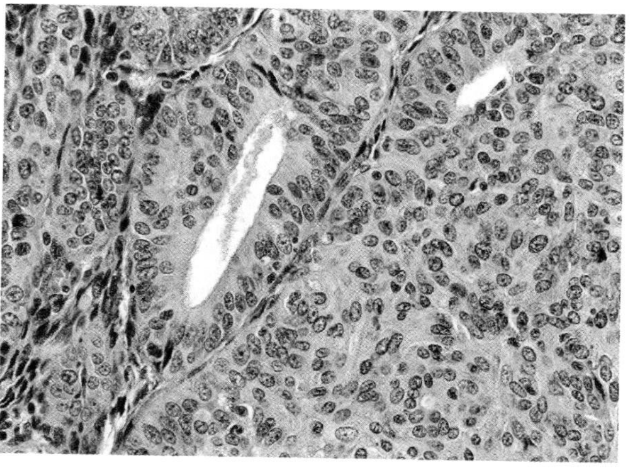

Fig. 9.11
Endometrioid carcinoma, FIGO grade 2 (architectural grade 2, nuclear grade 1). **Glandular and solid areas have generally uniform small, round to oval nuclei with granular chromatin**

Myoinvasion

Endometrial carcinoma may manifest different forms of myometrial invasion (*Figs. 9.17* and *9.18*). It can invade along a broad pushing front or it can infiltrate the myometrium diffusely as masses, cords, or clusters of cells, and individual glands. When it invades along a broad front it may be difficult to determine whether invasion is in fact present unless it can be compared to the adjacent uninvolved endomyometrium. When the tumor diffusely invades the myometrium the neoplastic glands usually elicit a reactive stromal response characterized by loose fibrous tissue accompanied by a chronic inflammatory infiltrate that surrounds the glands. Occasionally, well-differentiated carcinomas may be deeply invasive with glands directly in contact with surrounding myometrium in the absence of a stromal response (diffusely infiltrative or adenoma malignum pattern of invasion) [250, 256].

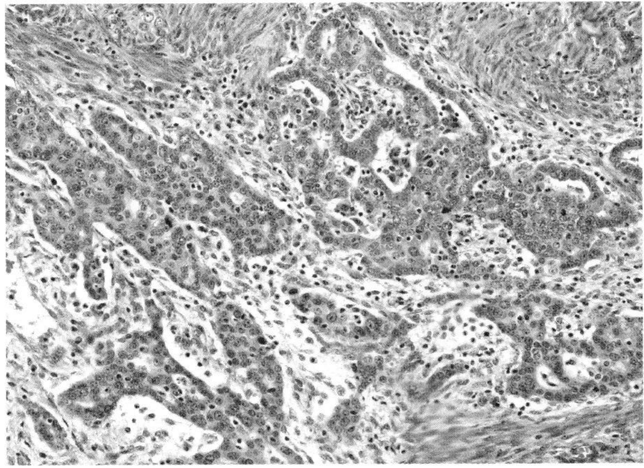

■ Fig. 9.12
Endometrioid carcinoma, FIGO grade 2 (architectural grade 2, nuclear grade 2). **Tumor is composed of intimately admixed glandular and solid nonsquamous epithelium within an edematous and inflamed altered stroma**

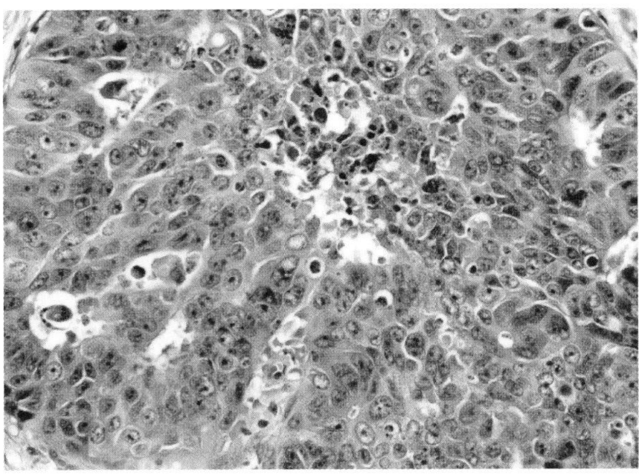

■ Fig. 9.14
Endometrioid carcinoma, FIGO grade 3 (architectural grade 3, nuclear grade 3). **Solid nonsquamous tumor with foci of necrosis and rare residual glandular lumens displays notable nuclear atypia characterized by nuclear enlargement and pleomorphism with vesicular chromatin and prominent nucleoli**

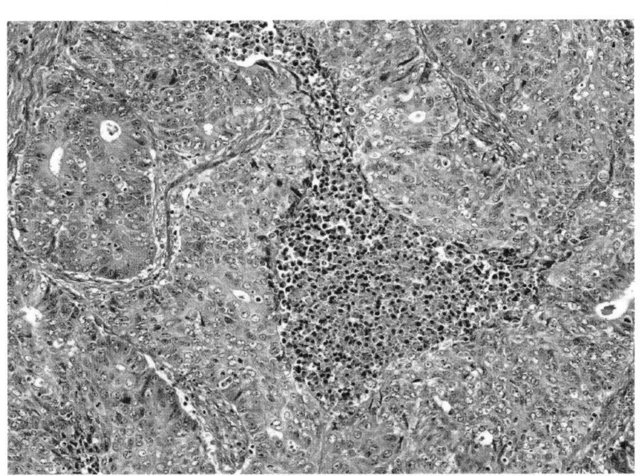

■ Fig. 9.13
Endometrioid carcinoma, FIGO grade 3 (architectural grade 3, nuclear grade 3). **A few residual glandular structures are present within an otherwise solid nonsquamous (>50%) tumor with areas of necrosis**

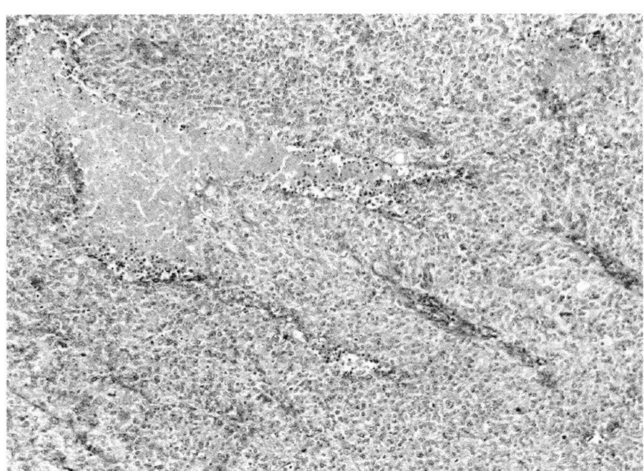

■ Fig. 9.15
Endometrioid carcinoma, FIGO grade 3 (architectural grade 3, nuclear grade 2). **Tumor is composed of solid nonsquamous epithelium with areas of necrosis**

In these cases, when myometrial invasion is superficial the presence of invasion can be identified if a haphazard glandular arrangement is present. Usually this pattern of invasion is found in deeply invasive tumors, however, and therefore recognizing myometrial invasion is not a problem. Endometrioid carcinomas with the diffusely infiltrative pattern of invasion share the same prognostic indicators of clinically aggressive disease as those having the more conventional pattern of myometrial invasion [250]. An unusual form of myoinvasion has been described that consists of outpouching of neoplastic glands that become detached and may be lined by flattened epithelium sometimes appearing as microcysts, which is associated with a fibromyxoid stromal reaction (● *Fig. 9.18*). This type of invasion has been termed MELF,

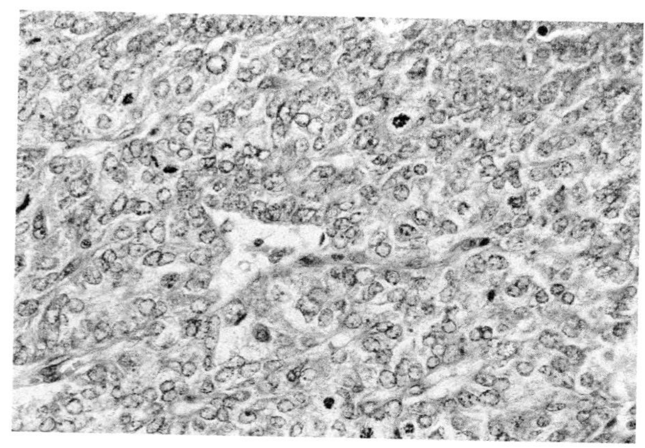

Fig. 9.16
Endometrioid carcinoma, FIGO grade 3 (architectural grade 3, nuclear grade 2). **Nuclei are only modestly pleomorphic, with vesicular chromatin and numerous mitotic figures. Spaces consistent with residual gland lumens favor endometrioid rather than undifferentiated carcinoma and clear cytoplasmic change in the absence of any other characteristic features of clear cell carcinoma is insufficient to diagnose the latter**

Table 9.3
Architectural grading of endometrial carcinoma

Grade	Description
Grade 1	No more than 5% of the tumor is composed of solid masses
Grade 2	6–50% of the tumor is composed of solid masses
Grade 3	More than 50% of the tumor is composed of solid masses

which stands for microcystic, elongated, and fragmented [279]. In the study cited, MELF invasion was associated with lymphovascular invasion, but not with poor prognosis in a multivariate analysis.

It may be difficult to distinguish myometrial invasion from the extension of the carcinoma into adenomyosis (*Fig. 9.19*). The distinction, however, is important because the presence of carcinoma in adenomyosis deeper than the maximum depth of true tumor invasion does not worsen the prognosis [164, 176, 195, 271]. When the carcinoma is surrounded by endometrial stroma and residual benign glands are present in these foci, the diagnosis of carcinoma extending into adenomyosis is straightforward. At times, however, the distinction from myometrial invasion may be extremely difficult, particularly in older women in whom adenomyosis may

Table 9.4
International Federation of Gynecology and Obstetrics Staging of Endometrial Cancer, 2009

Stage	Grade	Description
IA	G123	Tumor limited to the inner half of myometrium
IB	G123	Tumor invasion into the outer half of myometrium
II	G123	Tumor invades cervical stroma[a]
IIIA	G123	Tumor invades serosa and/or adnexa[b]
IIIB	G123	Vaginal and/or parametrial involvement
IIIC1	G123	Metastases to pelvic lymph nodes
IIIC2	G123	Metastases to paraaortic lymph nodes
IVA	G123	Tumor invasion of bladder and/or bowel mucosa
IVB	G123	Distant metastases including intraabdominal and/or inguinal lymph nodes

G1, 5% or less of a nonsquamous or nonmorular solid growth pattern; G2, 6–50% of a nonsquamous or nonmorular solid growth pattern; G3, more than 50% of a nonsquamous or nonmorular solid growth pattern.
Rules on staging:
1. Corpus cancer is now surgically staged. Those patients who do not undergo a surgical procedure should be staged according to the 1971 FIGO clinical staging.
2. Ideally, the thickness of the myometrium should be measured along with the depth of tumor invasion.
Notes on grading:
1. Notable nuclear atypia, inappropriate for the architectural grade, raises a grade 1 or grade 2 tumor by one grade.
2. In serous adenocarcinomas, clear cell adenocarcinomas, and squamous cell carcinomas, nuclear grading takes precedence.
3. Adenocarcinomas with squamous differentiation are graded according to the nuclear grade of the glandular component.
[a]Endocervical gland involvement should be considered stage I.
[b]Positive peritoneal fluid cytology should be reported separately, but does not affect the stage.

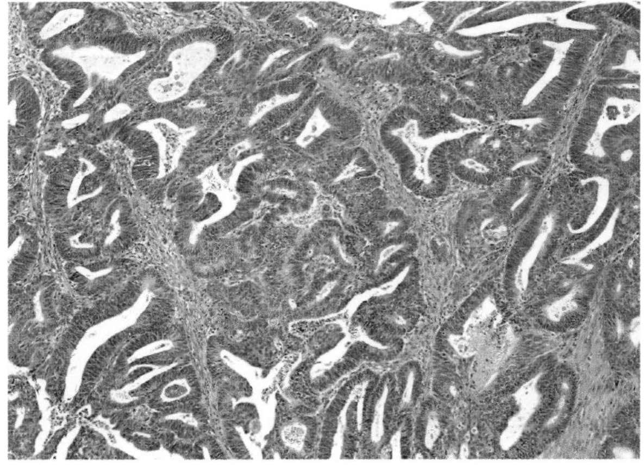

■ Fig. 9.17
Endometrioid carcinoma, FIGO grade 1, myoinvasive. **Myometrial invasion by carcinoma is characterized by islands of well-differentiated glands surrounded by smooth muscle**

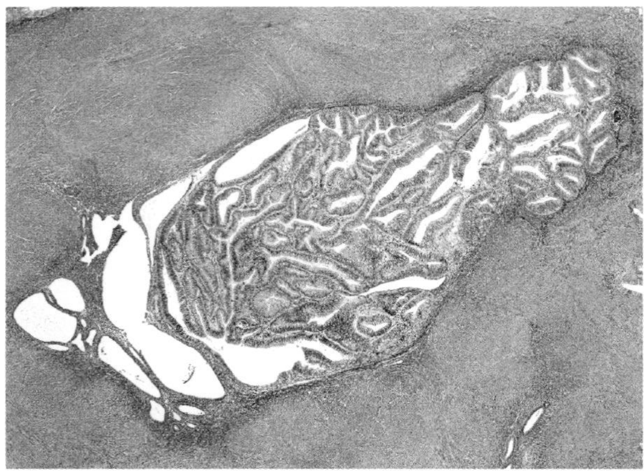

■ Fig. 9.19
Endometrioid carcinoma involving adenomyosis. **FIGO grade 1 carcinoma is present within an island of adenomyosis, identified by the residual benign endometrial glands and stroma along the periphery of the island**

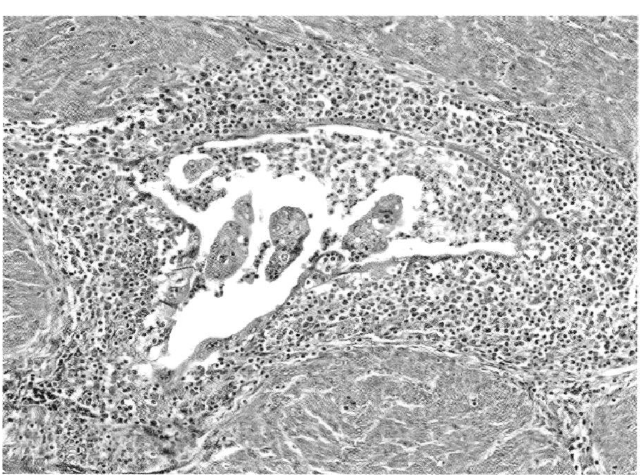

■ Fig. 9.18
Endometrioid carcinoma, FIGO grade 1, myoinvasive. **Some endometrioid carcinomas lose their characteristic columnar endometrioid features and invade myometrium insidiously as attenuated and dilated glands, often intimately associated with an inflammatory reaction**

have very minimal stroma as a result of fibrosis and atrophy. In these cases, it is necessary to evaluate additional features such as the presence of desmoplasia, surrounding edema and inflammation, and the shape of the glands [195]. In contrast to carcinoma involving adenomyosis, true myometrial invasion is usually characterized by desmoplasia or loosening of the myometrium surrounding the glands. Often there is accompanying chronic inflammation and the glandular outline is jagged and irregular, as compared to carcinoma involving adenomyosis in which the glands have a smooth, rounded outline, and desmoplasia, and inflammation are lacking (➋ *Fig. 9.19*). Since CD10 is normally expressed by endometrial stromal cells but not smooth muscle of the myometrium, it would seem that the presence of CD10 in the cells around an adenocarcinoma in the myometrium would indicate its presence in adenomyosis. Unfortunately, CD10 is also often (52% of cases) expressed focally in the cells surrounding clusters of tumor in the myometrium of women in whom adenomyosis is absent, thus eliminating its utility [281, 387]. A diagnosis of carcinoma involving adenomyosis should be made only when there is evidence of adenomyosis uninvolved by carcinoma or residual adenomyosis within foci involved by carcinoma in the uterus because some endometrioid carcinomas invade the myometrium without eliciting a stromal response (see foregoing). A recent study noted that adenocarcinoma involving adenomyosis frequently is associated with preceding estrogen use, low tumor grade, and an excellent prognosis [271].

The diagnosis of superficial myometrial invasion is often problematic due to irregularity of the normal endomyometrial junction, particularly in uteri from older women. The presence of residual nonneoplastic endometrial glands and stroma along the deep or peripheral aspect of rounded nests of carcinoma situated at the

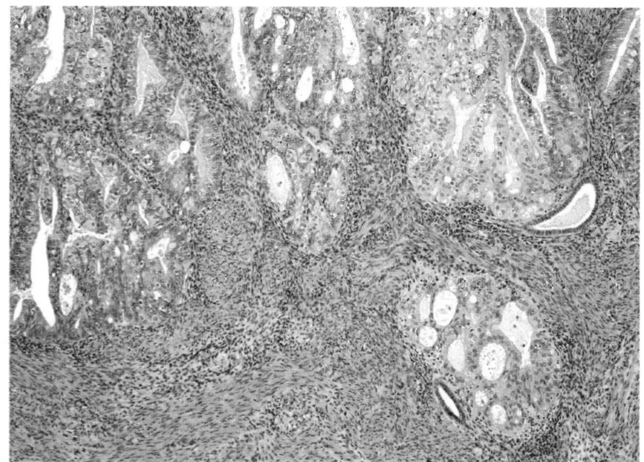

Fig. 9.20
Endometrioid carcinoma, FIGO grade 1, noninvasive. **Nests of carcinoma along an irregular endomyometrial junction suggest superficial myometrial invasion but preserved benign endometrial glands at the periphery of two nests indicate the tumor is still confined to the endometrium**

irregular endomyometrial junction is evidence that these nests are still within the endometrium proper and have not invaded superficial myometrium (Fig. 9.20).

Differential Diagnosis

The main problem in the differential diagnosis of low-grade endometrioid carcinoma is the distinction from atypical hyperplasia, atypical polypoid adenomyoma, hyperplasia with various types of cytoplasmic alterations (metaplasias), Arias–Stella reaction, and menstrual endometrium. The distinction from the first three conditions is discussed in Chap. 8, Precursor Lesions of Endometrial Carcinoma. At times an extremely atypical Arias–Stella reaction may simulate adenocarcinoma. In the reproductive age group, Arias–Stella reaction is much more likely than carcinoma, especially if the clinical history indicates a recent pregnancy. Nonetheless, carcinoma can occur in young women and also in pregnancy. In contrast to a carcinoma, the Arias–Stella reaction tends to be multifocal and is admixed with secretory glands and decidua. The glands in the Arias–Stella reaction may be complex and tortuous but lack confluent or papillary patterns. The stroma does not show a desmoplastic response. The nuclei in the glandular epithelium of the Arias–Stella reaction may be markedly enlarged, but the chromatin appears degenerated and smudged and mitotic figures are very unusual.

Menstrual endometrium can be confused with adenocarcinoma because of the extensive tissue breakdown characterized by tissue fragmentation and hemorrhage. The pattern of stromal breakdown results in fragmented glands of varying size and compact clusters of stromal cells haphazardly mixed with blood, which can appear ominous. The glandular epithelium, however, is bland and shows evidence of secretory activity. Adjacent intact fragments of endometrium with associated predecidual change usually can be identified and assist in the differential diagnosis.

Another problem in differential diagnosis is the distinction of primary endometrial carcinoma from endocervical adenocarcinoma. This is problematic because these carcinomas share morphologic features (endometrioid and mucinous differentiation). Distinction can be difficult even in hysterectomy specimens when the tumor involves both the lower uterine segment and endocervix and precursor lesions are lacking or obscured by carcinoma. The distinction is important because surgical management of these tumors often differs. See Immunohistochemical Findings for further discussion of markers that assist in this distinction.

A related problem is the distinction of a primary endometrial carcinoma from a metastasis from an extrauterine site, discussed in Tumors Metastatic to the Endometrium. A high-grade endometrioid carcinoma at times may be difficult to distinguish from a Malignant Mesodermal (Müllerian) mixed tumor (MMMT) (discussed in the section).

Immunohistochemical Findings

Endometrioid carcinoma expresses pan-cytokeratins, epithelial membrane antigen (EMA), and the glycoprotein associated markers CA125, Ber EP4, and B72.3, among others. The expression of carcinoembryonic antigen (CEA), which is uncommon, is almost always limited to apical membranes, although tumors showing extensive mucinous differentiation may express this antigen more diffusely. Nearly all endometrioid carcinomas are cytokeratin 7 positive and cytokeratin 20 negative [62, 418]. Occasional mucinous varieties express CDX2 [307, 419]. Unlike many other adenocarcinomas, endometrioid tumors frequently display strong staining for vimentin.

Studies of the molecular pathogenesis of endometrioid carcinoma have led to a better understanding of its immunophenotype. The preponderance of FIGO grades 1 and 2 endometrioid carcinomas express ER and PR and approximately one half of FIGO grade 3 endometrioid carcinomas without serous, clear cell or undifferentiated features are ER/PR positive [100, 225, 237, 328, 382, 413]. p53 overexpression resulting from *p53* mutation and accumulation of mutant p53 protein is not encountered in FIGO grade 1 adenocarcinomas and only in a minority of FIGO grade 2 adenocarcinomas, but is present in a significant number of FIGO grade 3 adenocarcinomas. However, when p53 staining is prominent, serous, clear cell, or undifferentiated tumors should be considered [100, 235–237, 362, 381, 395, 448]. Overexpression is defined as diffuse and strong expression in more than 50–75% of tumor cell nuclei. This should be distinguished from low-level expression of p53 in less than 50% of tumor cell nuclei, which is commonly found in endometrioid adenocarcinomas. β-catenin expression in tumor cell nuclei and cytoplasm (as opposed to cell membranes alone), as a consequence of *CTNNB1* mutation, is found in approximately one-third of FIGO grades 1 and 2 adenocarcinomas, especially those showing squamous or morular metaplasia [100, 352]. *PTEN* is frequently mutated in endometrioid carcinomas [54, 100, 298, 333, 373, 395, 435] and expression of this gene is sometimes silenced via hypermethylation of its promoter. Detecting these abnormalities with immunohistochemistry, however, is challenging [100, 303]. DNA MMR proteins are found to be lacking in tumor cell nuclei using immunohistochemistry in one-fifth to one-third of endometrioid carcinomas [101, 272, 308, 414]. In sporadic cases this most often results from *MLH1* promoter hypermethylation. Those that arise in the setting of HNPCC are due to mutations of *MSH6*, *MSH2*, *MLH1*, or *PMS2*, listed in descending order of prevalence. Interpreting DNA MMR protein immunohistochemistry relies on complete loss of expression in the setting of a valid positive internal control. Valid internal controls include nonneoplastic endometrial stroma and glands with reproducibly stained nuclei. Expression loss, when present, usually occurs in couplets (MLH1 with PMS2 and MSH2 with MSH6) due to the fact that these form protein–protein complexes and loss of one of the proteins leads to the destabilization of the other protein in the complex.

A panel of immunohistochemical markers comprised of ER, PR, and p16 has been shown to be useful for distinguishing endometrial endometrioid carcinomas from endocervical adenocarcinomas [26, 262, 269, 388, 434]. The vast majority of endocervical adenocarcinomas (~90%) are human papillomavirus (HPV)-related and exhibit diffuse/moderate to strong p16 expression due to complex molecular mechanisms by which high-risk HPV transforming proteins (E6, E7) interact with cell cycle regulatory proteins (p53, pRb) to generate a futile feedback loop resulting in p16 over-expression (see Chap. 6, Carcinoma and Other Tumors of the Cervix). Interestingly, these HPV-related endocervical adenocarcinomas also often lack hormone receptor expression (estrogen [ER] and progesterone [PR] receptors) [263, 335, 388, 434]. In contrast, endometrial endometrioid carcinomas are considered etiologically unrelated to HPV. They have been shown to exhibit generally patchy p16 expression of variable intensity, with mean/median extent of expression in 30–40% of tumor cells across all FIGO grades and only rare endometrioid tumors exhibiting diffuse/strong expression (*Fig. 9.21*) [433]. This patchy pattern is distinct from the diffuse/strong expression characteristic of HPV-related endocervical adenocarcinomas. In addition, most endometrial endometrioid carcinomas, particularly FIGO grades 1 and 2 tumors but also many FIGO grade 3 tumors, express hormone receptors [236, 263, 388]. Typical endometrial endometrioid carcinomas are p16 focal+/ER+/PR+, whereas typical endocervical adenocarcinomas are p16 diffuse+/ER−/PR−, with some of the latter retaining focal/limited expression of hormone receptors. We specifically recommend the use of PR in conjunction with ER based on our published [335, 388, 434] and unpublished experiences indicating that the subset of endocervical carcinomas that retains some expression of hormone receptors most often retains ER expression to some degree (often focal/weak to moderate) but entirely loses PR expression; thus, PR is the more discriminatory marker of the two when trying to distinguish endocervical adenocarcinomas from endometrial endometrioid carcinomas.

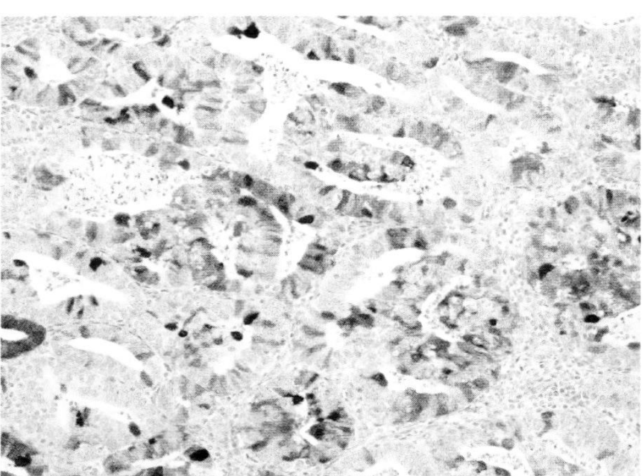

Fig. 9.21
Endometrioid carcinoma, FIGO grade 1. **Tumor exhibits patchy expression of p16**

Behavior and Treatment

Endometrioid adenocarcinoma spreads by lymphatic and vascular dissemination, direct extension to contiguous organs, and transperitoneal and transtubal seeding. Lymphatic metastasis is more common than hematogenous spread, but the involvement of the lungs without metastasis to mediastinal lymph nodes suggests that hematogenous spread may occur early in the course of disease. Endometrial carcinoma tends to spread to the pelvic lymph nodes before involving paraaortic lymph nodes. The relative frequency of metastasis to lymph node groups and various organs is shown in ➲ *Tables 9.5* and ➲ *9.6*, respectively.

The standard treatment for endometrial carcinoma is hysterectomy and bilateral salpingo-oophorectomy. Over the years, preoperative or postoperative radiotherapy and chemotherapy have been used in addition to hysterectomy. The current approach is to treat all patients when feasible by hysterectomy supplemented by surgical staging and to administer postoperative radiation to patients with poor prognostic factors that put them at high risk of recurrence. Postoperative estrogen replacement therapy has been advocated for patients with early-stage disease and no significant poor prognostic factors [93]. One study showed that survival is not compromised in patients with low tumor grade (grades 1 and 2), less than 50% myometrial invasion, and no metastases to lymph nodes or other organs [241]. Given the prognostic significance of pelvic and paraaortic lymph node status, these nodes should be sampled or dissected in patients when any of the following is present: greater than 50% myometrial invasion, grade 3 tumor, cervical involvement, extrauterine spread, serous, clear cell, or undifferentiated carcinoma, or palpably enlarged lymph nodes. In a GOG study only a quarter of patients had these findings, but they accounted for the majority of patients with positive aortic lymph nodes [277]. Several studies have shown that the depth of myometrial invasion can be assessed by gross inspection and intraoperative frozen section [106, 296, 367]. However, other studies have suggested that intraoperative assessments are not reproducible with discrepancies of up to 25% with the final diagnosis.

Postoperatively, patients are classified as low, intermediate, or high risk based on surgical pathologic staging. Patients with grade 1 or 2 tumors that are confined to the endometrium or are minimally invasive are defined as low risk and require no further therapy. Patients with pelvic or paraaortic lymph node metastases or involvement of the adnexa or intraperitoneal sites are high risk and receive postoperative radiation (vaginal cuff, pelvis, paraaortic area, or whole abdominal). Radiation appears to be of benefit because the 5-year survival rate for women with positive aortic lymph nodes who were treated with

Table 9.5

Sites of lymph node metastasis from endometrial carcinomas at autopsy (From Hendrickson E (1975) The lymphatic dissemination in endometrial carcinoma. A study of 188 necropsies. Am J Obstet Gynecol 123:570)

Lymph nodes	Relative frequency (%)
Paraaortic	64
Hypogastric	61
External iliac	48
Common iliac	40
Obturator	37
Sacral	22
Mediastinal	18
Inguinal	16
Supraclavicular	12

Table 9.6

Sites of metastasis from endometrial carcinoma at autopsy (From Hendrickson E (1975) The lymphatic dissemination in endometrial carcinoma. A study of 188 necropsies. Am J Obstet Gynecol 123:570)

Organ site	Relative frequency (%)
Lung	41
Peritoneum and omentum	39
Ovary	34
Liver	29
Bowel	29
Vagina	25
Bladder	23
Vertebra	20
Spleen	14
Adrenal	14
Ureter	8
Brain or skull	5
Vulva	4
Breast	4
Hand	
Femur	
Tibia	Rare
Pubic bone	
Skin	

postoperative radiation is nearly 40% [277]. Despite treatment with surgery and radiotherapy, 50% of stage III tumors recur. Half of these patients die with distant metastasis, although local control also is a major problem. About 4% of patients with endometrial carcinoma have stage IV disease. Spread to the lungs occurs in 36% of patients. Patients who do not qualify as low or high risk are intermediate in risk. A decision as to whether or not these patients should receive postoperative radiation should be individualized because there are no conclusive data demonstrating a survival benefit for these patients treated with postoperative radiotherapy. Studies evaluating the use of adjuvant hormonal or cytotoxic chemotherapy have shown no improvement in survival over surgery and radiation, and consequently these methods currently are not recommended as standard treatment. In contrast, radiation, hormone, and cytotoxic chemotherapy are used for management of patients with recurrent tumor; 50% of patients with isolated vaginal vault recurrence treated by irradiation are alive at 3 years [319].

Histologic Effects of Treatment

Radiation

The histologic changes in neoplastic tissues after intracavitary radiation are nonspecific and variable, showing minor to major alterations from their pre-irradiated state. Similarly, nonneoplastic endometrial or endocervical glands may be affected only minimally or show nuclear and cytoplasmic changes that are indistinguishable from those found in neoplastic cells. Because the cytologic changes in both neoplastic and nonneoplastic tissue are similar, the identification of carcinoma depends largely on the recognition of histologic patterns and signs of invasion. Irradiated carcinoma generally retains a haphazard glandular pattern, but nonirradiated, nonneoplastic glands tend to maintain their normal architectural arrangement despite radiation effects in the endometrial stroma and myometrium. When radiation effect is evident, nuclei tend to be enlarged, highly pleomorphic, and hyperchromatic, with coarsely clumped chromatin. The cytoplasm often is granular and swollen. Vacuolation can be present in both the nucleus and the cytoplasm. The nuclear changes result from the replication of DNA without cell division.

Cytoplasmic vacuolation results from the dilatation of various organelles and possible lysis caused by damaged lysosomal membranes. In some instances, radiation may enhance cellular differentiation. Occasionally, poorly differentiated carcinomas without squamous differentiation in the curettings may have nests of squamous epithelium in the resected uterus after radiation. It is in mitosis and the S phase of the cell cycle that a cell is most susceptible to radiation injury. Thus, the difference in radiosensitivity of tumor cells and benign cells is due largely to the increased mitotic activity of the neoplastic cells and the better reparative capacity of nonneoplastic cells. In view of the variable morphologic response to irradiation, it is often difficult to determine whether irradiated tumor cells are viable. On a practical basis, if tumor cells are evident after irradiation, it should be assumed that some retain the capacity to persist however abnormal they appear.

Radiation changes in the endometrial stroma and myometrium are greatest in the vicinity of the radiation source. The stromal cells are first converted to giant fibroblasts. Early vascular effects include damage to endothelial cells, resulting in thrombosis. The stroma undergoes progressive hyalinization, resulting in a collagenous scar. Elastic tissue often is fragmented and frayed, and blood vessels are thickened and sclerotic. Occasionally, changes similar to those found in atherosclerosis may be present in the intima of blood vessels. Foam cells occur in the intima, and myometrial cells may appear granular and swollen, especially in areas close to the radium source. Scarring, atrophy, and sclerosis of vessels characterize long-standing radiation effects. The endometrium is thin and easily traumatized, and small blood vessels in the stroma are thin walled and ectatic. Some blood vessels form plaques of lipid-filled clear cells in the media.

Progestins

Progestin-induced changes include secretory differentiation of glandular cells, mitotic arrest, conversion of spindle-shaped stromal cells to decidual cells, decrease in estrogen-related cellular changes such as ciliogenesis, and development or enlargement of squamous areas [331, 342]. The earliest evidence of progestin effect is subnuclear vacuolization, observed within 2–3 days of treatment. The vacuoles are a manifestation of glycoprotein synthesis, which is followed by an apocrine-type secretion in which the apical portion of the cytoplasm of the cell is discharged into the gland lumen, with reduction in the size of the cell. Longer term therapy aimed at eliminating the disease, at least until patients can become pregnant, results in a number of morphologic changes that can predict response to therapy. These include decreased glandular-to-stroma ratio, decreased to absent mitotic activity, decreased glandular cellularity, loss of cytologic atypia, and a variety of cytoplasmic changes including mucinous, secretory, squamous, and eosinophilic metaplasia. Persistent architectural abnormalities and/or cytologic atypia were predictive of treatment failure. Some architectural changes (cribriform and papillary patterns) induced by progestin treatment, are noteworthy as they may be confused with progression [424]. Importantly, biopsies taken after the initiation of treatment require a comparison to the pretreatment sample for correct interpretation and determination of treatment response (see Chap. 8, Precursor Lesions of Endometrial Carcinoma). It has been shown that patients with complex atypical hyperplasia and well differentiated carcinoma who were successfully treated with progestins had higher numbers of NK cells and lower numbers of regulatory T cells in post treatment specimens. These alterations in subpopulations of lymphocytes suggest that the effect of progestins goes beyond their direct growth regulatory effects on endometrial tissue [426].

Villoglandular Carcinoma

Villoglandular carcinoma is a variant of endometrioid carcinoma that displays a papillary architecture in which the papillary fronds are composed of a delicate fibrovascular core covered by columnar cells that generally contain bland nuclei [69, 174]. The median age is 61 years, similar to that of women with typical endometrioid carcinoma. In all other respects, women with these tumors are similar to patients with low-grade endometrioid carcinoma.

The microscopic appearance of villoglandular carcinoma is characterized by thin, delicate fronds covered by stratified columnar epithelial cells with oval nuclei that generally display mild to moderate (grade 1 or 2) atypia (*Figs. 9.22* and *9.23*). Occasionally, more atypical (grade 3) nuclei may be observed. Mitotic activity is variable, and abnormal mitotic figures are rare [69, 174]. Myometrial invasion usually is superficial.

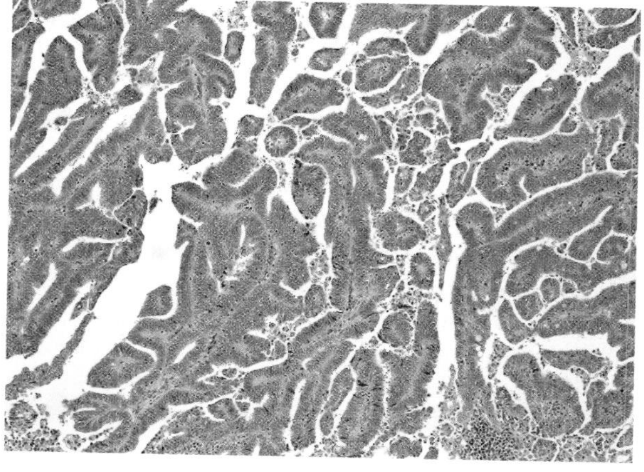

Fig. 9.22
Endometrioid carcinoma, villoglandular type. **Tumor has papillary architecture, which might lead to misclassification as serous carcinoma, but columnar epithelium with low-grade cytologic features (see *Fig. 9.23*) is consistent with endometrioid carcinoma**

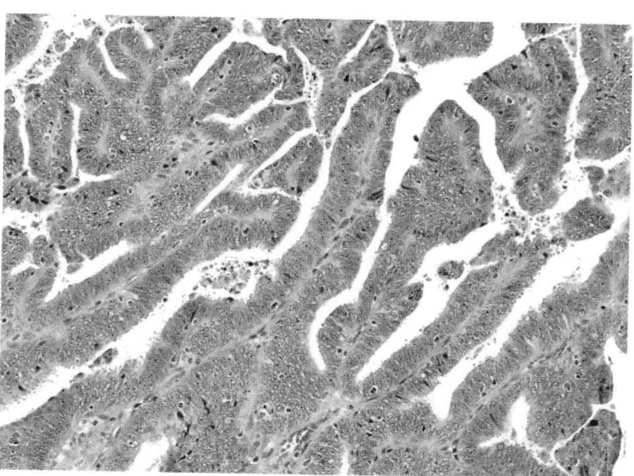

Fig. 9.23
Endometrioid carcinoma, villoglandular type. **Endometrioid differentiation is confirmed by the presence of columnar epithelium and low-grade cytologic features (elongated uniform nuclei)**

Differential Diagnosis

The main consideration in the differential diagnosis is serous carcinoma because both villoglandular and serous carcinomas have a prominent papillary pattern. In contrast to serous carcinomas, villoglandular carcinomas have long delicate papillary fronds and are covered by columnar cells with only mild to moderate nuclear atypia. The cells look distinctly endometrioid with a smooth, luminal border. To have significance as a distinctive entity, the diagnosis is reserved for tumors in which most of the neoplasm has a villoglandular appearance. In contrast to villoglandular carcinomas, serous carcinomas tend to have shorter, thick, densely fibrotic papillary fronds. The most important distinguishing feature is the cytologic appearance. The cells of serous carcinoma tend to be rounder, forming small papillary clusters that are detached from the papillary fronds, a finding that is often referred to as papillary tufts. As a consequence, the luminal border has a scalloped appearance. The nuclei of serous carcinomas are highly pleomorphic and atypical (grade 3). Cherry red macronucleoli typically are present and the cells have a hobnail appearance, often with smudged, hyperchromatic nuclei. It should be noted that considerable nuclear heterogeneity can be observed.

Villoglandular carcinomas are generally better differentiated than typical endometrioid carcinomas but are not significantly different with respect to depth of invasion or frequency of nodal metastases [442]. In addition, villoglandular carcinomas are frequently admixed with typical endometrioid carcinoma. In view of the frequent admixture of the two patterns and similar prognosis, villoglandular carcinoma is considered a variant of endometrioid carcinoma. Treatment is the same as for endometrioid carcinoma of comparable stage, grade, and depth of invasion.

Secretory Carcinoma

Secretory carcinoma is a variant of typical endometrial carcinoma in which the majority of cells exhibit subnuclear or supranuclear cytoplasmic vacuoles resembling early secretory endometrium. An unusual pattern, it represents only 1–2% of endometrial carcinomas [229, 402]. The age range is from 35 to 79 years, with a mean age of 55–58 [75, 402]. Most patients are postmenopausal and experience abnormal bleeding. This histologic subtype also may be seen after progestin treatment of an endometrioid carcinoma. In all other respects, including the association of obesity, hypertension, diabetes mellitus, and exogenous estrogen administration, patients with secretory carcinoma are similar to women with endometrioid carcinoma.

Microscopically, secretory carcinoma displays a well-differentiated glandular pattern and is composed of columnar cells, often unstratified, with subnuclear or supranuclear vacuolization closely resembling day 17–22 secretory endometrium (*Figs. 9.24–9.26*) [229, 402]. Usually the nuclei are grade 1. The secretory pattern may be focal or diffuse, and it is frequently admixed with endometrioid adenocarcinoma. The endometrium adjacent to secretory carcinoma in young women typically shows a secretory pattern that is more advanced than 17 days, and a corpus luteum is found in most premenopausal patients when a hysterectomy and bilateral salpingo-oophorectomy are performed. Nonetheless, a relationship to progesterone stimulation is not always demonstrable. In fact, secretory carcinoma may occur spontaneously in postmenopausal women without exogenous or abnormal levels of progesterone. The secretory activity in the tumor may be transient because it has been observed in curettings but not in the later hysterectomy specimen [75].

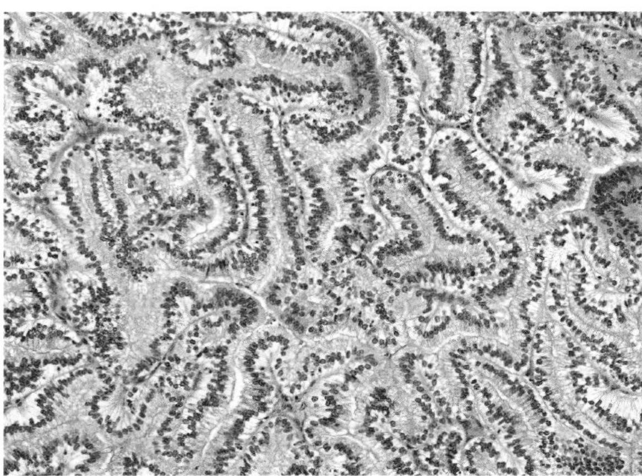

Fig. 9.24
Endometrioid carcinoma, secretory type, FIGO grade 1. **Endometrioid-type epithelium displays prominent sub- and supranuclear vacuolization, reminiscent of day 18 secretory endometrium**

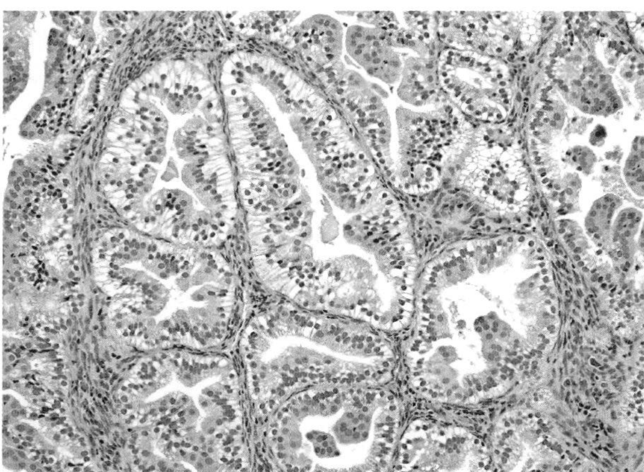

Fig. 9.25
Endometrioid carcinoma, secretory type, FIGO grade 1. **Endometrioid-type glands with secretory differentiation are present within a desmoplastic stroma. Prominent subnuclear vacuolization is reminiscent of day 17 secretory endometrium**

Differential Diagnosis

It is important to distinguish secretory carcinoma from clear cell carcinoma in view of the excellent prognosis of the former and unfavorable prognosis of the latter. Although both tumors are composed of cells with clear, glycogen-rich cytoplasm, the histologic features are distinctive. At times a secretory carcinoma that has a predominantly glandular

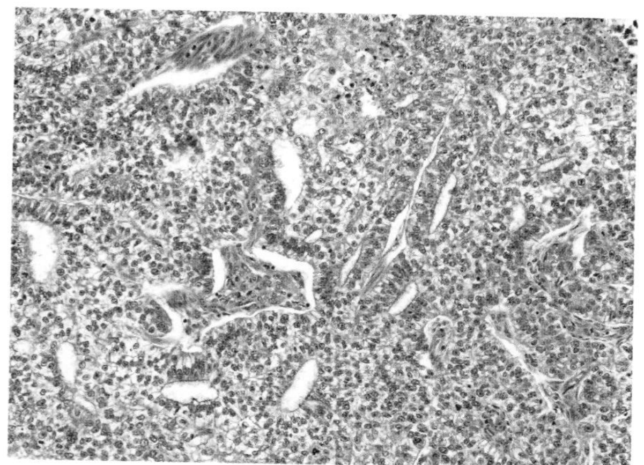

Fig. 9.26
Endometrioid carcinoma, secretory type, FIGO grade 2.
Endometrioid-type glands and solid nonsquamous epithelium exhibit diffuse secretory differentiation manifested as clear cytoplasmic change. Tumor has uniform low-grade cytologic features and lacks any of the characteristic architectural patterns of clear cell carcinoma, supporting a diagnosis of secretory type endometrioid carcinoma

pattern can become solid and simulate clear cell carcinoma. The tumors are distinguished by their architectural and cytologic appearance. Secretory carcinoma displays a glandular architecture like endometrioid carcinoma, is rarely papillary or cystic, and usually is not solid. The cells of secretory carcinoma are columnar, similar to those in endometrioid carcinoma, except that they have supranuclear or subnuclear vacuoles. In contrast, clear cell carcinoma often exhibits tubulocystic and/or papillary architecture but can be glandular. The cells usually have marked nuclear atypia (grade 3), with rounded cells having a variety of characteristic features including hobnail morphology, smudgy hyperchromasia, and prominent nucleoli. Cells with clear cytoplasm also may be seen in the squamous component of an endometrioid adenocarcinoma with squamous differentiation. The clear appearance of these cells is also due to the presence of glycogen. Clear squamous cells tend to be polygonal and usually merge with more typical squamous cells with abundant eosinophilic cytoplasm. The distinction of secretory carcinoma from atypical hyperplasia with secretory effect can be difficult and is based on the presence of stromal invasion in the carcinoma (see Chap. 8, Precursor Lesions of Endometrial Carcinoma). Treatment is the same as that for endometrioid carcinoma of the same stage and grade. Secretory carcinoma usually is low grade with a good prognosis [402]. Death from recurrent disease occurs rarely [75].

Ciliated Carcinoma

Ciliated carcinoma is a rare form of differentiation in low-grade endometrioid carcinoma [175]. It does not need to be classified separately from endometrioid carcinoma; its only importance is to remind the pathologist that endometrial proliferations with cilia may still be carcinomas. Estrogen induces cilia formation in the normal endometrium. Despite the prevalence of estrogen use, ciliated carcinoma is an extremely rare carcinoma, and most endometrial proliferations in which cilia are observed represent hyperplasias associated with eosinophilic or ciliated change. Patients range in age from 42 to 79 years, are often postmenopausal, and present with bleeding. Ciliated carcinoma has an association with exogenous estrogen treatment. Microscopically, ciliated carcinoma is almost always well differentiated and often displays a cribriform pattern. The gland lumens in the cribriform areas are lined by cells with prominent eosinophilic cytoplasm and cilia. The nuclei of ciliated cells generally have an irregular nuclear membrane and display coarse nuclear chromatin with prominent nucleoli. In most cases, ciliated carcinoma is admixed with nonciliated endometrioid carcinoma and occasionally areas of mucinous carcinoma. Although some ciliated carcinomas are moderately differentiated and invade to the middle third of the myometrium, none of the patients has developed recurrence or died of disease. Thus, the presence of cilia in a bona fide carcinoma identifies a low-grade neoplasm.

Endometrioid Carcinoma with Squamous Differentiation

Many endometrioid adenocarcinomas contain squamous epithelium, but the amount of squamous epithelium can vary widely. In a well-sampled neoplasm, the squamous element should constitute at least 10% of a tumor to qualify as an adenocarcinoma with squamous differentiation. Adenocarcinomas with squamous elements were formerly divided into those with benign-appearing squamous elements and favorable prognosis, designated adenoacanthoma (AA), and those with malignant-appearing squamous epithelium, and a worse prognosis, termed adenosquamous carcinoma (AS) [11, 284]. Recent studies indicate that the difference in behavior between AA and AS mainly reflects the difference in the grade of these respective neoplasms [4, 440, 441]. Thus, the categorization of carcinomas with squamous epithelium according to the depth of myometrial invasion and the grade of the glandular component provides more useful

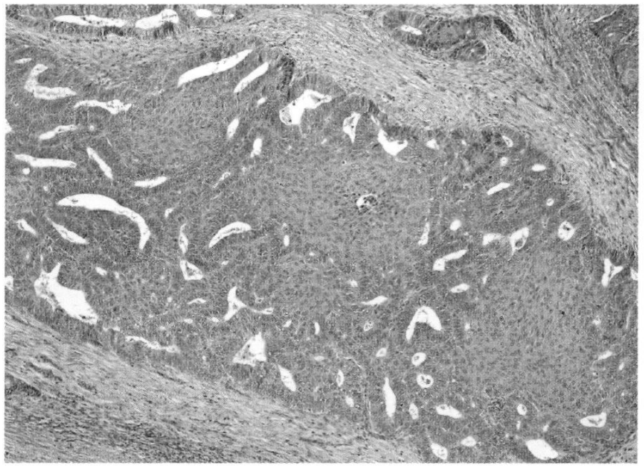

Fig. 9.27
Endometrioid carcinoma with squamous differentiation, FIGO grade 1. **Well-differentiated glands are intimately admixed with solid nests of low-grade squamous epithelium. Grading is based on the features of the glandular component alone**

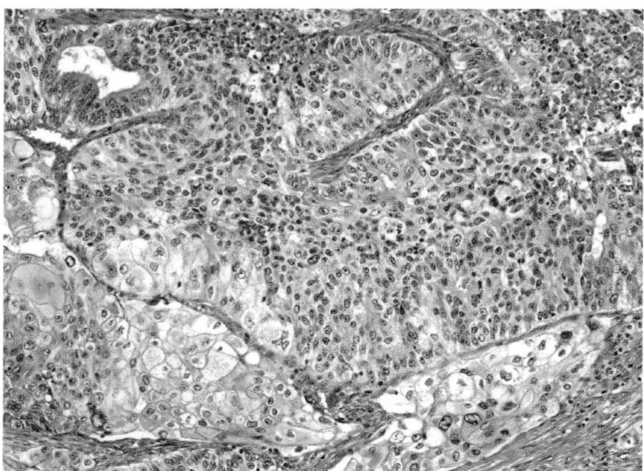

Fig. 9.28
Endometrioid carcinoma with focal squamous differentiation, FIGO grade 3. **Carcinoma has areas of squamous differentiation and is classified as high-grade endometrioid based on the solid nonsquamous epithelium (>50%) with focal residual glandular differentiation**

prognostic information than the division into AA or AS because the grade of the glandular component generally parallels that of the squamous element [440]. This understanding had led to the view that AA and AS reflect a continuum in the degree of differentiation of the squamous epithelium that parallels the differentiation of the glandular component. Accordingly, it is recommended that endometrioid carcinomas with squamous epithelium be classified simply as endometrioid carcinoma with squamous differentiation and graded, on the basis of the glandular component, as well, moderately, or poorly differentiated (grade 1, 2, or 3, respectively).

There are no differences in the clinical features of adenocarcinoma containing squamous epithelium and endometrioid adenocarcinoma. Thus, there are no differences in the frequency of obesity, hypertension, diabetes, and nulliparity among the large series in which this has been analyzed [11, 84].

Gross and Microscopic Findings

These tumors have no distinctive gross findings. Low-grade tumors (grade 1) are composed of glandular and squamous elements but generally the glandular component predominates; the nests of squamous epithelium are confined to gland lumens. The squamous epithelium resembles metaplastic squamous cells of the cervical transformation zone. Frequently, nests of cells with a prominent oval to spindle cell appearance, referred to as morules, are observed (*Fig. 9.27*). Intercellular bridges can be identified within the squamous epithelium, and keratin formation is common. The nuclei of the squamous cells are bland, uniform, and lack prominent nucleoli. Mitotic figures are rare. In higher-grade tumors, the squamous element is cytologically more atypical and is not confined to gland lumens but often extends out from the glands (*Fig. 9.28*). At times the squamous cells have a spindle appearance simulating a sarcoma. They may not be in direct continuity with the glandular epithelium, appearing in isolated nests within the myometrium or in vascular spaces. Keratinization and pearl formation occur to varying degrees.

Generally, the glandular component predominates, but masses of undifferentiated cells that may represent poorly differentiated glandular or squamous cells lie between glands. This undifferentiated epithelium should be considered glandular unless intercellular bridges are demonstrated or the cells have prominent eosinophilic cytoplasm, well-defined cytoplasmic borders, and a sheet-like proliferation without evidence of gland formation. Both the glandular and squamous components display grade 2 or 3 nuclear atypia, an increased nuclear cytoplasmic ratio, and increased mitotic activity. The glandular architecture usually is poorly differentiated. Tumors of intermediate differentiation are common. These neoplasms contain glandular and solid areas in which the squamous cells display a moderate degree of nuclear atypia, defying separation into a "benign" and "malignant" category.

A rare finding in patients with adenocarcinoma with squamous differentiation is the presence of keratin granulomas that may involve a wide variety of sites in the peritoneal cavity including the ovaries, tubes, omentum, and serosa of the uterus and bowel [70, 218]. Microscopically, these lesions consist of a central mass of keratin and necrotic squamous cells surrounded by a foreign body granulomatous reaction. A proliferation of mesothelial cells also may be present. The granulomas probably result from the exfoliation of necrotic cells from the tumor, followed by transtubal spread and implantation on peritoneal surfaces. It is important to distinguish pure keratin granulomas from lesions with both viable-appearing tumor cells and keratin accompanied by a foreign body-type giant cell reaction because the former lesions have not been associated with an unfavorable prognosis.

Differential Diagnosis

The most common problem in the differential diagnosis of the low-grade tumors is with atypical hyperplasia showing squamous metaplasia. To distinguish between the two, the criteria for identifying endometrial stromal invasion should be employed (see ➋ Chap. 8, Precursor Lesions of Endometrial Carcinoma). At times, a low-grade tumor may be confused with a high-grade carcinoma because the masses of squamous epithelium are misconstrued as a solid proliferation of neoplastic cells. The nuclear grade is high in poorly differentiated carcinoma, however. Occasionally, squamous morules may be confused with granulomas, but the presence of foreign body giant cells and an inflammatory infiltrate helps to identify the latter. For high-grade adenocarcinomas with squamous epithelium, the major problem in differential diagnosis in curettings is distinguishing a primary carcinoma of the endometrium from an adenosquamous carcinoma arising in the endocervix. In the cervix, the squamous component usually predominates, whereas in the endometrium the glandular component predominates. A profusion of cell types, especially mucinous or signet ring cells, is more characteristic of an endocervical neoplasm.

Behavior and Treatment

As already described, when stratified according to stage, grade, and depth of myometrial invasion, there are few differences in the behavior of carcinomas with squamous epithelium compared with endometrioid carcinomas without squamous epithelium [4, 440, 441]. As occurs with endometrioid carcinomas, the low-grade carcinomas with squamous epithelium tend to be only superficially invasive and seldom invade vascular channels. In contrast, high-grade tumors have a high frequency of deep myometrial invasion, vascular space involvement, and pelvic and paraaortic lymph node metastases. Metastasis of high-grade tumors occurs widely throughout the pelvis and abdomen, involving bowel, mesentery, liver, kidney, spleen, and lymph nodes. Distant metastasis may involve the lungs, heart, skin, and bones. Nearly two-thirds of metastases contain both glandular and squamous elements, but pure adenocarcinoma or squamous carcinoma is encountered in 20% and 8%, respectively [284]. Often it is the squamous component that is identified in vascular channels. Accordingly, the treatment for carcinomas with squamous epithelium is the same as that for endometrioid carcinomas of comparable stage.

Mucinous Carcinoma

This uncommon type of endometrial carcinoma has an appearance similar to mucinous carcinoma of the endocervix [98, 401]. Mucinous carcinoma represents the dominant cellular population in only 1–9% of endometrial carcinomas [267, 336]. To qualify as a mucinous carcinoma, more than one-half the cell population of the tumor must contain periodic acid–Schiff- (PAS-) positive, diastase-resistant intracytoplasmic mucin.

Judging from the few published cases, the clinical features of patients with mucinous carcinoma of the endometrium do not differ from those with endometrioid carcinoma. Patients range in age from 47 to 89 years and typically present with vaginal bleeding. In one study, more than 40% had a history of receiving exogenous estrogens [267]. Most patients present with stage I disease.

These tumors do not have distinctive gross features. The most frequent architectural pattern is glandular, often in a villoglandular configuration (➋ *Figs. 9.29* and ➋ *9.30*). The epithelial cells lining the glands and papillary processes tend to be uniform columnar cells with minimal stratification. Cribriform areas are unusual; cystically dilated glands filled with mucin and papillary fronds surrounded by extracellular lakes of mucin, containing neutrophils, are typical. Curiously, mucinous differentiation sometimes is associated with squamous differentiation. Nuclear atypia is mild to moderate, and mitotic activity is not prominent. Hyperplasia and mucinous metaplasia sometimes are present in the adjacent endometrium. One study reported that the carcinoma

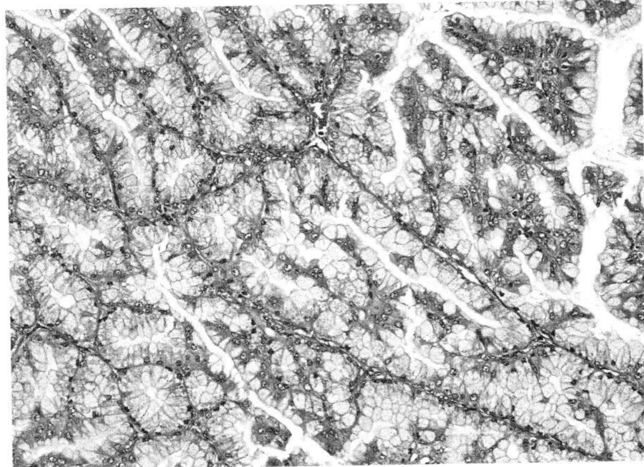

Fig. 9.29
Mucinous carcinoma, FIGO grade 1. **Confluent glands have abundant mucinous cytoplasm and small, basally situated nuclei**

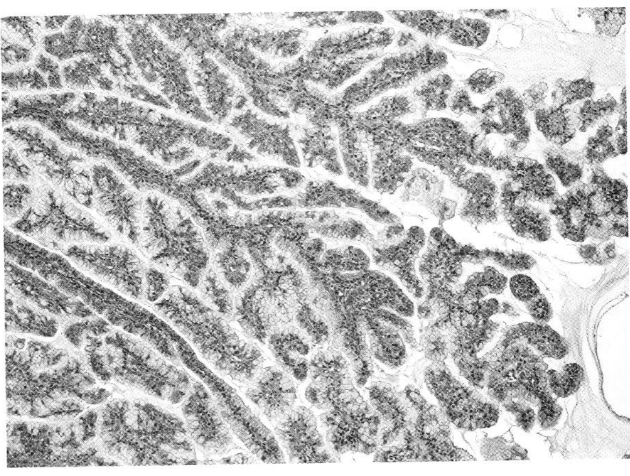

Fig. 9.30
Mucinous carcinoma, FIGO grade 1. **Tumor has extensive mucinous differentiation and confluent glandular and papillary growth; these architectural patterns allow for establishing a diagnosis of carcinoma**

was present in a polyp in 27% of the cases [267]. The presence of intracytoplasmic mucin can be identified on hematoxylin and eosin (H&E) stains by its distinctive granular, foamy, or bubbly appearance and can be confirmed by PAS, mucicarmine, or alcian blue stains. The intracytoplasmic mucin is variable in both the distribution of mucinous cells in the tumor and in the location of the mucin within individual cells. Mucin may be diffusely present in the cytoplasm, confined to the apical area, or show a combination of both patterns. Tumors dominated

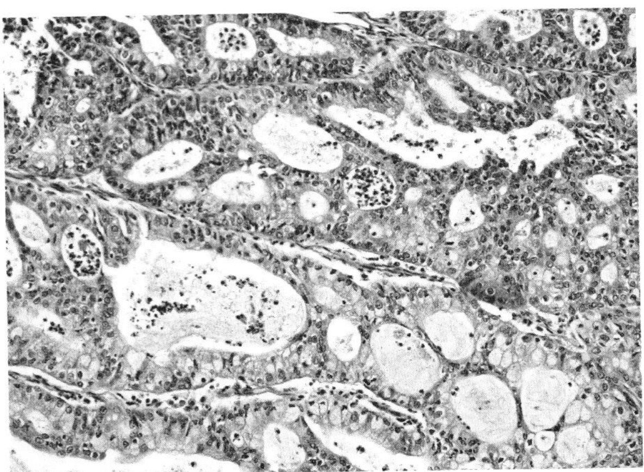

Fig. 9.31
Mucinous carcinoma, FIGO grade 1 (endometrioid carcinoma with mucinous differentiation). **Tumor exhibits a cribriform growth pattern and is comprised of glands with prominent mucinous cytoplasm as well as ones with a typical endometrioid appearance**

by typical endometrioid carcinoma with less than 50% of a mucinous component can be designated as endometrioid carcinomas with mucinous differentiation (*Fig. 9.31*).

Differential Diagnosis

Endocervical epithelium merges with the endometrium in the lower uterine segment, so it is not surprising that the distinction of primary endocervical from endometrial mucinous carcinoma in curettings can be difficult. There is no histochemical difference in the mucin at either site [336]. The distinction of endocervical from endometrial adenocarcinomas has been discussed earlier (see section Differential Diagnosis for endometrioid carcinoma).

The distinction of mucinous carcinoma of the endometrium from clear cell or secretory carcinoma is made on the basis of morphology and PAS and mucin stains. The cells in secretory carcinoma are clear (not granular or foamy) because of the presence of glycogen, which is PAS positive and is removed by diastase treatment. Mucin in these tumors is focal at most. Clear cell carcinoma is almost always papillary or solid in contrast to the glandular pattern of mucinous carcinoma. The cells in clear cell carcinoma tend to be polygonal rather than columnar and hobnail cells are almost invariably present, a cytologic feature that is absent in mucinous carcinoma.

Rarely, a mucinous carcinoma or a mixed mucinous and endometrioid carcinoma may contain areas that simulate microglandular hyperplasia of the cervix [436, 445].

Such foci are characterized by cells showing mucinous and eosinophilic change with microcystic spaces containing acute inflammatory cells. The patients are in their 50s and 60s, in contrast to women with microglandular hyperplasia, who are young. The complexity of the glandular pattern and the degree of cytologic atypia distinguish this type of carcinoma from microglandular hyperplasia.

Behavior and Treatment

When stratified by stage, grade, and depth of myometrial invasion, mucinous tumors behave as do endometrioid carcinomas [336]. Mucinous carcinomas, however, tend to be low grade and minimally invasive and therefore as a group have an excellent prognosis. The treatment is the same as for endometrioid carcinoma. Because most of the tumors are stage I, low grade, and minimally invasive, total abdominal hysterectomy and bilateral salpingo-oophorectomy usually suffice.

Serous Carcinoma

The existence of papillary patterns within endometrial carcinoma has been recognized since the turn of the century. In the past 2 decades, reports have described the morphologic similarity of serous carcinomas of the endometrium, which frequently display papillary architecture, to ovarian serous carcinomas and identified them as a highly aggressive type of endometrial carcinoma [75, 174, 233, 417]. Although papillary architecture is a common finding in serous carcinoma, most other types of endometrial carcinoma can display papillary architecture but are usually not highly aggressive tumors. What distinguishes serous carcinoma from these other types is the uniformly marked cytologic atypia. Thus, the designation "serous carcinoma," rather than "papillary serous carcinoma," is preferred so that cell type rather than architecture is emphasized.

Clinical Features

The prevalence of serous carcinomas reported from referral centers usually is about 10%; however, in a population-based study from Norway it was only 1% [5]. Patients with serous carcinoma range in age from 39 to 93 years but typically are postmenopausal and, in contrast to women with endometrioid carcinoma, are older (reported median and mean ages are in the late 60s). In addition, they are less likely to have received estrogen replacement therapy and are more likely to have abnormal cervical cytology. There are some data to suggest that women with this neoplasm are less likely to be obese and that a higher proportion of women are black [108]. In other respects, they appear similar.

Gross Findings

On gross examination, uteri containing these tumors often are small and atrophic. Generally the tumor is exophytic and has a papillary appearance. The depth of invasion is difficult to assess on macroscopic examination. It is not unusual to find a benign-appearing polyp containing the carcinoma in the hysterectomy specimen after a diagnosis of serous carcinoma or endometrial intraepithelial carcinoma has been made on a curetting because these tumors frequently develop within a polyp (see ➋ Chap. 8, Precursor Lesions of Endometrial Carcinoma) [58, 61, 361, 369, 380, 423].

Microscopic Findings

As experience with serous carcinoma has increased, it has become apparent that this neoplasm demonstrates considerable diversity in its architectural features (➋ *Figs. 9.32–9.42*). Although a papillary pattern typically predominates, glandular and solid patterns also occur [100, 174, 238, 361]. Serous carcinoma originally was described as having thick, short papillae, but subsequent studies have shown that thin papillae may be present in more than half of them. The cytologic features of these tumors also are quite varied. Polygonal cells

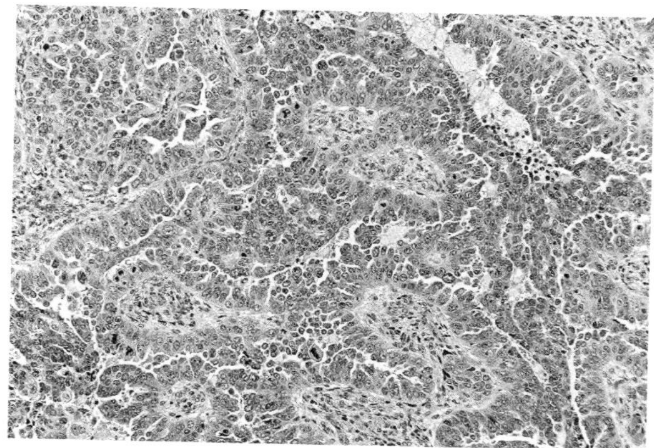

Fig. 9.32
Serous carcinoma. **Papillary tumor is lined by markedly atypical epithelium composed of cells with scalloped luminal borders, including hobnail type cells**

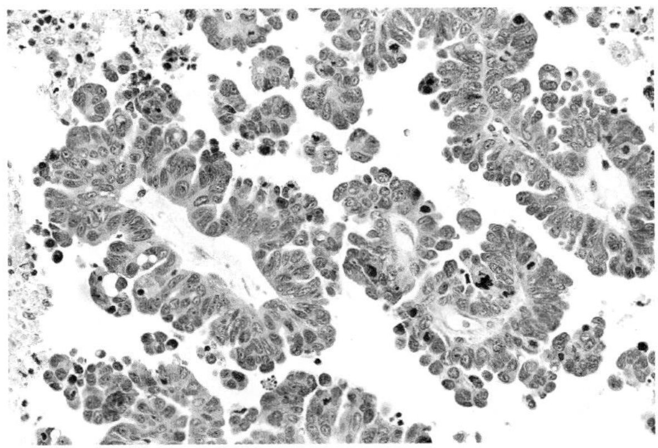

Fig. 9.33
Serous carcinoma. **Papillary structures and detached epithelial clusters have markedly atypical cells, including hobnail type cells**

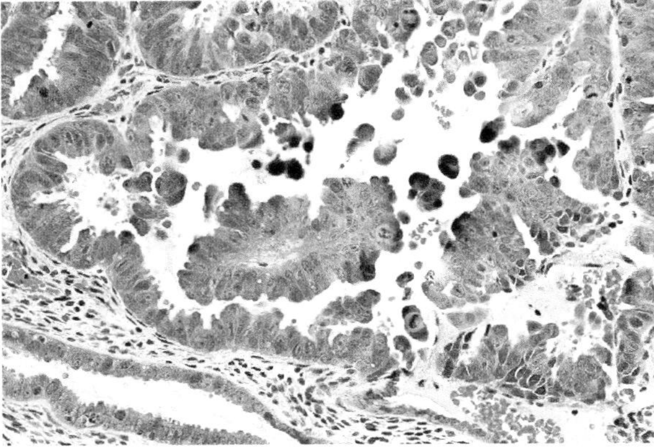

Fig. 9.35
Serous carcinoma. **Most nuclei are vesicular with prominent red nucleoli but some detached atypical cells have smudged hyperchromatic nuclei**

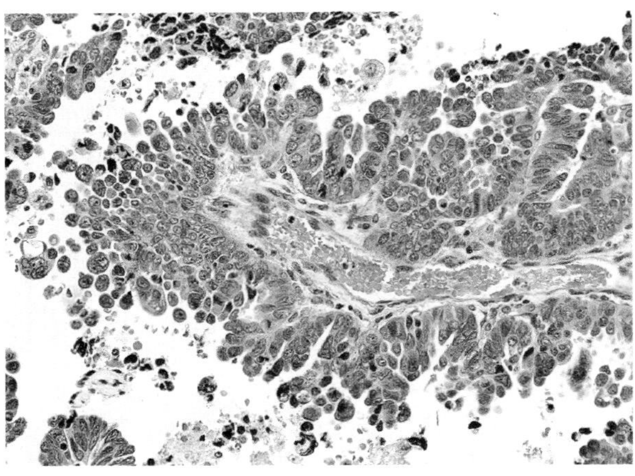

Fig. 9.34
Serous carcinoma. **Papillary structure is lined by markedly atypical hobnail type cells**

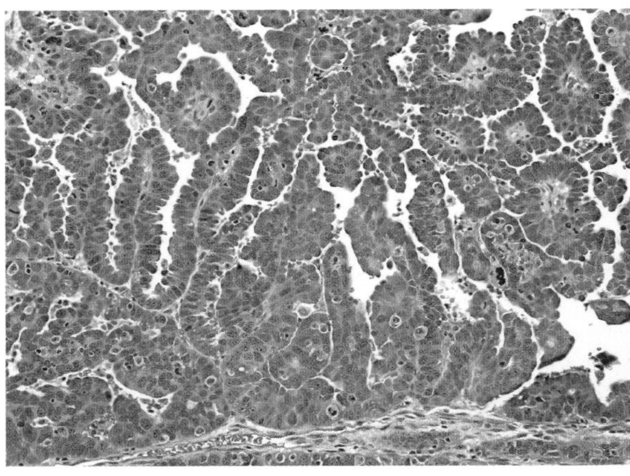

Fig. 9.36
Serous carcinoma. **Tumor is composed of papillae lined by epithelium having prominent scalloped luminal borders**

with eosinophilic and clear cytoplasm often are seen, but hobnail cells are among the most frequently observed cells. Marked nuclear atypia is always present and is required for a tumor to qualify as serous carcinoma (*Figs. 9.33, 9.35, 9.37, 9.40*). Thus, serous carcinoma is defined by the discordance between its architecture, which appears well differentiated (papillary or glandular pattern), and its nuclear morphology, which is high grade (grade 3 nuclei) [104]. Areas containing clear cells do not preclude the diagnosis of serous carcinoma.

Microscopically, the exophytic component of a serous carcinoma typically has a complex papillary architecture. The papillary fronds may be either short and densely fibrotic or thin and delicate. The cells covering the papillae and lining the glands form small papillary tufts, many of which are detached and float freely in spaces between the papillae and in gland lumens. The cells are cuboidal or hobnail shaped and contain abundant granular eosinophilic or clear cytoplasm. The cells tend to be loosely cohesive. There may be considerable cytologic variability throughout the tumor, as many cells tend to show marked cytologic atypia manifested by nuclear pleomorphism, hyperchromasia, and macronucleoli whereas others are small and not so ominous in appearance. Multinucleated cells, giant nuclei, and bizarre forms occur in half the tumors. Lobulated nuclei with smudged chromatin also

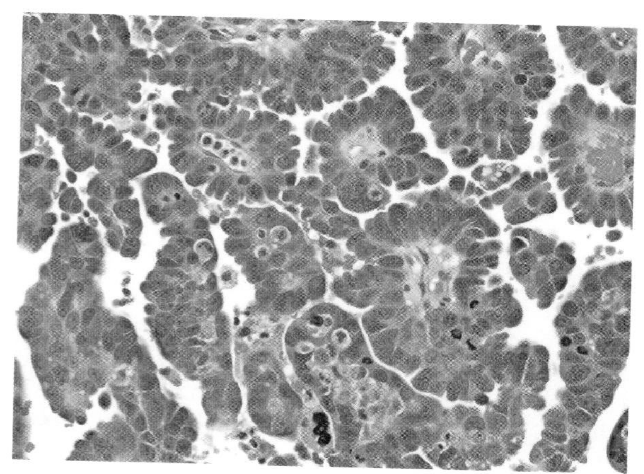

Fig. 9.37
Serous carcinoma. **Papillae are lined by cells with enlarged, vesicular nuclei with evident nucleoli. Several mitotic figures are present**

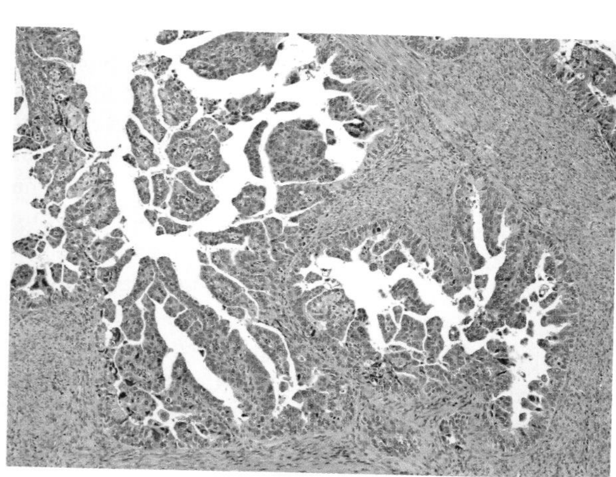

Fig. 9.38
Serous carcinoma. **Glands with prominent intraglandular papillary architecture infiltrate myometrium**

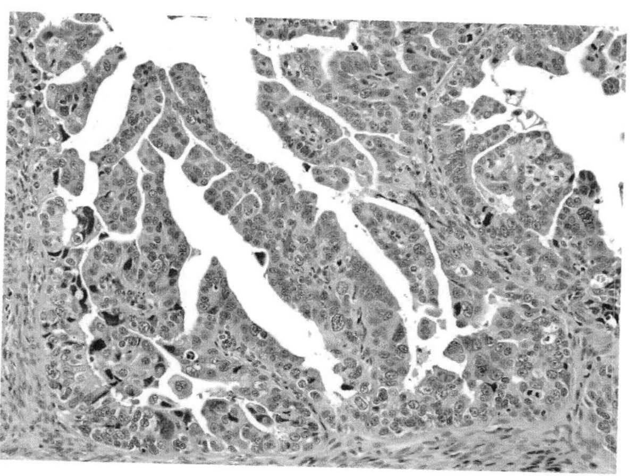

Fig. 9.39
Serous carcinoma. **Papillae are lined by markedly atypical epithelium**

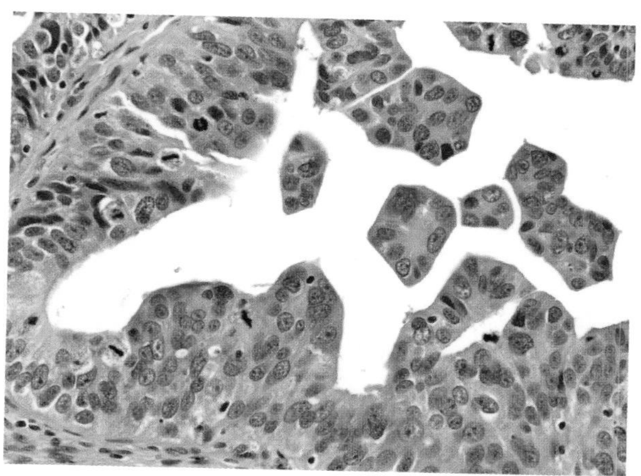

Fig. 9.40
Serous carcinoma. **Some glandular epithelium has smooth luminal borders but papillary epithelial tufts and marked nuclear atypia, with numerous mitotic figures, are characteristic of serous carcinoma**

are frequently encountered. Mitotic activity usually is high and abnormal mitotic figures are easily identified. Psammoma bodies are encountered in a third of cases. The invasive component of the neoplasm can show contiguous downgrowth; of papillary processes, or solid masses or glands, the latter often have a gaping appearance. Nests of cells within vascular spaces are commonly found (*Fig. 9.42*).

The adjacent endometrium in hysterectomy specimens with serous carcinoma is atrophic in almost all cases. Hyperplasia, generally without atypia, is present in less than 10% of cases [58, 361, 384]. In nearly 90% of cases, the surface endometrium adjacent to the carcinoma or at other sites away from the neoplasm is replaced by one or several layers of highly atypical cells that overlie atrophic endometrium and extend into normal glands. These cells are identical to those of the invasive carcinoma and at times form micropapillary processes. This lesion, which has been designated serous endometrial intraepithelial carcinoma (EIC; *Fig. 9.41*), is discussed in detail in Chap. 8, Precursor Lesions of Endometrial Carcinoma [23, 384]. The intraepithelial carcinoma can

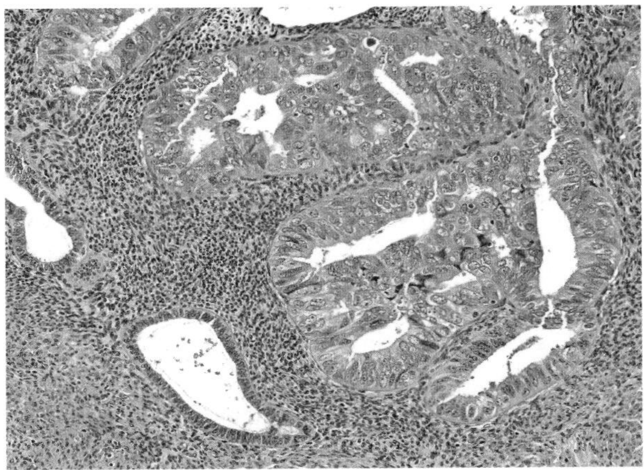

■ Fig. 9.41
Serous carcinoma. **An area of endometrial intraepithelial carcinoma (serous intraepithelial carcinoma) is present within a background of atrophic endometrium. Markedly atypical epithelium replaces preexisting endometrial glands**

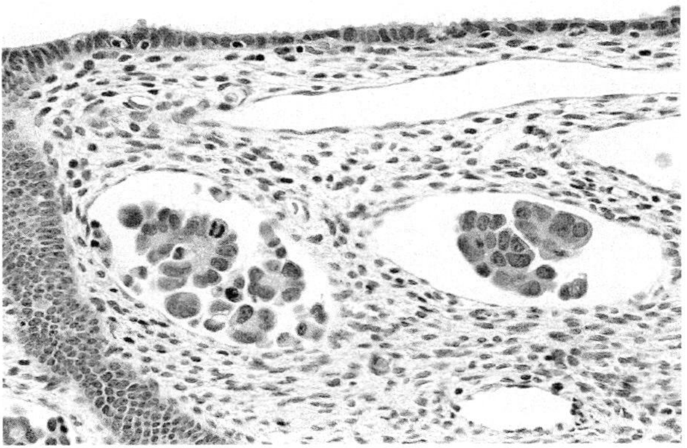

■ Fig. 9.42
Serous carcinoma. **Detached papillary epithelial cell clusters are present within lymphatic spaces of endometrium**

extensively replace the surface endometrium and underlying glands without stromal invasion. The clinicopathologic features and distinction of extensive EIC from early invasive serous carcinoma have been reported recently [423]. It has been proposed that EIC and serous carcinoma measuring 1 cm or less should be designated minimal uterine serous carcinoma because these lesions are difficult to distinguish and they behave in a similar fashion when confirmed as stage IA by meticulous surgical staging. It is important to recognize that patients whose uteri demonstrate only EIC, without evidence of invasive serous carcinoma in the completely sampled endometrium, can have metastatic serous carcinoma in the ovary, peritoneum, or omentum, presumably as a result of exfoliation and implantation of the loosely cohesive tumor cells [380, 423].

Differential Diagnosis

Serous carcinoma must be distinguished from villoglandular carcinoma, which also has papillary architecture. Unlike serous carcinoma, villoglandular carcinoma is characterized by the predominance of long, delicate papillary fronds that do not display papillary tufting. In addition, the cells are columnar, resembling cells in endometrioid carcinoma and lack high-grade nuclear atypia (see ➋ Villoglandular Carcinoma). A serous carcinoma with a prominent glandular pattern that lacks prominent papillary features may be confused with an endometrioid carcinoma. In this case, it is predominantly the nuclear morphology that aids in the distinction. The glands in an endometrioid carcinoma have a smooth luminal border and are lined by columnar cells with nuclei that are grade 1 or 2. Endometrioid carcinomas with grade 3 nuclei are almost always solid, not glandular. In contrast, the glands in a serous carcinoma are lined by cells with high-grade nuclei, some of which are hobnail shaped, thus imparting a scalloped luminal border to the glands. In addition, in most cases papillary tufts project or lie detached in the gland lumens. Immunohistochemical analysis can aid in the distinction of glandular serous carcinoma from endometrioid carcinoma. Several studies have demonstrated a very high frequency of strong, diffuse positivity for p53 in serous carcinomas, and this pattern of staining is correlated with the presence of mutations in the *p53* gene (see section ➋ Molecular Genetics) [227, 234, 273, 362, 396]. In addition, most serous carcinomas demonstrate a relative lack of expression of estrogen and progesterone receptors and very high proliferation indices as measured by immunohistochemical expression of Ki-67 compared to endometrioid carcinoma [59, 236]. In contrast, endometrioid carcinomas (particularly grades 1 and 2 tumors) frequently express hormone receptors and have lower proliferation indices [59, 236, 237]. In addition, strong, diffuse immunohistochemical expression of p53 is confined to a subset of grade 3 endometrioid carcinomas and is not encountered in lower-grade endometrioid carcinomas [236, 237]. Hence, glandular carcinomas with high-grade cytology for which the differential diagnosis includes grade 2 endometrioid carcinoma and serous carcinoma can be distinguished by immunohistochemistry for p53, Ki-67, and hormone receptors. The distinction of serous carcinoma from clear cell carcinoma is discussed later (see Clear Cell Carcinoma).

At times papillary syncytial eosinophilic change, particularly in a small curettage specimen in an older patient, may be difficult to distinguish from serous carcinoma. The papillary processes in eosinophilic change lack fibrovascular support and the cells that form these processes are small and lack significant nuclear atypia or mitotic activity. Typically, small microcystic spaces containing neutrophils are present in the syncytial masses (see Chap. 8, Precursor Lesions of Endometrial Carcinoma). At times it may not be clear if a serous carcinoma involving the endometrium is primary or metastatic from the ovary. More often than not the uterus is the primary site, even when invasion cannot be demonstrated in the hysterectomy specimen [420]. In these cases the ovarian involvement is typically bilateral and characterized by small foci of tumor on the ovarian surface or nodules of tumor in the parenchyma with clusters of tumor cells in hilar vascular spaces.

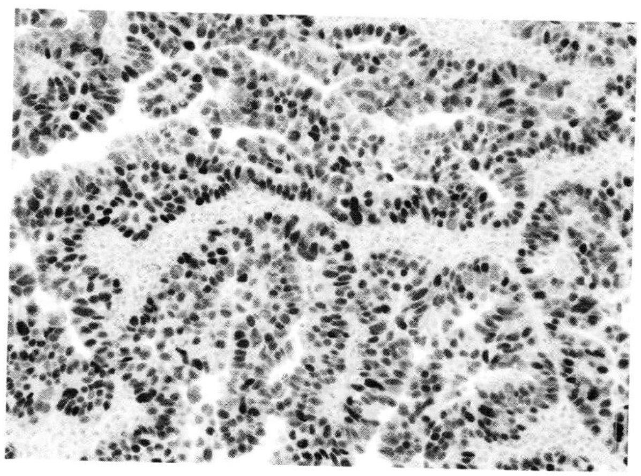

Fig. 9.43
Serous carcinoma. **Tumor exhibits diffuse/strong nuclear expression of p53 which correlates with a p53 mutation**

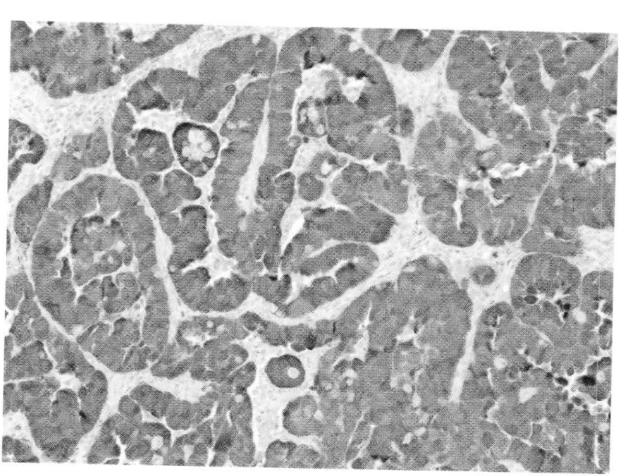

Fig. 9.44
Serous carcinoma. **Tumor exhibits diffuse/strong expression of p16**

Immunohistochemical Findings

Approximately 75% of endometrial serous carcinoma show p53 overexpression (intense expression in greater than 50–75% of tumor cell nuclei; *Fig. 9.43*) as a result of p53 mutation and the consequent accumulation of mutant protein [234, 362, 381, 396, 448]. Some of the remaining tumors, which show absolutely no p53 expression, have p53 mutations that result in a truncated p53 protein or a protein with conformational changes that cannot be detected using commercially available antibodies [396]. The Ki-67 labeling index is extremely high (i.e., greater than 50–75% of tumor cell nuclei) [236]. The typical serous carcinoma lacks diffuse ER and PR expression [59, 65, 100, 237, 380], although many carcinomas with hybrid endometrioid/serous features and admixtures of endometrioid and serous components express considerable amounts of ER [15]. PR is less frequently expressed, compared to ER. Diffuse/strong p16 is characteristic of serous carcinomas (*Fig. 9.44*) [73, 328, 433]. In contrast to most endocervical carcinomas, this does not imply HPV infection; rather, it may reflect disturbances in the cell cycle that favor hyperproliferative activity. In contrast to endometrioid adenocarcinomas, nuclear β-catenin expression and loss of PTEN, MLH1, MSH2, MSH6, and PMS2 are almost never encountered.

Despite important immunophenotypic differences that distinguish between clear-cut examples of serous, and endometrioid carcinomas of the endometrium, these tumors share some notable features. Like endometrioid carcinomas, endometrial serous carcinomas commonly express pan-cytokeratins, EMA, CA125, Ber EP4, B72.3, CK7, and vimentin, while they are usually negative for CK20 and lack diffuse, strong cytoplasmic expression of CEA.

Finally, there are some important differences between the immunophenotype of endometrial and ovarian, tubal and peritoneal serous carcinomas as a group. The most important is infrequent WT1 expression in endometrial serous carcinomas (seen in at most 20–30% of such cases) and the very common diffuse nuclear expression of WT1 in ovarian, tubal, and primary peritoneal examples (at least 70–80% of such cases) [9, 109, 152].

Behavior and Treatment

Serous carcinoma has a propensity for myometrial and lymphatic invasion. The hysterectomy specimen often discloses tumor in lymphatics extensively within the myometrium, cervix, broad ligament, fallopian tube, and ovarian hilus. In addition, intraepithelial carcinoma similar to that involving the endometrium has been reported on the surfaces of the ovaries, peritoneum, and mucosa of the endocervix and fallopian tube in the absence of gross disease in these sites [361, 423]. The involvement of peritoneal surfaces in the pelvis and abdomen, as in ovarian serous carcinoma, occurs early in the course of disease. Not surprisingly, most studies report that uterine serous carcinoma is clinically understaged in approximately 40% of cases [58, 108]. In addition to intraperitoneal spread, serous carcinoma can metastasize to the liver, brain, and skin.

The 5- and 10-year actuarial survival rates for all stages were 36% and 18%, respectively, in a study from Norway [5]; 5-year survival for pathologic stage I serous carcinoma was 40% in one study [58]. One study of stage I and II serous and clear cell carcinomas demonstrated a 5-year survival rate of 57% for patients with stage IA tumors, which was similar to that for patients with stage IB and IC tumors (53%) [81]. A recent retrospective study of stage I serous carcinoma evaluated outcomes in patients treated with different modalities. Patients who received chemotherapy, with our without radiation therapy, experienced more favorable outcomes when compared to patients treated with radiation or observation alone. Only 11.2% of patients treated with chemotherapy and radiation experienced recurrence, compared to 30.3% without therapy, and 25% when radiation was the sole treatment modality. The only subgroup that did not appear to benefit from chemotherapy included patients with stage IA serous carcinoma; only two of 27 such patients experienced recurrence [119].

In addition, prognostic factors for shorter survival included age greater than 60 years, vascular invasion, and greater than 50% myometrial invasion. Nearly half the serous carcinomas and 40% of the clear cell carcinomas in this study population that were thought to be early stage (clinical stage I and II) were upstaged to surgical stage III or IV despite the finding that the majority of these tumors had invaded only the inner third of the myometrium [80]. In addition, 13% of the serous carcinomas that were confined to the endometrium had paraaortic lymph node metastases. Patients with mixed endometrial carcinomas containing a component of serous carcinoma that accounted for at least 25% of the tumor have the same survival as patients with pure serous carcinoma, underscoring the importance of identifying areas of serous carcinoma in uterine carcinomas [361].

The current approach to treatment is hysterectomy and bilateral salpingo-oophorectomy along with omentectomy and careful surgical staging, including peritoneal cytology and pelvic and paraaortic lymph node sampling. In view of the highly aggressive behavior, adjuvant therapy should be considered for all tumors except those that qualify as minimal uterine serous carcinoma. In a study of 21 cases with pure EIC or minimal uterine serous carcinoma (less than 1 cm of carcinoma in the endometrium), all 14 patients whose tumors lacked myometrial or vascular invasion and who had no evidence of extrauterine disease at staging had an overall survival of 100% after a mean follow-up of 27 months [423]. The majority of these patients received no treatment after hysterectomy. Included among these cases were a few patients with the involvement of endocervical glands by EIC (stage IIA disease) who were also alive without evidence of disease at intervals ranging from 12 to 54 months. In contrast, the patients with either EIC or minimal serous carcinoma and evidence of extrauterine disease (even microscopic disease) all died of disease despite intensive chemotherapy. In another study of stage IA serous carcinoma, 11 of 13 patients were alive without evidence of disease after a median follow-up of 38 months [61]. Another study of 16 noninvasive serous carcinomas of the endometrium found that six tumors were stage IA and the remaining ten had metastases identified at staging [204]. Two of the six patients with stage IA disease experienced a recurrence but none died of disease during the follow-up period, which ranged from 2 to 73 months. Three patients with stage IIA disease also were alive without evidence of disease at intervals ranging from 37 to 61 months [119].

The finding of advanced-stage disease in the absence of myometrial invasion in ten patients emphasizes the need for complete staging of all patients with serous carcinoma. Another study of eight patients with serous or clear cell carcinoma confined to endometrial curettings without evidence of residual high-grade carcinoma (serous, clear cell, or FIGO grade 3 endometrioid) or vascular invasion in the hysterectomy specimen were without evidence of recurrence after a median follow-up of 3 years [27].

In a study evaluating cisplatin, doxorubicin (Adriamycin), and cyclophosphamide (PAC) chemotherapy, which has a 70% response rate in previously untreated ovarian serous carcinoma, the response rate for uterine serous carcinoma was only 20%, suggesting that there are inherent differences in uterine and ovarian serous carcinomas [244]. Another study of platinum-based chemotherapy found that eight of the 12 treated women were alive without evidence of disease, including four patients with advanced-stage disease and mean follow-up of 23 months, suggesting a possible role for chemotherapy [150]. More recent studies suggest that systemic platinum base therapies with or without taxane may be effective in the treatment of high stage serous carcinoma of the endometrium [212, 213]. These tumors are unresponsive to hormonal treatment because they almost always lack diffuse expression of hormone receptors.

In summary, it is very important for patients with serous carcinoma to be carefully staged as there may be extrauterine disease even if there is no or minimal myoinvasion. If there is no evidence of extrauterine disease after thorough staging the prognosis is favorable.

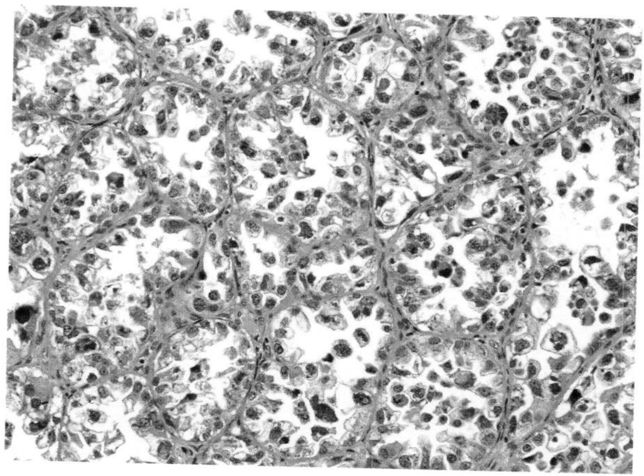

Fig. 9.45
Clear cell carcinoma. **Glands are lined by markedly atypical hobnail type cells with clear cytoplasm. This appearance is reminiscent of the Arias–Stella reaction in gestational endometrium**

Clear Cell Carcinoma

In the past, clear cell carcinoma was regarded as mesonephric in origin because of its resemblance to renal carcinoma, but the occurrence of clear cell carcinoma in the endometrium, a Müllerian derivative, is evidence of its Müllerian origin [229]. The prevalence of clear cell carcinoma ranges from 1% to 6% in most series. Almost all studies report that women with clear cell carcinoma are older than women with endometrioid carcinoma (mean age in late 60s) [2, 75, 208, 314, 379, 421]. Some studies have reported a higher likelihood of abnormal cytology, a lower frequency of some of the associated constitutional symptoms, such as obesity and diabetes mellitus, and a lack of association of estrogen replacement therapy compared with endometrioid carcinomas, but this has not been confirmed by other studies.

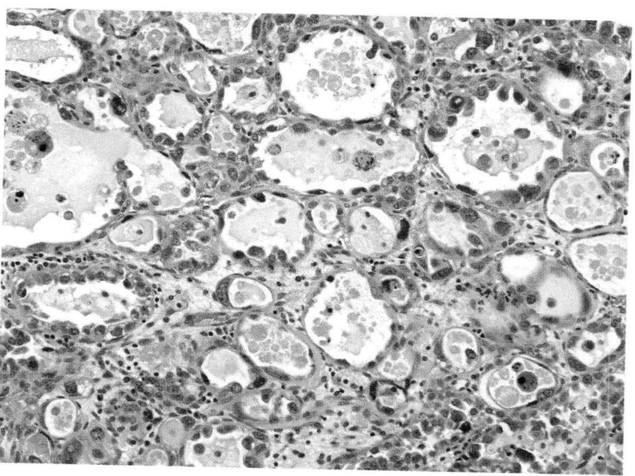

Fig. 9.46
Clear cell carcinoma. **Glands are lined by pleomorphic cells, some attenuated and others with prominent hobnail morphology**

These tumors do not have distinctive gross features. Clear cell carcinoma may exhibit solid, papillary, tubular, and cystic patterns (*Figs. 9.45–9.52*). The solid pattern is composed of masses of clear cells intermixed with eosinophilic cells, whereas papillary, tubular, and cystic patterns are composed predominantly of hobnail-shaped cells with interspersed clear and eosinophilic cells. Cystic spaces frequently are lined by flattened cells. Psammoma bodies can be found in association with papillary areas within the tumor. The cells typically are large, with clear or lightly stained eosinophilic cytoplasm. The clear cytoplasm results from the presence of glycogen, demonstrated with a PAS stain and diastase digestion. Cells that have discharged their glycogen and lost most of their cytoplasm are characterized by a naked nucleus, the hobnail cell. Nuclear atypia within a given tumor can be variable, ranging from mild to marked (*Figs. 9.50–9.52*). Almost always areas of marked atypia will be found, however. The atypia is manifested by pleomorphic, often large, multiple nuclei with prominent nucleoli. Mitotic activity is high, and

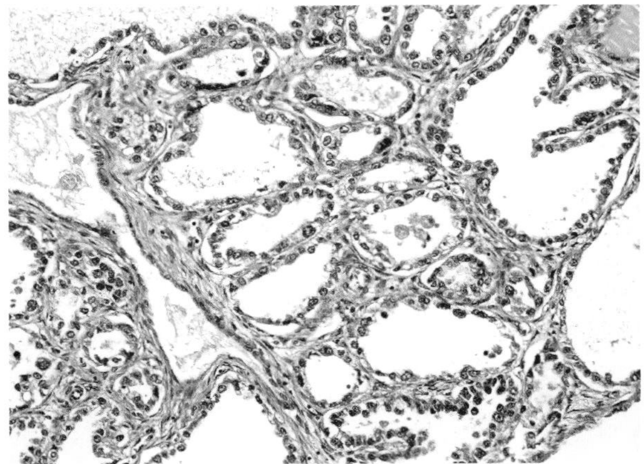

Fig. 9.47
Clear cell carcinoma. **Glands are lined by cells with clear cytoplasm and many uniform cuboidal cells with focal hobnail features**

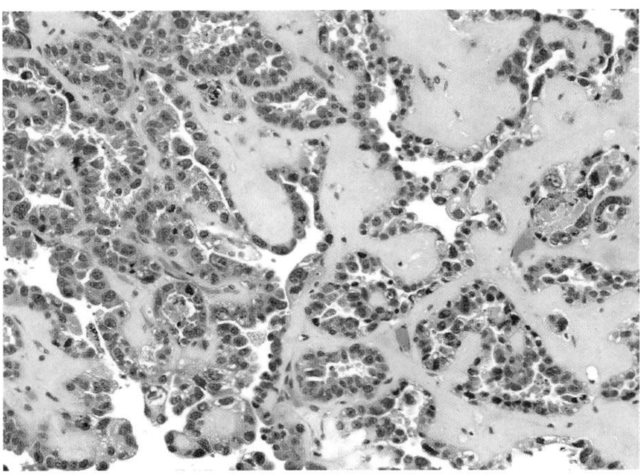

Fig. 9.48
Clear cell carcinoma. **Papillary tumor exhibits characteristic features, including hyalinized stroma and cells with clear to granular eosinophilic cytoplasm and hobnail morphology**

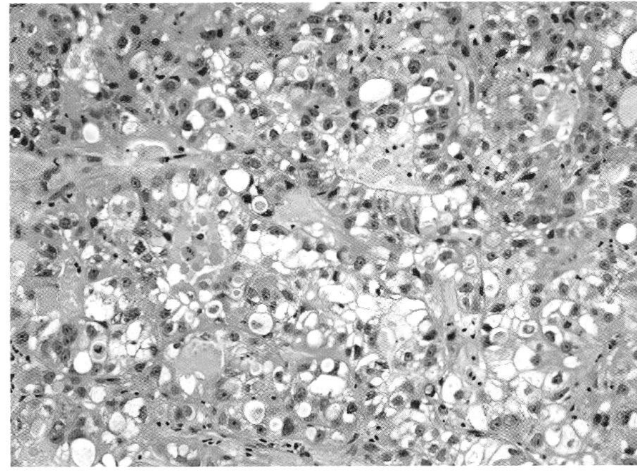

Fig. 9.49
Clear cell carcinoma. **Solid tumor is composed of cells with prominent clear cytoplasm and characteristic nuclei with vesicular chromatin and nucleoli**

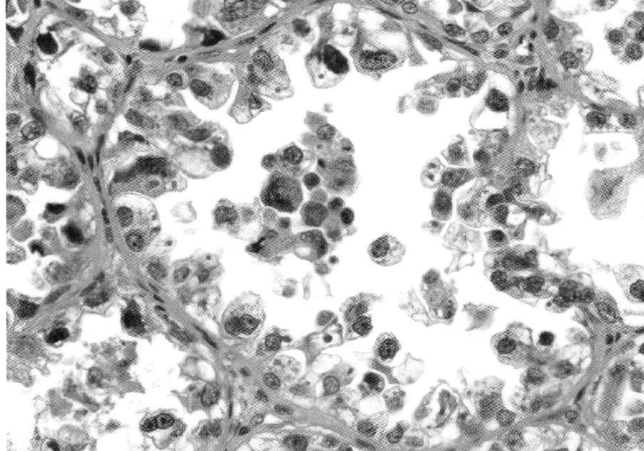

Fig. 9.50
Clear cell carcinoma. **Hobnail type cells protrude prominently into the gland lumen and are pleomorphic with hyperchromatic nuclei**

abnormal mitoses are readily seen. PAS-positive, diastase-resistant intracellular, and extracellular hyaline bodies, similar to those in endodermal sinus tumors, can be found in nearly two-thirds of clear cell carcinomas.

Differential Diagnosis

The differential diagnosis of clear cell carcinoma includes secretory carcinoma, serous carcinoma, and yolk sac tumor. The differential diagnosis of the first tumor has been discussed (see Secretory Carcinoma). Clear cell carcinoma can be distinguished from serous carcinoma by architectural and cytoplasmic rather than nuclear features because both tumors display similar high-grade nuclear features, including vesicular nuclei with prominent nucleoli, hobnail cells, and cells with hyperchromatic, smudged nuclei. Serous carcinomas do not display the tubulocystic or solid growth patterns, clear cytoplasm, and hyalinized stroma that are characteristic of clear cell

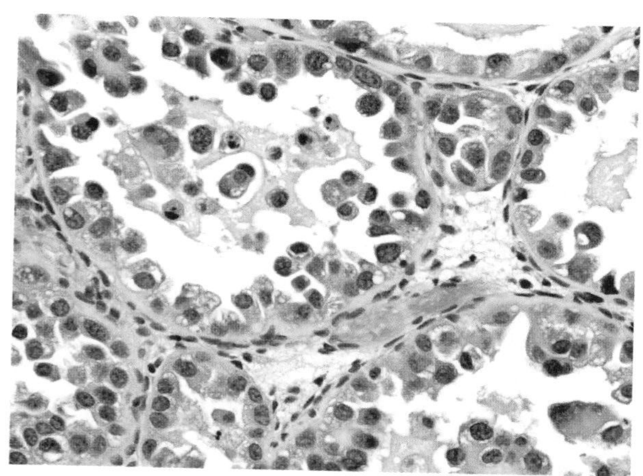

Fig. 9.51
Clear cell carcinoma. **Hobnail type cells have hyperchromatic nuclei and vacuolated clear cytoplasm**

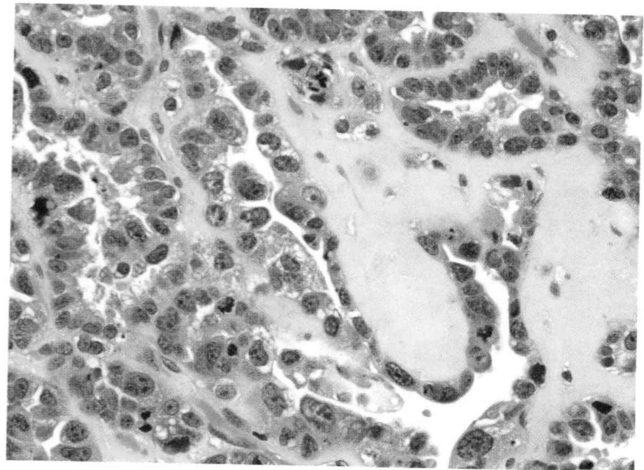

Fig. 9.52
Clear cell carcinoma. **Hyalinized papillae are lined by cells with clear to eosinophilic cytoplasm and pleomorphic nuclei**

carcinomas. In some cases, mixtures of both types are found. Yolk sac tumors occur rarely in the endometrium but the patients are young, in contrast to women with clear cell carcinoma, who are almost always postmenopausal. Microscopically, yolk sac tumors often have a microcystic pattern that can resemble the tubulocystic pattern of clear cell carcinoma. Characteristically, the yolk sac tumor contains Schiller–Duval bodies, which are lacking in clear cell carcinoma. Yolk sac tumors are associated with elevated serum alpha-fetoprotein (AFP) levels, and AFP can be identified in the tumor by immunohistochemistry.

Clear cell carcinoma tends to be high grade, deeply invasive, and to present in an advanced stage. Similar to serous carcinoma, clear cell carcinomas are more frequently associated with deep myometrial invasion, high nuclear grade, lymphovascular space invasion, and pelvic lymph node metastasis compared to low-grade endometrioid carcinomas [346]. Occasionally they are confined to a polyp [208]. The reported survival of patients with clear cell carcinoma differs considerably as reported in various series, ranging from 21% to 75% [2, 75, 229, 314, 421]. In one series, none of the patients with tumor beyond stage I survived for 5 years, and even in stage I the 5-year survival was only 44% [421]. Another report of low-stage tumors demonstrated better survival, with an estimated survival rate of 71% [258]. In a series of nearly 97 patients the 5-year crude survival was 42% and the 10-year survival, 31% [2]. One study reported 5- and 10-year actuarial disease-free survival rates of 43% and 39% [7], and in another study median survival for CC was 29 months and 5-year survival was 50% [379]. The wide range in survival reported in these different series suggests that different investigators may be applying different criteria for the diagnosis of clear cell carcinoma, resulting in a heterogeneous group of cases being studied. Treatment is variable and in some institutions chemotherapy is used irrespective of stage. The role of adjuvant radiation or chemotherapy is not established at present. In view of the poor prognosis and because these tumors often have high nuclear grade and invade the myometrium deeply, adjuvant therapy often is administered.

Immunohistochemical Findings

Like endometrioid and serous carcinomas, clear cell carcinomas usually express pan-cytokeratins, EMA, CA125, BerEP4, B72.3, CK7, and vimentin, while they are usually negative for CK20 and WT1 and lack diffuse, strong cytoplasmic expression of CEA.

Clear cell carcinomas are typically ER/PR negative and show p53, p16, and Ki-67 expression that are intermediate between endometrioid and serous carcinomas [237, 328, 413]. Notably, p53 overexpression and proliferation indices that mimic serous carcinomas are generally not seen in clear cell carcinoma. Although some clear cell carcinomas show abnormalities in *CTNNB1* (β-catenin) and *PTEN* pathways [24, 63], insufficient numbers of well-characterized cases have been studied. Clear cell carcinoma of the endometrium might represent a manifestation of HNPCC [60]; as such, there are rare clear cell carcinomas with loss of MSH2 and MSH6 expression, related to mutations in the corresponding genes.

Mixed Types of Carcinoma

An endometrial carcinoma may show combinations of two or more of the pure types. By convention, a mixed carcinoma has at least one other component comprising at least 10% of the tumor. For example, an endometrioid carcinoma containing a clear cell carcinoma that constitutes 10% of the tumor is classified as an endometrioid carcinoma with areas of clear cell carcinoma. Except for a few studies evaluating the significance of foci of serous carcinoma admixed with endometrioid carcinoma, there are no data that can be used as a basis for making valid recommendations concerning what proportion of an additional component justifies being separately classified. Mixed serous and endometrioid carcinomas containing at least 25% of a serous component behave as pure serous carcinomas [361]. Except for serous and possibly clear cell components, it is likely that the combination of other tumor types has little, if any, clinical significance.

Malignant Mesodermal (Müllerian) Mixed Tumor (Carcinosarcoma)

Malignant Mesodermal (Müllerian) mixed tumors (MMMTs) represent less than 5% of malignant neoplasms of the uterine corpus [372]. By definition, they are composed of malignant epithelial and mesenchymal components as recognized by light microscopy. Because of the biphasic appearance of carcinosarcomas (MMMTs), there has been considerable controversy about their histopathogenesis. Recent clinicopathologic, immunohistochemical, and molecular genetic studies have provided substantial evidence that most MMMTs likely represent carcinomas with a mesenchymal component as a consequence of metaplasia and/or tumor progression [132, 261]. Some MMMTs might also arise via progression from an adenosarcoma. This is supported by the recognition that as many as one-third of MMMTs contain zones that closely resemble adenosarcoma [357] and by studies that report metastases from adenosarcomas that resemble MMMT [82]. It is also possible that these tumors arise by a process of bidirectional differentiation from a single multipotent stem cell.

The risk factors for MMMT have been difficult to determine as robust epidemiologic studies have not been done due to the low prevalence of the disease. One small study suggested that MMMTs may share risk factors (body weight, exogenous estrogen use, and nulliparity) with endometrial carcinoma [446]. Tamoxifen therapy has also been noted as a possible contributor to the development of MMMTs [97, 332, 393]. The risk apparently persists and might even increase after cessation of treatment [124]. MMMTs, along with high-grade endometrial carcinomas, have been reported to arise in patients previously treated with pelvic irradiation for rectal or cervical carcinomas [163, 322]. Endometrial carcinomas and MMMTs also demonstrate similar genetic abnormalities including defective DNA mismatch repair and *p53* and *PTEN* gene mutation [20, 398, 399].

Endometrial carcinomas and MMMTs share many clinical features. Like carcinomas, MMMTs metastasize to pelvic and paraaortic lymph nodes, pelvic soft tissues, vagina, peritoneal surfaces, and lungs [78, 129, 294]. The histologic appearance of metastases is variable. Three studies on metastatic MMMT have demonstrated that invasive foci in lymphatic or vascular spaces are essentially always pure carcinoma and metastatic lesions are most commonly purely carcinoma; occasionally, mixtures of carcinoma and sarcoma are found and only rarely is pure sarcoma encountered [41, 372, 386]. Studies have also suggested that staging surgery usually performed for carcinomas, with omentectomy, peritoneal biopsies, and lymph node dissection, is better suited to detecting occult metastatic MMMT than are staging procedures commonly performed for sarcomas [125, 429]. Both carcinomas and MMMTs respond well to cisplatin-based chemotherapy [392, 412].

Clinical Features

The mean age of patients with MMMTs is in the seventh decade, but the age range spans from the fourth through tenth decades. The disease tends to present like other endometrial cancers, with vaginal bleeding being common. Another typical presentation of carcinosarcoma is a polypoid mass that protrudes through the cervical os.

Gross Findings

MMMTs are frequently polypoid and usually fill the entire endometrial cavity. Many invade the myometrium but some are confined to polyps. The tumors often protrude through the cervical os, simulating a cervical neoplasm. The protruding tip of the mass can be necrotic, making diagnosis based on biopsy of this portion of the tumor difficult. In approximately a quarter of the cases the uterine tumor extends into the endocervix. The tumors are variably soft to firm and tan with areas of necrosis and hemorrhage.

Microscopic Findings

MMMTs are composed of an admixture of histologically malignant epithelial and mesenchymal components but the epithelial component of MMMT is frequently difficult to subclassify (➋ *Figs. 9.53–9.59*). In the most recent clinicopathologic review of MMMT, the authors reported that serous carcinomas and high-grade carcinomas, not otherwise specified, were the most frequent carcinoma components in MMMT [125]. Older studies have reported endometrioid carcinomas to be more common. Clear cell, mucinous, squamous, and mesonephric carcinoma also can be found as the epithelial component, but this is less common [41, 231, 294, 295, 372]. Approximately half the cases demonstrate a homologous stromal component, which is high-grade spindle cell (like fibrosarcoma) or pleomorphic (like malignant fibrous histiocytoma) in most cases. The homologous stromal component only rarely resembles leiomyosarcoma or low-grade endometrial stromal sarcoma [123, 372]. When heterologous elements are present, rhabdomyosarcoma and chondrosarcoma are the most common types encountered [37, 125, 372] (➋ *Figs. 9.55–9.59*). Heterologous elements can usually be recognized easily by light microscopy. Immunohistochemical stains to establish the presence of such elements are not recommended unless such confirmation is needed after the review of hematoxylin- and eosin-stained slides. Rhabdomyosarcoma can often be identified by finding round or elongated cells with fibrillar eosinophilic cytoplasm. Striated rhabdomyoblasts are apparent on occasion. Some MMMTs are composed of cells that contain cytoplasmic eosinophilic globules that should not be misinterpreted as evidence of

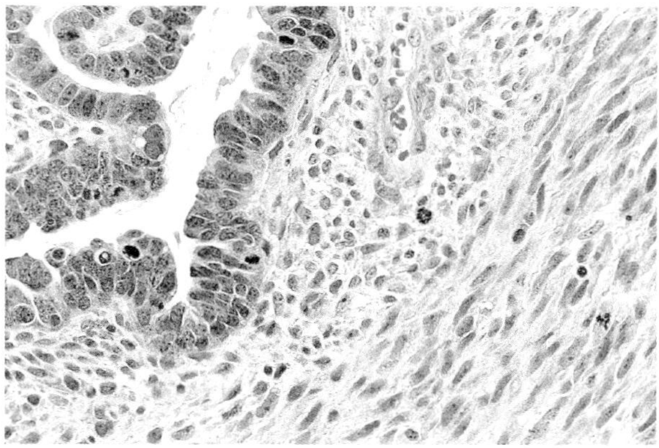

Fig. 9.54
Malignant mesodermal mixed tumor (carcinosarcoma).
Both carcinomatous and sarcomatous components have malignant cytologic features (nuclear pleomorphism and mitotic activity)

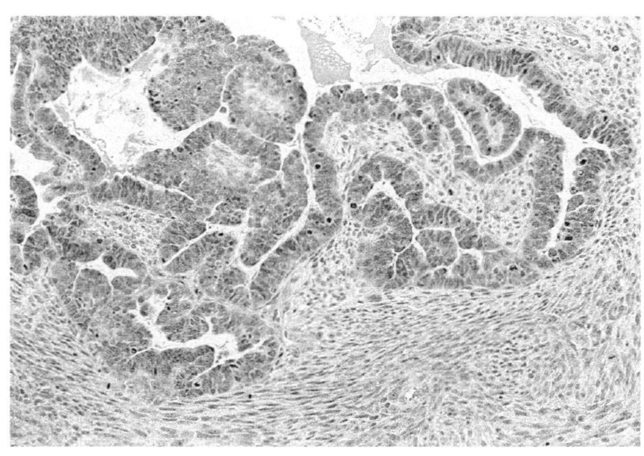

Fig. 9.53
Malignant mesodermal mixed tumor (carcinosarcoma).
High-grade adenocarcinoma with features of serous carcinoma is intimately admixed with a malignant spindle cell component (sarcoma)

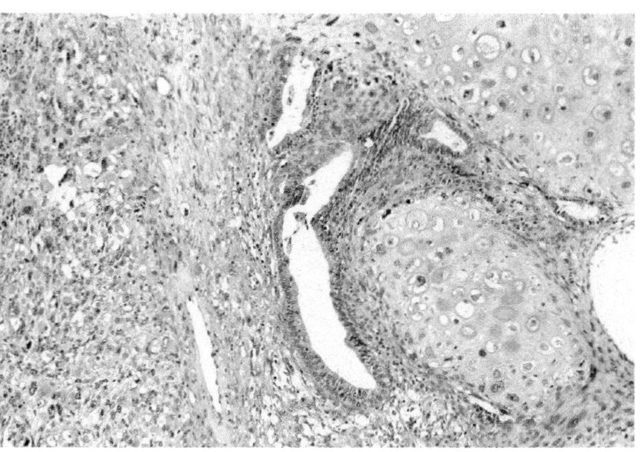

Fig. 9.55
Malignant mesodermal mixed tumor (carcinosarcoma).
Adenocarcinoma is intimately admixed with heterologous elements, including chondrosarcoma and rhabdomyosarcoma

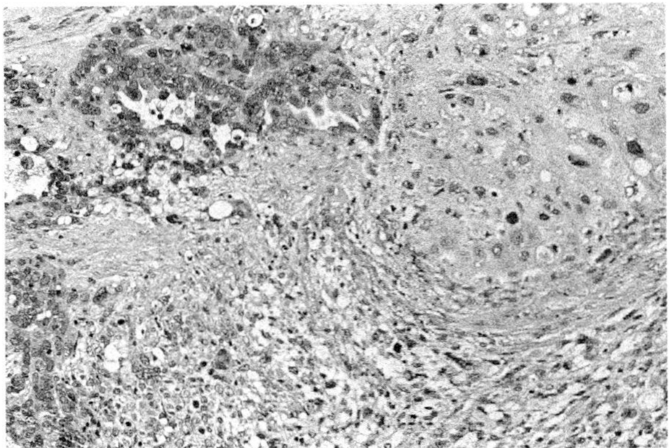

Fig. 9.56
Malignant mesodermal mixed tumor (carcinosarcoma).
Carcinoma is adjacent to spindle cell and chondroid components with malignant cytologic features

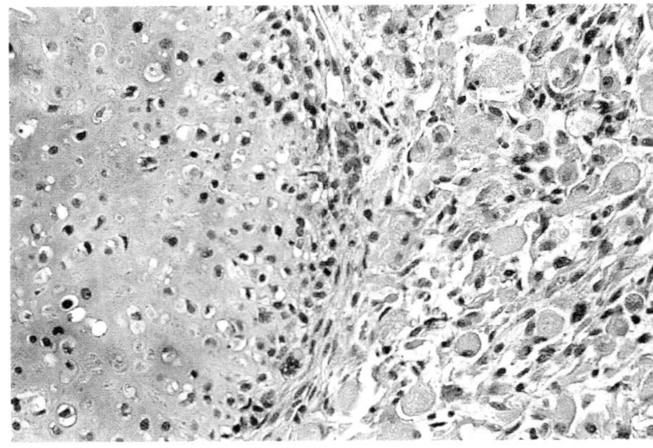

Fig. 9.58
Malignant mesodermal mixed tumor (carcinosarcoma).
Chondrosarcoma and rhabdomyosarcoma represent heterologous sarcomatous elements

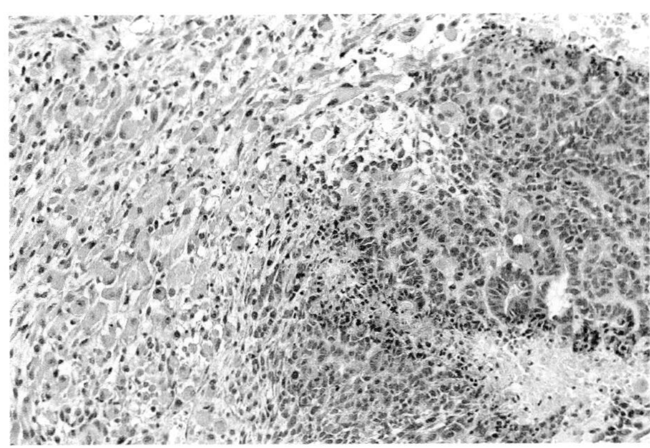

Fig. 9.57
Malignant mesodermal mixed tumor (carcinosarcoma).
Adenocarcinoma merges with rhabdomyosarcoma

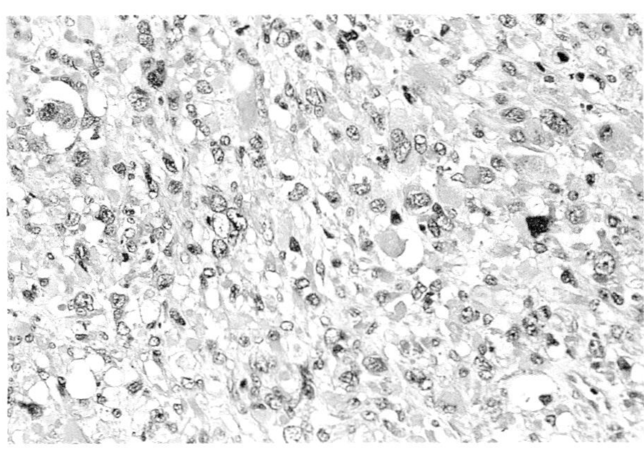

Fig. 9.59
Malignant mesodermal mixed tumor (carcinosarcoma).
Rhabdomyosarcoma is characterized by globoid pleomorphic cells with abundant eosinophilic cytoplasm

rhabdomyoblastic differentiation. Importantly, MMMTs as a group, are enriched for highly aggressive, biphasic, malignant mixed epithelial and mesenchymal neoplasms.

Differential Diagnosis

Monophasic tumors should not be diagnosed as a MMMT, although it is acknowledged that either the mesenchymal or epithelial components of MMMT might predominate in small samples such as biopsies and scant curettage specimens. Finding fragments of highly pleomorphic sarcoma, a high-grade carcinoma that is difficult to subclassify or heterologous elements in a small biopsy is usually sufficient to suggest that the biopsy might represent an incompletely sampled MMMT, but immunohistochemical results showing coexpression of epithelial and mesenchymal-associated markers are, by themselves, insufficient for a MMMT diagnosis.

The recently described dedifferentiated endometrial carcinoma is an example of a biphasic tumor containing differentiated and undifferentiated components [368].

However, unlike MMMTs the differentiated carcinoma is usually well-differentiated endometrioid and the undifferentiated component is composed of small, round cells of uniform size instead of spindle shaped or obviously pleomorphic cells (as discussed below with ➋ Undifferentiated Carcinomas). Endometrioid adenocarcinoma with spindle cell elements is another biphasic endometrial neoplasm that mimics MMMT; however, these tumors are composed of histologically low-grade elements and are less aggressive than typical MMMT and high-grade carcinoma [278]. In this tumor, the endometrioid elements, frequently showing squamous metaplasia, fuse imperceptibly with spindle cell elements that are never histologically high grade. In most cases, the endometrioid component is no more than FIGO grade 2 and the spindle cell component is cellular and sometimes mitotically active, but not markedly atypical. MMMT contains easily separable, high-grade epithelial, and mesenchymal elements whereas this type of endometrioid adenocarcinoma shows seamless fusion of the two. If there is confusion between this entity and MMMT, the tumor grade and the presence or absence of element fusion can be used to inform the decision. Endometrioid adenocarcinomas can contain chondroid and osteoid elements. Heterologous elements by themselves do not signify MMMT, although finding rhabdomyosarcoma along with adenocarcinoma almost always signifies MMMT.

Behavior and Treatment

Since MMMTs have been historically regarded as sarcomas, many studies have included patients with only clinical staging or incomplete surgical staging. Many older studies have also likely included histologic mimics of MMMT, particularly dedifferentiated carcinoma and endometrioid adenocarcinoma with spindle cell elements. Despite this, studies of comprehensively staged patients and others comprised of clinically staged patients agree that the behavior of MMMTs is significantly worse than FIGO grade 3 endometrial carcinomas, serous carcinomas, and clear cell carcinomas [19, 125, 148, 409]. Surgical stage is likely the most important prognostic factor.

Pathologically determined prognostic features in clinically staged MMMT patients are generally the same as for patients with suboptimally staged endometrial carcinoma. Extrauterine extension and/or deep myometrial invasion along with lymphovascular invasion are reported to be independent predictors of survival in numerous analyses [30, 37, 43, 136, 187, 289, 292, 337, 349, 429]. The presence of serous or clear cell carcinoma also is reported to have a significant tendency to be associated with metastatic disease, but the histologic appearance of the sarcomatous component does not appear to have any prognostic significance in many studies of clinically staged patients [136, 231, 292, 372, 383]. Advanced age may also be associated with poor outcome [187, 292]. The 5-year survival for patients with advanced-stage disease is only 15–30% [148, 289, 383].

A recent study looked at the clinical and pathologic features of comprehensively staged patients with FIGO stage I MMMT. This confirmed that stage I MMMT is a more aggressive disease when compared to a control group of comprehensively staged patients with FIGO stage I, FIGO grade 3 endometrioid, serous or clear cell carcinoma [125]. The 3-year disease-free survival was 87% for women with high-grade carcinoma compared with 42% for women with MMMT. Unlike studies of clinically staged patients, epithelial tumor type, lymphovascular invasion, depth of myometrial invasion, and predominance of carcinoma relative to sarcoma had no relationship to overall survival. The grade of the epithelial and mesenchymal components had no bearing on overall survival either, but they were almost always high-grade. The only clinical or pathologic factor found to have statistical significance with respect to clinical outcome was the presence of heterologous sarcomatous differentiation (principally rhabdomyoblastic), as assessed on the review of hematoxylin- and eosin-stained slides only. Heterologous sarcomatous elements were associated with very poor survivals [125]. When outcomes were stratified based on the presence of heterologous sarcomatous elements, the survival of patients with homologous MMMT was found to be indistinguishable from that of patients with high-grade endometrial carcinoma. Patients with heterologous MMMT had survivals that were significantly worse. The 3-year overall survival for surgical stage I MMMT was only 45% for heterologous tumors, compared with 93% for homologous tumors. This study evaluated the significance of heterologous sarcomatous elements in comprehensively staged FIGO stage I MMMT patients only, so it remains to be determined whether heterologous elements drive prognosis in patients with high stage disease. The clinical significance of heterologous elements had been noted previously [257], but studies of other clinically staged patients failed to support this view [136, 231, 252, 372, 425].

MMMTs metastasize to pelvic and paraaortic lymph nodes, pelvic soft tissues, vagina, peritoneal surfaces, and lungs [78, 129, 294]. MMMTs are treated by total hysterectomy and bilateral salpingo-oophorectomy with pelvic and paraaortic lymph node dissection, pelvic washings, and tumor debulking, if indicated. Older studies reported a decrease in local recurrences with external beam radiation therapy to the pelvis [182]. This was confirmed in a more recent retrospective study, but a convincing effect on overall survival was not appreciated [57]. In an analysis of recurrence patterns, this study also reported a 38% overall local recurrence rate and a 57% frequency of distant recurrences, most of which were peritoneal [57]. A Gynecologic Oncology Group (GOG) study of ifosfamide with or without cisplatin for the treatment of advanced, persistent, or recurrent MMMT demonstrated that the addition of cisplatin provided a small improvement in progression-free survival but no significant survival benefit [392]. Recently, the GOG published results that favored the use of combination chemotherapy (three cycles of cisplatin, ifosfamide, and mesna) over whole abdominal radiotherapy [427]. Although the estimated probability of recurrence in each arm of the study did not differ significantly, the recurrence rate was lower in the chemotherapy arm, when adjusted for stage and age, and the estimated death rate was lower in the chemotherapy group. In practice, many patients are offered combination therapy with carboplatin and taxol. Studies that address which, if any, MMMT patients are good candidates for targeted therapies are ongoing [79, 249, 326, 327, 351].

Undifferentiated Carcinoma

The World Health Organization (WHO) defines undifferentiated endometrial carcinoma as a tumor lacking any evidence of differentiation. The most common entity considered in the differential diagnosis of an undifferentiated tumor is FIGO grade 3 endometrioid adenocarcinoma, which should only be diagnosed when the tumor is obviously endometrioid in character. Confirmatory endometrioid features in this context include even focal glandular architecture, squamous metaplasia, or trabecular and nested growth patterns. Most FIGO grade 3 endometrioid carcinomas either contain focal glandular architecture and/or resemble non-keratinizing, poorly differentiated squamous cell carcinoma.

Different types of undifferentiated carcinomas can now be recognized, which means that tumors lacking differentiation on review of hematoxylin and eosin-stained slides probably represent a very heterogeneous group. Small cell carcinoma of neuroendocrine is one tumor that should be separated from the rest, as these tumors demonstrate a unique combination of immunohistochemical, ultrastructural, clinical, and biologic features. Another unique tumor is the undifferentiated carcinoma described recently [18].

Microscopic Findings

The recently described undifferentiated carcinoma [18] is a tumor composed predominately of a monotonous proliferation of small to intermediate-sized, discohesive cells arranged in sheets without an obvious nested or trabecular architecture or gland formation (*Figs. 9.60* and *9.61*).

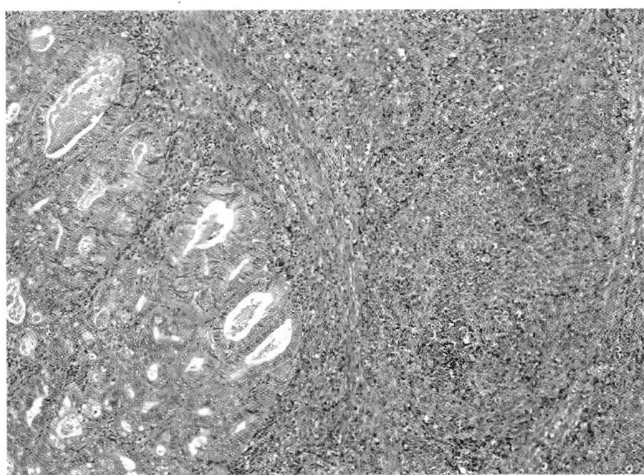

Fig. 9.60
Undifferentiated carcinoma. **Solid tumor lacking any differentiating features is present adjacent to, but not admixed with, FIGO grade 1 endometrioid carcinoma**

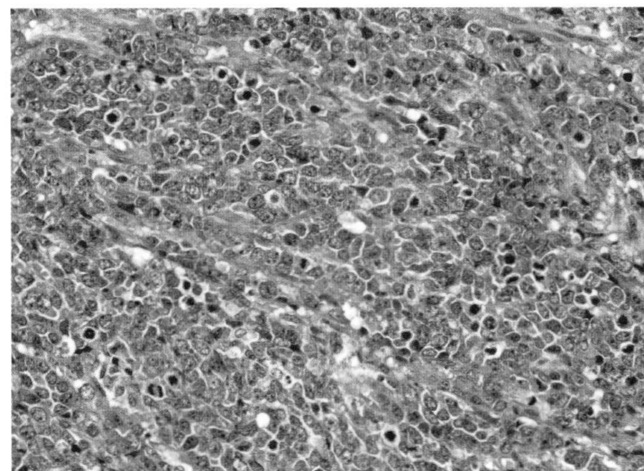

Fig. 9.61
Undifferentiated carcinoma. **Dyscohesive atypical cells lacking any differentiating features suggest a differential diagnosis of undifferentiated carcinoma versus lymphoma**

However, rare foci of abrupt keratinization are allowed. The low power appearance is reminiscent of endometrial stromal sarcoma, although the tongue-like pattern of myometrial infiltration and characteristic vasculature are lacking. The nuclear features, which often include vesicular chromatin with small chromocenters or nucleoli, along with the very high mitotic rate, are also incompatible with endometrial stroma sarcoma. In many cases, the cytologic appearance of this type of undifferentiated carcinoma recalls large cell lymphoma when the cytoplasm is scant and plasmacytoma when the cytoplasm is more abundant and rhabdoid. Although the tumor stroma is generally inapparent, some tumors display a myxoid matrix. Many examples also contain numerous tumor-infiltrating lymphocytes. When this feature is prominent, the tumor may resemble a lymphoepithelial-like carcinoma of the cervix or nasopharynx. Small cell carcinoma of neuroendocrine type is also a diagnostic consideration, but undifferentiated carcinoma does not typically demonstrate salt-and-pepper chromatin, nuclear molding, or neuroendocrine marker (chromogranin and synaptophysin) expression in greater than 10% of cells. Many endometrial carcinomas containing undifferentiated components also contain foci of well- or moderately differentiated endometrioid adenocarcinoma (➋ *Fig. 9.60*). These tumors have been called "de-differentiated endometrial carcinoma" [368]. In these tumors, the gland forming, or differentiated, components are superficial, adjacent to the endometrial cavity, whereas the undifferentiated areas are deeper in the endometrium and myometrium and sharply delimited from the differentiated areas. This accounts for the occasional scenario in which the well-differentiated endometrioid component is diagnosed on endometrial curettage, followed by recognition of the presence of a more deeply placed undifferentiated component on hysterectomy.

Immunohistochemical Findings

Immunohistochemically, the undifferentiated cells in general fail to express markers that would support a diagnosis of lymphoma, plasmacytoma, rhabdomyosarcoma, or a neuroendocrine tumor. Exceptions to this rule include CD138 expression in some examples and low-level expression of synaptophysin and chromogranin in others. The undifferentiated component characteristically shows only focal or weak keratin expression, but nearly every case exhibits intense EMA and cytokeratin 18 expression in a small minority of cells [18]. ER and PR staining is negative. Perhaps as many as one-half demonstrate abnormal DNA mismatch repair protein expression.

Clinical Features

Patients with undifferentiated and dedifferentiated carcinomas span a wide age range, from the third to eighth decade. Endometrial primaries are more common than ovarian primaries. Some patients have synchronous endometrial and ovarian endometrioid carcinomas, with the presence of the undifferentiated component recognizable in only one site. The most common presentation is vaginal bleeding. In many cases, patients are suspected of having lymphoma because of extensive, systemic lymph node involvement coupled with high serum LDH levels. Approximately one-half of patients have extrauterine disease at surgery. These are described as highly aggressive tumors and are almost always fatal. In some cases, a diagnosis of well-differentiated endometrioid adenocarcinoma may be followed by the emergence of undifferentiated carcinoma in a metastatic site. Recent data suggest that undifferentiated carcinomas frequently demonstrate an abnormal DNA mismatch repair gene expression profile that places some of them within the spectrum of tumors encountered among patients with Lynch syndrome/hereditary nonpolyposis colorectal carcinoma syndrome.

Prognostic Factors of Endometrial Carcinoma

Based largely on a series of Gynecologic Oncology Group (GOG) studies, it has been shown that the risk factors for the recurrence of endometrial carcinoma can be divided into uterine and extrauterine factors [46, 94, 277]. Uterine factors include (1) histologic type, (2) grade, (3) depth of myometrial invasion, (4) cervical involvement, (5) vascular invasion, (6) presence of atypical endometrial hyperplasia, (7) hormone receptor status, and (8) DNA ploidy and S-phase fraction. Extrauterine factors include (1) adnexal involvement, (2) intraperitoneal metastasis, (3) positive peritoneal cytology, and (4) pelvic and paraaortic lymph node metastasis. Patients with no evidence of extrauterine disease, no cervical involvement, and no evidence of vascular invasion are at a low overall risk of recurrence. For these patients the grade and depth of invasion are important prognostic factors. In contrast to this low-risk group of patients, women with evidence of extrauterine disease, cervical involvement, or vascular invasion constitute a high-risk group. If one of these three factors is positive, the frequency of recurrence is 20%, increasing to 43% for two positive factors, and 63% for three factors [277].

Clinical Factors

Age, race, and socioeconomic status are prognostic factors in endometrial cancer. Some studies have shown that age is the most important prognostic factor followed by FIGO stage, tumor grade, race, and socioeconomic status [142]. Younger women tend to have lower-grade and less invasive tumors, but age remains an important independent risk factor. It has also been demonstrated that women aged 45 or less have a better prognosis than women over age 45 because of a significantly higher proportion of early-stage disease and less myometrial invasion [431]. Another study also demonstrated that age is a significant prognostic factor, with decreased survival for women over age 50 unrelated to surgical stage or grade of carcinoma [122]. Although there is a lower prevalence of endometrial cancer in African–American women as compared with white women, white women have a significant survival advantage as compared with African–American women even after controlling for other clinicopathologic and socioeconomic factors [38, 83, 178]. Some studies have shown that African–American women have a higher proportion of high-grade tumors and less favorable histologic subtypes and tend to present with higher-stage tumors compared to white women [83, 178]. In addition, they are treated less often at every stage of disease. Another study showed that the incidence of high-risk tumors is the same in African–American and white women, whereas the incidence of low-risk tumors is significantly lower in African–American women [318]. Although an elevated body mass index (BMI) is associated with a lower stage and other better prognostic factors, when adjusted for these factors, survival was lower in overweight patients [143].

Histologic Grade

Numerous studies have confirmed the value of grading [6, 75, 111, 224, 240, 440, 444]. For example, FIGO data collected from almost 5,000 surgically staged patients indicate that the 5-year overall survival rates for women with surgical stage I endometrial carcinoma dropped from 92.1% for those with grade 1 tumors, to 87.5% for those with grade 2 tumors, to 74.5% for those with grade 3 tumors [95]. The survival difference is not limited to early-stage disease, and a 30% difference in survival was also found in the comparison of women with grade 1, stage III tumors (69.7%) to those with grade 3, stage III tumors (39.6%). In a study of more than 600 women with clinical stage I or occult stage II endometrioid adenocarcinoma, the 5-year relative survival was as follows: grade 1, 94%; grade 2, 84%; and grade 3, 72% [440]. According to a population-based study from the Norwegian Radium Hospital involving nearly 2,000 patients, the 5- and 10-year survival rates for patients with grade 1 tumors were 88% and 80%, respectively; with grade 2 tumors, 77% and 62%; and with grade 3 tumors, 60% and 49% [6].

A study of the reproducibility of the FIGO grading method found that interobserver reproducibility was acceptable for the architectural grade but unacceptably low for the assessment of notable nuclear atypia [288]. A more recent study comparing FIGO grading to pure nuclear grading of endometrioid carcinoma demonstrated fair interobserver reproducibility for FIGO grading but only poor interobserver reproducibility for nuclear grading [235]. Using a database of 715 patients with low clinical stage endometrial carcinomas (excluding serous and clear cell types), the utility of the FIGO grading system using arbitrary definitions for three nuclear grades was examined [444]. Patients with architectural grade 1 or 2 adenocarcinomas but with predominantly grade 3 nuclei were moved up one grade. This change resulted in upgrading 44 patients for whom the risk of recurrence and death from tumor was similar to that of the other patients in the grade into which they were reassigned. This study provided support for the FIGO modification of architectural grade based on inappropriate nuclear atypia and reinforced the need for a uniform definition of nuclear grade.

Histologic grade is highly correlated with other prognostic factors such as age, stage, and depth of myometrial invasion, so its prognostic utility must also be examined in multivariate analyses. In such studies, the significance of histologic grade in the prediction of survival or recurrence is diminished after adjustment for the other factors, suggesting that grade primarily provides information about the probability of local or disseminated spread of tumor [6, 443]. Nevertheless, even for patients with metastatic (stage III) tumor, the histologic grade is significant in predicting outcome after multivariate analysis [158].

Alternative methods of assignment of histologic grade have been proposed, including a two-tiered system for assessing uterine tumor grade, based on a study of 85 patients with stage I and II endometrial cancer [400]. Separation of tumors into two groups based on the amount of solid growth identified those that recurred as having greater than 20% solid growth. The two-tier grading system yielded a higher degree of interobserver agreement than the three-tier FIGO system. A binary architectural grading system based on the presence of greater than 50% solid growth, a diffusely infiltrative rather than pushing pattern of invasion, and tumor cell necrosis has been described [235]. Tumors displaying at least two of these three features were classified as high grade whereas those displaying one of those features was classified as low grade. The binary system stratified patients into three distinct prognostic groups (This study was done using the 1988 FIGO staging). Patients with stage I low-grade tumors with invasion confined to the inner half of the myometrium (stages IA and IB) had a 100% 5-year survival rate. Patients with low-grade tumors that invaded into the outer half of the myometrium or beyond (stages IC-IV) had a 5-year survival rate of 67%. Similarly, those with high-grade tumors with invasion confined to the myometrium (stages IA–IC) had a 5-year survival rate of 76%. Patients with advanced-stage (stages II–IV) high-grade tumors had a 26% 5-year survival rate. In addition, greater intra- and interobserver reproducibility were demonstrated for the binary system in comparison with the FIGO system and pure nuclear grading. There are several advantages of the binary system over the FIGO system. The assessment of solid growth does not require distinction of squamous from nonsquamous growth, small amounts of solid growth (around 5%) need not be recognized, and nuclear grading is not necessary. Five studies have subsequently compared the utility of this system to the current FIGO grading method [10, 103, 209, 344, 354]. In general, both methods provide for significant stratification of risk by univariate and multivariate analysis. The two grade system tended to result in a slightly reduced difference in survival between low and high grade as compared to grades 1 and 3 in the FIGO system, but it did eliminate the intermediate grade category. Interobserver and intraobserver reproducibility was often, but not always, found to be greater for the two grade system. Based on the relatively small difference in outcome between those patients with FIGO grade 1 and FIGO grade 2 tumors, some have suggested simply collapsing FIGO grades 1 and 2 into a single category. An additional binary grading scheme has been proposed and can be applied to any type of endometrial carcinoma present in biopsy, curettage, or hysterectomy specimens. This prognostically relevant scheme categorizes a tumor as high-grade when any two of the following three features are present: predominant papillary or solid architecture; high nuclear grade; and more than five mitotic figures per ten high power fields. This grading scheme can be used in practice when an endometrial carcinoma cannot be assigned a specific subtype. The group also tested the prognostic relevance of a revised FIGO grading scheme for endometrioid carcinomas specifically; this supported grouping together FIGO grades 1 and 2 endometrioid carcinomas as low-grade and FIGO grade 3 carcinoma as high-grade. This practice was found to be reproducible and prognostically relevant [14]. It is not clear whether any of the alternative systems would significantly improve upon the reproducibility, ease, or prognostic utility of the current method, and the three grade method continues to be used in the 2009 revised FIGO staging system.

Surgical–Pathological Staging (FIGO Staging)

The stage reflects the extent of disease at the time of diagnosis. It is useful to determine prognosis and plan treatment as well as to provide a standardized method of reporting data among different investigators. Complete staging requires hysterectomy and bilateral salpingo-oophorectomy, as well as assessment of the pelvic and paraaortic lymph nodes. At present, there is debate regarding the necessity for complete surgical staging of all women with endometrial adenocarcinoma, with some favoring restriction of lymphadenectomy to those at intermediate or high risk of nodal spread [67]. Others have argued that lymphadenectomy itself is a therapeutic procedure, based on retrospective survival data [8]. A new FIGO staging system has been adopted in 2009, with input from the International Society of Gynecological Pathologists [437], representing a refinement to the system last revised in 1988 (➋ *Table 9.4*). Major changes from the staging system of 1988 include the inclusion of tumors with no myometrial invasion and those with inner half myometrial invasion in stage IA, elimination of cervical gland involvement from stage II, elimination of positive peritoneal fluid cytology from stage IIIA, and separation of pelvic from paraaortic lymph node metastases within stage IIIC. Pathologic analysis includes evaluation of the grade of the tumor, depth of myometrial invasion, and determination of endocervical stromal involvement; therefore, it is essential that all this information be communicated clearly in the surgical pathology report. The prognostic utility of surgical–pathologic stage has been confirmed in multiple studies of large numbers of patients using both univariate and multivariate analysis [6, 46, 94, 137, 180, 224, 428, 438, 443, 444].

Myometrial Invasion

Effective in 2009, FIGO staging of endometrial carcinoma limited to the uterine corpus (stage I) is divided into those that are confined to the endometrium or involve the inner half of the myometrium, which are stage IA, and those involving more than half the uterine wall thickness, which are stage IB. The combination of tumors that lack any myoinvasion from those with inner half myometrial invasion is based on two pragmatic observations: first, there is diagnostic difficulty and low reproducibility in distinguishing true superficial myometrial invasion from those tumors involving the basal endometrium as it interdigitates normally with the myometrium [13, 371]; second, there is almost no difference in survival between those patients with carcinoma confined to the endometrium and those with superficial myometrial invasion (91% versus 90%) [95]. In addition, we recommend measuring the maximum depth of invasion in millimeters and expressing this as a percentage of the myometrial thickness. For example, 2 mm of myometrial invasion in a uterus measuring 1 cm thick would be 20% invasion. Tumor in vascular spaces beyond the deepest point of invasion should not be used for the measurement of the depth of invasion. The distance of the tumor from the serosa also has prognostic significance [355].

Myometrial invasion, independent of tumor grade, is an important predictor of prognosis. In fact, it is probably the single most important predictor of behavior in stages I and II disease and has been shown to be an independent predictor of outcome for women with early-stage endometrial carcinoma [5, 22, 46, 77, 112, 240, 277, 443]. For example, in the GOG experience, recurrence developed in only one of 99 (1%) patients with no myometrial invasion compared with 15 of 196 (7.7%) with inner-third, eight of 55 (14.5%) with middle-third, and six of 40 (15%) with outer-third invasion when grade was not corrected [277]. In another GOG study it was shown that the 5-year relative survival for endometrioid carcinoma confined to the endometrium was 94%; involving the inner third, 91%; involving the middle third, 84%; and involving the outer third, 59% [440]. The frequency of lymph node metastasis also is related to the depth of myometrial invasion. In clinical stage I endometrial carcinoma, inner-third myometrial invasion is associated with lymph node metastasis in 5% of cases, middle-third invasion with metastasis in 23%, and outer-third invasion with metastasis in 33%. When grade and myometrial invasion are analyzed together, grade 1 tumors invading the inner third of the myometrium do not have pelvic node metastasis, but with outer-third invasion, pelvic node metastasis occurs in 25%. A similar trend occurs with higher-grade tumors.

Cervical Involvement

According to the new FIGO staging system, tumors that are confined to the uterus but involving the cervical stroma are stage II. In contrast, neoplasms that are confined to the surface epithelium or glands of the endocervix are now considered to represent only stage I disease. Cervical stromal involvement is characterized by carcinoma that is not confined to the surface epithelium or preexisting endocervical glands and typically elicits a stromal reaction. However, not all tumors evoke a stromal desmoplastic response and it then may be difficult to distinguish whether the neoplastic glands represent preexisting or newly formed glands [394]. Cervical involvement is associated with a somewhat elevated risk of recurrence, with an overall relapse rate of 16% in the absence of extrauterine disease [266]. Since cervical involvement is often associated with increasing grade, depth of invasion, and tumor volume, the higher recurrence rate is not surprising. There is limited and conflicting data on the prognostic significance of cervical invasion by endometrial adenocarcinoma, after adjustment for other risk factors [33, 91, 120, 198, 325].

Peritoneal Cytology

Tumor cells in a peritoneal cytology specimen are often found in association with adnexal, nodal, or omental spread, but are rarely the only manifestation of extrauterine spread of endometrial adenocarcinoma. Previously, a positive peritoneal cytology was a basis for classification of the tumor as stage IIIA, however, it is no longer used in the staging of endometrial adenocarcinoma. The significance of a positive peritoneal cytology has been the subject of several studies [92, 159, 168, 201, 214, 384, 407, 432, 443]. Some studies have reported the significance of positive peritoneal cytology, including one in which almost 40% of clinical stage I patients with positive peritoneal cytology suffered tumor recurrence compared with 10% of those with negative washings [92, 168, 407]. Other studies, however, have reported a lack of significance of peritoneal cytology in predicting the probability of recurrence or death from endometrial adenocarcinoma [159, 432]. Positive peritoneal cytology has been associated with other risk factors for recurrence, such as high grade, deep myometrial invasion, or extrauterine spread [159, 168, 214]. One study, however, found that positive peritoneal cytology did not correlate with histologic subtype, FIGO grade, depth of myometrial invasion, or vascular invasion and was only significantly associated with stage III and IV disease [161]. Nonetheless, in a study of 567 patients with clinical stage I and II disease, a statistically significant difference in survival between patients with and without positive peritoneal cytology was found that persisted when the data were subjected to multivariate analysis [407]. Only 7% of patients with negative cytology recurred, while 32% of those with positive peritoneal cytology suffered a recurrence. Another study also found a threefold increase in the risk of death from tumor for a similar population using a multivariate analysis that adjusted for other risk factors [443]. In a review that included a total of 3,800 patients in 17 studies, in three of five studies in which multivariate analysis was performed, malignant cytology was associated with a significant, independent decrease in survival or an increase in the recurrence rate [268]. The weight of evidence supports the interpretation that the presence of malignant cells in peritoneal washings is a significant indicator of a worsened prognosis.

Vascular Invasion and Lymph Node Metastases

Venous or lymphatic invasion is defined by the presence of neoplastic cells within endothelial-lined channels. Although artifactual retraction of stroma around aggregates of neoplastic cells may simulate vascular invasion, vascular invasion can usually be reliably assessed in the myometrium peripheral to the bulk of the tumor mass. Occasionally, a subtle pattern of lymphatic space involvement by neoplasm may mimic intravascular histiocytes [265]. Also, the presence of perivascular lymphocytic infiltrates in the myometrium, but not lymphocytic infiltrate at the tumor–myometrial junction, is frequently associated with vascular invasion and hence is a useful marker of vascular invasion [10]. Vascular invasion is relatively uncommonly seen in endometrioid adenocarcinoma of the uterus (about 10–20% of cases) [291], but the frequency increases with deeper myometrial invasion, aggressive cell types, and decreasing histologic differentiation [3, 167, 375]. Nonetheless, some studies have revealed a significant correlation between vascular invasion and tumor recurrence independent of differentiation and depth of myometrial invasion. In one investigation of FIGO stage I endometrial adenocarcinomas, nine of 15 patients with lymphatic invasion died of tumor, while none of the 78 without identified vascular invasion died of cancer [138]. In a similar study of stage I cases, it was found that lymphatic invasion represented a strong predictor of tumor recurrence and extrapelvic metastasis, which was independent of depth of invasion or histologic differentiation [167].

In an analysis of stage I, grade 1 endometrioid adenocarcinomas with a poor outcome, vascular invasion in addition to myometrial invasion, mitotic index, and absence of progesterone receptor were significant factors that predicted aggressive behavior [403]. In another study aimed at comparing the significance of various pathologic risk factors in stage I endometrioid carcinoma, univariate analysis showed that vascular invasion was more important than grade and depth of myometrial invasion in predicting prognosis [21]. In a series of 513 consecutive cases of carcinoma limited to the uterus, multivariate analysis revealed lymphatic vascular invasion as the only predictor of distant recurrence [291]. Another study examined specimens with probable lymphatic invasion using immunoperoxidase with an antibody directed against factor VIII [240]. A greatly increased risk of recurrence was present in those with definite vascular invasion but not in those in whom the lining of the spaces failed to stain. Immunohistochemistry with antibody directed against CD31 increased the identification of vascular space invasion from 19% of cases (identified by H&E stains) to 50% of cases. Interestingly, recurrence was statistically related to the detection of vascular space invasion on H&E stained but not immunohistochemically stained sections [12]. Another study found that vascular invasion was a statistically significant indicator of death from tumor in early clinical stage tumors, but not for surgical stage I and II endometrial adenocarcinoma [443]. This finding suggests that lymphatic invasion may help to identify patients likely to have spread to lymph nodes or distant sites, but that its importance is diminished for those in whom thorough sampling of nodes has failed to identify metastases. Others have also found that vascular invasion was a significant prognosticator by univariate analysis but less important after adjusting for other variables [3]. Nevertheless, one study found that among women with lymph node metastases the presence or absence of vascular invasion in the primary tumor was associated with different survival rates [186].

About 10% of women with endometrioid endometrial adenocarcinoma have metastasis to pelvic lymph nodes [71]. Nearly a third of patients with pelvic lymph node spread also have positive paraaortic lymph nodes. Among the extrauterine risk factors, the presence of positive paraaortic lymph nodes is most important in predicting prognosis [277]. Only 36% of patients with positive paraaortic nodes were free of tumor at 5 years compared with 85% with negative paraaortic nodes. The highest correlation of positive paraaortic lymph nodes is with pelvic lymph nodes. Other features that correlate with positive aortic nodes are vascular invasion (19%), deep myometrial invasion (17%), positive peritoneal cytology (16%), cervical involvement (12%), and grade 3 tumors (8%). An increasing absolute number of lymph nodes containing metastatic carcinoma has also been associated with a decreasing survival [66]. Pelvic and paraaortic sentinel node identification has been attempted, successfully, in a pilot study, but it is currently not employed as a routine procedure for endometrial carcinoma [126].

Endometrial Hyperplasia and Metaplasia

Among nontumor risk factors, the presence of atypical endometrial hyperplasia and various metaplasias, especially ciliated cell and eosinophilic change, are important in identifying patients with a favorable prognosis. The presence of atypical hyperplasia and metaplasia correlates with low tumor grade and lack of myometrial invasion [38, 204]. In contrast, high-grade tumors are associated more often with an atrophic endometrium [74].

Ploidy

About two-thirds of endometrial adenocarcinomas are composed of cells that are diploid at the level of flow or static cytometry. This statement is qualified, as the sensitivity of the technique is limited and the addition or deletion of DNA equivalent to one average chromosome would not alter the assessment of a cell as diploid. Similar to many of the other prognostic factors, diploid tumors tend to be more frequently associated with less aggressive cell type, superficial invasion, and better histologic differentiation [51, 144, 193, 378, 389, 410]. Survival has generally been higher for women with diploid tumors [51, 193, 410]. One study of stage I patients demonstrated 94% progression-free survival for those with diploid tumors versus 64% for those with aneuploid cancers, but these results have not been universally reproducible [161, 162, 164, 167]. However, in more recent larger studies employing multivariate analysis, ploidy has almost always remained a strong predictor of outcome [165, 251, 293, 313, 315, 391, 404, 439]. Thus, DNA content can be considered a prognostic indicator of demonstrated utility for endometrial adenocarcinoma.

Steroid Receptors

The studies that have employed immunohistochemical methods to assess intranuclear receptor content in formalin-fixed paraffin-embedded tumor tissues have demonstrated that endometrioid carcinomas frequently express ER and PR whereas serous and clear cell carcinomas are usually negative [202, 236, 237, 328]. In most studies, the presence and quantity of steroid receptors have been correlated with histologic differentiation, FIGO stage, and survival [65, 102, 144, 145, 202, 260].

Several studies have reported variable results regarding the correlation of hormone receptor expression and prognosis. One study found that the presence of ER, but not PR, was predictive of survival [310]. Another study found that the presence of PR was a favorable prognosticator [403]. Yet another study found that both ER and PR were predictive of survival, but also strongly related to the clinical stage, histologic grade, and the absence of vascular invasion [144]. In contrast, another study reported that recurrence was related to the absence of ER or PR, and that response to progestin therapy was more common in PR-positive tumors, but noted that survival for patients with surgical stage I or II disease was not related to ER or PR [110]. Others have found that ER and PR were not independently predictive of lymph node metastasis [276]. However, PR persisted as a significant prognosticator of survival in two studies using multivariate analyses [134, 297]. Given the disparity in results and the relationship with other strong risk factors, hormone receptor expression is best considered a prognostic indicator of potential utility.

Our understanding of steroid receptor structure and function continues to grow, with the recognition of two isoforms for estrogen receptor (alpha and beta) and for progesterone receptor (A and B) [135], with various mRNA splice variants [88]. Each of the isoforms appears to induce different and sometimes opposing effects [49, 53, 64, 85, 149, 181, 194], and the expression of isoform specific antibodies is actively being investigated in endometrial cancer [29, 345].

BCL-2 and Markers of Apoptosis

BCL-2 is a proto-oncogene that inhibits programmed cell death, which is manifest morphologically as apoptosis. In the endometrium, BCL-2 expression assessed by immunohistochemistry varies during the menstrual cycle and is highly expressed in the proliferative phase, with downregulation during the secretory phase [153]. Given this cyclic regulation of endometrial growth, differentiation, and shedding, it is not surprising that during the past few years there has been significant interest in apoptosis-related events, with more than a dozen immunohistochemical studies of BCL-2 in abnormal endometrium. In general, the observations support the concept that BCL-2 protein expression persists at high levels in simple hyperplasia but progressively diminishes in atypical hyperplasia and with decreasing differentiation in invasive endometrial adenocarcinoma [68, 72, 146, 173, 188, 290, 347, 397, 430]. Apoptotic cells and apoptotic bodies are also increased in poorly differentiated endometrioid carcinomas, clear cell carcinomas, and serous carcinomas compared with well-differentiated endometrioid adenocarcinomas [171, 172]. Loss of BCL-2 expression has also been associated with other features of poor prognosis including increasing depth of invasion, negative PR status, increasing FIGO stage, and aggressive cell types [146, 276, 341, 397, 447]. In two studies that used multivariate analysis to adjust for other prognostic factors, loss of BCL-2 expression was significantly related to the probability of lymph node metastasis or tumor recurrence [146, 347].

Markers of Proliferation

Various aspects of proliferation within tissues can now be assessed directly or indirectly by a multitude of modalities in tissue sections and cell suspensions. These methods include the determination of mitotic indices; S-phase fraction; proliferating cell nuclear antigen (PCNA); and Ki-67-, Ki-S5-, or MIB-1-positive cell populations by immunohistochemistry. Each assessment provides slightly different information about the number and type of cells in different parts of the cell cycle. Standardized methods for detection, enumeration, and determination of levels of significance do not exist for most of these parameters, however, and need to be established before the assays can be considered clinically useful.

Antibodies (Ki-67, Ki-S5, and MIB-1) directed against the DNA-binding nuclear protein, Ki-67 antigen, identify cells in most of G_1 and all of S, G_2, and M phases of the cell cycle, but not in the G_0, or quiescent, phase. In one study, MIB-1 staining correlated with grade and mitotic activity but did not predict short-term outcome [287]. Ki-S5 staining has been shown to be a significant predictor of survival by univariate but not multivariate analysis [45]. However, in a prospective study of 115 women with endometrial adenocarcinoma, immunohistochemical staining with Ki-67 was related to FIGO stage, cell type, histologic subtype, and probability of survival by univariate analysis; and, in addition, using multivariate analysis, only Ki-67 expression and stage remained as significant independent prognosticators [348]. Thus, Ki-67 could be considered a prognosticator of potential utility, but further corroboration is needed.

Proliferating cell nuclear antigen (PCNA) is a nuclear protein that is expressed in the late G_1 phase, peaks in the S phase, and persists in the G_2M phases of the cycle. A high PCNA index has failed to discriminate outcome in several studies but has been predictive of decreased survival by univariate analysis in other studies, although not by multivariate analysis [141, 165, 207, 215].

Flow cytometry can be used to distinguish populations of cells in the S phase or G_2 and M phases of the cycle. The prognostic value of flow cytometry to identify endometrial cancers composed of increased percentages (either 10% or 20%) of cells in the S phase of the cell cycle also has been variable. One study demonstrated a nonsignificant trend toward decreased survival whereas others have shown either significance by univariate analysis alone or significance by multivariate analysis [205, 313, 316, 348].

Tumor Suppressor Genes and Oncogenes

As noted above in the section Molecular Genetics of endometrial carcinoma, an inactivating mutation of the tumor suppressor gene *PTEN* is the most frequent genetic alteration observed in endometrioid adenocarcinoma [333, 395]. It is common in low-grade endometrioid carcinomas (about 50% of cases) but not in serous carcinoma, and consequently it is associated with a generally good survival. Immunohistochemical detection is highly dependent on the specific antibody employed, and it is currently not considered a prognosticator in endometrioid adenocarcinoma.

The *p53* gene is also classified as a tumor suppressor gene, the product of which is a protein involved in the regulation of the cell cycle at the G_1 checkpoint. Mutations of the *p53* gene often result in a protein with a longer half-life that accumulates in the cell. Upregulation of wild type (i.e., nonmutated) *p53* may occur after DNA damage and also result in overexpression detected by immunohistochemistry. Mutations or overexpression of *p53* in endometrial carcinoma has been examined in more than two dozen studies. Overexpression of *p53* protein has been generally related to higher FIGO stage, aggressive cell types (particularly serous carcinoma), increased histologic grade, and depth of myometrial invasion [16, 87, 147, 165, 197, 215, 217, 222, 236, 251, 286, 293, 396, 397, 430]. There is a surprisingly high degree of concordance in the observation that p53 overaccumulation is associated with a decreased probability of survival by univariate analysis, and this is true even by multivariate analysis in at least eight studies [34, 147, 165, 190, 192, 197, 217, 221, 222, 251, 285, 286, 316, 430]. These results support the classification of p53 expression as a prognostic indicator of proven utility.

HER-2/neu is a proto-oncogene, the product of which is a transmembrane growth factor receptor, p185erb-2, which shares some homology with the epidermal growth factor receptor. It is normally expressed at low levels in the cycling endometrium. Gene amplification or overexpression occurs in about 20–40% of endometrial carcinomas. Overexpression of HER-2/neu protein has been associated with advanced stage, decreased differentiation, aggressive cell types, particularly including clear cell type, and increased depth of myometrial invasion [40, 215, 329, 334]. Reports of its utility as a predictor of survival have been mixed, with no apparent association of overexpression to outcome identified in several studies, but a statistically significant relationship was shown in most others [35, 165, 177, 251, 282, 285, 286, 316, 329, 334, 343]. In several investigations, the significance of HER-2/neu amplification or overexpression as a prognosticator has remained after adjusting for other known risk factors [165, 282, 334]. At present, HER-2/neu overexpression is a prognostic factor of potential utility.

The activation of *RAS* proto-oncogenes through either point mutations or gene amplification has been identified in various malignant tumors. Mutations in codon 12 of *KRAS* appear to occur in only 10–15% of endometrial carcinomas, and in most studies they have not been related to stage, grade, depth of invasion, or survival, although one study found mutations predictive of recurrence and death by univariate analysis [56, 117, 191, 197, 359]. *KRAS* mutations currently represent a prognostic marker of unlikely utility.

Low-level ribosomal DNA (rDNA) methylation has been associated with a diminished disease-free survival in women with early-stage endometrial carcinoma [324].

Angiogenesis and Vascular Endothelial Growth Factor

Angiogenesis in the form of proliferation of new capillaries from preexisting vessels is necessary to permit tumor growth. This neovascularization potentially could result from stimulation by a variety of factors released from neoplastic cells, host cells responding to the neoplasm, or supporting matrix. In the endometrium, it appears that stromal vascularity is greater in the secretory phase than proliferative phase, but it is greater in the stroma of carcinoma than in cycling endometrium [275]. This difference may reflect stimulation by vascular endothelial growth factor (VEGF) RNA and its protein product, which have been found in high concentration in neoplastic cells but not in benign atrophic endometrial glandular cells [162]. Although tumor vascularity has been associated with increased stage, decreased differentiation, and lymphatic invasion, high microvessel counts have been a statistically significant predictor of decreased survival independent of other common risk factors in several, but not all, studies [203, 300, 302, 416]. Microvessel density thus represents a prognostic marker of potential utility.

Models for Predicting Prognosis

Recent studies reveal that the behavior of a tumor is based on a complex interaction of a number of different factors. Accordingly, models have been developed that assess several factors and permit more accurate prognostication than simply considering one factor alone. For example, by multivariate analysis, the depth of invasion and presence of vascular invasion-associated changes were found to provide a highly reliable model for predicting outcome (see *Table 9.7*) [21]. The model was better able to define patients who were at low and high risk of recurrence as compared with the traditional risk factors using grade and depth of invasion. Inclusion of ploidy in the model permitted even better discrimination of high- and low-risk patients. In a subset of pathologic stage I endometrioid carcinoma in whom ploidy analysis was performed, multivariate analysis showed that only the depth of invasion, DNA ploidy, and vascular invasion-associated changes were significant risk factors [22]. A statistical model based on these features permitted stratification of patients into four risk groups with 93%, 67%, 38%, and 10% survival, respectively (*Table 9.8*).

In an analysis of 819 women with clinical stage I and occult stage II adenocarcinoma of the endometrium entered on a GOG protocol, multivariate analysis demonstrated that age, cell type, architectural grade, depth of myometrial invasion, vascular space involvement, and peritoneal cytology

Table 9.7

Statistical model of survival predicted by myometrial invasion and vascular invasion-associated changes (Reprinted with permission from Ambros RA and Kurman RJ [10])

		Survival	
Score	No. of cases	No.	%
1	20	19	95
1–2	45	39	87
2–2.6	17	12	70
2.6	20	7	35

Table 9.8

Statistical model of survival predicted by depth of myometrial invasion, vascular invasion-associated changes, and tumor ploidy (Reprinted with permission from Ambros RA and Kurman RJ [9])

		Survival	
Score	No. of cases	No.	%
<2.2	27	25	93
2.2–2.3	12	8	67
2.4–4.0	8	3	38
>4	10	1	10

were independent risk factors for recurrence and death from tumor [443]. From these data it appears possible to create a model for assignment of the relative risk of death from tumor for individual patients based solely on information gathered by pathologic examination of the hysterectomy specimen. For example, a woman with grade 1 endometrioid carcinoma, with tumor confined to the endometrium and no vascular invasion, is arbitrarily assigned a risk of 1. Relative to this baseline risk, a woman with a grade 2 endometrioid carcinoma that invades superficial myometrium and lacks vascular space involvement has a relative risk of 2.6. Similarly, a woman with a grade 3 endometrioid carcinoma, with middle-third myometrial invasion, and positive vascular space involvement, has a relative risk of 10. The probability of disease-free survival at 5 years for these three women would be approximately 95%, 90%, and 65%, respectively. Knowledge of the specific risk for each patient would allow better prognostication and, potentially, individually tailored therapy.

Miscellaneous Epithelial Tumors

A number of rare examples of unusual neoplasms arising in the endometrium have been reported, but the data consist largely of case reports precluding a detailed clinicopathologic analysis. Some of these are discussed next.

Squamous Cell Carcinoma

Squamous carcinoma develops in the endometrium, but it is extremely rare. In a population-based study from Norway the prevalence was 0.1% [6]. To qualify as primary squamous carcinoma of the endometrium, three criteria must be met: (1) adenocarcinoma is not present in the endometrium, (2) the squamous carcinoma in the endometrium does not have any connection with the squamous epithelium of the cervix, and (3) squamous carcinoma is not present in the cervix. By these criteria, only 56 cases of primary squamous carcinoma of the endometrium have been reported [154]. The mean age of patients is 67 years. There is a strong association with cervical stenosis, pyometra, chronic inflammation, and nulliparity. The tumor may arise from ichthyosis uteri, a condition in which the endometrium is replaced by keratinized squamous epithelium. In the past, this condition was considered a sequela of the use of steam as treatment for endometritis. With the abandonment of this procedure, ichthyosis uteri have become quite rare.

Microscopically, squamous carcinomas of the endometrium resemble those in the cervix; however, at times they can be extremely well-differentiated and therefore difficult to diagnose with certainty in curettings. Sometimes the diagnosis is not established until a hysterectomy is performed.

In addition to typical squamous cell carcinoma, verrucous carcinoma may arise as a primary tumor in the endometrium (*Fig. 9.55*) [340]. The prognosis of squamous cell carcinoma is related to stage at diagnosis. In a review of the reported cases, 80% of stage I patients survived whereas survival for patients with stage III disease was only 20% [154].

Glassy Cell Carcinoma

Glassy cell carcinoma is regarded as a variant of a mixed adenosquamous carcinoma and rarely occurs in the endometrium [28, 76]. First described in the cervix, glassy cell carcinoma is a poorly differentiated neoplasm with little or no glandular or squamous differentiation and is composed of masses and nests of characteristic polygonal cells separated by a fibrous stroma that often contains an abundance of inflammatory cells. The cells have well-defined borders and granular eosinophilic or amphophilic cytoplasm, giving a ground glass appearance. The nuclei are enlarged and round, with centrally placed, prominent, eosinophilic nucleoli. Mitotic activity, including the presence of abnormal mitotic figures, is high. The behavior, based on a small series of cases, is highly aggressive.

Yolk Sac Tumor

Four cases of primary yolk sac tumor of the endometrium have been reported [200]. Three of the patients have been in their 20s, and one was 42 years of age. Light microscopic, immunohistochemical, and ultrastructural studies have shown features similar to yolk sac tumor of the ovary. AFP is elevated in the serum preoperatively and is localized within the cytoplasm of tumor cells. It is thought that these tumors arise in the uterus as a result of aberrant migration of primordial germ cells. All four patients were treated with hysterectomy followed by adjuvant multiagent chemotherapy. Two patients are long-term survivors, and two died of disease.

Giant Cell Carcinoma

Rare primary endometrial carcinomas may contain multinucleated giant cells resembling giant cell carcinomas in other sites such as the lung, thyroid, pancreas, and gallbladder. In a report of six cases, the giant cells accounted for a substantial part of the tumor [196]. The remainder of the neoplasm contained undifferentiated carcinoma and areas of more differentiated endometrioid carcinoma. Immunohistochemical studies demonstrated positive immunoreactivity for cytokeratin and epithelial membrane antigen in the giant cell component. Vimentin, desmin, and smooth muscle actin were negative. Four of the six patients in whom the tumor invaded more than superficially developed recurrent tumor, and three patients died of disease within 3 years. Tumors with cells resembling osteoclast-like giant cells also have been observed in the endometrium.

Choriocarcinoma

Rarely, primary choriocarcinoma of the endometrium may develop in a postmenopausal woman, representing a form of differentiation of a carcinoma derived from somatic cells rather than germ cells or trophoblasts. Six patients ranging in age from 48 to 78 years have been reported [206, 311, 350, 406]. Most patients had elevated serum human chorionic gonadotropin (hCG) levels and/or hCG detected in the syncytiotrophoblastic element in the tumor. A case of choriocarcinoma associated with a carcinosarcoma (malignant mesodermal mixed tumor) has been reported, and we have observed one such case as well [216]. These tumors appear to behave in an aggressive fashion.

Transitional Cell Carcinoma

Ten cases of transitional cell carcinoma of the endometrium have been reported [248, 385]. Patients have ranged in age from 41 to 83 years, with a mean of 62. The tumors are typically polypoid and present with uterine bleeding. Transitional cell carcinomas often are papillary and resemble transitional cell carcinomas of other organs. They are invariably admixed with other patterns of endometrial carcinoma, including endometrioid, squamous, and serous components. The overall prognosis does not appear to be worse than expected for the stage of disease, but the transitional cell component seems to be the more aggressive subtype among the patterns with which it is admixed [248].

Other Rare Variants

Other rare types of carcinomas of the endometrium that have been reported include an oxyphilic variant of endometrioid carcinoma, a primary signet-ring cell carcinoma, and an alpha-fetoprotein-secreting hepatoid adenocarcinoma associated with endometrioid carcinoma [184, 274, 317]. In addition, an endometrioid carcinoma associated with Ewing sarcoma/peripheral primitive neuroectodermal tumor has been reported [374].

Tumors Metastatic to the Endometrium

Ovarian Carcinoma

Simultaneous cancers involving the endometrium and the ovary may represent (1) metastasis from the endometrium to the ovary, (2) metastasis from the ovary to the endometrium, or (3) independent primary tumors. The distinction is important because the prognosis and treatment differ. It has been suggested that when the endometrial carcinoma is small and minimally invasive, the two neoplasms should be considered independent. One study found that if the two carcinomas have an endometrioid pattern, the prognosis is good, and therefore the two neoplasms probably are independent [111]. When serous or clear cell carcinoma is found, the prognosis is poor and a primary tumor with metastasis is likely. The primary neoplasm is identified by its larger size or more advanced stage.

Another study proposed that tumors be classified as primary in the endometrium with metastasis to the ovaries when there is multinodular ovarian involvement or at least two of the following criteria are met: (1) small (5 cm) ovaries, (2) bilateral ovarian involvement, (3) deep myometrial invasion, (4) vascular invasion, or (5) fallopian tube involvement [408]. When these criteria are used, there is a significant difference in the frequency of distant metastasis in the group classified as metastatic versus the group classified as an independent primary. Metastasis from the endometrium to the ovary occurs more often than the reverse. About a third of the cases are independent tumors involving both sites simultaneously. Independent tumors display either well-differentiated endometrioid or nonendometrioid patterns, whereas grade 3 endometrioid carcinoma and MMMTs generally are primary in one organ and metastatic to the other when detected.

Carcinomas from Extragenital Sites

When an extragenital tumor metastasizes to the uterus, it usually is a manifestation of obvious dissemination. The diagnosis in curettings may, on rare occasion, be the first clue of an occult primary tumor. The mean age of patients is 60 years. Metastatic breast cancer is the most frequent extragenital tumor that metastasizes to the uterus (47%) (➲ *Fig. 9.62*), followed by stomach (29%), cutaneous melanoma (5%), lung (4%), colon (3%), pancreas (3%), and kidney (3%) [228]. Metastatic neoplasms to the endometrium frequently infiltrate the endometrium diffusely, sparing the glands. Most neoplasms metastatic to the endometrium are poorly differentiated and lack squamous differentiation, unlike primary endometrial carcinoma. The myometrium can contain metastatic nodules as well.

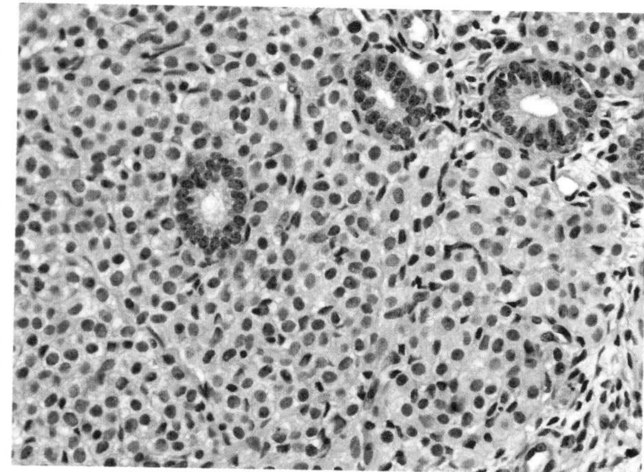

Fig. 9.62
Metastatic breast carcinoma. **Monotonous cells with uniform nuclei and pale eosinophilic cytoplasm replacing the stroma and surrounding residual inactive endometrial glands are consistent with metastatic lobular breast carcinoma**

References

1. The Cancer and Steroid Hormone Study of the Centers for Disease Control and the National Institute of Child Health and Human Development (1987) Combination oral contraceptive use and the risk of endometrial cancer. JAMA 257:796–800
2. Abeler VM, Kjorstad KE (1991) Clear cell carcinoma of the endometrium: a histopathological and clinical study of 97 cases. Gynecol Oncol 40:207–217
3. Abeler VM, Kjorstad KE (1991) Endometrial adenocarcinoma in Norway. A study of the total population. Cancer 67:3093–3103
4. Abeler VM, Kjorstad KE (1992) Endometrial adenocarcinoma with squamous cell differentiation. Cancer 69:488–495
5. Abeler VM, Kjorstad KE (1990) Serous papillary carcinoma of the endometrium: a histopathological study of 22 cases. Gynecol Oncol 39:266–271
6. Abeler VM, Kjorstad KE, Berle E (1992) Carcinoma of the endometrium in Norway: a histopathological and prognostic survey of a total population. Int J Gynecol Cancer 2:9–22
7. Abeler VM et al (1996) Clear cell carcinoma of the endometrium. Prognosis and metastatic pattern. Cancer 78:1740–1747
8. Abu-Rustum NR et al (2008) Is there a therapeutic impact to regional lymphadenectomy in the surgical treatment of endometrial carcinoma? Am J Obstet Gynecol 198:457 e1–e5; discussion 457 e5–e6
9. Acs G, Pasha T, Zhang PJ (2004) WT1 is differentially expressed in serous, endometrioid, clear cell, and mucinous carcinomas of the peritoneum, fallopian tube, ovary, and endometrium. Int J Gynecol Pathol 23:110–118
10. Al Kushi A et al (2002) Markers of proliferative activity are predictors of patient outcome for low-grade endometrioid adenocarcinoma but not papillary serous carcinoma of endometrium. Mod Pathol 15:365–371
11. Alberhasky RC, Connelly PJ, Christopherson WM (1982) Carcinoma of the endometrium. IV. Mixed adenosquamous carcinoma. A clinical-pathological study of 68 cases with long-term follow-up. Am J Clin Pathol 77:655–664
12. Alexander-Sefre F et al (2004) Clinical value of immunohistochemically detected lymphovascular invasion in endometrioid endometrial cancer. Gynecol Oncol 92:653–659
13. Ali A, Black D, Soslow RA (2007) Difficulties in assessing the depth of myometrial invasion in endometrial carcinoma. Int J Gynecol Pathol 26:115–123
14. Alkushi A et al (2005) Description of a novel system for grading of endometrial carcinoma and comparison with existing grading systems. Am J Surg Pathol 29:295–304
15. Alkushi A et al (2007) Identification of prognostically relevant and reproducible subsets of endometrial adenocarcinoma based on clustering analysis of immunostaining data. Mod Pathol 20:1156–1165
16. Alkushi A et al (2004) Interpretation of p53 immunoreactivity in endometrial carcinoma: establishing a clinically relevant cut-off level. Int J Gynecol Pathol 23:129–137
17. Allard JE, Maxwell GL (2009) Race disparities between black and white women in the incidence, treatment, and prognosis of endometrial cancer. Cancer Control 16:53–56
18. Altrabulsi B et al (2005) Undifferentiated Carcinoma of the Endometrium. Am J Surg Pathol 29:1316–1321
19. Amant F et al (2005) Endometrial carcinosarcomas have a different prognosis and pattern of spread compared to high-risk epithelial endometrial cancer. Gynecol Oncol 98:274–280

20. Amant F et al (2002) PTEN mutations in uterine sarcomas. Gynecol Oncol 85:165–169
21. Ambros RA, Kurman RJ (1992) Combined assessment of vascular and myometrial invasion as a model to predict prognosis in stage I endometrioid adenocarcinoma of the uterine corpus. Cancer 69:1424–1431
22. Ambros RA, Kurman RJ (1992) Identification of patients with stage I uterine endometrioid adenocarcinoma at high risk of recurrence by DNA ploidy, myometrial invasion, and vascular invasion. Gynecol Oncol 45:235–239
23. Ambros RA et al (1995) Endometrial intraepithelial carcinoma: a distinctive lesion specifically associated with tumors displaying serous differentiation. Hum Pathol 26:1260–1267
24. An HJ et al (2004) Molecular characterization of uterine clear cell carcinoma. Mod Pathol 17:530–537
25. Andersson M, Storm HH, Mouridsen HT (1991) Incidence of new primary cancers after adjuvant tamoxifen therapy and radiotherapy for early breast cancer. J Natl Cancer Inst 83:1013–1017
26. Ansari-Lari MA et al (2004) Distinction of endocervical and endometrial adenocarcinomas: immunohistochemical p16 expression correlated with human papillomavirus (HPV) DNA detection. Am J Surg Pathol 28:160–167
27. Aquino-Parsons C et al (1998) Papillary serous and clear cell carcinoma limited to endometrial curettings in FIGO stage 1a and 1b endometrial adenocarcinoma: treatment implications. Gynecol Oncol 71:83–86
28. Arends JW et al (1984) Adenocarcinoma of the endometrium with glassy-cell features – immunohistochemical observations. Histopathology 8:873–879
29. Arnett-Mansfield RL et al (2001) Relative expression of progesterone receptors A and B in endometrioid cancers of the endometrium. Cancer Res 61:4576–4582
30. Arrastia CD et al (1997) Uterine carcinosarcomas: incidence and trends in management and survival. Gynecol Oncol 65:158–163
31. Ashton KA et al (2009) Estrogen receptor polymorphisms and the risk of endometrial cancer. BJOG 116:1053–1061
32. Austin H, Drews C, Partridge EE (1993) A case-control study of endometrial cancer in relation to cigarette smoking, serum estrogen levels, and alcohol use. Am J Obstet Gynecol 169:1086–1091
33. Ayhan A et al (2004) The long-term survival of women with surgical stage II endometrioid type endometrial cancer. Gynecol Oncol 93:9–13
34. Backe J et al (1997) p53 protein in endometrial cancer is related to proliferative activity and prognosis but not to expression of p21 protein. Int J Gynecol Pathol 16:361–368
35. Backe J et al (1997) Immunohistochemically detected HER-2/neu-expression and prognosis in endometrial carcinoma. Arch Gynecol Obstet 259:189–195
36. Barakat RR et al (1994) Tamoxifen use in breast cancer patients who subsequently develop corpus cancer is not associated with a higher incidence of adverse histologic features. Gynecol Oncol 55:164–168
37. Barwick KW, LiVolsi VA (1979) Malignant mixed mullerian tumors of the uterus. A clinicopathologic assessment of 34 cases. Am J Surg Pathol 3:125–135
38. Beckner ME, Mori T, Silverberg SG (1985) Endometrial carcinoma: nontumor factors in prognosis. Int J Gynecol Pathol 4:131–145
39. Beral V et al (1999) Use of HRT and the subsequent risk of cancer. J Epidemiol Biostat 4:191–210; discussion 210–215
40. Berchuck A et al (1991) Overexpression of HER-2/neu in endometrial cancer is associated with advanced stage disease. Am J Obstet Gynecol 164:15–21
41. Bitterman P, Chun B, Kurman RJ (1990) The significance of epithelial differentiation in mixed mesodermal tumors of the uterus. A clinicopathologic and immunohistochemical study. Am J Surg Pathol 14:317–328
42. Boccardo F et al (1992) Chemotherapy versus tamoxifen versus chemotherapy plus tamoxifen in node-positive, oestrogen-receptor positive breast cancer patients. An update at 7 years of the 1st GROCTA (Breast Cancer Adjuvant Chemo-Hormone Therapy Cooperative Group) trial. Eur J Cancer 28:673–680
43. Bodner-Adler B et al (2001) Prognostic parameters in carcinosarcomas of the uterus: a clinico-pathologic study. Anticancer Res 21:3069–3074
44. Bokhman JV (1983) Two pathogenetic types of endometrial carcinoma. Gynecol Oncol 15:10–17
45. Bonatz G et al (1999) Prognostic significance of a novel proliferation marker, anti-repp 86, for endometrial carcinoma: a multivariate study. Hum Pathol 30:949–956
46. Boronow RC et al (1984) Surgical staging in endometrial cancer: clinical-pathologic findings of a prospective study. Obstet Gynecol 63:825–832
47. Borst MP et al (1990) Oncogene alterations in endometrial carcinoma. Gynecol Oncol 38:364–366
48. Boyd J, Risinger JI (1991) Analysis of oncogene alterations in human endometrial carcinoma: prevalence of ras mutations. Mol Carcinog 4:189–195
49. Brandenberger AW et al (1999) Oestrogen receptor (ER)-alpha and ER-beta isoforms in normal endometrial and endometriosis-derived stromal cells. Mol Hum Reprod 5:651–655
50. Brinton LA et al (1992) Reproductive, menstrual, and medical risk factors for endometrial cancer: results from a case-control study. Am J Obstet Gynecol 167:1317–1325
51. Britton LC et al (1989) Flow cytometric DNA analysis of stage I endometrial carcinoma. Gynecol Oncol 34:317–322
52. Broaddus RR et al (2006) Pathologic features of endometrial carcinoma associated with HNPCC: a comparison with sporadic endometrial carcinoma. Cancer 106:87–94
53. Bukulmez O et al (2008) Inflammatory status influences aromatase and steroid receptor expression in endometriosis. Endocrinology 149:1190–1204
54. Bussaglia E et al (2000) PTEN mutations in endometrial carcinomas: a molecular and clinicopathologic analysis of 38 cases. Hum Pathol 31:312–317
55. Byron SA et al (2008) Inhibition of activated fibroblast growth factor receptor 2 in endometrial cancer cells induces cell death despite PTEN abrogation. Cancer Res 68:6902–6907
56. Caduff RF, Johnston CM, Frank TS (1995) Mutations of the Ki-ras oncogene in carcinoma of the endometrium. Am J Pathol 146:182–188
57. Callister M et al (2004) Malignant mixed Mullerian tumors of the uterus: analysis of patterns of failure, prognostic factors, and treatment outcome. Int J Radiat Oncol Biol Phys 58:786–796
58. Carcangiu ML, Chambers JT (1992) Uterine papillary serous carcinoma: a study on 108 cases with emphasis on the prognostic significance of associated endometrioid carcinoma, absence of invasion, and concomitant ovarian carcinoma. Gynecol Oncol 47:298–305
59. Carcangiu ML et al (1990) Immunohistochemical evaluation of estrogen and progesterone receptor content in 183 patients with endometrial carcinoma. Part I: Clinical and histologic correlations. Am J Clin Pathol 94:247–254
60. Carcangiu ML et al (2006) HNPCC-related endometrial carcinomas show a high frequency of non-endometrioid types and of high FIGO grade endometrioid carcinomas. Mod Pathol 19:173A

61. Carcangiu ML, Tan LK, Chambers JT (1997) Stage IA uterine serous carcinoma: a study of 13 cases. Am J Surg Pathol 21:1507–1514
62. Castrillon DH, Lee KR, Nucci MR (2002) Distinction between endometrial and endocervical adenocarcinoma: an immunohistochemical study. Int J Gynecol Pathol 21:4–10
63. Catasus L et al (2004) Molecular genetic alterations in endometrioid carcinomas of the ovary: similar frequency of beta-catenin abnormalities but lower rate of microsatellite instability and PTEN alterations than in uterine endometrioid carcinomas. Hum Pathol 35:1360–1368
64. Chakravarty D et al (2007) Estrogen receptor beta1 and the beta2/betacx isoforms in nonneoplastic endometrium and in endometrioid carcinoma. Int J Gynecol Cancer 17:905–913
65. Chambers JT et al (1990) Immunohistochemical evaluation of estrogen and progesterone receptor content in 183 patients with endometrial carcinoma. Part II: Correlation between biochemical and immunohistochemical methods and survival. Am J Clin Pathol 94:255–260
66. Chan JK, Kapp DS (2007) Role of complete lymphadenectomy in endometrioid uterine cancer. Lancet Oncol 8:831–841
67. Chan JK et al (2007) The impact of the absolute number and ratio of positive lymph nodes on survival of endometrioid uterine cancer patients. Br J Cancer 97:605–611
68. Chan WK et al (1995) Nuclear and cytoplasmic bcl-2 expression in endometrial hyperplasia and adenocarcinoma. J Pathol 177:241–246
69. Chen JL, Trost DC, Wilkinson EJ (1985) Endometrial papillary adenocarcinomas: two clinicopathological types. Int J Gynecol Pathol 4:279–288
70. Chen KT, Kostich ND, Rosai J (1978) Peritoneal foreign body granulomas to keratin in uterine adenocanthoma. Arch Pathol Lab Med 102:174–177
71. Chi DS et al (2008) The incidence of pelvic lymph node metastasis by FIGO staging for patients with adequately surgically staged endometrial adenocarcinoma of endometrioid histology. Int J Gynecol Cancer 18:269–273
72. Chieng DC, Ross JS, Ambros RA (1996) bcl-2 expression and the development of endometrial carcinoma. Mod Pathol 9:402–406
73. Chiesa-Vottero AG et al (2007) Immunohistochemical overexpression of p16 and p53 in uterine serous carcinoma and ovarian high-grade serous carcinoma. Int J Gynecol Pathol 26:328–333
74. Christopherson WM, Alberhasky RC, Connelly PJ (1982) Carcinoma of the endometrium: I. A clinicopathologic study of clear-cell carcinoma and secretory carcinoma. Cancer 49:1511–1523
75. Christopherson WM, Alberhasky RC, Connelly PJ (1982) Carcinoma of the endometrium. II. Papillary adenocarcinoma: a clinical pathological study, 46 cases. Am J Clin Pathol 77:534–540
76. Christopherson WM, Alberhasky RC, Connelly PJ (1982) Glassy cell carcinoma of the endometrium. Hum Pathol 13:418–421
77. Christopherson WM, Connelly PJ, Alberhasky RC (1983) Carcinoma of the endometrium. V. An analysis of prognosticators in patients with favorable subtypes and Stage I disease. Cancer 51:1705–1709
78. Chuang JT, Van Velden DJ, Graham JB (1970) Carcinosarcoma and mixed mesodermal tumor of the uterine corpus. Review of 49 cases. Obstet Gynecol 35:769–780
79. Cimbaluk D et al (2007) Uterine carcinosarcoma: immunohistochemical studies on tissue microarrays with focus on potential therapeutic targets. Gynecol Oncol 105:138–144
80. Cirisano FD Jr et al (1999) Epidemiologic and surgicopathologic findings of papillary serous and clear cell endometrial cancers when compared to endometrioid carcinoma. Gynecol Oncol 74:385–394
81. Cirisano FD Jr et al (2000) The outcome of stage I-II clinically and surgically staged papillary serous and clear cell endometrial cancers when compared with endometrioid carcinoma. Gynecol Oncol 77:55–65
82. Clement PB, Scully RE (1990) Mullerian adenosarcoma of the uterus: a clinicopathologic analysis of 100 cases with a review of the literature. Hum Pathol 21:363–381
83. Connell PP et al (1999) Race and clinical outcome in endometrial carcinoma. Obstet Gynecol 94:713–720
84. Connelly PJ, Alberhasky RC, Christopherson WM (1982) Carcinoma of the endometrium. III. Analysis of 865 cases of adenocarcinoma and adenoacanthoma. Obstet Gynecol 59:569–575
85. Connor EE et al (2007) Regulation of gene expression in the bovine mammary gland by ovarian steroids. J Dairy Sci 90(Suppl 1):E55–E65
86. Cook LS et al (1995) Population-based study of tamoxifen therapy and subsequent ovarian, endometrial, and breast cancers. J Natl Cancer Inst 87:1359–1364
87. Coppola D et al (1998) Prognostic significance of p53, bcl-2, vimentin, and S100 protein-positive Langerhans cells in endometrial carcinoma. Hum Pathol 29:455–462
88. Cork DM, Lennard TW, Tyson-Capper AJ (2008) Alternative splicing and the progesterone receptor in breast cancer. Breast Cancer Res 10:207
89. Creasman WT (1989) Announcement. FIGO stages: 1988 revision. Gynecol Oncol 35:125–127
90. Creasman WT (1997) Endometrial cancer: incidence, prognostic factors, diagnosis, and treatment. Semin Oncol 24:S1-140–S1-150
91. Creasman WT et al (1999) Significance of true surgical pathologic staging: a Gynecologic Oncology Group Study. Am J Obstet Gynecol 181:31–34
92. Creasman WT et al (1981) Prognostic significance of peritoneal cytology in patients with endometrial cancer and preliminary data concerning therapy with intraperitoneal radiopharmaceuticals. Am J Obstet Gynecol 141:921–929
93. Creasman WT et al (1986) Estrogen replacement therapy in the patient treated for endometrial cancer. Obstet Gynecol 67:326–330
94. Creasman WT et al (1987) Surgical pathologic spread patterns of endometrial cancer. A Gynecologic Oncology Group Study. Cancer 60:2035–2041
95. Creasman WT et al (2003) Carcinoma of the corpus uteri. Int J Gynaecol Obstet 83(Suppl 1):79–118
96. Crissman JD et al (1981) Endometrial carcinoma in women 40 years of age or younger. Obstet Gynecol 57:699–704
97. Curtis RE et al (2004) Risk of malignant mixed mullerian tumors after tamoxifen therapy for breast cancer. J Natl Cancer Inst 96:70–74
98. Czernobilsky B et al (1980) Endocervical-type epithelium in endometrial carcinoma: a report of 10 cases with emphasis on histochemical methods for differential diagnosis. Am J Surg Pathol 4:481–489
99. Daniel AG, Peters WA 3rd (1988) Accuracy of office and operating room curettage in the grading of endometrial carcinoma. Obstet Gynecol 71:612–614
100. Darvishian F et al (2004) Serous endometrial cancers that mimic endometrioid adenocarcinomas: a clinicopathologic and immunohistochemical study of a group of problematic cases. Am J Surg Pathol 28:1568–1578
101. de Leeuw WJ et al (2000) Prediction of a mismatch repair gene defect by microsatellite instability and immunohistochemical analysis in endometrial tumours from HNPCC patients. J Pathol 192:328–335
102. Deligdisch L, Holinka CF (1986) Progesterone receptors in two groups of endometrial carcinoma. Cancer 57:1385–1388

103. Demczuk S et al (2003) The comparison of the agreement in determining the histological grade of uterine endometrial endometrioid carcinoma, using the three-grade FIGO classification and the two-grade system. Pol J Pathol 54:179–181
104. Demopoulos RI et al (1996) Papillary carcinoma of the endometrium: morphometric predictors of survival. Int J Gynecol Pathol 15:110–118
105. Dockerty MB, Lovelady SB, Foust GT Jr (1951) Carcinoma of the corpus uteri in young women. Am J Obstet Gynecol 61:966–981
106. Doering DL et al (1989) Intraoperative evaluation of depth of myometrial invasion in stage I endometrial adenocarcinoma. Obstet Gynecol 74:930–933
107. Duggan BD et al (1994) Microsatellite instability in sporadic endometrial carcinoma. J Natl Cancer Inst 86:1216–1221
108. Dunton CJ et al (1991) Uterine papillary serous carcinoma: a review. Obstet Gynecol Surv 46:97–102
109. Egan JA et al (2004) Differential expression of WT1 and p53 in serous and endometrioid carcinomas of the endometrium. Int J Gynecol Pathol 23:119–122
110. Ehrlich CE et al (1988) Steroid receptors and clinical outcome in patients with adenocarcinoma of the endometrium. Am J Obstet Gynecol 158:796–807
111. Eifel P et al (1982) Simultaneous presentation of carcinoma involving the ovary and the uterine corpus. Cancer 50:163–170
112. Eifel PJ et al (1983) Adenocarcinoma of the endometrium. Analysis of 256 cases with disease limited to the uterine corpus: treatment comparisons. Cancer 52:1026–1031
113. Enomoto T et al (1993) Alterations of the p53 tumor suppressor gene and its association with activation of the c-K-ras-2 protooncogene in premalignant and malignant lesions of the human uterine endometrium. Cancer Res 53:1883–1888
114. Enriori CL, Reforzo-Membrives J (1984) Peripheral aromatization as a risk factor for breast and endometrial cancer in postmenopausal women: a review. Gynecol Oncol 17:1–21
115. Eshleman JR, Markowitz SD (1995) Microsatellite instability in inherited and sporadic neoplasms. Curr Opin Oncol 7:83–89
116. Esteller M et al (1999) MLH1 promoter hypermethylation is an early event in human endometrial tumorigenesis. Am J Pathol 155:1767–1772
117. Esteller M et al (1997) The clinicopathological significance of K-RAS point mutation and gene amplification in endometrial cancer. Eur J Cancer 33:1572–1577
118. Esteller M et al (1998) MLH1 promoter hypermethylation is associated with the microsatellite instability phenotype in sporadic endometrial carcinomas. Oncogene 17:2413–2417
119. Fader AN et al (2009) Platinum/taxane-based chemotherapy with or without radiation therapy favorably impacts survival outcomes in stage I uterine papillary serous carcinoma. Cancer 115:2119–2127
120. Fanning J et al (1991) Prognostic significance of the extent of cervical involvement by endometrial cancer. Gynecol Oncol 40:46–47
121. Farhi DC, Nosanchuk J, Silverberg SG (1986) Endometrial adenocarcinoma in women under 25 years of age. Obstet Gynecol 68:741–745
122. Farley JH et al (2000) Age-specific survival of women with endometrioid adenocarcinoma of the uterus. Gynecol Oncol 79:86–89
123. Ferguson SE et al (2007) Clinicopathologic features of rhabdomyosarcoma of gynecologic origin in adults. Am J Surg Pathol 31:382–389
124. Ferguson SE et al (2006) Comparison of uterine malignancies that develop during and following tamoxifen therapy. Gynecol Oncol 101:322–326
125. Ferguson SE et al (2007) Prognostic features of surgical stage I uterine carcinosarcoma. Am J Surg Pathol 31:1653–1661
126. Fersis N et al (2004) Sentinel node identification and intraoperative lymphatic mapping. First results of a pilot study in patients with endometrial cancer. Eur J Gynaecol Oncol 25:339–342
127. Fisher B et al (1994) Endometrial cancer in tamoxifen-treated breast cancer patients: findings from the National Surgical Adjuvant Breast and Bowel Project (NSABP) B-14. J Natl Cancer Inst 86:527–537
128. Fisher B et al (1998) Tamoxifen for prevention of breast cancer: report of the National Surgical Adjuvant Breast and Bowel Project P-1 Study. J Natl Cancer Inst 90:1371–1388
129. Fleming WP et al (1984) Autopsy findings in patients with uterine sarcoma. Gynecol Oncol 19:168–172
130. Fornander T et al (1989) Adjuvant tamoxifen in early breast cancer: occurrence of new primary cancers. Lancet 1:117–120
131. Franks AL, Kendrick JS, Tyler CW Jr (1987) Postmenopausal smoking, estrogen replacement therapy, and the risk of endometrial cancer. Am J Obstet Gynecol 156:20–23
132. Fujii H et al (2000) Frequent genetic heterogeneity in the clonal evolution of gynecological carcinosarcoma and its influence on phenotypic diversity. Cancer Res 60:114–120
133. Fukuchi T et al (1998) Beta-catenin mutation in carcinoma of the uterine endometrium. Cancer Res 58:3526–3528
134. Fukuda K et al (1998) Prognostic significance of progesterone receptor immunohistochemistry in endometrial carcinoma. Gynecol Oncol 69:220–225
135. Fuqua SA, Cui Y (2004) Estrogen and progesterone receptor isoforms: clinical significance in breast cancer. Breast Cancer Res Treat 87(Suppl 1):S3–S10
136. Gagne E et al (1989) Morphologic prognostic factors of malignant mixed mullerian tumor of the uterus: a clinicopathologic study of 58 cases. Mod Pathol 2:433–438
137. Gal D, Recio FO, Zamurovic D (1992) The new International Federation of Gynecology and Obstetrics surgical staging and survival rates in early endometrial carcinoma. Cancer 69:200–202
138. Gal D et al (1991) Lymphvascular space involvement – a prognostic indicator in endometrial adenocarcinoma. Gynecol Oncol 42:142–145
139. Gambrell RD Jr, Bagnell CA, Greenblatt RB (1983) Role of estrogens and progesterone in the etiology and prevention of endometrial cancer: review. Am J Obstet Gynecol 146:696–707
140. Garg K et al (2009) Selection of endometrial carcinomas for DNA mismatch repair protein immunohistochemistry using patient age and tumor morphology enhances detection of mismatch repair abnormalities. Am J Surg Pathol 33:925–933
141. Garzetti GG et al (1996) Proliferating cell nuclear antigen in endometrial carcinoma: pretreatment identification of high-risk patients. Gynecol Oncol 61:16–21
142. Gasparini GS, Fea RP (1992) Multivariate analysis of prognostic factors in 232 patients with clinical stage I endometrial carcinoma using the new FIGO surgical staging system. Int J Oncol 1:665–672
143. Gates EJ et al (2006) Body mass index as a prognostic factor in endometrioid adenocarcinoma of the endometrium. J Natl Med Assoc 98:1814–1822
144. Geisinger KR et al (1986) Endometrial adenocarcinoma. A multiparameter clinicopathologic analysis including the DNA profile and the sex steroid hormone receptors. Cancer 58:1518–1525

145. Geisinger KR et al (1986) Correlation of female sex steroid hormone receptors with histologic and ultrastructural differentiation in adenocarcinoma of the endometrium. Cancer 58:1506–1517
146. Geisler JP et al (1998) Lack of bcl-2 persistence: an independent prognostic indicator of poor prognosis in endometrial carcinoma. Gynecol Oncol 71:305–307
147. Geisler JP et al (1996) p53 as a prognostic indicator in endometrial cancer. Gynecol Oncol 61:245–248
148. George E et al (1995) Malignant mixed mullerian tumor versus high-grade endometrial carcinoma and aggressive variants of endometrial carcinoma: a comparative analysis of survival. Int J Gynecol Pathol 14:39–44
149. Giangrande PH, McDonnell DP (1999) The A and B isoforms of the human progesterone receptor: two functionally different transcription factors encoded by a single gene. Recent Prog Horm Res 54:291–313; discussion 313–314
150. Gitsch G et al (1995) Uterine papillary serous carcinoma. A clinical study. Cancer 75:2239–2243
151. Gitsch G et al (1995) Endometrial cancer in premenopausal women 45 years and younger. Obstet Gynecol 85:504–508
152. Goldstein NS, Uzieblo A (2002) WT1 immunoreactivity in uterine papillary serous carcinomas is different from ovarian serous carcinomas. Am J Clin Pathol 117:541–545
153. Gompel A et al (1994) Bcl-2 expression in normal endometrium during the menstrual cycle. Am J Pathol 144:1195–1202
154. Goodman A et al (1996) Squamous cell carcinoma of the endometrium: a report of eight cases and a review of the literature. Gynecol Oncol 61:54–60
155. Gray LA Sr, Christopherson WM, Hoover RN (1977) Estrogens and endometrial carcinoma. Obstet Gynecol Surv 32:619–621
156. Greenblatt RB, Gambrell RD Jr, Stoddard LD (1982) The protective role of progesterone in the prevention of endometrial cancer. Pathol Res Pract 174:297–318
157. Greenwald P, Caputo TA, Wolfgang PE (1977) Endometrial cancer after menopausal use of estrogens. Obstet Gynecol 50:239–243
158. Greven KM et al (1993) Pathologic stage III endometrial carcinoma. Prognostic factors and patterns of recurrence. Cancer 71:3697–3702
159. Grimshaw RN et al (1990) Prognostic value of peritoneal cytology in endometrial carcinoma. Gynecol Oncol 36:97–100
160. Gronroos M et al (1993) Mass screening for endometrial cancer directed in risk groups of patients with diabetes and patients with hypertension. Cancer 71:1279–1282
161. Gu M et al (2000) Peritoneal washings in endometrial carcinoma. A study of 298 patients with histopathologic correlation. Acta Cytol 44:783–789
162. Guidi AJ et al (1996) Expression of vascular permeability factor (vascular endothelial growth factor) and its receptors in endometrial carcinoma. Cancer 78:454–460
163. Hagiwara T, Mori T, Kaku T (2005) Development of endometrial cancer following radiation therapy for cervical carcinoma. Eur J Gynaecol Oncol 26:191–195
164. Hall JB, Young RH, Nelson JH Jr (1984) The prognostic significance of adenomyosis in endometrial carcinoma. Gynecol Oncol 17:32–40
165. Hamel NW et al (1996) Prognostic value of p53 and proliferating cell nuclear antigen expression in endometrial carcinoma. Gynecol Oncol 62:192–198
166. Hampel H et al (2006) Screening for Lynch syndrome (hereditary nonpolyposis colorectal cancer) among endometrial cancer patients. Cancer Res 66:7810–7817
167. Hanson MB et al (1985) The prognostic significance of lymph-vascular space invasion in stage I endometrial cancer. Cancer 55:1753–1757
168. Harouny VR et al (1988) The importance of peritoneal cytology in endometrial carcinoma. Obstet Gynecol 72:394–398
169. Hayes MP, Douglas W, Ellenson LH (2009) Molecular alterations of EGFR and PIK3CA in uterine serous carcinoma. Gynecol Oncol 113:370–373
170. Hayes MP et al (2006) PIK3CA and PTEN mutations in uterine endometrioid carcinoma and complex atypical hyperplasia. Clin Cancer Res 12:5932–5935
171. Heatley MK (1997) A high apoptotic index occurs in subtypes of endometrial adenocarcinoma associated with a poor prognosis. Pathology 29:272–275
172. Heatley MK (1995) Association between the apoptotic index and established prognostic parameters in endometrial adenocarcinoma. Histopathology 27:469–472
173. Henderson GS et al (1996) bcl-2 is down-regulated in atypical endometrial hyperplasia and adenocarcinoma. Mod Pathol 9:430–438
174. Hendrickson M et al (1982) Uterine papillary serous carcinoma: a highly malignant form of endometrial adenocarcinoma. Am J Surg Pathol 6:93–108
175. Hendrickson MR, Kempson RL (1983) Ciliated carcinoma – a variant of endometrial adenocarcinoma: a report of 10 cases. Int J Gynecol Pathol 2:1–12
176. Hernandez E, Woodruff JD (1980) Endometrial adenocarcinoma arising in adenomyosis. Am J Obstet Gynecol 138:827–832
177. Hetzel DJ et al (1992) HER-2/neu expression: a major prognostic factor in endometrial cancer. Gynecol Oncol 47:179–185
178. Hicks ML et al (1998) The National Cancer Data Base report on endometrial carcinoma in African-American women. Cancer 83:2629–2637
179. Hoffman MS et al (1989) Adenocarcinoma of the endometrium and endometrioid carcinoma of the ovary associated with pregnancy. Gynecol Oncol 32:82–85
180. Homesley HD, Zaino R (1994) Endometrial cancer: prognostic factors. Semin Oncol 21:71–78
181. Hopp TA et al (2004) Breast cancer patients with progesterone receptor PR-A-rich tumors have poorer disease-free survival rates. Clin Cancer Res 10:2751–2760
182. Hornback NB, Omura G, Major FJ (1986) Observations on the use of adjuvant radiation therapy in patients with stage I and II uterine sarcoma. Int J Radiat Oncol Biol Phys 12:2127–2130
183. Horwitz RI et al (1981) Necropsy diagnosis of endometrial cancer and detection-bias in case/control studies. Lancet 2:66–68
184. Hoshida Y et al (1996) Hepatoid adenocarcinoma of the endometrium associated with alpha-fetoprotein production. Int J Gynecol Pathol 15:266–269
185. Ingle JN (1994) Tamoxifen and endometrial cancer: new challenges for an "old" drug. Gynecol Oncol 55:161–163
186. Inoue Y et al (1996) The prognostic significance of vascular invasion by endometrial carcinoma. Cancer 78:1447–1451
187. Inthasorn P et al (2002) Analysis of clinicopathologic factors in malignant mixed Mullerian tumors of the uterine corpus. Int J Gynecol Cancer 12:348–353
188. Ioffe OB, Papadimitriou JC, Drachenberg CB (1998) Correlation of proliferation indices, apoptosis, and related oncogene expression (bcl-2 and c-erbB-2) and p53 in proliferative, hyperplastic, and malignant endometrium. Hum Pathol 29:1150–1159

189. Ismail SM (1996) The effects of tamoxifen on the uterus. Curr Opin Obstet Gynecol 8:27–31
190. Ito K et al (1997) Correlations between p21 expression and clinicopathological findings, p53 gene and protein alterations, and survival in patients with endometrial carcinoma. J Pathol 183:318–324
191. Ito K et al (1996) K-ras point mutations in endometrial carcinoma: effect on outcome is dependent on age of patient. Gynecol Oncol 63:238–246
192. Ito K et al (1994) Prognostic significance of p53 overexpression in endometrial cancer. Cancer Res 54:4667–4670
193. Iversen OE (1986) Flow cytometric deoxyribonucleic acid index: a prognostic factor in endometrial carcinoma. Am J Obstet Gynecol 155:770–776
194. Jacobsen BM et al (2005) Progesterone-independent effects of human progesterone receptors (PRs) in estrogen receptor-positive breast cancer: PR isoform-specific gene regulation and tumor biology. Mol Endocrinol 19:574–587
195. Jacques SM, Lawrence WD (1990) Endometrial adenocarcinoma with variable-level myometrial involvement limited to adenomyosis: a clinicopathologic study of 23 cases. Gynecol Oncol 37:401–407
196. Jones MA, Young RH, Scully RE (1991) Endometrial adenocarcinoma with a component of giant cell carcinoma. Int J Gynecol Pathol 10:260–270
197. Jones MW et al (1997) Prognostic value of p53 and K-ras-2 topographic genotyping in endometrial carcinoma: a clinicopathologic and molecular comparison. Int J Gynecol Pathol 16:354–360
198. Jordan LB, Al-Nafussi A (2002) Clinicopathological study of the pattern and significance of cervical involvement in cases of endometrial adenocarcinoma. Int J Gynecol Cancer 12:42–48
199. Jordan VC, Morrow M (1994) Should clinicians be concerned about the carcinogenic potential of tamoxifen? Eur J Cancer 30A:1714–1721
200. Joseph MG, Fellows FG, Hearn SA (1990) Primary endodermal sinus tumor of the endometrium. A clinicopathologic, immunocytochemical, and ultrastructural study. Cancer 65:297–302
201. Kadar N, Homesley HD, Malfetano JH (1992) Positive peritoneal cytology is an adverse factor in endometrial carcinoma only if there is other evidence of extrauterine disease. Gynecol Oncol 46:145–149
202. Kadar N, Malfetano JH, Homesley HD (1993) Steroid receptor concentrations in endometrial carcinoma: effect on survival in surgically staged patients. Gynecol Oncol 50:281–286
203. Kaku T et al (1997) Angiogenesis in endometrial carcinoma. Cancer 80:741–747
204. Kaku T et al (1993) Association of endometrial epithelial metaplasias with endometrial carcinoma and hyperplasia in Japanese and American women. Int J Gynecol Pathol 12:297–300
205. Kaleli S et al (1997) A strong prognostic variable in endometrial carcinoma: flow cytometric S-phase fraction. Cancer 79:944–951
206. Kalir T et al (1995) Endometrial adenocarcinoma with choriocarcinomatous differentiation in an elderly virginal woman. Int J Gynecol Pathol 14:266–269
207. Kallakury BV et al (1998) Cell proliferation-associated proteins in endometrial carcinomas, including papillary serous and endometrioid subtypes. Int J Gynecol Pathol 17:320–326
208. Kanbour-Shakir A, Tobon H (1991) Primary clear cell carcinoma of the endometrium: a clinicopathologic study of 20 cases. Int J Gynecol Pathol 10:67–78
209. Kapucuoglu N et al (2008) Reproducibility of grading systems for endometrial endometrioid carcinoma and their relation with pathologic prognostic parameters. Int J Gynecol Cancer 18:790–796
210. Katase K et al (1998) The incidence of subsequent endometrial carcinoma with tamoxifen use in patients with primary breast carcinoma. Cancer 82:1698–1703
211. Kaufman DW et al (1980) Decreased risk of endometrial cancer among oral-contraceptive users. N Engl J Med 303:1045–1047
212. Kelly MG et al (2004) Patients with uterine papillary serous cancers may benefit from adjuvant platinum-based chemoradiation. Gynecol Oncol 95:469–473
213. Kelly MG et al (2005) Improved survival in surgical stage I patients with uterine papillary serous carcinoma (UPSC) treated with adjuvant platinum-based chemotherapy. Gynecol Oncol 98:353–359
214. Kennedy AW et al (1987) Experience with pelvic washings in stage I and II endometrial carcinoma. Gynecol Oncol 28:50–60
215. Khalifa MA et al (1994) Expression of EGFR, HER-2/neu, P53, and PCNA in endometrioid, serous papillary, and clear cell endometrial adenocarcinomas. Gynecol Oncol 53:84–92
216. Khuu HM et al (2000) Carcinosarcoma of the uterus associated with a nongestational choriocarcinoma. South Med J 93:226–228
217. Kihana T et al (1995) Mutation and allelic loss of the p53 gene in endometrial carcinoma. Incidence and outcome in 92 surgical patients. Cancer 76:72–78
218. Kim KR, Scully RE (1990) Peritoneal keratin granulomas with carcinomas of endometrium and ovary and atypical polypoid adenomyoma of endometrium. A clinicopathological analysis of 22 cases. Am J Surg Pathol 14:925–932
219. Klemi PJ, Alanen KA, Salmi T (1995) Detection of malignancy in endometrium by brush sampling in 1042 symptomatic patients. Int J Gynecol Cancer 5:222–225
220. Kobayashi K et al (1999) Mutations of the beta-catenin gene in endometrial carcinomas. Jpn J Cancer Res 90:55–59
221. Kohlberger P et al (1996) p53 protein overexpression in early stage endometrial cancer. Gynecol Oncol 62:213–217
222. Kohler MF et al (1996) p53 overexpression in advanced-stage endometrial adenocarcinoma. Am J Obstet Gynecol 175:1246–1252
223. Kommoss F et al (1998) Steroid receptor expression in endometria from women treated with tamoxifen. Gynecol Oncol 70:188–191
224. Kosary CL (1994) FIGO stage, histology, histologic grade, age and race as prognostic factors in determining survival for cancers of the female gynecological system: an analysis of 1973–87 SEER cases of cancers of the endometrium, cervix, ovary, vulva, and vagina. Semin Surg Oncol 10:31–46
225. Koshiyama M et al (1993) Immunohistochemical analysis of p53 protein over-expression in endometrial carcinomas: inverse correlation with sex steroid receptor status. Virchows Arch A Pathol Anat Histopathol 423:265–271
226. Koss LG et al (1984) Detection of endometrial carcinoma and hyperplasia in asymptomatic women. Obstet Gynecol 64:1–11
227. Kovalev S et al (1998) Loss of p53 function in uterine papillary serous carcinoma. Hum Pathol 29:613–619
228. Kumar NB, Hart WR (1982) Metastases to the uterine corpus from extragenital cancers. A clinicopathologic study of 63 cases. Cancer 50:2163–2169
229. Kurman RJ, Scully RE (1976) Clear cell carcinoma of the endometrium: an analysis of 21 cases. Cancer 37:872–882
230. Lacey JV Jr et al (2008) PTEN expression in endometrial biopsies as a marker of progression to endometrial carcinoma. Cancer Res 68:6014–6020
231. Larson B et al (1990) Mixed mullerian tumours of the uterus–prognostic factors: a clinical and histopathologic study of 147 cases. Radiother Oncol 17:123–132

232. Larson DM et al (1995) Comparison of D&C and office endometrial biopsy in predicting final histopathologic grade in endometrial cancer. Obstet Gynecol 86:38–42
233. Lauchlan SC (1981) Tubal (serous) carcinoma of the endometrium. Arch Pathol Lab Med 105:615–618
234. Lax SF et al (2000) The frequency of p53, K-ras mutations, and microsatellite instability differs in uterine endometrioid and serous carcinoma: evidence of distinct molecular genetic pathways. Cancer 88:814–824
235. Lax SF et al (2000) A binary architectural grading system for uterine endometrial endometrioid carcinoma has superior reproducibility compared with FIGO grading and identifies subsets of advance-stage tumors with favorable and unfavorable prognosis. Am J Surg Pathol 24:1201–1208
236. Lax SF et al (1998) Clear cell carcinoma of the endometrium is characterized by a distinctive profile of p53, Ki-67, estrogen, and progesterone receptor expression. Hum Pathol 29:551–558
237. Lax SF et al (1998) Comparison of estrogen and progesterone receptor, Ki-67, and p53 immunoreactivity in uterine endometrioid carcinoma and endometrioid carcinoma with squamous, mucinous, secretory, and ciliated cell differentiation. Hum Pathol 29:924–931
238. Lee KR, Belinson JL (1991) Recurrence in noninvasive endometrial carcinoma. Relationship to uterine papillary serous carcinoma. Am J Surg Pathol 15:965–973
239. Lee KR, Scully RE (1989) Complex endometrial hyperplasia and carcinoma in adolescents and young women 15 to 20 years of age. A report of 10 cases. Int J Gynecol Pathol 8:201–213
240. Lee KR, Vacek PM, Belinson JL (1994) Traditional and nontraditional histopathologic predictors of recurrence in uterine endometrioid adenocarcinoma. Gynecol Oncol 54:10–18
241. Lee RB, Burke TW, Park RC (1990) Estrogen replacement therapy following treatment for stage I endometrial carcinoma. Gynecol Oncol 36:189–191
242. Leiserowitz GS et al (1993) The proto-oncogene c-fms is overexpressed in endometrial cancer. Gynecol Oncol 49:190–196
243. Lesko SM et al (1985) Cigarette smoking and the risk of endometrial cancer. N Engl J Med 313:593–596
244. Levenback C et al (1992) Uterine papillary serous carcinoma (UPSC) treated with cisplatin, doxorubicin, and cyclophosphamide (PAC). Gynecol Oncol 46:317–321
245. Levi F et al (1993) Dietary factors and the risk of endometrial cancer. Cancer 71:3575–3581
246. Levine RL et al (1998) PTEN mutations and microsatellite instability in complex atypical hyperplasia, a precursor lesion to uterine endometrioid carcinoma. Cancer Res 58:3254–3258
247. Li J et al (1997) PTEN, a putative protein tyrosine phosphatase gene mutated in human brain, breast, and prostate cancer. Science 275:1943–1947
248. Lininger RA et al (1997) Transitional cell carcinoma of the endometrium and endometrial carcinoma with transitional cell differentiation. Cancer 79:1933–1943
249. Livasy CA et al (2006) EGFR expression and HER2/neu overexpression/amplification in endometrial carcinosarcoma. Gynecol Oncol 100:101–106
250. Longacre TA, Hendrickson MR (1999) Diffusely infiltrative endometrial adenocarcinoma: an adenoma malignum pattern of myoinvasion. Am J Surg Pathol 23:69–78
251. Lukes AS et al (1994) Multivariable analysis of DNA ploidy, p53, and HER-2/neu as prognostic factors in endometrial cancer. Cancer 73:2380–2385
252. Macasaet MA et al (1985) Prognostic factors in malignant mesodermal (mullerian) mixed tumors of the uterus. Gynecol Oncol 20:32–42
253. Mack TM et al (1976) Estrogens and endometrial cancer in a retirement community. N Engl J Med 294:1262–1267
254. MacMahon B (1997) Overview of studies on endometrial cancer and other types of cancer in humans: perspectives of an epidemiologist. Semin Oncol 24:S1-122–S1-139
255. Magriples U et al (1993) High-grade endometrial carcinoma in tamoxifen-treated breast cancer patients. J Clin Oncol 11:485–490
256. Mai KT et al (2002) Endometrioid carcinoma of the endometrium with an invasive component of minimal deviation carcinoma. Hum Pathol 33:856–858
257. Major FJ et al (1993) Prognostic factors in early-stage uterine sarcoma. A Gynecologic Oncology Group study. Cancer 71:1702–1709
258. Malpica A et al (1995) Low-stage clear-cell carcinoma of the endometrium. Am J Surg Pathol 19:769–774
259. Maxwell GL et al (1998) Mutation of the PTEN tumor suppressor gene in endometrial hyperplasias. Cancer Res 58:2500–2503
260. McCarty KS Jr et al (1979) Correlation of estrogen and progesterone receptors with histologic differentiation in endometrial adenocarcinoma. Am J Pathol 96:171–183
261. McCluggage WG (2002) Malignant biphasic uterine tumours: carcinosarcomas or metaplastic carcinomas? J Clin Pathol 55:321–325
262. McCluggage WG, Jenkins D (2003) p16 immunoreactivity may assist in the distinction between endometrial and endocervical adenocarcinoma. Int J Gynecol Pathol 22:231–235
263. McCluggage WG et al (2002) A panel of immunohistochemical stains, including carcinoembryonic antigen, vimentin, and estrogen receptor, aids the distinction between primary endometrial and endocervical adenocarcinomas. Int J Gynecol Pathol 21:11–15
264. McDonald TW et al (1977) Exogenous estrogen and endometrial carcinoma: case-control and incidence study. Am J Obstet Gynecol 127:572–580
265. McKenney JK, Kong CS, Longacre TA (2005) Endometrial adenocarcinoma associated with subtle lymph-vascular space invasion and lymph node metastasis: a histologic pattern mimicking intravascular and sinusoidal histiocytes. Int J Gynecol Pathol 24:73–78
266. Meis JM, Lawrence WD (1990) The immunohistochemical profile of malignant mixed mullerian tumor. Overlap with endometrial adenocarcinoma. Am J Clin Pathol 94:1–7
267. Melhem MF, Tobon H (1987) Mucinous adenocarcinoma of the endometrium: a clinico-pathological review of 18 cases. Int J Gynecol Pathol 6:347–355
268. Milosevic MF, Dembo AJ, Thomas GM (1992) The clinical significance of malignant peritoneal cytology in stage I endometrial carcinoma. Int J Gynecol Cancer 2:225–235
269. Missaoui N et al (2006) p16INK4A overexpression and HPV infection in uterine cervix adenocarcinoma. Virchows Arch 448:597–603
270. Mitchell H, Giles G, Medley G (1993) Accuracy and survival benefit of cytological prediction of endometrial carcinoma on routine cervical smears. Int J Gynecol Pathol 12:34–40
271. Mittal KR, Barwick KW (1993) Endometrial adenocarcinoma involving adenomyosis without true myometrial invasion is characterized by frequent preceding estrogen therapy, low histologic grades, and excellent prognosis. Gynecol Oncol 49:197–201
272. Modica I et al (2007) Utility of immunohistochemistry in predicting microsatellite instability in endometrial carcinoma. Am J Surg Pathol 31:744–751

273. Moll UM et al (1996) Uterine papillary serous carcinoma evolves via a p53-driven pathway. Hum Pathol 27:1295–1300
274. Mooney EE et al (1997) Signet-ring cell carcinoma of the endometrium: a primary tumor masquerading as a metastasis. Int J Gynecol Pathol 16:169–172
275. Morgan KG, Wilkinson N, Buckley CH (1996) Angiogenesis in normal, hyperplastic, and neoplastic endometrium. J Pathol 179:317–320
276. Morris PC et al (1995) Steroid hormone receptor content and lymph node status in endometrial cancer. Gynecol Oncol 56:406–411
277. Morrow CP et al (1991) Relationship between surgical-pathological risk factors and outcome in clinical stage I and II carcinoma of the endometrium: a Gynecologic Oncology Group study. Gynecol Oncol 40:55–65
278. Murray SK, Clement PB, Young RH (2005) Endometrioid carcinomas of the uterine corpus with sex cord-like formations, hyalinization, and other unusual morphologic features: a report of 31 cases of a neoplasm that may be confused with carcinosarcoma and other uterine neoplasms. Am J Surg Pathol 29:157–166
279. Murray SK, Young RH, Scully RE (2003) Unusual epithelial and stromal changes in myoinvasive endometrioid adenocarcinoma: a study of their frequency, associated diagnostic problems, and prognostic significance. Int J Gynecol Pathol 22:324–333
280. Mutter GL et al (1996) Allelotype mapping of unstable microsatellites establishes direct lineage continuity between endometrial precancers and cancer. Cancer Res 56:4483–4486
281. Nascimento AF et al (2003) The role of CD10 staining in distinguishing invasive endometrial adenocarcinoma from adenocarcinoma involving adenomyosis. Mod Pathol 16:22–27
282. Nazeer T et al (1995) Multivariate survival analysis of clinicopathologic features in surgical stage I endometrioid carcinoma including analysis of HER-2/neu expression. Am J Obstet Gynecol 173:1829–1834
283. Nelen MR et al (1999) Novel PTEN mutations in patients with Cowden disease: absence of clear genotype-phenotype correlations. Eur J Hum Genet 7:267–273
284. Ng AB et al (1973) Mixed adenosquamous carcinoma of the endometrium. Am J Clin Pathol 59:765–781
285. Nielsen AL, Nyholm HC (1994) p53 protein and c-erbB-2 protein (p185) expression in endometrial adenocarcinoma of endometrioid type. An immunohistochemical examination on paraffin sections. Am J Clin Pathol 102:76–79
286. Nielsen AL, Nyholm HC (1996) The combination of p53 and age predict cancer specific death in advanced stage (FIGO Ic-IV) of endometrial carcinoma of endometrioid type. An immunohistochemical examination of growth fraction: Ki-67, MIB-1 and PC10; suppressor oncogene protein: p53; oncogene protein: p185 and age, hormone treatment, stage, and histologic grade. Eur J Obstet Gynecol Reprod Biol 70:79–85
287. Nielsen AL, Nyholm HC, Engel P (1994) Expression of MIB-1 (paraffin ki-67) and AgNOR morphology in endometrial adenocarcinomas of endometrioid type. Int J Gynecol Pathol 13:37–44
288. Nielsen AL, Thomsen HK, Nyholm HC (1991) Evaluation of the reproducibility of the revised 1988 International Federation of Gynecology and Obstetrics grading system of endometrial cancers with special emphasis on nuclear grading. Cancer 68:2303–2309
289. Nielsen SN et al (1989) Clinicopathologic analysis of uterine malignant mixed mullerian tumors. Gynecol Oncol 34:372–378
290. Niemann TH et al (1996) bcl-2 expression in endometrial hyperplasia and carcinoma. Gynecol Oncol 63:318–322
291. Nofech-Mozes S et al (2008) Lymphovascular invasion is a significant predictor for distant recurrence in patients with early-stage endometrial endometrioid adenocarcinoma. Am J Clin Pathol 129:912–917
292. Nordal RR et al (1997) An evaluation of prognostic factors in uterine carcinosarcoma. Gynecol Oncol 67:316–321
293. Nordstrom B et al (1996) Carcinoma of the endometrium: do the nuclear grade and DNA ploidy provide more prognostic information than do the FIGO and WHO classifications? Int J Gynecol Pathol 15:191–201
294. Norris HJ, Roth E, Taylor HB (1966) Mesenchymal tumors of the uterus. II. A clinical and pathologic study of 31 mixed mesodermal tumors. Obstet Gynecol 28:57–63
295. Norris HJ, Taylor HB (1966) Mesenchymal tumors of the uterus. 3. A clinical and pathologic study of 31 carcinosarcomas. Cancer 19:1459–1465
296. Noumoff JS et al (1991) The ability to evaluate prognostic variables on frozen section in hysterectomies performed for endometrial carcinoma. Gynecol Oncol 42:202–208
297. Nyholm HC, Christensen IJ, Nielsen AL (1995) Progesterone receptor levels independently predict survival in endometrial adenocarcinoma. Gynecol Oncol 59:347–351
298. Obata K et al (1998) Frequent PTEN/MMAC mutations in endometrioid but not serous or mucinous epithelial ovarian tumors. Cancer Res 58:2095–2097
299. Obermair A et al (1999) Endometrial cancer: accuracy of the finding of a well differentiated tumor at dilatation and curettage compared to the findings at subsequent hysterectomy. Int J Gynecol Cancer 9:383–386
300. Obermair A et al (1999) Prognostic significance of tumor angiogenesis in endometrial cancer. Obstet Gynecol 93:367–371
301. Oda K et al (2005) High frequency of coexistent mutations of PIK3CA and PTEN genes in endometrial carcinoma. Cancer Res 65:10669–10673
302. Ozuysal S et al (2003) Angiogenesis in endometrial carcinoma: correlation with survival and clinicopathologic risk factors. Gynecol Obstet Invest 55:173–177
303. Pallares J et al (2005) Immunohistochemical analysis of PTEN in endometrial carcinoma: a tissue microarray study with a comparison of four commercial antibodies in correlation with molecular abnormalities. Mod Pathol 18:719–727
304. Parazzini F et al (1997) The epidemiology of female genital tract cancers. Int J Gynecol Cancer 7:169–181
305. Parazzini F et al (1991) The epidemiology of endometrial cancer. Gynecol Oncol 41:1–16
306. Parazzini F et al (1995) Smoking and risk of endometrial cancer: results from an Italian case-control study. Gynecol Oncol 56:195–199
307. Park KJMPB et al (2008) Immunoprofile of adenocarcinomas of the endometrium, endocervix, and ovary with mucinous differentiation. Appl Immunohistochemistry Mol Morphol 17:8–11
308. Peiro G et al (2002) Microsatellite instability, loss of heterozygosity, and loss of hMLH1 and hMSH2 protein expression in endometrial carcinoma. Hum Pathol 33:347–354
309. Persson I et al (1989) Risk of endometrial cancer after treatment with oestrogens alone or in conjunction with progestogens: results of a prospective study. BMJ 298:147–151
310. Pertschuk LP et al (1996) Estrogen receptor immunocytochemistry in endometrial carcinoma: a prognostic marker for survival. Gynecol Oncol 63:28–33

311. Pesce C et al (1991) Endometrial carcinoma with trophoblastic differentiation. An aggressive form of uterine cancer. Cancer 68:1799–1802
312. Peterson EP (1968) Endometrial carcinoma in young women. A clinical profile. Obstet Gynecol 31:702–707
313. Pfisterer J et al (1995) Prognostic value of DNA ploidy and S-phase fraction in stage I endometrial carcinoma. Gynecol Oncol 58:149–156
314. Photopulos GJ et al (1979) Clear cell carcinoma of the endometrium. Cancer 43:1448–1456
315. Pickar JH, Thorneycroft I, Whitehead M (1998) Effects of hormone replacement therapy on the endometrium and lipid parameters: a review of randomized clinical trials, 1985 to 1995. Am J Obstet Gynecol 178:1087–1099
316. Pisani AL et al (1995) HER-2/neu, p53, and DNA analyses as prognosticators for survival in endometrial carcinoma. Obstet Gynecol 85:729–734
317. Pitman MB et al (1994) Endometrioid carcinoma of the ovary and endometrium, oxyphilic cell type: a report of nine cases. Int J Gynecol Pathol 13:290–301
318. Plaxe SC, Saltzstein SL (1997) Impact of ethnicity on the incidence of high-risk endometrial carcinoma. Gynecol Oncol 65:8–12
319. Podczaski E et al (1992) Detection and patterns of treatment failure in 300 consecutive cases of "early" endometrial cancer after primary surgery. Gynecol Oncol 47:323–327
320. Podsypanina K et al (1999) Mutation of Pten/Mmac1 in mice causes neoplasia in multiple organ systems. Proc Natl Acad Sci USA 96:1563–1568
321. Pollock PM et al (2007) Frequent activating FGFR2 mutations in endometrial carcinomas parallel germline mutations associated with craniosynostosis and skeletal dysplasia syndromes. Oncogene 26:7158–7162
322. Pothuri B et al (2006) Radiation-associated endometrial cancers are prognostically unfavorable tumors: a clinicopathologic comparison with 527 sporadic endometrial cancers. Gynecol Oncol 103:948–951
323. Potischman N et al (1996) Case-control study of endogenous steroid hormones and endometrial cancer. J Natl Cancer Inst 88:1127–1135
324. Powell MA et al (2002) Ribosomal DNA methylation in patients with endometrial carcinoma: an independent prognostic marker. Cancer 94:2941–2952
325. Prat J (2004) Prognostic parameters of endometrial carcinoma. Hum Pathol 35:649–662
326. Raspollini MR et al (2006) Expression and amplification of HER-2/neu oncogene in uterine carcinosarcomas: a marker for potential molecularly targeted treatment? Int J Gynecol Cancer 16:416–422
327. Raspollini MR et al (2005) COX-2, c-KIT and HER-2/neu expression in uterine carcinosarcomas: prognostic factors or potential markers for targeted therapies? Gynecol Oncol 96:159–167
328. Reid-Nicholson M et al (2006) Immunophenotypic diversity of endometrial adenocarcinomas: implications for differential diagnosis. Mod Pathol 19:1091–1100
329. Reinartz JJ et al (1994) Expression of p53, transforming growth factor alpha, epidermal growth factor receptor, and c-erbB-2 in endometrial carcinoma and correlation with survival and known predictors of survival. Hum Pathol 25:1075–1083
330. Ribeiro G, Swindell R (1992) The Christie Hospital adjuvant tamoxifen trial. J Natl Cancer Inst Monogr 11:121–125
331. Richart RM, Ferenczy A (1974) Endometrial morphologic response to hormonal environment. Gynecol Oncol 2:180–197
332. Rieck GC, Freites ON, Williams S (2005) Is tamoxifen associated with high-risk endometrial carcinomas? A retrospective case series of 196 women with endometrial cancer. J Obstet Gynaecol 25:39–41
333. Risinger JI et al (1997) PTEN/MMAC1 mutations in endometrial cancers. Cancer Res 57:4736–4738
334. Rolitsky CD et al (1999) HER-2/neu amplification and overexpression in endometrial carcinoma. Int J Gynecol Pathol 18:138–143
335. Ronnett BM et al (2008) Endocervical adenocarcinomas with ovarian metastases: analysis of 29 cases with emphasis on minimally invasive cervical tumors and the ability of the metastases to simulate primary ovarian neoplasms. Am J Surg Pathol 32:1835–1853
336. Ross JC et al (1983) Primary mucinous adenocarcinoma of the endometrium. A clinicopathologic and histochemical study. Am J Surg Pathol 7:715–729
337. Rovirosa A et al (2002) Is vascular and lymphatic space invasion a main prognostic factor in uterine neoplasms with a sarcomatous component? A retrospective study of prognostic factors of 60 patients stratified by stages. Int J Radiat Oncol Biol Phys 52:1320–1329
338. Rutqvist LE et al (1995) Adjuvant tamoxifen therapy for early stage breast cancer and second primary malignancies. Stockholm Breast Cancer Study Group. J Natl Cancer Inst 87:645–651
339. Ryden S et al (1992) Long-term effects of adjuvant tamoxifen and/or radiotherapy. The South Sweden Breast Cancer Trial. Acta Oncol 31:271–274
340. Ryder DE (1982) Verrucous carcinoma of the endometrium – a unique neoplasm with long survival. Obstet Gynecol 59:78S–80S
341. Saegusa M et al (1996) Bcl-2 expression is correlated with a low apoptotic index and associated with progesterone receptor immunoreactivity in endometrial carcinomas. J Pathol 180:275–282
342. Saegusa M, Okayasu I (1998) Progesterone therapy for endometrial carcinoma reduces cell proliferation but does not alter apoptosis. Cancer 83:111–121
343. Saffari B et al (1995) Amplification and overexpression of HER-2/neu (c-erbB2) in endometrial cancers: correlation with overall survival. Cancer Res 55:5693–5698
344. Sagae S et al (2004) The reproducibility of a binary tumor grading system for uterine endometrial endometrioid carcinoma, compared with FIGO system and nuclear grading. Oncology 67:344–350
345. Saito S et al (2006) Progesterone receptor isoforms as a prognostic marker in human endometrial carcinoma. Cancer Sci 97:1308–1314
346. Sakuragi N et al (2000) Prognostic significance of serous and clear cell adenocarcinoma in surgically staged endometrial carcinoma. Acta Obstet Gynecol Scand 79:311–316
347. Sakuragi N et al (1998) Bcl-2 expression and prognosis of patients with endometrial carcinoma. Int J Cancer 79:153–158
348. Salvesen HB, Iversen OE, Akslen LA (1998) Identification of high-risk patients by assessment of nuclear Ki-67 expression in a prospective study of endometrial carcinomas. Clin Cancer Res 4:2779–2785
349. Sartori E et al (1997) Carcinosarcoma of the uterus: a clinicopathological multicenter CTF study. Gynecol Oncol 67:70–75
350. Savage J, Subby W, Okagaki T (1987) Adenocarcinoma of the endometrium with trophoblastic differentiation and metastases as choriocarcinoma: a case report. Gynecol Oncol 26:257–262
351. Sawada M et al (2003) Different expression patterns of KIT, EGFR, and HER-2 (c-erbB-2) oncoproteins between epithelial and mesenchymal components in uterine carcinosarcoma. Cancer Sci 94:986–991

352. Schlosshauer PW, Ellenson LH, Soslow RA (2002) Beta-catenin and E-cadherin expression patterns in high-grade endometrial carcinoma are associated with histological subtype. Mod Pathol 15:1032–1037
353. Schlosshauer PW et al (2000) Mutational analysis of the CTNNB1 and APC genes in uterine endometrioid carcinoma. Mod Pathol 13:1066–1071
354. Scholten AN et al (2004) Prognostic significance and interobserver variability of histologic grading systems for endometrial carcinoma. Cancer 100:764–772
355. Schwab KV et al (2009) Prospective evaluation of prognostic significance of the tumor-free distance from uterine serosa in surgically staged endometrial adenocarcinoma. Gynecol Oncol 112:146–149
356. Scully RE, Bonfiglio TA, Kurman RJ, Silverberg SG, Wilkinson EJ (1994) Histologic typing of female genital tract tumors (international histological classification of tumors), 2nd edn. Springer, New York, pp 1–189
357. Seidman JD, Chauhan S (2003) Evaluation of the relationship between adenosarcoma and carcinosarcoma and a hypothesis of the histogenesis of uterine sarcomas. Int J Gynecol Pathol 22:75–82
358. Seidman JD, Kurman RJ (1999) Tamoxifen and the endometrium. Int J Gynecol Pathol 18:293–296
359. Semczuk A et al (1998) K-ras gene point mutations in human endometrial carcinomas: correlation with clinicopathological features and patients' outcome. J Cancer Res Clin Oncol 124:695–700
360. Shapiro S et al (1980) Recent and past use of conjugated estrogens in relation to adenocarcinoma of the endometrium. N Engl J Med 303:485–489
361. Sherman ME et al (1992) Uterine serous carcinoma. A morphologically diverse neoplasm with unifying clinicopathologic features. Am J Surg Pathol 16:600–610
362. Sherman ME, Bur ME, Kurman RJ (1995) p53 in endometrial cancer and its putative precursors: evidence for diverse pathways of tumorigenesis. Hum Pathol 26:1268–1274
363. Sherman ME et al (1997) Risk factors and hormone levels in patients with serous and endometrioid uterine carcinomas. Mod Pathol 10:963–968
364. Shia J (2008) Immunohistochemistry versus microsatellite instability testing for screening colorectal cancer patients at risk for hereditary nonpolyposis colorectal cancer. Part I. The utility of immunohistochemistry. J Mol Diagn 10:293–300
365. Shia J et al (2008) Routinely assessed morphological features correlate with microsatellite instability status in endometrial cancer. Hum Pathol 39:116–125
366. Shia J et al (2009) Immunohistochemistry as first-line screening for detecting colorectal cancer patients at risk for hereditary nonpolyposis colorectal cancer syndrome: A two antibody panel may be as predictive as a four antibody panel. Am J Surg Pathol 33(11):1639–1645
367. Shim JU et al (1992) Accuracy of frozen-section diagnosis at surgery in clinical stage I and II endometrial carcinoma. Am J Obstet Gynecol 166:1335–1338
368. Silva EG et al (2006) Association of low-grade endometrioid carcinoma of the uterus and ovary with undifferentiated carcinoma: a new type of dedifferentiated carcinoma? Int J Gynecol Pathol 25:52–58
369. Silva EG, Jenkins R (1990) Serous carcinoma in endometrial polyps. Mod Pathol 3:120–128
370. Silva EG, Tornos CS, Follen-Mitchell M (1994) Malignant neoplasms of the uterine corpus in patients treated for breast carcinoma: the effects of tamoxifen. Int J Gynecol Pathol 13:248–258
371. Silverberg SG (2007) The endometrium. Arch Pathol Lab Med 131:372–382
372. Silverberg SG et al (1990) Carcinosarcoma (malignant mixed mesodermal tumor) of the uterus. A Gynecologic Oncology Group pathologic study of 203 cases. Int J Gynecol Pathol 9:1–19
373. Simpkins SB et al (1998) PTEN mutations in endometrial cancers with 10q LOH: additional evidence for the involvement of multiple tumor suppressors. Gynecol Oncol 71:391–395
374. Sinkre P et al (2000) Endometrial endometrioid carcinomas associated with Ewing sarcoma/peripheral primitive neuroectodermal tumor. Int J Gynecol Pathol 19:127–132
375. Sivridis E, Buckley CH, Fox H (1987) The prognostic significance of lymphatic vascular space invasion in endometrial adenocarcinoma. Br J Obstet Gynaecol 94:991–994
376. Smith DC et al (1975) Association of exogenous estrogen and endometrial carcinoma. N Engl J Med 293:1164–1167
377. Society AC (2000) 2000 cancer statistics. CA Cancer J Clin 50:1–64
378. Sorbe B, Risberg B, Frankendal B (1990) DNA ploidy, morphometry, and nuclear grade as prognostic factors in endometrial carcinoma. Gynecol Oncol 38:22–27
379. Soslow RA et al (2007) Clinicopathologic analysis of 187 high-grade endometrial carcinomas of different histologic subtypes: similar outcomes belie distinctive biologic differences. Am J Surg Pathol 31:979–987
380. Soslow RA, Pirog E, Isacson C (2000) Endometrial intraepithelial carcinoma with associated peritoneal carcinomatosis. Am J Surg Pathol 24:726–732
381. Soslow RA et al (1998) Distinctive p53 and mdm2 immunohistochemical expression profiles suggest different pathogenetic pathways in poorly differentiated endometrial carcinoma. Int J Gynecol Pathol 17:129–134
382. Soslow RA et al (2000) Cyclin D1 expression in high-grade endometrial carcinomas–association with histologic subtype. Int J Gynecol Pathol 19:329–334
383. Spanos WJ Jr et al (1984) Malignant mixed Mullerian tumors of the uterus. Cancer 53:311–316
384. Spiegel GW (1995) Endometrial carcinoma in situ in postmenopausal women. Am J Surg Pathol 19:417–432
385. Spiegel GW, Austin RM, Gelven PL (1996) Transitional cell carcinoma of the endometrium. Gynecol Oncol 60:325–330
386. Sreenan JJ, Hart WR (1995) Carcinosarcomas of the female genital tract. A pathologic study of 29 metastatic tumors: further evidence for the dominant role of the epithelial component and the conversion theory of histogenesis. Am J Surg Pathol 19:666–674
387. Srodon M, Klein WM, Kurman RJ (2003) CD10 immunostaining does not distinguish endometrial carcinoma invading myometrium from carcinoma involving adenomyosis. Am J Surg Pathol 27:786–789
388. Staebler A et al (2002) Hormone receptor immunohistochemistry and human papillomavirus in situ hybridization are useful for distinguishing endocervical and endometrial adenocarcinomas. Am J Surg Pathol 26:998–1006
389. Stendahl U et al (1991) Prognostic significance of proliferation in endometrial adenocarcinomas: a multivariate analysis of clinical and flow cytometric variables. Int J Gynecol Pathol 10:271–284

390. Stewart HJ (1992) The Scottish trial of adjuvant tamoxifen in node-negative breast cancer. Scottish Cancer Trials Breast Group. J Natl Cancer Inst Monogr 11:117–120
391. Susini T et al (1994) Prognostic value of flow cytometric deoxyribonucleic acid index in endometrial carcinoma: comparison with other clinical-pathologic parameters. Am J Obstet Gynecol 170:527–534
392. Sutton G et al (2000) A phase III trial of ifosfamide with or without cisplatin in carcinosarcoma of the uterus: a Gynecologic Oncology Group Study. Gynecol Oncol 79:147–153
393. Swerdlow AJ, Jones ME (2005) Tamoxifen treatment for breast cancer and risk of endometrial cancer: a case-control study. J Natl Cancer Inst 97:375–384
394. Tambouret R, Clement PB, Young RH (2003) Endometrial endometrioid adenocarcinoma with a deceptive pattern of spread to the uterine cervix: a manifestation of stage IIb endometrial carcinoma liable to be misinterpreted as an independent carcinoma or a benign lesion. Am J Surg Pathol 27:1080–1088
395. Tashiro H et al (1997) Mutations in PTEN are frequent in endometrial carcinoma but rare in other common gynecological malignancies. Cancer Res 57:3935–3940
396. Tashiro H et al (1997) p53 gene mutations are common in uterine serous carcinoma and occur early in their pathogenesis. Am J Pathol 150:177–185
397. Taskin M et al (1997) bcl-2 and p53 in endometrial adenocarcinoma. Mod Pathol 10:728–734
398. Taylor NP et al (2006) Defective DNA mismatch repair and XRCC2 mutation in uterine carcinosarcomas. Gynecol Oncol 100:107–110
399. Taylor NP et al (2006) DNA mismatch repair and TP53 defects are early events in uterine carcinosarcoma tumorigenesis. Mod Pathol 19:1333–1338
400. Taylor RR et al (1999) An analysis of two versus three grades for endometrial carcinoma. Gynecol Oncol 74:3–6
401. Tiltman AJ (1980) Mucinous carcinoma of the endometrium. Obstet Gynecol 55:244–247
402. Tobon H, Watkins GJ (1985) Secretory adenocarcinoma of the endometrium. Int J Gynecol Pathol 4:328–335
403. Tornos C et al (1992) Aggressive stage I grade 1 endometrial carcinoma. Cancer 70:790–798
404. Trere D et al (1994) Interphase AgNOR quantity and DNA content in endometrial adenocarcinoma. Gynecol Oncol 53:202–207
405. Tsuda H et al (1997) Prospective study to compare endometrial cytology and transvaginal ultrasonography for identification of endometrial malignancies. Gynecol Oncol 65:383–386
406. Tunc M et al (1998) Endometrium adenocarcinoma with choriocarcinomatous differentiation: a case report. Eur J Gynaecol Oncol 19:489–491
407. Turner DA et al (1989) The prognostic significance of peritoneal cytology for stage I endometrial cancer. Obstet Gynecol 74:775–780
408. Ulbright TM, Roth LM (1985) Metastatic and independent cancers of the endometrium and ovary: a clinicopathologic study of 34 cases. Hum Pathol 16:28–34
409. Vaidya AP et al (2006) Uterine malignant mixed mullerian tumors should not be included in studies of endometrial carcinoma. Gynecol Oncol 103:684–687
410. van der Putten HW et al (1989) Prognostic value of quantitative pathologic features and DNA content in individual patients with stage I endometrial adenocarcinoma. Cancer 63:1378–1387
411. van Leeuwen FE et al (1994) Risk of endometrial cancer after tamoxifen treatment of breast cancer. Lancet 343:448–452
412. van Rijswijk RE et al (1994) The effect of chemotherapy on the different components of advanced carcinosarcomas (malignant mixed mesodermal tumors) of the female genital tract. Int J Gynecol Cancer 4:52–60
413. Vang R et al (2001) Immunohistochemical analysis of clear cell carcinoma of the gynecologic tract. Int J Gynecol Pathol 20:252–259
414. Vasen HF et al (2004) Identification of HNPCC by molecular analysis of colorectal and endometrial tumors. Dis Markers 20:207–213
415. Voskuil DW et al (2007) Physical activity and endometrial cancer risk, a systematic review of current evidence. Cancer Epidemiol Biomarkers Prev 16:639–648
416. Wagatsuma S et al (1998) Tumor angiogenesis, hepatocyte growth factor, and c-Met expression in endometrial carcinoma. Cancer 82:520–530
417. Walker AN, Mills SE (1982) Serous papillary carcinoma of the endometrium. A clinicopathologic study of 11 cases. Diagn Gynecol Obstet 4:261–267
418. Wang NPSZ et al (1995) Coordinate expression of cytokeratins 7 and 20 defines unique subsets of carcinomas. Appl Immunohistochem 3:99–107
419. Wani Y et al (2008) Aberrant Cdx2 expression in endometrial lesions with squamous differentiation: important role of Cdx2 in squamous morula formation. Hum Pathol 39:1072–1079
420. Baergen RN et al (2001) Early uterine serous carcinoma: Clonal origin of extra uterine disease. Int J Gynecol Pathol 20:214–219
421. Webb GA, Lagios MD (1987) Clear cell carcinoma of the endometrium. Am J Obstet Gynecol 156:1486–1491
422. Weir HK, Sloan M, Kreiger N (1994) The relationship between cigarette smoking and the risk of endometrial neoplasms. Int J Epidemiol 23:261–266
423. Wheeler DT et al (2000) Minimal uterine serous carcinoma: diagnosis and clinicopathologic correlation. Am J Surg Pathol 24:797–806
424. Wheeler DT, Bristow RE, Kurman RJ (2007) Histologic alterations in endometrial hyperplasia and well-differentiated carcinoma treated with progestins. Am J Surg Pathol 31:988–998
425. Wheelock JB et al (1985) Uterine sarcoma: analysis of prognostic variables in 71 cases. Am J Obstet Gynecol 151:1016–1022
426. Witkiewicz AK, McConnell T, Potoczek M, Emmons RUB, Kurman RJ (2010) Increased natural killer cells and decreased regulatory T cells are seen in complex atypical hyperplasia and well-differentiated carcinoma treated with progestins. Hum Pathol 41:26–32
427. Wolfson AH et al (2007) A gynecologic oncology group randomized phase III trial of whole abdominal irradiation (WAI) vs. cisplatin-ifosfamide and mesna (CIM) as post-surgical therapy in stage I-IV carcinosarcoma (CS) of the uterus. Gynecol Oncol 107:177–185
428. Wolfson AH et al (1992) The prognostic significance of surgical staging for carcinoma of the endometrium. Gynecol Oncol 45:142–146
429. Yamada SD et al (2000) Pathologic variables and adjuvant therapy as predictors of recurrence and survival for patients with surgically evaluated carcinosarcoma of the uterus. Cancer 88:2782–2786
430. Yamauchi N et al (1996) Immunohistochemical analysis of endometrial adenocarcinoma for bcl-2 and p53 in relation to expression of sex steroid receptor and proliferative activity. Int J Gynecol Pathol 15:202–208
431. Yamazawa K et al (2000) Prognostic factors in young women with endometrial carcinoma: a report of 20 cases and review of literature. Int J Gynecol Cancer 10:212–222

432. Yazigi R, Piver MS, Blumenson L (1983) Malignant peritoneal cytology as prognostic indicator in stage I endometrial cancer. Obstet Gynecol 62:359–362
433. Yemelyanova A et al (2009) Utility of p16 expression for distinction of uterine serous carcinomas from endometrial endometrioid and endocervical adenocarcinomas: immunohistochemical analysis of 201 cases. Am J Surg Pathol 33:1504–1514
434. Yemelyanova A et al (2009) Endocervical adenocarcinomas with prominent endometrial or endomyometrial involvement simulating primary endometrial carcinomas: utility of HPV DNA detection and immunohistochemical expression of p16 and hormone receptors to confirm the cervical origin of the corpus tumor. Am J Surg Pathol 33:914–924
435. Yokoyama Y et al (2000) Expression of PTEN and PTEN pseudogene in endometrial carcinoma. Int J Mol Med 6:47–50
436. Young RH, Scully RE (1992) Uterine carcinomas simulating microglandular hyperplasia. A report of six cases. Am J Surg Pathol 16:1092–1097
437. Zaino RJ (2009) FIGO staging of endometrial adenocarcinoma: a critical review and proposal. Int J Gynecol Pathol 28:1–9
438. Zaino RJ (1995) Pathologic indicators of prognosis in endometrial adenocarcinoma. Selected aspects emphasizing the GOG experience. Gynecologic Oncology Group. Pathol Ann 30(Pt 1): 1–28
439. Zaino RJ et al (1998) DNA content is an independent prognostic indicator in endometrial adenocarcinoma. A Gynecologic Oncology Group study. Int J Gynecol Pathol 17:312–319
440. Zaino RJ et al (1991) The significance of squamous differentiation in endometrial carcinoma. Data from a Gynecologic Oncology Group study. Cancer 68:2293–2302
441. Zaino RJ, Kurman RJ (1988) Squamous differentiation in carcinoma of the endometrium: a critical appraisal of adenoacanthoma and adenosquamous carcinoma. Semin Diagn Pathol 5:154–171
442. Zaino RJ et al (1998) Villoglandular adenocarcinoma of the endometrium: a clinicopathologic study of 61 cases: a gynecologic oncology group study. Am J Surg Pathol 22:1379–1385
443. Zaino RJ et al (1996) Pathologic models to predict outcome for women with endometrial adenocarcinoma: the importance of the distinction between surgical stage and clinical stage – a Gynecologic Oncology Group study. Cancer 77:1115–1121
444. Zaino RJ et al (1995) The utility of the revised International Federation of Gynecology and Obstetrics histologic grading of endometrial adenocarcinoma using a defined nuclear grading system. A Gynecologic Oncology Group study. Cancer 75:81–86
445. Zaloudek C et al (1997) Microglandular adenocarcinoma of the endometrium: a form of mucinous adenocarcinoma that may be confused with microglandular hyperplasia of the cervix. Int J Gynecol Pathol 16:52–59
446. Zelmanowicz A et al (1998) Evidence for a common etiology for endometrial carcinomas and malignant mixed mullerian tumors. Gynecol Oncol 69:253–257
447. Zheng W et al (1996) p53 overexpression and bcl-2 persistence in endometrial carcinoma: comparison of papillary serous and endometrioid subtypes. Gynecol Oncol 61:167–174
448. Zheng W et al (1998) p53 immunostaining as a significant adjunct diagnostic method for uterine surface carcinoma: precursor of uterine papillary serous carcinoma. Am J Surg Pathol 22:1463–1473
449. Ziel HK, Finkle WD (1975) Increased risk of endometrial carcinoma among users of conjugated estrogens. N Engl J Med 293:1167–1170

10 Mesenchymal Tumors of the Uterus

Charles J. Zaloudek · Michael R. Hendrickson · Robert A. Soslow

R. J. Kurman, L. Hedrick Ellenson, B. M. Ronnett (eds.), *Blaustein's Pathology of the Female Genital Tract (6th ed.)*, DOI 10.1007/978-1-4419-0489-8_10,

This chapter deals with neoplasms of the uterus in which there is mesenchymal differentiation. Purely mesenchymal tumors, such as those derived from smooth muscle and endometrial stroma, are considered, as are some benign and malignant neoplasms in which there are mixtures of epithelium and connective tissues. We use a slightly modified version of the comprehensive classification of mesenchymal neoplasms of the uterus, developed by the World Health Organization (WHO; [409]) which is shown in ➲ *Table 10.1*.

Proper pathologic study of a mesenchymal tumor of the uterus is predicated on careful gross examination and adequate sectioning. The tumor should be examined thoroughly, and one block of tissue should be taken for each centimeter of tumor diameter, except from grossly typical leiomyomas; even the latter may have to be examined extensively if the microscopic appearance is unusual. Three major goals of the pathologic examination of potentially malignant mesenchymal tumors are to determine the type of tumor margin (expansile or infiltrating), to evaluate the depth of myometrial invasion, and to determine whether the tumor involves the serosa or extends beyond the uterus. Tissue samples should be taken with these requirements in mind.

Leiomyomas are common uterine tumors, but other types of benign and malignant mesenchymal tumors are uncommon. Malignant mesenchymal tumors comprise less than 3% of uterine malignancies. The tumor stage is the single most important prognostic factor. In the past, uterine sarcomas were staged using a staging system developed for endometrial carcinoma. This has not proven entirely satisfactory, and a new staging system has been developed for uterine sarcomas (➲ *Table 10.2*; [131]). The new staging system has two compartments, one for leiomyosarcoma and one for endometrial stromal sarcoma (ESS) and adenosarcoma. Carcinosarcoma, or malignant mixed Müllerian tumor (MMMT), which is discussed in ➲ Chap. 9, Endometrial Carcinoma, is a mixed epithelial–mesenchymal neoplasm in which both elements are malignant; it has much in common with endometrial carcinoma and is staged using the endometrial carcinoma staging system. The staging system for uterine tumors is a surgical–pathologic one, so pathologists must be familiar with the criteria for staging and make certain to provide all information necessary for staging in their surgical pathology reports. We complete a synoptic comment for every case that includes all information necessary for staging as well as the actual stage.

Table 10.1

Classification of mesenchymal and mixed tumors of the uterus

Smooth muscle tumors
Leiomyoma
Mitotically active leiomyoma
Cellular leiomyoma
Hemorrhagic cellular leiomyoma
Atypical leiomyoma (bizarre leiomyoma)
Epithelioid leiomyoma
Myxoid leiomyoma
Vascular leiomyoma
Lipoleiomyoma
Leiomyoma with other elements
Leiomyoma with hematopoietic cells
Diffuse leiomyomatosis
Dissecting leiomyoma
Smooth muscle tumor of uncertain malignant potential
Leiomyosarcoma
Epithelioid leiomyosarcoma
Myxoid leiomyosarcoma
Other smooth muscle tumors
Benign metastasizing leiomyoma
Intravenous leiomyomatosis
Disseminated peritoneal leiomyomatosis
PEComa
Angiomyolipoma
Lymphangioleiomyomatosis
Endometrial stromal tumors
Endometrial stromal nodule
Endometrial stromal sarcoma (low grade)
Undifferentiated endometrial sarcoma (high grade)
Mixed endometrial stomal–smooth muscle tumors
Uterine tumor resembling an ovarian sex cord tumor
Adenomatoid tumor
Other mesenchymal tumors (benign and malignant)
Homologous
Heterologous
Mixed epithelial–nonepithelial tumors
Benign
Adenofibroma
Adenomyoma
Atypical polypoid adenomyoma
Malignant
Adenosarcoma (homologous or heterologous)
Mixed müllerian tumor (carcinosarcoma), homologous or heterologous
Miscellaneous tumors
Neuroectodermal tumors
Lymphoma
Other

Smooth Muscle Tumors

Smooth muscle neoplasms of the uterus are extremely common, and most are leiomyomas. These tumors may

Table 10.2
Staging for uterine sarcomas (leiomyosarcomas, endometrial stromal sarcomas, adenosarcomas, and carcinosarcomas)

(1) Leiomyosarcoma	
Stage	Definition
I	Tumor limited to uterus
IA	<5 cm
IB	>5 cm
II	Tumor extends to the pelvis
IIA	Adnexal involvement
IIB	Tumor extends to extrauterine pelvic tissue
III	Tumor invades abdominal tissues (not just protruding into the abdomen)
IIIA	One site
IIIB	>One site
IIIC	Metastasis to pelvic and/or para-aortic lymph nodes
IV	
IVA	Tumor invades bladder and/or rectum
IVB	Distant metastasis
(2) Endometrial stromal sarcomas (ESS) and adenosarcoma[a]	
Stage	Definition
I	Tumor limited to uterus
IA	Tumor limited to endometrium/endocervix with no myometrial invasion
IB	Less than or equal to half myometrial invasion
IC	More than half myometrial invasion
II	Tumor extends to the pelvis
IIA	Adnexal involvement
IIB	Tumor extends to extrauterine pelvic tissue
III	Tumor invades abdominal tissues (not just protruding into the abdomen)
IIIA	One site
IIIB	>One site
IIIC	Metastasis to pelvic and/or para-aortic lymph nodes
IV	
IVA	Tumor invades bladder and/or rectum
IVB	Distant metastasis
(3) Carcinosarcomas	
Carcinosarcomas should be staged as carcinomas of the endometrium	

[a]Simultaneous tumors of the uterine corpus and ovary/pelvis in association with ovarian/pelvic endometriosis should be classified as independent primary tumors.

be incidental in uteri removed for other reasons, but they are also frequently responsible for a variety of common gynecologic and obstetric difficulties. Histologically, all but a small minority of leiomyomas is easily identified as having a smooth muscle phenotype and being benign. A small percentage of uterine smooth muscle neoplasms are leiomyosarcomas, which, using modern diagnostic criteria, are highly malignant neoplasms. Most leiomyosarcomas are easily recognized both as showing smooth muscle differentiation and as malignant. A small number of uterine smooth muscle proliferations pose difficult diagnostic challenges for a variety of reasons involving either problems of phenotype or anticipated clinical behavior (benign or malignant or something in between).

Our discussion of smooth muscle neoplasms first presents a general approach to the evaluation of uterine smooth muscle neoplasms, detailing the individual features that need to be assessed: the type of differentiation, the degree of cellularity, the mitotic index, the presence and degree of cytologic atypia, and the presence of necrosis and its pattern. Second, we gather the facts of epidemiology, pathology, molecular biology, cytogenetics, natural history, and treatment around a discussion of each of the named smooth muscle entities.

Evaluation of Smooth Muscle Neoplasms

The most effective way of distinguishing clinically benign from clinically malignant uterine smooth muscle neoplasms is through the use of multivariate criteria; that is, criteria that involve considering several microscopic features as an ensemble [32, 254]. These features include differentiated cell type within the smooth muscle group, the presence and type of tumor necrosis, the degree of cytologic atypia, the mitotic index, and the relationship of the process to surrounding normal structures, including extrauterine sites.

Differentiated Cell Type

The term usual smooth muscle differentiation denotes a pattern of differentiation recapitulating that of the constituent cells of the normal myometrium. Usual smooth muscle cells are elongated, possess distinct cell membranes, and have readily apparent eosinophilic, sometimes fibrillar cytoplasm. These cells grow in a fascicular arrangement.

Epithelioid smooth muscle cells are round or polygonal and have eosinophilic to colorless cytoplasm. They may have perinuclear cytoplasmic vacuoles or there may be a perinuclear rim of eosinophilic cytoplasm, although the rest of the cytoplasm is clear. When the cytoplasm is completely clear, the label "clear cell" is used. It is useful to do HMB45 stains when epithelioid tumors are encountered in the myometrium since some of these may fall into the category of PEComa (see section ➋ PEComa). Other considerations include metastatic (or locally invasive) carcinoma (cytokeratin positivity) and metastatic melanoma (S-100 positive). Some endometrial stromal neoplasms may have an epithelioid appearance. Recently, the use of histone deacetylase 8 (HDAC8) has been advocated as a specific marker for smooth muscle in this setting [100].

Myxoid smooth muscle proliferations feature widely spaced stellate cells with inapparent cytoplasm embedded in a myxoid matrix. Malignant myxoid smooth muscle neoplasms exhibit varying degrees of cytologic atypia and often have an appearance reminiscent of myxofibrosarcoma (myxoid malignant fibrous histiocytoma or myxofibrosarcoma) of the soft tissues.

Less common types of differentiation, such as fat and skeletal muscle, are discussed later (see ➋ Leiomyomas with Other Elements).

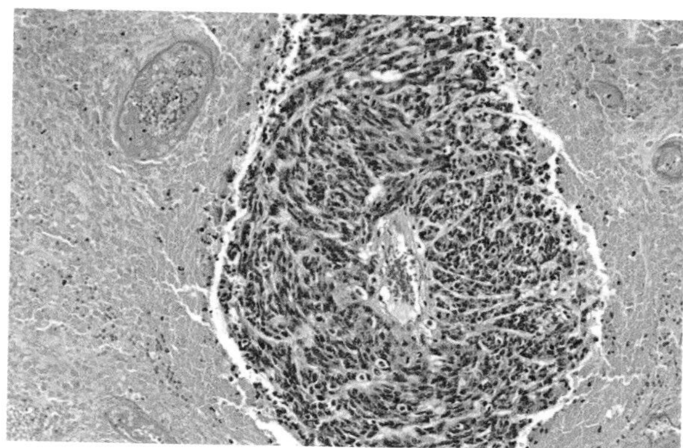

Fig. 10.1
Coagulative tumor cell necrosis. **Viable cells are present only around the blood vessel. Ghostlike outlines of necrotic atypical tumor cells can still be discerned in the surrounding tissue**

Patterns of Necrosis

The presence or absence and type of necrosis are powerful predictors of clinical behavior [32]. Two patterns of necrosis in uterine smooth muscle tumors are diagnostically important: coagulative tumor cell necrosis and hyalinizing (or "infarction-type") necrosis [32].

In coagulative tumor cell necrosis, there is an abrupt transition between necrotic and preserved cells (➋ *Fig. 10.1*). The hematoxyphilia of the nuclei is often retained in the necrotic cells, and usually there is no associated inflammation. The characteristic low-power microscopic pattern is one of blood vessels cuffed by viable cells surrounded by a sea of necrotic tumor [32, 69]. Coagulative tumor cell necrosis is commonly present in clinically malignant smooth muscle neoplasms. In contrast, hyalinizing necrosis has a distinctly zonal pattern with central necrosis, a more peripheral zone of granulation tissue, and, at the periphery, a variable amount of hyaline eosinophilic collagen interposed between the central degenerated region and peripheral preserved smooth muscle cells (➋ *Fig. 10.2*). This pattern is highly reminiscent of an infarction at various stages of evolution. When shadow cells or nuclei are discernible in the necrosis, there is little hyperchromasia or nuclear pleomorphism. Acute infarction produces a necrosis pattern indistinguishable from coagulative tumor cell necrosis; that is, the juxtaposition of preserved tumor adjacent to necrotic tumor. Strategies useful in distinguishing acute ischemic necrosis

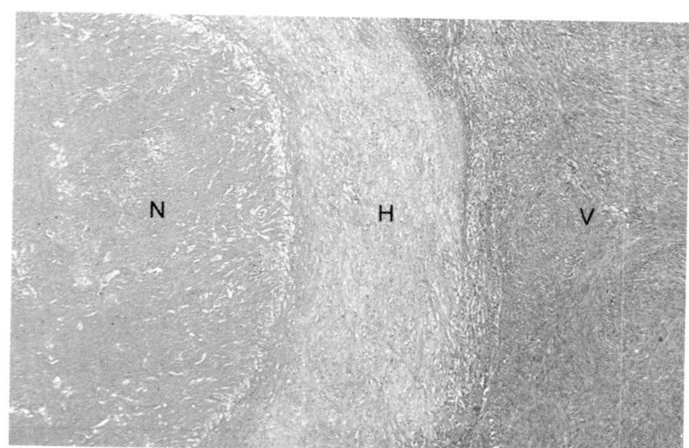

Fig. 10.2
Bland necrosis. **An area of bland necrosis (N) is separated from viable spindle-shaped tumor cells (V) by a zone of hyalinized collagen (H)**

from diagnostically useful tumor cell necrosis involve noting (1) the presence or absence of hyperchromasia and nuclear pleomorphism in the "shadow cells" of the necrotic tumor; and (2) (in the absence of these nuclear features) discerning a pattern of ongoing ischemia elsewhere in the problematic smooth muscle neoplasm. Trichrome preparations are useful in detecting patchy foci of healed ischemic damage of all stages beyond the acute phase of ischemia; the trichrome stain highlights a band of collagen between zones of necrotic and viable tumor. P16 immunostaining has been recommended for distinguishing between leiomyosarcoma and leiomyoma when the pattern of necrosis is ambiguous [23, 60].

Another pattern of necrosis that may be seen in ulcerated submucous leiomyomas features ulceration, acute inflammatory cells, and an associated zonal reparative process.

Cytologic Atypia

Several studies have demonstrated a relationship between cytologic atypia and clinical behavior in uterine smooth muscle neoplasms [32]. The problem, as always, is defining "significant atypia" in a way that is reproducible and can be communicated to others. Bell et al. found that a two-tiered scheme of absent to mild atypia and moderate to severe atypia is reasonably reproducible [32]. They defined moderate to severe atypia as follows: nuclear hyperchromatism and pleomorphism that is obvious at scanning power (➲ *Fig. 10.3*). Enlarged and sometimes abnormal mitotic figures (MF) are a frequent finding. Most commonly, moderate to severe atypia is diffusely present throughout the neoplasm, but it can, occasionally, be present only focally. In contrast, absent or mild atypia features uniform cells with no more than mild nuclear pleomorphism (➲ *Fig. 10.4*). The chromatin of the constituent cells is typically fine to granular. The nuclei may be enlarged in comparison to those of the cells comprising the surrounding myometrium, but the enlargement is uniform throughout the tumor. More than one or two enlarged abnormal MF place the tumor in the moderate to severe atypia group. The pattern of atypia described above is analogous to that found in malignant fibrous histiocytomas of the soft tissue (also known as pleomorphic undifferentiated sarcoma). A more difficult type of diffuse severe atypia to recognize features uniformly enlarged, hyperchromatic cells (➲ *Fig. 10.5*); this pattern is analogous to that seen, for example, in monophasic synovial sarcoma of the soft tissues. Recognition of this pattern involves a comparison of the constituent cells of the tumor to the surrounding normal myocytes and appreciating the nucleomegaly and hyperchromasia of the neoplastic cells relative to the surrounding normal myocytes. A helpful feature in diagnosing the uncommon neoplasms with this type of uniform severe atypia is the associated finding of diffuse, massive infiltration of the

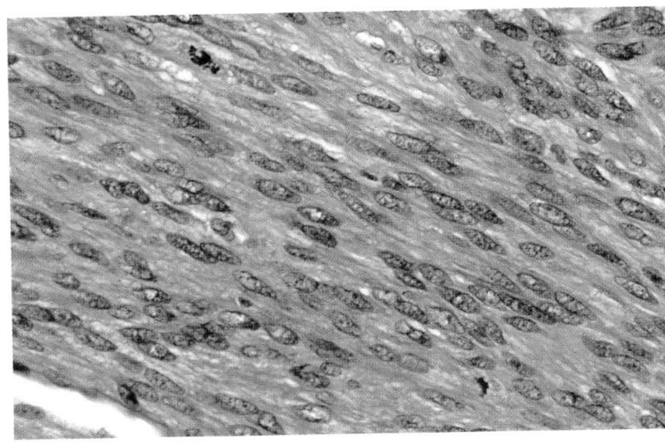

Fig. 10.4
Diffuse mild atypia. **Uniform mild atypia characterizes this infiltrating smooth muscle neoplasm**

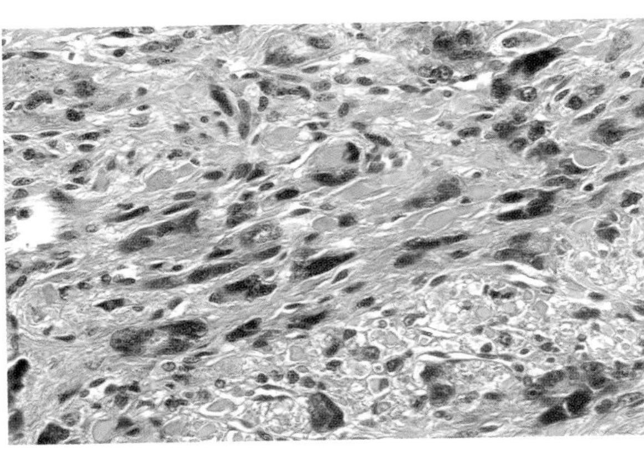

Fig. 10.3
Severe pleomorphic atypia. **Nuclear pleomorphism against a background of diffuse severe atypia of spindled cells**

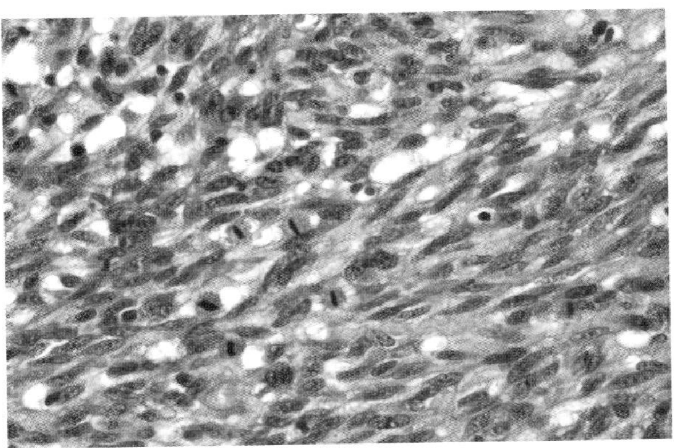

Fig. 10.5
Severe uniform atypia. **Relatively uniform malignant cells exhibiting nuclear hyperchromasia and a high mitotic index**

surrounding myometrium that leaves islands of normal myometrium in its wake.

Mitotic Index

The mitotic index is expressed in terms of the number of definite MF per 10 high-power fields (HPF; [180, 418]).

Compulsive mitosis counting, fortunately, is not always necessary; the required level of compulsiveness depends on associated features such as whether there is significant cytological atypia or whether there is tumor cell necrosis. In the absence of these two features, the precise mitotic index is of little managerial importance below 20 MF/10 HPF. The mitotic index is determined by first finding the area with the highest density of MF and then counting them in that area. The slide is searched at low magnification for the most mitotically active area. Then, mitotic counts are performed at high magnification in four sets of ten randomly chosen contiguous fields. The mitotic index is expressed as the average number of MF per 10 HPF. Care must be taken not to count lymphocytes, karyorrhectic debris, precipitated hematoxylin, or mast cells as MF. Most reliable are MF in metaphase, anaphase, or telophase. A critical review of mitotic counting has been presented [312]. Often the issue is not the statistical strategy used to count MF, but what exactly should be regarded as an MF.

Relationship to Surrounding Normal Structures and the Anatomic Distribution of the Process

It is important to note the relationship of the smooth muscle neoplasm to the surrounding myometrium and uterine vessels and to determine whether there is any extrauterine extension. Infiltrative margins, intravascular growth, and extrauterine spread, although commonly encountered in uterine malignancies, are not, when seen as isolated findings, diagnostic of sarcoma. It is important to be aware of some relatively rare smooth muscle proliferations that are either benign or clinically low-grade processes that mimic leiomyosarcoma by virtue of their relationship to normal uterine structures or their extrauterine extension.

Leiomyoma

Leiomyomas are the most common uterine neoplasms [330, 427]. They are noted clinically in 20–30% of women over 30 years of age, and are found in as many as 75% of uteri when a systematic search is conducted [86, 96, 330]. Most leiomyomas are detected in middle-aged women. They are uncommon in women less than 30 years of age; however, the youngest patient on record was 13 years old. Some leiomyomas apparently shrink after the menopause, but their frequency does not decrease. Leiomyomas are more common in African-American women than in white women [217].

The growth of leiomyomas is affected by the hormonal milieu [16, 261, 345, 391]. Leiomyomas contain estrogen and progesterone receptors, which can be demonstrated biochemically and immunohistochemically [426]. Leiomyomas may increase in size during estrogen therapy, and most decrease in size when the patient is treated with a gonadotropin-releasing hormone (GnRH) agonist [4, 349, 377, 396, 417]. Progestins, progesterone, hormone replacement therapy, clomiphene use, and pregnancy occasionally are associated with a rapid increase in the size of leiomyomas and sometimes produce hemorrhagic degeneration [376].

Clinical Features

The clinical presentation of leiomyomas depends on their size and location [51]. Leiomyomas cause many signs and symptoms, the most common of which are pain, a sensation of pressure, and abnormal uterine bleeding. Even small leiomyomas, when submucosal, can cause bleeding due to compression of the overlying endometrium and compromise of its vascular supply. In some instances, infertility is attributed to the presence of leiomyomas. Large tumors can be detected during pelvic examination because they produce uterine enlargement or an irregular uterine contour. Some leiomyomas are pedunculated and protrude through the cervical os. On rare occasions, subserosal pedunculated leiomyomas undergo torsion, infarction, and separation from the uterus. Secondary infection of leiomyomas can result in fever, leukocytosis, and an elevated sedimentation rate. Among the complications of pregnancy ascribed to leiomyomas are spontaneous abortion, premature rupture of membranes, dystocia, inversion of the uterus, and postpartum hemorrhage.

Gross Findings

Despite the variety of histologic subtypes of leiomyoma, all are grossly similar. Multiple leiomyomas are present in two thirds of women with these neoplasms [86]. Leiomyomas are spherical and firm; they bulge above the surrounding myometrium from which they are easily shelled out. The cut surfaces are white to tan, with a whorled trabecular pattern (➋ *Fig. 10.6*). Leiomyomas can be located anywhere in the myometrium. Submucosal leiomyomas compress the overlying endometrium. As they enlarge, they bulge into the endometrial cavity. Rare examples become pedunculated and prolapse through the cervix. Intramural leiomyomas are the most common. Subserosal leiomyomas can become pedunculated and, if there is torsion and necrosis of the pedicle, the leiomyoma can lose its connection with the uterus. Very rarely, some become attached to another pelvic structure (parasitic leiomyoma). The appearance of a leiomyoma is commonly altered by degenerative changes. Submucosal leiomyomas are frequently ulcerated and hemorrhagic. Hemorrhage and necrosis can be observed in leiomyomas, particularly if they are large or occur in women who are pregnant or undergoing high-dose progestin therapy. Dark red areas represent hemorrhage, and sharply demarcated yellow areas reflect necrosis. The damaged smooth muscle is replaced eventually by firm white or translucent collagenous tissue. Cystic degeneration also occurs, and some leiomyomas become extensively calcified. The imaging features of leiomyomas have been extensively studied [112, 425].

Microscopic Findings

Typical leiomyomas are composed of whorled, anastomosing fascicles of uniform fusiform smooth muscle cells. The spindle-shaped cells have indistinct borders and abundant fibrillar eosinophilic cytoplasm (➋ *Fig. 10.7*). Nuclei are elongated with blunt or tapered ends, and have finely dispersed chromatin and small nucleoli. MF usually are infrequent. Most leiomyomas are more cellular than the surrounding myometrium; those that are not are identified by their nodular circumscription and by the disorderly arrangement of the smooth muscle fascicles within them, which are out of alignment with the surrounding myometrium. Degenerative changes are common in leiomyomas. Hyaline fibrosis is present in more than 60%, particularly in postmenopausal women [85]. Edema is present in about 50% of leiomyomas and, on occasion, marked hydropic change can mimic the appearance of a myxoid smooth muscle tumor or produce a pattern that can be confused with intravenous leiomyomatosis (IVL) [78, 79]. There are significant areas of hemorrhage, which tend to be zonal and sharply demarcated in

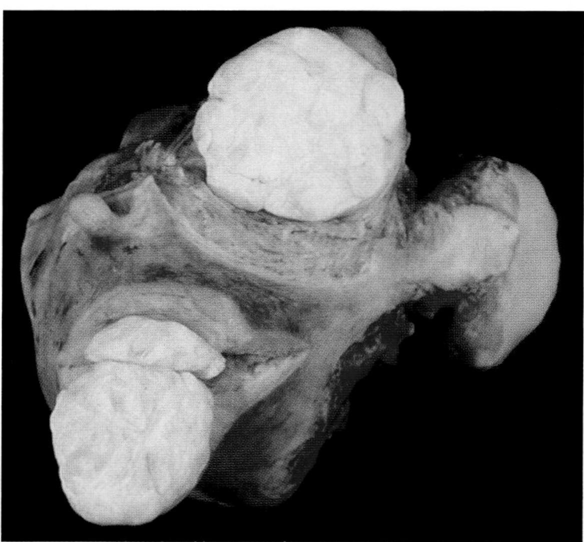

Fig. 10.6
Enlarged uterus containing multiple leiomyomas. **The leiomyomas have a whorled white-tan cut surface that bulges above the surrounding myometrium**

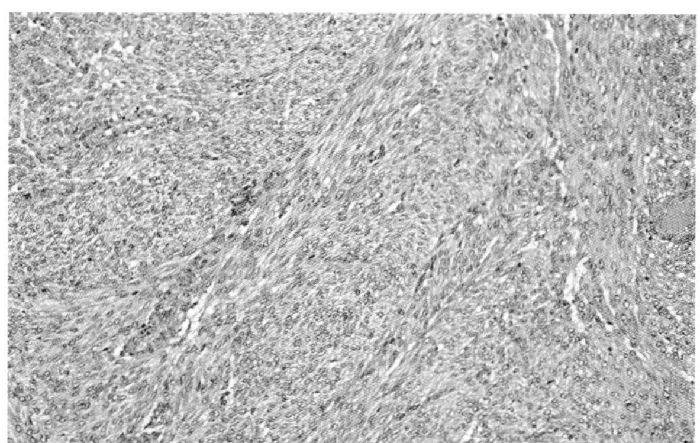

Fig. 10.7
Leiomyoma. **The spindle-shaped tumor cells have cytologically bland relatively uniform nuclei with fine chromatin and small nucleoli. The cytoplasm is abundant, eosinophilic, and fibrillar**

about 10% of leiomyomas, and cystic degeneration and microcalcification each occur in about 4%. Hemorrhage, edema, myxoid change, hypercellular foci, and cellular hypertrophy occur in leiomyomas in women who are pregnant or taking progestins (see section Hemorrhagic Cellular Leiomyoma and Hormone-Induced Changes). Progestational agents are associated with a slight increase in mitotic activity, but not to the level observed in a leiomyosarcoma.

The margins of most leiomyomas are microscopically circumscribed, but some benign tumors interdigitate with the surrounding myometrium, occasionally extensively (see section Dissecting Leiomyoma). Submucous leiomyomas, particularly if they protrude into the endometrial cavity, may display extensive necrosis, often with acute inflammatory cells. Not infrequently, there is increased mitotic activity in the tumor cells near areas of necrosis. On the other hand, the coagulative tumor cell necrosis common in leiomyosarcoma is not often associated with acute inflammation. In addition, the outlines of cells are prominent in the latter whereas they are inconspicuous or absent in submucous necrosis. Also, the MF seen in conjunction with inflammatory necrosis have normal morphology.

Immunohistochemistry

Smooth muscle cells in the myometrium and within smooth muscle tumors react with antibodies to muscle-specific actin, alpha-smooth muscle actin, desmin, and caldesmon [120]. There is immunoreactivity with vimentin, but the intensity of staining and the proportion of cells that stain are less than with the muscle-specific antibodies. Cytokeratin immunoreactivity is frequently observed in the myometrium and in smooth muscle tumors, the extent and intensity of reactivity depending on the antibodies used and the fixation of the specimen [49, 120, 163]. Epithelial membrane antigen (EMA) is usually negative in smooth muscle tumors.

Cytogenetics

Nonrandom inactivation of the X chromosome, demonstrated by glucose-6-phosphate dehydrogenase isoform expression and other techniques, indicates that leiomyomas are a proliferation of a single clone of smooth muscle cells. Each one of the multiple leiomyomas in a particular uterus appears to be a distinct clone [173, 253, 267, 342]. Cytogenetic studies provide further evidence of the clonal nature of the smooth muscle cell proliferation in many leiomyomas [342].

A large literature has appeared in recent years concerning the cytogenetic abnormalities in leiomyomas. Approximately 40% of uterine leiomyomas have chromosomal abnormalities detectable by conventional cytogenetic analysis, including t(12;14)(q15;q23–24), rearrangements involving the short arm of chromosome 6, and interstitial deletions of the long arm of chromosome 7 [253, 342, 389]. This growing body of literature may in time shed some light on the development of this extremely common neoplasm but to date has little diagnostic relevance. Of more general interest is the observation that the ordinary leiomyoma is almost certainly more than one neoplasm; in other words, the conventional light microscopic leiomyoma phenotype can be realized in a multitude of genotypic ways.

Clinical Behavior and Treatment

Most leiomyomas are asymptomatic, and only a minority requires treatment. Therapy is indicated only if leiomyomas are symptomatic, interfere with fertility, enlarge rapidly, or pose diagnostic problems [51, 325, 431]. Sometimes they can be excised (myomectomy), but if they are large or multiple, a hysterectomy may be required. Treatment with leuprolide acetate or another gonadotropin-releasing hormone agonist (GnRHa) results in shrinkage of leiomyomas, a decrease in uterine volume, and alleviation of the patient's symptoms [261, 345, 377]. The maximum effect is noted after 8 to 12 weeks. The leiomyomas increase in size again with cessation of the GnRH agonist therapy. Such therapy can be used before surgery to decrease uterine size (facilitating myomectomy or permitting treatment by vaginal rather than abdominal hysterectomy) and to reduce the risk of hemorrhage during surgery. Gonadotropin-releasing hormone antagonists may become available for this type of treatment in the future. Evidence suggests that they are effective and act rapidly without causing an initial flare in steroid levels, as is caused by GNRHa [134]. Finally, leiomyomas can be treated by uterine artery embolization, which leads to ischemia and involution of the leiomyomas [263, 385, 392]. This method of treatment is of potential interest to pathologists, because (1) if a hysterectomy is subsequently necessary there may be areas of ischemic necrosis in a leiomyoma that must be differentiated from the type of tumor cell necrosis seen in leiomyosarcoma, and (2) the embolic particles can be seen in microscopic sections and may cause confusion, unless the pathologist knows what they are [113, 274, 434].

Specific Subtypes of Leiomyoma

Most subtypes of leiomyoma are chiefly of interest in that they mimic malignancy in one or more respects. These subtypes are mitotically active leiomyoma, cellular leiomyoma, hemorrhagic cellular leiomyoma, leiomyoma with bizarre nuclei, epithelioid leiomyoma, and myxoid leiomyoma. Other leiomyoma variants – vascular leiomyoma, leiomyoma with other elements, and leiomyomas with hematopoietic elements are more curiosities than diagnostic problems.

Mitotically Active Leiomyoma

Occasionally, a typical-appearing leiomyoma in a premenopausal woman will have ≥5 MF/10 HPF (*Figs. 10.8a, b*); these are designated as mitotically active leiomyomas [32, 105, 311, 333, 341]. The number is usually 5–9 MF/10 HPF, but occasional mitotically active leiomyomas with 10–20 MF/10 HPF have been reported. The clinical evolution is benign, even if the neoplasm is treated by myomectomy. It is imperative that this diagnosis not be used for neoplasms that exhibit moderate to severe nuclear atypia, for those that contain abnormal MF, or for those that demonstrate zones of tumor cell necrosis. Leiomyomas removed during the secretory phase of the menstrual cycle have a significantly increased mitotic index compared to those removed during menses or during the proliferative phase [211]. Also, leiomyomas removed from women who are taking progestins have a higher mitotic rate than that observed in women who are taking a combination of estrogen and progestin or who are not taking any exogenous hormones [413]. The patient's hormonal status may play a role in the increased number of MF seen in mitotically active leiomyomas [341]. No studies of GnRHa have demonstrated a difference in mitotic index between treated and untreated patients, although an increase may be seen several weeks after cessation of treatment. In one study comparing leiomyomas removed from treated patients with tumors from untreated controls, cellular proliferation (Ki-67 and proliferating cell nuclear antigen [PCNA] labeling indices), estrogen receptors, and progesterone receptors were decreased in tumors from treated patients, but a statistically significant decrease in the mitotic index was not observed [428].

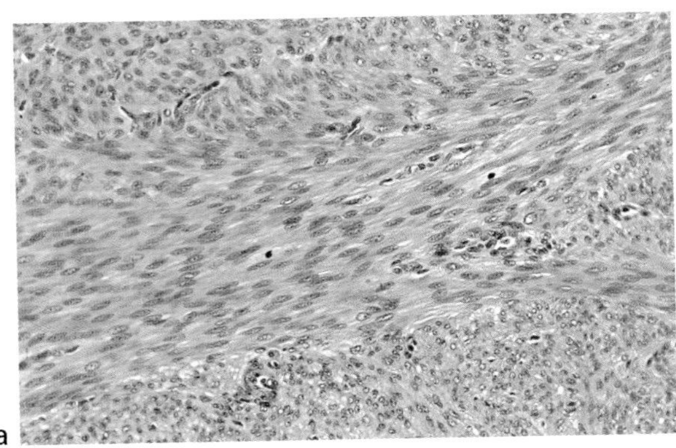

a

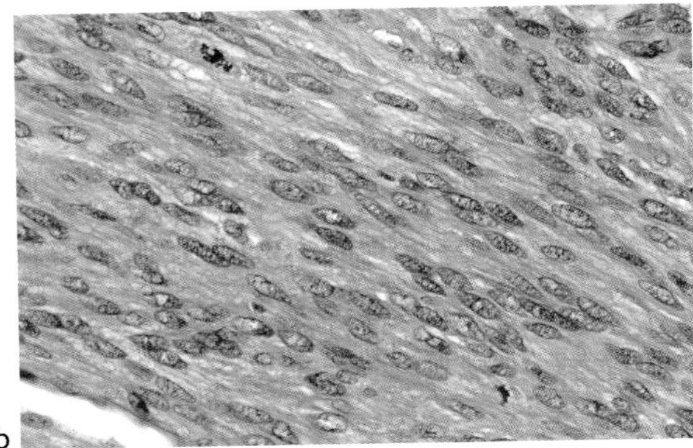

b

Fig. 10.8
Mitotically active leiomyoma. **(a)** The tumor is not hypercellular and there is no nuclear atypia, but two mitotic figures are present (*center*). **(b)** High magnification view of the central portion of *Fig. 10.8a*, showing two mitotic figures but bland tumor cell morphology and absence of necrosis

Cellular Leiomyoma

A cellular leiomyoma is one in which the cellularity is "significantly" greater than the surrounding myometrium; "significantly" translates, operationally, into a use of the modifier "cellular" in less than 5% of leiomyomas. The isolated finding of hypercellularity may suggest a diagnosis of leiomyosarcoma, but cellular leiomyoma lacks tumor cell necrosis, has few MF, and lacks the moderate to severe cytologic atypia seen in leiomyosarcoma. Palisading of nuclei, reminiscent of that seen in the Verocay bodies of a neurilemoma, is present in some cellular leiomyomas [154]. The ultrastructural appearance of these tumors,

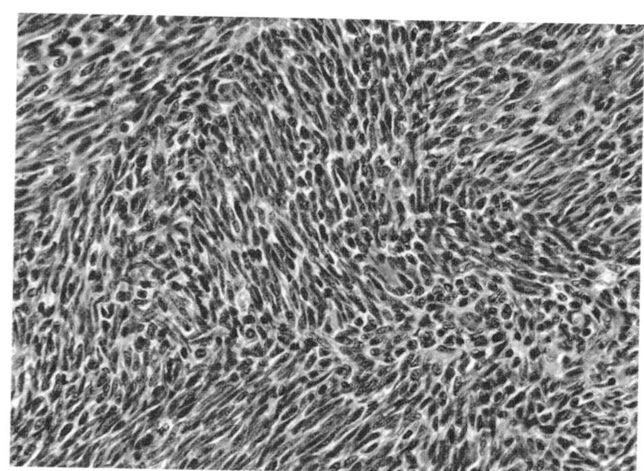

Fig. 10.9
Highly cellular leiomyoma. **The tumor is markedly cellular, and the cells are small and round to spindle shaped**

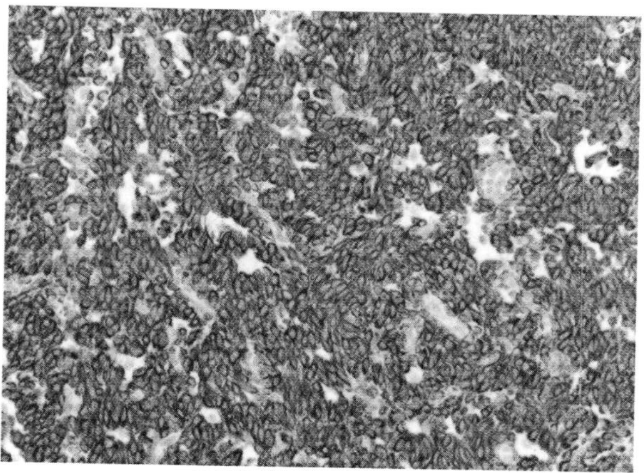

Fig. 10.10
Positive staining for desmin in highly cellular leiomyoma. **The tumor cells were also immunoreactive for smooth muscle actin and caldesmon, but staining for CD10 was negative**

however, is that of an ordinary leiomyoma [154]. Prolapse of submucosal leiomyomas may result in accentuated cellularity [271]. A cellular leiomyoma composed of small cells with scanty cytoplasm can be confused with an endometrial stromal tumor. This problem becomes particularly difficult with what has been termed a "highly cellular leiomyoma" (*Fig. 10.9*; [321]).

Features that help distinguish a cellular leiomyoma from a stromal tumor are the spindled shape of the cells, the fusiform shape of the nuclei, the reticulin pattern, and the absence of a plexiform vasculature. Reticulin fibers tend to parallel the fascicles of cells in a leiomyoma, but the reticulin network surrounds individual tumor cells in an endometrial stromal tumor. Additionally, Oliva et al. emphasized the presence of large thick-walled muscular vessels as features that serve to distinguish a highly cellular leiomyoma from a stromal proliferation [321]. Although some authors have reported that smooth muscle cells and stromal cells have immunophenotypic similarities, marked diffuse staining with muscle markers, particularly desmin (*Fig. 10.10*), is more suggestive of a smooth muscle tumor than of a stromal neoplasm [321]. In a hysterectomy specimen, the relationship of the proliferation to the surrounding normal structures can be appreciated. In the absence of myoinvasion or vascular invasion, the differential lies between two benign conditions: highly cellular leiomyoma and stromal nodule. When there is intravascular tumor, the distinction between endometrial stromal and smooth muscle differentiation becomes clinically relevant as the differential diagnosis lies between stromal sarcoma (a clinically low-grade malignancy) and IVL (clinically benign unless there are cardiac complications).

Care must be taken to consider benign alternatives to stromal sarcoma when a cellular mesenchymal proliferation is recovered in an endometrial sampling. Thus, three issues need to be considered in this setting: (1) what differentiation does the proliferation exhibit (smooth muscle or endometrial stromal); (2) are the criteria of malignancy evaluable; and, finally, (3) are the criteria of malignancy met? In a "low penalty" hysterectomy setting (an older woman or a young woman who has no interest in having children), the issue is usually resolved by what amounts to a diagnostic hysterectomy. In the "high penalty" hysterectomy setting (young woman wishing to retain her fertility or older woman who is a poor surgical candidate), diagnostic modalities that might clarify the situation without the need of hysterectomy (e.g., hysteroscopy, imaging studies, repeat sampling) should be considered. Again, the important point is that not all cellular, spindle cell proliferations recovered in a curettage are stromal sarcoma; the clinically innocuous cellular leiomyoma is a highly probable alternative. Rarely, some uterine neoplasms appear to be composed of a mixture of stromal and smooth muscle cells [32, 317, 318].

Hemorrhagic Cellular Leiomyoma and Hormone-Induced Changes

Hemorrhagic cellular leiomyoma, or "apoplectic" leiomyoma, is a form of cellular leiomyoma that is found in women who are taking oral contraceptives or who are either pregnant or postpartum [294, 306]. Multifocal stellate hemorrhages are present grossly (Fig. 10.11). Microscopically, the leiomyoma is cellular and contains patchy areas of hemorrhage and edema. Necrosis generally is not present. MF, which may be slightly increased in number, are detected mainly within a narrow zone resembling granulation tissue around areas of hemorrhage. In contrast to leiomyosarcoma, neither atypical MF nor significant cytologic atypia are present, and the neoplasm has a circumscribed, compressive margin.

With the advent of GnRHa therapy to shrink leiomyomata, a substantial body of literature has accumulated concerning the mechanism of shrinkage and the histologic correlates of this process. Some workers have found no differences between GnRHa-treated and untreated leiomyomas [167, 393], whereas others have been able to detect changes in tumor vasculature, pattern of necrosis, proliferation index, and cellularity [81, 83, 88, 103, 205, 361, 428]. None of these differences are sufficiently striking to be of practical importance in distinguishing leiomyoma from leiomyosarcoma. On rare occasions, leiomyosarcomas have been discovered in patients undergoing GnRHa therapy [278].

Leiomyoma with Bizarre Nuclei (Atypical Leiomyoma)

As an isolated finding, cytologic atypia, even when severe, is an unreliable criterion for the diagnosis of clinically malignant uterine smooth muscle tumors because it can be seen in clinically benign, otherwise banal smooth muscle neoplasms [32, 110]. A leiomyoma that exhibits moderate to severe cytologic atypia is designated an atypical leiomyoma. The atypical cells may be distributed throughout the leiomyoma or they may be focal; they have enlarged hyperchromatic nuclei with prominent chromatin clumping and, often, smudging (Fig. 10.12). Large cytoplasmic pseudonuclear inclusions are often present. Multinucleated tumor giant cells can be numerous and prompt the name "bizarre" or "symplastic" leiomyoma. These changes have been noted in leiomyomas excised from women taking progestins [124, 339]. By definition, MF cannot be present in numbers in excess of 10 MF/10 HPF in an atypical leiomyoma, and tumor cell necrosis must be absent. Most atypical leiomyomas have 0–4 MF/10 HPF. While tumors with 5–9 MF/10 HPF fall into the atypical leiomyoma category, it is prudent to view such tumors as smooth muscle tumors of uncertain malignant potential (STUMP), particularly if the mitotic count is at the upper end of the range or there are atypical MF. A mitotic index higher than 10 MF/10 HPF in a tumor with diffuse moderate to severe nuclear atypia is diagnostic of malignancy (Table 10.4; [32]). A smooth muscle tumor featuring diffuse moderate to severe atypia and coagulative tumor cell necrosis should be considered a leiomyosarcoma regardless of the mitotic index.

It is worth noting that leiomyosarcomas can vary greatly in appearance and may contain areas that lack the typical features of hypercellularity, cytologic atypia, and increased mitotic activity. Thus, extensive sampling is important to rule out leiomyosarcoma; atypical leiomyoma is a diagnosis of exclusion. The age of the patient must also be considered,

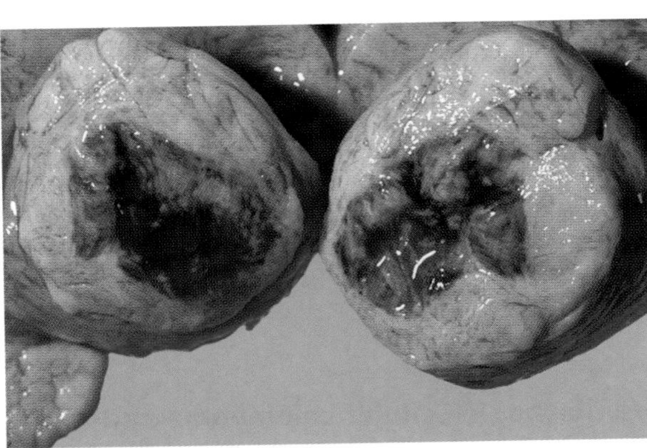

Fig. 10.11
Hemorrhagic cellular leiomyoma. **Multiple foci of hemorrhage are visible on the cut surfaces of a myomectomy specimen**

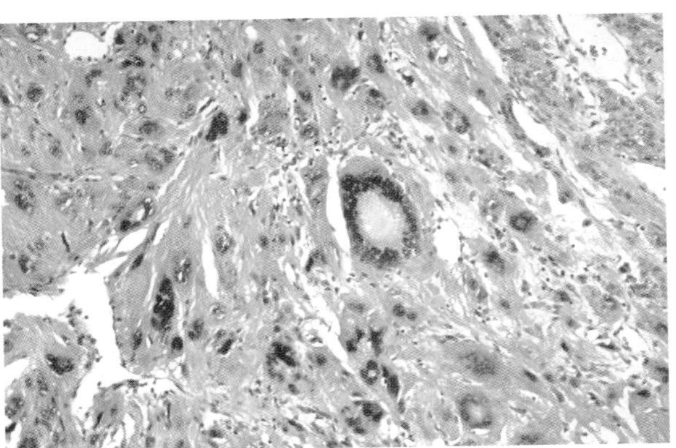

Fig. 10.12
Atypical leiomyoma. **Tumor cells have single or multiple pleomorphic nuclei with coarse, smudged chromatin**

as atypical leiomyoma is less common in postmenopausal women. A careful search for other features of leiomyosarcoma is indicated when a smooth muscle tumor containing atypical cells is detected in an older woman.

The natural history of smooth muscle neoplasms featuring mitotic indices of <10 MF/10 HPF that lack tumor cell necrosis, and that exhibit diffuse moderate to severe atypia remains controversial. Downes and Hart reported a benign clinical course in their series of 24 cases of atypical leiomyoma [110]. On the other hand, Bell et al. found 1 clinically malignant tumor in 43 cases (2%), all of which had at least 2 years follow-up [32]. The patient who failed did so over several years, a clinical course unlike that of the usual leiomyosarcoma. These workers considered the entire group of neoplasms with moderate to severe atypia, a mitotic index <10 MF/10 HPF, and without tumor cell necrosis as "atypical leiomyomas with a low risk of recurrence." A recent Mayo Clinic study of uterine leiomyosarcoma and leiomyoma variants reported similar findings: 3 of 18 patients with leiomyoma variants died of disease, but between 6 and 11 years after diagnosis [156]. Peters et al. reported a series of 15 STUMP and confirmed both the low failure rate in this category and the slow tempo of disease when recurrence did occur [334]. Although necrosis was not recorded, at least some of the tumors in their group would qualify as atypical leiomyomas using the Bell et al. criteria. Ip et al. reported similar findings in an analysis of 16 STUMPs [194]. Two of 16 tumors recurred at 15 and 51 months; both patients were alive at 40 and 74 months. Both tumors that recurred were atypical leiomyomas with multifocal moderate to severe nuclear atypia, 4–5 MF/10 HPF, and no tumor necrosis. The two tumors that recurred were the only ones that showed diffuse positive immunostaining for p16 and p53. The differences in reported experience are probably related to differences in patient sample size in studies of a neoplastic process with a very low clinical failure rate.

Epithelioid Leiomyoma

This category includes tumors formerly classified as leiomyoblastoma, clear cell leiomyoma, and plexiform leiomyoma [228]. Epithelioid smooth muscle tumors have the same histologic appearance in the uterus as in other sites in the body. The mean age of women with epithelioid leiomyoma is in the fifth decade, with a range of 30–78 years [228, 340]. Epithelioid leiomyomas are yellow or gray and may contain areas of hemorrhage. They tend to be softer than the usual leiomyoma. Most are solitary, and they can occur in any part of the uterus. The median diameter is 6–7 cm.

Microscopically, the cells are round or polygonal rather than spindle-shaped, and they are arranged in clusters or cords. The nuclei are round, relatively large, and centrally positioned. There are three basic subtypes of epithelioid leiomyoma: leiomyoblastoma, clear cell leiomyoma, and plexiform leiomyoma. Mixtures of the various patterns are common, providing the basis for designating all of these as epithelioid leiomyomas. Leiomyoblastoma is composed of round cells with eosinophilic cytoplasm (➋ *Fig. 10.13*) rather than spindle cells. The cells in clear cell leiomyoma are polygonal and have abundant clear cytoplasm and well-defined cell membranes (➋ *Fig. 10.14*). The cells may contain glycogen,

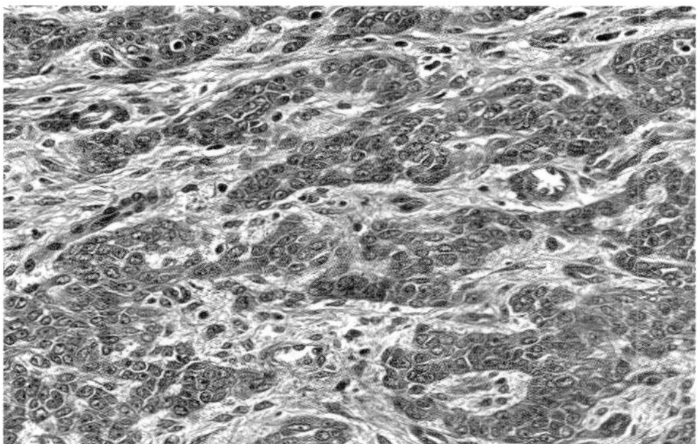

Fig. 10.13
Epithelioid smooth muscle tumor. **Cellular tumor composed of poorly cohesive polygonal cells with eosinophilic cytoplasm**

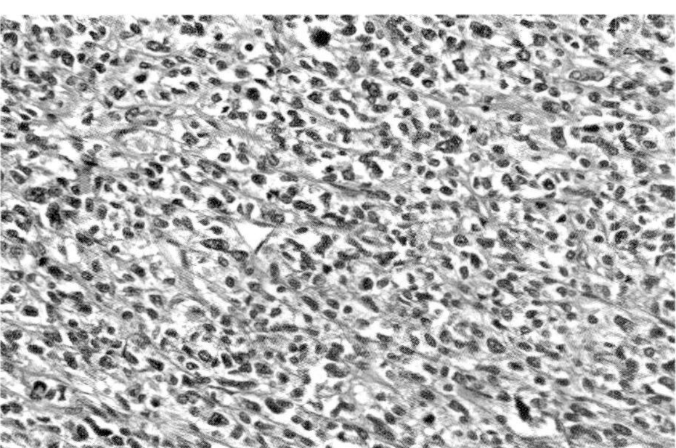

Fig. 10.14
Clear cell variant of epithelioid leiomyoma. **Nests of cells with abundant clear cytoplasm**

but there is minimal lipid and mucin is absent. The nucleus sometimes is displaced to the periphery of the cell, resulting in a signet-ring appearance. Plexiform leiomyoma is characterized by cords or nests of round cells with scanty to moderate amounts of cytoplasm. Transition to more typical spindled smooth muscle cells is often identified within an epithelioid leiomyoma. Immunohistochemical study confirms the myogenous phenotype of the tumor cells [47, 104, 192, 353]. Ultrastructural study reveals features of smooth muscle differentiation such as parallel cytoplasmic filaments, dense bodies, and basal lamina production [192, 196, 270]. The cells in some clear cell leiomyomas contain numerous mitochondria or cytoplasmic vacuoles.

Small plexiform leiomyomas that are detected only on microscopic examination are referred to as plexiform tumorlets (● *Fig. 10.15*; [206]). These lesions were formerly thought to be angiomas or endometrial stromal tumors, but ultrastructural examination revealed myofilaments and other features of smooth muscle cells [206, 310], and that the cells have a myogenous immunophenotype [104]. Plexiform tumorlets usually are solitary and submucosal, but they can occur anywhere in the myometrium and even in the endometrium. Multiple tumorlets are present in some patients [374].

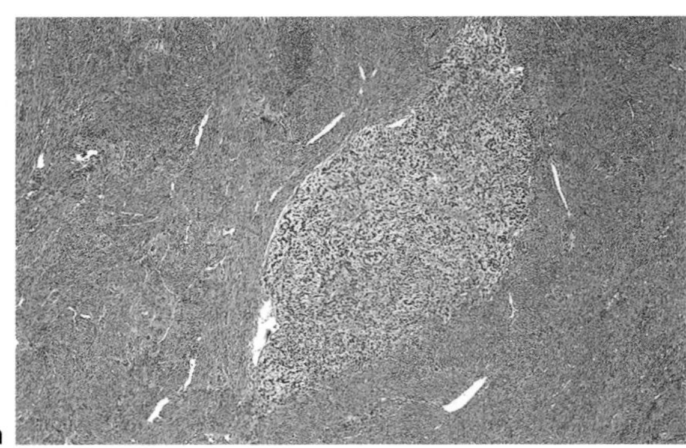

a

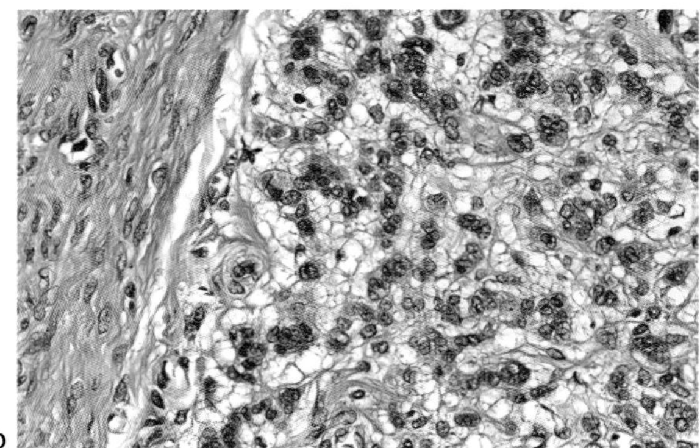

b

■ Fig. 10.15
Plexiform tumorlet. **This microscopic tumor is completely surrounded by normal myometrium (a) and consists of serpiginous cords of epithelioid smooth muscle cells (b)**

The behavior of epithelioid smooth muscle neoplasms of the uterus is difficult to predict [69, 228, 340]. Small tumors that lack cytologic atypia, tumor cell necrosis, and an elevated mitotic index can be safely regarded as benign. Plexiform tumorlets invariably are benign. Epithelioid leiomyomas with circumscribed margins, extensive hyalinization, and predominance of clear cells generally are benign. The behavior of epithelioid leiomyomas with two or more of the following features is not well established: large size (>6 cm), moderate mitotic activity (2–4 MF/10 HPF), moderate to severe cytologic atypia, and necrosis.

The accumulated experience with epithelioid tumors as a group is limited and discourages dogmatism in predicting clinical course. Those neoplasms with moderate to severe atypia, without necrosis, and fewer than 5 MF/10HPF should be classified as STUMP because experience is too limited to be certain about their aggressive potential. Careful follow-up is warranted. Neoplasms with ≥5 MF/10 HPF metastasize with sufficient frequency that all should be regarded as epithelioid leiomyosarcomas [228]. Epithelioid differentiation in more than just a few foci of a uterine smooth muscle tumor is a worrisome finding because the absence of cytologic atypia and tumor cell necrosis is no guarantee of a clinically benign course when the tumor contains ≥5 MF/10 HPF [199], although the failure rate is probably quite low. All epithelioid smooth muscle tumors with tumor cell necrosis reviewed at Stanford have been clinically malignant. On the other hand, seven epithelioid tumors with <5 MF/10 HPF, with at most minimal cytologic atypia, and without necrosis behaved in a benign fashion. Most malignant epithelioid smooth muscle tumors are of the leiomyoblastoma type, although clear cell leiomyosarcoma has been reported [381]. The epithelioid appearance of these neoplasms raises a broad differential including carcinoma and epithelioid variants of gestational trophoblastic disease.

Myxoid Leiomyoma

Myxoid leiomyomas are soft and translucent. Microscopically, there is abundant amorphous myxoid material between the smooth muscle cells [269]. The margins of a myxoid leiomyoma are circumscribed, and neither cytologic atypia nor MF are present. We diagnose leiomyoma with myxoid stroma when the cells are small and uniform, atypia is absent or at most mild, and there are no more than 2 MF/10 HPF. Areas of ordinary leiomyoma should be present focally. Large myxoid smooth muscle tumors and those in which an infiltrating margin, cytologic atypia, or mitotic activity are observed microscopically should be regarded with suspicion. Some myxoid smooth muscle tumors exhibiting these features are clinically malignant even though they do not meet standard criteria for a diagnosis of leiomyosarcoma. Myxoid differentiation coupled with enlarged and atypical cells is an ominous finding. Four of seven such uterine tumors studied at Stanford progressed. We diagnose myxoid leiomyosarcoma in the presence of moderate to marked atypia with or without necrosis and with any mitotic index. The tumor margins are usually infiltrating.

Vascular Leiomyoma

Vascular leiomyomas contain numerous large-caliber vessels with muscular walls. It can be difficult to distinguish a vascular leiomyoma from a hemangioma or an arteriovenous malformation if the vascular component predominates. Vascular leiomyomas are well defined, circumscribed neoplasms that contain at least foci of typical spindled smooth muscle cells. Hemangiomas are very rare in the uterus and are usually of the cavernous type. Hemangiomas and arteriovenous malformations tend to be poorly defined grossly and microscopically and lack the sharp circumscription of a leiomyoma.

Leiomyoma with Other Elements

Some benign uterine neoplasms are composed of a mixture of smooth muscle cells and other elements. Endometrial stromal cells are prominent in some mixed tumors [317]. The natural history of these rare neoplasms is incompletely documented, although it appears that the rules for assessing malignancy in endometrial stromal tumors applies to mixed tumors as well. Infiltrative margins and/or vascular invasion are associated with a malignant clinical course, and the absence of these features with a benign one [317].

It is not uncommon to find scattered adipocytes in an otherwise typical leiomyoma. A leiomyoma that contains a striking amount of fat is called a lipoleiomyoma (*Fig. 10.16*); if a vascular component is also present, it is designated as an angiolipoleiomyoma. Most such tumors occur in middle-aged or elderly women and may arise in any part of the uterus, including the cervix [432]. They average 6 cm in diameter and have soft yellow areas on the cut surface. Fat cells are generally found in circumscribed areas within the leiomyoma but may be present diffusely. Brown fat, skeletal muscle, and cartilage have been identified in leiomyomas [59, 137, 266, 440]. In most instances, the smooth muscle component predominates and is composed of spindled cells. Other types of leiomyoma, such as epithelioid leiomyoma [47], may also have a lipomatous component and fatty change is common in IVL. The vascular component of an angiolipoleiomyoma may be venous, arterial, or indeterminate. Only a few pure lipomas have been described in the uterus [106, 338]. Complex cytogenetic abnormalities have been described in a case of lipoleiomyoma [331].

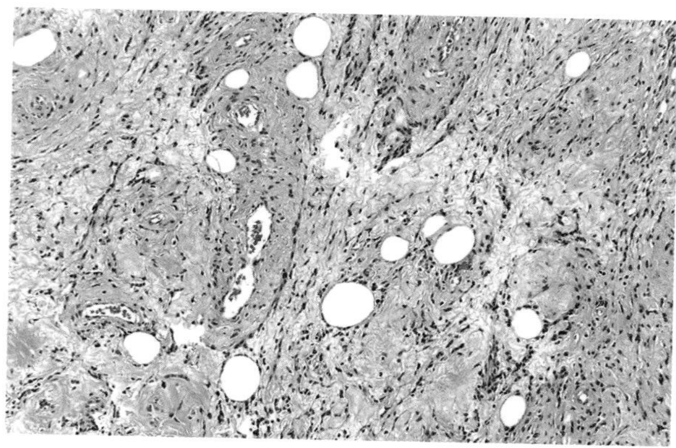

Fig. 10.16
Lipoleiomyoma. **The tumor is composed of an intermixture of fat cells, smooth muscle, and collagen**

Leiomyoma with Hematopoietic Cells

Large numbers of hematopoietic cells, which sometimes have no obvious etiology, may infiltrate leiomyomas. Leiomyomas may develop abscesses in the setting of bacterial infection. Peculiar infiltrates include extramedullary hematopoiesis in the absence of systemic disease [368], a prominent histiocytic infiltrate [5], a prominence of mast cells or eosinophils [89, 259, 324, 421], and, most importantly, a dense lymphoid infiltrate that can mimic lymphoma [130].

Smooth Muscle Proliferations with Unusual Growth Patterns, Diffuse Leiomyomatosis, and Myometrial Hypertrophy

Diffuse leiomyomatosis is an unusual condition in which innumerable small smooth muscle nodules produce symmetric enlargement of the uterus. The uterus may be greatly enlarged, weighing up to 1,000 g. The smooth muscle nodules range from microscopic to 3 cm in size, but most are less than 1 cm in diameter. They are composed of uniform, bland, spindled smooth muscle cells and are less circumscribed than typical leiomyomas. The clinical course may be complicated by hemorrhage, but the condition is benign [69, 166, 231, 291]. Myometrial hypertrophy is a condition in which the myometrium is thickened and the uterus is symmetrically enlarged. No specific gross or microscopic abnormality is noted; the uterus is abnormal in size only. Uterine weight increases with age and with increasing parity until the menopause. The average uterine weight decreases after the menopause. The weight beyond which the uterus is abnormally large, indicative of myometrial hypertrophy, is 130 g for the nulliparous uterus, 210 g for parity 1–3, and 250 g for parity of 4 and above [232].

Dissecting Leiomyoma

Dissecting leiomyoma refers to a benign smooth muscle proliferation with a border marked by the dissection of compressive tongues of smooth muscle into the surrounding myometrium and, occasionally, into the broad ligament and pelvis [357]. This pattern of infiltration may also be seen in IVL (see following). When edema and congestion are prominent, a uterine dissecting leiomyoma with extrauterine extension may resemble placental tissue, hence the name cotyledonoid dissecting leiomyoma [143, 358, 359].

Intravenous Leiomyomatosis and Leiomyoma with Vascular Invasion

IVL is a very rare smooth muscle tumor characterized by nodular masses of histologically benign smooth muscle cells growing within venous channels [67, 82, 292, 302, 307]. Women with IVL have a median age of 45 years; few are younger than 40 years. There is no racial predisposition, history of infertility, or decreased parity. The main symptoms are abnormal bleeding and pelvic discomfort. Most patients have a pelvic mass. Grossly, IVL is a complex coiled or nodular growth within the myometrium with convoluted, wormlike extensions into the uterine veins in the broad ligament or into other pelvic veins (➲ *Fig. 10.17*). The growth extends into the vena cava in more than 10% of patients, and in some it reaches as far as the heart [67, 82, 219, 399]. The wormlike masses vary from soft and spongy to rubbery and firm, and their color is pink-white or gray. Intravenous growth with an IVL-like pattern has been described in leiomyosarcoma [80], so it is important to carefully assess any such growth for features that might signify malignancy (high mitotic rate, significant nuclear atypia, and tumor cell necrosis).

Microscopically, tumor is found within venous channels lined by endothelium (➲ *Fig. 10.18*). Arteries are not involved. The histologic appearance is highly variable, even within the same tumor. The cellular composition of some examples of IVL is similar to a leiomyoma, but most contain prominent zones of fibrosis or hyalinization. Smooth muscle cells may be inconspicuous and difficult to identify. The intravenous growth is itself highly vascular (➲ *Fig. 10.19*), and in some cases contains so many small and large blood vessels that the process may resemble a vascular tumor. Any type of smooth muscle differentiation that occurs in a leiomyoma can be present in IVL [67]. Cellular, atypical, epithelioid, and lipoleiomyomatous growth patterns have all been described; these have the same behavior and prognosis as ordinary IVL [46, 67, 171].

IVL originates in vascular smooth muscle in some cases [307]. The tumor is predominantly or entirely intravascular in this situation, and there are many sites of attachment to the vein walls. Other examples develop by

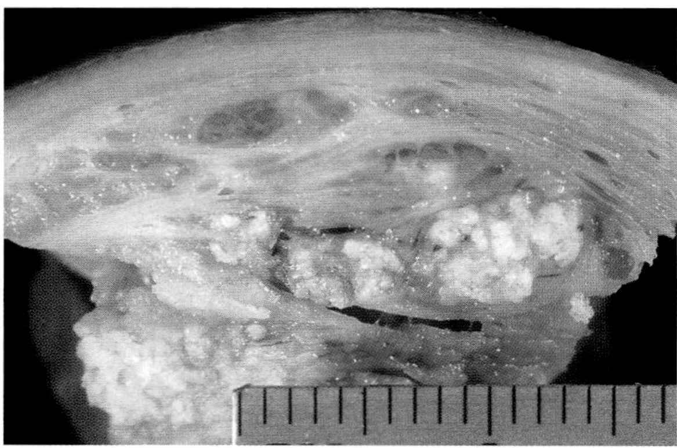

Fig. 10.17
Intravenous leiomyomatosis. **Brown and white plugs of intravascular tumor grow extensively in the myometrium**

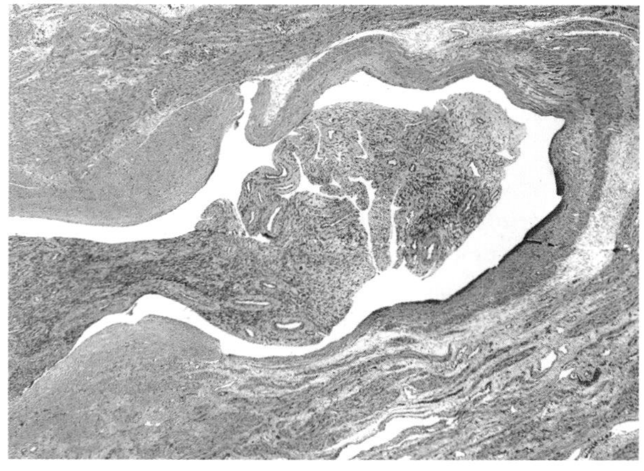

Fig. 10.18
Intravenous leiomyomatosis. **A plug of smooth muscle tumor grows within a large vein in the myometrium**

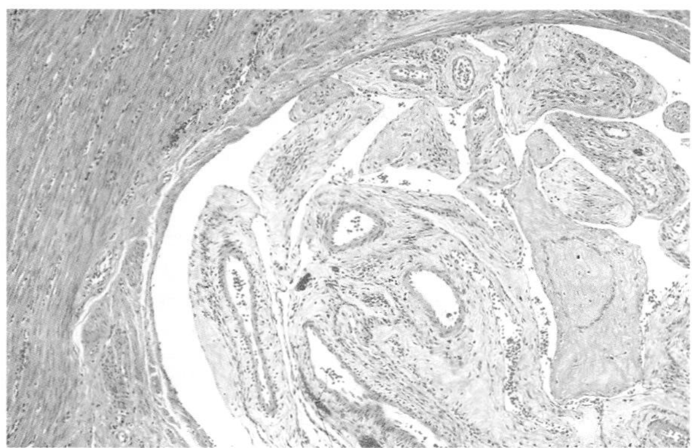

Fig. 10.19
Intravenous leiomyomatosis. **Nearly the entire tumor was within vascular spaces. Note that the intravascular tumor is highly vascular and extensively hyalinized**

intravascular extension from a leiomyoma [302, 307]. In these cases the bulk of the tumor is extravascular and sites of origin from a vein wall are not found. Treatment is by total abdominal hysterectomy and bilateral salpingo-oophorectomy together with excision of any extrauterine extensions. IVL has a favorable prognosis even when it is incompletely excised [292]. Pelvic recurrence is infrequent and usually is amenable to surgical excision [117, 307]. Residual pelvic tumor may remain stable but progressive growth is possible. IVL is a hormonally dependent tumor, and progression is more likely in women whose treatment does not include bilateral salpingo-oophorectomy. Long-term survival is possible after removal of plugs of tumor from the vena cava or right atrium or excision of nodules from the lung. In one case, leuprolide acetate induced tumor regression and rendered debulking surgery feasible in a patient with previously unresectable, widespread, retroperitoneal intravascular leiomyomatosis [416].

Benign Metastasizing Leiomyoma

Benign metastasizing leiomyoma is a nebulous condition in which "metastatic" smooth muscle tumor deposits in the lung, lymph nodes, or abdomen appear to be derived from a benign leiomyoma of the uterus. The lung is the most common site of involvement. One or multiple nodules of a low-grade smooth muscle tumor grow in an expansile pattern within the pulmonary parenchyma, often incorporating bronchioles (*Figs. 10.20a and b*). Reports of this condition are often difficult to assess. Almost all cases of benign metastasizing leiomyoma occur in women, most with a history of pelvic surgery. The primary neoplasm, typically removed years before the metastatic deposits are detected, often has been inadequately studied. In some cases, the primary tumor was not examined histologically by the reporting author and, in others, the cytologic appearance, including mitotic counts, is not recorded for either the primary tumor or the alleged metastasis. A few examples may represent deportation metastases from IVL that reach the lungs, where they become implanted and grow as multiple intrapulmonary nodules of smooth muscle [237]. Others may represent a multifocal smooth muscle proliferation involving the uterus and extrauterine sites [62]. Most examples of "benign metastasizing leiomyoma," however, appear to be either a primary benign smooth muscle lesion of the lung in a woman with a history of uterine leiomyoma or pulmonary metastases from a morphologically noninformative smooth muscle neoplasm of the uterus [32, 82, 147, 437]. The findings of a recent cytogenetic study were most consistent with a monoclonal origin of both uterine and pulmonary tumors and the interpretation that the pulmonary tumors were metastatic [412]. The hormone dependence of this proliferation is suggested by the finding of estrogen and progesterone receptors in metastatic deposits [197] and the regression of tumors during pregnancy [185], after the menopause, and after oophorectomy [3]. The imaging characteristics of BML have been recently reviewed [82]. The differential diagnosis includes a pulmonary metastasis from a low-grade ESS with smooth muscle or myofibroblastic differentiation [441].

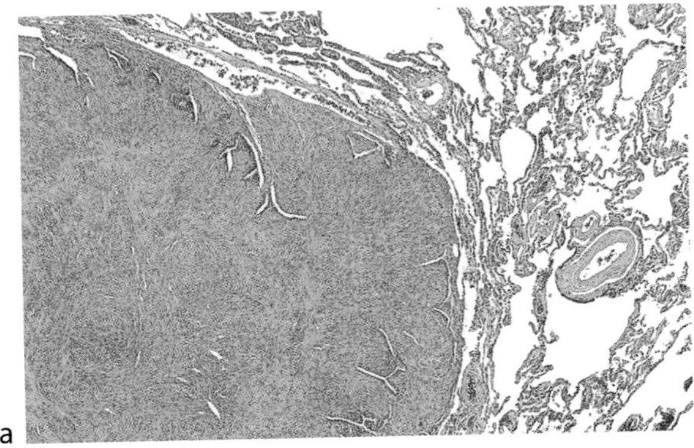
a

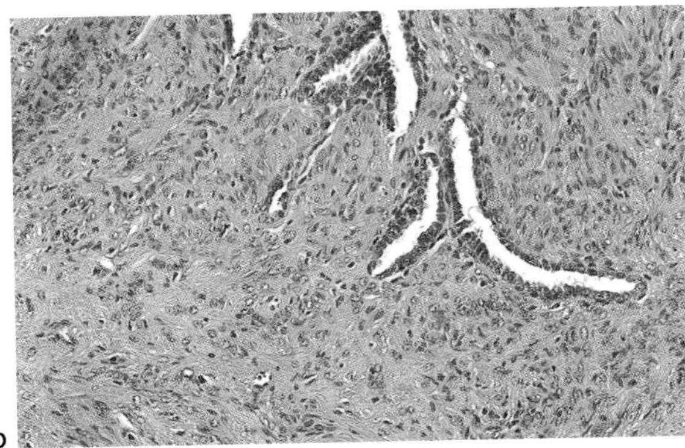
b

Fig. 10.20
Benign metastasizing leiomyoma. **A circumscribed smooth muscle tumor is present in the lung (a). At high magnification, incorporated bronchioles are surrounded by cytologically bland smooth muscle cells (b)**

Peritoneal Leiomyomas ("Parasitic" Leiomyomas)

On rare occasions, leiomyomas have been reported to "detach" from their initial subserosal location and "attach" to some other pelvic site. This improbable event presumably occurs through the mediation of a combination of infarction and inflammatory adhesions. A diagnosis of parasitic leiomyoma should be made with great caution because clinically malignant smooth muscle neoplasms arising in the retroperitoneum or gastrointestinal tract are notorious for being bland and having a low mitotic index. The plausibility of "parasitic leiomyomas" must be evaluated against the background of the infrequent occurrence of primary (single or multiple) smooth muscle neoplasms arising in other components of the female internal genitalia and the neighboring pelvic peritoneum [37, 242].

Disseminated Peritoneal Leiomyomatosis

Disseminated peritoneal leiomyomatosis (DPL) is a rare condition characterized by the presence of multiple smooth muscle, myofibroblastic, and fibroblastic nodules on the peritoneal surfaces of the pelvic and abdominal cavities in women of reproductive age [284, 411]. This condition is discussed in connection with leiomyoma of the uterus because it must be distinguished from metastatic leiomyosarcoma. Most cases are associated with pregnancy, an estrinizing granulosa tumor, or oral contraceptive use [411]. The most common presentation is as an unexpected finding at the time of cesarean section. DPL appears as multiple, small, granular white or tan nodules on the pelvic and abdominal peritoneum, on the surfaces of the uterus, adnexa, intestines, and in the omentum (*Figs. 10.21a and b*). The nodules are distributed randomly, and most of them are less than 1 cm in diameter; this contrasts with metastatic leiomyosarcoma, in which the nodules tend to be fewer, larger, and invasive into adjacent tissues. Microscopically, the nodules consist of collagen, fibroblasts, myofibroblasts, smooth muscle cells, and, in pregnancy or the postpartum period, decidual cells (*Fig. 10.22*). Spindle cells usually dominate, raising the possibility that disseminated peritoneal leiomyomatosis may be confused with a metastatic sarcoma. The clinical setting is quite different, however, as is the morphology of the cells. MF are infrequent in DPL, and nuclear atypia and pleomorphism are minimal or absent. Electron microscopic studies have shown that most nodules are composed of smooth muscle and decidual cells, although some are mixtures of decidua and fibroblasts or myofibroblasts [160, 301, 335, 411]. A cytogenetic study assessed the clonality of 42 tumorlets and 15 normal tissues from four women with DPL by analyzing X chromosome inactivation as indicated by the methylation status of the androgen receptor gene (HUMARA). In each of the four patients, the same parental X chromosome was nonrandomly inactivated in all tumorlets, consistent with a metastatic unicentric neoplasm or, alternatively, selection for an X-linked allele in clonal multicentric lesions [343]. Disseminated peritoneal leiomyomatosis is initiated or promoted by hormonal factors in most cases. Estrogen and progesterone receptors may be demonstrated within DPL by biochemical or immunohistochemical methods [111]. DPL generally regresses or remains static after removal of the hormonal stimulus (i.e., after delivery), so radical attempts at excision are unnecessary [411]. In keeping with a hormonally dependent process, DPL may regress during therapy with

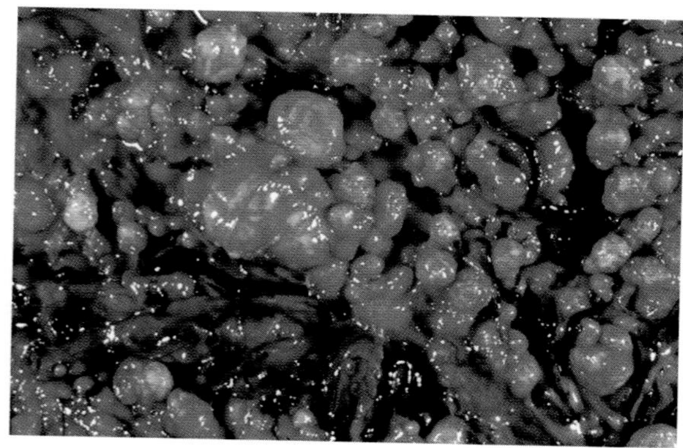

a

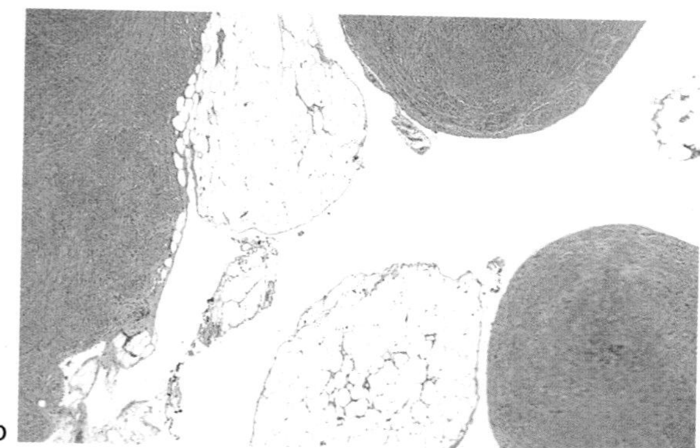

b

Fig. 10.21
Disseminated peritoneal leiomyomatosis. **Disseminated peritoneal leiomyomatosis presents grossly as multiple or numerous small nodules of smooth muscle in the omentum (a) or on the peritoneum. A low-power photomicrograph illustrates multiple nodules of smooth muscle cells surrounded by omental fat (b)**

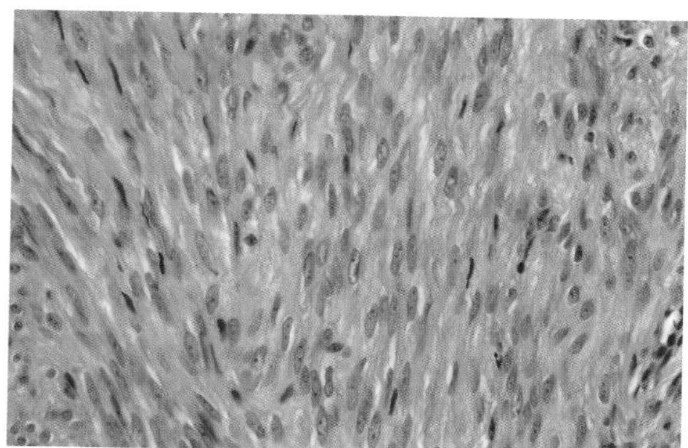

Fig. 10.22
Disseminated peritoneal leiomyomatosis. **The peritoneal nodules consist of histologically bland spindle-shaped smooth muscle cells; mitotic figures are absent**

a GnRH agonist [169]. The peritoneal smooth muscle nodules may enlarge again when the GnRH agonist is discontinued or if the patient becomes pregnant. A few cases of malignant DPL have been reported [31]. Several were distinguished from typical cases of DPL by not having an exposure to estrogen or associated uterine leiomyomas and by absence of estrogen and progesterone receptors in their tumors.

Leiomyosarcoma

Leiomyosarcoma represents about 1.3% of uterine malignancies and more than 50% of uterine sarcomas, excluding carcinosarcoma [1]. Approximately 1 of every 800 smooth muscle tumors of the uterus is a leiomyosarcoma, but less than 1% of women thought clinically to have leiomyoma prove to have leiomyosarcoma [238].

Clinical Features

The median age of women with leiomyosarcoma is 50–55 years [1, 157], nearly a decade older than women with leiomyomas, although the disease is well known to occur in women in the third decade of life. Leiomyosarcoma is more prevalent in African-American women than in white women [48]. There is no relationship with gravidity or parity. The clinical presentation is nonspecific. The main symptoms are abnormal vaginal bleeding, lower abdominal pain, or a pelvic or abdominal mass [157]. The average duration of symptoms before diagnosis is 5 months [233]. There appears to be little support for the clinical dictum that a rapidly enlarging uterine smooth muscle neoplasm is indicative of leiomyosarcoma. In one study, only 1 of 371 women with this finding proved to have a leiomyosarcoma [327]. Unlike MMMT, leiomyosarcoma is seldom associated with a history of pelvic radiation.

Gross Findings

Most leiomyosarcomas are intramural, and 50–75% are solitary masses [371]. A higher proportion involves the cervix than is the case with leiomyoma. Leiomyosarcoma averages 6–9 cm in diameter and is soft or fleshy with poorly defined margins [1]. The cut surface is gray-yellow or pink, often with areas of necrosis and hemorrhage (*Fig. 10.23*). Leiomyosarcoma tends to be larger and softer than leiomyoma; it has a more irregular margin, and it is more likely to be hemorrhagic and necrotic

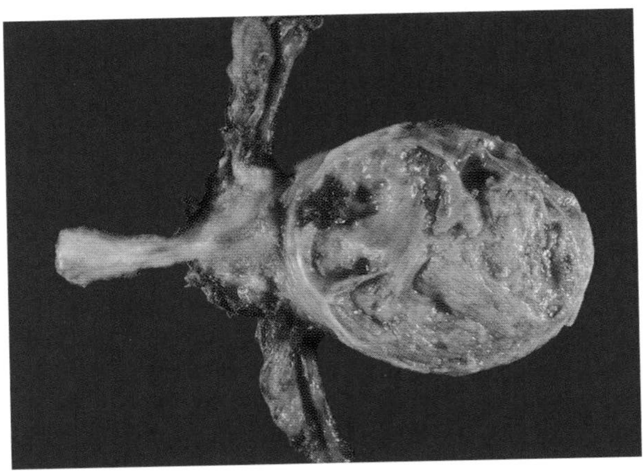

Fig. 10.23
Leiomyosarcoma. **Leiomyosarcoma is typically a solitary neoplasm, softer than the usual leiomyoma, and with areas of necrosis and hemorrhage on the cut surface**

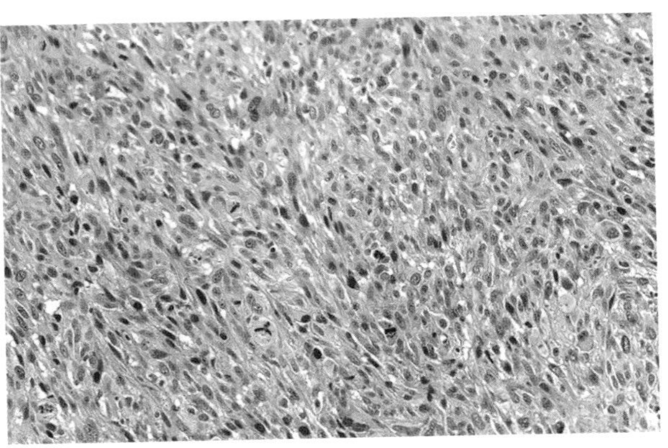

Fig. 10.24
Leiomyosarcoma. **The tumor cells are spindle-shaped with eosinophilic cytoplasm. The nuclei are fusiform, hyperchromatic, and atypical, and there are many mitotic figures**

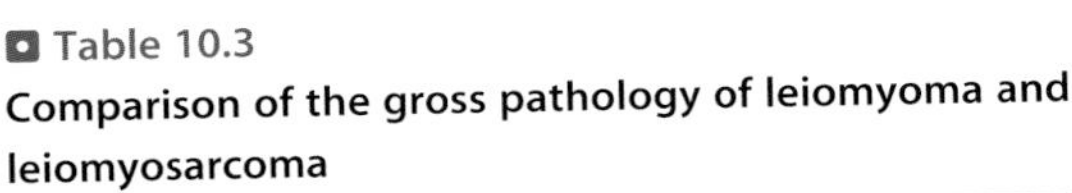

Table 10.3
Comparison of the gross pathology of leiomyoma and leiomyosarcoma

Leiomyoma	Leiomyosarcoma
Usually multiple	Usually solitary (50–75%)
Variable size, usually 3–5 cm	Large, usually 5–10 cm or larger
Firm, whorled cut surface	Soft, fleshy cut surface
White	Yellow or tan
Hemorrhage and necrosis (infarction-type) infrequent	Hemorrhage and necrosis (coagulative tumor cell-type) frequent

(*Table 10.3*). On the other hand, most smooth muscle neoplasms that have a peculiar gross appearance are found to be benign and to exhibit some form of "degeneration," usually ischemic. The diagnostic usefulness of imaging studies in separating benign from malignant smooth muscle neoplasms has recently been discussed [372].

Microscopic Findings

The usual leiomyosarcoma is composed of fascicles of spindle cells with abundant eosinophilic cytoplasm (*Fig. 10.24*). Longitudinal cytoplasmic fibrils, best appreciated with a trichrome stain, are frequently present. The nuclei are fusiform, usually have rounded ends, and are hyperchromatic with coarse chromatin and prominent

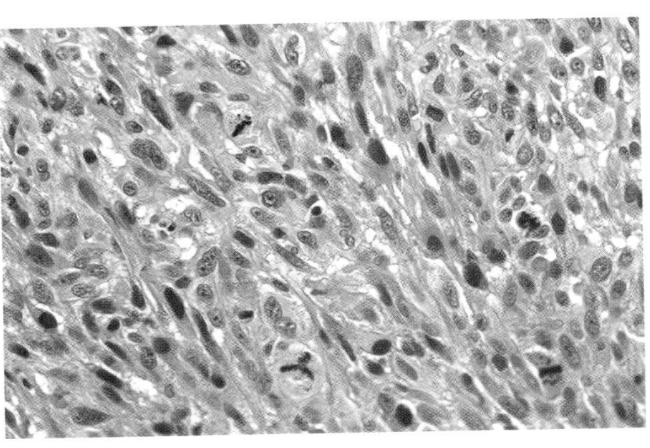

Fig. 10.25
Leiomyosarcoma. **The tumor cells vary in size and shape. Several mitotic figures are present including an abnormal one**

nucleoli (*Fig. 10.25*). Cellular pleomorphism can be marked in poorly differentiated neoplasms (*Fig. 10.26*). Multinucleated tumor cells are found in 50% of leiomyosarcomas. Giant cells resembling osteoclasts are occasionally present [95, 262, 328] and, rarely, xanthoma cells may be prominent [164]. Many leiomyosarcomas invade the surrounding myometrium, but a leiomyosarcoma with a circumscribed margin can give rise to metastases. Vascular invasion is identified in 10–22% of leiomyosarcomas. Tumor cell necrosis is typically prominent but need not be present. The mitotic index is typically in

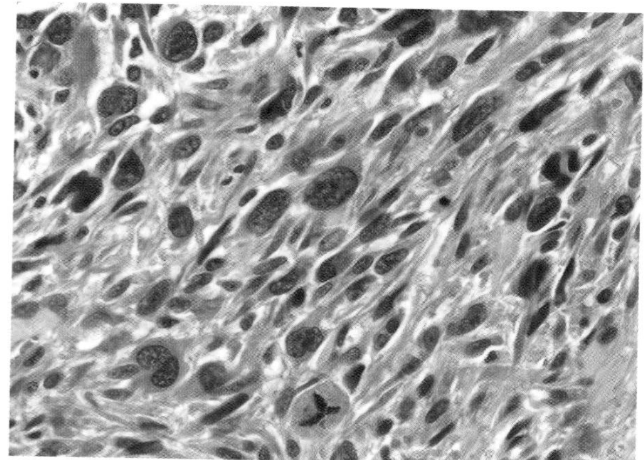

Fig. 10.26
Leiomyosarcoma. The tumor cell nuclei are pleomorphic, with some giant nuclei and an atypical mitotic figure

excess of 15 MF/10 HPF [332]. The main criteria used to diagnose leiomyosarcoma of the uterus are the presence of nuclear atypia, a high mitotic index, and coagulative tumor cell necrosis (*Table 10.4*).

Myxoid leiomyosarcoma is a large, gelatinous neoplasm that usually appears circumscribed on gross examination [226, 369]. Microscopically, the smooth muscle cells are usually widely separated by myxoid material (*Fig. 10.27*; [216]). The characteristic low cellularity partly accounts for the low mitotic index in most myxoid leiomyosarcomas. Sometimes, however, the mitotic index is high and there is a high degree of atypia. In addition to the myxoid appearance, other microscopic features that help identify the tumor as a leiomyosarcoma include myometrial infiltration and vascular invasion. One unusual myxoid leiomyosarcoma arose within a leiomyoma [286]. Despite the low mitotic counts, myxoid leiomyosarcoma has the same unfavorable prognosis as typical leiomyosarcoma. Myxoid smooth muscle tumors of the uterus must be regarded with suspicion, and any myxoid smooth muscle tumor with significant nuclear atypia, regardless of the mitotic count or the presence or absence of necrosis should be classified as a leiomyosarcoma. It is critical to distinguish the myxoid differentiation found in myxoid leiomyosarcomas from the vastly more prevalent hydropic changes seen in degenerating leiomyomas [78]. In addition, myxoid leiomyosarcoma must be differentiated from an inflammatory myofibroblastic tumor (IMT; see section Inflammatory Myofibroblastic Tumor; [344]). In myxoid leiomyosarcoma, not only is the stroma myxoid but the cells are enlarged with hyperchromatic nuclei and

Table 10.4
Histologic criteria for the diagnosis of uterine smooth muscle tumors with standard smooth muscle differentiation

Tumor cell necrosis	Atypia	MF/10 HPF	Diagnosis
Present	Diffuse moderate to severe	Any level	Leiomyosarcoma
Present	None to mild	≥10	Leiomyosarcoma
Present	None to mild	<10	STUMP (rule out infarcted leiomyoma)
Absent	Diffuse moderate to severe	≥10	Leiomyosarcoma
Absent	Diffuse moderate to severe	<5	Atypical leiomyoma with low risk of recurrence
Absent	Diffuse moderate to severe	5–9 or atypical mitotic figures	STUMP
Absent	None to mild	<5	Leiomyoma
Absent	None to mild	≥5	Mitotically active leiomyoma
Absent	Focal moderate to severe	≥5	STUMP
Absent	Focal moderate to severe	<5	Atypical leiomyoma

pleomorphism is usually obvious. The usual case of myxoid leiomyosarcoma bears a striking resemblance to soft tissue myxoid "malignant fibrous histiocytoma."

Epithelioid leiomyosarcomas are composed of round or polygonal cells and exhibit one of the patterns of epithelioid differentiation (*Fig. 10.28*). The leiomyoblastoma pattern is most common, although clear cell epithelioid leiomyosarcomas have also been reported [340, 380, 381]. The usual features of malignancy seen in more conventional leiomyosarcomas are generally present: cytologic atypia, tumor cell necrosis, and a high mitotic index [69, 212, 287]. Epithelioid smooth muscle tumors with significant nuclear atypia and either necrosis or ≥5 MF/10 HPF are classified as leiomyosarcomas [228, 340].

Finally, there is the rare, otherwise conventional smooth muscle tumor with a low mitotic count that proves to be clinically malignant. Unless the tumor is invasive or contains abnormal MF or areas of tumor cell necrosis, there are no good grounds for suspecting that it is a leiomyosarcoma until it announces itself by metastasizing. Doubtless, the pulmonary metastases from some "benign metastasizing leiomyomas" originate from neoplasms in this category.

Immunohistochemistry

Immunohistochemistry is generally not required for the diagnosis of leiomyosarcoma, but immunostains are occasionally necessary to differentiate leiomyosarcoma from other uterine malignancies such as undifferentiated endometrial sarcoma (UES) or sarcomatoid carcinoma. Immunostains can confirm that extrauterine sarcoma deposits show smooth muscle differentiation and hence are compatible with metastatic leiomyosarcoma. Recently published studies suggest that immunohistochemistry may play a role in the classification of atypical smooth muscle tumors that are difficult to recognize as leiomyosarcoma using standard criteria.

A variety of antibodies can be used to confirm that a uterine tumor exhibits smooth muscle differentiation (*Table 10.5*). Experience is greatest with smooth muscle actin, desmin, and caldesmon, but calponin and smooth muscle myosin are also occasionally used for this purpose. Cytoplasmic staining is observed in smooth muscle cells with all of these markers, although staining for one or more of them can be lost in poorly differentiated leiomyosarcomas. Myofibroblasts can also stain with smooth muscle markers, particularly smooth muscle actin, so positive staining with one of these markers is not conclusive evidence of smooth muscle differentiation. CD10 is generally used as a marker of endometrial stromal differentiation, but as experience with this antibody has accumulated it has become clear that some smooth muscle tumors are also CD10 positive, although staining is often weak and focal [277, 414]. Leiomyosarcoma appears more

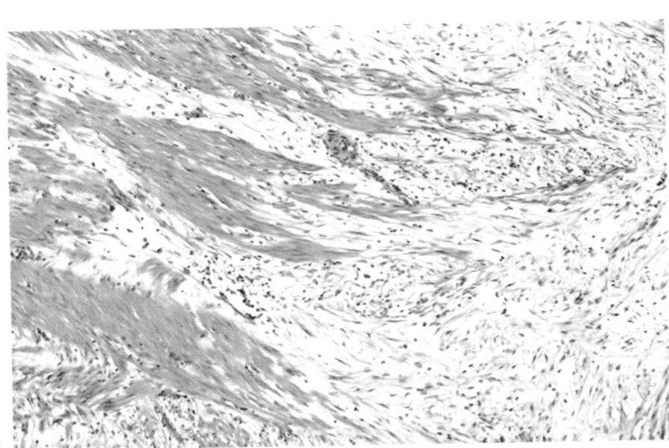
a

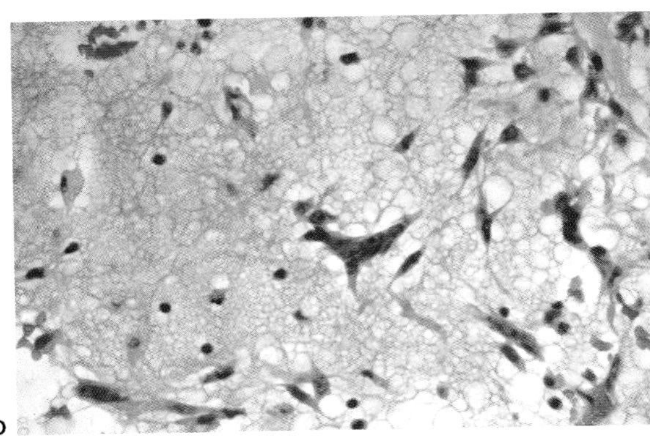
b

Fig. 10.27
Myxoid leiomyosarcoma. **The abundant myxoid stroma widely separates bundles of smooth muscle cells, resulting in a hypocellular appearance (a). As shown here (b), the degree of nuclear atypia can be deceptively bland, and, because the tumor cells are widely separated by myoid stroma, the number of mitotic figures per 10 HPF is often low**

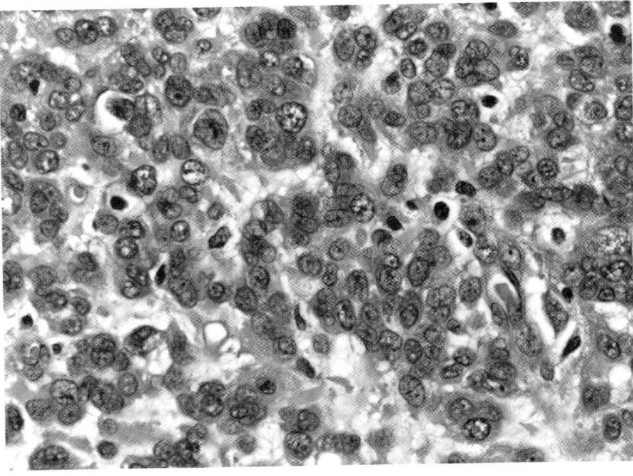

Fig. 10.28
Epithelioid leiomyosarcoma of the "leiomyoblastoma" type. **The tumor cells are polygonal with pale cytoplasm and atypical nuclei. Mitotic figures are not numerous, but there was extensive coagulative tumor cell necrosis**

Table 10.5

Immunohistochemical features of leiomyosarcoma and leiomyoma

	SMA	Desmin	Caldesmon	CD10	PR	P16	P53	MIB-1 PHH3
LMS	+	+	+/−	−/+	−	+	+/−	↑
LM[a]	+	+	+	−	+	−	−	−

[a]Many leiomyoma variants and STUMP show overlap with leiomyosarcoma.
LMS, Leiomyosarcoma; LM, Leiomyoma

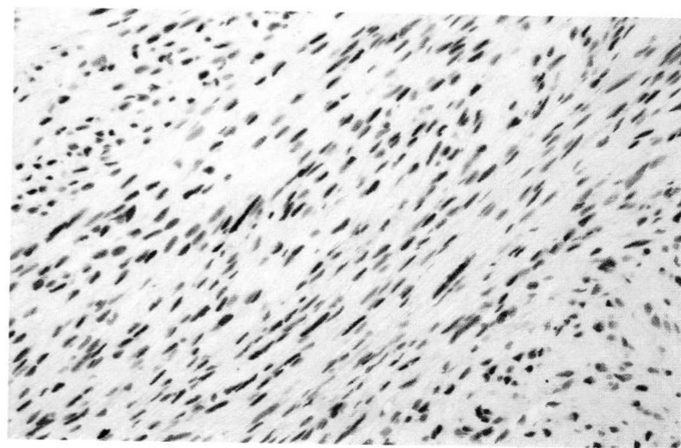

Fig. 10.29
Positive staining for p53 in leiomyosarcoma. **Most tumor cell nuclei show strong positive staining**

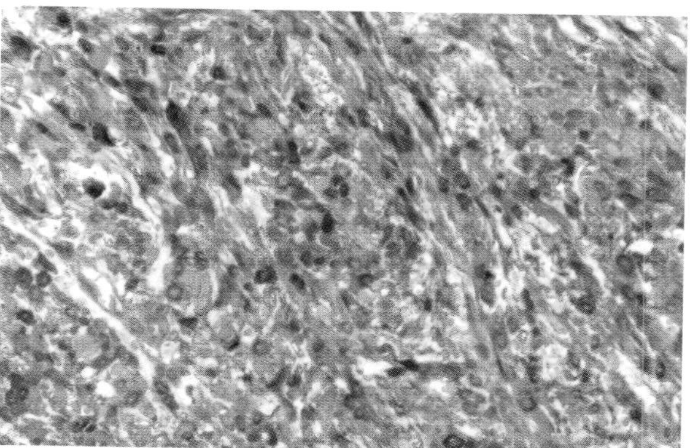

Fig. 10.30
Positive staining for p16 in leiomyosarcoma. **Nearly all tumor cells show strong nuclear and/or cytoplasmic staining. Staining must be strong and diffuse to be of significance**

likely than other types of smooth muscle tumors to stain for CD10. In one study, eight of nine leiomyosarcomas showed staining for CD10 (1+ to 3+ intensity, staining in 5–60% of tumor cells) [320]. Histone deacetylase 8 (HDAC8) has been proposed as a marker of smooth muscle differentiation and has been reported to stain leiomyosarcoma with a frequency similar to that obtained with other markers, although with less intensity; it does not appear to be widely used [100]. Myometrial smooth muscle cells are frequently immunoreactive for cytokeratin, so it is not surprising that occasional leiomyosarcomas show positive cytoplasmic staining for cytokeratin [320].

Immunohistochemistry can, in some cases, suggest that a problematic smooth muscle tumor is a leiomyosarcoma (*Table 10.5*). Mutation of the p53 gene or positive staining for p53 (strong nuclear staining in >50% of tumor cell nuclei) is reported mainly in leiomyosarcoma (*Fig. 10.29*), although unfortunately only a minority of tumors is p53 positive [149, 313]. Different results were reported in one study, in which atypical leiomyomas and STUMPs were reported to stain with the same frequency and intensity as leiomyosarcoma [60]. Reported results can be difficult to interpret because of differing criteria for leiomyosarcoma, use of different antibodies, failure to clearly report the intensity and extent of staining, acceptance of low levels of staining as positive, or lack of clinical follow-up [11, 41, 101, 170, 235, 239]. To ensure reproducible results strong nuclear staining (2–3+) should be present in >50% of tumor cell nuclei. More recently gene expression studies have shown overexpression of p16 in leiomyosarcoma [386], suggesting that immunostaining for p16 might be helpful in the differential diagnosis of problematic smooth muscle tumors. Studies of p16 staining in uterine smooth muscle tumors [23, 44, 60, 149, 313] have generally found diffuse strong staining in leiomyosarcoma (*Fig. 10.30*), despite differences in diagnostic criteria and antibodies. Staining is cytoplasmic or nuclear or is present in both sites. Some authors have found little staining for p16 in STUMPs and atypical leiomyomas, while others have shown considerable overlap in staining [60, 313]. Clinical follow-up has been reported in only a few cases, and some examples of p16 positive STUMPs have proven to be clinically malignant [23, 194], suggesting that diffuse strong staining for p16 may help to define a group of STUMPs that should be suspected of actually being leiomyosarcomas, particularly if p53 is also overexpressed. Loss of staining for progesterone receptors has been proposed as a possible marker for leiomyosarcoma [433]. Staining for progesterone receptors is lost in 40–80% of leiomyosarcomas, but it is retained in 70–100% of STUMPs and in most leiomyomas [43, 241, 285, 447]. Staining for estrogen receptors is more variable. Staining for hormone receptors tends to be positive in STUMPs, whether or not they subsequently recur or metastasize, so staining for hormone receptors does not appear to be helpful in subclassifying STUMPs into high- and low-risk categories [194]. In summary, immunohistochemistry may be helpful in the diagnosis of leiomyosarcoma. Diffuse strong staining for p16, especially when accompanied by diffuse strong staining for p53 supports a diagnosis of leiomyosarcoma. However, such staining is not an absolute criterion for a diagnosis of leiomyosarcoma, and the immunostain results must be interpreted in conjunction with the histologic findings. Light microscopic evaluation still forms the basis for classification of uterine smooth muscle tumors.

Cytogenetics

The cytogenetics of leiomyosarcoma are even more complicated and varied than those of leiomyoma. A wide variety of chromosomal changes have been described, but no specific diagnostically useful findings have emerged [363]. A translocation that is often present in leiomyomas, t(12;14), has not been identified in leiomyosarcoma, suggesting that leiomyosarcoma is generally not derived from a preexisting leiomyoma.

Clinical Behavior and Treatment

In the past, the staging system for uterine corpus carcinomas was used for uterine sarcomas. However, a new staging system designed to reflect the different biological behavior of sarcomas has been introduced (➲ *Table 10.2*; [131]).

A recent retrospective review of uterine leiomyosarcomas treated at the Mayo Clinic provides a clinicopathologic portrait of leiomyosarcoma as currently defined. Sixty-eight percent of the 208 patients reviewed presented with disease confined to the uterus. Six percent had cervical involvement; approximately half had cervical involvement only. Nine percent were Stage III and 20% Stage IV [157]. Patients with leiomyosarcoma relapse both loco-regionally and hematogenously. A recent review of 71 uterine leiomyosarcomas reports relapses in the following sites as the sole site: vagina, 22%; pelvis, 19%, lung, 22%; bone, 9%; and retroperitoneum, 12%. Relapse in both lung and pelvis occurred in 16% of patients [157].

The incidence of lymph node metastasis varies from series to series, but it is substantially lower than that found in clinical stage I and II high-risk endometrial carcinomas [157]. In a Gynecologic Oncology Group (GOG) study, 83% of 59 clinical stage I and II leiomyosarcoma patients were surgical stage I; 2 of 59 (3%) had lymph node involvement, 2 had adnexal involvement, and 1 had positive peritoneal cytology [258]. Three of 37 women studied at Memorial Sloan Kettering Cancer Center had positive lymph nodes, but no women with stage I or II tumors had lymph node metastases [240]. Lymph node involvement is higher in series reporting advanced-stage leiomyosarcoma, and figures as high as 44% are reported in autopsy series [133, 355]. Goff et al. found in their series of 15 surgically staged patients that lymph nodes were involved only when there was peritoneal disease [158]. Moreover, a high percentage of lymph node-negative patients failed. In view of this, there would appear to be little role for lymph node sampling in this disease.

Leiomyosarcoma is a highly malignant neoplasm with poor survival rates when tumors are classified with contemporary criteria. For postmenopausal women, primary therapy for early-stage leiomyosarcoma is total abdominal hysterectomy and bilateral salpingo-oophorectomy. Therapy in premenopausal women is more controversial. The ovaries are only rarely the site of metastatic disease in clinically low-stage leiomyosarcoma; in the GOG study, only 2 of 59 patients had this finding [258], and ovarian metastases were present in only 2 of 71 women studied at Memorial Sloan Kettering Cancer Center [240]. Moreover, there is no evidence that oophorectomy influences the results of therapy [151, 157, 233]. Accordingly, ovarian conservation is reasonable in premenopausal women. On the other hand, patients with low-grade smooth muscle neoplasms metastatic to the lung have responded to oophorectomy alone [3].

The literature provides conflicting reports on the efficacy of radiotherapy and chemotherapy in the management of leiomyosarcoma [144, 145, 155, 157, 178, 268, 402, 448]. Two series reported no effect of radiotherapy,

[33, 183], whereas the GOG series showed a lower relapse rate in patients with early-stage leiomyosarcoma when they were treated with combined radiation and surgery compared to patients treated with surgery alone (none versus 17%) [258]. Two recent reports on the use of radiation therapy to treat women with early stage (stage I or II) leiomyosarcoma detected no survival benefit for women who were treated with radiotherapy [348, 439]. The role of radiotherapy would appear to be limited given the conflicting reports on the radiosensitivity of leiomyosarcoma and its noncontroversial tendency to spread hematogenously. Advocates of adjuvant radiotherapy have argued that although survival is not changed, pelvic radiation prevents local and regional recurrences and thus is associated with an improvement in the quality of remaining life [151, 157, 183]. A recently reported randomized study that evaluated the value of adjuvant pelvic radiotherapy in women with stage I or II leiomyosarcoma found no increase in local control in radiated women [348].

Recurrent or metastatic leiomyosarcoma is very difficult to treat. A minority of patients responds to chemotherapy with doxorubicin [402, 403]. Localized pelvic or abdominal recurrences and solitary pulmonary metastases occasionally are amenable to surgical resection [108, 245]. Given the poor results obtained by surgery alone in early-stage leiomyosarcoma, there is an urgent need for effective adjuvant chemotherapy; unfortunately, no active regimen has been identified.

The variation in survival rates reported historically for leiomyosarcoma is largely a result of the use of different criteria for its diagnosis. Overall, 5-year survival rates in series using modern criteria range from 15% to 35% [41, 233, 332]. When only stage I and II tumors are considered, the 5-year survival rate is 40–70% [41, 145, 233, 268, 304, 305, 329, 332, 438]. The 3-year progression-free interval was 31% in a GOG series of 59 early-stage leiomyosarcomas; the first recurrence was in the pelvis in 14% of cases and in the lung in 41% [258].

The prognosis of leiomyosarcoma depends chiefly on stage. For stage I tumors, some investigators have found the size of the neoplasm to be an important prognostic factor [1]. In Evans' series, all patients with tumors larger than 5 cm died of disease, while only three of eight patients with tumors smaller than 5 cm died of disease [119]. In another series of metastasizing leiomyosarcomas, only 20% were less than 5 cm [199]. Premenopausal women have had a more favorable outcome in some series but not in others. Several series, including the large GOG study of early-stage leiomyosarcoma, have found mitotic index to be of prognostic significance [1, 145, 233, 258, 329, 332], whereas others have not [119]. A modification of the classification of [32] was employed as a grading scheme in one study and found to provide independent prognostic information [41]. A grading scheme designed for soft tissue neoplasms has been tested in uterine sarcomas and shown to have no prognostic significance [329, 332].

What should be incorporated in the pathology report in the face of these conflicting claims about prognostically relevant features? We do not grade leiomyosarcomas, as no universally agreed-upon grading scheme exists, but do comment on the features listed here: maximum tumor diameter, mitotic index, the presence or absence of necrosis and its extent if present, the nature of the tumor periphery (invasive or circumscribed), and the presence or absence of vascular space involvement.

A variety of practical issues relating to the management of leiomyosarcoma (including the problem of a diagnosis of leiomyosarcoma in a premenopausal patient after a myomectomy) has recently been presented [372].

Smooth Muscle Tumor of Uncertain Malignant Potential (STUMP)

This diagnosis is used when there is significant doubt about the failure rate associated with a particular combination of histologic features. With the acquisition of more clinicopathologic information about smooth muscle neoplasms, the size of this category has diminished. Some of the situations for which we currently employ this designation include the following:

1. The available clinicopathologic information about a differentiated type is scant, and there is, for whatever reason, some chance that the neoplasm might not be benign; this is true of myxoid and epithelioid neoplasms that lack tumor cell necrosis, have midrange atypia, and have moderately high mitotic indices.
2. There is uncertainty concerning the type of smooth muscle differentiation present, which would make a difference in the prediction of its clinical behavior.
3. There is uncertainty about the mitotic index, which would make a difference in the prediction made about the clinical behavior of the neoplasm. This situation most frequently occurs in smooth muscle neoplasms with standard smooth muscle differentiation that lack tumor cell necrosis, have moderate to severe atypia, have a mitotic index in the neighborhood of 10 MF/10 HPF, and have structures that could be regarded either as abnormal MF or smudged karyorrhectic nuclei, because counting them as MF would result in

a leiomyosarcoma diagnosis and as smudged nuclei would result in a diagnosis of atypical leiomyoma.

4. There is uncertainty about the presence or type of tumor cell necrosis. Sometimes the distinction between hyaline/infarction necrosis and tumor cell necrosis is ambiguous. There may be widespread individual cell necrosis or a pattern that could represent either early infarction or tumor cell necrosis [194].

Ip et al. recently reviewed cases of STUMP with adequate follow-up reported in the literature [194]. Depending on the subcategory of STUMP, 4–27% of tumors proved to be clinically malignant (i.e., they recurred or metastasized). In contrast to typical examples of leiomyosarcoma, recurrences in patients with STUMPs are often detected after a long interval, and long survival is possible after a recurrence. As discussed above in the section on leiomyosarcoma, histologic parameters together with the results of immunostaining for p16 and p53 may help to stratify patients with STUMPs into low- and high-risk categories. Diffuse strong staining for p16, especially when accompanied by diffuse strong staining for p53, appears to signify that a STUMP should be viewed as high risk [23, 194].

PEComa

PEComa is a rare, recently described neoplasm composed of cells showing "perivascular epithelioid cell" (PEC) differentiation [136, 419]. These cells, for which there is no known normal counterpart, have clear to eosinophilic cytoplasm and exhibit positive staining for smooth muscle and melanocytic markers [265]. In particular, HMB-45, Melan A, and microphthalmia transcription factor (MiTF) positivity is characteristic and smooth muscle markers (smooth muscle actin and desmin) are often positive. The PEC family of tumors includes, in addition to PEComa, angiomyolipoma and clear cell tumors of the lung and pancreas.

PEComas are neoplasms of adulthood, and when they involve the uterus they typically present either as a mass or cause uterine bleeding; they may be associated with lymphangioleiomyomatosis (LAM) and tuberous sclerosis. PEComas are usually solitary neoplasms ranging in size from 0.5 to 16.0 cm, although rarely multiple lesions are described. They may be either circumscribed or infiltrative with a nondistinctive texture and coloration. Microscopically, the low power impression is of either a compressive or, less commonly, an infiltrative neoplasm. Sometimes there is a tongue-like pattern of invasion of the myometrium reminiscent of the type of invasion seen in low-grade ESS (*Fig. 10.31*; [419]).

The tumor cells range from epithelioid to spindled, and they have moderate to abundant, clear-to-eosinophilic cytoplasm and well-defined cell borders (*Fig. 10.32*). The tumor cell cytoplasm sometimes has a distinctive granular or finely vacuolated bubbly

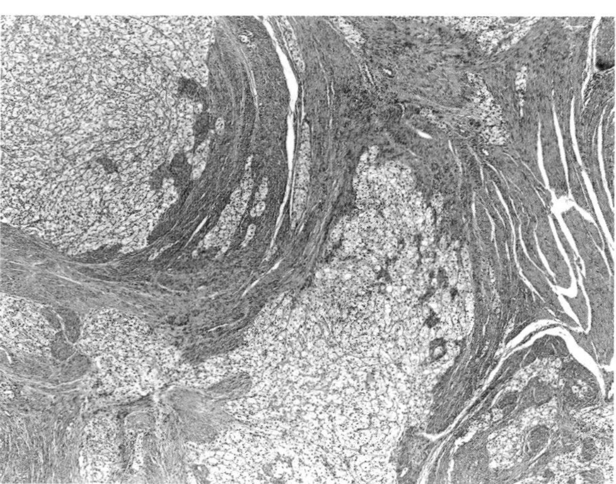

Fig. 10.31
PEComa. **In this uterine PEComa, tongues of pale tumors cells push through the myometrium in a pattern that is somewhat reminiscent of an endometrial stromal sarcoma**

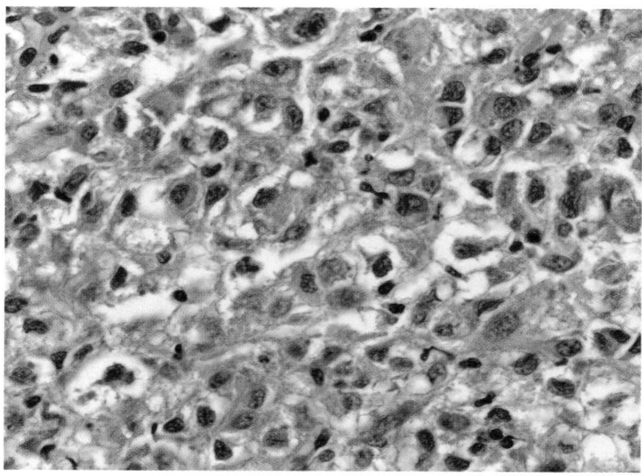

Fig. 10.32
PEComa. **The tumor is composed of nests and sheets of epithelioid tumor cells with flocculent eosinophilic cytoplasm and vesicular nuclei with coarse chromatin and conspicuous nucleoli**

appearance, particularly in spindle cells. The degree of nuclear atypia and the mitotic index are characteristically low and necrosis is uncommon, but tumors with significant atypia and frequent MF occur. A variant with abundant hyalinized stroma that can partially obscure the tumor cells has been reported [184].

Immunohistochemical study is essential to confirm the diagnosis. The most characteristic finding is patchy, positive HMB-45 staining of tumor cell cytoplasm (➋ *Fig. 10.33*). Other melanocytic markers such as Melan-A and microphthalmia transcription factor (MiTF) are also often positive; S-100 can be positive but it is more often negative [136]. Positive staining for smooth muscle markers is also typical. Smooth muscle actin is the smooth muscle marker that is most likely to be positive, but some tumors also stain for caldesmon or desmin [140]. Cytokeratin, CD117, and CD34 are generally negative. A minority of tumors shows positive staining for TFE3, a potential pitfall in the differential diagnosis with alveolar soft part sarcoma (ASPS; [136]). However, ASPS does not show staining for HMB-45 or smooth muscle actin. Electron microscopic study of one uterine PEComa that showed positive immunostaining for HMB-45 revealed premelanosomes in the tumor cells [326].

Both benign and malignant variants of PEComa (based on the extent of tumor at diagnosis or clinical follow-up) have been reported [107, 165]. In one recent review, 44% of corpus cases were classified as malignant and 56% as benign [121, 122]. Features proposed as being predictive of an unfavorable outcome include large size (>5 cm), high cellularity, significant nuclear atypia, mitotic activity (>1 MF/10 HPF), coagulative tumor cell necrosis, invasive growth, and lymphovascular space invasion [136]. Firm criteria for malignancy, as exist for uterine smooth muscle tumors, remain to be delineated. Benign tumors are those that are small (<5 cm), with low cellularity, a noninvasive periphery and absence of lymphovascular space invasion, a low mitotic count, and absence of nuclear atypia or tumor cell necrosis.

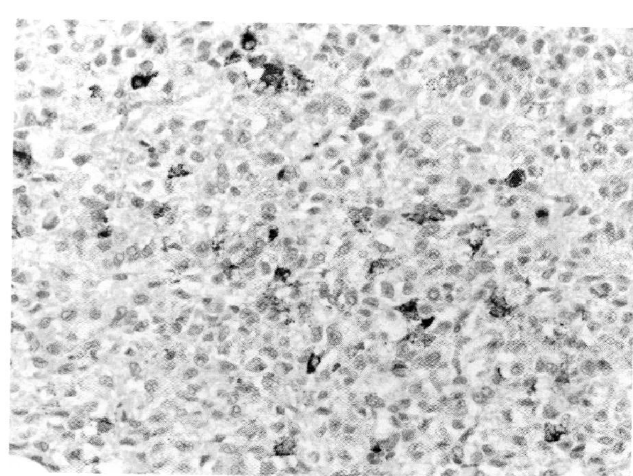

Fig. 10.33
Positive staining for HMB-45 in a uterine PEComa. Staining is typically patchy and often of medium intensity

The differential diagnosis includes ESS (HMB-45 negative), metastatic melanoma (S100 positive), and epithelioid smooth muscle neoplasms. In the uterus, there is dispute about whether PEComas are a distinct type of neoplasm or a variant of a smooth muscle neoplasm. Fueling this dispute is the non-specificity of HMB-45 positivity in mesenchymal neoplasms of the uterus. HMB-45 positivity has been reported in over one third of conventional uterine leiomyosarcomas [382], in epithelioid areas of otherwise conventional uterine leiomyosarcomas [190, 380], and in metastases from an epithelioid leiomyosarcoma [379]. It has been suggested that positive immunostaining for CD1a favors a diagnosis of PEComa over an epithelioid smooth muscle tumor [123], but the validity of this test needs to be verified by further study. Until the controversy is resolved, it is best to classify a tumor with the morphologic and immunohistochemical features of leiomyosarcoma as such, regardless of whether it stains for HMB-45, while noting the presence of features of a PEComa if present. Tumors that do not meet criteria for leiomyosarcoma and that exhibit the morphologic features of a PEComa, including positive staining for HMB-45, can be designated as PEComas, and grouped into benign and uncertain malignant potential groups based on the morphologic features noted above.

Lymphangioleiomyomatosis (LAM) and angiomyolipoma are two conditions in the same family as PEComa that are occasionally detected in the uterus. Angiomyolipoma is a benign tumor that contains abnormal blood vessels, fat, and spindled or epithelioid smooth muscle cells in varying proportions. HMB-45 positive tumor cells are present in the fat and among the smooth muscle cells. LAM is generally a microscopic finding in the uterus [168, 415]. It consists of dilated lymphovascular spaces associated with smooth muscle cells with flocculent eosinophilic cytoplasm (➋ *Fig. 10.34*), some of which show positive staining for HMB-45. There is a strong association between angiomyolipoma and LAM of the uterus and tuberous sclerosis, although not every patient with angiomyolipoma or LAM carries a diagnosis of tuberous sclerosis.

Endometrial Stromal Tumors

Endometrial stromal tumors are rare and can be benign or malignant (● *Table 10.6*). Benign endometrial stromal tumors are called stromal nodules; they are circumscribed, expansile, and do not invade the myometrium. Malignant stromal tumors are endometrial sarcomas. The more common low-grade sarcomas are called ESS, and the high-grade sarcomas are called UES. Endometrial sarcomas infiltrate the myometrium, invade vascular spaces, and have the capability to invade adjacent tissues and to metastasize. Several variants of endometrial stromal tumors exist, including tumors with histologic features reminiscent of ovarian sex cord–stromal tumors and tumors with smooth muscle differentiation. Most endometrial stromal tumors originate in the uterus, but rare examples arise outside the uterus, presumably in endometriosis [25, 58, 141, 220, 443].

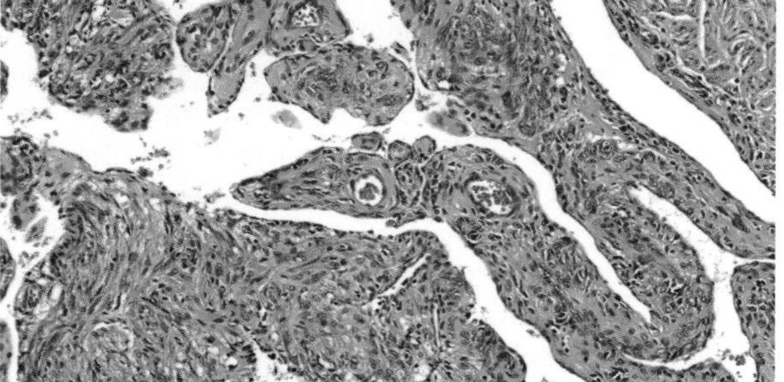

Fig. 10.34
Lymphangioleiomyomatosis involving the myometrium. The tumor cells are usually spindled with oval nuclei and flocculent eosinophilic cytoplasm. The growth is centered on dilated lymphovascular spaces, and intravascular growth is typically present, often at the periphery of the area of involvement. Sometimes, it mimics the appearance of intravascular endometrial stromal sarcoma

Endometrial Stromal Nodule

Endometrial stromal nodules are rare benign tumors composed mainly of endometrial stromal cells. [109, 126, 410] They represent less than a quarter of endometrial stromal tumors.

Clinical Features

Endometrial stromal nodules have been reported in women from 23 to 86 years of age. The average patient age is around 50 years, and about 75% of patients are premenopausal. There is no racial predisposition. The main symptom is abnormal uterine bleeding, which is occasionally severe enough to cause anemia. Pelvic or abdominal discomfort is a frequent complaint. Physical examination typically reveals uterine enlargement or a uterine mass. The average duration of symptoms before diagnosis is about 2 months. About 10% of patients are asymptomatic, and their tumors are found incidentally when hysterectomy is performed for another condition.

Gross Findings

Endometrial stromal nodules have a circumscribed contour and range from <1 cm to >20 cm in diameter; the average size is 5–6 cm (● *Fig. 10.35*). Many stromal nodules are polypoid and protrude into the uterine cavity.

Table 10.6
Classification of endometrial stromal tumors

Tumor	Category	Margin	Nuclear atypia	Nuclear pleomorphism	Usual mitotic activity (MF/10 HPF)
SN	Benign	Circumscribed	Minimal	Minimal	<3
ESS	Malignant, low grade	Invasive	Minimal	Minimal	<3
UES, monomorphic	Malignant, high grade	Invasive	Moderate to marked	Minimal to moderate	>10
UES, pleomorphic	Malignant, high grade	Invasive	Marked	Marked	>10

SN, Endometrial stromal nodule; ESS, Endometrial stromal sarcoma; UES, Undifferentiated endometrial sarcoma

Some of these are located entirely within the endometrium while others are submucosal. Nearly half of all stromal nodules are located entirely within the myometrium with no apparent connection to the endometrium. One unusual tumor was embedded in a term placenta [208]. Stromal nodules have fleshy-yellow or tan cut surfaces and they tend to bulge above the surrounding myometrium. Cystic changes are not uncommon and rare tumors contain foci of hemorrhage or necrosis. About 5% of patients have two or more nodules. The cervix is seldom involved.

Microscopic Findings

Stromal nodules have expansile, noninfiltrative margins that compress the surrounding endometrium and myometrium (➲ *Fig. 10.36*). Minor irregularities of the margin are common. Rarely one or a few fingerlike protrusions of tumor push into the adjacent myometrium, or small satellite nodules are present in the immediately adjacent myometrium (➲ *Fig. 10.37*). As long as these protrusions or satellites do not extend more than 3 mm from the main nodule and there is no vascular invasion the tumor is still regarded as a stromal nodule [109, 410]. More extensive invasion or vascular invasion indicates that the tumor is a stromal sarcoma, not a stromal nodule. It is important to be aware of the gross pathologic appearance of a stromal nodule and to know which sections are from the interior of the tumor and which show the interface with the surrounding myometrium. Alternating areas of stromal, fibrous, and smooth muscle differentiation within a stromal nodule can be misinterpreted as myoinvasion if endometrial stromal cells interdigitate with well-developed bundles of metaplastic smooth muscle.

Endometrial stromal nodules consist of cells that closely resemble normal proliferative-phase endometrial stromal cells. The tumor cells have uniform, small, darkly staining, round or oval nuclei with finely granular chromatin and inconspicuous nucleoli (➲ *Fig. 10.38*). The cytoplasm varies from scanty to moderate, and cell borders tend to be poorly defined. A reticulin network encircles individual cells. Mitotic activity ranges from none to more than 15 MF/10 HPF but it is usually low (<3 MF/10 HPF). MF cannot be identified in about 50% of stromal nodules, and >5 MF/10 HPF are detected in only 5–10% of them. Myxoid or fibrous stromal changes occasionally occur in stromal nodules, and if extensive they can obscure the diagnosis [322]. In such cases it is essential to thoroughly study the tumor to find foci of typical endometrial stromal differentiation. Smooth muscle differentiation is common in endometrial stromal nodules (➲ *Fig. 10.39*). The smooth muscle cells are typically spindle-shaped with fusiform blunt-ended nuclei and fibrillar eosinophilic cytoplasm, but they are occasionally epithelioid with rounded nuclei and moderate eosinophilic cytoplasm. Epithelioid smooth muscle cells are often embedded in aggregates of hyalinized collagen. In the past, endometrial stromal tumors with extensive smooth muscle

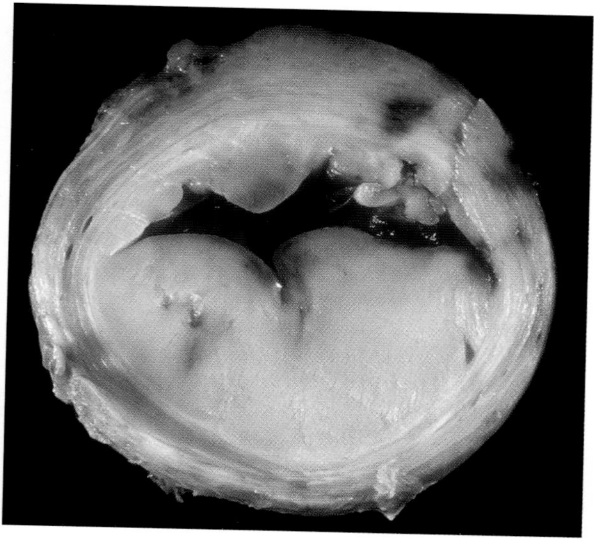

Fig. 10.35
Endometrial stromal nodule. **The nodule is circumscribed with no evidence of invasion into the surrounding myometrium. It has a homogeneous tan cut surface, quite different from a leiomyoma. There is central cystic change**

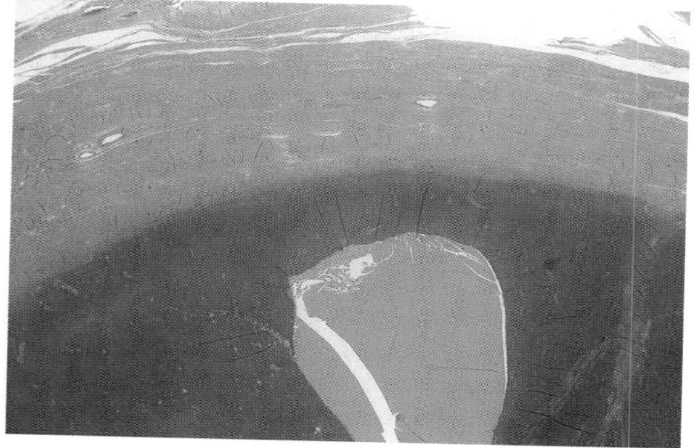

Fig. 10.36
Endometrial stromal nodule. **Note the circumscribed pushing margin. Expansile growth without invasion into the surrounding myometrium characterizes a stromal nodule**

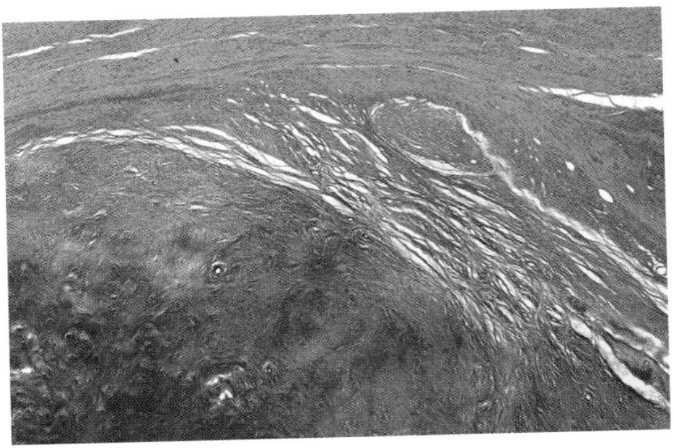

■ Fig. 10.37
Endometrial stromal nodule. **This nodule has a mainly circumscribed periphery, but there is a focal irregularity with a small satellite nodule. As long as irregularities or satellites extend no more than 3 mm from the main nodule and there is no vascular invasion, a diagnosis of stromal nodule is still appropriate. If the extent of invasion is >3 mm or there is vascular invasion, the tumor should be classified as an endometrial stromal sarcoma**

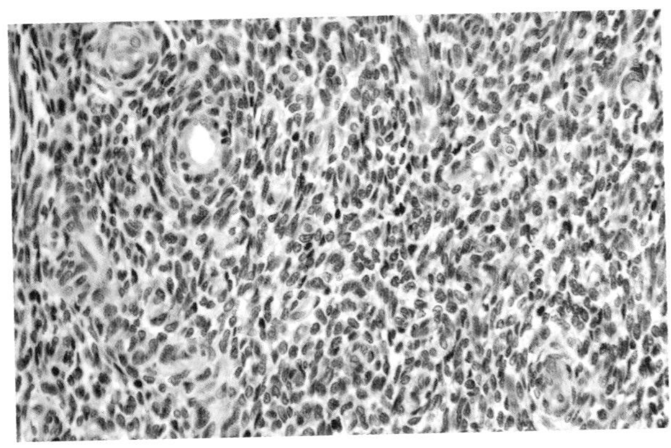

■ Fig. 10.38
Endometrial stromal nodule. **The tumor is cellular and is composed of uniform bland endometrial stromal cells with round to oval nuclei and scanty cytoplasm. Mitotic figures are infrequent. Note the conspicuous evenly distributed small arterioles**

differentiation (>30%) were classified as combined stromal–smooth muscle tumors [317], but since it appears that the endometrial stromal cell component determines the clinical behavior, it makes sense to classify all such tumors as endometrial stromal nodules with smooth muscle differentiation.

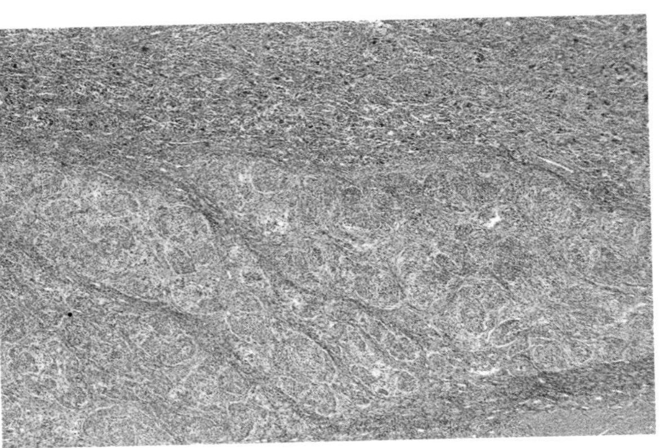

■ Fig. 10.39
Endometrial stromal nodule with smooth muscle differentiation. **Bundles of spindled smooth muscle cells (*bottom*) are juxtaposed with sheets of small dark stromal cells (*top*)**

Stromal nodules are highly vascular. Small uniformly distributed arterioles are invariably present and can be readily appreciated at low magnification in most, but not all, stromal nodules; sometimes it is necessary to search for them at higher magnification. Large thick-walled blood vessels are occasionally present, especially in areas of smooth muscle differentiation. Hyaline plaques and areas of hyaline fibrosis are common in stromal nodules. Epithelial or sex cord-like arrangements of cells, such as cords or trabeculae of tumor cells or gland-like structures, are sometimes seen in stromal nodules (➋ *Fig. 10.40*). If sex cord-like differentiation is especially prominent, a uterine tumor resembling an ovarian sex cord tumor (UTROSCT) should be considered. Uncommon findings that are occasionally noted in stromal nodules include predominance of epithelioid stromal cells with abundant eosinophilic cytoplasm [316], striated muscle cells [251], decidual changes, aggregates of foam cells, cysts, areas of infarction, and calcifications.

Immunohistochemistry and Molecular Pathology

Immunohistochemistry can help confirm the diagnosis of a stromal nodule and it is helpful in the differential diagnosis between a stromal nodule and a highly cellular leiomyoma. Stromal nodules exhibit variable staining for smooth muscle actin and other smooth muscle markers such as desmin and caldesmon [320, 321]. Staining is often weak and focal; staining for desmin and caldesmon is absent in most stromal tumors [104, 309]. Foci of

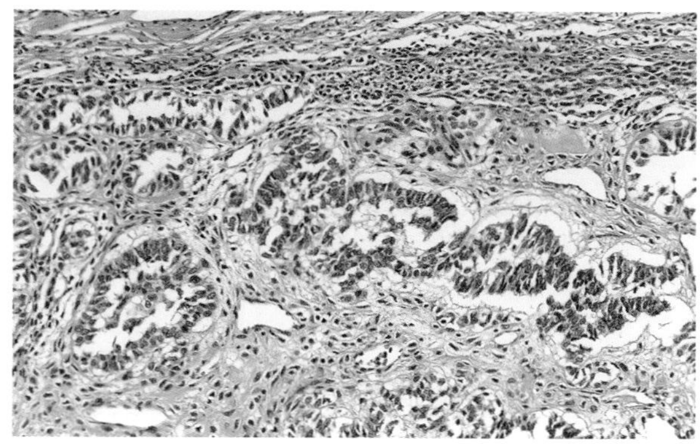

Fig. 10.40
Focal sex cord-like differentiation in an endometrial stromal nodule. **Cords and gland like arrangements of low columnar cells are surrounded by fibrous and endometrial-type stroma**

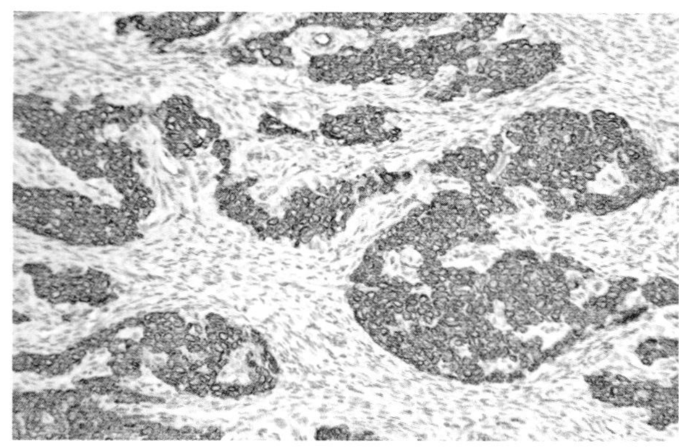

Fig. 10.41
Smooth muscle differentiation in an endometrial stromal nodule. **The bundles of smooth muscle cells show strong immunoreactivity for smooth muscle actin, while the surrounding endometrial stromal cells show no staining**

smooth muscle differentiation are of course usually positive for all smooth muscle markers (*Fig. 10.41*). CD10 is a good marker for endometrial stromal cells and is positive in nearly all stromal nodules [277]. In stromal nodules with smooth muscle differentiation, staining for CD10 is present in smooth muscle cells as well as in endometrial stromal cells [320]. Endometrial stromal cells show nuclear staining for WT-1 and the cells in stromal nodules are positive for this marker in a majority of cases [401]. Immunostains for estrogen and progesterone receptors are generally positive in endometrial stromal nodules, and some of them exhibit staining for androgen receptors as well [288].

Cytogenetic abnormalities occur in endometrial stomal neoplasms, including endometrial stromal nodules. The most common abnormality is a t(7;17)(p15q21) that results in a JAZF1–JJAZ1 gene fusion [221]. The translocation, which was present in four of four stromal nodules in a recent study [308], can be detected by traditional cytogenetics, as well as by molecular pathologic tests such as reverse transcriptase–polymerase chain reaction and fluorescence in situ hybridization. In stromal nodules with smooth muscle differentiation, the translocation is present both in the endometrial stromal component and in the smooth muscle component, suggesting a common cell of origin for both elements [318]. At present, testing for the translocation is a research procedure, not a clinical diagnostic test.

Differential Diagnosis

The main differential diagnostic considerations are low-grade ESS and highly cellular leiomyoma. Diagnosis of a low-grade ESS requires identification of more extensive myoinvasion than is allowable in a stromal nodule: invasion >3 mm from the periphery of the nodule or into blood vessels. The maximum allowable distance of invasion of 3 mm is an arbitrary one, chosen to minimize the likelihood that a tumor designated as a stromal nodule will prove to be malignant. When an endometrial stromal tumor is identified in an endometrial biopsy or curettage, it is difficult or impossible to determine whether it is invasive, since the tumor margin cannot be adequately evaluated. The likely diagnosis in such cases is a low-grade ESS, since stromal sarcomas are far more common than stromal nodules, but it is often necessary to make the nonspecific diagnosis of an "endometrial stromal tumor." It is then usually necessary for the patient to have a hysterectomy for diagnostic purposes to provide adequate visualization of the periphery of the tumor. In some cases, it is possible to identify myoinvasion or vascular invasion in curetted tissue fragments, indicating that the tumor is a stromal sarcoma. It is important to be cautious when considering a diagnosis of stromal sarcoma in curettings, since fragments of a stromal nodule with smooth muscle differentiation can simulate myoinvasion and prompt a mistaken diagnosis of stromal sarcoma [251].

Cellular leiomyomas, especially the variant designated as highly cellular leiomyoma, can be misdiagnosed as endometrial stromal nodules, which they closely resemble

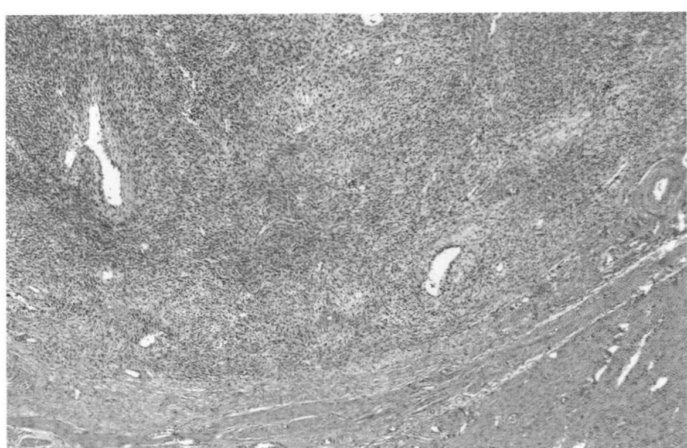

Fig. 10.42
Highly cellular leiomyoma. **The tumor is circumscribed and cellular like a stromal nodule, but the tumor cells are slightly larger and have more abundant eosinophilic cytoplasm. The blood vessels are larger than in a stromal nodule. The tumor cells showed strong positive staining for desmin, but were CD10 negative**

microscopically [321]. They are circumscribed tumors that are composed of small round to oval cells with scanty cytoplasm (*Fig. 10.42*). Highly cellular leiomyomas often interdigitate with the surrounding myometrium, and hence microscopically they sometimes appear less circumscribed than a stromal nodule. It is not uncommon to see a transition from round cells with scanty cytoplasm in the center of the tumor to short spindled cells with more abundant eosinophilic cytoplasm at the periphery, to easily recognizable spindle-shaped smooth muscle cells in the surrounding myometrium. Fascicular growth of tumor cells is usually present, at least focally. The cells in highly cellular leiomyomas tend to be larger than those in stromal nodules, and they may have a distinctive rim of eosinophilic cytoplasm. Leiomyomas lack the numerous arterioles that are present in stromal nodules, but they often contain conspicuous large thick-walled blood vessels. Immunohistochemistry can help in the differential diagnosis. Smooth muscle tumors tend to be positive for all commonly used smooth muscle markers, such as smooth muscle actin, smooth muscle myosin, desmin and caldesmon (*Table 10.7*). They are less likely than stromal nodules to stain for CD10, although some do; staining for CD10, when present, is likely to be weak or focal. Highly cellular leiomyoma shows positive nuclear staining for WT-1, so this marker is not helpful in the distinction between a stromal nodule and a highly cellular leiomyoma. Since the staining patterns of stromal nodules and highly cellular leiomyomas overlap, it is important to

Table 10.7
Immunohistochemical findings in endometrial stromal and smooth muscle tumors

Antibody	Stromal tumor	Smooth muscle tumor
Smooth muscle actin	0 to ++	++ to +++
Desmin	0 to +	++ to +++
Caldesmon	0	++ to +++
CD10	+ to +++	0 to +

perform a panel of immunostains, typically including CD10, smooth muscle actin, desmin, and caldesmon, and to interpret the results in conjunction with the histology of the tumor.

Clinical Behavior and Treatment

With one exception [214], which was probably an ESS, all stromal nodules reported to date have had a benign clinical evolution [57, 410]. Nevertheless, hysterectomy is usually the appropriate therapy because the periphery of the tumor must be thoroughly evaluated to be certain that it is completely circumscribed and noninvasive. In occasional cases, usually involving tumors occurring in young women, small nodules that can be completely excised by polypectomy or myomectomy may be treated by local excision rather than hysterectomy. Six of the 60 patients reported by Tavassoli and Norris were treated in this fashion and none had a recurrence [410]. In one case, excision of a stromal nodule was possible after a course of treatment with leuprolide acetate [367]. Neither minor irregularities of the margin nor the presence of frequent MF appear to imply an unfavorable prognosis. It is possible that patients with limited myoinvasion beyond 3 mm (i.e., 3 mm to 1 cm and no vascular invasion) may have a favorable outcome, but there is insufficient follow-up of such patients to be certain. It has been proposed that tumors of this type be designated "endometrial stromal tumors with limited infiltration" [109] or as "low grade endometrial stromal sarcoma with limited infiltration" [26].

Endometrial Stromal Sarcoma (ESS)

ESS is a tumor of endometrial stromal cells that invades the myometrium. ESS was traditionally divided into two categories, low-grade and high-grade ESS, but in the current WHO classification only low-grade stromal sarcoma (LGSS) is called ESS [409]. High-grade tumors are now designated as UES. In this chapter (➲ *Table 10.6*), we designate LGSS as "endometrial stromal sarcoma (ESS)" and high-grade tumors as "undifferentiated endometrial sarcoma (UES)." The prevalence of ESS is difficult to estimate because of diagnosis and classification issues. In a recent large study from Norway (which excluded carcinosarcoma), 20% of uterine sarcomas were ESS and 6% were UES [1].

Clinical Features

ESS occurs at an earlier age than most other uterine malignancies. The mean age is between 42 and 53 years [56, 236], and more than 50% of patients are premenopausal. Rare examples occur in young women or girls. There is no association with any of the endometrial carcinoma risk factors, but occasional patients have a history of prior pelvic irradiation. A few cases of ESS have been reported in women treated for breast cancer with tamoxifen. The main symptoms are abnormal vaginal bleeding and abdominal pain [215]. The uterus is typically enlarged and has an irregular contour. A few women have bulky polypoid tumors that protrude from the cervical os. The usual clinical impression is that the patient has a uterine leiomyoma that is causing an exceptional degree of bleeding. Occasional patients present with intra-abdominal or pulmonary metastases. ESS usually cannot be detected on Papanicolaou smears because the cells lack sufficient atypia to permit their differentiation from benign endometrial stromal cells [337].

Stromal tumors that involve the endometrium can be recognized in endometrial biopsies and curettings. A definitive diagnosis of stromal sarcoma can be made if myometrial invasion is identified in the tissue fragments or with imaging studies, but a hysterectomy is usually required to permit the thorough evaluation of the tumor margin necessary to distinguish an ESS from a benign stromal nodule. Because ESS are considerably more common than stromal nodules, a stromal tumor found in an endometrial biopsy or curettage is likely to be malignant. As discussed earlier, endometrial stromal tumors must be differentiated from highly cellular leiomyomas because the treatment of these tumors is quite different. At surgery, ESS may resemble IVL or a leiomyoma that has extended into the parametrium or broad ligament. These entities can usually be distinguished on frozen section examination.

Gross Findings

ESS usually involves the endometrium, sometimes extensively. It forms soft, tan, smooth-surfaced polyps that are occasionally partly infarcted and hemorrhagic (➲ *Fig. 10.43*). By definition, ESS invades the myometrium. There are three main patterns of growth within the myometrium. In the first, the myometrium is diffusely thickened, but a clearly defined tumor is not evident. In the second, there is a nodular tumor with soft, tan or yellow-orange cut surfaces, as opposed to the white, whorled, firm surface of a leiomyoma. In the third, and most frequent, pattern of growth the myometrium is permeated by poorly demarcated pink, tan, or yellow cords and nodules of tumor (➲ *Fig. 10.44*).

ESS grows beyond the uterus as infiltrating masses of tan or white tumor that can be palpated as firm cords in the parauterine tissues. Pink or tan strands of tumor protrude from the cut surface of the infiltrated tissues and sometimes can be pulled from tissue spaces and vessels. Intravenous growth extending into the inferior vena cava has been reported, and in very rare cases there is extension or metastasis to the heart [252, 404].

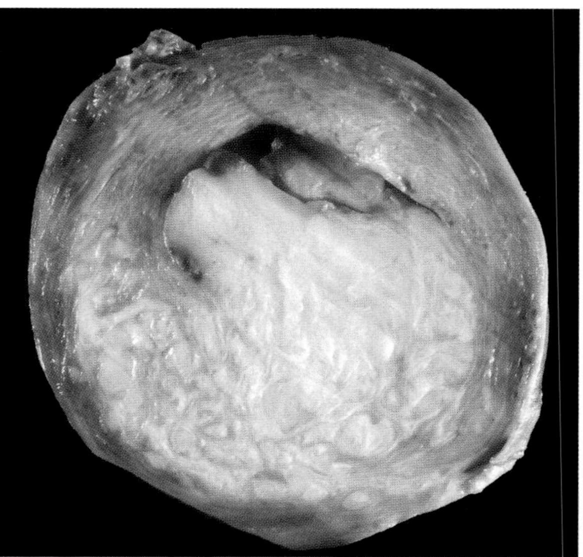

◘ Fig. 10.43
Endometrial stromal sarcoma. **Fleshy tan-white polypoid tumor grows into the endometrial cavity and cords of tumor extensively infiltrate the myometrium, resulting in a thickened uterine wall almost entirely infiltrated by tumor**

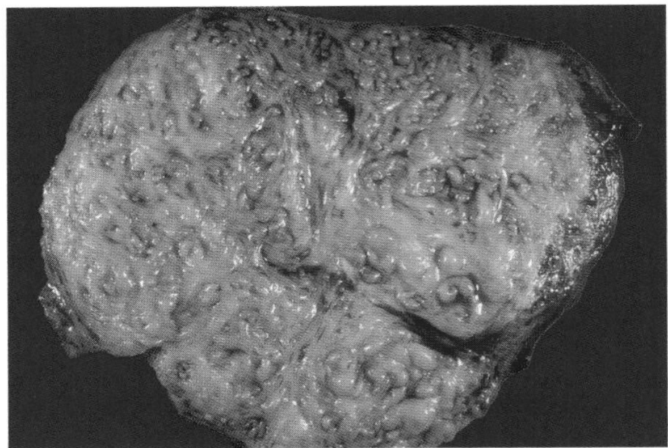

Fig. 10.44
Endometrial stromal sarcoma. **The cut surface of endometrial stromal sarcoma often has a trabeculated appearance caused by diffuse myometrial permeation by cords and nodules of yellow tan tumor. Sometimes, tumor can be grossly identified within vascular spaces. This appearance is quite different from what is seen on the cut surface of a leiomyoma**

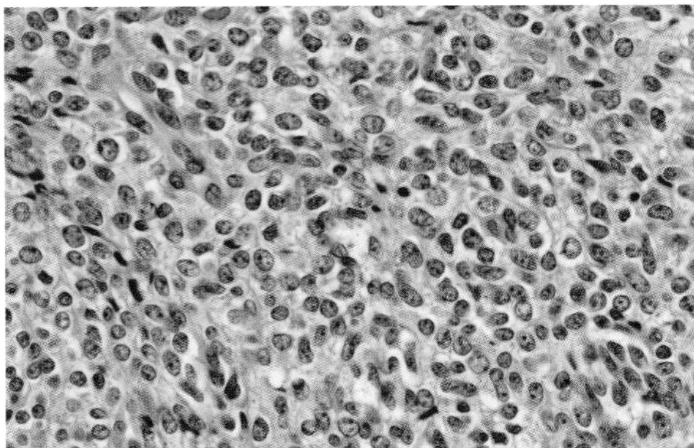

Fig. 10.45
Endometrial stromal sarcoma. **Endometrial stromal sarcoma is composed of cells that resemble the stromal cells in proliferative endometrium. They have uniform round or oval nuclei, finely granular chromatin, small or no nucleoli, and scanty cytoplasm with ill-defined cell borders**

Microscopic Findings

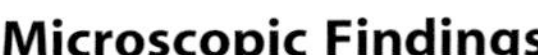

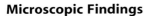

ESS cells resemble proliferative phase or hyperplastic endometrial stromal cells. ESS are low-grade tumors with cells of relatively uniform size and shape, imparting a monotonous appearance to the tumor. The tumor cells have round or ovoid nuclei with finely granular dispersed chromatin and small, inconspicuous nucleoli (➲ *Fig. 10.45*). The cytoplasm is amphophilic, and the cell borders are poorly defined. Rare tumors contain cells with bizarre or multiple nuclei; the nuclei can appear degenerated and have the type of smudged chromatin seen in "symplastic" leiomyomas [27]. Some ESS consist predominantly of spindle-shaped cells that are fibroblastic or myofibroblastic in appearance with fusiform nuclei and elongated cell bodies (➲ *Fig. 10.46*) [322, 441]. Such tumors have variable amounts of collagen in the background and at the extreme can appear fibrous. Other unusual variants include tumors in which the cells have clear cytoplasm, abundant eosinophilic cytoplasm resulting in an epithelioid appearance [316, 159], abundant granular eosinophilic cytoplasm resulting in an oxyphilic appearance, and hyaline perinuclear cytoplasmic inclusions resulting in a rhabdoid appearance [273]. Reticulin fibers surround individual cells or small groups of cells in a basket-weave pattern. Mitotic activity is low in most ESS. There are typically <3 MF/10 HPF, but there can be greater mitotic activity in neoplasms that are otherwise typical of ESS; occasionally there are >10 MF/10 HPF [118]. Proliferation of small vessels and arterioles resembling endometrial spiral arterioles is a characteristic finding (➲ *Fig. 10.47*) that is generally present at least focally in an ESS. The arterioles tend to be uniformly distributed among the stromal cells, and capillaries and small veins are often conspicuous as well. Occasionally whorls of tumor cells surround the arterioles.

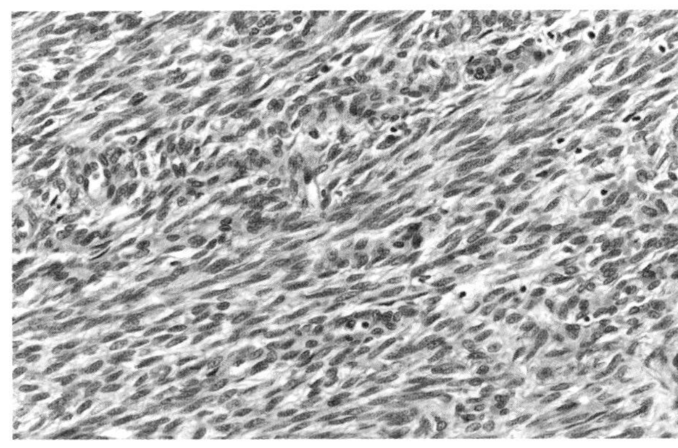

Fig. 10.46
Fibroblastic/myofibroblastic variant of endometrial stromal sarcoma. **The tumor cells have oval or fusiform nuclei and are spindled with eosinophilic cytoplasm. There is fibrillar collagenous matrix in the background**

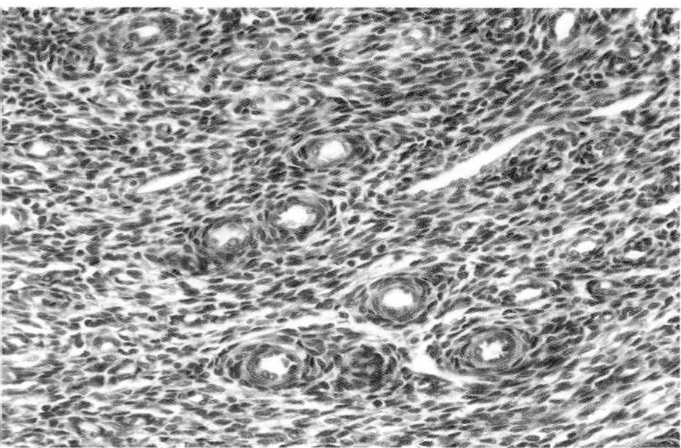

Fig. 10.47
Endometrial stromal sarcoma. **Note the numerous small blood vessels distributed relatively uniformly among the tumor cells**

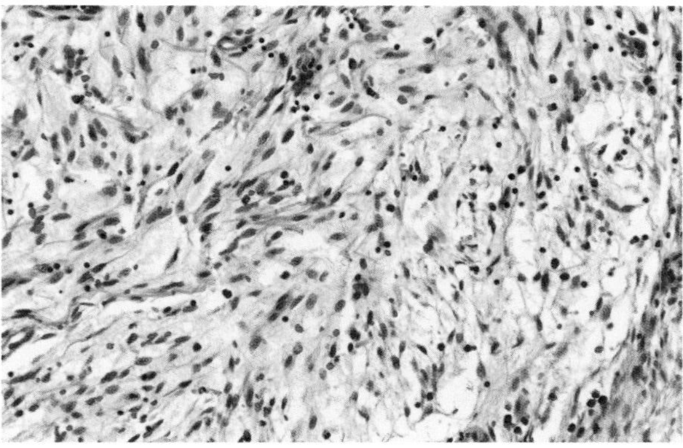

Fig. 10.49
Myxoid variant of endometrial stromal sarcoma. **Abundant pale myxoid stroma separates the tumor cells. Scattered inflammatory cells are also present**

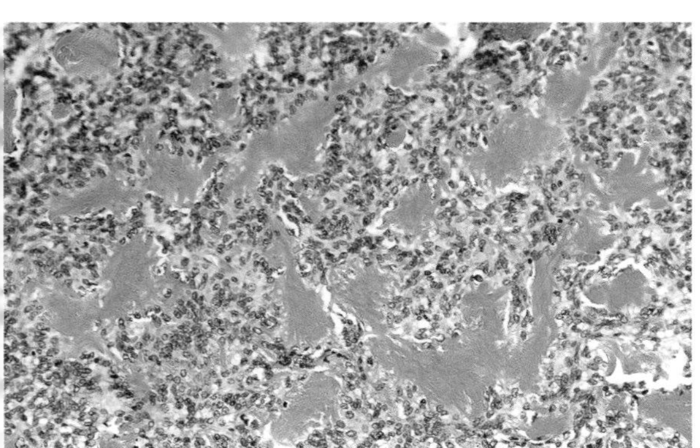

Fig. 10.48
Endometrial stromal sarcoma. **Eosinophilic hyaline material in an endometrial stromal sarcoma. Hyaline plaques and nodules are commonly present in endometrial stromal sarcomas and endometrial stromal nodules, and favor the diagnosis of a stromal tumor over a smooth muscle tumor**

Plaques and zones of hyaline fibrosis (*Fig. 10.48*) are common in LGSS, and aggregates of foam cells or foci of necrosis are occasionally noted. Rarely, abundant myxoid stroma widely separates the tumor cells (*Fig. 10.49*; [322]). Tumors with abundant myxoid stroma are classified as myxoid variants of ESS. The stromal cells can show focal or diffuse decidual changes in patients who are pregnant or taking exogenous progestins. Smooth muscle differentiation is not uncommonly present in ESS, as it is in stromal nodules. Tumors in which the proportion of smooth muscle cells exceeds 30% have been classified as combined stromal–smooth muscle tumors, but since the stromal component appears to determine the clinical behavior we favor classifying such tumors as ESS with smooth muscle differentiation. Smooth muscle differentiation can take the form of typical smooth muscle cells growing as bundles of spindle-shaped myoid cells with fibrillar eosinophilic cytoplasm, as epithelioid cells that are sometimes embedded in collagen resulting in a "starburst"-like appearance, or as whorls of cells resulting in a vaguely meningothelial appearance [446]. More unusual types of differentiation that occasionally occur in ESS include the presence of striated muscle cells and fat; the clinical significance of striated muscle cells in an ESS is unclear [27].

ESS invades the myometrium and may extensively permeate it (*Figs. 10.50* and *10.51*). Invasion of vascular channels is a characteristic finding (*Fig. 10.52*). Immunohistochemical staining for blood vascular and lymphovascular endothelial cells indicates that ESS mainly invades blood vessels. Rare ESS have been identified in association with placental tissues, usually in decidua adjacent to the placenta [210]. Epithelial-like differentiation occurs in about 25% of ESS. It is highly variable in its appearance and can take the form of trabecular cords of epithelioid cells, mesothelial-like tubules lined by cuboidal or low columnar cells with eosinophilic cytoplasm, endometrial-type glands, or glands lined by clear or vacuolated cells (*Fig. 10.53*). The epithelial-like pattern is cordlike or trabecular and reminiscent of an ovarian sex cord tumor in some instances. In other tumors, glands lined by columnar endometrial type cells are present focally or extensively within the ESS (*Fig. 10.54*) [77].

Endometrial glandular differentiation can make it difficult to recognize that the tumor is a stromal sarcoma, not florid adenomyosis [275]. Findings that favor an ESS with glandular differentiation include an invasive growth pattern, vascular invasion, and the absence of glands in parts of the tumor, which then have the typical appearance of ESS. Glandular differentiation can be present in the uterine primary or in metastatic sites [50, 77].

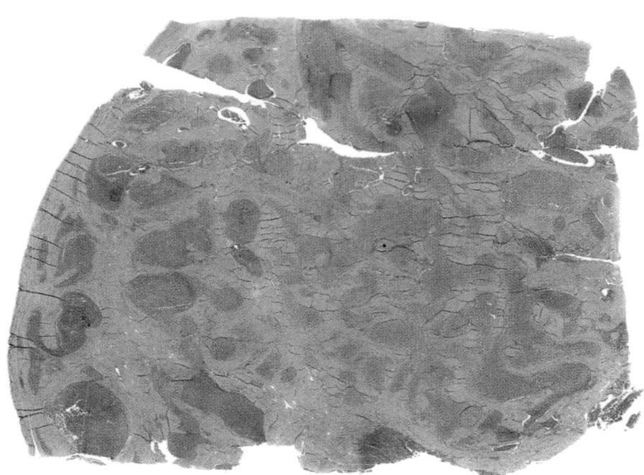

Fig. 10.50
Endometrial stromal sarcoma. **Whole mount showing extensive myometrial invasion by blue stained tongues and nests of tumor cells**

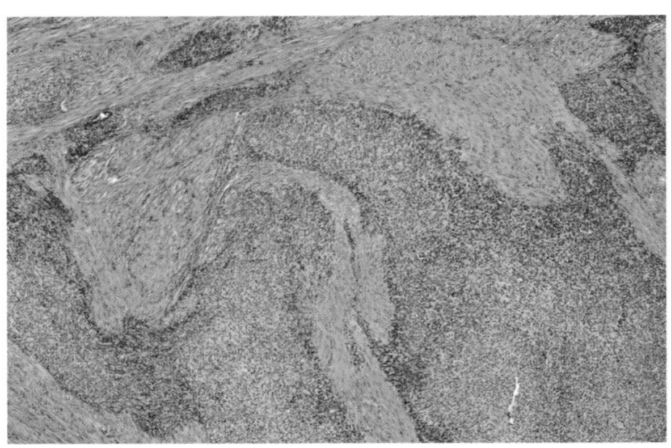

Fig. 10.51
Endometrial stromal sarcoma. **Irregular tongues and prongs of tumor cells invade the myometrium, pushing between bundles of smooth muscle cells**

Immunohistochemistry and Molecular Pathology

Immunostains for cytoplasmic thin and intermediate filaments can be useful in the diagnosis of ESS. Although stromal sarcoma cells are immunoreactive for vimentin, other tumors in the differential diagnosis, such as smooth muscle tumors, are also vimentin positive. Staining for vimentin is therefore mainly used to verify that a tumor is

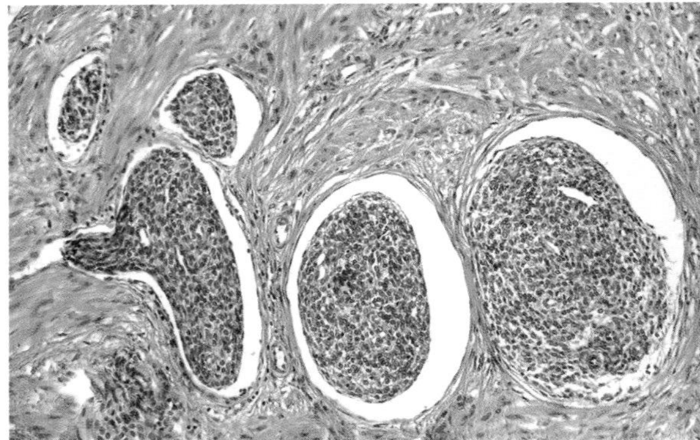

Fig. 10.52
Endometrial stromal sarcoma. **Vascular invasion is a common finding in endometrial stromal sarcoma. Immunohistochemical staining reveals that the vascular endothelial cells typically stain for CD31 but not for D2-40, suggesting that the invaded vessels are veins, not lymphatic vessels**

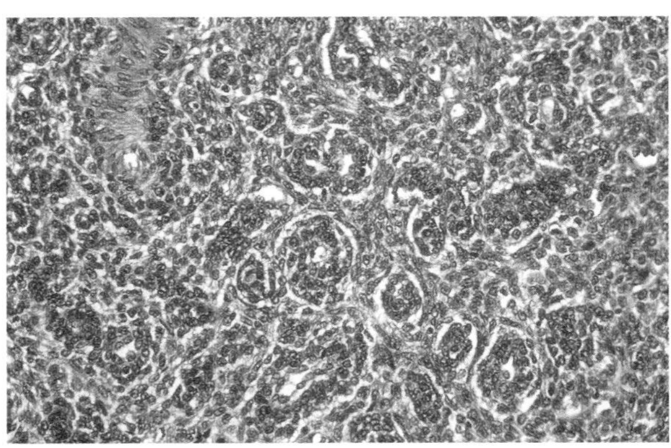

Fig. 10.53
Endometrial stromal sarcoma. **Epithelial-like differentiation in an endometrial stromal sarcoma. In this tumor, poorly formed tubules are lined by small polygonal cells with nuclei that are not unlike those in the surrounding stromal cells**

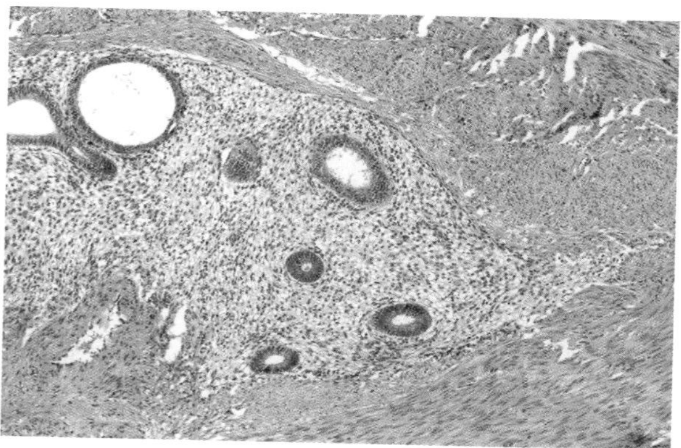

Fig. 10.54
Glands in endometrial stromal sarcoma. **Rare endometrial stromal sarcomas contain endometrial-type glands within myoinvasive nests of endometrial stromal cells**

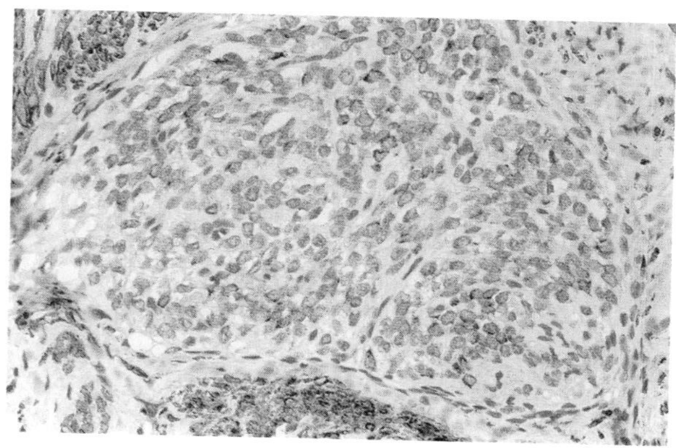

Fig. 10.56
Weak desmin staining in an endometrial stromal sarcoma. **The surrounding smooth muscle fascicles are strongly positive**

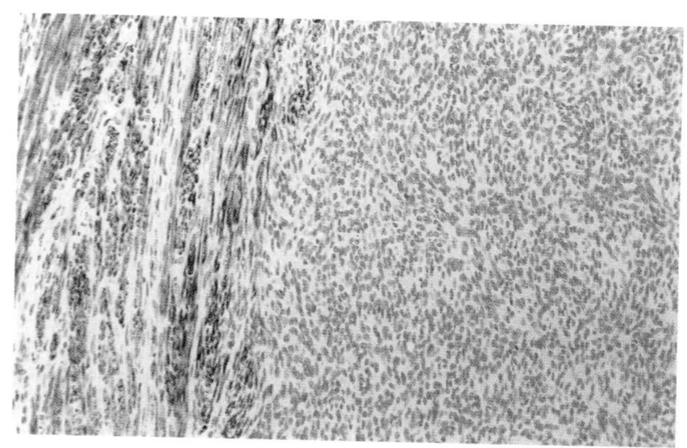

Fig. 10.55
No staining for desmin in this endometrial stromal sarcoma. **The myometrium, on the left, is strongly positive**

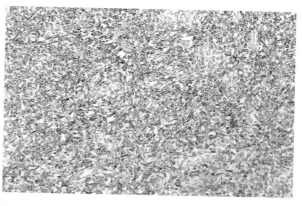

Fig. 10.57
Strong positive staining for cytokeratin in an endometrial stromal sarcoma. **A cytokeratin cocktail composed of AE1/AE3 and CAM5.2 was used**

adequately preserved for immunohistochemical testing. Immunoreactivity for actin and desmin has been reported in ESS, but our experience, like that of others, is that most ESS either lack these filaments or express them only weakly. Actin, as detected by antibodies to smooth muscle actin, is the more likely of the two to be expressed, and occasional tumors exhibit diffuse strong staining for actin filaments. ESS cells generally either do not stain for desmin (*Fig. 10.55*) or show only focal and weak reactivity (*Fig. 10.56*). Although occasional ESS exhibit diffuse or strong staining for desmin, this is uncommon and diffuse strong staining for both actin and desmin suggests that the tumor is a small cell smooth muscle tumor that simulates a stromal neoplasm or, particularly if the staining is focal, that there is smooth muscle differentiation in the tumor. Of the muscle markers, caldesmon is the one that is least likely to stain ESS tumor cells [360]; it usually stains only areas of smooth muscle differentiation. Staining for keratin is reported in 0–50% of ESS (*Fig. 10.57*; [6]). The frequency of staining depends in part on the keratin antibody that is used. A keratin cocktail that includes AE1/AE3 is most likely to show positive staining, which appears to be mainly due to staining for CK19 [6]. Some authors report that ESS are frequently cytokeratin positive [38], although our experience, like that of others [35], is that only occasional ESS are keratin

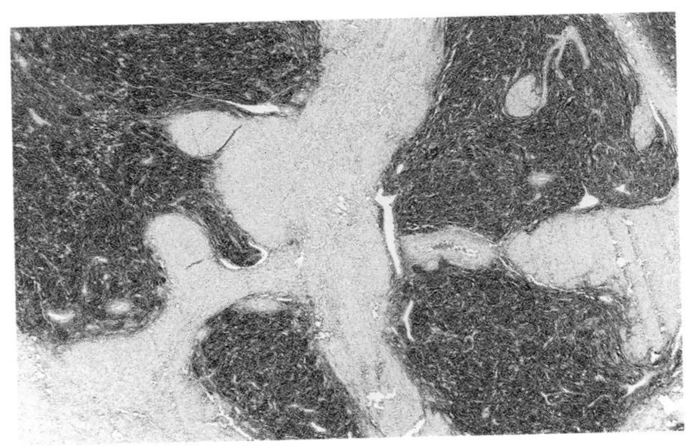

Fig. 10.58
Strong staining for CD10 in endometrial stromal sarcoma. **Invasive nests of endometrial stromal sarcoma are strongly CD10 positive, while the myometrium is completely CD10 negative**

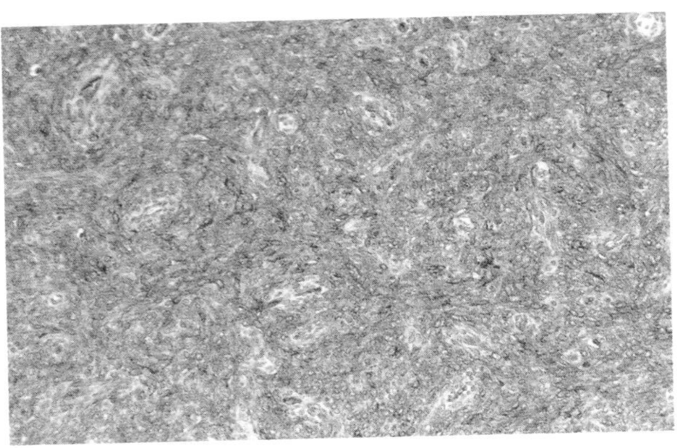

Fig. 10.59
Strong positive cytoplasmic staining for CD10 in endometrial stromal sarcoma. **This is a characteristic of endometrial stromal sarcomas**

positive. Positive staining can be diffuse or confined to the epithelial-like structures seen in some ESS. Staining for EMA is negative. CD10 is the most useful positive marker for ESS (*Fig. 10.58*; [8, 35, 64]). The tumor cell cytoplasm often shows strong positive staining for CD10 (*Fig. 10.59*), although in some tumors staining is variable and present only focally [277]. Smooth muscle tumors tend to be CD10 negative or show focal weak staining. WT-1 is positive in the tumor cell nuclei in most ESS [8, 84]. Nuclear staining for beta-catenin is reported to be present in ESS, but not in cellular leiomyomas, although the proportion of ESS that show positive staining is as low as 40% [201, 227, 298]. The epithelial or sex cord-like structures that are present in about a quarter of ESS have a mixed epithelial–myogenic phenotype [249]. They may stain for cytokeratin but staining for EMA is negative. They also tend to stain strongly for vimentin, muscle-specific actin, and, in some instances, desmin [315]. Occasionally, these epithelial-like structures stain for calretinin, and the ones that resemble sex cord derivatives can be immunoreactive for inhibin and CD99 (see section Uterine Tumors Resembling an Ovarian Sex Cord Tumor) [28]. ESS is not immunoreactive for CD34; this helps in the evaluation of extrauterine metastases, where the differential diagnosis may include such CD34-positive tumors as hemangiopericytoma and solitary fibrous tumor [35].

Immunostains for proliferation markers such as Ki-67 (MIB-1) stain the nuclei of cycling tumor cells; the percentage of positive nuclei generally correlates with the degree of mitotic activity, which in ESS tends to be low.

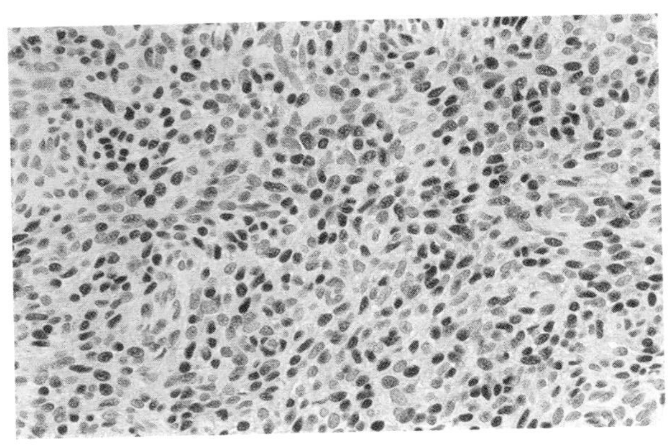

Fig. 10.60
Strong nuclear staining for progesterone receptors, in this endometrial stromal sarcoma. **Staining for estrogen receptors was also positive**

Estrogen and progesterone receptors can be demonstrated in most ESS (*Fig. 10.60*; [35, 351]), and some exhibit positive nuclear staining for androgen receptors [288]. Positive immunohistochemical staining for hormone receptors can be used to guide therapy in those instances in which the clinician is contemplating treatment with progestins or some other form of hormonal therapy. ESS rarely show staining for CD117 (c-KIT) or show c-kit mutations [218, 295, 320]. Nevertheless, a few responses to imatinib therapy have been reported.

A variety of cytogenetic abnormalities have been reported in ESS [364]. The most common is a recurrent translocation involving chromosomes 7 and

17 [t(7;17)(p15;q21)] [94]. Other abnormalities include rearrangements involving the short arm of chromosome 7, especially 7p21~p15 and the short arm of chromosome 6, particularly 6p21. As a result of the (7;17)(p15;q21) translocation, two genes JAZF1 at 7p15 and JJAZ1 (more recently designated as SUZ12) at 17q21 are fused [187, 221]. In the initial report, the fusion was detected in three of three stromal nodules and five of five ESS [221]. Subsequent studies have shown that the fusion can be identified in a majority of ESS but not all of them, and that it can be detected by fluorescence in situ hybridization as well as by reverse transcriptase–polymerase chain reaction testing [187, 189, 227, 308]. A JAZF1/JJAZ1 fusion is less likely to be found ESS variants such as fibrous, myxoid, or epithelioid ESS [189]. The mechanism by which the fusion is involved in the pathogenesis of ESS is unknown.

Chromosomal band 7~p21→p15 is rearranged with other chromosomes than 17 in some ESS [279]. In some tumors, rearrangement with 6p21 results in fusion of the PHD finger protein 1 (PHF1) gene at 6p21 with the JAZF1 gene at 7p15, leading to the formation of a JAZF1/PHF1 fusion gene [280]. Chromosomal band 6p21 is rearranged with translocation partners other than chromosome 7 in some tumors. In about a third of reported tumors no abnormality of 7p15 or 6p21 has been identified [279]. Thus, while alterations involving chromosomes 6, 7, and 17, presumably affecting the PHF1, JAZF1, and JJAZ1 genes, are common in ESS, they are not present in every tumor.

Differential Diagnosis

ESS must be differentiated from other types of endometrial stromal neoplasms. The differential diagnosis between an endometrial stromal nodule and an ESS is based on the presence of myometrial invasion in ESS. This is discussed above, in the section on endometrial stromal nodules. The criteria for differentiating between an ESS and a UES have shifted in recent years, and the differential diagnosis relies less on mitotic counts than in the past. We discuss differential diagnostic criteria in the next section, after we present the pathologic features of UES.

Several uncommon smooth muscle tumors have overlapping features with ESS. It is important to differentiate them from ESS, because their treatment and prognosis is different. Highly cellular leiomyoma is most often confused with an endometrial stromal nodule, but when it has an irregular interdigitating interface with the surrounding myometrium or is detected in an endometrial biopsy or curettage it can mimic an ESS. Highly cellular leiomyoma does not exhibit the type of infiltrative growth into the myometrium that is seen in ESS, nor does it invade vascular spaces. The tumor cells tend to be larger than endometrial stromal cells, and it is often possible to identify more typical spindle-shaped smooth muscle cells, particularly at the interface with the surrounding myometrium. Large thick-walled blood vessels are commonly present, and the small arterioles that are characteristic of ESS are generally not present. Immunohistochemistry can be helpful, since highly cellular leiomyoma tends to show strong diffuse staining for smooth muscle markers such as smooth muscle actin, smooth muscle myosin, desmin, and caldesmon, and extensive staining for CD10 is unusual [8, 65]. IVL can simulate a vascular invasive ESS, particularly when the tumor cells have an epithelioid appearance. However, IVL tends to be a predominantly intravascular tumor, while ESS is primarily extravascular. The tumor cells in IVL tend to be larger than stromal cells. They often have conspicuous eosinophilic cytoplasm, some may be spindle-shaped, and they stain for smooth muscle markers, but usually not for CD10. Prominent large blood vessels and hyalinization can be conspicuous in the intravenous tumor plugs in IVL. Rare tumors show features of both ESS and IVL [277].

Tumors of perivascular epithelioid cells (PEComas) occasionally occur in the uterus [121, 136, 419]. Most are relatively circumscribed neoplasms composed of epithelioid or spindle-shaped cells with moderate to abundant eosinophilic or clear cytoplasm. They tend to grow around or into lymphatic vessels in the myometrium. They often pose a differential diagnostic problem, but it is usually with smooth muscle tumors of various types. Rare perivascular epithelioid cell tumors show tongue-like infiltration of the myometrium, and these need to be differentiated from ESS [419]. The cells in perivascular epithelioid cell tumors have the appearance of modified smooth muscle cells. The tumor cells are larger and have more abundant pale or eosinophilic cytoplasm than the cells of an ESS, and the cytoplasm often has a granular or flocculent character. Immunohistochemistry is particularly helpful in this differential diagnosis, as PEComa cells show at least patchy staining for HMB-45 and various smooth muscle markers, and lack staining for CD10.

Finally, several benign conditions can potentially be confused with ESS. These include adenomyosis with sparse glands, "intravascular" adenomyosis, and intravascular menstrual endometrium. These are illustrated later in this chapter, in the section on adenomyosis. In older women, foci of adenomyosis can contain few or even no glands, resulting in findings that might be confused with ESS [161]. However, adenomyosis with sparse glands is a focal microscopic finding unassociated with a tumor mass, and it is usually seen in association with foci of typical adenomyosis in which glands are readily apparent. The stromal cells in adenomyosis with sparse glands are atrophic, and sometimes the foci have a fibrotic appearance. Distribution of the stromal cells tends to be zonal, with low cellularity centrally, resulting in a pale appearance, and greater cellularity at the periphery, resulting in a dark blue-purple rim. Occasionally, small foci of adenomyosis appear to be within vascular spaces [362]. Particularly when glands are sparse, this finding raises the differential diagnosis of ESS. Intravascular adenomyosis is a microscopic finding that is not associated with a tumor mass, glands are usually present among the stromal cells, and foci of typical adenomyosis are generally present in the adjacent myometrium. Rarely, fragments of menstrual or non-menstrual endometrium are detected within vascular spaces in a hysterectomy specimen [29]. These are likely an artifact associated with surgery or tissue processing. They are differentiated from ESS by the presence of glands among the stromal cells and absence of a tumor mass.

Clinical Behavior and Treatment

The extent of tumor, the type of surgical intervention, and, possibly, certain pathologic parameters determine the risk of recurrence. The tumor stage is the most significant prognostic factor. Hysterectomy and bilateral salpingo-oophorectomy is the standard treatment for stage I stromal sarcoma, with debulking of extrauterine tumor performed in more advanced cases. Some gynecologic oncologists remove the adnexa, even in young women, because adnexal spread is not always visible at surgery, ESS generally contain estrogen receptors and the residual tumor cells might be stimulated by estrogen secreted by the ovaries, and some studies have suggested that recurrence is more frequent when the adnexal structures are conserved [248]. A number of studies suggest, however, that salpingo-oophorectomy may not be necessary in young women whose adnexa appear normal, as an adverse outcome has not observed in patients whose ovaries have been conserved [12, 56, 57, 247]. Conservative approaches to treatment are sometimes considered in young women when preservation of fertility is an important consideration. If the uterus is small, and if the tumor is low grade and circumscribed or delimited on hysteroscopy or MRI, gynecologic oncologists sometimes attempt to treat ESS by local excision. Unfortunately, our experience has been that this is rarely successful and the tumor tends to recur within a year or two.

Even when the tumor appears confined to the uterus (stage I), there is a high risk of pelvic recurrence, ranging from 25% to 50% [42, 57, 146]. The risk of recurrence is even greater in patients with advanced-stage tumors [57]. Some oncologists recommend postoperative progestin therapy for ESS with the hope of reducing the risk of recurrence [63], but many patients are unable to tolerate long-term treatment; more recently aromatase inhibitors have been used as they are better tolerated [350]. ESS grows slowly, and recurrences are often not detected until many years after initial treatment. Most recurrences are in the pelvis and involve the pelvic soft tissues, ureters, bladder, vagina, or bowel [146]. Metastases in the abdomen involve the peritoneal surfaces or omentum. A few patients develop pulmonary metastases, which can be difficult to diagnose, especially if the interval between resection of the primary tumor and detection of the metastases is long [2, 24, 256, 365]. Recurrent or metastatic ESS can be stabilized or suppressed with progestational agents in more than 50% of patients [63, 93, 336]. Tumors with a high level of progesterone receptors are most likely to respond to progestin therapy. A few patients with recurrent tumors have been treated with GnRHa or aromatase inhibitors with favorable results in reported cases [52, 223, 243, 336]. Recurrent or metastatic ESS that do not respond to treatment with progestins can sometimes be treated surgically or with radiotherapy. Chemotherapy tends to be ineffective. ESS is a slowly progressive tumor and, in those patients who ultimately die of tumor, the median time from diagnosis to death ranges up to about 11 years. Despite the high frequency of recurrences, women with stage I low-grade ESS have a 5-year survival rate in excess of 80% [236]. The outcome is less favorable for women with advanced-stage tumors, for whom 5-year survival rates of 40–50% have been reported. Recurrent ESS occasionally transform into higher-grade sarcomas, with increased nuclear atypia and mitotic activity and loss of response to hormone therapy [15].

Undifferentiated Endometrial Sarcoma (UES)

Most monophasic endometrial sarcomas are low-grade tumors, classified, as indicated above, as ESS. Only about a quarter of endometrial sarcomas are high grade, based on their pathologic features and clinical behavior. In one recent study, 6% of uterine sarcomas were classified as high grade (UES) and 20% as low grade (ESS) [1]. Some high-grade endometrial sarcomas are composed of monotonous cells that bear at least some resemblance to endometrial stromal cells. Others consist of pleomorphic cells reminiscent of the cells in the mesenchymal component of a carcinosarcoma. The former were designated as high-grade ESS in the past, but in the current WHO classification of uterine tumors all high-grade endometrial sarcomas are grouped together in the UES category [409]. Nevertheless, the histology, immunohistochemistry, and molecular genetics of UES suggest a relationship between monomorphic UES and ESS, while pleomorphic UES appears to be unrelated to ESS.

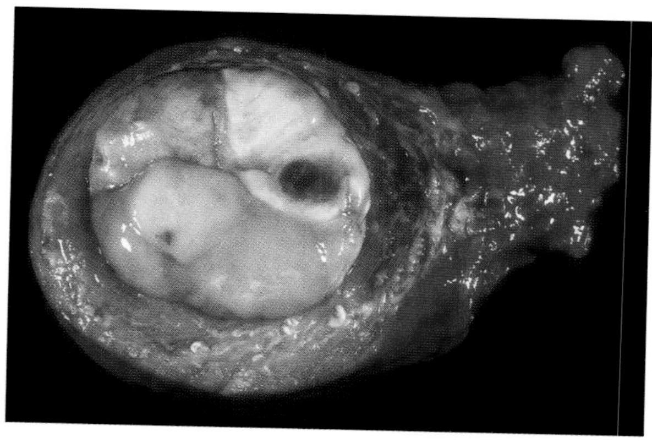

Fig. 10.61
Undifferentiated endometrial sarcoma. **The tumor is polypoid and fills the endometrial cavity. The cut surface is tan-white, and there are extensive zones of necrosis at the top**

Clinical Features

The average age of women with UES is 55–60 years [99]; in one study, monomorphic tumors occurred in younger patients than pleomorphic tumors [227]. The most common symptom is abnormal uterine bleeding. Uterine enlargement is the most common physical finding. In some patients the tumor prolapses through the cervical os. A significant proportion of patients have extrauterine tumor spread at diagnosis, either to the pelvic lymph nodes, the upper abdomen, or to distant sites such as the lungs (i.e., stage III or IV tumors) [236].

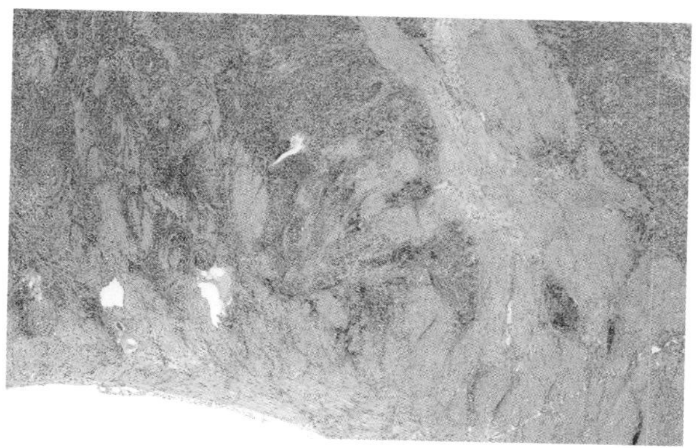

Fig. 10.62
Undifferentiated endometrial sarcoma. **There is extensive deep myoinvasion.**

Gross Findings

UES grow as soft, fleshy, polypoid tumors that bulge into, and often fill, the endometrial cavity (*Fig. 10.61*). Multiple masses of soft, white-to-tan tumor invade the underlying myometrium on a broad front. Hemorrhage and necrosis are frequently present.

Microscopic Findings

UES most often grows as a polypoid tumor that projects into the endometrial cavity and invades the underlying myometrium. Myometrial invasion tends to be along a broad front (*Fig. 10.62*), with destruction and replacement of involved areas of myometrium. Tumor cell necrosis is generally present and can be extensive (*Fig. 10.63*). The uniform proliferation of small blood vessels that is seen in ESS is not present in UES [118], where there is a haphazard distribution of variably sized blood vessels. Vascular invasion by tongues and plugs of tumor is present in most tumors (*Fig. 10.64*). UES can be divided into monomorphic and pleomorphic variants; the former were previously designated as high-grade ESS. Monomorphic UES are composed of relatively uniform tumor cells that bear some resemblance to endometrial stromal cells. However, the tumor cells are larger and have medium-sized atypical nuclei (*Fig. 10.65*). The chromatin ranges from finely granular to coarse and nucleoli are of small to medium size. Tumor cell cytoplasm is eosinophilic or amphophilic and cell borders are indistinct. MF tend to be numerous. Fibromyxoid patterns of growth in which the tumor cells are spindled or separated by myxoid

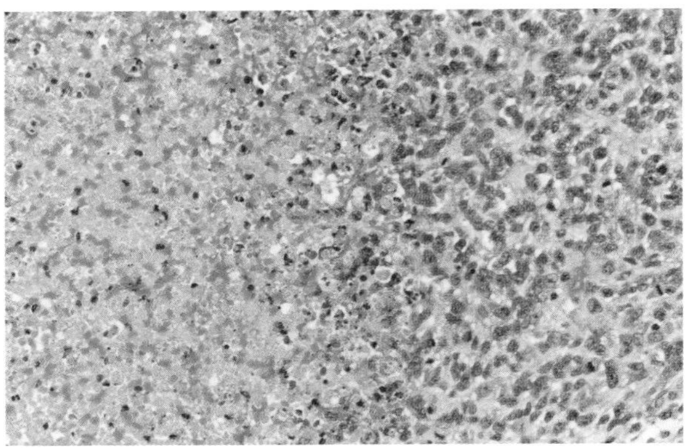

■ Fig. 10.63
Undifferentiated endometrial sarcoma with coagulative tumor cell necrosis, (on the left,) is often present. **Only ghostlike outlines of the degenerative tumor cells are visible in the necrotic zone**

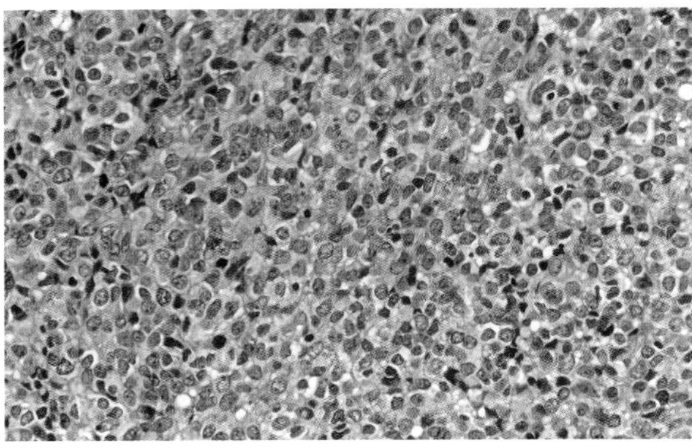

■ Fig. 10.65
Undifferentiated endometrial sarcoma, monomorphic type. **The cells have relatively uniform nuclei that bear some resemblance to endometrial stromal cells. However, they are larger and more atypical with coarse chromatin and small nucleoli. Mitotic figures are typically numerous**

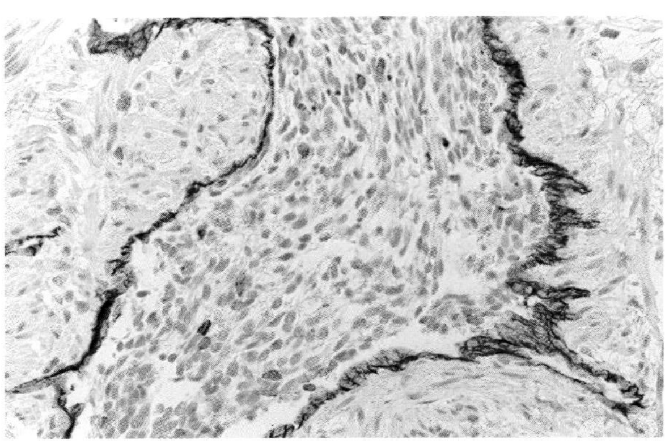

■ Fig. 10.64
Vascular invasion by an undifferentiated endometrial sarcoma. **The endothelial cells lining a vein are immunoreactive for CD31, while the tumor cells in the vein lumen show no staining**

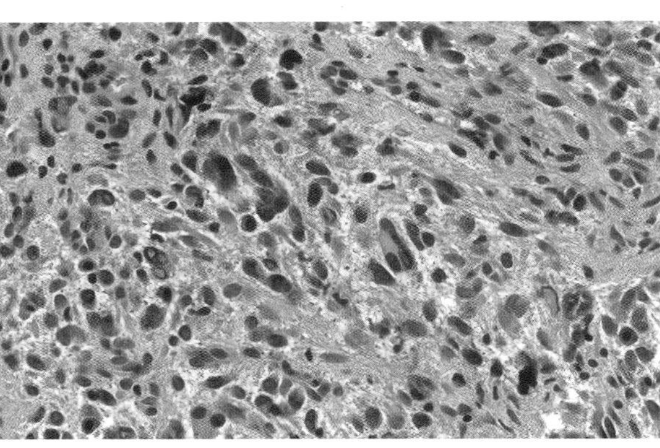

■ Fig. 10.66
Undifferentiated endometrial sarcoma, pleomorphic type. **The tumor cells vary greatly in size and shape. The nuclei are markedly atypical and range from medium-sized to large. Multinucleated cells are present. The cytoplasm is eosinophilic and varies from scant to abundant**

stroma are occasionally present in UES. In pleomorphic UES the tumor cells are large and atypical with considerable variation in nuclear size and shape and prominent nucleoli (➋ *Fig. 10.66*). Giant cells, some with multiple nuclei, are present in some tumors. MF are numerous, and atypical MF are often noted. Spindle-shaped cells tend to predominate in pleomorphic UES, but epithelioid or rhabdoid cells are present in many tumors and predominate in some of them. The cytoplasm, which ranges from eosinophilic to amphophilic, is more abundant and better delimited than in monomorphic UES. Mitotic activity is variable in both types of UES but there are usually $\geq$10 MF/10 HPF, and not uncommonly there are $\geq$20 MF/10 HPF in the most active areas. The finding of occasional cases in which there is an admixture of ESS and UES, usually of the monomorphic type, indicates that, at least occasionally, an ESS can evolve into a higher-grade sarcoma [61, 227].

Immunohistochemistry and Molecular Pathology

Immunohistochemistry is not as helpful in the evaluation of UES as it is in ESS. This is partly because UES comprises a heterogeneous group of neoplasms and partly because reactivity for many antigens, including hormone receptors, is lost in some of these poorly differentiated tumors. Some UES lack staining for CD10, while staining is present in others (➲ *Fig. 10.67*). When present, staining for CD10 tends to be focal and of variable intensity [8, 201]. Staining for smooth muscle markers is absent in most tumors, and when present it is weak and focal [8]. Staining for smooth muscle markers is seen less often in UES than in ESS. Nuclear staining for beta-catenin is reported to be present in a majority of UES, but this is not associated with beta-catenin mutations, which are not present [201]. Estrogen and progesterone receptors are present in about 50% of monomorphic UES, but they are rarely present in pleomorphic UES [227].

The (7;17)(p15;q21) translocation that is present in low-grade endometrial stromal tumors, in which two genes, JAZF1 at 7p15 and JJAZ1 (more recently designated as SUZ12) at 17q21 are fused, has also been detected in some UES. In the initial study reporting the JAZF1/JJAZ1 fusion, it was detected in three of seven high-grade stromal sarcomas [221]. The authors commented that two of the high-grade stromal sarcomas would be classified as "undifferentiated ESS" by some, and that of these two, one showed the fusion and the other did not. More recently, the fusion was detected in one of three monomorphic UES, but in none of three pleomorphic UES [227]. In the same study, the fusion transcript was detected in 50% of ESS. In another study, the fusion transcript was not detected in either of two UES [187]. A study of genes that are deregulated in endometrial sarcomas revealed that some of the most deregulated genes were those of secreted frizzled-related proteins, which are thought to be modulators of the Wnt-signaling pathway [188]. Decreased expression of secreted frizzled-related protein 4 was detected in both ESS and UES.

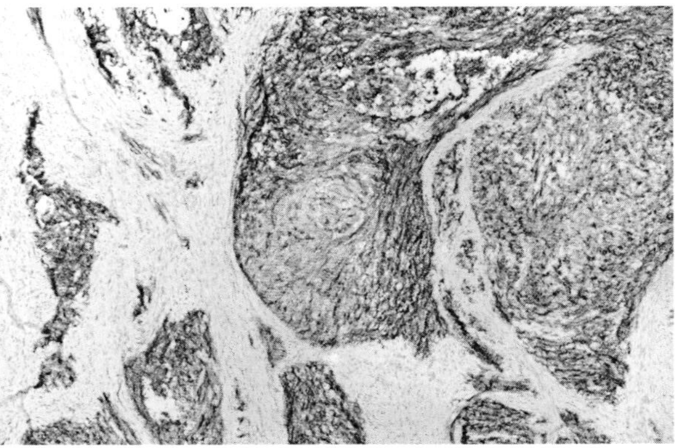

Fig. 10.67
Positive staining for CD10 in this undifferentiated endometrial sarcoma. **Note absence of staining in the myometrium. Other examples of UES show minimal or no staining for CD10**

Differential Diagnosis

Distinction between ESS and UES can be difficult, since the tumor cells can have a somewhat similar appearance. The tumor cells in UES tend to be larger and to exhibit greater nuclear atypia. Mitotic activity is no longer considered to be the only criterion for distinguishing between ESS and UES, as it once was. Occasional ESS have >10 MF/10 HPF and UES can have <10 MF/10 HPF. As a general rule, however, MF are infrequent in ESS and they are numerous, usually >10/10 HPF, in UES. The uniform distribution of small arterioles that is characteristic of ESS is absent in most UES. When ESS invades the myometrium tongues of tumor cells, often with smooth or rounded contours, appear to push between smooth muscle bundles. On the other hand, UES invades the myometrium on a broad front with destruction of the myometrium.

Leiomyosarcoma is almost always considered in the differential diagnosis of UES. Small cell and epithelioid variants of leiomyosarcoma can mimic monomorphic UES, and other types of leiomyosarcoma can resemble pleomorphic UES. The location of the tumor can help in the differential diagnosis. UES usually involves the endometrium as well as the myometrium, while leiomyosarcoma tends to be limited to the myometrium. The presence of areas typical of leiomyosarcoma, with tumor cells having fusiform nuclei with rounded ends and fibrillar eosinophilic cytoplasm favors a diagnosis of leiomyosarcoma. Staining for actin, desmin, and caldesmon can help in the differential diagnosis since leiomyosarcoma is often immunoreactive for these markers, whereas UES is typically negative. Strong positive staining for actin, desmin, and/or caldesmon therefore favors leiomyosarcoma, but negative staining is uninformative, because a significant proportion of poorly differentiated leiomyosarcomas also fail to stain for these filaments.

Rhabdomyosarcoma is uncommon in the uterus, but it does occur, usually in older women in the same age range as UES. If rhabdomyoblastic differentiation is not appreciated, the tumor is likely to be misdiagnosed as UES. Diagnostic rhabdomyoblasts range from round cells with round or oval nuclei and rims of eosinophilic cytoplasm to spindle cells with fusiform nuclei and abundant eosinophilic cytoplasm, in which cross striations can sometimes be identified. Less-differentiated rhabdomyoblasts cannot be differentiated from UES cells by routine microscopic examination. Immunohistochemistry is essential for the diagnosis of rhabdomyosarcoma. There is strong cytoplasmic staining for desmin, and there is nuclear staining for myogenin. Staining for both of these markers tends to be patchy within the tumor, and usually more cells stain for desmin than for myogenin. Myogenin is the more specific marker, as it stains only cells showing striated muscle differentiation, while desmin stains smooth muscle cells as well as rhabdomyosarcoma cells.

Adenosarcoma, especially when there is sarcomatous stromal overgrowth, and carcinosarcoma (MMMT) both enter the differential diagnosis of UES. These tumors both have epithelial as well as mesenchymal components. In adenosarcoma, the epithelium is histologically benign, while the epithelial component of a carcinosarcoma is a carcinoma. The mesenchymal components of these tumors frequently resemble UES, either of monomorphic or polymorphic type. The key to the correct diagnosis is to note that the tumor has an epithelial component. This is usually not difficult in an adequately sampled carcinosarcoma. Adenosarcoma poses greater diagnostic difficulty, since it is sometimes difficult to decide whether benign glands represent part of the tumor or entrapped glands where the tumor infiltrates the endometrium or foci of adenomyosis. When glands are distributed throughout the mesenchymal component, even in relatively small numbers, a diagnosis of adenosarcoma is appropriate.

Undifferentiated endometrial carcinoma must be differentiated from UES, especially monomorphic UES. Undifferentiated endometrial carcinoma has only been widely recognized as a distinct clinicopathologic entity for a few years [10], and it is likely that undifferentiated carcinomas have been misdiagnosed as undifferentiated sarcomas or high-grade ESS in the past. Undifferentiated carcinomas are composed of sheets of poorly cohesive, intermediate-sized cells, which sometimes have a rhabdoid appearance, with eosinophilic cytoplasm and eccentric nuclei [10]. They differ from UES in that the cells are rarely spindle-shaped or pleomorphic, at least some tumor cells express cytokeratins (especially CK18) and EMA, and lymph node metastases are frequently present at the time of diagnosis.

Clinical Behavior and Treatment

UES is relatively uncommon, and its clinical behavior is difficult to evaluate because differences in diagnostic criteria make it impossible to differentiate between treatment results for ESS and UES in many series. Also, some reports have included other types of high-grade sarcomas such as rhabdomyosarcoma or leiomyosarcoma.

Treatment includes hysterectomy and, in most cases, radiation therapy and/or chemotherapy depending on the stage of the tumor. Reported 5-year survival rates vary. In recent reports in which diagnostic criteria are clear, survival has been poor, and related to stage. Most women with extrauterine disease at diagnosis develop recurrences and die of tumor [42, 227]. Women with stage I tumors have a better prognosis, but a stage I tumor is no guarantee of survival, as shown in Evans' original study in which six of seven patients with UES, all confined to the uterus at diagnosis, died of tumor [118]. In a study of Italian women with UES, 55% of patients with disease confined to the uterus had a recurrence, as did 75% of those with extrauterine disease at diagnosis [146]. Overall survival is significantly lower for women with UES than for those with ESS [146, 236]. In one study, cytoreductive surgery improved survival for patients with extrauterine tumor spread [236]. Pelvic recurrences are fewer, and survival is better in patients with low-stage disease who are treated with combined surgery and radiotherapy. Recurrence outside the radiation field is the most common reason for treatment failure in a patient who has had combined therapy. An effective chemotherapy regimen is not available, and most UES do not express progesterone receptors or respond to hormonal therapy.

Endometrial Stromal Tumor Variants

There are two types of neoplasms containing endometrial stroma that can be viewed as variants of endometrial stromal nodules or sarcomas. One is a combined smooth muscle–stromal tumor and the other is a tumor that resembles, at least focally, an ovarian sex cord tumor.

Combined Stromal–Smooth Muscle Tumor

Focal areas of smooth muscle differentiation are commonly observed in endometrial stromal tumors, but tumors with extensive areas of both smooth muscle and endometrial stromal differentiation are rare. It is sometimes possible to demonstrate the (7;17)(p15;q21) translocation that characterizes endometrial stromal tumors in both the stromal and smooth muscle components of combined tumors [318]. Since smooth muscle cells are more differentiated than stromal cells, this likely indicates that the smooth muscle element of combined tumors is derived from the stromal component by a process of metaplasia. We currently classify combined tumors as endometrial stromal nodules or ESS with smooth muscle differentiation, depending on whether the tumor margin is circumscribed (stromal nodule) or invasive (stromal sarcoma), since the clinical behavior is determined by the stromal component. Tumors with prominent smooth muscle differentiation are discussed at greater length here. In the past, combined smooth muscle–stromal tumors were arbitrarily defined as neoplasms having at least 30% of each component [69, 317, 410]. The components tend to be sharply demarcated, although they occasionally merge into each other. Tumors with circumscribed margins are more common than those with infiltrating margins.

The stromal elements are typical of an endometrial stromal neoplasm and consist of uniform small cells with round nuclei and scanty cytoplasm. Small thin-walled blood vessels are scattered uniformly throughout the stromal component, and epithelial-like structures are present in some tumors. The immunophenotype of the stromal cells is identical to that observed in other endometrial stromal tumors. In most tumors, the stromal cells do not stain for desmin or caldesmon, or only scattered cells stain. Staining for smooth muscle actin shows a similar pattern, although in some tumors staining is more extensive or more intense. The smooth muscle elements grow in fascicles (*Fig. 10.68*), irregular circumscribed aggregates of spindle cells surrounded by stromal cells, or nodules within which the tumor cells are embedded in collagenous stroma, sometimes resulting in a "starburst"-like appearance (*Fig. 10.69*). The smooth muscle cells vary in appearance from typical spindle-shaped smooth muscle cells with abundant eosinophilic cytoplasm to rounded epithelioid cells with clear or amphophilic cytoplasm; the latter type predominate in the collagenous nodules. Despite their variable appearance, the smooth muscle cells have a typical immunophenotype and show uniform strong positive staining for smooth muscle actin (*Fig. 10.70*), desmin (*Fig. 10.71*), and caldesmon (*Fig. 10.72*). Large, thick-walled blood vessels are typically present in the smooth muscle areas.

The clinical evolution of combined smooth muscle–stromal tumors is poorly documented, but tumors with an infiltrative margin are ESS capable of recurrence or metastasis, whereas those with a circumscribed margin are benign endometrial stromal nodules [69, 317]. A tumor in which the smooth muscle elements show features of leiomyosarcoma such as significant nuclear atypia, a high mitotic rate, and necrosis presumably would have the potential to metastasize, but no case of this type with documented metastases has been reported to date. Some neoplasms that were reported as "stromomyomas" are endometrial stromal tumors in

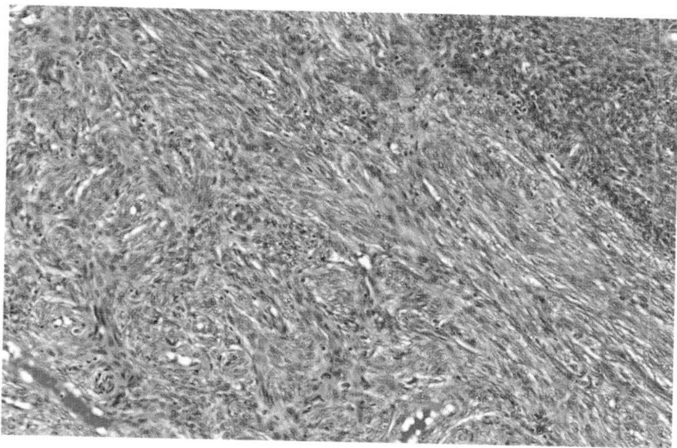

Fig. 10.68
Endometrial stromal tumor with smooth muscle differentiation. **In this example, the two components are separate. A small amount of the endometrial stromal component is present at the upper right. The smooth muscle component grows as fascicles of spindle-shaped cells with eosinophilic cytoplasm**

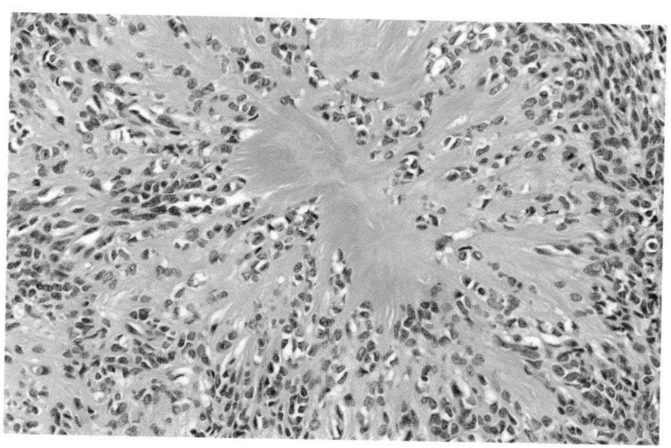

Fig. 10.69
Endometrial stromal tumor with starburst pattern and smooth muscle differentiation. **Epithelioid smooth muscle cells are embedded in a collagenous matrix and appear to radiate from the center. Smaller endometrial stromal cells surround this structure, and are best seen at the right**

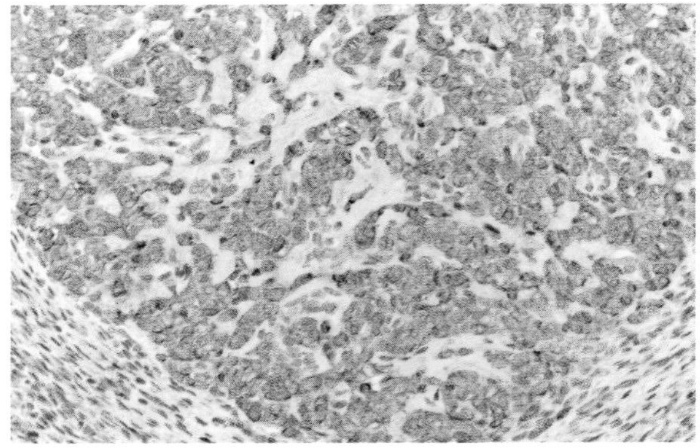

Fig. 10.70
Endometrial stromal tumor with smooth muscle differentiation. **Strong positive staining for smooth muscle actin differentiates the smooth muscle elements in this endometrial stromal tumor with smooth muscle differentiation from the surrounding stromal cells, which are SMA negative**

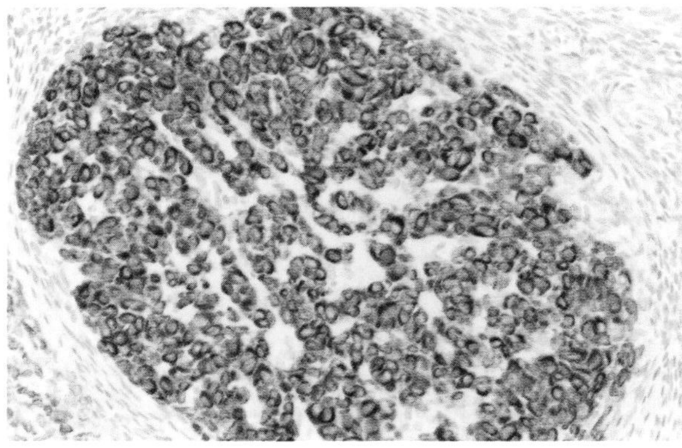

Fig. 10.71
Endometrial stromal tumor with smooth muscle differentiation. **The smooth muscle cells show strong desmin positivity, while the stromal cells do not stain for desmin**

which there are trabeculae and cords of cells that exhibit ultrastructural features of smooth muscle differentiation [408]. This finding is not surprising because the epithelial-like structures commonly seen in endometrial stromal tumors often have a myogenous immunophenotype, and such tumors are best classified as endometrial stromal tumors, not combined neoplasms. At present, the diagnosis of a combined tumor is based solely on the presence of significant amounts of both elements as recognized by routine light microscopy.

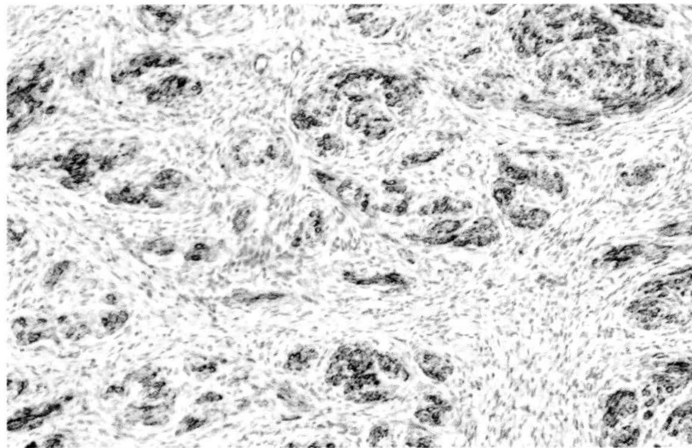

Fig. 10.72
Endometrial stromal nodule with extensive smooth muscle differentiation. **The smooth muscle cells are immunoreactive for caldesmon, while the stromal cells show no staining**

Uterine Tumors with Sex Cord-like Elements

The tumors in this category were initially described by Clement and Scully, who separated them into two types [72, 91]. Type I tumors are endometrial stromal nodules or sarcomas, some having been shown to harbor the JAZF1–JJAZ1 gene fusion [187, 318], in which there are significant areas (>10% of the tumor) of epithelial-like structures that have an appearance reminiscent of an ovarian sex cord–stromal tumor. Tumors of this type are commonly referred to as endometrial stromal tumors with sex cord-like elements (ESTSCLE). The sex cord-like cells range from small, cuboidal, or polygonal cells with scanty amphophilic or eosinophilic cytoplasm to plump polygonal cells with pale foamy or granular eosinophilic cytoplasm. Their nuclei often resemble those of the surrounding stromal cells. The sex cord-like cells grow in cords, trabeculae, or nests, or form tubules (➋ *Fig. 10.73*). Immunohistochemical tests to elucidate their nature yield variable results. There is most often a mixed epithelial–myoid phenotype, with immunoreactivity for cytokeratin and actin, and, in some cases, desmin [28, 249]. Immunostains for EMA are almost always negative. In accord with the resemblance to a sex cord tumor, immunoreactivity for sex cord markers such as calretinin, inhibin, and CD 99 are detected in the sex cord-like structures in about a third of type I tumors [28, 195].

Type II tumors, which consist predominantly or exclusively of sex cord-like elements, are often referred to as uterine tumors resembling ovarian sex cord tumors

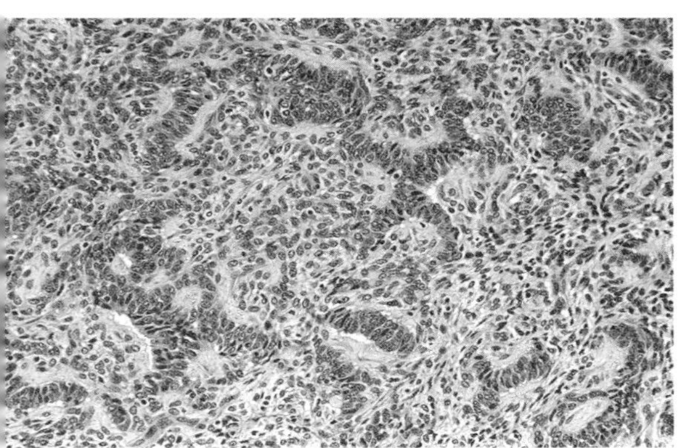

Fig. 10.73
Uterine tumor resembling an ovarian sex cord tumor (UTROSCT). **Trabeculae of darkly stained cells resemble ovarian sex cords. The nuclei of the cells in the cords resemble those in the surrounding stromal cells in this stromal tumor with prominent sex cord elements (ESTSCLE)**

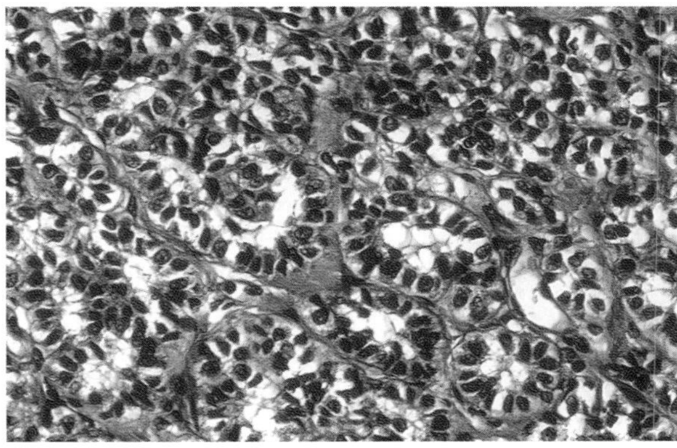

Fig. 10.74
Uterine tumor resembling an ovarian sex cord tumor (UTROSCT). **The low columnar tumor cells grow in a tubular pattern with scanty stroma**

(UTROSCT). UTROSCT are intramural or submucosal nodules surrounded by myometrium or polypoid tumors that grow into the endometrial cavity. They are yellow or tan and have a circumscribed or slightly irregular periphery. The average diameter is 6–7 cm. Microscopically, most are circumscribed, but examples with infiltrative margins and, rarely, vascular invasion have been reported [195, 395]. The tumor cells form plexiform cords, trabeculae, and nests, and may line well-formed tubules with lumens (➋ *Fig. 10.74*). Glomeruloid formations or tubules with a retiform appearance are occasionally present [92, 195]. In some tumors, retiform tubules dominate the histologic picture, and it has been proposed that these neoplasms should be designated as retiform uterine tumors resembling ovarian sex cord tumors (RUTROSCT) [303]. The tumor cells have uniform small bland nuclei with inconspicuous nucleoli, and MF are rare, typically <3 MF/10 HPF. The cytoplasm varies from scant to moderate and eosinophilic to abundant and foamy, and the cells are cuboidal or columnar in shape. Sertoliform cells, polygonal cells with eosinophilic or foamy cytoplasm (➋ *Fig. 10.75*), or cells resembling granulosa cells are present in some tumors. The stroma ranges from endometrial-like to hyaline or fibrous and smooth muscle is present in some type II tumors. Stroma accounts for less than 50% of the tumor and is often scanty in type II tumors. The histogenesis of type II tumors is unclear, with an origin from endometrial stroma or uncommitted cells in the uterus having been proposed. Recently, it has been shown that these tumors do not

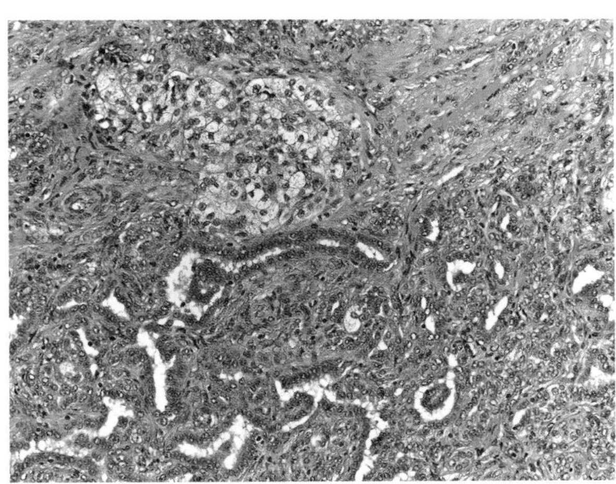

Fig. 10.75
Uterine tumor resembling an ovarian sex cord tumor (UTROSCT). **This tumor contains tubules lined by low columnar cells and nests of polygonal cells with abundant foamy cytoplasm**

harbor the JAZF1–JJAZ1 gene fusion that characterizes endometrial stromal tumors, indicating that they are unlikely to be endometrial stromal neoplasms [395]. Diverse immunohistochemical results have been described in tumors of this type, but the sex cord-like structures are usually immunoreactive for vimentin, cytokeratin, sex cord markers including calretinin (➋ *Fig. 10.76*), inhibin (➋ *Fig. 10.77*), CD 99, Melan-A, CD56, WT-1, and, often, smooth muscle actin or desmin [28, 191, 195, 224, 320]. Immunostains for EMA have been reported as negative in most tumors, but weak to moderate staining was reported in one study of four cases [191]. Positive staining for estrogen and progesterone receptors is often present [224]. Positive staining for two or more markers of sex cord differentiation is seen in most UTROSCT [195]. The immunophenotype, together with the absence of heterologous mesenchymal elements and clear-cut carcinoma, helps to differentiate these rare tumors from a MMMT.

Clinically, uterine tumors with sex cord-like elements occur in middle-aged women; the average age is around 50 [91, 395]. The main symptom is abnormal bleeding or pelvic pain. Most patients have an enlarged uterus or a palpable uterine mass. Although type I and II tumors have a similar presentation, the clinical behavior differs. Type I tumors (ESTSCLE) are endometrial stromal tumors with a focal sex cord pattern; those with circumscribed margins are benign, but those with infiltrating margins behave as low-grade ESS. In Clement and Scully's initial report, three of five patients with follow-up had recurrences and two died [72]. In their review of the literature, Baker et al. found that about 15% of reported cases were known to have recurred [28]. Type II tumors (UTROSCT), on the other hand, usually have a benign clinical evolution, although rare examples exhibit more aggressive behavior [36]. Conservative management may be possible in a young woman when conservation of fertility is a consideration [179].

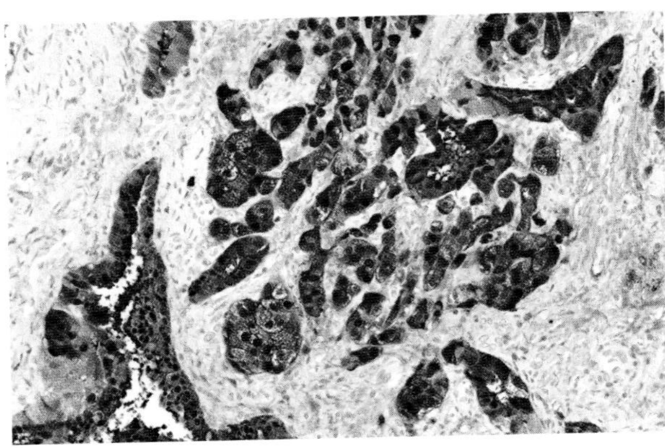

Fig. 10.76
Uterine tumor resembling an ovarian sex cord tumor (UTROSCT). **Sex cord-like tubules show strong positive staining for calretinin in this UTROSCT**

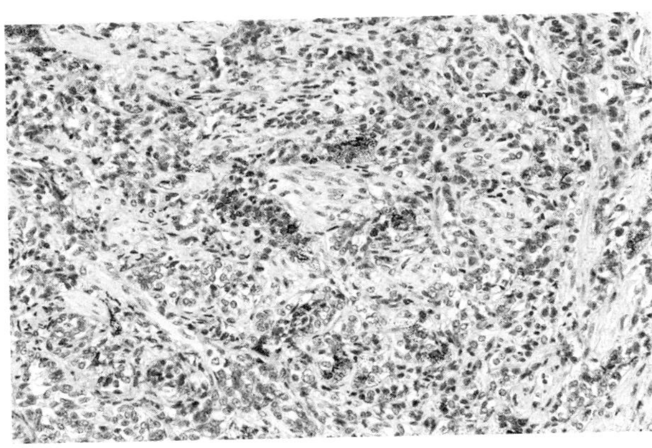

Fig. 10.77
Uterine tumor resembling an ovarian sex cord tumor (UTROSCT). **Cord-like arrangements of cells, many with foamy cytoplasm, show modest but definite staining for inhibin in this UTROSCT**

Mixed Epithelial–Mesenchymal Tumors

Mixed epithelial–mesenchymal tumors contain both epithelial and mesenchymal elements as active participants in the neoplastic process (*Table 10.8*). The tumors in this group are morphologically, but perhaps not histogenetically, related. The mixed epithelial–mesenchymal tumor group includes adenofibroma and adenosarcoma. MMMT, or carcinosarcoma, is included in this group in many classifications of uterine tumors, including the one published by the WHO [409]. Recent biologic and clinical

Table 10.8
Mixed epithelial–mesenchymal tumors of the uterus

Tumor	Malignant potential	Epithelium	Mesenchymal component
Adenofibroma	None; benign	Benign	Benign, homologous
Adenosarcoma	Low	Benign	Malignant, homologous or heterologous[a]
Carcinosarcoma (mixed müllerian tumor)	High	Carcinoma	Malignant, high grade, homologous or heterologous

[a]Usually low grade and homologous, but can be high grade and heterologous especially in cases with sarcomatous stromal overgrowth (see text).

studies, however, suggest a close relationship between MMMT and endometrial carcinoma, and MMMT is often considered to be a special type of sarcomatoid or metaplastic carcinoma. In this book, MMMT is discussed in ➋ Chap. 9, Endometrial Carcinoma.

Adenofibroma

Adenofibroma is a benign biphasic neoplasm that typically occurs in the endometrium, although occasionally it arises in the cervix or at an extrauterine location [445].

Clinical Features

Women with adenofibroma tend to be elderly [445]. The median age is 68 years, and most patients are peri- or postmenopausal. Despite a predilection for the elderly, adenofibroma occurs in women of all ages, from <20 years to >80 years. There is no known association with race, nor does adenofibroma have the epidemiologic features of endometrial carcinoma. Abnormal vaginal bleeding is the most frequent complaint. Less common findings include abdominal pain, abdominal enlargement, or a polypoid tumor projecting from the cervix. Some patients have a history of prior removal of polyps.

Gross Findings

Adenofibroma is a lobulated polypoid tumor that can arise anywhere in the uterus or in the cervix. It varies from soft to firm and is tan or brown. About 50% of adenofibromas contain small cysts that give the cut surface a spongy or mucoid appearance. The tumor ranges from 2 to 20 cm in maximum diameter, with a median of 7 cm. A large adenofibroma may fill the endometrial cavity and enlarge the uterus.

Microscopic Findings

Adenofibroma is composed of a mixture of histologically bland epithelium and mesenchyme. It originates in the endometrium or cervix. Broad papillary or polypoid stromal fronds covered by epithelium project from the surface of the neoplasm or extend into cystic spaces within it (➋ *Fig. 10.78*). Columnar or cuboidal epithelial cells, most often of endometrioid type, line cysts and cleft-like spaces. A mixture of various types of epithelia, including endocervical, tubal, and squamous, often occurs within the same neoplasm. The epithelium can be hyperplastic and stratified, but when this is the case the possibility that the tumor might be an atypical polypoid adenomyoma should be carefully considered. Endometrioid and serous carcinoma have both been reported in an adenofibroma; in such cases the behavior is determined by the carcinoma and the patient should be treated accordingly [282, 423].

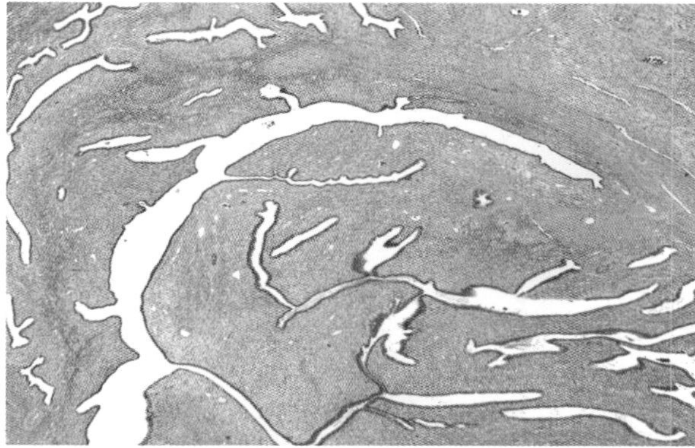

Fig. 10.78
Adenofibroma. **Cleft-like glands and polypoid stromal projections are lined by benign epithelium in adenofibroma**

The mesenchymal component is usually fibrous, consisting of fibroblasts and collagen (➋ *Fig. 10.79*), but mixtures of endometrial stromal cells and fibroblasts are present in some neoplasms. The cellularity of the stroma is generally low, and there is no periglandular condensation of stromal cells. The mesenchymal cells exhibit no nuclear atypia or mitotic activity. Rarely, histologically benign heterologous elements such as fat or skeletal muscle are present [182, 384]. Adenofibromas are usually confined to the endometrium or cervical mucosa, and do not invade the underlying myometrium or cervical stroma (➋ *Fig. 10.80*). Two unique adenofibromas that invaded the myometrium, and, in one case, myometrial veins, have, however, been reported [75].

Differential Diagnosis

It can be difficult to differentiate between an adenofibroma and a benign endometrial or endocervical polyp. A papillary configuration or a vaguely "phyllodes-like" pattern in which polypoid stromal cores covered by benign epithelium project from the surface or into cystically dilated glands favors an adenofibroma. The

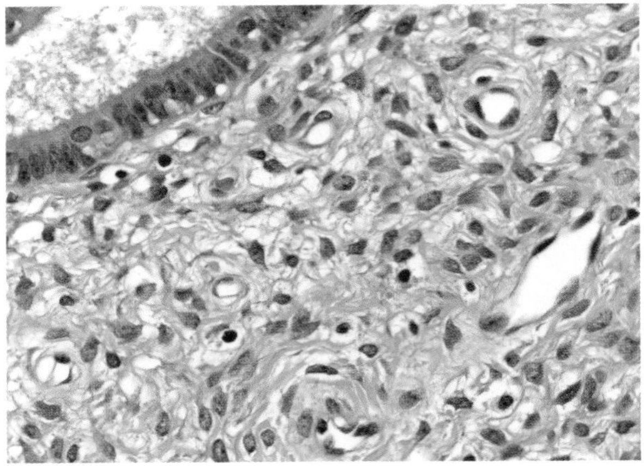

Fig. 10.79
Adenofibroma. **The epithelium in an adenofibroma is benign, and in this example it is of endometrioid type. The stromal cells are benign and have pale oval or fusiform nuclei and ill-defined cell borders. No mitotic figures are present. The background contains delicate collagen fibers and blood vessels are conspicuous**

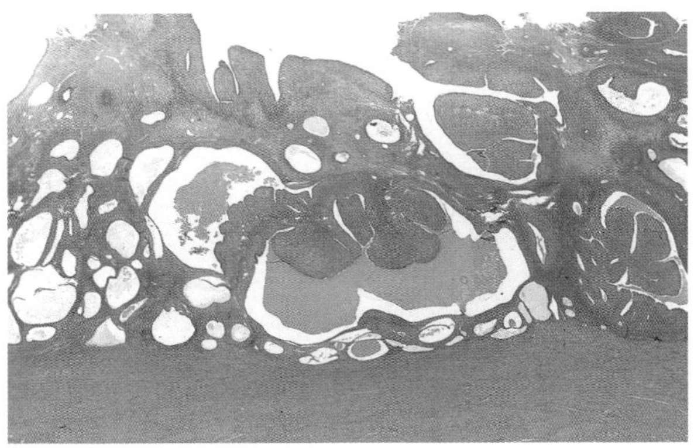

Fig. 10.80
Adenofibroma. **A typical superficial tumor that is limited to the endometrium and does not invade the myometrium**

stromal component of an adenofibroma tends to be more fibrous and more uniform than the stroma of a typical polyp.

The most important differential diagnosis is with adenosarcoma since these tumors have a somewhat similar appearance at low magnification. In the past, this differential diagnosis rested on finding hypercellular or atypical stroma with >4 MF/10 HPF in an adenosarcoma [204, 445]. Over time the diagnostic criteria for adenosarcoma have been broadened to the point that some authors now doubt the existence of adenofibromas [148]. We think that adenofibroma can be diagnosed, but it is necessary to examine the entire tumor to rule out the presence of abnormal areas indicative of adenosarcoma; this usually requires a hysterectomy. Features that are indicative of adenosarcoma include hypercellular periglandular stroma, stromal cell atypia, and virtually any detectable mitotic activity. A practical approach is to classify any tumor with the appropriate architecture, a cellular or atypical stroma, and more than a rare MF as an adenosarcoma. Occasionally, a problematic adenofibromatous tumor occurs in a young woman where conservation of fertility is an important consideration. Such tumors can be designated as "atypical adenofibromatous tumors," but the pathology report should contain a note cautioning that a recurrence could have fully developed features of an adenosarcoma.

Clinical Behavior and Treatment

Hysterectomy is the preferred treatment for an adenofibroma because the neoplasm may recur if it is incompletely curetted or excised. Hysterectomy ensures complete removal, and also permits the thorough sampling needed to exclude an adenosarcoma. Conservative therapy, such as hysteroscopy with repeat curettage, can be considered in situations in which hysterectomy is not the first choice of treatment, such as in a young woman who wishes to preserve her fertility. Adenofibroma is benign and no tumor-related deaths have been reported. Both of the previously mentioned patients with myoinvasive adenofibromas were well after hysterectomy [75], but the prognosis is less clear-cut when an adenofibroma exhibits unusual gross or microscopic features.

Adenosarcoma

Initially reported by Clement and Scully [71], adenosarcoma is a biphasic tumor with benign epithelial elements and a sarcomatous stroma. It most often occurs in the endometrium, but it is also found in the cervix and in extrauterine pelvic locations [73, 114, 148, 193, 198], such as the fallopian tube, ovary, and paraovarian tissues. Rarely, synchronous tumors occur in the uterus and an extrauterine site, such as the ovary.

Clinical Features

Adenosarcoma occurs in women of all ages. The median age is 50–59 years, with a range of 15–90 years [40, 76, 148, 204, 445]. Extrauterine adenosarcoma occurs in younger women and is more aggressive than its uterine counterpart.

There is no association of adenosarcoma with obesity or hypertension. A few patients have a history of prior pelvic radiation [76]. Occasional patients are diabetic. A few cases of adenosarcoma have been reported in women who have been treated for breast cancer with tamoxifen [19, 70, 148, 290]. Some patients have recurrent cervical or endometrial polyps and give a history of one or more prior polypectomies.

The most common presenting symptom is abnormal vaginal bleeding [424]. Vaginal discharge, pain, nonspecific urinary symptoms, a palpable pelvic mass, and a tumor protruding from the cervix are other common signs and symptoms. Most patients have stage I tumors at the time of diagnosis [40, 76, 148, 445].

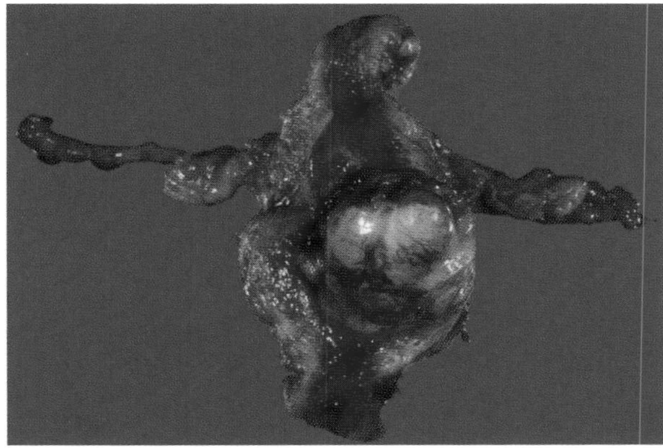

Fig. 10.81
Adenosarcoma. **A polypoid tumor arises in the endometrium and fills the endometrial cavity**

Gross Findings

Adenosarcoma most often arises in the endometrium and fills the uterine cavity, often resulting in an enlarged uterus [76]. Rare tumors grow as nodules in the myometrium, presumably arising in adenomyosis [162, 314]. Adenosarcoma arises in the cervix in 5–10% of cases [148, 198, 204, 213, 260]. Adenosarcoma is usually polypoid and averages 5–6 cm in maximum dimension (*Fig. 10.81*), although it occasionally grows as multiple papillary or polypoid masses. It can be either soft or firm. The cut surface is tan, brown, or gray, and zones of hemorrhage and necrosis are observed in about 25% of adenosarcomas. Small cysts are present in most tumors.

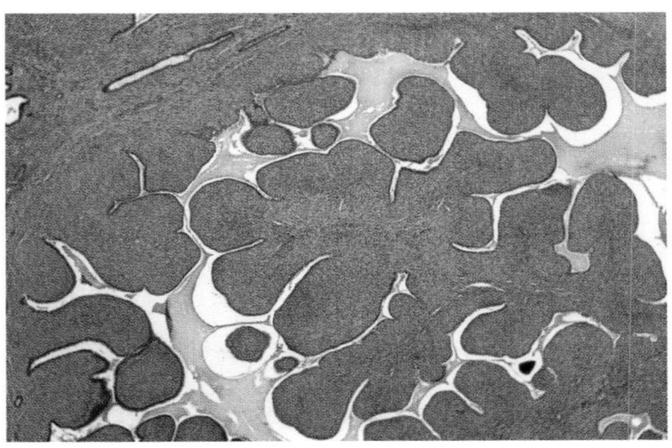

Fig. 10.82
Adenosarcoma. **Papillary stromal fronds are lined by benign epithelium. The stroma is hypercellular, and the cellularity is greatest beneath the epithelium**

Microscopic Findings

Tubular glands and cleft-like spaces are distributed throughout the tumor, and papillary stromal fronds covered by epithelium project from the surface and into cysts (*Fig. 10.82*), resulting in a phyllodes tumor-like appearance [76, 445]. The surface and glandular epithelium most often resembles inactive or proliferative endometrial epithelium. Many other types of epithelium also occur in adenosarcoma, including secretory, mucinous, squamous, and clear cell. The epithelium typically is cytologically bland, but hyperplastic and even atypical hyperplastic epithelium is occasionally noted [148]. By definition, carcinoma is not present in adenosarcoma (see *Table 10.8*), but cases have been reported in which adenocarcinoma is present in the endometrium adjacent to the adenosarcoma [76]. Glands are often present in areas of myometrial invasion, which are observed in 15–52% of adenosarcomas, suggesting that the epithelium is an actively proliferating part of the neoplasm.

The mesenchymal component of an adenosarcoma is generally a low-grade homologous sarcoma such as ESS or a fibroblastic/myofibroblastic sarcoma resembling the fibroblastic variant of ESS (*Fig. 10.83*; [76, 148, 390]),

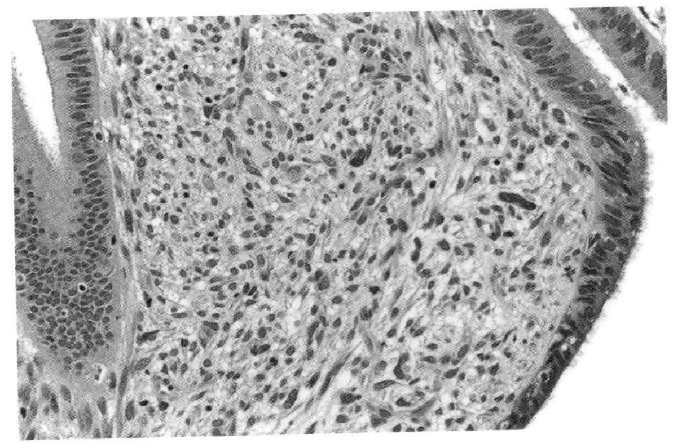

■ Fig. 10.83
Adenosarcoma. **The stroma of an adenosarcoma is more cellular than that of an adenofibroma, especially in the vicinity of the epithelial component. The stromal cells usually resemble endometrial stromal cells or fibroblasts. The nuclei can be relatively uniform but, as in this case, atypia and pleomorphism can be conspicuous**

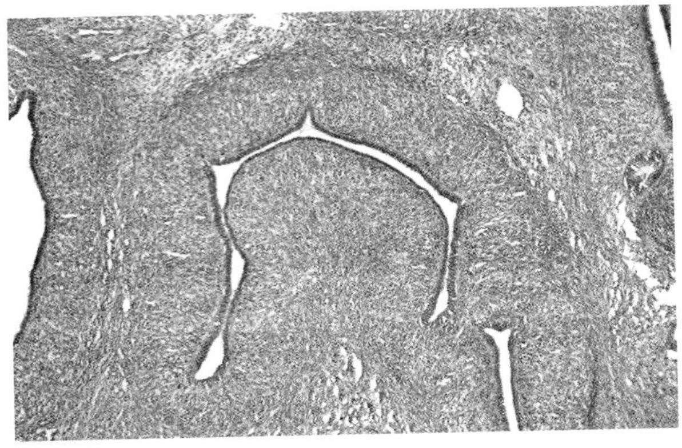

■ Fig. 10.84
Adenosarcoma. **Periglandular stromal hypercellularity is a characteristic of adenosarcoma**

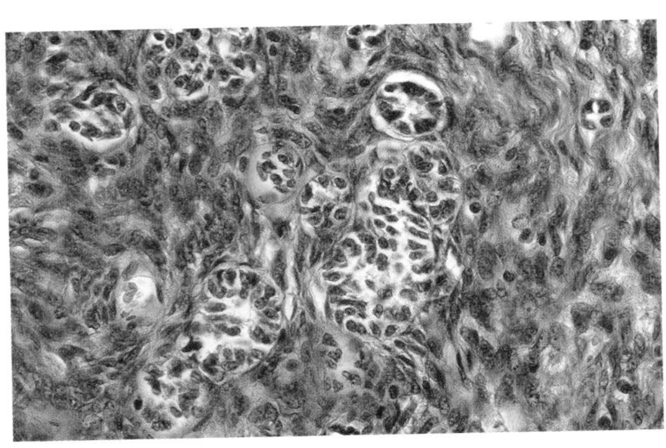

■ Fig. 10.85
Adenosarcoma. **Sex cord-like trabeculae or tubules are occasionally present in the stroma of an adenosarcoma**

although high-grade sarcoma can be present, even in cases without sarcomatous overgrowth. Smooth muscle is present in some tumors and can be conspicuous [125]. Periglandular stromal hypercellularity is a characteristic feature of adenosarcoma (➋ *Fig. 10.84*), and hypercellular stromal cuffs surround glands or form a band beneath the surface at least focally in almost every case. The degree of mesenchymal cell nuclear atypia is variable, but it is mild to moderate in most tumors. MF are readily identified in most tumors and generally number 2–4/10 HPF or more [76, 148, 204, 445]. MF tend to be most numerous in the cellular stromal cuffs around the glands. Neoplasms with the morphologic features of adenosarcoma (cellular stroma, periglandular cuffing, stromal cell atypia, and, in some cases, myometrial invasion), but in which mitotic activity is inconspicuous, can recur, or metastasize [76, 148]. Therefore, a neoplasm with the typical appearance of an adenosarcoma in which atypical, hypercellular stroma is condensed around the epithelial elements should be diagnosed as an adenosarcoma even if there are only 1–2 MF/10 HPF [76]. Adenosarcomas often contain bland areas indistinguishable from adenofibroma, so extensive microscopic study may be required to identify a sarcomatous component.

Trabecular, insular, or tubular arrangements of plump epithelial-like cells, some having abundant foamy cytoplasm, are present in about 5% of adenosarcomas (➋ *Fig. 10.85*) [74, 148, 181]. These structures, which are designated as sex cord-like elements, resemble the sex cord-like structures commonly seen in endometrial stromal tumors. Heterologous mesenchymal elements are present in 20–25% of adenosarcomas. Striated muscle (rhabdomyosarcoma) is the most common heterologous element, but cartilage, fat, and other elements are occasionally observed [229].

Sarcomatous overgrowth, which is present in about 10% of adenosarcomas, is said to occur when the sarcomatous component of the tumor occupies 25% or more of the total tumor volume [40, 68, 204]. Epithelial elements are absent in the region of sarcomatous overgrowth and the mesenchymal component is typically of high grade, with increased cellularity and mitotic activity and greater nuclear atypia (➋ *Fig. 10.86*) as compared to the appearance of the background adenosarcoma [68].

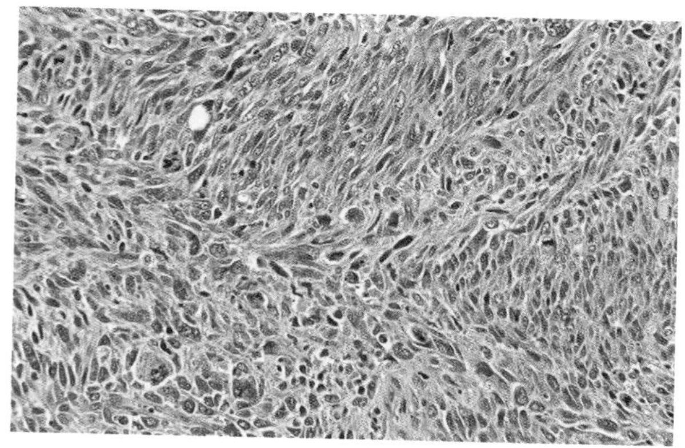

Fig. 10.86
Adenosarcoma with sarcomatous overgrowth. **A high-grade spindle cell sarcoma has developed in an adenosarcoma and comprises more than 25% of the tumor volume**

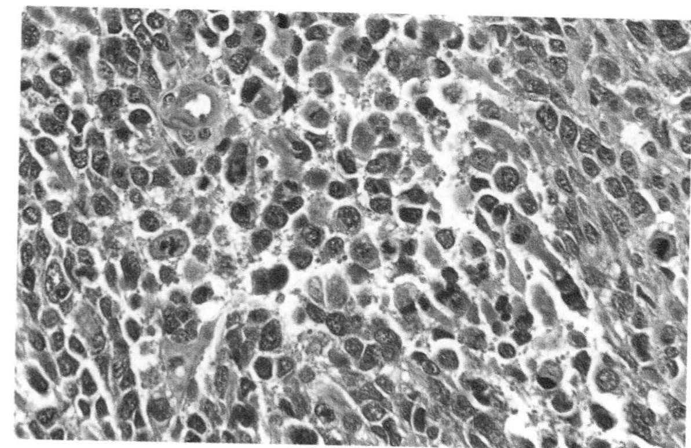

Fig. 10.87
Adenosarcoma with rhabdomyosarcoma in zones of sarcomatous overgrowth. **Rhabdomyoblasts are round or spindle-shaped and have prominent eosinophilic cytoplasm. It is sometimes possible to identify cross-striations, but these days immunohistochemistry is typically used to confirm the presence of rhabdomyoblasts**

The sarcoma can be stromal sarcoma, fibrosarcoma, or leiomyosarcoma, or a mixture of elements [204]. Heterologous elements, particularly rhabdomyosarcoma (*Fig. 10.87*), may occur in, and be limited to, the zone of sarcomatous overgrowth [148, 204]. The zones of pure sarcomatous growth can be present in or constitute the entire myoinvasive component of an adenosarcoma. Lymphovascular space invasion, which is rare in adenosarcoma, is most often found in zones of sarcomatous overgrowth [204].

Immunohistochemistry

The epithelial component of adenosarcoma is keratin positive, and it usually stains for estrogen and progesterone receptors. The mesenchymal component often resembles ESS, so it is not surprising that adenosarcoma and ESS share many immunophenotypic features. The mesenchymal cells in adenosarcoma typically show cytoplasmic staining for CD10, and there is nuclear staining for estrogen and progesterone receptors (ER and PR) and for WT-1 [13, 14, 148, 281, 390]. Staining is often most conspicuous in the periglandular stromal cuffs where the cell density is greatest. Staining for CD10 and hormone receptors is often weaker or lost in areas of high-grade sarcomatous overgrowth, which demonstrate increased levels of nuclear staining for the proliferation marker Ki-67 (MIB-1) and, often, for p53 [148, 390]. Focal staining for keratin, sometimes with a dot-like pattern, is occasionally noted and patchy weak staining for smooth muscle actin and/or desmin is present in many adenosarcomas. Areas of smooth muscle and rhabdomyosarcomatous differentiation show strong positive cytoplasmic staining for desmin [390], and the latter show positive nuclear staining for myogenin.

Differential Diagnosis

The differential diagnosis includes benign entities such as endometrial and endocervical polyps and adenofibroma, as well as various malignant tumors, including ESS, other uterine sarcomas, and, in young patients with cervical tumors, botryoid rhabdomyosarcoma.

Many patients with adenosarcoma give a history of prior removal of "polyps." In general, polyps are smaller than adenosarcomas. Microscopically, the stroma of benign polyps tends to be fibrous and few if any MF are present. Polyps often have conspicuous central blood vessels. Problems arise when large polyps have more cellular zones with endometrial type stroma, where mitotic activity can overlap with the lower end of the range seen in adenosarcoma [174]. However, polyps lack the characteristic architecture of an adenosarcoma, they do not have periglandular stromal hypercellularity, nuclear atypia is usually absent, and mitotic activity at the level commonly present in adenosarcoma (>4 MF/10 HPF) is not seen.

Bizarre stromal cells are occasionally present in polyps, but these appear to represent a degenerative phenomenon, since the cells have smudged nuclear chromatin and they are not mitotically active [406].

Adenofibroma is a rare benign tumor of the cervix or endometrium. The overall architecture is similar to adenosarcoma, but the stroma is predominantly fibrous and less cellular than that of an adenosarcoma, with no condensation of stromal cells around the epithelial elements. The stromal cells are bland, and MF are absent or difficult to find. Some adenosarcomas contain bland areas similar in appearance to an adenofibroma, so the diagnosis of an adenofibroma generally requires hysterectomy so that the entire tumor can be evaluated microscopically. Several authors have noted that it is occasionally difficult to differentiate between an adenofibroma and a low-grade adenosarcoma [76, 148].

The stroma of an adenosarcoma tends to resemble an ESS or one of its variants, so the differential diagnosis includes ESS. ESS can incorporate benign glands at its periphery, but glands tend to be absent away from the edges of the tumor, while in adenosarcoma glands are distributed throughout the tumor. Stromal sarcoma often contains epithelial or sex cord-like elements, but these do not resemble the type of epithelium present in adenosarcoma. Rare stromal sarcomas contain endometrial type glands. These are often irregularly distributed in the tumor such that many areas lack glands. Also, the stroma does not condense around the glands, and the phyllodes-like architecture of an adenosarcoma is not seen.

Other pure sarcomas of the uterus or cervix can incorporate benign glands at their periphery. However, no glands are present in most parts of the tumor and the sarcoma tends to be of significantly higher grade than the mesenchymal element of an adenosarcoma. A high-grade mesenchymal component is present in an adenosarcoma with stromal overgrowth, but such tumors invariably have areas with the typical architecture and low-grade mesenchymal elements that characterize an adenosarcoma.

In a young patient, a botryoid rhabdomyosarcoma of the cervix enters the differential diagnosis. Botryoid rhabdomyosarcomas have a polypoid surface contour similar to that seen in adenosarcoma and the hypercellular subsurface zone commonly referred to as the "cambium layer," which resembles the type of stromal hypercellularity that is seen around epithelial elements in an adenosarcoma [98, 127]. However, glands are usually not distributed throughout a rhabdomyosarcoma and the mesenchymal cells, some of which are usually recognizable as rhabdomyoblasts, tend to be more primitive and mitotically active than the stromal cells of an adenosarcoma. Immature cartilage is present in many cervical rhabdomyosarcomas.

Carcinosarcoma, like adenosarcoma, has both epithelial and mesenchymal components. However, in carcinosarcoma the epithelial component is an adenocarcinoma or an undifferentiated carcinoma and the mesenchymal component is a sarcoma, usually of high grade.

Clinical Behavior and Treatment

Adenosarcoma is usually treated by hysterectomy and bilateral salpingo-oophorectomy, although a few young patients have been treated by local excision of the tumor [76, 445]. Metastasis to lymph nodes is rare, although occasional patients whose tumors show sarcomatous overgrowth have pelvic lymph node metastases [204, 375]. The role of postoperative pelvic radiation and chemotherapy is unclear. Adenosarcoma is not as aggressive as MMMT, but it recurs in 25–40% of patients and occasionally follows an aggressive course. Recurrence is generally in the pelvis or vagina, but distant metastases occur in 5% of patients (Clement and Scully 1990). Recurrences typically consist exclusively of the sarcomatous component, but both epithelium and stroma are occasionally present. Pathologic features of the primary tumor that are associated with an increased risk of recurrence or metastasis are extrauterine spread at diagnosis; myometrial invasion, especially into the outer half of the myometrium; and sarcomatous overgrowth of the mesenchymal component [76, 148, 204, 225, 424, 445]. Patients with adenosarcoma with sarcomatous overgrowth of the mesenchymal component have a prognosis similar to that of women with carcinosarcoma [225]. Invasion of capillary–lymphatic spaces in the myometrium or the presence of rhabdomyosarcoma in zones of sarcomatous overgrowth also portend an unfavorable outcome. There is no clear correlation between the prognosis and the mitotic rate in the mesenchymal component. Extended clinical observation is necessary because there is typically a long (3.5–5 years) interval between treatment and recurrence. About a quarter of patients with adenosarcoma die of tumor, often more than 5 years after initial diagnosis.

Homologous and Heterologous Sarcomas

The tumors in this category are high-grade sarcomas that often resemble the mesenchymal component of a MMMT. Most pleomorphic homologous sarcomas arise in the endometrium and consist of round or spindled cells with variable amounts of cytoplasm and pleomorphic atypical nuclei. These are a type of undifferentiated endometrial sarcoma, and are discussed above in the section on Undifferentiated Endometrial Sarcoma. Some may result from sarcomatous stromal overgrowth in an adenosarcoma or carcinosarcoma or by dedifferentiation of a low-grade ESS. Although most undifferentiated sarcomas are of endometrial origin, a few appear to arise in the myometrium, either from nonspecific mesenchymal elements or by dedifferentiation of a leiomyosarcoma.

Pure heterologous sarcomas occasionally arise in the uterus. Some are assumed to represent complete heterologous stromal overgrowth in an adenosarcoma or carcinosarcoma. Rhabdomyosarcoma, which is discussed below, is by far the most common heterologous uterine sarcoma [127, 323], but chondrosarcoma [296], osteosarcoma [115], liposarcoma [30], and tumors containing mixtures of heterologous elements also occur. Histologically benign heterotopic bone, cartilage, and fat are occasionally found in the uterus, and rare benign tumors contain one or more of these elements [293, 356]. They should not be mistaken for heterologous sarcomas or carcinosarcomas, in which the mesenchymal elements are histologically malignant.

Rhabdomyosarcoma

Rhabdomyosarcoma is a malignant neoplasm that displays skeletal muscle differentiation. It is the most common soft tissue tumor in children and approximately 20% of pediatric rhabdomyosarcomas originate in the genital tract. In adults, rhabdomyosarcoma of the female genital tract is a rare tumor [129, 175, 250]. Most of the clinical and pathologic data about rhabdomyosarcoma derive from cooperative group trials assessing multimodality treatment for pediatric rhabdomyosarcoma at various anatomic locations, including the female genital tract [17, 87, 200, 264, 347].

Largely based on pediatric data, rhabdomyosarcoma is categorized into three major variants with significant differences in clinical behavior and prognosis. The most common and generally most favorable variant is embryonal rhabdomyosarcoma, which includes botryoid, spindle cell, and anaplastic histologic subtypes. The recently described sclerosing rhabdomyosarcoma may be related to embryonal rhabdomyosarcoma [135]. The other two types of rhabdomyosarcoma, alveolar and pleomorphic rhabdomyosarcoma, are less common and usually have a significantly less favorable clinical outcome.

Clinical Features

In adults, the median age at diagnosis of female genital tract rhabdomyosarcoma is in the fifth to seventh decade and the most common presenting symptom is abnormal vaginal bleeding [127, 323]. The majority of women, approximately 75%, present with local or regional disease. The primary site is the cervix in approximately one half of women, making it the most common site of origin of genital tract rhabdomyosarcoma in adults; only 20% of tumors are uterine. Children and young adults with cervical or uterine rhabdomyosarcoma present with vaginal bleeding or with a polypoid tumor that protrudes from the vagina.

Gross Findings

Cervical rhabdomyosarcomas are mainly polypoid gray-tan or red tumors. Botryoid rhabdomyosarcoma, the most common type in the cervix, is often described as resembling a cluster of grapes. Uterine rhabdomyosarcoma tends to be a polypoid endometrial tumor that grows into the uterine cavity and invades the myometrium. Some rhabdomyosarcomas are nodular tumors located entirely within the myometrium. The average tumor size at presentation is about 3 cm, but many tumors are larger and measure 10–15 cm or more.

Microscopic Findings

Rhabdomyosarcomas of the cervix are more common than those of the uterine corpus, and most are embryonal rhabdomyosarcomas of the botryoid subtype. Botryoid rhabdomyosarcomas are polypoid tumors that have a densely cellular zone of primitive cells beneath the surface epithelium (the "cambium layer"; ➋ *Fig. 10.88*; [98]). The substance of the polyps is generally myxoid or edematous, with varying cellularity. The tumor cells are rhabdomyoblasts that range from undifferentiated small round cells with hyperchromatic nuclei and scanty cytoplasm ("small round blue cells") to strap-shaped cells with eosinophilic cytoplasm and easily appreciated cross-striations. Interestingly, foci of immature-appearing cartilage are admixed with the rhabdomyoblasts in a significant minority of cases [98, 127]. The non-polypoid and infiltrative portions of the tumors are usually histologically indistinguishable from embryonal rhabdomyosarcomas of the usual (non-botryoid) sort with cellular zones that alternate with paucicellular zones with

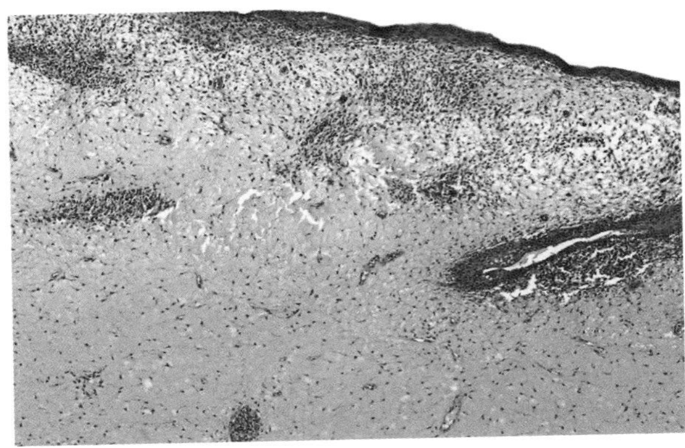

Fig. 10.88
Botryoid rhabdomyosarcoma. **These tumors are typically composed of grape-like tumors with a paucicellular matrix that appears myxoid or edematous. Condensation of primitive cells beneath the overlying epithelium and alongside any entrapped epithelium (so-called cambium layer) is common. Phyllodes-like architecture and intraglandular stromal papillae, seen in adenosarcoma, are lacking**

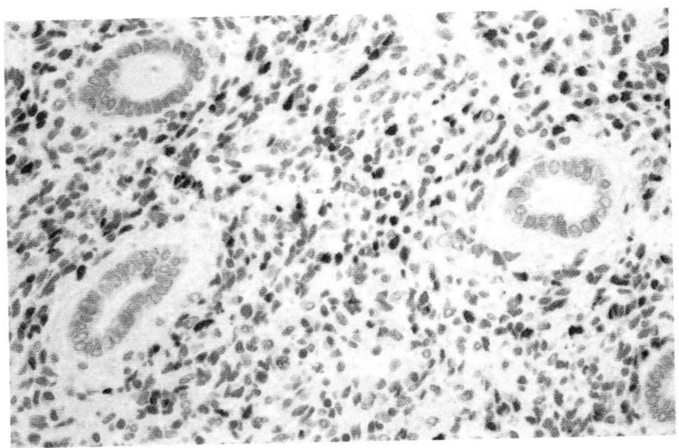

Fig. 10.89
Botryoid rhabdomyosarcoma. **Myogenin expression in tumor cell nuclei confirms rhabdomyoblastic differentiation**

a myxoid or edematous matrix. An unusual botryoid rhabdomyosarcoma that contained areas with a more pleomorphic pattern has been reported [186].

Rhabdomyosarcomas of the uterine body in older patients are often high-grade pleomorphic sarcomas composed of round, polygonal, or spindle-shaped cells admixed with aggregates of large rhabdomyoblasts [323]. The rhabdomyoblasts range from round cells with prominent perinuclear rims of eosinophilic cytoplasm to spindle- or tadpole-shaped cells with fibrillar eosinophilic cytoplasm.

In the female genital tract, alveolar rhabdomyosarcoma occurs most often in the vulva. Although occasionally reported, it is uncommon in the uterine body and cervix [54, 352]. The tumor cells tend to be larger than those in embryonal rhabdomyosarcoma. In some tumors round or irregular spaces are surrounded by tumor cells, resulting in an alveolar appearance. Tumor cells often seem to cling to the conspicuous fibrovascular septae that traverse sheets of tumor cells. In other tumors there is solid growth of tumor cells with no alveolar spaces. Regardless of the growth pattern, the tumor cells have a distinctive cytologic appearance with round nuclei, larger than those in embryonal rhabdomyosarcoma, and scanty cytoplasm. Multinucleated tumor cells are commonly present. Round and spindled cells with brightly eosinophilic cytoplasm are present in most cases and are important clues to the diagnosis. Tumor cells with cross striations can generally be identified.

Immunohistochemistry and Molecular Pathology

The typical immunophenotype includes expression of desmin, muscle-specific actin, myogenin, and Myo-D1 (*Fig. 10.89*). Staining for these markers is present in greater than 90% of rhabdomyosarcomas [55, 90]. Desmin and muscle-specific actin are not specific for rhabdomyosarcoma, as positive staining is also found in tissues demonstrating smooth muscle and myofibroblastic differentiation. Myogenin and Myo-D1 are nuclear regulatory proteins that are expressed early in skeletal muscle differentiation. Myogenin is the more widely used of the two because there are fewer technical problems associated with its use. In general, the expression of these markers is negatively correlated with differentiation; nuclear staining is widespread in tumors with numerous differentiated rhabdomyoblasts, but only scattered myogenin positive cells are found in rhabdomyosarcomas composed predominantly of undifferentiated cells with few histologically recognizable rhabdomyoblasts.

Expression of myogenin and Myo-D1 is common to all tumors demonstrating skeletal muscle differentiation, which means that tumors other than pure rhabdomyosarcoma (e.g., carcinosarcoma containing rhabdomyoblasts) must be excluded before using myogenin or Myo-D1 immunoreactivity to confirm a diagnosis of rhabdomyosarcoma. Rhabdomyosarcoma may rarely express markers that are more commonly expressed in its histologic mimics, including staining for CD99 (O13), cytokeratin, S100, or WT1. Occasional tumors show co-expression of neuroendocrine markers such as chromogranin and synaptophysin along with desmin and myogenin. Such neoplasms have been referred to as "ectomesenchymomas."

Immunohistochemistry may help with the subclassification of rhabdomyosarcoma. Staining for myogenin is likely to be strong and diffuse in alveolar rhabdomyosarcoma; staining is weaker and more focal in embryonal rhabdomyosarcoma [176, 289]. Positive nuclear staining for PAX-5 is reported to be present in about two thirds of alveolar rhabdomyosarcomas, but staining tends to be absent in embryonal rhabdomyosarcoma [400]. In a limited number of cases with genetic correlation, staining occurred only in tumors that had one of the characteristic translocations, but there was no correlation with a specific translocation [400]. A panel of four immunostains, AP2β, P-cadherin, epidermal growth factor receptor (EGFR), and fibrillin-2, is reported to differentiate between translocation positive alveolar rhabdomyosarcoma (positive for AP2β and P-cadherin) and embryonal rhabdomyosarcoma (positive for EGFR and fibrillin-2); translocation-negative alveolar rhabdomyosarcoma can be suspected if staining for all four markers is absent [429]. This immunohistochemical panel does not appear to be in widespread use.

A majority of alveolar rhabdomyosarcomas exhibit a clonal chromosomal translocation, either t(2;13)(q35;q14), resulting in a PAX3–FKHR fusion, or t(1;13)(p36;q14), resulting in a PAX7–FKHR fusion. There appears to be a survival difference between patients whose tumors have the PAX3–FKHR fusion and those whose tumors have the PAX7–FKHR fusion, with the former having a significantly worse prognosis, at least when metastatic disease develops [388].

Differential Diagnosis

Myxoid leiomyosarcoma may resemble embryonal rhabdomyosarcoma, and pleomorphic leiomyosarcoma can appear similar to pleomorphic rhabdomyosarcoma. Embryonal rhabdomyosarcoma, when spindled and growing in fascicles, frequently has a subtle moth-eaten appearance that results from a heterogeneous admixture of cells, some containing densely eosinophilic cytoplasm and others clear or amphophilic cytoplasm (*Fig. 10.90*). Round rhabdomyoblasts with bright-red cytoplasm are often haphazardly intermixed. The low-power appearance of leiomyosarcoma, in contrast, is generally more uniform. Most embryonal rhabdomyosarcomas with an infiltrative, spindle cell appearance underlie a botryoid tumor and/or are clearly epitheliotropic. Leiomyosarcomas, in contrast, are usually more deeply seated lesions.

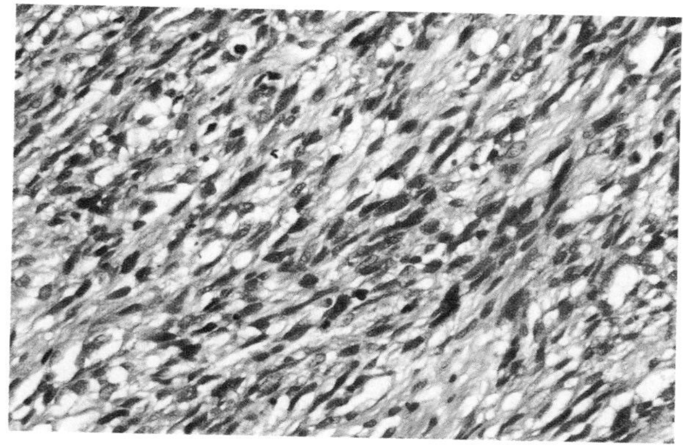

Fig. 10.90
Rhabdomyosarcomas with spindle cell morphology may mimic leiomyosarcoma. **As compared to leiomyosarcomas, rhabdomyosarcomas more frequently lack an eosinophilic appearance at low power and instead demonstrate a subtle moth-eaten look owing to the admixture of round and spindled rhabdomyoblasts**

Immunohistochemistry is useful for distinguishing rhabdomyosarcoma from leiomyosarcoma. Diffuse desmin expression is present in both, but only rhabdomyosarcoma shows staining for myogenin. Caldesmon can be positive in leiomyosarcoma, but it is generally negative in rhabdomyosarcoma.

Adenosarcoma and embryonal rhabdomyosarcoma both show polypoid growth and stromal condensation beneath epithelium, but botryoid rhabdomyosarcoma more typically contains conspicuous myxoid stroma, and has a sprinkling of small cellular aggregates of dark blue, primitive and mitotically active cells in a paucicellular background. These features can sometimes be appreciated macroscopically, such that gross inspection of a glass slide can suggest the correct diagnosis. In contrast to adenosarcoma, rhabdomyosarcoma does not exhibit phyllodes-like growth or intraglandular stromal papillae. Adenosarcomas with stromal overgrowth frequently contain rhabdomyoblastic foci. It is unclear whether there are significant clinical differences between such tumors and pure rhabdomyosarcoma. Some rhabdomyosarcomas might represent adenosarcomas with complete heterologous stromal overgrowth.

Stromal-predominant carcinosarcoma is excluded by a careful search for a malignant epithelial component. The presence of any type of carcinoma indicates that the tumor is a carcinosarcoma. It is generally assumed that some genital pleomorphic rhabdomyosarcomas represent carcinosarcomas in which the epithelial component is overgrown by the sarcomatous mesenchymal component.

Pleomorphic undifferentiated sarcoma can resemble rhabdomyosarcoma, as it is composed of mitotically active atypical round or spindle cells. However, rhabdomyoblasts with eosinophilic cytoplasm are not present, and there is no staining for myoid markers such as desmin and myogenin.

Undifferentiated carcinoma also enters the differential diagnosis as it consists of medium-sized round cells with scanty cytoplasm with no obvious glandular differentiation. Undifferentiated carcinoma may show areas of cellular cohesion, and the tumor cells show at least focal staining for keratin or EMA. Staining for markers of myoid differentiation is absent.

Clinical Behavior and Treatment

Most adult patients are treated surgically, with or without chemotherapy and radiation therapy. In a recent retrospective review of genital tract rhabdomyosarcoma in adults, the median time to progression was only 9 months and the median disease-specific survival was 21 months; the 5-year disease-specific survival was only 29% [127]. Neither age nor stage correlated with survival. Women with cervical rhabdomyosarcoma had a longer time to progression than women with disease at other gynecologic sites and women with an embryonal rhabdomyosarcoma had improved progression free survivals compared to those with non-embryonal types of rhabdomyosarcoma. Other authors have reported similar poor survival rates in adults with genital tract rhabdomyosarcoma [276, 323].

Children with genital tract rhabdomyosarcoma are generally treated by biopsy to establish the diagnosis, followed by chemotherapy and in some instances radiation. Primary surgical management, as used in adults, is very uncommon. The poor survival statistics for adults with genital tract rhabdomyosarcoma contrast sharply with the rather favorable survival rates in pediatric rhabdomyosarcoma: 5-year overall survival of 82%, with 94% survival for patients with the botryoid histologic subtype of rhabdomyosarcoma and 66% survival for those with non-embryonal variants of rhabdomyosarcoma [22, 244].

Alveolar Soft Part Sarcoma (ASPS)

ASPS is uncommon in the female genital tract, but it occasionally occurs in the vagina, cervix, or uterus. Uterine tumors have been described in the endometrium, lower uterine segment, and myometrium [209, 299, 346]. The average patient age is about 30 years, and most patients present because of abnormal bleeding [299].

ASPS is composed of cells with abundant clear to eosinophilic cytoplasm that grow in solid nests or, when there is loss of cellular cohesion, an alveolar pattern (➲ *Fig. 10.91*). The tumor cell cytoplasm is filled with granules and crystals that are PAS-positive and diastase-resistant. Nuclei are usually round with prominent nucleoli. The fibrovascular framework that supports the nests and alveoli can be conspicuous. ASPS that arise in the soft tissues frequently show vascular invasion, but this is uncommon in gynecologic cases. Alveolar soft part sarcomas are characterized by a chromosomal translocation, t(x;17)(p11;q25), in which the TFE3 transcription factor gene on chromosome Xp11 is fused to a novel gene on chromosome17q25 [230]. An immunohistochemical stain for the TFE3 protein, which is a nuclear antigen, can be used as a diagnostic adjunct to recognize tumors with this translocation or other abnormalities involving TFE3 [20, 21, 209, 354]. Alveolar soft part sarcomas show variable, but usually weak or negative immunoreactivity for keratins, desmin, smooth muscle actin, S100, and HMB45.

The differential diagnosis of ASPS includes adenocarcinoma, epithelioid smooth muscle tumor, PEComa, metastatic melanoma, and a uterine tumor resembling UTROSCT. Adenocarcinoma, epithelioid smooth muscle tumor, metastatic melanoma, and UTROSCT all have a different immunophenotype than ASPS, but the immunohistochemical features of PEComa and ASPS can sometimes be similar. This is because rare PEComas express

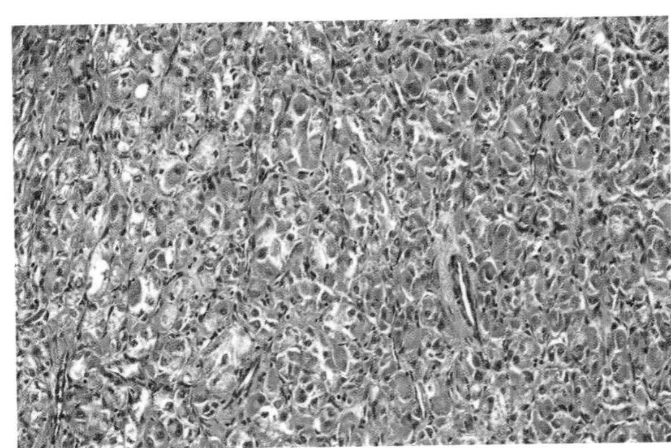

■ Fig. 10.91
Alveolar soft part sarcoma. **The tumor is formed of nested aggregates of epithelioid tumor cells with granular or crystalline cytoplasm**

TFE3 and, at the same time, show only weak HMB45 expression [136]. Any appreciable desmin staining or staining with markers such as tyrosinase, microphthalmia transcription factor, or Melan-A would support PEComa over ASPS.

Gynecologic ASPS has a relatively good prognosis compared to soft tissue ASPS, but the number of cases and the length of follow-up reported are insufficient to draw definitive conclusions. In the largest series of nine patients, one patient died of tumor but the other eight were alive with no evidence of tumor, 9 months to 17 years after diagnosis [299].

Primitive Neuroectodermal Tumor

Primitive neuroectodermal tumor (PNET) only rarely arises in the uterus [97, 138, 177, 387]. PNET can occur at any age, but most are found in postmenopausal women. The median age in the largest series was 58 years, and most patients had stage III or stage IV tumors [116]. The usual clinical presentation is with abnormal vaginal bleeding.

PNET is a soft, fleshy, gray or white polypoid mass that originates in the endometrium and invades the myometrium. Microscopically, PNET is composed of small cells with round to oval hyperchromatic nuclei and scanty cytoplasm (➲ *Fig. 10.92*). MF are usually numerous. Evidence of neuroectodermal differentiation includes the presence of a fibrillary background or the formation of rosettes or pseudo-rosettes.

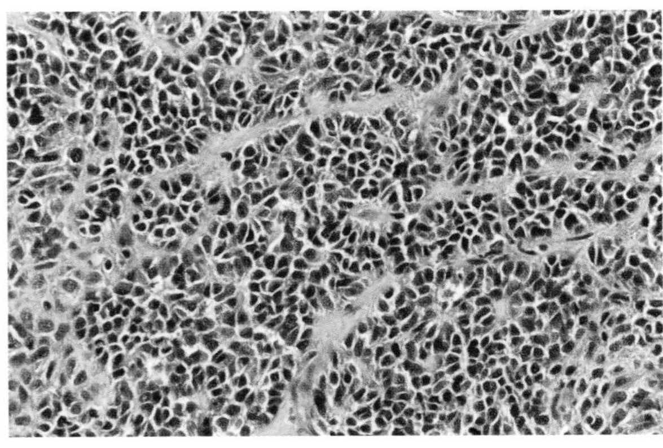

Fig. 10.92
Primitive neuroectodermal tumor of the uterus. **The tumor is composed of small cells with hyperchromatic nuclei, coarse chromatin, and scanty cytoplasm, arranged in nests and trabeculae. Rosettes or pseudorosettes are seen in some cases. This case was immunoreactive for CD56, chromogranin, and neurofilament**

Immunostains are generally positive for one or more neural or neuroendocrine marker, and staining for keratin is generally absent. The most useful immunostains are keratin, which is generally negative, and synaptophysin and neurofilament, which are usually positive. Staining for other neuroectodermal markers such as chromogranin, neuron-specific enolase, and CD56 is more variable but occasionally one or more are positive. Many uterine PNET, especially those with a t(11;22) express CD99 in a diffuse, membranous pattern, as well as FLI-1. Positive staining for CD99 is not proof that a tumor is a peripheral-type PNET, since tumors without evidence of a translocation frequently show CD99 staining [116].

Uterine PNET appear to fall into two categories. Some have a chromosomal translocation, usually t(11;22) resulting in a fusion between the EWS and FLI1 genes. These demonstrate histologic, immunohistochemical, and biologic similarities to peripheral PNET (pPNET; [39, 383, 422]). Other uterine PNET, including all tested tumors in the largest reported series, lack evidence of an EWSR1 rearrangement, and are thus more akin to the central type of PNET [116].

Mixtures of PNET and other tumor types are occasionally seen. PNET has been reported in association with various types of sarcoma, with carcinosarcoma and adenosarcoma and with endometrioid adenocarcinoma [116, 142, 383]. When associated with carcinosarcoma or adenosarcoma, PNET is viewed by some as a form of heterologous differentiation.

Too few patients have been studied to define the clinical behavior and most appropriate treatment for PNET of the uterus. Women with stage I neoplasms can be cured, but more advanced tumors are frequently fatal. In the only large series reported to date 7 of 13 patients with follow-up died of tumor and 6 were alive with no evidence of disease [116].

Miscellaneous Mesenchymal Tumors and Conditions: Inflammatory Myofibroblastic Tumor (IMT)

IMT, also known as inflammatory pseudotumor, is a benign but potentially locally aggressive proliferation of myofibroblasts [153, 344]. IMT occurs in all age groups, including premenopausal women and children. The presentation is with symptoms related to the presence of a mass, such as pain or pressure, but some patients have constitutional symptoms including fever, weight loss, and fatigue.

Grossly, the tumors range up to 12 cm in maximum diameter. They are firm or soft, and the cut surfaces are tan or white and often mucoid. Microscopically, the myofibroblasts are spindle-shaped or stellate and have pale eosinophilic cytoplasm (➲ *Fig. 10.93*). Their nuclei are granular or vesicular, and they may have prominent nucleoli. Mitotic activity is variable, but the mitotic index is generally <10/10 HPF and atypical MF are not present. The background is frequently edematous [378], and lymphocytes and plasma cells are scattered among the myofibroblasts. Immunohistochemical stains for smooth muscle actin or desmin typically are positive, although staining may be focal. Staining for specific markers of smooth muscle differentiation, such as caldesmon, tends to be absent. IMT may show cytoplasmic staining for ALK-1, a useful diagnostic feature.

IMT is a benign lesion that does not metastasize. Recurrences of uterine IMT have not been reported, but there is a local recurrence rate of about 15% in patients with extrauterine IMT. IMT were initially considered to be inflammatory pseudotumors, but the documentation of the clonal nature of some IMT and the demonstration of chromosomal rearrangements involving the ALK locus region indicate that it may be more appropriate to view them as true neoplasms [234, 398].

Adenomyosis and Adenomyoma

Adenomyosis is a common condition, detected in 15–30% of hysterectomy specimens [373]. It is characterized by the presence of endometrial glands and stroma within the myometrium [34]. Adenomyomas are uncommon tumor-like masses composed of endometrial glands, stroma, and smooth muscle. They differ from adenomyosis mainly in that they are circumscribed nodular masses.

Clinical Features

Patients are typically pre- or perimenopausal women who present with abnormal bleeding and dysmenorrhea. Symptoms tend to be more severe in women with deep myometrial involvement [246]. The uterus is enlarged and may harbor other lesions associated with hyperestrinism [203]. Adenomyosis is usually most extensive in the posterior wall, which may be thickened. A clinical diagnosis of adenomyosis can often be confirmed by imaging studies such as transvaginal ultrasonography or MRI.

Pathologic Findings

On gross examination, the cut surface of the myometrium is trabeculated and contains hemorrhagic foci, but a distinct tumor nodule is not present. Small blood-filled cysts may be noted.

Adenomyosis is a condition in which rounded or irregular foci of endometrial stroma and glands are present in the myometrium (➲ *Fig. 10.94*). The lower border of the endometrium is irregular and dips into the superficial myometrium. To avoid misclassifying a normal

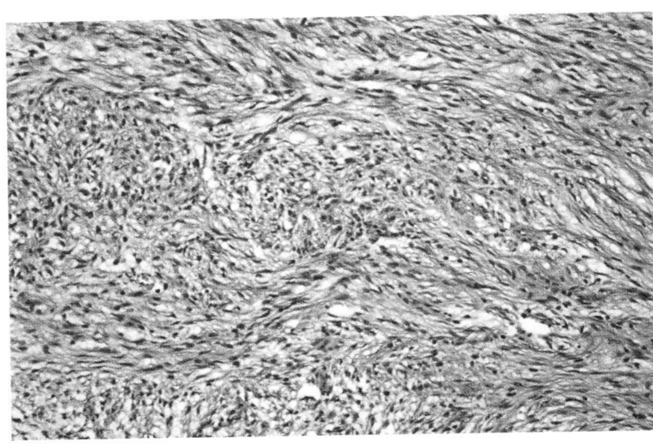

◘ Fig. 10.93
Inflammatory myofibroblastic tumor. **The tumor is a histologically low-grade spindle cell proliferation of largely mitotically inactive spindle cells set in a myxoid and inflammatory background (Courtesy of Joseph Rabban, M.D.)**

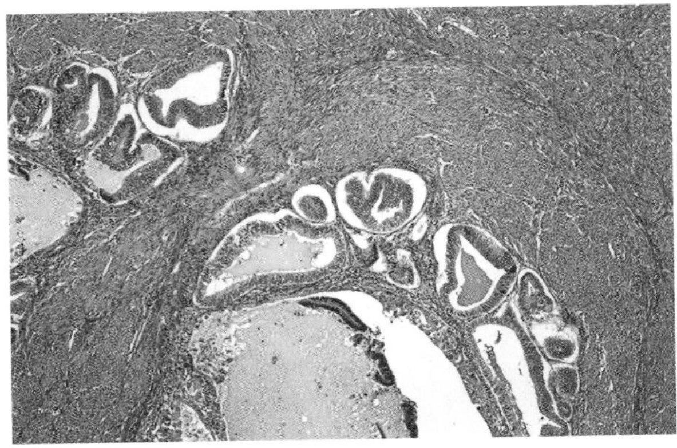

◘ Fig. 10.94
Adenomyosis. **The periphery of this focus of adenomyosis containing endometrial hyperplasia is relatively lacking in endometrial stroma. This focus can be recognized as adenomyosis because of its lobular shape and the circumferential smooth muscle hypertrophy that surrounds it**

histologic finding as adenomyosis, it is advisable to make the diagnosis only when the distance between the lower border of the endometrium and the adenomyosis exceeds one half of a low-power field (about 2.5 mm), an admittedly arbitrary measurement. Adenomyosis exhibits a varied functional response to ovarian hormones. Proliferative glands and stroma generally are observed in the first half of the menstrual cycle. Adenomyosis may not respond to physiologic levels of progesterone, and secretory changes frequently are absent or incomplete during the second half of the cycle.

There are variants of adenomyosis that pathologists should be aware of as they can suggest a malignant tumor. In one, endometrial tissue protrudes into myometrial vessels, simulating vascular invasion by a neoplasm, such as ESS (➲ *Fig. 10.95a*). Intravascular endometrial tissue, consisting of endometrial stroma and glands or endometrial stroma alone, can be found in as many as 20% of uteri with adenomyosis [362]. It usually appears to originate in the perivascular region and push into the vessel lumen; immunostains reveal the intravascular adenomyosis to be covered by a layer of CD31-positive endothelial cells (➲ *Fig. 10.95b*). Other problematic variants of adenomyosis include those where either the glandular or stromal component is altered or sparse. A low power key to recognizing these as adenomyosis is the circumferential muscular hypertrophy that surrounds foci of adenomyosis and the maintenance of a lobular appearance without surrounding stromal desmoplasia. In the gland-poor variant that tends to occur in elderly women, sometimes designated "adenomyosis with sparse glands," glands are few in number and some adenomyotic foci consist mainly or exclusively of endometrial stromal cells [161]. Careful evaluation reveals that these variants of adenomyosis lack features of malignancy and are almost always accompanied by foci of typical adenomyosis. The presence of the stroma-poor variant can be suspected at low-power examination, using the criteria discussed above. In this variant, the stroma is frequently less cellular centrally than at the periphery, resulting in a focus of adenomyosis with a pale center and a darkly stained peripheral zone (➲ *Fig. 10.96*). The stroma can be atrophic and fibrotic and may resemble the stroma of an atrophic endometrial polyp, with the acquisition of an eosinophilic, fibrillary appearance and loss of the monotonous, blue ovoid cells more typically associated with endometrial stroma. The eosinophilic, fibrillary appearance may superficially resemble myometrium, but high power examination can reveal a clear demarcation between the surrounding, hypertrophic, well-organized bundles of myometrium and the disorganized, thin fibrils of altered endometrial stroma [9].

a
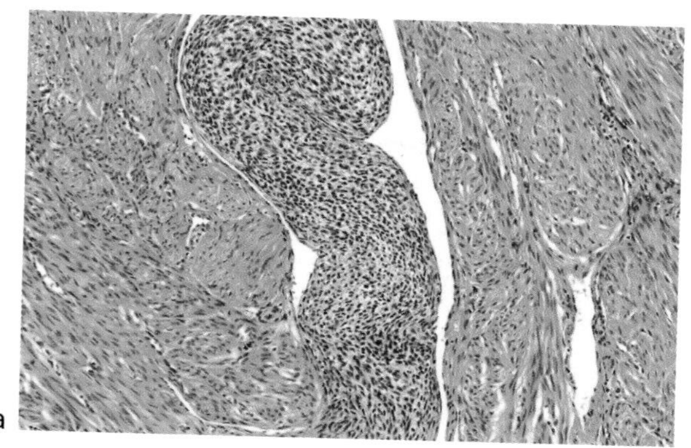

b
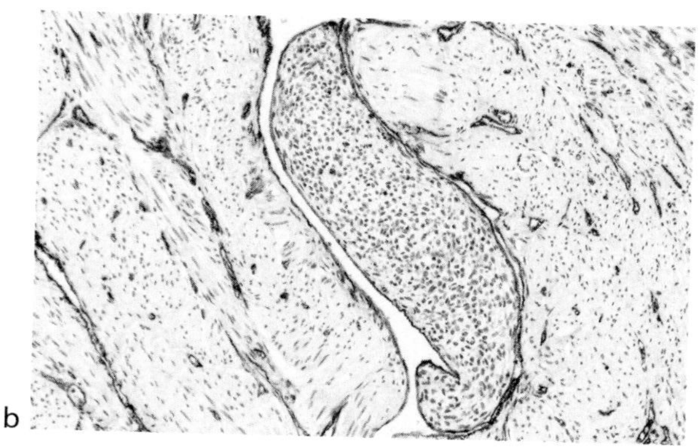

Fig. 10.95
(a) Intravascular endometrial tissue in a patient with adenomyosis. **In this example no glands are present, raising the possibility of endometrial stromal sarcoma. However, there was no mass and no myoinvasive stromal tumor was present. Typical foci of adenomyosis were widely present in the region. (b) Intravascular endometrial tissue in a patient with adenomyosis. An immunostain for CD31 reveals that the vein is lined by a layer of endothelial cells. The intravascular endometrial tissue is completely covered by a layer of CD31-positive endothelial cells, suggesting that it is actually extravascular and has protruded into the vein lumen, pushing the endothelium over it**

Most examples of adenomyosis contain endometrial stroma with a CD10-positive immunophenotype [297, 394]. The eosinophilic, fibrillary stroma described previously in atrophic adenomyosis frequently expresses CD10 only weakly or focally, so absent CD10 staining does not entirely exclude the presence of endometrial stroma and adenomyosis.

An adenomyoma is a circumscribed, nodular aggregate of smooth muscle, endometrial glands, and, usually,

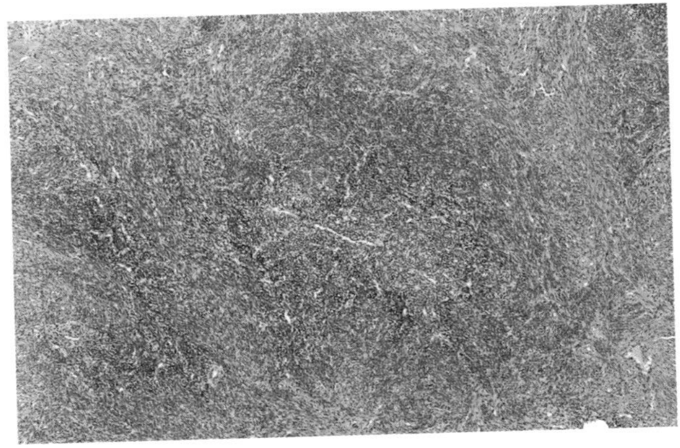

Fig. 10.96
Adenomyosis with sparse glands. **Nearby foci of adenomyosis contained both glands and stroma, but this one consists of stroma only. The center is less cellular and appears pale. The periphery is more cellular and therefore is more darkly stained**

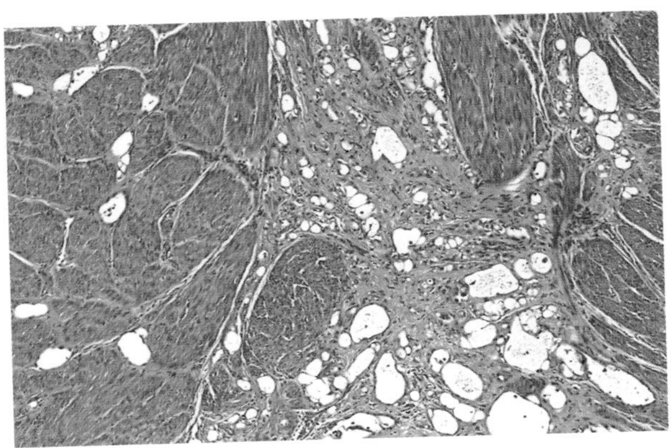

Fig. 10.97
Adenomatoid tumor within hypertrophic myometrium. **Variably sized tubules are lined by flattened or cuboidal mesothelial cells**

endometrial stroma [152, 202, 405]. It may be located within the myometrium, or it may involve or originate in the endometrium and grow as a polyp. About 2% of endometrial polyps are adenomyomas. A rare variant of an adenomyomatous polyp, the atypical polypoid adenomyoma, has atypical hyperplastic glands that usually contain foci of squamous metaplasia (see Chap. 7, Benign Diseases of the Endometrium).

Adenomatoid Tumor

Adenomatoid tumors are distinctive genital tract neoplasms of mesothelial origin that occur in both men and women [102, 300]. In women they occur in the uterus, the fallopian tube, and the ovary [444].

Clinical Features

Adenomatoid tumors typically occur in women of reproductive age; the median age is 42 years. There is no evidence that they impair fertility, and they are usually incidental findings in uteri removed for other causes. Adenomatoid tumors are found in about 1% of hysterectomy specimens, but no specific symptoms have been attributed to them. Adenomatoid tumors are benign. Rarely, an adenomatoid tumor merges with another type of mesothelioma that has the potential for recurrence.

Pathologic Findings

Adenomatoid tumors are usually located subserosally in the cornual myometrium. They are typically small, measuring 0.5–1 cm in diameter, but some are larger and giant and cystic adenomatoid tumors have been reported. Adenomatoid tumors are round and rubbery and are often thought to be leiomyomas. The cut surfaces are gray or tan and may have a spongy appearance due to the presence of uniform small cysts.

Microscopically, adenomatoid tumors tend to be circumscribed, although rare diffuse variants have been described. They consist of tubules and cords of varying size and shape that are lined by flat or cuboidal epithelial cells (*Fig. 10.97*). Collagen, elastic tissue, and smooth muscle surround the epithelial elements. The smooth muscle may predominate such that the tumor appears at first glance to be a leiomyoma or lipoleiomyoma. The cuboidal epithelial cells have cytologically bland, eccentric, round nuclei and abundant pale cytoplasm. The cytoplasm is often vacuolated, sometimes to the extent that some tumor cells resemble signet-ring cells. The growth of the epithelial cells between smooth muscle bundles and the presence of signet-ring-like cells may raise the suspicion of metastatic adenocarcinoma. Nuclear atypia, however, is absent or minimal, MF are infrequent, and stains for mucin are negative. When the cells lining the tubules are flattened, an adenomatoid tumor may resemble a hemangioma or lymphangioma. However, the lumens do not contain blood, and immunostains for such vascular markers as factor VIII-related antigen and CD 31 are negative. Ultrastructural and immunohistochemical studies reveal that the epithelial cells in adenomatoid tumors have a mesothelial phenotype. Immunostains are positive for cytokeratin and vimentin and for such mesothelial cell-associated antigens as calretinin, WT1, and D2-40 [370]. Stains for adenocarcinoma-associated antigens such as CD 15, CEA, B72.3, and Ber-EP4 are usually negative.

Vascular Tumors

Hemangiomas of the uterus, like those at other sites, are composed of neoplastic vessels lined by flat or cuboidal endothelial cells. The endothelial cells have bland nuclei and MF are rare or, most typically, absent. Uterine hemangiomas can be subclassified as capillary, cavernous, or venous, depending on the appearance of the vessels [255, 435]. There are no clinical differences between the subtypes. Capillary hemangiomas of the cervix are the most common vascular tumors of the uterus. Hemangiomas of the corpus are uncommon, and they vary considerably in size. Large hemangiomas can extend through the full thickness of the myometrium and can result in severe bleeding that requires a hysterectomy. Arteriovenous malformations can occur in the uterus [132, 257]. They are differentiated from venous hemangiomas by the presence of thick-walled vessels of both arterial and venous types. The histologic distinction between a hemangioma and a vascular malformation can be difficult, but it is not critical because their clinical features are similar. A few examples of angiosarcoma of the uterus have been reported [53, 229, 283, 366, 407, 436]. Angiosarcoma is a large, hemorrhagic, and often extensively necrotic tumor that grows in the myometrium. It consists of anastomosing vascular channels that are lined by atypical cuboidal or "tombstone"-shaped endothelial cells (*Fig. 10.98*). Many MF are usually present. Some high-grade angiosarcomas consist partly or completely of solid sheets of difficult-to-recognize epithelioid endothelial cells [407]. When these cells predominate, the nature of the tumor can be determined by identifying characteristic foci of vascular growth, often at the periphery of the tumor, and by positive immunohistochemical stains for markers of vascular differentiation such as factor VIII-related antigen or CD 31. Angiosarcoma extensively invades and replaces the myometrium and has a poor prognosis.

In the past, a few uterine tumors have been reported as hemangiopericytomas. Most of these appear to have been endometrial stromal nodules or low-grade ESS that were misdiagnosed as hemangiopericytomas. Whether true hemangiopericytomas occur in the uterus is unclear, but if they do, they are certainly very rare. Rare solitary fibrous tumors of the uterus have been reported, however [66, 430]. Whenever a diagnosis of hemangiopericytoma of the uterus is considered, the possibility that the tumor is an endometrial stromal tumor must be excluded. Occasional endometrial stroma sarcomas that metastasize to extra-uterine sites can resemble hemangiopericytoma and solitary fibrous tumor (*Fig. 10.99*); endometrial stromal

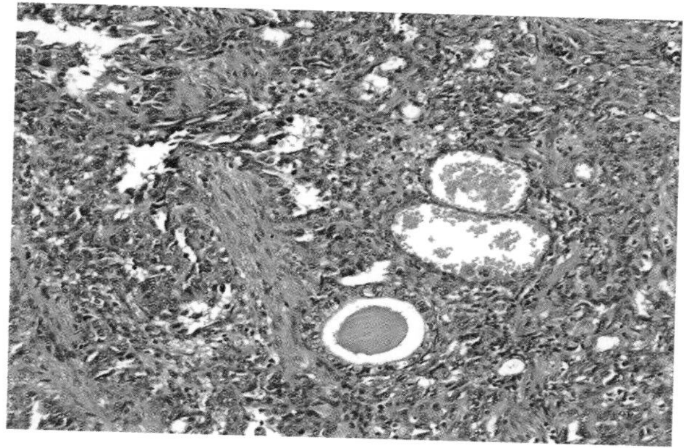

Fig. 10.98
Angiosarcoma of the uterus. **The growth is partly solid but vascular lumens are readily identified. The malignant cells are cuboidal or polygonal and have atypical hyperchromatic nuclei. Numerous mitotic figures were visible at higher magnification. A benign gland is surrounded by tumor (*lower center*)**

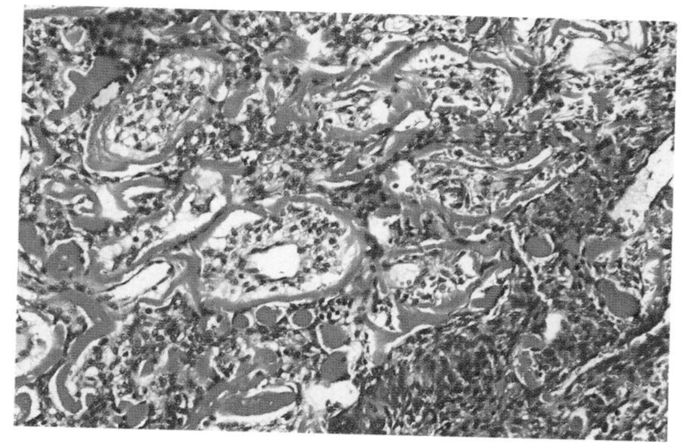

Fig. 10.99
Endometrial stromal tumor. **Many endometrial stromal tumors contain collagen bundles and stag horn vessels that recall hemangiopericytoma and solitary fibrous tumor. Immunohistochemical stains can be used to distinguish between these entities**

tumors express ER, PR, and CD10 and lack diffuse CD34, in contrast to hemangiopericytoma and solitary fibrous tumor, which express CD34 diffusely and can occasionally express weak CD10 and PR [35].

Lymphoma

Lymphoma rarely occurs with initial signs or symptoms suggestive of a uterine tumor, but when it does, the cervix is involved three times more often than is the endometrium [172]. Most patients are older than 20 years and present with an abdominal or pelvic mass, abnormal vaginal bleeding, a vaginal discharge, or pelvic discomfort. Diffuse large cell lymphomas of B-cell type are most common [18, 139, 222, 420]. An 80–90% survival rate has been reported for women with localized lymphomas of the uterus and vagina [172, 397, 420]. The differential diagnosis includes a leiomyoma with a heavy lymphocytic infiltrate and an inflammatory lymphoma-like lesion (pseudolymphoma). Rare leiomyomas contain a heavy lymphocytic infiltrate; however, these are circumscribed tumors in which there are recognizable areas of residual smooth muscle tumor [45, 130]. Additionally, the lymphocytic infiltrate consists of a mixture of cell types. Inflammatory "pseudolymphomas" mainly involve the cervical or endometrial surface or are just beneath it, whereas lymphoma is larger and more deeply situated [442]. Uterine involvement as a manifestation of leukemia is very rare [150, 172, 207, 319].

Inflammatory processes contain a heterogeneous population of lymphoid cells in contrast to the more monomorphic population seen in most lymphomas, and they are polyclonal. The differential diagnosis also includes neoplastic entities, including small cell carcinoma, undifferentiated carcinoma, and IMT, entities discussed elsewhere in this text.

References

1. Abeler VM, Royne O et al (2009) Uterine sarcomas in Norway. A histopathological and prognostic survey of a total population from 1970 to 2000 including 419 patients. Histopathology 54(3):355–364
2. Abrams J, Talcott J et al (1989) Pulmonary metastases in patients with low-grade endometrial stromal sarcoma. Clinicopathologic findings with immunohistochemical characterization. Am J Surg Pathol 13:133–140
3. Abu-Rustum NR, Curtin JP et al (1997) Regression of uterine low-grade smooth-muscle tumors metastatic to the lung after oophorectomy. Obstet Gynecol 89(5 PT 2):850–852
4. Adamson GD (1992) Treatment of uterine fibroids: Current findings with gonadotropin-releasing hormone agonists. Am J Obstet Gynecol 166:746–751
5. Adany R, Fodor F et al (1990) Increased density of histiocytes in uterine leiomyomas. Int J Gynecol Pathol 9(2):137–144
6. Adegboyega PA, Qiu S (2008) Immunohistochemical profiling of cytokeratin expression by endometrial stroma sarcoma. Hum Pathol 39(10):1459–1464
7. Agoff SN, Crispin DA et al (2001) Neoplasms of the ampulla of vater with concurrent pancreatic intraductal neoplasia: a histological and molecular study. Mod Pathol 14(3):139–146
8. Agoff SN, Grieco VS et al (2001) Immunohistochemical distinction of endometrial stromal sarcoma and cellular leiomyoma. Appl Immunohistochem Mol Morphol 9(2):164–169
9. Ali A, Black D et al (2007) Difficulties in assessing the depth of myometrial invasion in endometrial carcinoma. Int J Gynecol Pathol 26(2):115–123
10. Altrabulsi B, Malpica A et al (2005) Undifferentiated carcinoma of the endometrium. Am J Surg Pathol 29(10):1316–1321
11. Amada S, Nakano H et al (1995) Leiomyosarcoma versus bizarre and cellular leiomyomas of the uterus: a comparative study based on the MIB-1 and proliferating cell nuclear antigen indices, p53 expression, DNA flow cytometry, and muscle specific antigens. Int J Gynecol Pathol 14:134–142
12. Amant F, De Knijf A et al (2007) Clinical study investigating the role of lymphadenectomy, surgical castration and adjuvant hormonal treatment in endometrial stromal sarcoma. Br J Cancer 97(9):1194–1199
13. Amant F, Schurmans K et al (2004) Immunohistochemical determination of estrogen and progesterone receptor positivity in uterine adenosarcoma. Gynecol Oncol 93(3):680–685
14. Amant F, Steenkiste E et al (2004) Immunohistochemical expression of CD10 antigen in uterine adenosarcoma. Int J Gynecol Cancer 14(6):1118–1121
15. Amant F, Woestenborghs H et al (2006) Transition of endometrial stromal sarcoma into high-grade sarcoma. Gynecol Oncol 103(3):1137–1140
16. Andersen J (1998) Factors in fibroid growth. Baillières Clin Obstet Gynaecol 12(2):225–243
17. Andrassy RJ, Wiener ES et al (1999) Progress in the surgical management of vaginal rhabdomyosarcoma: a 25-year review from the Intergroup Rhabdomyosarcoma Study Group. J Pediatr Surg 34(5):731–734; discussion 734–735
18. Aozasa K, Saeki K et al (1993) Malignant lymphoma of the uterus. Report of seven cases with immunohistochemical study. Cancer 72(6):1959–1964
19. Arenas M, Rovirosa A et al (2006) Uterine sarcomas in breast cancer patients treated with tamoxifen. Int J Gynecol Cancer 16(2):861–865
20. Argani P, Antonescu CR et al (2001) Primary renal neoplasms with the ASPL-TFE3 gene fusion of alveolar soft part sarcoma – A distinctive tumor entity previously included among renal cell carcinomas of children and adolescents. Am J Pathol 159(1):179–192
21. Argani P, Lal P et al (2003) Aberrant nuclear immunoreactivity for TFE3 in neoplasms with TFE3 gene fusions: a sensitive and specific immunohistochemical assay. Am J Surg Pathol 27(6):750–761
22. Arndt CAS, Donaldson SS et al (2001) What constitutes optimal therapy for patients with rhabdomyosarcoma of the female genital tract? Cancer 91(12):2454–2468
23. Atkins KA, Arronte N et al (2008) The use of p16 in enhancing the histologic classification of uterine smooth muscle tumors. Am J Surg Pathol 32(1):98–102
24. Aubry MC, Myers JL et al (2002) Endometrial stromal sarcoma metastatic to the lung – a detailed analysis of 16 patients. Am J Surg Pathol 26(4):440–449

25. Baiocchi G, Kavanagh JJ et al (1990) Endometrioid stromal sarcomas arising from ovarian and extraovarian endometriosis: report of two cases and review of the literature. Gynecol Oncol 36:147–151
26. Baker P, Oliva E (2007) Endometrial stromal tumors of the uterus: a practical approach using conventional morphology and ancillary techniques. J Clin Pathol 60(3):235–243
27. Baker PM, Moch H et al (2005) Unusual morphologic features of endometrial stromal tumors: a report of 2 cases. Am J Surg Pathol 29(10):1394–1398
28. Baker RJ, Hildebrandt RH et al (1999) Inhibin and CD99 (MIC2) expression in uterine stromal neoplasms with sex-cord-like elements. Hum Pathol 30(6):671–679
29. Banks ER, Mills SE et al (1991) Uterine intravascular menstrual endometrium simulating malignancy. Am J Surg Pathol 15:407–412
30. Bapat K, Brustein S (1989) Uterine sarcoma with liposarcomatous differentiation: report of a case and review of the literature. Int J Gynaecol Obstet 28:71–75
31. Bekkers RL, Willemsen WN et al (1999) Leiomyomatosis peritonealis disseminata: does malignant transformation occur? A literature review. Gynecol Oncol 75(1):158–163
32. Bell SW, Kempson RL et al (1994) Problematic uterine smooth muscle neoplasms: a clinicopathologic study of 213 cases. Am J Surg Pathol 18:535–558
33. Berchuck A, Rubin SC et al (1988) Treatment of uterine leiomyosarcoma. Obstet Gynecol 71:845–850
34. Bergeron C, Amant F et al (2006) Pathology and physiopathology of adenomyosis. Best Pract Res Clin Obstet Gynaecol 20(4): 511–521
35. Bhargava R, Shia J et al (2005) Distinction of endometrial stromal sarcomas from "hemangiopericytomatous" tumors using a panel of immunohistochemical stains. Mod Pathol 18(1):40–47
36. Biermann K, Heukamp LC et al (2008) Uterine tumor resembling an ovarian sex cord tumor associated with metastasis. Int J Gynecol Pathol 27(1):58–60
37. Billings SD, Folpe AL et al (2001) Do leiomyomas of deep soft tissue exist? An analysis of highly differentiated smooth muscle tumors of deep soft tissue supporting two distinct subtypes. Am J Surg Pathol 25(9):1134–1142
38. Binder SW, Nieberg RK et al (1991) Histologic and immunohistochemical analysis of nine endometrial stromal tumors: an unexpected high frequency of keratin protein positivity. Int J Gynecol Pathol 10:191–197
39. Blattner JM, Gable P et al (2007) Primitive neuroectodermal tumor of the uterus. Gynecol Oncol 106(2):419–422
40. Blom R, Guerrieri C (1999) Adenosarcoma of the uterus: a clinicopathologic, DNA flow cytometric, p53 and mdm-2 analysis of 11 cases. Int J Gynecol Cancer 9:37–43
41. Blom R, Guerrieri C et al (1998) Leiomyosarcoma of the uterus: a clinicopathologic, DNA flow cytometric, p53, and mdm-2 analysis of 49 cases. Gynecol Oncol 68:54–61
42. Blom R, Malmstrom H et al (1999) Endometrial stromal sarcoma of the uterus: a clinicopathologic, DNA flow cytometric, p53, and mdm-2 analysis of 17 cases. Int J Gynecol Cancer 9:98–104
43. Bodner K, Bodner-Adler B et al (2004) Estrogen and progesterone receptor expression in patients with uterine smooth muscle tumors. Fertil Steril 81(4):1062–1066
44. Bodner-Adler B, Bodner K et al (2005) Expression of p16 protein in patients with uterine smooth muscle tumors: an immunohistochemical analysis. Gynecol Oncol 96(1):62–66
45. Botsis D, Koliopoulos C et al (2005) Frequency, histological, and immunohistochemical properties of massive inflammatory lymphocytic infiltration of leiomyomas of the uterus: an entity causing diagnostic difficulties. Int J Gynecol Pathol 24(4):326–329
46. Brescia RJ, Tazelaar HD et al (1989) Intravascular lipoleiomyomatosis: a report of two cases. Hum Pathol 20:252–256
47. Brooks JJ, Wells GB et al (1992) Bizarre epithelioid lipoleiomyoma of the uterus. Int J Gynecol Pathol 11:144–149
48. Brooks SE, Zhan M et al (2004) Surveillance, epidemiology, and end results analysis of 2677 cases of uterine sarcoma 1989–1999. Gynecol Oncol 93(1):204–208
49. Brown DC, Theaker JM et al (1987) Cytokeratin expression in smooth muscle and smooth muscle tumors. Histopathology 11:477–486
50. Brunisholz Y, Miller J et al (2004) Endometrial stromal sarcoma resembling adenomyosis and menstrual-phase endometrium. Gynecol Oncol 95(1):256–259
51. Bukulmez O, Doody KJ (2006) Clinical features of myomas. Obstet Gynecol Clin N Am 33(1):69–84
52. Burke C, Hickey K (2004) Treatment of endometrial stromal sarcoma with a gonadotropin-releasing hormone analogue. Obstet Gynecol 104(5 Pt 2):1182–1184
53. Cardinale L, Mirra M et al (2008) Angiosarcoma of the uterus: report of 2 new cases with deviant clinicopathologic features and review of the literature. Ann Diagn Pathol 12(3):217–221
54. Case AS, Kirby TO et al (2005) A case report of rhabdomyosarcoma of the uterus associated with uterine inversion. Gynecol Oncol 96(3):850–853
55. Cessna MH, Zhou H et al (2001) Are myogenin and MyoD1 expression specific for rhabdomyosarcoma? A study of 150 cases, with emphasis on spindle cell mimics. Am J Surg Pathol 25(9): 1150–1157
56. Chan JK, Kawar NM et al (2008) Endometrial stromal sarcoma: a population-based analysis. Br J Cancer 99(8):1210–1215
57. Chang KL, Crabtree GS et al (1990) Primary uterine endometrial stromal neoplasms. A clinicopathologic study of 117 cases. Am J Surg Pathol 14:415–438
58. Chang KL, Crabtree GS et al (1993) Primary extrauterine endometrial stromal neoplasms: a clinicopathologic study of 20 cases and a review of the literature. Int J Gynecol Pathol 12:282–296
59. Chen KT (1999) Uterine leiomyohibernoma. Int J Gynecol Pathol 18(1):96–97
60. Chen L, Yang B (2008) Immunohistochemical analysis of p16, p53, and Ki-67 expression in uterine smooth muscle tumors. Int J Gynecol Pathol 27(3):326–332
61. Cheung ANY, Ng WF et al (1996) Mixed low grade and high grade endometrial stromal sarcoma of uterus: differences on immunohistochemistry and chromosome in situ hybridisation. J Clin Pathol 49(7):604–607
62. Cho KR, Woodruff JD et al (1989) Leiomyoma of the uterus with multiple extrauterine smooth muscle tumors: a case report suggesting multifocal origin. Hum Pathol 20:80–83
63. Chu MC, Mor G et al (2003) Low-grade endometrial stromal sarcoma: hormonal aspects. Gynecol Oncol 90(1):170–176
64. Chu PG, Arber DA (2000) Paraffin-section detection of CD10 in 505 nonhematopoietic neoplasms – Frequent expression in renal cell carcinoma and endometrial stromal sarcoma. Am J Clin Pathol 113(3):374–382
65. Chu PG, Arber DA et al (2001) Utility of CD10 in distinguishing between endometrial stromal sarcoma and uterine smooth muscle tumors: an immunohistochemical comparison of 34 cases. Mod Pathol 14(5):465–471
66. Chu PW, Liu JY et al (2006) Solitary fibrous tumor of the uterus. Taiwan J Obstet Gynecol 45(4):350–352

67. Clement PB (1988) Intravenous leiomyomatosis of the uterus. Pathol Annu 23(Pt 2):153–183
68. Clement PB (1989) Mullerian adenosarcomas of the uterus with sarcomatous overgrowth. A clinicopathological analysis of 10 cases. Am J Surg Pathol 13:28–38
69. Clement PB (2000) The pathology of uterine smooth muscle tumors and mixed endometrial stromal-smooth muscle tumors: a selective review with emphasis on recent advances. Int J Gynecol Pathol 19(1):39–55
70. Clement PB, Oliva E et al (1996) Mullerian adenosarcoma of the uterine corpus associated with tamoxifen therapy: a report of six cases and a review of tamoxifen-associated endometrial lesions. Int J Gynecol Pathol 15:222–229
71. Clement PB, Scully RE (1974) Mullerian adenosarcoma of the uterus. A clinicopathologic analysis of ten cases of a distinctive type of mullerian mixed tumor. Cancer 34:1138–1149
72. Clement PB, Scully RE (1976) Uterine tumors resembling ovarian sex-cord tumors. A clinicopathologic analysis of 14 cases. Am J Clin Pathol 66:512–525
73. Clement PB, Scully RE (1978) Extrauterine mesodermal (Mullerian) adenosarcoma: a clinicopathologic analysis of five cases. Am J Clin Pathol 69:276–283
74. Clement PB, Scully RE (1989) Mullerian adenosarcomas of the uterus with sex cord-like elements. A clinicopathologic analysis of eight cases. Am J Clin Pathol 91:664–672
75. Clement PB, Scully RE (1990) Mullerian adenofibroma of the uterus with invasion of myometrium and pelvic veins. Int J Gynecol Pathol 9:363–371
76. Clement PB, Scully RE (1990) Mullerian adenosarcoma of the uterus: a clinicopathologic analysis of 100 cases with a review of the literature. Hum Pathol 21:363–381
77. Clement PB, Scully RE (1992) Endometrial stromal sarcomas of the uterus with extensive glandular differentiation: a report of three cases that caused problems in differential diagnosis. Int J Gynecol Pathol 11:163–173
78. Clement PB, Young RH et al (1992) Diffuse, perinodular, and other patterns of hydropic degeneration within and adjacent to uterine leiomyomas. Problems in differential diagnosis. Am J Surg Pathol 16:26–32
79. Coad JE, Sulaiman RA et al (1997) Perinodular hydropic degeneration of a uterine leiomyoma: a diagnostic challenge. Hum Pathol 28(2):249–251
80. Coard KC, Fletcher HM (2002) Leiomyosarcoma of the uterus with a florid intravascular component ("intravenous leiomyosarcomatosis"). Int J Gynecol Pathol 21(2):182–185
81. Cohen D, Mazur MT et al (1994) Hyalinization and cellular changes in uterine leiomyomata after gonadotropin releasing hormone agonist therapy. J Reprod Med 39:377–380
82. Cohen DT, Oliva E et al (2007) Uterine smooth-muscle tumors with unusual growth patterns: imaging with pathologic correlation. AJR Am J Roentgenol 188(1):246–255
83. Colgan TJ, Pendergast S et al (1993) The histopathology of uterine leiomyomas following treatment with gonadotropin-releasing hormone analogues. Hum Pathol 24:1073–1077
84. Coosemans A, Nik SA et al (2007) Upregulation of Wilms' tumour gene 1 (WT1) in uterine sarcomas. Eur J Cancer 43(10):1630–1637
85. Cramer SF, Horiszny J et al (1996) The relation of fibrous degeneration to menopausal status in small uterine leiomyomas with evidence for postmenopausal origin of seedling myomas. Mod Pathol 9:774–780
86. Cramer SF, Patel A (1990) The frequency of uterine leiomyomas. Am J Clin Pathol 94:435–438
87. Crist W, Gehan EA et al (1995) The third intergroup rhabdomyosarcoma study. J Clin Oncol 13:610–630
88. Crow J, Gardner RL et al (1995) Morphological changes in uterine leiomyomas treated by GnRH agonist goserelin. Int J Gynecol Pathol 14:235–242
89. Crow J, Wilkins M et al (1991) Mast cells in the female genital tract. Int J Gynecol Pathol 10(3):230–237
90. Cui S, Hano H et al (1999) Evaluation of new monoclonal anti-MyoD1 and anti-myogenin antibodies for the diagnosis of rhabdomyosarcoma. Pathol Int 49(1):62–68
91. Czernobilsky B (2008) Uterine tumors resembling ovarian sex cord tumors: an update. Int J Gynecol Pathol 27(2):229–235
92. Czernobilsky B, Mamet Y et al (2005) Uterine retiform sertoli-leydig cell tumor: report of a case providing additional evidence that uterine tumors resembling ovarian sex cord tumors have a histologic and immunohistochemical phenotype of genuine sex cord tumors. Int J Gynecol Pathol 24(4):335–340
93. Dahhan T, Fons G et al (2009) The efficacy of hormonal treatment for residual or recurrent low-grade endometrial stromal sarcoma. A retrospective study. Eur J Obstet Gynecol Reprod Biol 144:80–84
94. Dal Cin P, Sayed Aly M et al (1992) Endometrial stromal sarcoma t(7;17)(p15–21;q12–21) is a nonrandom chromosome change. Cancer Genet Cytogenet 63:43–46
95. Darby AJ, Papadaki L et al (1975) An unusual leiomyosarcoma of the uterus containing osteoclast-like giant cells. Cancer 36:495–504
96. Day Baird D, Dunson DB et al (2003) High cumulative incidence of uterine leiomyoma in black and white women: ultrasound evidence. Am J Obstet Gynecol 188(1):100–107
97. Daya D, Lukka H et al (1992) Primitive neuroectodermal tumors of the uterus: a report of four cases. Hum Pathol 23:1120–1129
98. Daya DA, Scully RE (1988) Sarcoma botryoides of the uterine cervix in young women: a clinicopathological study of 13 cases. Gynecol Oncol 29:290–304
99. De Fusco PA, Gaffey TA et al (1989) Endometrial stromal sarcoma: review of Mayo Clinic experience, 1945–1980. Gynecol Oncol 35:8–14
100. de Leval L, Waltregny D et al (2006) Use of histone deacetylase 8 (HDAC8), a new marker of smooth muscle differentiation, in the classification of mesenchymal tumors of the uterus. Am J Surg Pathol 30(3):319–327
101. de Vos S, Wilczynski SP et al (1994) p53 alterations in uterine leiomyosarcomas versus leiomyomas. Gynecol Oncol 54:205–208
102. Delahunt B, Eble JN et al (2000) Immunohistochemical evidence for mesothelial origin of paratesticular adenomatoid tumour. Histopathology 36(2):109–115
103. Demopoulos RI, Jones KY et al (1997) Histology of leiomyomata in patients treated with leuprolide acetate. Int J Gynecol Pathol 16:131–137
104. Devaney K, Tavassoli FA (1991) Immunohistochemistry as a diagnostic aid in the interpretation of unusual mesenchymal tumors of the uterus. Mod Pathol 4:225–231
105. Dgani R, Piura B et al (1998) Clinical-pathological study of uterine leiomyomas with high mitotic activity. Acta Obstet Gynecol Scand 77(1):74–77
106. Dharkar DD, Kraft JR et al (1981) Uterine lipomas. Arch Pathol Lab Med 105:43–45
107. Dimmler A, Seitz G et al (2003) Late pulmonary metastasis in uterine PEComa. J Clin Pathol 56(8):627–628

108. Dinh TA, Oliva EA et al (2004) The treatment of uterine leiomyosarcoma. Results from a 10-year experience (1990–1999) at the Massachusetts General Hospital. Gynecol Oncol 92(2):648–652
109. Dionigi A, Oliva E et al (2002) Endometrial stromal nodules and endometrial stromal tumors with limited infiltration – A clinicopathologic study of 50 cases. Am J Surg Pathol 26(5): 567–581
110. Downes KA, Hart WR (1997) Bizarre leiomyomas of the uterus: a comprehensive pathologic study of 24 cases with long-term follow-up. Am J Surg Pathol 21(11):1261–1270
111. Due W, Pickartz H (1989) Immunohistologic detection of estrogen and progesterone receptors in disseminated peritoneal leiomyomatosis. Int J Gynecol Pathol 8:46–53
112. Dueholm M, Lundorf E et al (2002) Accuracy of magnetic resonance imaging and transvaginal ultrasonography in the diagnosis, mapping, and measurement of uterine myomas. Am J Obstet Gynecol 186(3):409–415
113. Dundr P, Mara M et al (2006) Pathological findings of uterine leiomyomas and adenomyosis following uterine artery embolization. Pathol Res Pract 202(10):721–729
114. Eichhorn JH, Young RH et al (2002) Mesodermal (mullerian) adenosarcoma of the ovary: a clinicopathologic analysis of 40 cases and a review of the literature. Am J Surg Pathol 26(10): 1243–1258
115. Emoto M, Iwasaki H et al (1994) Primary osteosarcoma of the uterus: report of a case with immunohistochemical analysis. Gynecol Oncol 54:385–388
116. Euscher ED, Deavers MT et al (2008) Uterine tumors with neuroectodermal differentiation: a series of 17 cases and review of the literature. Am J Surg Pathol 32(2):219–228
117. Evans AT III, Symmonds RE et al (1981) Recurrent pelvic intravenous leiomyomatosis. Obstet Gynecol 57:260–264
118. Evans HL (1982) Endometrial stromal sarcoma and poorly differentiated endometrial sarcoma. Cancer 50:2170–2182
119. Evans HL, Chawla SP et al (1988) Smooth muscle neoplasms of the uterus other than ordinary leiomyoma. A study of 46 cases, with emphasis on diagnostic criteria and prognostic factors. Cancer 62:2239–2247
120. Eyden BP, Hale RJ et al (1992) Cytoskeletal filaments in the smooth muscle cells of uterine leiomyomata and myometrium: an ultrastructural and immunohistochemical analysis. Virchows Archiv A Pathol Anat Histopathol 420:51–58
121. Fadare O (2008) Perivascular epithelioid cell tumor (PEComa) of the uterus: an outcome-based clinicopathologic analysis of 41 reported cases. Adv Anat Pathol 15(2):63–75
122. Fadare O (2008) Uterine PEComa: appraisal of a controversial and increasingly reported mesenchymal neoplasm. Int Semin Surg Oncol 5:7
123. Fadare O, Liang SX (2008) Epithelioid smooth muscle tumors of the uterus do not express CD1a: a potential immunohistochemical adjunct in their distinction from uterine perivascular epithelioid cell tumors. Ann Diagn Pathol 12(6):401–405
124. Fechner RE (1968) Atypical leiomyomas and synthetic progestogen therapy. Am J Clin Pathol 49:697–703
125. Fehmian C, Jones J et al (1997) Adenosarcoma of the uterus with extensive smooth muscle differentiation: Ultrastructural study and review of the literature. Ultrastruct Pathol 21(1):73–79
126. Fekete PS, Vellios F (1984) The clinical and histologic spectrum of endometrial stromal neoplasms: a report of 41 cases. Int J Gynecol Pathol 3:198–212
127. Ferguson SE, Gerald W et al (2007) Clinicopathologic features of rhabdomyosarcoma of gynecologic origin in adults. Am J Surg Pathol 31(3):382–389
128. Ferguson SE, Tornos C et al (2007) Prognostic features of surgical stage I uterine carcinosarcoma. Am J Surg Pathol 31(11):1653–1661
129. Ferrari A, Dileo P et al (2003) Rhabdomyosarcoma in adults. A retrospective analysis of 171 patients treated at a single institution. Cancer 98(3):571–580
130. Ferry JA, Harris NL et al (1989) Uterine leiomyomas with lymphoid infiltration simulating lymphoma: a report of seven cases. Int J Gynecol Pathol 8:263–270
131. FIGO (2009) FIGO staging for uterine sarcomas. Int J Gynaecol Obstet 104(3):179
132. Fleming H, Ostor AG et al (1989) Arteriovenous malformations of the uterus. Obstet Gynecol 73:209–214
133. Fleming WP, Peters WA et al (1984) Autopsy findings in patients with uterine sarcoma. Gynecol Oncol 19:168–172
134. Flierman PA, Oberye JJ et al (2005) Rapid reduction of leiomyoma volume during treatment with the GnRH antagonist ganirelix. BJOG 112(5):638–642
135. Folpe AL, McKenney JK et al (2002) Sclerosing rhabdomyosarcoma in adults: report of four cases of a hyalinizing, matrix-rich variant of rhabdomyosarcoma that may be confused with osteosarcoma, chondrosarcoma, or angiosarcoma. Am J Surg Pathol 26(9): 1175–1183
136. Folpe AL, Mentzel T et al (2005) Perivascular epithelioid cell neoplasms of soft tissue and gynecologic origin: a clinicopathologic study of 26 cases and review of the literature. Am J Surg Pathol 29(12):1558–1575
137. Fornelli A, Pasquinelli G et al (1999) Leiomyoma of the uterus showing skeletal muscle differentiation: A case report. Hum Pathol 30(3):356–359
138. Fraggetta F, Magro G et al (1997) Primitive neuroectodermal tumour of the uterus with focal cartilaginous differentiation. Histopathology 30(5):483–485
139. Frey NV, Svoboda J et al (2006) Primary lymphomas of the cervix and uterus: the University of Pennsylvania's experience and a review of the literature. Leuk Lymphoma 47(9):1894–1901
140. Fukunaga M (2005) Perivascular epithelioid cell tumor of the uterus: report of four cases. Int J Gynecol Pathol 24(4):341–346
141. Fukunaga M, Ishihara A et al (1998) Extrauterine low-grade endometrial stromal sarcoma: report of three cases. Pathol Int 48(4): 297–302
142. Fukunaga M, Nomura K et al (1996) Carcinosarcoma of the uterus with extensive neuroectodermal differentiation. Histopathology 29(6):565–570
143. Fukunaga M, Ushigome S (1998) Dissecting leiomyoma of the uterus with extrauterine extension. Histopathology 32(2): 160–164
144. Gadducci A, Cosio S et al (2008) The management of patients with uterine sarcoma: a debated clinical challenge. Crit Rev Oncol Hematol 65(2):129–142
145. Gadducci A, Landoni F et al (1996) Uterine leiomyosarcoma: analysis of treatment failures and survival. Gynecol Oncol 62:25–32
146. Gadducci A, Sartori E et al (1996) Endometrial stromal sarcoma: analysis of treatment failures and survival. Gynecol Oncol 63: 247–253
147. Gal AA, Brooks JJ et al (1989) Leiomyomatous neoplasms of the lung: a clinical, histologic, and immunohistochemical study. Mod Pathol 2:209–216

148. Gallardo A, Prat J (2009) Mullerian adenosarcoma: a clinicopathologic and immunohistochemical study of 55 cases challenging the existence of adenofibroma. Am J Surg Pathol 33(2):278–288
149. Gannon BR, Manduch M et al (2008) Differential immunoreactivity of p16 in leiomyosarcomas and leiomyoma variants. Int J Gynecol Pathol 27(1):68–73
150. Garcia MG, Deavers MT et al (2006) Myeloid sarcoma involving the gynecologic tract: a report of 11 cases and review of the literature. Am J Clin Pathol 125(5):783–790
151. Gard GB, Mulvany NJ et al (1999) Management of uterine leiomyosarcoma in Australia. Aust N Z J Obstet Gynaecol 39(1):93–98
152. Gilks CB, Clement PB et al (2000) Uterine adenomyomas excluding atypical polypoid adenomyomas and adenomyomas of endocervical type: a clinicopathologic study of 30 cases of an underemphasized lesion that may cause diagnostic problems with brief consideration of adenomyomas of other female genital tract sites. Int J Gynecol Pathol 19(3):195–205
153. Gilks CB, Taylor GP et al (1987) Inflammatory pseudotumor of the uterus. Int J Gynecol Pathol 6:275–286
154. Gisser SD, Young I (1977) Neurilemoma-like uterine myomas: an ultrastructural reaffirmation of their non-Schwannian nature. Am J Obstet Gynecol 129:389–392
155. Giuntoli RL 2nd, Bristow RE (2004) Uterine leiomyosarcoma: present management. Curr Opin Oncol 16(4):324–327
156. Giuntoli RL 2nd, Gostout BS et al (2007) Diagnostic criteria for uterine smooth muscle tumors: leiomyoma variants associated with malignant behavior. J Reprod Med 52(11):1001–1010
157. Giuntoli RL, Metzinger DS et al (2003) Retrospective review of 208 patients with leiomyosarcoma of the uterus: prognostic indicators, surgical management, and adjuvant therapy. Gynecol Oncol 89(3):460–469
158. Goff BA, Rice LW et al (1993) Uterine leiomyosarcoma and endometrial stromal sarcoma: lymph node metastases and sites of recurrence. Gynecol Oncol 50:105–109
159. Goh SG, Chuah KL et al (2005) Uterine epithelioid endometrial stromal sarcoma presenting as a "cervical polyp". Ann Diagn Pathol 9(2):101–105
160. Goldberg MF, Hurt WG et al (1977) Leiomyomatosis peritonealis disseminata: report of a case and review of the literature. Obstet Gynecol 49:46s–52s
161. Goldblum JR, Clement PB et al (1995) Adenomyosis with sparse glands: a potential mimic of low-grade endometrial stromal sarcoma. Am J Clin Pathol 103:218–223
162. Gollard R, Kosty M et al (1995) Two unusual presentations of mullerian adenosarcoma: case reports, literature review, and treatment considerations. Gynecol Oncol 59(3):412–422
163. Gown AM, Boyd HC et al (1988) Smooth muscle cells can express cytokeratins of "simple" epithelium. Immunocytochemical and biochemical studies in vitro and in vivo. Am J Pathol 132:223–232
164. Grayson W, Fourie J et al (1998) Xanthomatous leiomyosarcoma of the uterine cervix. Int J Gynecol Pathol 17:89–90
165. Greene LA, Mount SL et al (2003) Recurrent perivascular epithelioid cell tumor of the uterus (PEComa): an immunohistochemical study and review of the literature. Gynecol Oncol 90(3):677–681
166. Grignon DJ, Carey MR et al (1987) Diffuse uterine leiomyomatosis: a case study with pregnancy complicated by intrapartum hemorrhage. Obstet Gynecol 69:477–480
167. Gutmann JN, Thornton KL et al (1994) Evaluation of leuprolide acetate treatment on histopathology of uterine myomata. Fertil Steril 61:622–626
168. Gyure KA, Hart WR et al (1995) Lymphangiomyomatosis of the uterus associated with tuberous sclerosis and malignant neoplasia of the female genital tract: a report of two cases. Int J Gynecol Pathol 14:344–351
169. Hales HA, Peterson CM et al (1992) Leiomyomatosis peritonealis disseminata treated with a gonadotropin- releasing hormone agonist. Am J Obstet Gynecol 167:515–516
170. Hall KL, Teneriello MG et al (1997) Analysis of Ki-ras, p53, and MDM2 genes in uterine leiomyomas and leiomyosarcomas. Gynecol Oncol 65:330–335
171. Han HS, Park IA et al (1998) The clear cell variant of epithelioid intravenous leiomyomatosis of the uterus: report of a case. Pathol Int 48(11):892–896
172. Harris NL, Scully RE (1984) Malignant lymphoma and granulocytic sarcoma of the uterus and vagina. A clinicopathologic analysis of 27 cases. Cancer 53:2530–2545
173. Hashimoto K, Azuma C et al (1995) Clonal determination of uterine leiomyomas by analyzing differential inactivation of the X-chromosome-linked phosphoglycerokinase gene. Gynecol Obstet Investig 40:204–208
174. Hattab EM, Allam-Nandyala P et al (1999) The stromal component of large endometrial polyps. Int J Gynecol Pathol 18(4):332–337
175. Hawkins WG, Hoos A et al (2001) Clinicopathologic analysis of patients with adult rhabdomyosarcoma. Cancer 91(4):794–803
176. Heerema-McKenney A, Wijnaendts LC et al (2008) Diffuse myogenin expression by immunohistochemistry is an independent marker of poor survival in pediatric rhabdomyosarcoma: a tissue microarray study of 71 primary tumors including correlation with molecular phenotype. Am J Surg Pathol 32(10): 1513–1522
177. Hendrickson MR, Scheithauer BW (1986) Primitive neuroectodermal tumor of the endometrium: report of two cases, one with electron microscopic observations. Int J Gynecol Pathol 5: 249–259
178. Hensley ML, Maki R et al (2002) Gemcitabine and docetaxel in patients with unresectable leiomyosarcoma: results of a phase II trial. J Clin Oncol 20(12):2824–2831
179. Hillard JB, Malpica A et al (2004) Conservative management of a uterine tumor resembling an ovarian sex cord-stromal tumor. Gynecol Oncol 92(1):347–352
180. Hilsenbeck SG, Allred DC (1992) Improved methods of estimating mitotic activity in solid tumors. Hum Pathol 23(6):601–602
181. Hirschfield L, Kahn LB et al (1986) Mullerian adenosarcoma with ovarian sex cord-like differentiation. A light- and electron-microscopic study. Cancer 57:1197–1200
182. Horie Y, Ikawa S et al (1995) Lipoadenofibroma of the uterine corpus: report of a new variant of adenofibroma (benign mullerian mixed tumor). Arch Pathol Lab Med 119:274–276
183. Hornback NB, Omura G et al (1986) Observations on the use of adjuvant radiation therapy in patients with stage I and II uterine sarcoma. Int J Radiat Oncol Biol Phys 12(12):2127–2130
184. Hornick JL, Fletcher CD (2008) Sclerosing PEComa: clinicopathologic analysis of a distinctive variant with a predilection for the retroperitoneum. Am J Surg Pathol 32(4):493–501
185. Horstmann JP, Pietra GG et al (1977) Spontaneous regression of pulmonary leiomyomas during pregnancy. Cancer 39:314–321
186. Houghton JP, McCluggage WG (2007) Embryonal rhabdomyosarcoma of the cervix with focal pleomorphic areas. J Clin Pathol 60(1):88–89
187. Hrzenjak A, Moinfar F et al (2005) JAZF1/JJAZ1 gene fusion in endometrial stromal sarcomas: molecular analysis by reverse

transcriptase-polymerase chain reaction optimized for paraffin-embedded tissue. J Mol Diagn 7(3):388–395
188. Hrzenjak A, Tippl M et al (2004) Inverse correlation of secreted frizzled-related protein 4 and beta-catenin expression in endometrial stromal sarcomas. J Pathol 204(1):19–27
189. Huang HY, Ladanyi M et al (2004) Molecular detection of JAZF1-JJAZ1 gene fusion in endometrial stromal neoplasms with classic and variant histology: evidence for genetic heterogeneity. Am J Surg Pathol 28(2):224–232
190. Hurrell DP, McCluggage WG (2005) Uterine leiomyosarcoma with HMB45+ clear cell areas: report of two cases. Histopathology 47(5):540–542
191. Hurrell DP, McCluggage WG (2007) Uterine tumour resembling ovarian sex cord tumour is an immunohistochemically polyphenotypic neoplasm which exhibits coexpression of epithelial, myoid and sex cord markers. J Clin Pathol 60(10):1148–1154
192. Hyde KE, Geisinger KR et al (1989) The clear-cell variant of uterine epithelioid leiomyoma. An immunohistologic and ultrastructural study. Arch Pathol Lab Med 113:551–553
193. Inoue M, Fukuda H et al (1995) Adenosarcomas originating from sites other than uterine endometrium. Int J Gynaecol Obstet 48:299–306
194. Ip PP, Cheung AN et al (2009) Uterine smooth muscle tumors of uncertain malignant potential (STUMP): a clinicopathologic analysis of 16 cases. Am J Surg Pathol 33(7):992–1005
195. Irving JA, Carinelli S et al (2006) Uterine tumors resembling ovarian sex cord tumors are polyphenotypic neoplasms with true sex cord differentiation. Mod Pathol 19(1):17–24
196. Ito H, Sasaki N et al (1986) Bizarre leiomyoblastoma of the cervix uteri. Immunohistochemical and ultrastructural study. Acta Pathol Jpn 36:1737–1745
197. Jautzke G, Muller-Ruchholtz E et al (1996) Immunohistological detection of estrogen and progesterone receptors in multiple and well differentiated leiomyomatous lung tumors in women with uterine leiomyomas (so-called benign metastasizing leiomyomas). A report on 5 cases. Pathol Res Pract 192:215–223
198. Jones MW, Lefkowitz M (1995) Adenosarcoma of the uterine cervix: a clinicopathological study of 12 cases. Int J Gynecol Pathol 14: 223–229
199. Jones MW, Norris HJ (1995) Clinicopathologic study of 28 uterine leiomyosarcomas with metastasis. Int J Gynecol Pathol 14:243–249
200. Joshi D, Anderson JR et al (2004) Age is an independent prognostic factor in rhabdomyosarcoma: a report from the Soft Tissue Sarcoma Committee of the Children's Oncology Group. Pediatr Blood Cancer 42(1):64–73
201. Jung CK, Jung JH et al (2008) Diagnostic use of nuclear beta-catenin expression for the assessment of endometrial stromal tumors. Mod Pathol 21(6):756–763
202. Jung WY, Shin BK et al (2002) Uterine adenomyoma with uterus-like features: a report of two cases. Int J Surg Pathol 10(2): 163–166
203. Kairi-Vassilatou E, Kontogianni K et al (2004) A clinicopathological study of the relationship between adenomyosis and other hormone-dependent uterine lesions. Eur J Gynaecol Oncol 25(2):222–224
204. Kaku T, Silverberg SG et al (1992) Adenosarcoma of the uterus: a Gynecologic Oncology Group clinicopathologic study of 31 cases. Int J Gynecol Pathol 11:75–88
205. Kalir T, Goldstein M et al (1998) Morphometric and electron-microscopic analyses of the effects of gonadotropin-releasing hormone agonists on uterine leiomyomas. Arch Pathol Lab Med 122(5):442–446
206. Kaminski PF, Tavassoli FA (1984) Plexiform tumorlet: a clinical and pathologic study of 15 cases with ultrastructural observations. Int J Gynecol Pathol 3:124–134
207. Kapadia SB, Krause JR et al (1978) Granulocytic sarcoma of the uterus. Cancer 41:687–691
208. Karpf EF, Poetsch B et al (2007) Endometrial stromal nodule embedded into term placenta. APMIS 115(11):1302–1305
209. Kasashima S, Minato H et al (2007) Alveolar soft part sarcoma of the endometrium with expression of CD10 and hormone receptors. APMIS 115(7):861–865
210. Katsanis WA, O'Connor DM et al (1998) Endometrial stromal sarcoma involving the placenta. Ann Diagn Pathol 2(5):301–305
211. Kawaguchi K, Fujii S et al (1989) Mitotic activity in uterine leiomyomas during the menstrual cycle. Am J Obstet Gynecol 160:637–641
212. Kempson RL, Hendrickson MR (2000) Smooth muscle, endometrial stromal, and mixed Mullerian tumors of the uterus. Mod Pathol 13(3):328–342
213. Kerner H, Lichtig C (1993) Mullerian adenosarcoma presenting as cervical polyps: a report of seven cases and review of the literature. Obstet Gynecol 81:655–659
214. Kim KR, Jun SY et al (2005) Endometrial stromal tumor with limited infiltration and probable extrauterine metastasis: report of a case. Ann Diagn Pathol 9(1):57–60
215. Kim WY, Lee JW et al (2008) Low-grade endometrial stromal sarcoma: a single center's experience with 22 cases. Int J Gynecol Cancer 18(5):1084–1089
216. King ME, Dickersin GR et al (1982) Myxoid leiomyosarcoma of the uterus: a report of six cases. Am J Surg Pathol 6:589–598
217. Kjerulff KH, Langenberg P et al (1996) Uterine leiomyomas. Racial differences in severity, symptoms and age at diagnosis. J Reprod Med 41(7):483–490
218. Klein WM, Kurman RJ (2003) Lack of expression of c-kit protein (CD117) in mesenchymal tumors of the uterus and ovary. Int J Gynecol Pathol 22(2):181–184
219. Kokawa K, Yamoto M et al (2002) Postmenopausal intravenous lelomyomatosis with high levels of estradiol and estrogen receptor. Obstet Gynecol 100(5 PT 2):1124–1126
220. Kondi-Paphitis A, Smyrniotis B et al (1998) Stromal sarcoma arising on endometriosis. A clinicopathological and immunohistochemical study of 4 cases. Eur J Gynaecol Oncol 19(6):588–590
221. Koontz JI, Soreng AL et al (2001) Frequent fusion of the JAZF1 and JJAZ1 genes in endometrial stromal tumors. Proc Natl Acad Sci USA 98(11):6348–6353
222. Kosari F, Daneshbod Y et al (2005) Lymphomas of the female genital tract: a study of 186 cases and review of the literature. Am J Surg Pathol 29(11):1512–1520
223. Krauss K, Bachmann C et al (2007) Management of late recurrence of a low-grade endometrial stromal sarcoma (LGESS): treatment with letrozole. Anticancer Res 27(5B):3477–3480
224. Krishnamurthy S, Jungbluth AA et al (1998) Uterine tumors resembling ovarian sex-cord tumors have an immunophenotype consistent with true sex-cord differentiation. Am J Surg Pathol 22(9):1078–1082
225. Krivak TC, Seidman JD et al (2001) Uterine adenosarcoma with sarcomatous overgrowth versus uterine carcinosarcoma: comparison of treatment and survival. Gynecol Oncol 83(1):89–94
226. Kunzel KE, Mills NZ et al (1993) Myxoid leiomyosarcoma of the uterus. Gynecol Oncol 48:277–280
227. Kurihara S, Oda Y et al (2008) Endometrial stromal sarcomas and related high-grade sarcomas: immunohistochemical and molecular genetic study of 31 cases. Am J Surg Pathol 32(8):1228–1238

228. Kurman RJ, Norris HJ (1976) Mesenchymal tumors of the uterus. VI. Epithelioid smooth muscle tumors including leiomyoblastoma and clear cell leiomyoma: a clinical and pathological analysis of 26 cases. Cancer 37:1853–1865
229. Lack EE, Bitterman P et al (1991) Mullerian adenosarcoma of the uterus with pure angiosarcoma: case report. Hum Pathol 22: 1289–1291
230. Ladanyi M, Lui MY et al (2001) The der(17)t(X;17)(p11;q25) of human alveolar soft part sarcoma fuses the TFE3 transcription factor gene to ASPL, a novel gene at 17q25. Oncogene 20(1): 48–57
231. Lai FM, Wong FW et al (1991) Diffuse uterine leiomyomatosis with hemorrhage. Arch Pathol Lab Med 115:834–837
232. Langlois PL (1970) The size of the normal uterus. J Reprod Med 4:220–228
233. Larson B, Silfversward C et al (1990) Prognostic factors in uterine leiomyosarcoma. A clinical and histopathological study of 143 cases. The Radiumhemmet series 1936–1981. Acta Oncol 29:185–191
234. Lawrence B, Perez-Atayde A et al (2000) TPM3-ALK and TPM4-ALK oncogenes in inflammatory myofibroblastic tumors. Am J Pathol 157(2):377–384
235. Layfield LJ, Liu K et al (2000) Uterine smooth muscle tumors – Utility of classification by proliferation, ploidy, and prognostic markers versus traditional histopathology. Arch Pathol Lab Med 124(2):221–227
236. Leath CA III, Huh WK et al (2007) A multi-institutional review of outcomes of endometrial stromal sarcoma. Gynecol Oncol 105(3):630–634
237. Lee HJ, Choi J et al (2008) Pulmonary benign metastasizing leiomyoma associated with intravenous leiomyomatosis of the uterus: clinical behavior and genomic changes supporting a transportation theory. Int J Gynecol Pathol 27(3):340–345
238. Leibsohn S, d'Ablaing G et al (1990) Leiomyosarcoma in a series of hysterectomies performed for presumed uterine leiomyomas. Am J Obstet Gynecol 162:968–974
239. Leiser AL, Anderson SE et al (2006) Apoptotic and cell cycle regulatory markers in uterine leiomyosarcoma. Gynecol Oncol 101(1):86–91
240. Leitao MM, Sonoda Y et al (2003) Incidence of lymph node and ovarian metastases in leiomyosarcoma of the uterus. Gynecol Oncol 91(1):209–212
241. Leitao MM, Soslow RA et al (2004) Tissue microarray immunohistochemical expression of estrogen, progesterone, and androgen receptors in uterine leiomyomata and leiomyosarcoma. Cancer 101(6):1455–1462
242. Lerwill MF, Sung R et al (2004) Smooth muscle tumors of the ovary: a clinicopathologic study of 54 cases emphasizing prognostic criteria, histologic variants, and differential diagnosis. Am J Surg Pathol 28(11):1436–1451
243. Leunen M, Breugelmans M et al (2004) Low-grade endometrial stromal sarcoma treated with the aromatase inhibitor letrozole. Gynecol Oncol 95(3):769–771
244. Leuschner I, Harms D et al (2001) Rhabdomyosarcoma of the urinary bladder and vagina. A clinicopathologic study with emphasis on recurrent disease: a report from the Kiel pediatric tumor registry and the German CWS study. Am J Surg Pathol 25(7):856–864
245. Levenback C, Rubin SC et al (1992) Resection of pulmonary metastases from uterine sarcomas. Gynecol Oncol 45:202–205
246. LevGur M, Abadi MA et al (2000) Adenomyosis: Symptoms, histology, and pregnancy terminations. Obstet Gynecol 95(5): 688–691
247. Li AJ, Giuntoli RL et al (2005) Ovarian preservation in stage I low-grade endometrial stromal sarcomas. Obstet Gynecol 106(6): 1304–1308
248. Li N, Wu LY et al (2008) Treatment options in stage I endometrial stromal sarcoma: a retrospective analysis of 53 cases. Gynecol Oncol 108(2):306–311
249. Lillemoe TJ, Perrone T et al (1991) Myogenous phenotype of epithelial-like areas in endometrial stromal sarcomas. Arch Pathol Lab Med 115:215–219
250. Little DJ, Ballo MT et al (2002) Adult rhabdomyosarcoma – Outcome following multimodality treatment. Cancer 95(2):377–388
251. Lloreta J, Prat J (1992) Endometrial stromal nodule with smooth and skeletal muscle components simulating stromal sarcoma. Int J Gynecol Pathol 11(4):293–298
252. Lo KW, Yu MY et al (2008) Low-grade endometrial stromal sarcoma with florid intravenous component. Gynecol Obstet Invest 66(1): 8–11
253. Lobel MK, Somasundaram P et al (2006) The genetic heterogeneity of uterine leiomyomata. Obstet Gynecol Clin N Am 33(1):13–39
254. Longacre TA, Hendrickson MR et al (1997) Predicting clinical outcome for uterine smooth muscle neoplasms with a reasonable degree of certainty. Adv Anat Pathol 4(2):95–104
255. Lotgering FK, Pijpers L et al (1989) Pregnancy in a patient with diffuse cavernous hemangioma of the uterus. Am J Obstet Gynecol 160:628–630
256. Mahadeva R, Stewart S et al (1999) Metastatic endometrial stromal sarcoma masquerading as pulmonary lymphangioleiomyomatosis. J Clin Pathol 52(2):147–148
257. Majmudar B, Ghanee N et al (1998) Uterine arteriovenous malformation necessitating hysterectomy with bilateral salpingo-oophorectomy in a young pregnant patient. Arch Pathol Lab Med 122(9):842–845
258. Major FJ, Blessing JA et al (1993) Prognostic factors in early-stage uterine sarcoma: a gynecologic oncology group study. Cancer 71(Suppl):1702–1709
259. Maluf HM, Gersell DJ (1994) Uterine leiomyomas with high content of mast cells. Arch Pathol Lab Med 118:712–714
260. Manoharan M, Azmi MA et al (2007) Mullerian adenosarcoma of uterine cervix: report of three cases and review of literature. Gynecol Oncol 105(1):256–260
261. Marsh EE, Bulun SE (2006) Steroid hormones and leiomyomas. Obstet Gynecol Clin N Am 33(1):59–67
262. Marshall RJ, Braye SG et al (1986) Leiomyosarcoma of the uterus with giant cells resembling osteoclasts. Int J Gynecol Pathol 5: 260–268
263. Marshburn PB, Matthews ML et al (2006) Uterine artery embolization as a treatment option for uterine myomas. Obstet Gynecol Clin N Am 33(1):125–144
264. Martelli H, Oberlin O et al (1999) Conservative treatment for girls with nonmetastatic rhabdomyosarcoma of the genital tract: a report from the Study Committee of the International Society of Pediatric Oncology. J Clin Oncol 17(7):2117–2122
265. Martignoni G, Pea M et al (2008) PEComas: the past, the present and the future. Virchows Archiv 452(2):119–132
266. Martin-Reay DG, Christ ML et al (1991) Uterine leiomyoma with skeletal muscle differentiation. Report of a case. Am J Clin Pathol 96(3):344–347
267. Mashal RD, Fejzo ML et al (1994) Analysis of androgen receptor DNA reveals the independent clonal origins of uterine leiomyomata and the secondary nature of cytogenetic aberrations in the development of leiomyomata. Genes Chromosom Cancer 11(1):1–6

268. Mayerhofer K, Obermair A et al (1999) Leiomyosarcoma of the uterus: a clinicopathologic multicenter study of 71 cases. Gynecol Oncol 74(2):196–201
269. Mazur MT, Kraus FT (1980) Histogenesis of morphologic variations in tumors of the uterine wall. Am J Surg Pathol 4:59–74
270. Mazur MT, Priest JB (1986) Clear cell leiomyoma (leiomyoblastoma) of the uterus: ultrastructural observations. Ultrastruct Pathol 10:249–255
271. McCluggage WG, Alderdice JM et al (1999) Polypoid uterine lesions mimicking endometrial stromal sarcoma. J Clin Pathol 52(7): 543–546
272. McCluggage WG, Cromie AJ et al (2001) Uterine endometrial stromal sarcoma with smooth muscle and glandular differentiation. J Clin Pathol 54(6):481–483
273. McCluggage WG, Date A et al (1996) Endometrial stromal sarcoma with sex cord-like areas and focal rhabdoid differentiation. Histopathology 29(4):369–374
274. McCluggage WG, Ellis PK et al (2000) Pathologic features of uterine leiomyomas following uterine artery embolization. Int J Gynecol Pathol 19(4):342–347
275. McCluggage WG, Ganesan R et al (2009) Endometrial stromal sarcomas with extensive endometrioid glandular differentiation: report of a series with emphasis on the potential for misdiagnosis and discussion of the differential diagnosis. Histopathology 54(3):365–373
276. McCluggage WG, Lioe TF et al (2002) Rhabdomyosarcoma of the uterus: report of two cases, including one of the spindle cell variant. Int J Gynecol Cancer 12(1):128–132
277. McCluggage WG, Sumathi VP et al (2001) CD10 is a sensitive and diagnostically useful immunohistochemical marker of normal endometrial stroma and of endometrial stromal neoplasms. Histopathology 39(3):273–278
278. Mesia AF, Williams FS et al (1998) Aborted leiomyosarcoma after treatment with leuprolide acetate. Obstet Gynecol 92(4 Pt 2): 664–666
279. Micci F, Heim S (2007) Pathogenetic mechanisms in endometrial stromal sarcoma. Cytogenet Genome Res 118(2–4):190–195
280. Micci F, Panagopoulos I et al (2006) Consistent rearrangement of chromosomal band 6p21 with generation of fusion genes JAZF1/PHF1 and EPC1/PHF1 in endometrial stromal sarcoma. Cancer Res 66(1):107–112
281. Mikami Y, Hata S et al (2002) Expression of CD10 in malignant Mullerian mixed tumors and adenosarcomas: an immunohistochemical study. Mod Pathol 15(9):923–930
282. Miller KN, McClure SP (1992) Papillary adenofibroma of the uterus: report of a case involved by adenocarcinoma and review of the literature. Am J Clin Pathol 97:806–809
283. Milne DS, Hinshaw K et al (1990) Primary angiosarcoma of the uterus: a case report. Histopathology 16:203–205
284. Minassian SS, Frangipane W et al (1986) Leiomyomatosis peritonealis disseminata. A case report and literature review. J Reprod Med 31: 997–1000
285. Mittal K, Demopoulos RI (2001) MIB-1 (Ki-67), p53, estrogen receptor, and progesterone receptor expression in uterine smooth muscle tumors. Hum Pathol 32(9):984–987
286. Mittal K, Popiolek D et al (2000) Uterine myxoid leiomyosarcoma within a leiomyoma. Hum Pathol 31(3):398–400
287. Moinfar F, Azodi M et al (2007) Uterine sarcomas. Pathology 39(1):55–71
288. Moinfar F, Regitnig P et al (2004) Expression of androgen receptors in benign and malignant endometrial stromal neoplasms. Virchows Archiv 444(5):410–414
289. Morotti RA, Nicol KK et al (2006) An immunohistochemical algorithm to facilitate diagnosis and subtyping of rhabdomyosarcoma: the Children's oncology group experience. Am J Surg Pathol 30(8):962–968
290. Mourits MJE, Hollema H et al (1998) Adenosarcoma of the uterus following tamoxifen treatment for breast cancer. Int J Gynecol Cancer 8:168–171
291. Mulvany NJ, Ostor AG et al (1995) Diffuse leiomyomatosis of the uterus. Histopathology 27:175–179
292. Mulvany NJ, Slavin JL et al (1994) Intravenous leiomyomatosis of the uterus: a clinicopathologic study of 22 cases. Int J Gynecol Pathol 13:1–9
293. Murray SK, Clement PB et al (2005) Endometrioid carcinomas of the uterine corpus with sex cord-like formations, hyalinization, and other unusual morphologic features: a report of 31 cases of a neoplasm that may be confused with carcinosarcoma and other uterine neoplasms. Am J Surg Pathol 29(2):157–166
294. Myles JL, Hart WR (1985) Apoplectic leiomyomas of the uterus. A clinicopathologic study of five distinctive hemorrhagic leiomyomas associated with oral contraceptive usage. Am J Surg Pathol 9:798–805
295. Nakayama M, Mitsuhashi T et al (2006) Immunohistochemical evaluation of KIT expression in sarcomas of the gynecologic region. Int J Gynecol Pathol 25(1):70–76
296. Namizato CS, Muriel-Cueto P et al (2008) Chondrosarcoma of the uterus: case report and literature review. Arch Gynecol Obstet 278(4):369–372
297. Nascimento AF, Hirsch MS et al (2003) The role of CD10 staining in distinguishing invasive endometrial adenocarcinoma from adenocarcinoma involving adenomyosis. Mod Pathol 16(1):22–27
298. Ng TL, Gown AM et al (2005) Nuclear beta-catenin in mesenchymal tumors. Mod Pathol 18(1):68–74
299. Nielsen GP, Oliva E et al (1995) Alveolar soft-part sarcoma of the female genital tract: a report of nine cases and review of the literature. Int J Gynecol Pathol 14:283–292
300. Nogales FF, Isaac MA et al (2002) Adenomatoid tumors of the uterus: an analysis of 60 cases. Int J Gynecol Pathol 21(1):34–40
301. Nogales FF, Matilla A et al (1978) Leiomyomatosis peritonealis disseminata: an ultrastructural study. Am J Clin Pathol 699:452–457
302. Nogales FF, Navarro N et al (1987) Uterine intravascular leiomyomatosis: an update and report of seven cases. Int J Gynecol Pathol 6:331–339
303. Nogales FF, Stolnicu S et al (2009) Retiform uterine tumors resembling ovarian sex cord tumors. A comparative immunohistochemical study with retiform structures of the female genital tract. Histopathology 54(4):471–477
304. Nola M, Babic D et al (1996) Prognostic parameters for survival of patients with malignant mesenchymal tumors of the uterus. Cancer 78(12):2543–2550
305. Nordal RR, Kristensen GB et al (1995) The prognostic significance of stage, tumor size, cellular atypia and DNA ploidy in uterine leiomyosarcoma. Acta Oncol 34:797–802
306. Norris HJ, Hilliard GD et al (1988) Hemorrhagic cellular leiomyomas ("apoplectic leiomyoma") of the uterus associated with pregnancy and oral contraceptives. Int J Gynecol Pathol 7:212–224
307. Norris HJ, Parmley T (1975) Mesenchymal tumors of the uterus. V. Intravenous leiomyomatosis. A clinical and pathologic study of 14 cases. Cancer 36:2164–2178
308. Nucci MR, Harburger D et al (2007) Molecular analysis of the JAZF1-JJAZ1 gene fusion by RT-PCR and fluorescence in situ hybridization in endometrial stromal neoplasms. Am J Surg Pathol 31(1):65–70

309. Nucci MR, O'Connell JT et al (2001) h-Caldesmon expression effectively distinguishes endometrial stromal tumors from uterine smooth muscle tumors. Am J Surg Pathol 25(4):455–463
310. Nunez-Alonso C, Battifora HA (1979) Plexiform tumors of the uterus: ultrastructural study. Cancer 44:1707–1714
311. O'Connor DM, Norris HJ (1990) Mitotically active leiomyomas of the uterus. Hum Pathol 21:223–227
312. O'Leary TJ, Steffes MW (1996) Can you count on the mitotic index? Hum Pathol 27:147–151
313. O'Neill CJ, McBride HA et al (2007) Uterine leiomyosarcomas are characterized by high p16, p53 and MIB1 expression in comparison with usual leiomyomas, leiomyoma variants and smooth muscle tumors of uncertain malignant potential. Histopathology 50(7):851–858
314. Oda Y, Nakanishi I et al (1984) Intramural mullerian adenosarcoma of the uterus with adenomyosis. Arch Pathol Lab Med 108(10): 798–801
315. Ohta Y, Suzuki T et al (2003) Low-grade endometrial stromal sarcoma with an extensive epithelial-like element. Pathol Int 53(4):246–251
316. Oliva E, Clement PB et al (2002) Epithelioid endometrial and endometrioid stromal tumors: a report of four cases emphasizing their distinction from epithelioid smooth muscle tumors and other oxyphilic uterine and extrauterine tumors. Int J Gynecol Pathol 21(1):48–55
317. Oliva E, Clement PB et al (1998) Mixed endometrial stromal and smooth muscle tumors of the uterus – A clinicopathologic study of 15 cases. Am J Surg Pathol 22:997–1005
318. Oliva E, de Leval L et al (2007) High frequency of JAZF1-JJAZ1 gene fusion in endometrial stromal tumors with smooth muscle differentiation by interphase FISH detection. Am J Surg Pathol 31(8):1277–1284
319. Oliva E, Ferry JA et al (1997) Granulocytic sarcoma of the female genital tract: a clinicopathologic study of 11 cases. Am J Surg Pathol 21(10):1156–1165
320. Oliva E, Young RH et al (2002) An immunohistochemical analysis of endometrial stromal and smooth muscle tumors of the uterus – A study of 54 cases emphasizing the importance of using a panel because of overlap in immunoreactivity for individual antibodies. Am J Surg Pathol 26(4):403–412
321. Oliva E, Young RH et al (1995) Cellular benign mesenchymal tumors of the uterus: a comparative morphologic and immunohistochemical analysis of 33 highly cellular leiomyomas and six endometrial stromal nodules, two frequently confused tumors. Am J Surg Pathol 19:757–768
322. Oliva E, Young RH et al (1999) Myxoid and fibrous endometrial stromal tumors of the uterus: a report of 10 cases. Int J Gynecol Pathol 18(4):310–319
323. Ordi J, Stamatakos MD et al (1997) Pure pleomorphic rhabdomyosarcomas of the uterus. Int J Gynecol Pathol 16:369–377
324. Orii A, Mori A et al (1998) Mast cells in smooth muscle tumors of the uterus. Int J Gynecol Pathol 17(4):336–342
325. Ouyang DW, Economy KE et al (2006) Obstetric complications of fibroids. Obstet Gynecol Clin N Am 33(1):153–169
326. Park SH, Ro JY et al (2003) Perivascular epithelioid cell tumor of the uterus: immunohistochemical, ultrastructural and molecular study. Pathol Int 53(11):800–805
327. Parker WH, Fu YS et al (1994) Uterine sarcoma in patients operated on for presumed leiomyoma and rapidly growing leiomyoma. Obstet Gynecol 83:414–418
328. Patai K, Illyes G et al (2006) Uterine leiomyosarcoma with osteoclast like giant cells and long standing systemic symptoms. Gynecol Oncol 102(2):403–405
329. Pautier P, Genestie C et al (2000) Analysis of clinicopathologic prognostic factors for 157 uterine sarcomas and evaluation of a grading score validated for soft tissue sarcoma. Cancer 88(6):1425–1431
330. Payson M, Leppert P et al (2006) Epidemiology of myomas. Obstet Gynecol Clin N Am 33(1):1–11
331. Pedeutour F, Quade BJ et al (2000) Dysregulation of HMGIC in a uterine lipoleiomyoma with a complex rearrangement including chromosomes 7, 12, and 14. Genes Chromosom Cancer 27(2): 209–215
332. Pelmus M, Penault-Llorca F et al (2009) Prognostic factors in early-stage leiomyosarcoma of the uterus. Int J Gynecol Cancer 19(3):385–390
333. Perrone T, Dehner LP (1988) Prognostically favorable "mitotically active" smooth-muscle tumors of the uterus. A clinicopathologic study of ten cases. Am J Surg Pathol 12:1–8
334. Peters WA III, Howard DR et al (1994) Uterine smooth-muscle tumors of uncertain malignant potential. Obstet Gynecol 83: 1015–1020
335. Pieslor PC, Orenstein JM et al (1979) Ultrastructure of myofibroblasts and decidualized cells in leiomyomatosis peritonealis disseminata. Am J Clin Pathol 72:875–882
336. Pink D, Lindner T et al (2006) Harm or benefit of hormonal treatment in metastatic low-grade endometrial stromal sarcoma: single center experience with 10 cases and review of the literature. Gynecol Oncol 101(3):464–469
337. Policarpio-Nicolas ML, Cathro HP et al (2007) Cytomorphologic features of low-grade endometrial stromal sarcoma. Am J Clin Pathol 128(2):265–271
338. Pounder DJ (1982) Fatty tumors of the uterus. J Clin Pathol 35:1380–1383
339. Prakash S, Scully RE (1964) Sarcoma-like pseudopregnancy changes in uterine leiomyomas. Report of a case resulting from prolonged norethindrone therapy. Obstet Gynecol 24:106–110
340. Prayson RA, Goldblum JR et al (1997) Epithelioid smooth-muscle tumors of the uterus – A clinicopathologic study of 18 patients. Am J Surg Pathol 21(4):383–391
341. Prayson RA, Hart WR (1992) Mitotically active leiomyomas of the uterus. Am J Clin Pathol 97:14–20
342. Quade BJ (1995) Pathology, cytogenetics and molecular biology of uterine leiomyomas and other smooth muscle lesions. Curr Opin Obstet Gynecol 7(1):35–42
343. Quade BJ, McLachlin CM et al (1997) Disseminated peritoneal leiomyomatosis - Clonality analysis by X chromosome inactivation and cytogenetics of a clinically benign smooth muscle proliferation. Am J Pathol 150(6):2153–2166
344. Rabban JT, Zaloudek CJ et al (2005) Inflammatory myofibroblastic tumor of the uterus: a clinicopathologic study of 6 cases emphasizing distinction from aggressive mesenchymal tumors. Am J Surg Pathol 29(10):1348–1355
345. Rackow BW, Arici A (2006) Options for medical treatment of myomas. Obstet Gynecol Clin N Am 33(1):97–113
346. Radig K, Buhtz P et al (1998) Alveolar soft part sarcoma of the uterine corpus. Report of two cases and review of the literature. Pathol Res Pract 194:59–63
347. Raney RB, Anderson JR et al (2001) Rhabdomyosarcoma and undifferentiated sarcoma in the first two decades of life: a selective

review of intergroup rhabdomyosarcoma study group experience and rationale for Intergroup Rhabdomyosarcoma Study V. J Pediatr Hematol Oncol 23(4):215–220

348. Reed NS, Mangioni C et al (2008) Phase III randomised study to evaluate the role of adjuvant pelvic radiotherapy in the treatment of uterine sarcomas stages I and II: an European Organisation for Research and Treatment of Cancer Gynaecological Cancer Group Study (protocol 55874). Eur J Cancer 44(6):808–818
349. Regidor PA, Schmidt M et al (1995) Estrogen and progesterone receptor content of GnRH analogue pretreated and untreated uterine leiomyomata. Eur J Obstet Gynecol Reprod Biol 63:69–73
350. Reich O, Regauer S (2007) Hormonal therapy of endometrial stromal sarcoma. Curr Opin Oncol 19(4):347–352
351. Reich O, Regauer S et al (2000) Expression of oestrogen and progesterone receptors in low-grade endometrial stromal sarcomas. Br J Cancer 82(5):1030–1034
352. Rivasi F, Botticelli L et al (2008) Alveolar rhabdomyosarcoma of the uterine cervix. A case report confirmed by FKHR break-apart rearrangement using a fluorescence in situ hybridization probe on paraffin-embedded tissues. Int J Gynecol Pathol 27(3):442–446
353. Rizeq MN, Van de Rijn M et al (1994) A comparative immunohistochemical study of uterine smooth muscle neoplasms with emphasis on the epithelioid variant. Hum Pathol 25:671–677
354. Roma AA, Yang B et al (2005) TFE3 immunoreactivity in alveolar soft part sarcoma of the uterine cervix: case report. Int J Gynecol Pathol 24(2):131–135
355. Rose PG, Piver MS et al (1989) Patterns of metastasis in uterine sarcoma. An autopsy study. Cancer 63:935–938
356. Roth E, Taylor HB (1966) Heterotopic cartilage in the uterus. Obstet Gynecol 27:838–844
357. Roth LM, Reed RJ (1999) Dissecting leiomyomas of the uterus other than cotyledonoid dissecting leiomyomas: a report of eight cases. Am J Surg Pathol 23(9):1032–1039
358. Roth LM, Reed RJ (2000) Cotyledonoid leiomyoma of the uterus: report of a case. Int J Gynecol Pathol 19(3):272–275
359. Roth LM, Reed RJ et al (1996) Cotyledonoid dissecting leiomyoma of the uterus – The Sternberg tumor. Am J Surg Pathol 20(12): 1455–1461
360. Rush DS, Tan JY et al (2001) h-caldesmon, a novel smooth muscle-specific antibody, distinguishes between cellular leiomyoma and endometrial stromal sarcoma. Am J Surg Pathol 25(2):253–258
361. Rutgers JL, Spong CY et al (1995) Leuprolide acetate treatment and myoma arterial size. Obstet Gynecol 86:386–388
362. Sahin AA, Silva EG et al (1989) Endometrial tissue in myometrial vessels not associated with menstruation. Int J Gynecol Pathol 8:139–146
363. Sandberg AA (2005) Updates on the cytogenetics and molecular genetics of bone and soft tissue tumors: leiomyosarcoma. Cancer Genet Cytogenet 161(1):1–19
364. Sandberg AA (2007) The cytogenetics and molecular biology of endometrial stromal sarcoma. Cytogenet Genome Res 118(2–4): 182–189
365. Satoh Y, Ishikawa Y et al (2003) Pulmonary metastases from a low-grade endometrial stromal sarcoma confirmed by chromosome aberration and fluorescence in-situ hybridization approaches: a case of recurrence 13 years after hysterectomy. Virchows Archiv 442(2):173–178
366. Schammel DP, Tavassoli FA (1998) Uterine angiosarcomas – A morphologic and immunohistochemical study of four cases. Am J Surg Pathol 22(2):246–250
367. Schilder JM, Hurd WW et al (1999) Hormonal treatment of an endometrial stromal nodule followed by local excision. Obstet Gynecol 93(5 Pt 2):805–807
368. Schmid C, Beham A et al (1990) Haematopoiesis in a degenerating uterine leiomyoma. Arch Gynecol Obstet 248(2):81–86
369. Schneider D, Halperin R et al (1995) Myxoid leiomyosarcoma of the uterus with unusual malignant histologic pattern – a case report. Gynecol Oncol 59:156–158
370. Schwartz EJ, Longacre TA (2004) Adenomatoid tumors of the female and male genital tracts express WT1. Int J Gynecol Pathol 23(2):123–128
371. Schwartz LB, Diamond MP et al (1993) Leiomyosarcomas: clinical presentation. Am J Obstet Gynecol 168:180–183
372. Schwartz PE, Kelly MG (2006) Malignant transformation of myomas: myth or reality? Obstet Gynecol Clin N Am 33(1):183–198
373. Seidman JD, Kjerulff KH (1996) Pathologic findings from the Maryland Women's Health Study: practice patterns in the diagnosis of adenomyosis. Int J Gynecol Pathol 15:217–221
374. Seidman JD, Thomas RM (1993) Multiple plexiform tumorlets of the uterus. Arch Pathol Lab Med 117:1255–1256
375. Seidman JD, Wasserman CS et al (1999) Cluster of uterine mullerian adenosarcoma in the Washington, DC metropolitan area with high incidence of sarcomatous overgrowth. Am J Surg Pathol 23(7):809–814
376. Sener AB, Seckin NC et al (1996) The effects of hormone replacement therapy on uterine fibroids in postmenopausal women. Fertil Steril 65(2):354–357
377. Shaw RW (1998) Gonadotrophin hormone-releasing hormone analogue treatment of fibroids. Baillières Clin Obstet Gynaecol 12(2):245–268
378. Shintaku M, Fukushima A (2006) Inflammatory myofibroblastic tumor of the uterus with prominent myxoid change. Pathol Int 56(10):625–628
379. Silva EG, Bodurka DC et al (2005) A uterine leiomyosarcoma that became positive for HMB45 in the metastasis. Ann Diagn Pathol 9(1):43–45
380. Silva EG, Deavers MT et al (2004) Uterine epithelioid leiomyosarcomas with clear cells: reactivity with HMB-45 and the concept of PEComa. Am J Surg Pathol 28(2):244–249
381. Silva EG, Tornos C et al (1995) Uterine leiomyosarcoma with clear cell areas. Int J Gynecol Pathol 14:174–178
382. Simpson KW, Albores-Saavedra J (2007) HMB-45 reactivity in conventional uterine leiomyosarcomas. Am J Surg Pathol 31(1): 95–98
383. Sinkre P, Albores-Saavedra J et al (2000) Endometrial endometrioid carcinomas associated with Ewing sarcoma/peripheral primitive neuroectodermal tumor. Int J Gynecol Pathol 19(2):127–132
384. Sinkre P, Miller DS et al (2000) Adenomyofibroma of the endometrium with skeletal muscle differentiation. Int J Gynecol Pathol 19(3):280–283
385. Siskin GP, Shlansky-Goldberg RD et al (2006) A prospective multicenter comparative study between myomectomy and uterine artery embolization with polyvinyl alcohol microspheres: long-term clinical outcomes in patients with symptomatic uterine fibroids. J Vasc Interv Radiol 17(8):1287–1295
386. Skubitz KM, Skubitz AP (2003) Differential gene expression in leiomyosarcoma. Cancer 98(5):1029–1038
387. Sorensen JB, Schultze HR et al (1998) Primitive neuroectodermal tumor (PNET) of the uterine cavity. Eur J Obstet Gynecol Reprod Biol 76(2):181–184

388. Sorensen PH, Lynch JC et al (2002) PAX3-FKHR and PAX7-FKHR gene fusions are prognostic indicators in alveolar rhabdomyosarcoma: a report from the children's oncology group. J Clin Oncol 20(11):2672–2679
389. Sornberger KS, Weremowicz S et al (1999) Expression of HMGIY in three uterine leiomyomata with complex rearrangements of chromosome 6. Cancer Genet Cytogenet 114(1):9–16
390. Soslow RA, Ali A et al (2008) Mullerian adenosarcomas: an immunophenotypic analysis of 35 cases. Am J Surg Pathol 32(7):1013–1021
391. Sozen I, Arici A (2006) Cellular biology of myomas: interaction of sex steroids with cytokines and growth factors. Obstet Gynecol Clin N Am 33(1):41–58
392. Spies JB, Ascher SA et al (2001) Uterine artery embolization for leiomyomata. Obstet Gynecol 98(1):29–34
393. Sreenan JJ, Prayson RA et al (1996) Histopathologic findings in 107 uterine leiomyomas treated with leuprolide acetate compared with 126 controls. Am J Surg Pathol 20(4):427–432
394. Srodon M, Klein WM et al (2003) CD10 immunostaining does not distinguish endometrial carcinoma invading myometrium from carcinoma involving adenomyosis. Am J Surg Pathol 27(6):786–789
395. Staats PN, Garcia JJ et al (2009) Uterine tumors resembling ovarian sex cord tumors (UTROSCT) lack the JAZF1-JJAZ1 translocation frequently seen in endometrial stromal tumors. Am J Surg Pathol 33(8):1206–1212. doi:10.1097/PAS.0b013e3181a7b9cf
396. Stovall TG, Ling FW et al (1991) A randomized trial evaluating leuprolide acetate before hysterectomy as treatment for leiomyomas. Am J Obstet Gynecol 164:1420–1423
397. Stroh EL, Besa PC et al (1995) Treatment of patients with lymphomas of the uterus or cervix with combination chemotherapy and radiation therapy. Cancer 75:2392–2399
398. Su LD, Atayde-Perez A et al (1998) Inflammatory myofibroblastic tumor: cytogenetic evidence supporting clonal origin. Mod Pathol 11:364–368
399. Suginami H, Kaura R et al (1990) Intravenous leiomyomatosis with cardiac extension: successful surgical management and histopathologic study. Obstet Gynecol 76:527–529
400. Sullivan LM, Atkins KA et al (2009) PAX immunoreactivity identifies alveolar rhabdomyosarcoma. Am J Surg Pathol 33(5):775–780
401. Sumathi VP, Al-Hussaini M et al (2004) Endometrial stromal neoplasms are immunoreactive with WT-1 antibody. Int J Gynecol Pathol 23(3):241–247
402. Sutton G, Blessing J et al (2005) Phase II evaluation of liposomal doxorubicin (Doxil) in recurrent or advanced leiomyosarcoma of the uterus: a Gynecologic Oncology Group study. Gynecol Oncol 96(3):749–752
403. Sutton G, Blessing JA et al (1996) Ifosfamide and doxorubicin in the treatment of advanced leiomyosarcomas of the uterus: a Gynecologic Oncology Group study. Gynecol Oncol 62:226–229
404. Tabata T, Takeshima N et al (1999) Low-grade endometrial stromal sarcoma with cardiovascular involvement – a report of three cases. Gynecol Oncol 75(3):495–498
405. Tahlan A, Nanda A et al (2006) Uterine adenomyoma: a clinicopathologic review of 26 cases and a review of the literature. Int J Gynecol Pathol 25(4):361–365
406. Tai LH, Tavassoli FA (2002) Endometrial polyps with atypical (bizarre) stromal cells. Am J Surg Pathol 26(4):505–509
407. Tallini G, Price FV et al (1993) Epithelioid angiosarcoma arising in uterine leiomyomas. Am J Clin Pathol 100:514–518
408. Tang CK, Toker C et al (1979) Stromomyoma of the uterus. Cancer 43:308–316
409. Tavassoli FA, Devilee P et al (2003) Pathology and genetics of tumors of the breast and female genital organs. Lyon, International Agency for Research on Cancer
410. Tavassoli FA, Norris HJ (1981) Mesenchymal tumors of the uterus. VII. A clinicopathological study of 60 endometrial stromal nodules. Histopathology 5:1–10
411. Tavassoli FA, Norris HJ (1982) Peritoneal leiomyomatosis (leiomyomatosis peritonealis disseminata): a clinicopathologic study of 20 cases with ultrastructural observations. Int J Gynecol Pathol 1:59–74
412. Tietze L, Guenther K et al (2000) Benign metastasizing leiomyoma: A cytogenetically balanced but clonal disease. Hum Pathol 31(1):126–128
413. Tiltman AJ (1985) The effect of progestins on the mitotic activity of uterine fibromyomas. Int J Gynecol Pathol 4:89–96
414. Toki T, Shimizu M et al (2002) CD10 is a marker for normal and neoplastic endometrial stromal cells. Int J Gynecol Pathol 21(1): 41–47
415. Torres VE, Bjornsson J et al (1995) Extrapulmonary lymphangioleiomyomatosis and lymphangiomatous cysts in tuberous sclerosis complex. Mayo Clin Proc 70:641–648
416. Tresukosol DR, Kudelka AP et al (1995) Leuprolide acetate and intravascular leiomyomatosis. Obstet Gynecol 86:688–692
417. Upadhyaya NB, Doody MC et al (1990) Histopathological changes in leiomyomata treated with leuprolide acetate. Fertil Steril 54: 811–814
418. Van Diest PJ, Baak JP et al (1992) Reproducibility of mitosis counting in 2,469 breast cancer specimens: results from the Multicenter Morphometric Mammary Carcinoma Project. Hum Pathol 23(6):603–607
419. Vang R, Kempson RL (2002) Perivascular epithelioid cell tumor ("PEComa") of the uterus: a subset of HMB-45-positive epithelioid mesenchymal neoplasms with an uncertain relationship to pure smooth muscle tumors. Am J Surg Pathol 26(1):1–13
420. Vang R, Medeiros LJ et al (2000) Non-Hodgkin's lymphomas involving the uterus: a clinicopathologic analysis of 26 cases. Mod Pathol 13(1):19–28
421. Vang R, Medeiros LJ et al (2001) Uterine leiomyomas with eosinophils: a clinicopathologic study of 3 cases. Int J Gynecol Pathol 20(3):239–243
422. Varghese L, Arnesen M et al (2006) Primitive neuroectodermal tumor of the uterus: a case report and review of literature. Int J Gynecol Pathol 25(4):373–377
423. Venkatraman L, Elliott H et al (2003) Serous carcinoma arising in an adenofibroma of the endometrium. Int J Gynecol Pathol 22(2): 194–197
424. Verschraegen CF, Vasuratna A et al (1998) Clinicopathologic analysis of mullerian adenosarcoma: the M.D. Anderson Cancer Center experience. Oncol Rep 5(4):939–944
425. Vitiello D, McCarthy S (2006) Diagnostic imaging of myomas. Obstet Gynecol Clin N Am 33(1):85–95
426. Viville B, Charnock-Jones DS et al (1997) Distribution of the A and B forms of the progesterone receptor messenger ribonucleic acid and protein in uterine leiomyomata and adjacent myometrium. Hum Reprod 12(4):815–822
427. Vollenhoven B (1998) Introduction: the epidemiology of uterine leiomyomas. Baillières Clin Obstet Gynaecol 12(2):169–176
428. Vu K, Greenspan DL et al (1998) Cellular proliferation, estrogen receptor, progesterone receptor, and bcl-2 expression in GnRH agonist-treated uterine leiomyomas. Hum Pathol 29(4): 359–363

429. Wachtel M, Runge T et al (2006) Subtype and prognostic classification of rhabdomyosarcoma by immunohistochemistry. J Clin Oncol 24(5):816–822
430. Wakami K, Tateyama H et al (2005) Solitary fibrous tumor of the uterus producing high-molecular-weight insulin-like growth factor II and associated with hypoglycemia. Int J Gynecol Pathol 24(1): 79–84
431. Wallach EE, Vlahos NF (2004) Uterine myomas: an overview of development, clinical features, and management. Obstet Gynecol 104(2):393–406
432. Wang X, Kumar D et al (2006) Uterine lipoleiomyomas: a clinicopathologic study of 50 cases. Int J Gynecol Pathol 25(3):239–242
433. Watanabe K, Suzuki T (2006) Uterine leiomyoma versus leiomyosarcoma: a new attempt at differential diagnosis based on their cellular characteristics. Histopathology 48(5):563–568
434. Weichert W, Denkert C et al (2005) Uterine arterial embolization with tris-acryl gelatin microspheres: a histopathologic evaluation. Am J Surg Pathol 29(7):955–961
435. Weissman A, Talmon R et al (1993) Cavernous hemangioma of the uterus in a pregnant woman. Obstet Gynecol 81:825–827
436. Witkin GB, Askin FB et al (1987) Angiosarcoma of the uterus: a light microscopic, immunohistochemical, and ultrastructural study. Int J Gynecol Pathol 6:176–184
437. Wolff M, Silva F et al (1979) Pulmonary metastases (with admixed epithelial elements) from smooth muscle neoplasms: report of nine cases, including three males. Am J Surg Pathol 3:325–342
438. Wolfson AH, Wolfson DJ et al (1994) A multivariate analysis of clinicopathologic factors for predicting outcome in uterine sarcomas. Gynecol Oncol 52:56–62
439. Wright JD, Seshan VE et al (2008) The role of radiation in improving survival for early-stage carcinosarcoma and leiomyosarcoma. Am J Obstet Gynecol 199(5):536.e1–536.e8
440. Yamadori I, Kobayashi S et al (1993) Uterine leiomyoma with a focus of fatty and cartilaginous differentiation. Acta Obstet Gynecol Scand 72:307–309
441. Yilmaz A, Rush DS et al (2002) Endometrial stromal sarcomas with unusual histologic features: a report of 24 primary and metastatic tumors emphasizing fibroblastic and smooth muscle differentiation. Am J Surg Pathol 26(9):1142–1150
442. Young RH, Harris NL et al (1985) Lymphoma-like lesions of the lower female genital tract: a report of 16 cases. Int J Gynecol Pathol 4:289–299
443. Young RH, Prat J et al (1984) Endometrioid stromal sarcomas of the ovary. A clinicopatholgic analysis of 23 cases. Cancer 53:1143–1155
444. Young RH, Silva EG et al (1991) Ovarian and juxtaovarian adenomatoid tumors: a report of six cases. Int J Gynecol Pathol 10:364–372
445. Zaloudek CJ, Norris HJ (1981) Adenofibroma and adenosarcoma of the uterus: a clinicopathologic study of 35 cases. Cancer 48:354–366
446. Zamecnik M, Sultani K (2007) Meningothelial-like nodules: additional pattern of myoid differentiation in endometrial stromal tumors. Pathol Int 57(9):632–633
447. Zhai YL, Kobayashi Y et al (1999) Expression of steroid receptors, Ki-67, and p53 in uterine leiomyosarcomas. Int J Gynecol Pathol 18(1):20–28
448. Zivanovic O, Leitao MM et al (2009) Stage-specific outcomes of patients with uterine leiomyosarcoma: a comparison of the international Federation of gynecology and obstetrics and american joint committee on cancer staging systems. J Clin Oncol 27(12): 2066–2072

11 Diseases of the Fallopian Tube and Paratubal Region

Russell Vang · James E. Wheeler

R. J. Kurman, L. Hedrick Ellenson, B. M. Ronnett (eds.), *Blaustein's Pathology of the Female Genital Tract (6th ed.)*, DOI 10.1007/978-1-4419-0489-8_11,

The Italian physician and anatomist Gabriele Falloppio provided the first detailed and accurate description of the oviducts in humans in 1561 A.D. and designated it the "*Uteri Tuba*" [88]. This organ was eventually named after him. Since that time, a wide variety of non-neoplastic and neoplastic diseases of the fallopian tube has become recognized, but it is only recently that the pathogenesis of fallopian tube carcinoma is beginning to be understood.

Surgical specimens removed specifically for lesions of the fallopian tube are much less common than specimens from other sites in the gynecologic tract; nonetheless, the fallopian tube is frequently examined by the surgical pathologist because it accompanies specimens that were removed for lesions of other gynecologic organs, and the tube plays an important role in reproduction, including problems related to infertility. The majority of fallopian tube lesions examined by the surgical pathologist are non-neoplastic. Benign and malignant tumors of the fallopian tube are uncommon, but, as discussed below, early carcinomas of the fimbriated end of the fallopian tube are becoming more frequently recognized because of complete examination of all fallopian tube tissue submitted as part of prophylactic bilateral salpingo-oophorectomy specimens or major resections for ovarian carcinoma.

This chapter provides a detailed discussion of normal fallopian tube (embryology, gross anatomy, and histology) and gross examination, non-neoplastic lesions, benign and malignant tumors, and gestational trophoblastic disease of the fallopian tube. Paratubal/para-ovarian and pelvic ligament lesions are presented as well.

Normal Fallopian Tube and Gross Examination

Embryology

Regardless of genetic sex, the paired müllerian (paramesonephric) ducts develop on the anterolateral surface of the paired urogenital ridges in both females and males beginning in the sixth week of embryonic life [171, 172, 199]. At the cranial end of the urogenital ridge, the peritoneum gives rise to a population of epithelial cells, which segregate from the peritoneal layer [91]. This new population proliferates and forms the longitudinally oriented müllerian ducts [91, 175]. The mesenchyme surrounding the luminal epithelial layer of the müllerian duct is also derived from the peritoneum. Cranially, the ducts open into the peritoneal cavity. Each of the paired ducts grows caudally in the urogenital ridge immediately lateral to and using the wolffian (mesonephric) duct as a guide. Spatially lateral to the cranial aspect of the wolffian ducts, the müllerian ducts then ventrally cross the wolffian ducts. The longitudinally oriented and caudal portions of the müllerian ducts now lie medial to the wolffian ducts as they enter the pelvis. The caudal ends of the müllerian ducts abut on the posterior wall of the urogenital sinus immediately between the two wolffian ducts. In the eighth week of embryonic life, these caudal ends of the paired müllerian ducts fuse with each other but are still separated by a septum (➲ *Figs. 11.1* and ➲ *11.2*). All these developments occur in both female and male fetuses and are completed before the testis (if the embryo is male) begins to secrete müllerian inhibiting substance (MIS), also known as anti-müllerian hormone (In the absence of MIS, the müllerian ducts develop passively to form the fallopian tubes, uterus, and vaginal wall. Likewise, in the absence of testosterone, the wolffian ducts regress.). In the development of the female, the first two parts of the müllerian duct (the cranial longitudinal segment, which opens into the peritoneal cavity and the transverse portion, which crosses the wolffian duct) form the fallopian tube. The cranial-most aspect of the first part forms the fimbriated end, and the caudal-most segment of the müllerian duct (the fused portion) forms the uterus. During the growth of the second portion of the müllerian duct (the transverse segment that crosses the wolffian duct), the urogenital ridges form a transverse pelvic fold. After the fusion of the caudal segment of the müllerian duct, the transverse pelvic fold extends laterally from the fused müllerian duct toward the pelvic sidewall (➲ *Fig. 11.2*). This pelvic fold forms the broad ligament to which the fallopian tube is attached.

The lumen of the fallopian tube is initially oval to round and lined by immature columnar epithelium, but the mucosa forms plicae at week 14. In week 16, the fallopian tube begins an active growth phase and starts to coil. Smooth muscle appears in the walls of the genital canal between 18 and 20 weeks. The fallopian tube muscular wall develops only around the müllerian duct, so that the wolffian duct remnants are external to the true wall of the canal. From the 22nd to 36th week, there is an increase in the growth and coiling of the fallopian tube at a rate of approximately 3 mm/week [108]. Fimbriae do not develop until the 20th week, at which time only three to four are present in each fallopian tube [226]. The fimbriae increase in number throughout gestation, and at term, six to eight are present in each tube. The number continues to increase after birth.

Important genes in the embryologic development of the müllerian duct include the *Wnt* family, *Lim1*, *Pax2*, and *Emx2* [243]. In addition, the *Hox* family of genes (*Hox*

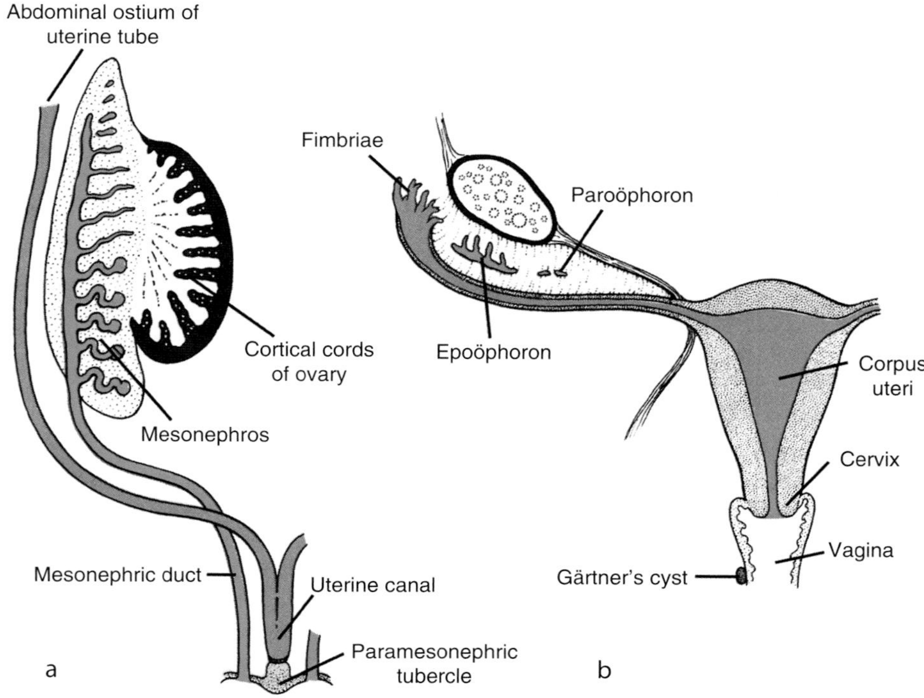

Fig. 11.1
(**a**) Diagram of ventral aspect of coronal section through female embryo at the end of the eighth week. **The arrangement of the müllerian (*red*) and wolffian (mesonephric) (*blue*) ducts is shown. The cranial portion of the müllerian duct is lateral to the wolffian duct. The former grows in a caudal direction and crosses ventral to the latter and is in a medial position at the caudal end. The caudal ends of the müllerian ducts fuse, which eventually form the uterus. (b) The developed fallopian tube with accompanying wolffian remnants. The *red* and *blue* structures correspond to their precursors in (a) (From Sadler TW. *Langman's Medical Embryology, 6th Edition.* Baltimore: Williams & Wilkins; 1990:Figs. 15–22. *Printed with permission from Lippincott Williams & Wilkins*)**

in mice, *HOX* in humans) is particularly essential for development of this anatomic structure [65, 228, 243]. The *Hox* family represents four clusters of genes (*Hoxa* through *Hoxd*), which encode transcription factors that direct embryogenesis. Their main function is to control patterning and positional identity along a developing axis, such as the hindbrain, axial skeleton, and limbs. One of the anatomic sites controlled by the *Hoxa* cluster during embryogenesis is the müllerian duct, in which each *Hoxa* gene controls the morphogenesis of different segments along the developing axis of the müllerian duct. *Hoxa-9* through *Hoxa-13* are sequentially located in tandem with one another in the same region of the chromosome. It has been shown in mice that the physical order of the *Hoxa* genes on the chromosome corresponds to the same spatial order of the different segments of the developing müllerian duct (i.e., *Hoxa-9* is expressed in the fallopian tube, *Hoxa-10 and -11* in the uterine corpus, *Hoxa-11* in the uterine cervix, and *Hoxa-13* in the upper vagina). This same spatial organization of *Hoxa* genes with their respective derivatives of the different segments of the müllerian duct is also maintained in humans [228]. Thus, interaction between *HOXA-9* and presumably several other non-HOX genes determines the proper development of the human fallopian tube.

Gross Anatomy

The fallopian tube is located anterior to the ovary. The tube extends medially from the area of its corresponding ovary to its origin in the posterosuperior aspect of the uterine fundus. In an adult during the reproductive years, its length is usually between 9 and 12 cm. The tube at the ovarian end opens to the peritoneal cavity and is composed of about 25 finger-like extensions of the tube – the

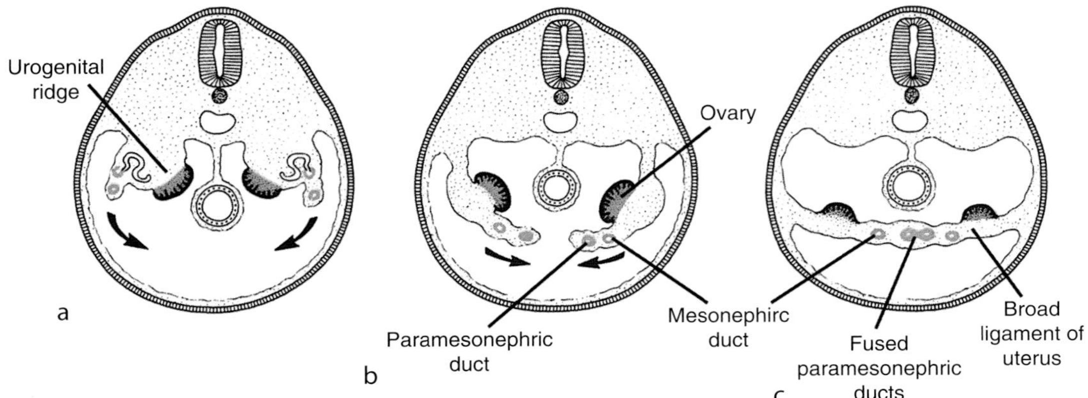

Fig. 11.2
Diagram of transverse section of female embryo. (a) through (c) show progressively lower levels through urogenital ridge. The müllerian (paramesonephric) ducts (*orange*) eventually fuse and are then located medial to the wolffian ducts (*blue*). The fusion of the müllerian ducts creates a transverse fold, which becomes the broad ligament (c) (From Sadler TW. *Langman's Medical Embryology, 6th Edition.* Baltimore: Williams & Wilkins; 1990:Figs. 15–23. *Printed with permission from Lippincott Williams & Wilkins*)

fimbriae. The fallopian tube consists of five main segments. From medial to lateral, they are the intramural (interstitial) portion, isthmus, ampulla, infundibulum, and fimbriated end (*Fig. 11.3*). The fimbriae attach to the expanded end of the tube, the infundibulum, which is about 1 cm long and 1 cm in diameter. The infundibulum lies within a few millimeters of the lateral or tubal end of the ovary. It narrows gradually to about 4 mm in diameter and merges medially with the ampullary portion of the tube, which extends about 6 cm, passing anteriorly around the ovary. At a point characterized by relative thickening of the muscular wall along with a smaller diameter compared with the ampulla, the isthmic portion begins and extends about 2 cm toward the uterus. Within the myometrium, the tube extends as a 1 cm-long intramural segment until it joins the extension of the endometrial cavity at the uterotubal junction. Throughout its extrauterine course, the tube lays in a peritoneal fold along the superior margin of the broad ligament – the mesosalpinx.

The arterial blood supply has a dual origin from branches of the ovarian and uterine arteries. Tubal branches of the uterine artery pass in the mesosalpinx laterally from the cornu of the uterus to anastomose with tubal branches of the ovarian artery. Venous drainage parallels the arterial supply via anastomosing tubal branches of uterine and ovarian veins, also located in the mesosalpinx. The arterial and venous distributions for lateral portions of the tube are supplied by the ovarian vessels whereas the uterine vessels supply the medial portions of the tube. Drainage from the ovarian veins is to the inferior vena cava on the right and renal vein on the left. Drainage from the uterine plexus is to the internal iliac vein. Tubal lymphatics typically drain into ovarian and uterine vessels. The former and latter drain into the para-aortic and internal iliac lymph nodes, respectively.

The nerve supply of the tube is both sympathetic and parasympathetic. Sympathetic fibers from T10 through L2 synapse in the celiac, aortic, renal, inferior mesenteric, cervicovaginal, and possibly presacral plexuses. Sensory pain fibers pass along with the sympathetic nerves to the spinal cord at the level of T10–T12. Parasympathetic fibers from the vagus nerve supply the lateral portion of the tube via postganglionic fibers from the ovarian plexus whereas the medial portion is innervated via S2–S4 parasympathetic fibers synapsing in the pelvic plexuses.

Histology

A mucosa, wall of smooth muscle (muscularis or myosalpinx), and serosa constitute the three layers of the fallopian tube. The mucosal layer lies directly on the muscularis. It consists of a luminal epithelial lining and a scanty underlying lamina propria containing vessels and spindle or oval mesenchymal cells. Although the lamina propria may be small in area, this is the site of decidua in 5–12% of postpartum tubes (*Fig. 11.4*), and decidua

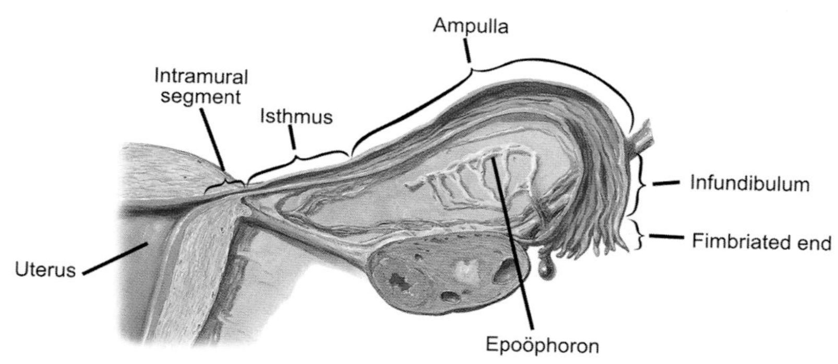

Fig. 11.3
Posterior aspect (*upper*) and coronal section (*lower*) of fallopian tube including anatomic relationships with adjacent structures. **All five segments of the fallopian tube (intramural segment, isthmus, ampulla, infundibulum, and fimbriated end) are illustrated (From Netter FH. *Atlas of Human Anatomy*. West Caldwell: CIBA-GEIGY Corporation; 1989:Plate 350. *Printed with permission from Elsevier, Inc. All rights reserved*)**

may be seen in 80% of tubes removed for ectopic pregnancy [89]. The stroma of the plicae of the fallopian tube tends to be more fibrotic in the postmenopausal years. The mucosa increases significantly in its gross structural complexity as the lumen enlarges from the uterine to the ovarian ends. The interstitial/intramural portion contains a mostly flat mucosa with minimal undulation. It is lined by endometrium in the most proximal portion at the junction of the endometrial cavity and tubal ostium. Farther away from the tubal ostium, the mucosa of the interstitial/intramural portion is lined by an epithelial lining that is more typical of distal portions of the tube but with lesser numbers of ciliated cells. The isthmus shows slightly greater undulation than is seen in the interstitial/intramural portion and contains a limited number of blunted plicae (*Fig. 11.5*). In the ampulla, the plicae are frond-like and delicate, and both secondary and tertiary branches may be appreciated (*Fig. 11.6*). The infundibular and fimbriated end plical patterns are similar to that of the ampulla except that the plicae of the fimbriated end are essentially exophytic and have no underlying smooth muscle wall. A distinct fimbria, the *fimbria ovarica*, runs from the tubal ostium to one pole of the ovary and is involved in ovum pick-up, in which there appears to be a realignment of fimbriae in their relationship to the ovary itself.

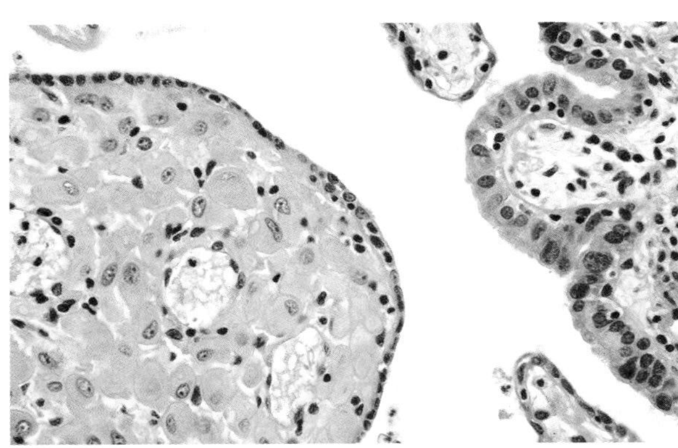

◘ Fig. 11.4
Decidua. **The plicae are expanded due to decidual change within the lamina propria. The decidual cells have cytologic features similar to those of endometrial decidua. Scattered lymphocytes are present in the background**

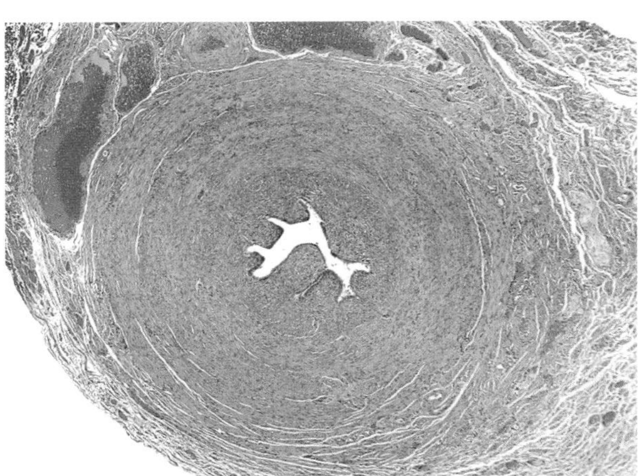

◘ Fig. 11.5
Isthmus. **The appearance is similar to the interstitial (intramural) segment except that the mucosa shows slightly more undulation with a limited number of blunted plicae**

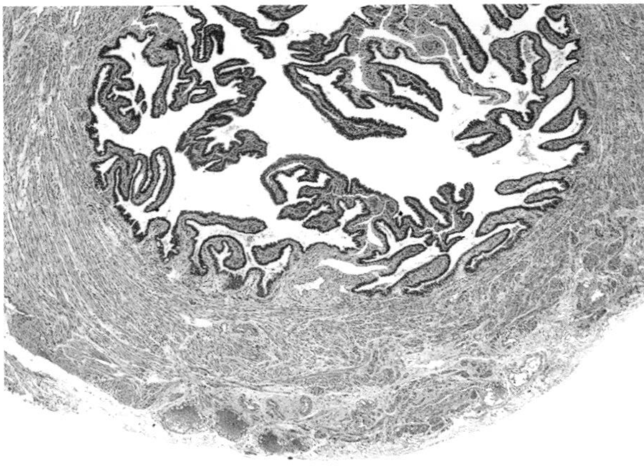

◘ Fig. 11.6
Ampulla. **In comparison with the interstitial (intramural) segment and isthmus, the ampulla has a greater diameter of the entire cross section of the tube, greater diameter of the lumen, and thinner muscularis. The plical architecture of the ampulla is more complex than that of the interstitial (intramural) segment and isthmus**

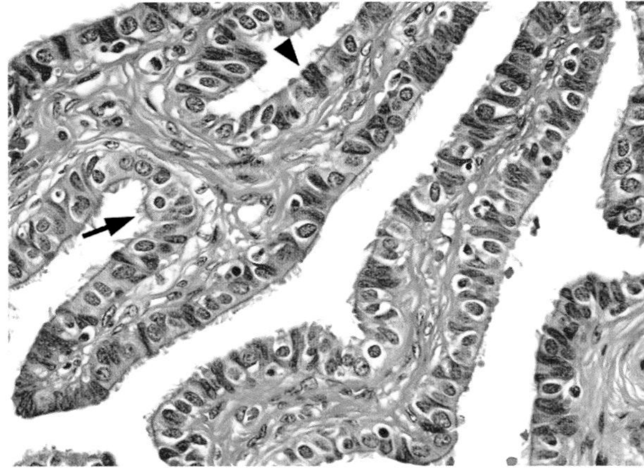

◘ Fig. 11.7
Mucosa of the fallopian tube. **The epithelium contains a mixture of ciliated (*arrow*) and secretory (*arrowhead*) cells**

The epithelium of the mucosa is composed of a single layer of cells, or it may be pseudostratified. It predominantly consists of ciliated and secretory cells; the latter are more numerous (◐ *Fig. 11.7*). A third cell, the intercalated ("peg") cell, is thought to exist. Some believe that this is a variant of the secretory cell, but it is not reliably identified on H&E sections. Ciliated cells are more abundant in the lateral portions of the tube, and the secretory cells are more numerous in the medial portions. The ciliated cell is columnar or round and has a mild to moderate amount of eosinophilic or clear cytoplasm. The nucleus is oval to round, and the chromatin is moderately granular and slightly basophilic. Ultrastructurally, each of the cilia is composed of a central pair of microtubules that is surrounded by nine outer doublet microtubules. In Kartagener's syndrome, where cilia are scanty and structurally/functionally defective, fertility is impaired but not abolished [94]. The reader is referred elsewhere for additional details regarding the structure and physiology of fallopian tube cilia [147].

The secretory cell also is columnar and approximately the same height as the ciliated cell but often narrower with scant eosinophilic cytoplasm. Its nucleus is columnar, and it is thinner and slightly darker than the nucleus of the ciliated cell. Immunohistochemically, the normal mucosal epithelium of the fallopian tube frequently and diffusely expresses WT-1, ER, and PR, and the Ki-67 labeling index is typically <5%. The secretory cell exhibits the immunophenotype HMFG2(+)/PAX8(+)/p73(−) [28, 140, 201].

The morphologic characteristics of the tubal epithelium change during life. Ciliated cells appear during early fetal development and persist until the postmenopausal years. At this time, as circulating estrogen levels drop, the cilia are gradually lost. Estrogen therapy in postmenopausal women, however, restores both the cilia and the ability to transport particulate matter. The presence of estrogen receptor in the fallopian tube also supports that estrogen is involved with ciliogenesis. The characteristics of the tubal epithelium change during the course of the menstrual cycle [61]. Early in the cycle, the cells are of low height, and the secretory cells appear relatively inactive. As ovulation approaches, probably under the influence of an increasing amount of estrogen, the secretory cells become prominent and actually project above the luminal border of the ciliated cells. In association with the effects of estrogen and progesterone, changes in cilial maturity and repeated ciliation and deciliation occur during the menstrual cycle, including maximal ciliation around the time of ovulation [61, 235]. Additional details of fallopian tube physiology are available elsewhere [112].

In addition to the three epithelial cell types described above, scattered lymphocytes may be seen located basally above the basement membrane. Immunohistological analysis of these lymphocytes indicates a preponderance of the T-cytotoxic/suppressor subtype, consistent with formation of mucosal-associated lymphoid tissue (MALT) [163].

The tubal muscularis generally has two layers: an inner circular layer and outer longitudinal layer. The circular layer forms the major muscle mass of the tube. Its thickness varies, being greater in the isthmus and lesser in the ampulla/infundibulum. The outer longitudinal layer is easily overlooked, as it is composed of inconspicuous bundles of smooth muscle interspersed with loose connective tissue containing numerous small blood vessels. At the uterine end, beginning in the intramural tube and

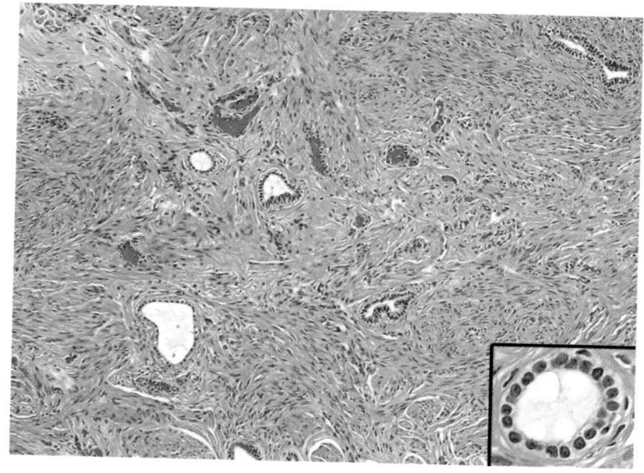

Fig. 11.8
Wolffian (mesonephric) duct remnants. **The tubules are invested by abundant muscular stroma.** ***Inset:*** **They are round and lined by a single layer of bland cuboidal cells. This example is non-ciliated, but other cases may contain cilia**

extending laterally about 2 cm, there is, in addition, an inner longitudinal layer. The serosa is lined by flattened mesothelial cells. Beneath the mesothelium lies a small amount of connective tissue containing a few collagen fibers and blood vessels.

The wolffian or mesonephric duct develops in close proximity to the fallopian tube, and remnants from it normally persist throughout adult life. These remnants consist of 10–15 mesonephric tubules lying within abundant muscular stroma just peripheral to the fallopian tube. The tubules (epoöphoron) are lined by a single layer of low-columnar or cuboidal epithelium containing non-ciliated or ciliated cells (*Fig. 11.8*).

Gross Examination

Salpingectomy for Benign Disease, with or Without Hysterectomy

In hysterectomies with benign disease, both fallopian tubes should be measured in the longitudinal and transverse dimensions. The serosa should be examined for gross lesions. The patency of the fimbriated end can be determined with a blunt probe. If a lesion is present, it should be measured, its location (corneal/intramural, isthmic, ampullary, infundibular, or fimbriated end) noted, and its relationship to the lumen and serosa described. The entire length of the tube should be transversely cut ("bread loafed") to identify lesions within the lumen. Grossly visible lesions should be sampled. For grossly unremarkable tubes, standard sections include ≥1 block from each side.

Hysterectomy and/or Oophorectomy with Salpingectomy for Non-fallopian Tube Malignant Disease

In hysterectomies for malignant disease, attention should be given to identifying involvement of the fallopian tubes, especially since focal disease may upstage the patient. The tubes should be examined, measured, and cut as described above. In cases of ovarian, peritoneal, or endometrial serous carcinomas, it is advisable to submit all tissue from both fallopian tubes for histologic examination to identify tubal intraepithelial carcinoma (TIC), especially in the fimbriated end (see Carcinoma section below).

Total or Partial Salpingectomy for Tubal Ectopic Pregnancy

The external appearance of the specimen should be carefully examined, and blood distending the lumen should be sought and sampled. If the tubal pregnancy is apparent, its site and location should be noted as described previously and sampled. A rupture site if present should be described and sampled. If the ectopic pregnancy is not obvious, extensive sampling may be necessary. Even a tubal abortion leaves foci of trophoblast at the implantation site. Blood clot in the tube or as a separate specimen should be sampled for microscopic examination to identify trophoblastic cells or chorionic villi.

Bilateral Partial Salpingectomy for Tubal Sterilization

The most important thing in this setting is to document that the tube has been completely transected. This requires complete cross sectioning of the entire tube, and submitting the entire specimen for histologic examination.

Prophylactic Bilateral Salpingo-Oophorectomy

Measurements should be made as specified above. The fimbriated end should be amputated from the rest of the tube and serially sectioned at 2-mm intervals along the long axis. The entire length of the remaining tube should be cut perpendicular to the long axis ("bread loafed") at 2-mm intervals (*Fig. 11.9*). The ovary should also be cut perpendicular to the long axis ("bread loafed") at 2-mm intervals. All fallopian tube and ovarian tissue should be submitted for histologic examination. Although there is no standard in terms of how many H&E slides need to be prepared from each block, our routine practice is one H&E slide per block; however, it has been recognized that in anecdotal cases, additional deeper H&E levels may identify a small tubal intraepithelial carcinoma not present on the initial H&E level.

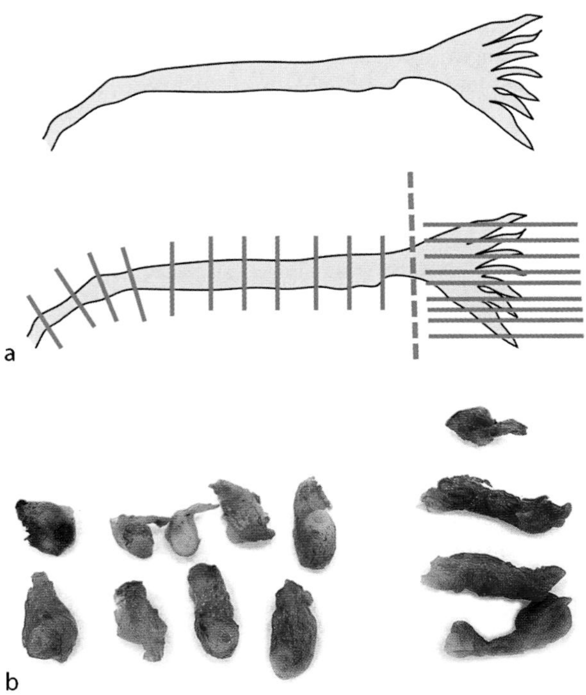

Fig. 11.9
Sectioning of fallopian tube from a prophylactic bilateral salpingo-oophorectomy specimen. (a) Diagram of fallopian tube prior to (*upper*) and during (*lower*) sectioning. From the proximal-most end of the fallopian tube to the beginning of the fimbriated end, transverse sections (*solid, vertical/diagonal, and red lines*) should be cut at 2-mm intervals. The fimbriated end should be amputated (*dashed, vertical, and red lines*). The fimbriated end should be cut at 2-mm intervals parallel to the long axis of the fallopian tube (*solid, horizontal, and red lines*). All gross tissue should be submitted for histologic examination. (b) Gross photograph of fallopian tube after complete sectioning as per (a)

Salpingectomy for Tubal Neoplasms, with or Without Hysterectomy and/or Oophorectomy

A protocol for gross examination of a tube with carcinoma has been developed by the Association of Directors of Anatomic and Surgical Pathology [146]. This protocol also lists the essential clinical, gross, and histologic information which should be included in the pathology report. The size of the specimen and tumor should be recorded, as should the exact location of the tumor within the tube. The external surface should be examined for visible disease, and any lesions should be sampled. It is important to note whether the fimbriated end is open or closed, the latter being determined by having a hydrosalpinx-like, hematosalpinx-like, or pyosalpinx-like gross appearance. At least three sections from the tumor should be obtained. Sections should show the relationship of the tumor with mucosa, depth of invasion, and serosa.

Non-neoplastic Lesions of Fallopian Tube

Metaplasia, Hyperplasia, and Other Epithelial/Non-Epithelial Changes

The tubal epithelium may undergo various metaplastic changes, including squamous, transitional, mucinous, or oncocytic type (➲ *Fig. 11.10*) [68, 193, 214]. Mucinous metaplasia may be associated with Peutz–Jeghers syndrome and can also accompany chronic inflammation. Arias-Stella reaction can occur with intrauterine pregnancy. Mucosal hyperplasia of variable degree and extent, which may be bilateral, is frequent [162, 200, 241, 242]. It is nonspecific, without clinical significance, and can be associated with various conditions and lesions. The hyperplastic epithelium can show stratification, loss of cell polarity, crowding of cells, and small papillary tufts; however, mitotic activity is usually low. In the setting of inflammation, mucosal distortion (including plical blunting and stromal fibrosis) may be seen. Nuclear atypia can be present but is typically mild [107]. In some cases, particularly those associated with marked salpingitis, the degree of hyperplasia (including cribriform architecture)

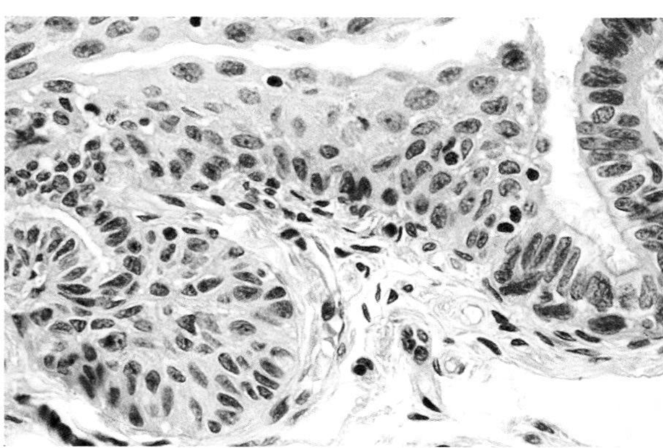

Fig. 11.10
Squamotransitional cell metaplasia. he upper center portion shows more squamous differentiation while the lower left portion shows more transitional cell differentiation. Other cases may be of pure squamous or transitional cell type

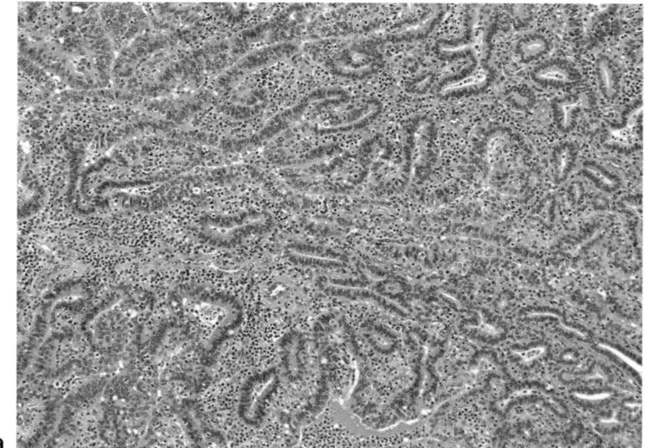

a

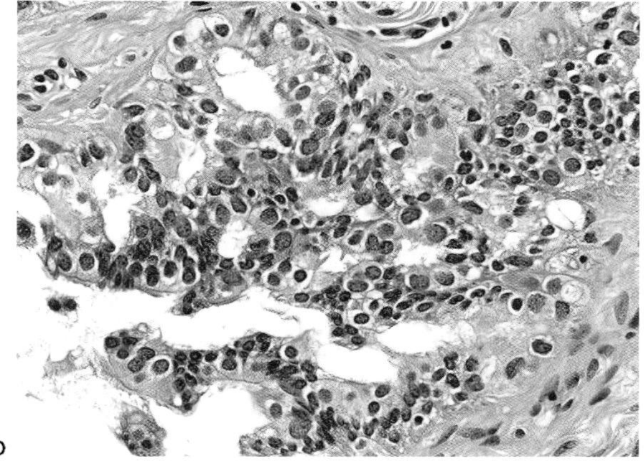

b

Fig. 11.11
Epithelial hyperplasia. In the setting of inflammation, mucosal distortion may be seen. (**a**) Marked distortion of the plicae is present in this case of florid salpingitis. Other foci (**b**) show glandular epithelium with cribriform architecture. The nuclei exhibit only mild atypia and are mitotically inactive. Ciliated cells can still be identified

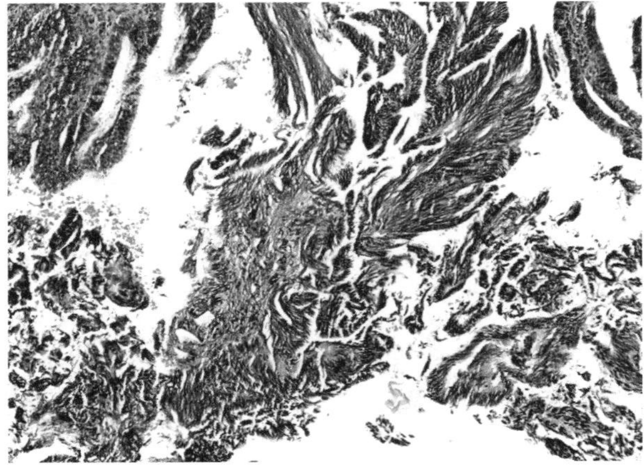

Fig. 11.12
Thermal artifact. **This appearance may falsely suggest adenocarcinoma because of the distorted and stratified epithelium with darkly staining nuclei. However, closer magnification will show nuclei with the streaming effect that is characteristic of thermal injury**

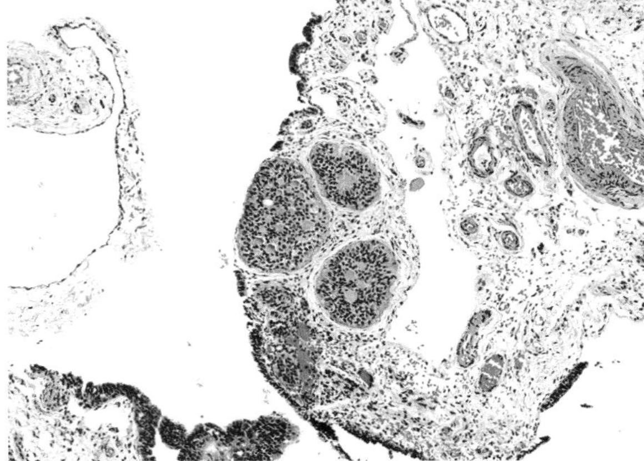

Fig. 11.13
Sex cord inclusions in the fimbriated end of the fallopian tube. **Immunohistochemical stains for inhibin and calretinin were diffusely positive. The ovaries were thoroughly sampled, and an ovarian mass was not present. Photo courtesy of Dr. Kathleen Cho (Univ. of Michigan Medical School)**

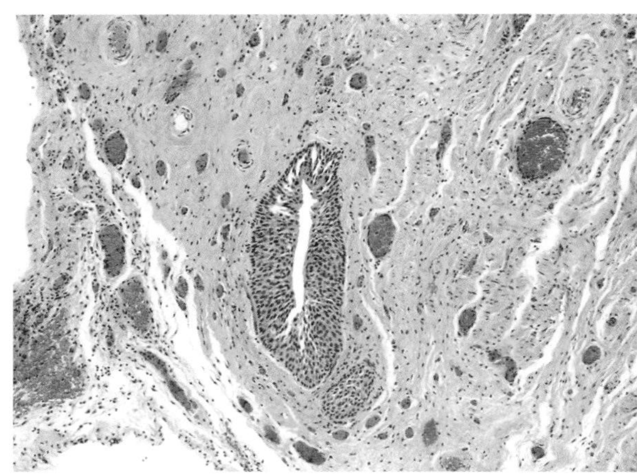

Fig. 11.14
Walthard nests. **Walthard nests may be either solid or cystic. Closer magnification will show nuclei which are bland with transitional (urothelial) cell differentiation**

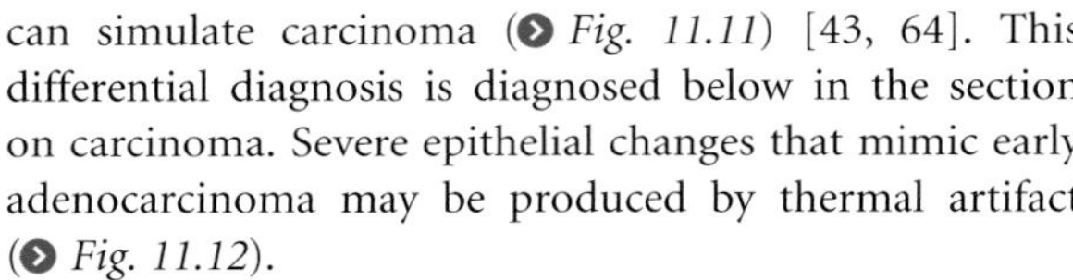

can simulate carcinoma (➲ *Fig. 11.11*) [43, 64]. This differential diagnosis is diagnosed below in the section on carcinoma. Severe epithelial changes that mimic early adenocarcinoma may be produced by thermal artifact (➲ *Fig. 11.12*).

Psammoma bodies ("salpingoliths") are an occasional finding. They are nonspecific and can be seen with normal-appearing epithelium or in various miscellaneous settings, such as chronic salpingitis associated with IgG antibodies to *Chlamydia*, ovarian serous tumors, or otherwise normal epithelium [152, 216].

Nests of cells morphologically similar to ovarian hilus cells have been described in the mid-portion of the tube. In the absence of either Reinke crystals or close association with nonmyelinated nerve fibers, it is difficult to exclude the possibility of an adrenal rest. Hilus cell nests with Reinke crystals may be seen, however, in fimbrial stroma. Ectopic pancreatic tissue or sex cord inclusions (➲ *Fig. 11.13*) can rarely occur.

The tubal serosa, by invagination, may give rise to a number of benign inclusion cysts. The simplest is a 1- to 2-mm unilocular cyst lying directly beneath the serosal surface lined by one or more layers of mesothelial cells – a mesothelial inclusion cyst. By a process of transitional cell metaplasia, small Walthard nests can arise as 1- to 2-mm yellow-white nodules beneath the serosa. Histologically, the Walthard nest may be solid or cystic and resemble urothelium (➲ *Fig. 11.14*). The cells have nuclei that are irregularly ovoid with a longitudinal nuclear groove, giving them a coffee-bean appearance. Both mesothelial inclusion cysts and Walthard nests are common incidental findings of no clinical importance.

Endometriosis and Endosalpingiosis

Normally, endometrial tissue can be found within the mucosa of the intramural and isthmic portions of the fallopian tube. The presence of endometrial tissue within the lumen has been referred to as "endometrial colonization"; however, it is unclear whether this is a variant of normal as opposed to true endometriosis. Endometriosis of the tube can be found within the lumen or myosalpinx or on the serosa. In occasional cases, the configuration of endometriosis may produce a mass clinically or grossly simulating a tumor ("polypoid endometriosis") [180]. A form of endometriosis designated "post-salpingectomy endometriosis" occurs in the tip of the proximal stump of the fallopian tube years after tubal ligation [44]. This form is apparently common. Endosalpingiosis is ectopic tubal-type epithelium involving the serosal surface of the tube. Both endometriosis and endosalpingiosis are discussed in detail in Chap. 13, Diseases of the Peritoneum.

Salpingitis Isthmica Nodosa

Salpingitis isthmica nodosa (SIN) is a pseudoinfiltrative lesion consisting of diverticula of tubal epithelium in the isthmus. It occurs in women between the ages of 25 and 60 years (average, 30 years). SIN is often bilateral. The external gross appearance is that of one or more nodularities in the isthmus, ranging up to 1–2 cm in diameter. The serosa is smooth. Grossly, the tissue is firm, and careful inspection may disclose some of the dilated diverticula.

Histologically at low-power magnification, round to elongated dilated glands proliferate through the muscularis, which is usually accompanied by nodular smooth muscle hyperplasia and mural thickening (*Fig. 11.15*). The glands proliferate in a circumferential and swirling pattern around the centrally dilated lumen of the fallopian tube. In some sections, it may be possible to appreciate a communication with the central lumen, indicating a diverticular process. The glands are composed of a single layer of bland tubal-type epithelium. An altered stromal reaction is typically absent. However, SIN is frequently associated with chronic salpingitis [132]. Endometrioid stromal cells lying beneath the diverticula may be abundant; however, they are usually sparse or absent. If both glands and stroma are present, it may be difficult to distinguish SIN from tubal endometriosis in some cases.

The etiology is unknown, but post-inflammatory distortion and an adenomyosis-like process are possibilities. An important complication of SIN is infertility, and there is a strong association with ectopic tubal pregnancy

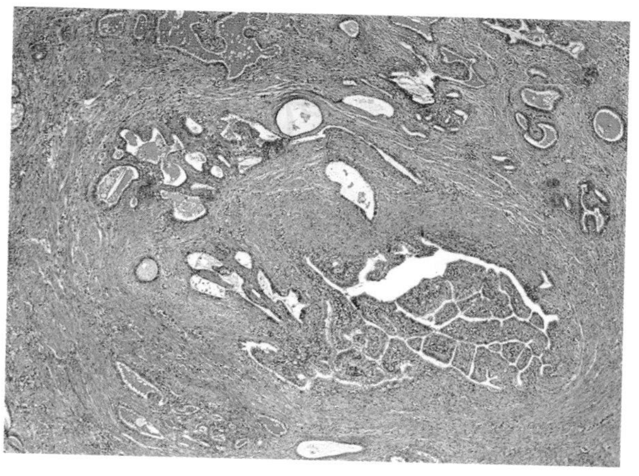

Fig. 11.15
Salpingitis isthmica nodosa. **Glands infiltrate the wall in a circumferential and swirling manner around the central lumen in the fallopian tube. The glands are mostly rounded, and some are cystically dilated. Occasional glands show mild contour irregularities. Some glands contain blood within the lumens. Closer magnification will show glands lined by a single layer of bland tubal epithelium**

[89, 104, 149, 183, 206]. A rare complication that we have seen is rupture of a deep diverticulum through the serosa, with subsequent mild intra-abdominal bleeding and pelvic pain.

Ectopic Pregnancy

An ectopic pregnancy occurs when the developing blastocyst implants at a site other than the endometrium of the fundus or lower uterine segment. Because more than 95% of ectopic pregnancies occur in the fallopian tube, the terms ectopic pregnancy and tubal pregnancy are nearly synonymous. However, implantation on both tubal fimbriae and ovary or in the interstitial segment of the fallopian tube (intramural pregnancy) or cornu, abdominal cavity, cervix, or retroperitoneum also may occur, in descending order of frequency [29]. Hepatic, diaphragmatic, and splenic pregnancies are extremely rare [56].

Etiology

The mechanisms responsible for ectopic pregnancy are largely unknown, but any disease process that alters the normal tubal anatomy seems to increase the frequency. Although delay in entering the uterine cavity may predispose the blastocyst to tubal nidation, experimentally delayed conceptuses in rabbit, guinea pig, and mouse oviducts degenerate and fail to implant. However, ectopic pregnancy is reported uncommonly in nonhuman primates. As many as 88% and 43% of carefully studied tubes with an ectopic pregnancy will show chronic salpingitis and salpingitis isthmica nodosa, respectively [89]. Ultrastructural studies have demonstrated that the mucosa of fallopian tubes in women with ectopic pregnancies have lower numbers of ciliated cells compared with women who have intrauterine pregnancies [234]. Risk factors for ectopic pregnancy are (in descending order of magnitude) prior ectopic pregnancy, prior tubal surgery, smoking (>20 cigarettes/day), pelvic inflammatory disease, multiple spontaneous abortions (≥3), increasing age (>40 years), prior medically induced abortion, infertility (>1 year), multiple sexual partners (>5), and previous intrauterine contraceptive device (IUD) use [27].

Clinical Features

Currently, ectopic pregnancy accounts for 1–2% of clinically known pregnancies [3, 70, 232]. Simultaneous ectopic and intrauterine implantations (heterotopic pregnancy) used to occur in 1 in 30,000 pregnancies decades ago; however, the frequency now can be as high as 0.75–1% of pregnancies after undergoing assisted reproductive technology [92, 150]. The classic presentation of ectopic pregnancy includes amenorrhea with subsequent vaginal bleeding and/or abdominal pain. Tubal rupture is associated with intra-abdominal hemorrhage. The frequency of left- versus right-sided ectopic tubal pregnancies is similar, but they are slightly more common on the right [29, 30]. Rare cases are bilateral.

Serial serum beta-human chorionic gonadotropin (β-hCG) measurements and transvaginal ultrasonography are important parts of the clinical evaluation. Management typically consists of either surgery (salpingectomy or salpingostomy) or medical therapy (methotrexate). Incomplete removal of trophoblastic tissue may result in persistent ectopic pregnancy, which occurs in 2–11% and 4–20% of cases after laparotomy with salpingostomy and laparoscopic salpingostomy, respectively [70, 79]. These figures are similar to the frequency of failure with systemic methotrexate therapy. In some cases, persistent ectopic pregnancy may be a result of spillage of gestational tissue from disruption/morcellation of the specimen after salpingostomy or salpingectomy. In such instances, the lesional tissue may be found as nodules/implants on pelvic, omental, or uterine serosal surfaces [39, 63].

Pathologic Features

The unruptured tubal pregnancy is characterized grossly by a somewhat irregular elongated dilatation of the tube, with a blue discoloration caused by hematosalpinx (*Fig. 11.16*). Within the tube, most ectopic pregnancies are found in the ampulla (~80%), isthmus (12%), and fimbriae (5%) [29].

Nearly two thirds of cases contain a grossly or microscopically identifiable embryo. Chorionic villi usually are found in the blood-filled and dilated tubal lumen and, in 75% of cases, appear viable. Implantation is deeper and more apt to be associated with a viable pregnancy when the placentation occurs on the mesosalpingeal side of the tube as compared with the anti-mesosalpingeal side [121]. The extra-villous intermediate trophoblast of the conceptus penetrates deep in the tubal wall. On occasion, this proliferation may exhibit diffuse sheet-like architecture, which can raise concern for a gestational trophoblastic neoplasm or hydatidiform mole [33, 211]; however, this appearance is within the range of proliferation that can be encountered in ectopic pregnancies (*Fig. 11.17*). Perhaps because of the limited ability of the endosalpingeal stroma to undergo decidualization, and analogous to a placenta increta, the chorionic villi invade muscularis and then serosa [181]. Another major difference compared with uterine implantation is the failure of tubal trophoblast to differentiate into chorion frondosum and chorion laeve [196], but a gestational sac can be seen [181]. Vascular changes in mid-sized tubal arteries adjacent to ectopic pregnancies are similar to those found in the vessels near uterine implantations, with invasion by intermediate trophoblast, proliferation of the vascular intima, and accumulation of foam cells in the intima.

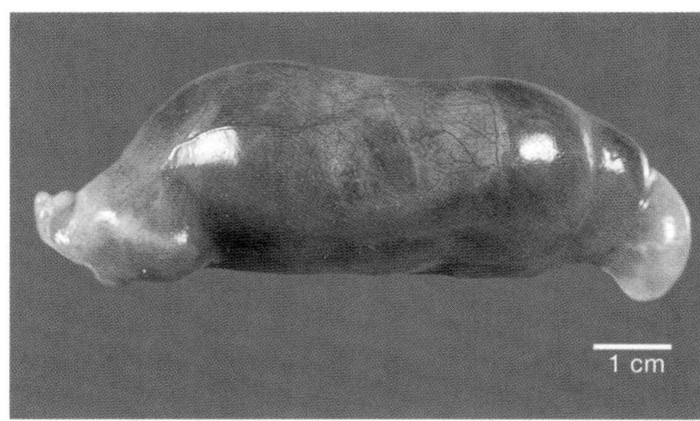

Fig. 11.16
Ectopic pregnancy. **External view of dilated fallopian tube containing an ectopic pregnancy. The cross section will show a hemorrhagic cut surface**

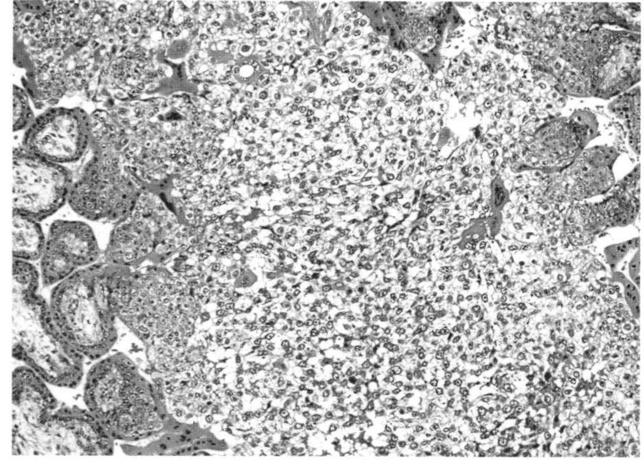

Fig. 11.17
Exuberant intermediate trophoblast proliferation in an ectopic pregnancy. **The sheet-like architecture and atypical epithelioid cells should not be mistaken for a gestational trophoblastic neoplasm or hydatidiform mole. Chorionic villi are present on the left side of the photograph**

Chronic salpingitis is found in nearly half the patients, with a reported range of 29–88% [89]. Salpingitis isthmica nodosa may also be present. Arias-Stella reaction can be seen in the fallopian tube mucosa [159]. Clear cell hyperplasia has been reported [230].

The clinicopathologic features of extratubal ectopic pregnancy vary according to the site [173]. Cornual or interstitial pregnancies may expand up to about 12 weeks, when rupture may lacerate one of the uterine arteries as well as the entire side of the uterus. Cervical ectopic pregnancy presents with bleeding similar to an incomplete abortion. Because of the nature of the cervical tissue underlying placental implantation, control of bleeding may be difficult. Ovarian pregnancy is clinically similar to tubal pregnancy, including frequent preoperative rupture. More than half the patients in one series had a history of previous reproductive tract disease or infertility [90]. Macroscopic examination typically reveals a hemorrhagic mass replacing the ovary. Pathologic criteria for ovarian pregnancy have been proposed as follows: (1) the tube must be intact and separate from the ovary; (2) the gestational sac must occupy the normal position of the ovary; (3) the gestational sac must be connected to the uterus by the utero-ovarian ligament; and (4) ovarian tissue must be demonstrated within the wall of the sac [90]. Pathologic documentation of ovarian tissue within the pregnancy may be difficult or impossible if treatment consists of conservative resection or if the pregnancy has extensively replaced the ovarian tissue.

Sequelae

The natural history of tubal ectopic pregnancy includes spontaneous expulsion from the fimbriated end (tubal abortion), as well as embryonal death and involution of the conceptus. Typically, however, continued growth of the trophoblast leads to increasing dilatation and weakening of the muscularis, with rupture at about the eighth week. About 25% of tubal pregnancies have ruptured by the time of diagnosis [69]. Hemorrhage due to rupture may be massive, and ectopic pregnancy is a major cause of maternal mortality during pregnancy. Rare ectopic pregnancies have proceeded to term with fetal viability.

In grossly normal fallopian tubes, chorionic villi or placental site nodules may be found, indicative of a prior unsuspected ectopic pregnancy [111, 168]. A subset of tubal pregnancies forms a mass that, with involution of trophoblast and reestablishment of the menstrual cycle, may present problems in differential diagnosis. This convoluted, blood-filled tube (including organization, variable inflammation, and adhesions), often with involved ipsilateral ovary, may simulate a tumor or an endometrioma. Most, but not all, patients will have detectable serum β-hCG. Extensive microscopic sampling of this so-called chronic ectopic pregnancy may be required to demonstrate trophoblastic tissue, which may consist of nonviable chorionic villi [231]. In more advanced pregnancy, death of the fetus with retention in the extrauterine location may be followed by calcification of the fetus (lithopedion) or both membranes and fetus (lithokelyphopedion).

Polyps

Polyps of the fallopian tube have been classified as tumors in the WHO Classification of fallopian tube neoplasms and in other textbooks on gynecologic pathology; however, they are included in the non-neoplastic section of this chapter for conceptual purposes. They are found in approximately 1–3% of women undergoing hysterosalpingography for infertility and may cause proximal tubal occlusion [50, 71]. Their causality of and relationship with infertility has been debated in the literature. They are typically small and preferentially occur in the intramural segment of the fallopian tube, particularly at the tubal ostium. Polyps are frequently bilateral. Although they are removed for microscopic examination only rarely, histologically they are of endometrioid type and resemble endometrial polyps [145]. Given that endometriosis of the tubal mucosa is found in some patients, it is possible that tubal polyps might represent a microscopic form of polypoid endometriosis.

Infertility

Most of the diseases discussed in this chapter may result in sufficient anatomic distortion to cause tubal infertility. In contrast, purely physiologic tubal dysfunction is not well defined but may be illustrated by the immotile cilia of Kartagener's syndrome that can lead to reduced fertility – only 3 of 12 women in one series succeeded in becoming pregnant [5]. Paratubal or fimbrial adhesions secondary to endometriosis, prior pelvic inflammatory disease, or appendicitis may interfere with normal tubal motility and ovum pick-up. For a detailed discussion of the pathophysiology of fallopian tube cilia in various diseases in relation to infertility, the reader is referred elsewhere [147]. Obliterative fibrosis (possibly secondary to inflammation within the uterus) or polyps at the uterine tubal ostium may lead to obstruction at the uterotubal junction [76, 139].

Issues Related to Sterilization Procedures

Sterilization by interference with tubal function involves procedures designed to damage or obstruct the mucosa or lumen of the fallopian tube by surgical removal of a segment of the tube (bilateral partial salpingectomy), rings/clamps, electrocoagulation, intratubal chemical methods (e.g., silicone plugs and methylcyanoacrylate), or intratubal mechanical devices (e.g., Essure system) [62, 223]. Tubal resection should be confirmed by histologic demonstration of a cross section of the fallopian tube including the entire lumen. On occasion, histologic sections may only show fibromuscular/fibrovascular tissue without fallopian tube mucosa. Such cases may represent pelvic ligaments or vessels that were clinically mistaken for a fallopian tube. In order to completely evaluate those cases, it may be necessary to cut deeper levels from the paraffin block, including the possibility of re-orienting and re-embedding the tissue in the block so as to entirely cut through it and find a fallopian tube lumen. The above protocol also applies to cases in which a fallopian tube is definitely present histologically but for which a complete cross section of the lumen is not seen on the H&E slide.

In women who were initially treated by surgical resection, spontaneous re-anastomosis or fistula formation, which may lead to fertilization and ectopic or intrauterine pregnancy, are common mechanisms of sterilization failure [221]. To identify the cause of failure of tubal sterilization procedures, careful gross examination of the specimen, occasionally specimen salpingography, longitudinal orientation of the tubal segment in the paraffin block, and meticulous sectioning techniques may be necessary.

Salpingitis

Salpingitis consists of three major types: acute, chronic, and granulomatous/histiocytic. On occasion, some cases will have mixed features, but this section is arranged according to the predominant histologic appearance.

Acute Salpingitis

Acute salpingitis is a purulent inflammatory process usually secondary to the passage of bacteria from the cervix and uterine cavity into the tubal lumen [137, 154]. It is the pathologic correlate of the clinical entity, pelvic inflammatory disease. It typically occurs in young, sexually active, and reproductive-age women. Important risk factors include patterns of sexual behavior and contraceptive use.

Grossly, the fallopian tube is enlarged and edematous (Fig. 11.18). The serosa is erythematous and may be covered with fibrinopurulent exudates. Pus may also fill the lumen. Histologically, the fallopian tube lumen,

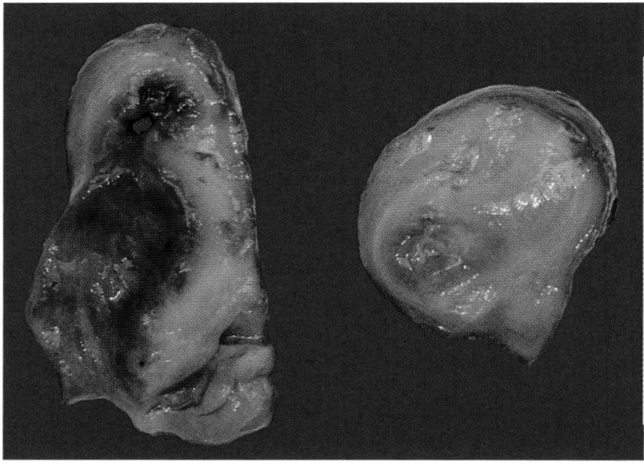

Fig. 11.18
Fallopian tube with acute salpingitis. **The tube is enlarged with a dilated lumen and erythematous mucosa. The wall is edematous and thickened. Other examples may contain pus in the lumen**

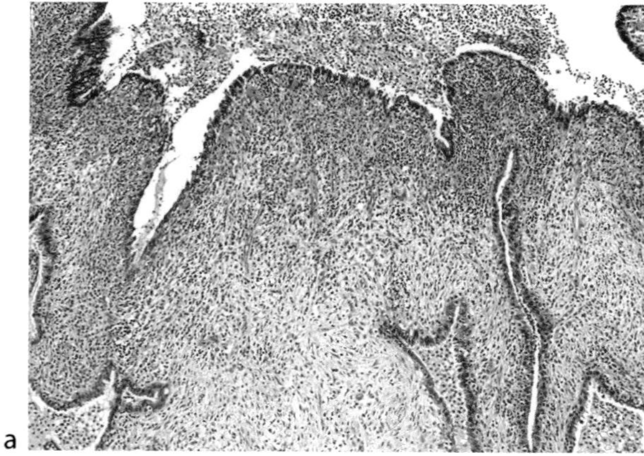

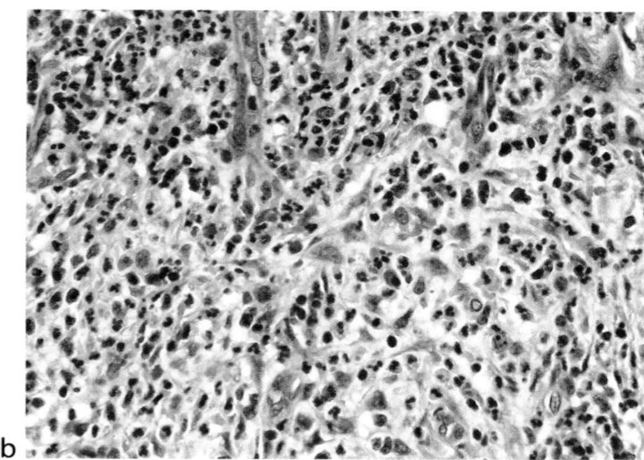

Fig. 11.19
Acute salpingitis. **(a) The mucosa shows distorted architecture and abundant inflammation, including pus in the overlying lumen. (b) The inflammatory component is mixed but mostly composed of abundant neutrophils**

mucosa, and wall contain neutrophils, fibrinous debris, and ulceration (*Fig. 11.19*). Edema and lymphocytes may be present as well. Mucosal hyperplasia and distortion can be seen. The histologic appearance varies according to the severity and phase of the disease. The appearance may also vary somewhat based on the specific causative microbial agent, as discussed below. Significant fallopian tube-specific sequelae include infertility and ectopic pregnancy.

It is not clear if organisms are carried upward by sperm or trichomonads as vectors or whether some form of passive transport is in effect [120]. The bacteria implicated in acute salpingitis appear to be from two sources: sexual transmission and lower genital tract flora. Although *Neisseria gonorrhoeae* and *Chlamydia trachomatis* have been considered the most common causative organisms, meticulous bacteriologic studies indicate that most cases are polymicrobial and that anaerobic bacteria, especially *Bacteroides* species and peptostreptococci, frequently are present, as well as aerobes such as *Escherichia coli.* The presence of serum antibodies against gonococcal pili in some of these women, however, suggests that gonococci may initiate the process, only to be supplanted by anaerobes. The role of mycoplasmas in acute salpingitis is controversial, and viruses do not appear to be etiologic. However, Herpes simplex virus infection involving the mucosa of a prolapsed tube with mixed acute and chronic inflammation has been reported [141].

The gonococcus gains access to the tube most readily at the time of menstruation. This situation corresponds to the typical clinical presentation in which the onset of acute pain occurs a few days after menses. The onset of non-gonococcal, non-chlamydial acute salpingitis is not, however, clearly related to the recent onset of menses [227]. Elegant *in vitro* studies by Ward et al. [237] have clarified the likely initial steps in gonococcal infection, and the molecular mechanisms involved have been reviewed elsewhere [67, 147]. *N. gonorrhoeae* perfused through the lumen of cultured whole tubes attach only to non-ciliated cells. Within 3 h, microvilli from the cells appear to embrace the gonococci and adhere to them. The bacteria then penetrate both the cells and intercellular junctions, with cell lysis and sloughing. Adjacent ciliated cells are also destroyed but are not invaded directly. Gonococcal lipopolysaccharide and gonococcal-induced tumor necrosis factor-alpha and various other cytokines cause much of the epithelial damage [148, 156], and the degree of pathogenicity likely depends on the bacterial as well as the host genome [11]. After cell lysis, the bacteria penetrate the subepithelial connective tissue. *In vivo,* this process is considerably modified by the host response.

N. gonorrhoeae spreads via the epithelial surface and thus causes mucosal damage. A brisk diapedesis of granulocytes from capillaries into the mucosa and lumen occurs, and there is vascular engorgement and edema of all tubal layers. As the lumen fills with granulocytes and cellular debris, and as the tube distends, pus may be seen dripping from the fimbriated end in patients undergoing laparoscopy. In severe cases, transudation of plasma proteins results in a fibrinous exudate on the serosal surface, which is erythematous because of vascular dilatation. The cell necrosis, distension of the tube, and focal peritonitis account for the symptoms of abdominal and pelvic pain. Over time, repeated infections result in recurrent symptoms as well as the anatomic changes of chronic salpingitis, discussed below.

Chlamydia trachomatis is cultured frequently from the cervix, uterus, and fallopian tubes in women with acute salpingitis [131, 151]. It is thought that the damage of the fallopian tube by *Chlamydia* is due to the 60-kDa chlamydial heat shock protein (hsp60), as well as other various cytokines [147]. The histologic appearance of tubes removed during the acute or subacute phase of chlamydial salpingitis is virtually identical to that caused by the gonococcus. There is an initial transmural and mucosal infiltration of neutrophils with an intraluminal exudate. Subsequently, there is a lymphoplasmacytic response with variable numbers of residual granulocytes. Chlamydial inclusion bodies have been identified within the epithelial cells [240]. On occasion, the lymphofollicular response may be so florid as to suggest lymphoma [236].

As a result of acute salpingitis (usually in the context of gonococcal or chlamydial disease), fibrinous adhesions develop between the fallopian tube serosa and surrounding peritoneal surfaces. Peritoneal inflammation may be widespread, and thin so-called violin-string adhesions may form between the liver and the anterior abdominal wall as part of the Fitz-Hugh–Curtis syndrome.

In severe cases of acute salpingitis (as well as with chronic or granulomatous salpingitis) with involvement of the ovary regardless of the specific microorganism, both the ovary and the tube are attached to one another by adhesions and create a mass in the form of a tubo-ovarian abscess (*Fig. 11.20*). Tubo-ovarian abscesses can be unilateral or bilateral. Histologically, the inflammatory component may be predominantly composed of neutrophils or contain a mixture of neutrophils, lymphocytes, histiocytes, and plasma cells. Widespread necrosis is common. The background fallopian tube and ovarian parenchyma will be markedly distorted, and abundant fibrous and edematous stroma may be present. Although *N. gonorrhoeae* and *C. trachomatis* are common bacterial causes of acute salpingitis, they are isolated in culture only rarely from tubo-ovarian abscesses. Both aerobic and anaerobic cultures of any tubo-ovarian abscess should be obtained in the operating room or laboratory. Prior treatment with antibiotics possibly may eliminate culturable organisms, but anaerobes are commonly isolated. *E. coli*, *Bacteroides fragilis*, and other *Bacteroides* species, *Peptostreptococcus*, *Peptococcus*, and aerobic streptococci are the most commonly found organisms [136]. Typically, these infections are polymicrobial.

Another organism that can result in tubo-ovarian abscess is *Actinomyces israelii*, which is part of the indigenous female genital tract flora [184]. Actinomycotic infections of the tube are associated with intrauterine contraceptive devices (IUDs) (see Chap. 7, Benign Diseases of the Endometrium) [60]. Anaerobic culture is necessary to permit growth of *Actinomyces israelii*. Microscopically, fragments of gram-positive filaments and sulfur granules may be recognized within pus. Pseudoactinomycotic radiate granules should not be mistaken for the sulfur granules of actinomycosis [24, 192].

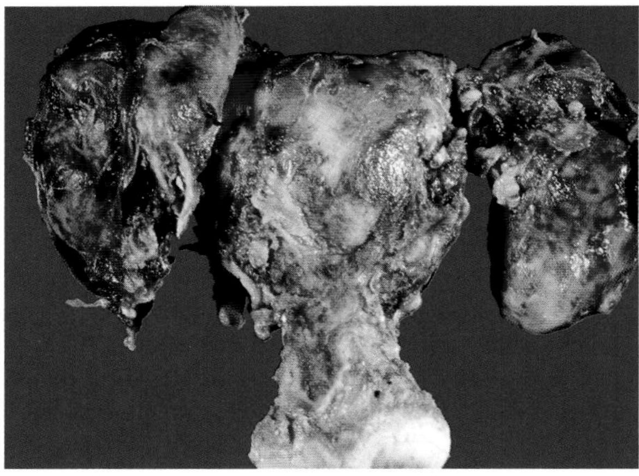

Fig. 11.20
Tubo-ovarian abscess. **In this case, bilateral tubo-ovarian abscesses are composed of fibroinflammatory masses, and the ovary and fallopian tube on each side are attached to one another by adhesions. The cut surface will show distorted fibrous tissue with edema, hemorrhage, and necrosis**

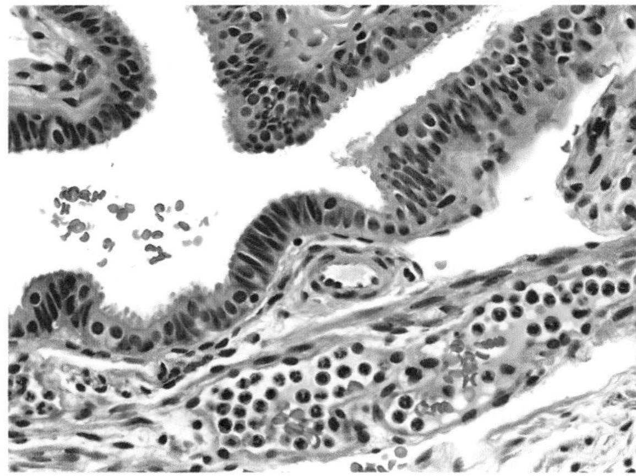

Fig. 11.21
Physiologic salpingitis. **A mild amount of acute inflammation is present within the vascular spaces in the mucosa. Other cases may have mild acute inflammation within the mucosal epithelium or lamina propria**

An asymptomatic form of acute salpingitis ("physiologic salpingitis") is seen in tubes removed during postpartum ligation. Beginning about 5 h after delivery and present up to 7–10 days later, a small number of acute or mixed acute and chronic inflammatory cells are found in the mucosa or lumen of 10% or more of specimens (➲ *Fig. 11.21*). Attempts to culture aerobic or anaerobic bacteria have been almost uniformly unsuccessful. The process may be secondary to the trauma of delivery or intrauterine tissue necrosis and is apparently of no clinical significance.

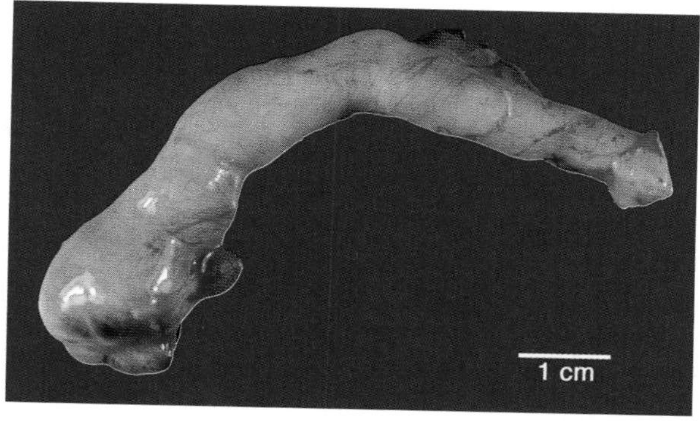

Fig. 11.22
Clubbed tube. **The fimbriated end is closed because of fimbrial adhesions, creating a blunted end**

Chronic Salpingitis

As a result of acute salpingitis, the proximity of the ovary to the fimbriae allows multiple tubo-ovarian adhesions to form, which may also cause occlusion of the tubal ostium. If the fimbriae close before the ovary is involved as part of a tubo-ovarian abscess, the inflamed and dilated tube can form a pyosalpinx full of acute and chronic inflammatory cells. When acute salpingitis resolves, the acute and most of the chronic inflammatory cells gradually disappear, and the patient is left with either a severely scarred tube in the form of chronic salpingitis or a hydrosalpinx. *C. trachomatis* DNA has even been detected in fallopian tubes in a subset of cases that contained only chronic salpingitis [103]. Thus, the finding of chronic salpingitis may imply previous pelvic inflammatory disease in some patients.

In chronic salpingitis, the mucosal plicae are often adherent to one another secondary to surface fibrin deposition from acute salpingitis. This may be focal or extensive. If it is severe enough, the bases of the fimbriae may coalesce in the center with the fimbriae radiating outward, or the tips of the fimbriae may adhere blocking the lumen and causing a blunted end – the so-called clubbed tube (➲ *Fig. 11.22*). Healing and organization in the non-fimbriated portions of the tube also lead to permanent bridging between folds. Classically, this results in so-called follicular salpingitis (➲ *Fig. 11.23*); however, that term is a misnomer as it suggests a pattern of inflammation characterized by lymphoid follicles. In chronic salpingitis, plicae may retain much of their size and shape, but plasma cells, lymphocytes, or both are still present in the mucosa (➲ *Fig. 11.24*). Often the height of the folds appears reduced, and the plicae may become blunted and have fibrous stroma. Therefore, the once orderly pattern of the mucosa becomes distorted. The mucosa may also be hyperplastic.

Hydrosalpinx is characterized by obliteration of the fimbriated end and dilation of the tube, usually the ampullary and infundibular portions (➲ *Fig. 11.25*). If the ovary is first involved by tubo-ovarian adhesions, the ovary may be compressed by the dilated tube. Because a luminal communication usually can be demonstrated between dilated and non-dilated portions of the tube, the etiology of the dilatation can be obscure. The dilated tube can become cystic and filled with serous fluid, and the wall is generally white, thin, and translucent with occasional fibrous adhesions on the external surface. The muscle wall is either thin and atrophic or replaced by fibrous tissue. Most of the epithelial lining consists of low-cuboidal cells, but an occasional plica may persist with columnar epithelium containing histologically normal

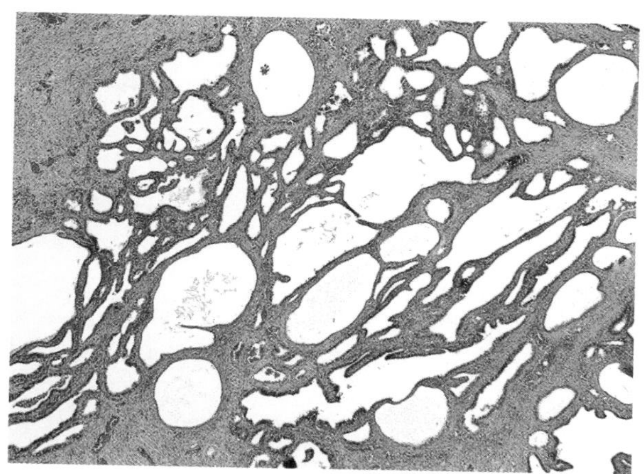

Fig. 11.23
Follicular salpingitis. **The plicae are adherent to one another, creating follicle-like spaces in the setting of chronic salpingitis**

ciliated and secretory cells (Fig. 11.26). A few lymphocytes may be found in the wall of the hydrosalpinx but are more commonly absent.

Granulomatous/Histiocytic Salpingitis and Foreign Bodies

Granulomatous and histiocytic inflammation of the fallopian tube may result from infection by a number of different organisms or be induced by a variety of noninfectious processes, some of which include tissue reactions due to microscopic foreign bodies.

Pseudoxanthomatous/Xanthogranulomatous Salpingitis

Pseudoxanthomatous salpingitis (variably referred to as "pigmentosis tubae") is characterized by lipofuscin- and hemosiderin-laden macrophages within the lamina propria of the mucosa of the fallopian tube, including distension of the plicae, and is associated with endometriosis (Fig. 11.27) [45, 78, 101, 164, 215]. The tubes may be enlarged and edematous, with the mucosa having a dark brown polypoid gross appearance. Despite the association with endometriosis, this process also might result from salpingitis with associated bleeding [45, 215]. It has been suggested that pseudoxanthomatous salpingitis should be distinguished from xanthogranulomatous salpingitis because of the latter's association with pelvic inflammatory disease and lack of association with

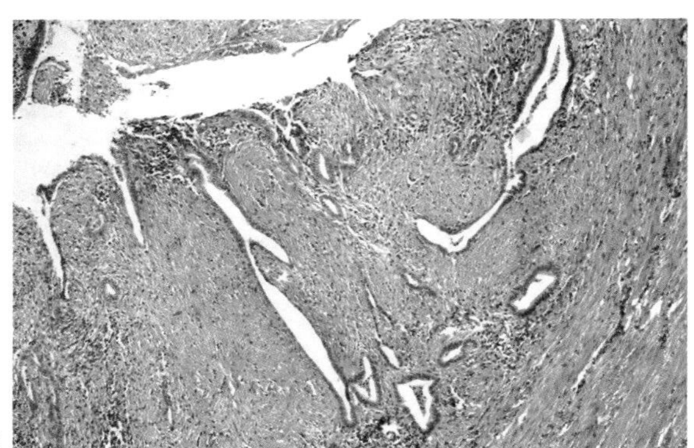

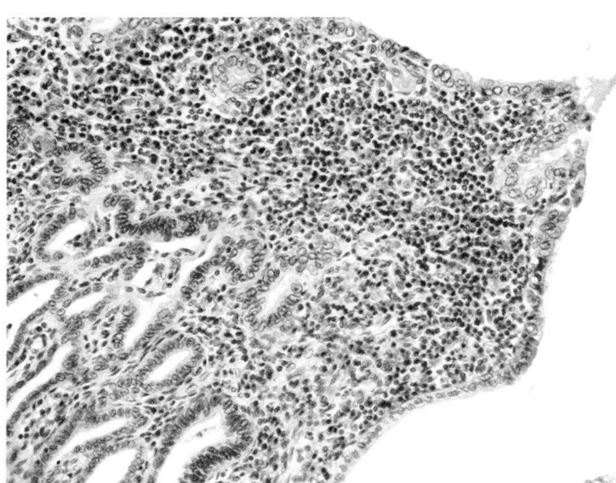

Fig. 11.24
Chronic salpingitis. **(a) Fibrotic and blunted plicae. (b) The distorted plicae show the lamina propria filled with lymphocytes and plasma cells**

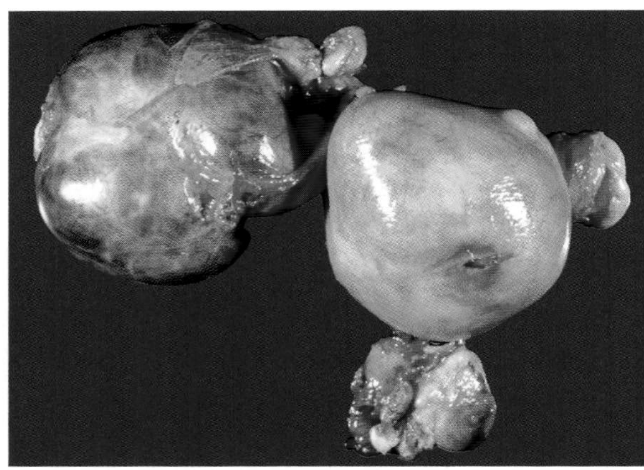

Fig. 11.25
Hydrosalpinx. **The fallopian tube is massively dilated, producing a large cystic mass**

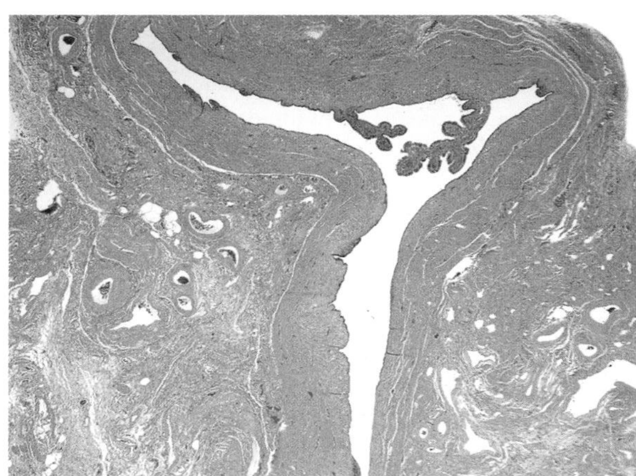

Fig. 11.26
Hydrosalpinx. **Most of the dilated fallopian tube contains a thin wall and atrophic mucosa. Residual small plicae are present. Note the smooth muscle within the wall**

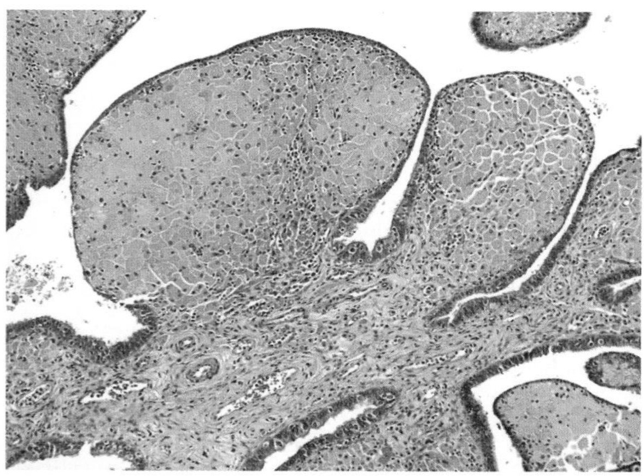

■ Fig. 11.27
Pseudoxanthomatous salpingitis. **The plicae are expanded and distorted due to sheets of histiocytes with eosinophilic cytoplasm in the lamina propria. This should not be mistaken for decidualization**

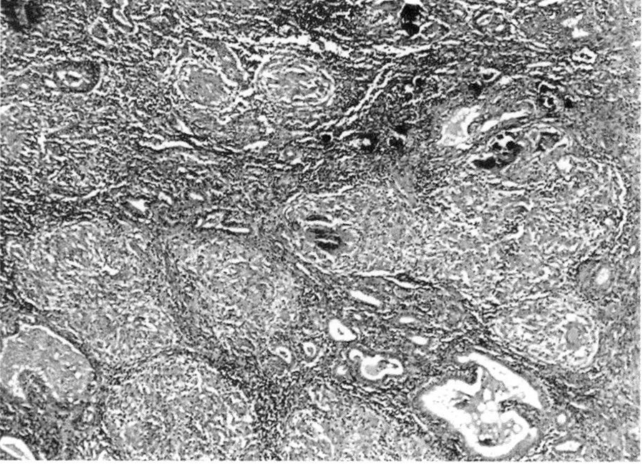

■ Fig. 11.28
Granulomatous salpingitis due to tuberculosis. **Noncaseating granulomas are present in the mucosa. Note calcifications and multinucleated giant cells. Other cases may contain caseating granulomas**

endometriosis [78]. In contrast with pseudoxanthomatous salpingitis, xanthogranulomatous salpingitis has mucosa which is usually grossly yellow and purulent, macrophages which are foamy (as opposed to the dark brown macrophages in pseudoxanthomatous salpingitis), and other types of inflammatory cells, including multinucleated giant cells [78, 133]. A potentially related lesion that has been described in the tube is xanthelasma [41].

Tuberculous Salpingitis

Mycobacterium tuberculosis historically has been the predominant etiologic agent of granulomatous salpingitis. The frequency of tuberculous salpingitis in women studied for tubal causes of infertility ranges from much less than 1% in the USA to nearly 40% in India [178]. Twenty percent of women who die of tuberculosis have tubal involvement [208]. Primary infection of the genitalia, as by coitus with a partner with genitourinary tuberculosis, is extremely rare. Secondary spread via a hematogenous route, usually from a primary pulmonary infection, is the usual route of infection. For unclear reasons, the bloodborne organism prefers the tubes rather than other parts of the female genital tract. The primary pulmonary lesion may not be radiologically evident, but extrapulmonary involvement of the peritoneum, kidneys, or other sites may be present. Lymphatic spread from primary intestinal tuberculosis or direct spread from the urinary bladder or gastrointestinal tract may occur. Tubal involvement is usually bilateral. Although the earliest pathologic lesions are microscopic, with advancing disease the tube increases in diameter and may become nodular, mimicking salpingitis isthmica nodosa. In the more common adhesive form of the disease, multiple dense adhesions may form between the tube and ovary, and the fimbriae and ostium may be obliterated [93]. With the exudative form of disease, progressive distension mimics bacterial pyosalpinx. Hematosalpinx, hydrosalpinx, tubo-ovarian abscesses, or a so-called frozen pelvis may be found late in the disease process [178]. In either form, serosal tubercles may be present.

In early disease, microscopic lesions are mucosal based with a typical granulomatous reaction of epithelioid histiocytes and lymphocytes arranged in a nodular configuration. Multinucleated giant cells are often seen, and focal or massive central caseation may be present (➔ *Fig. 11.28*). Immunosuppression can modify cellular immunity to a point where granulomas fail to form, and with this clinical information, the mere finding of acute and chronic inflammatory cells should lead to consideration of staining for acid-fast organisms. From the mucosa, extension to the muscularis and serosa may occur. As the tubercles enlarge and coalesce, they may erode through the mucosa and discharge their contents into the tubal lumen, and the tube may then become dilated. The mucosal inflammatory reaction leads to progressive scarring, with plical distortion and agglutination. Calcification can occur in areas of fibrosis. Because tubercles may not be present in a given section, the presence of caseation, fibrosis, or calcification in a tube may be the only histologic finding that suggests the need for more thorough evaluation. Notable mucosal distortion may result in hyperplasia mimicking carcinoma.

There are several complications of tuberculous salpingitis. Alteration in function is expected, and sterility is almost universal because of the common bilaterality of the disease. Because of repeated seeding of the endometrium from the infected tubes, the mycobacterial culture and the histologic finding of endometrial granulomas on curettage are diagnostically useful (see Chap. 7, Benign Diseases of the Endometrium).

Parasitic Salpingitis

Pinworm (Oxyuriasis) The pinworm, *Enterobius vermicularis,* may migrate up the female genital tract, embed in the tube, and cause an inflammatory reaction. The tube can be involved with the ovary as a tubo-ovarian abscess, or a fibrous nodular area may be present. Acute and chronic inflammatory cells may be found together with eosinophils and portions of a gravid female worm. Ova can be released into the tissue, where they provoke a granulomatous reaction (*Fig. 11.29*), but identification of ova can be obscured by calcification and granulomas.

Schistosomiasis (Bilharziasis) Although tubal schistosomiasis may be one of the more common causes of granulomatous salpingitis worldwide, it is rare in the USA. In Africa, the fallopian tube is involved by schistosomiasis in 22% of all infected women [84]. The ova of *Schistosoma haematobium* are most common, but *Schistosoma mansoni* eggs may be present in some women. Gross findings appear to be related to fibrosis surrounding the ova, producing a nodular or fibrotic tube. Histologically, the inflammatory reaction is typically granulomatous and may contain eosinophils, neutrophils, plasma cells, lymphocytes, and macrophages, including multinucleated giant cells. Some granulomas may be present within the stroma of the plicae and produce plical expansion. Ectopic pregnancy has been reported as occurring synchronously with tubal schistosomiasis in some patients.

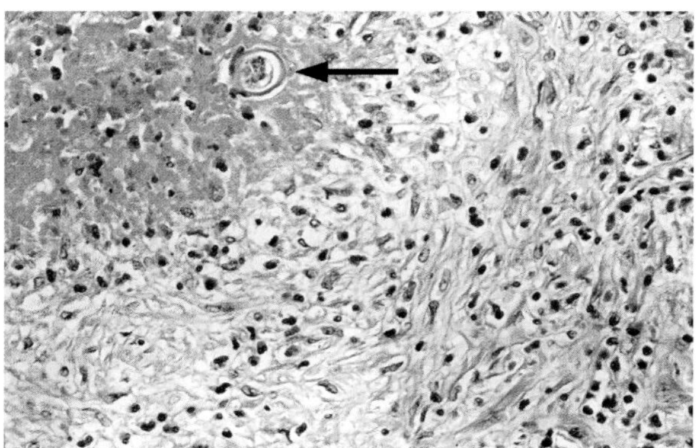

Fig. 11.29
Granulomatous salpingitis due to pinworm. **This caseating granuloma contains abundant eosinophils. A pinworm egg (*arrow*) is present within the necrotic zone**

Other Parasites Where the condition is common, hydatid disease secondary to *Echinococcus granulosus* infection may involve the female genital tract, including the adnexa. Cysticercosis (*Taenia solium*) also has been described in the tube [2]. Other rare parasites that have been reported in the fallopian tube include *Entamoeba histolytica* (amebiasis). Liesegang rings should not be mistaken for parasites [46].

Fungal Salpingitis

Other fungi that rarely can cause tubo-ovarian abscesses or granulomatous salpingitis include *Blastomyces dermatitidis, Coccidioides immitis, Candida,* and *Aspergillus.* These may be secondary to hematogenous spread or disseminated disease.

Sarcoidosis

Sarcoidosis of the tube is rare [25]. Histologically, noncaseating granulomas may be seen in the mucosa. Culture, histochemical stains, and clinical information are necessary to exclude other granulomatous diseases.

Crohn's Disease

Crohn's disease of the ileum, colon, or appendix may secondarily involve the tube and ovary to produce a granulomatous salpingitis and tubo-ovarian abscess. Noncaseating granulomas can involve the entire thickness of the tubal muscularis as well as the mucosa. The mucosa may exhibit hyperplasia with reactive atypia [32]. Fistulas from bowel to tube also can occur.

Other Types of Granulomatous/Histiocytic Lesions and Foreign Bodies

Malakoplakia has rarely been reported in the fallopian tube. Some vasculitides have a granulomatous pattern (see Vasculitis section below) [20]. Foreign body granulomas due to starch and talc, as well as pulse granulomas [197] can occur in the tube. In order to detect some foreign bodies, granulomatous or histiocytic reactions should be examined under polarized light. Extruded keratin from endometrioid carcinomas with squamous differentiation of the endometrium or ovary can produce keratin granulomas on the serosa or fimbriated end of the tube, as well as within the tubal lumen [124]. It should be noted, however, that not all foreign bodies produce a significant granulomatous or histiocytic response. Gelatin microsphere embolization particles (Embospheres®/EmboGold®) used in uterine artery embolization for treatment of uterine leiomyomas may sometimes be found in the fallopian tubes or ovaries because of the vascular anastomosis between the uterine and ovarian arteries [123]. In the fallopian tube, these particles are typically found within arterial lumens in the outer wall of the tube or para-tubal locations. They usually elicit only a mild lymphocytic response with rare multinucleated giant cells as opposed to the marked multinucleated giant cell reaction with a granulomatous or histiocytic component seen with other foreign bodies.

Torsion, Prolapse, and Intussusception

Among the various anatomic displacements of the tube, torsion is the most common. The usual predisposing factor is cystic enlargement of the ipsilateral ovary. A benign ovarian cyst or tumor is present in the majority of patients, but in a minority, a malignant ovarian tumor is the cause. Para-ovarian cysts also are associated with torsion. Tubal enlargement secondary to hydrosalpinx or pyosalpinx, or previous gynecologic surgery (especially sterilization), are additional etiologies, but torsion may occur in the absence of apparent adnexal disease [22]. The typical patient is in the reproductive years, occasionally pregnant, and complains of the sudden onset of lower abdominal pain. At operation, the adnexa on one side is twisted, usually once or twice. Venous outflow is compromised early, and the resulting congestion may lead to arterial compression. The adnexa often are enlarged, edematous, and dark and show hemorrhagic infarction. If surgical intervention is prompt, the tube may be preserved. Asymptomatic or undiagnosed torsion can occur.

Tubal prolapse into the vagina may occur rarely as a complication of vaginal or abdominal hysterectomy (see Chap. 3, Diseases of the Vagina) [195]. Clinically, this is characterized by dyspareunia, vaginal bleeding/discharge, or abdominal pain beginning a few days to several years after hysterectomy. However, some women may be asymptomatic. On clinical examination, an excrescence is seen in the vaginal vault, suggestive of granulation tissue or carcinoma. Fimbriae may be apparent grossly. Severe acute and chronic inflammation can be present microscopically, and papillary architecture or pseudogland formation by the tubal epithelium can mimic adenocarcinoma. Due to admixed granulation tissue, it may be difficult to recognize the lesional tissue as a distorted segment of fallopian tube; however, close scrutiny should reveal papillae lined by benign tubal epithelium. Depending on the specific differential diagnosis, immunohistochemical staining for WT-1, ER/PR, CK7, CK20, p16, and/or Ki-67 may be of help.

Intussusception of the tube is rare. In one case, a para-ovarian cyst was engulfed by the end of the tube, and the fimbriated end was pulled into the ampulla [4].

Congenital Anomalies

Structural congenital anomalies of the fallopian tube are rare. Diethylstilbestrol (DES) use during pregnancy was discontinued decades ago, but surgical specimens from patients who were born during the DES era may still be examined today. *In utero* exposure to DES produces shortened, sacculated, and convoluted fallopian tubes. The fimbriae are constricted, and the os is pinpoint [54]. The mucosa may be absent, or when it is present, the plicae do not develop [199].

Tubal duplication and accessory fallopian tubes are uncommon, but the latter occur more frequently [23, 47, 51, 83]. Absence of various segments of the fallopian tube (also variably referred to as atresia, hypoplasia, or interruption), absence of the ampullary muscularis, and complete absence of the tube have been described. These may be unilateral or bilateral, and they can occur with or without uterine anomalies, such as unicornuate or bicornuate uterus (reviewed in Nawroth et al. [167]).

Vasculitis

The fallopian tube can be involved by vasculitis as part of localized or systemic disease, and involvement of the tube is less frequent compared with other sites within the gynecologic tract. Vasculitis involving the female genital

Table 11.1
Histologic classification for neoplasms of the fallopian tube, including gestational trophoblastic disease: Modified 2003 WHO Classification

Epithelial
Benign, including mixed epithelial–mesenchymal tumors
Papilloma
Cystadenoma/cystadenofibroma (specify histologic type)
Metaplastic papillary tumor
Other
Borderline tumor (atypical proliferative, low malignant potential)
Serous
Mucinous
Endometrioid
Other histologic types
Malignant
Non-invasive carcinoma
Tubal intraepithelial carcinoma (specify histologic type when possible)
Invasive carcinoma
Serous
Mucinous
Endometrioid
Clear cell
Transitional cell
Squamous cell
Undifferentiated
Other histologic types
Mixed epithelial–mesenchymal
Adenofibroma (specify histologic type)
Adenosarcoma
Malignant müllerian mixed tumor (MMMT; carcinosarcoma)
Soft Tissue
Leiomyoma
Leiomyosarcoma
Mesothelial
Adenomatoid tumor
Germ cell
Teratoma
Mature
Immature
Other histologic types
Gestational trophoblastic disease
Placental site nodule
Hydatidiform mole
Choriocarcinoma
Placental site trophoblastic tumor
Other histologic types
Secondary involvement
Gynecologic and non-gynecologic carcinomas
Hematolymphoid
Lymphoma
Leukemia
Malignant mesothelioma
Other histologic types

tract can be of polyarteritis nodosa or giant cell arteritis types, but the former is more common [82, 105]. Either one or multiple arterioles/small arteries may be involved. Clinical correlation is needed to determine whether or not vasculitis is localized to the gynecologic tract; however, it is uncommon for patients with vasculitis involving the female genital tract to have either a previous diagnosis of systemic disease or subsequent development of systemic disease [82, 105].

Neoplasms of the Fallopian Tube

The neoplasms arising in the fallopian tube include benign and malignant types, but malignant tumors are more common than benign ones; however, both are infrequent. They are commonly mistaken for chronic salpingitis or pyosalpinx, both preoperatively and during the operative procedure itself. Many benign tumors are small enough to be incidental findings at laparotomy. The WHO Classification of fallopian tube tumors is listed in Table 11.1. Most of these are nonspecific histologic types since the same ones can be seen in other gynecologic sites, especially the ovary.

Benign Neoplasms

Adenomatoid Tumor

Adenomatoid tumor (benign mesothelioma) is the most frequent type of benign tubal tumor. Previously reported lymphangiomas probably represent examples of this entity. They are usually only 1–2 cm in diameter, appearing as a nodule beneath the tubal serosa, and are yellow or white-gray on cross section. Rare cases are bilateral. Similar lesions may be found in the uterus, cul-de-sac, or ovary (see Chap. 10, Mesenchymal Tumors of the Uterus). Their origin is presumed to be from the cells of the serosal mesothelium. A fortuitous section may demonstrate a connection between serosa and tumor, but usually the serosa covers the lesion.

Microscopically, the tumor may be large enough to displace the tubal lumen eccentrically and may grow into the supporting stroma of the luminal folds in an infiltrating manner. Multiple, small, slit-like, or ovoid tubules proliferate through the muscular wall of the fallopian tube; however, the stroma may be fibrous or hyalinized (➋ *Fig. 11.30*). Foci of chronic inflammation can also be present. A single layer of low-cuboidal or flattened epithelial-like cells, which contain abundant eosinophilic cytoplasm with variably sized vacuoles and round and bland nuclei line the tubules. Mitotic figures are rare. The tubules may be empty or contain pale fluid. Infarction may occur in adenomatoid tumor. When it occurs, and when marked, there is the potential for confusion with other lesions, such as adenocarcinoma, because of the obscured junction between adenomatoid tumor and non-neoplastic tissue, pseudoinfiltration, solid patterns in viable tumor, and reactive atypia [218].

Histochemical studies have shown Alcian blue-positive, hyaluronidase-digestible material in the cells and spaces; however, this material may be absent after routine processing for histologic sections. No significant glycogen or intracellular epithelial mucin is present, as might be found in a tumor of müllerian origin. Immunohistochemically, tumors express mesothelial markers (WT-1, calretinin, CK5/6, D2-40) and are usually negative for epithelial-specific markers (Ber-EP4, B72.3, MOC-31, ER, PR). Electron microscopic studies also support a mesothelial origin for these lesions. Clinically, they are asymptomatic, and recurrences after adequate excision are rare.

The most important lesion to be considered in the differential diagnosis, particularly at the time of frozen section, is metastatic signet ring cell carcinoma. Clinical data such as prior history of a carcinoma (some primary tumors may be occult, and such a history will not be known), extra-fallopian tube tumor seen intraoperatively (especially if multifocal), bilaterality, and histologic presence of a combination of glands, papillae, and solid sheets of tumor help favor a diagnosis of carcinoma. Nuclear atypia and mitotic activity should raise suspicion for carcinoma, but some signet ring cell carcinomas may lack these features. A source of confusion may be the presence of the Alcian blue-positive, hyaluronidase-digestible material within the lumens of the tubules in adenomatoid tumor. At the time of intraoperative consultation, this material resembles epithelial-type mucin on H&E frozen section slides; however, it is lost during routine processing and, as a result, is not present in permanent H&E sections.

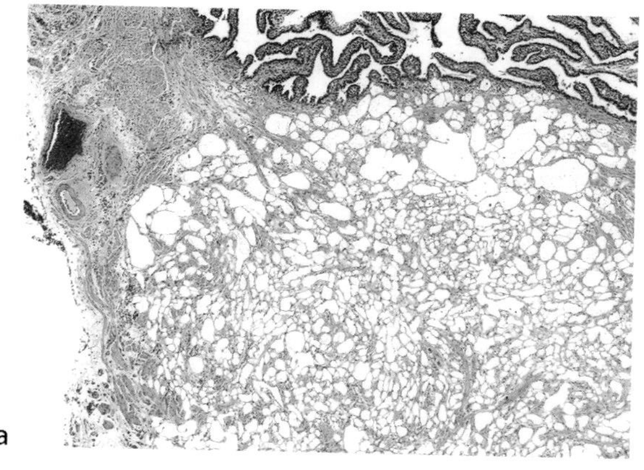

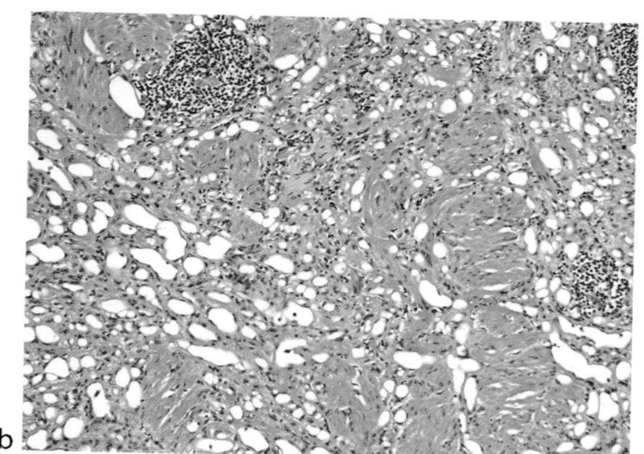

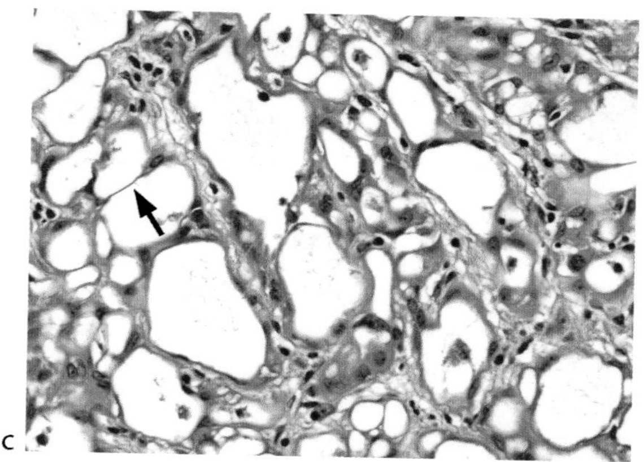

Fig. 11.30
Adenomatoid tumor. (a) Nodular configuration in the wall of the fallopian tube. (b) Diffuse proliferation of tubules that infiltrate the myosalpinx. Foci of chronic inflammation are also present. (c) The tubules are lined by a single layer of flat eosinophilic cells with cytoplasmic vacuoles and bland nuclei. The lumens of the tubules are empty. An intraluminal thin cytoplasmic strand, which can be focally seen in some cases, is present (*arrow*)

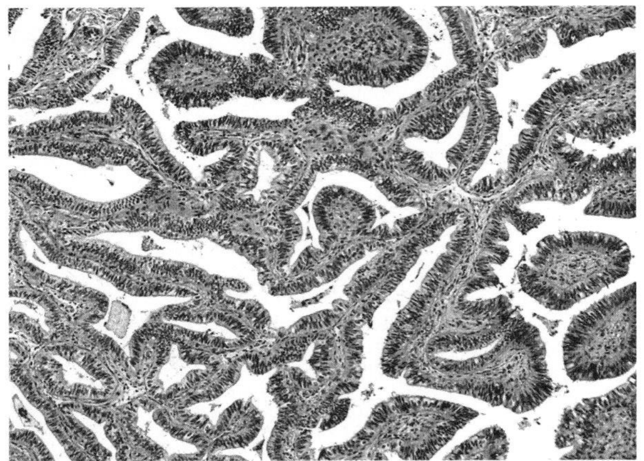

Fig. 11.31
Fallopian tube papilloma. **Abundant papillae with complex branching resemble the plicae of normal fallopian tube. Closer magnification will show the same type of epithelium seen in normal fallopian tube**

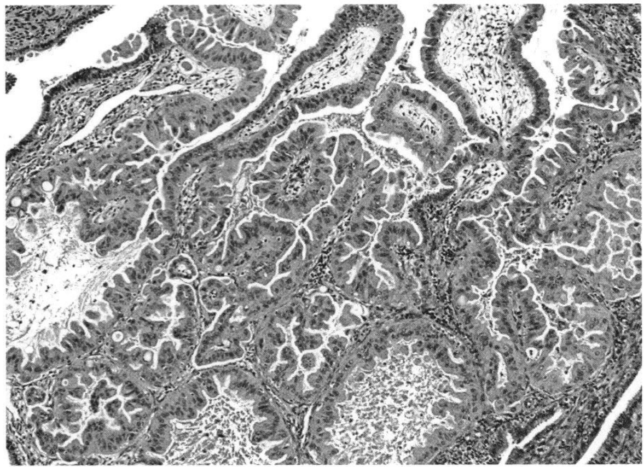

Fig. 11.32
Metaplastic papillary tumor. **The tumor is small and characteristically located within the lumen of the fallopian tube. It contains a limited number of medium-sized papillae. Closer magnification will show papillae lined by columnar to cuboidal cells that have abundant, dense, and eosinophilic cytoplasm with nuclei, which are bland or have, at most, mild atypia. Only a limited degree of stratification is present**

After frozen section analysis, immunohistochemical stains specific for mesothelial and epithelial markers will help aid distinction.

Epithelial Tumors

Papilloma is rare [87]. It is composed of an intraluminal mass with an "adenomatous" and very complex papillary proliferation. At low power, the proliferation resembles an exaggerated pattern of tubal mucosa with fine stromal fibrovascular cores, and the quantity of papillae is much greater than in the normal fallopian tube (*Fig. 11.31*). At higher power, the epithelium resembles normal fallopian tube mucosa, including the presence of ciliated and secretory cells. The nuclei are bland, and mitotic activity is not seen. In our anecdotal experience, fallopian tube papilloma diffusely expresses ER and WT-1, and the Ki-67 proliferation index is low. Because of the complex papillary proliferation, this tumor may be confused with atypical proliferative (borderline) serous tumor, low-grade serous carcinoma, or a villoglandular variant of endometrioid carcinoma. Although very complex, the orderly degree of papillary branching of papilloma is in contrast to a greater degree of complexity and hierarchical papillary branching with cellular stratification and tufting of atypical proliferative (borderline) serous tumor. The fine micropapillary tufting, associated psammoma bodies, and stromal invasion of low-grade serous carcinoma are not seen in papilloma. At low power, papilloma can resemble a villoglandular endometrioid carcinoma, but closer examination at high power shows endosalpingeal cell types and an absence of endometrioid differentiation. Furthermore, squamous metaplasia, endometriosis, and foci with solid growth would favor endometrioid carcinoma.

Metaplastic papillary tumor is rare and found as an incidental finding in the lumen of the fallopian tube during the postpartum period [19, 119, 203]. It is of microscopic size and composed of broad papillae lined by stratified and tufted epithelium with cells showing abundant eosinophilic cytoplasm (*Fig. 11.32*). The nuclei do not exhibit malignant features. It is not clear whether this lesion is a papillary metaplastic proliferation or small atypical proliferative (borderline) serous tumor associated with pregnancy. Regardless, the behavior appears benign.

Cystadenomas have been reported but are rare. Although the topic of whether or not atypical proliferative (borderline) tumors are benign has been debated in the literature, these tumors are included in the benign neoplasms section of this chapter for simplicity. Rare atypical proliferative (borderline) serous, endometrioid, and clear cell tumors of the fallopian tube have been reported. The literature is too limited to predict their outcome; however, behavior similar to their ovarian counterparts would be anticipated. Atypical proliferative (borderline) mucinous tumors have been described, but such cases should be rigorously evaluated to exclude the likely possibility that they represent secondary involvement of the fallopian tubes from a non-ovarian site.

Leiomyoma and Adenomyoma

Leiomyoma is the most common mesenchymal tumor of the fallopian tube; however, these tumors are much less common than uterine leiomyomas. They are usually small and grossly and microscopically similar to those found in the uterus and other gynecologic sites, and they can undergo similar degenerative changes. Rarely, benign glands and smooth muscle may be so intimately involved in a tumor that a diagnosis of adenomyoma may be warranted; however, these may arguably represent endometriosis with smooth muscle metaplasia ("endomyometriosis") or the so-called uterine-like mass.

Other Benign Mesenchymal and Mixed Epithelial–Mesenchymal Tumors

Although adenofibromas producing clinical masses are uncommon, those of microscopic size are not infrequent. In one consecutive series of fallopian tubes unassociated with tubo-ovarian malignancy or inflammatory disorders, and in which all tubal tissue was submitted for histologic examination, adenofibromas were found in 30% of cases [26]. In that study, the majority were <0.3 cm in size, and only a small subset were >1 cm. All arose in the fimbria. Some may be synchronously associated with an ovarian adenofibroma. Histologically, fallopian tube adenofibromas resemble their ovarian counterparts, with admixed epithelial and mesenchymal components (➲ *Fig. 11.33*). The epithelial component may contain papillary clefting and is frequently cystic or composed of small round tubules. Most tumors are of serous histologic type, but a minority of the tumors are of endometrioid type [7]. The mesenchymal component is hypercellular, densely fibrotic, or hyalinized. In lesions <0.1 cm in size, an epithelial component may be absent, and the diagnosis of an early adenofibroma may be suggested because of a patch of cellular spindled stroma with a subepithelial arrangement.

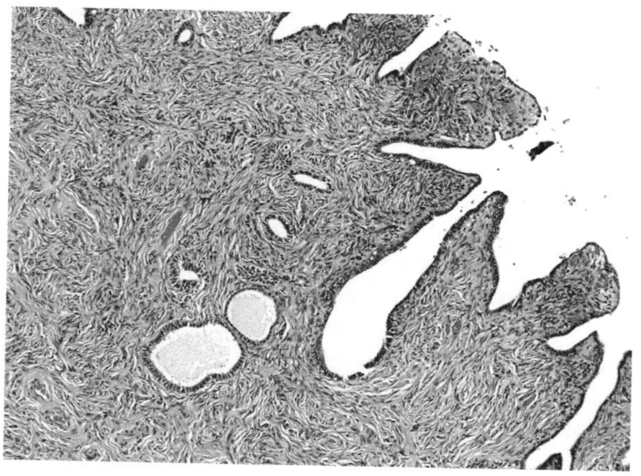

◘ Fig. 11.33
Adenofibroma. **Note the biphasic architecture with cellular fibromatous stroma and round glands lined by a single layer of bland cuboidal epithelium. Other cases may be predominantly composed of round and blunted papillae with cleft-like architecture or have an abundant component of tubules**

Cystadenofibroma, hemangioma, lipoma, chondroma, angiomyofibroblastoma, angiomyolipoma, and neural tumors are rare but have been reported. Their microscopic appearances are similar to their counterparts elsewhere in the body.

Teratoma

Tubal teratomas are rare. Clinically, a patient with a tubal teratoma usually is nulliparous and in the fourth decade. Grossly, the tumors are located most frequently in the lumen, often attached by a pedicle to the inner tubal wall. They may, however, be intramural or attached to the serosa. On section, they are more often cystic than solid and may be small (1–2 cm in diameter) or large (10–20 cm in diameter). As with their ovarian counterparts, ectodermal, mesodermal, and endodermal tissues are represented by mature elements. Most are in the form of a dermoid cyst. Rare teratomas consisting entirely of mature thyroid tissue have been described in the tube of women without clinical hyperthyroidism. Only rare cases of immature teratoma of the fallopian tube have been reported, including a mixed germ cell tumor in which one of the components was an immature teratoma [144]. Although ovarian teratomas appear to originate from abnormally developing ova, the pathogenesis of fallopian tube teratomas is unclear.

Malignant Neoplasms

Carcinoma

The history of the discovery and evolution about knowledge of carcinoma of the fallopian tube during the nineteenth and twentieth centuries has been reviewed elsewhere [244] and will not be repeated here. In the recent past, "carcinoma *in situ*" of the fallopian tube was considered uncommon since the majority of patients with fallopian tube carcinoma presented with advanced stage disease. Therefore, at the time of presentation, most tumors were of bulky size, and patients had symptomatic disease. Over the last several years, early tubal carcinomas (i.e., those that are commonly of microscopic size and clinically occult) have become diagnosed more frequently due to complete histologic examination of all fallopian tube tissue from prophylactic bilateral salpingo-oophorectomy specimens.

Clinical Features

Primary adenocarcinoma of the tube is uncommon, and it has been estimated to account for 0.7–1.5% of invasive malignancies of the gynecologic tract [21, 190]. However, the true frequency is difficult to determine, partly because some fallopian tube carcinomas might be misclassified as "ovarian" (*see below*). The incidence of fallopian tube carcinoma is 0.41 per 100,000 women in the USA [222].

Tumors with "carcinoma *in situ*"/intraepithelial carcinoma and small tumors with microscopic invasion are usually asymptomatic and more commonly seen as occult findings in prophylactic bilateral salpingo-oophorectomy specimens (see Occult Disease in ➋ Prophylactic Bilateral Salpingo-Oophorectomy Specimens section below for details regarding clinical presentation). They may be occasionally detected when tumor cells exfoliate into the fallopian tube lumen and are then found in endometrial or endocervical biopsies/curettages or Pap smears. In such instances, a fallopian tube origin may not be clinically evident at first (and sometimes not even grossly evident at the time of hysterectomy), and further clinical evaluation is needed to eventually identify the true origin in the tube. Likewise, in rare cases, occult invasive tubal carcinoma may present as a distant metastasis (e.g., malignant pleural effusion or metastatic carcinoma of unknown primary site in a supraclavicular lymph node).

Most women with symptomatic tumors are between 50 and 80 years of age, with the mean age in large studies ranging from 56 to 63 years [8, 98, 202, 222]. Tubal malignancies in women younger than age 40 years are very uncommon. Ninety percent of patients are white, non-Hispanic. A substantial proportion of women are nulliparous or have a previous history of infertility or pelvic inflammatory disease. Some patients have had a previous malignancy, usually breast carcinoma. A small percentage of patients have a synchronous tumor in another gynecologic site. The most common symptoms and signs are abnormal uterine bleeding/vaginal discharge, abdominal/pelvic mass, abdominal distention, and abdominal pain; however, a small subset of cases will be detected as an incidental finding as part of another gynecologic disorder [8, 17, 185]. Between 5% and 14% of women have ascites at the time of presentation [17, 66]. The classic symptom complex *hydrops tubae profluens* (intermittent colicky abdominal pain relieved by sudden discharge of watery fluid per vagina) is only present in a very small percentage of patients. Serum CA-125 is elevated in most but not all patients. Some patients have an elevated serum β-hCG level, which has been attributed to ectopic production. A subset of patients have tumor in endometrial biopsies/curettages or Pap smears. Because of the rarity of fallopian tube carcinoma, as well as the clinical presentation that simulates an ovarian tumor, a correct preoperative diagnosis of fallopian tube carcinoma is uncommon. Rare patients can have an associated paraneoplastic syndrome [153, 213].

In symptomatic cases, women with *BRCA*-associated tumors present at an age slightly younger than those with sporadic tumors, and both patient groups have similar clinicopathologic features; however, information in the literature is too limited to make definitive conclusions regarding prognostic differences [38, 143].

FIGO Stage

The staging system for fallopian tube carcinoma is that of the International Federation of Gynecology and Obstetrics (FIGO), which is primarily based on surgical pathology findings. Tubal intraepithelial carcinoma (TIC) represented stage 0 disease prior to the Seventh Edition of the AJCC Cancer Staging Manual; however, stage 0 no longer exists in the current system. With stage I tumors, disease is confined to the fallopian tube (➋ *Fig. 11.34*). Involvement of other pelvic sites represents stage II, and with stage III, tumor involves the peritoneum outside of the pelvis. Finally, distant metastases are classified as stage IV. Details are listed in ➋ *Table 11.2.*

The staging terminology for cases with TIC and only positive washings is unclear. Some clinicians consider this scenario FIGO stage 0 (prior staging system) while other authors have designated this stage IC. As TIC can be associated with disease on ovarian or peritoneal surfaces

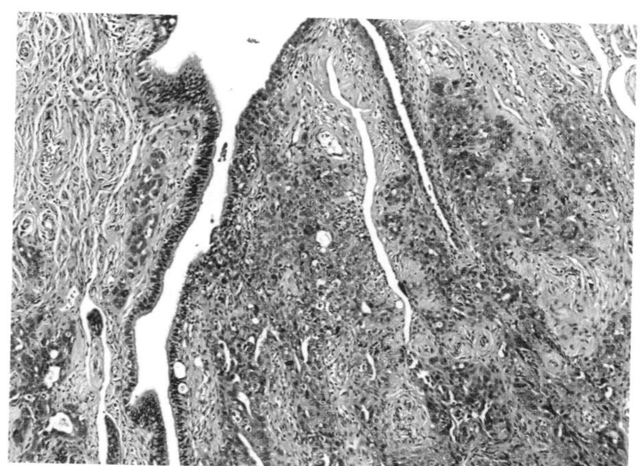

Fig. 11.34
Stage IA fallopian tube carcinoma. **Carcinoma invades into the underlying lamina propria**

(especially, since many TICs are located in the fimbriated end of the tube and, therefore, have direct access to the peritoneal cavity), one can speculate whether TICs with only positive washings should be considered greater than stage 0 (prior staging system).

It has been suggested that intraluminal masses without invasion qualify as neither stage 0 (prior staging system) nor stage IA [8]. Also, because of observed differences in prognosis for stage I fallopian tube carcinomas with different depths of invasion into the wall (similar to other abdominal/pelvic organs with a muscular wall), it has been recommended that the FIGO stage should be modified since such cases are not appropriately represented by the current version of the FIGO staging system. Alvarado-Cabrero et al. have proposed that stage I cases should be divided into substages IA-0 (intraluminal masses without invasion into lamina propria), IA-1 (invasion into lamina propria but not muscularis), and IA-2 (invasion of muscularis) [8]. As it has also been suggested that carcinomas in the fimbriated end without invasion have a worse prognosis than carcinomas invading the wall of the tube because of direct access to the peritoneal cavity, it has been proposed that the FIGO system should be modified since the former are not represented by the current version [7, 8]. This proposed stage would be designated I(F).

The majority of patients with symptomatic disease have advanced stage disease at presentation (stage >I). In the largest clinicopathologic study using hospital-based cases by Baekelandt et al., the distribution of stage was as follows: stage 0 (6%) (prior staging system), stage I (27%), stage II (22%), stage III (35%), and stage IV (12%) [17]. These results are similar to those of other large hospital-based or population-based studies, which have found the percentage of stage I cases to be 30–56% [96, 98, 202, 222].

Table 11.2
International Federation of Gynecology and Obstetrics (FIGO) staging system for fallopian tube carcinoma[a]

Stage	Description
Stage I	Growth limited to fallopian tubes
	IA: Growth limited to one tube with extension into submucosa[b] and/or muscularis but not penetrating serosal surface; no ascites
	IB: Growth limited to both tubes with extension into submucosa and/or muscularis but not penetrating serosal surface; no ascites
	IC: Tumor either Stage IA or Stage IB with extension through or onto tubal serosa or with positive ascites/peritoneal washings
Stage II	Growth involving one or both fallopian tubes with pelvic extension
	IIA: Extension and/or metastases to uterus and/or ovaries
	IIB: Extension to other pelvic tissues
	IIC: Tumor either Stage IIA or IIB and with positive ascites/peritoneal washings
Stage III	Tumor involving one or both fallopian tubes with peritoneal implants outside pelvis and/or positive retroperitoneal or inguinal lymph nodes. Superficial liver metastasis equals stage III. Tumor appears limited to true pelvis but with histologically proven malignant extension to small bowel or omentum
	IIIA: Tumor grossly limited to true pelvis with negative lymph nodes but with histologically confirmed microscopic involvement of abdominal peritoneal surfaces
	IIIB: Tumor involving one or both tubes with histologically confirmed implants of abdominal peritoneal surfaces, none exceeding 2 cm in diameter. Lymph nodes are negative
	IIIC: Abdominal implants >2 cm in diameter and/or positive retroperitoneal or inguinal lymph nodes
Stage IV	Growth involving one or both fallopian tubes with distant metastases. If pleural effusion is present, tumor cells must be present to be Stage IV. Parenchymal liver metastasis equals Stage IV

From Pettersson with slight modifications [186]
[a] Stage 0 does not exist in the 7th Edition of the AJCC Cancer Staging Manual
[b] "Submucosa" is interpreted as meaning lamina propria

The true stage distribution of all fallopian tube carcinomas in the general population is difficult to determine because of the existence of two patient populations, which are usually not included together in the same studies – patients with asymptomatic tumors (i.e., occult tubal carcinomas in prophylactic bilateral salpingo-oophorectomy specimens from women with an increased genetic risk for carcinoma) and those with symptomatic tumors (i.e., women with bulky tumors and advanced stage disease who may not be suspected of having an increased genetic risk for carcinoma).

Intraoperative and Gross Features

Bilaterality is infrequent (3–13% of cases) [8, 17, 98, 222]. The average tumor size is 5 cm (range, 0.2–10 cm) [8]. The fallopian tube is dilated in slightly over one half of cases, which intraoperatively can be mistaken for a hydrosalpinx, hematosalpinx, or pyosalpinx [8]. The tumor can appear as one or more yellow to tan nodules or a mass that fills the lumen (Fig. 11.35). Hemorrhage or necrosis is frequent. Most tumors are within the tubal portion (usually the distal two thirds), but a small percentage is located in the fimbriated end.

Histologic Features

Intraepithelial Carcinoma Noninvasive carcinomas of the fallopian tube have traditionally been considered "carcinoma *in situ*." With recognition of early carcinomas without invasion of underlying fallopian tube stroma in prophylactic bilateral salpingo-oophorectomy specimens, the term tubal intraepithelial carcinoma (TIC) has become popular in recent years. Given the ability of TIC to spread beyond the fallopian tube without invasion of underlying stroma (*see below*), the term carcinoma *in situ* should be abandoned because it implies that there is no potential for metastasis.

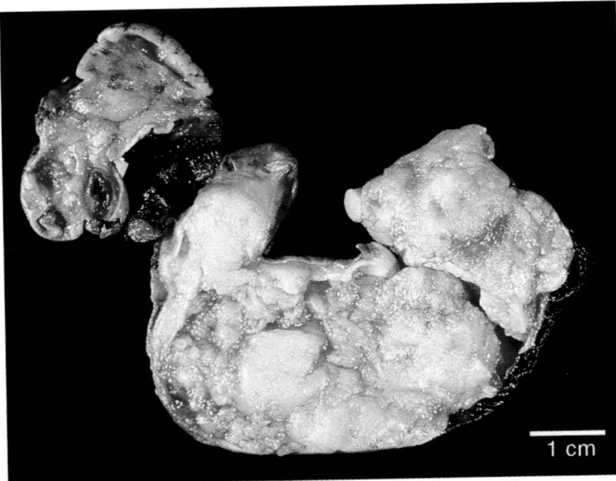

Fig. 11.35
Fallopian tube carcinoma. **The cut surface is slightly heterogeneous, nodular, irregular, and yellow-tan. For comparison, the structure at the upper left is the ovary uninvolved by tumor**

Histologically, TIC is the earliest morphologically recognizable form of carcinoma. It is characterized by absence of invasion of underlying fallopian tube stroma and the presence of cytologic abnormalities that result in the fallopian tube epithelium appearing darker than adjacent normal epithelium at low-power magnification (*Fig. 11.36*). In cases with invasive carcinoma in the same tube, TIC may be found directly adjacent to invasion. TIC may occur as a single focus or multifocally. The lesional epithelium is typically flat, but some degree of stratification may be seen. The luminal border may be straight or exhibit variable amounts of irregular contours and hobnail morphology. With increased stratification, small tufts of detached cells can be found within the tubal lumen. At high-power magnification, the lesional cells lack cilia and show variable combinations of nuclear enlargement, increased nuclear-to-cytoplasmic ratios, hyperchromasia or irregular chromatin distribution, loss of polarity, prominent nucleoli, and mitotic figures (*Fig. 11.37*). Nuclei may be oval or columnar but are frequently round.

The lesional cells of TIC show secretory cell differentiation [140]. Also, they cytologically resemble the cells of high-grade serous carcinoma. For these reasons, as well as what is known about the pathogenic relationship between TIC and invasive high-grade serous carcinoma (*see below*), most TICs should be considered as being of serous histologic type. Therefore, the diagnostic terms "tubal serous intraepithelial carcinoma" and "tubal intraepithelial carcinoma" should usually be considered synonymous. However, rare endometrioid TICs have been reported [113].

Before diagnosing an incidental lesion as TIC in a routine specimen, it is necessary to submit all remaining fallopian tube tissue for histologic examination as invasive carcinoma can be of small size.

Tubal dysplasias have been described in the literature, and the clinical significance of such lesions is unclear. Furthermore, standardized criteria and terminology, as well as reproducibility studies, have not been published. Accordingly, use of the diagnostic term "dysplasia" is discouraged. For worrisome atypical mucosal lesions of the fallopian tube which do not entirely qualify as TIC based on a combination of histologic and immunohistochemical

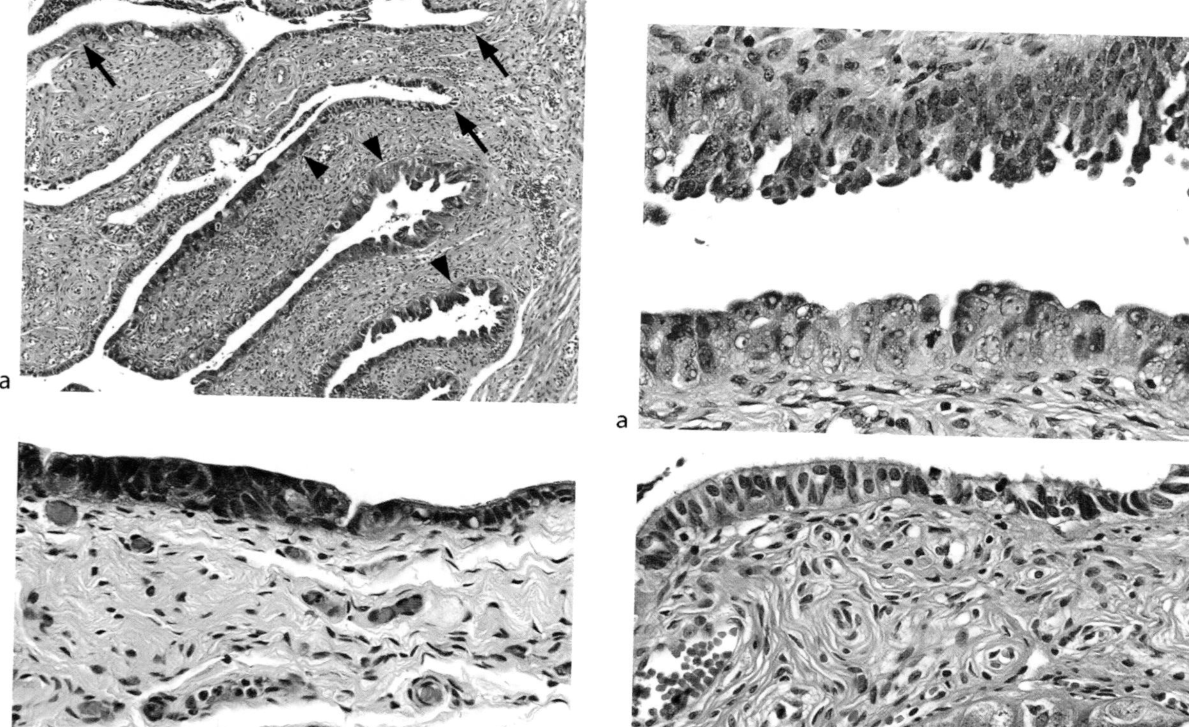

Fig. 11.36
Serous tubal intraepithelial carcinoma (STIC). (**a**) STIC is composed mostly of a flat proliferation of cells. However, at low-power magnification, STIC is visible because of the thicker and darker epithelium (*arrowheads*) compared with adjacent normal tubal epithelium (*arrow*). (**b**) Abrupt transition between STIC and normal tubal epithelium

Fig. 11.37
Serous tubal intraepithelial carcinoma (STIC). (**a**) The lesional cells can be hyperchromatic with high nuclear-to-cytoplasmic ratios, stratification, and loss of polarity (*upper half of photograph*), or they may show enlarged and round nuclei with vesicular chromatin, nucleoli, and mitotic figures (*lower half of photograph*). (**b**) Comparison between normal tubal epithelium (*upper half of photograph*) and STIC (*lower half of photograph*)

features (*see below*), one option for handling such problematic cases is to use a descriptive diagnosis with a comment that the lesion is concerning for but not sufficiently diagnostic of TIC.

Invasive Carcinoma Some otherwise conventional-appearing high-grade serous carcinomas within the lumen of the fallopian tube may be small without enlargement of the fallopian tube and lack invasion of the underlying tubal stroma. Such morphology in occasional cases can overlap with the upper morphologic limit of TIC, especially when the latter shows an increased degree of stratification. In such cases, the diagnostic threshold between TIC versus a small intraluminal high-grade serous carcinoma without invasion of underlying fallopian tube stroma is subjective and varies between authors [113, 244]. However, some authors have suggested that intraluminal masses without invasion qualify as neither stage 0 (prior staging system) nor stage IA (*see FIGO Stage above*) [8].

Some invasive carcinomas may be of small volume. As these may not be clinically evident, and in order to assess the possibility of the fallopian tube being a primary site of occult disease, it is important to submit all remaining fallopian tube tissue from grossly unremarkable tubes for histologic examination in women presenting with metastatic high-grade adenocarcinoma of unknown primary site.

The histologic types and appearances of invasive fallopian tube carcinoma are similar to its ovarian counterparts. In the largest clinicopathologic study using hospital-based cases, the distribution of histologic types was as follows: serous (80%), adenocarcinoma, not otherwise specified (10%), endometrioid (7%), clear cell (2%), mucinous (2%), and mixed serous-mucinous (1%) [17]. Most fallopian tube carcinomas are poorly differentiated, and well-differentiated tumors are very uncommon. Standardized grading schemes for fallopian tube carcinoma have not been implemented. However, we apply the same grading schemes as used for the ovary (i.e., low-versus high-grade for serous, FIGO uterine criteria for endometrioid, etc.).

The majority, if not all, tubal serous carcinomas are histologically indistinguishable from high-grade serous carcinomas of the ovary and include broad papillae with epithelial stratification, irregular slit-like spaces with micropapillary tufting, invasion by solid nests of variable size or sheets of tumor cells, necrosis, and psammoma bodies (*Fig. 11.38*) [8]. The nuclei are high grade, characterized by nuclear enlargement, hyperchromasia or irregular chromatin distribution with prominent nucleoli, irregular nuclear membranes, and abundant mitotic figures. TIC may be found adjacent to invasive carcinoma.

Most endometrioid carcinomas are grade 2 or 3, but some are grade 1 [166, 194]. They may resemble conventional endometrioid carcinomas as seen in the endometrium, including squamous differentiation and villoglandular architecture, but oxyphilic types, sex cord-like appearances, and spindled epithelial cells may be seen. In some cases, associated endometriosis is present. Benign stromal osseous metaplasia can be seen in a minority of cases. Almost one half of cases have an appearance resembling female adnexal tumor of wolffian origin (FATWO-like type) [53, 166]. Independent primary endometrioid carcinomas can synchronously arise in the fallopian tube and uterus [49].

Clear cell and transitional cell carcinomas resemble those seen in the ovary [8, 130]. Other rare histologic types include undifferentiated, small cell neuroendocrine, lymphoepithelioma-like, mixed serous-transitional cell, squamous cell, adenosquamous, hepatoid, glassy cell, and giant cell carcinomas [8, 10, 42, 99]. Mucinous carcinomas with a synchronous endocervical adenocarcinoma have been described, but such cases should be rigorously evaluated to exclude the likely possibility that they represent secondary involvement of the fallopian tubes from the endocervix. Unlike the ovary, low-grade serous carcinomas typically are not seen in the fallopian tube.

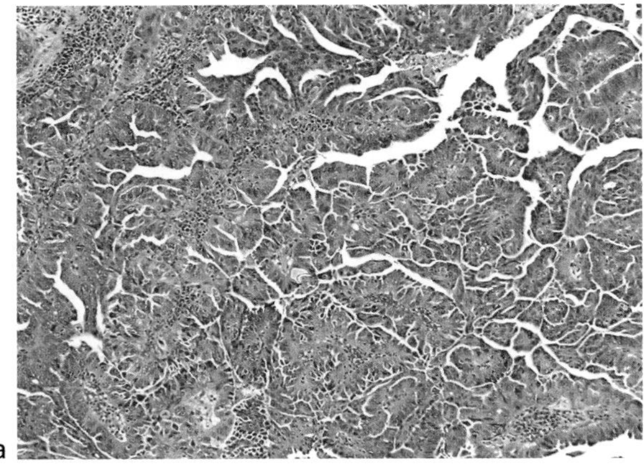

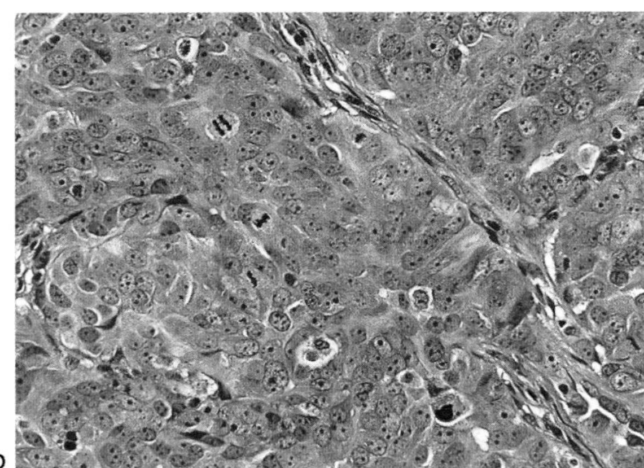

Fig. 11.38
Invasive high-grade serous carcinoma. **(a) Complex papillae with stratified epithelium producing irregular slit-like spaces and small epithelial tufts. (b) The nuclei are high-grade with abundant mitotic figures. Note enlarged nuclei with vesicular chromatin and nucleoli. In other cases, the nuclei may be hyperchromatic rather than vesicular**

Immunohistochemical Features

Although some cases of TIC may be diagnosed solely on histologic features without the need for immunohistochemistry, immunostains are helpful in establishing the diagnosis in problematic cases. TIC diffusely and strongly expresses p53 (*Fig. 11.39*); however, 21% of TICs did not overexpress p53 in one study [217]. The Ki-67 proliferation index is usually markedly elevated (*Fig. 11.39*). In one study, the mean Ki-67 labeling index was 72% (range: 40–95%) [113]. Also, p16, which is diffusely and

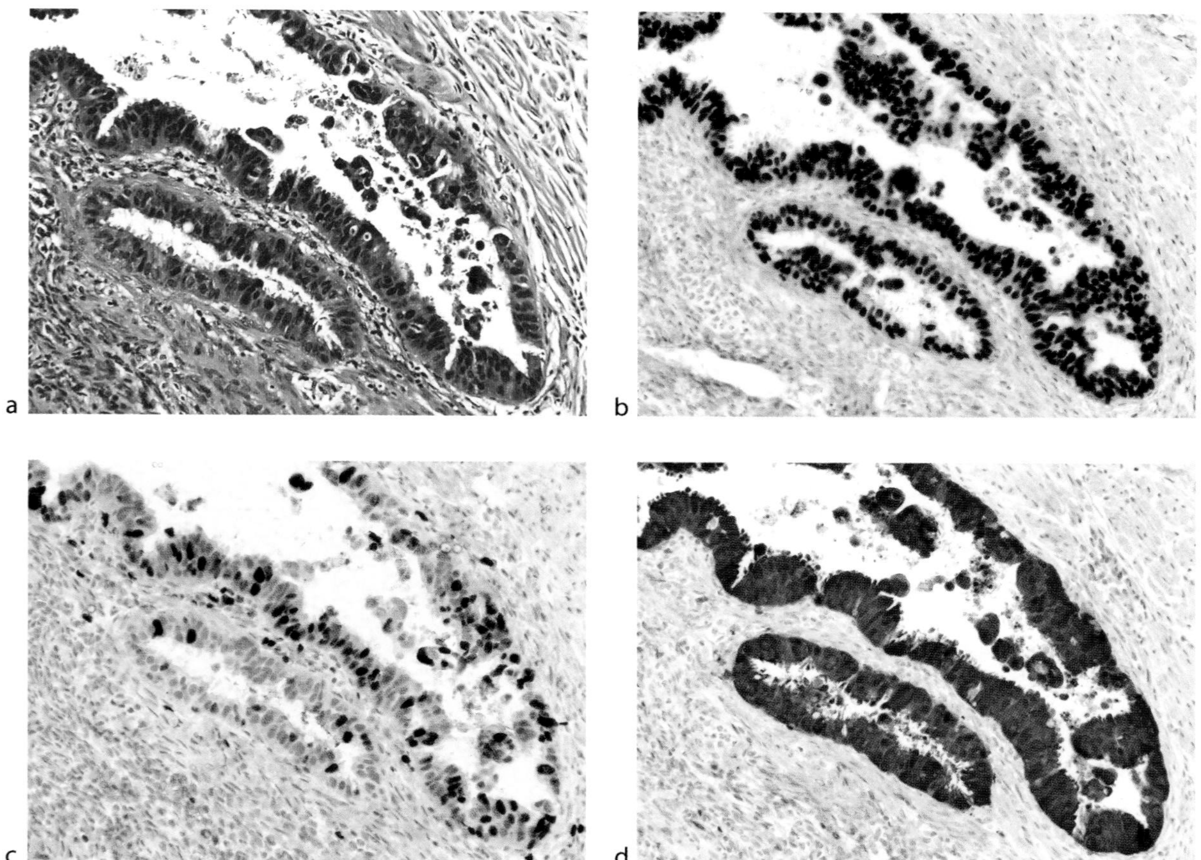

Fig. 11.39

Immunohistochemical features of serous tubal intraepithelial carcinoma. (a) H&E. (b) Diffuse expression of p53. (c) Elevated Ki-67 proliferation index. (d) Diffuse expression of p16

strongly expressed in endometrial serous carcinomas and many ovarian high-grade serous carcinomas, is occasionally expressed with a strong diffuse pattern in TIC in our experience. Of note, the diffuse patterns of expression of p53 and p16 show nearly all lesional cells being positive as opposed to a patchy pattern of staining in which substantial numbers of both negative and positive cells are present.

Invasive high-grade serous carcinomas usually show diffuse expression of WT-1. It should be noted, however, that expression is not restricted to invasive carcinomas, as normal fallopian tube epithelium and TIC also show WT-1 expression. Expression of ER and PR is variable. Although most cases overexpress p53, the exact extent of expression has not been adequately detailed in the literature. Immunohistochemical data are limited for endometrioid carcinomas, but in our experience, WT-1 and p53 can be diffusely expressed in some cases.

Treatment and Prognosis

Tumor usually spreads in an intraperitoneal, lymphatic, and hematogenous manner. At presentation, lymph node metastases are frequent, the lymph node groups most frequently involved are those in para-aortic and pelvic sites, and inguinal and supraclavicular lymph nodes can be involved as well; however, lymph node metastases may be present even when it appears that the tumor is limited to the tube [8, 17, 55, 59, 127, 128].

In the largest studies of fallopian tube carcinoma, patients have been treated in various fashions, but the most important prognostic factor is stage [8, 17, 98, 185, 198, 202]. The overall 5-year survivals for fallopian tube carcinoma for all stages combined range from 43% to 56% between studies [17, 96, 202]. In the largest clinicopathologic study using hospital-based cases, the 5-year survivals were as follows: stage 0 (88%) (prior staging system), stage I (73%), stage II (37%), stage III (29%), and stage IV (12%) [17]. These 5-year survivals are similar to those of other large studies [96, 98, 161, 185, 202]. It is also noteworthy that stage 0 disease (prior staging system) does not guarantee a cure, as the 5-year survivals for stage 0 (prior staging system) range from 75% to 91% between studies [17, 66, 209]. However, these studies do not provide details specifying whether the entire fallopian tube was submitted for histologic examination in those cases in order to exclude microscopic invasion (i.e., stage IA). For details regarding behavior of stage 0 cases (prior staging system) in the context of prophylactic bilateral salpingo-oophorectomy specimens, see the respective section below.

Alvarado-Cabrero et al. showed that subcategorization of stage I cases based on depth of invasion was prognostically significant [8]. In their study, patients with substages IA/B-0 (intraluminal masses without invasion into lamina propria) and IA/B-1 (invasion into lamina propria but not muscularis) had a better disease-free survival than those with substage IA-2 (invasion of muscularis), which was a statistically significant difference. They also demonstrated that patients with stage I(F) (carcinomas in the fimbriated end without invasion) had a poorer survival than those with substages IA/B-0 and IA/B-1, as well as that the survival for stage I(F) was similar to stages IA-2 and IC. These aspects have not been extensively studied in the literature. Two other studies also showed that differences in depth of invasion in the wall of the fallopian tube in stage I cases were prognostically significant while another study demonstrated that it was not [14, 17, 185].

Presence/amount of residual disease after surgery is a poor prognostic factor [17, 185, 202]. Closure of the fimbriated end (hydrosalpinx-like, hematosalpinx-like, or pyosalpinx-like gross appearance) has been shown to be a favorable prognostic factor on univariate but not multivariate analysis [8, 17]. Disagreement exists between studies regarding whether or not histologic grade, vascular invasion, age, or ascites is prognostically significant [8, 17, 98, 185, 202]. Histologic type has not been shown to be of prognostic importance [8, 17].

Treatment of fallopian tube carcinoma should consist of cytoreductive surgery and combination platinum/taxane chemotherapy, and as response to this chemotherapy regimen is analogous to that in patients with ovarian carcinoma, fallopian tube carcinoma should be treated similarly to ovarian carcinoma [17, 161, 177, 198]. In patients with a pre-chemotherapy elevated serum CA-125 level, this marker can be used to monitor disease for response and progression. In the study by Baekelandt et al., the median progression-free survival for the entire cohort was 32 months [17]. In that study, patients were not postoperatively treated in a uniform fashion. In a study of patients who received postoperative combination platinum/taxane chemotherapy, carcinoma recurred in 74% of patients with stage III or IV disease by 33 months [161]. In the study by Baekelandt et al., the pelvis was the most common site of recurrence, followed by upper abdomen, retroperitoneal lymph nodes, liver, pleura, vagina, lungs, supraclavicular lymph nodes, groin lymph nodes, brain, bone, breast, and adrenal gland in descending order [17].

Given the association of fallopian tube carcinoma with germline *BRCA* mutations, genetic counseling should be considered for all new diagnoses of fallopian tube carcinoma. For treatment and prognosis of occult fallopian tube carcinoma in prophylactic bilateral salpingo-oophorectomy specimens, see the respective section below.

Occult Disease in Prophylactic Bilateral Salpingo-Oophorectomy Specimens

At least 10% of ovarian carcinomas are hereditary rather than sporadic, and approximately 90% of the former have mutations of the *BRCA1* or *BRCA2* gene. Carriers of germline *BRCA1* and *BRCA2* mutations have 39–62% and 11–27% lifetime risks for ovarian carcinoma, respectively, and those risks (cumulative risk) increase over time from ages 40 to 80 years [9, 72, 75, 126]. Women with such mutations are also at risk for peritoneal and fallopian tube carcinoma. The exact proportion of fallopian tube carcinomas that is hereditary is not clear; however, 16–43% of patients with tubal carcinoma have shown *BRCA* germline mutations [16, 38, 143]. Given the significant risk of ovarian carcinoma for patients with *BRCA* mutations, prophylactic salpingo-oophorectomy is recommended by age 40 years, and such surgical procedures have been shown to significantly reduce the risk of pelvic carcinoma [1, 117]. This risk is not reduced to 0% since a small percentage of patients subsequently develop peritoneal carcinomas.

➋ *Table 11.3* highlights important features of patients with carcinomas detected in prophylactic salpingo-oophorectomy specimens. The frequency of finding a malignancy of the ovary, fallopian tube, or peritoneum during surgery or in the surgical specimen varies from 0% to 14% between studies. However, among 1,662 patients from 13 studies, carcinoma is found in 4% of cases (mean). The majority of carcinomas are primary tumors in the fallopian tube or ovary, but a very small proportion is due to primary peritoneal carcinomas or metastatic breast carcinoma in the ovary. Comparing just carcinomas in the fallopian tube and ovary, more are found in the tube compared with the ovary (64% versus 36%, respectively).

The percentage of carcinomas in the tube is even greater when considering only studies that submitted all tubal tissue (81% fallopian tube versus 19% ovary). Some of the earliest studies on occult carcinoma in prophylactic specimens did not remove the fallopian tube, and data from those studies are not presented here.

The mean age of patients with fallopian tube carcinoma is 53 years, which is slightly older than that of the

Table 11.3

Occult carcinoma in prophylactic bilateral salpingo-oophorectomy specimens:[a] Clinical features, pathologic sampling, and frequency

Reference[b,c]	n	Mean age (years) of patients who had surgery	Mean age (years) of patients with FT Ca	BRCA distribution of patients who had surgery	BRCA distribution of patients with FT Ca	All FT tissue submitted for histology	Total with Ca	Site distribution
[72]	490	48	56	374, BRCA 1 113, BRCA 2 3, BRCA 1+2	1, BRCA 1 2, BRCA 2	NR	11 (2%)	7, ovary 3, FT 1, malignant cytology without definitive primary
[73]	159	48	50	94, BRCA 1 65, BRCA 2	4, BRCA 1	–	7 (4%)	2, ovary 4, FT 1, primary peritoneal
[158]	133	45	51	NR	1, BRCA 1	NR[d]	2 (2%)	1, FT 1, metastatic breast Ca in ovary
[34]	122	47	58	60, BRCA 1 60, BRCA 2	4, BRCA 1 3, BRCA 2	+	7 (6%)	7, FT
[135]	113	47	54	40, BRCA 1 22, BRCA 2	4, BRCA 1 1, BRCA 2	+	6 (5%)	5, FT 1, primary peritoneal
[80]	101	NR	N/A	NR	N/A	+	0 (0%)	N/A
[118]	98	48	NR	56, BRCA 1 42, BRCA 2	NR	NR	3 (3%)	2, ovary 1, FT
[174]	90	46	41	58, BRCA 1 6, BRCA 2	2, BRCA 1	NR	5 (6%)	2, ovary 2, FT 1, ovary vs. FT indeterminate
[134]	89	49	50	56, BRCA 1 33, BRCA 2	2, BRCA 1	+	4 (4%)	1, ovary 2, FT 1, ovary vs. FT indeterminate
[100]	85	48	NR	NR	NR	NR	3 (4%)	3, FT
[191]	67	47	52	43, BRCA 1 24, BRCA 2	1, BRCA 1 2, BRCA 2	+	6 (9%)	3, ovary 3, FT
[210]	65	46	N/A	37, BRCA 1 28, BRCA 2	N/A	NR	2 (3%)	1, ovary 1, malignant cytology without definitive primary

Table 11.3 (Continued)

Reference[b,c]	n	Mean age (years) of patients who had surgery	Mean age (years) of patients with FT Ca	BRCA distribution of patients who had surgery	BRCA distribution of patients with FT Ca	All FT tissue submitted for histology	Total with Ca	Site distribution
[35]	50	50	NR	37, BRCA 1 13, BRCA 2	4, BRCA 1	–	7 (14%)	2, ovary 4, FT 1, metastatic breast Ca in ovary
Total (13 studies)	**1,662**	**47**	**53**	**855, BRCA 1 406, BRCA 2**	**23, BRCA 1 8, BRCA 2**	**30% of all patients[e]**	**Mean, 4% Range, 0–14%**	**Ovary-to-FT ratio = 36%:64%[f] (19%:81%)[g]**

Ca, Carcinoma
FT, Fallopian tube
n, Number of patients who underwent prophylactic surgery
N/A, Not applicable
NR, Not reported
+, Yes
–, No
[a] Patients with *BRCA* mutations or other increased risk for ovarian carcinoma
[b] When possible, cases that were apparently reported in more than one publication are listed only once here
[c] Series in which only ovaries were removed as part of the prophylactic surgery (or if it was not stated that fallopian tubes were removed) are not listed in this table
[d] Fallopian tubes not removed in all patients
[e] Percentage of all patients in table who definitively had all fallopian tube tissue submitted for histologic examination
[f] All series
[g] Only series that definitively had all fallopian tube tissue submitted for histologic examination

entire cohort undergoing prophylactic surgery (mean, 47 years). The mean age of *BRCA2* mutation-positive patients with fallopian tube carcinoma (59 years) is slightly older than that of *BRCA1* mutation-positive patients (50 years) [34, 72, 73, 95, 134, 135, 155, 158, 174, 176, 187, 191]. The proportion of patients with *BRCA1* mutations who undergo surgery is essentially twice that of those with mutations of *BRCA2*. Three percent and 2% of patients with *BRCA1* and *BRCA2* mutations, respectively, had carcinoma of the fallopian tube in the surgical specimen.

The vast majority of these carcinomas are occult, being of microscopic size and not seen intraoperatively. Most are either "carcinoma *in situ*"/intraepithelial carcinoma or invasive high-grade serous carcinoma, and in some cases TIC is found adjacent to the invasive carcinoma. Frequently, the carcinoma is located in the fimbriated end [6, 35, 73, 95, 157, 176, 187, 217]. A small proportion of carcinomas are of endometrioid histologic type. Clear cell carcinoma has been reported but is rare [95].

The invasive fallopian tube carcinomas are of variable stage but frequently stage I. Issues of interest are the behavior for cases with only TIC (+/− positive washings) and whether such patients should be treated with chemotherapy. *Table 11.4* lists features of patients with TIC in prophylactic bilateral salpingo-oophorectomy specimens. Only a limited number of such cases have been reported, and the available follow-up in many is short. Of the reported cases in the literature, some have been treated with chemotherapy, including those in which the peritoneal washings were negative for tumor. Based on the few cases with available follow-up, these do not appear to behave aggressively, but more cases with longer follow-up are needed.

Since many of the invasive fallopian tube carcinomas are occult and of small volume, an important question is whether the behavior of such cases is similar to symptomatically detected carcinomas that have bulky disease. The behavior of carcinomas (other than "carcinoma *in situ*"/intraepithelial carcinoma) in prophylactic bilateral salpingo-oophorectomy specimens is listed in *Table 11.5*. Stage IA tumors in prophylactic specimens with available follow-up in the literature have not shown aggressive behavior; however, too few cases have been reported, and

Table 11.4

Fallopian tube "carcinoma *in situ*"/intraepithelial carcinoma in prophylactic bilateral salpingo-oophorectomy specimens:[a] *pathologic features, treatment, and outcome*

Reference[b]		Located in fimbriated end[c]	Peritoneal washings[d]	Chemotherapy[c]	Follow-up
[6]	Case 4	+	–	–	No evidence of disease at 2.5 years
[34]	Case 1	+	+	+	NR
	Case 2	–	–	+	NR
	Case 4	+	–	+	NR
[35]	Case 4	NR	NR	–	Alive and well at 7.3 years
	Case 5	NR	–	–	Alive and well at 3.2 years
	Case 6	NR	–	–	Alive and well at 7 months
[48]	Case 48	+	NR	NR	Alive and well, <12 months
[135]	Case 2	NR	+	+	No evidence of disease at 4 years (follow-up from [6])
	Case 4	NR	–	+	No evidence of disease at 3 years (follow-up from [6])
	Case 6	NR	–	–	No evidence of disease (follow-up interval NR)
	Case 7	NR	–	–	No evidence of disease (follow-up interval NR)

NR, not reported
[a] Patients with *BRCA* mutations or other increased risk for ovarian carcinoma
[b] When possible, cases that were apparently reported in more than one publication are listed only once here
[c] Yes (+) or no (–)
[d] Positive (+) or negative (–) for malignant cells

the available follow-up is short. Advanced-stage tumors in prophylactic specimens show potential for aggressive behavior.

A portion of the fallopian tube (chiefly, the intramural segment) remains in the uterus after prophylactic bilateral salpingo-oophorectomy. In one study, it was shown that the segment of fallopian tube remaining in the hysterectomy specimen after prophylactic bilateral salpingo-oophorectomy had a median length of 1.2 cm (range: 0.6–1.5 cm) [85]. Despite the fact that not all tubal mucosa is removed during the prophylactic procedure, the risk for development of carcinoma in the remaining tube is probably minimal since (1) tubal carcinomas are not frequently found in the intramural segment, (2) follow-up studies of women after prophylactic bilateral salpingo-oophorectomy show a low frequency of subsequent pelvic carcinoma (in one study, the estimated risk of peritoneal carcinoma at 20 years after prophylactic surgery was only 4% [72]), and (3) most occult tubal carcinomas arise in the fimbriated end. Details regarding handling of prophylactic bilateral salpingo-oophorectomy specimens are provided in the section on Gross Examination above.

Pathogenesis, Including Molecular Features

Serous Carcinoma Gene expression profiles of fallopian tube and ovarian serous carcinomas have been shown to be similar, implying that tumorigenesis in both organs shares related molecular pathways [229]. *p53* has been identified as an important gene in the development of fallopian tube carcinoma. Mutations have been observed in serous carcinoma, but the frequency differs between studies [97, 245]. *p53* mutations have been detected in early stage carcinoma and TIC, suggesting that mutation of this gene is an early event in carcinogenesis [140, 245].

Opinions regarding the role of *HER-2/neu* in the pathogenesis of fallopian tube carcinoma vary. One study did not detect amplification in any cases and concluded that this gene does not play a role in pathogenesis [224]. However, overexpression has been shown in other studies. One study in particular demonstrated a correlation between overexpression and advanced stage, suggesting that *HER-2/neu* may be involved in tumor progression [169]. *K-ras* mutations are frequent [160]. This finding is of interest, as mutations of *K-ras* are infrequent in

Table 11.5

Behavior of fallopian tube carcinomas (other than "carcinoma *in situ*"/intraepithelial carcinoma) in prophylactic bilateral salpingo-oophorectomy specimens with available follow-up[a]

Reference[b]		Histologic type[c]	Stage	Chemotherapy	Follow-up
[35]	Case 3	High-grade serous carcinoma	IIB	+	Recurrence at 1.6 years; Alive with disease at 1.7 years
[72]	Case 5	NR	IA	NR	Alive at 1 year
	Case 8	NR	IA	NR	Alive at 6 years
	Case 9	NR	IIIC	NR	Alive at 2 years
[134]	Case 1	"Adenocarcinoma"	IA	NR	Dead from breast carcinoma 1 year after bilateral salpingo-oophorectomy
	Case 3	"Adenocarcinoma"	IA	NR	Alive without evidence of disease at 3.2 years
[135]	Case 3	High-grade serous carcinoma	NR	+	Recurrence at 1.4 years; alive with disease at 5.8 years (follow-up from [6])
[155]	Case report	NR	IA	–	Alive without evidence of disease at 3 months
[174]	Case 1	Grade 2 endometrioid carcinoma	IA	NR	Alive without evidence of disease at 3.8 years
	Case 2	High-grade serous carcinoma	IIIB	+	Recurrence at 1.7 years

NR, not reported
+, Yes
–, No
[a] Patients with *BRCA* mutations or other increased risk for ovarian carcinoma
[b] When possible, cases that were apparently reported in more than one publication are listed only once here
[c] Histologic type modified based on available details in cited reference

ovarian high-grade serous carcinoma; therefore, further study is warranted.

DNA cytometry and molecular genetic studies have shown that fallopian tube carcinomas are aneuploid and have a high degree of chromosomal instability, characterized by multiple gains and losses of genetic material at various loci on all chromosomes [102, 170, 182, 219]. One study demonstrated that epithelial atypia/dysplasia of the fallopian tube and TIC in risk-reducing prophylactic specimens contained chromosomal abnormalities, which implies that chromosomal instability is an early event in the pathogenesis of serous carcinoma [204]. The results of molecular genetic studies have also suggested multiple potential candidate oncogenes involved in the development of fallopian tube carcinoma [170, 219, 229].

An important molecular event involved in the development of hereditary fallopian tube carcinoma is germline mutation of *BRCA1* or *BRCA2*. These tumor suppressor genes are located on chromosomes 17 and 13, respectively. They are normally involved in transcriptional regulation of gene expression, cell cycle control, and recognition/repair of DNA damage. *BRCA*-associated carcinomas appear to follow the "2-hit model" of tumorigenesis, as seen in other organs (i.e., patients inherit a germline *BRCA* mutation [first hit], and with somatic loss of the wild-type allele [second hit], carcinoma develops).

In one report of two patients with a *BRCA1* germline mutation and serous carcinoma of the fallopian tube, both patients showed loss of the wild-type *BRCA1* allele in the tumors [246]. In another report, a patient with a *BRCA1* germline mutation and dysplasia of the fallopian tube exhibited loss of the wild-type *BRCA1* allele [188]. Two patients in a third report had *BRCA1* germline mutations and serous carcinoma of the fallopian tube, and loss of heterozygosity at multiple loci was observed on chromosome 13q, indicating that this chromosomal arm may contain tumor suppressor genes involved in the evolution of hereditary fallopian tube carcinoma [115]. Furthermore, the small number of samples of histologically normal fallopian tube epithelium from women with *BRCA* mutations that were analyzed in one study showed that the gene expression profile during the luteal phase of the menstrual cycle more closely resembled that of serous carcinoma compared with histologically normal samples from the follicular phase [229]. These findings suggest that the hormonal milieu during the menstrual cycle might play a role in carcinogenesis for women with *BRCA* mutations.

The pathogenesis of invasive high-grade serous carcinoma of the fallopian tube appears to begin with TIC as the first histologically identifiable lesion in this pathway. However, a precursor lesion of TIC has recently been proposed – the p53 signature [113, 140]. This lesion is composed of histologically normal mucosal epithelium and characterized by immunohistochemical overexpression of p53, which has been defined as a linear extent of $\geq$12 consecutive secretory cells showing strong expression (according to this definition, intervening p53-negative ciliated cells are allowed) (➲ *Fig. 11.40*). In one study, 57% of p53 signatures contained a *p53* mutation [140]. p53 signatures, however, have a low Ki-67 proliferation index. The mean Ki-67 proliferation index in one study was 3% (range: 0–30%) [113]. They show evidence of DNA damage, as manifested by immunohistochemical expression of γ-H2AX [113, 140]. When present, p53 signatures are usually located in the fimbriated end of the tube, and their frequency in women with *BRCA* mutations is similar to that of controls (10–38% versus 17–33%, respectively); however, p53 signatures are more frequent and multifocal in tubes with TIC [74, 140, 217].

A model has been suggested linking the p53 signature with TIC in which the p53 signature is the earliest step in the pathogenesis of fallopian tube carcinoma [113]. This is supported by the following: (1) p53 signatures are more common in tubes with TIC; (2) the p53 signature preferentially occurs in the same portion of the tube as TIC (fimbriated end); (3) both the p53 signature and TIC are thought to arise from the secretory cell; (4) the p53 signature, like TIC, shows p53 overexpression, *p53* mutations, and evidence of DNA damage; (5) direct continuity of the p53 signature with TIC has been reported (including an identical *p53* mutation in both components in one case [140]); (6) lesions histologically and immunohistochemically (Ki-67) intermediate between the p53 signature and TIC have been described; and (7) identical *p53* mutations in a p53 signature and peritoneal serous carcinoma in one case have been reported [37]. In this model, the fallopian tube mucosa in the fimbriated end undergoes injury, and as a result, the secretory cell experiences DNA damage with overaccumulation of p53 protein (p53 signature). With the development of a *p53* mutation, along with further cell proliferation and malignant transformation in a very small subset of women, the p53 signature then evolves into TIC. Although the p53 signature would be a common lesion in the general population regardless of *BRCA* status, it would, therefore, be in this

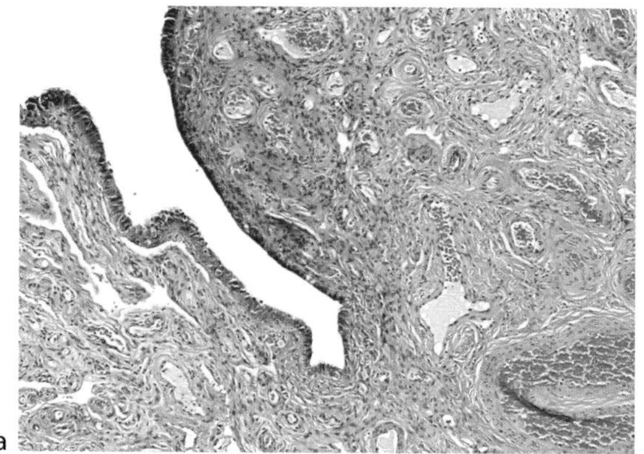

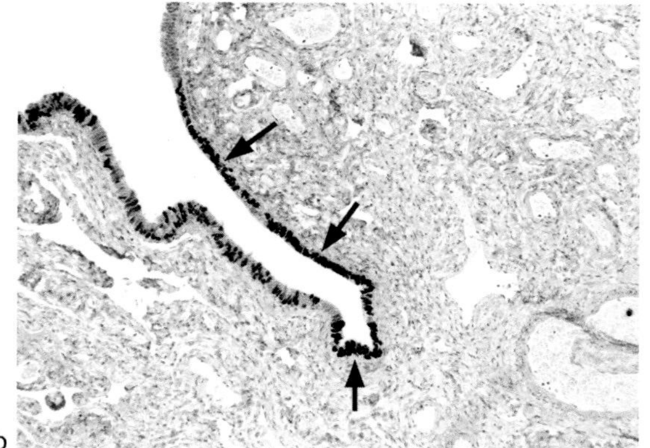

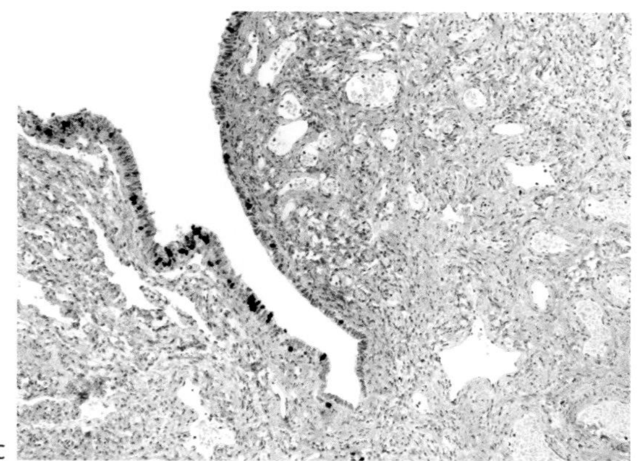

Fig. 11.40
p53 signature. **(a)** The tubal mucosa lacks morphologic features of intraepithelial carcinoma. **(b)** p53 expression is diffuse in three small segments of the mucosa (*arrows*), corresponding to (a). **(c)** The Ki-67 proliferation index is low in the three segments of diffuse p53 expression shown in (b). If these foci of diffuse p53 expression represented intraepithelial carcinoma, then the Ki-67 proliferation index would have been much higher (*compare with* ➲ *Fig. 11.39c*)

setting that further molecular alterations would allow for the possible development of a malignant clone with the potential to transform into TIC. Women without *BRCA* mutations can have a p53 signature, but it is possible that germline mutations of *BRCA* act as a promoter for the development of TIC [74]. It should also be noted that TIC and invasive carcinoma may arise independently of a *BRCA* mutation. In one study, the frequency of TIC in women with a *BRCA* mutation was not statistically different from that of controls (8% versus 3%, respectively) [217]. At this stage of growth, the TIC is of microscopic size, but with continued cell proliferation and growth of the tumor, malignant tumor cells eventually exfoliate into the peritoneal cavity (or proximally along the lumen of the tube) or infiltrate underlying tubal stroma in the form of invasive high-grade serous carcinoma. Progressive tumor growth eventually results in increasing tumor stage and volume of disease, peritoneal spread, and metastases, including involvement of lymph nodes.

Some evidence suggests that chronic salpingitis could be an etiology and that serous carcinomas may develop on a background of atrophy [57]. Unlike the ovary, serous carcinomas of the fallopian tube do not appear to follow a dualistic model as proposed for the ovary. Thus, a low-grade pathway, in which serous adenofibroma/cystadenofibroma evolves into atypical proliferative (borderline) serous tumor/noninvasive micropapillary (low-grade) serous carcinoma and then invasive low-grade serous carcinoma, typically is not seen in the fallopian tube.

Endometrioid Carcinoma As endometrioid carcinoma can evolve from endometriosis and atypical proliferative (borderline) endometrioid tumors in the ovary, these pathways are plausible in the fallopian tube. In one study of 26 endometrioid carcinomas of the fallopian tube, 23% of cases were associated with adjacent endometriosis [166]. In that study, direct continuity between carcinoma and endometriosis was not observed, but that does not exclude the possibility that carcinoma arose from endometriosis and obliterated any direct connection between the two. Although the fallopian tube is not an uncommon location for endometriosis, atypical (proliferative) borderline tumors occur only rarely in this anatomic site [7].

Differential Diagnosis

Non-neoplastic Lesions Pseudocarcinomatous hyperplasia can histologically simulate carcinoma because of cribriform architecture, pseudoinvasion of the muscularis, papillae within lymphatics, and subserosal mesothelial hyperplasia (*Fig. 11.11*) [43]. Patients with hyperplasia are usually premenopausal while those with carcinoma are typically postmenopausal. The tube can be enlarged in hyperplasia but does not show a mass on cross section unlike most cases of carcinoma; thus, the epithelial proliferation in hyperplasia is a microscopic finding. In contrast with carcinoma, hyperplasia usually exhibits a low mitotic index, absence of solid architecture, and a substantially lesser degree of nuclear atypia and nucleolar prominence. Acute or chronic salpingitis is usually present in hyperplasia, but some carcinomas can have an inflammatory component.

Determination of Site of Origin of Serous Carcinoma: Distinction from Ovarian/Peritoneal Primary Origin Traditionally, when carcinoma involves both the fallopian tube and ovary, the ovary has been considered the primary site given the much more frequent occurrence of primary ovarian carcinomas compared with fallopian tube primaries. Similarly, in the context of what would be conventionally considered a primary peritoneal carcinoma, involvement of the fallopian tube would generally be thought to represent secondary disease. Previously, criteria have been proposed for determining fallopian tube origin for tumors synchronously involving the tube and ovary. These criteria of Hu et al. (and subsequently modified by Sedlis) are as follows: (1) tumor arises from the endosalpinx, (2) histology of the tumor resembles tubal mucosa, (3) transition from benign to malignant epithelium, and (4) size of the fallopian tube tumor is larger than the ovarian tumor [106, 212]. As will be seen below, these criteria are nonspecific and unreliable.

It has been suggested that a subset of cases which appear to represent a primary ovarian or peritoneal high-grade serous carcinoma may actually be fallopian tube in origin. The finding of a synchronous TIC, in the setting of a synchronous ovarian or peritoneal high-grade serous carcinoma, has been proposed as indicating a fallopian tube origin [113, 125]. Lines of evidence supporting this include the following: (1) the fimbriated end of the tube is the preferred site of TIC; (2) the fimbriated end of the tube is in close proximity to the ovarian surface/peritoneal cavity; (3) intraepithelial carcinoma in the ovary or peritoneum is a rare finding; (4) early serous carcinomas in prophylactic bilateral salpingo-oophorectomy specimens from women with *BRCA* mutations (i.e., women who are at an increased risk for "ovarian" carcinoma) are commonly found in the fallopian tube (especially the fimbriated end) without disease in the ovary; (5) identical *p53* mutations have been reported in TIC and synchronous ovarian/peritoneal high-grade serous carcinomas; and (6) identical *p53* mutations in a p53 signature (see Pathogenesis, Including Molecular Features section above) and peritoneal serous carcinoma in one case have been reported [37].

It is possible that a small fallopian tube carcinoma can exfoliate cells onto the ovary or peritoneum, and preferential tumor growth in these secondary sites may overgrow the fallopian tube and obliterate any clues to a true fallopian tube origin in cases that do not initially appear as having arisen from the fallopian tube. Thus, the true frequency of "ovarian" carcinomas that really originated in the tube may be underestimated. In one study of consecutively accessioned pelvic serous carcinomas by Kindelberger et al. in which all fallopian tube tissue was submitted for histologic examination, 48% of cases initially interpreted as ovarian in origin contained a TIC, suggesting that a significant proportion of "ovarian" carcinomas could be of fallopian tube origin [125]. In that study, identical *p53* mutations were identified in the TIC and corresponding ovarian carcinoma in five of five cases tested. Interestingly, cases with a dominant mass in the ovary have a low frequency of TIC (11%) whereas TIC is much more common (45%) in cases in which involvement of the ovary did not create a dominant mass [201]. In a study by Carlson et al., nearly half of cases that would have originally been classified as primary peritoneal serous carcinoma contained a TIC [37]. In that study, identical *p53* mutations were identified in the TIC and corresponding peritoneal carcinoma in four of four cases tested.

Three possibilities may exist for cases with high-grade serous carcinoma in the ovary/peritoneum and TIC: (1) the fallopian tube is the primary lesion with secondary involvement of the ovary/peritoneum; (2) the ovary/peritoneum is the primary site with secondary involvement of the fallopian tube in the form of intraepithelial spread; and (3) both sites may be independent primaries. In cases where the primary site cannot be determined, this distinction usually will not be critical since most cases will typically be high stage, and the treatment and prognosis for a high-grade serous carcinoma simultaneously involving these sites will be similar regardless of which site is designated the primary origin [17, 161].

Determination of Site of Origin of Serous Carcinoma: Distinction from Endometrial Primary Origin Endometrial serous intraepithelial carcinoma (EIC) has been observed in association with TIC [114]. We have encountered cases of synchronous TIC and uterine malignant müllerian mixed tumor (MMMT) with a component of serous carcinoma. In these situations, the relationship between the fallopian tube and uterine tumors is not clear. Three possibilities may also exist, similar to that mentioned above: (1) the fallopian tube is the primary lesion with secondary involvement of the uterus; (2) the uterus is the primary site with secondary involvement of the fallopian tube; and (3) both sites may be independent primaries.

Other Fallopian Tube and Paratubal Neoplasms Because of the admixture of spindle cells in the epithelial component in some endometrioid carcinomas, the differential diagnosis can include malignant müllerian mixed tumor (MMMT). In general, the epithelial and mesenchymal components of MMMT, while admixed, do not show a histologic transition as opposed to the gradual transition between endometrioid glands and spindle cells in endometrioid carcinoma, and the latter has more of an orderly growth than MMMT. The degree of nuclear atypia and mitotic activity is greater in MMMT. The presence of malignant heterologous tissues would favor MMMT.

Endometrioid carcinomas with a female adnexal tumor of wolffian origin-like (FATWO-like) growth pattern can be confused with FATWO. Location within the lumen of the fallopian tube typically favors carcinoma since FATWO is usually in a paratubal location, but rare FATWOs can arise within the wall of the tube (see section Wolffian Adnexal Tumor ("Female Adnexal Tumor of Probable Wolffian Origin"; FATWO) below); however, the latter is predominantly within the muscularis as opposed to mostly occupying the lumen as in an endometrioid carcinoma. Villoglandular architecture, squamous differentiation, and endometriosis would favor carcinoma. Also, carcinoma contains larger, more conventional-appearing endometrioid glands. The degree of glandular confluence and nuclear atypia are usually greater in carcinoma than FATWO. The latter typically has more of an admixture of patterns, including open or closed tubules and sieve-like, solid, and spindled architecture; however, these features can be seen in FATWO-like endometrioid carcinomas. Calretinin is often positive in FATWO but occasionally may be negative; however, most carcinomas are negative. Carcinomas would be expected to express CK7, EMA, ER, and PR and be negative for inhibin. FATWO occasionally expresses CK7 and inhibin. ER, PR, and EMA are frequently negative in FATWO, but expression may occasionally be seen.

Sarcomas and Mixed Epithelial–Mesenchymal Tumors

Pure sarcomas of the tube may occur, and the mesenchymal component of mixed epithelial–mesenchymal tumors can be sarcomatous. Mixed epithelial–mesenchymal neoplasms in which the mesenchymal component is malignant and the epithelial component is benign are designated adenosarcoma whereas those in which both components are malignant are classified as malignant müllerian mixed tumor (MMMT; carcinosarcoma).

Pure sarcomas may be histologically subtyped if sufficient differentiation is present. Leiomyosarcomas are perhaps the most common type and may arise from the tube or broad ligament [110]. However, some may actually represent gastrointestinal stromal tumors arising outside of the gastrointestinal tract [77]. Other gynecologic-specific sarcomas, such as primary endometrioid stromal sarcoma arising in the tube, are rare [40]. Chondrosarcoma, malignant fibrous histiocytoma, and embryonal rhabdomyosarcoma have been described.

There are only a small number of tubal MMMTs in the literature, most of which are individual case reports [36, 77, 109]. Nearly all women are postmenopausal. They may have watery or bloody vaginal discharge and abdominal pain with signs of peritoneal spread. Grossly, the tumors distend the tube, and by the time of discovery, the majority of women have a pelvic mass with spread to adjacent pelvic and abdominal structures. The ovary must be identified clearly to rule out an origin in that organ. The grossly dilated tube when opened reveals an irregular mucosal surface with areas of necrosis and hemorrhage. Microscopically, distinct carcinoma and sarcoma components should be identifiable and intimately admixed with one another. The histologic appearance (➋ *Fig. 11.41*) is essentially identical to MMMTs of the uterus and ovary. Malignant glandular or squamous foci (or both) lie in an atypical mitotically active spindle or round cell background of sarcoma. In about half the cases, the sarcoma component may consist only of malignant elements homologous to the tube, such as smooth muscle or stromal

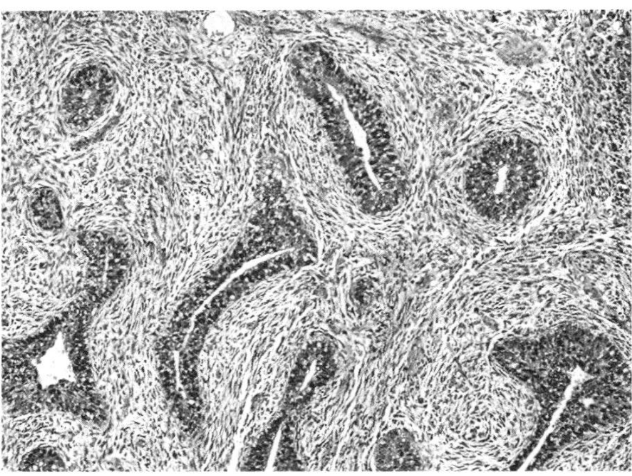

Fig. 11.41
Malignant müllerian mixed tumor. Intimate admixture of malignant epithelial and mesenchymal components

cells, but commonly there are foci of malignant cartilage, osteosarcoma, or rhabdomyosarcoma. Areas of TIC may be present adjacent to the main tumor mass, especially in the fimbriated end [36, 81]. The histology of metastases from MMMTs may be composed of carcinoma, sarcoma, or a mixture of both. The main tumor in the differential diagnosis of MMMT is a poorly differentiated endometrioid carcinoma with spindle cell features (see above section on ➋ Differential Diagnosis of ➋ Carcinoma). MMMT of the fallopian tube behaves aggressively, but prognosis is dependent on stage. Given that the experience is limited with tubal MMMT and that patients have been treated variably in the literature, standardized current treatment recommendations are not available. Other biphasic malignant tumors, such as adenosarcoma, are rare.

Metastatic Tumors/Secondary Involvement

Secondary involvement of the fallopian tube by carcinoma is much more common than primary tubal carcinoma, and metastatic carcinomas involving the tube are usually of ovarian or endometrial origin; however, metastases from the endocervix occur as well. Metastatic gynecologic or non-gynecologic carcinomas involving the pelvis typically involve the tubal serosal surface. Secondary involvement of the serosa in the form of implants from an ovarian atypical proliferative (borderline) serous tumor or by disseminated peritoneal adenomucinosis in the clinical syndrome of pseudomyxoma peritonei can occur too. In addition, lymphatic metastases may involve the mucosa or muscularis. Low-grade endometrial stromal sarcoma may involve the tubes by the extension of worm-like tongues of tumor along tubal lymphatics. Hematogenous metastases from breast carcinomas or other extra-pelvic tumors also may occur. Rarely, displaced benign endometrial tissue can be seen in the veins of the fallopian tube and should not be mistaken for metastatic carcinoma. On occasion, squamous carcinoma of the uterine cervix may spread in an *in situ* manner to involve the endometrial cavity, tubes, and even the ovarian surface [189]. The presence of tumor in the lumen of the fallopian tube in cases of endometrial serous carcinoma with metastases in the peritoneum (without myoinvasion or lymph-vascular space invasion in the uterus) suggests that the tubal lumen serves as a conduit for tumor spread [220]. In primary ovarian carcinoma, luminal groups of tumor cells may implant onto endosalpingeal surfaces and simulate TIC or early invasive primary tubal carcinoma. The distinction of fallopian tube versus ovarian origin for serous carcinoma is discussed in the above section on differential diagnosis of carcinoma.

Lymphoma

Primary tubal lymphoma is rare and is associated almost invariably with simultaneous involvement of the ipsilateral ovary [233]. Undifferentiated carcinoma and other small round blue cell tumors must be ruled out with appropriate immunohistochemical stains. For details, see ➋ Chap. 21, Hematologic Neoplasms.

Gestational Trophoblastic Disease of the Fallopian Tube

Trophoblastic tubal lesions are exceedingly uncommon. Patients have risk factors for ectopic pregnancy such as prior salpingitis and tubal occlusion [165]. The clinical presentation of a tubal hydatidiform mole or choriocarcinoma is similar to that of a tubal ectopic pregnancy; thus, rarely, an apparent ectopic pregnancy will prove to be a mole or choriocarcinoma. Hydatidiform moles usually occur as isolated growths but may be associated with intrauterine pregnancy. The histologic appearance resembles complete or partial moles as seen in the uterus. However, tubal moles are frequently overdiagnosed because ectopic pregnancies in the fallopian tube commonly have an exuberant extra-villous trophoblastic proliferation [33, 211]. Intraoperatively, the appearance of a tubal choriocarcinoma may be that of a large, hemorrhagic, and fleshy mass mostly destroying the tube. Histologically, the malignant trophoblastic proliferation resembles uterine choriocarcinoma. Response to modern chemotherapy in general has been excellent. Lesions of intermediate trophoblast, including placental site nodule, placental site trophoblastic tumor, and epithelioid trophoblastic tumor, are rare (see ➋ Chap. 20, Gestational Trophoblastic Tumors and Related Tumor-Like Lesions) [18, 111, 168, 179, 225].

Paratubal Lesions

Adrenal Rests

If a careful search is made, adrenal cortical rests may be found in the broad ligament in more than 20% of women. They lie adjacent to the ovarian vein and just beneath the peritoneum. Grossly, they appear as yellow nodules, but they may be obscured by fat. Medullary tissue is absent, but microscopically all three cortical layers are recognizable (➋ *Fig. 11.42*). This accessory tissue may hypertrophy secondary to adrenal destruction or may, rarely, give rise to a functional or nonfunctional cortical adenoma [207, 239].

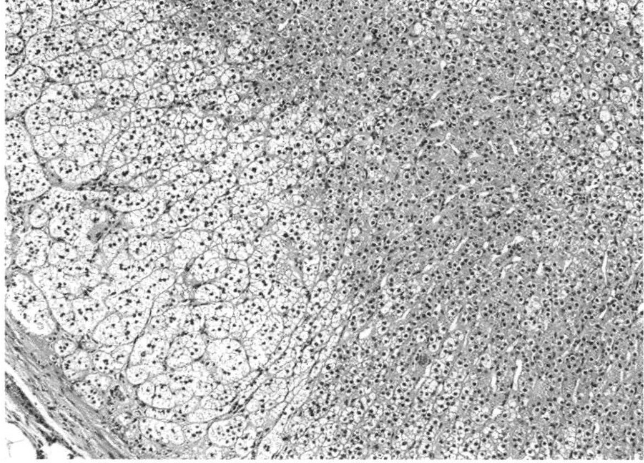

◻ Fig. 11.42
Adrenal rests. **They typically show similar cortical architecture and cells types as seen in the adrenal gland**

Paratubal Cysts

Paratubal cysts can be small or large. They have been classified based on their presumed origin: paramesonephric (müllerian), mesothelial, or mesonephric (wolffian). Differentiation may be difficult because of compression and atrophy of the lining cells. Those of paramesonephric type are the most common. In one study of paratubal cysts, 76% were paramesonephric, 24% were mesothelial, and none of the cysts were mesonephric [205]. The hydatid of Morgagni is by far the most common paramesonephric cyst. Grossly, it is attached to one of the fimbriae (➋ *Fig. 11.3*). It is ovoid or round, 2–10 mm in diameter, and contains clear serous fluid surrounded by a thin translucent wall. Microscopically, it is lined by epithelium resembling fallopian tube mucosa (including ciliated and non-ciliated cells), may have small epithelial-covered plicae projecting into the lumen, and may contain a thin smooth muscle wall (➋ *Fig. 11.43*). However, the cells lining the cyst can be flattened. Mesothelial cysts typically are lined by cuboidal or flattened cells and have a thin wall containing fibrous stroma. They lack the ciliated cells and thin plicae seen in paramesonephric cysts. Based on the available literature, it is not entirely clear what the specific histologic features of mesonephric cysts are.

Common differential diagnostic problems, which are usually of no clinical importance, are distinguishing a hydatid cyst of Morgagni from a serous cystadenoma and hydrosalpinx. In some cases, distinction from a serous cystadenoma may not be possible; however, hydatid cysts frequently contain a smooth muscle wall while the wall of a serous cystadenoma contains more fibromatous stroma than is typically seen in a hydatid cyst. Thin fallopian tube-like plicae, if present, favor a hydatid cyst rather than cystadenoma. In cases where the fallopian tube cannot be clearly discerned, distinction of a hydatid cyst from hydrosalpinx in which the fallopian tube is markedly distorted might be impossible since both can contain a thin smooth muscle wall and thin plicae lined by epithelium resembling that of the fallopian tube.

Wolffian Adnexal Tumor ("Female Adnexal Tumor of Probable Wolffian Origin"; FATWO)

This small group of distinctive tumors is described as located either within the leaves of the broad ligament, the mesosalpinx, or in the ovarian hilus (these tumors are also discussed in Chap. 17, Nonspecific Tumors of the Ovary Including Mesenchymal Tumors) [58, 116]. However, rare tumors can arise within the wall of the fallopian tube without growth in the lumen (*Fig. 11.44*). Patients range in age from 19 to 83 years (mean ranges from 42 to 45 years between studies). Either they have abdominal pain and a palpable mass, or the tumor is discovered as an incidental finding. The tumor is typically unilateral and localized without disseminated disease. The lesions measure from 0.8 to 20 cm in greatest dimension (mean, 6 cm) and are solid and lobulated with gross encapsulation. The cut surface is gray-yellow or tan, and the consistency may be firm, rubbery, or friable. Cysts or calcification may be present.

The microscopic appearance is variable. The tumors usually show a combination of growth patterns, including tubular (open or solid tubules), cystic, diffuse/solid, lobulated, sieve-like/retiform, and adenomatoid (*Fig. 11.45*). The tubal lumens and sieve-like spaces frequently contain eosinophilic, colloid-like material. The cells are cuboidal, flat, and/or spindled and have scant cytoplasm. The nuclei are typically bland, and the mitotic index is usually low. The stroma is either fibrous or hyalinized. FATWO typically expresses pan-cytokeratin and CD10. Calretinin, low molecular weight cytokeratin (CAM5.2), and androgen receptor are often positive but

Fig. 11.43
Paratubal cyst. **The cyst is thin and lined by bland tubal epithelium as seen in normal fallopian tubes. Focal residual plicae may be present**

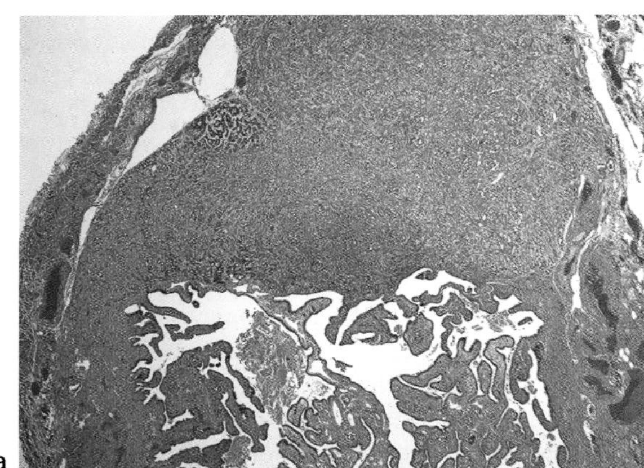

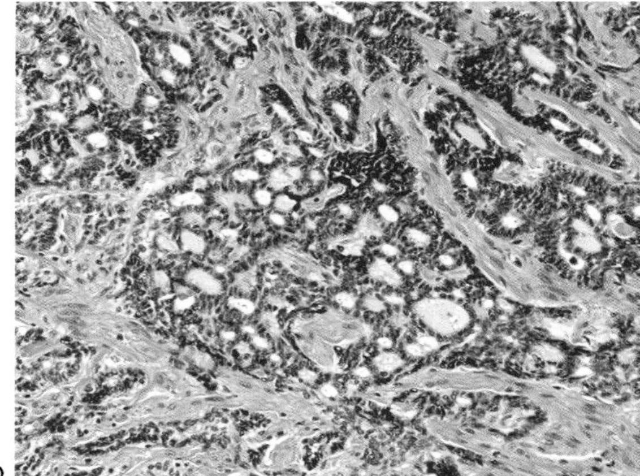

Fig. 11.44
Female adnexal tumor of wolffian origin (FATWO) in nonclassic location. **(a) The tumor is located within the wall of the fallopian tube rather than in a paratubal site but is not intraluminal. (b) The tumor exhibits the same architectural patterns seen in paratubal locations**

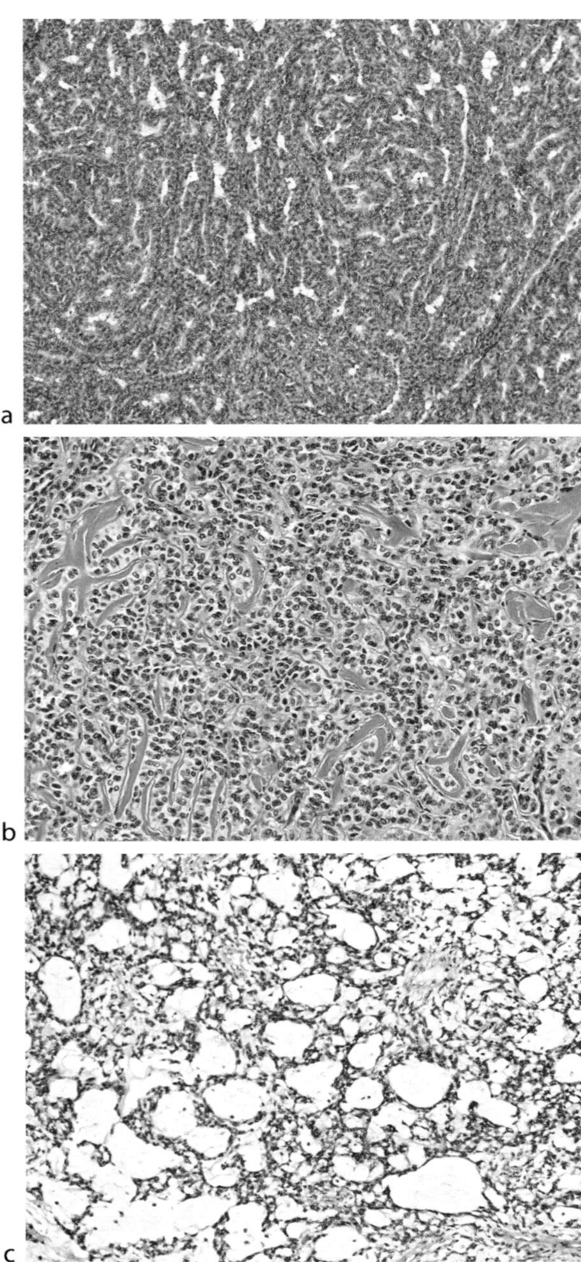

Fig. 11.45
Female adnexal tumor of wolffian origin (FATWO). **(a)** Open tubules. **(b)** Closed elongated tubules (note focally hyaline stroma). **(c)** Sieve-like pattern

occasionally may be negative. Expression of calretinin is usually diffuse. Tumors occasionally express CK7 and inhibin. Expression of CK7 is typically focal while the pattern with inhibin is variable, but the latter can be focal too. ER, PR, and EMA are frequently negative but expression may be seen on occasion. CK20 is typically negative.

Patients have been treated surgically, usually with a benign outcome. Malignant behavior is uncommon and includes multiple local recurrences and fatal metastases [31, 52]. It is difficult to predict which cases will exhibit malignant behavior. The tumors that demonstrate malignant behavior generally have nuclear atypia and mitotic activity; however, bland histology has been noted in some FATWOs that exhibit malignant behavior.

The differential diagnosis includes the FATWO-like variant of tubal endometrioid carcinoma (see above section on Differential Diagnosis of Carcinoma). Many of the histologic and immunohistochemical features of FATWO overlap with those of Sertoli cell tumor; however, the admixture of multiple growth patterns (particularly cystic architecture with a sieve-like pattern) and cell types in FATWO is generally greater than that is typically seen in Sertoli cell tumor, and sex cord-stromal tumors are rare in extra-ovarian sites.

Papillary Cystadenoma Associated with Von Hippel–Lindau Disease

These epithelial tumors are rare and characteristically arise in the broad ligament [15, 86, 129, 238]. Most of them are thought to be of mesonephric origin, but a müllerian origin has been suggested in one case [238]. In some cases, patients have a known history of the autosomal dominant disorder, von Hippel–Lindau disease; however, in other cases, the tumor in the broad ligament may be the first manifestation of the disease. Patients range in age from the third to fifth decades of life. Tumors may be unilateral or bilateral. They vary in size and are composed of cysts that contain a complex papillary proliferation (*Fig. 11.46*). The papillae are generally short and blunted. The stroma of the papillae varies in cellularity and may be hyalinized or fibrous. The papillae are usually lined by a single layer of low-cuboidal, non-ciliated cells that have eosinophilic or clear cytoplasm, but ciliated cells have been reported in one case [238]. The nuclei are bland, and the tumors are mitotically inactive. These tumors typically lack epithelial stratification and psammoma bodies. They are thought to be benign.

The importance of diagnosing this tumor (or suggesting it as a diagnostic possibility in ambiguous cases) is because of the association with von Hippel–Lindau disease (and, hence, various tumors of other organs, including renal cell carcinoma) and to not confuse it with other histologically similar neoplasms that do not have this association. The

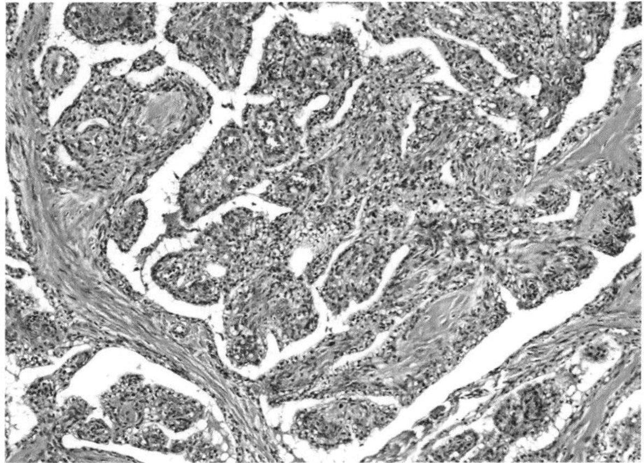

Fig. 11.46
Papillary cystadenoma associated with von Hippel–Lindau disease. **Cysts contain a complex papillary proliferation. The papillae are short and blunted. Closer magnification will show papillae lined by a single layer of cuboidal, non-ciliated cells with bland nuclei and clear to eosinophilic cytoplasm**

differential diagnosis includes cystadenofibromas of müllerian type with prominent papillary architecture that are not associated with von Hippel–Lindau disease. Those generally contain papillae which are much larger and less complex and contain cilia. They should also have areas which appear more conventionally adenofibromatous, including distinctive cleft-like architecture. Histologic overlap can also occur with atypical proliferative (borderline) serous tumor, but this tumor exhibits a hierarchical degree of papillae branching with epithelial stratification (including cellular tufts), ciliated cells, and psammoma bodies. Papillary cystadenomas associated with von Hippel–Lindau disease that are predominantly of clear cell type can mimic metastatic renal cell carcinoma [15]. In contrast with the latter, papillary cystadenoma diffusely expresses CK7 and is negative for RCC marker. CD10 is usually negative, but expression can be seen in some cases.

Other Paratubal/Para-ovarian and Pelvic Ligament Lesions

Atypical proliferative (borderline) tumor occurs more commonly in the broad ligament and paratubal/para-ovarian locations compared with carcinoma. Most of the atypical proliferative (borderline) tumors are of serous type [12]. These patients range in age from 19 to 67 years (mean, 32 years). The tumors are typically unilateral, and they range in size from 1 to 13 cm. They are usually confined to the broad ligament and histologically similar to their ovarian counterparts. The behavior appears to be favorable. Primary carcinoma of the broad ligament is rare [13]. Many of the patients are relatively young, and the tumors are usually unilateral. Some are associated with pelvic endometriosis. In most cases, disease is limited to the broad ligament. Various histologic types have been described, including endometrioid and clear cell.

Most mesenchymal tumors in paratubal/para-ovarian locations and pelvic ligaments are leiomyomas. Criteria for classification of benign, atypical, and malignant smooth muscle tumors in paratubal/para-ovarian locations have not been developed; however, some authors have advocated using the same criteria as used for uterine locations [122, 138]. It should be noted that criteria have been suggested for classifying smooth muscle tumors in the ovary [142]. For additional details regarding extra-uterine smooth muscle tumors, see Chap. 22, Soft Tissue Lesions Involving the Female Reproductive Organs. Sarcomas (leiomyosarcoma being the most common one) are rare.

Other primary lesions, some of which are rare, that may occur in paratubal/para-ovarian locations and pelvic ligaments include endometriosis, uterus-like mass, ectopic hilus cell nests, benign epithelial tumors (including serous cystadenoma and Brenner tumor; cystadenofibromas are occasional, usually incidental findings), adenomyoma, benign mesenchymal tumors (including lipoma, benign mesenchymoma, neurofibroma, and schwannoma), sex cord-stromal tumors (including fibroma, thecoma, and steroid cell tumor), ependymoma, teratoma, pheochromocytoma, carcinoid, perivascular epithelioid cell tumor (PEComa), malignant mesenchymal tumors (including extra-skeletal Ewing's sarcoma/PNET, adenosarcoma, endometrioid stromal sarcoma, rhabdomyosarcoma, "mixed mesenchymal sarcoma," liposarcoma, and alveolar soft part sarcoma), yolk sac tumor, and choriocarcinoma [138]. Various gynecologic and non-gynecologic tumors may secondarily involve paratubal/para-ovarian locations and pelvic ligaments. Such mesenchymal gynecologic tumors in particular include intravenous leiomyomatosis, diffuse uterine leiomyomatosis, cotyledenoid dissecting leiomyoma ("Sternberg tumor"), uterine leiomyosarcoma, and endometrial stromal sarcoma.

References

1. ACOG Practice Bulletin No. 89 (2008) Elective and risk-reducing salpingo-oophorectomy. Obstet Gynecol 111:231–241
2. Abraham JL, Spore WW, Benirschke K (1982) Cysticercosis of the fallopian tube: histology and microanalysis. Hum Pathol 13:665–670

3. ACOG (2008) ACOG Practice Bulletin No. 94: medical management of ectopic pregnancy. Obstet Gynecol 111:1479–1485
4. Adams BE (1969) Intussusception of a fallopian tube. Am J Surg 118:591–592
5. Afzelius BA, Eliasson R (1983) Male and female infertility problems in the immotile-cilia syndrome. Eur J Respir Dis Suppl 127:144–147
6. Agoff SN, Garcia RL, Goff B et al (2004) Follow-up of in situ and early-stage fallopian tube carcinoma in patients undergoing prophylactic surgery for proven or suspected BRCA-1 or BRCA-2 mutations. Am J Surg Pathol 28:1112–1114
7. Alvarado-Cabrero I, Navani SS, Young RH et al (1997) Tumors of the fimbriated end of the fallopian tube: a clinicopathologic analysis of 20 cases, including nine carcinomas. Int J Gynecol Pathol 16:189–196
8. Alvarado-Cabrero I, Young RH, Vamvakas EC et al (1999) Carcinoma of the fallopian tube: a clinicopathological study of 105 cases with observations on staging and prognostic factors. Gynecol Oncol 72:367–379
9. Antoniou A, Pharoah PD, Narod S et al (2003) Average risks of breast and ovarian cancer associated with BRCA1 or BRCA2 mutations detected in case series unselected for family history: a combined analysis of 22 studies. Am J Hum Genet 72:1117–1130
10. Aoyama T, Mizuno T, Andoh K et al (1996) Alpha-fetoprotein-producing (hepatoid) carcinoma of the fallopian tube. Gynecol Oncol 63:261–266
11. Arvidson CG, Kirkpatrick R, Witkamp MT et al (1999) Neisseria gonorrhoeae mutants altered in toxicity to human fallopian tubes and molecular characterization of the genetic locus involved. Infect Immun 67:643–652
12. Aslani M, Ahn GH, Scully RE (1988) Serous papillary cystadenoma of borderline malignancy of broad ligament. A report of 25 cases. Int J Gynecol Pathol 7:131–138
13. Aslani M, Scully RE (1989) Primary carcinoma of the broad ligament. Report of four cases and review of the literature. Cancer 64:1540–1545
14. Asmussen M, Kaern J, Kjoerstad K et al (1988) Primary adenocarcinoma localized to the fallopian tubes: report on 33 cases. Gynecol Oncol 30:183–186
15. Aydin H, Young RH, Ronnett BM et al (2005) Clear cell papillary cystadenoma of the epididymis and mesosalpinx: immunohistochemical differentiation from metastatic clear cell renal cell carcinoma. Am J Surg Pathol 29:520–523
16. Aziz S, Kuperstein G, Rosen B et al (2001) A genetic epidemiological study of carcinoma of the fallopian tube. Gynecol Oncol 80:341–345
17. Baekelandt M, Jorunn NA, Kristensen GB et al (2000) Carcinoma of the fallopian tube. Cancer 89:2076–2084
18. Baergen RN, Rutgers J, Young RH (2003) Extrauterine lesions of intermediate trophoblast. Int J Gynecol Pathol 22:362–367
19. Bartnik J, Powell WS, Moriber-Katz S et al (1989) Metaplastic papillary tumor of the fallopian tube. Case report, immunohistochemical features, and review of the literature. Arch Pathol Lab Med 113:545–547
20. Bell DA, Mondschein M, Scully RE (1986) Giant cell arteritis of the female genital tract. A report of three cases. Am J Surg Pathol 10:696–701
21. Benoit MF, Hannigan EV (2006) A 10-year review of primary fallopian tube cancer at a community hospital: a high association of synchronous and metachronous cancers. Int J Gynecol Cancer 16:29–35
22. Bernardus RE, Van der Slikke JW, Roex AJ et al (1984) Torsion of the fallopian tube: some considerations on its etiology. Obstet Gynecol 64:675–678
23. Beyth Y, Kopolovic J (1982) Accessory tubes: a possible contributing factor in infertility. Fertil Steril 38:382–383
24. Bhagavan BS, Ruffier J, Shinn B (1982) Pseudoactinomycotic radiate granules in the lower female genital tract: relationship to the Splendore-Hoeppli phenomenon. Hum Pathol 13:898–904
25. Boakye K, Omalu B, Thomas L (1997) Fallopian tube and pulmonary sarcoidosis. A case report. J Reprod Med 42:533–535
26. Bossuyt V, Medeiros F, Drapkin R et al (2008) Adenofibroma of the fimbria: a common entity that is indistinguishable from ovarian adenofibroma. Int J Gynecol Pathol 27:390–397
27. Bouyer J, Coste J, Shojaei T et al (2003) Risk factors for ectopic pregnancy: a comprehensive analysis based on a large case-control, population-based study in France. Am J Epidemiol 157:185–194
28. Bowen NJ, Logani S, Dickerson EB et al (2007) Emerging roles for PAX8 in ovarian cancer and endosalpingeal development. Gynecol Oncol 104:331–337
29. Breen JL (1970) A 21 year survey of 654 ectopic pregnancies. Am J Obstet Gynecol 106:1004–1019
30. Brenner PF, Roy S, Mishell DR Jr (1980) Ectopic pregnancy. A study of 300 consecutive surgically treated cases. JAMA 243:673–676
31. Brescia RJ, Cardoso de Almeida PC, Fuller AF Jr et al (1985) Female adnexal tumor of probable Wolffian origin with multiple recurrences over 16 years. Cancer 56:1456–1461
32. Brooks JJ, Wheeler JE (1977) Granulomatous salpingitis secondary to Crohn's disease. Obstet Gynecol 49:31–33
33. Burton JL, Lidbury EA, Gillespie AM et al (2001) Over-diagnosis of hydatidiform mole in early tubal ectopic pregnancy. Histopathology 38:409–417
34. Callahan MJ, Crum CP, Medeiros F et al (2007) Primary fallopian tube malignancies in BRCA-positive women undergoing surgery for ovarian cancer risk reduction. J Clin Oncol 25:3985–3990
35. Carcangiu ML, Peissel B, Pasini B et al (2006) Incidental carcinomas in prophylactic specimens in BRCA1 and BRCA2 germ-line mutation carriers, with emphasis on fallopian tube lesions: report of 6 cases and review of the literature. Am J Surg Pathol 30:1222–1230
36. Carlson JA Jr, Ackerman BL, Wheeler JE (1993) Malignant mixed mullerian tumor of the fallopian tube. Cancer 71:187–192
37. Carlson JW, Miron A, Jarboe EA et al (2008) Serous tubal intraepithelial carcinoma: its potential role in primary peritoneal serous carcinoma and serous cancer prevention. J Clin Oncol 26:4160–4165
38. Cass I, Holschneider C, Datta N et al (2005) BRCA-mutation-associated fallopian tube carcinoma: a distinct clinical phenotype? Obstet Gynecol 106:1327–1334
39. Cataldo NA, Nicholson M, Bihrle D (1990) Uterine serosal trophoblastic implant after linear salpingostomy for ectopic pregnancy at laparotomy. Obstet Gynecol 76:523–525
40. Chang KL, Crabtree GS, Lim-Tan SK et al (1993) Primary extrauterine endometrial stromal neoplasms: a clinicopathologic study of 20 cases and a review of the literature. Int J Gynecol Pathol 12:282–296
41. Chetty R, Reddy I, Batitang S (2003) Xanthelasma or xanthoma of the fallopian tube. Arch Pathol Lab Med 127:e417–e419
42. Cheung AN, So KF, Ngan HY et al (1994) Primary squamous cell carcinoma of fallopian tube. Int J Gynecol Pathol 13:92–95
43. Cheung AN, Young RH, Scully RE (1994) Pseudocarcinomatous hyperplasia of the fallopian tube associated with salpingitis. A report of 14 cases. Am J Surg Pathol 18:1125–1130

44. Clement PB (2007) The pathology of endometriosis: a survey of the many faces of a common disease emphasizing diagnostic pitfalls and unusual and newly appreciated aspects. Adv Anat Pathol 14:241–260
45. Clement PB, Young RH, Scully RE (1988) Necrotic pseudoxanthomatous nodules of ovary and peritoneum in endometriosis. Am J Surg Pathol 12:390–397
46. Clement PB, Young RH, Scully RE (1989) Liesegang rings in the female genital tract. A report of three cases. Int J Gynecol Pathol 8:271–276
47. Coddington CC, Chandler PE, Smith GW (1990) Accessory fallopian tube. A case report. J Reprod Med 35:420–421
48. Colgan TJ, Murphy J, Cole DE et al (2001) Occult carcinoma in prophylactic oophorectomy specimens: prevalence and association with BRCA germline mutation status. Am J Surg Pathol 25:1283–1289
49. Culton LK, Deavers MT, Silva EG et al (2006) Endometrioid carcinoma simultaneously involving the uterus and the fallopian tube: a clinicopathologic study of 13 cases. Am J Surg Pathol 30:844–849
50. David MP, Ben-Zwi D, Langer L (1981) Tubal intramural polyps and their relationship to infertility. Fertil Steril 35:526–531
51. Daw E (1973) Duplication of the uterine tube. Obstet Gynecol 42:137–138
52. Daya D (1994) Malignant female adnexal tumor of probable wolffian origin with review of the literature. Arch Pathol Lab Med 118:310–312
53. Daya D, Young RH, Scully RE (1992) Endometrioid carcinoma of the fallopian tube resembling an adnexal tumor of probable wolffian origin: a report of six cases. Int J Gynecol Pathol 11:122–130
54. DeCherney AH, Cholst I, Naftolin F (1981) Structure and function of the fallopian tubes following exposure to diethylstilbestrol (DES) during gestation. Fertil Steril 36:741–745
55. Deffieux X, Morice P, Thoury A et al (2005) Anatomy of pelvic and para-aortic nodal spread in patients with primary fallopian tube carcinoma. J Am Coll Surg 200:45–48
56. Delabrousse E, Site O, Le MA et al (1999) Intrahepatic pregnancy: sonography and CT findings. AJR Am J Roentgenol 173:1377–1378
57. Demopoulos RI, Aronov R, Mesia A (2001) Clues to the pathogenesis of fallopian tube carcinoma: a morphological and immunohistochemical case control study. Int J Gynecol Pathol 20:128–132
58. Devouassoux-Shisheboran M, Silver SA, Tavassoli FA (1999) Wolffian adnexal tumor, so-called female adnexal tumor of probable Wolffian origin (FATWO): immunohistochemical evidence in support of a Wolffian origin. Hum Pathol 30:856–863
59. di Re E, Grosso G, Raspagliesi F et al (1996) Fallopian tube cancer: incidence and role of lymphatic spread. Gynecol Oncol 62:199–202
60. Dische FE, Burt LJ, Davidson NJ et al (1974) Tubo-ovarian actinomycosis associated with intrauterine contraceptive devices. J Obstet Gynaecol Br Commonw 81:724–729
61. Donnez J, Casanas-Roux F, Caprasse J et al (1985) Cyclic changes in ciliation, cell height, and mitotic activity in human tubal epithelium during reproductive life. Fertil Steril 43:554–559
62. Donnez J, Casanas-Roux F, Ferin J (1979) Macroscopic and microscopic studies of fallopian tube after laparoscopic sterilization. Contraception 20:497–509
63. Doss BJ, Jacques SM, Qureshi F et al (1998) Extratubal secondary trophoblastic implants: clinicopathologic correlation and review of the literature. Hum Pathol 29:184–187
64. Dougherty CM, Cotten NM (1964) Proliferative epithelial lesions of the uterine tube. I. Adenomatous hyperplasia. Obstet Gynecol 24:849–854
65. Du H, Taylor HS (2004) Molecular regulation of mullerian development by Hox genes. Ann N Y Acad Sci 1034:152–165
66. Eddy GL, Copeland LJ, Gershenson DM et al (1984) Fallopian tube carcinoma. Obstet Gynecol 64:546–552
67. Edwards JL, Apicella MA (2004) The molecular mechanisms used by Neisseria gonorrhoeae to initiate infection differ between men and women. Clin Microbiol Rev 17:965–981
68. Egan AJ, Russell P (1996) Transitional (urothelial) cell metaplasia of the fallopian tube mucosa: morphological assessment of three cases. Int J Gynecol Pathol 15:72–76
69. Falcone T, Mascha EJ, Goldberg JM et al (1998) A study of risk factors for ruptured tubal ectopic pregnancy. J Womens Health 7:459–463
70. Farquhar CM (2005) Ectopic pregnancy. Lancet 366:583–591
71. Fernstrom I, Lagerlof B (1964) Polyps in the intramural part of the fallopian tubes. A radiologic and clinical study. J Obstet Gynaecol Br Commonw 71:681–691
72. Finch A, Beiner M, Lubinski J et al (2006) Salpingo-oophorectomy and the risk of ovarian, fallopian tube, and peritoneal cancers in women with a BRCA1 or BRCA2 Mutation. JAMA 296:185–192
73. Finch A, Shaw P, Rosen B et al (2006) Clinical and pathologic findings of prophylactic salpingo-oophorectomies in 159 BRCA1 and BRCA2 carriers. Gynecol Oncol 100:58–64
74. Folkins AK, Jarboe EA, Saleemuddin A et al (2008) A candidate precursor to pelvic serous cancer (p53 signature) and its prevalence in ovaries and fallopian tubes from women with BRCA mutations. Gynecol Oncol 109:168–173
75. Ford D, Easton DF, Stratton M et al (1998) Genetic heterogeneity and penetrance analysis of the BRCA1 and BRCA2 genes in breast cancer families. The Breast Cancer Linkage Consortium. Am J Hum Genet 62:676–689
76. Fortier KJ, Haney AF (1985) The pathologic spectrum of uterotubal junction obstruction. Obstet Gynecol 65:93–98
77. Foster R, Solano S, Mahoney J et al (2006) Reclassification of a tubal leiomyosarcoma as an eGIST by molecular evaluation of c-KIT. Gynecol Oncol 101:363–366
78. Furuya M, Murakami T, Sato O et al (2002) Pseudoxanthomatous and xanthogranulomatous salpingitis of the fallopian tube: a report of four cases and a literature review. Int J Gynecol Pathol 21:56–59
79. Fylstra DL (1998) Tubal pregnancy: a review of current diagnosis and treatment. Obstet Gynecol Surv 53:320–328
80. Gaarenstroom KN, van der Hiel B, Tollenaar RA et al (2006) Efficacy of screening women at high risk of hereditary ovarian cancer: results of an 11-year cohort study. Int J Gynecol Cancer 16(Suppl 1):54–59
81. Gagner JP, Mittal K (2005) Malignant mixed Mullerian tumor of the fimbriated end of the fallopian tube: origin as an intraepithelial carcinoma. Gynecol Oncol 97:219–222
82. Ganesan R, Ferryman SR, Meier L et al (2000) Vasculitis of the female genital tract with clinicopathologic correlation: a study of 46 cases with follow-up. Int J Gynecol Pathol 19:258–265
83. Gardner GH, Greene RR, Peckham BM (1948) Normal and cystic structures of broad ligament. Am J Obstet Gynecol 55: 917–939
84. Gelfand M, Ross MD, Blair DM et al (1971) Distribution and extent of schistosomiasis in female pelvic organs, with special reference to the genital tract, as determined at autopsy. Am J Trop Med Hyg 20:846–849
85. Gerritzen LH, Grefte JM, Hoogerbrugge N et al (2006) A substantial part of the fallopian tube is left after standard prophylactic bilateral salpingo-oophorectomy. Int J Gynecol Cancer 16:1940–1944
86. Gersell DJ, King TC (1988) Papillary cystadenoma of the mesosalpinx in von Hippel-Lindau disease. Am J Surg Pathol 12:145–149
87. Gisser SD (1986) Obstructing fallopian tube papilloma. Int J Gynecol Pathol 5:179–182

88. Graham H (1951) Eternal Eve; the history of gynaecology & obstetrics. Doubleday, Garden City, NY, pp 160–162
89. Green LK, Kott ML (1989) Histopathologic findings in ectopic tubal pregnancy. Int J Gynecol Pathol 8:255–262
90. Grimes HG, Nosal RA, Gallagher JC (1983) Ovarian pregnancy: a series of 24 cases. Obstet Gynecol 61:174–180
91. Guioli S, Sekido R, Lovell-Badge R (2007) The origin of the mullerian duct in chick and mouse. Dev Biol 302:389–398
92. Habana A, Dokras A, Giraldo JL et al (2000) Cornual heterotopic pregnancy: contemporary management options. Am J Obstet Gynecol 182:1264–1270
93. Haines M (1958) Tuberculous salpingitis as seen by the pathologist and the surgeon. Am J Obstet Gynecol 75:472–481
94. Halbert SA, Patton DL, Zarutskie PW et al (1997) Function and structure of cilia in the fallopian tube of an infertile woman with Kartagener's syndrome. Hum Reprod 12:55–58
95. Hartley A, Rollason T, Spooner D (2000) Clear cell carcinoma of the fimbria of the fallopian tube in a BRCA1 carrier undergoing prophylactic surgery. Clin Oncol (R Coll Radiol) 12:58–59
96. Heintz AP, Odicino F, Maisonneuve P et al (2006) Carcinoma of the fallopian tube. FIGO 6th Annual Report on the Results of Treatment in Gynecological Cancer. Int J Gynaecol Obstet 95(Suppl 1): S145–S160
97. Hellstrom AC, Blegen H, Malec M et al (2000) Recurrent fallopian tube carcinoma: TP53 mutation and clinical course. Int J Gynecol Pathol 19:145–151
98. Hellstrom AC, Silfversward C, Nilsson B et al (1994) Carcinoma of the fallopian tube. A clinical and histopathologic review. The Radiumhemmet series. Int J Gynecol Cancer 4:395–400
99. Herbold DR, Axelrod JH, Bobowski SJ et al (1988) Glassy cell carcinoma of the fallopian tube. A case report. Int J Gynecol Pathol 7:384–390
100. Hermsen BB, van Diest PJ, Berkhof J et al (2006) Low prevalence of (pre) malignant lesions in the breast and high prevalence in the ovary and fallopian tube in women at hereditary high risk of breast and ovarian cancer. Int J Cancer 119:1412–1418
101. Herrera GA, Reimann BE, Greenberg HL et al (1983) Pigmentosis tubae, a new entity: light and electron microscopic study. Obstet Gynecol 61:80S–83S
102. Heselmeyer K, Hellstrom AC, Blegen H et al (1998) Primary carcinoma of the fallopian tube: comparative genomic hybridization reveals high genetic instability and a specific, recurring pattern of chromosomal aberrations. Int J Gynecol Pathol 17:245–254
103. Hinton EL, Bobo LD, Wu TC et al (2000) Detection of Chlamydia trachomatis DNA in archival paraffinized specimens from chronic salpingitis cases using the polymerase chain reaction. Fertil Steril 74:152–157
104. Homm RJ, Holtz G, Garvin AJ (1987) Isthmic ectopic pregnancy and salpingitis isthmica nodosa. Fertil Steril 48:756–760
105. Hoppe E, de Ybarlucea LR, Collet J et al (2007) Isolated vasculitis of the female genital tract: a case series and review of literature. Virchows Arch 451:1083–1089
106. Hu CY, Taymor ML, Hertig AT (1950) Primary carcinoma of the fallopian tube. Am J Obstet Gynecol 59:58–67
107. Hunt JL, Lynn AA (2002) Histologic features of surgically removed fallopian tubes. Arch Pathol Lab Med 126:951–955
108. Hunter RH (1930) Observations on the development of the human female genital tract. Contrib Embryol 22:91–107
109. Imachi M, Tsukamoto N, Shigematsu T et al (1992) Malignant mixed Mullerian tumor of the fallopian tube: report of two cases and review of literature. Gynecol Oncol 47:114–124
110. Jacoby AF, Fuller AF Jr, Thor AD et al (1993) Primary leiomyosarcoma of the fallopian tube. Gynecol Oncol 51:404–407
111. Jacques SM, Qureshi F, Ramirez NC et al (1997) Retained trophoblastic tissue in fallopian tubes: a consequence of unsuspected ectopic pregnancies. Int J Gynecol Pathol 16:219–224
112. Jansen RP (1984) Endocrine response in the fallopian tube. Endocr Rev 5:525–551
113. Jarboe E, Folkins A, Nucci MR et al (2008) Serous carcinogenesis in the fallopian tube: a descriptive classification. Int J Gynecol Pathol 27:1–9
114. Jarboe EA, Miron A, Carlson JW et al (2009) Coexisting intraepithelial serous carcinomas of the endometrium and fallopian tube: frequency and potential significance. Int J Gynecol Pathol 28:308–315
115. Jongsma AP, Piek JM, Zweemer RP et al (2002) Molecular evidence for putative tumour suppressor genes on chromosome 13q specific to BRCA1 related ovarian and fallopian tube cancer. Mol Pathol 55:305–309
116. Kariminejad MH, Scully RE (1973) Female adnexal tumor of probable Wolffian origin. A distinctive pathologic entity. Cancer 31:671–677
117. Kauff ND, Barakat RR (2007) Risk-reducing salpingo-oophorectomy in patients with germline mutations in BRCA1 or BRCA2. J Clin Oncol 25:2921–2927
118. Kauff ND, Satagopan JM, Robson ME et al (2002) Risk-reducing salpingo-oophorectomy in women with a BRCA1 or BRCA2 mutation. N Engl J Med 346:1609–1615
119. Keeney GL, Thrasher TV (1988) Metaplastic papillary tumor of the fallopian tube: a case report with ultrastructure. Int J Gynecol Pathol 7:86–92
120. Keith LG, Berger GS, Edelman DA et al (1984) On the causation of pelvic inflammatory disease. Am J Obstet Gynecol 149:215–224
121. Kemp B, Kertschanska S, Handt S et al (1999) Different placentation patterns in viable compared with nonviable tubal pregnancy suggest a divergent clinical management. Am J Obstet Gynecol 181:615–620
122. Kempson RL, Fletcher CDM, Evans HL et al (2001) Tumors of the soft tissues. Atlas of tumor pathology, series 3, fascicle 30. Armed Forces Institute of Pathology, Washington, DC, pp 244–245
123. Kim HS, Thonse VR, Judson K et al (2007) Utero-ovarian anastomosis: histopathologic correlation after uterine artery embolization with or without ovarian artery embolization. J Vasc Interv Radiol 18:31–39
124. Kim KR, Scully RE (1990) Peritoneal keratin granulomas with carcinomas of endometrium and ovary and atypical polypoid adenomyoma of endometrium. A clinicopathological analysis of 22 cases. Am J Surg Pathol 14:925–932
125. Kindelberger DW, Lee Y, Miron A et al (2007) Intraepithelial carcinoma of the fimbria and pelvic serous carcinoma: evidence for a causal relationship. Am J Surg Pathol 31:161–169
126. King MC, Marks JH, Mandell JB (2003) Breast and ovarian cancer risks due to inherited mutations in BRCA1 and BRCA2. Science 302:643–646
127. Klein M, Rosen A, Lahousen M et al (1994) Lymphogenous metastasis in the primary carcinoma of the fallopian tube. Gynecol Oncol 55:336–338
128. Klein M, Rosen AC, Lahousen M et al (1999) Lymphadenectomy in primary carcinoma of the fallopian tube. Cancer Lett 147:63–66
129. Korn WT, Schatzki SC, DiSciullo AJ et al (1990) Papillary cystadenoma of the broad ligament in von Hippel-Lindau disease. Am J Obstet Gynecol 163:596–598

130. Koshiyama M, Konishi I, Yoshida M et al (1994) Transitional cell carcinoma of the fallopian tube: a light and electron microscopic study. Int J Gynecol Pathol 13:175–180
131. Kristensen GB, Bollerup AC, Lind K et al (1985) Infections with Neisseria gonorrhoeae and Chlamydia trachomatis in women with acute salpingitis. Genitourin Med 61:179–184
132. Kutluay L, Vicdan K, Turan C et al (1994) Tubal histopathology in ectopic pregnancies. Eur J Obstet Gynecol Reprod Biol 57: 91–94
133. Ladefoged C, Lorentzen M (1988) Xanthogranulomatous inflammation of the female genital tract. Histopathology 13:541–551
134. Laki F, Kirova YM, This P et al (2007) Prophylactic salpingo-oophorectomy in a series of 89 women carrying a BRCA1 or a BRCA2 mutation. Cancer 109:1784–1790
135. Lamb JD, Garcia RL, Goff BA et al (2006) Predictors of occult neoplasia in women undergoing risk-reducing salpingo-oophorectomy. Am J Obstet Gynecol 194:1702–1709
136. Landers DV, Sweet RL (1983) Tubo-ovarian abscess: contemporary approach to management. Rev Infect Dis 5:876–884
137. Lareau SM, Beigi RH (2008) Pelvic inflammatory disease and tubo-ovarian abscess. Infect Dis Clin North Am 22:693–708
138. Lax SF, Vang R, Tavassoli FA (2003) Tumours of the fallopian tube and uterine ligaments: tumours of the uterine ligaments. In: Tavassoli FA, Deville P (eds) World Health Organization classification of tumors. Pathology and genetics of tumours of the breast and female genital organs. IARC Press, Lyon, pp 212–216
139. Lee A, Ying YK, Novy MJ (1997) Hysteroscopy, hysterosalpingography and tubal ostial polyps in infertility patients. J Reprod Med 42:337–341
140. Lee Y, Miron A, Drapkin R et al (2007) A candidate precursor to serous carcinoma that originates in the distal fallopian tube. J Pathol 211:26–35
141. Lefrancq T, Orain I, Michalak S et al (1999) Herpetic salpingitis and fallopian tube prolapse. Histopathology 34:548–550
142. Lerwill MF, Sung R, Oliva E et al (2004) Smooth muscle tumors of the ovary: a clinicopathologic study of 54 cases emphasizing prognostic criteria, histologic variants, and differential diagnosis. Am J Surg Pathol 28:1436–1451
143. Levine DA, Argenta PA, Yee CJ et al (2003) Fallopian tube and primary peritoneal carcinomas associated with BRCA mutations. J Clin Oncol 21:4222–4227
144. Li S, Zimmerman RL, LiVolsi VA (1999) Mixed malignant germ cell tumor of the fallopian tube. Int J Gynecol Pathol 18:183–185
145. Lisa JR, Gioia JD, Rubin IC (1954) Observations on the interstitial portion of the fallopian tube. Surg Gynecol Obstet 99:159–169
146. Longacre TA, Oliva E, Soslow RA (2007) Recommendations for the reporting of fallopian tube neoplasms. Hum Pathol 38: 1160–1163
147. Lyons RA, Saridogan E, Djahanbakhch O (2006) The reproductive significance of human fallopian tube cilia. Hum Reprod Update 12:363–372
148. Maisey K, Nardocci G, Imarai M et al (2003) Expression of proinflammatory cytokines and receptors by human fallopian tubes in organ culture following challenge with Neisseria gonorrhoeae. Infect Immun 71:527–532
149. Majmudar B, Henderson PH III, Semple E (1983) Salpingitis isthmica nodosa: a high-risk factor for tubal pregnancy. Obstet Gynecol 62:73–78
150. Marcus SF, Macnamee M, Brinsden P (1995) Heterotopic pregnancies after in-vitro fertilization and embryo transfer. Hum Reprod 10:1232–1236
151. Mardh PA, Ripa T, Svensson L et al (1977) Chlamydia trachomatis infection in patients with acute salpingitis. N Engl J Med 296:1377–1379
152. Martin DC, Khare VK, Miller BE (1995) Association of Chlamydia trachomatis immunoglobulin gamma titers with dystrophic peritoneal calcification, psammoma bodies, adhesions, and hydrosalpinges. Fertil Steril 63:39–44
153. Matsushita H, Kodama S, Aoki Y et al (1998) Paraneoplastic cerebellar degeneration with anti-Purkinje cell antibody associated with primary tubal cancer. Gynecol Obstet Invest 45:140–143
154. McCormack WM (1994) Pelvic inflammatory disease. N Engl J Med 330:115–119
155. McEwen AR, McConnell DT, Kenwright DN et al (2004) Occult cancer of the fallopian tube in a BRCA2 germline mutation carrier at prophylactic salpingo-oophorectomy. Gynecol Oncol 92: 992–994
156. McGee ZA, Jensen RL, Clemens CM et al (1999) Gonococcal infection of human fallopian tube mucosa in organ culture: relationship of mucosal tissue TNF-alpha concentration to sloughing of ciliated cells. Sex Transm Dis 26:160–165
157. Medeiros F, Muto MG, Lee Y et al (2006) The tubal fimbria is a preferred site for early adenocarcinoma in women with familial ovarian cancer syndrome. Am J Surg Pathol 30:230–236
158. Meeuwissen PA, Seynaeve C, Brekelmans CT et al (2005) Outcome of surveillance and prophylactic salpingo-oophorectomy in asymptomatic women at high risk for ovarian cancer. Gynecol Oncol 97:476–482
159. Milchgrub S, Sandstad J (1991) Arias-Stella reaction in fallopian tube epithelium. A light and electron microscopic study with a review of the literature. Am J Clin Pathol 95:892–895
160. Mizuuchi H, Mori Y, Sato K et al (1995) High incidence of point mutation in K-ras codon 12 in carcinoma of the fallopian tube. Cancer 76:86–90
161. Moore KN, Moxley KM, Fader AN et al (2007) Serous fallopian tube carcinoma: a retrospective, multi-institutional case-control comparison to serous adenocarcinoma of the ovary. Gynecol Oncol 107:398–403
162. Moore SW, Enterline HT (1975) Significance of proliferative epithelial lesions of the uterine tube. Obstet Gynecol 45:385–390
163. Morris H, Emms M, Visser T et al (1986) Lymphoid tissue of the normal fallopian tube – a form of mucosal-associated lymphoid tissue (MALT)? Int J Gynecol Pathol 5:11–22
164. Munichor M, Kerner H, Cohen H et al (1997) The lipofuscin-iron association in pigmentosis tubae. Ultrastruct Pathol 21:273–280
165. Muto MG, Lage JM, Berkowitz RS et al (1991) Gestational trophoblastic disease of the fallopian tube. J Reprod Med 36:57–60
166. Navani SS, Alvarado-Cabrero I, Young RH et al (1996) Endometrioid carcinoma of the fallopian tube: a clinicopathologic analysis of 26 cases. Gynecol Oncol 63:371–378
167. Nawroth F, Nugent W, Ludwig M (2006) Congenital partial atresia of the fallopian tube. Reprod Biomed Online 12:205–208
168. Nayar R, Snell J, Silverberg SG et al (1996) Placental site nodule occurring in a fallopian tube. Hum Pathol 27:1243–1245
169. Nowee ME, Dorsman JC, Piek JM et al (2007) HER-2/neu and p27Kip1 in progression of fallopian tube carcinoma: an immunohistochemical and array comparative genomic hybridization study. Histopathology 51:666–673
170. Nowee ME, Snijders AM, Rockx DA et al (2007) DNA profiling of primary serous ovarian and fallopian tube carcinomas with array comparative genomic hybridization and multiplex ligation-dependent probe amplification. J Pathol 213:46–55

171. O'Rahilly R (1989) Prenatal human development. In: Wynn RM, Jollie WP (eds) Biology of the uterus, 2nd edn. Plenum, New York, pp 37–43
172. O'Rahilly R (1983) The timing and sequence of events in the development of the human reproductive system during the embryonic period proper. Anat Embryol (Berl) 166:247–261
173. Oliver R, Malik M, Coker A et al (2007) Management of extra-tubal and rare ectopic pregnancies: case series and review of current literature. Arch Gynecol Obstet 276:125–131
174. Olivier RI, van Beurden M, Lubsen MA et al (2004) Clinical outcome of prophylactic oophorectomy in BRCA1/BRCA2 mutation carriers and events during follow-up. Br J Cancer 90:1492–1497
175. Orvis GD, Behringer RR (2007) Cellular mechanisms of mullerian duct formation in the mouse. Dev Biol 306:493–504
176. Paccagnella GL, Cocco A, Ruggio F (2008) Microinvasive fimbrial fallopian tube carcinoma in a BRCA-2 mutation carrier. Int J Gynaecol Obstet 101:200
177. Papadimitriou CA, Peitsidis P, Bozas G et al (2008) Paclitaxel- and platinum-based postoperative chemotherapy for primary fallopian tube carcinoma: a single institution experience. Oncology 75:42–48
178. Parikh FR, Nadkarni SG, Kamat SA et al (1997) Genital tuberculosis – a major pelvic factor causing infertility in Indian women. Fertil Steril 67:497–500
179. Parker A, Lee V, Dalrymple C et al (2003) Epithelioid trophoblastic tumour: report of a case in the fallopian tube. Pathology 35:136–140
180. Parker RL, Dadmanesh F, Young RH et al (2004) Polypoid endometriosis: a clinicopathologic analysis of 24 cases and a review of the literature. Am J Surg Pathol 28:285–297
181. Pauerstein CJ, Croxatto HB, Eddy CA et al (1986) Anatomy and pathology of tubal pregnancy. Obstet Gynecol 67:301–308
182. Pere H, Tapper J, Seppala M et al (1998) Genomic alterations in fallopian tube carcinoma: comparison to serous uterine and ovarian carcinomas reveals similarity suggesting likeness in molecular pathogenesis. Cancer Res 58:4274–4276
183. Persaud V (1970) Etiology of tubal ectopic pregnancy. Radiologic and pathologic studies. Obstet Gynecol 36:257–263
184. Persson E, Holmberg K (1984) A longitudinal study of Actinomyces israelii in the female genital tract. Acta Obstet Gynecol Scand 63:207–216
185. Peters WA III, Andersen WA, Hopkins MP et al (1988) Prognostic features of carcinoma of the fallopian tube. Obstet Gynecol 71:757–762
186. Pettersson F (1992) Staging rules for gestational trophoblastic tumors and fallopian tube cancer. Acta Obstet Gynecol Scand 71:224–225
187. Peyton-Jones B, Olaitan A, Murdoch JB (2002) Incidental diagnosis of primary fallopian tube carcinoma during prophylactic salpingo-oophorectomy in BRCA2 mutation carrier. BJOG 109:1413–1414
188. Piek JM, van Diest PJ, Zweemer RP et al (2001) Dysplastic changes in prophylactically removed fallopian tubes of women predisposed to developing ovarian cancer. J Pathol 195:451–456
189. Pins MR, Young RH, Crum CP et al (1997) Cervical squamous cell carcinoma in situ with intraepithelial extension to the upper genital tract and invasion of tubes and ovaries: report of a case with human papilloma virus analysis. Int J Gynecol Pathol 16:272–278
190. Platz CE, Benda JA (1995) Female genital tract cancer. Cancer 75:270–294
191. Powell CB, Kenley E, Chen LM et al (2005) Risk-reducing salpingo-oophorectomy in BRCA mutation carriers: role of serial sectioning in the detection of occult malignancy. J Clin Oncol 23:127–132
192. Pritt B, Mount SL, Cooper K et al (2006) Pseudoactinomycotic radiate granules of the gynaecological tract: review of a diagnostic pitfall. J Clin Pathol 59:17–20
193. Rabban JT, Crawford B, Chen LM et al (2009) Transitional cell metaplasia of fallopian tube fimbriae: a potential mimic of early tubal carcinoma in risk reduction salpingo-oophorectomies from women with BRCA mutations. Am J Surg Pathol 33:111–119
194. Rabczynski J, Ziolkowski P (1999) Primary endometrioid carcinoma of fallopian tube. Clinicomorphologic study. Pathol Oncol Res 5:61–66
195. Ramin SM, Ramin KD, Hemsell DL (1999) Fallopian tube prolapse after hysterectomy. South Med J 92:963–966
196. Randall S, Buckley CH, Fox H (1987) Placentation in the fallopian tube. Int J Gynecol Pathol 6:132–139
197. Rhee DD, Wu ML (2006) Pulse granulomas detected in gallbladder, fallopian tube, and skin. Arch Pathol Lab Med 130:1839–1842
198. Riska A, Leminen A (2007) Updating on primary fallopian tube carcinoma. Acta Obstet Gynecol Scand 86:1419–1426
199. Robboy SJ, Taguchi O, Cunha GR (1982) Normal development of the human female reproductive tract and alterations resulting from experimental exposure to diethylstilbestrol. Hum Pathol 13:190–198
200. Robey SS, Silva EG (1989) Epithelial hyperplasia of the fallopian tube. Its association with serous borderline tumors of the ovary. Int J Gynecol Pathol 8:214–220
201. Roh MH, Kindelberger D, Crum CP (2009) Serous tubal intraepithelial carcinoma and the dominant ovarian mass: clues to serous tumor origin? Am J Surg Pathol 33:376–383
202. Rosen AC, Klein M, Hafner E et al (1999) Management and prognosis of primary fallopian tube carcinoma. Austrian Cooperative Study Group for Fallopian Tube Carcinoma. Gynecol Obstet Invest 47:45–51
203. Saffos RO, Rhatigan RM, Scully RE (1980) Metaplastic papillary tumor of the fallopian tube – a distinctive lesion of pregnancy. Am J Clin Pathol 74:232–236
204. Salvador S, Rempel A, Soslow RA et al (2008) Chromosomal instability in fallopian tube precursor lesions of serous carcinoma and frequent monoclonality of synchronous ovarian and fallopian tube mucosal serous carcinoma. Gynecol Oncol 110:408–417
205. Samaha M, Woodruff JD (1985) Paratubal cysts: frequency, histogenesis, and associated clinical features. Obstet Gynecol 65:691–694
206. Saracoglu FO, Mungan T, Tanzer F (1992) Salpingitis isthmica nodosa in infertility and ectopic pregnancy. Gynecol Obstet Invest 34:202–205
207. Sasano H, Sato S, Yajima A et al (1997) Adrenal rest tumor of the broad ligament: case report with immunohistochemical study of steroidogenic enzymes. Pathol Int 47:493–496
208. Schaefer G (1970) Tuberculosis of the female genital tract. Clin Obstet Gynecol 13:965–998
209. Schiller HM, Silverberg SG (1971) Staging and prognosis in primary carcinoma of the fallopian tube. Cancer 28:389–395
210. Schmeler KM, Sun CC, Bodurka DC et al (2006) Prophylactic bilateral salpingo-oophorectomy compared with surveillance in women with BRCA mutations. Obstet Gynecol 108:515–520
211. Sebire NJ, Lindsay I, Fisher RA et al (2005) Overdiagnosis of complete and partial hydatidiform mole in tubal ectopic pregnancies. Int J Gynecol Pathol 24:260–264
212. Sedlis A (1978) Carcinoma of the fallopian tube. Surg Clin North Am 58:121–129
213. Seeber J, Reimer D, Muller-Holzner E et al (2008) Fallopian tube cancer associated with paraneoplastic dermatomyositis – asymptomatic multivisceral exacerbated dermatomyositis mimicking

recurrent widespread malignant disease: case report. Eur J Gynaecol Oncol 29:168–170
214. Seidman JD (1994) Mucinous lesions of the fallopian tube. A report of seven cases. Am J Surg Pathol 18:1205–1212
215. Seidman JD, Oberer S, Bitterman P et al (1993) Pathogenesis of pseudoxanthomatous salpingiosis. Mod Pathol 6:53–55
216. Seidman JD, Sherman ME, Bell KA et al (2002) Salpingitis, salpingoliths, and serous tumors of the ovaries: is there a connection? Int J Gynecol Pathol 21:101–107
217. Shaw PA, Rouzbahman M, Pizer ES et al (2009) Candidate serous cancer precursors in fallopian tube epithelium of *BRCA1/2* mutation carriers. Mod Pathol 22:1133–1138
218. Skinnider BF, Young RH (2004) Infarcted adenomatoid tumor: a report of five cases of a facet of a benign neoplasm that may cause diagnostic difficulty. Am J Surg Pathol 28:77–83
219. Snijders AM, Nowee ME, Fridlyand J et al (2003) Genome-wide-array-based comparative genomic hybridization reveals genetic homogeneity and frequent copy number increases encompassing CCNE1 in fallopian tube carcinoma. Oncogene 22:4281–4286
220. Snyder MJ, Bentley R, Robboy SJ (2006) Transtubal spread of serous adenocarcinoma of the endometrium: an underrecognized mechanism of metastasis. Int J Gynecol Pathol 25:155–160
221. Soderstrom RM (1985) Sterilization failures and their causes. Am J Obstet Gynecol 152:395–403
222. Stewart SL, Wike JM, Foster SL et al (2007) The incidence of primary fallopian tube cancer in the United States. Gynecol Oncol 107:392–397
223. Stock RJ (1983) Histopathologic changes in fallopian tubes subsequent to sterilization procedures. Int J Gynecol Pathol 2:13–27
224. Stuhlinger M, Rosen AC, Dobianer K et al (1995) HER-2 oncogene is not amplified in primary carcinoma of the fallopian tube. Austrian Cooperative Study Group for Fallopian Tube Carcinoma. Oncology 52:397–399
225. Su YN, Cheng WF, Chen CA et al (1999) Pregnancy with primary tubal placental site trophoblastic tumor – a case report and literature review. Gynecol Oncol 73:322–325
226. Sulak O, Malas MA, Esen K et al (2005) Uterine tube-ovary relationship and fimbrial development during the fetal period. Saudi Med J 26:1080–1084
227. Sweet RL, Blankfort-Doyle M, Robbie MO et al (1986) The occurrence of chlamydial and gonococcal salpingitis during the menstrual cycle. JAMA 255:2062–2064
228. Taylor HS, Vanden Heuvel GB, Igarashi P (1997) A conserved Hox axis in the mouse and human female reproductive system: late establishment and persistent adult expression of the Hoxa cluster genes. Biol Reprod 57:1338–1345
229. Tone AA, Begley H, Sharma M et al (2008) Gene expression profiles of luteal phase fallopian tube epithelium from BRCA mutation carriers resemble high-grade serous carcinoma. Clin Cancer Res 14:4067–4078
230. Tziortziotis DV, Bouros AC, Ziogas VS et al (1997) Clear cell hyperplasia of the fallopian tube epithelium associated with ectopic pregnancy: report of a case. Int J Gynecol Pathol 16:79–80
231. Ugur M, Turan C, Vicdan K et al (1996) Chronic ectopic pregnancy: a clinical analysis of 62 cases. Aust NZ J Obstet Gynaecol 36:186–189
232. Van Den Eeden SK, Shan J, Bruce C et al (2005) Ectopic pregnancy rate and treatment utilization in a large managed care organization. Obstet Gynecol 105:1052–1057
233. Vang R, Medeiros LJ, Fuller GN et al (2001) Non-Hodgkin's lymphoma involving the gynecologic tract: a review of 88 cases. Adv Anat Pathol 8:200–217
234. Vasquez G, Winston RM, Brosens IA (1983) Tubal mucosa and ectopic pregnancy. Br J Obstet Gynaecol 90:468–474
235. Verhage HG, Bareither ML, Jaffe RC et al (1979) Cyclic changes in ciliation, secretion and cell height of the oviductal epithelium in women. Am J Anat 156:505–521
236. Wallace TM, Hart WR (1991) Acute chlamydial salpingitis with ascites and adnexal mass simulating a malignant neoplasm. Int J Gynecol Pathol 10:394–401
237. Ward ME, Watt PJ, Robertson JN (1974) The human fallopian tube: a laboratory model for gonococcal infection. J Infect Dis 129:650–659
238. Werness BA, Guccion JG (1997) Tumor of the broad ligament in von Hippel-Lindau disease of probable mullerian origin. Int J Gynecol Pathol 16:282–285
239. Wild RA, Albert RD, Zaino RJ et al (1988) Virilizing paraovarian tumors: a consequence of Nelson's syndrome? Obstet Gynecol 71:1053–1056
240. Winkler B, Reumann W, Mitao M et al (1985) Immunoperoxidase localization of chlamydial antigens in acute salpingitis. Am J Obstet Gynecol 152:275–278
241. Yanai-Inbar I, Silverberg SG (2000) Mucosal epithelial proliferation of the fallopian tube: prevalence, clinical associations, and optimal strategy for histopathologic assessment. Int J Gynecol Pathol 19:139–144
242. Yanai-Inbar I, Siriaunkgul S, Silverberg SG (1995) Mucosal epithelial proliferation of the fallopian tube: a particular association with ovarian serous tumor of low malignant potential? Int J Gynecol Pathol 14:107–113
243. Yin Y, Ma L (2005) Development of the mammalian female reproductive tract. J Biochem 137:677–683
244. Young RH (2007) Neoplasms of the fallopian tube and broad ligament: a selective survey including historical perspective and emphasising recent developments. Pathology 39:112–124
245. Zheng W, Sung CJ, Cao P et al (1997) Early occurrence and prognostic significance of p53 alteration in primary carcinoma of the fallopian tube. Gynecol Oncol 64:38–48
246. Zweemer RP, van Diest PJ, Verheijen RH et al (2000) Molecular evidence linking primary cancer of the fallopian tube to BRCA1 germline mutations. Gynecol Oncol 76:45–50

12 Nonneoplastic Lesions of the Ovary

Julie A. Irving · Philip B. Clement

R. J. Kurman, L. Hedrick Ellenson, B. M. Ronnett (eds.), *Blaustein's Pathology of the Female Genital Tract (6th ed.)*, DOI 10.1007/978-1-4419-0489-8_12,

Nonneoplastic lesions of the ovary frequently form a pelvic mass and are often associated with abnormal hormonal manifestations, thus potentially mimicking an ovarian neoplasm on clinical examination, at operation, or on pathologic examination. Many occur in the reproductive years and may be associated with infertility. Their proper recognition is, therefore, important to allow appropriate, usually conservative therapy, thereby avoiding unnecessary oophorectomy. This chapter begins with a very brief overview of the embryology and gross anatomy of the normal ovary, and key aspects of normal ovarian histology are featured in the discussion of relevant nonneoplastic lesions.

Embryology and Gross Anatomy

Embryology

During the development of both male and female human embryos, primordial germ cells migrate from the yolk sac to the urogenital ridges via the hindgut approximately 3 weeks post fertilization. In the absence of sex-determining region Y, the germ cells are incorporated into a proliferating mass of surface epithelial cells. From the second to the early third trimester, this thickened cortical mass of proliferating epithelial and germ cells divides into small groups demarcated by strands of stromal tissue extending from the medulla to the cortex. The small groups of germ cells and epithelial cells are further subdivided into primordial follicles composed of single germ cells surrounded by a layer of epithelial cells, the primitive granulosa cells. Interstitial (Leydig) cells develop within the stroma of the second-trimester female gonad, but most of these cells degenerate by term. The few found in the hilum of the adult ovary are called hilus cells. Early epithelial proliferations, which in males contribute to the connection between the sex cords and the mesonephric tubules, undergo degeneration in gonads destined to become ovary, leaving a few tubular remnants in the ovarian hilum, the rete ovarii.

Gross Anatomy

The newborn ovary is a tan, elongated, and flat structure that lies above the true pelvis. It may have a lobulated appearance with irregular edges [162]. Its approximate dimensions are 1.3 × 0.5 × 0.3 cm, and its weight is less than 0.3 g [162]. The ovary enlarges, increases in weight 30-fold, and changes in shape throughout infancy and childhood, and at puberty, has the size and shape of an adult ovary and lies within the true pelvis.

Adult ovaries are ovoid, approximately 3–5 × 1.5–3 × 0.6–1.5 cm, and weigh 5–8 g. Their size and weight, however, vary considerably depending on their content of follicular derivatives. Their pink-white exterior in early reproductive life is usually smooth but becomes increasingly convoluted thereafter. Thin-walled, fluid-filled cystic follicles and bright yellow corpora lutea may be partially visible from the external aspect. Three poorly defined zones are discernible on the sectioned surface: an outer cortex, an inner medulla, and the hilus. Follicular structures (cystic follicles, corpora lutea, and corpora albicantia) are usually visible in the cortex and medulla [28].

After the menopause, the ovaries typically shrink to a size approximately one half their size during the reproductive era. Their size varies considerably, however, depending on their content of ovarian stromal cells and the number of unresorbed corpora albicantia. Most postmenopausal ovaries have a shrunken, gyriform, external appearance, but some have a smooth surface. The sectioned surface is usually firm and predominantly solid, although occasional cysts several millimeters in diameter (inclusion cysts) may be visible within the cortex. Small white scars (corpora albicantia) are typically present within the medulla. Thick-walled blood vessels may be appreciable within the medulla and hilus [28].

In the adult, the ovaries lie on either side of the uterus close to the lateral pelvic wall, behind the broad ligament and anterior to the rectum. Each ovary is attached along its anterior (hilar) margin by a double fold of peritoneum, the mesovarium, to the posterior aspect of the broad ligament. Each ovary is also attached at its medial pole to the ipsilateral uterine cornu by the ovarian (utero-ovarian) ligament and from the superior aspect of its lateral pole to the lateral pelvic wall by the infundibulopelvic (suspensory) ligament.

The blood supply of the ovary is derived from anastamoses formed by the ovarian artery, a branch of the aorta, and the ovarian branch of the uterine artery. Approximately ten arterial branches from this arcade penetrate the ovarian hilus and course through the medulla, becoming markedly coiled and branched [166]. At the corticomedullary junction, the medullary arteries and arterioles form a plexus from which smaller, straight cortical arterioles arise and penetrate the cortex in a radial fashion. These cortical arterioles branch and anastomose, forming sets of interconnecting vascular arcades that give rise to dense capillary networks within the theca layers of the ovarian follicles [166]. The veins within the ovary accompany the arteries and become large and tortuous in the medulla. The veins join together in the hilus, forming a plexus that drains into the ovarian veins [166]; the left and right ovarian veins drain into the left renal vein and the inferior vena cava, respectively. Ovarian lymphatics originate predominantly within the theca layers of the follicles, and traverse the ovarian stroma to form a plexus at the hilus. Efferent lymphatics enter the mesovarium and form the subovarian plexus with branches from the fallopian tube and uterine fundus. Leaving the plexus, they pass along the free border of the infundibulopelvic ligament enmeshed with the ovarian veins and drain into the upper paraaortic lymph nodes at the level of the lower pole of the kidney [158]. Accessory channels can bypass the subovarian plexus, passing through the broad ligament to the internal iliac, external iliac, and interaortic lymph nodes, or via the round ligament to the iliac and inguinal lymph nodes [158]. When the pelvic and paraaortic lymph nodes are extensively replaced by tumor, retrograde lymphatic flow may provide a rare route of tumor spread to the ovaries.

Congenital Lesions and Ectopic Tissues

Absent Ovary

In phenotypic females, absence of both ovaries usually is associated with an abnormal karyotype and a syndrome of gonadal dysgenesis. In such cases, bilateral streak gonads or a unilateral streak gonad and a contralateral intraabdominal testis are usually found. However, rare cases of truly agonadal individuals have been reported, usually with a karyotype that is 46XY, but rarely, 46XX [152]. Rare patients with ataxia telangiectasia have had no evidence of ovarian tissue at laparotomy.

Rarely, one ovary may be absent in an otherwise normal woman, usually representing an incidental finding at operation or postmortem examination. Associated findings frequently include agenesis or malformation of the ipsilateral fallopian tube, round ligament, kidney, or ureter, alone or in various combinations. The differential diagnosis includes: (1) ectopic ovary, which may lie at the level of the liver, close to the kidney, within the omentum [152], or within an inguinal hernia and (2) adnexal torsion with atrophy or autoamputation.

Lobulated, Accessory, and Supernumerary Ovary

Examples of lobulated, accessory, and supernumerary ovary are among the rarest of gynecologic abnormalities. A lobulated ovary is a normally situated ovary divided by one or several fissures into two or more lobes. The lobes may be completely separate or connected by fibrous tissue or ovarian stroma; rarely both ovaries may be affected. A closely related anomaly is an accessory ovary, a structure containing normal ovarian tissue located in the vicinity of a normal, eutopic ovary with which it has a direct or ligamentous attachment. A supernumerary ovary is a similar structure but located at some distance from, and not connected to, a eutopic ovary [65]. It may be pelvic, attached to the uterus, bladder, or pelvic walls, or retroperitoneal, within the omentum, periaortic area, or mesentery, or inguinal. In most cases, the accessory or supernumerary ovary is less than 1 cm in size, and smaller examples may go unrecognized at operation or autopsy; they are multiple and bilateral in some cases [65]. The ectopic ovarian tissue possesses the functional potential, as evidenced by persistent menses after bilateral oophorectomy, as well as the pathologic potential of normal ovaries. The presence of a supernumerary ovary therefore is one histogenetic mechanism for ovarian-type tumors in extraovarian sites. This derivation is even more likely for nonepithelial tumors such as a granulosa-theca tumors within the broad ligament, which are unlikely to have a mesothelial or secondary müllerian origin (➔ Chap. 13, Diseases of the Peritoneum).

Lobulated and accessory ovary are closely related embryonically. The former results from lobulation of the ovarian anlage, whereas the latter presumably develops from a slightly separated part of the otherwise normally developing and migrating ovarian anlage. Pathogenetic theories for supernumerary ovary include aberrent migration of part of the gonadal ridge after incorporation of the germ cells or, alternatively, arrest of some of the migrating germ cells in an ectopic location with inductive transformation of the surrounding tissue into ovarian stroma. As many as one third of patients with lobulated ovaries, accessory ovary, and supernumerary ovary have other congenital genitourinary abnormalities.

Adrenal Cortical Rests

Although accessory adrenal cortical tissue frequently is observed within the wall of the fallopian tube and the broad ligament, it is an extremely rare finding in the ovary [199]. The adrenal rests are typically yellow, spherical, and encapsulated nodules several millimeters in size (➔ *Fig. 12.1*). Adrenal cortical ectopia in these sites can be explained by the close proximity of the anlage of the adrenal cortex to the gonadal ridge during embryonic development. Ovarian adrenal cortical rests may be the

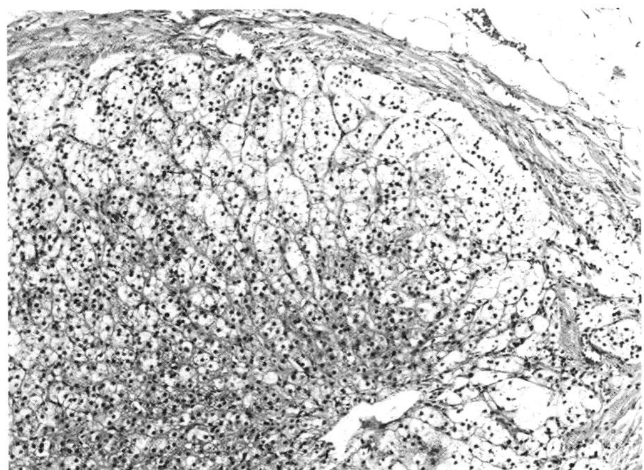

Fig. 12.1
Adrenal cortical rest within mesovarium

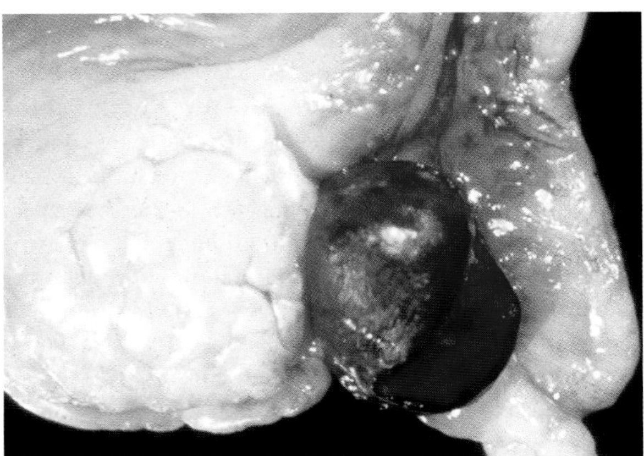

Fig. 12.2
Splenic–gonadal fusion. **A nodule of splenic tissue is contiguous with the surface of the ovary**

origin of occasional steroid cell tumors of the ovary that resemble adrenal cortical tissue in both their histologic appearance and endocrine manifestations.

Uterus-Like Ovarian Mass

Approximately ten reported examples of a uterus-like ovarian mass have been reported [150, 165, 190]. They have occurred in adult and occasionally early adolescent females (11–50 years of age) and were characterized by a central cavity lined by endometrial tissue and a thick wall of smooth muscle [150]. Additional findings have included an elevated CA-125 level (two cases), an associated breast carcinoma (two cases), and a contiguous endometrioid adenocarcinoma (one case). Although the lesion can be explained on the basis of an ovarian endometriotic cyst with smooth muscle metaplasia of its stromal component (endomyometriosis; see Chap. 13, Diseases of the Peritoneum), in some cases it may may be caused by a congenital malformation of the ipsilateral müllerian duct, an origin supported by the presence of congenital abnormalities of the urinary tract in three of the reported cases. In several other cases, however, residual ovarian parenchyma was identified at the periphery of the mass.

Splenic–Gonadal Fusion

Splenic–gonadal fusion (*Fig. 12.2*) is an extremely rare anomaly resulting from the fusion of the anlage of both organs during embryonic development. The male/female ratio is 9:1. Three examples have been described in newborn female infants, two of which were associated with partially undescended ovaries, as well as other, multiple, congenital anomalies [163]. All three cases were of the continuous type in which a cord-like structure connected the spleen to the left ovary or surrounding structures. In one of these cases, several intraovarian splenic nodules were found. A case of discontinuous splenic–gonadal fusion has been reported in a 19-year-old woman with no other apparent congenital abnormalities [126]. In an additional case, a 44-year-old woman had a septate uterus and a cluster of splenic nodules surrounding the otherwise normal left ovary; multiple adhesions made it difficult to ascertain if a splenic–ovarian cord was present [7]. The differential diagnosis in the discontinuous cases is with traumatic splenosis. Affected women usually have a history of trauma, and at laparotomy, splenic nodules are widely dispersed throughout the peritoneal cavity (Chap. 13, Diseases of the Peritoneum).

Prostatic Tissue

One case of ovarian ectopic prostatic tissue has been reported in a 70-year-old woman, postulated to arise from hilar mesonephric rests [192]. Prostatic tissue has also been described in mature cystic teratomas (Chap. 16, Germ Cell Tumors of the Ovary).

Infections

Common Bacterial Infections

Pelvic inflammatory disease (PID) of bacterial origin accounts for most ovarian infections in the western world. Although some studies have indicated that the presence of an intrauterine device (IUD) increases the risk of infection, other studies have shown that when the number of sexual partners are controlled for, IUDs do not increase the risk of PID [89]. Ovarian involvement by PID is almost always secondary to salpingitis and typically takes the form of a tuboovarian abscess (➋ *Fig. 12.3*), which usually is bilateral. The typical clinical manifestations are abdominal or pelvic pain, and, less often, fever, vaginal discharge or bleeding, and urinary symptoms [101]. An adnexal mass is palpable, demonstrable with imaging techniques, or visible at laparoscopy. A history of an acute infectious episode is present in only one third to one half of patients, suggesting that the subclinical infections are common [101]. A mixed flora with a preponderance of anaerobic organisms is typically recovered from the contents of the abscess [101]. With resolution, the only sequelae may be tuboovarian fibrous adhesions, but occasionally a healed abscess becomes a cyst.

A unilateral or bilateral ovarian abscess without tubal involvement is much rarer than a tuboovarian abscess. The former usually is secondary to direct or lymphatic spread of organisms from a nongynecologic pelvic inflammatory process, such as diverticulitis, appendicitis, inflammatory bowel disease, or postoperative pelvic infection. Rarely, an ovarian abscess is the result of a blood-borne infection. The external ovarian surface in such cases often is unremarkable, and the process may not be apparent until the organ is sectioned. Uncommonly, rupture of an ovarian or tuboovarian abscess leads to secondary peritonitis or, rarely, fistulas involving the colon, bladder, or vagina [191].

Milder, chronic, or recurrent forms of ovarian involvement by PID may take the form of a chronic perioophoritis, with periovarian and tuboovarian adhesions; sclerocystic ovarian changes may also be present. Rarely, a chronic ovarian abscess may result in a tumor-like mass, variably designated ovarian xanthogranuloma, xanthogranulomatous oophoritis, or inflammatory pseudotumor. The involved ovary in such cases is replaced by a solid or cystic, yellow, lobulated mass (➋ *Fig. 12.4*), characterized microscopically by foamy histiocytes admixed with multinucleated giant cells, plasma cells, fibroblasts, neutrophils, foci of necrosis, and fibrosis (➋ *Fig. 12.5*). Several additional examples of pseudotumorous xanthogranulomatous inflammation with a more diffuse involvement of the adnexa have been described [98].

Rare Bacterial Infections

Actinomycosis

Pelvic actinomyces infection is uncommon and usually represents a complication of an IUD, although most cases of IUD-related PID are nonactinomycotic [131, 179]. Almost 85% of cases have occurred in women who

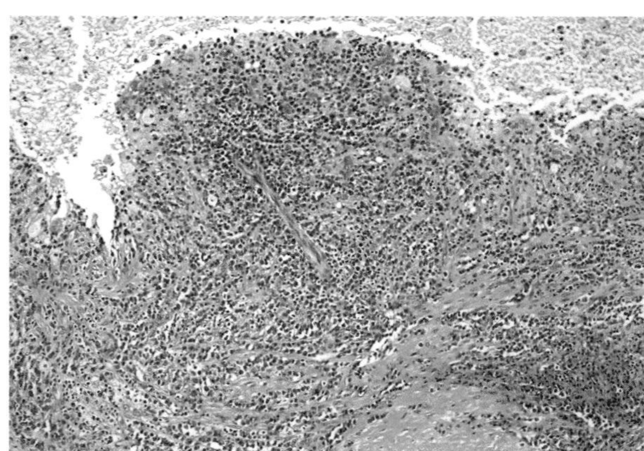

Fig. 12.3
Tuboovarian abscess. **Lining consists of inflammatory debris with subjacent granulation tissue**

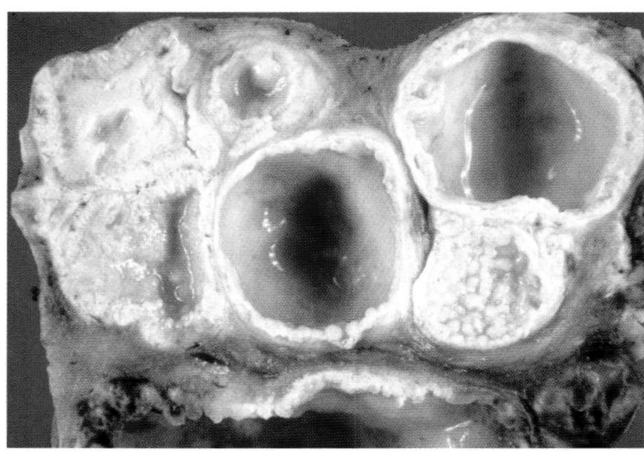

Fig. 12.4
Ovarian xanthogranuloma, sectioned surface

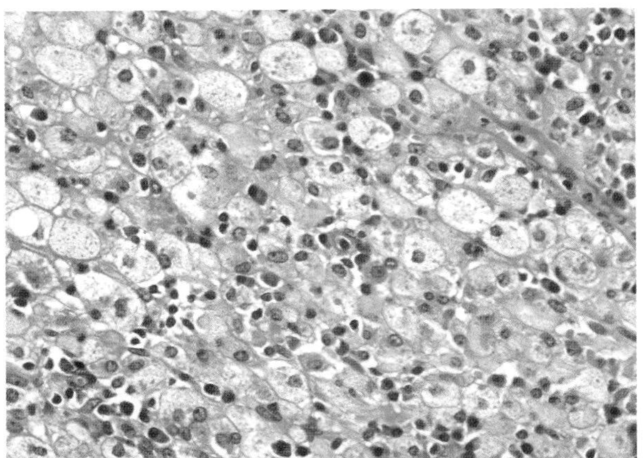

Fig 12.5
Xanthogranuloma of ovary. **Inflammatory reaction consists predominantly of foamy histiocytes**

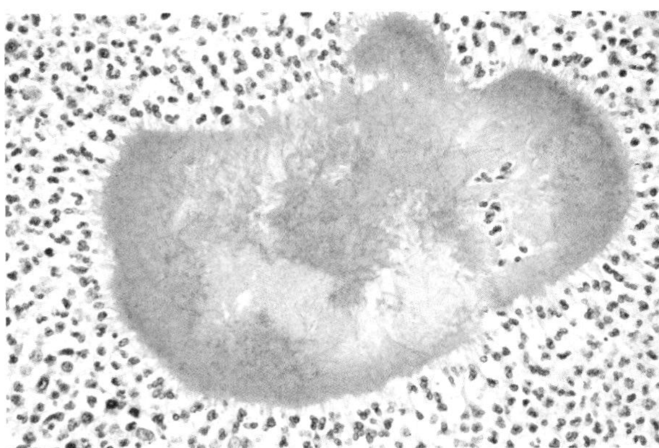

Fig. 12.6
Actinomycosis of ovary. **A colony of actinomyces (sulfur granule) is surrounded by a purulent exudate**

have had an IUD in place for 3 or more years [179], and the infection may be more common in women using plastic, rather than copper, IUDs. There is a high likelihood of subsequent sterility [179].

The adnexal involvement usually is unilateral, with destructive, often multiple, abscesses involving the ovary and fallopian tube (Chap. 11, Diseases of the Fallopian Tube and Paratubal Region) that may clinically mimic a pelvic malignancy [4]. Rarely, the characteristic actinomycotic (sulfur) granules are grossly visible within the abscess cavities. Microscopic examination typically reveals a nonspecific inflammatory response composed predominantly of neutrophils and foamy histiocytes sometimes admixed with lymphocytes and plasma cells. A specific diagnosis can be made only by finding the sulfur granules within the inflammatory exudate, but numerous blocks may be necessary to find them. The granules are composed of circumscribed rounded masses of basophilic, gram-positive, and argyrophilic bacteria growing as branching filaments with a characteristic radial or palisading pattern at the periphery of the granule (*Fig. 12.6*). A silver stain or fluorescent antibody stain may facilitate their detection [156], and negative modified acid-fast staining aids in the distinction from nocardia [161]. A diagnosis of actinomycosis may be made before salpingo-oophorectomy in some cases by finding the granules within endometrial curettings or cervico-vaginal smears. In one study, almost 90% of patients with actinomyces demonstrated by the latter method were found to have a tubo-ovarian abscess [22]. Sulfur granules should be distinguished from noninfectious, pseudoactinomyocotic radiate granules, which may be encountered in endometrial samples as a tisssue response to intrauterine devices (Chap. 7, Benign Diseases of the Endometrium) [161].

Tuberculosis

Tuberculous oophoritis is uncommon and usually secondary to tuberculous salpingitis (Chap. 11, Diseases of the Fallopian Tube and Paratubal Region). The tubes are almost always involved in tuberculosis of the female genital tract, but the ovarian parenchyma is affected in only 10% of cases [143]. Unilateral or bilateral adnexal masses, in some cases accompanied by an elevated CA-125 level, may clinically simulate an ovarian tumor. On macroscopic inspection, the ovaries are typically adherent to the tubal ampullae. Grossly visible caseation is rare. On histologic examination, the tuberculosis is typically confined to the cortex. In cases in which the ovary is enlarged, granulomas on the adjacent peritoneum may simulate metastatic ovarian cancer at operation [51, 143].

Malacoplakia

Of approximately 25 reported cases of gynecologic malacoplakia, only 4 have involved the ovary [27, 92]. Friable, yellow, focally hemorrhagic, and necrotic masses involve one or both ovaries and the ipsilateral fallopian tube. In one case, the process also involved contiguous portions of the small and large bowel, simulating a malignant ovarian tumor at operation [92]. Histologic examination reveals the typical features of malacoplakia

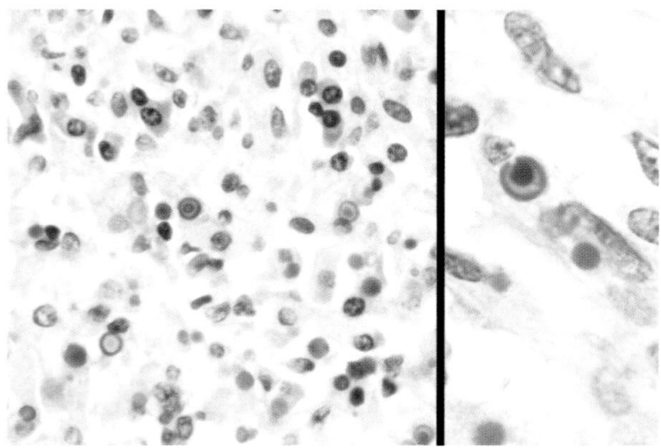

Fig. 12.7
Malacoplakia of ovary. **Mixed inflammatory infiltrate with epithelioid histiocytes, some containing Michaelis–Guttman bodies, shown at higher magnification in right image**

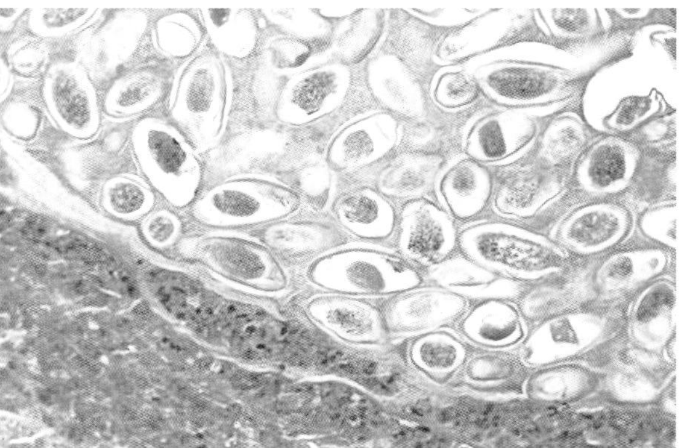

Fig. 12.8
Ovarian involvement by *Enterobius vermicularis*. **Note numerous and characteristically flat ova**

(*Fig. 12.7*). Organisms (*Escherichia coli* and/or *Enterococcus faecalis*) were demonstrated by culture in two of the cases [27, 92].

Leprosy

Although leprosy rarely involves the female genital tract, the ovary is the most commonly involved gynecologic site [19]. In one well-documented case, microscopic examination of the grossly normal ovaries revealed numerous vacuolated histiocytes within the ovarian stroma that contained *Mycobacterium leprae*. In chronic forms of leprous oophoritis, a chronic inflammatory cell infiltrate and fibrosis are seen, and bacilli usually are demonstrable.

Syphilis

For unknown reasons, syphilitic involvement of the ovary is very rare. Luetic oophoritis has been described in congenital, secondary, and tertiary forms of the disease. The pathology of these various stages is similar to those in extraovarian sites.

Parasitic Infections

Parasitic infestations of the ovary are extremely rare in most parts of the world. Ovarian schistosomiasis, however, is common in endemic areas; the fallopian tube is typically also involved [111]. Patients usually have lower abdominal pain, a pelvic mass, and occasionally irregular menses and infertility. The typical operative findings are an enlarged tube and ovary, numerous adhesions, and scattered peritoneal nodules that may simulate the implants of a malignant tumor. On histologic examination, granulomas, often containing eosinophils, surround schistosoma ova. Dense fibrosis frequently is seen in the later stages of the disease. We have seen an ovarian endometriotic cyst containing schistosoma ova, similar to a reported case of schistosomiasis involving intestinal endometriosis [1].

Ovarian involvement by *Enterobius vermicularis* usually is an incidental operative finding on the external surface, or, rarely, within the ovary [125, 159]. In several cases, there has been simultaneous involvement of the pelvic peritoneum, simulating a metastatic tumor [159]. The granulomas, which may undergo caseation and contain eosinophils, surround the adult female worms and ova (*Fig. 12.8*) [125]. The worms probably reach the peritoneal cavity by migration from the perineum through the lumen of the genital tract.

Rare cases of ovarian echinococcosis have been described [219]. In one of them, a typical hydatid cyst 12 cm in diameter involved the ovary.

Viral Infections

Oophoritis secondary to cytomegalovirus (CMV) can occur as an incidental finding in surgical or autopsy specimens in immunosuppressed patients, usually as part of a generalized infection [212]. On macroscopic examination, the ovaries are usually of normal size but contain foci of superficial cortical hemorrhagic necrosis several millimeters in size. Microscopic examination reveals foci of coagulative necrosis, with variable numbers of neutrophils, nuclear debris, and hemorrhage, as well as lymphocytes, plasma cells, and vascular dilatation in the surrounding stroma. Ovarian stromal and endothelial cells, even at a distance from the necrotic foci, contain typical intranuclear and occasional intracytoplasmic inclusion bodies. Immunohistochemical staining for CMV may facilitate the diagnosis in some cases [212], and intranuclear and intracytoplasmic herpes-type viral particles have been found on ultrastructural examination.

Mumps oophoritis as a clinical entity occurs much less commonly than mumps orchitis; clinical evidence of the lesion occurs in 5% of females with mumps. The pathology of the acute stage has not been well described. It is postulated that germ cell depletion secondary to mumps oophoritis may result in premature menopause and possibly an increased risk of ovarian cancer [39].

In view of the frequency of human papillomavirus (HPV) infection in the lower female genital tract, it is perhaps surprising that histologically documented examples of HPV infection of the ovary are exceptionally rare. We are aware of only one report in which HPV 16 DNA was detected by polymerase chain reaction (PCR) analysis with E6 and E7 primers in synchronous ovarian and cervical squamous cell carcinoma in situ lesions, the former presumably arising in an endometriotic cyst [112]. Lai et al. have found HPV-16 or HPV-18 DNA sequences by PCR in five of ten histologically normal ovaries [100].

Fungal Infections

Fungal infections of the ovary are extremely rare, even in patients with disseminated mycoses. Extremely rare examples of tuboovarian abscess due to *Blastomyces dermatitidis* have been reported [132]. In one case, the abscesses were bilateral and associated with miliary nodules involving the pelvic peritoneum, probably secondary to hematogenous spread from the lungs, while in another case, the infection was sexually transmitted.

Seven of 11 patients with coccidioidomycosis of the upper female genital tract had tuboovarian and peritoneal involvement; 2 of the 7 had concomitant coccidioidal endometritis [23]. One case of tuboovarian abscess caused by Aspergillus has been reported in an IUD user [94]. Rupture of the abscess led to generalized peritonitis.

Noninfectious Inflammatory Disorders

A variety of noninfectious, typically granulomatous, inflammatory disorders may involve the ovary. In addition, granulomas may be seen rarely in autoimmune oophoritis (page 35).

Foreign Body Granulomas

A variety of foreign materials may evoke a granulomatous reaction on the ovarian and extraovarian peritoneal surfaces, potentially mimicking a malignant tumor at operation. Examples include suture material, lipid material used in hysterosalpingographic contrast material, crystalline material such as talc, and keratin (➲ *Figs. 12.9* and ➲ *12.10*) from cystic teratomas and the squamous elements of endometrial and ovarian endometrioid adenocarcinomas (peritoneal and ovarian keratin granulomas are discussed in more detail in ➲ Chap. 13, Diseases of the Peritoneum) [120]. A foreign body reaction also occurs in response to starch granules from surgical gloves, starch-containing douche fluid, and lubricants. An 8-cm mass mimicking a primary ovarian tumor was due to a florid granulomatous reaction to oxidized cellulose (Surgicel™) [60]. Rarely, the starch granulomas are of the tuberculoid type, with or without caseous necrosis, and mimic tuberculosis on microscopic examination. Granulomatous oophoritis is occasionally a response to bowel contents

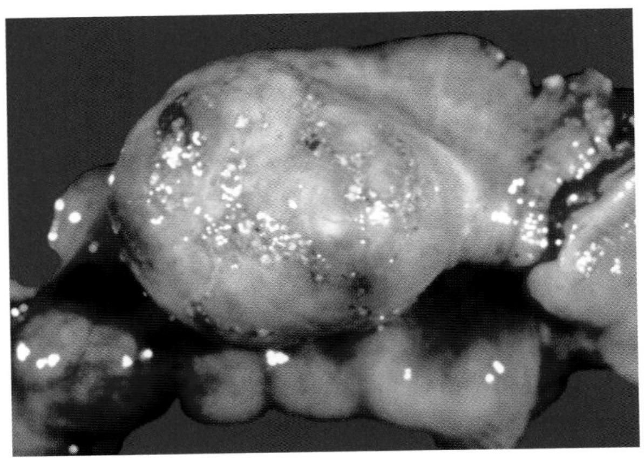

Fig. 12.9
Granulomatous reaction on ovarian surface potentially mimicking a malignant tumor. **Yellowish-brown granular deposits on ovarian surface, representing implants of keratin derived from an endometrial adenocarcinoma with squamous differentation**

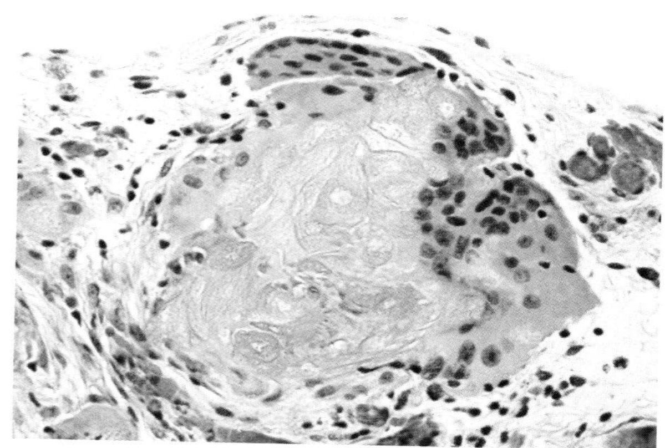

Fig. 12.10
Foreign body reaction to keratin implants on ovarian serosal surface. **There was a coexistent endometrial adenocarcinoma with squamous differentiation, confined to the uterus**

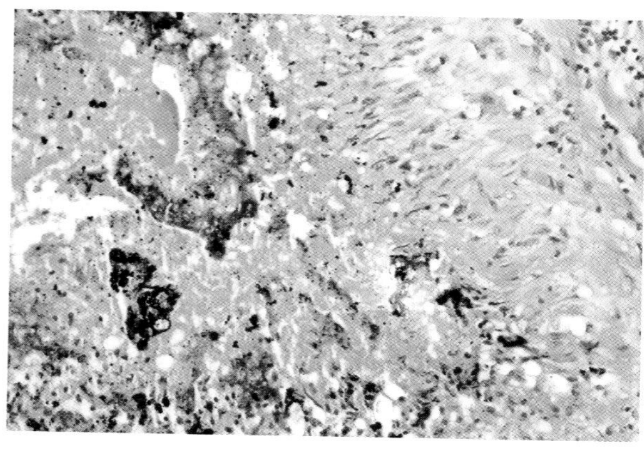

Fig. 12.11
Postcautery carbon pigment granuloma in ovary. **Note black carbon pigment. Palisading histiocytes are seen at the bottom and right**

that reach the ovary via a coloovarian fistula [61]. Foreign body-type granulomas containing brown to black carbon pigment have been described in the ovary secondary to laser or electrocautery treatment (*Fig. 12.11*) [201]. Implantation of gallstones on the peritoneum and ovarian surface ("ovarian cholelithiasis," *Fig. 12.12*; see also Fig. 13.3) may occur as a complication of laparoscopic cholecystectomy. It is also discussed in (Chap. 13, Diseases of the Peritoneum, page 3).

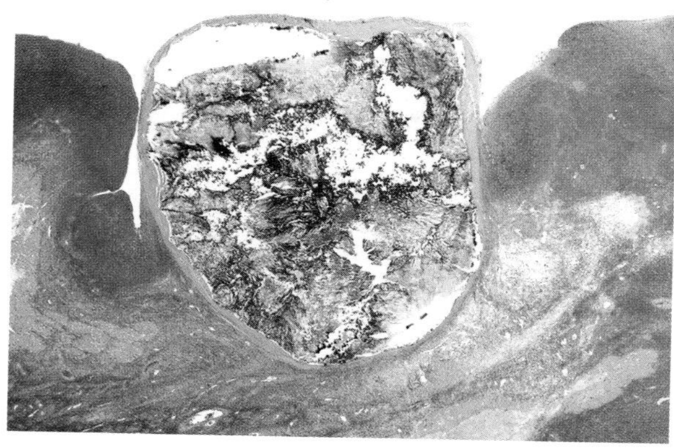

Fig. 12.12
Gallstone implanted on ovarian surface

Necrobiotic (Palisading) Granulomas

Necrobiotic granulomas have been encountered in the ovary, usually as an incidental microscopic finding [91, 120, 201]. In most cases, there is a history of an operation or cauterization involving the same ovary months to years earlier. The granulomas can be multiple and occasionally bilateral. A central zone of fibrinoid necrosis or hyalinization is usually surrounded by palisading, sometimes multinucleated, histiocytes and variable numbers of other inflammatory cells including lymphocytes, plasma cells, and eosinophils; a fibrous pseudocapsule forms in some of the cases (*Fig. 12.13*). Brown to black carbon pigment (as already noted) is typically present in multinucleated giant cells in postcautery palisading granulomas [201]. The differential diagnosis of palisading granulomas includes the other ovarian granulomas discussed in this chapter as well as necrotic pseudoxanthomatous nodules of endometriosis (Chap. 13, Diseases of the Peritoneum).

Granulomas Secondary to Systemic Diseases

In rare cases of ovarian involvement by sarcoidosis, the sarcoid granulomas were usually an incidental microscopic finding; in one case, findings of an elevated CA-125, an adnexal mass, and pelvic lymphadenopathy were clinically suspicious for malignancy [151]. Patients with systemic sarcoidosis may have involvement of other gynecologic sites or paraaortic lymph nodes. The finding of sarcoid-like granulomas in the ovary should alert the

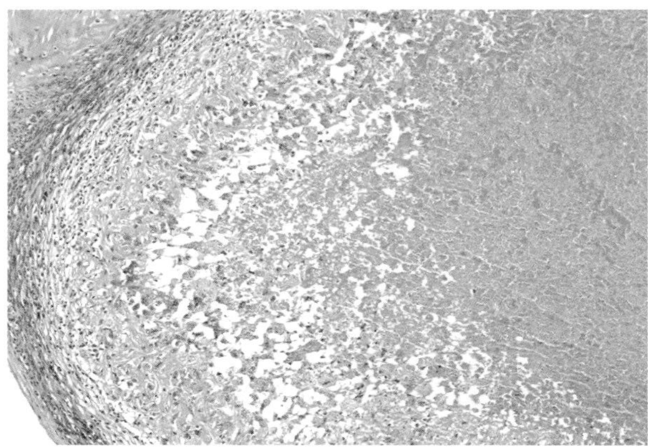

Fig. 12.13
Isolated palisading granuloma of ovary

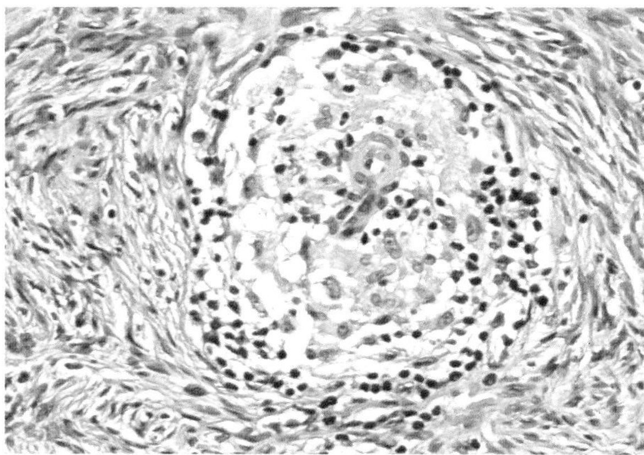

Fig. 12.14
Cortical granuloma. **Circumscribed collection of lymphocytes, spindle cells, and an occasional multinucleated giant cell lie within the ovarian stroma**

pathologist to the possibility of a rare dysgerminoma with a granulomatous reaction sufficiently extensive to obscure the malignant tumor cells. Crohn's disease is another rare cause of granulomatous oophoritis, usually caused by direct extension of the inflammatory process from the bowel [120]. The ipsilateral fallopian tube is also involved in most cases. Although not strictly granulomatous, mucicarminophilic histiocytosis can occasionally involve the ovary (Chap. 13, Diseases of the Peritoneum).

Cortical Granulomas

Cortical granulomas are common, incidental, microscopic findings within the ovarian cortex. The granulomas are spherical, well circumscribed, 100–500 μm in diameter, and are composed of spindle cells, epithelioid cells, lymphocytes, and, in some, multinucleated giant cells; occasional anisotropic fat crystals also may be seen (*Fig. 12.14*) [77, 120]. Hughesdon suggested that the granulomas become fibrotic with time, potentially accounting for at least some of the spherical, cloud-like, hyaline scars commonly encountered in the cortical stroma of postmenopausal women [77]. These scars resemble corpora fibrosa but usually are distinguishable from the latter by their more superficial location within the cortex, greater cellularity, weaker eosinophilia, and the presence of a reticulin framework [77]. It also has been suggested that hyaline scars may represent foci of atrophic stromal endometriosis, luteinized stromal cells, or ectopic decidua [77].

The frequency of cortical granulomas appears to be related to age. They are not usually encountered before the age of 30 years, but Hughesdon found active lesions in 40% of women over the age of 40 years; the number of lesions per cross section of ovary increased in successive decades [77]. The clinical significance, if any, of cortical granulomas is unknown. Possible associations with ovarian stromal hyperplasia, endometrial carcinoma, or both have been suggested but not demonstrated consistently.

Surface Proliferative Lesions

The Surface Epithelium, Inclusion Glands and Cysts, and Metaplasias

The normal ovarian surface epithelium consists of a single, focally pseudostratified layer of modified mesothelial cells. The cells vary from flat to cuboidal to columnar, and several types may be seen in different areas of the same ovary. Squamous metaplasia of the surface epithelium has been recently described in patients on long-term peritoneal dialysis [76]. The surface cells are separated from the underlying stroma by a distinct basement membrane. In oophorectomy specimens, the epithelium is almost always denuded as a result of handling by the surgeon and pathologist, as well as drying artifact as a result of delayed fixation. Preserved epithelium is usually confined to sulci and areas protected by surface adhesions. The surface epithelial cells are immunoreactive for cytokeratin, Ber-EP4, calretinin, desmoplakin, vimentin, and receptors for estrogen, progesterone, and epidermal growth factor receptors, but not desmin [47, 102].

Surface epithelial inclusion (SEI) glands and their cystic counterparts, SEI cysts, arise from cortical invaginations of the ovarian surface epithelium that have lost their connection with the surface. SEI glands and cysts can be found in ovaries from females of all ages, including fetuses, infants, and adolescents [16, 18]. With advancing age, their frequency increases to the extent that they are common in the late-reproductive and postmenopausal age groups.

SEI cysts may be visible on gross inspection of the ovary (*Fig. 12.15*), although most SEI glands and cysts are appreciable only on microscopic examination; cysts greater than 1 cm in diameter are designated a cystadenoma (Chap. 14, Surface Epithelial Tumors of the Ovary). SEI glands and cysts are usually multiple, scattered singly or in small clusters throughout the superficial cortex (*Fig. 12.16*); less commonly, they extend into the deeper cortical or medullary stroma. They are typically lined by a single layer of columnar cells that in postmenopausal patients is often ciliated, mimicking tubal (endosalpingeal) epithelium. Psammoma bodies may be seen within the cysts and the adjacent stroma (*Fig. 12.16*) and, rarely, within cervicovaginal Papanicolaou smears [108]. Similar glands, with or without associated psammoma bodies, encountered on the ovarian surface, within periovarian adhesions, and elsewhere on the peritoneum and in the omentum, are designated endosalpingiosis (Chap. 13, Diseases of the Peritoneum).

Less commonly, the lining of the glands and cysts consists of other müllerian cell types (endometrioid, mucinous) or nonspecific, flat, cuboidal, or columnar cells; rarely, apocrine metaplasia may be seen within a SEI cyst. An Arias–Stella-like reaction has been described within SEI glands in pregnant patients [18]. One study found that hyperplastic and metaplastic changes within SEI glands are more common in women with polycystic ovarian disease or endometrial carcinoma, suggesting a possible hormonal basis for these changes (*Fig. 12.17*) [167]. A rare pseudoneoplastic alteration in SEI glands is a striking vacuolar, presumably hydropic, cytoplasmic change of the lining cells. In such cases, abundant clear cytoplasm displaces the nucleus, potentially mimicking signet-ring cell carcinoma, especially when the cells proliferate to form solid nests (*Fig. 12.18*). Awareness of this phenomenon, additional sectioning (if necessary) to

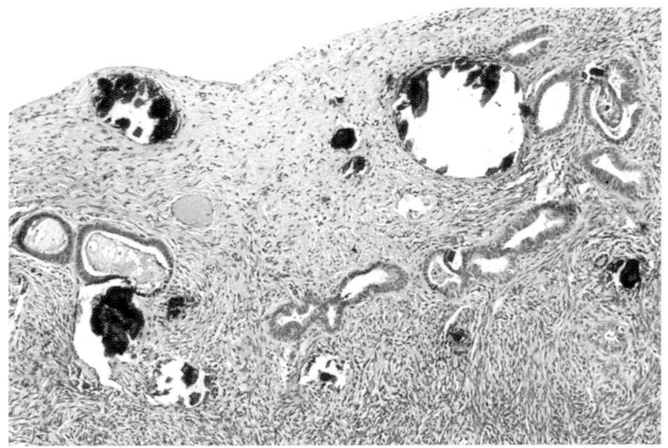

Fig. 12.16
Epithelial inclusion glands and small cysts, lined by a single layer of columnar cells. **Psammoma bodies are present within an occasional gland or cyst but are mostly in the adjacent stroma**

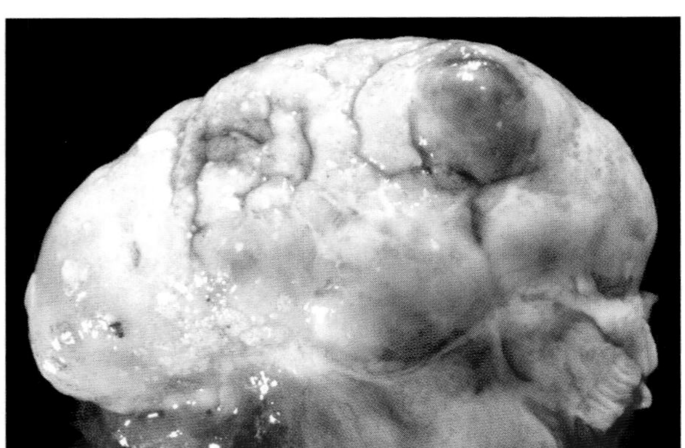

Fig. 12.15
Several epithelial inclusion cysts bulge from the ovarian surface

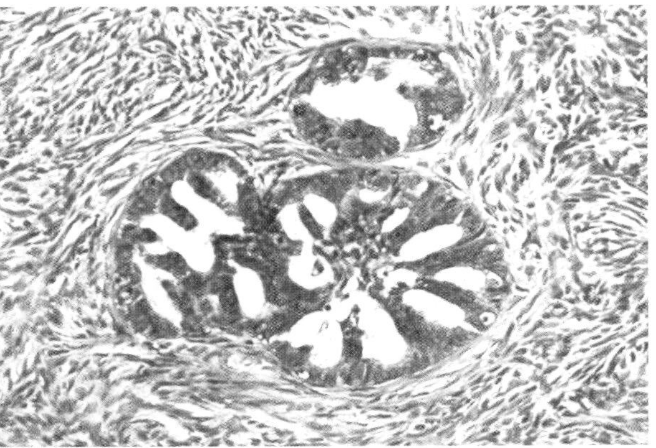

Fig. 12.17
Atypical epithelial inclusion cyst. **A cribriform pattern is present**

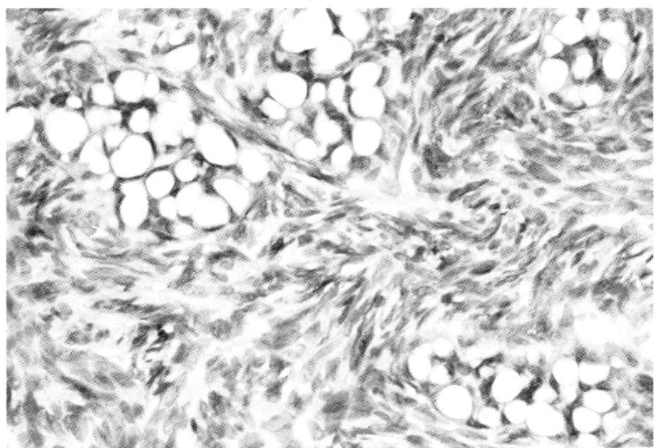

Fig. 12.18
Vacuolar change within surface epithelial inclusion glands. **The change results in solid nests within the ovarian stroma simulating signet-ring cells**

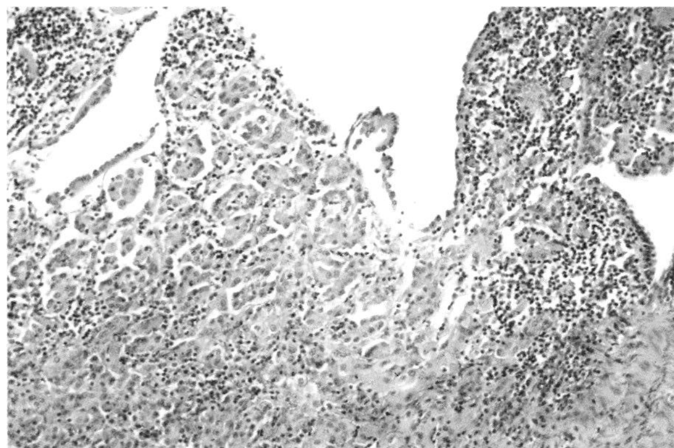

Fig. 12.19
Mesothelial proliferation on ovarian surface. **Mesothelial cells, growing in papillary pattern, are admixed with lymphocytes. The mesothelial cells exhibit mild nuclear pleomorphism and occasional multinucleation**

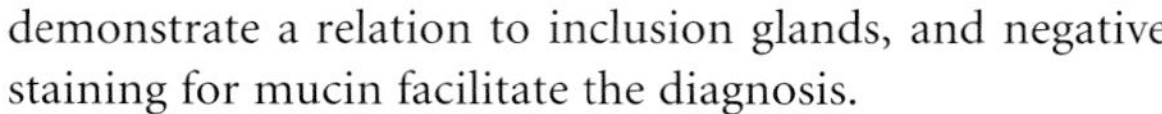

demonstrate a relation to inclusion glands, and negative staining for mucin facilitate the diagnosis.

SEI glands and cysts are likely the site of origin for most common epithelial tumors of the ovary. Several studies have found that patients with ovarian carcinoma have an increased number of SEI cysts (or surface epithelial invaginations, their precursors) in the contralateral ovary compared to controls [128, 205]. Additional support for this hypothesis is provided by the occasional presence of dysplastic changes within their linings [42, 183] as well as immunoreactivity for a variety of ovarian epithelial tumor markers including WT-1, epithelial membrane antigen, CA-125, CA-19-9, CEA, human chorionic gonadotropin (hCG), and placental alkaline phosphatase [17, 26, 79, 188]. SEI cysts are distinguished from cystadenomas by their smaller size (see earlier). The differential diagnosis also includes other unilocular ovarian cysts.

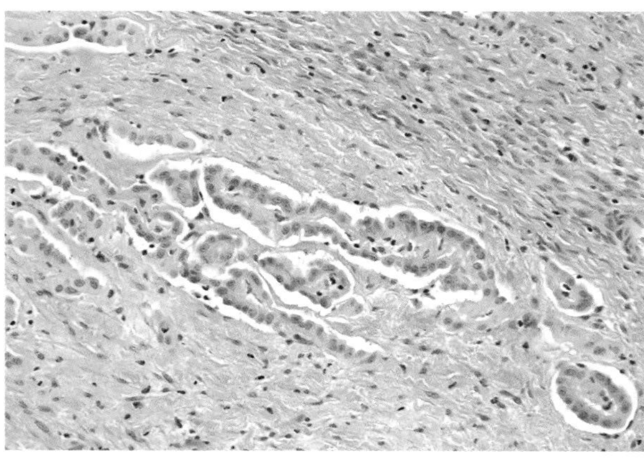

Fig. 12.20
Mural mesothelial hyperplasia within the wall of an ovarian serous borderline tumor

Mesothelial Proliferations

Proliferation of mesothelial cells on the ovarian surface, within periovarian fibrous adhesions or elsewhere on the pelvic peritoneum, is usually a response to pelvic inflammation but also occurs in response to ovarian tumors and endometriosis. Florid examples may be associated with complex glandular and papillary proliferations of mesothelial cells that may exhibit mild to moderate atypia (*Fig. 12.19*). Such a process may simulate stromal invasion in a borderline ovarian tumor (*Fig. 12.20*) or simulate a metastatic carcinoma, primary serous surface carcinoma, or malignant mesothelioma. This subject is discussed in more detail in Chap. 13, Diseases of the Peritoneum.

Surface Stromal Proliferations

Nodular, polypoid, and papillary stromal projections from the ovarian surface are a common incidental microscopic finding in women of late-reproductive and postmenopausal age. These projections are composed of ovarian stroma, exhibiting varying degrees of hyalinization covered

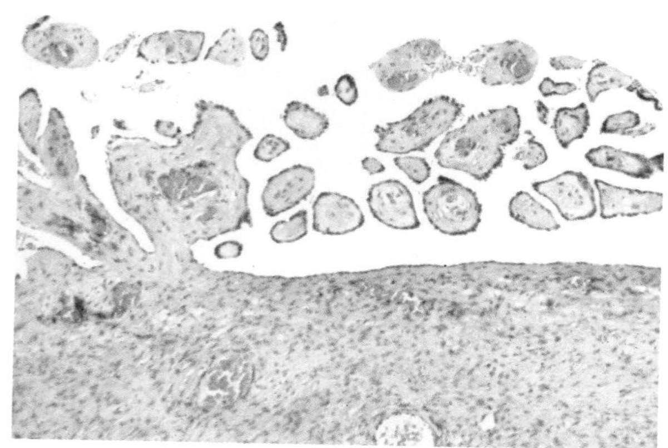

Fig. 12.21
Ovarian surface stromal proliferation. **Papillary and nodular stromal proliferation involves ovarian surface**

by a single layer of surface epithelium (Fig. 12.21). Detachment of these structures may give rise to "collagen balls" occasionally found in peritoneal washings [214]. Surface stromal proliferations are typically 1–3 mm in maximal dimension and do not exceed 1 cm, the arbitrary dividing line between this type of proliferation and a serous surface papilloma.

Nonneoplastic Lesions of the Follicular and Stromal Elements

This section describes the wide spectrum of nonneoplastic lesions that arise from the ovarian follicles and stroma. Many of them are secondary to ovarian stimulation by pituitary or chorionic gonadotropins and may be associated with excessive production of estrogens, androgens, or both. Although most nonneoplastic proliferations of Leydig cells are not of stromal origin, these lesions are most conveniently discussed in this section.

Solitary Follicle Cysts and Corpus Luteum Cysts

Solitary follicle cysts and corpus luteum cysts are nonneoplastic lesions derived from their normal counterparts.

For details regarding normal folliculogenesis, the reader is referred elsewhere, but a brief overview is provided here [28]. Normal follicular maturation begins during the luteal phase and continues throughout the follicular phase of the next cycle. Each month, usually only one developing follicle is dominant and achieves ovulation. The other developing follicles undergo atresia, and continued shrinkage and hyalinization of an atretic follicle produces the corpus fibrosum, a small scar consisting of a wavy strand of hyaline tissue. In the absence of fertilization, the collapsed ovulatory follicle becomes the corpus luteum of menstruation (CLM), a 1.5- to 2.0-cm round structure with a festooned contour and a center filled with a gray, focally hemorrhagic coagulum, and a color that changes during the luteal phase from brown to orange-yellow as it acquires more lipid. Occasionally, the CLM is cystic, but this feature is more characteristic of the corpus luteum of pregnancy (which may be indistinguishable from the CLM but is usually larger and bright yellow). During a period of several months, the CLM involutes by progressive fibrosis and shrinkage, with conversion to a corpus albicans. Most corpora albicantia and corpora fibrosa are resorbed.

Clinical Features

Solitary follicle cysts (FCs) are most common in nonpregnant women of reproductive age, particularly around the menarche and menopause. FCs may also occur during fetal life, in newborns, throughout childhood, and rarely after the onset of the menopause [104, 198]. Solitary or multiple FCs can be a component of the McCune–Albright syndrome (polyostotic fibrous dysplasia, cutaneous melanin pigmentation, and endocrine organ hyperactivity), as discussed later, and postpubertal women with cystic fibrosis may be predisposed to the development of solitary FCs [186]. Corpus luteum cysts (CLCs) usually occur during the reproductive era but rarely are found in neonates or follow sporadic ovulation in a postmenopausal woman.

The proportion of FCs and CLCs associated with clinical manifestations is unknown, because many are incidentally discovered by pelvic ultrasononography, laparoscopy, or laparotomy. Patients with clinically evident FCs and CLCs typically have either a palpable adnexal mass or manifestations related to increased estrogen production that may include isosexual precocity or pseudoprecocity, menstrual disturbances including amenorrhea and postmenopausal bleeding, or endometrial hyperplasia. A CLC is the most common finding in the ovarian remnant syndrome (see page 39). An uncommon clinical presentation of FCs and CLCs is rupture, which may cause abdominal pain, hemoperitoneum [67], and rarely exsanguination. Rupture is more likely to occur in patients receiving anticoagulant therapy or in those with bleeding diatheses [210]. Additionally, FCs occurring in utero or during the neonatal period may be complicated by adnexal torsion as well as hemorrhage and rupture; most regress during the first 4 months of life.

Gross Findings

Solitary follicle cysts (FCs) and corpus luteum cysts (CLCs) are thin walled and unilocular, ranging from 3 to 8 cm in diameter, although larger examples occur rarely (➲ *Fig. 12.22*), especially during pregnancy and the puerperium (see following). They usually have smooth surfaces and thin walls. CLCs are characterized by the presence of a convoluted yellow lining (➲ *Fig. 12.23*). The contents of FCs and CLCs vary from serous or serosanguineous fluid to clotted blood.

Microscopic Findings

FCs are lined by an inner layer of granulosa cells that may be focally denuded and an outer layer of theca interna cells (➲ *Fig. 12.24a*). The cells in either layer may be luteinized. Distinction between the two layers can be facilitated by a reticulin stain, which reveals dense reticulum surrounding the theca cells but sparse or absent reticulum in the granulosa layer (➲ *Fig. 12.24b*). CLCs exhibit a convoluted lining composed of large luteinized granulosa cells

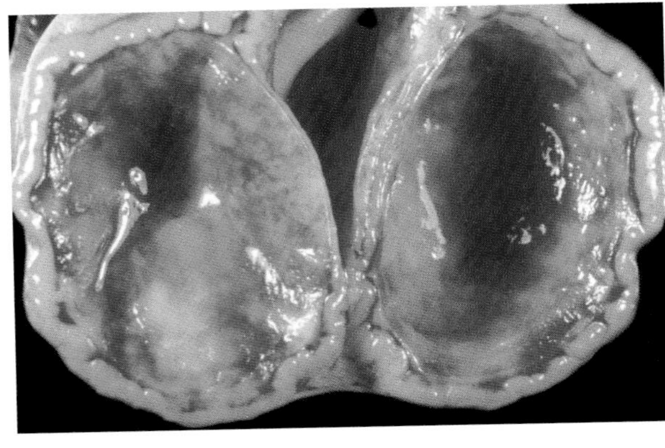

Fig. 12.23
Corpus luteum cyst. **Note the convoluted yellow lining**

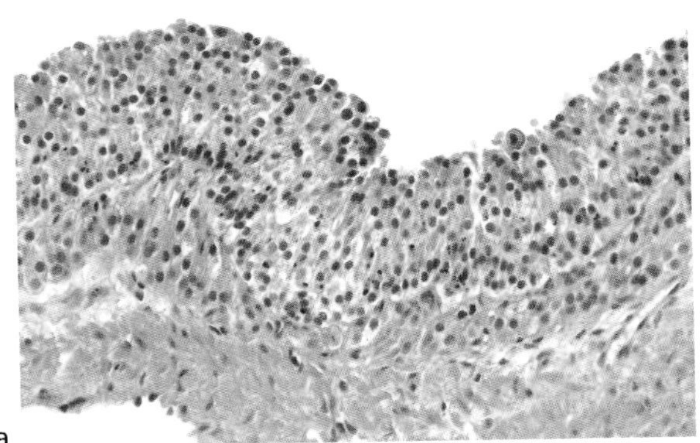

a

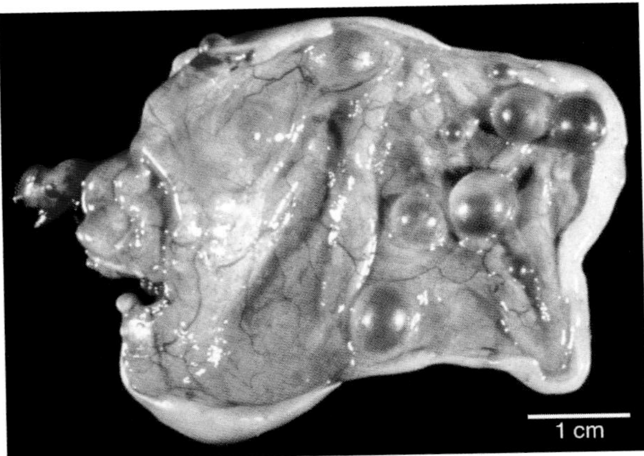

Fig. 12.22
Follicle cyst

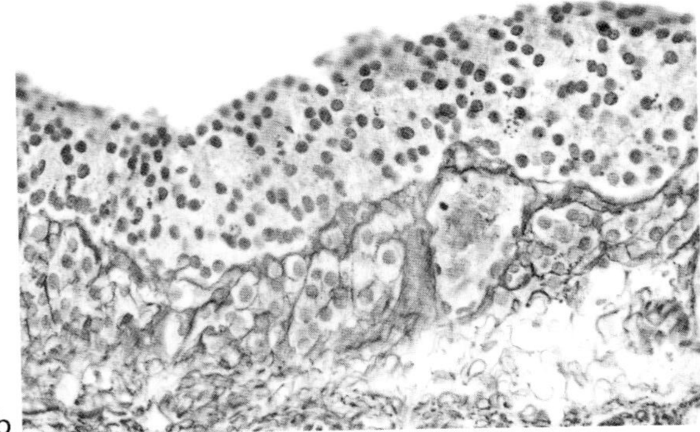

b

Fig. 12.24
Follicle cyst. **(a) Lining consists of an inner layer of granulosa cells and an outer layer of theca interna cells. (b) Distinction between the two layers is enhanced with a reticulin stain, showing a reticulum network within the theca interna layer and an absence of reticulin within the granulosa layer**

and an outer layer of smaller luteinized theca interna cells, with a prominent inner layer of connective tissue (➋ *Fig. 12.25*). CLCs associated with pregnancy typically have characteristic hyaline bodies and calcific foci within the granulosa cells. Focal infarction of a CLC, possibly secondary to inadequate hCG production, has been encountered in association with tubal pregnancy. Involution of FCs and CLCs usually leads to the formation of corpora fibrosa and corpora albicantia, respectively; rarely, the latter may be cystic.

A rare type of solitary FC, designated "large solitary luteinized follicle cyst of pregnancy and the puerperium" with distinctive clinical and pathologic features, occurs during pregnancy and the puerperium and is presumably related to hCG stimulation [29]. Patients present with a palpable adnexal mass (most commonly at the first postpartum visit) or are found to have a unilateral ovarian cyst at cesarean section. No endocrine disturbances have been reported to date. On gross inspection, the cyst resembles a typical FC except for its large size (median diameter 25 cm). On microscopic examination, the cyst is lined by one to many layers of luteinized granulosa and theca cells that are usually indistinguishable. Nests of luteinized cells may be embedded within the fibrous tissue of the cyst wall. The cells have abundant vacuolated to eosinophilic cytoplasm, vary considerably in size and shape, and in all the reported cases have exhibited focal marked nuclear pleomorphism and hyperchromasia; mitotic figures have been absent (➋ *Fig. 12.26*).

Pathogenesis

The pathogenesis of some FCs is probably related to abnormalities in the release of anterior pituitary gonadotropins, such as a failure of the normal preovulatory luteinizing hormone surge. FCs occurring in females with abnormalities in gonadotropin release can be multiple, bilateral, recurrent, and in some cases are accompanied by corpora lutea and the possibility of pregnancy. Other FCs appear to be autonomous and do not recur following removal. Girls with the McCune–Albright syndrome and precocious

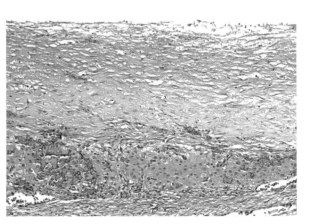

Fig. 12.25
Corpus luteum cyst. **A prominent inner layer of connective tissue is present**

a
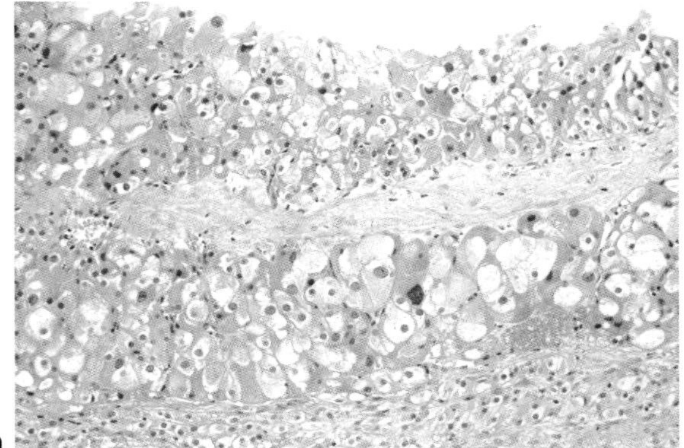

b
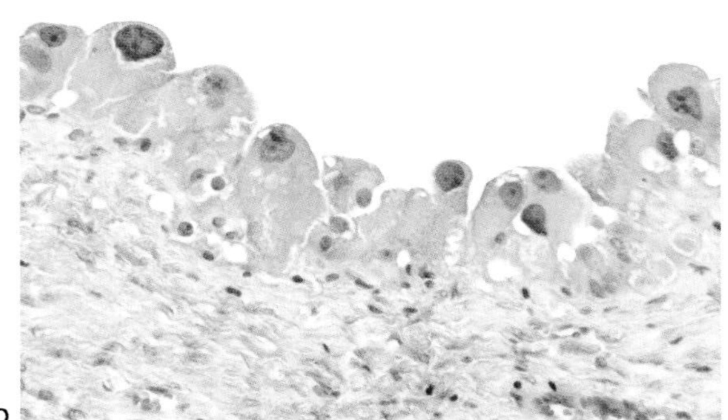

Fig. 12.26
Large solitary luteinized follicle cyst of pregnancy and puerperium. **(a) Luteinized cells with abundant eosinophilic to clear cytoplasm line a cyst (*upper*) and lie within its fibrous wall (*lower*). Note focal nuclear atypicality. (b) Higher-power view of lining cells showing marked nuclear hyperchromasia and atypicality**

puberty secondary to a FC may have elevated gonadotropin levels, whereas in others with this syndrome, the FCs appears to be mediated by a gonadotropin-independent mechanism [211]. Treatment with low-dose phasic oral contraceptives [24], gonadotropin-releasing hormone analogues [14], and tamoxifen [33] may also stimulate the development of FCs.

Clinical Behavior and Treatment

Most cases of FC and CLC regress spontaneously within 2 months; observation of small ovarian cysts in women of reproductive age is justifiable for this period. Regression in some cases can be accelerated by administration of a high-dose, combined estrogen–progestogen preparation. FCs associated with isosexual pseudoprecocity can sometimes be treated by cyst puncture; others may require surgical removal. Persistence of a cyst suggests that it is neoplastic, and in these cases laparotomy or laparoscopy is necessary.

Differential Diagnosis of Solitary Follicle Cysts

Solitary cysts of follicular origin should be distinguished on microscopic examination from other solitary unilocular ovarian cysts. Cysts otherwise identical to FCs and CLCs but less than 3 cm in diameter are generally regarded as physiologic, that is, cystic follicles and cystic corpora lutea, respectively. A simple cyst is of unknown origin because its lining has disappeared, was destroyed by rubbing or dessication after its removal, or because the lining consists of a thin layer of nonspecific epithelial-like cells. Additional sections may reveal theca lutein cells in its wall or foci of serous, endometrioid, or another type of epithelial lining, allowing a more specific diagnosis. Even a rare cystic struma ovarii may be misdiagnosed as a simple cyst if inconspicuous follicles in its wall are overlooked or not sampled.

Cysts of surface epithelial origin that are usually small, incidental microscopic findings are designated inclusion cysts. Otherwise, similar cysts measuring more than 1 cm are considered neoplastic and designated serous, endometrioid, or mucinous cystadenoma, depending on the nature of their lining (➲ Chap. 14, Surface Epithelial Tumors of the Ovary). Epidermoid cysts are those lined exclusively by mature squamous epithelium and are considered either monodermal teratomas or of surface epithelial origin [142, 217]. The finding of Walthard nests in the walls of some of these cysts favor the latter origin in at least some cases [217]. Endometriotic cysts are readily distinguishable by their characteristic lining of endometrial epithelium and stroma and pigmented histiocytes within their walls (➲ Chap. 13, Diseases of the Peritoneum). Solitary FCs should also be distinguished from those of rete origin that are located within the hilus (see page 40) [174].

Differentiating large FCs from unilocular cystic granulosa cell tumors of either the adult or juvenile type (➲ Chap. 15, Sex Cord-Stromal, Steroid Cell, and Other Ovarian Tumors with Endocrine, Paraendocrine, and Paraneoplastic Manifestations) may be difficult, especially if such a tumor has an orderly arrangement of granulosa and theca cells in its wall. Cystic granulosa cell tumors, however, are usually considerably larger than FCs, and the two cell types usually have a more disorderly pattern that may include obvious penetration of the cyst wall. In contrast to the large solitary luteinized FC of pregnancy, cystic granulosa cells tumors rarely have cells with bizarre nuclei.

Hyperreactio Luteinalis

Hyperreactio luteinalis (HL) is characterized by bilateral ovarian enlargement caused by the presence of multiple luteinized follicle cysts secondary to hCG stimulation [129].

Clinical Features

Hyperreactio luteinalis most commonly occurs with disorders resulting in high levels of hCG such as hydatidiform moles, choriocarcinoma, fetal hydrops (usually secondary to Rh sensitization but rarely of nonimmunologic type), and multiple gestations. Sixty percent of cases unassociated with gestational trophoblastic disease (GTD), however, have accompanied a singleton pregnancy. The frequency of HL in women with GTD ranges from 10% to 50% depending on whether it is detected by clinical examination or sonography. The presence of HL in these patients may indicate an increased risk for persistent or metastatic GTD (➲ Chap. 20, Gestational Trophoblastic Tumors and Related Tumor-Like Lesions) [129]. Rarely, HL has been preceded by the polycystic ovary syndrome (PCOS) [15].

HL can be detected as a pelvic mass during any trimester, at cesarean section, or rarely during the puerperium. Symptoms are usually absent, but hemorrhage into the cysts may cause abdominal pain. Rarely, the involved ovary undergoes torsion or rupture, sometimes with intraabdominal bleeding, which can be fatal. In contrast to patients with the ovarian hyperstimulation syndrome (see following), ascites is rare. In patients with HL accompanying GTD, HL is detected at the time of the diagnostic curettage or during the postoperative follow-up period [157]. In approximately 15% of cases unassociated with trophoblastic disease, there has been virilization of the patient but not the female infant [15]. Plasma testosterone levels have been elevated in these patients as well as nonvirilized patients with trophoblastic disorders, with the levels proportional to the degree of ovarian enlargement.

Pathological Findings

On macroscopic examination, multiple, usually bilateral, thin-walled cysts cause moderate to massive ovarian enlargement (up to 35 cm) (➲ *Fig. 12.27*). The cysts are filled with clear or hemorrhagic fluid. Microscopic examination reveals FCs with prominent luteinization of the theca interna cells and, in some cases, the granulosa cells (➲ *Fig. 12.28*). Occasionally, the latter have bizarre nuclei. There is usually marked edema of the theca layer and the intervening stroma; the latter frequently contains luteinized stromal cells.

Pathogenesis

Because HL occasionally occurs in patients with otherwise normal pregnancies and normal hCG levels, and because HL does not occur in all women with high hCG levels, factors other than the latter likely play a role in the pathogenesis of HL. An increased ovarian sensitivity to hCG in patients with the disorder has been suggested [21]. One study found elevated levels of other hormones, specifically progesterone, prolactin, and estradiol, in patients with HL and GTD, possibly implicating these hormones in the pathogenesis or maintenance of HL [148].

Clinical Behavior and Treatment

The cysts of HL typically involute during the puerperium, but occasionally regression is incomplete until 6 months postpartum. In exceptional cases, the cysts regress spontaneously during pregnancy. In cases associated with

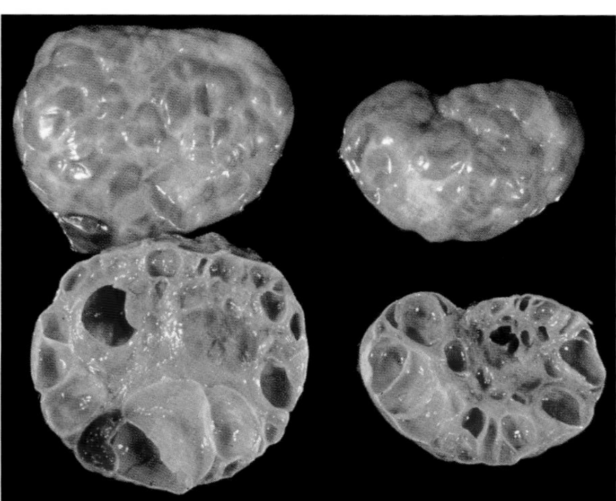

■ Fig. 12.27
Hyperreactio luteinalis. **Multiple thin-walled follicle cysts are present within the cortex**

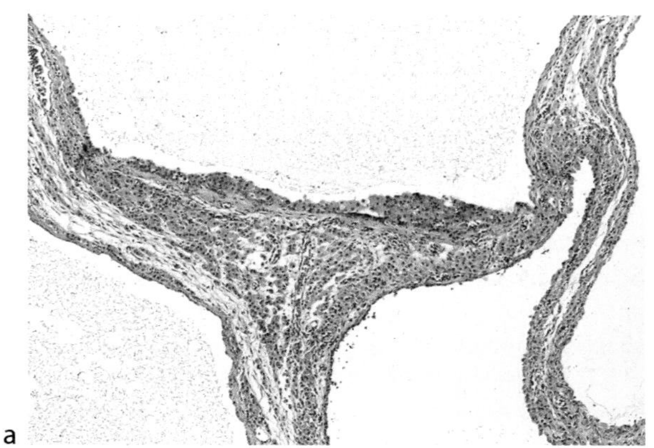

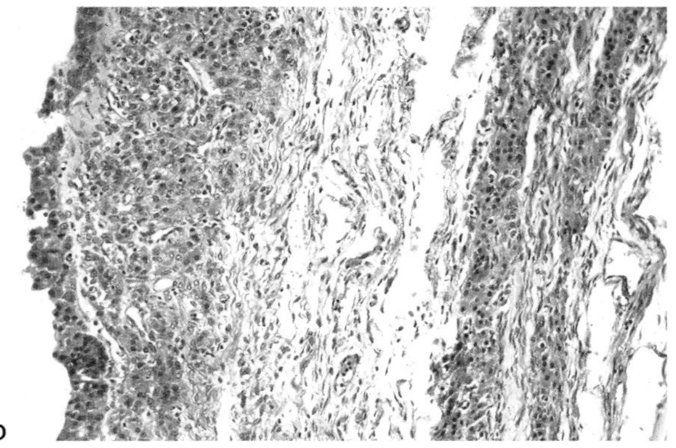

■ Fig. 12.28
Hyperreactio luteinalis. **Fluid-filled, thin-walled follicle cysts (a), lined by granulosa and theca layers, both of which exhibit marked luteinization and shown at higher magnification in (b)**

trophoblastic disease, gradual regression typically occurs 2–12 weeks after uterine evacuation, but occasionally the cysts persist for months or even enlarge after the hCG level has returned to normal [129, 157]. Operative treatment of HL is needed only to remove infarcted tissue, control hemorrhage, or reduce ovarian size to diminish androgen production in virilized patients. Rarely, HL recurs in subsequent pregnancies.

Differential Diagnosis

Lack of knowledge of the gross appearance of the enlarged ovaries of hyperreactio luteinalis and their resultant misinterpretation as cystic ovarian tumors occasionally leads to an unwarranted bilateral oophorectomy. If doubt exists, a frozen section examination of the cyst wall should solve the problem. Rarely, pregnancy luteomas coexist with HL, heightening the suspicion of a neoplastic process on gross examination.

Ovarian Hyperstimulation Syndrome

An iatrogenic form of HL, the ovarian hyperstimulation syndrome (OHS), occurs in a variable proportion of women undergoing ovulation induction, typically after the administration of follicle-stimulating hormone (FSH) followed by hCG, or rarely clomiphene alone [68]. The frequency of OHS has varied widely in the literature; it has been suggested that some degree of the syndrome exists in all patients undergoing ovulation induction, with a frequency of 0.5–5% for severe forms [86]. OHS occurs only after ovulation, is more severe in patients who conceive, and is particularly prone to occur if the ovaries were polycystic before the institution of therapy. Several cases of spontaneous OHS unassociated with ovulation induction have been reported, usually in the setting of high hCG levels, for example, with molar or multiple gestations [3, 49, 86]. There have been several reports of OHS occurring in association with severe hypothyroidism, usually in pregnant but occasionally in nonpregnant patients [49]. Careful selection of patients and regulation of drug dosage by monitoring estrogen levels and ovarian size have reduced the frequency of OHS. Current evidence has identified hCG to be a potent inducer of vascular endothelial growth factor; the latter is thought to have a major role in the increased vascular permeability associated with severe OHS [124, 209]. Recently, a mutation in the FSH receptor was found to be associated with recurrent, familial OHS [193].

In severe cases, the ovaries become massively enlarged, and ascites, sometimes with hydrothorax, (acute Meigs' syndrome) develops as a result of increased serosal permeability. Elevation of serum estrogens, progesterone, and testosterone typically occurs [68]. Hemoconcentration with secondary oliguria and thromboembolic phenomena is a life-threatening complication. High plasma levels of renin, aldosterone, and antidiuretic hormone may occur [68]. Patients usually respond to conservative therapy, such as cyst aspiration under ultrasonic guidance, and the cysts usually regress within 6 weeks. Operative intervention is only necessary in the rare instance of cyst torsion or rupture. Histologic examination of the ovaries reveals changes identical to those seen in HL, with the additional finding of one or more corpora lutea.

Rare Disorders Characterized by Multiple Follicle Cysts

Depending on the method of detection, as many as 75% of girls with juvenile hypothyroidism have multicystic ovaries [105, 168]. Rarely, the ovarian enlargement may be the presenting sign leading to a diagnosis of hypothyroidism. The clinical features, in addition to ovarian enlargement and manifestations of hypothyroidism, include varying degrees of sexual precocity in more than half the patients and galactorrhea. The sexual precocity and galactorrhea appear to be caused by increased secretion of pituitary gonadotropins and prolactin, respectively. A similar clinical picture can occur rarely in adults. Histologic examination, which has been performed in only a few cases, has revealed FCs, some with luteinization of the theca interna layer. In two cases, a depletion of primordial follicles was also noted. Treatment with thyroxin has resulted in regression of the hypothyroidism, the ovarian cysts, and sexual precocity, and a decline in the elevated gonadotropin and prolactin levels.

Multiple, bilateral FCs associated with estradiol production have been described in infants born before the 30th week of gestation [184]. The cysts, which are secondary to elevated levels of FSH and luteinizing hormone (LH), appear at a postconception age that slightly precedes the expected time of delivery. It is postulated that marked prematurity is associated with relative insensitivity of the hypothalamus and anterior pituitary to negative feedback by estradiol.

Congenital deficiency of 17-hydroxylase, an enzyme required for both cortisol and estrogen synthesis, results in low estrogen levels and secondarily elevated levels of FSH and LH [202]. The rare patients with this disorder have congenital adrenal hyperplasia, hypokalemia, hypertension, primary amenorrhea, absence of sexual maturation, and ovarian enlargement due to multiple, bilateral FCs. A late onset of the disorder can mimic idiopathic hirsutism or polycystic ovary syndrome (PCOS).

Polycystic Ovary Syndrome

Polycystic ovary syndrome (PCOS) is an idiopathic disorder, which can have a signficant impact on the health of affected women, with respect to potential reproductive, metabolic, cardiovascular, and neoplastic sequelae [50, 103, 144]. It is characterized by inappropriate gonadotropin secretion, chronic anovulation, hyperandrogenism, increased peripheral conversion of androgens to estrogens, and sclerocystic ovaries. Many patients also have abnormal glucose tolerance and hyperinsulinemia. The current clinical spectrum of PCOS is broader than that initially defined by Stein and Leventhal in 1935 (as the Stein–Leventhal syndrome), and as is discussed here, PCOS may be the result of multiple potential etiologies and be associated with variable clinical presentations [50, 144]. Some patients with PCOS have the HAIR-AN syndrome of hyperandrogenism (HA), insulin resistance (IR), and acanthosis nigricans (AN), a syndrome discussed after the section on stromal hyperthecosis, a closely related disorder that overlaps both clinically and pathologically with PCOS.

Clinical Features

PCOS has been estimated to affect 5–10% of the female population [93], making it the most common endocrinopathy in women of reproductive age [58]. The clinical diagnosis of PCOS can be challenging, as presenting signs and symptoms are heterogeneous. Recently, an international consensus group has provided updated diagnostic criteria, requiring at least two of the following: oligomenorrea/amenorrhea, hyperandrogenism/hyperandrogenemia, and polycystic ovaries on ultrasonography; other possible medical diagnoses must also be excluded [204]. Notably, the diagnosis of PCOS can be made in the absence of polycystic ovaries [50]. The affected women are typically in their third decade with a history of dysfunctional uterine bleeding related to anovulatory cycles and typically of peripubertal onset, or less commonly, secondary amenorrhea as well as subfertility or infertility; 80% exhibit evidence of hyperandrogenism, usually in the form of hirsutism [58, 202]. A significant proportion of women with PCOS are overweight or obese, which can exacerbate the underlying metabolic and reproductive abnormalities [50]. In addition to hirsutism, cutaneous manifestations include acne, androgenetic alopecia, and acanthosis nigricans (➋ HAIR-AN syndrome) [103]. Hyperinsulinemia, insulin resistance, and impaired glucose tolerance are present in the majority of patients, particularly in those who are obese, although these features may not appear until later in life [50, 144]. Frank virilization (clitoromegaly, deep voice, temporal baldness, male habitus) is rare, and if of sudden onset, suggests stromal hyperthecosis or a virilizing ovarian tumor rather than PCOS. The ovaries may or may not be palpably enlarged. Pelvic ultrasonography may help in establishing the diagnosis, as discussed below. Patients with PCOS have an increased risk for cardiovascular disease secondary to obesity, impaired glucose tolerance, and in some cases, hypertension and dyslipidemias [50].

Studies indicate that PCOS has a strong familial component and may be the most common endocrinopathy causing familial hirsutism. Single-gene mutations may rarely be implicated, but more likely the syndrome is multigenic; candidate genes involved in regulation of the hypothalamic–pituitary–ovarian axis are the major focus in current studies, including microarray analysis of target tissues [46, 50, 215].

Manifestations of unopposed estrogenic stimulation that occur in a significant proportion of patients include endometrial hyperplasia or, in approximately 1% of patients, endometrial carcinoma. The tumors typically occur in obese patients under the age of 40; conversely, up to one quarter of patients with endometrial carcinoma under 40 have PCOS [37]. The tumors are almost always grade 1 endometrioid adenocarcinomas that are confined to the endometrium or invade the myometrium superficially [37]. The carcinomas are rarely, if ever, fatal, and many are reversible with progesterone therapy or by ovulation induction (➋ Chap. 8, Precursor Lesions of Endometrial Carcinoma and ➋ Chap. 9, Endometrial Carcinoma). A wide variety of extrauterine tumors have also been described in patients with PCOS, but their association is probably coincidental [37]. One study, however, has found a 2.5-fold-increased risk of epithelial ovarian cancer in women with PCOS [177].

Gross Findings

Both ovaries, or rarely only one, are typically rounded and two to five times the normal size; the ovarian volume can be three times that of control subjects [107]. Occasionally, however, the ovaries may be of normal size. Superficial cortical cysts are usually visible beneath the white ovarian surface. Examination of the sectioned ovarian surface reveals a thickened, white, capsule-like superficial cortex and numerous subjacent cysts, typically of similar size and usually less than 1 cm in diameter (*Fig. 12.29*). There is usually a central zone of stroma with only rare or no stigmata of ovulation (corpora lutea or albicantia).

Ovarian tissue from patients with PCOS is rarely encountered, as treatment by ovarian wedge resection is no longer used. Polycystic ovaries are defined ultrasonographically by the presence of 12 or more follicles measuring 2–9 mm in diameter or increased ovarian volume (>10 cm^3) [9]. The typical gross or ultrasonographic ovarian morphology, however, is unnecessary to make the diagnosis of PCOS, and in the absence of the typical clinical findings, is not diagnostic of the syndrome (Differential Diagnosis) [202].

Microscopic Findings

The superficial cortex is fibrotic and hypocellular, resembling a capsule (*Fig. 12.30a*) and may contain prominent thick-walled blood vessels [78]. Tongues of similarly fibrotic stroma may extend from the superficial cortex into the deeper cortex and medulla. The cysts are atretic cystic follicles and have an inner lining of several layers of nonluteinized, focally exfoliated granulosa cells. There is a prominent outer layer of luteinized theca interna cells (*Fig. 12.30b*), giving rise to the term follicular hyperthecosis, but other studies have found that cystic follicles in women with PCOS differ from those in normal women only in their increased number [107]. Maturing follicles up to midantral stage and atretic follicles exhibiting prominent luteinization of the theca interna may be twice as numerous as in normal ovaries [78]. Primordial follicles are normal in number and appearance [78]. As noted, stigmata of prior ovulation are typically absent, but corpora lutea have been described in as many as 30% of otherwise typical cases of PCOS [78]. The deeper cortical and medullary stroma may have as much as a fivefold increase in volume. The stroma contains luteinized stromal cells in 80% of cases and, less commonly, foci of smooth muscle [78]. Nests of ovarian hilus (Leydig) cells may be more numerous in patients with PCOS than in age-matched controls.

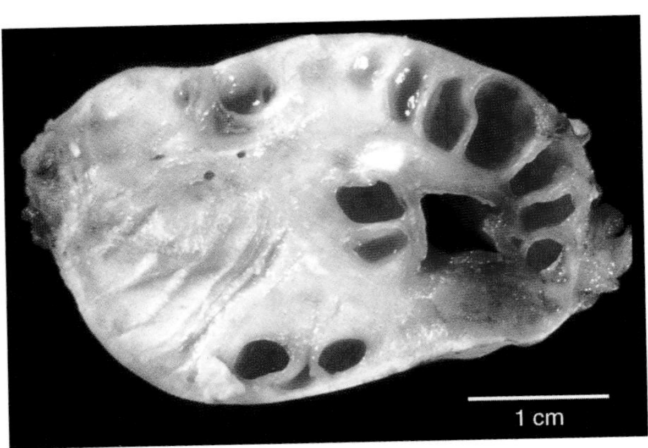

Fig. 12.29
Polycystic ovary disease. **Superficial cortical fibrosis and multiple cystic follicles are present**

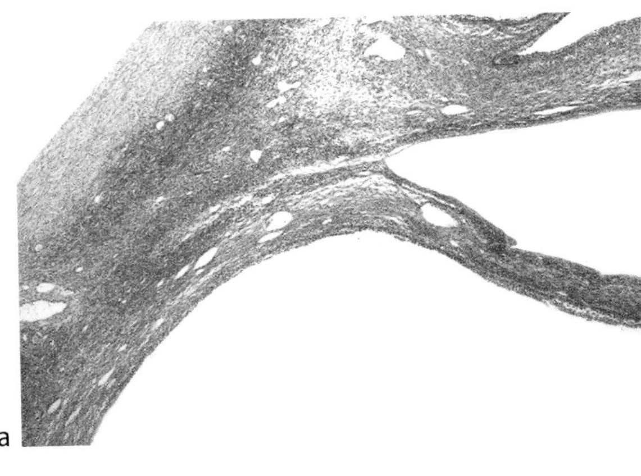

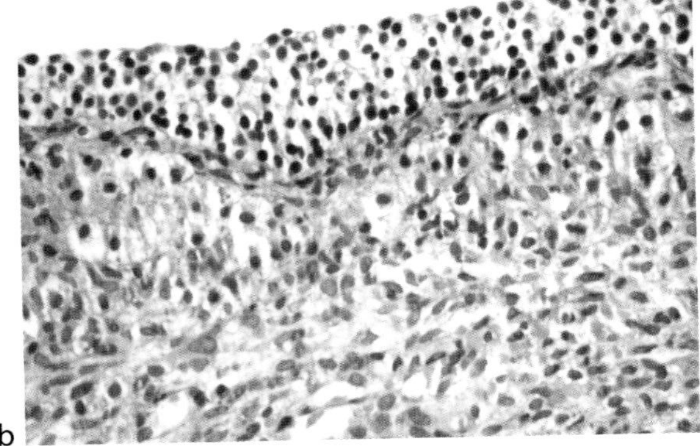

Fig. 12.30
Polycystic ovary disease. **(a) Multiple cystic follicles lie beneath the superficially fibrotic cortex. (b) A cystic follicle is lined by nonluteinized granulosa cells and an outer, thicker layer of luteinized theca interna cells**

Pathophysiology

The pathophyiology of PCOS is complex, and the initiating factor(s) is (are) not yet completely understood [202]. A cardinal finding is an elevation of the serum level of LH or an elevated LH:FSH ratio; of note, documentation of abnormal gonadotropin levels is not required for the diagnosis of PCOS in routine clinical practice, since their release is pulsatile and concentrations vary throughout the menstrual cycle [50]. LH stimulates the follicular theca interna cells to produce androstenedione, which is converted peripherally, primarily within adipose tissue, to estrone (E_1), and to a lesser extent, testosterone. More importantly, ovarian follicular production of testosterone is also increased, leading to the small increases in serum testosterone concentrations that are present in PCOS. Estradiol (E_2) levels remain normal or low normal, resulting in an elevated E_1/E_2 ratio. Elevated E_1 levels, and in some patients an increased secretion of inhibin, a nonsteroidal peptide produced by granulosa cells [200], inhibit secretion of FSH. An elevated LH:FSH ratio is thus a characteristic finding in PCOS. Ovarian estrogen production in PCOS is markedly diminished, probably a result of inactivity of the FSH-dependent aromatase system within the granulosa cells. Inadequate intrafollicular estrogen synthesis, increased intrafollicular androgens, and an elevated LH:FSH ratio result in cessation of follicle growth at the midantral stage, anovulation, and sclerocystic ovaries.

A number of interlinked factors potentially play a role in initiating or perpetuating PCOS. According to Taylor [202], "there are correlations between gonadotropin secretion, insulin secretion, and androgen secretion across the spectrum of patients with PCOS such that it remains impossible to determine the primary etiologic factor in the vast majority of patients." Obesity-related factors including hyperestronemia due to conversion of androstenedione to E_1 and hyperinsulinemia play a role in the pathogenesis of PCOS, and the increase in obesity in the United States has been postulated as an explanation for the reported increased incidence of PCOS [50]. An estimated 20–30% of patients with PCOS have adrenal androgen excess, as manifested by an elevated androgen dehydroepiandrosterone sulfate (DHES) and abnormal adrenal androgen responses to ACTH [169, 216]. The increased adrenal androgens can lead to hyperestronemia and consequently an elevated LH:FSH ratio. Although some investigators believe that the adrenal abnormalities (which may include late-onset congenital adrenal hyperplasia) are a primary disturbance, others have concluded that they are secondary to the hormonal milieu of PCOS [25].

Insulin resistance and hyperinsulinemia are present in most obese and nonobese women with PCOS, although these features tend to be more severe in the former group [140]. Despite peripheral insulin resistance, ovarian tissues remain responsive to insulin in women with PCOS. Insulin appears to amplify LH action, enhancing production of estradiol and progesterone from the follicular granulosa cells and possibly contributing to the arrest of follicle growth [64]. As discussed later (➋ HAIR-AN syndrome), insulin and insulin-like growth factor stimulate proliferation of ovarian stromal cells and their production of androgen. Hyperinsulinemia thus can increase circulating androgen levels (and by peripheral conversion, estrone) in patients with PCOS. The resultant hyperandrogenism may in turn increase insulin resistance.

Hyperprolactinemia is present in approximately 15–25% of patients with PCOS, but recent evidence indicates that they are distinct entities, with galactorrhea a feature of hyperprolactinemia but not PCOS; in one recent study, elevated plasma prolactin levels were attributable to pituitary adenomas and drug-related effect in 19% and 23% of cases, respectively [50, 54].

Differential Diagnosis

PCOS is a clinicopathologic syndrome, and the finding of polycystic ovaries with little or no evidence of prior ovulation does not warrant the diagnosis per se in the absence of the usual clinical findings. Polycystic ovaries that resemble those of PCOS are seen occasionally in prepubertal children and in otherwise normal girls during the first few years after the onset of puberty. Similarly, ultrasonographic studies have revealed that ovulating women with minor evidence of hyperandrogenism, but without menstrual irregularity, can have polycystic ovaries similar to those of patients with overt clinical manifestations except that the ovaries also contain corpora lutea and albicantia [160]. Thus, the boundary between the clinical syndrome of PCOS and normality is not clear cut.

Although PCOS does not cause a problem in differential diagnosis with a neoplasm for the pathologist, the clinical manifestations may suggest the possibility of an androgenic or estrogenic ovarian tumor, particularly in the exceptional cases in which the disease coexists with a nonfunctioning ovarian neoplasm. In some cases, in which the associated ovarian tumor is capable of function, such as a Sertoli–Leydig cell tumor, it may be difficult to determine which lesion was responsible for the endocrine manifestations.

The differential diagnosis includes a wide variety of other disorders that result in abnormal gonadotropin release, chronic anovulation, and sclerocystic ovaries. Sclerocystic ovaries are a nonspecific morphologic expression of chronic anovulation in the premenopausal patient and can accompany (1) adrenal lesions such as Cushing's syndrome, congenital adrenal hyperplasia (most commonly 21-hydroxylase or 11-beta-hydroxylase deficiency), and virilizing adrenal tumors; (2) primary hypothalamic–pituitary disorders; and (3) ovarian lesions that produce excessive quantities of estrogens or androgens, including sex cord-stromal tumors, steroid cell tumors, and nonneoplastic lesions such as Leydig cell hyperplasia and stromal hyperthecosis. As previously noted, the latter overlaps both clinically and pathologically with PCOS, and the two disorders may represent opposite poles of a single disease spectrum. Sclerocystic ovaries have also been described in patients with autoimmune oophoritis [10], after long-term use of oral contraceptives, in association with periovarian adhesions, and after long-term androgen therapy in female to male transsexuals [149]. An association between a PCOS-like syndrome and the use of the antiepileptic drug valproate has been found [80].

Stromal Hyperplasia and Stromal Hyperthecosis

Normal, spindle-shaped stromal cells, which have scant cytoplasm and resemble fibroblasts, are typically arranged in whorls or a storiform pattern within a dense reticulum network and a variable amount of collagen, which is most abundant in the superficial cortex. Stromal cells are typically immunoreactive for CD56, WT-1, vimentin, and estrogen and progesterone receptors [8, 69, 122]. In many women of late-reproductive and postmenopausal age, there is a decrease in stromal volume and cellularity, with an increase in collagen. A variety of other cells may be found within the ovarian stroma, most of which are probably derived from the spindle-shaped stromal cells, including luteinized stromal cells, enzymatically active stromal cells, decidual cells, endometrial stromal-type cells (stromal endometriosis, "ovarian stromatosis") (➲ Chap. 13, Diseases of the Peritoneum), smooth muscle cells, fat cells, stromal Leydig cells, and rare cells of neuroendocrine or APUD (amino precursor uptake and decarboxylation) type [28]. Stromal hyperplasia (SH) is characterized by varying degrees of proliferation of the ovarian stromal cells. Stromal hyperthecosis (HT) refers to the presence of luteinized cells within the stroma at a distance from the follicles; it is usually accompanied by at least a moderate degree of SH.

Clinical Features

The clinical manifestations are variable. Moderate to severe SH is most commonly encountered in women in their sixth and seventh decades and has been documented in more than one third of autopsied patients in this age group [194]. Similar degrees of SH are found less commonly in patients in the eighth decade, suggesting that it may be a reversible process. A strong negative association with parity was found in one study [194]. SH of moderate to severe degree may be found in women with disorders associated with androgenic or estrogenic manifestations including endometrial carcinoma, obesity, hypertension, and glucose intolerance, but these findings are less frequent and less obtrusive than in HT.

HT is most frequent in patients in the sixth to ninth decades. Some familial cases of HT have been reported [84]. The process has been documented in one third of autopsied patients over the age of 55, and exhaustive microscopic sampling may reveal that rare luteinized stromal cells are even more common in this age group [28]. In postmenopausal women, HT is usually mild and of doubtful clinical significance.

Clinically florid examples of HT are more common in patients in the younger reproductive age group, although rare cases occur in adolescents and postmenopausal patients [109]. The findings include marked virilization, obesity, hypertension, hyperinsulinemia, and decreased glucose tolerance. In addition, a small subset of women with HT (or occasionally PCOS) have the HAIR-AN syndrome (see following). The clinical picture of HT typically evolves gradually, but occasionally there is an abrupt onset, potentially suggesting the presence of an androgenic tumor, especially if the process is unilateral and associated with ovarian enlargement. Less commonly, the clinical findings are more characteristic of PCOS. In some patients with HT, especially postmenopausal women, estrogenic findings predominate and may include endometrial hyperplasia or even well-differentiated adenocarcinoma [109, 135, 176, 194]. Conversely, women with endometrial hyperplasia or carcinoma in some studies have had a high frequency of HT on microscopic examination of their ovaries [135, 176]. HT-related virilization has been present in two cases of placental site trophoblastic tumor, and in one case it was the presenting manifestation of the tumor [133, 138].

Gross Findings

SH and HT are almost invariably bilateral, and the ovaries range from normal size to 8 cm in maximum dimension, thus potentially mimicking an ovarian neoplasm [109]. The sectioned surfaces are usually solid, firm, homogenous, and white to yellow (➲ *Fig. 12.31*). In cases of nodular hyperthecosis, multiple yellow nodules may be appreciable. In premenopausal women, sclerocystic changes similar to those seen in PCOS may also be present [78]. HT rarely coexists with a neoplasm, usually a stromal luteoma, which may also have hormone-secreting potential [180].

Microscopic Findings

In both SH and HT, a variable degree of nodular or diffuse cortical and medullary proliferation of ovarian stromal cells is present (➲ *Fig. 12.32a*). A mild degree of SH cannot be reliably distinguished from the normal appearance. Follicular derivatives may lie within the hyperplastic stroma but may be rare or absent in advanced cases (➲ *Fig. 12.32b*). The stromal cells in SH are plumper than normal postmenopausal ovarian stromal cells, and have oval to fusiform, vesicular nuclei, and, frequently, cytoplasmic lipid. The luteinized stromal cells of HT are more common in the medulla but may also be present in the cortex. They appear as single cells, small nests, or nodules of polygonal cells with abundant eosinophilic to vacuolated cytoplasm, containing variable amounts of lipid (➲ *Fig. 12.33*). The round nucleus of the luteinized cells typically has a central small nucleolus. As noted, in premenopausal women including those with the HAIR-AN syndrome, sclerocystic changes characteristic of PCOS are also commonly present. In cases of HT accompanying the HAIR-AN syndrome (see following), edema and fibrosis of the ovarian stroma, rather than SH, are frequently a prominent change [117].

Other ovarian findings occasionally encountered in HT include an increased number of atretic follicles, small stromal nodules of metaplastic smooth muscle, hilus cell hyperplasia, hilus cell tumors, stromal luteomas, and thecomas [170, 181, 196, 220]. SH in the absence of HT has also been associated with thecomas [220]. Some cases of HT may be associated with massive ovarian edema.

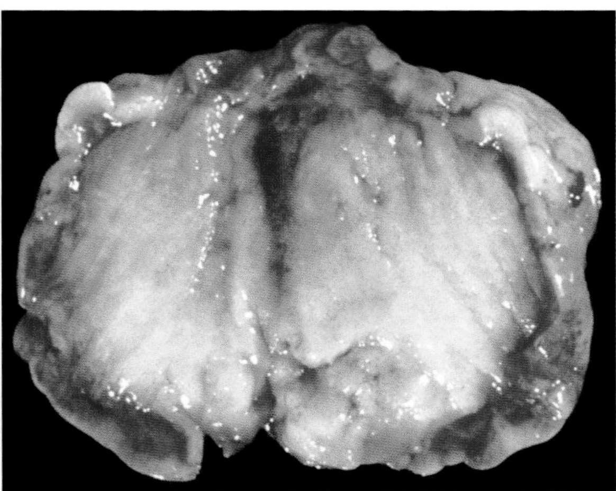

Fig. 12.31
Stromal hyperplasia and stromal hyperthecosis. **Solid, homogeneous, yellow sectioned surface**

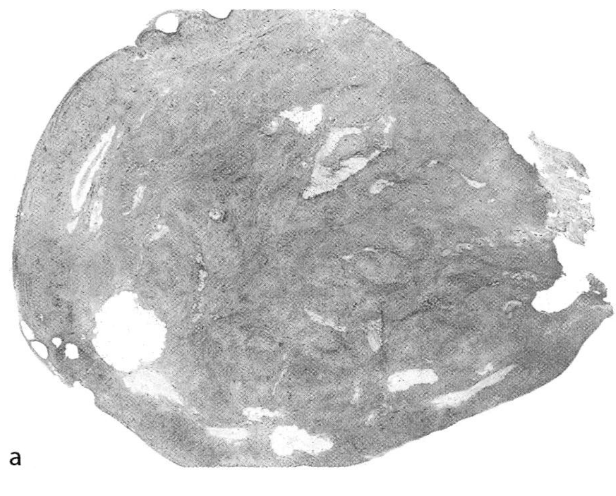

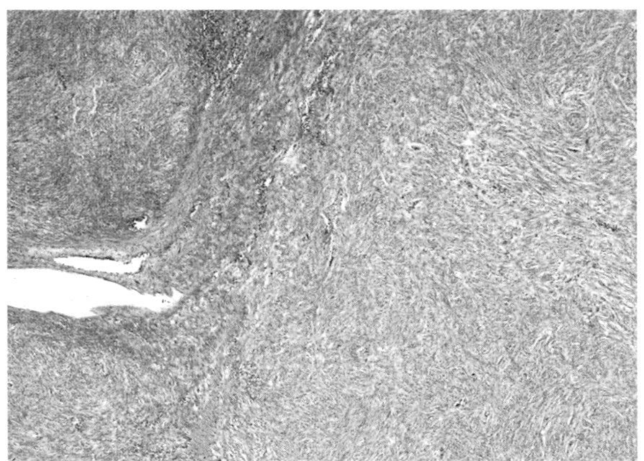

Fig. 12.32
Stromal hyperplasia. **(a) A diffuse proliferation of ovarian stromal cells within the cortex and medulla is seen. (b) Note absence of follicular derivatives**

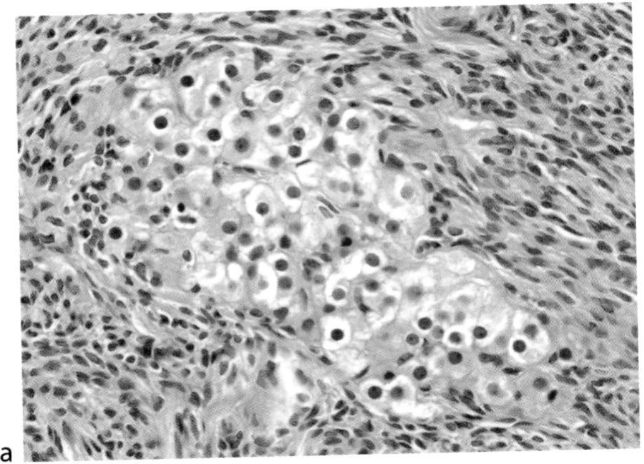

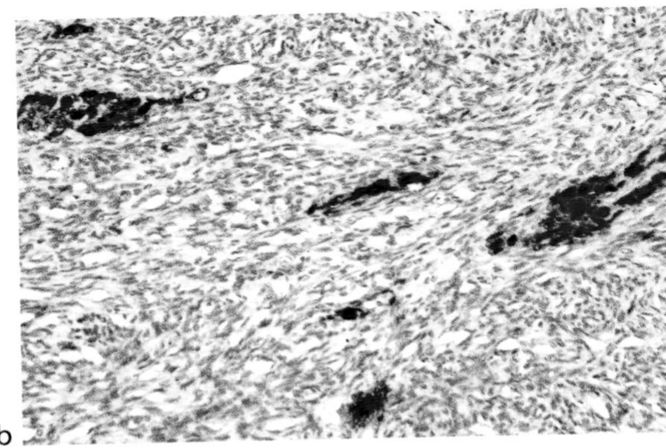

Fig. 12.33
Stromal hyperthecosis. (a) A nest of luteinized stromal cells is present within the ovarian stroma. (b) Calretinin immunostain highlights luteinized stromal cells

Histochemical analyses have shown that nonluteinized and luteinized stromal cells and cells transitional in appearance between the two have oxidative activity important in steroid hormone production [182]. The luteinized cells were immunoreactive for cytochrome P-450-17-alpha, which catalyzes androgen synthesis, in approximately 50% of the cases of SH in one series [176]. Luteinized stromal cells are also immunoreactive for inhibin, calretinin (Fig. 12.33), testosterone, estradiol, and follicle-stimulating hormone (FSH) [109, 121, 135, 154].

Pathophysiology

In vitro and in vivo studies have shown that ovaries with SH secrete more androstenedione, estrone, and estradiol than normal ovaries [43]. Similar studies using ovarian tissue from patients with HT [136] as well as in vivo studies in these patients have shown, respectively, markedly increased production rates and serum levels of ovarian testosterone, dihydrotestosterone, and androstenedione, usually in the male range [109]. As already noted, immunohistochemical staining for various enzymes involved in the conversion of cholesterol to steroid hormones in cases of HT has been consistent with androgen synthesis not only in the luteinized stromal cells characteristic of the disorder but also in the adjacent spindle-shaped stromal cells [176]. As in PCOS, the predominant estrogen in patients with SH and HT is estrone, derived predominantly from peripheral aromatization of ovarian androgens, resulting in an increased estrone/estradiol ratio [176].

Unlike patients with PCOS, most premenopausal patients with HT have normal gonadotropin levels [84]. That gonadotropins may play a role in SH and HT, however, is suggested by (1) elevated LH levels in occasional premenopausal women with HT and most postmenopausal patients with SH and HT; (2) immunoreactivity for FSH and LH receptors within ovarian stromal cells [139]; (3) in vitro incubation studies showing that FSH and LH stimulate proliferation of the ovarian stroma of pre- and postmenopausal women [194]; (4) studies showing that androgen production by the ovarian stromal cells in patients with and without HT is enhanced by LH [43, 136]; (5) the often prominent stromal luteinization during pregnancy; (6) cases of symptomatic HT complicating pregnancy and trophoblastic disease [133, 138]; and (7) the increase in pituitary amphophils in some cases of severe HT [109]. As noted, insulin resistance and hyperinsulinemia occur in as many as 90% of patients with HT and likely play a role in the pathogenesis of the stromal luteinization in these patients (HAIR-AN syndrome) [137].

Differential Diagnosis

In contrast to a fibroma, SH is almost always bilateral and is characterized by cells with smaller nuclei, scanty collagen, and nodules that commonly coalesce. The lesion is distinguished from a low-grade endometrioid stromal sarcoma by the spindle shape of its cells and by an absence of mitotic figures and regularly distributed arterioles.

The differential diagnosis of HT includes other nonneoplastic and neoplastic solid proliferations of luteinized cells, most of which are also virilizing. The nonneoplastic category includes pregnancy luteoma and Leydig cell hyperplasia (discussed elsewhere in this chapter) and the neoplasms include luteinized thecoma and steroid cell tumors (➋ Chap. 15, Sex Cord-Stromal, Steroid Cell, and Other Ovarian Tumors with Endocrine, Paraendocrine, and Paraneoplastic Manifestations). These neoplasms, in contrast to HT, are almost always unilateral and typically form distinct tumors or nodules appreciable on gross examination. Luteinized stromal cells, histologically similar to those present in HT, may also be encountered within the nonneoplastic stroma of a variety of benign and malignant ovarian tumors, including primary surface epithelial and germ cell tumors as well as metastatic tumors, that is, "tumors with functioning stroma" (➋ Chap. 15, Sex Cord-Stromal, Steroid Cell, and Other Ovarian Tumors with Endocrine, Paraendocrine, and Paraneoplastic Manifestations).

Clinical Behavior and Treatment

In contrast to patients with PCOS, those with HT usually exhibit little or no response to clomiphene treatment [84]. Many patients require bilateral oophorectomy to halt progressive virilization. Such treatment may also result in disappearance of hypertension and abnormalities in glucose tolerance. More recently, successful treatment of HT has been achieved with gonadotropin-releasing hormone (GnRH) agonists [195].

HAIR-AN Syndrome

In addition to the common occurrence of insulin resistance and hyperinsulinemia in patients with HT, some patients with HT have the HAIR-AN syndrome, a syndrome estimated to occur in as many as 5% of all women with hyperandrogenism [11, 48, 115]. The syndrome consists of hyperandrogenism (HA), typically of early, sometimes premenarcheal, onset; insulin resistance (IR); and acanthosis nigricans (AN) [11]. Striking degrees of masculinization are present in some patients with the HAIR-AN syndrome and may be disproportionate to the degree of hyperandrogenism [48]. Some patients have a normal glucose tolerance whereas others have symptomatic diabetes [85].

The syndrome has been most frequently described in patients with PCOS, although it appears likely that most, if not all, such patients also have HT [48, 117]. Unusual histologic findings in patients with HT and the HAIR-AN syndrome have included prominent follicular atresia, large numbers of degenerating oocytes, medullary stromal fibrosis, and numerous small nests of granulosa cells forming Call–Exner bodies [115]. Dermoid cysts and stromal luteoma have been rarely described in patients with the HAIR-AN syndrome in association with HT, sclerocystic ovaries, or both.

The typical laboratory findings include hyperinsulinemia and increased production rates and elevated serum levels of testosterone and androstendione [48]. In some patients, the severity of the insulin resistance is proportional to the testosterone elevation. Proposed mechanisms of insulin resistance have included a decreased number or functional capacity of insulin receptors, which may be associated with obesity, or in other cases, genetic alterations in the structure of the receptors (type A); antiinsulin receptor antibodies that decrease insulin receptor affinity for insulin and which are often associated with autoimmune diseases (type B); and postreceptor defects in insulin action or clearance (type C) [12, 85].

It has been postulated that the primary defect in the HAIR-AN syndrome is insulin resistance leading to hyperinsulinemia and the other findings in the syndrome. Thus, any cause of insulin resistance leading to hyperinsulinemia can produce the HAIR-AN syndrome. The hyperandrogenism itself may increase the severity of the insulin resistance, and thus a self-perpetuating cycle that increases in severity may result [11]. The acanthosis nigricans is probably an epiphenomenon secondary to the hyperandrogenism, hyperinsulinemia, or both.

Bilateral oophorectomy in patients with the HAIR-AN syndrome decreases hyperandrogenism but usually does not ameliorate insulin resistance [115, 137]. Gonadotropin suppression with oral contraceptives has been successful in decreasing ovarian androgen production in some patients. Marked improvement of acanthosis nigricans may follow correction of the hyperandrogenism.

Massive Edema and Ovarian Fibromatosis

Tumor-like enlargement of one, or occasionally, both ovaries secondary to an accumulation of edema fluid within the ovarian stroma is referred to as massive ovarian edema. Over 100 cases of this disorder have been reported [141, 171, 218]. A rarer lesion designated ovarian fibromatosis [218], characterized by diffuse ovarian fibrosis, is closely related to massive edema and is therefore considered in this section.

Clinical Features

Patients with massive edema are typically young, with a mean age of 21 years (range, 6–37 years) and have abdominal or pelvic pain, menstrual irregularities, and abdominal distension. The pain may be of several years duration or have a sudden onset and mimic the pain of acute appendicitis. Androgenic manifestations are present in approximately 20% of patients and are nearly always associated with the presence of luteinized stromal cells. Of these, two thirds are masculinized and the rest exhibit only hirsutism [218]. Serum testosterone has been elevated in some cases. Rare patients have had estrogenic manifestations, manifested by isosexual pseudoprecocity [141, 171, 218]. Pelvic examination typically reveals a palpable adnexal mass, which in 70% of cases has been right-sided. Abdominal exploration reveals unilateral involvement in 90% of cases, and in approximately half the patients, partial or complete torsion of the involved ovary. In one patient, the contralateral ovary had a twisted pedicle and was infarcted. Intraperitoneal fluid is not usually present, although rare patients have had an associated Meigs' syndrome. Rare cases of ovarian edema secondary to lymphatic permeation by metastatic cervical carcinoma have also been reported [95].

Patients with ovarian fibromatosis have ranged in age from 13 to 39 years, with an average of 25 years [218]. Clinical manifestations include menstrual abnormalities or amenorrhea, abdominal pain, and rarely hirsutism or virilization. The majority of patients have a palpable adnexal mass. Occasionally, the ovarian enlargement is an incidental finding late in pregnancy or during cesarean section. In some cases, the involved ovary was found twisted on its pedicle at the time of operation. The endocrine manifestations, including, in several cases, infertility, disappear after oophorectomy, indicating that the lesion produces steroid hormones.

Gross Findings

The involved ovary in massive edema is enlarged, soft, and fluctuant, ranging from 5.5 to 35 cm in maximum dimension (mean, 11.5 cm). The heaviest ovary weighed 2,400 g [218]. The ovary has a shiny, white, smooth exterior as a result of a white and fibrotic superficial cortex and a sectioned surface that is edematous or gelatinous and exudes watery fluid (*Fig. 12.34*). Occasional superficial FCs may be present. The ipsilateral fallopian tube may also be edematous.

In ovarian fibromatosis, there is usually complete or almost complete ovarian involvement by a fibromatous process [218]. In 20% of cases, the process is bilateral. The ovaries are 8–14 cm in maximum dimension with white and typically smooth or lobulated external surfaces. The cut surfaces are firm, white to gray, and solid except for the presence of cystic follicles in one third of cases (*Fig. 12.35*).

Microscopic Findings

The striking finding on low magnification in massive edema is marked, diffuse, stromal edema that separates and sometimes involves the follicular structures but typically spares the superficial cortex (*Fig. 12.36*). The latter is usually thickened and fibrotic. Higher magnification

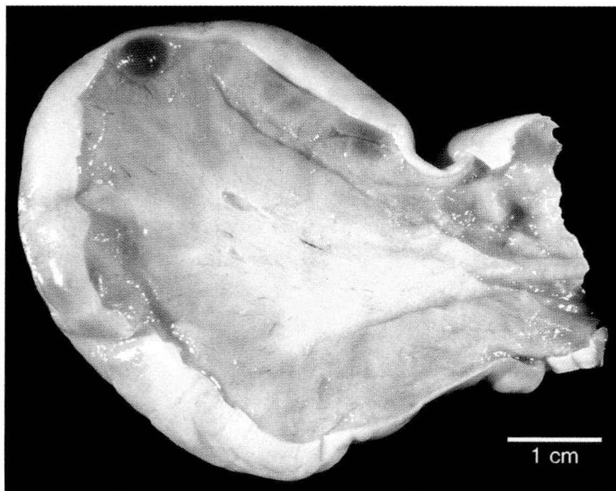

Fig. 12.34
Massive ovarian edema. **The ovary is enlarged and markedly edematous**

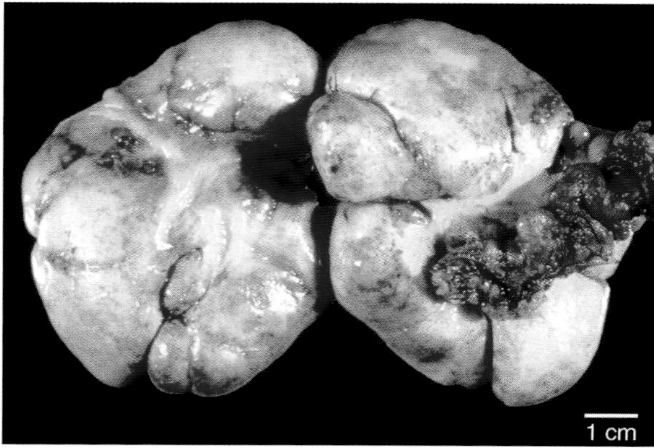

Fig. 12.35
Bilateral ovarian fibromatosis. **Convoluted external surface with patchy areas of white, fibrous tissue (right ovary)**

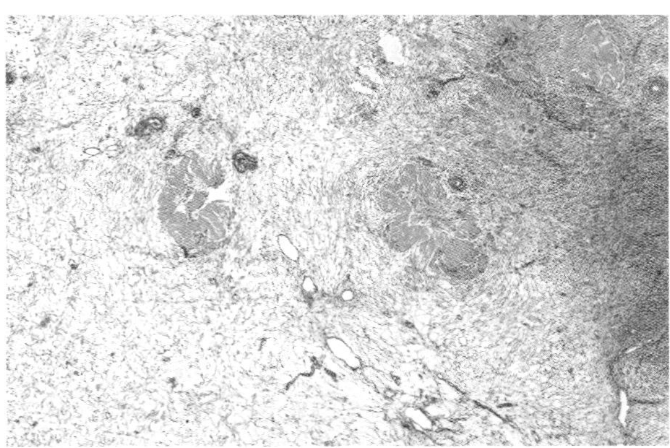

Fig. 12.36
Massive ovarian edema. **The edematous ovarian stroma separates several corpora fibrosa**

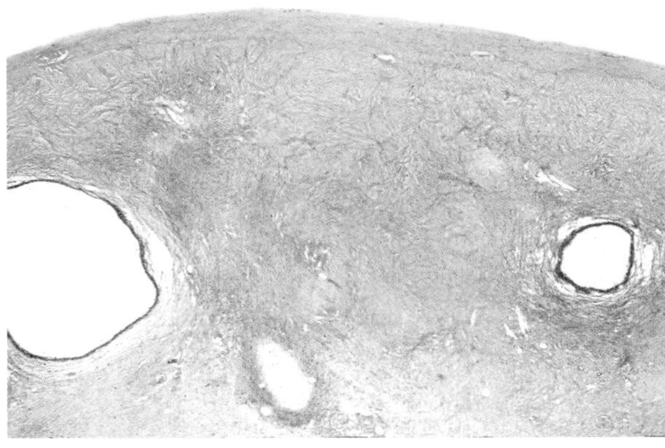

Fig. 12.38
Ovarian fibromatosis. **Fibrotic spindle cell proliferation invests follicular structures within the cortex**

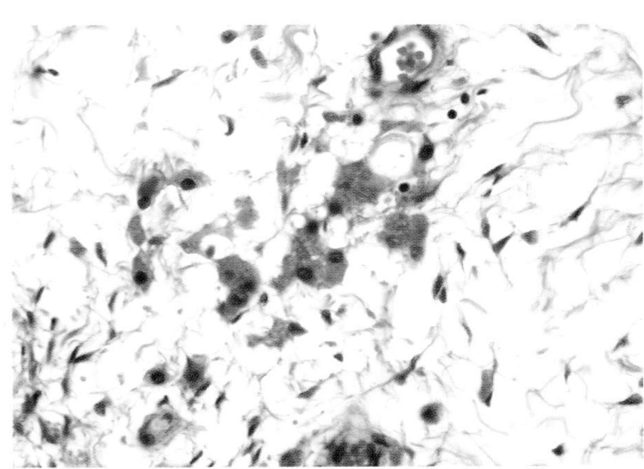

Fig. 12.37
Massive ovarian edema. **Luteinized stromal cells are present**

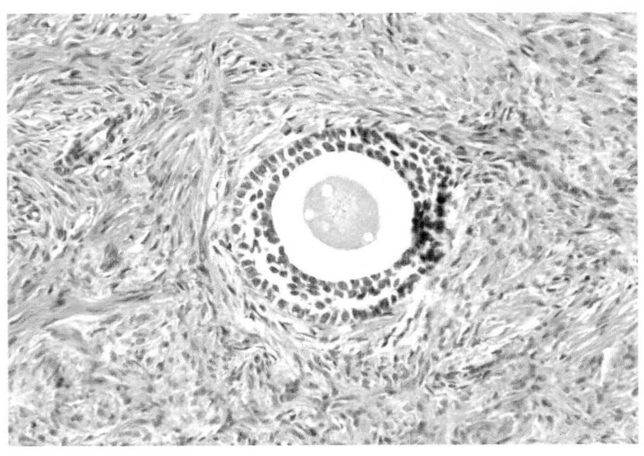

Fig. 12.39
Ovarian fibromatosis. **Fibrotic ovarian stroma surrounds a preantral follicle**

reveals spindle-shaped ovarian stromal cells separated by abundant pale-staining fluid that focally may impart a microcystic appearance. In nonedematous areas, the stroma has the appearance of normal stroma, hyperplastic stroma, or ovarian fibromatosis [218]. In approximately 40% of cases, foci of luteinized cells are present (➋ *Fig. 12.37*). Associated nonspecific findings include vascular and lymphatic dilatation within the ovary and occasionally the mesosalpinx, focal necrosis, extravasated erythrocytes, hemosiderin-laden macrophages, and mast cells [171, 218]. The contralateral ovary is normal in more than 75% of cases; in the rest, it is enlarged and edematous, or is nonedematous but altered by stromal hyperthecosis or sclerocystic changes.

Ovarian fibromatosis is characterized by a fibromatoid proliferation of collagen-producing spindle cells (➋ *Fig. 12.38*) that typically surrounds normal follicular structures and thickens the superficial cortex (➋ *Fig. 12.39*) [218]. In most cases of fibromatosis, the process is diffuse but it may be localized, and occasionally it is confined to or predominantly involves the cortex ("cortical fibromatosis"). The process varies from moderately cellular fascicles of spindle cells with a focal storiform pattern to relatively acellular bands of dense collagen. Small foci of uninvolved ovarian stroma are usually present. In rare cases, luteinized cells are seen within the lesion or the adjacent nonfibrotic stroma. Minor foci of stromal edema and microscopic foci of sex cord elements within the fibromatous tissue, alone or in combination, have been encountered in occasional cases [218].

Pathogenesis

The pathogenesis of massive edema is thought to be intermittent torsion of the ovary on its pedicle, causing partial obstruction of venous and lymphatic drainage. Torsion is observed in half the cases of massive edema, and a few cases of massive edema have been reported in association with obstruction of ovarian lymphatics secondary to metastatic carcinoma within pelvic and paraaortic lymph nodes [95, 218]. Luteinization of the ovarian stromal cells is considered a secondary phenomenon.

In at least some cases, massive edema likely occurs in an ovary with an underlying stromal proliferation, either fibromatosis or stromal hyperthecosis, that enlarges the ovary, promoting torsion with subsequent edema [218]. This interpretation is supported by the clinical similarities and pathologic overlap between massive edema and ovarian fibromatosis. Young and Scully suggest that massive edema is simply ovarian fibromatosis following torsion and accumulation of edema fluid [218]. Similarly, some examples of massive edema in which luteinized stromal cells are present in the same ovary and in the contralateral, edematous or nonedematous ovary may represent cases of stromal hyperthecosis in which one or both ovaries have undergone torsion.

Rather than accepting that fibromatosis is a precursor of massive edema, Russell and Farnsworth [173] hypothesized that the fibromatoses described by Young and Scully represent the "burned-out" stage of a reactive fibroblastic proliferation that at one end of the spectrum is represented by massive edema and at the other by a variety of highly cellular fibroblastic tumor-like lesions.

Differential Diagnosis

The differential diagnosis of massive edema includes ovarian neoplasms that may exhibit an edematous or myxoid appearance, most commonly fibroma, but also sclerosing stromal tumor, Krukenberg tumor, luteinized thecoma associated with sclerosing peritonitis, and the rare ovarian myxoma. Recognition of massive edema is therefore of great importance to prevent unnecessary oophorectomy in a young female. Fibromatosis also may be confused with a fibroma, or if sex cord-like nests are prominent, a Brenner tumor.

Massive edema and fibromatosis are distinguished from a neoplasm by the presence of follicular derivatives visible on both macroscopic and microscopic examination. A neoplasm may be surrounded by a rim of normal ovarian tissue in contrast to massive edema and fibromatosis, which usually diffusely involve the ovarian tissue. Additionally, ovarian fibromas occur in an older age group and are hormonally inactive, and Krukenberg tumors, in contrast to massive edema and fibromatosis, are characterized by signet-ring cells. Finally, the sex cord-like nests in fibromatosis are distinguishable from those of a Brenner tumor in their number, shape, and cell type.

Clinical Behavior and Treatment

Although most of the reported patients with massive edema have been successfully treated by oophorectomy, the condition should be managed conservatively, especially if the patient is young, because there is a strong likelihood that the condition will resolve. After an intraoperative frozen section of a wedge biopsy to exclude a neoplasm, an ovarian suspension procedure should be performed, with fixation of the involved ovary.

Pregnancy Luteoma

Pregnancy luteoma is a distinctive, nonneoplastic lesion of pregnancy, characterized by solid proliferations of luteinized cells, resulting in tumor-like ovarian enlargement that regresses during the puerperium [145].

Clinical Features

The patients are usually in their third or fourth decades, are multiparous in 80% of the cases, and a similar proportion are black. Most patients are asymptomatic, and the ovarian enlargement is discovered incidentally at cesarean section or postpartum tubal ligation. Rarely, a pelvic mass is palpable or obstructs the birth canal. In approximately 25% of cases, hirsutism or virilization appears or worsens during the latter half of pregnancy. Seventy percent of female infants born to virilized mothers are born with clitoromegaly and labial fusion. Plasma testosterone and other androgens may reach levels 70 times normal in virilized patients; increased values have also been demonstrated in nonvirilized patients [134]. Androgen levels in the infants may be increased but are usually lower than maternal levels or normal [134]. Regression of the luteomas usually begins within days after delivery and is complete within several weeks. Simultaneously, elevated androgen levels decrease rapidly, usually normalizing within 2 weeks postpartum. In rare cases, pregnancy luteomas occur in consecutive pregnancies. The diagnosis is made by excisional biopsy and frozen section examination of one nodule.

Gross Findings

Pregnancy luteomas are solid, fleshy, circumscribed, red to brown nodules ranging from microscopic up to 20 cm in diameter (median, 6.6 cm) (➲ *Fig. 12.40*) [145]. Hemorrhagic foci are common. The lesions are multiple in almost half the cases and bilateral in at least one third. A separate corpus luteum of pregnancy may also be visible. Examination of the ovaries days to weeks postpartum reveals brown puckered scars.

Microscopic Findings

The lesions are composed of sharply circumscribed, rounded masses of cells (➲ *Fig. 12.41*), that are also occasionally arranged in a trabecular or follicular pattern, the latter associated with spaces containing colloid-like material (➲ *Fig. 12.42a*). The cells are intermediate in size between the luteinized granulosa cells and luteinized theca cells of adjacent follicles and have abundant eosinophilic cytoplasm that contains little or no stainable lipid and central nuclei (➲ *Fig. 12.42b*). The nuclei may vary slightly in size and are hyperchromatic; nucleoli may be

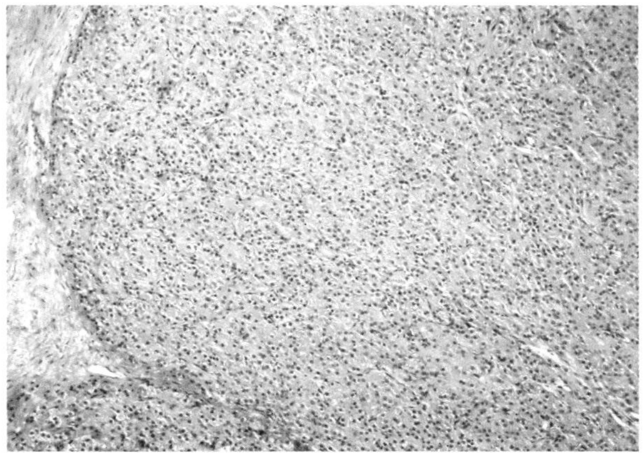

◘ Fig. 12.41
Pregnancy luteoma. **Solid, circumscribed nodule of luteinized cells replaces the normal parenchyma**

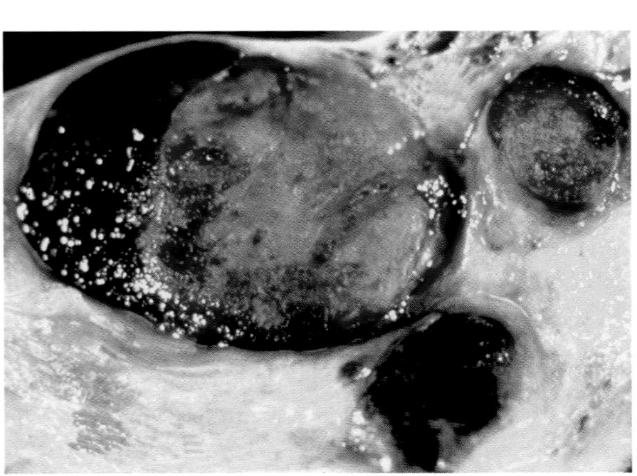

◘ Fig. 12.40
Pregnancy luteoma. **Multiple, solid, circumscribed, reddish-brown and hemorrhagic nodules replace the normal parenchyma**

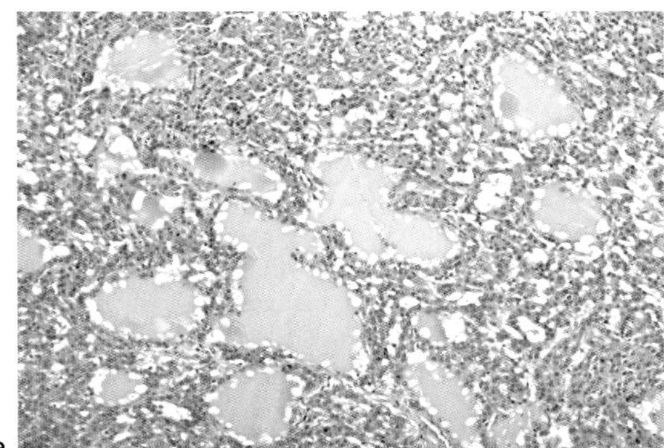

a

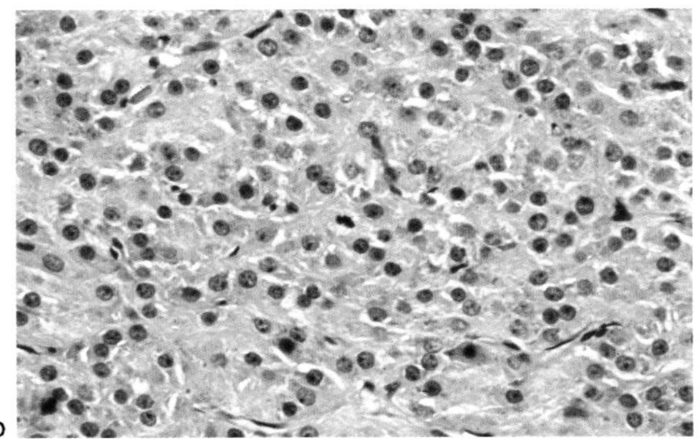

b

◘ Fig. 12.42
Pregnancy luteoma. **(a) Follicular pattern; (b) Solid growth pattern of polygonal luteinized cells**

prominent. Mitotic figures may range up to seven per ten high-power fields, with an average of two or three, and may be atypical [145]. Less common features include focal balloon-like cytoplasmic degeneration and colloid droplets similar to those seen in the corpus luteum of pregnancy. The stroma is scanty, and reticulin fibrils surround groups of cells. Examination of lesions removed postpartum shows shrunken aggregates of degenerating lipid-filled luteoma cells with pyknotic nuclei, infiltration by lymphocytes, and fibrosis.

Pathogenesis

Pregnancy luteomas most likely arise from hCG-induced proliferations of luteinized ovarian stromal cells. Some authors, however, have favored origin from luteinized follicular granulosa and theca cells [145]. The exclusive occurrence of the lesion in pregnancy suggests a role for hCG in its pathogenesis, and augmentation of steroidogenesis by pregnancy luteomas in response to hCG, both in vitro and in vivo, supports this interpretation. However, the rarity of pregnancy luteomas in association with gestational trophoblastic disease, which is typically accompanied by very high levels of hCG, and the almost exclusive recognition of the lesions during the third trimester when hCG levels are lower than earlier in pregnancy, indicate that hCG is not the only factor in their development. The occasional history of hirsutism, sometimes familial, antedating the pregnancy suggests that a preexistent endocrinopathy, such as stromal hyperthecosis or PCOS, may predispose to the development of the lesion in some patients.

Differential Diagnosis

When pregnancy luteomas are multiple, intraoperative inspection may suggest nodules of metastatic tumor. Such a diagnosis can usually be excluded by frozen section examination of one of the nodules, but the distinction may be difficult if the patient has a history or clinical evidence of an oxyphilic malignant tumor such as a malignant melanoma. When the luteoma is a single nodule, the microscopic differential diagnosis includes a number of lesions composed of luteinized cells occurring during pregnancy. However, the typical gross appearance of the pregnancy luteoma readily distinguishes it from a large solitary luteinized follicle cyst of pregnancy and puerperium, hyperreactio lueinalis, and corpus luteum of pregnancy. Solid primary neoplasms composed partially or entirely of luteinized cells such as granulosa tumors, thecomas, and steroid cell tumors may occur during pregnancy and enter the differential diagnosis. Such tumors are almost always unilateral and solitary compared to the more frequent bilaterality and multinodularity of the pregnancy luteoma. The partly luteinized group, that is, luteinized granulosa cell tumors and luteinized thecomas, contain typical nonluteinized foci and usually have denser reticulum patterns and more abundant intracellular lipid than seen in pregnancy luteoma. Entirely luteinized tumors belonging to the steroid cell category may closely resemble pregnancy luteoma histologically. Features favoring a steroid cell neoplasm include a dense reticulum pattern, intracellular lipid, lipochrome pigment, and in Leydig cell tumors, a hilar location and the presence of Reinke crystals (➲ Chap. 15, Sex Cord-Stromal, Steroid Cell, and Other Ovarian Tumors with Endocrine, Paraendocrine, and Paraneoplastic Manifestations). Differentiation of a solitary pregnancy luteoma from a lipid-poor steroid cell tumor may be impossible, but such a lesion in a pregnant woman is generally considered a pregnancy luteoma until proven otherwise.

Clinical Behavior and Treatment

Because the pregnancy luteoma is a benign, self-limited condition, no treatment is required.

Granulosa Cell Proliferations of Pregnancy

General and Pathologic Features

Granulosa cell proliferations that simulate small neoplasms have been encountered as incidental findings in the ovaries of pregnant women [31]. The older literature documented the presence of similar lesions in the ovaries of nonpregnant women, and we have encountered them in the ovary of a newborn that also contained a corpus luteum. The lesions in pregnant women are usually multiple and lie within atretic follicles, which are typically enveloped by a thick layer of luteinized theca cells. The granulosa cells may be arranged in solid, insular, microfollicular (➲ *Fig. 12.43*), or trabecular patterns, mimicking similar patterns in clinically evident granulosa cell tumors. In one case, a solid tubular pattern was identical to that seen in some Sertoli cell tumors. The granulosa cells typically contain scanty cytoplasm and grooved nuclei, resembling the cells of the adult-type granulosa cell tumor and in the case with a sertoliform pattern, the cells contained moderate amounts of finely vacuolated cytoplasm, suggesting the presence of lipid. In one case, there were large nodules of luteinized granulosa

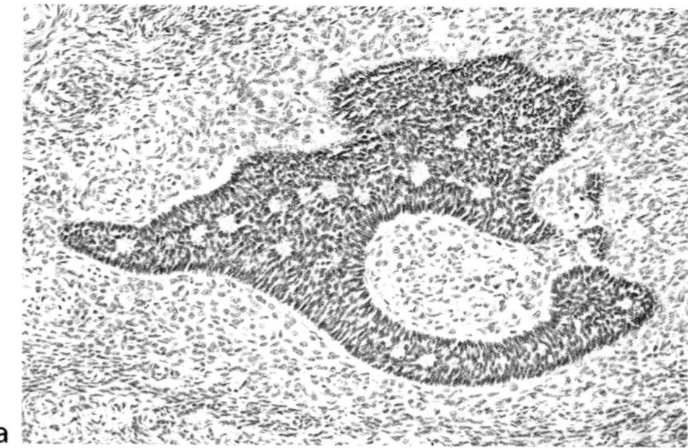

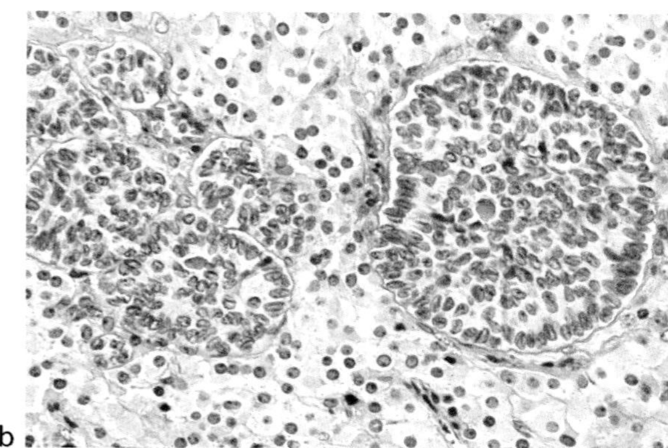

Fig. 12.43
Granulosa cell proliferations of pregnancy mimicking a small granulosa cell tumor. **The proliferations are within the center of an atretic follicle and are surrounded by the luteinized cells of the theca interna. (a) The proliferating cells form an irregular island containing Call-Exner formations. (b) In a different case, the granulosa cells form small nests and contain nuclear grooves**

cells with variably sized, round, nongrooved nuclei, resembling pregnancy luteomas except for their obvious origin in granulosa cells and the larger size of their cells.

Differential Diagnosis

The differential diagnosis in most of the cases is with a small granulosa or Sertoli cell tumor. Although similar proliferations have been previously interpreted as small tumors, the frequency of the lesions during pregnancy suggests an unusual nonneoplastic response to the hormonal milieu, possibly to the FSH-like property of hCG. The microscopic size of the lesions, their multifocality, and their confinement to atretic follicles support this interpretation.

Leydig Cell Hyperplasia

Leydig cells typically occur in the ovarian hilus, where they are also referred to as hilus cells and can be found in virtually all adult ovaries, typically intermingled with nonmyelinated nerves. Rarely, Leydig cells occur in nonhilar locations, either within the ovarian stroma or in extraovarian sites such as the lamina propria or adventitia of the fallopian tube [74]. Stromal (nonhilar) Leydig cell hyperplasia, in which Reinke crystal-containing Leydig cells are present within the ovarian stroma, is much less common than hilar Leydig cell hyperplasia. One recent report documented bilateral stromal Leydig cell hyperplasia in a postmenopausal woman who presented with virilization; hilus cell hyperplasia was absent [203].

Stromal Leydig cells are likely the origin of the rare Leydig cell tumors encountered within the ovarian stroma (Chap. 15, Sex Cord-Stromal, Steroid Cell, and Other Ovarian Tumors with Endocrine, Paraendocrine, and Paraneoplastic Manifestations). In one such case, there was also bilateral hilar Leydig cell hyperplasia and bilateral hilar Leydig cell tumors [196]. Stromal Leydig cells have also been rarely encountered within the nonneoplastic stroma of a variety of ovarian neoplasms and cysts, including mucinous and serous cystadenomas, Brenner tumors, struma ovarii, and strumal carcinoid tumors [175].

Hilar Leydig cell hyperplasia is difficult to define because hilus cell nests are typically widely separated and cannot be quantitated adequately without sectioning both ovaries extensively. Also, hilus cell proliferation can occur physiologically as a result of elevated hCG or LH levels, such as during pregnancy and after the menopause (*Fig. 12.44*) [28]. In such cases, the proliferation is often mild and generally not accompanied by a clinical endocrine disturbance, although such proliferations may account for at least some of the hirustism that is frequently observed during pregnancy. Severe degrees of hyperplasia, often associated with virilization, may occur in both pregnant and nonpregnant women. In some cases, elevated serum testosterone levels have been documented [41]. Hilus cell hyperplasia is characterized by an increased number of cells in a nodular or, less commonly, a diffuse arrangement, increased cell size, the presence of mitotic figures, cellular and nuclear pleomorphism, hyperchromasia, and multinucleation; crystals of Reinke may or may not be apparent by light microscopy (*Figs. 12.44* and *12.45*) [196].

Hilar Leydig cell hyperplasia may be associated with other ovarian lesions, including stromal hyperplasia, stromal hyperthecosis, stromal Leydig cell hyperplasia, rete cysts (Miscellaneous Lesions), and hilus cell neoplasia

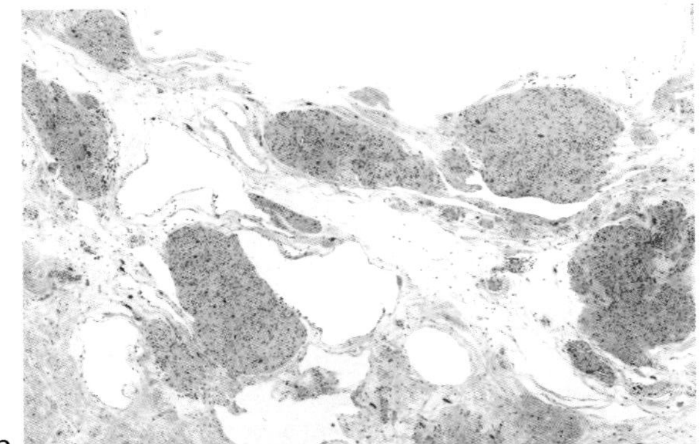

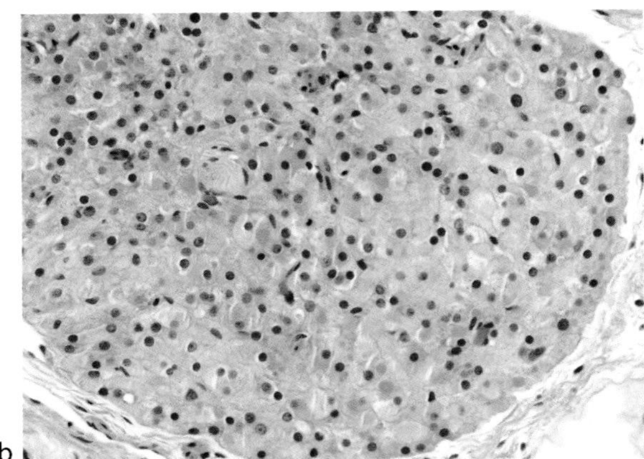

Fig. 12.44
Hilar Leydig cell hyperplasia in a postmenopausal woman. **(a) Nodular proliferation of hilar Leydig cells; (b) The hilus cells have abundant eosinophilic cytoplasm. No crystals are seen in this field, but spherical hyaline globules are present (*lower right*), likely representing crystal precursors**

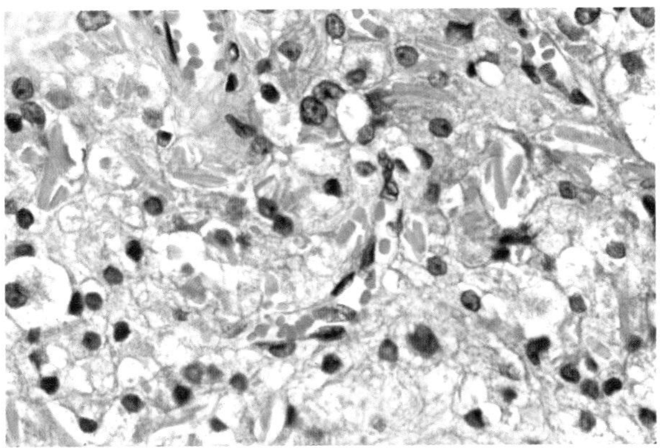

Fig. 12.45
Hilar Leydig cell hyperplasia. **Some nuclei are enlarged and hyperchromatic. Many crystals are seen in this field**

[196]. One case of hilus cell hyperplasia has been associated with the resistant ovary syndrome and other cases have been associated with gonadal dysgenesis [83]; in both disorders, LH levels are elevated. From a pathologic point of view, the distinction between a large hyperplastic nodule of hilus cells and a hilus cell tumor is arbitrary; we diagnose neoplasia when the nodule is more than 1 cm in diameter.

Ovarian "Tumor" of the Adrenogenital Syndrome

One ovarian example of this lesion has been reported [5]. A 36-year-old woman with congenital adrenal hyperplasia presented with an abrupt aggravation of her virilizing symptoms, relieved by bilateral salpingo-oophorectomy. Ovarian or paraovarian soft brown masses were present in both adnexae, which on microscopic examination were identical to the testicular tumor of the adrenogenital syndrome [5].

Ovarian Stromal Metaplasias Including Decidual Reaction

The ovarian stromal cell has the potential to differentiate, presumably by a process of metaplasia, into a variety of other mesenchymal cell types, most commonly decidua, but rarely smooth muscle, fat, and bone.

Ovarian Decidual Reaction

An ectopic decidual reaction may be encountered within the ovarian stroma as an isolated finding or as part of a more widespread decidual transformation of the subperitoneal pelvic mesenchyme (Chap. 13, Diseases of the Peritoneum) [20]. As in other sites of the secondary müllerian system, an ovarian decidual reaction usually represents a response of the indigenous stromal cells to the hormonal milieu of pregnancy. Ectopic decidua may be seen as early as the ninth week of gestation and is present in almost all ovaries at term. Less commonly, the decidua is associated with trophoblastic disease, in patients treated with progestagens, in the vicinity of a corpus luteum, and in association with hormonally active neoplastic and nonneoplastic lesions of the ovaries and adrenal glands [20, 146]. Prior ovarian radiation may be a predisposing factor by increasing the sensitivity of the stromal cells to hormonal stimulation [146]. Foci of ectopic decidua occasionally may occur within the ovaries of pre- and postmenopausal women with no obvious cause [146].

The decidual foci are usually seen only microscopically but in some cases, may be visible on macroscopic examination as variably sized, soft, tan to hemorrhagic nodules, or patches. The decidual cells typically occur singly, as small nodules, or confluent sheets in the superficial cortical stroma and the ovarian surface, often within periovarian adhesions (*Fig. 12.46*). The cells are indistinguishable from eutopic decidua on light microscopic and ultrastructural examination. Smooth muscle cells, probably derived from submesothelial fibroblasts or the ovarian stroma, may be admixed. A rich vascular network of distended capillaries and a sprinkling of lymphocytes are typically found within the decidual foci. Focal nuclear pleomorphism and hyperchromasia, sometimes in association with hemorrhagic necrosis, should not be misinterpreted as evidence of a malignant tumor. Occasionally, ectopic decidual cells may have vacuoles and eccentric nuclei simulating signet-ring cells [32]. The bland appearance of most of the nuclei, the absence of mitotic figures, the PAS negativity of the vacuolar contents, and the association with pregnancy should facilitate the correct diagnosis. Ectopic decidua in postpartum patients may undergo hyalinization.

Rarer Ovarian Stromal Metaplasias and Calcification

Foci of metaplastic smooth muscle (*Fig. 12.47a*) may be rarely encountered in the ovarian stroma of otherwise normal ovaries, within hyperplastic ovarian stroma (as in stromal hyperthecosis or polycystic ovaries), or within the walls of nonneoplastic or neoplastic cysts [78, 181]. Foci of mature fat have been described as a rare incidental histologic finding within the superficial ovarian stroma in obese women (*Fig. 12.47b*) [75]. Heterotopic bone formation in the ovary in the absence of an ovarian neoplasm is also unusual, typically occurring within periovarian adhesions or the walls of endometriotic cysts but rarely within otherwise normal ovaries [189].

In one case, extensive idiopathic calcification resulted in a stony hard consistency of both ovaries, which were of normal size [30]. Microscopic examination showed numerous spherical, laminated, calcific foci without accompanying epithelial cells (*Fig.12.48*). This process must be distinguished from a serous borderline tumor or carcinoma with confluent psammoma bodies, in which at least occasional neoplastic epithelial cells should be

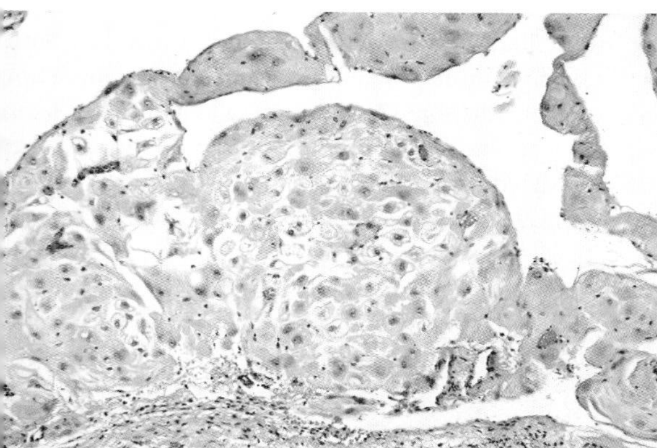

Fig. 12.46
Ectopic decidua. **Small nodules of decidual cells involving ovarian surface adhesions**

a
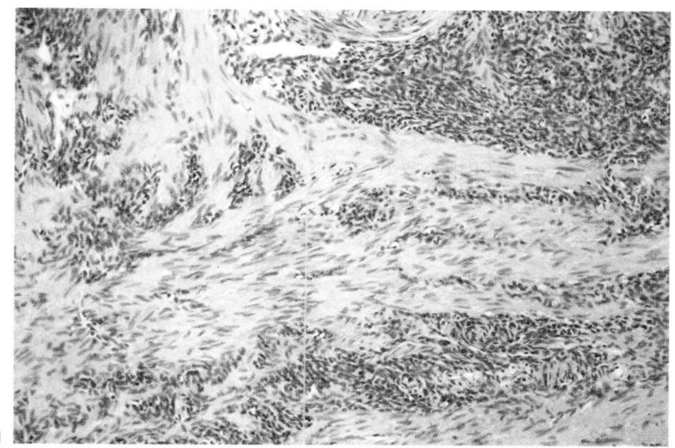

b
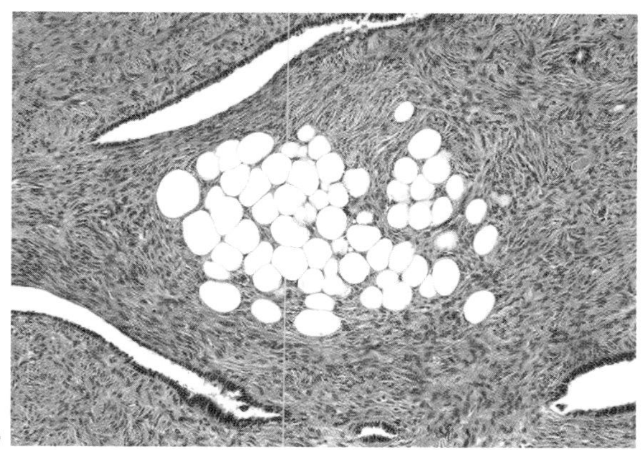

Fig. 12.47
Ovarian stromal metaplasia. **(a) Foci of smooth muscle are separated by ovarian stromal cells. (b) A focus of adipose tissue lies within the ovarian stroma, surrounded by epithelial inclusion glands**

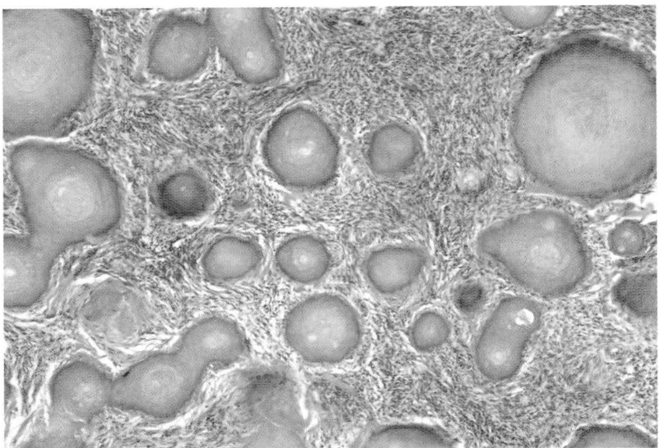

Fig. 12.48
Idiopathic ovarian calcification. **Numerous spherical, laminated, and calcific foci without accompanying epithelial cells occupy the ovarian stroma. Both ovaries were stony hard on gross examination**

identified, and from a "burned-out" gonadoblastoma replaced by laminated calcified masses. In cases of the latter type, the patient almost always has evidence of abnormal gonadal development and Y-chromosome material in her karyotype as well as residual typical gonadoblastoma in the same or contralateral gonad.

Disorders of Ovarian Failure

Premature ovarian failure (POF) or premature menopause is a result of a variety of disorders that lead to the onset of amenorrhea and infertility before the age of 35 years, or according to others, 40 years [164, 172, 206]. POF is uncommon, affecting an estimated 1% of women under the age of 40 [87] and accounting for only 4–10% of patients with secondary amenorrhea [172]. The ovarian failure is usually permanent, but occasionally it is reversible, at least temporarily, as manifested by subsequent ovulation and even conception [164, 206].

Patients with POF typically have a 46XX karyotype, normal secondary sexual characteristics, and secondary amenorrhea, although rarely prepubertal ovarian failure causes primary amenorrhea or oligomenorrhea and incompletely developed secondary sexual features. POF, therefore, probably represents a continuum in which individuals may be affected at any age before the expected age of menopause [164]. In contrast to patients with POF, patients with gonadal dysgenesis usually have an abnormal karyotype, streak gonads or abdominal testes, primary amenorrhea, ambiguous internal and external genitalia, and somatic abnormalities. The absence or decline in follicular activity in patients with POF typically results in low serum estrogen levels, often accompanied by estrogen withdrawal symptoms. Because of the failure of negative feedback, the low estrogen levels lead to elevated levels of pituitary gonadotropins, a feature that differentiates POF from central causes of amenorrhea related to hypothalamic or pituitary dysfunction.

Although three histologic patterns have been recognized, specifically premature follicular depletion (true premature menopause), resistant ovary syndrome, and autoimmune oophoritis, it is not known with certainty if each represents a distinct disorder or a nonspecific morphologic manifestation of a number of different disorders [172].

Premature Follicular Depletion

This disorder is characterized by ovaries that are typically small on gross inspection, resembling streak gonads. On microscopic examination, there is premature follicular depletion, with the ovaries resembling normal peri- or postmenopausal ovaries with complete, or nearly complete, absence of primordial and developing follicles [172]. Follicles in varying stages of atresia and stigmata of prior ovulation are typically present, excluding a streak gonad.

Postulated pathogenetic mechanisms include a decreased number of ovarian germ cells at birth, acceleration of normal follicular atresia, or prepubertal or postpubertal destruction of germ cells. With respect to the last, there is strong evidence, including the presence of antiovarian antibodies, autoimmune disorders, or both, implicating immune factors in a substantial proportion of women with POF. As some or all these cases likely represent an end stage of autoimmune oophoritis, they are considered further in that section (see page 35) [172]. Additionally, postnatal destruction of germ cells may be caused by cytotoxic drugs or radiation (Ovarian Changes Secondary to Cytotoxic Drugs and Radiation) and mumps oophoritis (Viral Infections). Because mumps oophoritis is probably clinically occult in the majority of cases, it may be a more frequent cause of premature menopause, including familial cases, than is generally suspected.

The occurrence of familial cases of POF, in a pattern consistent with an autosomal dominant mode of inheritance [119], implicates genetic factors in some cases; familial POF may account for 12–28% of cases of this disorder [87]. Occasional patients with an otherwise typical presentation have had chromosomal abnormalities, usually 47XXX, pure or mosaic, but occasionally 45XO/46XX [207]. In some familial cases, the affected women were 46XX but had an interstitial deletion of the long arm of the X chromosome [96]. A proportion of these patients have fragile X syndrome, with a premutation in the *FMR1* gene found in 14% of cases [187]. Some authors, however, exclude cases with chromosomal abnormalities from the category of POF so that it includes only "chromosomally competent" patients.

The presence of galactosemia in some patients with POF suggests that it may play a pathogenetic role. Approximately two thirds of females with galactosemia in one study had POF [90]. In many such patients dietary treatment of galactosemia had been delayed. One galactosemic patient with POF had the pattern of the resistent ovary syndrome (see following) on ovarian biopsy, but in a series of galactosemic patients who were not biopsied, some patients had severely atrophic ovaries, suggesting premature follicular depletion [52]. Similarly, experimental studies indicate that galactose or its metabolites may interefere with normal prenatal oogenesis. Depletion of primordial follicles has been described in several women with ataxia telangiectasia, which may be related to their severe immunosuppression or to their athymic state [57].

Resistant Ovary Syndrome

This rare syndrome, also known as Savage syndrome, is found in approximately 20% of patients with POF and characterized by primary or secondary amenorrhea, endogenous hypergonadotropinemia, and resistance to exogenous gonadotropins, often in massive doses [116, 172]. The resistance to endogenous and exogenous gonadotropins may be relative or absolute, episodic or chronic.

The ovaries typically have a normal prepubertal or adult appearance on macroscopic inspection. Microscopic examination reveals an appropriate number of normal-appearing primordial follicles but a complete, or nearly complete, absence of developing follicles. Atretic follicles and stigmata of prior ovulation may be present. In occasional patients, the space normally occupied by the ovum in some of the atretic follicles contains calcified material. In another case, numerous abnormal preantral follicles were found that contained multiple nodules of basement membrane material [116]. A histologic pattern similar to that in the resistant ovary syndrome occurs in morbid obesity, Cushing's syndrome, and hypogonadotropic ovarian failure secondary to hypothalamic–pituitary dysfunction.

The pathogenesis of this disorder is not yet established, but a possible deficiency of FSH and LH receptors within the ovary, the presence of antibodies to these receptors, or a postreceptor defect have been postulated. An IgG-like substance that alters FSH receptors and thereby impairs binding of this hormone was present in the serum of several patients with associated myasthenia gravis [52]. In another patient with the resistent ovary syndrome, lupus erythematosus appeared while the ovarian failure was evolving, and a serum antibody specific for the FSH receptor was found [116]. In another study, circulating autoimmune antibodies to thyroglobulin and smooth muscle were found in some patients [172]. As noted earlier, one patient with the resistent ovary syndrome had galactosemia [172].

Autoimmune Oophoritis

Clinical and Pathogenetic Features

Approximately 25 cases of autoimmune oophoritis have been documented pathologically [10, 106, 172, 185]. The patients, who have ranged in age from 17 to 48 years (mean, 31), typically present with oligomenorrhea or amenorrhea, or symptoms relating to multiple follicular cysts, including pelvic pain, adnexal torsion, or estrogenic manifestations, such as abnormal bleeding, and in one case endometrial adenocarcinoma [10, 106]. Most patients have steroid cell antibodies in their sera; Addison's disease, Hashimoto's thyroiditis, or Sjogren's disease have been additionally present in some cases [10, 53]. The Addison's disease may arise at the same time or subsequent to the ovarian failure and is associated at least in some cases with a lymphocytic adrenalitis. The steroid cell antibodies, which are rare in the general population, belong to a group of antibodies reactive with a range of antigens in steroid-producing cells. They are typically reactive against adrenal cortex, but in some cases also to theca interna, corpus luteum, thyroid epithelium and thyroglobulin, parathyroid cells, gastric parietal cells, and thymocytes, alone or in combination [40, 172].

There is also evidence supporting a role for cell-mediated immune mechanisms in the pathogenesis of autoimmune oophoritis. Studies have shown expression of major histocompatibility class II antigens by granulosa cells in autoimmune oophoritis, a phenomenon inducible by interferon gamma, a product of activated T cells [72]. Additionally, there have been reports of occasional patients with POF, including some with documented autoimmune oophoritis, in whom menses and ovulation resumed after administration of corticosteroids [38]. All the foregoing observations suggest that a complex immune process with an interplay of humoral and cellular mechanisms is involved in the pathogenesis of autoimmune oophoritis [185].

Autoimmune oophoritis is almost certainly more common than the small number of histologically documented cases would suggest. In two studies of women with POF who were not biopsied or in whom a biopsy revealed an afollicular pattern, two thirds [153] and 90% [127] of patients, respectively, had some evidence of autoimmune phenomena with immunologic testing. In a third study, some women with POF had a decreased ratio of inducer/helper lymphocytes to suppressor/cytotoxic lymphocytes as well as a decreased concentration of serum IgA, suggesting a mild suppression of immune competence [57]. Similarly, as many as one half of patients with POF in some series have or subsequently develop one or more associated autoimmune disorders; an average figure calculated from the literature is 20% [97]. Addison's disease or thyroid disease (Hashimoto's thyroiditis, Grave's disease) is the most common of these disorders and is typically accompanied or preceded by the presence of steroid cell antibodies [36]. Conversely, as many as 25% of patients with idiopathic Addison's disease may have POF, the latter usually preceding the former by several, but occasionally many, years [97]. Other autoimmune diseases that occur less commonly in these patients include rheumatoid arthritis, hypoparathyroidism, myasthenia gravis, diabetes mellitus, atrophic gastritis, pernicious anemia, hemolytic anemia, idiopathic thrombocytopenia purpura, alopecia, vitiligo, and sicca syndrome [36, 97]. POF occurs frequently in patients with two or more such diseases (polyglandular endocrinopathy) [97].

Additionally, a subgroup of patients with POF have chronic mucocutaneous candidiasis or chronic vaginal candidiasis, suggesting a defect in T-cell function, possibly secondary to circulating antibodies against T lymphocytes demonstrable in some of these patients [118]. Patients with these two types of candidiasis also frequently have anti-Candida, antithymocyte, and antiovarian antibodies, suggesting a shared antigen on these cells [118].

A partial genetic basis is suggested by a family history of an autoimmune disease in approximately one fifth of patients who have both POF and an autoimmune disease. Similarly, a prevalence of certain HLA antigens has been found in some patients with autoimmune endocrine disease [208].

The foregoing findings suggest that a substantial proportion of patients with the histologic pattern of premature follicular depletion likely represent an end stage of autoimmune oophoritis that is no longer recognizable on histologic examination.

Gross Findings

On gross examination, the ovaries may be small or normal in size, but in one third of cases one or both are enlarged by multiple follicular cysts, potentially simulating cystic neoplasms [10, 106]. The cysts are more common in the earlier phases of the disease and are likely caused by elevated gonadotropin levels. Small ovaries presumably reflect a late- or end stage of the disorder, after complete destruction of the follicles.

Microscopic Findings

The cardinal feature of autoimmune oophoritis on microscopic examination is a folliculotropic lymphoid infiltrate that affects developing follicles with a theca layer, corpora lutea, and atretic follicles (➋ *Fig. 12.49*). The intensity of the infiltrate increases with the degree of follicular maturation. The theca interna layer is typically more intensely infiltrated than the granulosa layer and may be focally destroyed; the granulosa layer may be focally disrupted with sloughing of its cells. The inflammatory infiltrate consists predominantly of lymphocytes and plasma cells, but eosinophils, histiocytes, and, rarely, sarcoid-like granulomas are also present, and may predominate [10]. Primordial follicles are typically present but uninvolved. Additionally, perivascular and perineural lymphoid infiltrates may be found in the hilus, and in some such cases, there has been an absence of Leydig cells, suggesting destruction of the latter by the inflammatory process [63]. Nonspecific findings have included the presence of abnormal "dysplastic" follicles, follicle cysts (as noted earlier), and superficial cortical fibrosis [10]. Immunophenotyping of the inflammatory infiltrate has revealed, variously, B and T lymphocytes, polyclonal plasma cells, macrophages, and natural killer cells [63, 106].

Vascular Lesions

Ovarian Hemorrhage

Rupture of a normal corpus luteum or a corpus luteum cyst may occasionally result in hemorrhage and, rarely, fatal hemoperitoneum. Although hemorrhage may occur

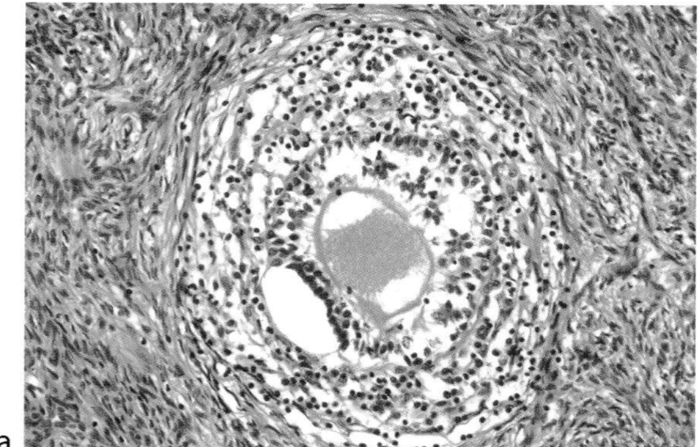

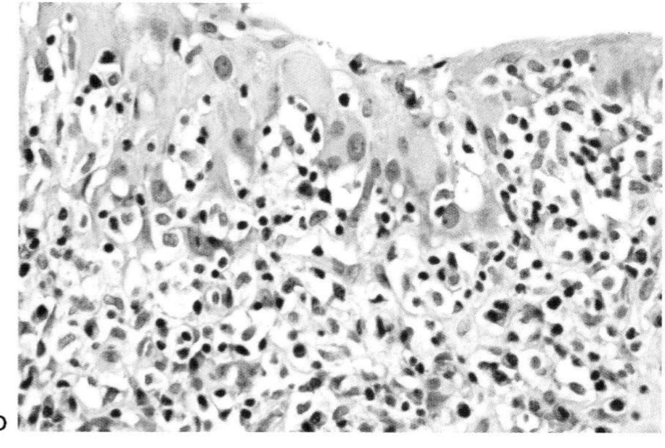

Fig. 12.49
Autoimmune oophoritis. **(a)** A maturing follicle is infiltrated by mononuclear inflammatory cells. **(b)** Corpus luteum partially destructed by intense lymphoplasmacytic infiltrate

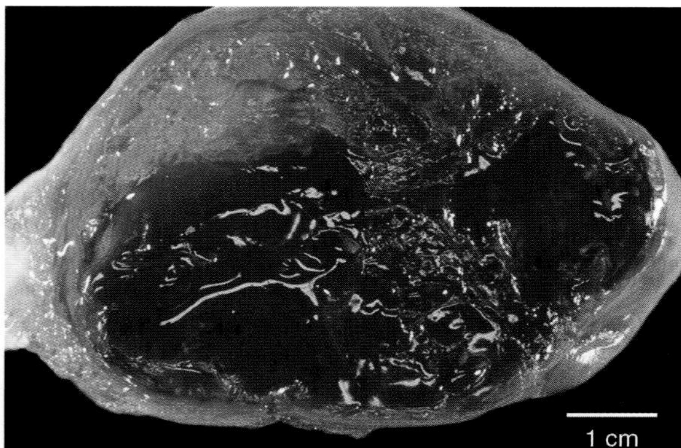

Fig. 12.50
Ovarian hemorrhage. Ovary from a patient being treated with anticoagulation therapy is replaced by a large hematoma

in otherwise normal women, it is observed more often in women receiving anticoagulant therapy (*Fig. 12.50*) [67]. The right ovary is the source of the hemorrhage in almost two thirds of patients, and the clinical manifestations frequently resemble acute appendicitis [67].

Ovarian Torsion and Infarction

Ovarian or adnexal torsion is most frequently a complication of an underlying ovarian lesion, usually a nonneoplastic cyst, abscess, or benign tumor but occasionally a malignant neoplasm [71]. Torsion of a normal ovary occurs rarely, especially in infants or children but also in adults. Bilateral adnexal torsion, synchronous or asynchronous, has been reported.

The patients present with clinical findings similar to those of acute appendicitis or with recurrent episodes of abdominal pain; occasionally, an adnexal mass is palpable. Laparotomy reveals a swollen, hemorrhagic, and in some cases, infarcted, tuboovarian mass twisted on its pedicle. Where possible, detorsion is advocated, rather than oophorectomy, to preserve ovarian function [147]. In rare cases, the torsion and infarction may be asymptomatic, and autoamputation can result in a mass, which is occasionally calcified, lying free in the peritoneal cavity or attached to adjacent structures. The differential diagnosis in such cases, as noted earlier (Congenital Lesions and Ectopic Tissues), is with congenital unilateral absence of the ovary and tube.

It is crucial to examine thoroughly any hemorrhagic infarcted ovarian mass to exclude a neoplasm. A search should be made for viable foci at the periphery of the lesion, and the necrotic tissue should be scrutinized for shadows of neoplastic cells.

Ovarian Vein Thrombophlebitis

Ovarian vein thombosis or thrombophlebitis is an uncommon but potentially fatal disorder that most often occurs postpartum but may follow pelvic operations or pelvic trauma or complicate other pelvic disorders such as pelvic inflammatory disease [213]. Patients usually present with fever and lower abdominal pain and an abdominal mass, almost always on the right side. The clinical picture may simulate acute appendicitis or pyelonephritis. The marked right-sided predominance in the puerperal cases is explained on the basis of retrograde venous flow in the left ovarian vein during the puerperium, protecting that side from bacterial spread from the uterus. Sonography, computed tomography (CT), and magnetic resonance imaging studies may be useful in establishing the diagnosis preoperatively, thus avoiding unnecessary laparotomy, as the mainstays of treatment are anticoagulation and antibiotic therapy [44].

If surgery is undertaken, the involved ovarian vein will be markedly enlarged and the thrombus usually extends to the inferior vena cava on the right or to the renal vein on the left. Rarely, one or both of the latter structures are also thrombosed. There is marked edema and inflammation of the surrounding retroperitoneal tissues. The ipsilateral ovary is usually congested but not infarcted, although asymptomatic bilateral ovarian infarction in a postpartum patient secondary to massive pelvic venous thrombosis has been reported. Some cases may be associated with the ovarian vein syndrome (➤ Rare Vascular Lesions).

Rare Vascular Lesions

Giant cell arteritis can rarely involve the female genital tract, including the ovaries [2, 13, 114]. The patients are almost invariably postmenopausal, and some patients with ovarian involvement have had systemic manifestations, such as a history of polymyagia rheumatica or temporal arteritis, an elevated erythrocyte sedimentation rate (ESR), or both. Less commonly, the arteritis is an incidental microscopic finding in an asymptomatic patient. Treatment is probably unnecessary in this group of patients, but they should be followed carefully, including repeated determinations of the ESR [13, 114]. Rare examples of vasculitis of polyarteritis nodosa type involving the ovaries or ovarian hilus have also been reported (➤ *Fig. 12.51*). Rarely, the finding is a reflection of systemic involvement, but usually polyarteritis in the female genital tract (typically the cervix) is an isolated finding without systemic manifestations on follow-up [2, 56, 59].

A rare cause of retroperitoneal hemorrhage is rupture of an ovarian artery or vein, typically during pregnancy or the puerperium [62]. In some cases, the rupture represents a complication of an aneurysm of the ovarian artery.

Varicosities of the ovarian vein, almost always on the right side, may occur in pregnant or parous women and cause ipsilateral ureteric compression and pyelonephritis, constituting the so-called ovarian vein syndrome. Ovarian arteriovenous fistulas have been reported as a rare complication of gynecologic surgery.

Ovarian Pregnancy

Up to 1–3% of all ectopic pregnancies are ovarian [66, 81]. The diagnosis of ovarian pregnancy should be restricted to cases in which there is no involvement of the fallopian tube. There is an increased frequency of ovarian pregnancy in patients with an intrauterine contraceptive device. The typical clinical presentation is severe pain with hemoperitoneum, and at laparotomy and on gross pathologic examination, the enlarged hemorrhagic ovary may mimic a hemorrhagic neoplasm (➤ *Fig. 12.52*). In a minority of the cases, gross identification of an embryo is indicative of the diagnosis, and in other cases, microscopic examination is diagnostic. One placental site nodule of the ovary has been described in a 61-year-old

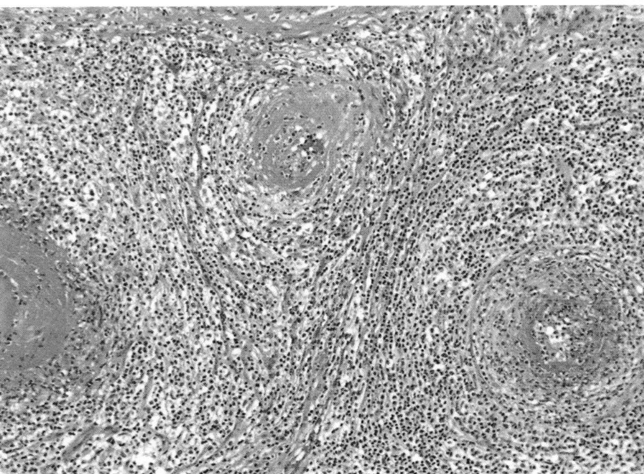

Fig. 12.51
Vasculitis of polyarteritis nodosa type in a postmenopausal woman. **Three ovarian hilar vessels are involved in this field. Polyarteritis also involved the uterine cervix in this case**

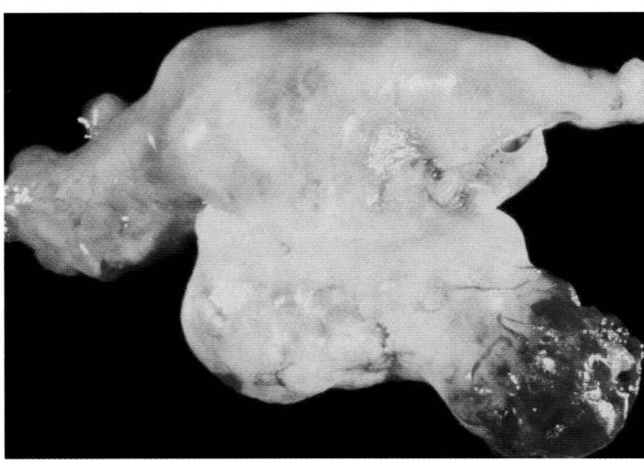

Fig. 12.52
Ovarian pregnancy. **A nodule of hemorrhagic placental tissue protrudes from the ovarian surface (*lower right*)**

woman, presumably representing the remnants of an old ovarian pregnancy [6]. Distinction between an ovarian pregnancy and the very rare examples of primary ovarian gestational trophoblastic disease (➲ Chap. 20, Gestational Trophoblastic Tumors and Related Tumor-Like Lesions) is made by applying criteria similar to those used in the uterus.

Ovarian Changes Secondary to Metabolic Diseases

Amyloidosis may rarely involve the ovaries, usually as an incidental microscopic finding in patients with systemic amyloidosis (➲ *Fig. 12.53*) [35]. There are several reports of tumor-like ovarian enlargement secondary to systemic or presumably localized amyloidosis [130].

Rare cases of ovarian enlargement secondary to involvement by systemic storage disorders (lipidoses, mucopolysaccharidoses) have been reported [45]. In such cases, the stored material is typically within macrophages, allowing histologic distinction from a steroid cell tumor or foci of fat within the ovarian stroma. An autopsy study in patients with diabetes mellitus revealed atrophic and fibrotic changes in the ovaries more frequently than in ovaries from control patients, although the differences were not statistically significant [55].

In contrast to frequent testicular involvement in hemochromatosis, in which hemosiderin is typically seen within walls of testicular blood vessels, pathologic changes in the ovary secondary to this disorder appear to be rare or nonexistent.

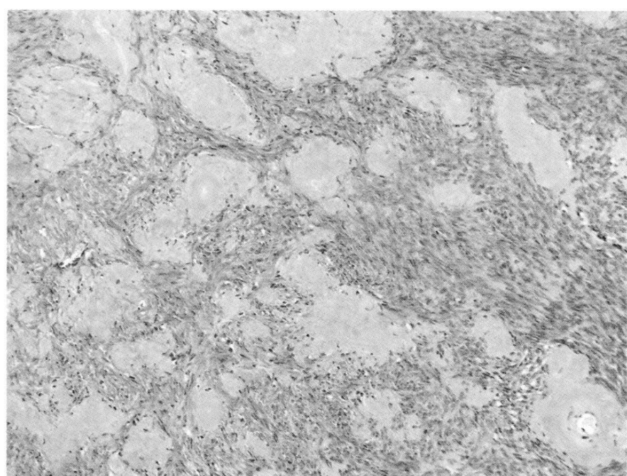

Fig. 12.53
Ovarian amyloidosis. **Amyloid involves the ovarian stroma and vessels**

Ovarian Changes Secondary to Cytotoxic Drugs and Radiation

Cytotoxic Drugs

Cytotoxic drugs may cause a variety of histologic changes in the ovaries of prepubertal and postpubertal patients, including focal or diffuse cortical fibrosis, impaired follicular maturation, and a reduction or depletion in follicle numbers [34, 73, 113]. Some studies have shown a direct correlation between the severity of these changes and the duration of the chemotherapy, the number of drugs, and malnourishment of the patients. These morphologic findings are consistent with clinical observations of diminished ovarian endocrine function or ovarian failure in some of these patients [178]. The risk of ovarian failure appears to be greater in patients who received higher doses and in whom treatment is begun after the age of 25 [34, 178]. In rare cases, the ovarian failure has reversed after cessation of the therapy.

Radiation

The ovary is among the most radiosensitive of organs. Relatively low doses of radiation (500–600 R) to the ovaries cause complete or nearly complete disappearance of primordial and developing follicles, fibrosis of the ovarian stroma, and vascular sclerosis in more than 90% of patients (➲ *Fig. 12.54*) [34, 73]. Follow-up studies of both children and adults who received pelvic radiation have shown that ovarian failure occurs in the majority of such patients [73, 197]. The ovarian stroma appears to be more radioresistant than the follicles and may continue to secrete androgens after radiation [82].

Miscellaneous Lesions

Ovarian Remnant Syndrome

Ectopic, accessory, and supernumerary ovary (➲ Congenital Lesions and Ectopic Tissues) should be distinguished from examples of the ovarian remnant syndrome (ORS), which is also known as the ovarian implant syndrome [88, 99, 110, 155]. The ORS should in turn be distinguished from the residual ovary syndrome, in which pelvic symptoms originate from ovaries preserved at the time of

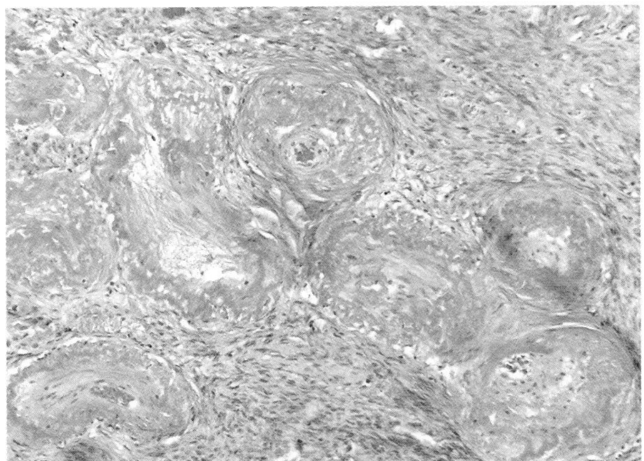

Fig. 12.54
Radiation changes. **Blood vessels are hyalinized, and the ovarian stroma is fibrotic**

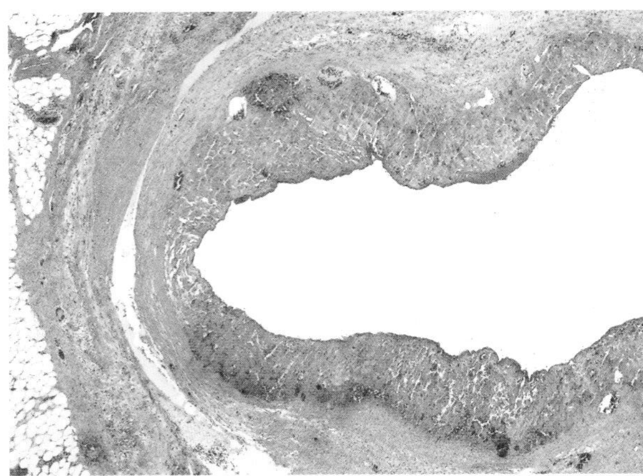

Fig. 12.55
Ovarian remnant syndrome. **A corpus luteum cyst is surrounded by congested fibroadipose tissue**

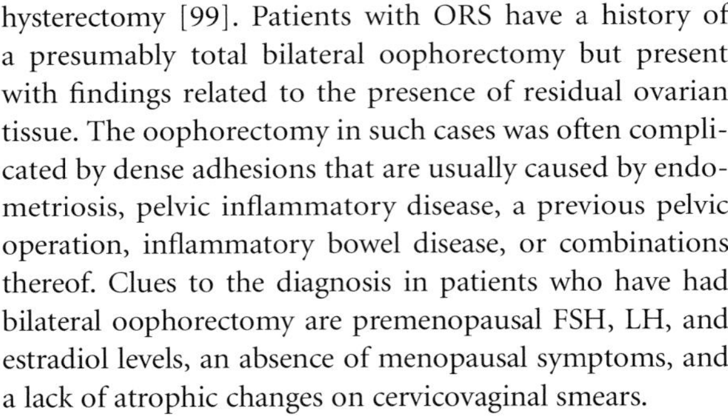

hysterectomy [99]. Patients with ORS have a history of a presumably total bilateral oophorectomy but present with findings related to the presence of residual ovarian tissue. The oophorectomy in such cases was often complicated by dense adhesions that are usually caused by endometriosis, pelvic inflammatory disease, a previous pelvic operation, inflammatory bowel disease, or combinations thereof. Clues to the diagnosis in patients who have had bilateral oophorectomy are premenopausal FSH, LH, and estradiol levels, an absence of menopausal symptoms, and a lack of atrophic changes on cervicovaginal smears.

Within weeks to months, but occasionally years, after the oophorectomy, women with ORS usually present with chronic or cyclic pelvic pain and, in about half the cases, a palpable pelvic mass. Ultrasonography or computed tomographic (CT) scanning may aid preoperative detection of nonpalpable symptomatic remnants [155], and stimulation of the residual ovarian tissue with clomiphene citrate therapy can facilitate their intraoperative localization [88]. Reoperation typically reveals a 3- to 4-cm cystic mass, covered by dense adhesions on the pelvic side wall, or less commonly, the mesentery; bilateral ovarian remnants rarely have been encountered. Obstruction or compression of the ureter, the colon, the small intestine, or the bladder may occur [155]. Pathologic examination usually reveals one or several follicular or corpus luteum cysts within a remnant of ovarian tissue surrounded by chronically inflamed fibrous tissue (*Fig. 12.55*). Less common findings have included endometriosis, benign neoplasms, or normal ovarian tissue. Excision of the remnants may be difficult and require multiple operations.

Rete Cysts

The rete ovarii, the ovarian analogue of the rete testis, which is present in the hilus of all ovaries, consists of a network of anastomosing branching tubules with intraluminal polypoid projections, lined by an epithelium that varies from flat to cuboidal to columnar. Solid cords of similar cells may also be seen. The rete is surrounded by a cuff of spindle cell stroma morphologically similar to, but discontinuous from, the ovarian stroma. The rete lies adjacent to and may communicate with mesonephric tubules within the mesovarium. The rete epithelium may undergo transitional metaplasia.

Occasional hilar cysts originate from the rete, and small tumor-like proliferations of the rete have been referred to as rete adenomas. Rete cysts are typically located in the ovarian hilus, and in one series, the cysts had a mean diameter of 8.7 cm (range, 1–24 cm) [174]. Most are unilocular, although occasionally they are multilocular. Rete cysts typically are lined by a single layer of nonciliated epithelium that varies from flat to cuboidal to columnar. In addition to their hilar location, clues to the origin of the cysts are an irregular contour of their inner surface with small crevice-like outpouchings and a wall that often contains bundles of smooth muscle and hyperplastic hilus cells (*Fig. 12.56*). A lesion interpreted as adenomatous hyperplasia of the rete ovarii has been reported, which formed a 3-mm nodule in the ovarian hilus of a 43-year-old woman. The lesion consisted of a poorly circumscribed proliferation of benign appearing tubules with scanty fibromuscular stroma, merging with the normal rete [70].

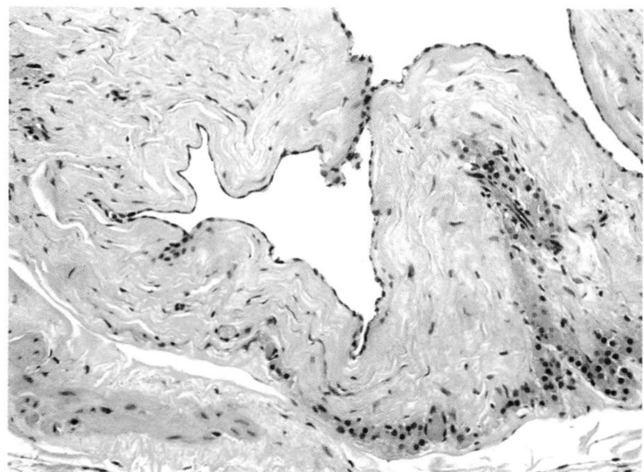

Fig. 12.56
Rete cyst. **The lining is composed of a single layer of flattened cells which line crevices. Note smooth muscle and nests of Leydig cells in the wall**

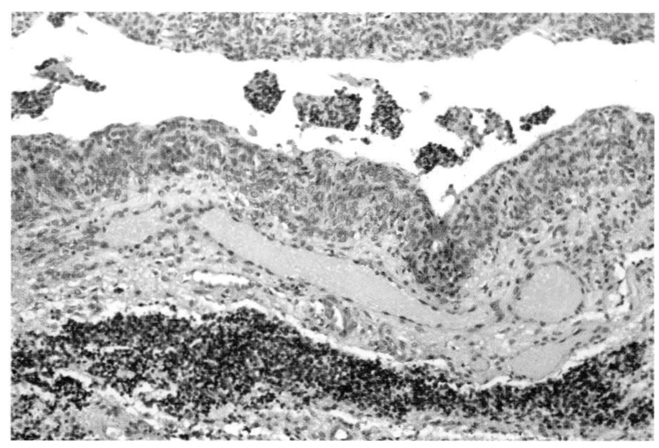

Fig. 12.57
Artifactual displacement of granulosa cells. **Nests of granulosa cells occupy an artifactual space in the ovarian stroma (*bottom*). Note adjacent cystic follicle (*top*) with detached granulosa cells similar to those in the stroma**

Artifacts and Normal Findings

The granulosa cells of normal follicles can be artifactually introduced into tissue spaces or vascular channels during sectioning (*Figs. 12.57* and *12.58*). This finding, especially when the displaced cells are shrunken or crushed, is occasionally misinterpreted as small cell carcinoma [123]. Awareness of this artifact, the bland nuclear features of the cells, and their similarity to cells lining nearby follicles are

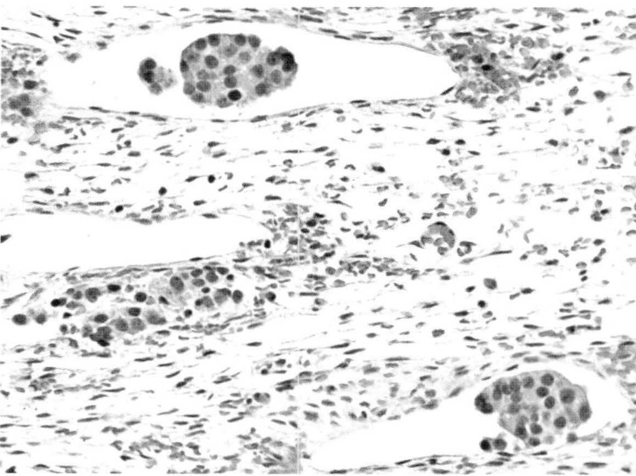

Fig. 12.58
Displaced luteinized granulosa cells in ovarian lymphatics

helpful clues to the correct diagnosis. Granulosa cells that appear to be deposited on the surface of the ovary secondary to follicle rupture may be misinterpreted as mesothelial cells and when numerous, may even suggest the possible diagnosis of a mesothelioma. Immunohistochemical staining for inhibin may confirm their presence in difficult cases.

Normal findings that may be misinterpereted as neoplastic include the occasionally highly mitotic granulosa cells and the theca externa cells of the normal developing follicle. Similarly, the corpus luteum of late pregnancy and the puerperium may contain numerous calcific deposits; we have encountered one case in which their presence in a patient with a history of a serous borderline tumor was misinterpreted as recurrent tumor.

Lesions that can involve the ovary, but which are more appropriately discussed in Chap. 13, Diseases of the Peritoneum, include mucicarminophilic histiocytosis and infarcted appendix epiploica.

References

1. Abrao MS, Dias JA Jr, Podgaec S et al (2006) Bowel endometriosis and schistosomiasis: a rare but possible association. Fertil Steril 85:1060
2. Abu-Farsakh H, Mody D, Brown RW et al (1994) Isolated vasculitis involving the female genital tract: clinicopathologic spectrum and phenotyping of inflammatory cells. Mod Pathol 7:610–615
3. Abu-Louz SK, Ahmed AA, Swan RW (1997) Spontaneous ovarian hyperstimulation syndrome with pregnancy. Am J Obstet Gynecol 177:476–477
4. Akhan SE, Dogan Y, Akhan S et al (2008) Pelvic actinomycosis mimicking ovarian malignancy: three cases. Eur J Gynaecol Oncol 29:294–297

5. Al-Ahmadie HA, Stanek J, Liu J et al (2001) Ovarian "tumor" of the adrenogenital syndrome. The first reported case. Am J Surg Pathol 25:1443–1450
6. Al-Hussaini M, Lioe TF, McCluggage WG (2002) Placental site nodule of the ovary. Letter. Histopathology 41:471–472
7. Almenoff IA (1966) Splenic-gonadal fusion. N Y State J Med 66:1679–1691
8. Al-Timimi A, Buckley CH, Fox H (1985) An immunohistochemical study of the incidence and significance of sex steroid hormone binding sites in normal and neoplastic human ovarian tissue. Int J Gynecol Pathol 4:24–41
9. Balen AH, Laven JS, Tan SL et al (2003) Ultrasound assessment of the polycystic ovary: international consensus definitions. Hum Reprod Update 9:505–514
10. Bannatyne P, Russell P, Shearman RP (1990) Autoimmune oophoritis: a clinicopathologic assessment of 12 cases. Int J Gynecol Pathol 9: 191–207
11. Barbieri RL, Ryan KJ (1983) Hyperandrogenism, insulin resistance, and acanthosis nigricans syndrome: a common endocrinopathy with distinct pathophysiologic features. Am J Obstet Gynecol 147:90–101
12. Barbieri RL, Smith S, Ryan KJ (1988) The role of hyperinsulinemia in the pathogenesis of ovarian hyperandrogenism. Fertil Steril 50:197–212
13. Bell DA, Mondschein M, Scully RE (1986) Giant cell arteritis of the female genital tract. A report of three cases. Am J Surg Pathol 10:696–701
14. Ben-Rafael Z, Bider D, Menashe Y et al (1990) Follicular and luteal cysts after treatment with gonadotropin-releasing hormone analogue for in vitro fertilization. Fertil Steril 53:1091–1094
15. Berger NG, Repke JT, Woodruff JD (1984) Markedly elevated serum testosterone in pregnancy without fetal virilization. Obstet Gynecol 63:260–262
16. Blaustein A (1981) Surface cells and inclusion cysts in fetal ovaries. Gynecol Oncol 12:222–233
17. Blaustein A, Kaganowicz A, Wells J (1982) Tumor markers in inclusion cysts of the ovary. Cancer (Phila) 49:722–726
18. Blaustein A, Kantius M, Kaganowicz A et al (1982) Inclusions in ovaries of females aged day 1–30 years. Int J Gynecol Pathol 1: 145–153
19. Bonar BE, Rabson AS (1957) Gynecologic aspects of leprosy. Obstet Gynecol 9:33–43
20. Boss JH, Scully RE, Wegner KH et al (1965) Structural variations in the adult ovary: clinical significance. Obstet Gynecol 25:747–764
21. Bradshaw KD, Santos-Ramos R, Rawlins SC et al (1986) Endocrine studies in a pregnancy complicated by ovarian theca lutein cysts and hyperreactio luteinalis. Obstet Gynecol 67:66S–69S
22. Burkman R, Schlesselman S, McCaffrey L et al (1982) The relationship of genital tract actinomycetes and the development of pelvic inflammatory disease. Am J Obstet Gynecol 143:585–589
23. Bylund DJ, Nanfro JJ, Marsh WL Jr (1986) Coccidioidomycosis of the female genital tract. Arch Pathol Lab Med 110:232–235
24. Caillouette JC, Koehler AL (1987) Phasic contraceptive pills and functional ovarian cysts. Am J Obstet Gynecol 156:1538–1542
25. Carmina E, Gonzalez F, Chang L et al (1995) Reassessment of adrenal androgen secretion in women with polycystic ovary syndrome. Obstet Gynecol 85:971–976
26. Charpin C, Bhan AK, Zurawski VR Jr et al (1982) Carcinoembryonic antigen (CEA) and carbohydrate determinant 19–9 (CA 19–9) localization in 121 primary and metastatic ovarian tumors: an immunohistochemical study with the use of monoclonal antibodies. Int J Gynecol Pathol 1:231–245
27. Chou SC, Wang JS, Tseng HH (2002) Malacoplakia of the ovary, fallopian tube and uterus: a case associated with diabetes mellitus. Pathol Int 52:789–793
28. Clement PB (2007) Ovary. In: Mills SE (ed) Histology for pathologists. Lippincott, Williams, and Wilkins, Philadelphia, PA, pp 1663–1694
29. Clement PB, Scully RE (1980) Large solitary luteinized follicle cyst of pregnancy and puerperium: A clinicopathological analysis of eight cases. Am J Surg Pathol 4:431–438
30. Clement PB, Cooney TP (1992) Idiopathic multifocal calcification of the ovarian stroma. Arch Pathol Lab Med 116:204–205
31. Clement PB, Young RH, Scully RE (1988) Ovarian granulosa cell proliferations of pregnancy. A report of nine cases. Hum Pathol 19:657–662
32. Clement PB, Young RH, Scully RE (1989) Nontrophoblastic pathology of the female genital tract and peritoneum associated with pregnancy. Semin Diagn Pathol 6:372–406
33. Cohen I, Figer A, Tepper R et al (1999) Ovarian overstimulation and cystic formation in premenopausal tamoxifen exposure: comparison between tamoxifen-treated and nontreated breast cancer patients. Gynecol Oncol 72:202–207
34. Cohen LE (2008) Cancer treatment and the ovary: the effects of chemotherapy and radiation. Ann N Y Acad Sci 1135:123–125
35. Copeland W Jr, Hawley PC, Teteris NJ (1985) Gynecologic amyloidosis. Am J Obstet Gynecol 153:555–556
36. Coulam CB (1983) The prevalence of autoimmune disorders among patients with primary ovarian failure. Am J Reprod Immunol 4: 63–66
37. Coulam CB, Annegers JF, Kranz JS (1983) Chronic anovulation syndrome and associated neoplasia. Obstet Gynecol 61:403–407
38. Cowchock FS, McCabe JL, Montgomery BB (1988) Pregnancy after corticosteroid administration in premature ovarian failure (polyglandular endocrinopathy syndrome). Am J Obstet Gynecol 158:118–119
39. Cramer DW, Welch WR, Cassells S et al (1983) Mumps, menarche, menopause, and ovarian cancer. Am J Obstet Gynecol 147:1–6
40. Damewood MD, Zacur HA, Hoffman GJ et al (1986) Circulating antiovarian antibodies in premature ovarian failure. Obstet Gynecol 68:850–854
41. Delibasi T, Erdogan MF, Serinsöz E et al (2007) Ovarian hilus-cell hyperplasia and high serum testosterone in a patient with postmenopausal virilization. Endocr Pract 13:472–475
42. Deligdisch L, Einstein AJ, Guera D et al (1995) Ovarian dysplasia in epithelial inclusion cysts. A morphometric approach using neural networks. Cancer (Phila) 76:1027–1034
43. Dennefors BL, Janson PO, Knutson F et al (1980) Steroid production and responsiveness to gonadotropin in isolated stromal tissue of human postmenopausal ovaries. Am J Obstet Gynecol 136:997–1002
44. Dessole S, Capobianco G, Arru A et al (2003) Postpartum ovarian vein thrombosis: an unpredictable event: two case reports and review of the literature. Arch Gynecol Obstet 267:242–246
45. Dincsoy HP, Rolfes DB, McGraw CA et al (1984) Cholesterol ester storage disease and mesenteric lipodystrophy. Am J Clin Pathol 81:263–269
46. Draper R, Walker EA, Bujalska IJ et al (2003) Mutations in the genes encoding 11beta-hydroxysteroid dehydrogenase type 1 and hexose-6-phosphate dehydrogenase interact to cause cortisone reductase deficiency. Nat Genet 34:434–439
47. Drapkin R, Crum CP, Hecht JL (2004) Expression of candidate tumor markers in ovarian carcinoma and benign ovary: evidence for a link between epithelial phenotype and neoplasia. Hum Pathol 35:1014–1021

48. Dunaif A, Hoffman AR, Scully RE et al (1985) Clinical, biochemical, and ovarian morphologic features in women with acanthosis nigricans and masculinization. Obstet Gynecol 66:545–552
49. Edwards-Silva RN, Han CS, Hoang Y et al (2008) Spontaneous ovarian hyperstimulation in a naturally conceived pregnancy with uncontrolled hypothyroidism. Obstet Gynecol 111:498–501
50. Ehrmann DA (2005) Polycystic ovary syndrome. N Engl J Med 352:1223–1236
51. Elmore RG, Li AJ (2007) Peritoneal tuberculosis mimicking advanced-stage epithelial ovarian cancer. Obstet Gynecol 110:1417–1419
52. Escobar ME, Cigorraga SB, Chiauzzi VA et al (1982) Development of gonadotropin resistant ovary syndrome in myasthenia gravis: suggestion of similar autoimmune mechanisms. Acta Endocrinol 99:431–436
53. Euthymiopoulou K, Aletras AJ, Ravazoula P et al (2007) Antiovarian antibodies in primary Sjogren's syndrome. Rheumatol Int 27: 1149–1155
54. Filho RB, Domingues L, Naves L (2007) Polycystic ovary syndrome and hyperprolactinemia are distinct entities. Gynecol Endocrinol 23:267–272
55. Fraley DS, Totten RS (1968) An autopsy study of endocrine organ changes in diabetes mellitus. Metabolism 17:896–900
56. Francke M, Mihaescu A, Chaubert P (1998) Isolated necrotizing arteritis of the female genital tract: a clinicopathologic and immunohistochemical study of 11 cases. Int J Gynecol Pathol 17:193–200
57. Friedman CI, Neff J, Kim MH (1984) Immunologic parameters in premature follicular depletion: T and B lymphocytes, T-cell subpopulations, cutaneous reactivity, and serum immunoglobulin concentrations. Diagn Immunol 2:48–52
58. Futterweit W (1999) Polycystic ovary syndrome: clinical perspectives and management. Obstet Gynecol Surv 54:403–413
59. Ganesan R, Ferryman SR, Meier L, Rollason TP (2000) Vasculitis of the female genital tract and its clinicopathologic correlation: a study of 46 cases with follow-up. Int J Gynecol Pathol 19:258–265
60. Gao HW, Lin CK, Yu CP et al (2002) Oxidized cellulose (Surgicel™) granuloma mimicking a primary ovarian tumor. Int J Gynecol Pathol 21:422–423
61. Gilks CB, Clement PB (1987) Colo-ovarian fistula: a report of two cases. Obstet Gynecol 69:533–537
62. Ginsburg KA, Valdes C, Schnider G (1987) Spontaneous utero-ovarian vessel rupture during pregnancy: three case reports and a review of the literature. Obstet Gynecol 69:474–476
63. Gloor E, Hurlimann J (1984) Autoimmune oophoritis. Am J Clin Pathol 81:105–109
64. Granks S, Gilling-Smith C, Watson H, Willis D (1999) Insulin action in the normal and polycystic ovary. Endocrinol Metab Clin N Am 28:361–378
65. Hahn-Pedersen J, Munkholm Larsen P (1984) Supernumerary ovary. Acta Obstet Gynecol Scand 63:365–366
66. Hallatt JG (1982) Primary ovarian pregnancy: a report of twenty-five cases. Am J Obstet Gynecol 143:55–60
67. Hallatt JG, Steele CH Jr, Snyder M (1984) Ruptured corpus luteum with hemoperitoneum: a study of 173 surgical cases. Am J Obstet Gynecol 149:5–9
68. Haning RV Jr, Strawn EY, Nolten WE (1985) Pathophysiology of the ovarian hyperstimulation syndrome. Obstet Gynecol 66:220–224
69. He H, Luthringer DJ, Hui P et al (2008) Expression of CD56 and WT1 in ovarian stroma and ovarian stromal tumors. Am J Surg Pathol 32:884–890
70. Heatley MK (2000) Adenomatous hyperplasia of the rete ovarii. Letter. Histopathology 36:383–384
71. Hibbard LT (1985) Adnexal torsion. Am J Obstet Gynecol 152: 456–461
72. Hill JA, Welch WR, Faris HM et al (1990) Induction of class II major histocompatibility complex antigen expression in human granulosa cells by interferon gamma: a potential mechanism contributing to autoimmune ovarian failure. Am J Obstet Gynecol 162:534–540
73. Himelstein-Braw R, Peters H, Faber M (1977) Influence of irradiation and chemotherapy on the ovaries of children with abdominal tumours. Br J Cancer 36:269–275
74. Honoré LH, O'Hara KE (1979) Ovarian hilus cell heterotopia. Obstet Gynecol 53:461–464
75. Honoré LH, O'Hara KE (1980) Subcapsular adipocytic infiltration of the human ovary: a clinicopathological study of eight cases. Eur J Obstet Gynaecol Reprod Biol 10:13–20
76. Hosfield EM, Rabban JT, Chen L et al (2008) Squamous metaplasia of the ovarian surface epithelium and subsurface fibrosis: Distinctive pathologic findings in the ovaries and fallopian tubes of patients of peritoneal dialysis. Int J Gynecol Pathol 27:465–474
77. Hughesdon PE (1976) The endometrial identity of benign stromatosis of the ovary and its relation to other forms of endometriosis. J Pathol 119:201–209
78. Hughesdon PE (1982) Morphology and morphogenesis of the Stein-Leventhal ovary and of so-called "hyperthecosis". Obstet Gynecol Surv 37:59–77
79. Hutson R, Ramsdale J, Wells M (1995) p53 protein expression in putative precursor lesions of epithelial ovarian cancer. Histopathology (Oxf) 27:367–371
80. Isojärvi JIT, Laatikainen TJ, Pakarinen AJ et al (1993) Polycystic ovaries and hyperandrogenism in women taking valproate for epilepsy. N Engl J Med 329:1383–1388
81. Ito H, Ishihara A, Koita H et al (2003) Ovarian pregnancy: report of four cases and review of the literature. Pathol Int 53:806–809
82. Janson PO, Jansson I, Skryten A et al (1981) Ovarian endocrine function in young women undergoing radiotherapy for carcinoma of the cervix. Gynecol Oncol 11:218–223
83. Judd HL, Scully RE, Atkins L et al (1970) Pure gonadal dysgenesis with progressive hirsutism. Demonstration of testosterone production by gonadal streaks. N Engl J Med 282:881–885
84. Judd HL, Scully RE, Herbst AL et al (1973) Familial hyperthecosis: comparison of endocrinologic and histologic findings with polycystic ovarian disease. Am J Obstet Gynecol 117:976–982
85. Kahn CR, Flier JS, Bar RS et al (1976) The syndromes of insulin resistance and acanthosis nigricans: insulin-receptor disorders in man. N Engl J Med 294:739–745
86. Kaiser UB (2003) The pathogenesis of the ovarian hyperstimulation syndrome. N Engl J Med 349:729–732
87. Kalu E, Panay N (2008) Spontaneous premature ovarian failure: management challenges. Gynecol Endocrinol 24:273–279
88. Kaminski PF, Sorosky JI, Mandell MJ et al (1990) Clomiphene citrate stimulation as an adjunct in locating ovarian tissue in ovarian remnant syndrome. Obstet Gynecol 76:924–926
89. Kaufman DW, Shapiro S, Rosenberg L et al (1980) Intrauterine contraceptive device use and pelvic inflammatory disease. Am J Obstet Gynecol 136:159–162
90. Kaufman FR, Kogut MD, Donnell GN et al (1981) Hypergonadotropic hypogonadism in female patients with galactosemia. N Engl J Med 304:994–998
91. Kernohan NM, Best PV, Jandial V, Kitchener HC (1991) Palisading granuloma of the ovary. Histopathology (Oxf) 19:279–280
92. Klempner LB, Giglio PG, Niebles A (1987) Malacoplakia of the ovary. Obstet Gynecol 69:537–540

93. Knochenhauer ES, Key TJ, Kahsar-Miller M et al (1998) Prevalence of the polycystic ovary syndrome in unselected black and white women in the Southeastern United States: a prospective study. J Clin Endocrinol Metab 83:3078–3082
94. Kostelnik FV, Fremount HN (1976) Mycotic tubo-ovarian abscess associated with the intrauterine device. Am J Obstet Gynecol 125:272–274
95. Krasević M, Haller H, Rupcić S et al (2004) Massive edema of the ovary: a report of two cases due to lymphatic permeation by metastatic carcinoma from the uterine cervix. Gynecol Oncol 93:564–567
96. Krauss CM, Turksoy N, Atkins L et al (1987) Familial premature ovarian failure due to an interstitial deletion of the long arm of the X chromosome. N Engl J Med 317:125–131
97. LaBarbera AR, Miller MM, Ober C et al (1988) Autoimmune etiology in premature ovarian failure. Am J Reprod Immunol Microbiol 16:115–122
98. Ladefoged C, Lorentzen M (1988) Xanthogranulomatous inflammation of the female genital tract. Histopathology (Oxf) 13: 541–551
99. Lafferty HW, Angioli R, Rudolph J et al (1996) Ovarian remnant syndrome: experience at Jackson Memorial Hospital, University of Miami, 1985 through 1993. Am J Obstet Gynecol 174: 641–645
100. Lai C, Hsueh S, Lin C et al (1992) Human papillomavirus in benign and malignant ovarian and endometrial tissues. Int J Gynecol Pathol 11:210–215
101. Landers DV, Sweet RL (1985) Current trends in the diagnosis and treatment of tuboovarian abscess. Am J Obstet Gynecol 151: 1098–1110
102. Latza U, Niedobitek G, Schwarting R et al (1990) Ber-EP4: new monoclonal antibody which distinguishes epithelia from mesothelia. J Clin Pathol 43:213–219
103. Lee AT, Zane LT (2007) Dermatologic manifestations of polycystic ovary syndrome. Am J Clin Dermatol 8:201–219
104. Liapi C, Evain-Brion D (1987) Diagnosis of ovarian follicular cysts from birth to puberty: a report of twenty cases. Acta Pediatr Scand 76:91–96
105. Lindsay AN, Voorhess ML, MacGillivray MH (1983) Multicystic ovaries in primary hypothyroidism. Obstet Gynecol 61:433
106. Lonsdale RN, Roberts PF, Trowell JE (1991) Autoimmune oophoritis associated with polycystic ovaries. Histopathology (Oxf) 19:77–81
107. Lunde O, Hoel PS, Sandvik L (1988) Ovarian morphology in patients with polycystic ovaries and in an age-matched reference material. Gynecol Obstet Invest 25:192–201
108. Luzzatto R, Brucker N (1981) Benign inclusion cysts of the ovary associated with psammoma bodies in vaginal smears. Acta Cytol 25:282–284
109. Madeido G, Tieu TM, Aiman J (1985) Atypical ovarian hyperthecosis in a virilized postmenopausal woman. Am J Clin Pathol 83:101–107
110. Magtibay PM, Nyholm JL, Hernandez JL et al (2005) Ovarian remnant syndrome. Am J Obstet Gynecol 193:2062–2066
111. Mahmood K (1975) Granulomatous oophoritis due to Schistosoma mansoni. Am J Obstet Gynecol 123:919–920
112. Manolitsas TP, Lanham SA, Hitchcock A et al (1998) Synchronous ovarian and cervical squamous intraepithelial neoplasia: an analysis of HPV status. Gynecol Oncol 70:428–431
113. Marcello MF, Nuciforo G, Romeo R et al (1990) Structural and ultrastructural study of the ovary in childhood leukemia after successful treatment. Cancer (Phila) 66:2099–2104
114. Marrogi AJ, Gersell DJ, Kraus FT (1991) Localized asymptomatic giant cell arteritis of the female genital tract. Int J Gynecol Pathol 10:51–58
115. Massachusetts General Hospital Case Records (1982) Case 25–1982. Ovarian stromal hyperthecosis. Acanthosis nigricans. N Engl J Med 306:1537–1544
116. Massachusetts General Hospital Case Records (1986) Case 46–1986. Resistant-ovary syndrome, with hyalinization of preantral follicles. N Engl J Med 315:1336–1344
117. Massachusetts General Hospital Case Records (1988) Case 22–1988. Ovarian stromal hyperthecosis, with virilization, insulin resistance, and acanthosis nigricans. N Engl J Med 318:1449–1457
118. Mathur S, Melchers JT III, Ades EW et al (1980) Anti-ovarian and anti-lymphocyte antibodies in patients with chronic vaginal candidiasis. J Reprod Immunol 2:247–262
119. Mattison DR, Evans MI, Schwimmer WB et al (1984) Familial premature ovarian failure. Am J Hum Genet 36:1341–1348
120. McCluggage WG, Allen DC (1997) Ovarian granulomas: a report of 32 cases. J Clin Pathol 50:324–327
121. McCluggage WG, Maxwell P (2001) Immunohistochemical staining for calretinin is useful in the diagnosis of ovarian sex cord-stromal tumours. Histopathology 38:403–408
122. McCluggage WG, McKenna M, McBride HA (2007) CD56 is a sensitive and diagnostically useful immunohistochemical marker of ovarian sex cord-stromal tumors. Int J Gynecol Pathol 26: 322–327
123. McCluggage WG, Young RH (2004) Non-neoplastic granulosa cells within ovarian vascular channels: a rare potential diagnostic pitfall. J Clin Pathol 57:151–154
124. McClure N, Healy DL, Rogers PA (1994) Vascular endothelial growth factor as capillary permeability agent in ovarian hyperstimulation. Lancet 344:235–236
125. McMahon JN, Connolly CE, Long SV et al (1984) Enterobius granulomas of the uterus, ovary and pelvic peritoneum. Two case reports. Br J Obstet Gynaecol 91:289–290
126. Meneses MF, Ostrowski ML (1989) Female splenic-gonadal fusion of the discontinuous type. Hum Pathol 20:486–488
127. Mignot MH, Schoemaker J, Kleingeld M et al (1989) Premature ovarian failure. I: The association with autoimmunity. Eur J Obstet Gynecol Reprod Biol 30:59–66
128. Mittal KR, Zeleniuch-Jacquotte A, Cooper JL et al (1993) Contralateral ovary in unilateral ovarian carcinoma: a search for preneoplastic lesions. Int J Gynecol Pathol 12:59–63
129. Montz FJ, Schlaerth JB, Morrow CP (1988) The natural history of theca lutein cysts. Obstet Gynecol 72:247–251
130. Mount SL, Eltabbakh GH, Hardin NJ (2002) Beta-2 microglobulin amyloidosis presenting as bilateral ovarian masses. A case report and review of the literature. Am J Surg Pathol 26:130–133
131. Muller-Holzner E, Ruth NR, Abfalter E et al (1995) IUD-associated pelvic actinomycosis: a report of five cases. Int J Gynecol Pathol 14:70–74
132. Murray JJ, Clark CA, Lands RH et al (1985) Reactivation blastomycosis presenting as a tuboovarian abscess. Obstet Gynecol 64: 828–830
133. Nagamani H, Kaspar HG, Van Dinh T et al (1990) Hyperthecosis of the ovaries in a woman with a placental site trophoblastic tumor. Obstet Gynecol 76:931–935
134. Nagamani M, Gomez LG, Garza J (1982) In vivo steroid studies in luteoma of pregnancy. Obstet Gynecol 59:105S–111S
135. Nagamani M, Hannigan EV, Van Dinh T et al (1988) Hyperinsulinemia and stromal luteinization of the ovaries in

postmenopausal women with endometrial cancer. J Clin Endocrinol Metab 67:144–148
136. Nagamani M, Stuart CA, Doherty MG (1992) Increased steroid production by the ovarian stromal tissue of postmenopausal women with endometrial cancer. J Clin Endocrinol Metab 74:172–176
137. Nagamani M, Van Dinh T, Kelver ME (1986) Hyperinsulinemia in hyperthecosis of the ovaries. Am J Obstet Gynecol 154:384–389
138. Nagelberg SB, Rosen SW (1985) Clinical and laboratory investigation of a virilized woman with placental-site trophoblastic tumor. Obstet Gynecol 65:527–534
139. Nakano R, Shima K, Yamoto M et al (1989) Binding sites for gonadotropins in human postmenopausal ovaries. Obstet Gynecol 73:196–200
140. Nestler JE, Clore JN, Blackard WG (1989) The central role of obesity (hyperinsulinemia) in the pathogenesis of the polycystic ovary syndrome. Am J Obstet Gynecol 161:1095–1097
141. Nogales FF, Martin-Sances L, Mendoza-Garcia E et al (1996) Massive ovarian edema. Histopathology (Oxf) 28:229–234
142. Nogales FF, Silverberg SG (1976) Epidermoid cysts of the ovary: a report of five cases with histogenetic considerations and ultrastructural findings. Am J Obstet Gynecol 124:523–528
143. Nogales-Ortiz F, Taracon I, Nogales FF (1979) The pathology of female genital tract tuberculosis. Obstet Gynecol 53:422–428
144. Norman RJ, Dewailly D, Legro RS et al (2007) Polycystic ovary syndrome. Lancet 370:685–697
145. Norris HJ, Taylor HB (1967) Nodular theca-lutein hyperplasia of pregnancy (so-called “pregnancy luteoma”). A clinical and pathologic study of 15 cases. Am J Clin Pathol 47:557–566
146. Ober WB, Grady HG, Schoenbucher AK (1957) Ectopic ovarian decidua without pregnancy. Am J Pathol 33:199–217
147. Oelsner G, Shashar D (2006) Adnexal torsion. Clin Obstet Gynecol 49:459–463
148. Osathanondh R, Berkowitz RS, de Cholnoky C et al (1986) Hormonal measurements in patients with theca lutein cysts and gestational trophoblastic disease. J Reprod Med 31:179–183
149. Pache TD, Chadha S, Goorens LJG et al (1991) Ovarian morphology in long-term androgen-treated female to male transsexuals A human model for the study of polycystic ovary syndrome? Histopathology (Oxf) 19:445–452
150. Pai SA, Desai SB, Borges AM (1998) Uterus-like masses of the ovary associated with breast cancer and raised serum CA 125. Am J Surg Pathol 22:333–337
151. Parveen AS, Elliott H, Howells R (2004) Sarcoidosis of the ovary. J Obstet Gynaecol 24:465
152. Peer E, Peretz BA, Makler A et al (1981) Bilateral adnexal agenesis with an ectopic ovary: case report and review of the literature. Eur J Obstet Gynecol Reprod Biol 12:37–42
153. Pekonen F, Seigberg R, Makinen T et al (1986) Immunological disturbances in patients with premature ovarian failure. Clin Endocrinol 25:1–6
154. Pelkey TJ, Frierson HF Jr, Mills SE et al (1998) The diagnostic utility of inhibin staining in ovarian neoplasms. Int J Gynecol Pathol 17:97–105
155. Pettit PD, Lee RA (1988) Ovarian remnant syndrome: diagnostic dilemma and surgical challenge. Obstet Gynecol 71:580–583
156. Pine L, Curtis EM, Brown JM (1985) Actinomyces and the intrauterine contraceptive device: aspects of the fluorescent antibody stain. Am J Obstet Gynecol 152:287–290
157. Planner RS, Abell DA, Barbaro CA et al (1982) Massive enlargement of the ovaries after evacuation of hydatidiform moles. Aust NZ J Obstet Gynaecol 22:96–100
158. Plentl AA, Friedman EA (1971) Lymphatic system of the female genitalia. Saunders, Philadelphia, PA
159. Podgajski M, Kukura V, Duic Z et al (2007) Ascites, high CA-125 and chronic pelvic pain in an unusual clinical manifestation of Enterobius vermicularis ovarian and sigmoid colon granuloma. Eur J Gynaecol Oncol 28:513–515
160. Polson DW, Wadsworth J, Adams J et al (1988) Polycystic ovaries – a common finding in normal women. Lancet ii:870–872
161. Pritt B, Mount SL, Cooper K et al (2006) Pseudoactinomycotic radiate granules of the gynaecological tract: review of a diagnostic pitfall. J Clin Pathol 59:17–20
162. Pryse-Davies J (1974) The development, structure and function of the female pelvic organs in childhood. Clin Obstet Gynaecol 1:483–508
163. Putschar WGJ, Manion WC (1956) Splenic-gonadal fusion. Am J Pathol 32:15–33
164. Rebar RW, Erickson GF, Yen SSC (1982) Idiopathic premature ovarian failure: clinical and endocrine characteristics. Fertil Steril 37:35–41
165. Redman R, Wilksonson EJ, Massoll NA (2005) Uterine-like mass with features of an extrauterine adenomyoma presenting 22 years after total abdominal hysterectomy-bilateral salpingo-oophorectomy: a case report and review of the literature. Arch Pathol Lab Med 129:1041–1043
166. Reeves G (1971) Specific stroma in the cortex and medulla of the ovary. Cell types and vascular supply in relation to follicular apparatus and ovulation. Obstet Gynecol 37:832–844
167. Resta L, Scordari MD, Colucci GA et al (1989) Morphological changes of the ovarian surface epithelium in ovarian polycystic disease or endometrial carcinoma and a control group. Eur J Gynaecol Oncol 10:39–41
168. Riddlesberger MM Jr, Kuhn JP, Munschauer RW (1981) The association of juvenile hypothyroidism and cystic ovaries. Radiology 139:77–80
169. Rodin A, Thakkar H, Taylor N et al (1994) Hyperandrogenism in polycystic ovary syndrome. Evidence of dysregulation of 11-beta-hydroxysteroid dehydrogenase. N Engl J Med 330:460–465
170. Roth LM, Sternberg WH (1973) Ovarian stromal tumors containing Leydig cells. II. Pure Leydig cell tumor, non-hilar type. Cancer (Phila) 32:952–960
171. Roth LM, Deaton RL, Sternberg WH (1979) Massive ovarian edema. A clinicopathologic study of five cases including ultrastructural observations and review of the literature. Am J Surg Pathol 3:11–21
172. Russell P, Bannatyne P, Shearman RP et al (1982) Premature hypergonadotropic ovarian failure: clinicopathological study of 19 cases. Int J Gynecol Pathol 1:185–201
173. Russell P, Farnsworth A (1997) Massive edema and fibromatosis. In: Russell P, Farnsworth A (eds) Surgical pathology of the ovaries. Churchill Livingstone, New York, pp 147–154
174. Rutgers JL, Scully RE (1988) Cysts (cystadenomas) and tumors of the rete ovarii. Int J Gynecol Pathol 7:330–342
175. Rutgers JL, Scully RE (1986) Functioning ovarian tumors with peripheral steroid cell proliferation: a report of twenty-four cases. Int J Gynecol Pathol 5:319–337
176. Sasano H, Fukunaga M, Rojas M et al (1989) Hyperthecosis of the ovary. Clinicopathologic study of 19 cases with immunohistochemical analysis of steroidogenic enzymes. Int J Gynecol Pathol 8:311–320
177. Schildkraut J, Schwingl PJ, Bastos E et al (1996) Epithelial ovarian cancer risk among women with polycystic ovary syndrome. Obstet Gynecol 88:554–559

178. Schilsky RL, Sherins RJ, Hubbard SM et al (1981) Long-term follow-up of ovarian function in women treated with MOPP chemotherapy for Hodgkin's disease. Am J Med 71:552–556
179. Schmidt WA (1982) IUDs, inflammation, and infection: assessment after two decades of IUD use. Hum Pathol 13:878–881
180. Scully RE (1964) Stromal luteoma of the ovary. Cancer (Phila) 17:769–778
181. Scully RE (1981) Smooth-muscle differentiation in genital tract disorders [Editorial]. Arch Pathol Lab Med 105:505–507
182. Scully RE, Cohen RB (1964) Oxidative-enzyme activity in normal and pathologic human ovaries. Obstet Gynecol 24:667–681
183. Scully RE (1986) Ovary. In: Henson DE, Albores-Saavedra J (eds) The pathology of incipient neoplasia. Saunders, Philadelphia, PA, pp 279–293
184. Sedin G, Bergquist C, Lindgren PG (1985) Ovarian hyperstimulation syndrome in preterm infants. Pediatr Res 19:548–551
185. Sedmak DD, Hart WR, Tubbs RR (1987) Autoimmune oophoritis: a histopathologic study of involved ovaries with immunologic characterization of the mononuclear cell infiltrate. Int J Gynecol Pathol 6:73–81
186. Shawker TH, Hubbard VS, Reichert CM et al (1983) Cystic ovaries in cystic fibrosis: an ultrasound and autopsy study. J Ultrasound Med 2:439–444
187. Sherman SL (2000) Permature ovarian failure in the fragile X syndrome. Am J Med Genet 97:189–194
188. Shimizu M, Toki T, Takagi Y et al (2000) Immunohistochemical detection of the Wilm's tumor gene (WT-1) in epithelial ovarian tumors. Int J Gynecol Pathol 19:158–163
189. Shipton EA, Meares SD (1965) Heterotopic bone formation in the ovary. Aust N Z J Obstet Gynaecol 5:100–102
190. Shutter J (2005) Uterus-like ovarian mass presenting near menarche. Int J Gynecol Pathol 24:382–384
191. Simstein NL (1981) Colo-tubo-ovarian fistula as complication of pelvic inflammatory disease. South J Med 74:512–513
192. Smith CET, Toplis PJ, Nogales FF (1999) Ovarian prostatic tissue originating from hilar mesonephric rests. Am J Surg Pathol 23:232–236
193. Smits G, Olatunbosun O, Delbaere A (2003) Ovarian hyperstimulation syndrome due to a mutation in the follicle-stimulating hormone receptor. N Engl J Med 349:760–766
194. Snowden JA, Harkin PJR, Thornton JG et al (1989) Morphometric assessment of ovarian stromal proliferation: a clinicopathological study. Histopathology (Oxf) 14:369
195. Steingold KA, Judd HL, Nieberg RK et al (1986) Treatment of severe androgen excess due to ovarian hyperthecosis with a long-acting gonadotropin-releasing hormone agonist. Am J Obstet Gynecol 154:1241–1248
196. Sternberg WH, Roth LM (1973) Ovarian stromal tumors containing Leydig cells. I. Stromal-Leydig cell tumor and non-neoplastic transformation of ovarian stroma to Leydig cells. Cancer (Phila) 32:940–951
197. Stillman RJ, Schinfeld JS, Schiff I et al (1981) Ovarian failure in long-term survivors of childhood malignancy. Am J Obstet Gynecol 139:62–66
198. Strickler RC, Kelly RW, Askin FB (1984) Postmenopausal ovarian follicle cyst: an unusual cause of estrogen excess. Int J Gynecol Pathol 3:318–322
199. Symonds DA, Driscoll SG (1973) An adrenal cortical rest within the fetal ovary: report of a case. Am J Clin Pathol 60:562–564
200. Tanabe K, Gagliano P, Channing CP et al (1983) Levels of inhibin-F activity and steroids in human follicular fluid from normal women and women with polycystic ovarian disease. J Clin Endocrinol Metab 57:24–31
201. Tatum ET, Beattie JF Jr, Bryson L (1996) Postoperative carbon pigment granuloma. A report of eight cases involving the ovary. Hum Pathol 27:1008–1011
202. Taylor AE (1998) Polycystic ovary syndrome. Endocrinol Metab Clin N Am 27:877–902
203. Taylor HC, Pillay I, Setrakian S (2000) Diffuse stromal Leydig cell hyperplasia: a unique cause of postmenopausal hyperandrogenism and virilization. Mayo Clin Proc 75:288–292
204. The Rotterdam ESHRE/ASRM-Sponsored PCOS consensus workshop group (2004) Revised 2003 consensus on diagnostic criteria and long-term health risks related to polycystic ovary syndrome. Hum Reprod 19:41–47
205. Tressera F, Grases PJ, Labastida R et al (1998) Histological features of the contralateral ovary in patients with unilateral ovarian cancer: a case control study. Gynecol Oncol 71:437–441
206. van Karseren YM, Schoemaker J (1999) Premature ovarian failure: a systematic review on therapeutic interventions to restore ovarian function and achieve pregnancy. Hum Reprod Update 5:483–492
207. Villanueva AL, Rebar RW (1983) Triple-X syndrome and premature ovarian failure. Obstet Gynecol 62:70S–73S
208. Walfish PG, Gottesman IS, Shewchuk AB et al (1983) Association of premature ovarian failure with HLA antigens. Tissue Antigens 21:168–169
209. Wang TH, Horng SG, Chang CL et al (2002) Human chorionic gonadotropin-induced ovarian hyperstimulation syndrome is associated with up-regulation of vascular endothelial growth factor. J Clin Endocrinol Metab 87:3300–3308
210. Weinstein D, Rabinowitz R, Malach D et al (1983) Ovarian hemorrhage in women with Von Willebrand's disease. A report of two cases. J Reprod Med 28:500–502
211. Wierman ME, Beardsworth DE, Mansfield MJ et al (1985) Puberty without gonadotropins. A unique mechanism of sexual development. N Engl J Med 312:65–72
212. Williams DJ, Connor P, Ironside JW (1990) Pre-menopausal cytomegalovirus oophoritis. Histopathology (Oxf) 16:405–407
213. Witlin AG, Sibai BM (1995) Postpartum ovarian vein thrombosis after vaginal delivery: a report of 11 cases. Obstet Gynecol 85:775–780
214. Wojcik EM, Naylor B (1992) "Collagen balls" in peritoneal washings. Acta Cytol 36:466–470
215. Wood JR, Nelson VL, Ho C (2003) The molecular phenotype of polycystic ovary syndrome (PCOS) theca cells and new candidate PCOS genes defined by microarray analysis. J Biol Chem 278:26380–26390
216. Yildiz BO, Azziz R (2007) The adrenal and polycystic ovary syndrome. Rev Endocr Metab Disord 8:331–342
217. Young RH, Prat J, Scully RE (1980) Epidermoid cyst of the ovary. A report of three cases with comments on histogenesis. Am J Clin Pathol 73:272–276
218. Young RH, Scully RE (1984) Fibromatosis and massive edema of the ovary, possibly related entities: a report of 14 cases of fibromatosis and 11 cases of massive edema. Int J Gynecol Pathol 3:153–178
219. Zergeroğlu S, Küçükah T, Koç Ö (2004) Primary ovarian echinococcosis. Arch Gynecol Obstet 270:285–286
220. Zhang J, Young RH, Arseneau J (1982) Ovarian stromal tumors containing lutein or Leydig cells (luteinized thecomas and stromal Leydig cell tumors): a clinicopathological analysis of fifty cases. Int J Gynecol Pathol 1:270–285

13 Diseases of the Peritoneum

Julie A. Irving · Philip B. Clement

R. J. Kurman, L. Hedrick Ellenson, B. M. Ronnett (eds.), *Blaustein's Pathology of the Female Genital Tract (6th ed.)*, DOI 10.1007/978-1-4419-0489-8_13,

This chapter considers the wide range of nonneoplastic and neoplastic lesions that involve the peritoneum, and in some cases the retroperitoneal lymph nodes, of females. The first half of the chapter covers inflammatory lesions, tumor-like lesions (including mesothelial hyperplasia), mesothelial neoplasms, miscellaneous primary tumors, and metastatic tumors. The final half of the chapter is devoted to a large group of lesions that exhibit müllerian differentiation on microscopic examination and share a potential origin from the secondary müllerian system, the prototypical example of which is endometriosis.

Inflammatory Lesions

Acute Peritonitis

Acute diffuse peritonitis, characterized by a serosal fibrinopurulent exudate, is most commonly associated with a perforated viscus, and is usually bacterial or chemical (bile or gastric or pancreatic juice) in origin. The lipases in pancreatic juice typically produce fat necrosis. Spontaneous bacterial peritonitis occurs most often in children and in adults who are immunocompromised or have cirrhosis of the liver [242]. Rare infectious causes of acute peritonitis include Candida [15], Actinomycetes, and amoebas [111]. Recurrent attacks of acute peritonitis are an almost constant feature of familial Mediterranean fever (recurrent polyserositis; periodic disease) [220]. Localized acute peritonitis may be associated with infection (or infarction) of specific organs, as in pelvic inflammatory disease.

Granulomatous Peritonitis

A variety of infectious and noninfectious agents can cause granulomatous peritonitis. The peritoneum may be studded with nodules, which can mimic disseminated tumor at operation. The diagnosis rests on the histologic, and in some cases, microbiologic, identification of the causative agent.

Infectious

Tuberculous peritonitis, which is increasing in frequency, particularly among immunosuppressed patients, may be secondary to spread from a focus within the abdominopelvic cavity or be a manifestation of miliary spread [122]. The granulomas are characterized by caseous necrosis and Langhans type giant cells; mycobacteria may be demonstrated by acid-fast stains or immunofluorescence methods. Rarely, granulomatous peritonitis is a complication of fungal infections, including histoplasmosis, coccidioidomycosis, and cryptococcosis, and parasitic infestations, including schistosomiasis, oxyuriasis, echinococcosis, ascariasis, and strongyloidiasis.

Noninfectious

Foreign material, typically recognizable on histologic examination, can elicit a granulomatous reaction on the peritoneum. Starch granules from surgical gloves, douche fluid, and lubricants typically incite a granulomatous and fibrosing peritonitis; in occasional cases, the inflammatory reaction may be of tuberculoid type with caseous necrosis [162]. The periodic acid–Schiff (PAS) positive starch granules exhibit a characteristic Maltese-cross configuration under polarized light. Talc was once an important cause of granulomatous and fibrosing peritonitis because of its use as a lubricant on surgical gloves, and talc-induced peritonitis has also been described in drug abusers. Other iatrogenic causes of granulomatous peritonitis include cellulose and cotton fibers from surgical pads and drapes, microcrystalline collagen hemostat (Avitene) [175], and oily materials such as hysterosalpingographic contrast medium, which can be associated with a lipogranulomatous reaction. In one described case, a foreign body reaction to Surgicel™ resulted in a pelvic mass that mimicked recurrent ovarian cancer [63].

Contamination of the peritoneal cavity by bowel contents, including vegetable matter, food-derived starch, and barium sulfate, can produce a peritoneal foreign body reaction. Sebaceous material and keratin from ruptured dermoid cysts typically evoke an intense granulomatous, lipogranulomatous, and fibrosing peritoneal inflammatory reaction that may mimic a neoplasm at operation (*Fig. 13.1*). Granulomatous inflammation to keratin derived from uterine and ovarian endometrioid carcinomas with squamous differentiation is discussed later in Tumor-Like Lesions.

Spillage of amniotic fluid at cesarean section, with its content of vernix caseosa (keratin, squames, sebum, and lanugo hair) and meconium (bile, pancreatic, and intestinal secretions), produces a granulomatous peritonitis [86]. Meconium peritonitis caused by bowel perforation in utero can also be a problem in newborn infants. In contrast to vernix caseosa peritonitis, calcification rather than granulomatous inflammation dominates the microscopic picture, which in some cases is associated with striking radiographic findings. In boys, the process may

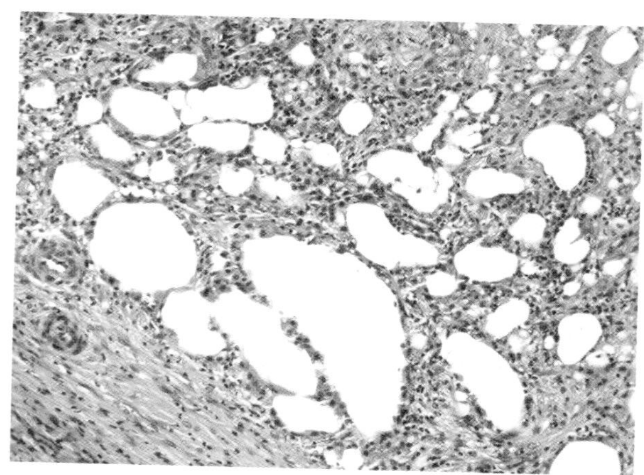

Fig. 13.1
Lipogranulomatous peritonitis due to ruptured ovarian dermoid cyst

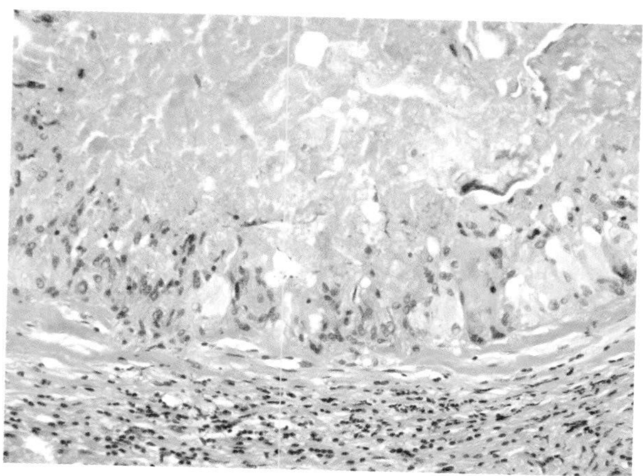

Fig. 13.2
Peritoneal granuloma secondary to diathermy ablation for endometriosis. **Histiocytes surround a necrotic center containing wisps of brown pigment**

involve the tunica vaginalis and result in a tumor-like scrotal mass [79]. Rare cases of meconium peritonitis are associated with disseminated intravascular spread of the meconium.

Granulomatous peritonitis has also been described secondary to Crohn's disease, sarcoidosis, and Whipple's disease. Necrotizing peritoneal granulomas have been described following diathermy ablation of endometriosis (*Fig. 13.2*) [37]. Necrotic pseudoxanthomatous nodules of endometriosis, which can resemble necrotic granulomas, are described on page 28.

Granulomatous inflammation can occur in the peritoneum secondary to spillage of bile or gallstones during laparoscopic cholecystectomy, with subsequent implantation of gallstones on peritoneal surfaces, including the ovaries ("ovarian cholelithiasis"; see also Chap. 12, Nonneoplastic Lesions of the Ovary, Fig. 12.12) [238]. The embedded gallstones may cause abdominal pain, be associated with a foreign body granulomatous reaction and fibrosis or act as a nidus for infection; the reddish-brown, pigmented lesions visible at laparoscopy can mimic endometriosis [146]. Cholesterol crystals and bile pigment may be identifiable within the foreign body giant cells (*Fig. 13.3*). Positive Fouchet's staining for bile and awareness of the history of a previous cholecystectomy will facilitate the correct diagnosis.

Nongranulomatous Histiocytic Lesions

The peritoneum can be occasionally involved by histiocytic infiltrates rather than discrete granulomas.

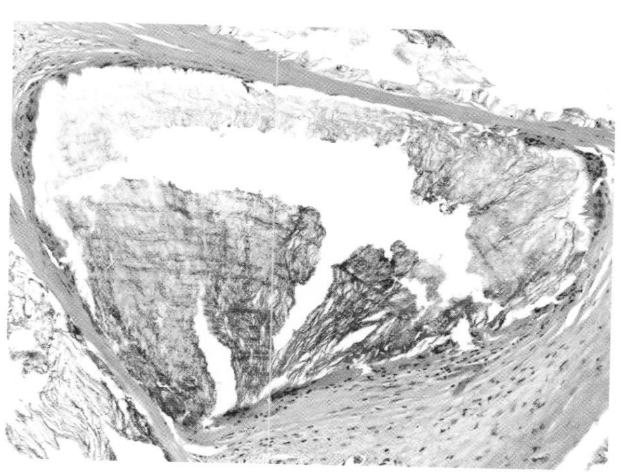

Fig. 13.3
Gallstone peritonitis. **Gallstones are embedded in the pelvic peritoneum. Note the rim of foreign body giant cells and surrounding fibrosis. Laparoscopic cholecystectomy had been performed 18 months earlier**

Ceroid- and lipid-rich histiocytes involving the peritoneum and omentum can be secondary to endometriosis [49] or can occur in association with a peritoneal decidual reaction [244]. Peritoneal lesions consisting of pigment-laden histiocytes have been referred to as peritoneal melanosis. Reported cases of melanosis have usually been associated with ovarian dermoid cysts, sometimes with preoperative rupture [108]; association with a serous cystadenoma has also been reported. At laparotomy, focal or diffuse, tan to black, peritoneal staining, or similarly pigmented, tumor-like nodules are encountered within the pelvis and in the omentum. Some of the cysts within the ovarian tumors exhibit pigmentation of their contents and lining. On histologic examination, the ovarian and peritoneal pigmentation consists of pigment-laden histiocytes within a fibrous stroma (➋ *Fig. 13.4*). In at least three of the reported cases and in a fourth case we have encountered, gastric mucosa was prominent within an otherwise typical dermoid cyst. No obvious source for the pigment could be identified in most of the cases; Jaworski et al. demonstrated the pigment to have neither the histochemical features of melanin nor hemosiderin, but was rich in iron, and postulated that the pigment was derived from hemorrhage secondary to peptic ulceration of gastric mucosa [108]. These cases of benign peritoneal melanosis should obviously be distinguished from metastatic malignant melanoma, a distinction that is straightforward because of the bland nuclear features and absence of mitotic figures of the pigmented histiocytes.

Nonpigmented histiocytes can occasionally occur as a nonspecific peritoneal inflammatory response in the form of nodular, plaque-like, or more extensive aggregates that may appear as small grossly visible peritoneal nodules at operation, or more commonly as a microscopic finding. Histologically, the aggregates are composed of a monotonous population of histiocytes with moderate amounts of pale eosinophilic cytoplasm; the nuclei may be reniform and/or contain a groove, reminiscent of Langerhans-type histiocytes (➋ *Fig 13.5*). We are aware of one such case from a patient with a granulosa cell tumor in which the histiocytes were initially misinterpreted microscopically as metastatic granulosa cell tumor. Admixed mesothelial cells may also be present ("nodular histiocytic/mesothelial hyperplasia"). A recent report has described a diffuse histiocytic proliferation of the pelvic peritoneum associated with endocervicosis [199]. In these cases, immunohistochemical staining for CD68 and cytokeratin can aid the distinction of histiocytes from mesothelial cells (➋ *Fig. 13.5*).

Mucicarminophilic histiocytosis is characterized by histiocytes that contain polyvinylpyrrolidone (PVP), a substance that has been used as a blood substitute [124]. These cells can be found in many sites, both within and outside the female reproductive organs, including the ovary, the pelvic lymph nodes, and the omentum. The histiocytes have vacuolated basophilic to lavender

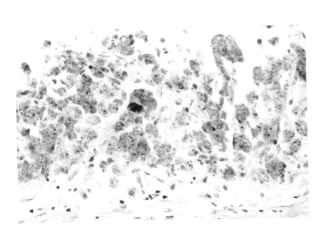

Fig. 13.4
Peritoneal melanosis. **Histiocytes are laden with brown pigment**

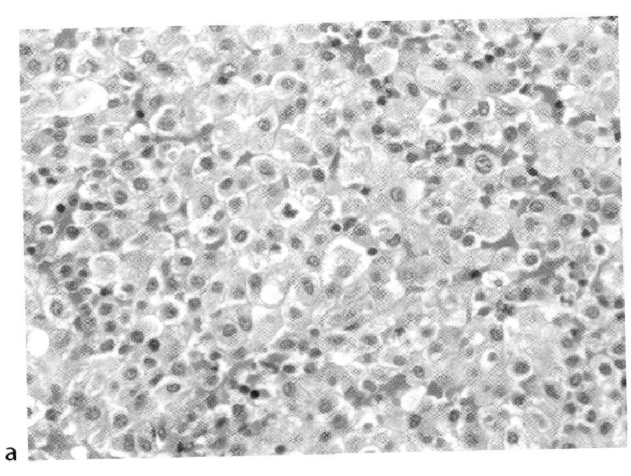

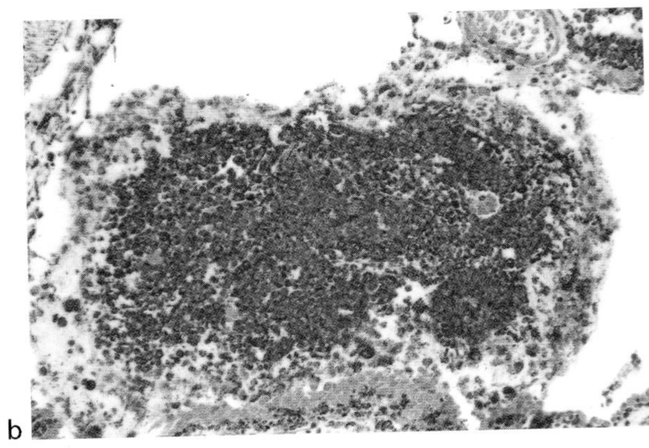

Fig. 13.5
Nodule of histiocytes involving the peritoneal surface. **(a) The cells have moderate pale eosinophilic cytoplasm, some with reniform nuclei. (b) Positive immunostaining of histiocytes with CD68**

cytoplasm and an eccentric nucleus, an appearance that may suggest the diagnosis of signet-ring cell adenocarcinoma (➋ *Fig. 13.6*). The histiocytes are mucicarminophilic, but in contrast to neoplastic signet-ring cells, are PAS negative; a variety of other stains are also helpful in the differential diagnosis [124].

Peritoneal collections of mucicarmine-positive histiocytes have also been described associated with topical administration of oxidized regenerated cellulose, a hemostatic agent [119]. The cytoplasm of these cells is PAS positive, diastase resistant, CD 68 positive, and S-100 and cytokeratin negative.

Peritoneal Fibrosis

Reactive peritoneal fibrosis, often accompanied by fibrous adhesions, is a common sequela of prior peritoneal inflammation and a frequent complication of a surgical procedure. The fibrosis can on occasion take the form of well-circumscribed fibrous nodules. Some reactive peritoneal fibrous lesions may contain spindle cells that are immunoreactive for vimentin, smooth muscle actin, and cytokeratin, referred to as multipotential subserosal cells by Bolen et al. [20]. Rarely, reactive fibrous proliferations of the peritoneum can form tumor-like nodules, in contrast to the more widespread peritoneal thickening of sclerosing peritonitis. In one case we have seen, three of these nodules, which we refer to as peritoneal fibrous nodules [38], were found in the cul-de-sac in a woman with an ovarian mucinous cystadenocarcinoma. Similar nodules involved the serosal aspect of the tumor. The nodules were composed of moderately cellular fascicles of benign-appearing spindle cells resembling fibroblasts and myofibroblasts that contained occasional mitotic figures. Some of the spindle cells had the immunoprofile of the multipotential subserosal cells noted earlier.

Localized hyaline plaques are a common incidental finding on the splenic capsule and are probably related to splenic congestion [241]. Nonspecific fibrous thickening of the peritoneum may be seen in patients with hepatic cirrhosis and ascites. The designation sclerosing peritonitis has been applied to a clinically significant, potentially fatal lesion that represents a reactive hyperplasia of the submesothelial mesenchymal cells to a variety of stimuli. The first description, by Concato, was that of pearly white thickening of the visceral peritoneum, either as discrete plaques or continuous sheets involving the hepatic, splenic, and diaphragmatic peritoneum. The process often encases the small bowel ("abdominal cocoon"), causing bowel obstruction. Sclerosing peritonitis occurs in an idiopathic form, which most frequently, but not invariably, affects adolescent girls in tropical countries [78]. Known causes include practolol therapy, chronic ambulatory peritoneal dialysis, the use of a peritoneovenous (LeVeen) shunt, bacterial or mycobacterial infection, sarcoidosis, the carcinoid syndrome, familial Mediterranean fever, and fibrogenic foreign materials as seen in drug users. Additionally, sclerosing peritonitis has an enigmatic association with luteinized thecomas of the ovary (➋ *Fig. 13.7*; see ➋ Chap. 15, Sex Cord-Stromal

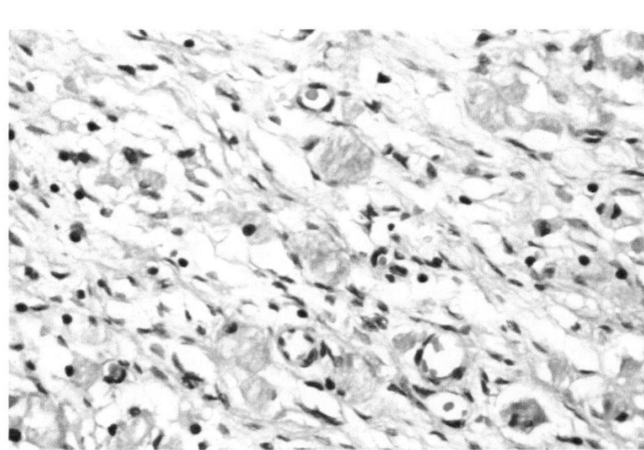

Fig. 13.6
Mucicarminophilic histiocytosis. **Note multiple vacuolated histiocytes, some with a signet-ring-cell appearance**

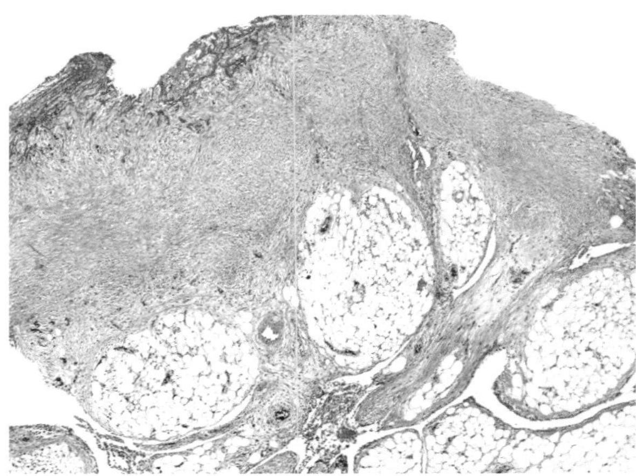

Fig. 13.7
Sclerosing peritonitis associated with bilateral luteinized thecomas of the ovary. **Omentum shows surface involvement by cellular, reactive fibrous tissue**

Steroid Cell, and Other Ovarian Tumors with Endocrine, Paraendocrine, and Paraneoplastic Manifestations) [47, 222]. Some patients with sclerosing peritonitis have been successfully treated utilizing antiestrogens and/or GnRH agonists. Sclerosing peritonitis should be distinguished from the rarer "peritoneal encapsulation," a congenital malformation in which an accessory peritoneal membrane encases loops of small bowel in a saclike structure. The latter condition is largely asymptomatic and is usually found incidentally at laparotomy or autopsy. Confusion arises when the two terms are used interchangeably or even together, as in "encapsulating peritonitis."

Reactive nodular fibrous pseudotumor is a term that has been applied to single or multiple lesions ranging up to 6 cm involving the gastrointestinal tract or mesentery in adults; some have been associated with bowel wall infiltration but all have had a benign clinical course [251]. Microscopically, the lesions are composed of a low to moderate cellular proliferation of fibroblasts, collagen, and mononuclear inflammatory cells that are usually sparse. The fibroblastic cells show variable immunoreactivity for vimentin, CD117, muscle specific actin, smooth muscle actin, and desmin, with negative staining for CD34 and ALK-1. Sclerosing mesenteritis (mesenteric panniculitis, mesenteric lipodystrophy) usually occurs as a localized mass in the small bowel mesentery, and is characterized by variable fibrosis, inflammation, and fat necrosis [70].

In occasional cases, it may be difficult to differentiate between markedly reactive peritoneal fibrosis and a desmoplastic mesothelioma lacking frankly sarcomatoid areas, particularly in a small biopsy specimen. These tumors, however, are very rare in the peritoneal cavity, especially in women. Features favoring a diagnosis of mesothelioma include nuclear atypia, necrosis, organized patterns of collagen deposition (fascicular, storiform), and infiltration of adjacent tissues [136].

Rare Types of Peritonitis

Eosinophilic peritonitis is seen rarely in cases of eosinophilic gastroenteritis and the hypereosinophilic syndrome [1]. Isolated cases of eosinophilic ascites have been associated with childhood atopy, peritoneal dialysis, vasculitis, lymphoma or metastatic carcinoma, and ruptured hydatid cysts [1]. Rare cases of peritonitis may be secondary to peritoneal involvement by collagen vascular diseases, including systemic lupus erythematosus and Degos' disease.

Tumor-Like Lesions

Mesothelial Hyperplasia

Hyperplasia of mesothelial cells is a common response to inflammation (including pelvic inflammatory disease), and chronic effusions (*Figs. 13.8* and *13.9*). Hyperplastic lesions may be noted at operation as solitary or multiple small nodules, but more commonly are incidental findings on microscopic examination [36]. Mesothelial hyperplasia often involves the adnexal areas in cases of chronic salpingitis and endometriosis [117] and is occasionally encountered, particularly in the omentum, in association with ovarian tumors [44]. Mesothelial hyperplasia can also occur within the superficial ovarian stroma overlying a borderline epithelial tumor and in such cases can be misinterpreted as invasive tumor (*Fig. 13.10*) [44]. Mesothelial hyperplasia may be confined to a hernia sac, and in such cases may be caused by trauma or incarceration [196]. Hyperplastic mesothelial cells occasionally are an incidental microscopic finding within pelvic and intra-abdominal lymph nodes, and in such cases are usually associated with mesothelial hyperplasia of the peritoneum (*Fig. 13.11*) [48]. The mesothelial cells may be misinterpreted as metastatic tumor, particularly in a woman with a known primary pelvic tumor. The appearance of the cells on routine stains suggests the correct diagnosis, and can be confirmed by histochemical and immunohistochemical staining (see following).

In florid examples, solid, trabecular, tubular, papillary, or tubulopapillary patterns (*Figs. 13.8* and *13.9*) and limited degrees of extension of the mesothelial cells into the underlying reactive fibrous tissues or the walls of

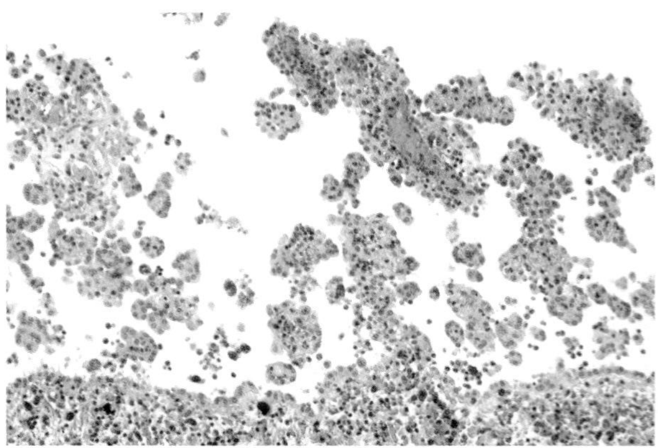

Fig. 13.8
Mesothelial hyperplasia with a papillary pattern

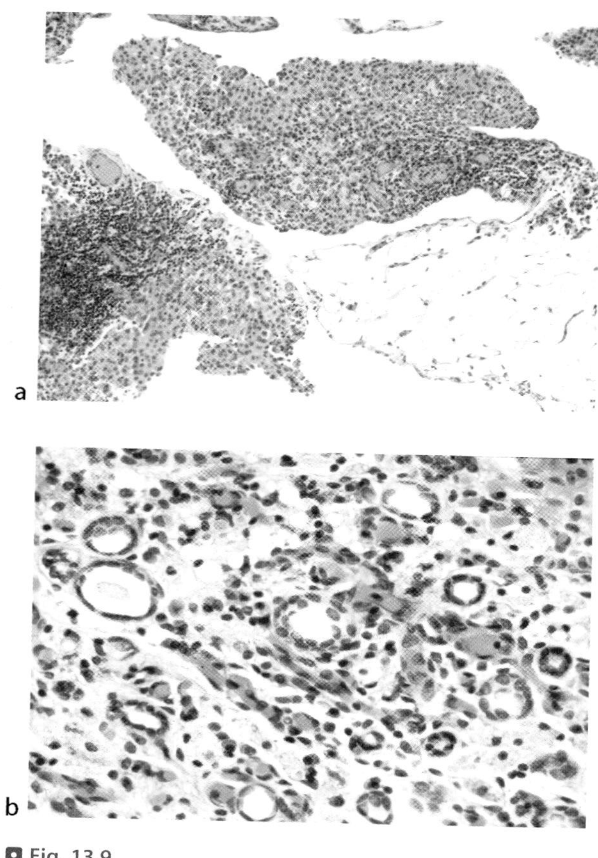

■ Fig. 13.9
Mesothelial hyperplasia. **(a) Nodular pattern. (b) Tubular pattern**

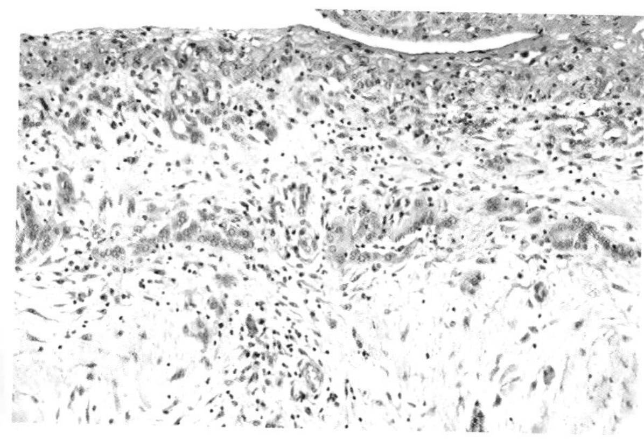

■ Fig. 13.10
Mesothelial hyperplasia within superficial ovarian stroma. **An underlying borderline epithelial tumor was present**

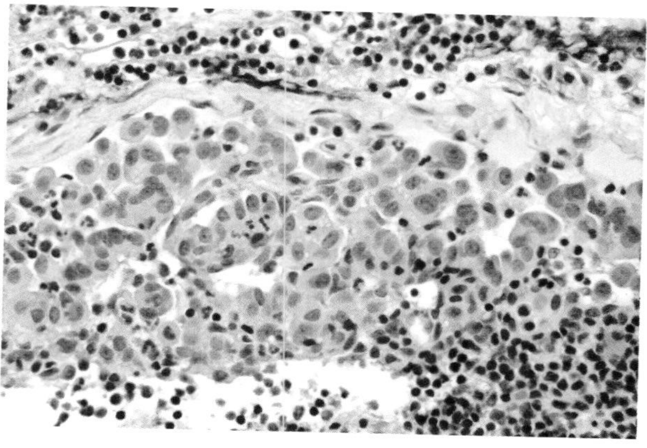

■ Fig. 13.11
Hyperplastic mesothelial cells within the subcapsular sinus of a pelvic lymph node

ovarian tumors, endometriotic cysts, and peritoneal inclusion cysts (see below) may be seen ("mural mesothelial proliferation"). The cells are often focally disposed in linear, sometimes parallel, thin layers, separated by fibrin or fibrous tissue (➋ *Fig. 13.10*). The mesothelial cells may have cytoplasmic vacuoles containing acid mucin (predominantly hyaluronic acid) or, less commonly, exhibit marked cytoplasmic clearing. Mild to moderate nuclear pleomorphism, mitotic figures, and occasional multinucleated cells may be seen. Psammoma bodies are encountered in occasional cases, and rarely, eosinophilic strap-shaped cells resembling rhabdomyoblasts have been described.

The major differential diagnosis is with peritoneal malignant mesothelioma (PMM). The presence of grossly visible nodules, necrosis, conspicuous large cytoplasmic vacuoles, marked nuclear pleomorphism, and deep infiltration favor PMM over mesothelial hyperplasia [36]. Some of these features, however, such as marked nuclear atypia, are not always present or may be present only focally within a PMM. Immunostains may facilitate the differential diagnosis. Immunoreactivity for p53 [109] and intense cytoplasmic immunoreactivity for epithelial membrane antigen (EMA) [97] are characteristic of the cells of PMM but not hyperplastic mesothelial cells; reactive mesothelial cells, in contrast to PMMs, tend to be desmin-positive [10]. Application of proliferative markers Ki67 and repp86 have recently been shown to be of diagnostic utility in differentiating PMM from reactive mesothelial hyperplasia (approximately 25% versus 5% labeling index, respectively) [232]. Despite these differential features, in occasional cases the distinction between a hyperplastic and malignant mesothelial lesion may be difficult or impossible, particularly in a biopsy specimen. If the lesion in question is a PMM, follow-up usually reveals its nature within several months because of its typical rapid growth. In contrast, an atypical mesothelial proliferation occasionally persists for years without an apparent cause. An apparently benign, otherwise typical mesothelial proliferation, however, occasionally precedes the appearance of a PMM [36]. Some cases of "atypical mesothelial hyperplasia" evolving into PMM, however, likely represent PMM ab initio [173].

The differential diagnosis of mesothelial hyperplasia also includes borderline serous tumors of primary peritoneal or ovarian origin. Grossly visible ovarian or peritoneal tumor, columnar cells with or without cilia, the presence of intracellular or extracellular neutral mucin, and numerous psammoma bodies all favor a serous tumor. Immunohistochemical markers for epithelial differentiation (see section on PMM) may also be of value in the differential diagnosis.

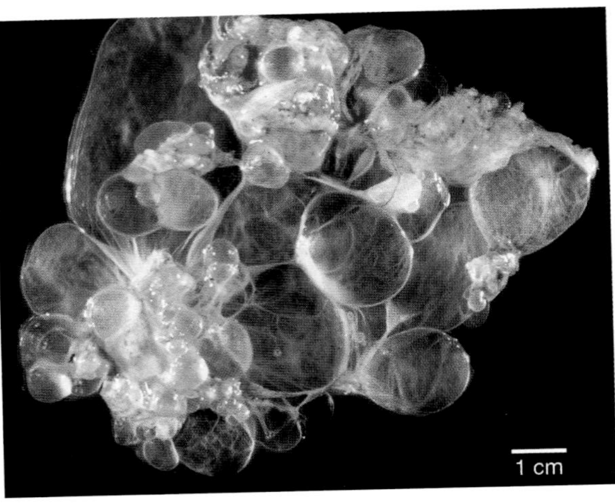

Fig. 13.12
Peritoneal inclusion cyst. **Multilocular cystic mass consists of thin-walled cysts with a smooth lining**

Peritoneal Inclusion Cysts

Peritoneal inclusion cysts typically occur in the peritoneal cavity of women in the reproductive age group [145, 197]. Rarely, they occur in males and in the pleural cavity. Unilocular peritoneal inclusion cysts are usually incidental findings at laparotomy in the form of single or multiple, small, thin-walled, translucent, unilocular cysts that may be attached or lie free in the peritoneal cavity. Occasionally, they may involve the round ligament simulating an inguinal hernia [95]. The cysts have a smooth lining, and contents that vary from yellow and watery to gelatinous. Although most of these unilocular mesothelial cysts are probably reactive in origin, some of those located in the mesocolon, mesentery of the small intestine, retroperitoneum, and splenic capsule may be developmental [197].

Multilocular peritoneal inclusion cysts (MPICs) may form large bulky masses (*Fig. 13.12*); these lesions have also been referred to as benign cystic mesotheliomas, inflammatory cysts of the peritoneum, or postoperative peritoneal cysts. MPICs are usually associated with clinical manifestations, most commonly lower abdominal pain, a palpable mass, or both. They are usually adherent to pelvic organs and may simulate a cystic ovarian tumor on clinical examination, at laparotomy [145], or even on pathologic examination; the upper abdominal cavity, the retroperitoneum, or hernia sacs may also be involved [197]. Unlike the smaller unilocular cysts, the septa and walls of MPICs may contain considerable amounts of fibrous tissue. Their contents may resemble those of the unilocular cysts or be serosanguineous or bloody.

On microscopic examination, MPICs are typically lined by a single layer of flat to cuboidal, occasionally hobnail-shaped, mesothelial cells with generally bland nuclear features, although a degree of reactive atypia is not infrequent (*Figs. 13.13* and *13.14*). The lining cells occasionally form small papillae and cribriform patterns or undergo squamous metaplasia. In some cases, mural proliferations of typical or atypical mesothelial cells arranged singly, as gland-like structures or nests (*Figs. 13.15* and *13.16*) [145], or in patterns resembling those in adenomatoid tumors may be encountered. Occasional vacuolated mesothelial cells in the stroma may simulate signet-ring cells [197]. The septa typically consist of a loose, fibrovascular connective tissue with a sparse inflammatory infiltrate. In some cases, marked acute and chronic inflammation, abundant fibrin, broad bands of granulation and fibrous tissue, and evidence of recent and remote hemorrhage are present in the cyst walls. The mesothelial cells are typically immunoreactive for calretinin, and some cases are positive for estrogen (ER), progesterone receptors (PR), or both [208].

A history of a prior abdominal operation, pelvic inflammatory disease, endometriosis, or combinations thereof was present in 84% of patients in one series [197], suggesting a role for inflammation in the pathogenesis of the cysts. An inflammatory pathogenesis is also supported by the occurrence of cases in which the

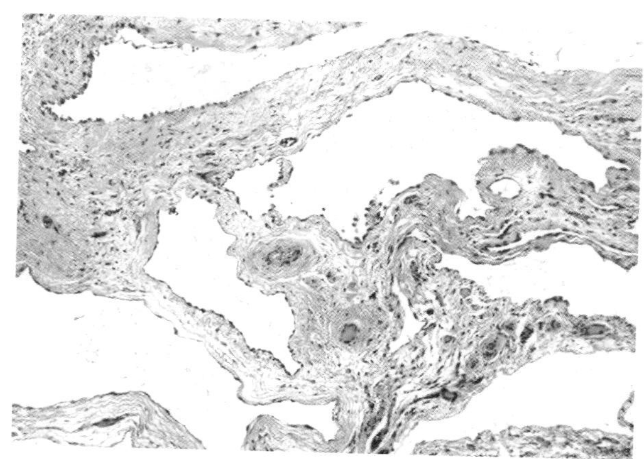

Fig. 13.13
Multilocular peritoneal inclusion cyst (MPIC). **Cystic spaces are lined by a single layer of flat mesothelial cells and are separated by thin fibrous septa**

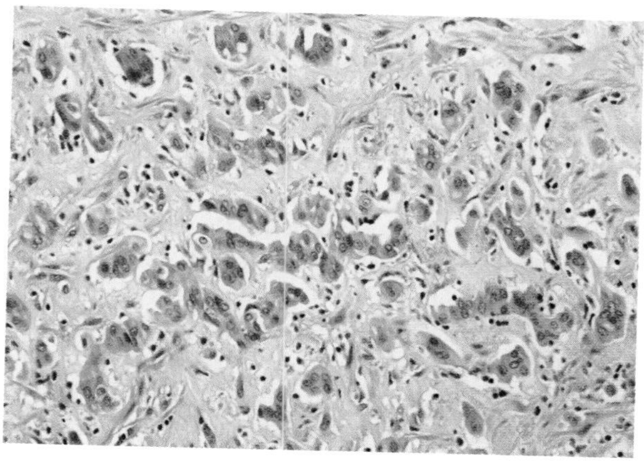

Fig. 13.15
Multilocular peritoneal inclusion cyst with mural mesothelial proliferation. **Cord-like arrangements within a reactive fibrous stroma create an infiltrative pattern**

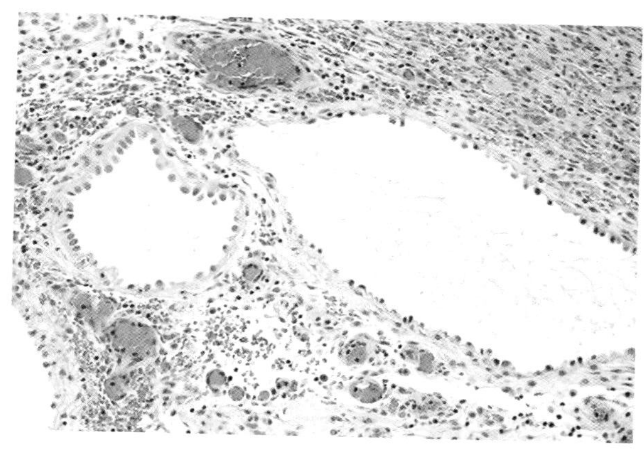

Fig. 13.14
Multilocular peritoneal inclusion cyst. **Cystic spaces are lined by cells with mild reactive nuclear atypia**

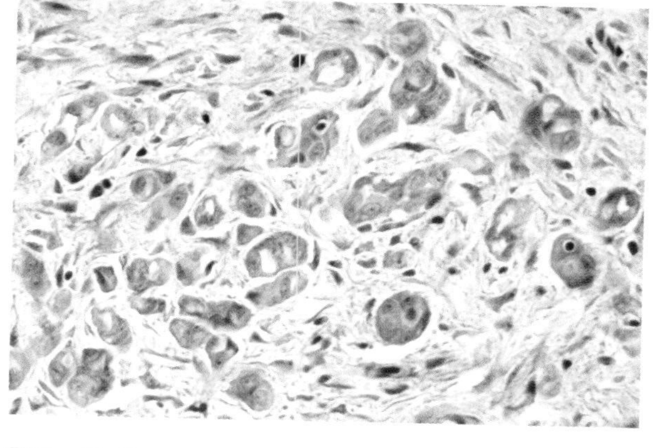

Fig. 13.16
Multilocular peritoneal inclusion cyst with mural mesothelial proliferation. **High power view showing benign-appearing mesothelial cells forming small nests and lining small tubules**

dividing line between florid adhesions associated with inflammation and a MPIC may be difficult. With rare exceptions, there has been no association with asbestos exposure. Follow-up examinations have not disclosed malignant behavior in cases that we consider MPICs, but in as many as one half of these, the lesions have recurred from months to many years postoperatively [197]. It is likely, however, that at least some of these "recurrences" are the result of newly formed postoperative adhesions. Some patients have responded favorably to treatment with GnRH agonists or tamoxifen [208]. For these reasons – although accepting that low-grade cystic mesotheliomas occur rarely (see page 12) – we prefer the designation multilocular peritoneal inclusion cyst to benign cystic mesothelioma for such lesions, until there is convincing evidence for their neoplastic nature.

Aside from the contentious problem of their distinction from "true" cystic mesotheliomas (see page 12), MPICs are confused most often with multilocular cystic lymphangiomas. In contrast to MPICs, the latter typically occur in children, more frequently in boys. In addition, they are usually extrapelvic, being almost always localized to the mesentery of the small intestine, omentum, mesocolon, or retroperitoneum. Their contents may be chylous, and on histologic examination lymphoid aggregates and smooth muscle, which are rare findings in MPICs, are typically present within their walls. In problematic cases, immunohistochemical stains are useful in distinguishing endothelial from mesothelial cells. Another lesion that merits consideration in the differential diagnosis of MPICs is the rare multicystic adenomatoid tumor. In contrast to MPICs, the latter typically involve the myometrium, contain foci of typical adenomatoid tumor, and lack prominent numbers of inflammatory cells. A detailed discussion of other lesions in the differential diagnosis of MPICs has been presented elsewhere [197].

Splenosis

Splenosis, which results from implantation of splenic tissue, is typically an incidental finding at laparotomy or autopsy months to years after splenectomy for traumatic splenic rupture [27]. A few to innumerable, red-blue, peritoneal nodules, ranging from punctate to 7 cm in diameter, are scattered widely throughout the abdominal cavity and, less commonly, over the pelvic cavity. The intraoperative appearance may mimic endometriosis, benign or malignant vascular tumors, or metastatic cancer.

Trophoblastic Implants

Implants of trophoblast on the pelvic or omental peritoneum may complicate the operative treatment of tubal pregnancy [29, 66, 194, 233]. The implants are more likely to occur in cases managed by laparoscopy (1.9% of cases) than those managed by laparotomy (0.6% of cases) and are more likely to occur after salpingotomy than salpingectomy. The clinical presentation in such cases includes an initial decline in the serum human chorionic gonadotropin (hCG) level after removal of the ectopic pregnancy, followed by a rising level, abdominal pain, and in some cases intra-abdominal hemorrhage. Microscopic examination of the implants reveals viable trophoblastic tissue that may include chorionic villi. Some lesions resemble a placental site nodule or plaque (➋ *Fig. 13.17*).

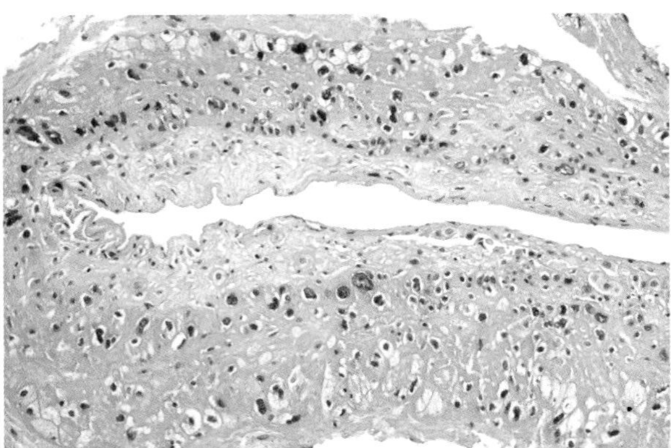

Fig. 13.17
Placental site plaque of the peritoneum

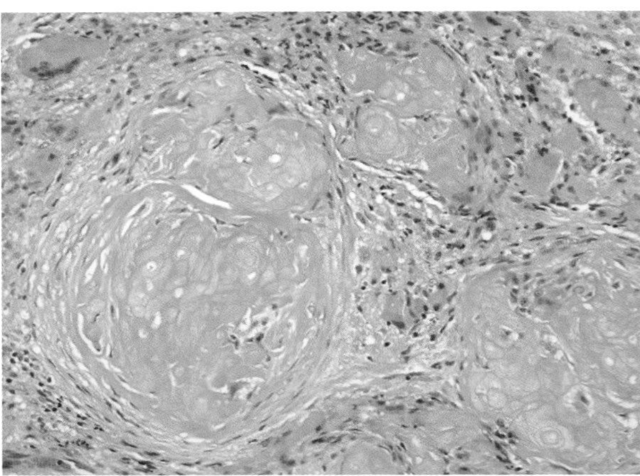

Fig 13.18
Peritoneal keratin granuloma

Peritoneal Keratin Granulomas

Peritoneal granulomas that form in response to implants of keratin derived from neoplasms of the female reproductive tract may be confused with metastatic tumor [121]. The tumors are most commonly endometrioid carcinomas with squamous differentiation originating in the endometrium or ovary, or, rarely, squamous cell carcinomas of the cervix or atypical polypoid adenomyomas of the uterus. The granulomas consist of laminated deposits of keratin, sometimes with ghost squamous cells, surrounded by foreign body giant cells and fibrous tissue (see ➋ *Fig. 13.18*; see also ➋ Chap. 12, Nonneoplastic Lesions of the Ovary, Figs. 12.9 and 12.10). Follow-up data on these patients suggest that the granulomas have no prognostic significance, although they should be thoroughly sampled by the gynecologist and carefully examined microscopically to exclude the presence of viable tumor. The differential diagnosis includes peritoneal granulomas in response to keratin derived from other sources, as discussed earlier in this chapter.

Infarcted Appendix Epiploica

Appendices epiploicae may undergo torsion and infarction [239]. Subsequent calcification can result in a hard tumor-like mass that may be found attached or loose in the peritoneal cavity. In the late stages, these structures are typically composed of layers of hyalinized connective tissue surrounding a central necrotic and calcified zone in which infarcted adipose tissue is usually recognizable (*Fig. 13.19*).

Mesothelial Neoplasms

Adenomatoid Tumor

This benign tumor of mesothelial origin, adenomatoid tumor, rarely arises from extragenital peritoneum, such as the omentum or mesentery, but is much more commonly encountered within the fallopian tube and myometrium (see Chap. 10, Mesenchymal Tumors of the Uterus, and Chap. 11, Diseases of the Fallopian Tube and Paratubal Region), and, in the male, the epididymis.

Well-Differentiated Papillary Mesothelioma

Well-differentiated papillary mesotheliomas (WDPMs) of the peritoneum are uncommon lesions [62, 88]. Eighty percent of the cases have occurred in women, who are usually of reproductive age; occasional patients are postmenopausal. WDPMs are usually an incidental finding at operation, but rare cases have been associated with abdominal pain or ascites. Occasional patients, including two who were sisters, have had possible exposure to asbestos [62].

At laparotomy and on gross examination, WDPMs may be solitary but are usually multiple, and appear as gray to white, firm, papillary or nodular lesions measuring less than 2 cm in diameter. The omental and pelvic peritoneum are typically involved; several examples have also been encountered on the gastric, intestinal, or mesenteric peritoneum. Microscopic examination reveals fibrous papillae covered by a single layer of flattened to cuboidal mesothelial cells (*Fig. 13.20*) with occasional basal vacuoles; the nuclear features are bland, and mitotic figures are rare or absent. Uncommon patterns include tubulopapillary, adenomatoid-like, branching cords, or solid sheets. The stroma of some tumors may be extensively fibrotic. Multinucleated stromal giant cells and psammoma bodies are encountered in occasional cases. When multiple lesions are present, they should each be sampled histologically as lesions with the appearance of a WDPM may rarely be associated with others that have the appearance of malignant mesothelioma and progressive disease [88]. The diagnosis of WDPM should be strictly reserved for tumors with bland nuclear features and no evidence of invasion.

With the exception of one case that appeared to evolve into a diffuse malignant mesothelioma, follow-up studies suggest that most WDPMs are benign. Occasional examples, however, have persisted for as many as 29 years [62].

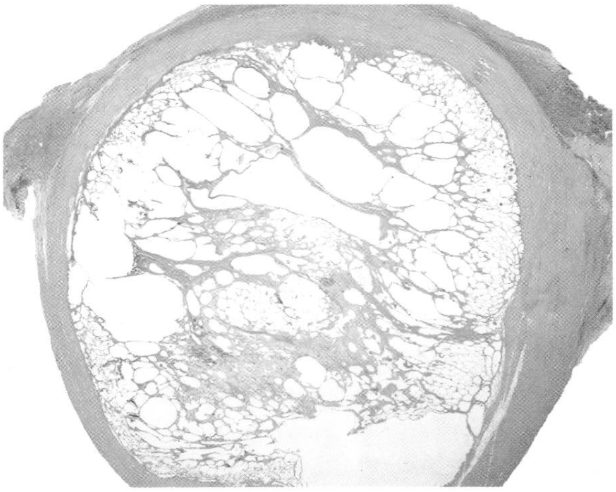

Fig 13.19
Infarcted appendix epiploica

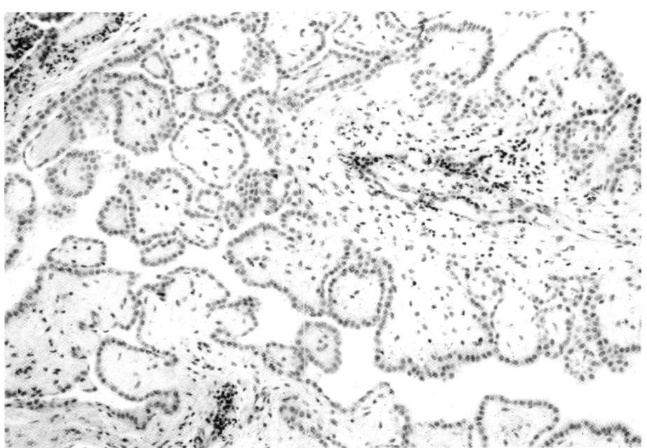

Fig 13.20
Well-differentiated papillary mesothelioma (WDPM).
Fibrous papillae are lined by a single layer of uniform, flat to cuboidal, mesothelial cells

Several patients with WDPM have died, although the adjuvant therapy used in such cases possibly was a contributory factor [62].

Low-Grade Cystic Mesothelioma

Although we believe that most multilocular cystic mesothelial lesions are MPICs, we have seen very rare cases of what appear to be bona fide multicystic mesotheliomas. In contrast to MPICs, the cysts are lined, at least focally, by markedly atypical mesothelial cells, and the tumors may contain areas of conventional malignant mesothelioma on histologic examination.

Malignant Mesothelioma

Clinical Features

Peritoneal malignant mesotheliomas (PMMs) are much less common than similar tumors in the pleural cavity, and account for only 10–20% of all mesotheliomas [9, 12, 88, 118]. These tumors are particularly rare in women, in whom most malignant papillary neoplasms of the peritoneum are extraovarian papillary serous carcinomas (see ➋ Lesions of the Secondary Müllerian System).

About two thirds of the patients with PMM are male, usually middle aged or elderly; occasional PMMs occur in young adults or children. The patients typically present with nonspecific manifestations, including abdominal discomfort and distension, digestive disturbances, and weight loss. Ascites is present in the majority of cases, and cytologic examination of the ascitic fluid may be diagnostic of PMM in some cases. The diagnosis, however, usually requires laparotomy or laparoscopy and biopsy. PMMs may rarely present within a hernia or hydrocele sac, as a retroperitoneal, umbilical, intestinal, or pelvic tumor, or as cervical or inguinal lymphadenopathy [229]. Rarely there is prominent ovarian involvement, the intraoperative appearance mimicking that of a primary ovarian tumor with peritoneal spread [52].

More than 80% of the patients in one large series had a history of asbestos exposure, but most of them were identified because of an occupational exposure to asbestos. In contrast, two series of PMMs in women found no association with a history of asbestos exposure [88, 118]. Asbestos fibers, however, have been identified with special techniques in some of these women [96]. Aside from asbestos, radiation, chronic inflammation, organic chemicals, and nonasbestos mineral fibers may be etiologic agents in some cases.

Most males with PMMs reported in the literature survived less than 2 years after diagnosis, although there have been occasional long-term survivors. A recent study of PMMs in women [118], however, found that 40% of the patients survived longer than 4 years. Increasing nuclear and nucleolar size has been shown to correlate with shorter survival in epithelial tumors [31]. The histopathological subtype (see below) is of prognostic significance, as biphasic PMMs are associated with a much shorter survival than pure epithelial tumors [31]; deciduoid mesotheliomas are usually rapidly fatal [214]. Two recent studies have identified a number of favorable prognostic factors including an age less than 60 years, low nuclear grade, low mitotic count, minimal residual disease after cytoreduction, and an absence of deep invasion [75, 163]. Localized mesotheliomas, although very uncommon, may also be associated with a better prognosis.

Pathologic Findings

At laparotomy, the visceral and parietal peritoneum are diffusely thickened or extensively involved by nodules and plaques. The viscera are often encased by tumor (➋ *Fig. 13.21*) and may be invaded, although local invasion and metastases to lymph nodes, liver, lungs, and pleura are less frequent than in association with carcinomas with comparable degrees of peritoneal involvement. Significant degrees of invasion or metastatic involvement of abdominal viscera, however, may be encountered at autopsy, such as transmural invasion of bowel wall or massive replacement of the pancreas. Some tumors incite

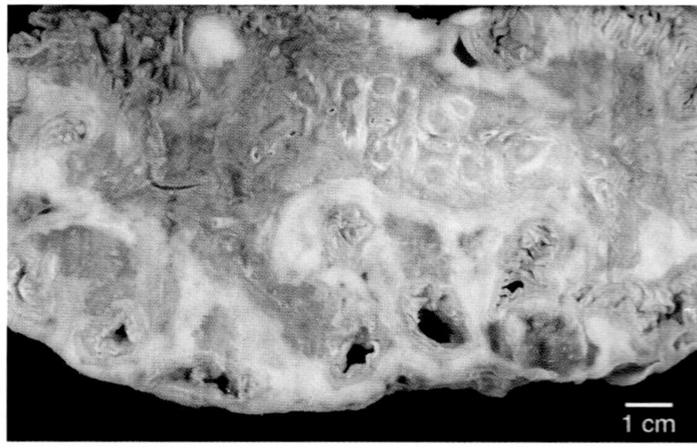

Fig 13.21
Peritoneal malignant mesothelioma (PMM). **The tumor encases loops of bowel (Courtesy of J. Prat, M.D., Barcelona, Spain)**

a striking desmoplastic reaction. As noted earlier, rare PMMs form localized solitary masses.

The typical histologic features (➋ *Figs. 13.22–13.25*) are identical to malignant mesotheliomas involving the pleura. Most tumors are composed of epithelial cells arranged in tubulopapillary and solid patterns; areas of necrosis may be present. There is usually evidence of invasion of subperitoneal tissues, such as the omentum. As already noted, intra-abdominal lymph nodes may be involved. The tumor cells usually retain some resemblance to mesothelial cells, with a cuboidal shape and eosinophilic cytoplasm. Usually there are mild to moderate degrees of nuclear atypicality and variably prominent nucleoli. Mitotic figures usually are present but are not numerous. Rare tumors with an exclusively solid pattern of polygonal cells with abundant eosinophilic cytoplasm and prominent nucleoli ("deciduoid" PMMs) (➋ *Fig. 13.26*), with one exception, have arisen in the peritoneum [214]. Two thirds of such tumors have occurred in females, some of whom were adolescents or young adults. Biphasic and sarcomatoid PMMs occur, but are less common than their pleural counterparts, accounting for only 5 of

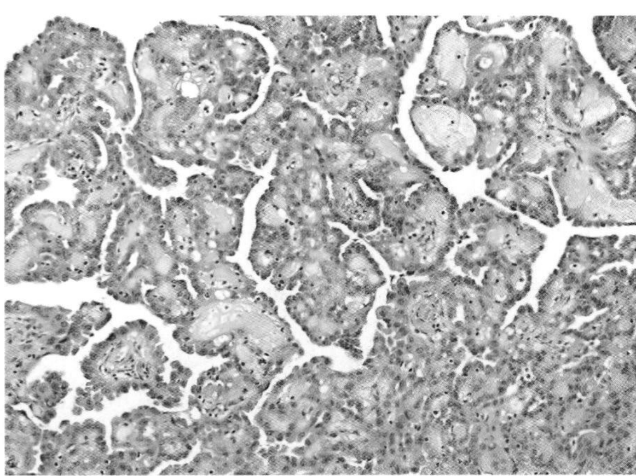

Fig 13.22
Peritoneal malignant mesothelioma. **Papillary pattern**

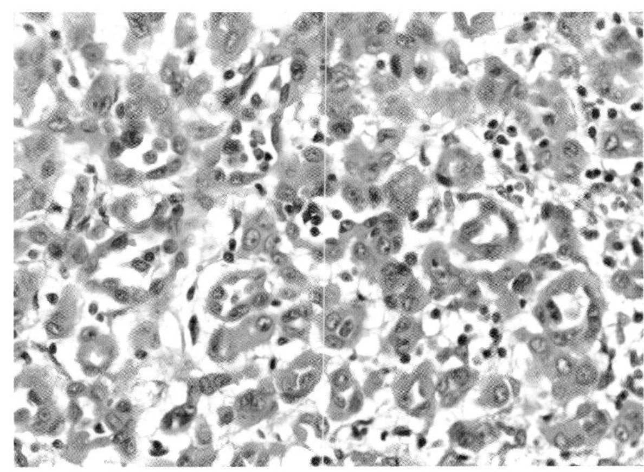

Fig 13.24
Peritoneal malignant mesothelioma. **Tumor cells are arranged as small tubules and nests**

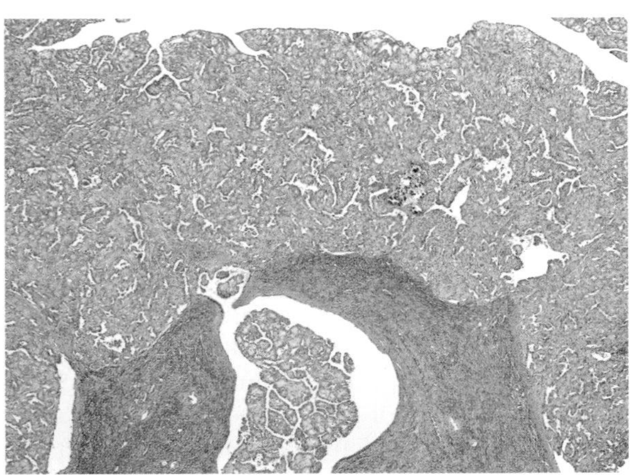

Fig 13.23
Peritoneal malignant mesothelioma. **Tubulopapillary pattern, with prominent involvement of ovarian surface**

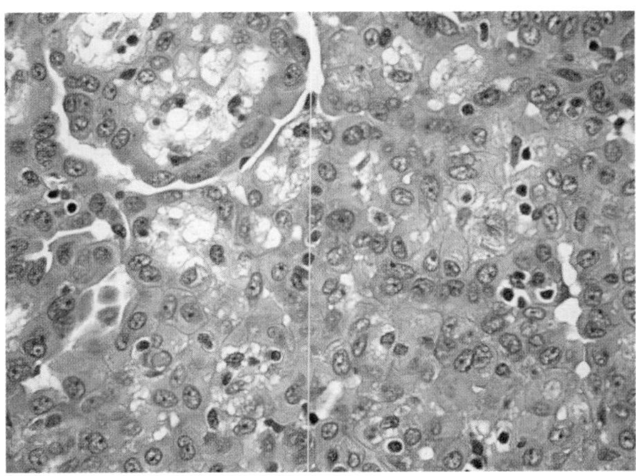

Fig 13.25
Peritoneal malignant mesothelioma. **The cells are cuboidal or polygonal, with eosinophilic cytoplasm and moderate nuclear atypia**

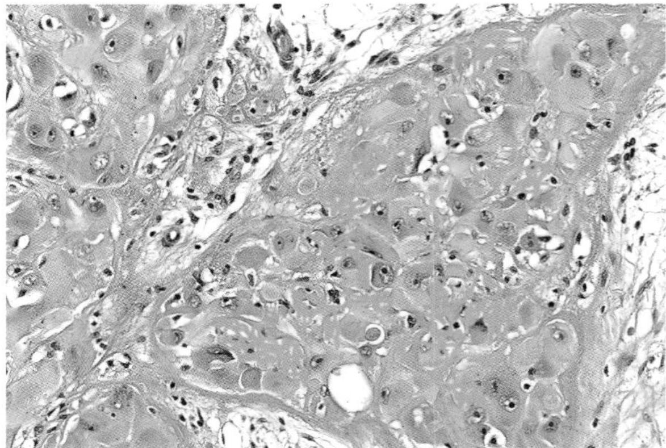

Fig 13.26
Peritoneal malignant mesothelioma. **Solid growth pattern composed of cells with abundant eosinophilic cytoplasm (deciduoid PMM)**

75 PMMs in one recent study [12]. Psammoma bodies are present in approximately one third of cases, but are usually less prominent than in serous neoplasms. Occasional tumors contain a prominent inflammatory infiltrate, such as a dense lymphocytic infiltrate with lymphoid follicles, granulomas, or large numbers of foamy lipid-rich histiocytes. Some tumors consisting predominantly of cells with clear cytoplasm, rich in glycogen or occasionally lipid, have also been reported [168]. The immunohistochemical (see next section) and ultrastructural features of PMMs are similar to their pleural counterparts.

Differential Diagnosis

The differential diagnoses of PMM with atypical mesothelial hyperplasia (see Mesothelial Hyperplasia) and of desmoplastic PMM versus reactive fibrosis (see Peritoneal Fibrosis) have been previously discussed. Another frequently problematic lesion in the differential diagnosis is adenocarcinoma with diffuse peritoneal involvement, including metastatic adenocarcinomas (see Metastatic Tumors) and adenocarcinomas of primary peritoneal origin (see Lesions of the Secondary Müllerian System). Features favoring a diagnosis of PMM include a prominent tubulopapillary pattern, polygonal cells with moderate amounts of eosinophilic cytoplasm, only mild to moderate nuclear atypia, a paucity of mitotic figures, and the presence of acid mucin (alcianophilic material) rather than neutral (PASD) mucin.

PMMs usually lack immunoreactivity for a variety of "epithelial" antigens, including carcinoembryonic antigen, B72.3, Leu-M1 (CD 15), MOC-31, CA 19–9, S-100 protein, Ber-EP4, and placental alkaline phosphatase. Positive immunoreactivity for MOC-31, Ber-EP4, and estrogen receptors favors serous carcinoma; positive staining with calretinin, cytokeratin 5/6, podoplanin, and D2–40 favors PMM, but these markers are less discriminatory as they may be positive in a minor proportion of serous carcinomas [14, 54, 168–170]. Comin has found that an h-caldesmon+/calretinin+/estrogen receptor–/Ber-EP4– immunophenotype strongly favors PMM over serous carcinoma [54]. However, no single immunohistochemical stain is diagnostic in the separation of PMM from adenocarcinoma, and the results of a panel of antibodies should be interpreted in conjunction with the hematoxylin and eosin (H&E) and mucin stains.

"Deciduoid" PMMs must be distinguished from an ectopic decidual reaction involving the peritoneum. Prominent nucleoli, often brisk mitotic activity, and cytokeratin immunoreactivity in the deciduoid tumors exclude an ectopic decidual reaction.

Lin et al. have reported peritoneal epithelioid hemangioendotheliomas or epithelioid angiosarcomas that have mimicked PMM [134]. Features that suggested the diagnosis of PMM in some of the cases included epithelioid cells in a tubulopapillary pattern and the presence of reactive or neoplastic spindle cells resulting in a focal biphasic pattern. Variable degrees of vascular differentiation and immunoreactivity of the neoplastic cells for endothelial antigens (and negative or weak cytokeratin staining) excluded the diagnosis of PMM.

Miscellaneous Primary Tumors

Intra-abdominal Desmoplastic Small Round Cell Tumor

Clinical Features

This rare tumor (desmoplastic small round cell tumor, DSRCT) is of uncertain histogenesis, but it may ultimately prove to be a primitive tumor of mesothelial origin ("mesothelioblastoma") [126, 165–167, 255]. Although most of the tumors are intra-abdominal, similar tumors have also been described in the pleura and rarely at a distance from a mesothelium-lined surface (parotid gland, tentorium, and hand). DSRCTs exhibit a reciprocal translocation [t(11;22) (p13;q12)], resulting in fusion of the EWS1 gene on chromosome 22 and the Wilm's tumor suppressor gene (WT1) on chromosome 11 that appears to be unique for this tumor [165]. This fusion results in the expression of the EWS/WT1 chimeric transcript detectable by reverse transcriptase polymerase chain reaction (PCR). The EWS/ERG fusion gene characteristic of Ewing's sarcoma/peripheral neuroectodermal tumors has been found in rare DSRCTs, suggesting some overlap between the two groups of tumors.

DSRCTs have a strong male predilection (M:F ratio, 4:1) and are most common in adolescents and young adults (range, 5–76 years) who usually have abdominal distension, pain, and a palpable abdominal, pelvic, or scrotal mass, sometimes in association with ascites. Some patients have had an elevated serum level of CA-125 or neuron-specific enolase (NSE). Laparotomy typically discloses variably sized but usually large, intra-abdominal masses associated with smaller peritoneal "implants" of similar appearance. The tumor is sometimes confined to the pelvis, and prominent involvement of the tunica vaginalis or the ovaries may mimic a primary testicular or ovarian tumor [255]. The retroperitoneum is involved in some cases. One tumor appeared to originate within the liver.

After initial treatment (debulking and postoperative chemotherapy, irradiation, or both), there may be an initial response, but more than 90% of patients die of tumor progression. The bulk of the tumor tends to remain within the peritoneal cavity, although extraabdominal metastases occur in some patients.

Pathologic Findings

On gross examination, the tumors, which may reach 40 cm in maximal dimension, have smooth or bosselated outer surfaces and firm to hard, gray-white, focally myxoid, and necrotic sectioned surfaces. Direct invasion of intra-abdominal or pelvic viscera may occur.

Microscopic examination reveals sharply circumscribed aggregates of small epithelioid cells delimited by a cellular desmoplastic stroma (*Fig. 13.27*). The aggregates vary from tiny clusters (or even single cells) to rounded or irregularly shaped islands. Other common features include rounded rosette-like or gland-like spaces, peripheral palisading of basaloid cells in some of the nests, and central necrosis with or without calcification. The tumor cells are typically uniform with scanty cytoplasm and indistinct cell borders (*Fig. 13.28*), although tumor cells with eosinophilic cytoplasmic "inclusions" and an eccentric nucleus, resulting in a rhabdoid appearance, are frequently also present. Small to medium-sized, round, oval, or spindle-shaped hyperchromatic nuclei have clumped chromatin and nucleoli that are usually inapparent. Mitotic figures and single necrotic cells are numerous.

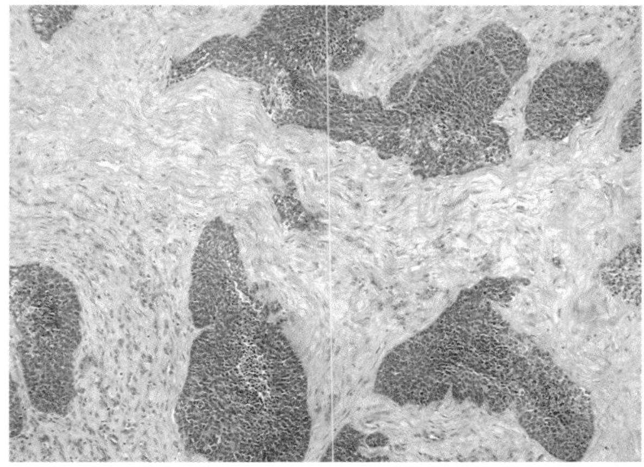

Fig 13.27
Intra-abdominal desmoplastic small round cell tumor (DSRCT). **The cellular nests of tumor are sharply circumscribed and separated by a fibrous stroma. Focal necrosis of the tumor is seen**

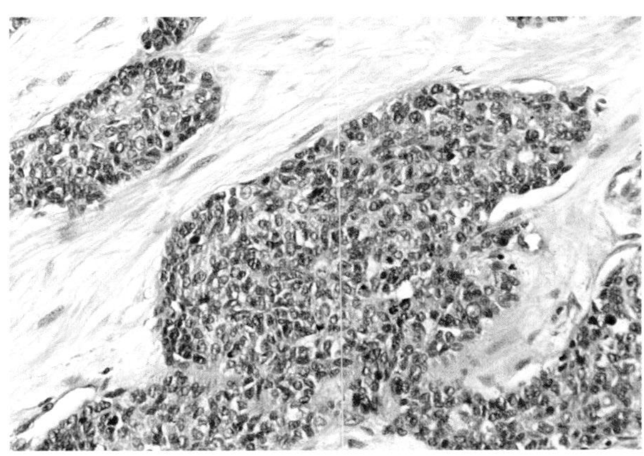

Fig. 13.28
Intra-abdominal desmoplastic small round cell tumor. **The tumor cells have scant cytoplasm and malignant nuclear features**

Architectural features noted in a minority of cases, which can occasionally predominate and lead to diagnostic problems, include tubules, glands (sometimes with luminal mucin), cysts, papillae, anastomosing trabeculae, cords of cells mimicking lobular breast carcinoma, adenoid cystic-like foci, and only a sparse desmoplastic stroma. Cytologic features noted in a minority of cases, which can occasionally predominate, include spindle cells, cells with abundant eosinophilic or clear cytoplasm, which may create a biphasic pattern, signet-ring-like cells, and cells with marked nuclear pleomorphism [166]. Invasion of vascular spaces, especially lymphatics, is a common feature. Lymph nodes are occasionally involved by tumor.

Immunohistochemical and Ultrastructural Findings

The usual immunoreactivity for epithelial (low molecular weight cytokeratins, epithelial membrane antigen [EMA]), neural/neuroendocrine (neuron-specific enolase [NSE], CD57/Leu-7), and muscle (desmin) markers, as well as vimentin, suggests divergent differentiation. Desmin and vimentin immunoreactivity is typically paranuclear and globular and is particularly intense in the rhabdoid cells. Immunoreactivity for other antigens has been present in a variable proportion of cases, including Wilms' tumor protein (WT1), Leu-M1 (CD 15), S-100, B72.3, CA-125, MIC-2 protein, actin (MSA, SMA), desmoplakin, CD 99, MOC-31, NB84, Ber-EP4, chromogranin, and synaptophysin, but not HBA 71 (Ewing's sarcoma/PNET antigen) [126, 167, 258]. The stroma is typically immunoreactive for vimentin and muscle specific actin.

Ultrastructural variability suggests a range of differentiation. Cell junctions have varied from scant and primitive to more prominent ones including intermediate, desmosomal, and tight types. Paranuclear intermediate cytoplasmic filaments and basal lamina surrounding the nests of tumor have been prominent features in most of the cases [167].

Differential Diagnosis

The typical age of the patient, the absence of an extraperitoneal primary tumor, the distribution of the tumor, and its typical microscopic features and immunoprofile facilitate the distinction from other malignant small blue cell tumors in most cases. Identification of the unique reciprocal translocation is diagnostic in problem cases.

Solitary Fibrous Tumor

Although once referred to as fibrous mesotheliomas, these tumors are now designated solitary fibrous tumors and are believed to originate from submesothelial fibroblasts [23, 254]. The clinical and pathologic features are similar to their much more common pleural counterparts, including immunoreactivity for CD34 and lack of immunoreactivity for cytokeratin, an immunoprofile that is useful in distinguishing these tumors from desmoplastic mesotheliomas [23]. Typical tumors are clinically benign. One peritoneal solitary fibrous tumor that was focally sarcomatous was clinically malignant [82].

Inflammatory Myofibroblastic Tumor

Day et al. reviewed the features of seven cases of abdominal "inflammatory pseudotumor," [61] a lesion that has also been referred to as plasma cell granuloma or, more recently, inflammatory myofibroblastic tumor [182]. Various anatomical locations have been reported but most tumors arise in the lung, mesentery, omentum, or retroperitoneum. The abdominal lesions are typically encountered in patients younger than 20 years of age, often in the first decade, who present with a mass, fever, growth failure or weight loss, hypochromic anemia, thrombocytosis, and polyclonal hypergammaglobulinemia. Laparotomy typically reveals a solid mesenteric mass that on microscopic examination consists of myofibroblastic spindle cells, mature plasma cells, and small lymphocytes. The spindle cells often show positive cytoplasmic immunoreactivity for ALK-1, with associated chromosomal translocations detected in approximately 50% of cases. Inflammatory myofibroblastic tumors are regarded as neoplasms of low-grade or intermediate biologic behavior, which can be associated with favorable outcome, but have a tendency for local recurrence and generally a low risk of distant metastasis. Coffin et al. recently reported that abdominopelvic tumors had a higher rate of recurrence relative to other anatomical sites and that ALK-negative tumors were more likely to be associated with distant metastases [53].

Calcifying Fibrous Tumor

The rare lesion known as calcifying fibrous tumor, initially considered a pseudotumor, is likely neoplastic, with a predilection for children and young adults but which can occur over a wide age range and in a variety of anatomical sites including the subcutaneous or deep soft tissues and the pleura [159, 217]. In the peritoneum, the calcifying fibrous tumor is usually an incidental finding involving the visceral peritoneum of the small intestine or stomach. The tumors are often small (less than 5 cm) but can be larger and sometimes multiple. Microscopically, they are hypocellular, composed of bland spindle cells, hyalinized collagen, a chronic lymphoplasmacytic inflammatory infiltrate, and psammomatous or dystrophic calcifications. The spindle cells are typically CD34-positive and ALK-negative, the latter regarded as evidence that these lesions are distinct from the inflammatory myofibroblastic tumor; rare cells may show positive staining with muscle actin and desmin [159, 217].

Omental–Mesenteric Myxoid Hamartoma

The omental–mesenteric myxoid hamartoma designation was applied by Gonzalez-Crussi et al. to a lesion in infants characterized by multiple omental and mesenteric nodules composed of plump mesenchymal cells in a myxoid, vascularized stroma [89]. The diagnosis of the referring pathologists was usually that of some type of sarcoma, but the follow-up was uneventful. The lesions may be hamartomatous or a variant of inflammatory myofibroblastic tumor.

Sarcomas

The majority of intra-abdominal sarcomas are of non-peritoneal origin and arise in the retroperitoneum or gastrointestinal tract; they include leiomyosarcomas, liposarcomas, and gastrointestinal stromal tumors, and are not discussed further here. Rarely, malignant vascular tumors may arise from the peritoneum (epithelioid hemangioendothelioma, epithelioid angiosarcoma) and are briefly discussed above in the differential diagnosis with malignant mesothelioma [134].

Gestational Trophoblastic Disease

Rarely, gestational trophoblastic disease (including placental site trophoblastic tumor, hydatidiform mole, and choriocarcinoma) may arise in the peritoneum, presumably secondary to an intra-abdominal pregnancy.

Metastatic Tumors

Peritoneal involvement by metastatic tumor is typically a result of seeding from a primary tumor arising within the abdomen or pelvis, most commonly the ovary. Peritoneal serous tumors in which the ovaries are normal or only minimally involved may arise directly from the peritoneum (see ➲ Lesions of the Secondary Müllerian System) or rarely are metastatic from a serous papillary carcinoma of the endometrium or fallopian tube. Other tumors that may be associated with peritoneal seeding include carcinomas of the breast and gastrointestinal tract, especially the colon and stomach, and the pancreas. In such cases, the metastatic tumor may take the form of signet-ring cells widely scattered in a fibrous stroma (➲ *Fig. 13.29*). Occasionally, the signet-ring cells can have relatively bland nuclear features, resulting in a deceptively benign appearance.

Pseudomyxoma Peritonei

Pseudomyxoma peritonei, which is a clinical term referring to the presence of masses of jelly-like mucus in the pelvis and often the abdomen, is usually a result of peritoneal spread from a typically low-grade mucinous

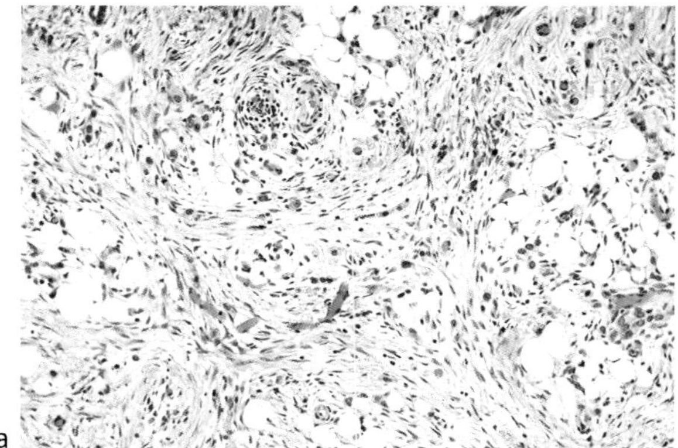

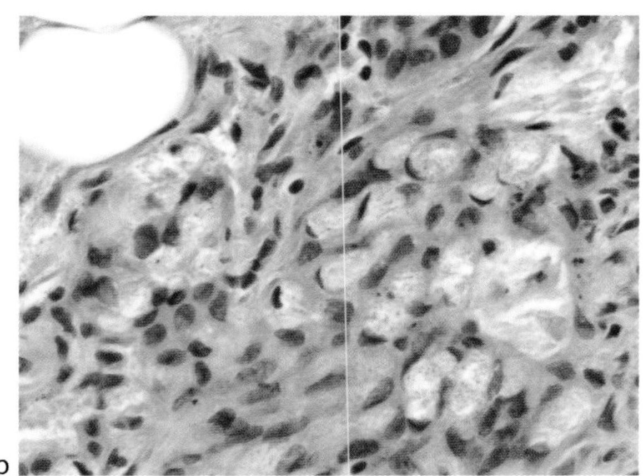

Fig 13.29
Poorly differentiated adenocarcinoma with signet-ring cells involving the peritoneum. **(a)** Deceptively bland, malignant cells infiltrate omental fat lobules, with an associated desmoplastic stromal reaction. **(b)** High-power view of signet-ring cells

neoplasm, usually originating within the appendix or, less commonly, from a primary tumor elsewhere in the gastrointestinal tract. Ovarian involvement is common in such cases and this topic is discussed in detail in ➲ Chap. 14, Surface Epithelial Tumors of the Ovary, and ➲ Chap. 18, Metastatic Tumors of the Ovary.

Lesions of the Secondary Müllerian System

These peritoneal lesions are characterized by müllerian differentiation on microscopic examination and share an origin from the so-called secondary müllerian system, that is, the pelvic and lower abdominal mesothelium and the subjacent mesenchyme of females [128]. The müllerian potential of this layer is consistent with its close embryonic relation to the müllerian ducts that arise by invagination of the coelomic epithelium. Displacement of coelomic epithelium and subcoelomic mesenchyme during embryonic development could account for the presence of identical lesions within pelvic and abdominal lymph nodes. The origin of many of these lesions, however, is not known with certainty, and other proposed histogenetic mechanisms are discussed where appropriate.

Lesions of the secondary müllerian system include those containing endometrioid, serous, and mucinous epithelium, simulating normal or neoplastic endometrial, tubal, and endocervical epithelium. The metaplastic potential of the pelvic peritoneum also includes differentiation toward cells of transitional (urothelial) type, exemplified most commonly by Walthard nests. Proliferation of the subjacent mesenchyme may accompany epithelial differentiation of the mesothelium or may give rise to a variety of pure mesenchymal lesions composed of endometrial stromal-type cells, decidua, or smooth muscle.

Endometriosis in Usual Sites

Endometriosis is defined as the presence of endometrial tissue outside the endometrium and myometrium. Usually both epithelium and stroma are seen, but occasionally the diagnosis of endometriosis can be made when only one component is present, as discussed below.

Etiology and Pathogenesis

Two theories have been proposed for the pathogenesis of endometriosis: (1) metastases of endometrial tissue to its ectopic location (metastatic theory); and (2) metaplastic development of endometrial tissue at the ectopic site (metaplastic theory). The metastatic theory explains the majority of cases, but a metaplastic origin likely accounts for occasional cases in which metastatic spread of endometrial tissue is unlikely or impossible (see following).

Metastatic Theory

Sampson [205] proposed that endometriosis was caused by reflux of endometrial tissue through the fallopian tubes by a process of retrograde menstruation, with subsequent implantation and growth on peritoneal surfaces. Implantation of menstrual endometrium has also been proposed to explain endometriosis within surgical scars, on traumatized cervical and vaginal mucosa, and within perineal and vulvar scars following vaginal delivery. Passage of refluxed menstrual endometrium from the peritoneal cavity through diaphragmatic defects, diaphragmatic lymphatics, or both may explain pleural endometriosis.

Observations supporting the menstrual implantation hypothesis include the following: (1) endometriotic lesions are most common in areas closest to the tubal ostia and occur in a distribution that appears dependent on gravity and uterine position [104]; (2) lateral predisposition of ovarian endometriomas, which are more commonly left-sided than right-sided, a phenomenon attributed to reduced flow of peritoneal fluid due to the presence of the sigmoid colon in the left pelvis [230] (3) retrograde menstruation through the fallopian tubes is a common physiologic process, occurring in 90% of menstruating women with patent tubes [93]; (4) endometriosis is more common in women with early menarche, heavy menstrual flow, long menstrual flow (greater than 7 days), and frequent menses (cycle less than 27 days); (5) menstrual endometrium is viable, capable of growth in tissue culture and after subcutaneous or intrapelvic injection [65]; (6) endometriosis is more frequent in females with congenital obstruction to menstrual flow [164]; and (7) endometriosis may follow uteropelvic or utero-abdominal wall fistulas in experimental animals and humans.

Although endometriosis in some scars may be a result of menstrual implantation, endometriosis within scars after uterine operations may be secondary to intraoperative implantation of endometrial tissue [34, 224]. Supporting this theory is the greater frequency of scar endometriosis after abdominal hysterotomy than after cesarean section in some studies, consistent with the greater viability of transplanted early-pregnancy endometrium compared to late-pregnancy endometrium. Also, the occurrence of endometriosis within an episiotomy scar is much higher if uterine curettage is performed immediately after delivery than in patients without postdelivery curettage [177].

The presence of endometriosis in distant sites (e.g., lungs, extremities, and brain) is most easily explained by hematogenous spread from the uterus. Similarly, endometriosis within lymph nodes is likely a result of lymphatic spread. Evidence supporting the origin of endometriosis from lymphatic or hematogenous spread includes (1) the presence of normal endometrial tissue within endothelium-lined spaces as an incidental histologic finding within the myometrium, most often associated with adenomyosis; (2) the presence of intraluminal vascular involvement in rare endometriotic lesions; (3) the presence of intravascular or perivascular trophoblastic tissue and "decidua" as an incidental microscopic finding within the lungs of pregnant patients [223]; (4) the occurrence of pulmonary endometriosis almost exclusively in women who have had prior uterine operations that could predispose to the embolization of endometrial tissue; (5) the experimental production of pulmonary endometriosis by intravenous injection of endometrial tissue in rabbits; and (6) the observations that tumor cells, blood, dye, and radiographic material can migrate from the pelvis to the umbilicus by retrograde lymphatic flow.

Metaplastic Theory

The origin of pelvic endometriosis by a process of metaplasia from the pelvic peritoneum is consistent with the putative müllerian potential of this tissue, which, as noted earlier, has been referred to as the secondary müllerian system [128]. Evidence for the metaplastic theory includes (1) the demonstration of endometriosis in subjects in whom metastasis of normally situated endometrium could not occur or is highly unlikely, such as those with Turner's syndrome and pure gonadal dysgenesis who are amenorrheic and have hypoplastic uteri [179], and in males; (2) the experimental induction of peritoneal endometriosis adjacent to millipore filters that contain endometrial tissue but that prevent cellular transfer; (3) the observation that autologous endometrial implants in rabbits degenerate but are associated with the subsequent development of endometriosis in adjacent tissues; and (4) the juxtaposition of endometriosis with other putative metaplastic lesions of the peritoneum, such as diffuse peritoneal leiomyomatosis [91].

Other Etiologic Factors

Endometriosis is an idiopathic disease in most patients, and why only a minority of females are affected despite the common occurrence of retrograde menstruation is unknown. Some potential etiologic factors have been discussed (congenital obstruction, iatrogenic implantation); others are summarized in the following section.

Familial and Genetic Factors Several studies concluded that the prevalence of endometriosis is greater in mothers and sisters of women with endometriosis than in the mothers and sisters of their husbands [127, 218]. Lamb et al. calculated the overall risk for first-degree relatives to be 4.9% [127]. Genetic studies suggest a polygenic mode of inheritance (influenced by several different genes) or one that is multifactorial (a result of interaction between genetic and environmental factors). In opposition to the foregoing, Houston et al. [102] concluded that there were methodologic flaws in these studies [127, 218] and that an inherited tendency to endometriosis has not yet been substantiated.

Molecular genetic analysis has elucidated a number of intriguing theories regarding the pathogenesis of endometriosis [24]. By microarray analysis, Wu et al. have shown that in patients with endometriosis, the ectopic and eutopic endometria have different gene expression profiles [247]. Putative endometrial progenitor/stem cells, which are thought to reside in the basalis endometrium and possibly in the bone marrow, have recently been characterized by in vitro and in vivo assays [206]. It has been shown that patients with endometriosis shed significantly more basalis layer during menstruation compared with normal controls, supporting the hypothesis that endometriotic implants develop from endometrial progenitor/stem cells, which are in turn derived from retrograde menstrual flow, known to be higher in women with endometriosis [93, 132, 206].

Hormonal Factors Because endometriosis occurs almost exclusively in women of reproductive age, hormonal factors may play an etiologic role. The rare examples of endometriosis in phenotypic females with gonadal dysgenesis and in males have usually been associated with the use of exogenous estrogens [138, 179]. Similarly, smoking and exercise, which are inversely correlated with endogenous estrogen levels, appear to be protective factors for the development of endometriosis. In a recent large epidemiologic study, factors associated with an increased risk of endometriosis included low body weight, alcohol use, and certain menstrual characteristics (early menarche, short cycle length, and heavy menstrual cycles) [140].

It has been suggested that the progestational milieu of pregnancy may inhibit the development of endometriosis. Many studies have indicated that endometriosis is more likely to occur in women who have delayed pregnancy and is less common in multiparous women [192]. Similarly, in some studies, patients with endometriosis are much less likely to have used oral contraceptives than similar patients without endometriosis.

Some studies have found an increased frequency of the luteinized unruptured follicle syndrome (LUFS) in patients with endometriosis. In normal women, the ruptured corpus luteum releases its progesterone-rich fluid into the peritoneal cavity. It has been postulated that this fluid may inhibit implantation and growth of refluxed endometrial fragments at the time of menstruation [123]. In patients with LUFS, a corpus luteum is formed, but rupture and fluid release do not occur, resulting in lowered luteal-phase levels of progesterone in the peritoneal fluid [123]. This local hormonal imbalance may be critical in allowing endometrial cells to implant on the peritoneum. Other studies, however, have shown no difference in the luteal-phase peritoneal fluid hormone values in women with and without endometriosis.

Immune Factors One study has demonstrated a reduced T-lymphocyte-mediated cytotoxicity to autologous endometrial cells and a decreased lymphocyte stimulation response to autologous endometrial antigens in patients with endometriosis [225]. The degree of depressed cellular immunity was directly proportional to the severity of the disease. The authors of this study suggested that certain cell-mediated immune mechanisms that may be operative in limiting the growth of endometriotic tissue may be impaired in patients with endometriosis. Other authors have suggested that the growth of endometriotic implants may be stimulated by activated macrophages. Recent evidence has shown that local production of interleukin-4, a cytokine involved in the Th2 immune response, induces proliferation of endometriotic stromal cells [172]. Cyclo-oxygenase-2, which is involved in the biosynthesis of prostaglandin E2, is highly expressed in ectopic endometria relative to eutopic endometria, and is thought to play a promotory role in the development of endometriosis [13].

Clinical Features

Epidemiologic Factors

The highest risk of the disease has traditionally been considered to be in the upper socioeconomic levels of developed societies, especially among women who delay pregnancy, although, according to Houston, these associations have not been proven statistically [102]. Although endometriosis was once considered to be more common in Caucasians, recent studies showing a similar frequency of the disease in Orientals and blacks cast doubt on this view.

The true prevalence of endometriosis is unknown as many patients are asymptomatic; estimates for the prevalence of the disease in women of reproductive age are 10–15% [147]. Prevalence figures, however, have varied widely, depending on the population studied and the method of diagnosis (clinical, operative, or pathologic). Similarly, a study of the incidence rates of pelvic endometriosis in white females of reproductive age in Rochester, Minnesota (USA), found that the overall incidence of the disease more than doubled (from 108.8 to 246.9 cases per 100,000 person-years) as the definition of a case was extended from histologically confirmed cases to clinically and surgically diagnosed cases [101].

More than 80% of affected patients are in the reproductive age group. In one study, the age-specific incidence rates increased in successive age groups through age 44 and then declined for women 45–49 years [101]. Less than 5% of cases occur in postmenopausal women, and in these patients the disease is frequently not diagnosed premenopausally [115]. Endometriosis can be clinically significant in this age group, with 20–30% of affected patients requiring operative management [115, 189]. In some postmenopausal patients with endometriosis, an association with obesity and endometrial carcinoma has been noted, suggesting that hyperestrinism may play a role, but in other series, a majority of patients have had no obvious exogenous or endogenous source of estrogen [115]. Almost 10% of patients with endometriosis are adolescents [32]. Endometriosis was found at laparoscopy in approximately 50% of teenage patients with dysmenorrhea or chronic pelvic pain in three studies [32]. In some studies, adolescents with endometriosis have a particularly high frequency of a congenital obstruction to menstrual flow.

Symptoms and Signs

The recurrent cyclic menstrual, inflammatory, and fibrotic changes within endometriotic lesions are likely responsible for most of the symptomatology of endometriosis, although there is often no direct relationship between the extent of the disease and the severity of the symptoms [32]. An exception to the foregoing applies to women with deeply infiltrating endometriosis, a clinical term used for patients with deep pelvic pain, usually in the form of severe dyspareunia and dysmenorrhea, which is often associated with rectovaginal lesions or involvement of bowel, ureter, or bladder [56]. One study has shown significant reduction in painful symptoms obtained with complete surgical excision of deep lesions [35]. Hormonal responsiveness of the lesions as judged histologically also does not correlate with symptoms, and microscopic examination of symptomatic endometriosis in postmenopausal patients typically reveals atrophic changes [115]. Age generally does not appear to affect disease severity in most studies [102]. An exception to the foregoing is one study in which women in the age group of 26–52 years had less extensive disease than women 16–25 years of age [192]. A higher frequency of nulliparity in the younger women appeared to account for part of this difference [102]. Another recent study found that endometriosis in postmenopausal patients was morphologically less extensive and less active in appearance relative to endometriosis in premenopausal women, but that the endometriotic foci retained the same immunoprofile by estrogen and progesterone receptor immunostaining [58].

The typical symptoms that are attributed to pelvic endometriosis are acquired dysmenorrhea, lower abdominal, pelvic, and back pain, dyspareunia, irregular bleeding, and infertility. Infertility is present in up to 30% of women with endometriosis, although the putative association between mild endometriosis and infertility has been challenged and remains controversial. The subject of endometriosis-related infertility has been reviewed elsewhere [92, 147] and is not considered in detail here. Potential pathogenetic factors include tubal factors (adhesions, luminal obstruction), ovarian factors (anovulation, luteal-phase dysfunction, LUFS), immune factors (antiendometrial antibodies), peritoneal factors (increased prostaglandins, increased macrophages), and an increased risk of spontaneous abortion.

Pelvic examination may reveal tender nodules in the cul-de-sac and uterosacral ligaments, tender, semifixed, cystic ovaries, and a fixed, retroverted uterus. The rectovaginal septum may also be tender and indurated. The endometriotic lesions frequently enlarge and become more painful during menses. The clinical manifestations also vary according to the site of the endometriosis, as is discussed later in this chapter. As the clinical manifestations of endometriosis are frequently nonspecific, vary widely between patients, and may be absent in a high proportion of patients, a definitive diagnosis requires direct visualization by laparoscopy (or laparotomy) and, ideally, biopsy. Hormonal suppression and surgical ablation remain commonly employed therapeutic modalities, and while treatment of endometriosis is not discussed here, it is important to note that with advances in the understanding of the pathogenesis of endometriosis, future methods may include molecular-targeted drug therapies such as cyclo-oxygenase inhibitors and immunomodulators in an attempt to minimize the need for surgical intervention [24, 92].

Laparoscopic Findings

A number of recent studies have stressed that endometriotic foci, especially early ones, are frequently nonpigmented and may have a wide variety of laparoscopic appearances, including clear, white, and red lesions [107, 137, 226]. Sequential laparoscopic examinations indicate that nonpigmented endometriotic implants eventually evolve into the typical pigmented lesions [107]. Even in patients with laparoscopically typical disease, biopsy may yield only nondiagnostic tissue, and thus, in the opinion of some authors, diagnosis and treatment should not always depend on microscopic confirmation [33]. Other authors have found that 25% of laparoscopically atypical lesions prove to be endometriosis on histological examination, and therefore advocate that all lesions suggestive of endometriosis, both typical and atypical, should be excised if eradication is the surgical objective [3]. In another study, only 50% of all laparoscopic biopsies from clinically suspicious foci were proven microscopically to be endometriosis [240].

Laparoscopically detectable defects or "pockets" involving the pelvic peritoneum are frequently associated with, and likely caused by, endometriosis [193]. In one study, 80% of women with pelvic peritoneal defects had endometriosis, and in another, the endometriotic foci were often located along the edges of the defects [193]. Conversely, 18–28% of women with endometriosis had peritoneal defects [193].

Serum Markers

Levels of CA-125 may be elevated in the serum and peritoneal fluid of patients with endometriosis [74]. The concentrations of serum CA-125 correlate with both the severity and the clinical course of the disease. The serum test has low sensitivity, however, and is not appropriate for general screening purposes. In contrast, CA-125 levels have acceptable sensitivities and very high specificities in populations with a relatively high prevalence of the disease and are useful in monitoring response to treatment.

Antiendometrial antibodies have been found in up to 83% of women with laparoscopically confirmed endometriosis. In one study, the antibody titers in women who had had a good response to hormonal treatment were lower than in those with untreated endometriosis or in whom there had been a poor response to treatment, and in another study, sequential determination of antibody levels showed that they were lowered by hormonal treatment.

Effects of Pregnancy

Although rare cases of endometriosis undergo permanent regression during pregnancy, the ameliorative effect of pregnancy noted in many cases of endometriosis is only temporary. The behavior of endometriosis during pregnancy is extremely variable among different patients and between one pregnancy and another in the same patient. During pregnancy, visible endometriotic lesions frequently undergo initial enlargement, with occasional ulceration and bleeding, followed by shrinkage. In most sites, there is a decrease in the associated pain.

A rare complication of endometriosis during pregnancy is intrapartum or postpartum rupture of the lesion, most probably caused by a softening of the lesion secondary to stromal decidualization, pressure from the expanding uterus, or both. Rupture occurs most frequently in the ovaries or bowel, typically resulting in perforation and an acute abdomen. Rarely, hemoperitoneum, sometimes fatal, is caused by hemorrhage from decidualized endometriotic lesions at term.

Rare Complications

Massive, sometimes serosanguineous, ascites can occur in patients with pelvic endometriosis; a right pleural effusion is also present in one third of such patients [157]. If one or both ovaries are involved, the operative findings may simulate those of an ovarian carcinoma. The pathogenesis of the ascites is not clear. Possible sources include production by endometriotic cysts, irritated peritoneal mesothelial cells, or the ovarian serosa (Meigs-like syndrome). Other rare complications include hemorrhage from an endometriotic focus and spontaneous rupture of ovarian endometriotic cysts, resulting in an acute abdomen.

Gross Features of Peritoneal and Ovarian Endometriosis

The most common anatomical sites of endometriosis are the ovaries, the uterosacral, broad, or round ligaments, the rectovaginal septum and cul-de-sac, and the serosa of the uterus, fallopian tubes, or other pelvic organs (see ➋ *Table 13.1*). Less common sites include the serosa of the large bowel, small bowel, and appendix, the mucosa of the female genital tract, the skin, the urinary tract, and pelvic lymph nodes. These sites and other additional rare sites of involvement are discussed separately below.

Depending on their duration and their superficial or deep location in relation to the peritoneal surface, endometriotic foci may appear as punctate, red, blue, brown, or white spots or patches with either a slightly raised or a puckered surface (➋ *Fig. 13.30*). Ecchymotic or brown areas have sometimes been described as "powder burns." The endometriotic foci are frequently associated with dense fibrous adhesions. The lesions may form nodules or cysts or both. Rarely, endometriosis can take the form of polypoid masses that project from the serosal surfaces, into the lumens of endometriotic cysts, or from the mucosa of the bowel (➋ *Fig. 13.31*) or bladder. In some of these cases, there is a history of exogenous estrogen use and hyperplastic changes are found on microscopic examination [176]. This appearance, which we refer to as polypoid endometriosis, can simulate a malignant tumor on clinical, intraoperative, or pathologic examination [155, 176].

Endometriotic cysts (endometriomas) most commonly involve the ovaries, where they can partially or almost completely replace the normal tissue; bilateral

Table 13.1
Sites of endometriosis

Common	Less common	Rare
Ovaries Uterine ligaments (uterosacral, round, broad) Rectovaginal septum Cul-de-sac Peritoneum of uterus, tubes, rectosigmoid, ureter, bladder	Large bowel, small bowel, appendix Mucosa of cervix, vagina, and fallopian tubes Skin (scars, umbilicus, vulva, perineum, inguinal region) Ureter, bladder Omentum, pelvic lymph nodes Inguinal (noncutaneous)	Lungs, pleura Soft tissues, breast Bone Upper abdominal peritoneum Stomach, pancreas, liver Urethra, kidney, prostate, paratesticular Sciatic nerve, subarachnoid space, brain

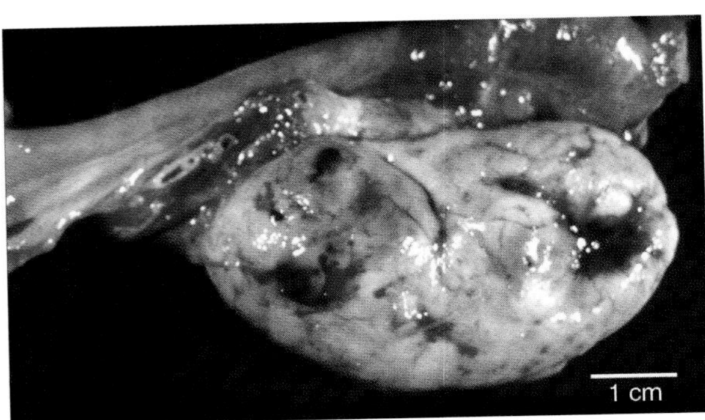

Fig. 13.30
Endometriosis of ovary. **Multiple, hemorrhagic lesions involve the ovarian surface (Courtesy of R.E. Scully, M.D., Boston, MA)**

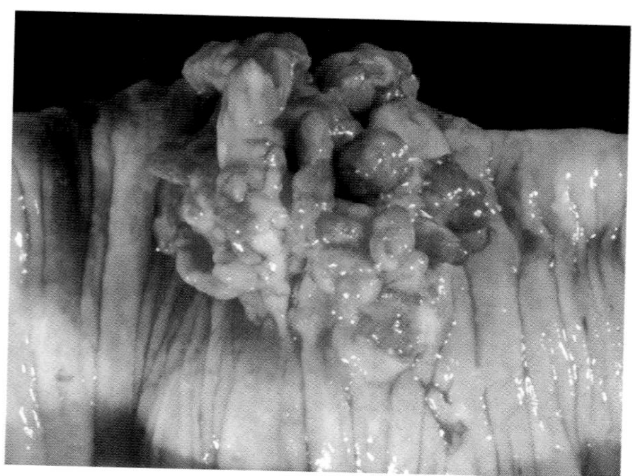

Fig. 13.31
Polypoid endometriosis. **A polypoid mass projects from the mucosa of the large bowel**

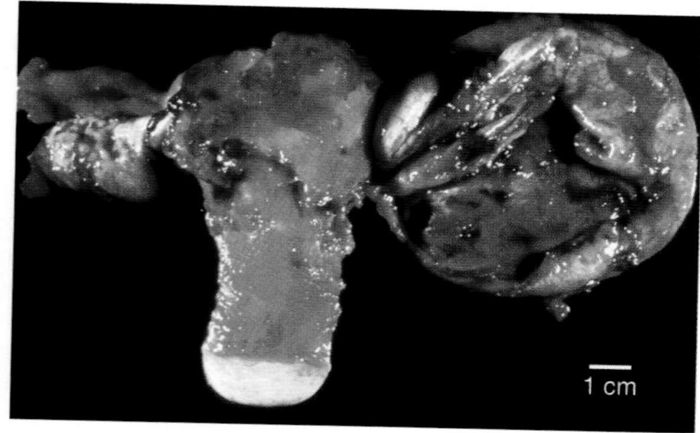

Fig. 13.32
Endometriotic cyst of ovary. **The cyst has been opened to reveal a focally hemorrhagic lining. Multiple hemorrhagic lesions also involve the uterine serosal surface**

involvement occurs in one third to one half of the cases [67]. The cysts rarely exceed 15 cm in diameter; larger examples are more likely to harbor a neoplasm. Endometriotic cysts are commonly covered by dense fibrous adhesions, which may result in fixation to adjacent structures. The cyst walls are usually thick and fibrotic, with a smooth or shaggy, brown to yellow lining (*Fig. 13.32*). The cyst contents typically consist of altered, semifluid or inspissated, chocolate-colored material; rarely, the cyst is filled with watery fluid. Any solid areas in the cyst wall or intraluminal polypoid projections should be sampled histologically to exclude a neoplasm originating in the cyst (see page 37).

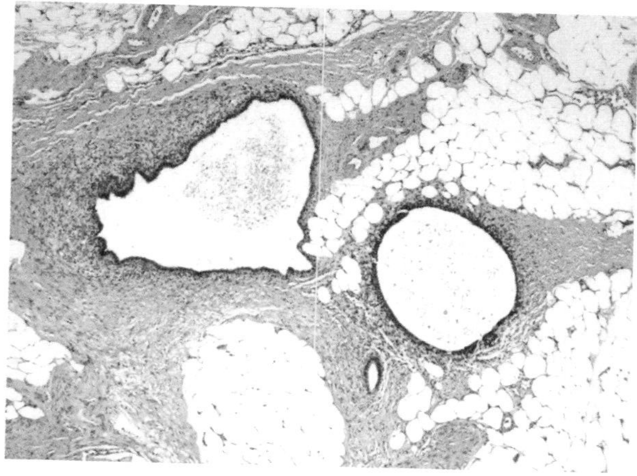

Fig. 13.33
Endometriosis of cul-de-sac. **Cystic endometrial glands with a cuff of endometrial stroma are surrounded by fibrous and adipose tissue**

Typical Microscopic Findings

Many of the problems and pitfalls encountered in the histological diagnosis of endometriosis have been addressed in detail in a recent comprehensive review [39]. The typical appearance in reproductive age women, in whom the disease is usually diagnosed, is of one or more glands lined by endometrioid epithelium, surrounded by a mantle of densely packed small fusiform cells with scanty cytoplasm and bland cytology, typical of nonneoplastic endometrial stromal cells (*Figs. 13.33* and *13.34*). Small blood vessels, which may be engorged, are present and sometimes draw attention to the lesion on low-power examination. When seen in the ovary, the most common site encountered by the surgical pathologist, endometriosis varies from simple to microscopically dilated glands (*Fig. 13.35*) to grossly recognizable endometriotic cysts. This spectrum is seen at extraovarian sites, although striking cysts are less common to rare, depending on the site. Endometriosis may occur anywhere in the ovary but is most common in the cortex. Sometimes it is very superficial and may occur on the surface as small nodules, irregularly shaped aggregates, or even have a plaque-like configuration (*Fig. 13.35*). Surface endometriosis is typically associated with fibrous tissue and inflammatory cells and, if prominent and of significant duration, there may be conspicuous adhesions. Glands, which can sometimes be cystic, may hang off the surface of the ovary, tethered to it by the associated stroma and fibrous tissue. Endometriotic glands in the cortex of the ovaries of perimenopausal or

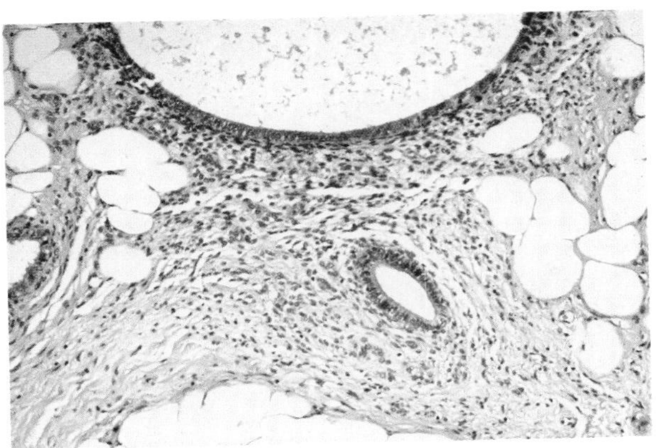

Fig. 13.34
Endometriosis of cul-de-sac (higher magnification of Fig. 13.33). **Endometriotic glands are lined by inactive epithelium and surrounded by a thin rim of endometrial stroma**

postmenopausal women, or glands that are atrophic for any reason, may be mistaken for inclusion glands and cysts if the often subtle, sometimes barely perceptible, cuffs of stroma are overlooked or obscured by hemorrhage or histiocytes (see *Fig. 13.35*). Immunostaining for CD10 can facilitate the recognition of the stromal cells, particularly when sparse and when glandular epithelium is minimal or absent (*Fig. 13.35c*) [227].

The appearance of endometriotic tissue varies with the extent of its response to the normal hormonal fluctuations of the menstrual cycle and the duration of the process. When the appearances of simultaneous samples of eutopic endometrium and endometriotic foci from reproductive age women are compared, cyclic changes are seen in the endometriosis in 44–80% of the cases, with considerable variability in glandular morphology [149, 252]. When more than one endometriotic focus is examined in the same patient, the appearance of the specimens does not differ significantly from one to another [18]. In most postmenopausal patients, the endometriotic tissue is atrophic with glands, that are occasionally cystic, lined by flattened epithelial cells surrounded by a dense fibrotic stroma with sometimes a barely perceptible tendency for the stroma to be more cellular close to the gland, a feature that may be a diagnostic clue; the appearance is similar to that of simple or cystic atrophy of the endometrium (*Fig. 13.36*) [115]. In a minority of cases, however, the endometriotic tissue has an active appearance, with or without the metaplastic and hyperplastic changes that are more commonly present in premenopausal women.

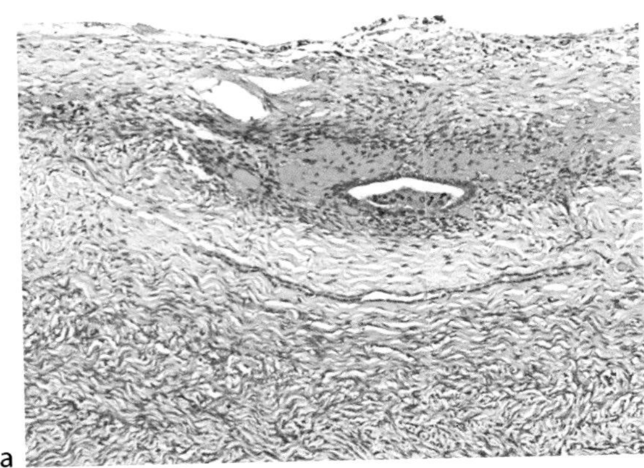

a

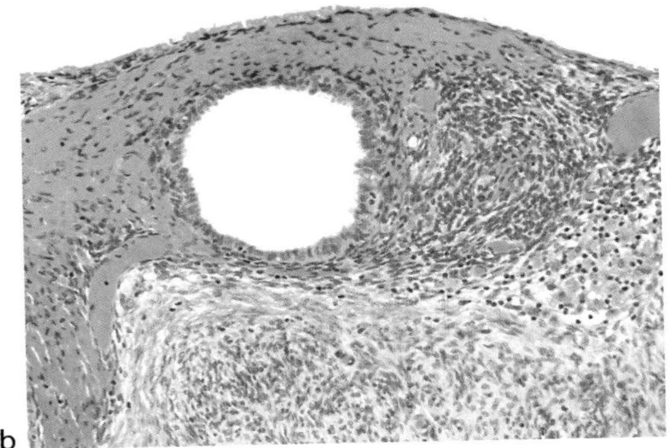

b

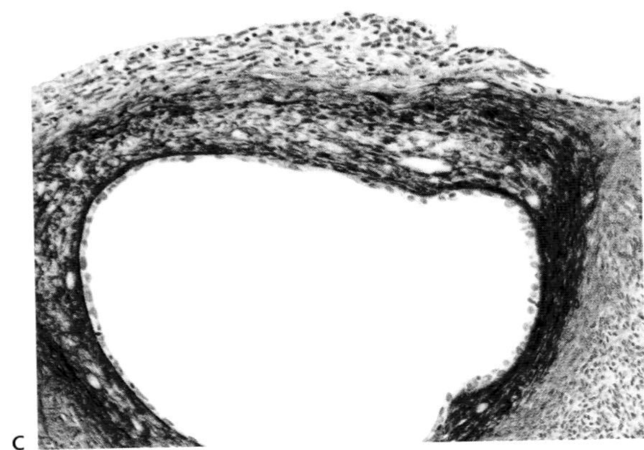

c

Fig. 13.35
Subtle endometriosis involving the ovarian surface. **(a) The periglandular endometriotic stroma is only focal and less cellular than usual. (b) The periglandular endometriotic stroma is obscured by hemorrhage. In both examples, failure to recognize the endometriotic stroma could result in the diagnosis of endometriosis being missed and the endometriotic glands being misinterpreted as epithelial inclusion glands. (c) Endometrial stromal cells highlighted by positive CD10-immunoreactivity**

At the time of menstruation, hemorrhage may occur within the stroma and glandular lumens of endometriotic foci, as well as a secondary inflammatory response consisting predominantly of a diffuse infiltration of histiocytes. The histiocytes typically convert the extravasated red blood cells into glycolipid and granular brown pigment, becoming so-called pseudoxanthoma cells (➲ *Figs. 13.37* and ➲ *13.38*) that can replace most or all the endometriotic stroma [49]. Most of the pigment is ceroid (lipofuscin, hemofuscin), and hemosiderin is typically present to a much lesser extent [49]. The amount of pigment in an endometriotic lesion appears to increase with its age, and early lesions are frequently nonpigmented [107]. Variable numbers of lymphocytes and smaller numbers of other inflammatory cells may be present. Large numbers of neutrophils with microabscess formation should raise the possibility of secondary bacterial infection [210].

As already mentioned, a common manifestation of ovarian endometriosis is striking cystification resulting in an endometriotic cyst. The epithelial and stromal lining of an endometriotic cyst frequently becomes attenuated, and the former may be reduced to a single layer of cuboidal cells that may retain some endometrial characteristics but which are often devoid of specific features. In such circumstances, recognition of the cyst as endometriotic may only be possible if a rim of subjacent endometrial stroma persists. Commonly, the cyst lining of endometrial epithelium and stroma is totally lost, and replaced by granulation tissue, dense fibrous tissue containing fibroblasts with particularly small nuclei, and variable numbers of pseudoxanthoma cells (presumptive endometriosis) (➲ *Fig. 13.38*). In some "old" endometriotic cysts, ossification, calcification, and old luminal blood clot can produce striking gross and microscopic appearances. The epithelial cells lining endometriotic cysts are often focally large and cuboidal with abundant eosinophilic cytoplasm and large atypical nuclei (➲ *Fig. 13.39*) [39, 212]. The significance of such nuclear atypia is unclear. Although it may be reactive, cells with these features may merge with clear cell adenocarcinomas and endocervical-like mucinous borderline tumors (EMBLTs) [83, 200, 201]. When this atypia is an isolated finding in an endometriotic cyst, however, the follow-up is typically uneventful [212].

Endometriosis that involves smooth muscle in the uterine ligaments or the walls of hollow viscera differs significantly in its appearance from that of endometriosis

Fig. 13.36
Endometriosis in a postmenopausal woman. The glands are cystic, atrophic, and separated by a fibrous stroma

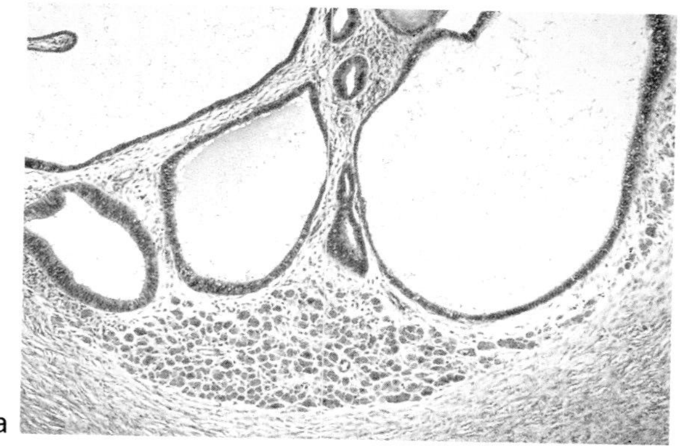

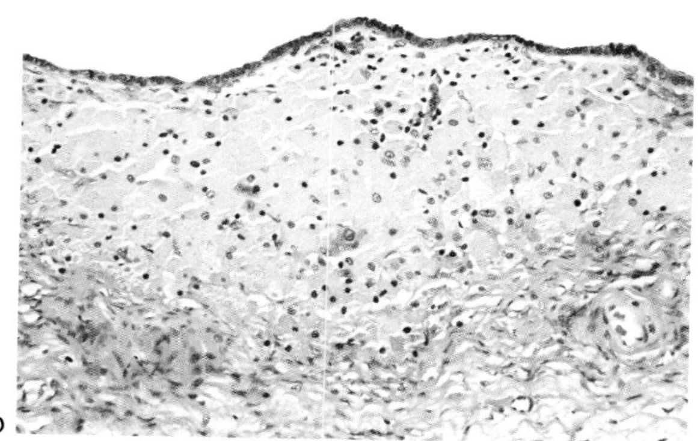

Fig. 13.37
Lining of ovarian endometriotic cyst. (a) The lining consists of cystically dilated endometrial glands and numerous pigment-laden histiocytes within the subjacent stroma. (b) Endometriotic surface epithelial lining with underlying, lightly pigmented histiocytes

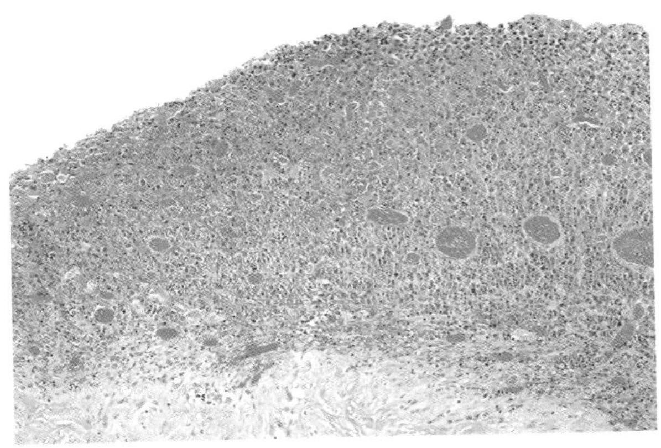

Fig. 13.38
Lining of ovarian endometriotic cyst. **In this field, the lining consists only of fibrotic granulation tissue and pigment-laden histiocytes (presumptive endometriosis)**

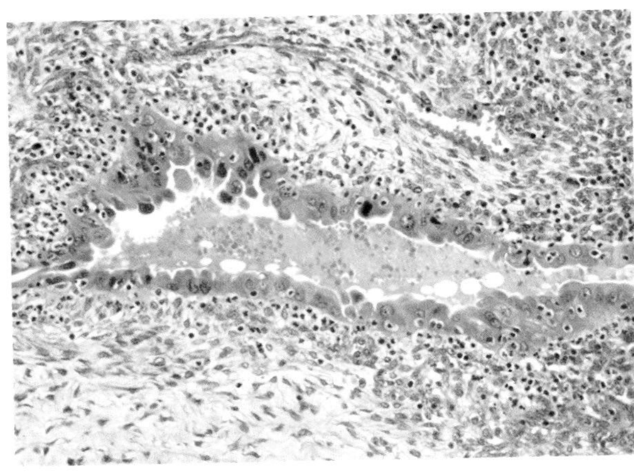

Fig. 13.39
Lining of ovarian endometriotic cyst. **The epithelial cells show notable nuclear atypia**

in the ovaries and the peritoneal surfaces. In the former, there is typically a striking proliferation of the indigenous smooth muscle, often resulting in a firm, solid, tumor-like mass. The appearance is similar to that of adenomyosis with secondary striking myometrial hypertrophy.

Unusual Microscopic Findings

Metaplastic Glandular Changes

Metaplastic changes similar to those occurring in eutopic endometrial glands have been described in endometriotic glands [84]. These changes include ciliated, eosinophilic,

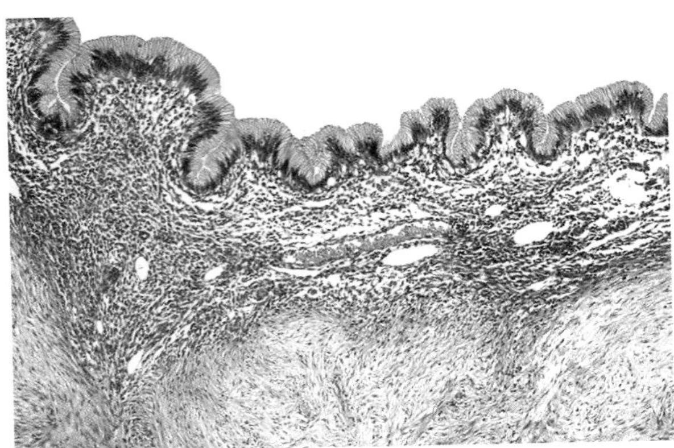

Fig. 13.40
Mucinous metaplasia in endometriosis

hobnail, and, rarely, squamous and mucinous metaplasia (*Fig. 13.40*); the latter may be characterized by the presence of endocervical-type cells or, less often, goblet cells. In one study of ovarian endometriosis [84], there was a significant association between the presence of metaplasia in the endometriosis and a synchronous ovarian epithelial cancer. Additionally, all four endocervical-like mucinous borderline tumors (EMBLTs) in the same study were associated with foci of ovarian endometriosis that exhibited both mucinous metaplasia and hyperplasia. In some cases of endometriosis, the distinction between papillary mucinous metaplasia and an early EMBLT may be arbitrary.

Unusual Hormonal Changes

Endometriotic tissue usually exhibits striking progestational changes (*Fig. 13.41*) during pregnancy or progestin therapy. In such cases, examination reveals a decidual reaction with atrophy of the endometrial glands, which are small and lined by cuboidal or flattened epithelial cells (*Fig. 13.41a*). In pregnancy the glands can rarely exhibit the Arias–Stella reaction (*Fig. 13.41b*), optically clear nuclei, or both. Necrosis of the decidual cells, foci of marked stromal edema, and infiltration by lymphocytes are additional findings in patients receiving progestational agents. Inactive or atrophic changes similar to those that are seen typically in the endometriotic foci of postmenopausal patients may be present in premenopausal patients treated with hormones [161]. Additionally, endometriotic foci often disappear or are replaced by fibrous tissue after danazol therapy.

Hyperplastic Glandular Changes

A variety of hyperplastic and atypically hyperplastic changes similar to those occurring in the endometrium have been described in endometriotic glands, sometimes related to an endogenous or exogenous estrogenic stimulus (*Fig. 13.42*) [83, 205, 249] or tamoxifen therapy [142, 209]. Hyperplastic changes are particularly common in cases of polypoid endometriosis [176]. It is logical to conclude that such atypical changes have a malignant potential similar to those in the endometrium, and indeed, rare cases of hyperplastic endometriosis have preceded the development of an adenocarcinoma in the same area or have coexisted with carcinoma in the same specimen (*Fig. 13.42*; see also *Fig. 13.56*, later in this chapter) [125].

Stromal Changes

The endometriotic stroma may also undergo metaplasia, typically smooth muscle metaplasia, which is encountered most often within the walls of ovarian endometriotic cysts but occasionally elsewhere (*Fig. 13.43*) [80, 81, 211]. Extensive amounts of smooth muscle within the endometriotic stroma can result in "endomyometriosis" or uterus-like masses, which have been described within an obturator lymph node, the ovary, the small bowel, the broad ligament, and lumbosacral region, and in males, in the scrotum [174, 191, 257]. In some cases, a uterus-like mass in the region of the ovary may possibly represent a congenital malformation rather than an unusual

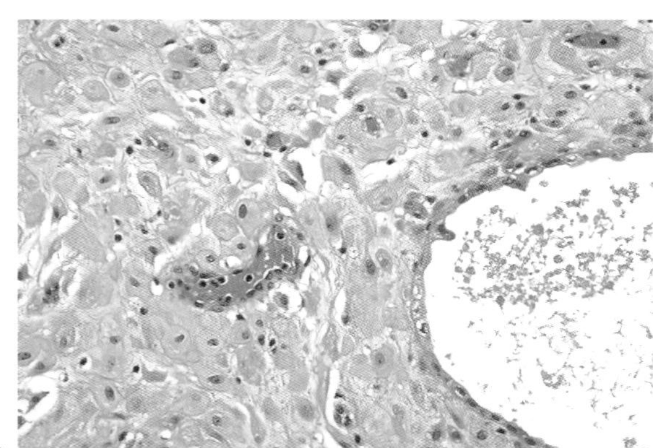
a

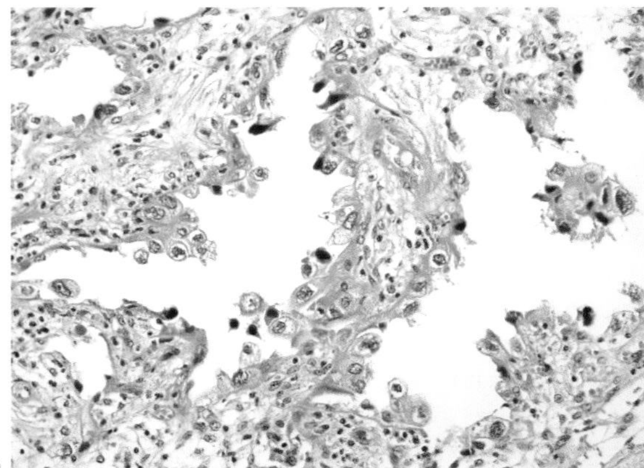
b

Fig. 13.41
Pregnancy-induced changes within endometriosis. **(a) The endometriotic gland is atrophic, and the stroma exhibits marked decidual transformation. (b) The endometriotic glands exhibit the Arias–Stella reaction**

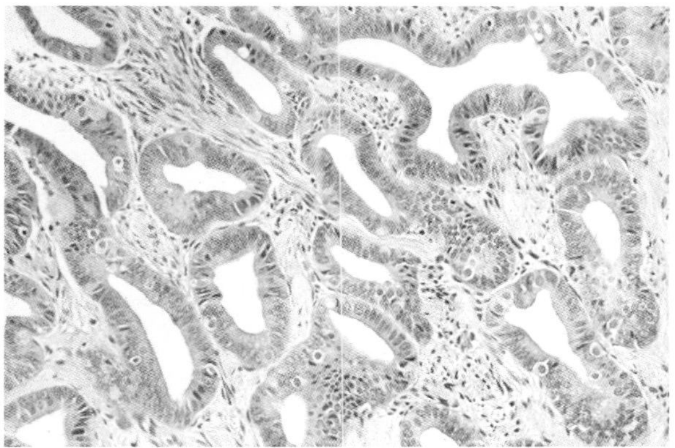

Fig. 13.42
Hyperplasia within endometriosis. **Endometriotic glands exhibit architectural and cytologic atypia. Endometrioid carcinoma was found elsewhere in the specimen (see *Fig. 13.56*)**

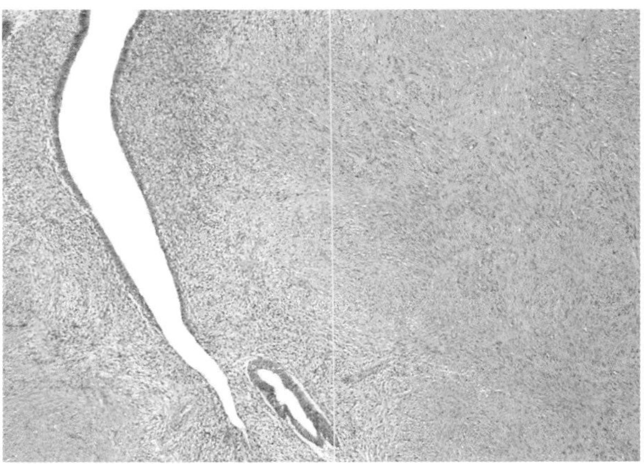

Fig. 13.43
Endometriosis with smooth muscle metaplasia. **Endometriotic glands and stroma surrounded by extensive, metaplastic smooth muscle**

manifestation of endometriosis [188]. Occasional cases of endometriosis can elicit a striking periglandular myxoid [40] (➲ *Fig. 13.44*) or elastotic [46] response (➲ *Fig. 13.45*), which in both situations can focally obliterate the endometriotic stroma. In two cases, extensive myxoid change in endometriosis was misinterpreted as pseudomyxoma peritonei and/or metastatic adenocarcinoma, one at the time of frozen section [40, 94].

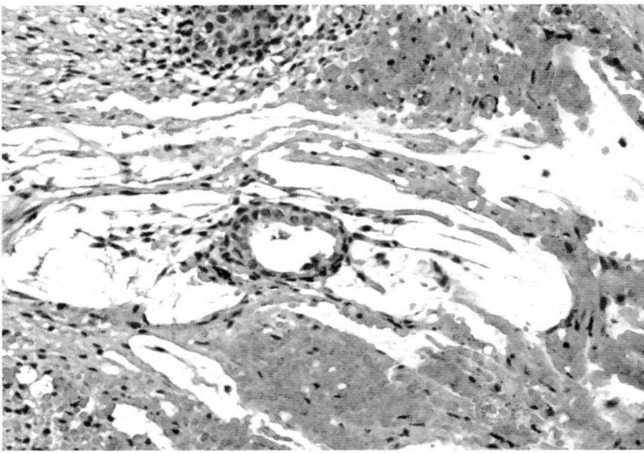

■ Fig. 13.44
Endometriosis with prominent myxoid stroma. **A small endometriotic gland with a periglandular rim of endometriotic stroma is surrounded by loose fibrous tissue and pools of acellular mucin. This appearance was misinterpreted as pseudomyxoma peritonei on frozen section examination**

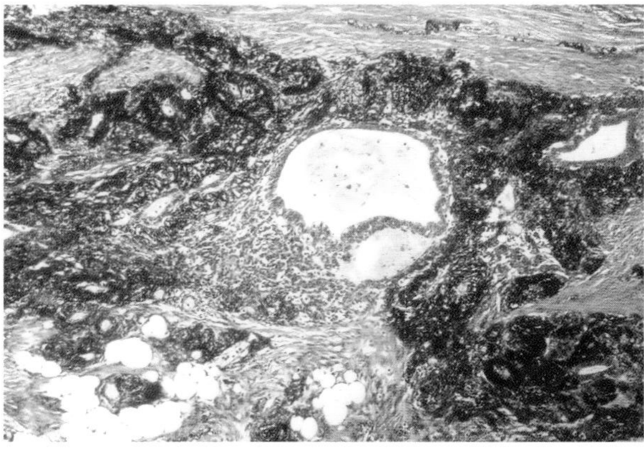

■ Fig. 13.45
Endometriosis with prominent elastotic stroma. **Large masses of elastic tissue replace the normal endometriotic stroma. (Elastic tissue stain)**

Anatomical location and hormonal factors appear to be predisposing factors, as there is a propensity for myxoid change to occur in endometriosis of the skin or superficial soft tissues, and also during pregnancy or the puerperium; the latter situation may be further confounded by the presence of decidual change of the stromal cells [39].

Stromal Endometriosis

Some cases of endometriosis are characterized by an absence or rarity of glands, so-called stromal endometriosis [21, 46, 51]; the same term was used in the older literature to refer to what is now designated low-grade endometrial stromal sarcoma (ESS). Stromal endometriosis is most commonly encountered in the ovary, where it is typically an incidental microscopic finding within the ovarian stroma ("benign stromatosis"). There is usually no associated pelvic endometriosis, and the process likely represents a metaplastic response of the ovarian stromal cells. A disproportionate number of cases of stromal endometriosis are seen within the superficial stroma of the uterine cervix (see page 30) [51]. Endometriosis involving the pelvic peritoneum can take the form of multiple small nodules of endometriotic stroma in which endometriotic glands are absent or rare, a finding referred to as micronodular stromal endometriosis [21, 46]. (➲ *Fig. 13.46*). As noted above, immunostaining for CD10 may be of assistance in confirming the presence of endometriotic stromal cells, but this marker is less useful in cases of stromal endometriosis involving the cervix, as normal cervical stroma may be strongly CD10-positive [143].

Necrotic Pseudoxanthomatous Nodules

Occasionally, ovarian and extraovarian endometriosis take the form of "necrotic pseudoxanthomatous nodules," which typically occur in postmenopausal women [49]. Multiple nodules can be attached to the peritoneum or, less commonly, lie free in the peritoneal cavity. When associated with enlargement of one or both ovaries, the intraoperative findings can mimic those of carcinoma with peritoneal spread. The nodules are characterized by a central zone of necrosis surrounded by pseudoxanthoma cells, often in a palisaded arrangement, hyalinized fibrous tissue, or both (➲ *Fig. 13.47*). Typical endometriotic glands and stroma are sparse or absent within the nodules and their immediate vicinity, but foci of recognizable endometriosis are usually present in the ovaries. The typical postmenopausal age group of the patient and the appearance of the nodules suggest that they represent end-stage or burned-out foci of endometriosis that should be distinguished from other necrotic peritoneal and ovarian granulomas, as well as necrotic tumor, on histologic examination.

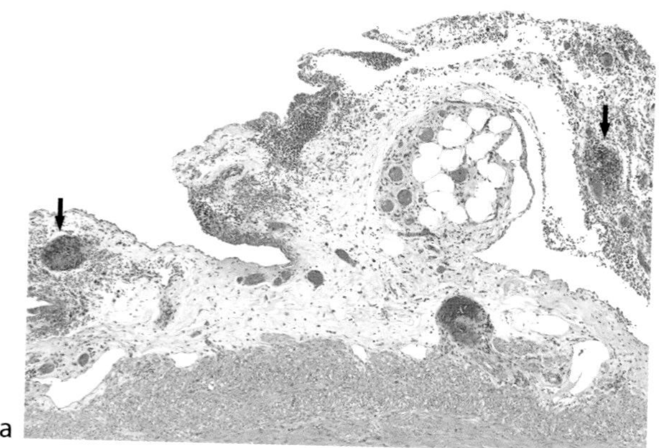

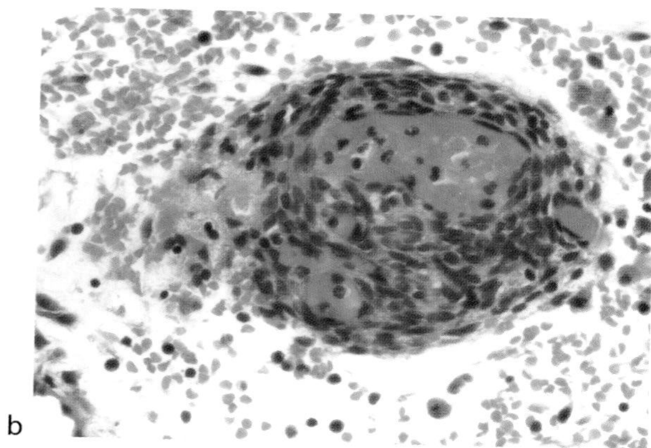

◘ Fig. 13.46
Micronodular stromal endometriosis involving the appendiceal serosa. (**a**) Two stromal nodules (arrows) are evident at far left and far right. (**b**) High-power view of one nodule

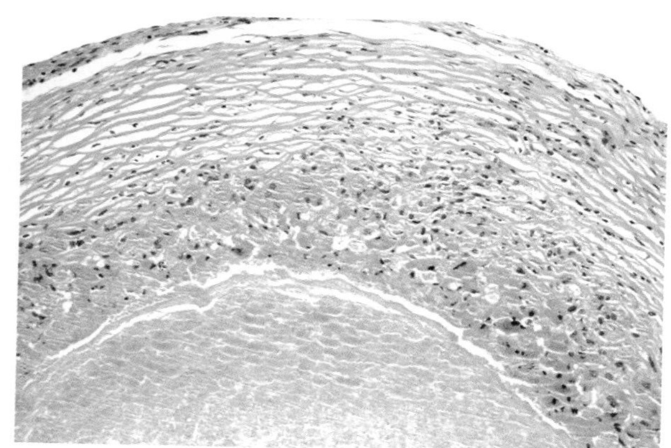

◘ Fig. 13.47
Necrotic pseudoxanthomatous nodule of endometriosis. A central area of necrosis is surrounded by pseudoxanthoma cells and an outer zone of fibrous tissue

Rare Miscellaneous Findings

Rare examples of endometriosis have been encountered in intimate association with foci of peritoneal leiomyomatosis, glial implants of ovarian teratomas, and nodules of splenosis. Perineural and vascular invasion can occur rarely in otherwise typical, benign endometriotic lesions, findings that may incorrectly suggest the diagnosis of malignancy [198].

Liesegang rings are eosinophilic, acellular, ringlike structures composed of periodic precipitation zones from colloidal solutions that are supersaturated in vitro or in vivo. They are typically encountered within necrotic, inflamed, or fibrotic tissues and have been found on microscopic examination within endometriotic cysts (➲ *Fig. 13.48*) [180]. These structures have been confused with, and should be distinguished from, parasites and foreign material on histologic examination [50].

Microscopic examination of the fallopian tubes in patients with endometriosis has revealed nonspecific chronic salpingitis in as many as one third of cases [59]. A less common lesion, so-called pseudoxanthomatous salpingitis or pseudoxanthomatous salpingiosis, characterized by infiltration of the tubal mucosa by pseudoxanthoma cells, is almost always associated with pelvic endometriosis [49, 59].

Ultrastructural, Histochemical, and Steroid Receptor Studies

Endometriotic glands typically exhibit ultrastructural features that represent a response, but an incomplete one, to the prevailing hormonal milieu of the particular phase of

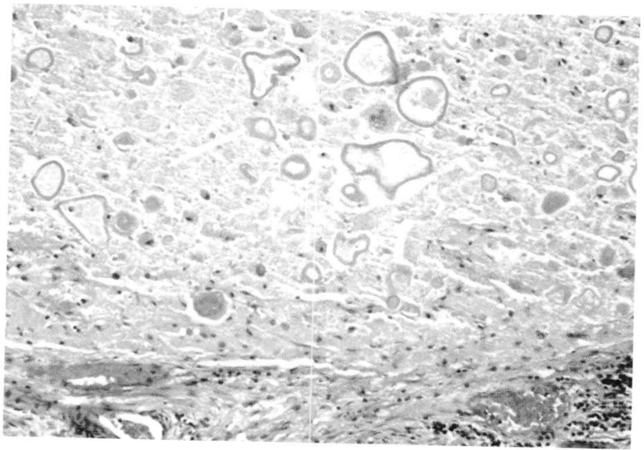

◘ Fig. 13.48
Liesegang rings in an endometriotic cyst

the menstrual cycle. In contrast to eutopic endometrial glands, it is usually not possible to date the glands precisely within the secretory phase because of marked interglandular and intraglandular variability. Ultrastructural examination of endometriotic tissue following danazol treatment shows either arrest of the endometriotic glandular epithelium in the early proliferative phase or disorganization of the epithelial cells with atrophic changes.

Estrogen (ER) and progesterone receptors (PR) are present in endometriotic glands and stroma but usually in lower concentrations than in eutopic endometrium [25]. In a variable number of cases, one or both receptors are absent. Moreover, the normal variation in the quantity of both receptors exhibited by eutopic endometrium during the menstrual cycle is diminished or absent within foci of endometriosis [131]. Differences in receptor concentrations between eutopic endometrium and endometriotic epithelium in response to danazol have also been noted. No correlation has been found between receptor levels and severity of symptoms.

In summary, the findings of these studies are consistent with the incomplete and variable hormonal response of endometriotic foci observed on microscopic examination. They indicate a greater degree of autonomy of endometriotic tissue from the mechanisms controlling eutopic endometrium and may explain the failure of hormonal therapy in some patients [148].

Differential Diagnosis

Endometriosis may be accompanied by, and should be distinguished from, endosalpingiosis, which is characterized by glands lined by benign tubal-type epithelium, unassociated with endometrial stroma or the usual histiocytic inflammatory reaction of endometriosis (see ➋ Endosalpingiosis). A misdiagnosis of endosalpingiosis or, if in the ovary, an epithelial inclusion gland (see ➋ Chap. 12, Nonneoplastic Lesions of the Ovary) is likely when the endometriotic stroma is sparse or obscured by hemorrhage (see ➋ *Fig. 13.35*).

Necrotic pseudoxanthomatous nodules should be distinguished from other ovarian and peritoneal necrotic nodules, such as infectious granulomas and isolated palisading granulomas of the ovary (see ➋ Chap. 12, Nonneoplastic Lesions of the Ovary), and as noted earlier, peritoneal granulomas related to diathermy [37]. Such lesions, in addition to having characteristic features, lack the numerous pseudoxanthoma cells that are typical of endometriotic lesions.

Rare low-grade endometrial stromal sarcomas (ESSs) contain numerous benign-appearing or atypical endometrial glands, to the extent that confusion with endometriosis may occur [42]. Indeed, it is likely that at least some cases referred to as aggressive endometriosis are examples of ESS with prominent glandular differentiation [42]. These tumors, however, in contrast to typical endometriosis, contain foci of more typical ESS devoid of glands, and in some cases, prominent mitotic activity of the stromal cells, sex-cord-like elements, and prominent vascular invasion.

A diagnosis of adenosarcoma was initially considered in some cases of polypoid endometriosis. Adenosarcomas, in contrast to polypoid endometriosis, are characterized by a stromal component that usually exhibits dense periglandular cellularity, atypia (albeit mild in many cases), intraglandular papillae, and increased mitotic activity.

Cervical and Vaginal Endometriosis

Superficial endometriosis of the uterine cervix is more common than is generally appreciated [11, 51, 85]. The predilection for sites of trauma and the usual absence of associated pelvic endometriosis suggest implantation as the most likely pathogenetic mechanism. The condition may be an incidental finding in an asymptomatic patient or be associated with premenstrual or postcoital spotting or menorrhagia. The solitary or multiple lesions typically involve the ectocervix; endocervical lesions have been described only rarely. The endometriotic foci appear as friable, ecchymotic streaks, patches, nodules, or cysts measuring from 1 mm to 2 cm in diameter. Rare lesions have been puckered secondary to fibrosis within the lesion, or papillary, simulating a carcinoma. In patients who have had a recent cone biopsy or extensive cautery, the entire transformation zone may be involved [105]. Before menses, the lesions typically enlarge and change from bright red to blue; during menses they may rupture, leaving an irregular ulcer. Because a punch biopsy may yield nondiagnostic tissue due to the size of the lesion (which is frequently small), tissue crushing, and fragmentation, aspiration cytology may be useful in establishing the diagnosis. Cervical endometriosis may be the source of abnormal gland cells identified on cervicovaginal smears [231].

On histologic examination, the endometriotic focus is usually confined to the superficial lamina propria (➋ *Fig. 13.49*). The diagnosis can be missed when the endometriotic stromal component is sparse or obscured by edema, hemorrhage, or inflammatory cells [11]. In such cases, the endometriotic glands, particularly when they show atypia or mitotic activity, can be misinterpreted as endocervical glandular dysplasia, adenocarcinoma in situ, or even invasive adenocarcinoma (➋ *Fig. 13.50*). As

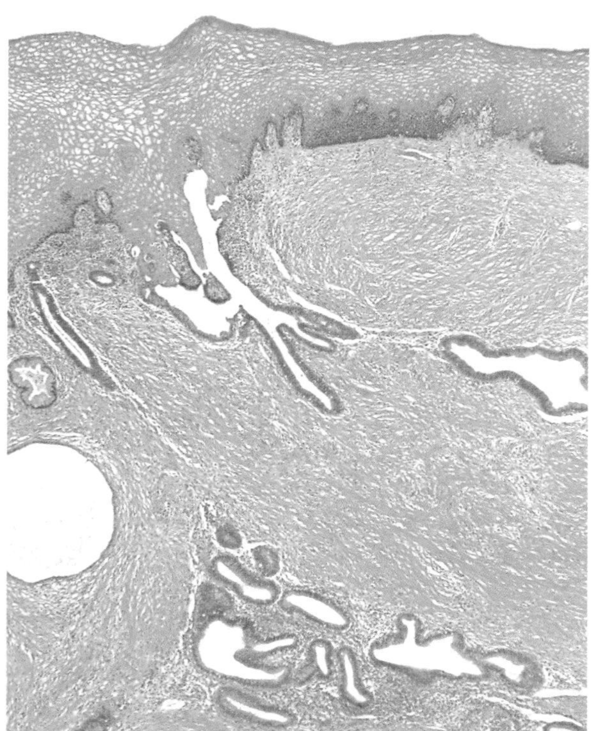

Fig. 13.49
Superficial cervical endometriosis. **Endometriotic glands and surrounding stroma lie beneath squamous epithelium**

previously noted, only endometrial stroma (stromal endometriosis) is found in occasional cases of superficial cervical endometriosis, even after serial sectioning (*Fig. 13.51*) [51].

In contrast to superficial cervical endometriosis, deep cervical endometriosis is usually an extension of cul-de-sac involvement in association with more widespread pelvic endometriosis. It may be palpable as deep, firm nodules or cysts in the posterior wall of the cervix [85]. The diagnosis is made by biopsy or pathologic examination of the hysterectomy specimen. The differential diagnosis includes downgrowth of adenomyosis from the uterine corpus.

Superficial vaginal endometriosis, which typically involves the vault, is rarer than cervical endometriosis but is similar to the latter macroscopically, both in its predilection for involving sites of prior trauma and in its lack of associated pelvic endometriosis [85]. Deep vaginal endometriosis is more common, is typically associated with pelvic endometriosis, and appears as nodular or polypoid masses involving the posterior vaginal fornix (*Fig. 13.52*) [85]. The differential diagnosis of vaginal endometriosis, particularly of the superficial type, includes vaginal adenosis of the tuboendometrial variety; the latter, however, lacks endometrial stroma and the characteristic inflammatory response of endometriosis. Endometriosis of the vulva is discussed in a subsequent section (see Cutaneous Endometriosis).

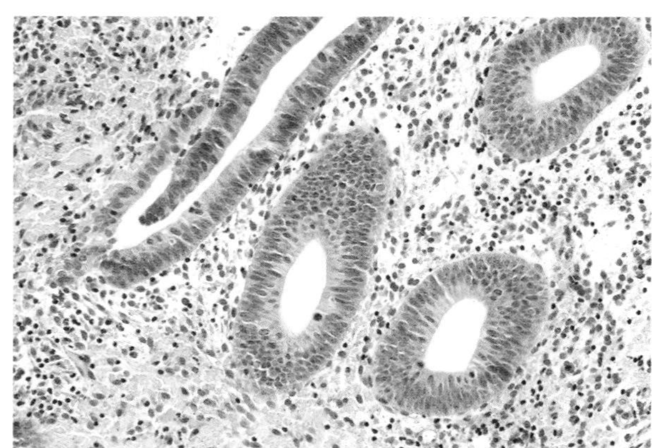

Fig. 13.50
Superficial endometriosis of the uterine cervix. **The endometriotic glands show cellular stratification and mitotic figures. If the scanty endometriotic stroma and histiocytes had not been appreciated, these glands may have been misinterpreted as endocervical glandular adenocarcinoma in situ**

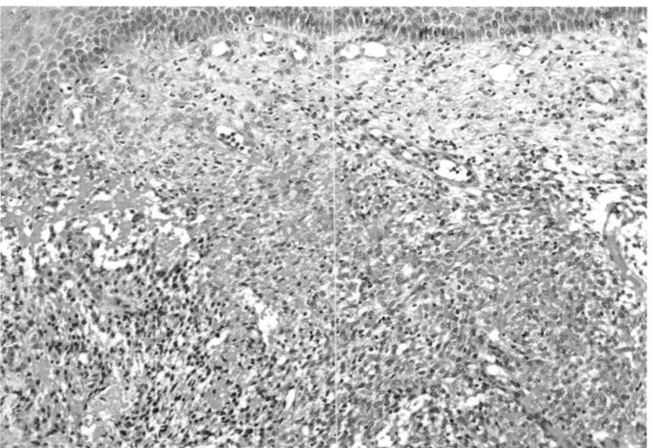

Fig. 13.51
Stromal endometriosis of uterine cervix. **A cellular sheet of hemorrhagic, endometriotic stroma lies below the exocervical squamous epithelium**

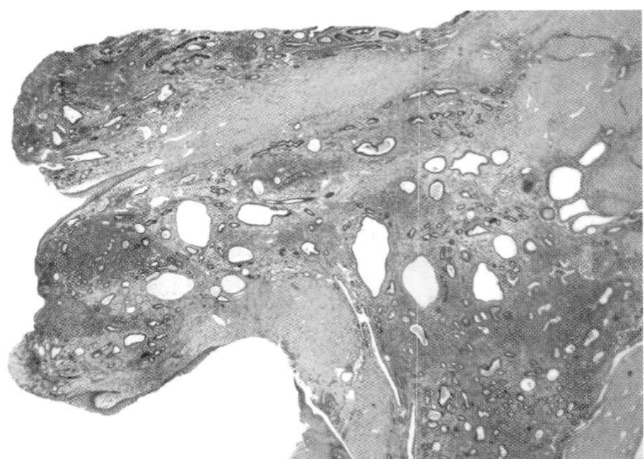

Fig. 13.52
Polypoid endometriosis of vagina

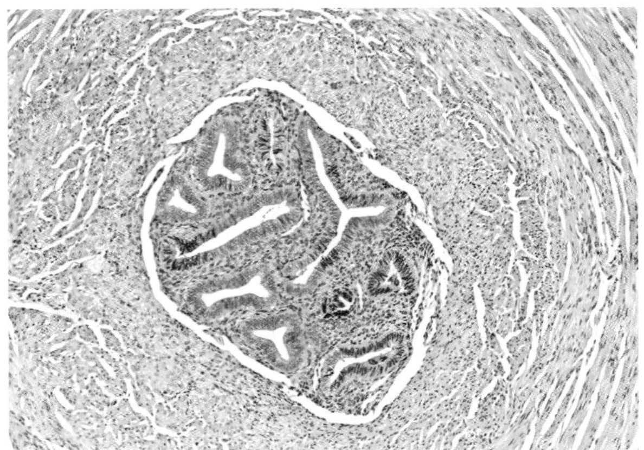

Fig. 13.53
Endometriosis (colonization) of the fallopian tube. **The tubal lumen is occluded by endometrial glands and stroma. Spaces at the junction of endometrial tissue and myosalpinx represent dilated lymphatic channels**

In a recent study of vaginal endometrioid adenocarcinoma, a strong association with vaginal endometriosis was found, with the latter present in 14 of 18 cases [221]. As the vagina is a common site for recurrence of endometrial adenocarcinomas, identification of endometriosis is an important observation in establishing a vaginal origin [39, 221].

Tubal Endometriosis

The term "tubal endometriosis" has been applied to at least three different unrelated lesions of the fallopian tube. The most common type is serosal or subserosal endometriosis, typically associated with endometriosis elsewhere in the pelvis; the myosalpinx is usually not involved.

Endometrial tissue may extend directly from the uterine cornu and replace the mucosa of the interstitial and isthmic portions of the tube in as many as 25% and 10% of women in the general population, respectively [39]. This finding is considered to represent a normal morphologic variation, although in some cases the ectopic endometrial tissue may give rise to intratubal polyps [60]. In occasional cases, the endometrial tissue may occlude the tubal lumen, that is, intraluminal endometriosis ("endometrial colonization") (➲ *Fig. 13.53*); involvement may be bilateral. Intraluminal endometriosis is typically unassociated with endometriosis elsewhere. The disorder accounts for 15–20% of tubal-related infertility; it may also be associated with tubal pregnancy.

The third type of endometriosis involving the fallopian tube has been designated postsalpingectomy endometriosis. It occurs in the tip of the proximal tubal stump, typically 1–4 years following tubal ligation [195]. It is closely related to, and may be associated with, salpingitis isthmica nodosa. The lesion is analogous to uterine adenomyosis, consisting of endometrial glands and stroma extending from the endosalpinx into the myosalpinx and frequently to the serosal surface. Hysterosalpingography or India ink injection of the specimen may show tuboperitoneal fistulous tracts; postligation pregnancies are a rare complication. Postsalpingectomy endometriosis has been documented in 20–50% of tubes examined following ligation. The frequency of this complication is increased with the electrocautery method of ligation, with short proximal stumps, and with increasing postligation intervals.

Intestinal Endometriosis

Intestinal involvement has been documented in as many as 37% of patients with endometriosis undergoing laparotomy [245], although the average frequency appears to be approximately 12%. In the majority of such cases, the involvement is confined to the serosa or subserosa and is unassociated with clinical manifestations referable to the intestinal tract. In contrast, from 0.7% to 2.5% of patients with endometriosis require bowel resection for symptomatic lesions [187]. In some series, as many as half the patients with symptomatic intestinal endometriosis have no extraintestinal involvement; the endometriotic nature of the intestinal lesions in such cases is more likely to be unrecognized preoperatively or at the time of laparotomy. Misdiagnosis is also common in postmenopausal patients because of a decreased index of suspicion, even though the intestine is one of the more common sites of clinically significant endometriosis in this age group [115]. As many as 7% of patients with symptomatic intestinal endometriosis are postmenopausal.

Intestinal sites of involvement include, in descending order of frequency, the rectum and sigmoid, the appendix, the terminal ileum, the cecum, and other parts of the large and small bowel, including Meckel's diverticulum [250]. In one large study [187], 15% of patients had more than one site of involvement. The presenting symptoms include, alone or in combination, acute or chronic abdominal pain, diarrhea, constipation, hematochezia, and decrease in stool caliber. Although the frequently catamenial nature of the symptoms may suggest the correct diagnosis, the clinical presentation can mimic acute appendicitis, bowel obstruction due to adhesions or a hernia, a neoplasm, or even inflammatory bowel disease. Endoscopic and radiographic studies typically demonstrate an extramucosal stenosing lesion; endoscopic biopsies are usually of no diagnostic value.

Endometriosis of the rectosigmoid area is usually a solitary lesion, involving a segment several centimeters in length, whereas ileal involvement is frequently multifocal and may involve segments of bowel up to 45 cm in length [250]. On gross examination, the segment of bowel is indurated and often angulated by a poorly defined, usually noncircumferential mass; the serosal surface may be puckered and covered by adhesions. Sectioning typically reveals a firm, gray-white, solid, mural mass, the bulk of which represents markedly thickened muscularis propria; the latter often has a radiating fanlike appearance. Small cystic spaces containing altered blood may be seen but are uncommon. In contrast to a primary adenocarcinoma, the overlying mucosa is usually intact, despite the high frequency of symptomatic bleeding in some series of patients. However, rare cases of polypoid endometriosis have involved the intestinal mucosa; such lesions can grossly mimic an adenocarcinoma (see ➲ *Fig. 13.31*) [176]. On microscopic examination of symptomatic intestinal endometriosis, islands of endometriotic tissue are typically scattered throughout the hyperplastic muscularis propria, with or without involvement of other layers (➲ *Fig. 13.54*) [250].

A complication of intestinal endometriosis is perforation, which is usually associated with pregnancy; a marked decidual reaction is typically seen with the endometriotic stroma in such cases. Other complications include volvulus, intussusception, acute appendicitis, appendiceal mucocele, intramural hematoma, and the development of a malignant neoplasm (see below) [155, 249].

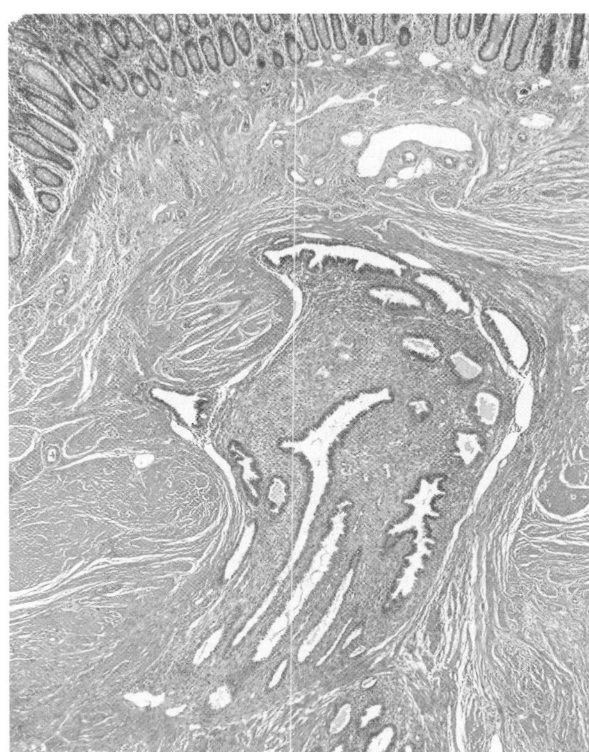

Fig. 13.54
Colonic endometriosis. **A nest of endometriotic glands and stroma lie in the muscularis propria**

Urinary Tract Endometriosis

Urinary tract involvement has been documented at laparotomy in from 16% to 20% of patients with endometriosis [192, 245]. In most of these cases, the endometriosis is found on the serosa of the urinary bladder or that overlying the ureter and is without local clinical manifestations. Similarly, high-volume intravenous urography has demonstrated subtle, clinically insignificant abnormalities in 15% of women with proven pelvic endometriosis before therapy. In contrast, only 0.5–1% of patients with endometriosis have clinically significant urinary tract involvement; approximately 30% of such patients ultimately require nephrectomy for a hydronephrotic or nonfunctioning kidney. Most reported cases of urinary tract endometriosis have involved the urinary bladder or the ureters (with approximately equal frequency); the kidneys and the urethra are involved much less commonly. Urinary tract involvement is usually associated with endometriosis elsewhere in the pelvis, although the symptoms relating to the urinary tract may be the initial or sole manifestations of the disease in such patients [223]. In some series, however, as many as half the patients with ureteral involvement have disease restricted to the ureter and the adjacent uterosacral ligament [110]. Patients with renal endometriosis typically do not have endometriosis elsewhere, suggesting an embolic, likely blood-borne, origin.

From one third to one half of the affected patients are over 40 years of age and almost 5% of the patients are postmenopausal, some of whom had received estrogen replacement therapy. A preoperative diagnosis may be suspected by the catamenial nature of the symptoms, which include suprapubic or flank pain, frequency, urgency, dysuria, and hematuria; chills and fever secondary to a urinary tract infection have been the presenting symptoms in occasional cases. A tender suprapubic or flank mass may be palpable. Many patients, however, particularly those with ureteric involvement, have nonspecific manifestations or present with a silent obstructive uropathy, occasionally complicated by hypertension, renal failure (in cases of bilateral involvement), or both [110, 223]. In patients with bladder involvement, urography may reveal a filling defect; a stricture in the lower ureter with hydroureter and hydronephrosis or a nonfunctioning kidney is the typical urographic finding in those with ureteral involvement. All seven patients with ureteral endometriosis in one recent study had hydroureter, in most cases accompanied by hydronephrosis, two with superimposed pyelonephritis [4]. Endoscopy may confirm vesical or even ureteral involvement, and the lesions may exhibit catamenial enlargement, darkening, and bleeding. Endoscopy and biopsy, however, are often nondiagnostic [223].

Symptomatic endometriosis of the bladder is usually a result of mural involvement, and the lesions are typically located on the trigone, the floor of the bladder, or low on the posterior wall [223]. Involvement is rarely confined to the lateral walls, the dome, or the ureterovesical junction. Gross examination typically reveals a solitary, blue, red, gray, or brown multicystic mass that thickens the wall and sometimes projects into the bladder lumen; the lesions have ranged from several millimeters to 14 cm in diameter. The mucosa is usually intact, but occasionally may be ulcerated and bleeding, particularly during menses. Histologic examination reveals fibrosis and proliferation of the muscularis around the foci of endometriosis; the lamina propria was also involved in 60% of the cases in one study [223]. Obstruction of both ureteric orifices, vesicocolic fistula, and malignant transformation have been rare complications.

With rare exceptions, endometriosis of the ureter is confined to its lower one third, usually involving a segment less than 2 cm in length that lies 2–5 cm from the ureterovesical junction; involvement has been bilateral in approximately 10% of the cases [4, 223]. Six of seven cases in the study cited above involved the left ureter only [4]. Ureteral endometriosis has been traditionally divided into extrinsic and intrinsic forms, although this distinction has not been possible in many of the reported cases because the affected segment of ureter was not removed for microscopic examination. Also, it is likely that at least some intrinsic cases were initially of extrinsic type. In the latter, endometriosis of the uterosacral ligament or ureteral adventitia causes ureteral luminal narrowing by compression, fibrosis, or both; in some such cases, there is transmural scarring of the ureter. Intrinsic involvement is characterized by endometriotic tissue within a typically hyperplastic and fibrotic muscularis; in some cases, the lamina propria is also involved. Mucosal involvement rarely takes the form of a polypoid mass projecting into the lumen [223].

On gross examination, endometriosis of the kidney is typically a solitary, well-circumscribed, hemorrhagic, solid and cystic mass that focally replaces the renal parenchyma; the lesions in the ten reported cases have measured from 1.5 to 13 cm in diameter. In occasional cases, polypoid masses have projected into the renal pelvis. Foci of smooth muscle have been found admixed with the endometriotic tissue on microscopic examination in some of the cases.

Only rare cases of urethral endometriosis have been described [59]. In one, a caruncle-like nodule projected from the urethral orifice in a 38-year-old woman with dysuria. In others, a 24-year-old woman with dysuria and dyspareunia was found to have endometriosis in the wall of a large urethral diverticulum, and a 35-year-old woman with left lower abdominal pain had endometriosis involving a left mid-urethral diverticulum as well as a vaginal endometriotic cyst.

Cutaneous Endometriosis

The majority of the reported cases of cutaneous endometriosis have occurred within surgical scars [34, 100, 113, 153, 224], or rarely within needle tracts; the remainder are spontaneous. Both types are associated with pelvic endometriosis in only a minority of cases [34, 224].

Because scar-related endometriosis typically occurs after operations on the uterus or fallopian tubes, the site most commonly involved is the lower abdominal wall; the umbilicus is involved less commonly. Similarly, most cases of endometriosis of the lower vagina, vulva, Bartholin's gland, perineum, and perianal region involve areas of obstetric or surgical trauma, most commonly episiotomy scars [34, 85, 177, 224]. The overall frequency of post-Cesarean scar endometriosis was 0.08% in one recent study, and the authors hypothesized that an increased risk of incisional endometriomas may result from failure to close the parietal and visceral peritoneum with sutures [153]. Scar-related cases occur less commonly after nongynecologic procedures, such as an appendectomy or inguinal hernia repair [224]. Spontaneous cutaneous endometriosis typically involves the umbilicus [224] and, less commonly, the inguinal [224] and perianal regions.

The most common symptoms are those relating to a cutaneous mass or nodule that, in the scar-related cases, appears weeks to years following surgery [100, 224]; the average postoperative interval from the time of Cesarean section in the study cited above was 3.2 years [153]. A catamenial increase in size and tenderness, and occasionally bleeding from the lesion, suggest the diagnosis. Patients with perianal lesions may have involvement of the external sphincter producing anorectal pain and irritation simulating an anal fistula, abscess, or thrombosed hemorrhoid. Umbilical endometriosis may simulate an umbilical hernia on physical examination. The lesions occasionally recur following excision; the recurrence rate of 445 cases of abdominal wall endometriosis after surgical excision was 4.3% [100].

On clinical examination, the lesions are firm, solitary nodules, varying up to 6–12 cm in diameter, and pink to brown to blue-black depending on the age of the lesion and the depth within the skin. The cut surface of the scar-related lesions is typically gray-white, with or without focal areas of recent or old hemorrhage [34]. On microscopic examination, the endometriosis may involve the dermis (*Fig. 13.55*), the subcutis, or both [224] and, in occasional cases, underlying skeletal muscle. Metaplastic glandular and stromal changes may be present, similar to those observed in endometriotic lesions elsewhere, most commonly tubal metaplasia, in addition to oxyphilic, hobnail, mucinous, and papillary syncytial metaplasia [113]. In one study, which evaluated 71 cases of cutaneous and superficial soft tissue endometriosis, smooth muscle metaplasia was found in one third of cases, and 25% of lesions showed reactive epithelial atypia [113]. There is typically no continuity between the cutaneous and peritoneal lesions in patients with associated pelvic endometriosis.

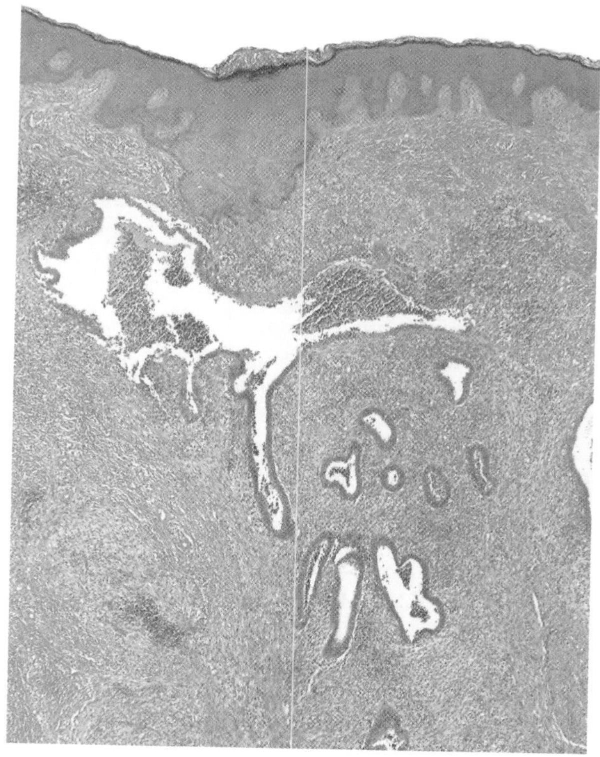

Fig. 13.55
Cutaneous endometriosis. **Endometriotic foci are present within the dermis**

The association of abdominal scar-related endometriosis and episiotomy scar-related endometriosis with uterine operations and episiotomies, respectively, suggests implantation of endometrial tissue as the most likely pathogenesis. The risk of implantation appears to be much higher after hysterotomy than after cesarean section or vaginal delivery, suggesting that the decidua of late pregnancy has a reduced ability to implant. When curettage is performed immediately after vaginal term delivery, however, the frequency of endometriosis in the episiotomy scar becomes much higher [177]. In nonpregnant patients, implantation of endometrium during endometrial curettage or spontaneous implantation of menstrual endometrium has also been implicated in occasional cases of scar-related endometriosis. Lymphatics have been demonstrated between the pelvis and umbilicus that may explain cases of spontaneous endometriosis in the latter site.

Inguinal Endometriosis

Noncutaneous inguinal endometriosis, secondary to involvement of the extraperitoneal portion of the round ligament, occurs in less than 1% of patients with endometriosis [26]. The usual presentation is that of a painful, typically right-sided, hernia-like inguinal mass, with catamenial exacerbation in some cases. In approximately one third of the reported cases, an inguinal hernia may also be present. The lesion can impinge on the pubic tubercle and mimic arthritis, bursitis, or tendinitis. Rarely, endometriosis in the inguinal region has also been described in inguinal or femoral hernia sacs or the canal of Nuck [190].

Endometriosis of Lymph Nodes

Lymph node involvement by endometriosis is uncommon, and many examples reported as such, particularly in the older literature, are lymph nodes involved by benign müllerian (usually endosalpingiotic) glands devoid of an endometrial stromal component. The involved lymph nodes may be visibly or palpably enlarged at operation. On microscopic examination, in contrast to glandular inclusions, endometriotic foci are characterized by a more central location within the node, an endometrial stromal component, and the frequent presence of erythrocytes and pseudoxanthoma cells. Endosalpingiosis and endometriosis may coexist, however, in the same lymph node. As in other sites, decidual transformation of the endometriotic stroma has been encountered during pregnancy. As previously noted, one case of intranodal endomyometriosis has been reported.

Pleuropulmonary Endometriosis

Pathologically documented cases of endometriosis involving the lungs or pleura are rare. Some reported examples interpreted as pulmonary endometriosis have taken the form of microscopic foci of "decidua" found at autopsy in pregnant or recently pregnant women. Most such lesions would likely be interpreted by current criteria as foci of embolic intermediate trophoblast, although one case of bona fide deciduosis of the lung has been documented [77]. Many cases of purported pleuropulmonary endometriosis have been diagnosed solely on the basis of clinical manifestations or in conjunction with nonspecific histologic or cytologic findings. Coverage here is based on the 38 pathologically documented cases of thoracic endometriosis in the literature, 21 of which were pleural and 17 of which were parenchymal [77].

The affected patients are usually in the reproductive age group, although rare patients are postmenopausal. The clinical manifestations of pleural endometriosis usually differ from those associated with parenchymal involvement. In the former, the characteristic presentation is one of recurrent catamenial shortness of breath related to catamenial pneumothorax, typically right sided. Less common presentations include recurrent right-sided, typically hemorrhagic effusions, hemoptysis, or catamenial pain. Chest X-rays usually reveal a pneumothorax, or occasionally, a hemothorax, pleural effusion, or a pleural lesion. Coexistent intra-abdominal endometriosis has been demonstrated in approximately one third of cases, although in another one third of cases, its presence or absence was not confirmed. In contrast, patients with parenchymal endometriosis typically present with catamenial hemoptysis or blood-tinged cough; other patients are asymptomatic and the lesion is an incidental radiographic finding. Chest X-ray typically shows a nodule, infiltrates, or opacification of an entire lobe [77]. Only one patient has had documented peritoneal endometriosis, although in most patients the peritoneum has not been visualized. The majority of patients with parenchymal endometriosis have had prior uterine operations.

Pleural endometriosis is almost invariably confined to the right side; one case with bilateral involvement has been reported. The lesions are typically multiple, dark red or blue nodules or cysts on the diaphragmatic pleura; parietal, visceral, and pericardial pleural surfaces are also affected less commonly. Associated pathologic changes have included diaphragmatic fenestrations in 50% of the cases and occasionally pleural blebs. Parenchymal endometriotic lesions are typically solitary, tan to gray, focally hemorrhagic nodules or thin-walled cysts measuring up to 6 cm in diameter. Several lesions have been subpleural or have involved bronchial walls and lumina. Parenchymal lesions lack the almost exclusively right-sided location of pleural endometriosis; one case had a bilateral miliary distribution. In additional contrast to pleural lesions, associated diaphragmatic fenestrations have not been described.

The clinicopathologic differences between pleural endometriosis and parenchymal endometriosis of the lung suggest that they differ in their histogenesis. The distribution of the parenchymal lesions and their strong association with prior uterine trauma strongly suggest an embolic origin. In contrast, most if not all pleural lesions are likely a result of passage of endometriotic tissue from the peritoneal cavity through diaphragmatic defects or diaphragmatic lymphatics, consistent with the right-sided predominance of both structures. The catamenial pneumothorax in these patients, and in those with catamenial pneumothorax unassociated with pleural endometriosis, may be related to the diaphragmatic defects that allow passage of air from the peritoneal into the pleural cavity. The escape of air from defects in the visceral pleura produced by the endometriotic lesions or from preexistent blebs is another possible explanation for the pneumothorax in these patients. It has been suggested that prostaglandins produced by eutopic endometrium or endometriotic tissue at the time of the menses may predispose to alveolar rupture.

Soft Tissue and Skeletal Endometriosis

Rarely, typical endometriomas have occurred in skeletal muscle or deep soft tissues in distant sites. The presentation is usually that of a mass associated with catamenial pain, tenderness, and enlargement. The involved sites have included the trapezius, extensor carpi radialis, thumb, biceps femoris, thigh, and the knee. A unique endometrioma occurred in the breast of a patient with a 2-year history of catamenial bloody nipple discharge [154]. Rare pelvic endometriotic cysts have eroded lumbar vertebrae, causing catamenial lumbar pain.

Upper Abdominal Endometriosis

Endometriotic implants may occasionally occur on the omentum; omental endometriosis was only one eighth as common as omental endosalpingiosis in one study [259]. Rarely, endometriotic implants may involve the peritoneal surfaces of the liver or the diaphragm. As with pleural diaphragmatic involvement, implants on the peritoneal side of the diaphragm have occasionally been associated with diaphragmatic defects and catamenial pneumothorax. Rare endometriomas of the epigastrium, the tail of the pancreas, and the liver parenchyma have been reported.

Endometriosis of the Nervous System

Approximately 30 cases of endometriosis of the sciatic nerve sheath at the level of the sciatic notch have been described, typically associated with catamenial sciatica [183]. Some cases have been associated with a visible peritoneal evagination attached to the involved portion of the nerve ("pocket sign"). A case of subarachnoid endometriosis of the lumbar spinal cord caused catamenial radicular pain and recurrent subarachnoid hemorrhage [135]. In another case, a cerebral endometrioma was discovered in the parietal lobe of a patient who had a 3-year history of episodic headaches that culminated in a generalized seizure [234].

Endometriosis in Males

Rare examples of endometriosis have been described in men receiving long-term estrogen therapy for prostatic carcinoma. With the exception of one case involving the abdominal wall [138], the sites of involvement have been confined to the genitourinary tract, specifically the urinary bladder, prostate, and paratesticular region [257]. The two paratesticular lesions were endomyometriotic in composition.

Neoplasms Arising from Endometriosis

Recent studies evaluating consecutive cases of endometriosis found that a malignant tumor was associated with ovarian and pelvic endometriosis in 4% and 10% of cases, respectively [185]. However, exact frequencies of malignancy arising from pelvic endometriosis in the general population are not known, as some tumors likely overgrow and obliterate the endometriotic foci from which they arose [155]. Coexistence of endometriosis and a mullerian-type tumor is not definitive evidence that the tumor has arisen from the endometriosis, unless merging of the two lesions is histologically identified. In most cases, the term "endometriosis-associated" tumor is preferable.

For stage I epithelial ovarian cancers, up to 30% have associated ovarian endometriosis, with an even higher frequency for endometrioid and clear cell carcinomas. Studies to determine putative precursor lesions in such cases have shown that hyperplastic changes ("atypical endometriosis," discussed above), similar to those that arise in eutopic endometrium, may occur in endometriotic lesions. Such morphologic findings may be observed in the setting of endogenous or exogenous estrogenic stimuli or tamoxifen therapy (see *Fig. 13.42*). Atypical ovarian endometriosis was found in approximately 60% of endometriosis-associated carcinomas, but in only 2% of cases of ovarian endometriosis not associated with carcinoma [83]. Some endometriotic lesions, including atypical endometriosis, and the synchronous carcinoma share similar molecular genetic alterations, including *PTEN* mutations, loss of heterozygosity

(LOH), and over-expression of p53 and c-erb-2 [185, 186, 203, 204, 207]. Recently, it has been shown that women with carcinomas arising in endometriosis tend to be younger (and premenopausal), obese, and have a history of unopposed estrogens, in comparison to women with uncomplicated endometriosis. Furthermore, endometriosis-associated tumors are more often lower grade and lower stage, and have a better prognosis than similar tumors without associated endometriosis [71]. Approximately 75% of tumors complicating endometriosis arise within the ovary. The most common extraovarian site is the rectovaginal septum; less frequent sites include the vagina, colon and rectum [249], urinary bladder, and other sites in the pelvis and abdomen. In some cases, there is a history of prolonged unopposed estrogen replacement therapy [249]. As previously noted, hyperplastic and metaplastic changes within endometriosis may precede or be found synchronously with the neoplasm. Tumors arising in endometriosis in unusual sites are more likely to be misdiagnosed than similar tumors arising in ovarian endometriosis, such as an endometrioid adenocarcinoma arising in colonic endometriosis being mistaken for a primary colonic adenocarcinoma (see below), an error that could result in inappropriate staging and treatment [249].

Endometrioid carcinoma (➋ *Fig. 13.56*) is the most common tumor arising within ovarian endometriosis, accounting for almost 75% of such cases. Direct origin of endometrioid carcinoma from endometriotic tissue has been demonstrated in as many as 24% of cases in some series [155]. At least 90% of the carcinomas arising from extraovarian endometriosis have been of endometrioid type [155]. Rarely, endometrioid tumors arising in ovarian and extraovarian endometriosis may exhibit a benign or borderline adenofibromatous pattern [249]. Endometrioid carcinoma is the most common tumor to arise in intestinal endometriosis; the majority of endometriosis-associated intestinal tumors occur in the rectosigmoid colon, with most of the remainder in the ileum and the cecum [39, 181, 219]. The following features are in favor of endometrioid adenocarcinoma over a primary colonic adenocarcinoma: Atypical gross features, the presence of endometriosis, an absence of mucosal involvement, lower grade nuclei than expected for colonic adenocarcinoma, squamous metaplasia, an absence of dirty necrosis, and a cytokeratin 7+/cytokeratin 20-/CDX2- immunoprofile [39, 114, 219]. Other tumors arising in intestinal endometriosis include endometrioid stromal sarcoma, mullerian adenosarcoma, carcinosarcoma, clear cell carcinoma, squamous cell carcinoma, and mixed germ cell tumor [39].

Clear cell carcinoma (➋ *Figs. 13.57* and ➋ *13.58*) is the second most common tumor originating in endometriosis, accounting for approximately 15% of such cases. In some studies, the frequency of endometriosis coexisting with clear cell carcinoma of the ovary is even higher than with endometrioid carcinoma; pelvic endometriosis has been reported in 24–49% of cases of ovarian clear cell carcinoma [200, 235]. A few examples of clear cell carcinoma arising within extraovarian endometriosis have also

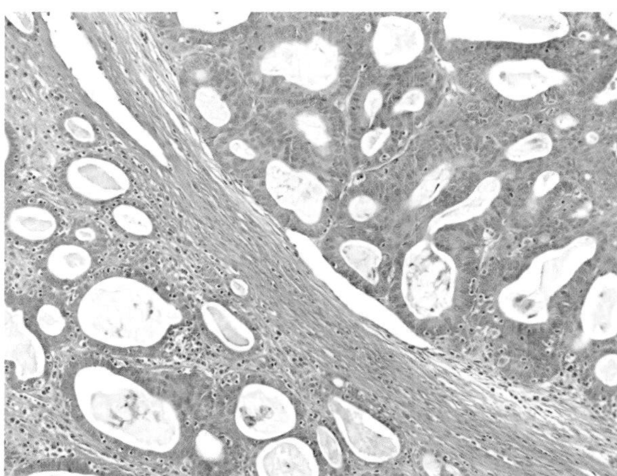

Fig. 13.56
Endometrioid carcinoma arising within endometriosis. **Benign endometriotic glands (*left*) with adjacent carcinomatous glands (*right*)**

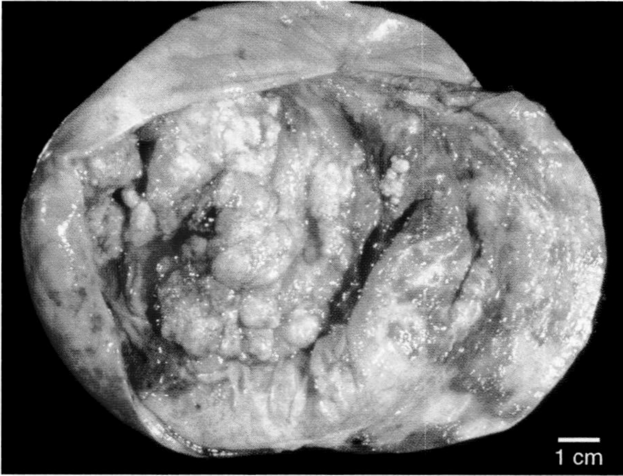

Fig. 13.57
Clear cell carcinoma arising within an endometriotic cyst. **Fleshy pale tumor nodules protrude into the cyst lumen**

been described [2, 98]. A recent study, which utilized the polymerase chain reaction and loss of heterozygosity (LOH) analysis using laser-microdissected tumor tissue, has indicated that ovarian clear cell adenofibroma may be a clonal precursor for clear cell carcinoma, shown by high concordance rates of allelic patterns between clear cell carcinoma and benign and borderline clear cell adenofibromatous components, with 95% of cases showing an identical LOH pattern [248]. Patients with endometriosis-associated clear cell carcinomas of the ovary have also recently been found to have improved progression free and overall survival rates in comparison to those without endometriosis [171].

Ovarian and extraovarian epithelial tumors of other types arising from endometriosis include endometrioid adenofibromas and borderline tumors of endocervical-like and mixed cell type, as well as serous borderline tumors and squamous cell carcinomas [158, 200, 201, 249]. Endometrioid stromal sarcomas (ESSs), malignant mesodermal mixed tumors, and adenosarcomas (both typical and with sarcomatous overgrowth) (➲ *Fig. 13.59*) account for approximately 10% and 20% of tumors arising in ovarian and extraovarian endometriosis, respectively [41, 215, 249, 256]. Approximately one quarter of tumors arising in colonic endometriosis are adenosarcomas [219, 250]. In one study, 60% of ESSs apparently arising within the ovary were associated with ovarian endometriosis [256]. Rare examples of yolk sac tumor have arisen in association with endometriosis [202], and in one unique case, a sex cord tumor with annular tubules was intimately associated with endometriosis of the tubal serosa [90].

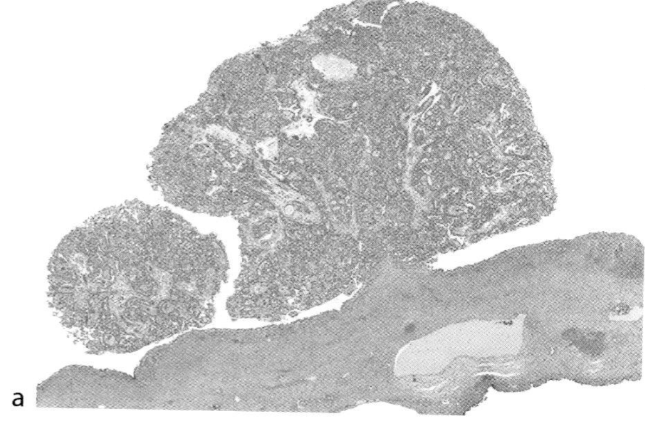

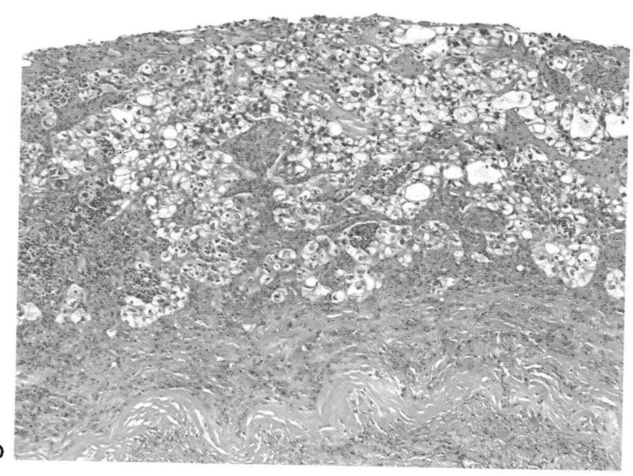

◘ Fig. 13.58
Clear cell carcinoma arising within an endometriotic cyst. **(a)** Low-power view showing nodules of clear cell carcinoma protruding into the cyst lumen. **(b)** High-power view of a different case, showing clear cell carcinoma with background pigmented histiocytes

Peritoneal Endometrioid Lesions Other Than Endometriosis

Benign glands lined by endometrial epithelium (but lacking endometrial stroma) with the peritoneal distribution of endosalpingiosis occasionally occur [128]; some may represent foci of endometriosis in which the stromal component has undergone atrophy. Benign endometrioid peritoneal "implants" lacking an endometrial stromal

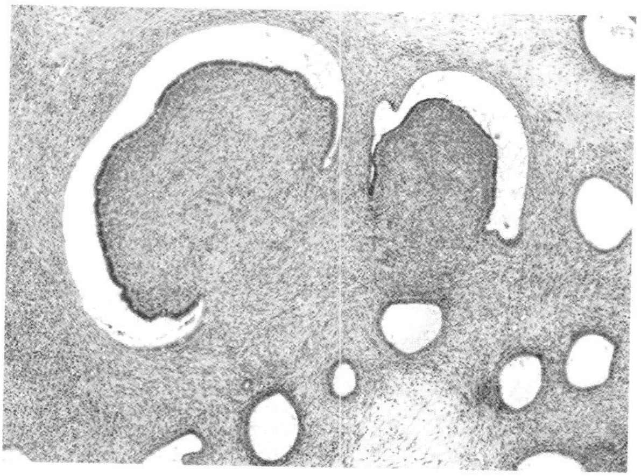

◘ Fig. 13.59
Mesodermal adenosarcoma arising in ovarian endometriosis. Low-grade sarcomatous stroma forms periglandular cuffs and intraglandular papillae

component have also been reported in association with a borderline ovarian endometrioid tumor [200]. The peritoneal lesions were interpreted as having arisen directly from the peritoneum.

A variety of extrauterine, extraovarian, pelvic, or retroperitoneal neoplasms of endometrioid type occur in the absence of demonstrable endometriosis. These tumors have generally been considered to arise directly from the mesothelium or submesothelial stroma, or possibly from foci of endometriosis that have been obliterated by the tumor. They have included endometrioid cystadenofibroma and cystadenocarcinoma, endometrioid stromal sarcoma, homologous and heterologous types of malignant mesodermal mixed tumor, and mesodermal adenosarcoma.

Peritoneal Serous Lesions

Serous lesions of the peritoneum include those that are nonneoplastic (endosalpingiosis) and neoplastic, which are morphologically analogous to their ovarian counterparts.

Endosalpingiosis

Clinical Findings

Endosalpingiosis typically refers to the presence of benign glands lined by tubal-type epithelium involving the peritoneum and subperitoneal tissues; the term may also be used to refer to similar glands within retroperitoneal lymph nodes (see ➲ Benign Intranodal Glands of Müllerian Type). This disorder occurs almost exclusively in females, typically during their reproductive years, with a mean age of 29.7 years in one study [259], although occasional cases have been described in postmenopausal women. Endosalpingiosis is almost always an incidental finding at either the time of operation or more commonly on microscopic examination. Zinsser and Wheeler found endosalpingiosis in 12.5% of surgically removed omenta in a retrospective study, but this figure doubled when omenta were examined more thoroughly in a prospective study [259]. Endosalpingiosis may be detected as multiple fine pelvic calcifications on X-ray examination or as psammoma bodies within cul-de-sac fluid, peritoneal washings [216], the lumen of the fallopian tube, or cervical Papanicolaou smears [116].

An origin from the secondary müllerian system is favored by most investigators, but the association of endosalpingiosis with chronic salpingitis implicates implantation of sloughed tubal epithelium as a possible histogenetic mechanism in some cases [259]. A similar association with serous tumors of borderline malignancy suggests that some endosalpingiotic foci may represent tumor implants that have undergone maturation [141]. Endosalpingiosis in the absence of residual tumor at the time of second-look laparotomy in patients with ovarian epithelial neoplasms does not justify additional treatment [55].

Pathologic Findings

Endosalpingiosis is most commonly encountered on the pelvic peritoneum covering the uterus, fallopian tubes, ovaries, and cul-de-sac [259]. Less frequent sites include the pelvic parietal peritoneum, omentum [259], bladder and bowel serosa, paraaortic area, and skin, including laparotomy scars. Endosalpingiosis is usually inapparent at the time of operation or on gross inspection of the involved tissues but may be visible as multiple, punctate (1–2 mm), white to yellow, opaque or translucent, fluid-filled cysts, which impart a vesicular or granular appearance to the involved surface; rarely larger cysts may be seen [45]. Rare examples of cystic endosalpingiosis have involved the wall of the uterus, resulting in grossly apparent transmural cysts [45].

Microscopic examination reveals multiple, simple glands, often cystically dilated and lined by a single layer of epithelium resembling that of the normal fallopian tube (➲ *Figs. 13.60* and ➲ *13.61*). The glands are frequently surrounded by a loose or dense connective tissue stroma that may contain a sparse mononuclear inflammatory cell infiltrate. The glands may exhibit irregular contours, crowding, and intraluminal stromal papillae. The three

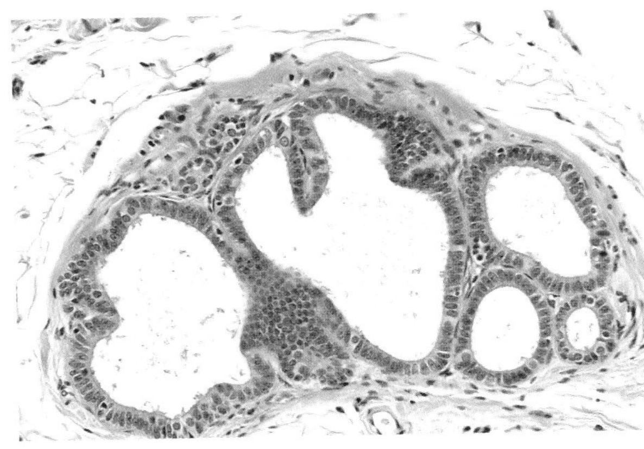

Fig. 13.60
Endosalpingiosis. **Complex glandular structure lies beneath uterine serosa. Glands are lined by a single layer of benign endosalpingeal epithelium**

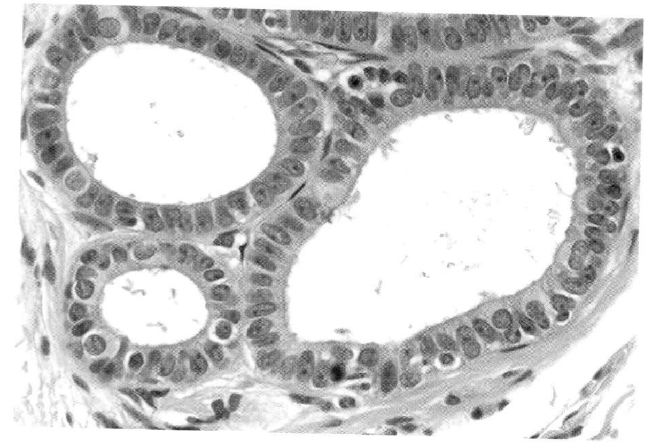

Fig. 13.61
Endosalpingiosis. **Glands within the omentum are lined by benign endosalpingeal epithelium**

cell types of the normal fallopian tube epithelium are found in varying numbers: pale ciliated cells, secretory cells, and dark rodlike, intercalated or "peg" cells. The cells have prominent luminal margins, distinct borders, and basal nuclei. Focal cellular pseudostratification may be present. The nuclei have fine chromatin and delicate nuclear membranes and typically lack significant atypia or mitotic activity. Psammoma bodies are frequently present within the lumens or in the adjacent stroma, and, in occasional cases, numerous psammoma bodies are embedded in subserosal connective tissue. Endosalpingiotic glands can rarely extend into the underlying tissues, such as the wall of the appendix or, as noted earlier, the uterus [45]. Staining with the PAS method reveals a basement membrane surrounding each gland and PAS-positive, diastase-resistant material in the apices of the lining cells and within the glandular lumens. Estrogen and progesterone receptors have been identified immunohistochemically within the cells.

The term atypical endosalpingiosis has been applied to endosalpingiotic lesions in which there is cellular stratification, including cellular buds, cribriform patterns, and varying degrees of cellular atypia, occurring in the absence of a serous tumor of borderline malignancy. Such lesions merge histologically with peritoneal serous tumors of borderline malignancy (see next section). Bell and Scully use the latter term if the "lesions composed of tubal-type epithelium exhibit papillarity, tufting, or detachment of cell clusters … . even when they arise on a background of endosalpingiosis." [16] Endosalpingiotic glands should be differentiated from mesonephric remnants, which are common incidental microscopic findings in the region of the fallopian tube. Mesonephric tubules are typically located more deeply than endosalpingiosis and characteristically have a collar of smooth muscle under the epithelial lining, which is typically a single layer of nonciliated, low columnar to cuboidal cells. Rare extraovarian borderline and malignant serous tumors have been shown to arise from endosalpingiosis [28, 144].

Peritoneal Serous Tumors

The full spectrum of serous neoplasms arising within the ovary may also arise directly from the extraovarian peritoneum. These tumors are considered only briefly here because their clinicopathologic features closely resemble those of their ovarian counterparts. Primary peritoneal serous borderline tumors are usually associated with widespread extraovarian peritoneal involvement and normal-sized ovaries that are free of disease or which have serosal involvement similar to that involving the extraovarian peritoneum [16, 19]. The most common presenting features in patients with these tumors, who are typically under the age of 35 years (range, 16–67), are infertility and chronic pelvic or abdominal pain. Many cases, however, are discovered incidentally at laparotomy for other conditions. At operation, focal or diffuse miliary granules, fibrous adhesions, or both involve the pelvic peritoneum and omentum and, less commonly, the abdominal peritoneum. Microscopic examination reveals superficial tumor that resembles noninvasive epithelial or desmoplastic implants of borderline serous tumors of ovarian origin. Coexistent endosalpingiosis has been found in 85% of cases. The prognosis of peritoneal serous borderline tumors is favorable; approximately 85% of patients have had no clinically persistent or progressive disease on follow-up. In rare cases, transformation to an invasive low-grade peritoneal serous carcinoma (LGPSC) may occur, although in a proportion of these, the invasive tumor may have been present but not sampled at the time of the initial operation.

Although most primary peritoneal serous carcinomas are high grade (see following paragraph), some have low-grade nuclear features and are distinguished from peritoneal serous borderline tumors by the presence of invasion. Low-grade peritoneal serous carcinomas (LGPSCs) resemble invasive implants of serous borderline tumors (*Fig. 13.62*) [243]. Some may have a micropapillary pattern [68]. They lack high-grade nuclear atypia, invade tissue or lymphovascular spaces or both, and have appreciable solid epithelial proliferation. Peritoneal psammocarcinomas [87, 141, 243] are a subtype of

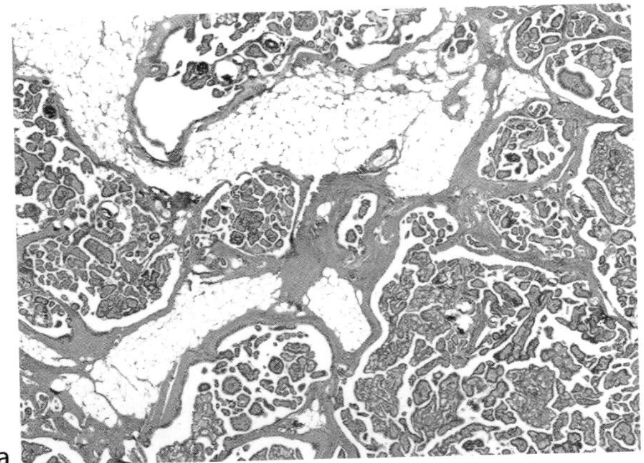

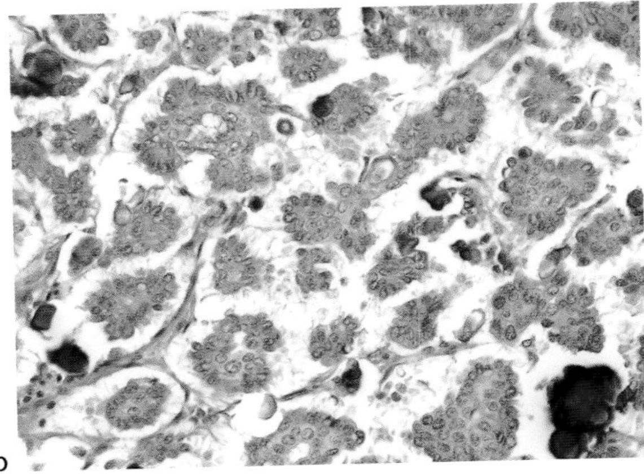

Fig. 13.62
Low-grade primary papillary serous carcinoma of the peritoneum. **(a) The tumor is infiltrating the omental fat. (b) The papillae are lined by tumor cells resembling serous borderline neoplasia. Note the psammoma bodies**

LGPSCs with psammoma bodies in most of the tumor nests and absent or rare solid epithelial proliferation (see Chap. 14, Surface Epithelial Tumors of the Ovary); lymphatic invasion is often conspicuous. The average ages of patients in one study were 57 years (LGPSC of usual type) and 40 years (peritoneal psammocarcinomas) [243]. Features present in both tumors are usually abdominal pain, mass, or both, but approximately 40% are incidental findings. Operative and gross findings vary from nodules to adhesions to a dominant mass. Short-term outcomes for LGPSCs and peritoneal psammocarcinomas are favorable, but follow-up is too limited in the reported cases to determine long-term outcomes. These tumors should be distinguished from peritoneal serous borderline tumors, which are very similar except for an absence of invasion. Adequate sampling is necessary to identify invasion, with highest yields of invasive foci in the omentum.

Typical peritoneal serous carcinomas have high-grade nuclear features and have been referred to as serous surface papillary carcinomas, serous papillary carcinomas of the peritoneum, or extraovarian peritoneal serous papillary carcinoma [5, 17, 69, 236]. The typical intraoperative appearance of a primary peritoneal serous carcinoma, with widespread peritoneal tumor associated with ovaries of normal size, may mimic that of a diffuse malignant mesothelioma or peritoneal carcinomatosis associated with an unknown primary tumor. The ovaries are often involved by small surface "implants" but retain their normal size and shape. In some series, the patients have had an average age that is a decade older than patients with similar tumors of ovarian origin. Some tumors have occurred in women who had had bilateral oophorectomy performed as prophylactic treatment for BRCA-related familial ovarian cancer [30], suggesting that some peritoneal serous carcinomas may be a phenotypic variant of familial ovarian cancer [112]. The risk of peritoneal serous carcinoma in BRCA1 mutation carriers is about 4% at 20 years after prophylactic salpingo-oophorectomy [30, 76].

Primary peritoneal serous carcinomas resemble their ovarian counterparts on microscopic and immunohistochemical examination; their distinction from malignant mesothelioma has been previously discussed. Criteria for their separation from primary ovarian serous carcinomas with peritoneal spread have been proposed by the Gynecologic Oncology Group: (1) both ovaries are either normal in size or enlarged by a benign process; (2) in the judgment of the surgeon and the pathologist, the bulk of the tumor is in the peritoneum and the extent of tumor involvement at one or more extraovarian sites is greater than on the surface of either ovary; (3) microscopic examination of the ovaries reveals no tumor, tumor confined to the surface epithelium with no evidence of cortical invasion, tumor involving the ovarian surface and the underlying cortical stroma but less than 5 mm in area, or tumor less than 5 mm in diameter within the ovarian substance, with or without surface involvement; and (4) the histologic and cytologic characteristics of the tumor are predominantly serous and similar or identical to those of ovarian serous papillary adenocarcinomas of any grade. In most series, these tumors have a prognosis similar to that of high-stage ovarian serous carcinomas with a similar volume of residual tumor and similar postoperative treatment [106].

The differential diagnosis includes metastatic serous carcinoma from an occult primary tubal or endometrial serous carcinoma (see ➲ Chap. 11, Diseases of the Fallopian Tube and Paratubal Region, and ➲ Chap. 9, Endometrial Carcinoma). Peritoneal serous carcinomas, like their ovarian and tubal counterparts but unlike endometrial serous carcinomas, are typically immunoreactive for WT1 [72]. If serous carcinoma involves the tubes or endometrium as well as the peritoneum, it may not be possible, short of clonality studies, to determine if they are independent primaries or if one is metastatic from the other.

Rare extraovarian serous tumors take the form of localized, typically cystic masses, usually within the broad ligament and less commonly within the retroperitoneum. Serous papillary cystadenomas and adenofibromas, serous borderline tumors, and serous carcinomas have been described in these sites [7, 8, 237].

Endocervicosis (including Mullerianosis)

Benign glands of endocervical type involving the peritoneum, so-called endocervicosis, are rare, but examples involving the posterior uterine serosa, cul-de-sac, vaginal apex, outer wall of the uterine cervix, and the urinary bladder have been documented [43, 128, 139, 160, 253]. In the last site, the lesions usually formed tumor-like masses that involved the posterior wall or posterior dome of the bladder in women of reproductive age. On microscopic examination, benign endocervical-type glands were located predominantly within the smooth muscle of the muscularis propria (➲ *Fig. 13.63*) [43, 160]. In several cases, the infiltrative pattern of the glands, mild epithelial atypia, and a reactive periglandular stroma, alone or in combination, resulted in an initial misdiagnosis of well-differentiated adenocarcinoma. In such cases, the absence of a mucosal-based tumor and no more than mild atypia facilitate the diagnosis of endocervicosis, The differential diagnosis also includes mullerianosis, a term applied to lesions composed of an admixture of mullerian glandular epithelia (tubal, endocervical, and endometrioid), sometimes with foci of endometriotic stroma. Examples of mullerianosis have been reported in the urinary bladder, mesosalpinx, and inguinal lymph nodes [133, 252].

Extraovarian Mucinous Tumors

Ovarian-type mucinous neoplasms, in the absence of a primary tumor within the ovary, have been described in extraovarian sites, typically in the retroperitoneum (➲ *Fig. 13.64*) [64, 128, 129, 178]; a single case has been described in the inguinal region [228]. These tumors form large cystic masses that on histologic examination resemble ovarian mucinous cystadenomas, borderline tumors, or cystadenocarcinomas (➲ *Fig. 13.65*); some tumors contain ovarian-type stroma in their walls. Mural nodules, usually consisting of anaplastic carcinoma, similar to those in ovarian mucinous tumors, have been present in several cases [151]. Although it is possible that some of these tumors originate within a supernumerary ovary, the great rarity of the latter, the absence of follicles or their derivatives within the ovarian-like stroma, and the rare occurrence of similar tumors in males strongly support a peritoneal origin. It has been recently suggested that, in some cases of pseudomyxoma peritonei associated with ovarian and appendiceal mucinous tumors, the peritoneal lesions may arise directly from the peritoneum as part of a multifocal neoplastic process [150, 213].

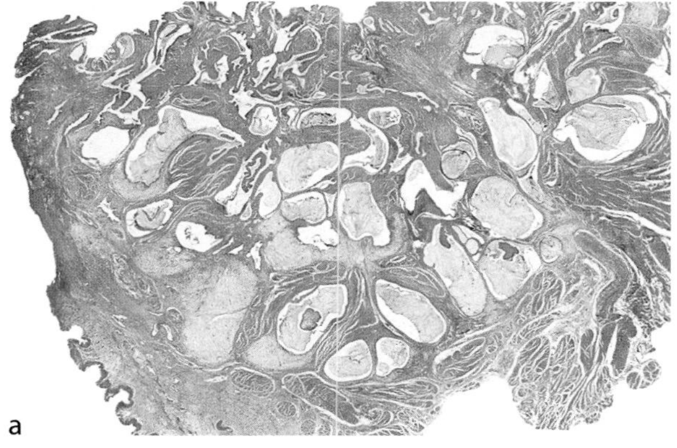
a

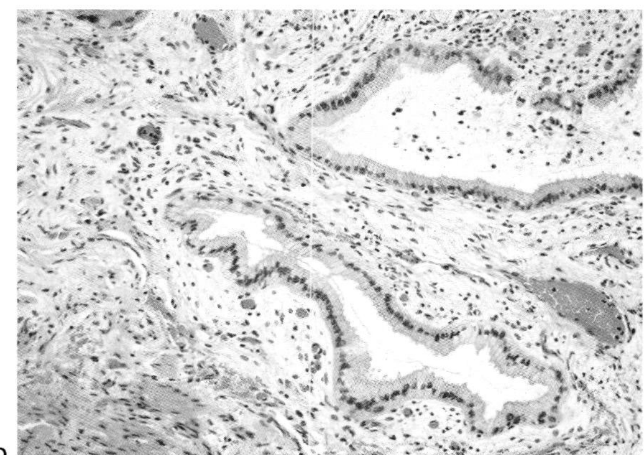
b

Fig. 13.63
Endocervicosis of urinary bladder. **(a) Benign endocervical-type glands lie within the muscularis propria. (b) High-power view of glands with cytologically bland, endocervical-type mucinous epithelium**

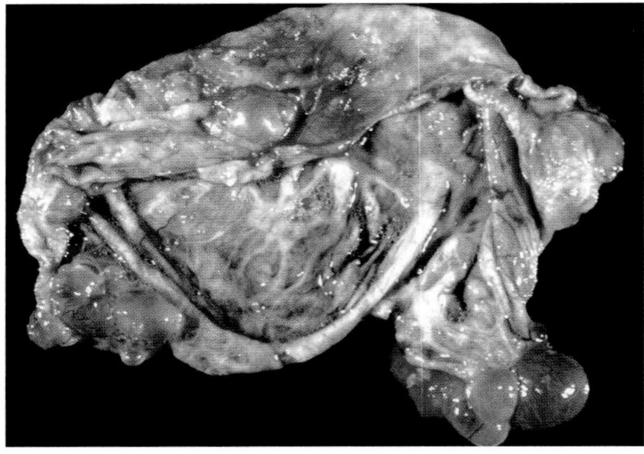

Fig. 13.64
Retroperitoneal mucinous tumor. **The specimen has been opened to reveal multiple locules with mucinous contents (Courtesy of R.E. Scully, M.D., Boston, MA)**

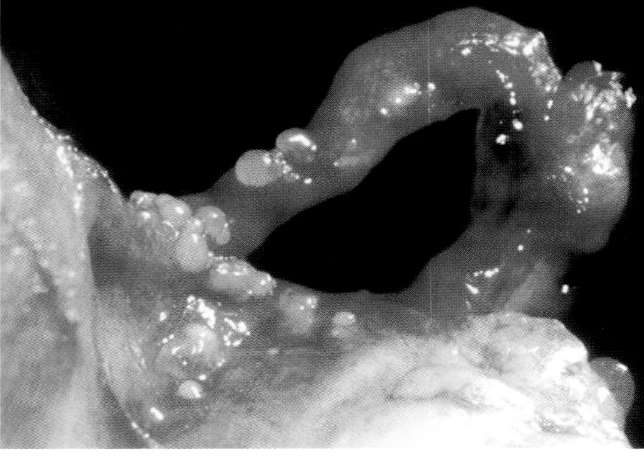

Fig. 13.66
Walthard nests. **Multiple small cysts cover the serosa of fallopian tube and mesosalpinx**

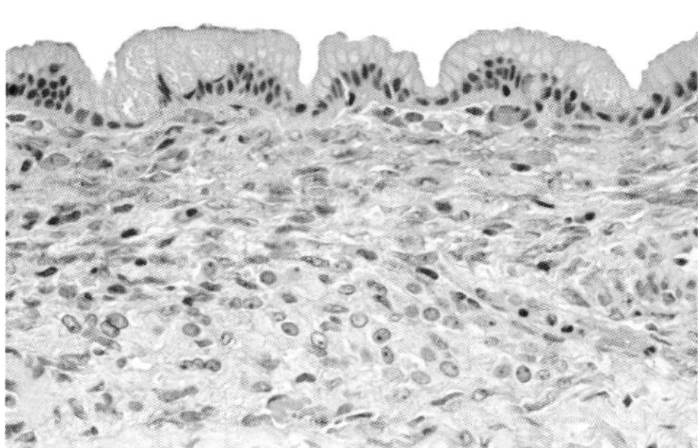

Fig. 13.65
Retroperitoneal mucinous cystadenoma

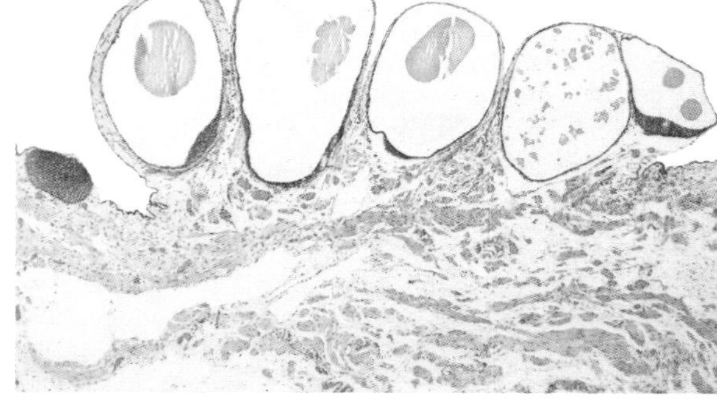

Fig. 13.67
Walthard nests on fallopian tube serosa. **A nest (far left) and multiple cysts are formed or lined by benign transitional-type cells**

Peritoneal Transitional, Squamous, and Clear Cell Lesions

Nests of transitional (urothelial) epithelium referred to as Walthard nests are commonly present on the pelvic peritoneum in women of all ages, typically involving the serosal surfaces of the fallopian tubes (*Figs. 13.66* and *13.67*), mesosalpinx, and mesovarium [22]. Walthard nests are uncommon on the ovarian surface but may be seen in the hilus, probably originating from the peritoneum of the mesovarium; they are most common on the tubal serosa (see Chap. 11, Diseases of the Fallopian Tube and Paratubal Region). Rare extraovarian Brenner tumors have been encountered, most commonly in the broad ligament. In contrast to Walthard nests, squamous metaplasia of the peritoneum is rare; it is usually an incidental microscopic finding but in one case it resulted in tiny, but grossly visible, nodules [156]. Two clear cell carcinomas of apparent peritoneal origin have been reported. One was a localized mass within the sigmoid mesocolon [73] whereas the other diffusely involved the peritoneum [130]; no endometriosis was identified in either case.

Peritoneal Decidual Reaction

Clinical and Operative Findings

An ectopic decidual reaction similar to that seen in the lamina propria of the fallopian tube, cervix, and vagina may also be seen within the submesothelial stroma of the peritoneal cavity. Frequent sites of ectopic decidua include the submesothelial stroma of the fallopian tubes, uterus and uterine ligaments, appendix and omentum, and within pelvic adhesions. Rare sites have included the serosal surfaces of the diaphragm, liver, spleen, and the renal pelvis.

Submesothelial decidua is typically an incidental microscopic finding, but florid lesions may be visible at the time of cesarean section or postpartum tubal ligation as multiple, gray to white, focally hemorrhagic nodules or plaques studding the peritoneal surfaces and simulating a malignant tumor. Several cases have been associated with massive, occasionally fatal, intraperitoneal hemorrhage during the third trimester, labor, or the puerperium. Other rare clinical presentations include abdominal pain, which may simulate that of appendicitis, and hydronephrosis and hematuria secondary to renal pelvic involvement.

Microscopic Findings

Microscopic examination discloses submesothelial decidual cells disposed individually or arranged in nodules or plaques (*Fig. 13.68*). Smooth muscle cells, probably derived from submesothelial myofibroblasts, may be admixed. The decidual foci are typically vascular and contain a sprinkling of lymphocytes. Focal hemorrhagic necrosis and varying degrees of nuclear pleomorphism and hyperchromasia of the decidual cells may suggest a tumor such as a deciduoid malignant mesothelioma [214], but their bland appearance and mitotic inactivity militate against such a diagnosis. We have seen several cases of an omental decidual reaction in which most of the decidual cells exhibited striking vacuolization with basophilic mucin and an eccentric location of the nucleus. The appearance of the cells raised the possibility of metastatic signet-ring cell carcinoma, but in contrast to the cells of the latter, the vacuoles within the decidual cells contain acid rather than neutral mucin, and their cytoplasm lacks immunoreactivity for cytokeratin.

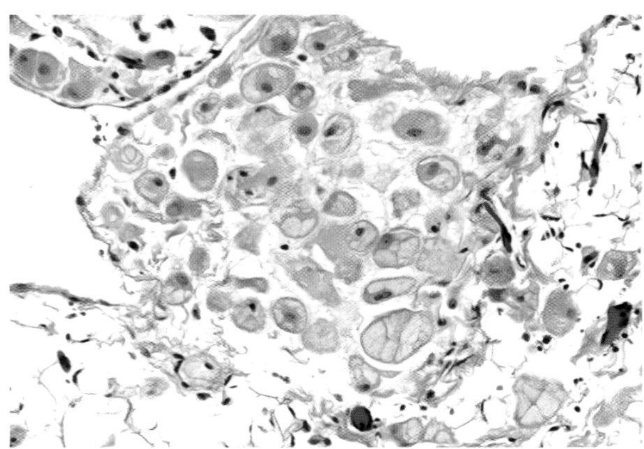

Fig. 13.68
Ectopic decidua beneath pelvic peritoneum. Note the prominent cytoplasmic vacuoles

Diffuse Peritoneal Leiomyomatosis

Diffuse peritoneal leiomyomatosis is a rare disorder characterized by the presence of multiple submesothelial nodules of cytologically benign smooth muscle, frequently associated with uterine leiomyomas and, rarely, ovarian leiomyomas. The nodules are generally considered to arise from multipotential submesothelial mesenchymal cells. This disorder is discussed elsewhere (see Chap. 10, Mesenchymal Tumors of the Uterus).

Benign Intranodal Glands of Müllerian Type

Clinical Features

Benign glands of müllerian type are most commonly encountered within the pelvic and paraaortic lymph nodes of females [99, 120], and less often in inguinal and femoral lymph nodes. Because these glands are almost always incidental microscopic findings in lymph nodes removed in cases of pelvic carcinoma, their reported frequency, which has varied from 2% to 41%, depends on the number of lymph nodes removed and the extent of the histologic sampling. Almost all the patients have been adults, although rare examples have been reported in children. In males, the presence of similar glands has been recorded rarely within lymph nodes in the pelvis, abdomen, and mediastinum. Although typically without clinical or intraoperative manifestations, rare examples of lymph nodes containing müllerian-type glands have been associated with a false-positive lymphangiogram, ureteral obstruction secondary to lymph node enlargement, or visible enlargement at the time of operation.

In a number of patients, intranodal glandular inclusions have been accompanied by endosalpingiosis of the peritoneum, salpingitis isthmica nodosa, or acute and chronic salpingitis [120]. Other patients have had coexistent ovarian serous tumors, which have been benign, borderline tumors, or carcinomas [184].

Pathologic Findings

On gross examination, the glands are usually not apparent, although rarely they are recognizable as cysts measuring up to a few millimeters in diameter. The glands are typically located in the periphery of the node, most commonly within its capsule or between the lymphoid follicles in the superficial cortex (➲ *Fig. 13.69*); rarely, they lie free within the subcapsular sinuses [120]. In florid cases, they can be diffusely distributed throughout the lymph node. Intraglandular or periglandular psammoma bodies are commonly present. Intranodal glands may be surrounded by a thin rim of fibrous tissue or abut directly on the surrounding lymphoid cells.

The glands may be round and cystically dilated or exhibit an irregular contour as a result of infolding. They are most commonly lined by a single layer of cuboidal to columnar tubal-type epithelium, with an admixture of ciliated, secretory, and intercalated cell types (➲ *Fig. 13.70*). With special stains, mucin can be demonstrated in the apical portion of the secretory cells and within the gland spaces. The cells have a benign appearance with regular, basally oriented or pseudostratified, oval to round nuclei, fine nuclear chromatin, and occasional small nucleoli; mitotic figures are typically absent. In rare cases, the cells can exhibit varying degrees of atypia and stratification; the latter can produce an intraglandular cribriform pattern or luminal obliteration by sheets of cells (➲ *Fig. 13.71*). These cases of atypical endosalpingiosis may rarely be the origin of intranodal serous neoplasms (see following).

Examples of intranodal glandular inclusions lined by benign endometrioid epithelium, mucinous epithelium of endocervical or goblet cell type, or metaplastic squamous epithelium have been reported [128, 152].

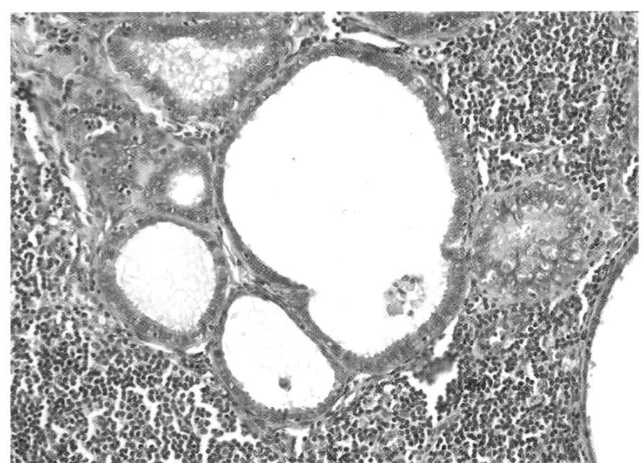

◘ Fig. 13.70
Endosalpingiotic glands within pelvic lymph node. **The glands are lined by benign cells of multiple types, including ciliated cells**

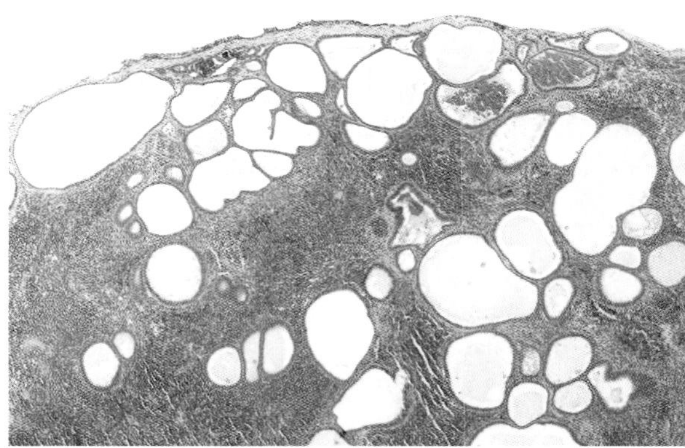

◘ Fig. 13.69
Endosalpingiotic glands within pelvic lymph node. **The glands are located within and immediately beneath the node capsule as well as deeper within the node**

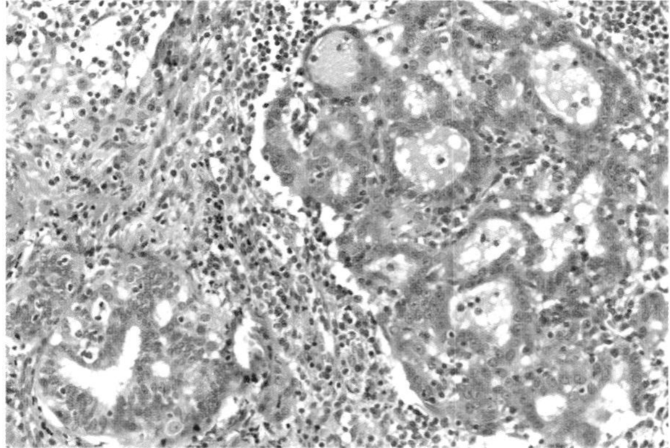

◘ Fig. 13.71
Atypical endosalpingiotic glands within pelvic lymph node. **Some of the glands exhibit luminal obliteration by cells growing in solid and cribriform patterns**

Differential Diagnosis

In most cases the distinction between glandular inclusions and metastatic adenocarcinoma is not difficult unless a primary ovarian serous tumor of low malignant potential is present, in which case the distinction may be difficult or impossible. Features favoring a benign diagnosis include a capsular or interfollicular location of the glands, lining cells of multiple types including ciliated forms, a lack of significant cellular atypia and mitotic activity, and an absence of a desmoplastic stromal reaction. Complicating the differential diagnosis is the very rare development of borderline or frankly malignant change in müllerian glandular inclusions in lymph nodes. This diagnosis is suggested in cases in which the intranodal neoplasm merges with foci of atypical endosalpingiosis. Intranodal nests of benign squamous epithelium should not be mistaken for metastatic squamous cell carcinoma. Features favoring a benign diagnosis include bland cytologic features, mitotic inactivity, and, in some cases, an origin within benign glands.

Intranodal Ectopic Decidua

Ectopic decidua unassociated with endometriosis has been described as a rare, incidental microscopic finding in paraaortic and pelvic lymph nodes, usually removed as part of a radical hysterectomy for carcinoma of the cervix in pregnant patients [6, 152, 246]. A subserosal ectopic decidual reaction may be present elsewhere in the pelvis. In some cases, the decidual tissue has been recognized on careful macroscopic examination as tiny, gray, subcapsular nodules. On microscopic examination, the decidual nests typically occupy the subcapsular sinus and superficial cortex (➋ *Fig. 13.72*), although more central parts of the lymph node may also be involved. The cells appear benign, but may contain occasional bizarre, hyperchromatic nuclei, mimicking metastatic squamous cell carcinoma. The absence of mitotic activity, keratinization, and stromal desmoplasia facilitate the diagnosis. Metastatic squamous cell carcinoma, however, may be present in the same node.

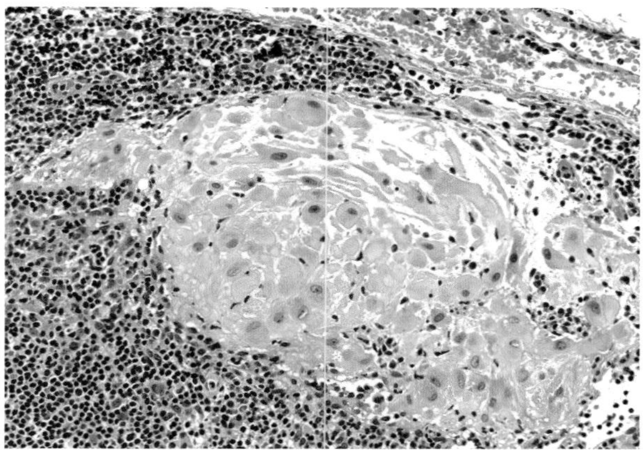

Fig. 13.72
Ectopic decidua within pelvic lymph node. **The nodal architecture is focally replaced by sheets of decidualized cells**

Intranodal Leiomyomatosis

Rare cases of lymph node involvement by mitotically inactive, cytologically benign smooth muscle have been described (➋ *Fig. 13.73*) [57, 103]. Most patients have had concurrent typical uterine leiomyomas or, less commonly, diffuse peritoneal leiomyomatosis [103] or similar nodules within the lungs [57]. In pregnant patients, the process may merge with intranodal decidua [103]. The finding in most cases likely is secondary to lymphatic spread from uterine leiomyomas ("benign metastasizing leiomyoma"; see ➋ Chap. 10, Mesenchymal Tumors of the Uterus), but in some cases the intranodal smooth muscle may arise from entrapped subcoelomic mesenchyme or myofibroblastic organization of intranodal decidua. The presence of benign-appearing smooth muscle in a lymph node should also bring into consideration the diagnosis of lymphangioleiomyomatosis. This disorder is usually, but not invariably, associated with pulmonary involvement. Benign intranodal smooth muscle should also be distinguished from metastatic

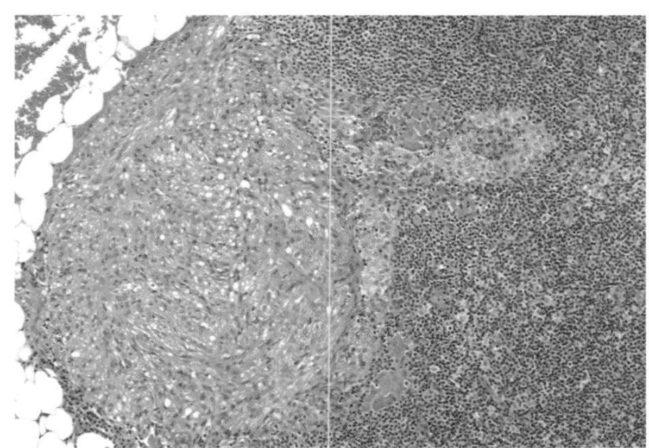

Fig. 13.73
Benign smooth muscle within pelvic lymph node

well-differentiated leiomyosarcoma of uterine origin. Patients with the latter usually have a large uterine mass, and on histologic examination the intranodal tumor is cellular and exhibits evidence of cellular atypicality and mitotic activity.

References

1. Adams HW, Mainz DL (1977) Eosinophilic ascites. A case report and review of the literature. Digest Dis 22:40–42
2. Ahn GH, Scully RE (1991) Clear cell carcinoma of the inguinal region arising from endometriosis. Cancer (Phila) 67:116–120
3. Albee RB Jr, Sinervo K, Fisher DT (2008) Laparoscopic excision of lesions suggestive of endometriosis or otherwise atypical in appearance: relationship between visual findings and final histologic diagnosis. J Minim Invasive Gynecol 15:32–37
4. Al-Khawaja M, Tan PH, MacLennan GT et al (2008) Ureteral endometriosis: clinicopathological and immunohistochemical study of 7 cases. Hum Pathol 39:954–959
5. Altaras MM, Aviram R, Cohen I et al (1991) Primary peritoneal papillary serous adenocarcinoma: clinical and management aspects. Gynecol Oncol 40:230–236
6. Ashraf M, Boyd CB, Beresford WA (1984) Ectopic decidual reaction in para-aortic and pelvic lymph nodes in the presence of cervical squamous cell carcinoma during pregnancy. J Surg Oncol 26:6–8
7. Aslani M, Ahn G, Scully RE (1988) Serous papillary cystadenoma of borderline malignancy of broad ligament. Int J Gynecol Pathol 7:131–138
8. Aslani M, Scully RE (1989) Primary carcinoma of the broad ligament. Report of four cases and review of the literature. Cancer (Phila) 64:1540–1545
9. Attanoos R, Gibbs AR (1997) Pathology of malignant mesothelioma. Histopathology (Oxf) 30:403–418
10. Attanoos RL, Griffin A, Gibbs AR (2003) The use of immunohistochemistry in distinguishing reactive from neoplastic mesothelium. A novel use for desmin and comparative evaluation with epithelial membrane antigen, p53, platelet-derived growth factor-receptor, P-glycoprotein and bcl-2. Histopathology 43:231–238
11. Baker PM, Clement PB, Bell DA et al (1999) Superficial endometriosis of the uterine cervix: a report of 20 cases of a process that may be confused with endocervical glandular dysplasia or adenocarcinoma in situ. Int J Gynecol Pathol 18:198–205
12. Baker PM, Clement PB, Young RH (2005) Malignant peritoneal mesotheliomas in women: A study of 75 cases with emphasis on their morphologic spectrum and differential diagnosis. Am J Clin Pathol 123:724–737
13. Banu SK, Lee J, Speights VO Jr et al (2008) Cyclooxygenase-2 regulates survival, migration, and invasion of human endometriotic cells through multiple mechanisms. Endocrinology 149:1180–1189
14. Barnetson RJ, Burnett RA, Downie I et al (2006) Immunohistochemical analysis of peritoneal mesothelioma and primary and secondary serous carcinoma of the peritoneum. Antibodies to estrogen and progesterone receptors are useful. Am J Clin Pathol 125:67–76
15. Bayer AS, Blumenkrantz MJ, Montgomerie JZ et al (1976) Candida peritonitis. Report of 22 cases and review of the English literature. Am J Med 61:832–840
16. Bell DA, Scully RE (1990) Serous borderline tumors of the peritoneum. Am J Surg Pathol 14:230–239
17. Ben-Baruch G, Sivan E, Moran O et al (1996) Primary peritoneal serous papillary carcinoma: a study of 25 cases and comparison with stage III-IV ovarian papillary serous carcinoma. Gynecol Oncol 60:393–396
18. Bergqvist A, Ljungberg O, Myhre E (1984) Human endometrium and endometriotic tissue obtained simultaneously: a comparative histological study. Int J Gynecol Pathol 3:135–145
19. Biscotti CV, Hart WR (1992) Peritoneal serous micropapillomatosis of low malignant potential (serous borderline tumors of the peritoneum). A clinicopathologic study of 17 cases. Am J Surg Pathol 16:467–475
20. Bolen JW, Hammar SP, McNutt MA (1986) Reactive and neoplastic serosal tissue. A light microscopic, ultrastructural and immunohistochemical study. Am J Surg Pathol 10:34–47
21. Boyle DP, McCluggage WG (2009) Peritoneal stromal endometriosis: a detailed morphological analysis of a large series of cases of a common and under-recognized form of endometriosis. J Clin Pathol 62:530–533
22. Bransilver BR, Ferenczy A, Richart RM (1974) Brenner tumors and Walthard cell nests. Arch Pathol Lab Med 98:76–86
23. Brunnemann RG, Ro JY, Ordonez NG et al (1999) Extrapleural solitary fibrous tumor: a clinicopathologic study of 24 cases. Mod Pathol 12:1034–1042
24. Bulun SE (2009) Mechanisms of disease: endometriosis. N Engl J Med 360:268–279
25. Bur ME, Greene GL, Press MF (1987) Estrogen receptor localization in formalin-fixed, paraffin-embedded endometrium and endometriotic tissues. Int J Gynecol Pathol 6:140–151
26. Candiani GB, Vercellini P, Fedele L et al (1991) Inguinal endometriosis: pathogenetic and clinical implications. Obstet Gynecol 78:191–194
27. Carr NJ, Turk EP (1992) The histological features of splenosis. Histopathology (Oxf) 21:549–553
28. Carrick KS, Milvenan JS, Albores-Saavedra J (2003) Serous tumor of low malignant potential arising in inguinal endosalpingiosis. Int J Gynecol Pathol 22:412–415
29. Cartwright PS (1991) Peritoneal trophoblastic implants after surgical management of tubal pregnancy. J Reprod Med 36:523–524
30. Casey MJ, Synder C, Bewtra C et al (2005) Intra-abdominal carcinomatosis after prophylactic oophorectomy in women of hereditary breast ovarian cancer syndrome kindreds associated witih *BRCA1* and *BRCA2* mutations. Gynecol Oncol 97:457–467
31. Ceruto CA, Brun EA, Chang D et al (2006) Prognostic significance of histomorphologic parameters in diffuse malignant peritoneal mesothelioma. Arch Pathol Lab Med 130:1653–1661
32. Chatman DL, Ward AB (1982) Endometriosis in adolescents. J Reprod Med 27:156–160
33. Chatman DL, Zbella EA (1987) Biopsy in laparoscopically diagnosed endometriosis. J Reprod Med 32:855–857
34. Chatterjee SK (1980) Scar endometriosis: a clinicopathologic study of 17 cases. Obstet Gynecol 56:81–84
35. Chopin N, Vieira M, Borghese B et al (2005) Operative management of deeply infiltrating endometriosis: results on pelvic pain symptoms according to a surgical classification. J Minim Invasive Gynecol 12:106–112
36. Churg A, Cagle PT, Roggli VL (2006) Tumors of the serosal membranes. Atlas of tumor pathology, ser IV. Armed Forces Institute of Pathology, Washington, DC
37. Clarke TJ, Simpson RHW (1990) Necrotizing granulomas of peritoneum following diathermy ablation of endometriosis. Histopathology (Oxf) 16:400–402

38. Clement PB (1995) Reactive tumor-like lesions of the peritoneum (Editorial). Am J Clin Pathol 103:673–676
39. Clement PB (2007) The pathology of endometriosis: a survey of the many faces of a common disease emphasizing diagnostic pitfalls and unusual and newly appreciated aspects. Adv Anat Pathol 14:241–260
40. Clement PB, Granai CO, Young RH et al (1994) Endometriosis with myxoid change: a case simulating pseudomyxoma peritonei. Am J Surg Pathol 18:849–853
41. Clement PB, Scully RE (1978) Extrauterine mesodermal (müllerian) adenosarcoma. A clinicopathologic analysis of five cases. Am J Clin Pathol 69:276–283
42. Clement PB, Scully RE (1992) Endometrial stromal sarcomas of the uterus with extensive endometrioid glandular differentiation. A report of three cases that caused problems in differential diagnosis. Int J Gynecol Pathol 11:163–173
43. Clement PB, Young RH (1992) Endocervicosis of the urinary bladder: a report of six cases of a benign müllerian lesion that may mimic adenocarcinoma. Am J Surg Pathol 16:533–542
44. Clement PB, Young RH (1993) Florid mesothelial hyperplasia associated with ovarian tumors: a possible source of error in tumor diagnosis and staging. Int J Gynecol Pathol 12:51–58
45. Clement PB, Young RH (1999) Tumor-like manifestations of florid cystic endosalpingiosis: a report of four cases including the first reported cases of mural endosalpingiosis of the uterus. Am J Surg Pathol 23:166–175
46. Clement PB, Young RH (2000) Two previously unemphasized features of endometriosis: micronodular stromal endometriosis and endometriosis with stromal elastosis. Int J Surg Pathol 8:223–227
47. Clement PB, Young RH, Hanna W et al (1993) Sclerosing peritonitis associated with luteinized thecomas of the ovary: a clinicopathological analysis of six cases. Am J Surg Pathol 18:1–13
48. Clement PB, Young RH, Oliva E et al (1996) Hyperplastic mesothelial cells within abdominal lymph nodes: a mimic of metastatic ovarian carcinoma and serous borderline tumor. A report of two cases associated with ovarian neoplasms. Mod Pathol 9:879–886
49. Clement PB, Young RH, Scully RE (1988) Necrotic pseudoxanthomatous nodules of the ovary and peritoneum in endometriosis. Am J Surg Pathol 12:390–397
50. Clement PB, Young RH, Scully RE (1989) Liesegang rings in endometriosis. A report of three cases. Int J Gynecol Pathol 8:271–276
51. Clement PB, Young RH, Scully RE (1990) Stromal endometriosis of the uterine cervix. A variant of endometriosis that may simulate a sarcoma. Am J Surg Pathol 14:449–455
52. Clement PB, Young RH, Scully RE (1996) Malignant mesotheliomas presenting as ovarian masses. Am J Surg Pathol 20:1067–1080
53. Coffin CM, Hornick JL, Fletcher CD (2007) Inflammatory myofibroblastic tumor: comparison of clinicopathologic, histologic, and immunohistochemical features including ALK expression in atypical and aggressive cases. Am J Surg Pathol 31:509–520
54. Comin CE, Saieva C, Messerini (2007) h-caldesmon, calretinin, estrogen receptor, and Ber-EP4: A useful combination of immunohistochemical markers for differentiating epithelioid peritoneal mesothelioma from serous papillary carcinoma of the ovary. Am J Surg Pathol 31:1139–1148
55. Copeland LJ, Silva EG, Gershenson DM et al (1988) The significance of müllerian inclusions found at second-look laparotomy in patients with epithelial ovarian neoplasms. Obstet Gynecol 71:763–770
56. Cornillie FJ, Oosterlynck D, Lauweryns JM et al (1990) Deeply infiltrating pelvic endometriosis: histology and clinical significance. Fertil Steril 53:978–983
57. Cramer SF, Meyer JS, Kraner JF et al (1980) Metastasizing leiomyoma of the uterus. S-phase fraction, estrogen receptor, and ultrastructure. Cancer (Phila) 45:932–937
58. Cumiskey J, Whyte P, Kelehan P et al (2008) A detailed morphologic and immunohistochemical comparison of pre- and postmenopausal endometriosis. J Clin Pathol 61:455–459
59. Czernobilsky B, Silverstein A (1978) Salpingitis and ovarian endometriosis. Fertil Steril 30:45–49
60. David MP, Ben-Zwi D, Langer L (1981) Tubal intramural polyps and their relationship to infertility. Fertil Steril 35:526–531
61. Day DL, Sane S, Dehner LP (1986) Inflammatory pseudotumor of the mesentery and small intestine. Pediatr Radiol 16:210–215
62. Daya D, McCaughey WTE (1990) Well-differentiated papillary mesothelioma of the peritoneum. A clinicopathologic study of 22 cases. Cancer (Phila) 65:292–296, 185–195
63. Deger RB, LiVolsi VA, Noumoff JS (1995) Foreign body reaction (gossypiboma) masking as recurrent ovarian cancer. Gynecol Oncol 56:94–96
64. de Peralta MN, Delahoussaye PM, Tornos CS et al (1994) Benign retroperitoneal cysts of müllerian type: a clinicopathologic study of three cases and review of the literature. Int J Gynecol Pathol 13:273–278
65. D'Hooghe T, Bambra CS, Raeymaekers BM et al (1995) Intrapelvic injection of menstural endometrium causes endometriosis in baboons (Papio cynocephalus and Papio anubis). Am J Obstet Gynecol 173:125–134
66. Doss BJ, Jacques SM, Qureshi F et al (1998) Extratubal secondary trophoblastic implants: clinicopathologic correlation and review of the literature. Hum Pathol 29:184–187
67. Egger H, Weigmann P (1982) Clinical and surgical aspects of ovarian endometriotic cysts. Arch Gynecol 233:37–45
68. Elmore LW, Sherman ME, Seidman JD et al (2000) p53 expression and mutational status of primary peritoneal micropapillary serous carcinoma (abstract). Mod Pathol 13:124A
69. Eltabbakh GH, Werness BA, Piver S et al (1998) Prognostic factors in extraovarian primary peritoneal carcinoma. Gynecol Oncol 71:230–239
70. Emory TS, Monihan JM, Carr NJ et al (1997) Sclerosing mesenteritis, mesenteric panniculitis and mesenteric lipodystrophy: a single entity? Am J Surg Pathol 21:392–398
71. Erzen M, Rakar S, Klancar B et al (2001) Endometriosis-assocaited ovarian carcinoma: An entity distinct from other ovarian carcinomas as suggested by a nested case-control study. Gynecol Oncol 83:100–108
72. Euscher ED, Malpica A, Deavers MT et al (2005) Differential expression of WT-1 in serous carcinomas in the peritoneum with or without associated serous carcinoma in endometrial polyps. Am J Surg Pathol 29:1074–1078
73. Evans H, Yates WA, Palmer WE et al (1990) Clear cell carcinoma of the sigmoid mesocolon: a tumor of the secondary müllerian system. Am J Obstet Gynecol 162:161--163
74. Fedele L, Vercellini P, Arcaini L et al (1988) CA 125 in serum, peritoneal fluid, active lesions, and endometrium of patients with endometriosis. Am J Obstet Gynecol 158:166–170
75. Feldman AL, Libutti SK, Pingpank JF et al (2003) Analysis of factors associated with outcome in patients with malignant peritoneal mesothelioma undergoing surgical debulking and intraperitoneal chemotherapy. J Clin Oncol 24:4560–4567
76. Finch A, Beiner M, Lubinski J et al (2006) Salpingo-oophorectomy and the risk of ovarian, fallopian tube, and peritoneal cancers in women with a *BRCA1* or *BRCA2* mutation. JAMA 296:185–192

77. Flieder DB, Moran CA, Travis WD et al (1998) Pleuro-pulmonary endometriosis and pulmonary ectopic deciduosis: a clinicopathologic and immunohistochemical study of 10 cases with emphasis on diagnostic pitfalls. Hum Pathol 29:1495–1503
78. Foo KT, Ng KC, Rauff A et al (1978) Unusual small intestinal obstruction in adolescent girls: the abdominal cocoon. Br J Surg 65:427–430
79. Forouhar F (1982) Meconium peritonitis. Pathology, evolution, and diagnosis. Am J Clin Pathol 78:208–213
80. Fredericks S, Russell P, Cooper M et al (2005) Smooth muscle in the female pelvic peritoneum: a clinicopathological analysis of 31 women. Pathology 37:14–21
81. Fukunaga M (2000) Smooth muscle metaplasia in ovarian endometriosis. Histopathology 36:348–352
82. Fukunaga M, Naganuma H, Ushigome S et al (1996) Malignant solitary fibrous tumour of the peritoneum. Histopathology (Oxf) 28:463–466
83. Fukunaga M, Nomura K, Ishikawa E et al (1997) Ovarian atypical endometriosis: Its close association with malignant epithelial tumors. Histopathology (Oxf) 30:249–255
84. Fukunaga M, Ushigome S (1998) Epithelial metaplastic changes in ovarian endometriosis. Mod Pathol 11:784–788
85. Gardner HL (1966) Cervical and vaginal endometriosis. Clin Obstet Gynecol 9:358–372
86. George E, Leyser S, Zimmer HL et al (1995) Vernix caseosa peritonitis: an infrequent complication of cesarean section with distinctive histopathologic features. Am J Clin Pathol 103:681–684
87. Gilks CB, Bell DA, Scully RE (1990) Serous psammocarcinoma of the ovary and peritoneum. Int J Gynecol Pathol 9:110–121
88. Goldblum J, Hart WR (1995) Localized and diffuse mesotheliomas of the genital tract and peritoneum in women. A clinicopathological study of nineteen true mesothelial neoplasms, other than adenomatoid tumors, multicystic mesotheliomas and localized fibrous tumors. Am J Surg Pathol 19:1124–1137
89. Gonzalez-Crussi F, deMello DE, Sotelo-Avila C (1983) Omental-mesenteric myxoid hamartomas. Am J Surg Pathol 7:567–578
90. Griffith LM, Carcangiu M (1991) Sex cord tumor with annular tubules associated with endometriosis of the fallopian tube. Am J Clin Pathol 96:259–262
91. Guarch R, Puras A, Ceres R et al (2001) Ovarian endometriosis and clear cell carcinoma, leiomyomatosis peritonealis disseminata, and endometrial adenocarcinoma: an unusual, pathogenetically related association. Int J Gynecol Pathol 20:267–270
92. Gupta S, Goldberg JM, Aziz N et al (2008) Pathogenic mechanisms in endometriosis-associated infertility. Fertil Steril 90:247–257
93. Halme J, Hammond MG, Hulka JF et al (1984) Retrograde menstruation in healthy women and in patients with endometriosis. Obstet Gynecol 64:151–154
94. Hameed A, Jafri N, Copeland LJ et al (1996) Endometriosis with myxoid change simulating mucinous adenocarcinoma and pseudomyxoma peritonei. Gynecol Oncol 62:317–319
95. Harper GB Jr, Awbrey BJ, Thomas CG Jr et al (1986) Mesothelial cysts of the round ligament simulating inguinal hernia. Report of four cases and review of the literature. Am J Surg 151:515–517
96. Heller DS, Gordon RE, Clement PB et al (1999) Presence of asbestos in peritoneal mesotheliomas in women. Int J Gynecol Cancer 9:452–455
97. Henderson DW, Shilkin KB, Whitaker D (1998) Reactive mesothelial hyperplasia vs. mesothelioma, including mesothelioma in situ. Am J Clin Pathol 110:397–404
98. Hitti IF, Glasberg SS, Lubicz S (1990) Clear cell carcinoma arising in extraovarian endometriosis: report of three cases and review of the literature. Gynecol Oncol 39:314–320
99. Horn L-C, Bilek K (1995) Frequency and histogenesis of pelvic retroperitoneal lymph node inclusions of the female genital tract. An immunohistochemical study of 34 cases. Path Res Pract 191:991–996
100. Horton JD, Dezee KJ, Ahnfeldt EP et al (2008) Abdominal wall endometriosis: a surgeon's perspective and review of 445 cases. Am J Surg 196:207–212
101. Houston DE, Noller KL, Melton J et al (1987) Incidence of pelvic endometriosis in Rochester, Minnesota, 1970–1979. Am J Epidemiol 125:959–969
102. Houston DE, Noller KL, Melton J III et al (1988) The epidemiology of pelvic endometriosis. Clin Obstet Gynecol 31:787–800
103. Hsu YK, Rosenshein NB, Parmley TH et al (1981) Leiomyomatosis in pelvic lymph nodes. Obstet Gynecol 57:91S–93S
104. Ishimaru T, Masuzaki H (1991) Peritoneal endometriosis: endometrial tissue implantation as its primary etiologic mechanism. Am J Obstet Gynecol 165:210–214
105. Ismail SM (1991) Cone biopsy causes cervical endometriosis and tubo-endometrioid metaplasia. Histopathology (Oxf) 18:107–114
106. Jaaback KS, Ludeman L, Clayton NL et al (2006) Primary peritoneal carcinoma in a UK cancer center: comparison with advanced ovarian carcinoma over a 5-year period. Int J Gynecol Cancer 16(suppl 1): 123–128
107. Jansen RPS, Russell P (1986) Nonpigmented endometriosis: clinical, laparoscopic, and pathologic definition. Am J Obstet Gynecol 155:1154–1159
108. Jaworski RC, Boadle R, Greg J et al (2001) Peritoneal "melanosis" associated with a ruptured ovarian dermoid cyst: report of a case with electron-probe energy dispersive X-ray analysis. Int J Gynecol Pathol 20:386–389
109. Kafiri G, Thomas DM, Shepherd NA et al (1992) p53 expression is common in malignant mesotheliomas. Histopathology (Oxf) 21:331–334
110. Kane C, Drouin P (1985) Obstructive uropathy associated with endometriosis. Am J Obstet Gynecol 151:207–211
111. Kapoor OP, Nathwani BN, Joshi VR (1972) Amoebic peritonitis. A study of 73 cases. J Trop Med Hyg 75:11–15
112. Karlan BY, Baldwin RL, Lopez-Luevanos E et al (1999) Peritoneal serous papillary carcinoma, a phenotypic variation of familial ovarian cancer: Implications for ovarian cancer screening. Am J Obstet Gynecol 180:917–928
113. Kazakov DV, Ondic O, Zamecnik M et al (2007) Morphological variations of scar-related and spontaneous endometriosis of the skin and superficial soft tissue: a study of 71 cases with emphasis on atypical features and types of müllerian differentiations. J Am Acad Dermatol 57:134–146
114. Kelly P, McCluggage WG, Gardiner KR et al (2008) Intestinal endometriosis morphologically mimicking colonic adenocarcinoma. Histopathology 52:510–514
115. Kempers RD, Dockerty MB, Hunt AB et al (1960) Significant postmenopausal endometriosis. Surg Gynecol Obstet 111: 348–356
116. Kern SB (1991) Prevalence of psammoma bodies in Papanicolaou-stained cervicovaginal smears. Acta Cytol 35:81–88
117. Kerner H, Gaton E, Czernobilsky B (1981) Unusual ovarian, tubal and pelvic mesothelial inclusions in patients with endometriosis. Histopathology (Oxf) 5:277–282

118. Kerrigan SAJ, Turnnir RT, Clement PB et al (2002) Diffuse malignant epithelial mesotheliomas of the peritoneum in women: a clinicopathologic study of 25 cases. Cancer 94:378–385
119. Kershisnik MM, Ro JY, Cannon GH et al (1994) Histiocytic reaction in pelvic peritoneum associated with oxidized regenerated cellulose. Am J Clin Pathol 103:27–31
120. Kheir SM, Mann WJ, Wilkerson JA (1981) Glandular inclusions in lymph nodes. The problem of extensive involvement and relationship to salpingitis. Am J Surg Pathol 5:353–359
121. Kim K, Scully RE (1990) Peritoneal keratin granulomas with carcinomas of endometrium and ovary and atypical polypoid adenomyoma of endometrium. A clinicopathological analysis of 22 cases. Am J Surg Pathol 14:925–932
122. Koc S, Beydilli G, Tulunay G et al (2006) Peritoneal tuberculosis mimicking advanced ovarian cancer: a retrospective review of 22 cases. Gynecol Oncol 103:565–569
123. Koninckx PR, Ide P, Vandenbroucke W et al (1980) New aspects of the pathophysiology of endometriosis and associated infertility. J Reprod Med 24:257–260
124. Kuo T, Hsueh S (1984) Mucicarminophilic histiocytosis. A polyvinylpyrrolidone (PVP) storage disease simulating signet-ring cell carcinoma. Am J Surg Pathol 8:419–428
125. LaGrenade A, Silverberg SG (1988) Ovarian tumors associated with atypical endometriosis. Hum Pathol 19:1080–1084
126. Lae ME, Roche PC, Jin L et al (2002) Desmoplastic small round cell tumor. A clinicopathological, immunohistochemical, and molecular study of 32 tumors. Am J Surg Pathol 26:823–835
127. Lamb K, Hoffmann RG, Nichols TR (1986) Family trait analysis: a case-control study of 43 women with endometriosis and their best friends. Am J Obstet Gynecol 154:596–601
128. Lauchlan SC (1972) The secondary müllerian system. Obstet Gynecol Surv 27:133–146
129. Lee I, Ching K, Pang M, Ho T (1996) Two cases of primary retroperitoneal mucinous cystadenocarcinoma. Gynecol Oncol 63: 145–150
130. Lee KR, Verma U, Belinson J (1991) Primary clear cell carcinoma of the peritoneum. Gynecol Oncol 41:259–262
131. Lessey BA, Metzger DA, Haney AF et al (1989) Immunohistochemical analysis of estrogen and progesterone receptors in endometriosis: comparison with normal endometrium during the menstrual cycle and the effect of medical therapy. Fertil Steril 51:409–415
132. Leyendecker G (2002) Endometriosis results from the dislocation of basalis endometrium. Hum Reprod 17:2736
133. Lim S, Kim JY, Park K et al (2003) Mullerianosis of the mesosalpinx: a case report. Int J Gynecol Pathol 22:209–212
134. Lin BT-Y, Colby T, Gown AM et al (1996) Malignant vascular tumors of the serous membranes mimicking mesothelioma. A report of 14 cases. Am J Surg Pathol 20:1431–1439
135. Lombardo L, Mateos JH, Barroeta FF (1968) Subarachnoid hemorrhage due to endometriosis of the spinal canal. Neurology 18:423–426
136. Mangano WE, Cagle PT, Churg A et al (1998) The diagnosis of desmoplastic malignant mesothelioma and its distinction from fibrous pleurisy. A histologic and immunohistochemical analysis of 31 cases including p53 immunostaining. Am J Clin Pathol 110:191–199
137. Martin DC, Hubert GD, Vander Zwaag R et al (1989) Laparoscopic appearances of peritoneal endometriosis. Fertil Steril 51:63–67
138. Martin JD Jr, Hauck AE (1985) Endometriosis in the male. Am Surg 51:426–430
139. Martinka M, Allaire C, Clement PB (1999) Endocervicosis presenting as a painful vaginal mass: a case report. Int J Gynecol Pathol 18:274–276
140. Matalliotakis TM, Cakmak H, Fragouli YG et al (2008) Epidemiological characteristics in women with and without endometriosis in the Yale series. Arch Gynecol Obstet 277:389–393
141. McCaughey WTE, Kirk ME, Lester W et al (1984) Peritoneal epithelial lesions associated with proliferative serous tumours of the ovary. Histopathology (Oxf) 8:195–208
142. McCluggage WG, Bryson C, Lamki H et al (2000) Benign, borderline, and malignant endometrioid neoplasia arising in endometriosis in association with tamoxifen therapy. Int J Gynecol Pathol 19:276–279
143. McCluggage WG, Oliva E, Herrington CS et al (2003) CD10 and calretinin staining of endocervical glandular lesions, endocervical stroma and endometrioid adenocarcinomas of the uterine corpus: CD10 positivity is characteristic of, but not specific for, mesonephric lesions and is not specific for endometrial stroma. Histopathology 43:144–150
144. McCoubrey A, Houghton O, McCallion K et al (2005) Serous adenocarcinoma of the sigmoid mesentery arising in cystic endosalpingiosis. J Clin Pathol 58:1221–1223
145. McFadden DE, Clement PB (1986) Peritoneal inclusion cysts with mural mesothelial proliferation. A clinicopathological analysis of six cases. Am J Surg Pathol 10:844–854
146. Merchant SH, Haghir S, Gordon GB (2000) Granulomatous peritonitis after laparoscopic cholecystectomy mimicking pelvic endometriosis. Obstet Gynecol 96:830–831
147. Metzger DA, Haney AF (1988) Endometriosis: etiology and pathophysiology of infertility. Clin Obstet Gynecol 31:801–812
148. Metzger DA, Lessey BA, Soper JT et al (1991) Hormone-resistant endometriosis following total abdominal hysterectomy and bilateral salpingo-oophorectomy: correlation with histology and steroid receptor content. Obstet Gynecol 78:946–950
149. Metzger DA, Olive DL, Haney AF (1988) Limited hormonal responsiveness of ectopic endometrium: histologic correlation with intrauterine endometrium. Hum Pathol 19:1417–1424
150. Michael H, Sutton G, Roth LM (1987) Ovarian carcinoma with extracellular mucin production: reassessment of "pseudomyxoma ovarii et peritonei". Int J Gynecol Pathol 6:298–312
151. Mikami M, Tei C, Takehara K et al (2003) Retroperitoneal primary mucinous adenocarcinoma with a mural nodule of anaplastic tumor: a case report and literature review. Int J Gynecol Pathol 22:205–208
152. Mills SE (1983) Decidua and squamous metaplasia in abdominopelvic lymph nodes. Int J Gynecol Pathol 2:209–215
153. Minaglia S, Mishell DR Jr, Ballard CA (2007) Incisional endometriomas after Cesarean section: a case series. J Reprod Med 52:630–634
154. Moloshok AA, Ivanko AI (1984) Endometriosis of the breast (an observation). Vopr Onkol 30:88–89
155. Mostoufizadeh M, Scully RE (1980) Malignant tumors arising in endometriosis. Clin Obstet Gynecol 23:951–963
156. Mourra N, Nion I, Parc R et al (2004) Squamous metaplasia of the peritoneum: a potential diagnostic pitfall. Histopathology 44:621–622
157. Muneyyirci-Delale O, Neil G, Serur E et al (1998) Endometriosis with massive ascites. Obstet Gynecol 69:42–46
158. Naresh KN, Ahuja VK, Rao CR et al (1991) Squamous cell carcinoma arising in endometriosis of the ovary. J Clin Pathol 44:958–959

159. Nascimento AF, Ruiz R, Hornick JL et al (2002) Calcifying fibrous 'pseudotumor': clinicopathologic study of 15 cases and analysis of its relationship to inflammatory myofibroblastic tumor. Int J Surg Pathol 10:189–196
160. Nazeer T, Ro JY, Tornos C et al (1996) Endocervical type glands in urinary bladder: a clinicopathologic study of six cases. Hum Pathol 27:816–820
161. Nisolle-Pochet M, Casanas-Roux F, Donnez J (1988) Histologic study of ovarian endometriosis after hormonal therapy. Fertil Steril 49:423
162. Nissim F, Ashkenazy M, Borenstein R et al (1981) Tuberculoid cornstarch granulomas with caseous necrosis. Arch Pathol Lab Med 105:86–88
163. Nonaka D, Kasamura S, Baratti D et al (2005) Diffuse malignant mesothelioma of the peritoneum. A clinicopathologic study of 35 patients treated locoregionally at a single institution. Cancer 104:2181–2188
164. Olive DL, Henderson DY (1987) Endometriosis and müllerian anomalies. Obstet Gynecol 69:412–415
165. Ordi J, de Alava E, Torné A et al (1998) Intraabdominal desmoplastic small round cell tumor with EWS/ERG fusion transcript. Am J Surg Pathol 22:1026–1032
166. Ordonez NG (1998) Desmoplastic small round cell tumor. I: A histopathologic study of 39 cases with emphasis on unusual histologic patterns. Am J Surg Pathol 22:1303–1313
167. Ordonez NG (1998) Desmoplastic small round cell tumor. II: An ultrastructural and immunohistochemical study with emphasis on new histochemical markers. Am J Surg Pathol 22:1303–1313
168. Ordóñez NG (2005) Mesothelioma with clear cell features: an ultrastructural and immunohistochemical study of 20 cases. Hum Pathol 36:465–473
169. Ordóñez NG (2005) Value of estrogen and progesterone receptor immunostaining in distinguishing between peritoneal mesotheliomas and serous carcinomas. Hum Pathol 36:1163–1167
170. Ordóñez NG (2006) Value of immunohistochemistry in distinguishing peritoneal mesothelioma from serous carcinoma of the ovary and peritoneum. A review and update. Adv Anat Pathol 13:16–25
171. Orezzoli JP, Russell AH, Oliva E et al (2008) Prognostic implication of endometriosis in clear cell carcinoma of the ovary. Gynecol Oncol 110:336–344
172. OuYang Z, Hirota Y, Osuga Y et al (2008) Interleukin-4 stimulates proliferation of endometriotic stromal cells. Am J Pathol 173:463–469
173. Padmanabhan V, Mount SL, Eltabbakh GH (2003) Peritoneal atypical mesothelial proliferation with progression to invasive mesothelioma: a case report and review of the literature. Pathology 35:260–263
174. Pai SA, Desai SB, Borges AM (1998) Uterus-like masses of the ovary associated with breast cancer and raised serum CA 125. Am J Surg Pathol 22:333–337
175. Park SA, Giannattasio C, Tancer ML (1981) Foreign body reaction to the intraperitoneal use of avitene. Obstet Gynecol 58:664–668
176. Parker RL, Dadmanesh F, Young RH et al (2004) Polypoid endometriosis: a clinicopathologic analysis of 24 cases and a review of the literature. Am J Surg Pathol 28:285–297
177. Paull T, Tedeschi LG (1972) Perineal endometriosis at the site of episiotomy scar. Obstet Gynecol 40:28–34
178. Pearl ML, Valea F, Chumas J et al (1996) Primary retroperitoneal mucinous cystadenocarcinoma of low malignant potential: a case report and literature review. Gynecol Oncol 61:150–152
179. Peress MR, Sosnowski JR, Mathur RS et al (1982) Pelvic endometriosis and Turner's syndrome. Am J Obstet Gynecol 144:474–476
180. Perrotta PL, Ginsburg FW, Siderides CI et al (1998) Liesegang rings and endometriosis. Int J Gynecol Pathol 17:358–362
181. Peterson VC, Underwood JCE, Wells M et al (2002) Primary endometrioid adenocarcinoma of the large intestine arising in colorectal endometriosis. Histopathology 40:171–176
182. Pettinato G, Manivel JC, De Rosa N et al (1990) Inflammatory myofibroblastic tumor (plasma cell granuloma). Clinicopathologic study of 20 cases with immunohistochemical and ultrastructural observations. Am J Clin Pathol 94:538–546
183. Possover M, Chiantera V (2007) Isolated infiltrative endometriosis of the sciatic nerve: a report of three patients. Fertil Steril 87(417):e17–e19
184. Prade M, Spatz A, Bentley R et al (1995) Borderline and malignant serous tumor arising in pelvic lymph nodes: evidence of origin in benign glandular inclusions. Int J Gynecol Pathol 14:87–91
185. Prefumo F, Venturini PL, Fulcheri E (2002) Analysis of p53 and c-erb-2 expression in ovarian endometrioid carcinomas arising in endometriosis. Int J Gynecol Pathol 22:83–88
186. Prowse AH, Manek S, Varma S et al (2006) Molecular genetic evidence that endometriosis is a precursor of ovarian cancer. Int J Cancer 119:556–562
187. Prystowsky JB, Stryker SJ, Ujiki GT et al (1988) Gastrointestinal endometriosis. Incidence and indications for resection. Arch Surg 123:855–858
188. Pueblitz-Peredo S, Luevano-Flores E, Rincon-Taracena R et al (1985) Uteruslike mass of the ovary: endomyometriosis or congenital malformation? A case with a discussion of histogenesis. Arch Pathol Lab Med 109:361–364
189. Punnonen R, Klemi PJ, Nikkanen V (1980) Postmenopausal endometriosis. Eur J Obstet Gynecol Reprod Biol 11:195–200
190. Quagliarello J, Coppa G, Bigelow B (1985) Isolated endometriosis in an inguinal hernia. Am J Obstet Gynecol 152:688–689
191. Rahilly MA, Al-Nafusi A (1991) Uterus-like mass of the ovary associated with endometrioid carcinoma. Histopathology (Oxf) 18:549–551
192. Redwine DB (1987) The distribution of endometriosis in the pelvis by age groups and fertility. Fertil Steril 47:173–175
193. Redwine DB (1989) Peritoneal pockets and endometriosis. Confirmation of an important relationship, with further observations. J Reprod Med 34:270–272
194. Reich H, De Caprio J, McGlynn F et al (1989) Peritoneal trophoblastic tissue implants after laparoscopic treatment of tubal ectopic pregnancy. Fertil Steril 52:337
195. Rock JA, Parmley TH, King TM et al (1981) Endometriosis and the development of tuboperitoneal fistulas after tubal ligation. Fertil Steril 35:16–20
196. Rosai J, Dehner LP (1975) Nodular mesothelial hyperplasia in hernia sacs. A benign reactive condition stimulating a neoplastic process. Cancer (Phila) 35:165–175
197. Ross MJ, Welch WR, Scully RE (1989) Multilocular peritoneal inclusion cysts (so-called cystic mesotheliomas). Cancer (Phila) 64:1336–1346
198. Roth LM (1973) Endometriosis with perineural involvement. Am J Clin Pathol 59:807–809
199. Ruffolo R, Suster S (1993) Diffuse histiocytic proliferation mimicking mesothelial hyperplasia in endocervicosis of the female pelvic peritoneum. Int J Surg Pathol 1:101–106
200. Rutgers JL, Scully RE (1988) Ovarian müllerian mucinous papillary cystadenomas of borderline malignancy. A clinicopathological analysis. Cancer (Phila) 61:340–348

201. Rutgers JL, Scully RE (1988) Ovarian mixed-epithelial papillary cystadenomas of borderline malignancy of mullerian type. A clinicopathological analysis. Cancer (Phila) 61:546–554
202. Rutgers JL, Young RH, Scully RE (1987) Ovarian yolk sac tumor arising from an endometrioid carcinoma. Hum Pathol 18:1296–1299
203. Sainz de la Cuesta R, Eichhorn JH, Rice LW et al (1996) Histologic transformation of benign endometriosis to early epithelial ovarian cancer. Gynecol Oncol 60:238–244
204. Sainz de al Cuesta R, Izquierdo M, Cañamero M et al (2004) Increased prevalence of p53 overexpression from typical endomteriosis to atypical endometriosis and ovarian cancer associated with endometriosis. Eur J Obstet Gynecol Reprod Biol 113:87–93
205. Sampson JA (1927) Peritoneal endometriosis due to the menstrual dissemination of endometrial tissue into the peritoneal cavity. Am J Obstet Gynecol 14:422–469
206. Sasson IE, Taylor HS (2008) Stem cells and the pathogenesis of endometriosis. Ann N Y Acad Sci 1127:106–115
207. Sato N, Tsunoda H, Nishida M et al (2000) Loss of heterozygosity on 10q.23.3 and mutation of the tumor suppressor gene PTEN in benign endometrial cysts of the ovary: possible sequence progression from benign endometrial cyst to endometrioid carcinoma and clear cell carcinoma of the ovary. Cancer Res 60:7052–7056
208. Sawh RN, Malpica A, Deavers MT et al (2003) Benign cystic mesothelioma of the peritoneum: a clinicopathologic study of 17 cases and immunohistochemical analysis of estrogen and progesterone receptor status. Hum Pathol 34:369–374
209. Schlesinger C, Silverberg SG (1999) Tamoxifen-associated polyps (basalomas) arising in multiple endometriotic foci: a case report and review of the literature. Gynecol Oncol 73:305–311
210. Schmidt CL, Demopoulos RI, Weiss G (1981) Infected endometriotic cysts: clinical characterization and pathogenesis. Fertil Steril 36:27–30
211. Scully RE (1981) Smooth-muscle differentiation in genital tract disorders (Editorial). Arch Pathol Lab Med 105:505–507
212. Seidman JD (1996) Prognostic importance of hyperplasia and atypia in endometriosis. Int J Gynecol Pathol 15:1–9
213. Seidman JD, Elsayed AM, Sobin LH et al (1993) Association of mucinous tumors of the ovary and appendix. A clinicopathologic study of 25 cases. Am J Surg Pathol 17:22–34
214. Shia J, Erlandson R, Klimstra DS (2002) Deciduoid mesothelioma: a report of 5 cases and literature review. Ultrastruct Pathol 26:355–363
215. Shiraki M, Otis CN, Powell JL (1991) Endometrial stromal sarcoma arising from ovarian and extraovarian endometriosis: report of two cases and review of the literature. Surg Pathol 4:333–343
216. Sidaway MK, Silverberg SG (1987) Endosalpingiosis in female peritoneal washings: a diagnostic pitfall. Int J Gynecol Pathol 6:340–346
217. Sigel JE, Smith TA, Reith JD et al (2001) Immunohistochemical analysis of anaplastic lymphoma kinase expression in deep soft tissue calcifying fibrous pseudotumor: evidence of a late sclerosing stage of inflammatory myofibroblastic tumor? Ann Diagn Pathol 5:10–14
218. Simpson JL, Elias S, Malinak LR et al (1980) Heritable aspects of endometriosis. I. Genetic studies. Am J Obstet Gynecol 137: 327–331
219. Slavin RE, Krum R, Van Dinh T (2000) Endometriosis-associated intestinal tumors: a clinical and pathological study of 6 cases with a review of the literature. Hum Pathol 31:456–463
220. Sohar E, Gafni J, Pras M et al (1967) Familial Mediterranean fever. A survey of 470 cases and review of the literature. Am J Med 43:227–253
221. Staats PN, Clement PB, Young RH (2007) Primary endometrioid adenocarcinoma of the vagina: a clinicopathologic study of 18 cases. Am J Surg Pathol 31:1490–1501
222. Staats PN, McCluggage WG, Clement PB et al (2008) Luteinized thecomas (thecomatosis) of the type typically associated with sclerosing peritonitis: a clinical, histopathologic, and immunohistochemical analysis of 27 cases. Am J Surg Pathol 32:1273–1290
223. Stanley KE, Utz DC, Dockerty MB (1965) Clinically significant endometriosis of the urinary tract. Surg Gynecol Obstet 120:491–498
224. Steck WD, Helwig EB (1966) Cutaneous endometriosis. Clin Obstet Gynecol 9:373–383
225. Steele RW, Dmowski WP, Marmer DJ (1984) Immunologic aspects of human endometriosis. Am J Reprod Immunol 6:33–36
226. Stripling MC, Martin DC, Chatman DL et al (1988) Subtle appearance of pelvic endometriosis. Fertil Steril 49:427–431
227. Sumathi VP, McCluggage WG (2002) CD10 is useful in demonstrating endometrial stroma at ectopic sites and confirming a diagnosis of endometriosis. J Clin Pathol 55:391–392
228. Sun CJ, Toker C, Masi JD et al (1979) Primary low grade adenocarcinoma occurring in the inguinal region. Cancer (Phila) 44:340–345
229. Sussman J, Rosai J (1990) Lymph node metastasis as the initial manifestation of malignant mesothelioma. Report of six cases. Am J Surg Pathol 14:818–828
230. Sznurkowski JJ, Emerich J (2008) Endometriomas are more frequent on the left side. Acta Obstet Gynecol Scand 87:104–106
231. Szyfelbein WM, Baker PM, Bell DA (2004) Superficial endometriosis of the cervix: a source of abnormal glandular cells on cervicovaginal smears. Diagn Cytopathol 30:88–91
232. Taheri ZM, Mehrafza M, Mohammadi F et al (2008) The diagnostic value of Ki-67 and repp 86 in distinguishing between benign and malignant mesothelial proliferations. Arch Pathol Lab Med 132:694–697
233. Thatcher SS, Grainger DA, True LD et al (1989) Pelvic trophoblastic implants after laparoscopic removal of a tubal pregnancy. Obstet Gynecol 74:514–515
234. Thibodeau LL, Prioleau GR, Manuelidis EE et al (1987) Cerebral endometriosis. J Neurosurg 66:609–610
235. Toki T, Fujii S, Silverberg SG (1996) A clinicopathologic study of the association of endometriosis and carcinoma of the ovary using a scoring system. Int J Gynecol Cancer 6:68–75
236. Truong LD, Maccato ML, Awalt H et al (1990) Serous surface carcinoma of the peritoneum: a clinicopathologic study of 22 cases. Hum Pathol 21:99–110
237. Ulbright TM, Morley DJ, Roth LM et al (1983) Papillary serous carcinoma of the retroperitoneum. Am J Clin Pathol 79:633–637
238. Vadlamudi G, Graebe R, Khoo M et al (1997) Gallstones implanting in the ovary. A complication of laparoscopic cholecystectomy. Arch Pathol Lab Med 121:155–158
239. Vuong PN, Guyot H, Moulin G et al (1990) Pseudotumoral organization of a twisted epiploic fringe or 'hard-boiled egg' in the peritoneal cavity. Arch Pathol Lab Med 114:531–533
240. Walter AJ, Hentz JG, Magtibay PM et al (2001) Endometriosis: correlation between histologic and visual findings at laparoscopy. Am J Obstet Gynecol 184:1407–1413

241. Wanless IR, Bernier V (1983) Fibrous thickening of the splenic capsule. Arch Pathol Lab Med 107:595–599
242. Weinstein MP, Iannini PB, Stratton CW et al (1978) Spontaneous bacterial peritonitis. A review of 28 cases with emphasis on improved survival and factors influencing prognosis. Am J Med 64:592–598
243. Weir M, Bell DA, Young RH (1998) Grade 1 peritoneal serous carcinomas. A report of 14 cases and comparison with 7 peritoneal serous psammocarcinomas and 19 peritoneal serous borderline tumors. Am J Surg Pathol 22:849–862
244. White J, Chan Y-F (1994) Lipofuscinosis peritonei associated with pregancy-related ectopic decidua. Histopathology (Oxf) 25:83–85
245. Williams TJ, Pratt JH (1977) Endometriosis in 1,000 consecutive celiotomies: incidence and management. Am J Obstet Gynecol 129:245–250
246. Wu DC, Hirschowit S, Natarajan S (2005) Ectopic decidua of pelvic lymph nodes: a potential diagnostic pitfall. Arch Pathol Lab Med 129:e117–e120
247. Wu Y, Strawn E, Basir Z et al (2006) Genomic alterations in ectopic and eutopic endometria of women with endometriosis. Gynecol Obstet Invest 62:148–159
248. Yamamoto S, Tsuda H, Takano M et al (2008) Clear-cell adenofibroma can be a clonal precursor for clear-cell adenocarcinoma of the ovary: a possible alternative ovarian clear-cell carcinogenic pathway. J Pathol 216(1):103–110
249. Yantiss RK, Clement PB, Young RH (2000) Neoplastic and pre-neoplastic changes in gastrointestinal endometriosis: A study of 17 cases. Am J Surg Pathol 24:513–524
250. Yantiss RK, Clement PB, Young RH (2001) Endometriosis of the intestinal tract. A study of 44 cases of a disease that may cause diverse challenges in clinical and pathological evaluation. Am J Surg Pathol 25:445–454
251. Yantiss RK, Nielsen GP, Lauwers GY et al (2003) Reactive nodular fibrous pseudotumor of the gastrointestinal tract and mesentery. Am J Surg Pathol 27:532–540
252. Young RH, Clement PB (1996) Müllerianosis of the urinary bladder. Mod Pathol 9:731–737
253. Young RH, Clement PB (2000) Endocervicosis involving the uterine cervix: a report of four cases of a benign process that may be confused with deeply invasive endocervical adenocarcinoma. Int J Gynecol Pathol 19:322–328
254. Young RH, Clement PB, McCaughey WTE (1990) Solitary fibrous tumors ("fibrous mesotheliomas") of the peritoneum: a report of three cases. Arch Pathol Lab Med 114:493–495
255. Young RH, Eichhorn JH, Dickersin GR et al (1992) Ovarian involvement by the intra-abdominal desmoplastic small round cell tumor with divergent differentiation: a report of three cases. Hum Pathol 23:454–464
256. Young RH, Prat J, Scully RE (1984) Endometrioid stromal sarcomas of the ovary. A clinicopathologic analysis of 23 cases. Cancer (Phila) 53:1143–1155
257. Young RH, Scully RE (1986) Testicular and paratesticular tumors and tumor-like lesions of ovarian common epithelial and müllerian types. A report of four cases and review of the literature. Am J Clin Pathol 86:146–152
258. Zhang PJ, Goldblum JR, Pawel BR et al (2003) Immunophenotype of desmoplastic small round cell tumors as detected in cases with EWS/WT1 gene fusion product. Mod Pathol 16:229–235
259. Zinsser KR, Wheeler JE (1982) Endosalpingiosis in the omentum. A study of autopsy and surgical material. Am J Surg Pathol 6:109–117

14 Surface Epithelial Tumors of the Ovary

Jeffrey D. Seidman · Kathleen R. Cho · Brigitte M. Ronnett · Robert J. Kurman

R. J. Kurman, L. Hedrick Ellenson, B. M. Ronnett (eds.), *Blaustein's Pathology of the Female Genital Tract (6th ed.)*, DOI 10.1007/978-1-4419-0489-8_14,

Epidemiology

Geographic Distribution, Incidence and Mortality

Worldwide, ovarian cancer is the sixth most common cancer in women and the seventh most common cause of cancer death. There are about 204,000 new cases and 125,000 deaths annually [29]. In most Western countries, ovarian carcinoma is the fifth most common malignancy and ranks fourth in cancer mortality. In the Western hemisphere, it accounts for 4% of cancer in women and is the most frequent cause of death due to gynecological cancer. In US women, ovarian cancer ranks ninth in incidence and fifth in mortality, and accounts for 3% of cancers diagnosed and 5% of cancer deaths. It is estimated that in the United States in 2010, there were 21,880 new ovarian cancer cases and 13,850 deaths [137]. Approximately 1.4% of American women will develop ovarian cancer in their lifetime. In general, the disease is more common in industrialized countries where parity is lower, but there are notable exceptions such as Japan which has a low parity and low rate of ovarian cancer. The incidence varies widely among different ethnic groups. The lifetime risk varies widely from 0.45% in Japan to 1.7% in Sweden. Annual incidence rates of ovarian cancer range from less than 5 per 100,000 women in The Gambia, Brazil, Thailand, Algeria, and India, to greater than 13 per 100,000 in the United Kingdom, United States, Germany, and Scandinavia. In the United States, based on SEER (Surveillance, Epidemiology, and End Results (US National Cancer Institute)) data, the rate is 13.5 per 100,000 (2000–2004) [340]. Scandinavia has one of the highest annual incidence rates at greater than 16 per 100,000 women [337]. There has been little change in incidence over the past few decades with a few exceptions: in Korea, the age-standardized incidence increased by 25% from 3.8 to 4.7 per 100,000 from 1993 to 2002 [57], and over the same period, the incidence in Israel decreased by nearly one third from 9.6 to 6.6 per 100,000 [217]. The extent to which changes in diagnostic criteria or calculation methods may account for these changes is unclear. However, in the United States, changing the age-adjustment to the 2000 standard has artificially increased the incidence of ovarian cancer by about 20% [9]. In addition, the incidence of ovarian carcinoma appears to have decreased as peritoneal and tubal carcinomas have increased [110]. This may reflect a recent increase in the awareness of peritoneal and particularly tubal carcinomas among pathologists. Accordingly, relatively small changes in the incidence of ovarian carcinoma are probably due to these factors. Migration studies have shown that ovarian cancer rates approach those of the place of immigration rather than the place of emigration, suggesting a significant environmental component to ovarian cancer risk.

Ovarian cancer rates vary among different ethnic groups. White women have higher rates than blacks and Asians; in the United States, African-American women have a rate two thirds that of white women, and Asians have a 48% lower death rate than whites [340]. In Israel, Jewish women have a risk eightfold that of non-Jewish women as 1 of 40 Jewish women have a *BRCA1* mutation [184].

Epidemiologic studies of ovarian cancer rely on accurate tumor classification. It has become apparent that a large proportion of mucinous carcinomas involving the ovaries are actually metastatic from elsewhere. The specific association of smoking with ovarian mucinous carcinoma is interesting, since some smoking-associated extraovarian mucinous carcinomas such as pancreatic cancer can mimic primary ovarian mucinous tumors when they metastasize to the ovary. This suggests that misclassification of ovarian mucinous tumors has had an effect on epidemiological studies (see ➲ Mucinous Tumors, later in this chapter).

The large volume of literature on atypical proliferative (borderline) tumors belies their low prevalence. Large institutions such as Stanford University [190] and Washington Hospital Center encounter only about three atypical proliferative serous tumors (APSTs) per year in-house. Two general hospitals in Barcelona had fewer than 5 per year combined [262]. Population-based incidence data on borderline tumors are scant; in the United States, the annual incidence is 2.5 per 100,000 (1.5 per 100,000 for serous tumors in white women) [222] and in Sweden, 6.6 per 100,000 (all borderline tumors) [111].

Etiology and Risk Factors

Age

Ovarian cancer rates increase with age. In the United States, the annual incidence steadily increases from less than 3 per 100,000 in women age less than 30, and plateaus at 54 per 100,000 in the 75–79-year age group. In the United States, the median age of women with ovarian cancer is about 63 years at diagnosis, and the median age at death 71 years [340]. In the 40–59-year and 60–79-year age groups, ovarian cancer ranks fourth and fifth, respectively, in cancer deaths in US women [136]. The mean age varies substantially among subgroups, a reflection of differences in hereditary syndromes and differences in the pathogenesis of different types of ovarian carcinoma

Table 14.1
Mean age in subgroups of ovarian cancer (years)

Lynch syndrome II-associated carcinoma	40
Well-differentiated (micropapillary) serous carcinoma	43–45
Endometrioid carcinoma arising in endometriosis	50
BRCA1-associated carcinoma	53
FIGO stage I carcinoma	53
Clear cell carcinoma	50–53
Endometrioid carcinoma	55–58
BRCA2-associated carcinoma	59
FIGO stage III high-grade serous carcinoma	59–64
Carcinosarcoma (malignant mixed müllerian tumor (MMMT))	64–66

(*Table 14.1*) (See Morphologic and Molecular Pathogenesis, later in this chapter).

Many studies have shown that age is an independent prognostic factor [106, 377], but these data are difficult to evaluate as there are multiple interacting factors involved. To some extent, age-related prognostic differences are largely explained by higher proportions of low-grade, low-stage, optimally debulked, and Type I tumors (see Morphologic and Molecular Pathogenesis, later in this chapter) in younger patients, who are also generally healthier than older patients, who are more likely to have a lower performance status, more comorbid conditions, and have a lower likelihood of responding to chemotherapy [8, 350]. Older women are also treated less aggressively than younger women; in the SEER database, over 40% of American women older than 85 years did not receive definitive treatment.

The risk of death in the presence of comorbid conditions is 30–40% higher than those without such conditions [8]. A population-based study in Maryland showed that women aged more than 50 years are more than twice as likely as younger women to die within 30 days after surgery (mortality rates of 2.6% and 1.2%, respectively; $p = 0.010$) [348]. Accordingly, younger women with invasive ovarian cancer on average do have a more favorable stage distribution and other prognostically favorable features and thus a better prognosis, even when stratified by stage.

Reproductive Factors

Evidence suggests that reproductive factors are important in ovarian cancer risk. Established protective factors include increasing parity and oral contraceptive use [62]. Early menarche and late menopause are significant risk factors. Pregnancies appear to be more strongly protective for endometrioid and clear cell carcinoma as compared to serous carcinoma [166]. High socioeconomic status is associated with an increased ovarian cancer risk and lower fertility. Several recent meta-analyses of hormone replacement therapy and ovarian cancer risk have shown a slightly but significantly elevated risk with odds ratios of 1.1–1.3 [397]. The protective effect of increased parity and oral contraceptive use applies only to non-mucinous tumors. However, as noted earlier, data on mucinous carcinomas of the ovary prior to the mid- to late-1990s are unreliable because a large proportion of apparent primary ovarian mucinous carcinomas have now been recognized to be metastatic (see Mucinous Tumors, later in this chapter, and Chap. 18, Metastatic Tumors of the Ovary).

Surgically induced protective factors include hysterectomy, tubal ligation, and bilateral salpingo-oophorectomy. The mechanism for risk reduction with hysterectomy and tubal ligation is unclear, although both can prevent passage of endometrial tissue via retrograde menstruation, which is one of the proposed mechanisms for the development of endometriosis, and endometriosis is a precursor of some ovarian cancers [345] (See Endometrioid Carcinoma Arising in Endometriosis, later in this chapter). This mechanism is further supported by the finding that the frequency of clear cell carcinoma is inversely related to tubal ligation to a stronger degree than other cell types, and clear cell carcinoma, among all types of ovarian carcinomas, has the highest association with endometriosis [166, 255, 256]. In addition, hysterectomy and tubal ligation prevent the introduction of a variety of potential environmental carcinogens from entering the peritoneal cavity and thereby coming into contact with tubal and ovarian tissue.

Ovulation and Hormonal Factors

The most commonly cited hormonal mechanism for the etiology of ovarian cancer is the incessant ovulation hypothesis. It was hypothesized that ovulation repeatedly traumatizes the ovarian surface epithelium and thus stimulates proliferation, creating a milieu that predisposes the actively proliferating epithelium to malignant transformation. This hypothesis is supported by epidemiologic observations of a direct correlation between the number of ovulations, i.e., the length of the reproductive years uninterrupted by pregnancies or oral contraceptive use, and the risk of ovarian cancer. Most of these studies report a 50% reduction of ovarian cancer in women who have been on oral contraceptives. Moreover, the longer the duration of usage, the greater is the protective effect. The gonadotropin hypothesis, which is less favored than the incessant ovulation hypothesis, proposes that high levels of circulating gonadotropins increase the risk of ovarian cancer either directly by altering estrogen levels or via mechanisms that cause primary ovarian failure. Another hypothesis proposes that androgen levels are important. At present, no clear-cut hormonal explanation for ovarian carcinogenesis is known.

Inflammation

It has been suggested that inflammation, potentially incited by ovulation-induced surface damage [233], by retrograde menstruation-induced salpingitis [287], or by the introduction of foreign material through the vagina and uterine cavity, plays an important role in ovarian carcinogenesis. Evidence of a proinflammatory microenvironment in endometriosis supports this hypothesis for Type I tumors [95]. High-grade serous carcinomas are associated with chronic salpingitis in 53% of cases, significantly more often than 23% seen with non-serous tumors, lending circumstantial support to this hypothesis [309].

Other Risk Factors

Other potential risk factors have been studied, but associations with ovarian cancer risk are weak or inconclusive. These include body mass index, age at birth of first child, breastfeeding, weight, diet, talc, smoking, certain types of viral infections in childhood, and ionizing radiation. A study of 49,000 women showed a reduction in ovarian cancer risk in postmenopausal women on a low-fat diet, with a hazard ratio of 0.6 [264].

Morphologic and Molecular Pathogenesis

Ovarian carcinogenesis can be divided into two broad phases: malignant transformation and peritoneal dissemination. Until recently, some investigators believed that benign, "borderline," and malignant ovarian tumors reflect sequential steps in malignant transformation, regardless of their type of differentiation (i.e., serous, mucinous, endometrioid, or clear cell). Accordingly, many studies in the cell and molecular biology literature juxtaposed these entities in an attempt to elucidate the events in ovarian carcinogenesis, and often considered the different histological types of ovarian tumors essentially interchangeable. Further, the traditional view of peritoneal dissemination was that carcinoma begins in the ovary, undergoes progressive dedifferentiation from a well to a poorly differentiated tumor, and then spreads through the peritoneal cavity before metastasizing to distant sites. These time-honored views now do not appear to be valid for the majority of ovarian cancers as described below.

A New Model of Ovarian Cancer Pathogenesis

Advances in molecular biology correlated with morphologic studies aimed at investigating the relationship of borderline tumors to invasive carcinoma have shed new light on the pathogenesis of ovarian carcinoma and have challenged many of the time-honored concepts of ovarian neoplasia. These studies have led to the proposal of a new model of carcinogenesis, which has important clinical implications. In addition, recent studies have provided evidence that what has traditionally been regarded as the origin of ovarian carcinoma, namely the surface epithelium, may rather be the fallopian tube in many cases. Accordingly, the view that ovarian cancer begins in the ovary and spreads systematically to the pelvis, abdomen, and then distant sites is being challenged and the concept that ovarian carcinoma, over time, progresses from well to poorly differentiated does not appear to be valid. This section will summarize these new developments in our understanding of ovarian carcinogenesis and are discussed in greater detail in the individual sections on the different cell types later in the chapter.

Mounting clinicopathologic and molecular genetic data have led to the proposal of a new model of ovarian carcinogenesis that reconciles the differing relationships of borderline and malignant tumors that exist among the different cell types of ovarian cancer. This model divides surface epithelial tumors into two broad categories: Type I and Type II, based on their clinicopathologic features and characteristic molecular genetic changes [56, 167, 168, 170]. Type I and Type II refer to tumorigenic pathways and are not histopathologic diagnostic terms (➲ *Fig. 14.1* and ➲ *Table 14.2*). This classification system will undoubtedly continue to evolve, particularly as the molecular changes that characterize the less common types of ovarian carcinomas and the distinction between morphologically overlapping categories (e.g., high-grade serous versus high-grade endometrioid) become more clearly defined.

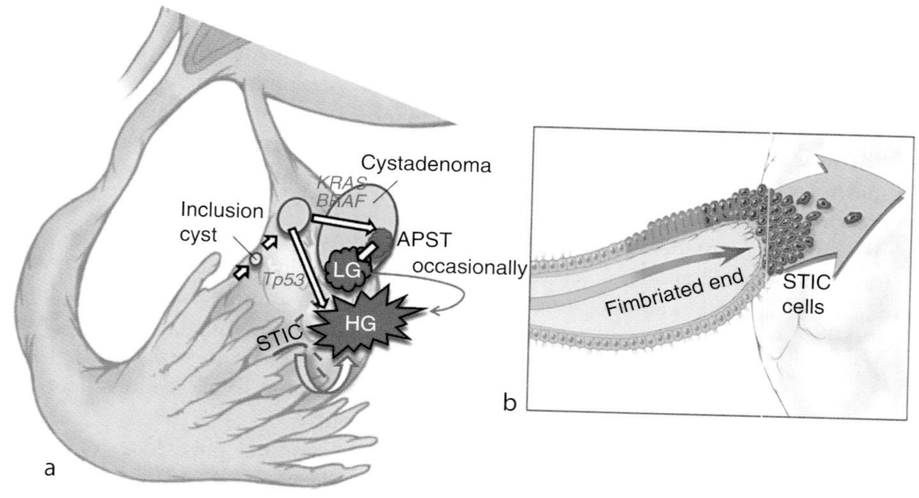

Fig. 14.1a
Schematic of proposed origin of high-grade serous carcinoma. **(a) STIC cells from fimbrial epithelium and occasionally cells from ovarian surface epithelial inclusions via cystadenomas and atypical proliferative serous tumors (APST) can develop into high-grade serous carcinoma (b) STIC cells implanting on ovarian surface**

Table 14.2
Type 1 versus type 2 ovarian carcinoma: precursors and molecular features

	Common precursors	Most frequent mutations	Chromosomal instability[a]
Type I tumors			
Low-grade serous CA	APST, noninvasive MPSC	KRAS, BRAF	Low
Low-grade endometrioid CA	Endometriosis	CTNNB1, PTEN	Low
Clear cell CA[b]	Endometriosis	PIK3CA	Low
Mucinous CA	APMT	KRAS	Low
Type II tumors			
High-grade serous CA	U[c]	TP53	High
High-grade endometrioid CA	U	TP53	High
Undifferentiated CA	U	U	U
Carcinosarcoma	U	TP53	U

[a]Low versus high chromosomal instability refers to comparison between low-grade and high-grade carcinomas within the same histologic type.
[b]Criteria for classification of clear cell carcinoma into type I versus type II subsets are uncertain (see text).
[c]Some high-grade carcinomas may be associated with tubal intraepithelial serous carcinomas.
APMT, atypical proliferative mucinous tumor; APST, atypical proliferative serous tumor; CA, carcinoma; MPSC, micropapillary serous carcinoma; U, unknown.
Modified with permission of the author [56].

Type I tumors are low grade, relatively indolent neoplasms that arise from well-characterized precursor lesions (atypical proliferative (borderline) tumors and endometriosis), and usually present as large stage I neoplasms. This group includes low-grade serous (invasive micropapillary serous carcinoma (MPSC)), low-grade endometrioid, mucinous, and tentatively clear cell carcinomas. Clear cell carcinoma, although it exhibits most of the features of the Type I tumors such as association with a well-established precursor (endometriosis) and frequent presentation in stage I, is typically high grade unlike the other Type I tumors. Nonetheless, preliminary molecular genetic data show a greater similarity of clear cell carcinoma to Type I as compared to Type II tumors.

Type I tumors often harbor somatic mutations of genes encoding protein kinases including *KRAS, BRAF, PIK3CA*, and *ERBB2*, as well as other signaling molecules including *PTEN* and *CTNNB1* (β-catenin). The atypical proliferative or borderline serous and mucinous tumors in turn appear to develop from cystadenomas, while the atypical proliferative endometrioid and clear cell tumors arise from endometriosis, typically endometriotic cysts (endometriomas) (*Fig. 14.1b*).

In contrast, Type II tumors, of which the vast majority are high-grade serous carcinomas, are aggressive, high-grade neoplasms from the outset; in the past, they have been said to arise "de novo." Recent data, however, suggest that high-grade serous carcinomas arise from intraepithelial carcinomas, the majority of which have been detected in the tubal fimbriae (see Chap. 11, Diseases of the Fallopian Tube and Paratubal Region). At this time it is not clear as to what proportion of high-grade serous carcinomas arise from the tube. More than 75% of Type II carcinomas have *TP53* mutations. Interestingly, the few examples of stage I high-grade serous carcinomas that have been studied have been shown to harbor mutations of *TP53* [183]. Therefore, it appears that conventional high-grade serous carcinoma even in its earliest stage of development resembles advanced-stage serous carcinoma at both the morphologic and molecular level. Of further interest has been the detection of *TP53* mutations in tubal intraepithelial carcinomas, and in a recently described putative precursor lesion of tubal intraepithelial carcinoma designated "p53 signature." This lesion appears morphologically normal but overexpresses p53, and can harbor a p53 mutation. These findings highlight the importance of p53 mutation in the early development of high-grade serous carcinoma [149]. These findings have important clinical implications (see Screening and Prevention).

The anatomical progression of ovarian carcinoma is poorly understood. It is generally assumed that carcinoma originates in the ovary, is confined to the ovary for a period of time, and then disseminates to the pelvis, followed by the abdominal cavity before spreading to distant sites. This view underlies the basis of the International Federation of Gynecology and Obstetrics (FIGO) staging system in which tumors confined to the ovary are stage I, those involving the pelvic organs stage II, with involvement of abdominal organs stage III, and when spread occurs to distant sites stage IV (*Table 14.3*). There are, however, significant problems with this assumption. Clinicopathologic comparison of stage I with stage III carcinomas shows that stage I tumors are predominantly Type I and non-serous, while stage III tumors are predominantly Type II and most often high-grade serous; furthermore, stage I tumors tend to be significantly larger, an observation that would suggest that ovarian carcinomas get smaller with progression [389].

It is important to recognize that Type II ovarian carcinomas account for the vast majority of ovarian cancer deaths. Most Type II tumors are high-grade serous carcinomas, and, at the time of diagnosis, most are widely disseminated throughout the peritoneum (FIGO stage III and IV), with the largest volume of tumor outside the ovaries. Serous carcinoma and its variants (peritoneal serous carcinoma, carcinosarcoma, undifferentiated carcinoma, and mixed carcinomas with a high-grade serous component) account for 87% of cases of carcinomatosis from ovarian carcinoma and accordingly the vast majority of ovarian cancer deaths [107, 114, 301] (*Table 14.4*). These data that analyze stage distribution by histologic type suggest that early and advanced stage tumors are fundamentally different diseases, and provide further support for the dualistic model [154, 168, 389].

Like other cancers, ovarian carcinomas arise through a multistep process in which clonal selection acts on

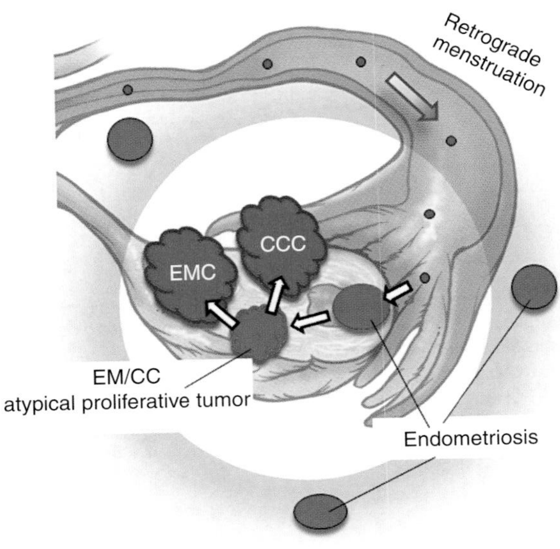

Fig. 14.1b
Schematic of the proposed origin of type I tumors. **Retrograde menstruation leads to the development of endometriosis and atypical proliferative tumors which can give rise to endometrioid and clear cell carcinomas**

Table 14.3

Carcinoma of the ovary: International Federation of Gynecology and Obstetrics (FIGO) nomenclature (Rio de Janeiro 1988)

Stage I	Growth limited to the ovaries
Ia	Growth limited to one ovary; no ascites present containing malignant cells. No tumor on the external surface; capsule intact
Ib	Growth limited to both ovaries; no ascites present containing malignant cells. No tumor on the external surfaces; capsules intact
Ic[a]	Tumor either stage Ia or Ib, but with tumor on surface of one or both ovaries, or with capsule ruptured, or with ascites present containing malignant cells, or with positive peritoneal washings
Stage II	Growth involving one or both ovaries with pelvic extension
IIa	Extension and/or metastases to the uterus and/or tubes
IIb	Extension to other pelvic tissues
IIc[a]	Tumor either stage IIa or IIb, but with tumor on surface of one or both ovaries; or with capsule(s) ruptured; or with ascites present containing malignant cells or with positive peritoneal washings
Stage III	Tumor involving one or both ovaries with histologically confirmed peritoneal implants outside the pelvis and/or positive retroperitoneal or inguinal nodes. Superficial liver metastases equals stage III. Tumor is limited to the true pelvis, but with histologically proven malignant extension to small bowel or omentum
IIIa	Tumor grossly limited to the true pelvis, with negative nodes, but with histologically confirmed microscopic seeding of abdominal peritoneal surfaces, or histologic-proven extension to small bowel or mesentery
IIIb	Tumor of one or both ovaries with histologically confirmed implants, peritoneal metastasis of abdominal peritoneal surfaces, none exceeding 2 cm in diameter; nodes are negative
IIIc	Peritoneal metastasis beyond the pelvis; 2 cm in diameter and/or positive retroperitoneal or inguinal nodes
Stage IV	Growth involving one or both ovaries with distant metastases. If pleural effusion is present, there must be positive cytology to allot a case to stage IV; parenchymal liver metastasis equals stage IV

[a]To evaluate the impact on prognosis of the different criteria for allotting cases to stage Ic or IIc; it would be of value to know if rupture of the capsule was spontaneous, or caused by the surgeon; and if the source of malignant cells detected was peritoneal washings, or ascites.
From Heintz et al.

cells with somatic mutations and altered gene expression to allow outgrowth of progeny with increasingly aggressive growth properties. The genes mutated in cancer are not selected randomly, but frequently encode proteins that function in highly conserved signaling pathways. Over the past several years, a number of studies have evaluated ovarian epithelial tumors for molecular genetic alterations such as point mutations, gene amplifications, deletions, and translocations. The molecular biology and genetics of ovarian cancer have been recently reviewed [56]. Although a detailed cataloguing of the genetic alterations identified to date in ovarian epithelial tumors is beyond the scope of this chapter, some useful themes have emerged. First, while few if any changes appear to be unique to ovarian cancer, studies have shown that certain alterations appear to be particularly characteristic of specific histological types of ovarian carcinomas. Second, for carcinomas with serous or endometrioid differentiation, specific genetic alterations distinguish low-grade from high-grade carcinomas. Third, identification of shared genetic alterations in some histological types of ovarian carcinomas and their putative precursor lesions has provided useful insights into the pathogenetic pathways leading to ovarian cancer. Details of the molecular biology of the different cell types of ovarian carcinoma are reviewed in their respective sections later in this chapter.

Putative Histopathologic Precursor Lesions

The study of precursors of ovarian carcinoma is difficult because the ovaries are not readily accessible for screening, and ovarian carcinomas typically present in advanced stage, obliterating or rendering unrecognizable any precursor lesion that may have been present. Furthermore, identification of a putative precursor lesion is based on microscopic examination of a complete resection, and therefore the natural history of the lesion cannot be observed. Studies on ovaries removed prophylactically

Table 14.4
Distribution of ovarian carcinoma by cell type and FIGO stage, Washington Hospital Center, 1991–2009 (% in parentheses)

	I[a] no. (%)	II no. (%)	III no. (%)	IV no. (%)	Total no. (%)
Serous, high grade	10 (2.5)	7 (1.5)	148 (34)	49 (11)	214 (49)
Serous, low grade[d]	0	0	14 (3)	3 (0.5)	17(4)
Serous peritoneal	0	1 (0)	43 (10)	18 (4)	62 (14)
Endometrioid	16 (3.5)	6 (1.5)	8 (2)	2 (0.5)	32 (7.5)
Clear cell	13 (3)	8 (2)	11 (2.5)	5 (1)	37 (8.5)
Mucinous	11 (2.5)	0	2 (0.5)	0	13 (3)
Seromucinous	3 (0.5)	1 (0)	1 (0)	0	5 (1)
Transitional	2 (0.5) [1[b]]	0	[6[b]]	0	2 (0.5)
Mixed	4 (1)	2 (0.5)	9 (2)	3 (0.5)	18 (4.0)
Undifferentiated	0	0	1 (0)	0	1 (0)
Carcinosarcoma	1 (0)	3 (0.5)	23 (5.5)[c]	5 (1)	32 (7.5)
Squamous	0	0	0	2 (0.5)	2 (0.5)
Total	60 (14)	28 (6.5)	260 (60)	87 (20)	435

[a]Only 41 (68%) of stage I tumors were comprehensively staged, including 5 high-grade serous carcinomas.
[b]There were two stage I malignant Brenner tumors. We classify transitional cell carcinomas (TCCs) as serous carcinoma; the remaining seven cases are included under the serous category.
[c]Four stage III carcinosarcomas were primary peritoneal tumors.
Percentages under 10% are rounded to the nearest 0.5%. Sum of percentages is not 100% due to rounding.
[d]Serous, low grade are invasive carcinomas.

from high-risk women, and normal-appearing ovaries contralateral to stage I carcinomas, have generated conflicting data [312].

Surface Epithelial Dysplasia

Investigators have studied ovarian surface epithelium in the vicinity of carcinomas in an attempt to define the putative entity of "ovarian dysplasia," and have reported atypical cellular and nuclear features that appear more frequently in ovarian surface epithelium near or contralateral to carcinomas in comparison to control ovaries. Much of these data derive from one group of investigators and have not been independently validated [308]. Some investigators have reported that, although not identifiable by light microscopy, subtle nuclear changes identified by image analysis are detectable in the surface epithelium of ovaries prophylactically removed from high-risk women in comparison to controls. In contrast, another group of investigators examined high-risk ovaries under oil immersion and found only subtle atypical features that were not significantly more common in cases than controls [308].

Surface Epithelial Inclusions

The superficial ovarian cortex often contains simple glands and cysts lined by a single layer of flat or nondescript cuboidal epithelium, which often undergoes metaplasia to tubal-type epithelium. These are termed surface epithelial or cortical (formerly "germinal") inclusions, and they are more common in older women (see also Chap. 12, Non-neoplastic Lesions of the Ovary). Their origin is unknown. Historically they have been considered to arise after post-ovulatory repair of the damaged ovarian surface; however the evidence for this is weak [121]. It has been stated that they arise when invaginations or clefts of the ovarian cortex lined by surface epithelium lose their connection to the surface. However, this circumstantial observation may be based on confusion of tangentially sectioned clefts with inclusions [312]. Conceivably, the origin of inclusions could be the fimbrial epithelium, which is in close apposition with the ovarian surface epithelium [168, 258] (*Fig. 14.1c*). Ovarian surface adhesions may also play a role.

Some studies on prophylactic oophorectomy specimens in high-risk women and normal-appearing ovaries contralateral to stage I carcinomas have shown a higher number of these cortical inclusions in comparison to controls, but others have not confirmed these findings. These studies have also evaluated a variety of other features including cortical invaginations (clefts) and surface papillomatosis, and some have found the latter two to be more common in cancer-prone ovaries than in controls, but these findings have not been confirmed by other investigators [258, 312]. Many of these studies have significant drawbacks and are not strictly comparable to one another. For example, the method of quantitation of cortical inclusions and clefts is variable [312].

Endometriosis

Although the precursors of ovarian carcinoma are for the most part unknown, endometriosis is the best documented and most easily recognized precursor. This is because carcinomas arising in endometriosis are Type I tumors, which grow slowly; therefore there is a greater window of opportunity for discovery prior to obliteration of the precursor lesion by the carcinoma. Endometriosis is common and found in 10% of reproductive-age women, but the risk of malignant transformation in an individual patient is very low. Nonetheless, endometriosis is associated with up to about 20% of ovarian cancers and is acknowledged to be the precursor of many endometrioid and clear cell carcinomas and an occasional mucinous carcinoma [392]. Serous carcinomas may be found coincidentally in women with endometriosis, but do not appear to be histogenetically related.

The plausibility of endometriosis as an ovarian cancer precursor is supported by our understanding of endometrial cancer precursors. Atypical endometrial hyperplasia in the uterus is a well-defined precursor of endometrial adenocarcinoma (see Chap. 8, Precancerous Lesions of the Endometrium), and changes similar to this lesion are occasionally observed in endometriosis. In addition, atypical changes are also seen in endometriosis in the vicinity of endometrioid adenocarcinomas of the ovary, and even more frequently in association with clear cell carcinoma. On occasion, the full morphologic spectrum from

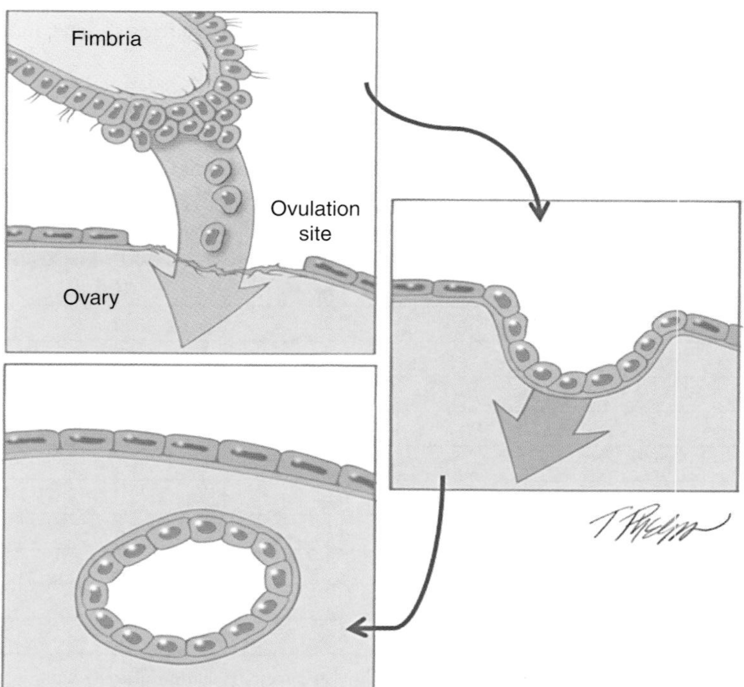

Fig. 14.1c
Schematic of proposed mechanism for the origin of ovarian surface epithelial inclusions from fimbrial epithelium. **Epithelial cells from fimbria implant on site of rupture on the ovary where ovulation occurred. These epithelial cells can conceivably invaginate to form a cortical inclusion cyst**

endometriosis with hyperplasia to atypical hyperplasia and well-differentiated endometrioid adenocarcinoma can be observed. The risk of neoplastic transformation appears to be low [298]. Further support for the premalignant potential of endometriosis comes from molecular biologic studies that have demonstrated molecular alterations, including LOH in the *PTEN* gene and microsatellite instability [6, 374], as well as chromosomal aberrations including trisomies and monosomies [159], all indicative of a neoplastic process [351]. Therefore, a significant proportion of endometriotic lesions have the potential to undergo additional genetic changes and malignant transformation. Parenthetically, if ovarian endometriotic cysts were classified as benign epithelial neoplasms, which some certainly are, this would radically change the distribution of ovarian surface epithelial tumors. More specifically, in our series (➋ *Table 14.5*), endometriomas would be at least as common as serous cystadenoma and therefore would be the most common benign ovarian neoplasm. Alternatively, since endometriosis is probably of endometrial origin, it can be argued that tumors arising in endometriosis are ultimately not of ovarian origin.

It has been estimated that carcinoma develops in 0.3–3% of cases of endometriosis [6, 336] but this is very likely an overestimate since a large number of cases of endometriosis never come to biopsy. The true figure is probably closer to 0.3% or lower. Ovarian endometriosis appears to be significantly more likely to undergo malignant transformation than extraovarian endometriosis [336]. As noted earlier, the relative proportion of endometrioid and clear cell carcinomas that are associated with endometriosis is much higher than that for the other cell types.

Further evidence that endometriosis is a precursor of ovarian carcinoma is provided by large studies from Sweden and Japan. In a Swedish study of over 20,000 women hospitalized with endometriosis, after a mean follow-up of 11.4 years, the risk of ovarian cancer in comparison to the control population was 1.9. Patients with a long-standing history of endometriosis (10 years or longer) had a relative risk of 4.2 [308]. In a study in Japan of 6,398 women with endometriosis, the standardized incidence ratio was 9.0 after 17 years of follow-up, with a risk of 13.2 in women diagnosed after age 50 [152]. In the latter study, the mean age at diagnosis of ovarian carcinoma was 51, a reflection of the significantly younger age of women with endometriosis-associated cancers (see ➋ *Table 14.1* and "Endometrioid adenocarcinoma associated with endometriosis," later in this chapter).

Table 14.5
Distribution of 1,000 ovarian epithelial tumors by cell type. Washington Hospital Center, 1999–2008

	Benign (%)	Atypical proliferative (%)[a]	Malignant (%)[b]	Total (%)
Serous	48.9[c]	1.8	16.6	67.3
Endometrioid	0.9[d]	0.2	1.9	3
Clear cell	0	0.2	2.2	2.4
Mucinous	7.4[e]	0.9	0.6	8.9
Seromucinous	1.7	0.4	0.4	2.5
Transitional	9.8[f]	0.1	0.6	10.5
Mixed	0.6[g]	0	1.0	1.6
Undifferentiated	–	–	0	0
Carcinosarcoma	–	–	2.3	2.3
Squamous	1.4	–	0.1	1.5
Total	70.7	3.6	25.7	100

[a]Also referred to as "borderline" tumors, and includes those with intraepithelial carcinoma and/or microinvasion.
[b]Includes peritoneal primaries.
[c]Includes 1.7% with focal atypia.
[d]Includes 0.2% proliferative endometrioid tumors.
[e]Includes 0.6% with focal atypia.
[f]Includes metaplastic Brenner tumors.
[g]0.5% serous-endometrioid and 0.1% mucinous-endometrioid.

Benign and Atypical Proliferative Neoplasms

Although the natural history of benign ovarian tumors cannot be observed since they must be completely removed for accurate diagnosis, the observation of morphologically benign areas within carcinomas, and recent molecular data, strongly suggest that borderline tumors are precursors of low-grade serous, endometrioid and mucinous carcinomas (Type I tumors in the dualistic model). The evidence supporting these conclusions is discussed in their respective sections.

Serous Tubal Intraepithelial Carcinoma (STIC) and p53 Signature

It has recently been proposed that the origin of some serous carcinomas is the tubal fimbriae [168, 287]. The fimbriae normally extend over, and are in close contact with, the ovarian surface. As noted earlier, the origin of surface epithelial inclusions is unknown. Reported associations of chronic salpingitis with both ovarian serous tumors and tubal carcinomas [71, 309] suggest the possibility of incorporation of fimbrial epithelium into the ovarian cortex via adhesions or a role of salpingitis in tubal carcinogenesis [258, 287].

The typical fallopian tube carcinoma is a high-grade serous carcinoma and, until recently, was felt to be characterized by a dilated tubal lumen containing grossly obvious tumor. However, a fimbrial carcinoma might not lead to a dilated tubal lumen and could be misinterpreted as ovarian in origin. Epithelial atypia, carcinoma in situ, and small high-grade serous tubal carcinomas have been found in prophylactic specimens from women with *BRCA* mutations (➋ *Table 14.6*). In addition, it is frequently impossible to completely separate the ovary and tube for evaluation in serous carcinoma. All of these observations suggest the possibility that some apparent ovarian cancers are in fact tubal in origin [59, 168, 258, 287]. Carcinoma involving the tubal mucosa is generally regarded as secondary when there is also tumor in the ovary, peritoneum, and/or endometrium [191, 287]; however this is an assumption. Many of the dominant tumorous adnexal masses appear to be paraovarian and/or extensively involve the fallopian tube in a manner consistent with peritoneal or tubal origin. Sometimes the fallopian tube cannot be identified, perhaps in some cases because a large cystic carcinoma is actually an unrecognizable tube filled with carcinoma. The identification of *TP53* mutations in TICs as well as in high-grade serous carcinomas provide further support for the tubal origin of many high-grade serous carcinomas (see ➋ Chap. 11, Diseases of the Fallopian Tube and Paratubal Region).

Meticulous examination of risk-reducing salpingo-oophorectomy (RRSO) specimens has disclosed occult invasive carcinomas in 3% of cases: 53% ovarian, 39% tubal, and 8% peritoneal (➋ *Table 14.6*), and it has been suggested that some apparent primary peritoneal carcinomas after RRSO reflect undetected microscopic ovarian carcinomas [44]. It has also been suggested that some apparent peritoneal carcinomas in women who have undergone oophorectomy but not salpingectomy may reflect metastases from primary tubal carcinomas [88]. Foci of tubal carcinoma in situ and atypical hyperplasia have been reported in RRSO specimens, and the tubal fimbria seems to be a preferred site [42, 43, 149, 212, 287] (See ➋ Chap. 11, Diseases of the Fallopian Tube and Paratubal Region). The reported frequency of occult invasive carcinomas in prophylactic specimens varies widely; 0–12% among 16 series including 1,750 patients (➋ *Table 14.6*). This wide range could reflect differing thresholds for the diagnosis of tubal carcinoma, particularly carcinoma in situ. In addition, there are several potential sources of bias in these types of studies [151].

In light of the above findings, the search for precursors of Type II ovarian carcinomas has shifted to the fimbriae of the fallopian tubes, where serous tubal intraepithelial carcinomas (STICs) have been identified in association with a high proportion of high-grade serous carcinomas. STICs contain *TP53* mutations and are cytologically malignant, but are confined to the tubal epithelium. More recently it has been found that that there are short stretches of morphologically normal tubal epithelium that are immunohistochemically positive for p53, and that have a Ki-67 proliferation index higher than normal tubal epithelium but lower than STICs. A minimum of 12 tubal secretory epithelial cells that are p53 positive has been proposed as a definition for a "p53 signature," which is a candidate for a STIC precursor. p53 signatures have been associated with STICs as well as apparent ovarian serous carcinoma, but are also found in the general population. *TP53* mutations have been found in a majority of p53 signatures. These findings have led to the proposal that the p53 signature is the long-sought precursor of a subset of ovarian high-grade serous carcinomas. Much of these data derive from one group of investigators and await confirmation in larger series and by other investigators. Nonetheless, this is an attractive hypothesis that fits much of the data that have hitherto been difficult to reconcile regarding the origin of ovarian cancer. A more comprehensive discussion can be found in ➋ Chap. 11, Diseases of the Fallopian Tube and Paratubal Region.

Table 14.6
Incidental carcinomas found in prophylactic salpingo-oophorectomy specimens

Series	Year	No. cases	No. invasive carcinomas (ovarian/tubal/ peritoneal)	Serous tubal intraepithelial carcinoma
Lu [193]	2000	50	3 (2/0/1)	0
Colgan [61]	2001	60	4 (2/2/0)	1
Leeper [180]	2002	30	2 (0/1/1)	2
Kauff [143]	2002	98	3 (2/1/0)	0
Rebbeck [269]	2002	259	6 (6/0/0)	0
Olivier [245]	2004	128	5 (3/2/0)	0
Meeuwissen [214]	2005	133	1 (0/1/0)	0
Powell [261]	2005	67	4 (3/1/0)	3
Casey [44]	2005	238	0	0
Lamb [172]	2006	113	2 (0/1/1)	4
Carcangiu [42]	2006	50	6 (2/4/0)	3
Finch [88]	2006	159	6 (4/1/1)	1
Gaarenstroom [96]	2006	127	0	0
Medeiros [212]	2006	13	2 (0/2/0)	3
Schmeler [294]	2006	47	0	0
Laki [171]	2007	89	4 (2/2/0)	0
Hermsen [122]	2007	89	3 (1/2/0)	0
Total		1750	51 (27/20/4)	17

Some incidental carcinomas that are reported to have involved both ovary and tube were assigned as primary ovarian unless a clear histologic description permitted assignment as a tubal primary or a clear gross description described a dominant tubal mass. Some incidental ovarian surface carcinomas could reflect a peritoneal primary.

The importance of the fimbriae in carcinogenesis is highlighted by a recent study which describes the junction of the peritoneum with the fimbrial epithelium (tubal-peritoneal junction (TPJ)) [314]. Since junctions between different types of epithelium are known to be hot spots for carcinogenesis (e.g., the gastroesophageal and anorectal junctions), the presence of the TPJ in and around the fimbriae suggests that this junction is in fact the source of serous carcinomas. That study also found transitional metaplasia to be common and perhaps normal at the TPJ. In light of the above findings, it can be argued that since serous carcinomas are usually of fimbrial origin, endometrioid and clear cell carcinomas are ultimately of endometrial origin, and Brenner and mucinous tumors may also arise in the fimbriae via transitional metaplasia [168], it may be the case that no "ovarian surface epithelial tumors" are of ovarian origin. This would make gonadal stromal and germ cell tumors the only true ovarian (gonadal) tumors, just as in the testis, and is consistent with the fact that men do not have fallopian tubes to give rise to these epithelial tumors.

Familial (Hereditary) Ovarian Cancer

BRCA and Other Genes

At least 10% of ovarian carcinomas arise in the setting of highly penetrant, autosomal dominant genetic predisposition. Hereditary ovarian cancer has been recently reviewed [263, 284]. Three major types of genetic predisposition to ovarian cancer have been identified, including site-specific ovarian cancer, hereditary breast/ovarian cancer, and hereditary non-polyposis colorectal cancer (HNPCC, Lynch syndrome II). Notably, the increased frequency of ovarian cancer in relatives of women with ovarian cancer is not paralleled by an increase among relatives of women with "borderline" or mucinous ovarian tumors.

Site-specific ovarian cancer is recognized in families in which two or more first- or first- and second-degree relatives have ovarian carcinoma. The lifetime risk of ovarian carcinoma is approximately threefold higher in these families than in the general population. This type of hereditary predisposition is currently considered an "ovarian-specific" variant of hereditary breast/ovarian cancer, as no susceptibility gene other than *BRCA1* and *BRCA2* has been identified.

Hereditary breast and ovarian cancer is associated with germline mutations of either *BRCA1* or *BRCA2*. The risk of developing ovarian carcinoma by age 70 years for *BRCA1* and *BRCA2* carriers is estimated as 40% and 18%, respectively [53]. The *BRCA1* and *BRCA2* genes map to chromosome 17q and 13q, respectively, and encode proteins that play important roles in DNA repair, cell cycle checkpoint control, protein ubiquitinization, and chromatin remodeling [284]. Germline mutations of these genes include small deletions, insertions, point mutations, and gene rearrangements that typically lead to prematurely truncated protein products. Mutations are widely distributed throughout both genes. Given the genes' large size and the absence of mutational "hotspots," mutation screening based on traditional sequencing approaches is cumbersome and has been largely supplanted by new automated technologies allowing rapid mutation detection. Studies suggest the site of the mutation within these genes may correlate with risk for ovarian cancer. For example, mutations between nucleotides 2,401 and 4,190 in *BRCA1* increase the risk of ovarian cancer, but reduce the risk of breast cancer [268]. Mutations involving nucleotides 4,075–6,503 of *BRCA2* exon 11 are also associated with increased risk of ovarian cancer, and hence, this region has been referred to as the "ovarian cancer cluster region"[100]. Mutations of *BRCA1* and *BRCA2* are uncommon in sporadic cases of ovarian carcinomas, but these genes are functionally inactivated in a substantial fraction of cases through allelic deletions and/or silencing due to promoter hypermethylation.

Increased risk for developing ovarian cancer has also been observed in patients affected by HNPCC, and this accounts for about 2% of ovarian cancers [195]. This autosomal dominant syndrome is associated with elevated risk of colon carcinoma without polyposis, endometrial carcinoma, and less frequently, carcinomas of other organs, including the ovary. HNPCC is caused by mutations in genes that encode proteins involved in DNA mismatch repair. Over 70% of individuals with HNPCC harbor germline mutations of *hMSH2* or *hMLH1*, with mutations of *hPMS1*, *hPMS2*, and *hMSH6* being less common. Studies of ovarian carcinomas arising in the setting of HNPCC are rather limited, but in one retrospective series of 80 affected patients including 31 known and 35 presumptive mutation carriers, ovarian cancers were found to arise at an earlier age than sporadic cases and tended to be well or moderately differentiated and relatively low stage (FIGO stage I or II) at diagnosis [373].

Clinicopathologic Features of Familial Ovarian Cancers

Ovarian cancer in women with familial ovarian cancer occurs at a younger age than sporadic ovarian cancer. For *BRCA1*-associated ovarian cancer, the age at diagnosis is about 53 years, and for Lynch syndrome II, 40 years (➋ *Table 14.1*). In the largest series with centralized pathology review [375], cancers in *BRCA* carriers were compared to those in noncarriers. Among 220 women, mutation-associated tumors were of significantly higher grade and stage as compared to non-mutation-associated tumors. No mucinous and no borderline tumors were found in the mutation-associated group. Primary peritoneal carcinoma occurred rarely in both groups. Nearly all mutation-associated tumors appear to be high-grade high-stage serous carcinomas, slightly but significantly different from the distribution in the general population [317]. Despite the unfavorable stage and grade distribution, the prognosis for germline *BRCA*-mutation-associated familial cases appears to be somewhat better than for sporadic cases. In sporadic ovarian cancer, absent or reduced *BRCA1* protein expression is more common in high-stage, high-grade serous carcinomas as compared to low-stage and non-serous carcinomas [352].

Mouse Models of Ovarian Cancer and Implications for Treatment

Genetically engineered mouse (GEM) models of each major subtype of ovarian cancer will undoubtedly prove useful for improving knowledge of ovarian cancer biology and for preclinical testing of signal transduction inhibitors as novel therapeutics. Historically, most animal models of ovarian cancer were based on xenografting human ovarian cancer cells into immunodeficient mice. Such models have limitations, including incomplete recapitulation of tumor–host interactions and inability to replicate early stages of tumor development. Recently described GEM models of ovarian cancer appear to overcome some weaknesses of the xenograft models as tumors arise orthotopically in immunologically intact animals and more closely mimic the behavior of human ovarian cancers. One approach involves ex vivo genetic modification of primary murine ovarian surface epithelium (MOSE) [249]. In this model, MOSE cells were removed from $p53^{-/-}$ transgenic mice expressing the cell surface avian retroviral receptor (ARR) under the control of the keratin-5 promoter and cultured in vitro for several generations. The cultured MOSE were infected, via the ARR, with replication-competent avian leucosis-derived vectors carrying oncogenes, such as c-*MYC*, *KRAS*, or *AKT*. MOSE cells expressing various combinations of oncogenes were then surgically transplanted under the ovarian bursa of recipient mice. The addition of any two of the oncogenes was sufficient to induce tumor formation when infected cells were injected at subcutaneous, intraperitoneal, or ovarian sites. In another model, a promoter element from the murine Müllerian Inhibitory Substance II Receptor (*MISIIR*) gene was used to drive expression of SV40 T-Ag (large and small) in MOSE [64]. In this model, approximately 50% of female mice develop bilateral poorly differentiated ovarian carcinomas. Flesken-Nikitin and colleagues used an alternative approach to conditionally inactivate the p53 and Rb tumor suppressors in the mouse ovarian surface epithelium [89]. A single ovarian intrabursal injection of recombinant adenovirus-expressing Cre recombinase (AdCre) in female mice homozygous for conditional (floxed) *p53* and *Rb* alleles led to development of ovarian carcinomas. Mice from all three models develop poorly differentiated papillary carcinomas of the ovary with greatest resemblance to human serous carcinomas. The tumors disseminate intraperitoneally and are frequently accompanied by bloody ascites.

Given the morphological and molecular heterogeneity of ovarian carcinomas described above, a goal for researchers in the field is the development of mouse models that recapitulate each major histological type of ovarian cancer. Toward that end, Dinulescu and colleagues used ovarian bursal injection of AdCre to coordinately activate an oncogenic *KRas* allele and inactivate *Pten* in the MOSE [75]. Although ovarian carcinomas resembling endometrioid adenocarcinomas developed, as described above, *KRAS* mutations in human ovarian endometrioid carcinomas are rather uncommon, and data supporting cooperation between mutant *KRAS* and *PTEN* loss in human tumors are lacking [383]. In light of the data identifying frequent co-occurrence of canonical Wnt and PI3K/Pten/Akt signaling defects in the human tumors, Wu and colleagues employed ovarian bursal injection of AdCre to conditionally inactivate the *Pten* and *Apc* tumor suppressor genes in the ovarian surface epithelium of $Apc^{flox/flox}$; $Pten^{flox/flox}$ mice [383]. The injected ovaries uniformly and rapidly developed tumors with similar morphology to human ovarian endometrioid cancers. In addition, the mouse tumors exhibited biological behavior and gene expression patterns similar to their human tumor counterparts with comparable signaling pathway defects. It is expected that mouse models of ovarian cancer will yield new insights into ovarian cancer pathogenesis, particularly with respect to putative precursor lesions and mechanisms by which tumors develop and progress.

Implications for Treatment

Mouse models that faithfully recapitulate their human tumor counterparts may prove especially useful for preclinical testing of novel therapeutics that target specific molecular defects in the tumor cells. Animal models such as this are expected to accelerate the translation of promising new therapies from the laboratory to the clinic. The readily recognizable aberrations of specific signaling pathways in many Type I tumors including low-grade serous carcinomas, low-grade endometrioid carcinomas, and mucinous carcinomas suggest that inhibitors targeting specific components of these pathways may be effective for treating patients with advanced-stage disease that is refractory to current chemotherapy. For example, MEK inhibitors such as CI-1040 and Quercetin from red wine extract deserve consideration as therapeutic agents for patients with low-grade serous carcinomas [175]. This notion is supported by studies of Pohl et al., who demonstrated that treatment of ovarian serous carcinoma cells harboring *KRAS* or *BRAF* mutations with a MEK inhibitor, CI-1040, resulted in significant growth inhibition in vitro as compared to tumor cells with wild-type *KRAS* and *BRAF* [259]. Since low-grade serous carcinoma and its presumptive precursor, APST, have a high frequency of mutations in *KRAS* and *BRAF*, future clinical trials should help to determine if MEK inhibitors can prolong disease-free interval and overall survival in patients with advanced-stage low-grade serous carcinomas. Similarly, the observation that growth of murine ovarian carcinomas with PI3K/Pten signaling pathway defects is profoundly inhibited by drugs that target this pathway provides further support for testing such agents in women with disseminated low-grade (Type I) endometrioid carcinomas.

Finally, the high level of genetic instability that characterizes the majority of ovarian epithelial cancers (i.e., Type II tumors) presents a tremendous challenge with respect to the development of effective screening programs and therapeutic strategies that target the particular molecular defects present in a given patient's tumor. The lack of shared aberrations of cellular signaling pathways (except those mediated by p53) in high-grade serous and endometrioid carcinomas makes it difficult to design target-based therapies for these tumors at present. Clearly, a major goal of ongoing work in the field is to identify additional "hallmark" genetic alterations that characterize the Type II tumors. As our understanding of the molecular pathogenesis of each major type of ovarian carcinoma improves, the design of "personalized" therapeutic regimens based on the particular alterations present in a given patient's tumor may become a reality. It is reasonable to hope that drugs targeting specific molecular defects in tumor cells could be used alone or in combination with existing treatment modalities to substantially improve the clinical outcome for women with ovarian cancer.

Table 14.7

Recent screening trials based primarily on pelvic ultrasound

Series	Year	No. of patients	Stage I or low-stage cancers[b]	High-stage cancers
Rufford [283][a]	2004	110,317	31	16
Buys [38]	2005	28,816	1	18
Van Nagell [360]	2007	25,327	14	15
Kobayashi [153]	2008	41,688	17	10
Partridge [253]	2009	34,261	17	43
Menon [219]	2009	98,308	28	32
Total		338,717	108	134

[a]Compiled from a 1983–2000 review.
[b]Some series grouped stage II with stage I as "low stage."
Atypical proliferative (borderline), germ cell, and stromal tumors are excluded. All invasive carcinomas, including those of tubal or peritoneal origin, are included.

Screening and Prevention

Screening Tests

An understanding of the new model of ovarian cancer pathogenesis has important implications for ovarian cancer screening. A presumptive goal of screening should be to detect high-grade serous carcinoma in stage I. Since high-grade serous carcinomas, which account for the vast majority of ovarian cancer deaths, are usually relatively small at their site of origin even when they are widely disseminated, both vaginal ultrasound and serum CA125 lack sufficient sensitivity and specificity to effectively detect them at a curable stage, if one even exists. Screening trials have generally identified stage I non-serous tumors, borderline tumors, nonepithelial tumors, and advanced-stage serous carcinomas, with the identification of stage I high-grade serous carcinoma an exceedingly rare event, even in series focusing on high-risk women [214, 359]. In a compilation of some recent series, among over 338,000 women screened, there were only 242 invasive cancers detected, the majority of which were already in advanced stage (*Table 14.7*). Over 3,100 women had to be screened to detect each low-stage carcinoma. Furthermore, advanced-stage serous carcinomas have been detected during intervals after a normal screen in several large studies [219], providing further evidence that the time course of progression of typical ovarian cancer is not amenable to effective screening by transvaginal sonography.

The fact that many ovarian cancer patients in retrospect have had symptoms, sometimes chronic, prior to diagnosis, has led to efforts to develop a symptom index for early diagnosis [10]. Unfortunately, this is unlikely to be effective because the early symptoms of ovarian cancer are too nonspecific and very common. Moreover, the relatively low prevalence of ovarian cancer in the general population makes the development of an effective screen test extremely challenging [127].

In contrast to Type II tumors, only about 20% of ovarian carcinomas are Type I tumors. These appear to grow slowly from benign cystadenomas, atypical proliferative tumors, and endometriomas, which become quite large before undergoing malignant transformation. As a result, most patients with these tumors are diagnosed with large pelvic masses on pelvic examination without the need of ultrasound before the neoplasms have undergone malignant transformation or peritoneal dissemination. This sequence of events with delayed transformation and dissemination accounts for the high proportion of FIGO stage I, low-grade cases among Type I carcinomas (mucinous and endometrioid) as compared to high-grade serous carcinomas.

Prevention

Few data are available regarding prevention of ovarian cancer. In the Nurse's Health Study of over 80,000 women, there was a modest inverse association between caffeine intake and ovarian cancer risk in women not using hormones, while alcohol and smoking had no effect, with the exception of smoking, which increased the risk of mucinous carcinoma [358]. A large review found that smoking doubles the risk of mucinous carcinoma [141]; however, data on mucinous tumors prior to the mid- to late-1990s are unreliable because it is now recognized that most mucinous carcinomas involving the ovary are metastatic (see Epidemiology, earlier in this chapter, and Mucinous Tumors, later in this chapter).

RRSO is often performed in patients at high risk of ovarian cancer. Unfortunately, the reduction in risk is not complete and appears to be only about 95–98%. The risk of primary peritoneal serous carcinoma is significant and estimated at 0.2–0.35% per year after salpingo-oophorectomy [44, 88] with a slightly higher risk for BRCA1 carriers [44]. Nearly all reported cases have occurred within 10 years of prophylactic surgery; however, longer follow-up might reveal a more extended period of increased risk.

Prognostic Factors

The only universally accepted prognostic factors for patients with ovarian cancer are FIGO stage and, in stage IIIC and IV patients, volume of residual disease after surgical staging (with or without debulking). Age is a strong prognostic factor in many studies but may not be independent, as already discussed (see Etiology and Risk Factors; Age, earlier in this chapter). Other factors that may be important but about which there is continued debate include cell type, histopathologic grade, and tumor rupture.

Cell Type and Histologic Grade

The issue of the prognostic importance of cell type and grade is complex because these features are interdependent, making it difficult to analyze them separately. The vast majority of serous and clear cell carcinomas are high grade regardless of the grading system used, while endometrioid and mucinous carcinomas are more often low grade [106, 313].

On reviewing the literature, histologic grade is reported to be a significant prognostic factor in many studies and in literature reviews. However, most of these data are not useful because of the number of different grading systems, the failure to specify which system was used, the lack of uniform pathologic review, and the fact that grade is among the most poorly reproducible observations among pathologists. Two recent large studies with uniform expert pathology review found that grade was not an independent prognostic factor on multivariate analysis: a Canadian population-based study of 575 patients [106], and a review of 1,895 stage III patients from a compilation of Gynecologic Oncology Group (GOG) studies [378].

For all major cell types of ovarian carcinoma, histologic subtype is not an independent prognostic factor when stage is taken into account, with the possible exception of clear cell carcinoma, which historically has portended a very poor outcome. However, many large recent series have not confirmed this [49, 182, 239, 255, 313, 329, 353, 369, 393] (see Clear Cell Carcinoma, later in this chapter). Some recent large studies suggest that advanced-stage endometrioid carcinomas have a better progression free and overall survival as compared to stage-stratified serous carcinoma [338, 378]. This could reflect a higher proportion of low-grade tumors among the endometrioid carcinomas as noted above.

At present, grading of ovarian carcinoma is clinically important only for stage IA, IB, and IIA patients because chemotherapy can be withheld for low-grade tumors in view of their excellent prognosis when untreated. Stage IA and IB, grade 1 carcinomas have survival rates as high as 97% [106]. However, stage I ovarian cancer is a heterogeneous group with only a small minority being serous carcinomas. Since the decision to treat or not to treat is a binary one, the data suggest that the binary system can be used, with chemotherapy withheld for low-grade stage I, i.e., Type I tumors (see High-Grade Serous Carcinoma for further information on grading, later in this chapter). There are insufficient data available to determine whether the binary system is appropriate for non-serous tumors; furthermore, even for serous tumors, only advanced stage cases have been tested.

Stage, Patterns of Spread, and Survival

The most recent version of the FIGO staging of gynecological cancers is shown in *Table 14.3* [119]. FIGO stage is so powerful a predictor of outcome in ovarian cancer that most other putative prognostic factors are of little importance in comparison to stage, with the exception of volume of residual disease after staging and debulking in stages IIIC and IV.

Standard procedures for surgical staging have evolved over the past 3 decades. In the early 1980s, it became clear that approximately one third of ovarian cancer patients with apparent stage I disease (confined to the ovaries) were upstaged at subsequent complete staging laparotomy. The extent of surgical exploration and tissue sampling are currently quite thorough when performed by a gynecological oncologist, but suboptimal staging often still occurs when performed by nonspecialists. Survival rates for the lower stages gradually improved in the 1970s and 1980s as occult advanced-stage tumors were detected and properly categorized.

Comprehensive staging as described later in this chapter ("Treatment"; "Surgery") will generally be sufficient surgical treatment for patients in stages I and II. Patients with advanced-stage disease often require debulking, or cytoreductive surgery, as well. Although cure is uncommon, cytoreductive surgery improves survival. Other benefits include improved patient comfort, reduction in the adverse metabolic consequences due to tumor including enhanced ability to maintain nutrition, enhanced ability to tolerate chemotherapy, and enhanced responsiveness of residual tumor to chemotherapy. Aggressive primary cytoreductive surgery has a low morbidity and mortality rate and is supported by an improved survival rate in multiple studies. The median survival is about 3–4 years or longer after optimal cytoreduction as compared to about 1–2 years after suboptimal cytoreduction. Systematic lymphadenectomy as compared to removal of only clinically suspicious nodes improves progression-free survival by a few months but does not improve overall survival in optimally debulked patients [48, 341]. Many patients with bulky disease cannot be optimally cytoreduced at primary surgery. It has been found that two to three cycles of chemotherapy followed by interval debulking significantly increases the proportion of patients who can be successfully cytoreduced.

Staging takes both surgical and pathological findings into account, hence the term, "surgicopathologic stage." Stage can usually be deduced solely from the histopathologic and cytologic findings. However, limited evidence suggests that dense adhesions of an apparent stage I tumor that require sharp dissection, leaving a raw area following dissection, or when dissection results in tumor rupture, are associated with a prognosis similar to that of a more advanced stage tumor [250]. At present, it is not clear whether upstaging based on dense adhesions is warranted, although one recent study suggests that it is not [299]. This and other problems in assigning stage are summarized in *Table 14.8.*

Table 14.8
Problems and pitfalls in staging ovarian carcinoma

Problem	Solution
What constitutes ovarian surface involvement?	Tumor cells directly exposed to the peritoneal cavity, generally manifested as exophytic surface papillae
Does slight leakage warrant substage C?	Yes
Does rupture of a benign component of a heterogeneous tumor warrant substage C?	No guidelines or data are available
Does sigmoid colon involvement indicate stage II or III?	II. The sigmoid colon is a pelvic structure
Does invasion of skeletal muscle of diaphragm, posterior abdominal wall (psoas muscles), or anterior abdominal wall (rectus muscles) warrant stage IV?	No. This is stage III
Does invasion of the diaphragm indicate stage IV?	Invasion through to the pleural surface of the diaphragm or into the parietal pleura warrants stage IV
Does abdominal wall involvement indicate stage III or IV?	Invasion through the anterior rectus sheath, or into subcutis or skin, warrants stage IV
Does splenic parenchymal involvement indicate stage III or IV?	No guidelines are available
Does dense adherence to extraovarian structures warrant upstaging in the absence of histologic confirmation of extraovarian disease?	Unresolved. Practices vary and FIGO guidelines are not clear [299]
Are chest CT and other extra-abdominal evaluations for apparent stage III patients needed to rule out stage IV?	No

The stage distribution of ovarian cancer varies by histological type (*Table 14.4*). The highest proportion of FIGO stage I cases is found among Type I tumors. The vast majority of mucinous carcinomas are stage I, as are one-third to one-half of clear cell carcinomas and nearly half of endometrioid carcinomas. Only 3% of serous carcinomas are diagnosed in stage I. Low-grade serous carcinoma, a Type I tumor, is rarely diagnosed in stage I, although the morphologically noninvasive form of MPSC is somewhat more often diagnosed in stage I. In our series, only 14% of ovarian cancers were stage I, and

Table 14.9
Five-year survival by stage (%), in four continents

FIGO stage	FIGO [119]	The USA [340]	Korea [57]	The Netherlands [370]	Australia [213]
I	86		91.4	81.2	88
IA	89.6	94			
IB	86.1	91.1			
IC	83.4	79.8			
II	70		75.6	60	65
IIA	70.7	76.4			
IIB	65.5	66.9			
IIC	71.4	57			
III	34		45.7	24.5	27
IIIA	46.7	45.3			
IIIB	41.5	38.6			
IIIC	32.5	35.2			
IV	18.6	17.9	20.4	11.7	12

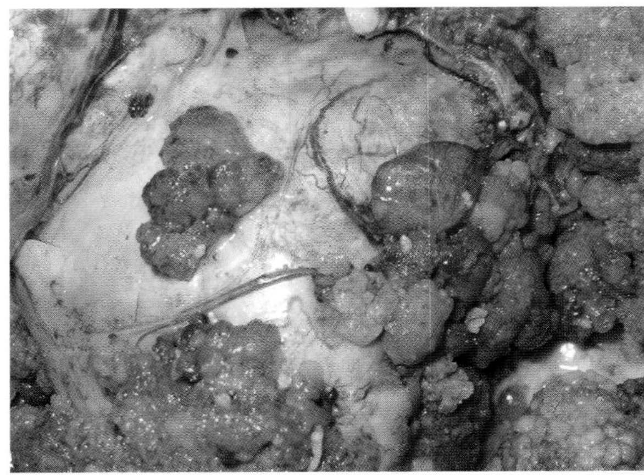

Fig. 14.2
Low grade (micropapillary) serous carcinoma. **The outer surface displays exophytic papillary excrescences reflecting ovarian surface involvement**

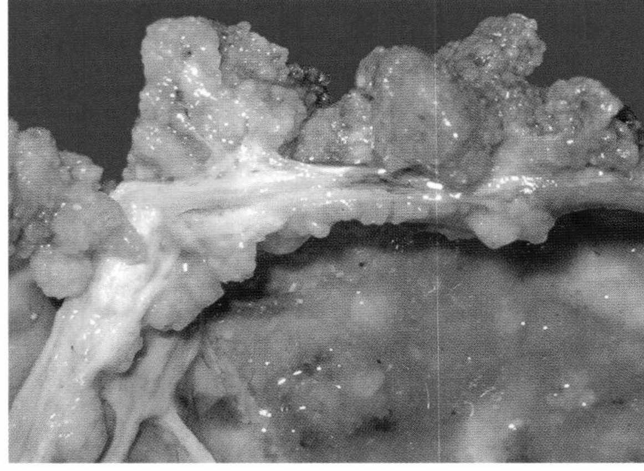

Fig. 14.3
Low grade (micropapillary) serous carcinoma. **Sectioning reveals papillary excrescences on both inner and outer surfaces (same tumor as *Fig. 14.2*)**

one third of these were not comprehensively staged. Five-year survival rates by stage are shown in *Table 14.9.*

Stage I ovarian cancer is confined to the ovaries and peritoneal fluid or washings. Tumor rupture or tumor cells in peritoneal washings or ascitic fluid warrant a stage of IC. Ovarian surface involvement by tumor is also considered to reflect stage IC disease. We consider ovarian surface involvement to be present only when tumor cells are exposed to the peritoneal cavity. Thus, surface involvement is characterized by exophytic papillary tumor on the surface of the ovary or on the outer surface of a cystic neoplasm replacing the ovary (*Figs. 14.2* and *14.3*); rarely a smooth ovarian tumor surface will be shown to have an exposed single layer of neoplastic epithelium. Assessment of surface involvement requires careful gross examination and cooperation between the surgeon and the pathologist. Poor prognostic factors in stage I have historically been grade 3, clear cell type, and IC substage (including rupture). However, this is controversial [313, 369]. Several large recent studies have shown that stage IC tumors do not have a poorer outcome than IA, nor does clear cell histology or rupture portend a poor outcome [50, 182, 239, 313, 353]. Occasionally a large ovarian tumor that is stage IB is associated with a contralateral normal size ovary with small tumor foci on the surface suggesting that the latter is metastatic. Among stage I tumors with bilateral involvement, one third have this appearance [313]. Stage IB is quite uncommon and is found in only 1–5% of stage I cases [119, 182, 389]. Data from several studies suggest that stage I clear cell carcinoma is more frequently IC as compared to the other cell types [313, 329], possibly because of an increased risk of rupture [353].

Stage II ovarian carcinoma is a small and heterogeneous group, and comprises less than 10% of ovarian cancers, 6.5% in our series. It is defined as extension or metastasis to extraovarian pelvic organs. As such, it includes examples of direct extension to the tubes and pelvic sidewall, as well as metastatic seeding of the pelvic peritoneum, and therefore may include curable tumors that have directly extended to adjacent organs but have not yet metastasized, as well as tumors that have seeded the pelvic peritoneum by metastasis and therefore have a poor prognosis. Of note, the sigmoid colon is within the pelvis, and therefore, sigmoid involvement is stage II (➲ *Table 14.8*). As noted earlier, some "pathologic stage I" tumors are considered "surgical stage II" by many surgeons [299]. Although stage II is subclassified into three substages, these do not separate direct extension from metastasis.

Ovarian cancer most commonly presents in stage III and the vast majority of these (84%) are stage IIIC [119]. These tumors characteristically spread along peritoneal surfaces involving both pelvic and abdominal peritoneum including the omentum, surfaces of the small and large bowel, mesentery, paracolic gutters, diaphragm, and peritoneal surfaces of the liver and spleen. Less often, there is a solitary dominant primary ovarian tumor that directly invades bowel or other abdominal structures without the usual features of peritoneal studding. Ascites is found in two thirds and its presence correlates with suboptimal cytoreduction and a higher number of positive lymph nodes [16]. Metastases to retroperitoneal or pelvic lymph nodes are found in the majority of patients who undergo node sampling or dissection and in up to 78% of advanced-stage patients [117, 135]. Inguinal lymph nodes are less commonly involved. Nodal metastasis indicates stage IIIC even in the absence of peritoneal metastasis. Nodal metastasis without peritoneal metastasis is relatively uncommon and seems to portend a better outcome as compared to stage IIIC patients with bulky abdominal disease, even those who have been optimally cytoreduced [58]. The majority of these have positive para-aortic nodes. Isolated positive pelvic nodes with negative para-aortics is very uncommon (0–3%) [117]. Palpable suspicious nodes are positive in 75% while 32% of non-suspicious nodes are positive [117]. In node-positive stage IIIC cases, about one fourth of resected lymph nodes are positive. Patients with tumors that otherwise appear to be stage I have lymph node metastases in about 9% of cases; the corresponding figures for stages II, III, and IV are 36%, 55%, and 88%, respectively. Most studies have shown that the number of positive nodes has no prognostic significance [15]. Rarely, inguinal (stage III), or supraclavicular (stage IV) node metastases will be the presenting manifestation of ovarian carcinoma [87].

Bowel involvement is grossly evident in 72% of stage III patients, and 40% require bowel resection [135]. This is manifested as serosal and subserosal involvement that is frequently extensive and often forms large tumorous masses. More than half of patients have multiple bowel segments involved. The rectosigmoid is the most common site and is involved in 80% of those with bowel involvement. Focal invasion of the outer layer of muscularis propria is not uncommon. Invasion into the submucosa or transmural invasion with mucosal ulceration occurs much less often.

Volume of residual disease is an important prognostic factor in most studies, but this applies only to stages IIIC and IV, as stages IIIA and IIIB have low-volume disease by definition (➲ *Table 14.3*). Regrettably, there is no standard definition of optimal versus suboptimal debulking, the latter group being those considered to have high volume of residual disease. Criteria used rely on the size of the largest nodule remaining. Eighty-seven percent of gynecologic oncologists use 0, 0.5, or 1.0 cm as the threshold, with 1.0 cm the most widely used. Most studies show that the complete elimination of macroscopic disease (i.e., a zero threshold) is associated with the most favorable prognosis [83].

Stage IV is defined as distant metastasis and includes patients with parenchymal liver metastases and extraabdominal metastases; 12–21% of patients present in stage IV [119, 300]. A complete extraabdominal evaluation to exclude distant metastases such as CT of the chest and other studies is not required to assign stage III (➲ *Table 14.8*). The median survival for stage IV is 23 months. Liver and lungs/pleurae are the most common metastatic sites, and anterior abdominal wall metastasis including periumbilical skin and subcutis is frequent. A solitary distant metastasis is a favorable prognostic factor as compared to multiple metastases [347].

Lung and pleural metastases have been reported in up to 45% of ovarian cancer patients [347], and respiratory failure is one of the most common clinical causes of death. In one large series, at presentation, 15% of ovarian cancer patients had pulmonary metastases, and an additional 30% developed pulmonary metastases after a mean of 9 months. During the course of the disease, one third of patients had pleural effusions, and three quarters of these contained malignant cells on cytopathological examination. Among patients with pulmonary involvement, malignant pleural effusion is three times as common as solid parenchymal lung metastasis. A few studies have shown that women with malignant pleural effusion do worse than those with other distant metastases. Historically, the 5-year survival has been 6% after pulmonary metastasis; however, this has improved to 17–36% as surgical resection of metastases has been widely performed.

Hepatic metastases have been found in half of ovarian cancer patients at autopsy. The median survival of stage IV patients with liver metastases is about 1 year. With surgical resection of metastases, the survival improves to a median of about 2 years [347]. As with pulmonary metastases, solitary lesions and those resected with a tumor-free margin are associated with a better outcome. In a study of 29 patients with liver metastases, the median time to recurrence in the liver was 29 months. The median survival for those having undergone resection of a solitary nodule was 25 months as compared to 10 months for those with multiple nodules [189].

Anterior abdominal wall metastases frequently involve periumbilical subcutis and skin. Extraperitoneal abdominal wall involvement warranting the stage IV designation occurs when tumor has invaded through the anterior rectus sheath (➋ *Table 14.8*). Invasion of the rectus muscle alone is considered stage III. When carcinoma is present in a specimen labeled "abdominal wall," if skin is not present for orientation, review of the operative report or discussion with the surgeon is needed to determine whether a stage IV designation is warranted. The pathology report should be explicit in this regard.

Splenic parenchymal metastases are found in 20% of patients at autopsy. There are no specific guidelines for changing the stage based on splenic parenchymal metastasis and it is not clear whether splenic involvement is an adverse prognostic factor in patients who are otherwise stage IIIC. Among ovarian cancer patients who undergo splenectomy, only about half have splenic metastases [14].

Diaphragmatic metastases are usually confined to the peritoneal surface. On occasion, tumor will invade into or penetrate through the diaphragm and the depth of invasion or extent of involvement may necessitate partial diaphragm resection. Penetration of the parietal pleural surface of the diaphragm warrants designation as stage IV.

As survival rates have improved in the taxane era, previously rare sites of distant metastasis such as bone and brain are being diagnosed more often. Brain metastases are present in 0.1% of patients at presentation [216], and are found in up to 6% of patients at autopsy. CNS recurrence is clinically manifested as carcinomatous meningitis in 4–6% of patients, and the median survival is less than 5 months. About half of patients have multiple brain lesions, and in 30–40%, the brain is the only site of distant metastasis. Among patients who develop brain parenchymal involvement after diagnosis, the median time after diagnosis is about 20 months, and the subsequent survival is less than 6 months [216, 347]. The absence of extracranial metastases is prognostically favorable. Bone metastases occur in 1–2% of patients during the course of the disease and are found in up to 15% at autopsy. The median survival after bone metastasis is diagnosed is 4 months. Interestingly, among women with a history of ovarian carcinoma who present with a breast or axillary mass, one third have metastatic ovarian carcinoma and two thirds have a primary breast carcinoma [142].

Cytopathology

Ovarian epithelial neoplasms are usually evaluated in two types of cytopathological specimens: fine-needle aspirates (FNA) of ovarian cysts and peritoneal fluids (obtained by peritoneal washing or by aspiration of ascitic fluid). Intraoperative smears of ovarian tumors can also be useful adjuncts to, or replacements for, frozen section examination. Once disseminated, ovarian cancers may also be examined in FNA specimens or effusions from sites of distant metastasis. Rarely, the presence of psammoma bodies in a Pap smear will be the first sign of primary or recurrent ovarian or peritoneal serous carcinoma, more commonly when associated with atypical glandular cells of undetermined significance (AGUS) or in older women with symptoms and signs suggesting malignancy [223]. In a review of over 200,000 Pap smears, psammoma bodies were found in six patients, two of whom proved to have ovarian carcinoma [266]. In a review of 138 cases of AGUS, 5 (3.6%) proved to have ovarian cancers [344].

Fine-Needle Aspiration of Ovarian Cysts

FNA may be useful in patients who appear to have inoperable ovarian cancer or who cannot undergo surgery fo[r] other reasons. Unsatisfactory specimens from ovarian cys[t] aspirates are common and limit the usefulness of th[e] procedure.

FNA specimens from most carcinomas are cellular an[d] contain cytologically malignant cells, but accurate subclas[-]sification is often difficult and may be impossible base[d] solely on cytologic material. Features useful in subclassifi[-]cation of epithelial neoplasms include psammoma bodie[s] and papillary structures, which suggest serous differentia[-]tion, elongated cells, and focal squamous features tha[t] suggest endometrioid differentiation and cells with abun[-]dant clear, frothy, cytoplasm, and prominent enlarge[d] nucleoli, which suggest clear cell differentiation. Colum[-]nar cells with large cytoplasmic vacuoles containin[g] basophilic cytoplasmic mucin suggest mucinous differen[-]tiation and, if malignant nuclear features are presen[t] should immediately raise the question of metastatic carc[i]noma to the ovaries (see ➋ Mucinous Tumors, later in th[is] chapter, and ➋ Chap. 18, Metastatic Tumors of t[he] Ovary). FNA specimens from serous carcinomas are us[u]ally very cellular and display malignant cells, singly and [in] clusters, with nuclear enlargement, hyperchromasia, irre[g]ular chromatin clumping, and prominent nucleoli. Bizar[re] tumor giant cells are common. Mucinous carcinom[as] yield mucus and high cellularity with single cells, cluste[rs] and syncytial fragments displaying pleomorphism, coarse chromatin, prominent nucleoli, and vacuolated cytoplasm. Exclusion of metastatic mucinous carcinoma is generally not possible in cytologic material, but if sufficient material is available for immunoperoxidase stains, the differential diagnosis can be narrowed. Cytologic material from endometrioid carcinomas resembles that from serous carcinomas but with scanty, more granular cytoplasm, nuclear crowding, and microacini. Squamous differentiation may be present. Clear cell carcinomas display cells with abundant pale vacuolated cytoplasm. Nuclear features often include pleomorphism and macronucleoli.

FNA of benign epithelial neoplasms usually produces a paucicellular specimen. Most of the material consists of macrophages and lymphocytes with few epithelial cells. The background is generally clean, unless torsion or necrosis has occurred. Benign serous tumors may display cohesive sheets of uniform cells with round to oval nuclei, moderate amounts of cytoplasm with well-defined cell borders, and occasionally cilia. The nuclei have finely granular chromatin and small nucleoli. Cystadenofibromas also may display spindled stromal cells without atypia. Mucinous cystadenomas display tall columnar cells with basal nuclei without atypia and occasionally signet ring-like cells. Since any ovarian tumor more than a few centimeters in diameter requires careful gross examination and directed sampling of different areas, a diagnosis of a benign epithelial neoplasm on FNA is likely to have a significant false-negative rate. Atypical proliferative epithelial tumors of all types may display a degree of cytologic atypia that overlaps with invasive well-differentiated carcinoma, and therefore this distinction requires tissue examination in all cases.

Peritoneal Fluid Cytology

Cytological samples of peritoneal fluid are routinely obtained during staging procedures for ovarian cancer. Washings are performed or ascites aspirated upon entering the peritoneal cavity, prior to surgical manipulation that could dislodge tumor cells. Cytological findings are important in substaging early (FIGO I and II) ovarian cancer; malignant cells in peritoneal washings or ascites warrants assignment of tumors to stage IC or IIC. Cytology is more sensitive in detecting ovarian carcinoma in ascites than in peritoneal washes, as well as in patients with peritoneal metastases measuring >0.5 cm as compared to those with smaller volume disease. Malignant cells are more often present in ascites as compared to washings, and their presence correlates positively with volume of ascites, serous histology, stage, and positive lymph nodes [16]. Peritoneal serous carcinoma more commonly yields positive cytologic specimens as compared to ovarian serous carcinoma [22]. The cytologic features of tumor cells generally resemble those in FNA specimens (see above) but may be more degenerate. The prognosis of patients with stage IC ovarian cancer based on positive peritoneal cytology is poorer than for stages IA and IB. In addition, patients with stage III disease with positive cytology have a poorer prognosis than stage III patients with negative cytology.

Peritoneal lavage is often performed at the time of RRSO in high-risk women. Occult carcinomas can be identified in these cytology specimens. Colgan and associates found malignant cells in 3 of 35 such specimens. One microscopic ovarian surface carcinoma and one in situ tubal carcinoma were found; no carcinoma could be identified in the third patient. Endosalpingiosis was found in 22% [60]. Rarely, malignant cells have been reported in washings at RRSO without an identifiable carcinoma by histology [88], and in two studies, positive cytology specimens led to the discovery of early-stage tubal carcinomas [2, 212].

The main component of benign peritoneal washings is mesothelial cells arranged singly and in sheets. In Papanicolou stains, mesothelial cells appear as round or polygonal cells with dense, cyanophilic cytoplasm and centrally placed, round nuclei with smooth contours and finely granular chromatin. Degenerate and reactive mesothelial cells often display fine or course cytoplasmic vaculation and a lightly stained perinuclear zone.

The presence of epithelial cells in peritoneal fluid samples from patients with atypical proliferative ("borderline") epithelial ovarian tumors has been highlighted in the past as a problematic area of cytopathology. This problem no longer exists because much more accurate histological subclassification of these neoplasms into benign and malignant types (see ➋ Serous Tumors and ➋ Mucinous Tumors sections below) renders the peritoneal fluid cytology specimens in the vast majority of these patients who have benign tumors of no importance. The small proportion of patients who have bona fide carcinomas (patients with invasive MPSCs or APSTs with invasive implants) can be substaged based on the presence or absence of epithelial cells resembling the primary ovarian tumor in the cytology specimens. This situation is rarely encountered since most of these latter tumors are stages III and IV.

The most important pitfall in the examination of peritoneal cytology specimens in women involves benign epithelial proliferations. Women with or without cancer can have endometriosis and/or endosalpingiosis involving peritoneal surfaces. These lesions often shed epithelial fragments into peritoneal washings or ascites; in addition, benign fallopian tube epithelium, particularly if salpingitis is present, and benign eutopic endometrial tissue via expulsion through the fallopian tubes may also be shed into the fluid. If the cells in the fluid are not obviously malignant, comparison of the cytologic features of the epithelium in the fluid with those of the tissue sections are essential in arriving at the correct diagnosis. It is also important to be aware of the cytological abnormalities that may be caused by intraperitoneal chemotherapy as well as radiation, as they may mimic malignancy.

Treatment

Surgery

Initial surgical management of ovarian cancer includes staging, which is aimed at defining the extent of disease, and debulking, which is aimed at reducing tumor burden. In addition to removing the primary tumor intact, total abdominal hysterectomy, bilateral salpingo-oophorectomy, and omentectomy are performed. Fertility-sparing surgery can be performed in selected young patients. Random peritoneal biopsies including the diaphragm, and para-aortic and often pelvic lymph node sampling are essential unless there is obvious disseminated peritoneal disease.

Comprehensive staging will generally be sufficient surgical treatment for patients in stages I and II. Patients with advanced-stage disease often require debulking, or cytoreductive surgery, as well. Cytoreductive surgery, both primary (at presentation) and secondary (after recurrence), prolongs survival and progression-free interval. The median survival after first recurrence followed by secondary cytoreduction is 2–4 years in optimally cytoreduced patients and about 1 year in suboptimally cytoreduced patients. Patients operated on by gynecological oncologists have superior survival rates as compared to those operated on by general surgeons [79].

Chemotherapy

The survival for patients with stage IA and IB, low-grade tumors is 90% or better, and there is no demonstrable benefit from adjuvant chemotherapy. Stage IC is generally regarded as a negative prognostic indicator, but some recent studies have not confirmed this. It is possible that the inability to demonstrate a prognostic difference between stages IA and IC in recent studies is due to a beneficial effect of chemotherapy on stage IC patients. For low-stage ovarian cancer with prognostic features that are generally considered adverse (high-grade and stages IC and IIA), it is not clear whether adjuvant chemotherapy is superior to no treatment. Although there certainly exists a group of low-stage patients that are cured without any further treatment, identification of this group has been difficult as studies of low-stage patients have evaluated a wide variety of features and many of the results are conflicting [313]. Management options for this group include platinum-based chemotherapy (PBC) with or without a taxane, or no treatment.

Patients with advanced stage (FIGO III and IV) disease benefit from chemotherapy using platinum with or without a taxane. PBC has resulted in a significant improvement in response rate, response duration, time to progression, and overall survival. Long-term survival (>5 years) can be achieved with platinum-based combination chemotherapy in over 50% of patients with stage III small-volume residual disease. A recent autopsy study analyzing patients treated with PBC found that 49% of all PBC-treated patients had metastases confined to the abdomen as compared to only 16% of those treated with older chemotherapeutic regimens. There was a higher frequency of liver metastases and fewer lung and pleural metastases. It was therefore suggested that PBC can help prevent extraabdominal spread [114]. At present, a platinum compound in combination with paclitaxel is the best first-line chemotherapy for advanced-stage ovarian cancer. Recent data on platinum-based intraperitoneal chemotherapy for first-line treatment of optimally debulked stage III disease have shown about 20% improvement in both progression-free and overall survival [123], with the median survival increasing by about 12 months. An NC Clinical Announcement in 2006 established a combination of intraperitoneal and intravenous platinum with o without a taxane as standard treatment for optimall debulked stage III patients. However, the optimal regime is still not clear and significant toxicity issues remain. Th advantages of the intraperitoneal route include highe drug concentrations, prolonged tumor exposure, an reduced systemic toxicity [97].

Occasionally, a cytoreductive procedure is abandone due to unresectable disease or inability of the patient t tolerate the procedure. These patients generally underg neoadjuvant chemotherapy to reduce the extent of disea or improve performance status, followed by interv debulking surgery. This management does not appear have an appreciable effect on survival if there is a concerted upfront attempt at cytoreduction. If there is no initial attempt at cytoreduction, the survival is inferior [32, 33, 188].

Second-look laparotomy has no demonstrated effect on survival. In recurrent ovarian cancer, platinum with or without a taxane can be of value. Paclitaxel is active in many patients whose tumors are platinum-resistant.

Other Therapeutic Modalities

Radiation and hormonal therapy may be alternatives in patients who cannot tolerate surgery or chemotherapy. Long-term follow-up of patients who received consolidation radiation therapy and those treated with radiation and melphalan in the 1970s have shown long-term survival rates comparable to those currently treated with PBC; however radiation toxicity rates are high [78, 257]. Hyperthermic intraperitoneal chemotherapy combined with aggressive cytoreduction is used in some centers, but there are no prospective randomized trials demonstrating its efficacy [199].

Up to one third of ovarian cancers have amplification or overexpression of the *HER2/neu* proto-oncogene; however, recent success in treating *HER2*-positive breast cancer with trastuzumab has not been repeated in ovarian cancer [174]. Similarly, immunohistochemical expression of c-kit (CD117) has been variable, but generally low, suggesting that imatinib will not be of value [145]. Amplification and immunoreactivity for EGFR have been reported in 20% and 28% of ovarian cancers, respectively, and clinical responses to gefitinib, an EGFR inhibitor, have been variable but generally low [335]. The VEGF inhibitor, bevacizumab, has shown some activity in ovarian cancer, but the data are preliminary [163]. In vitro drug-resistance assays are sometimes used to guide therapy, more often with recurrent tumor, but data are limited.

Table 14.10
The World Health Organization (WHO) classification of ovarian tumors

Serous tumors
Serous cystadenoma, adenofibroma
Serous tumor of borderline malignancy (of low malignant potential)
Serous adenocarcinoma
Mucinous tumors, endocervical-like and intestinal types
Mucinous cystadenoma
Mucinous tumor of borderline malignancy (of low malignant potential)
Mucinous adenocarcinoma
Endometrioid tumors
Endometrioid cystadenoma, adenofibroma
Endometrioid tumor of borderline malignancy (of low malignant potential)
Endometrioid adenocarcinoma
Clear cell tumors
Clear cell adenofibroma, cystadenoma
Clear cell tumor of borderline malignancy (of low malignant potential)
Clear cell adenocarcinoma
Transitional cell tumors
Brenner tumor
Brenner tumor of borderline malignancy (proliferating)
Malignant Brenner tumor
Transitional cell carcinoma (TCC) (non-Brenner type)
Squamous cell tumors
Mixed epithelial tumors (specify components)
Benign
Of borderline malignancy (of low malignant potential)
Malignant
Undifferentiated carcinoma

Modified from [297]

Pathology of Ovarian Epithelial Neoplasms

The World Health Organization (WHO) classification of surface epithelial tumors is summarized in *Table 14.10*, and the distribution of ovarian surface epithelial tumors is shown in *Table 14.5*. Ovarian epithelial tumors comprise about half of all ovarian tumors, and account for about 40% of benign tumors and nearly 90% of malignant tumors. A uniform series using standard histologic criteria to assess the distribution of ovarian tumors has not been reported since Russell's review of 1,000 surface epithelial tumors in the late 1970s [308]. We have recently evaluated 1,000 consecutive ovarian surface epithelial tumors accessioned at the Washington Hospital Center from 1999 to 2009 (*Table 14.5*). Although not population-based, our data on carcinomas are very similar to population-based data from Canada [107] and Sweden [4], with the exception of a somewhat higher frequency of mucinous carcinoma in the latter study.

The apparent cell-type distribution has changed significantly in the past 2 decades as metastatic mucinous carcinomas have been recognized and properly categorized. Primary invasive mucinous carcinoma now appears to be quite uncommon, comprising only 3% of ovarian carcinomas and less than 1% of advanced-stage carcinomas (➲ *Table 14.4*) [104, 301], although they appear to be somewhat more common in Asia with 6.7% found in a recent Thai study [147]. Carcinosarcoma (malignant mixed müllerian tumor – MMMT), previously regarded as a rare primary ovarian tumor, now appears to comprise over 7% of ovarian carcinomas in the United States and 2.5% in Thailand. This apparent increase in frequency may be due to more thorough sampling with the identification of small sarcomatous components in otherwise typical high-grade serous carcinomas.

Accurate pathologic classification is predicated on examination of histological sections that are representative of the entire neoplasm. Intratumoral heterogeneity is a common phenomenon of many sites and it is particularly common in ovarian tumors. Since volume is exponentially related to a spherical tumor diameter, small tumors measuring up to about 5–7 cm can easily be thoroughly sampled, while larger tumors cannot. A 15 cm solid tumor, for example, would require hundreds of sections to achieve the same sampling per unit volume as a 5 cm tumor examined with five sections. Type II tumors, usually high-grade serous carcinoma, are relatively uniform. In contrast, Type I tumors display a wide variety of patterns and degrees of epithelial proliferation in different areas. Although extensive sampling is not generally needed for invasive carcinomas, noninvasive tumors need careful gross examination and directed sampling of papillary, solid, and any unusual areas to make certain that invasive foci are not overlooked. This is particularly important for the atypical proliferative (borderline) endometrioid, mucinous, clear cell, and low-grade serous cell types, i.e., the precursors of Type I carcinomas.

CAP and WHO Recommendations

The College of American Pathologists (CAP) has issued guidelines for the reporting of ovarian cancer [243]. Complete reporting with the CAP cancer checklist requires assessment of ovarian surface involvement and tumor rupture for stages I and II. It is therefore important that the pathologist communicate with the surgeon or review the operative report to provide these data. For advanced stage, the size of the largest peritoneal nodule needs to be assessed, and although this is often evident from the gross pathologic examination, the surgeon's input may be required since the tumor may be incompletely resected. In apparent stage III patients, clinical or pathologic information may be needed to determine whether distant metastases have been diagnosed (stage IV).

The CAP does not recommend any specific grading system. There are features found in the checklist that are not routinely reported: (1) For bilateral tumors, which one is the primary (this is possible in only a small minority of cases); (2) The presence of venous or lymphatic invasion; (3) specimen type (requiring, e.g., distinguishing an omental biopsy, partial omentectomy, and complete omentectomy). Some of the data are considered optional. Required elements include specimen type, specimen integrity, primary site, tumor size, histologic type, grade, and TNM stage. There is a separate CAP checklist for peritoneal tumors [244]. This should not be used for primary peritoneal serous carcinomas as it is incomplete for this purpose. The ovary checklist is more appropriate.

The status of peritoneal implants is required for the reporting of borderline tumors. However, it is not necessary to use the CAP checklist for borderline tumors unless carcinoma (invasive implants or invasive MPSC) is present.

In the most recent edition of the WHO classification of ovarian tumors [297], there are some differences from the classification used in this chapter (➲ *Table 14.10*). The most notable difference is division of serous borderline tumors (SBT) into APST (benign) and noninvasive MPSC (low-grade malignant), while WHO uses SBT with micropapillary pattern for the latter tumor. In addition, we do not use the modifiers "cystadeno," "papillary," "surface," "fibroma," and "adeno" for serous carcinomas, as these create multiple different names for the most common type of ovarian cancer. Because of this multiplicity of names, the International Classification of Diseases for Oncology contains at least four different codes for synonyms for serous carcinoma [90]. This leads to confusion in cancer registries as well as difficulties in the interpretation of population-based data. Regarding microinvasion, the WHO recommends a cutoff of 3 mm for microinvasion for APST, whereas we prefer 5 mm for all cell types. The category of intraepithelial carcinoma, which WHO uses for mucinous tumors, we use on rare occasion for endometrioid and clear cell tumors as well. Finally, we require 25% of a second epithelial component for diagnosis of a mixed epithelial tumor, whereas WHO uses 10%.

Serous Tumors

The classification of serous neoplasms of the ovary has been mired in confusion and controversy due to the widely misunderstood intermediate category between benign and malignant. The borderline group has now been successfully subclassified into benign (APST) and low-grade malignant (noninvasive MPSC or APST with invasive peritoneal implants) categories and is therefore no longer needed. The terminology is summarized in *Table 14.11*.

Serous Cystadenoma and Adenofibroma

Benign serous tumors include cystadenomas, adenofibromas, cystadenofibromas, and surface papillomas. These tumors are common and account for two thirds of benign ovarian epithelial tumors and the majority of ovarian serous tumors. They occur in adults of all ages, with reported mean ages varying widely from 40 to 60 years. The symptoms and signs associated with large tumors are nonspecific and most commonly include pelvic pain, discomfort, or an asymptomatic pelvic mass. Tumors measuring 1–3 cm are usually incidental findings. Bilaterality rates are variable depending upon both the thoroughness with which an apparently uninvolved ovary is examined as well as the threshold for diagnosis of a small serous neoplasm. Accordingly, 12–23% of cystadenomas are bilateral.

Table 14.11
Terminology of serous tumors

Old Terminology	New terminology
Ovarian	
Serous borderline tumor (SBT)	Atypical proliferative serous tumor (APST)
Serous tumor of low malignant potential	
Micropapillary serous borderline tumor	Noninvasive micropapillary serous carcinoma (MPSC)
Well-differentiated serous carcinoma	Low grade (invasive) micropapillary serous carcinoma
Microinvasion	Microinvasion[a]
	Microinvasive carcinoma[b]
Peritoneal	
Noninvasive epithelial implant	Implant[c]
Noninvasive desmoplastic implant	Implant[c]
Noninvasive implant with micropapillary pattern	Metastatic low-grade serous carcinoma[c]
Invasive implant	Metastatic low-grade serous carcinoma[c]

[a]Usual type characterized by small clusters of eosinophilic cells just beneath the surface epithelium.
[b]Less common type characterized by micropapillae and or small solid nests of cells surrounded by a space, identical in appearance to invasive low-grade micropapillary serous carcinoma.
[c]Proposed new terminology.

Benign serous tumors are equally distributed among unilocular cysts, multilocular cysts, and cystadenofibromas [307]. They are composed of cysts filled with clear watery (serous) fluid or thin mucoid material. Occasionally, they contain thicker mucus-like material more typical of mucinous neoplasms. The external surfaces of the cysts are smooth and glistening. Occasionally, papillary excrescences are found on the external surface of the cyst. The tumors vary widely in size up to 30 cm, with a mean of 5–8 cm. The lining of the cyst is either flat or may have a varying number of coarse papillary projections. Such papillary excrescences rarely cover the entire inner surface of the cyst. Adenofibromas are solid neoplasms composed of tough, rubbery tissue with interspersed glandular spaces.

Normal-sized ovaries often have small surface papillary projections with a fibrotic stromal component resembling a microscopic adenofibroma or cystadenofibroma; these have been termed surface papillomas, and when multiple, surface papillomatosis (see Chap. 12, Nonneoplastic Lesions of the Ovaries). In addition, surface epithelial inclusions may become cystically dilated. It has been suggested that a serous neoplasm be diagnosed only if the lesion is >1 cm in diameter. This is arbitrary and therefore unlikely to distinguish neoplastic growth from simple serous cysts or non-neoplastic hyperplasias of the ovarian cortex.

The vast majority of lesions classified as serous cystadenoma display a serous epithelial lining lacking proliferation. In a recent study, only 7% of serous cystadenomas had greater than 1 mm of epithelial proliferation [307]. Accordingly, most serous cystadenomas are not true neoplasms, but rather represent cystically dilated inclusions.

Cystadenomas are lined by pseudostratified, tubal-type epithelium, with the characteristic elongated (secretory cell) and rounded (ciliated cell) nuclei (*Fig. 14.4*). A single layer of flattened to cuboidal cells with uniform basal nuclei is also common. Although the cells often

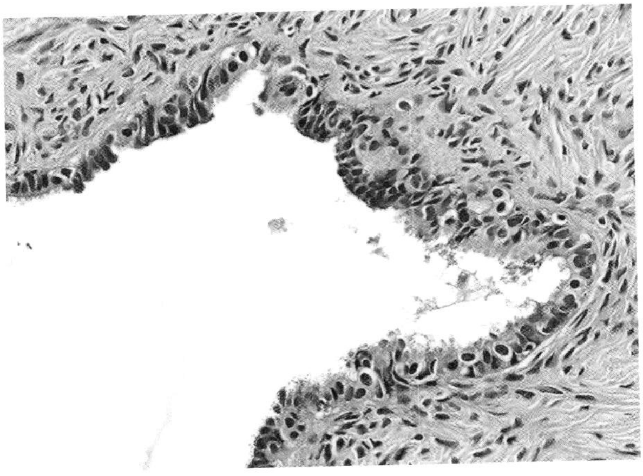

Fig. 14.4
Serous cystadenoma. **A single layer of serous epithelium characterized by ciliated, secretory, and intercalated cells as in the normal fallopian tube**

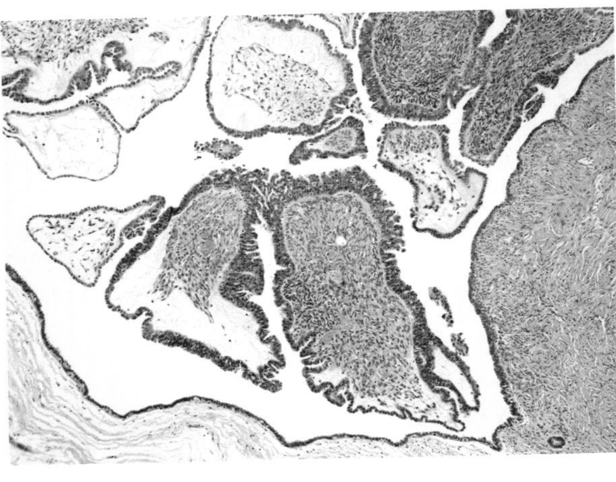

Fig. 14.5
Serous cystadenoma with focal proliferation and atypia. **Epithelial stratification and tufting are present in less than 10% of this otherwise ordinary serous cystadenoma**

produce mucin, which is secreted into the cystic spaces, they do not contain basophilic cytoplasmic vacuoles or granules characteristic of mucinous neoplasms. In large cysts, the epithelium often becomes attenuated. Mitoses and atypia are generally absent. Psammoma bodies are present in the stroma in 15% of cystadenomas. There is a broad spectrum of epithelial proliferation in benign serous tumors, which is manifested by variation in the prominence and complexity of the papillae, from a simple, single layer and blunt papillae to focal epithelial stratification and detachment of cell clusters approaching the degree of proliferation seen in APSTs. Identification of these features in 10% of the tumor separates serous cystadenoma from APST. If these features are focal (<10%), a diagnosis of serous cystadenoma with focal atypia is used (*Fig. 14.5*) [7, 310].

The stroma of benign serous tumors can resemble normal ovarian stroma, but is generally more fibrous or edematous. When the stroma is highly cellular and fibrous and forms large solid areas containing scattered glands or thick papillary projections lined by serous epithelium, the tumor is designated an adenofibroma, or if cystic, cystadenofibroma (*Fig. 14.6*). Pseudoxanthoma cells with granular, light-brown cytoplasmic pigment beneath the epithelium can be seen on occasion.

The immunohistochemical profile of serous cystadenoma is similar to that of normal ovarian surface epithelium and tubal epithelium. In addition to positivity with most commonly used epithelial markers, p63 is positive in most cases [260].

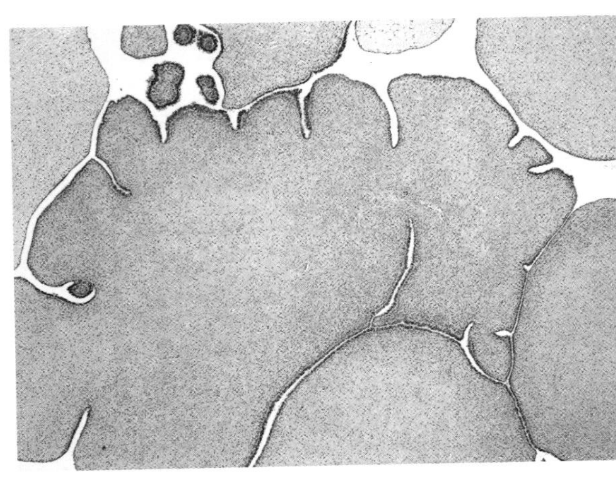

Fig. 14.6
Serous cystadenofibroma. **Broad fibrous papillae lined by a single layer of tubal-type epithelium protrude into a cys**

A variety of benign cysts may occur in and around th ovary and broad ligament and may simulate serou cystadenomas both grossly and microscopically. Func tional ovarian cysts may have a denuded or attenuate lining. Similarly, an endometriotic cyst on occasion wi mimic a serous cystadenoma if it lacks hemorrhage, an endometriotic stroma is inconspicuous. Broad ligame cysts, such as hydatid cysts of Morgagni, mesonephr cysts, and mesothelial (peritoneal) cysts, often mim a serous cystadenoma. Mesonephric cysts are lined b cuboidal cells and are usually surrounded by concentric smooth muscle bundles. Peritoneal cysts are very common, are lined by mesothelial cells, and frequently arise via ovarian surface adhesions. Occasionally, hydrosalpinx will mimic a serous cystadenoma grossly and microscopically. Careful gross examination and discussion with the surgeon helps in the recognition that the apparent cyst represents a dilated fallopian tube.

A recent report indicates that the cells lining the cysts in most serous cystadenomas are polyclonal and therefore non-neoplastic [54]. Unilateral salpingo-oophorectomy or ovarian cystectomy is adequate treatment. Clinical recurrence is uncommon and reflects either incomplete resection or a new primary tumor.

Low Grade Serous Tumors Atypical Proliferative Serous Tumor (APST); Serous Borderline Tumor (SBT)

The "borderline" category of ovarian epithelial tumors was introduced in the early 1970s in order to describe a group of tumors that did not display invasion, but that occasionally appeared to behave in a malignant fashion. Their behavior appeared to be intermediate between benign cystadenomas and frank serous carcinomas. The classification was intended as provisional, but with its continued use over the past 3 decades, the borderline category has become entrenched and regarded as a specific entity. Recent studies have documented a wide histologic spectrum encompassed by the borderline category that correlates with behavior. Tumors at the lower end of the spectrum behave in a benign fashion and display a papillary architecture in which papillae have a hierarchical branching pattern. These tumors are termed "APST." Tumors at the upper end of the spectrum behave like low-grade carcinomas, display a more complex nonhierarchical branching pattern characterized by delicate micropapillae, and are classified as "noninvasive MPSC." APSTs comprise about 50% of atypical proliferative (borderline) ovarian tumors of all histologic types (➋ *Table 14.5*). The atypical proliferative terminology has been accepted by the WHO since 2000 [90], and was accepted as synonymous with "borderline" at the 2003 Borderline Ovarian Tumor conference, while "low malignant potential" was not recommended at the latter meeting [310].

Clinical Findings

The clinical features of patients with APSTs are similar to those for serous cystadenomas; the mean age is 42 years. The risk factors are similar to those for ovarian cancer with notable exceptions of a higher frequency of infertility and a lower frequency of *BRCA* mutations.

Operative Findings

Thirty-seven percent of APSTs are bilateral in the older literature; the recent Stanford series showed a 55% bilaterality rate [190]. This difference probably reflects more diligent examination of normal-sized ovaries with the identification of small serous proliferations. Exophytic papillae reflecting ovarian surface involvement are common, and are more often found in patients who also have peritoneal implants. Tumors with an exophytic component are associated with implants in 49–69% of cases as compared to 4–27% tumors that are completely intracystic [190, 262].

Gross Findings

APSTs tend to have fine, friable, and exuberant papillary projections in contrast to the smooth-walled cysts of serous cystadenoma. Papillae are nearly always present on the internal surfaces of the cyst, and are present on the external surfaces in up to 70% of cases. The adenofibromatous variant of APST is unusual.

Peritoneal endosalpingiosis in patients with APST is grossly inconspicuous. Noninvasive desmoplastic implants are firm and fibrotic, and are covered by an inflammatory exudate in 20% of cases. Invasive implants (metastatic low-grade serous carcinoma) resemble typical serous carcinoma, but are often less bulky and more calcified.

Thorough sampling of the primary tumor for histological examination is needed to rule out invasion. Previous recommendations of one section per centimeter of maximum tumor diameter will not identify invasion in a significant minority of cases in which invasion is actually present. Recent data suggest that at least two sections per centimeter are needed to confidently exclude invasion [303] (see ➋ Microinvasion below).

Microscopic Findings

APSTs display extensive epithelial stratification, tufting (budding), and detachment of individual cells and cell clusters in addition to hierarchical branching with successively smaller papillae emanating from the larger, more centrally located papillae (➋ *Figs. 14.7–14.9*). Stratification and budding in at least 10% of the tumor warrants a diagnosis of APST. Complex papillary patterns often display stromal invaginations cut tangentially that must be distinguished from stromal invasion (➋ *Fig. 14.8*).

Focal areas of fusion of the epithelial buds may create a roman bridge or cribriform pattern (➋ *Figs. 14.10* and ➋ *14.11*). Similarly, foci of nonhierarchical branching with

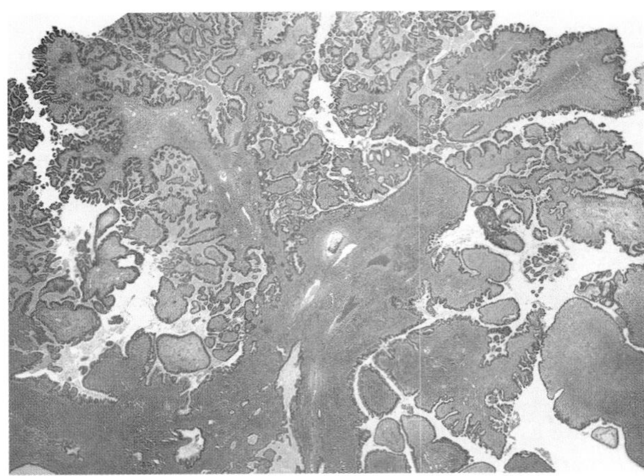

Fig. 14.7
Atypical proliferative (borderline) serous tumor (APST). **A complex hierarchical branching pattern is present**

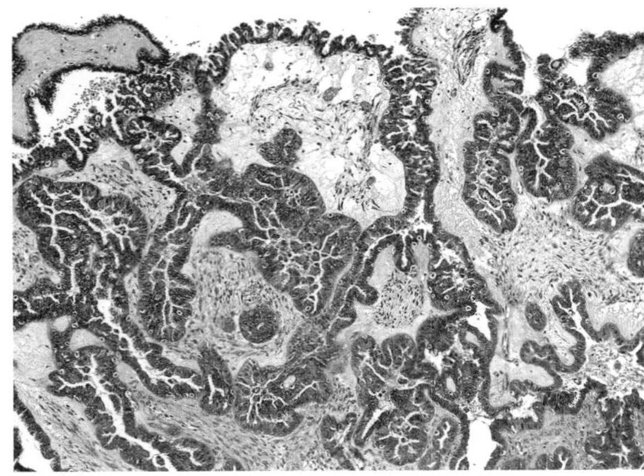

Fig. 14.9
Atypical proliferative (borderline) serous tumor. **The stroma is edematous. Detached cell clusters are present between small and large papillae**

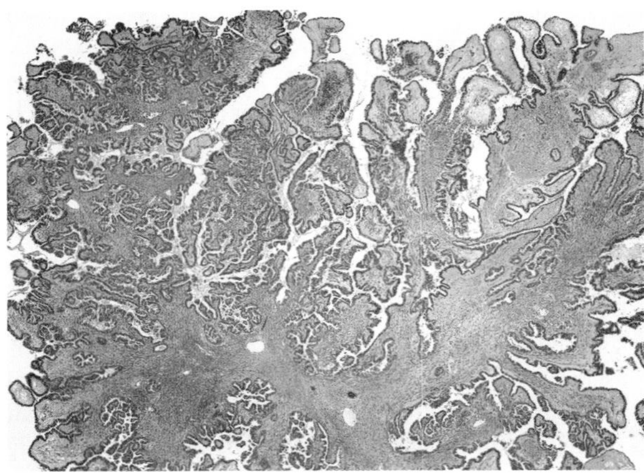

Fig. 14.8
Atypical proliferative (borderline) serous tumor. **Gland-like structures within the stroma reflect tangential sectioning of a complex papillae and are not indicative of invasion**

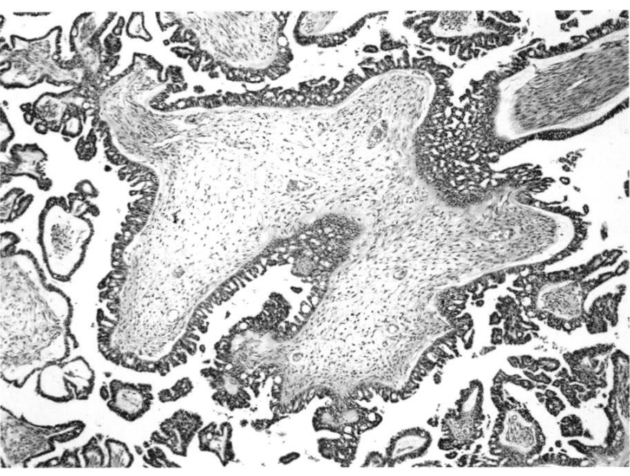

Fig. 14.10
Atypical proliferative (borderline) serous tumor. **Fusion of surface papillae create a roman bridge or cribriform pattern**

fine elongated micropapillae emanating directly from large central papillae are seen not infrequently (*Fig. 14.12*). When cribriform and/or micropapillary patterns constitute either a 5 mm or greater confluent area, or 10% or greater proportion, the tumor warrants classification as noninvasive MPSC (see "Malignant serous tumors" below).

The cells in APSTs show features of epithelial and occasionally mesothelial differentiation. Ciliated cells resembling fallopian tube epithelium are present in about one third of tumors. Hobnail-type cells may be present (*Figs. 14.11* and *14.13*) and occasionally the epithelium becomes attenuated and resembles mesothelium. In addition, cells with abundant eosinophilic cytoplasm and rounded nuclei, occasionally resembling mesothelial cells, may be present, particularly on the tips of the papillae. The nuclei of APSTs resemble those in cystadenomas but tend to display slightly more atypia. Nuclei are basally located and tend to be ovoid or rounded. The chromatin is usually fine and nucleoli are

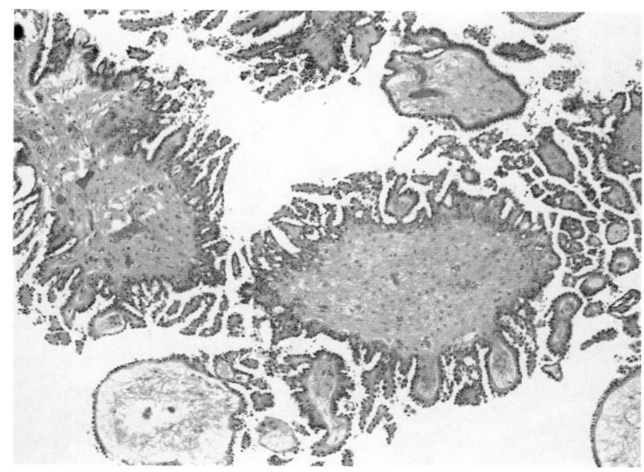

Fig. 14.11
Atypical proliferative (borderline) serous tumor. **Numerous hobnail cells line papillae. Detached cell clusters are present**

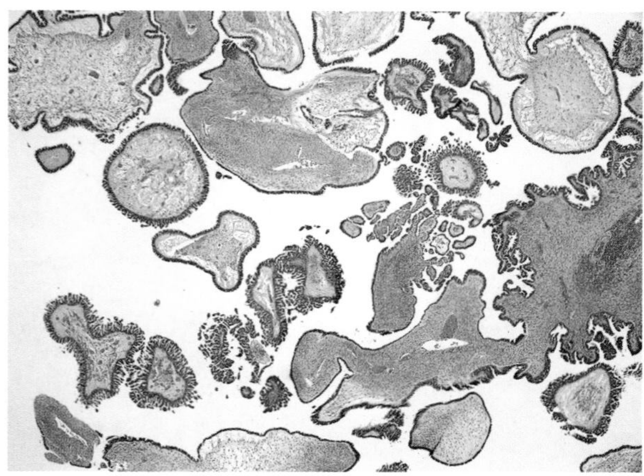

Fig. 14.12
Atypical proliferative (borderline) serous tumor.
A micropapillary architecture is present in less than 10% of the tumor

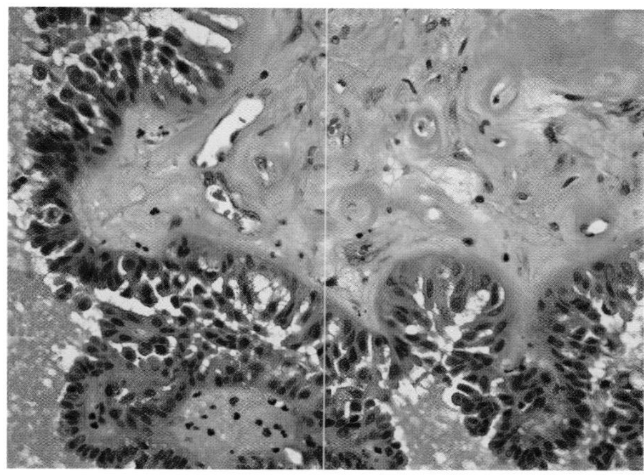

Fig. 14.13
Atypical proliferative (borderline) serous tumor. **Hobnail cells with abundant eosinophilic cytoplasm are prominent**

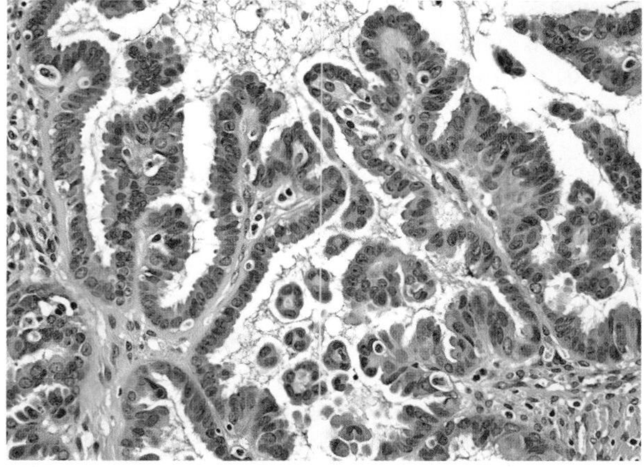

Fig. 14.14
Atypical proliferative (borderline) serous tumor. **Small clusters of cells and small papillae appear detached from the larger papillae**

occasionally prominent (*Figs. 14.14* and *14.15*). Mitoses are not common and rarely exceed four per ten high-power fields (HPF). Psammoma bodies are present in up to half of APSTs.

Occasionally, foci resembling noninvasive desmoplastic peritoneal implants (see Noninvasive Peritoneal Implants below) are found on the surfaces of the ovarian tumor. This has been referred to as "autoimplantation." Autoimplants are found on the ovarian surface or between exophytic surface papillae. They are multifocal in two thirds of cases and range from 0.1 to 2.5 cm in size. They have a well-delineated border with adjacent tissue. Microscopically they are identical to noninvasive desmoplastic implants. Infarcted tumor papillae are found in about one third of cases. In all advanced-stage cases, noninvasive desmoplastic peritoneal implants are present. Postulated mechanisms for the origin of this lesion include adhesion of the ovarian tumor to desmoplastic implants and infarction of tumor papillae [275]. The term "autoimplant" suggests that such lesions might arise by detachment of papillae from the tumor surface and subsequent reattachment back to itself, but there is no evidence for this phenomenon. This lesion has no known clinical significance.

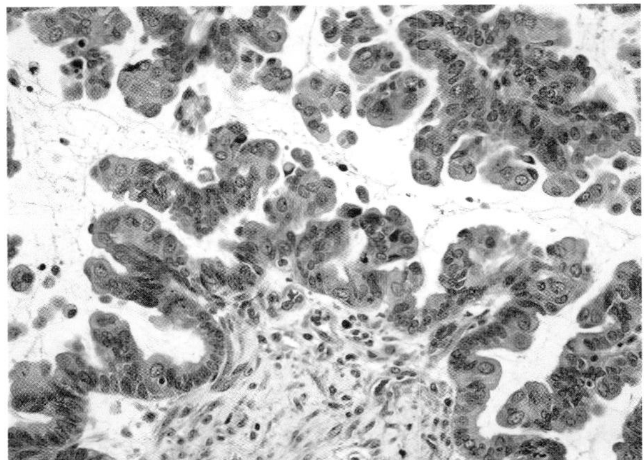

Fig. 14.15
Atypical proliferative (borderline) serous tumor. **There is mild cytologic atypia and small prominent nucleoli**

Microinvasion Two distinct types of lesions have been designated "microinvasion" in APSTs. In most published reports, the two types have not been specifically distinguished or correlated with outcome.

Usual Type of Microinvasion (Eosinophilic Type) This type of microinvasion accounts for the vast majority of reported cases. It is characterized by isolated cells and small cell clusters with abundant eosinophilic cytoplasm that appear to be budding from the epithelium into the superficial stromal cores of the papillae (*Figs. 14.16–14.20*). The lesion must be smaller than 5 mm, and can be multiple. The true nature of these eosinophilic cells is not clear. In most cases, they do not evoke a host stromal response and they bear little resemblance to invasive carcinoma. We remain unconvinced that this lesion is a manifestation of invasive carcinoma.

When carefully sought, 10% of reported APSTs contain microinvasion; however, microinvasion was specifically noted in only 1.3% of reported APSTs up to 1999 [305]. However, two recent series suggest that microinvasion may be found in 25% of cases [126, 226], and in one study of APST with noninvasive implants, 56% had microinvasion [326]. A high proportion of APSTs diagnosed during pregnancy show microinvasion [210]. A recent study demonstrated a significant association of microinvasion with papillary infarction [160].

Microinvasive Carcinoma The second type of microinvasion occurs less commonly and is characterized by a haphazard infiltrative pattern of small solid nests of cells and micropapillae, often surrounded by a clear space and associated with an identifiable stromal response (i.e., desmoplasia; *Figs. 14.20–14.23*). Occasionally the nests display a cribriform pattern. This second pattern of invasion closely resembles primary ovarian invasive low-grade serous carcinomas as well as the peritoneal lesions that have been designated "invasive implants." Accordingly we refer to this second type of microinvasion as "microinvasive carcinoma," because the evidence, albeit limited, indicates that it is a manifestation

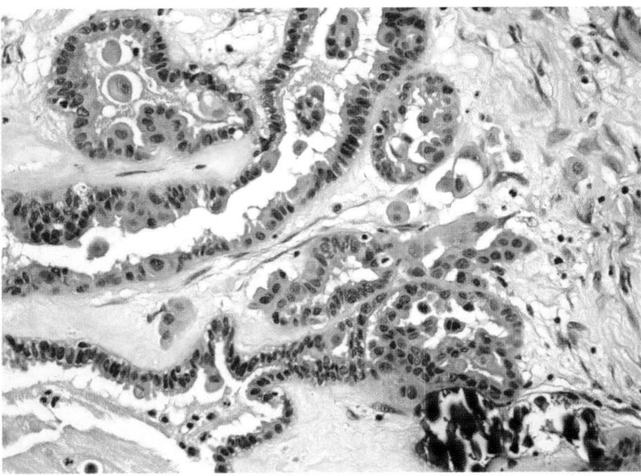

Fig. 14.16
Atypical proliferative (borderline) serous tumor with microinvasion. **Single cells with abundant eosinophilic cytoplasm are present in the stroma. Note the similarity to eosinophilic cells on the surface of the papillae**

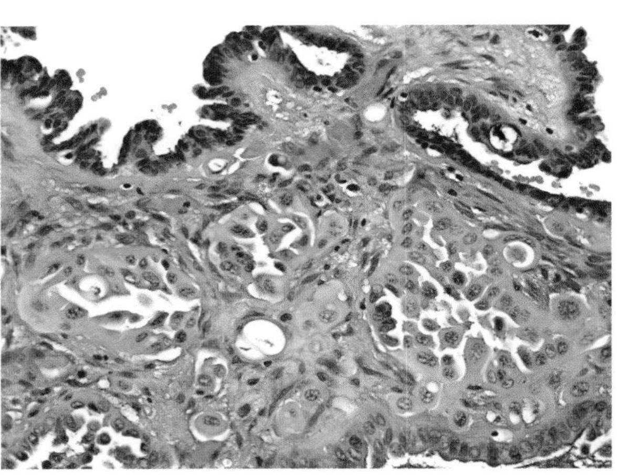

Fig. 14.17
Atypical proliferative (borderline) serous tumor with microinvasion. **Single cells and cell clusters with abundant eosinophilic cytoplasm within the stroma**

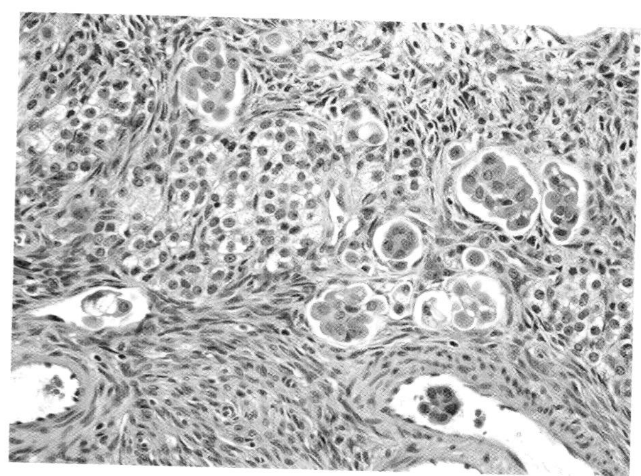

Fig. 14.18
Atypical proliferative (borderline) serous tumor with microinvasion. **Eosinophilic cell clusters of about 3–12 cells are surrounded by a space. Compare to cluster of luteinized ovarian stromal cells in the center, which have paler cytoplasm and are not surrounded by a space**

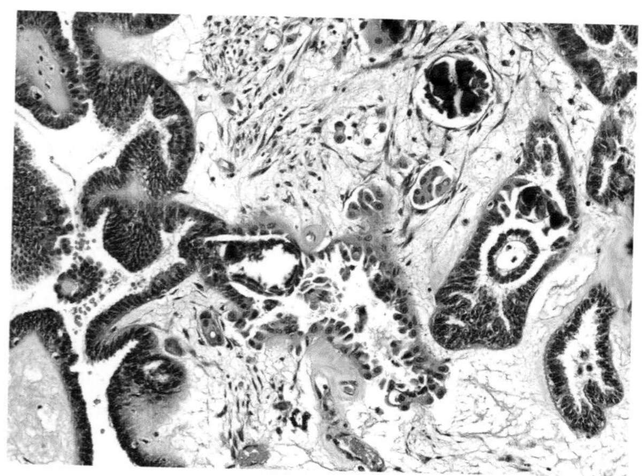

Fig. 14.19
Atypical proliferative (borderline) serous tumor with microinvasion. **Single eosinophilic cells and cell clusters in the stroma, adjacent to a noninvasive gland-like structure lined by similar eosinophilic cells with a hobnail pattern. Note psammomatous calcification in the stroma and within the epithelium**

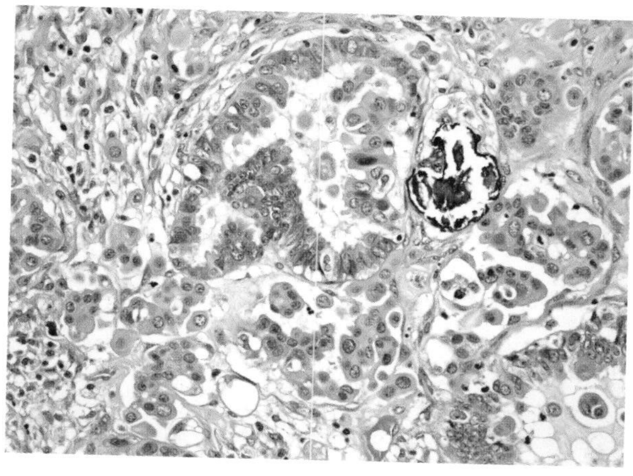

Fig. 14.20
Atypical proliferative (borderline) serous tumor with microinvasion. **Single eosinophilic cells and cell clusters infiltrate the stroma**

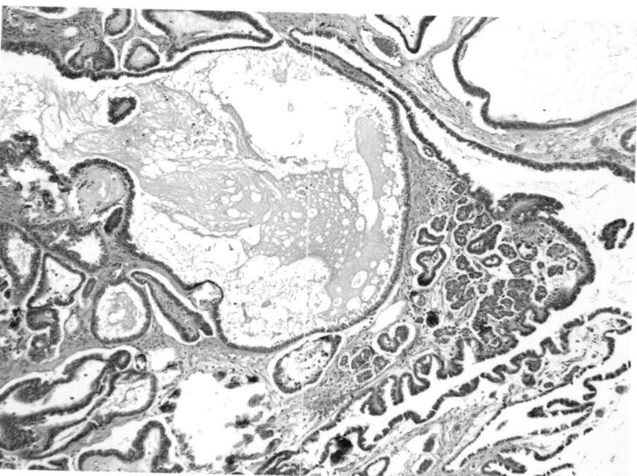

Fig. 14.21
Atypical proliferative (borderline) serous tumor with microinvasive carcinoma. **Small papillae on the *right side* are surrounded by spaces and display an infiltrative pattern**

of true invasive carcinoma. To qualify as microinvasive carcinoma, the lesion should be smaller than 5 mm. Multiple foci are permitted.

Microinvasion has been associated with a higher frequency of bilaterality, exophytic growth, and peritoneal implants [262]. Recent evidence suggests that the identification of microinvasion or microinvasive carcinoma is a clue that further sampling might disclose more extensive invasion. A minimum of two sections per centimeter of maximum tumor diameter are needed to maximize detection of occult invasion [303].

The clear space surrounding most nests and micropapillae, and occasionally surrounding single cells

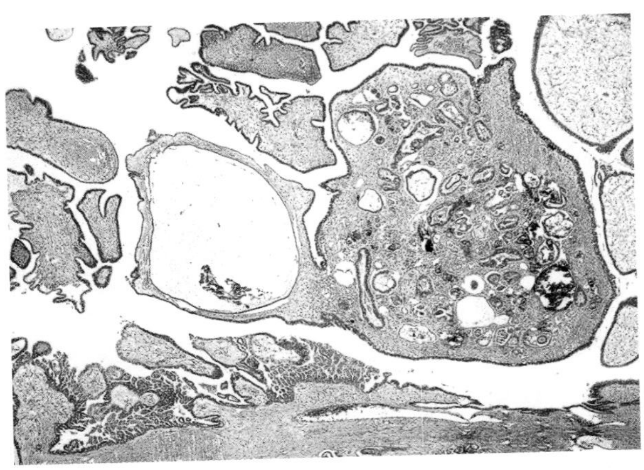

◘ Fig. 14.22
Atypical proliferative (borderline) serous tumor with microinvasive carcinoma. **A large papilla occupies the *right* half of the photograph and contains both micropapillae and macropapillae surrounded by spaces and display an infiltrative pattern. This focus is about 5 mm, and is therefore at the boundary between APST with microinvasive carcinoma and invasive low-grade serous carcinoma**

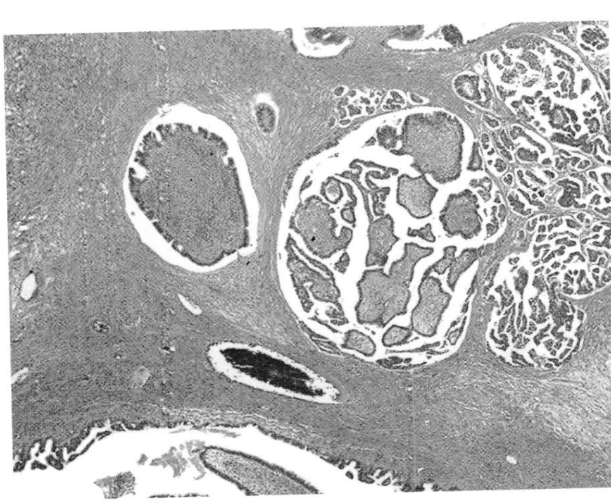

◘ Fig. 14.23
Atypical proliferative (borderline) serous tumor with microinvasive carcinoma. **Invasive papillae of varying sizes, from micropapillae surrounded by spaces on the *right* side, to a single macropapillae on the *left***

and small clusters, have generally been considered artifactual due to tissue retraction. However, recent work using a lymphatic endothelium-specific antibody, D2-40, has demonstrated that many of these spaces represent lymphatics and therefore lymphatic invasion [289]. Among 20 SBT (19 APST and 1 noninvasive MPSC) with microinvasion, 60% had lymphatic invasion as compared to none of 20 (18 APST and 2 noninvasive MPSC) without microinvasion. In this study, lymphatic invasion correlated with microinvasion but not with age, stage, autoimplantation, micropapillary architecture, or pattern/extent of microinvasion.

Clinical Behavior and Treatment A review of 94 patients with microinvasion reported up to 1999 showed 100% survival [305]. More recently, Longacre and associates found that microinvasion was a significant predictor of survival on univariate but not multivariate analysis [190, 210]. Although more data are needed, from the standpoint of prognosis and patient management, microinvasion does not appear to have any clinical relevance. On the other hand, limited data suggest that microinvasive carcinoma is associated with a higher risk of recurrence [210]. Whether or not staging is needed for a woman with microinvasive carcinoma is unclear. There are no data at present suggesting that follow-up or any treatment will influence recurrence or survival.

Associated Peritoneal Lesions: Endosalpingiosis and "Implants" APSTs are often associated with serous lesions involving the peritoneum. Endosalpingiosis, or benign glandular inclusions, are found in 40% of patients. At present, 40% of reported APSTs are associated with peritoneal implants in contrast to 25% in the pre-1980 literature [305]. However, in population-based and hospital-based material, the figure is closer to 10–20% [17, 68, 252, 380], suggesting a referral bias to large specialized centers in favor of tumors with implants as compared to those without. In the Stanford study, 59% had implants [190]. Among those with implants, about three fourths were noninvasive, and one fourth were invasive. It is important to note that the origin of peritoneal "implants" is unknown and the purported mechanism of "detachment and implantation" is an assumption (see ➲ Pathogenesis of Peritoneal Implants below).

Endosalpingiosis Endosalpingiosis, or benign glandular inclusions, may involve the peritoneal surfaces in patients with or without benign or malignant serous ovarian tumors (see ➲ Chap. 13, Diseases of the Peritoneum). These glands typically are lined by simple columnar epithelium, often displaying tubal-type differentiation. The epithelium may display minor degrees of cytologic atypia and form simple papillary structures [20] (➲ *Fig. 14.24*); psammoma bodies are sometimes prese

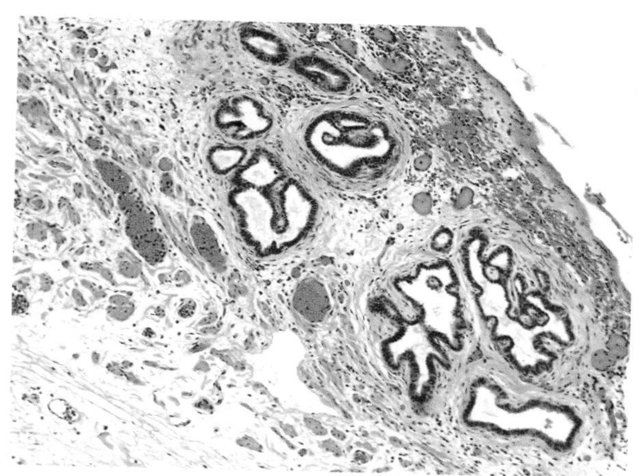

Fig. 14.24
Endosalpingiosis. **Simple glands, some with small blunt papillae, are lined by benign tubal-type epithelium**

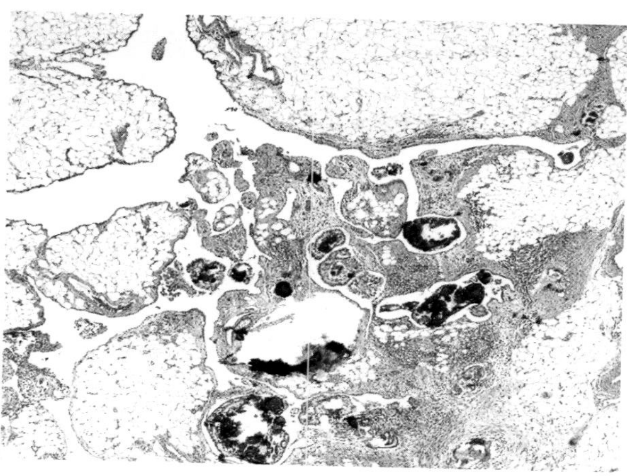

Fig. 14.25
Noninvasive epithelial implant (implant). **Papillary structures on the surface of the peritoneum and also within clefts of peritoneum**

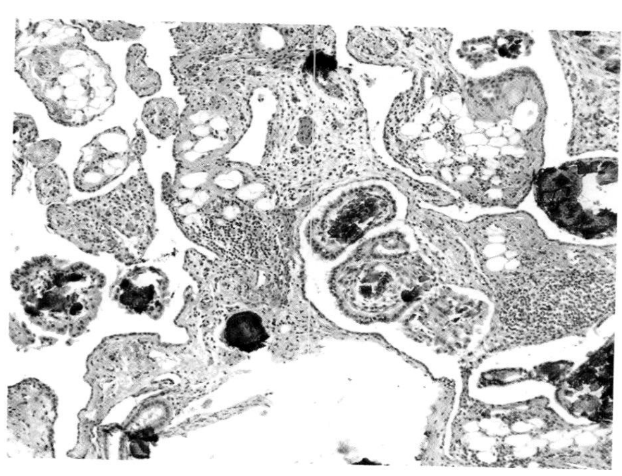

Fig. 14.26
Noninvasive epithelial implant (implant). **Psammoma bodies and chronic inflammation are present; there is no invasion of underlying tissue**

and may persist after degeneration of the associated epithelial structures. Mitotic figures are absent.

Noninvasive Peritoneal Implants Among women with APSTs, 31% (78% of all patients with implants) have peritoneal epithelial lesions that display a degree of proliferation beyond that usually seen in endosalpingiosis, but that lack features of invasion. These have been designated "noninvasive implants" and have two morphological forms: epithelial and desmoplastic. Some patients have both types of noninvasive implants.

Epithelial implants are papillary and resemble the ovarian APST to some extent (➲ *Figs. 14.25–14.29*). The cores of the papillae have fibrovascular support, and the epithelial cells resemble those in endosalpingiosis. Thus, mild atypia is often present, but mitoses are usually absent (➲ *Figs.14.28* and ➲ *14.29*). Calcification in the form of psammoma bodies is common and frequently is extensive (➲ *Figs. 14.25–14.26*). This type of implant often resembles a mucosal lesion of the fallopian tube that has been termed "salpingolith," which is characterized by psammomatous calcification surrounded by a single layer of tubal-type epithelium. Salpingoliths are found in 51% of advanced-stage APST/MPSC as compared to 24% of stage I cases [309]. Their significance is unknown (see ➲ Chap. 11, Diseases of the Fallopian Tube).

The desmoplastic noninvasive implant is a plaque-like thickening overlying peritoneal surfaces and may extend into the septae that separate omental lobules creating a low-power appearance that suggests invasion (➲ *Figs. 14.30* and ➲ *14.31*). These implants display an exuberant fibroblastic proliferation in which gland-like or papillary structures lined by epithelial cells are present. Psammoma bodies are usually present. The epithelium typically shows minimal and occasionally more marked cytologic atypia (➲ *Figs. 14.32–14.34*). The fibroblastic proliferation often has a granulation tissue-like appearance characterized by edematous fascicles of plump fibroblasts, often with interspersed small vascular channels (➲ *Figs. 14.31* and ➲ *14.32*). Typically, the cells forming the gland-like structures merge with the surrounding fibroblasts, which surround the glands, making

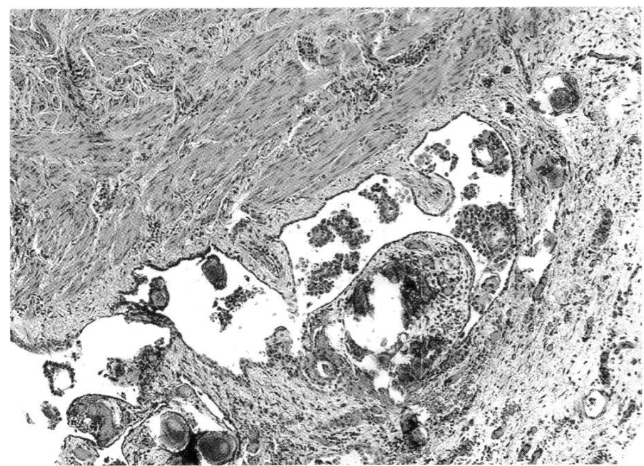

Fig. 14.27
Noninvasive epithelial implant (implant). **An adhesion on the uterine serosa is lined by mesothelial cells and displays surface papillae. Note psammoma bodies, chronic inflammation, and absence of invasion of underlying tissue**

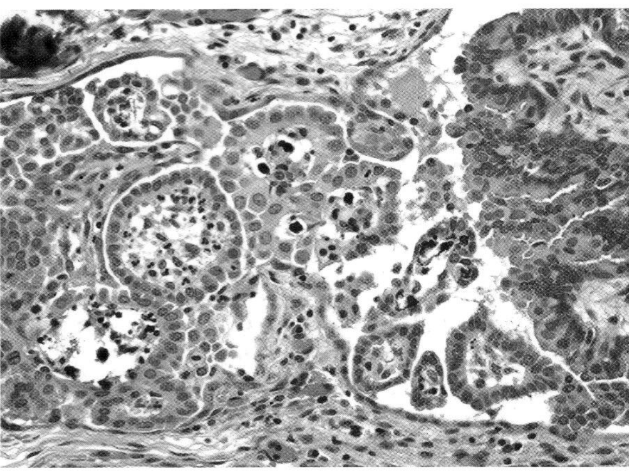

Fig. 14.29
Noninvasive epithelial implant (implant). **Mild cytologic atypia and small prominent nucleoli are present**

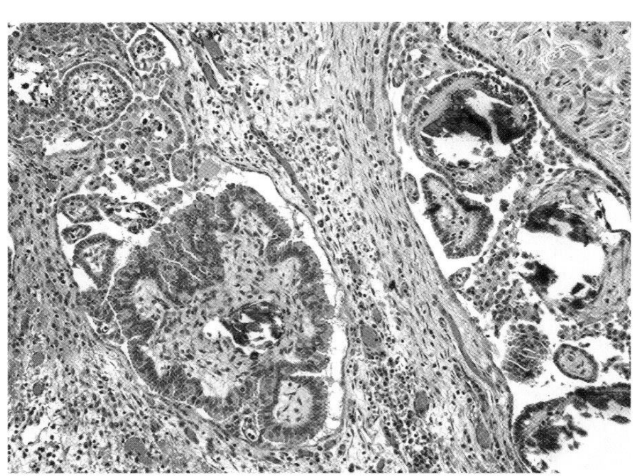

Fig. 14.28
Noninvasive epithelial implant (implant). **Papillae resembling primary ovarian atypical proliferative serous tumor**

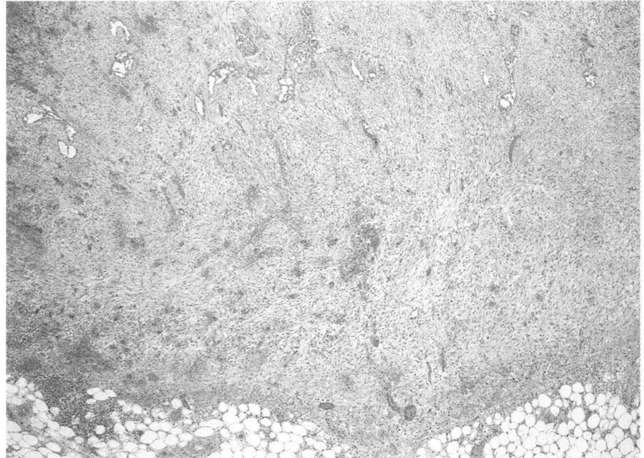

Fig. 14.30
Noninvasive desmoplastic implant (implant). **Low power view showing a plaque-like lesion with fibrosis, inflammation, and an irregular interface with underlying adipose tissue. Note gland-like structures at the top of the field displaying a linear orientation**

distinction between the two cell populations difficult at times, reminiscent of a reactive mesothelial proliferation (*Fig. 14.32*). The gland-like structures tend to be parallel to one another and can appear parallel or perpendicular to the peritoneal surface (*Figs. 14.30* and *14.31*). Notably, desmoplastic implants bear little resemblance to the associated ovarian tumor, suggesting that they arise in situ and reflect a reactive mesothelial process. Scattered cells with abundant eosinophilic cytoplasm may be seen in the stroma (*Fig. 14.34*). These resemble the eosinophilic cells of the usual type of microinvasion (see above). Previously, some experts had considered this a reflection of early invasion, but these cells do not appear to alter prognosis and therefore are considered part of the desmoplastic noninvasive implant [25]. Mitotic figures are usually absent, and psammoma bodies are present in over 90% of cases.

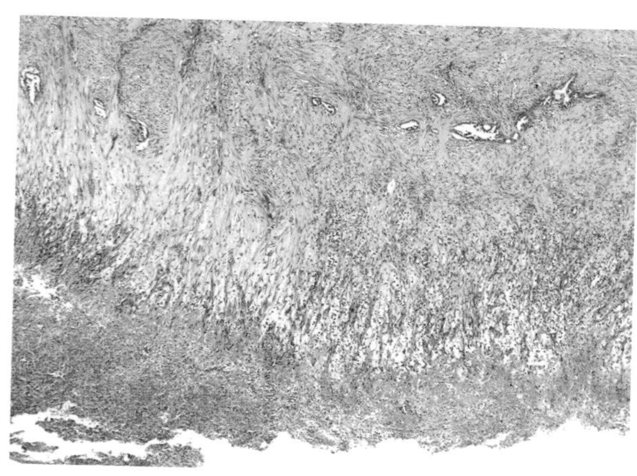

Fig. 14.31
Noninvasive desmoplastic implant (implant). **Low power view showing a plaque-like lesion with granulation tissue and an acute inflammatory exudate. Note gland-like structures at the top of the field are oriented parallel to the surface**

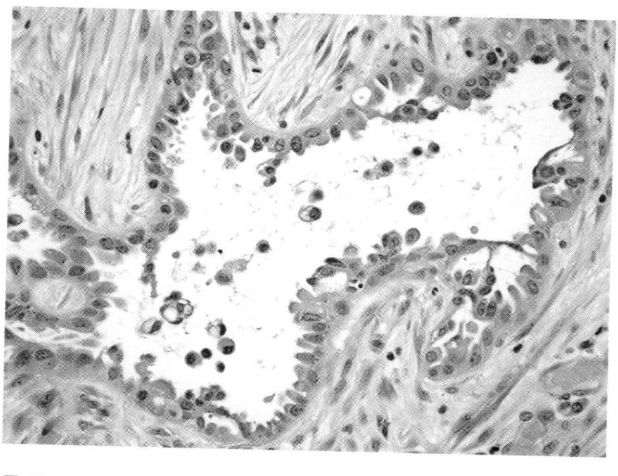

Fig. 14.33
Noninvasive desmoplastic implant (implant). **The cells lining the gland-like spaces display abundant eosinophilic cytoplasm and mild cytologic atypia**

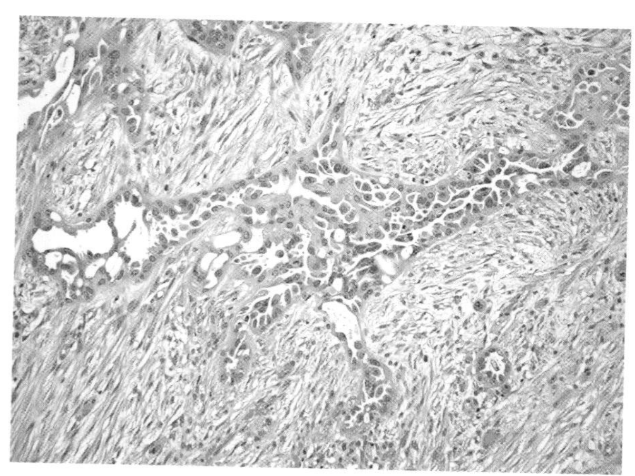

Fig. 14.32
Noninvasive desmoplastic implant (implant). **The gland-like structures are surrounded by a granulation tissue-like stroma**

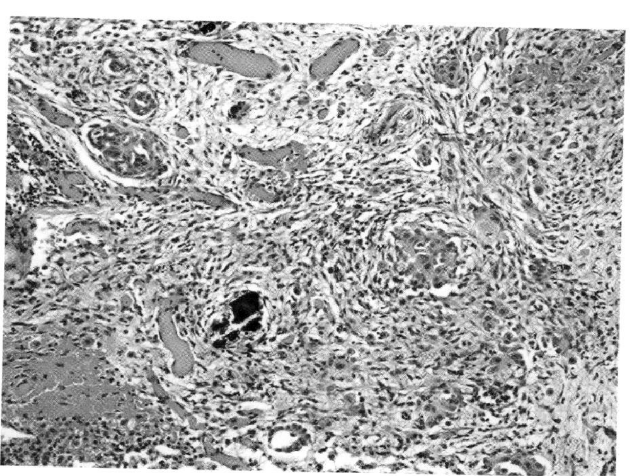

Fig. 14.34
Noninvasive desmoplastic implant (implant). **Single cells with abundant eosinophilic cytoplasm are in the stroma. This is not indicative of invasion. Note the inflamed and edematous stroma**

Inflammation is frequent in implants of all types. In noninvasive desmoplastic implants, chronic inflammation is nearly always present (*Figs. 14.30* and *14.34*), and in 20% of cases, an acute inflammatory exudate overlies the implant (*Fig. 14.31*). Salpingitis is associated with 60% of APST and noninvasive MPSC and is not stage-dependent. The presence and type of inflammation in the implants do not seem to correlate with the presence and type of salpingitis [309].

Invasive Peritoneal Implants Among patients with APST or noninvasive MPSC, 9% (22% of those with implants) have invasive implants. In a population-based study from Canada, 12% of stage III patients had invasive implants [105]. About three fourths of patients with invasive implants have noninvasive MPSC; the finding of invasive implants with APST is very unusual and warrants further sampling of the ovarian tumor to identify occult areas of MPSC or invasion (➲ *Table 14.12*).

The characteristic architectural feature of an invasive implant is a haphazard infiltrative growth pattern (➲ *Figs. 14.35–14.38*). A confluent or cribriform glandular pattern may be present. An exophytic pattern is not uncommon (➲ *Fig. 14.39*) and usually displays a micropapillary pattern. Typically, micropapillae are haphazardly arranged and small solid nests of cells embedded in fibrous stroma and surrounded by a clear space or cleft are present (➲ *Figs. 14.35* and ➲ *14.40*). Sometimes, micropapillae are present within glands, and may appear to fuse with one another to create a web-like appearance (➲ *Fig. 14.41*). Invasive implants often display only mild cytologic atypia (➲ *Fig. 14.40*), but occasionally atypia is moderate. If severe atypia is present, high-grade serous

Table 14.12

Frequency of invasive implants associated with atypical proliferative serous tumor (APST) compared to noninvasive micropapillary serous carcinoma (MPSC)

Series	Year	APST	niMPSC
Seidman [304]	1996	3/54	10/11
Eichorn [80]	1999	0/15	3/18
Goldstein [108]	2000	–	2/5
Slomovitz [330]	2002	0/16	0/6
Prat [262]	2002	5/32	1/14
Deavers [70]	2002	5/81	3/18
Smith-Sehdev [331]	2003	–	44/56
Longacre [190]	2006	9/100	5/11
Chang [51]	2008	4/57	3/18
Total		26/355[a]	71/157[a]
		(7%)	(45%)

[a] $p < 0.0001$ (chi square).
Modified from [311].

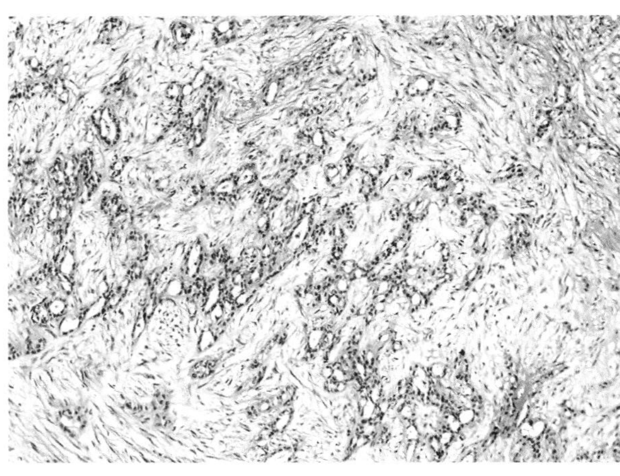

Fig. 14.36
Metastatic low grade serous carcinoma (invasive implant). **A haphazard infiltrative pattern of angulated glands is present**

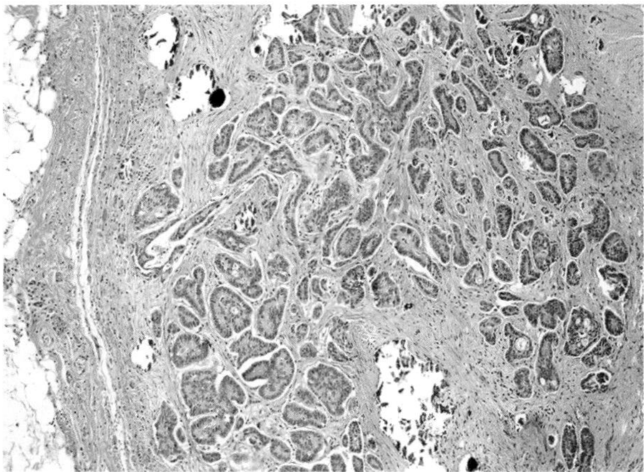

Fig. 14.35
Metastatic low grade serous carcinoma (invasive implant). **Low power view displaying a haphazard infiltrative pattern of micropapillae**

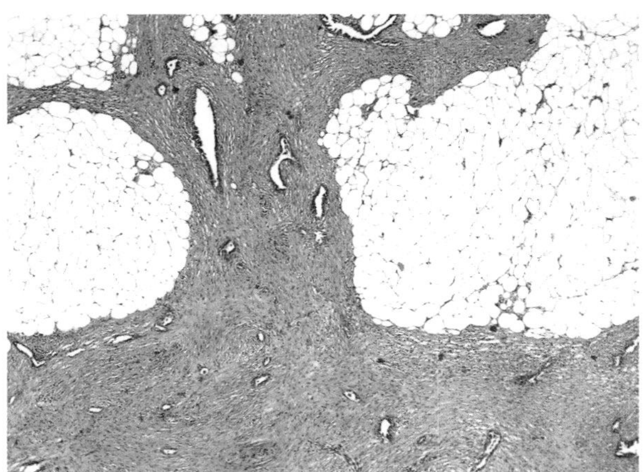

Fig. 14.37
Metastatic low grade serous carcinoma (invasive implant). **Although the glands are relatively sparsely distributed, they have an infiltrative pattern that is best appreciated at low power**

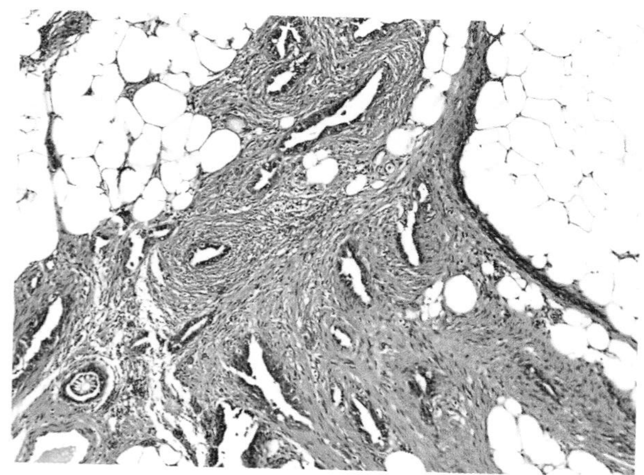

■ Fig. 14.38
Metastatic low grade serous carcinoma (invasive implant). **Angulated glands infiltrate omentum**

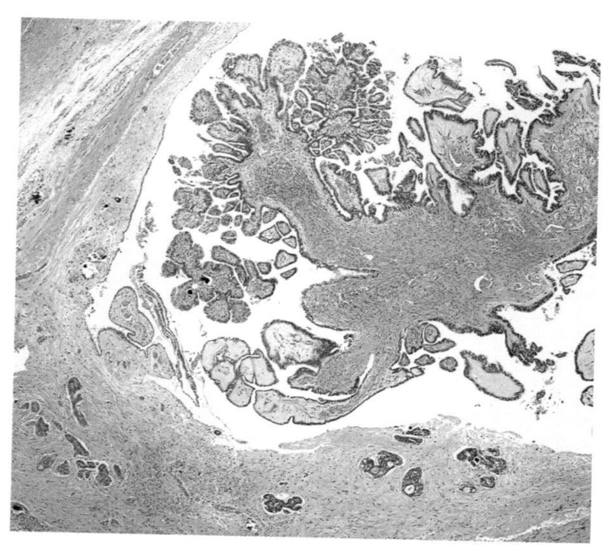

■ Fig. 14.39
Metastatic low grade serous carcinoma (invasive implant). **An exophytic noninvasive papillary pattern resembling the primary ovarian tumor is accompanied by invasive nests and micropapillae under the peritoneal surface**

carcinoma should be diagnosed. Mitotic figures are occasionally present.

The distinction of noninvasive desmoplastic implants from invasive low-grade serous carcinoma (invasive implants) may be very difficult at times, but is important since it is this feature that is the best predictor of outcome for tumors with extraovarian disease. Useful features that

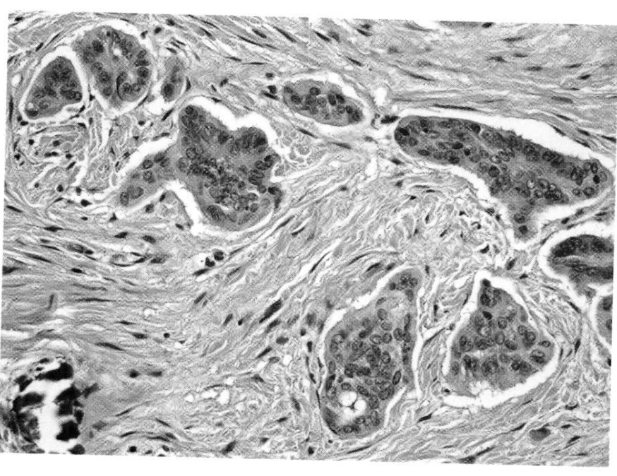

■ Fig. 14.40
Metastatic low grade serous carcinoma (invasive implant). **Solid nests and micropapillae are surrounded by a space**

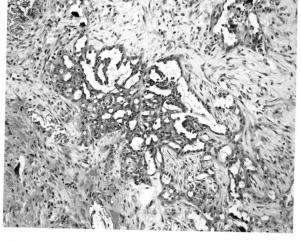

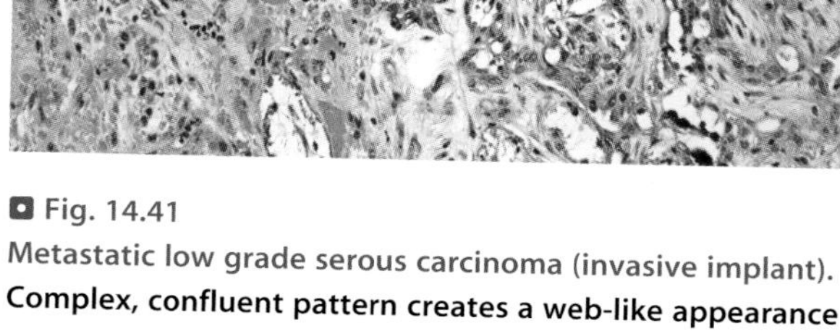

■ Fig. 14.41
Metastatic low grade serous carcinoma (invasive implant). **Complex, confluent pattern creates a web-like appearance**

distinguish invasive from noninvasive desmoplastic implants are summarized in ➲ *Table 14.13*. A helpful feature in distinguishing a desmoplastic noninvasive implant from an invasive implant is that the fibroblastic reaction associated with the noninvasive implant is generally much more extensive than the gland-like proliferation, which tends to be sparse (➲ *Figs. 14.30* and ➲ *14.31*); this creates an appearance suggestive of sclerosing peritonitis with florid reactive mesothelial proliferation. In contrast, the

Table 14.13
Morphologic features distinguishing invasive from noninvasive peritoneal implants

Feature	Invasive implants	Noninvasive implants	
		Desmoplastic	Epithelial
Growth pattern	Haphazard infiltration	Orderly arrangement	Exophytic or in submesothelial invaginations beneath the peritoneal surface
	High ratio of epithelium to stroma	Low ratio of epithelium to stroma	
Epithelial component	Small rounded nests containing serous and mesothelial-type cells with high nuclear: cytoplasmic ratio, surrounded by a clear space	Irregular gland-like structures lined by one or two layers of nondescript epithelial and mesothelial-type cells, often with abundant eosinophilic cytoplasm	Papillary structures with thick papillae displaying a hierarchical pattern similar to primary ovarian APST
	Endophytic micropapillae displaying a confluent pattern	The lining epithelial cells of the gland-like structures often appear to merge with the surrounding stromal cells	
	Exophytic micropapillae resembling MPSC of the ovary		
Stromal component	Loose or dense fibrous tissue	Frequent appearance of granulation tissue	No stromal reaction
Psammoma bodies	Generally infrequent and sparse, but may at times be extensive	Frequent and can be extensive	Frequent
Cytologic atypia	Generally mild to moderate	Mild to moderate	Mild to moderate
Inflammation	Generally minimal	Frequent and occasionally marked; fibrinopurulent exudate may be present	Minimal

MPSC, micropapillary serous carcinoma; APST, atypical proliferative serous tumor.

ratio of epithelium to stroma is much higher in the invasive implant (➲ *Fig. 14.35*). At times, the gland-like structures are more crowded, but the proliferation lacks the haphazard infiltrative pattern of carcinoma. It has been suggested that a small implant without underlying tissue be classified as noninvasive based on the assumption that it had been easily removed [24, 105]. There are no data to support this view.

At the 2006 annual meeting of the International Society of Gynecological Pathologists, five experts independently classified implants from photomicrographs. Despite prior concerns about the reproducibility of implant subclassification, the high level of interobserver agreement confirmed the accuracy of the diagnostic criteria. The critical issue for the general pathologist is recognition of the noninvasive desmoplastic implant. This type of implant has a very specific appearance as discussed and illustrated above, and once this is recognized, the noninvasive epithelial implants are easily recognized as noninvasive and the invasive implants as carcinoma.

A study in which implants designated as invasive were associated with a 65% recurrence rate compared with a recurrence rate of 14% for implants designated as noninvasive confirmed that the presence of individual cells within the stroma was not helpful in separating invasive from noninvasive implants [25]. That study found that the vast majority of invasive implants could be identified in the absence of overt invasion of underlying normal tissue and yet still accurately predict poor outcome. Features found to be useful in diagnosing these lesions in the absence of invasion were the presence of solid nests surrounded by a clear space or cleft, or micropapillae sometimes displaying a confluent arrangement.

Pathogenesis of Peritoneal Implants The pathogenesis of the peritoneal lesions associated with APSTs and noninvasive MPSCs is unknown. As noninvasive epithelial implants to some degree resemble the ovarian tumors, these are the ones most likely to arise by the detachment–implantation mechanism, althoug evidence for this is only circumstantial. In contrast, noninvasive desmoplastic implants more closely resemble a reactive mesothelial process, and are likely to be independent of the primary ovarian tumor. Molecular data are conflicting in resolving whether noninvasive implants represent independent primary peritoneal lesions or arise from exfoliation or detachment from the ovarian tumor with subsequent attachment to the peritoneal surface. Molecular analysis of implants associated with APSTs or noninvasive MPSCs is particularly challenging because the lesions may be quite small, isolation of epithelial cells within highly desmoplastic stroma requires relatively sophisticated and laborious techniques such as laser capture microdissection, and proper histological classification of implant type (invasive versus noninvasive versus endosalpingiosis) is essential for reaching meaningful conclusions [319]. PCR-based assays for loss of heterozygosity and nonrandom X-chromosome inactivation patterns have been used to assess the clonal relationships of APSTs with associated invasive and noninvasive implants, but the studies were based on very few cases, particularly of invasive implants, and reached different conclusions about the clonal relationship of the implants to the ovarian APST [112, 192, 322]. Analysis of shared *KRAS* mutations in APSTs and associated implants concluded that most implants are probably derived from the ovarian tumor, but that some may reflect multifocal origin [74]. Details regarding the nature of the implants studied were not provided. Clearly, additional molecular analysis of greater numbers of carefully classified and microdissected implants will be necessary to definitively address this issue.

Invasive implants are rare, and bona fide invasive implants reflect peritoneal metastases of MPSCs (some with undetected occult invasion) or, less likely, independent primary peritoneal serous carcinomas. Since MPSCs are often exophytic, even in the absence of invasion malignant cells can be shed from the surface of the tumor and implant on peritoneal surfaces. The Borderline Ovarian Tumor Conference participants agreed that the terms invasive implants and invasive carcinoma are synonymous [310].

Lymph Nodes Forty five percent of patients with APST/noninvasive MPSC, in whom lymph nodes are examined, have nodal endosalpingiosis, in comparison to about 10% of women who have nodes removed for other reasons. Up to 42% of these patients have nodes containing serous lesions with proliferative features beyond endosalpingiosis. The mean number of involved nodes is three, and nearly half of patients have at least one node with diffuse involvement. There is a strong association with invasive peritoneal implants [209] and micropapillary architecture [51]. In the Stanford series [209], 42% of patients with APST and lymph node resection had lymph node lesions, but this is likely an overestimate due to consultation bias and may also be related to the higher frequency of node sampling in patients with peritoneal implants. In a recent study from Korea, noninvasive MPSCs were significantly more likely to have lymph node lesions as compared to APSTs ($p = 0.037$, Fisher's exact test) [51].

Proliferative serous lesions have been reported in over 100 cases of APSTs [51, 209, 226, 305]. Although these lesions have been referred to as "metastases," it is preferable to refer to them as "associated serous lesions in lymph nodes" or "lymph node involvement," as they may or may not be related to the ovarian tumor.

Lymph node lesions apart from endosalpingiosis can be divided into two types. One is characterized by individual cells and clusters of cells with abundant eosinophilic cytoplasm in the sinuses, predominantly subcapsular sinuses (➲ *Fig. 14.42*). The nature of these cells is unclear, but it has been suggested that some of them may be mesothelial in origin. When associated with simple papillae with serous features, they are not mesothelial and correspond to "individual cells, cell clusters and simple papillae" as described in the Stanford series [209]. Cells with abundant eosinophilic cytoplasm are nearly always present on the surface of primary APSTs, and are often present in the stroma of noninvasive desmoplastic implants. It is plausible that these cells exfoliate and are

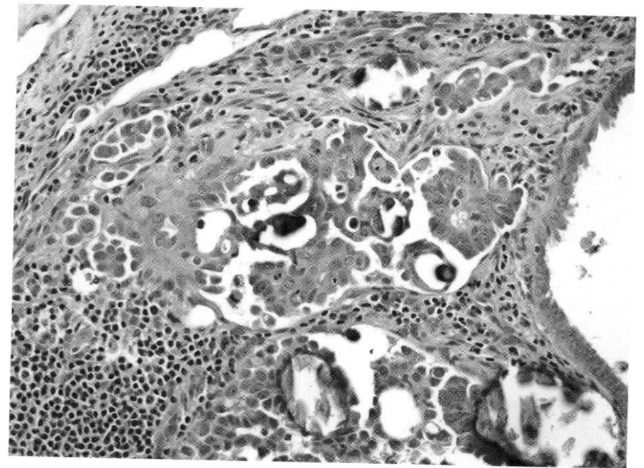

Fig. 14.42
Lymph node lesion associated with atypical proliferative serous tumor. **Single eosinophilic cells and cell clusters are seen in a subcapsular sinus**

filtered from the peritoneal fluid by regional lymph nodes – so-called deportation.

The second type of lymph node lesion is characterized by glandular inclusions and papillary serous structures, usually within or just beneath the capsule of the lymph node, that resemble the ovarian APST (➋ *Figs. 14.43* and ➋ *14.44*). The majority of these papillary serous lesions are also associated with endosalpingiosis in the same lymph node [226]. Cytologic atypia is mild or moderate and mitotic figures are rarely seen. The observation of papillary proliferations arising within endosalpingiosis, and the rare reports of APSTs and carcinomas arising within lymph nodes from endosalpingiosis suggest an independent origin of this second type of lymph node lesion. Bona fide metastatic low-grade serous carcinoma typically displays numerous papillae packing the sinuses or with a haphazard pattern (➋ *Figs. 14.45* and ➋ *14.46*).

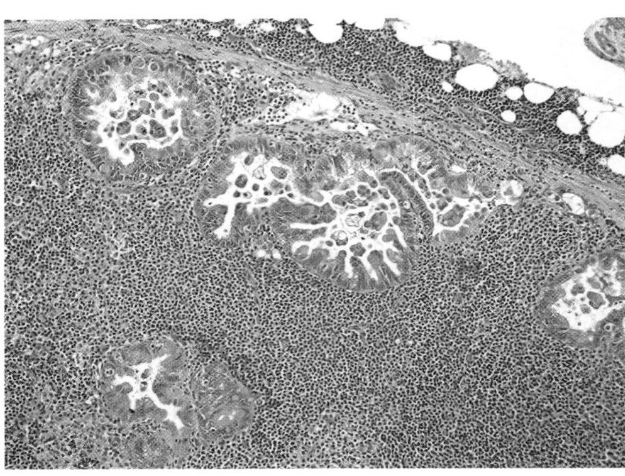

Fig. 14.43
Lymph node lesion associated with atypical proliferative serous tumor. **Note detachment of cell clusters at the tips of papillae as occurs in the primary atypical proliferative serous tumor**

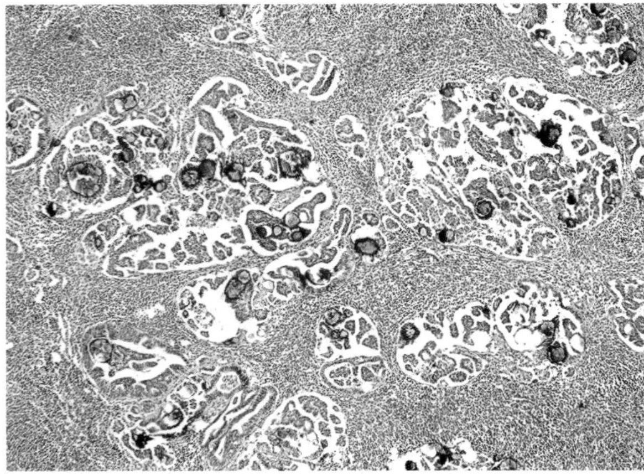

Fig. 14.45
Lymph node with metastatic low-grade serous carcinoma. **In contrast to involvement limited to lymphatic sinuses there is infiltration of lymph node parenchyma**

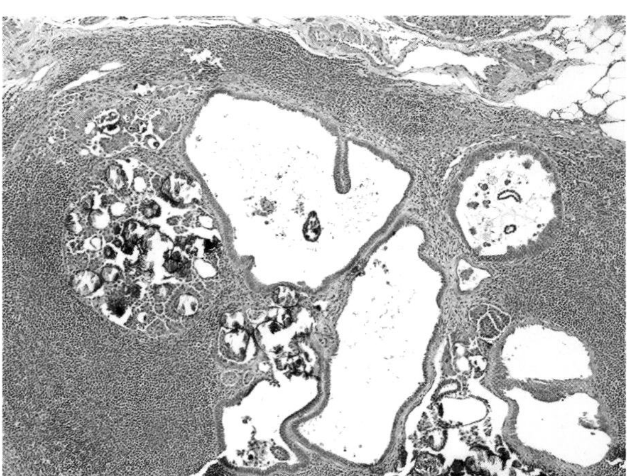

Fig. 14.44
Lymph node lesion associated with atypical proliferative serous tumor. **There is an admixture of endosalpingiosis and papillary structures resembling a noninvasive implant**

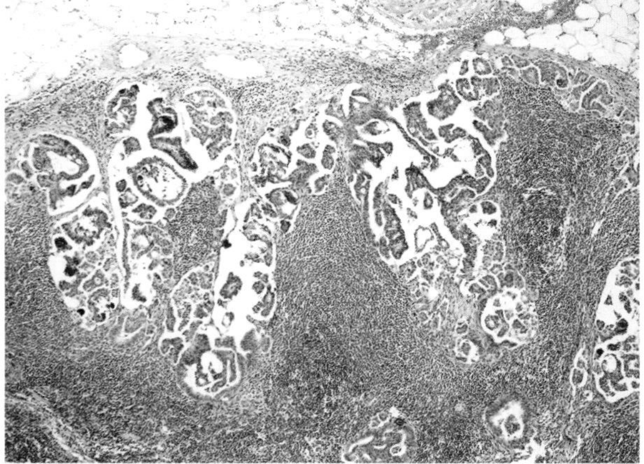

Fig. 14.46
Lymph node with metastatic low-grade serous carcinoma. **Some of the papillae are thin and elongated, resembling the primary ovarian invasive micropapillary serous carcinoma**

In the 2006 Stanford series, 8 of 31 patients (26%) with lymph node involvement had invasive peritoneal implants. Among 22 patients with follow-up, 4 were alive with disease and there were two deaths, one of a patient with indeterminate peritoneal implants. The presence of nodular aggregates of cells in the nodes was found to be an adverse prognostic factor.

Immunohistochemistry

Limited data on the immunohistochemistry of APSTs indicate that they are positive for CK7 and OC-125. About half the cases are positive for Leu M1. Focal positivity for CK20 is seen in a small minority of cases. WT1 is weakly positive [385]. Most cases express estrogen and progesterone receptors. They are also positive for other epithelial markers including EMA and cytokeratins. Patchy nuclear staining for p53 may occur, but such positivity does not correlate strongly with p53 mutation [328].

There are few studies examining the immunostaining of peritoneal implants. Lee and associates found that invasive implants and metastatic carcinoma show loss of calretinin-positive mesothelial cells and CD-34-positive fibroblasts, while they were preserved in noninvasive implants. Smooth muscle actin-positive myofibroblasts were present in both invasive and noninvasive implants [176].

Differential Diagnosis

Most papillary neoplasms in the ovary that are not serous cystadenomas or APSTs are obviously malignant, and are discussed below ("Malignant serous tumors, differential diagnosis"). Benign epithelial neoplasms that may display a papillary pattern resembling APST include atypical proliferative seromucinous tumor (APSMT; müllerian or endocervical-like type mucinous tumor) and atypical proliferative endometrioid tumor. These tumors are discussed in their respective sections below.

The distinction of a serous cystadenoma from an APST is not of major importance because both lesions are biologically benign. More importantly, the distinction of a noninvasive MPSC from an APST separates benign from a malignant neoplasm. Either a 5 mm confluent area or 10% of the tumor displaying micropapillary growth is required for a diagnosis of noninvasive MPSC (see "Malignant serous tumors" below).

Intraoperative Consultation Low-grade serous neoplasms are heterogeneous, and carcinomas nearly always have benign-appearing areas resembling a cystadenoma or an APST. It should therefore come as no surprise that approximately 20–30% of ovarian tumors diagnosed as atypical proliferative ("borderline") at the time of frozen section examination prove to be carcinomas on further sampling. Accordingly, it is important that the surgeon perform a thorough exploration when the frozen section is diagnosed as an APST. Since only 15% of unilateral tumors are associated with extraovarian disease, formal staging is probably not necessary for a unilateral ovarian tumor unless suspicious peritoneal lesions are found. In contrast, 56% of bilateral tumors are associated with extraovarian disease and therefore staging in this setting is advisable.

Clinical Behavior and Treatment

In six prospective randomized trials including 373 patients with SBTs followed for a mean of 6.7 years, the survival was 100% [305], and large studies, some population-based, in the United States, Korea, and Sweden show a 10-year survival of 96–100% [5, 65, 160, 252, 320]. The disease-specific survival rate of patients with SBTs (APSTs and noninvasive MPSCs) confined to the ovaries after a mean of approximately 6.7 years, based on over 2,000 reported cases, exceeds 99.5% [305]. Essentially all fatal cases have been shown to have not been comprehensively staged or sufficiently sampled. If patients with invasive implants (carcinoma) or indeterminate implants (histologically indeterminate or slides unavailable) are excluded, then the overall survival for patients with lymph node lesions other than endosalpingiosis is 98–99% [51, 76, 209, 305]. The survival for patients with microinvasion or microinvasive carcinoma unassociated with invasive implants is 100% [305].

The behavior of SBTs with extraovarian lesions is based on the type of implants that are present. In the older literature, survival for SBTs with peritoneal implants ranged from 70% to 90%. Now, after excluding noninvasive MPSCs, nontumor deaths, and invasive peritoneal implants, it is clear that the survival rate of patients with APSTs with noninvasive implants approaches 100% after a mean follow-up of 7.4 years [305]. Recurrences and deaths reported in the literature are poorly documented in the majority of cases. When carefully documented, most deaths are either treatment-related or are the result of complications from adhesions and bowel obstruction rather than carcinoma [169]. A literature review of over 18,000 borderline tumors, which included over 4,000 SBTs with clinical follow-up, failed to identify a single well-documented case of an SBT with noninvasive peritoneal implants, whose primary ovarian tumor had been adequately sampled to exclude invasion (at that time, one section per centimeter of maximum tumor diameter) that had progressed to documented invasive carcinoma. Among 27 published cases that reportedly progressed to invasive carcinoma, none were documented to have been adequately sampled for pathological examination [305]. Since that review, progression to invasive low-grade serous carcinoma has been reported in a few additional cases; however, these reports suffer from the same problems associated with older reports of fatalities including completeness of staging and extent of histological sampling [190, 326].

In general, the noninvasive serous tumors, SBTs, associated with invasive implants are noninvasive MPSCs, not APSTs. Based on a literature review of 467 noninvasive serous tumors, which included both invasive and noninvasive implants, the survival rate for patients with invasive implants was 66% after a mean follow-up of 7.4 years, compared to 95% for patients with noninvasive implants ($p < 0.0001$) [305]. The survival rate for patients with invasive implants is similar to that for patients with invasive low-grade (micropapillary) serous carcinoma [103].

Except for patients with invasive implants, conservative treatment, i.e., cystectomy or unilateral salpingo-oophorectomy, is sufficient therapy. Many women have had successful pregnancies after such treatment. Even though many women with APST have not had formal staging, if the primary tumor has been adequately sampled and there is no evidence of invasion or a micropapillary pattern (see "Micropapillary serous carcinoma" below), it is probably unnecessary to go back and do formal staging, although data addressing this question are scant. Limited data suggest that chemotherapy is of little, if any, value and may be detrimental [169]. For women with invasive peritoneal implants, i.e., low-grade serous carcinoma, there are insufficient data on upfront treatment for evaluation, but limited data suggest that surgery but not chemotherapy is of value after recurrence [34].

Low-Grade Serous Carcinoma; Micropapillary Serous Carcinoma, Invasive and Noninvasive Types; Micropapillary Serous Borderline Tumor; Psammocarcinoma

In 1996, it was observed that a characteristic micropapillary pattern in SBTs was associated with invasive implants and a worse prognosis than typical SBTs [37, 304]. Despite the lack of demonstrable invasion, these tumors behaved like low-grade carcinomas in contrast to the other tumors in this group that had nearly 100% survival. It was therefore proposed that they be designated MPSC [304]. The term "micropapillary serous carcinoma" has been accepted by the WHO since 2000 [90]. Others have preferred the term "micropapillary serous borderline tumor"[310].

Unfortunately, the term MPSC has been used for two morphologically distinct, albeit related, entities and this has caused some confusion among clinicians [311]. The noninvasive form of MPSC is a variant of serous borderline tumor. The invasive form of MPSC has been classified as well-differentiated serous carcinoma. Thus, invasive MPSC is synonymous with low-grade serous carcinoma [103].

There are several possible explanations for the low-grade malignant behavior of a noninvasive tumor. MPSCs that do not display destructive infiltrative growth are morphologically noninvasive, but it is conceivable that the complex exophytic micropapillary pattern may be a form of invasion. Occult invasion may be missed due to sampling factors. Alternatively, it is possible that the exophytic micropapillary pattern is a form of intraepithelial carcinoma, or "carcinoma in situ," which, when exposed to the peritoneum, may exfoliate malignant cells which implant on peritoneal surfaces and subsequently invade. Any one of these explanations would account for the strong association of this pattern with invasive implants (metastatic carcinoma). When areas of stromal invasion exceeding 5 mm (the size limit for microinvasion; see ➋ Microinvasion above) are present, the neoplasm is interpreted as the invasive form of MPSC and is also referred to as low-grade serous carcinoma.

Noninvasive MPSCs comprise 14% of SBTs in consultation-based material; 10% in stage I and 19% in advanced stage. In a population-based study from Canada, Gilks et al. found that 26% of advanced-stage SBTs were noninvasive MPSCs [105]. Invasive MPSCs are quite uncommon and comprise only 4% of ovarian carcinomas and 6% of serous carcinomas (➋ *Table 14.4*); 6–9% of advanced stage serous carcinomas are invasive MPSCs [103, 106, 300].

Clinical Findings The mean age of patients with the noninvasive form of MPSC is 42 years, the invasive form 45, and the psammomatous variant (psammocarcinoma) 54. The most common presentation is an asymptomatic pelvic mass, but abdominal pain, fullness, or distention are common symptoms in advanced stage [331].

Operative Findings For noninvasive MPSC, two thirds are bilateral as compared to only one third with APST. Half of patients are stage I and the remainder are stages II and III. For invasive MPSC, 80–90% are bilateral and 94%

are advanced stage [103, 331]. Bilateral tumors and those with an exophytic component are more likely to be associated with advanced-stage disease; 74% of intracystic tumors are advanced stage as compared to nearly all of those with exophytic tumors [331]. The psammomatous variant of invasive MPSC is more likely to be primary in the peritoneum.

Gross Findings The mean tumor size for the noninvasive form is about 8 cm, and for the invasive form about 11 cm [303, 331]. Surface involvement is present in 54% of cases (➲ *Figs. 14.2* and ➲ *14.3*). As these tumors are very well differentiated, they tend to have a more papillary and cystic gross appearance like APSTs, and little if any necrosis, in contrast to many typical high-grade serous carcinomas, which often have solid areas and extensive necrosis. Bilaterality, exophytic growth, and peritoneal implants are more common with noninvasive MPSCs as compared to APST [70, 262]. The psammomatous variant is more likely to adhere to and invade the myometrium via the uterine serosa.

Microscopic Findings Noninvasive MPSC is a proliferating serous neoplasm that displays a high degree of epithelial proliferation and complexity but is noninvasive. The tumor displays a characteristic pattern of papillary branching (➲ *Figs. 14.47–14.52*). The distal papillary branches are thin and delicate with minimal fibrovascular support, and emanate abruptly from thick, more centrally located papillae without intervening branches of successive intermediate sizes, unlike the hierarchical branching pattern of APSTs (➲ *Figs. 14.47* and ➲ *14.48*). When the papillae fuse, a cribriform pattern or a roman bridge-like pattern results on the surfaces of the large papillae (➲ *Figs. 14.49* and ➲ *14.50*). Both micropapillary and cribriform patterns may be present (➲ *Fig. 14.51*). A 5 mm diameter area of a confluent micropapillary pattern [310], or 10% of the tumor occupied by the micropapillary pattern [190, 276] is required for the

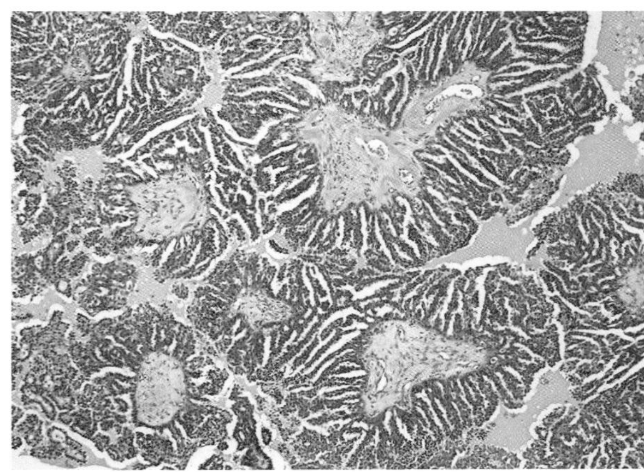

Fig. 14.48
Noninvasive micropapillary serous carcinoma. **The papillae are long and thin with scanty fibrovascular support and arise abruptly from large papillae**

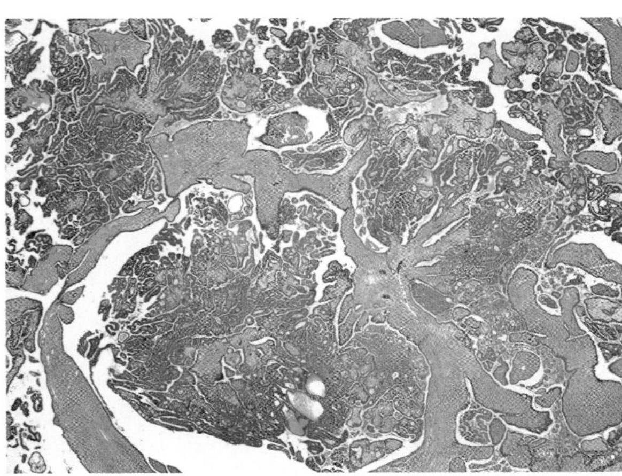

Fig. 14.47
Noninvasive micropapillary serous carcinoma. **Low power view. Large papillae are surrounded by numerous thin micropapillae**

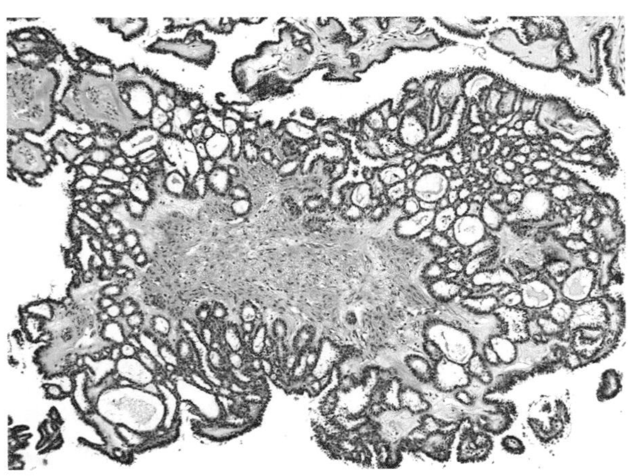

Fig. 14.49
Noninvasive micropapillary carcinoma. **A cribriform pattern is created by the apparent fusion of micropapillae on the surfaces of large papillae**

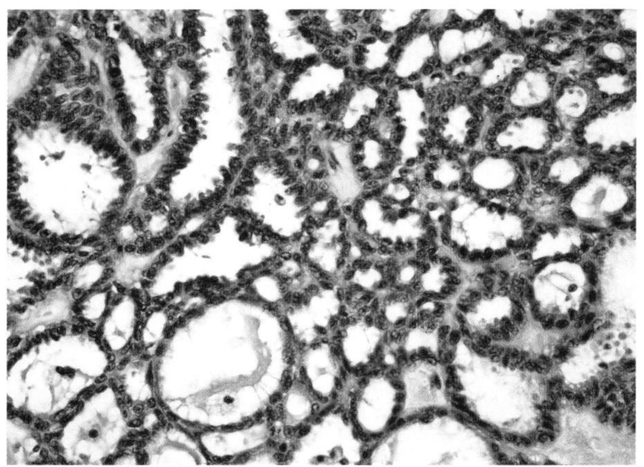

Fig. 14.50
Noninvasive micropapillary carcinoma. **Mild cytologic atypia and a cribriform pattern are present**

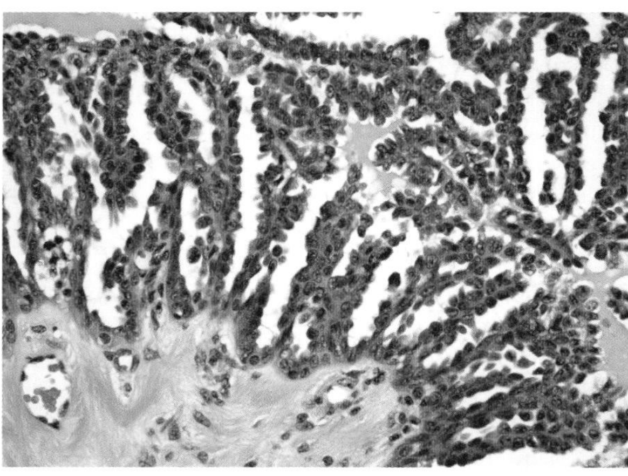

Fig. 14.52
Noninvasive micropapillary serous carcinoma. **The epithelium lining micropapillae displays mild cytologic atypia**

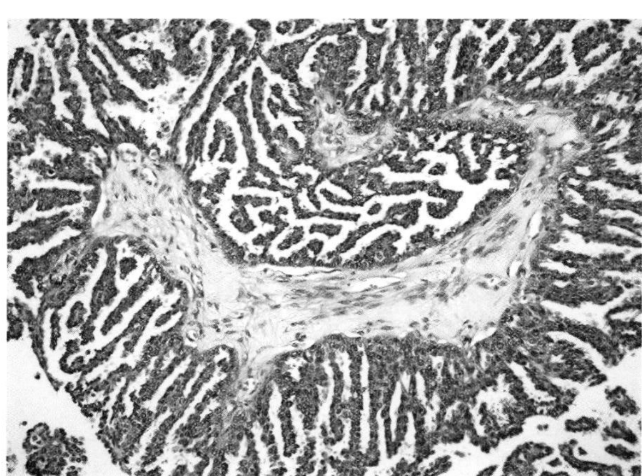

Fig. 14.51
Noninvasive micropapillary serous carcinoma. **Thin micropapillae with minimal fibrovascular support fuse to form a cribriform pattern in lower part of the field**

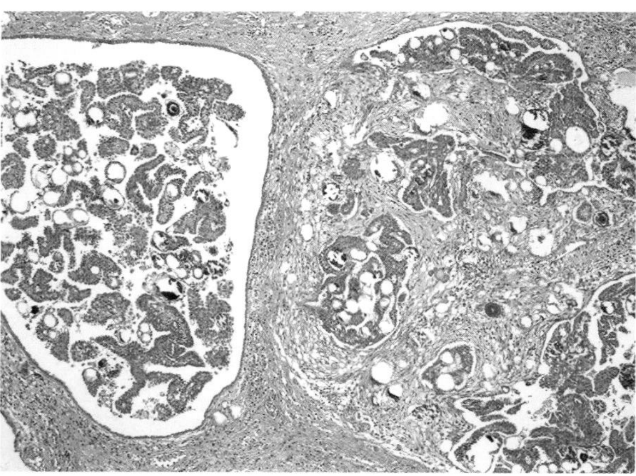

Fig. 14.53
Invasive micropapillary serous carcinoma. **Noninvasive pattern on the *left* is accompanied by infiltrative growth on the *right***

diagnosis. The majority of noninvasive MPSCs have areas of typical APST [304, 330, 331] in contrast to only 2% of high-grade serous carcinoma [103]. In cases associated with metastases (invasive implants), invasion has been found in the primary tumor after exhaustive histologic sampling [303].

Noninvasive MPSC displays no invasion of the stromal cores of the papillae. Invasion in MPSC is recognized by haphazard infiltrative growth composed of solid nests or complex gland-like structures displaying micropapillae (*Figs. 14.53–14.59*). The nests and gland-like structures are often surrounded by a clear space or cleft. Psammoma bodies are common. The psammomatous variant of invasive MPSC, so-called psammocarcinoma, is characterized by a myriad of psammoma bodies occupying >75% of the papillae (*Fig. 14.60*). An uncommon pattern of invasion designated "macropapillary" is characterized by large papillae invading the stroma, also surrounded by clear

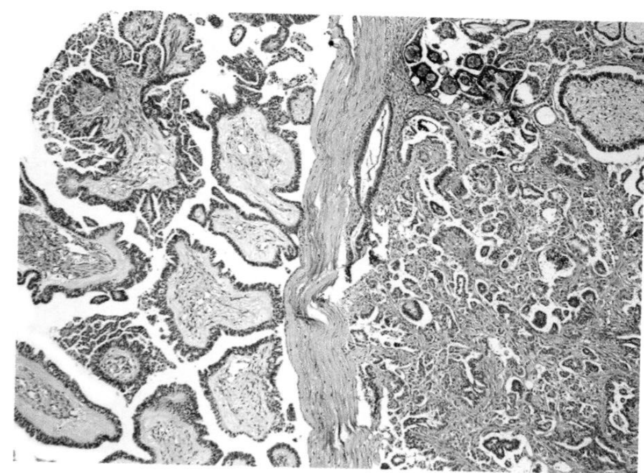

Fig. 14.54
Invasive micropapillary serous carcinoma. **This tumor displays a spectrum of proliferation from areas resembling serous cystadenoma and atypical proliferative serous tumor with focal micropapillary features on the *left*, and invasive low-grade serous carcinoma on the *right***

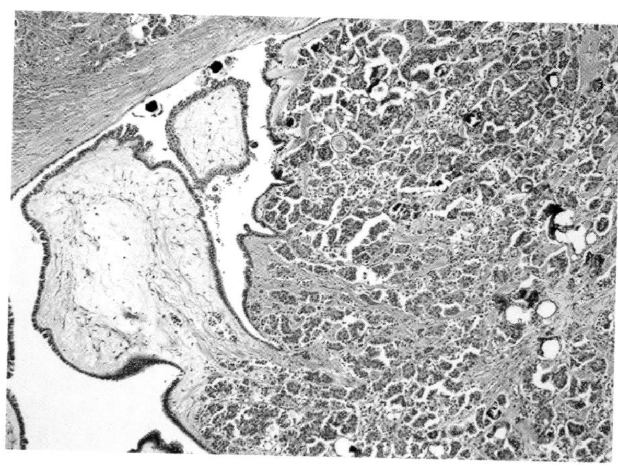

Fig. 14.56
Invasive micropapillary serous carcinoma. **Large edematous papillae contain numerous small micropapillae displaying haphazard infiltrative growth**

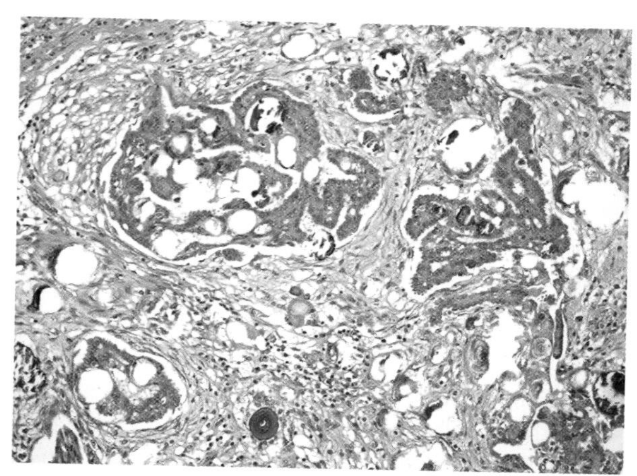

Fig. 14.55
Invasive micropapillary serous carcinoma. **Confluent glandular and cribriform patterns with haphazard infiltration of the stroma**

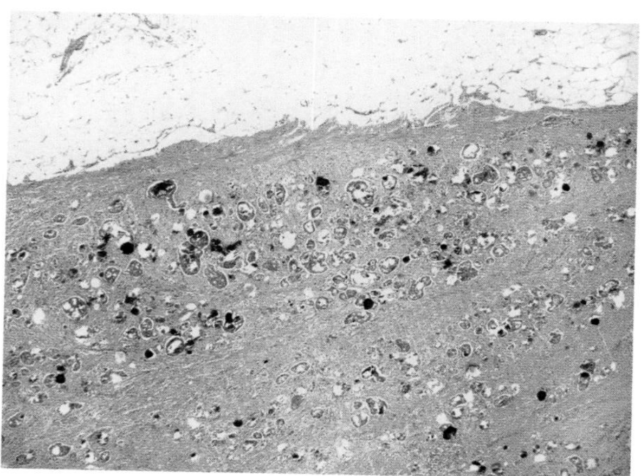

Fig. 14.57
Metastatic micropapillary serous carcinoma (invasive implant). **Haphazard infiltrative pattern of glands and nests within the omentum. Fibrosis and psammoma bodies are present**

spaces [390] (*Figs. 14.22* and *14.23*). The nature of these clefts is unknown, but as noted earlier, some probably reflect lymphatic spaces. Intratumoral lymphatic invasion is seen in about one third of cases [289]. It has also been suggested that the spaces are generated by the contraction of stromal myofibroblasts, particularly in peritoneal implants [176].

MPSCs with or without invasion display similar cytologic features. Cells tend to be rounded with scant cytoplasm, and there is mild or moderate nuclear atypia, often with prominent small nucleoli (*Figs. 14.50* and *14.52*). These cytologic features differ somewhat from APST; however the mean nuclear area appears to be similar in both groups [132]. The cells in APSTs tend to be

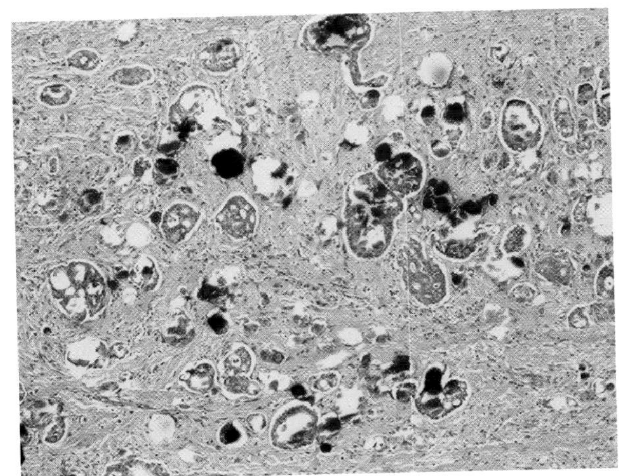

Fig. 14.58
Metastatic micropapillary serous carcinoma (invasive implant). **Small and medium size nests of epithelium with a cribriform pattern invade the omentum**

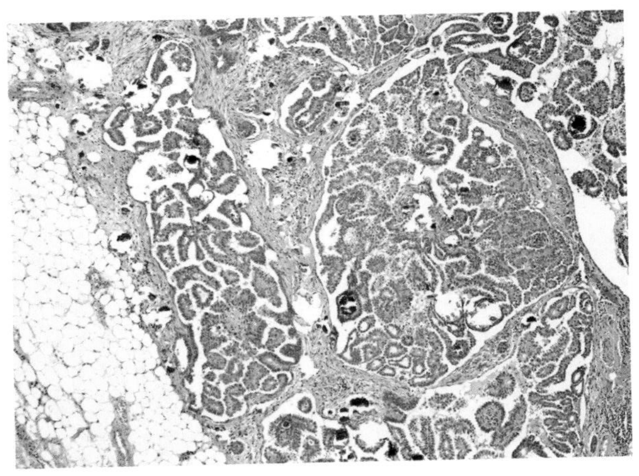

Fig. 14.59
Metastatic micropapillary serous carcinoma. **Complex micropapillary pattern involves the peritoneal surfaces**

columnar, are often ciliated, and have less nuclear atypia. Mitotic activity tends to be low. Severe nuclear atypia warrants a designation of high-grade serous carcinoma even in the absence of overt invasion.

The peritoneal implants associated with MPSC are frequently invasive (i.e., carcinoma). Among 157 reported cases of advanced-stage noninvasive MPSC, 45% of the implants were invasive, in comparison to 7% of the implants associated with APSTs ($p < 0.0001$; *Table 14.12*). Noninvasive MPSCs also are more likely to be associated with serous lesions in lymph nodes that

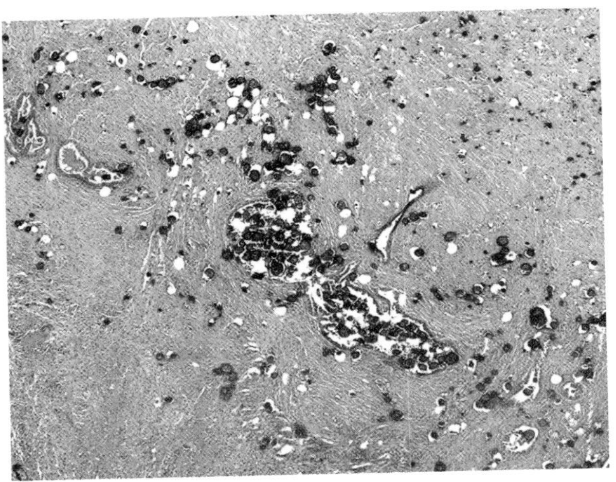

Fig. 14.60
Invasive micropapillary serous carcinoma, psammomatous variant. **Numerous psammoma bodies have obliterated most of the carcinomatous glands**

replace the node parenchyma, supporting the view that these are invasive carcinomas with metastatic potential [51] (see Low Grade Serous Tumors Atypical Proliferative Serous Tumor (APST); Serous Borderline Tumor (SBT); Lymph Nodes).

Immunohistochemistry There are few published data on the immunohistochemistry of MPSC. p53 is usually negative but can be focally positive in up to 43% [237, 381]. However, only strong diffuse nuclear p53 positivity correlates with missense *TP53* mutation [328]. WT1 is usually positive (nuclear staining) [237]. ER and PR show nuclear positivity in about 50%, significantly more often than in high-grade serous carcinomas [381]. EMA, cytokeratin 7, and CA125 are also positive, with EMA showing membranous staining and the other two a cytoplasmic pattern of staining.

Differential Diagnosis A 5 mm diameter area of confluent micropapillary architecture distinguishes noninvasive MPSCs from APSTs, which often have scattered small foci of a micropapillary pattern. Ten percent of the tumor displaying the micropapillary pattern is also a valid cutoff [190, 276]. Either criterion can be used, as it is rare for less than 5 mm of confluent micropapillary growth to be more than 10% of the tumor [190]. Anything less than this, in the absence of other features of invasion, should be classified as an APST. The distinguishing morphologic features of serous neoplasms, including the invasive and noninvasive variants of MPSC, are shown in *Table 14.14*.

Table 14.14
Distinguishing morphologic features of serous ovarian neoplasms

Diagnosis	Atypia	Stratification and detachment	Micropapillary pattern	Stromal invasion
Serous cystadenoma	Absent, or present in <10%	Absent, or present in <10%	Absent	Absent
APST	Present in ≥10%	Present in ≥10%	May be present, <5 mm of confluence	Absent
MPSC, noninvasive	Present	Usually present	Present, ≥5 mm of confluence	Absent
MPSC, invasive	Present	Usually present	Present	Present
Serous carcinoma	Present	May be present	May be present	Present

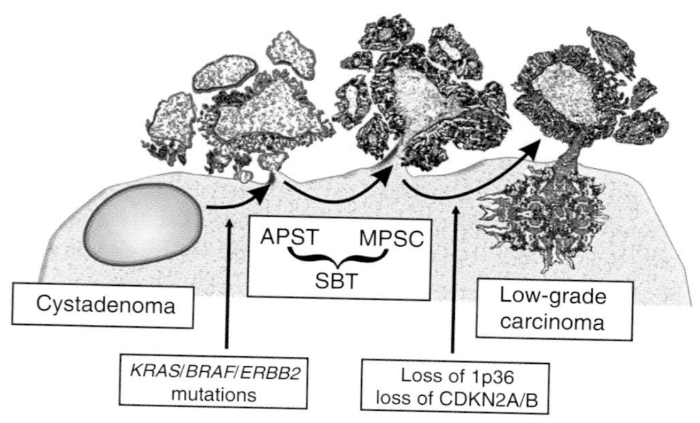

Fig. 14.61
Schematic of the pathogenesis of low-grade serous carcinoma. **Modified from reference [328]**

Molecular Biology Activating mutations in *KRAS* and one of its downstream effectors, *BRAF*, have been identified in a variety of human cancers and mutations of either *KRAS* or *BRAF* lead to constitutive activation of MAPK signaling [371]. Molecular genetic studies have highlighted the importance of the Ras/Raf/MEK/MAPK signaling pathway in the pathogenesis of low-grade ovarian serous carcinomas. Frequent *KRAS* mutations in APST/serous borderline tumors were first reported by Mok and colleagues [225]. Several subsequent studies verified the original finding and further demonstrated that mutations in *KRAS* and *BRAF* characterize both APSTs and low-grade serous carcinomas [203, 323, 327]. Specifically, activating mutations in codon 12 and less commonly in codon 13 of *KRAS* or in codon 600 of *BRAF* occur in approximately two thirds of APSTs and low-grade serous carcinomas. Mutations in *KRAS* and *BRAF* are mutually exclusive insofar as tumors with mutant *KRAS* do not have mutant *BRAF* and vice versa. Furthermore, a 12 bp insertion mutation of *ERBB2* (*HER2/neu*), which activates an upstream regulator of K-Ras, has been found in 9% of APSTs and these mutations are only observed in tumors lacking mutant *KRAS* and *BRAF* [231]. These studies illustrate how different mutational defects can serve to deregulate the same signaling pathway in cancer cells. In contrast to APSTs and low-grade serous carcinomas, *KRAS* and *BRAF* mutations are very uncommon in high-grade serous carcinomas [327]. Collectively these data indicate that *KRAS* and *BRAF* mutations are largely confined to low-grade serous carcinomas and APSTs and suggest that APSTs are likely precursors of low-grade serous carcinomas, but not the more common high-grade serous carcinomas (*Fig. 14.61*). *KRAS* and *BRAF* mutations are lacking in isolated serous cystadenomas, putative precursors of APSTs [54]. However, identical *KRAS* or *BRAF* mutations have been detected the APSTs and adjacent cystadenoma epithelium in serous cystadenomas associated with small APSTs [125]. These findings suggest that mutations of *KRAS* and *BRAF* are early events associated with serous tumor initiation and that a small subset of serous cystadenomas that acquire *KRAS* or *BRAF* mutations may progress to APST. Perhaps, not surprisingly, *TP53* mutations are uncommon in low-grade serous carcinomas and APSTs [328].

Overall, 70–80% of low-grade serous carcinomas and APSTs express active MAPK [131]. Activated MAPK signaling has been observed in a substantial fraction (41%) of high-grade serous carcinomas as well [131], presumably through mechanisms other than activating mutations of *KRAS* and *BRAF,* such as mutation of *NF1,* which is mutated in over 20% of these tumors [288]. Nf1 acts as a Ras-GTPase activating protein (Ras-GAP), which catalyzes hydrolysis of Ras-GTP to Ras-GDP, with resultant downregulation of downstream signaling through Raf, Ral/Cdc42, PLC, and PI3K. These findings are likely to have therapeutic relevance in the near term. Although published studies on the response of low-grade serous carcinomas to traditional chemotherapy are few, some investigators have noted poor response of low-grade (micropapillary) serous carcinomas to platinum-based therapeutic regimens [34, 331]. A number of anticancer agents targeting the Ras/Raf/MEK/ERK pathway are being developed and a few have been tested in clinical trials [379]. Molecularly targeted agents may provide an effective alternative or adjunct to platinum/taxane-based chemotherapy for low-grade serous carcinomas or for treatment of platinum-resistant high-grade serous carcinomas with activated MAPK signaling.

In contrast to high-grade serous carcinoma, discrete regions of chromosomal gains have not been reproducibly detected in low-grade serous carcinoma or its putative precursor lesion, APST. However, based on studies using a limited number of polymorphic markers, a few sub-chromosomal regions (e.g., 1p and 9q) show frequent deletion in low-grade serous neoplasms [161]. In a recent study using high-density SNP arrays to assess DNA copy number changes in tumor cells isolated from affinity purified borderline, low-grade, and high-grade serous ovarian neoplasms, Kuo and colleagues identified frequent allelic deletions of 1p36 and 9p21 in low-grade serous carcinomas, but not in serous borderline tumors. The 1p36 region contains several candidate tumor suppressors, including *miR-34a,* which encodes a p53-regulated microRNA that mimics p53's effects on growth arrest and apoptosis. 9p21 harbors the *CDKN2A* locus, which encodes p16, p15, and p14 (Arf) [27, 164].

Clinical Behavior and Treatment Despite the absence of destructive infiltrative growth in the noninvasive variant of MPSC, the data indicate that it behaves as a low-grade serous carcinoma [51, 70, 80, 108, 190, 262, 304, 330, 331]. Stage I noninvasive MPSC appears to be cured by adnexectomy alone. Since the disease-specific survival for >2,000 stage I SBTs was 99.5% prior to the separation of APST from noninvasive MPSC [305], and 10% of these are expected to be MPSCs, it is reasonable to conclude that stage I noninvasive MPSC has virtually 100% survival as well [311, 331]. In contrast to noninvasive MPSCs, invasive MPSCs are rarely stage I. The 5- and 10-year survival rates for patients with advanced-stage noninvasive MPSC are approximately 75–85% and 40–60%, respectively. After recurrence as invasive carcinoma, the outcome of noninvasive MPSC is similar to that of invasive MPSC, with a progression-free survival of about 2 years and a median survival of 6–7 years [103, 321, 331].

Invasive MPSC is synonymous with invasive low-grade serous carcinoma. Although the patterns of spread are similar to ordinary high-grade serous carcinoma, low-grade serous carcinoma has a better prognosis. Stage III low-grade serous carcinoma is more likely to be stage IIIA (small volume peritoneal disease) as compared to high-grade serous carcinoma, which is nearly always stage IIIC (bulky peritoneal disease) [300]. The natural history of low-grade serous carcinoma is characterized by indolent growth that is resistant to chemotherapy, and recurrences that maintain the well-differentiated histological appearance of the primary tumor, even decades later. Rare exceptions show transformation to high-grade serous carcinoma [104].

A comparison of survival of 75 women with invasive and noninvasive MPSC found no significant survival difference between the two groups [331]. The strong association of noninvasive MPSC with invasive implants is a highly significant difference from APSTs (➋ *Table 14.12*). These findings indicate that noninvasive MPSCs are in fact carcinomas. Further sampling of apparent noninvasive MPSCs may reveal invasion in some, and perhaps most cases.

Low-grade serous carcinoma does not respond appreciably to platinum-taxane therapy in the first-line or neoadjuvant setting [103, 295]. Primary cytoreduction, and with recurrence, secondary cytoreduction, appear to be more effective approaches, but data are limited [34].

High-Grade Serous Carcinoma

Clinical Findings

High-grade serous carcinoma is the most common type of ovarian cancer and accounts for approximately 50% of ovarian carcinomas; however, if the clinically and pathologically identical peritoneal serous carcinomas are included (see below), the frequency is about 63% (➋ *Table 14.4*). Serous carcinoma most often occurs in the sixth and seventh decades, and the reported mean age varies from 57 to 63 years. Nearly all comprehensively staged patients present in advanced stage with tumor usually disseminated throughout the abdominal and pelvic cavities. The most common presenting symptoms are abdominal pain and distention due to ascites or bulky abdominal tumor. A slightly older age, larger volume of ascites, and a lower frequency of a palpable pelvic mass occurs with peritoneal serous carcinomas as compared to ovarian serous carcinoma [19, 22, 26]. Gastrointestinal symptoms are also common. Other symptoms include urinary frequency, dysuria, and vaginal bleeding. Stage I tumors may present as an asymptomatic mass on a routine pelvic examination, but as noted above, stage I serous carcinoma is very rare. Importantly, three fourths of women with a history of breast cancer who subsequently develop peritoneal carcinomatosis are found to have new primary ovarian or peritoneal serous carcinomas [99]. Therefore, a woman with a history of breast carcinoma who develops peritoneal carcinomatosis should not be assumed to have a breast carcinoma recurrence.

Operative Findings

Two thirds of advanced-stage cases involve both ovaries. Nearly all advanced-stage ovarian carcinomas involve peritoneal surfaces, including the pelvic peritoneum (stage II) and the surfaces of the bowel and other abdominal organs (stage III). Both pelvic and abdominal spread can be by direct extension or metastasis. For example, direct extension to the rectosigmoid, broad ligament, or uterus can occur by contiguous growth, or by exfoliation of malignant cells resulting in seeding of the peritoneal surfaces of the bowel or pelvic peritoneum. Operative findings are described in more detail earlier in this chapter (see ➋ Prognostic Factors, Stage above).

In 10–20% of women with advanced stage serous carcinoma, the ovaries are small and display predominantly surface involvement. These findings warrant a diagnosis of primary peritoneal serous carcinoma (see ➋ Differential Diagnosis below, and ➋ Chap. 13, Diseases of the Peritoneum). It has been suggested recently that some of these may be tubal carcinomas of fimbrial origin.

On rare occasions, typical primary serous carcinomas arise in extraperitoneal locations including pelvic or retroperitoneal lymph nodes, broad ligament, retroperitoneum, or endocervix. More commonly, serous carcinomas arise in the endometrium (see ➋ Chap. 9, Endometrial Carcinoma).

Gross Findings

Serous carcinomas range from microscopic to about 20 cm in greatest dimension. They are typically multilocular, cystic and solid, with soft, friable papillae filling the cyst cavities, and occasionally may be completely solid. The cysts also contain serous, turbid, or bloody fluid. The external surfaces may be smooth or bosselated and often display papillae. Solid areas on cut surface are pink to gray, and may be soft or firm depending on the character of the tumor stroma. Hemorrhage and necrosis are often present. Omental metastases are characterized by firm nodules of variable size with white or gray cut surfaces, which may coalesce to form an omental cake. A grossly normal omentum contains microscopic tumor in 22% of cases.

Microscopic Findings

High-grade serous carcinomas display complex papillary and solid patterns and marked cytologic atypia (➋ *Figs. 14.62–14.71*). Frequently they display a lace-like or labyrinthine pattern (➋ *Figs. 14.64* and ➋ *14.65*) characterized by extensive bridging and coalescence of papillae resulting in slit-like spaces. Areas of solid growth, and

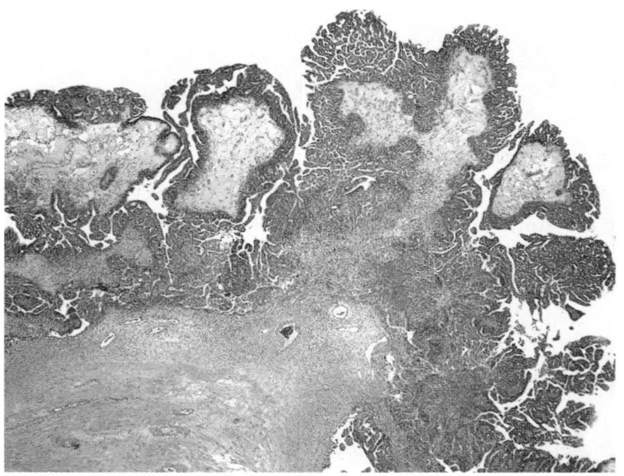

Fig. 14.62
High-grade serous carcinoma. **Low power view displaying absence of stromal invasion. Despite absence of invasion, the tumor should not be classified as borderline since the tumor cells are high grade (see ➋ *Fig. 14.63*)**

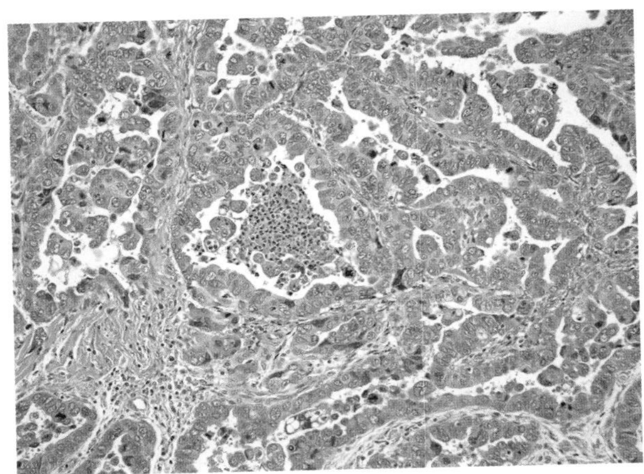

■ Fig. 14.63
High-grade serous carcinoma (same tumor as in ➋ *Fig. 14.62*). **Markedly atypical nuclei, high mitotic index, and abnormal mitotic figures**

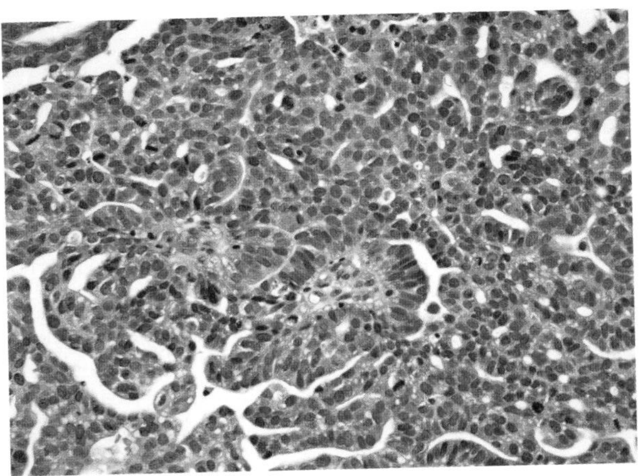

■ Fig. 14.65
High-grade serous carcinoma. **Slit-like spaces are very characteristic of this neoplasm**

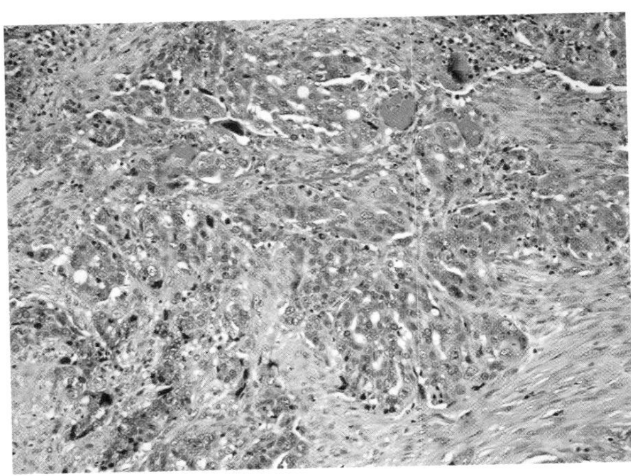

■ Fig. 14.64
High-grade serous carcinoma. **Slit-like spaces create a labyrinthine pattern. Nuclei are markedly atypical**

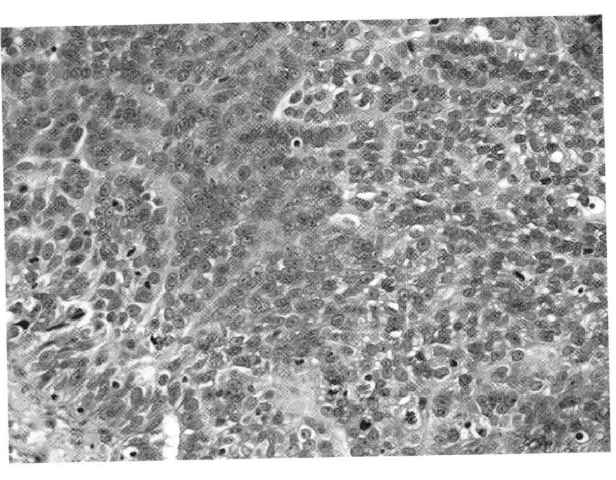

■ Fig. 14.66
High-grade serous carcinoma. **Solid growth, marked cytologic atypia and high mitotic activity**

glandular and cribriform patterns are common (➋ *Figs. 14.66* and ➋ *14.69*). A villoglandular-type papillary pattern can be seen; the high-grade nuclear atypia, often with bizarre nuclei, identifies it as serous rather than endometrioid, and this pattern typically merges with other characteristic serous features. Cytoplasmic clear cell change may occur, but characteristic architectural patterns of clear cell carcinoma are not present (see ➋ Differential Diagnosis, and ➋ Clear Cell Carcinoma below; ➋ *Fig. 14.70*). The cells may be small and uniform focally, but nearly all cases display areas of large, pleomorphic nuclei with obvious malignant features. Multinucleated tumor giant cells may be present (➋ *Figs. 14.67* and ➋ *14.68*). Bizarre nuclei greater than 50 μm in diameter are characteristic, and occur in 86% of advanced stage tumors [300] (➋ *Fig. 14.67*).

Serous carcinomas that are predominantly solid are composed of sheets of cells with high-grade nuclei and usually contain isolated bizarre mononuclear giant cells or syncytial-like aggregates. Mitoses, including abnormal mitoses, are numerous and necrosis is often pronounced (➋ *Fig. 14.67*). There are focal areas with papillary or

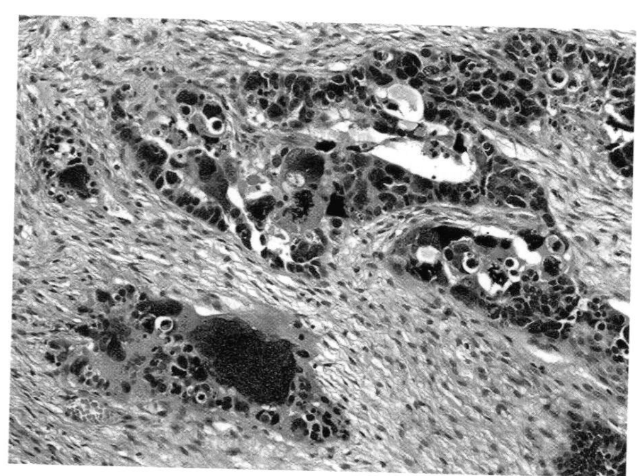

Fig. 14.67
High-grade serous carcinoma. **Bizarre nuclei with multinucleated tumor giant cells and atypical mitotic figures**

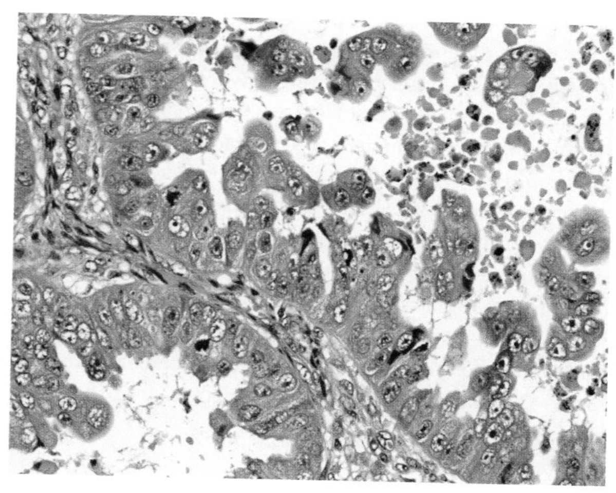

Fig. 14.68
High-grade serous carcinoma. **Marked cytologic atypia, tufting, and detached cell clusters**

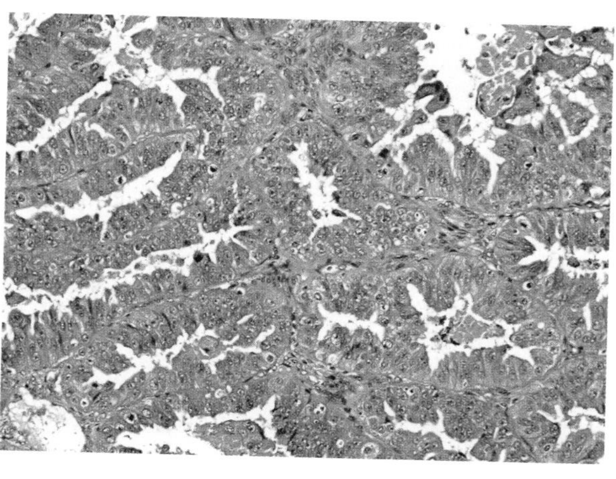

Fig. 14.69
High-grade serous carcinoma. **Characteristic high-grade cytologic features of serous carcinoma**

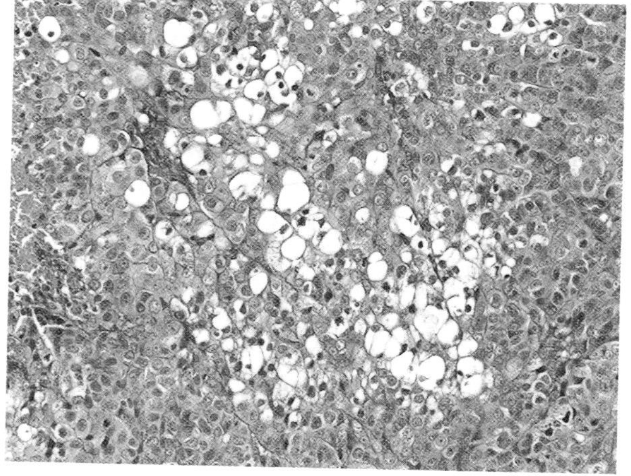

Fig. 14.70
High-grade serous carcinoma with focal cytoplasmic clearing and signet ring-like cells. **This tumor should not be described as having clear cell carcinoma features as the architectural features of clear cell carcinoma are not present**

glandular architecture that permit the diagnosis of a serous carcinoma rather than undifferentiated carcinoma. Psammoma bodies are present in 25% of cases. Rarely, a completely solid carcinoma without any evidence of glands, papillae, or other recognizable patterns occurs; this is probably a variant of high-grade serous carcinoma but is designated undifferentiated carcinoma (see Undifferentiated Carcinoma below). Intratumoral lymphatic vascular invasion is seen in about one third of cases, and hilar lymphatic invasion in two thirds [289].

Grade Morphometric measurement of nuclear area and direct measurement of nuclear size show a bimodal distribution for serous carcinoma that separates serous carcinomas into a small group of low-grade carcinomas and a much larger group of high-grade serous carcinomas [132, 300]. These findings along with the distinctly different molecular genetic profile that distinguish low- from high-grade serous carcinoma support the use of a two-tier

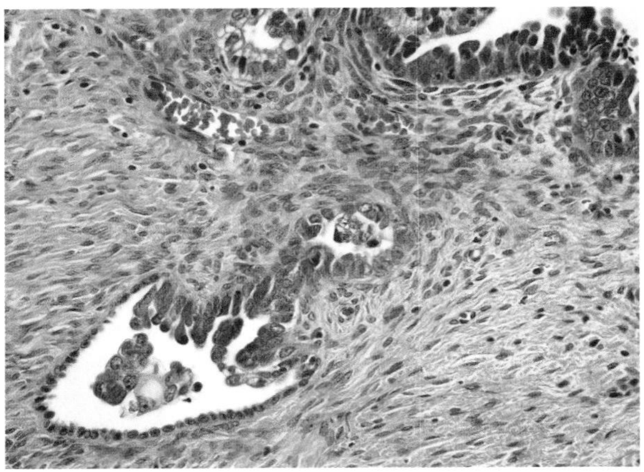

Fig. 14.71
High-grade serous carcinoma. **This small focus of high-grade serous carcinoma partially involves an ovarian surface epithelial inclusion. This could be an intraepithelial precursor of serous carcinoma or more likely extension of an established invasive serous carcinoma to an adjacent inclusion**

grading system instead of the traditional three tier systems of well, moderate, and poorly differentiated serous carcinomas. Unlike the two-tier system proposed by Malpica and colleagues from MD Anderson (MDACC), the three-tier system as advocated by Shimizu and associates [196, 197, 308] does not have a histological or molecular basis to separate grades II and III [104, 367]. It has been shown that in the unusual cases where the nuclear grade, which is the basis of the binary system, does not clearly appear to be low or high grade, i.e., grade II, these tumors lack KRAS and BRAF mutations (the hallmark of low-grade serous carcinoma) and display p53 mutations (the hallmark of high-grade serous carcinomas) in over 90% of cases [18]. Accordingly, these tumors that appear to be midway between low and high grade should be considered high grade. Such tumors of intermediate nuclear grade qualify as high grade in the MDACC system. Besides the morphometric and molecular underpinning that support the binary grading system, it more consistently separates prognostic groups [196, 197, 300]. The two-tier system has been validated to be reproducible among generalists and specialists [197]. The system does not require mitotic counting which is time-consuming and has poor reproducibility.

The MDACC system distinguishes low grade from high grade as follows. Low-grade serous carcinoma is characterized by uniform cells with mild to moderate nuclear atypia, whereas high-grade tumors have pleomorphic cells with marked nuclear atypia (>3:1 variation in nuclear size and shape). Low-grade tumors have a mitotic index <12 per 10 HPF, and usually much lower (<5 per 10 HPF), while high-grade tumors usually display >12 per 10 HPF.

This binary grading system effectively separates typical high-grade serous carcinoma from low-grade (micropapillary) serous carcinoma (see below) with 5-year survival rates of about 35% and 75%, respectively, for FIGO stage III. However, it is possible that patient's age and comorbidity have as much to do with this survival difference as grade. Women with high-grade serous carcinoma are nearly 2 decades older and consequently have more comorbid conditions and a shorter life expectancy as compared to those with low-grade serous carcinoma. In a population-based study of ovarian cancer in Denmark [350], ovarian cancer patients with severe comorbidity were about a decade older, and within each stage grouping, patients with more comorbidity had increased mortality. In one study of stage III ovarian serous carcinoma [300], the postoperative mortality (<2 months) in patients with high-grade tumors was 11% as compared to 0% for low grade. Thus, the high mortality rates in high-grade ovarian cancer may be disproportionately related to comorbid conditions as compared to low-grade ovarian cancer. In addition, low-grade serous carcinoma (invasive MPSC) is more likely to be stage IIIA or IIIB as compared to high-grade, which is nearly always IIIC, further confounding grade-stratified prognostication [103, 300]. It can therefore be argued that grade is at best a covariate, and at worst, not meaningful. A recent large population-based study on maximally debulked patients from Vancouver, Canada, found that stage and cell type are independent prognostic factors and grade is not [106].

Histologic Effects Induced by Chemotherapy Limited data are available on the histologic appearance of serous carcinoma shortly after chemotherapy [221]. Interval debulking specimens (after neoadjuvant chemotherapy) frequently show masses of psammoma bodies with scanty epithelium. Large omental cakes are often reduced to a normal size omentum with extensive fat necrosis and fibrosis, and with scattered foci of carcinoma throughout. Lymphocytes, foamy histiocytes, hemosiderin, and cholesterol clefts are often present. Scattered tumor cells show typical high-grade serous features, often with even more bizarre nuclear forms. In addition, they may show abundant clear, vacuolated, or eosinophilic cytoplasm and huge nucleoli. Sassen and associates found that the presence of scattered solitary tumor cells, fibrosis, foamy macrophages, and foreign body-type giant cells were highly specific (80–100%) but not sensitive indicators of neoadjuvant chemotherapy. Inflammation, hemosiderin, and isolated psammoma bodies were also associated with chemotherapy but were less specific [291].

Immunohistochemistry

Cytoplasmic immunopositivity is seen with CAM 5.2 and cytokeratin 7 in 100% of cases; BER-EP4, 95% [63], cytokeratin 20, 34%; vimentin, 45%; B72.3, 73% (usually weak)[63]; carcinoembryonic antigen, 19%; OC-125, 91%; gross cystic disease fluid protein-15 (GCDFP-15), 2%; and S-100, 30%. Membranous positivity is seen with epithelial membrane antigen (EMA) in 100% of cases. Nuclear positivity is seen for WT1 in 90% and for ER in 88–95% [63, 247] but some studies show that only a minority are ER-positive [381]. Nuclear staining for PR is usually absent or only weakly positive [63, 221] but can be strongly positive in up to 25% [178, 381]. The CK7/20 panel shows CK7+/CK20− in the majority of serous, endometrioid, and clear cell ovarian carcinomas, while the remainder are CK7+/CK20+. CK7 cytoplasmic positivity is nearly always strong and diffuse. When CK20 is positive, it is generally cytoplasmic and focal or patchy. p53, BRCA1, and WT1 nuclear stains and p16 (cytoplasmic, usually with concomitant nuclear staining) are positive in most high-grade serous carcinomas [12, 36, 47, 55, 229, 237, 352, 364, 385]. To be considered significant, p16 and p53 staining should be strong and diffuse. WT1-positive tumors are more often high-stage, high-grade, bcl-2 positive and have a higher proliferation index based on increased nuclear staining for Ki-67, as compared to WT1 negative tumors [385].

Calretinin displays weak cytoplasmic positivity in up to one quarter of serous carcinomas [47, 227] and moderate to strong positivity in 5–10% [63, 194]. CK5/6 is weakly positive in about one fourth of cases [63]. bcl-2 is positive in one third [385]. TTF-1, a marker for lung and thyroid carcinomas, is focally or weakly positive (nuclear reactivity) in 24–37% of serous carcinomas, but occasionally can be diffusely positive [20, 162]. CD99 is often positive. Inhibin, a marker of sex cord–stromal tumors, is usually negative but can be focally positive [47, 206]. p63 is usually negative [260]. Other markers that are reliably negative include h-caldesmon and thrombomodulin. CA19-9, CD 15, and D2-40 are negative or only weakly positive [63]. One study comparing pre- and post-neoadjuvant chemotherapy tumor specimens showed that the immunophenotype of high-grade serous carcinoma does not change significantly after carboplatin–paclitaxel treatment [221].

Differential Diagnosis Although metastatic carcinomas to the ovary, particularly colorectal tumors, most often mimic mucinous or endometrioid ovarian carcinomas, metastases may display a wide variety of patterns, and metastatic colorectal carcinomas can rarely resemble serous carcinoma [185]. In addition to CK7 and CK20, a few investigators have found monoclonal CEA useful in this differential [206] (see ➲ Mucinous Tumors below, and ➲ Chap. 18, Metastatic Tumors of the Ovary).

The distinction of serous from endometrioid carcinoma is generally not important in practice because the stage-stratified prognosis and treatment are similar. Although there is morphologic overlap, many experts believe that high-grade nonpapillary adenocarcinomas with glandular and cribriform patterns (non-clear cell, non-mucinous) most often represent serous carcinomas and should not be diagnosed as mixed or as endometrioid carcinoma unless the classic patterns of endometrioid adenocarcinoma of the uterine corpus are clearly recognizable [154, 207, 333]. Diffuse strong ER and PR reactivity and negative staining for WT1, p53, and p16 favor an endometrioid carcinoma, while the opposite findings are more common in serous carcinoma [206]. Molecular studies have not yet resolved whether the nonspecific high-grade adenocarcinomas have genetic features of endometrioid or serous carcinoma. The contrasting features of high-grade serous and endometrioid carcinomas are shown in ➲ *Table 14.15.*

Serous carcinomas often invade the fallopian tubes, and, on occasion, the distinction of an ovarian from a primary tubal carcinoma may be difficult (See ➲ Chap. 11, Diseases of the Fallopian Tube and Paratubal Region, and ➲ Chap. 18, Metastatic Tumors of the Ovary). Meticulous sectioning of the fallopian tube, which is typically dilated and filled with tumor when primary, can be helpful in making the distinction, but carcinomas involving the fimbriae are more difficult to clearly assign. Microscopically, the presence of carcinoma in situ in uninvolved tubal epithelium (serous tubal intraepithelial carcinoma – STIC) is helpful. It can be difficult to distinguish carcinoma in situ of the tube from hyperplasia and reactive changes [191]. Not infrequently, a primary tubal carcinoma is associated with metastases larger than 5 mm in the ovary. Since the 5 mm criterion is intended to separate ovarian from peritoneal tumors (see below), classification as primary tubal carcinoma is warranted if the tube shows the features of a primary tubal carcinoma.

Population-based studies have shown that approximately 10% of patients with apparent advanced-stage serous carcinoma have normal sized or slightly enlarged ovaries with only surface involvement [22], although

Table 14.15

Distinction between poorly differentiated serous adenocarcinoma and poorly differentiated endometrioid adenocarcinoma

Morphology	Serous	Endometrioid
Glandular spaces	Slit-like	Round, punched out
Psammoma bodies	Common	Rare
Tumor giant cells	Common	Rare
Papillae	Small, complex with budding	Longer and broader
Adenofibromatous growth pattern	Rare	Common
Squamous elements	Rare	Common
Endometriosis	Rare	Common
Immunohistochemistry		
WT1	Diffuse positive	Negative or focally positive
P53	Diffuse positive	Negative, focally or diffuse positive
P16	Diffuse positive	Negative or focally positive
Vimentin	Negative	Sometimes positive
Beta-catenin	Membranous	Membranous and, in some cases, nuclear positivity

Modified from [207]

recent series have shown a higher proportion ranging from 18% to 29% [115, 134, 301]. These are classified as primary peritoneal serous carcinomas. The following criteria for this distinction have been proposed by the GOG [26]: (1) both ovaries must be either physiologically normal in size or enlarged by a benign process; (2) the involvement in the extraovarian sites must be greater than the involvement on the surface of either ovary; (3) microscopically, the tumor in the ovary must be one of the following: (a) nonexistent, (b) confined to the ovarian surface epithelium with no evidence of cortical invasion, (c) involving ovarian surface epithelium and/or underlying cortical stroma but with no tumor nodule measuring greater than 5 × 5 mm; (4) the histological and cytological characteristics of the tumor must be predominantly of the serous type that is similar or identical to ovarian serous carcinoma, any grade.

From a practical standpoint, the distinction of ovarian from peritoneal carcinoma is not critical since the behavior and treatment are similar, but the distinction is important in epidemiologic, histopathologic, and molecular studies. Although widely used, the above criteria are arbitrary and too restrictive, and as such very likely underestimate the frequency of tubal as well as peritoneal carcinoma. In some cases, the ovaries display multiple small nodules of tumor, a feature characteristic of primary peritoneal carcinoma, but if only one nodule exceeds 5 mm, it must be classified as ovarian. Thus, primary peritoneal and tubal carcinomas are more common than previously realized.

The uterus is removed as part of the staging procedure for ovarian and peritoneal serous carcinomas. When the tumor appears to be primary peritoneal, the pathologist should meticulously examine the endometrium. Serous carcinoma of the endometrium and its putative precursor, endometrial intraepithelial carcinoma, can disseminate throughout the peritoneum even when microscopic and lacking myometrial invasion (see Chap. 9, Endometrial Carcinoma). It is possible that a small proportion of apparent primary peritoneal serous carcinomas reflect disseminated endometrial serous carcinomas with an occult primary endometrial tumor.

When a large endometrial serous carcinoma lacking myometrial invasion is associated with carcinomatosis, it can be difficult to assign a primary site to the ovarian and peritoneal lesions using morphology alone. If the ovarian involvement is multinodular and bilateral, metastatic disease to the ovaries and peritoneum is likely. WT1 can be of value, as peritoneal serous carcinomas are positive like their ovarian counterparts, whereas endometrial serous carcinomas are usually negative or weakly positive [1, 86, 118, 205, 206]. p53 is not as useful as it is positive in ovarian, peritoneal, and endometrial serous carcinomas. Independent serous carcinomas of the ovary and endometrium are possible but rare, and diagnostic criteria for this situation have not been well defined.

Primary ovarian epithelial tumors of non-serous types may occasionally mimic serous carcinoma: typically clear cell and endometrioid carcinomas. Clearing of the cytoplasm is not uncommon focally in serous carcinoma and is not indicative of clear cell carcinoma unless the typical architectural patterns of clear cell carcinoma are present (*Fig. 14.70*) [116, 207]. Similarly, glandular and cribriform patterns are common in serous carcinoma and should not be interpreted as endometrioid unless other characteristic features of eutopic endometrial carcinoma are present (*Table 14.15*). More importantly, malignant germ cell tumors, particularly embryonal carcinoma and yolk sac tumor, often have solid and papillary patterns, respectively, which may mimic serous carcinoma. The age of the patient is an important clue, as malignant germ cell tumors almost always occur in much younger patients. Immunohistochemistry utilizing antibodies against alpha fetoprotein, which reliably stains yolk sac tumors, can be useful in this distinction (see Chap. 16, Germ Cell Tumors of the Ovary). Clinical correlation with serum levels of AFP may also be of value. On occasion, distinction of serous carcinoma from the retiform variant of Sertoli–Leydig cell tumor (SLCT) is difficult. Positive inhibin and negative EMA staining in the latter tumors, as well as the younger age of these patients, are useful distinguishing features (see Chap. 15, Sex Cord-Stromal, Steroid Cell, and Other Ovarian Tumors with Endocrine, Paraendocrine, and Paraneoplastic Manifestations).

Diffuse malignant mesothelioma, particularly those with a papillary pattern, may on rare occasion be difficult to distinguish from serous carcinoma. At the Washington Hospital Center from 1999 to 2009, one diffuse malignant mesothelioma was diagnosed in the same population as over 300 ovarian and peritoneal carcinomas. The best markers for distinguishing mesothelioma from serous carcinoma include calretinin, CK5/6, and thrombomodulin, which are positive in mesotheliomas, and ER and BER-EP4 which are negative. ER appears to be more sensitive and specific than other stains that are typically negative in mesotheliomas in women [247]. The panel of ER, calretinin, and BER-EP4 (or MOC 31) has been recommended for a clear distinction in most cases [206, 248] with some recommending the addition of h-caldesmon, which stains mesotheliomas [63]. Of note, OC-125 is often positive in mesothelioma [20].

Ovarian carcinoma is often considered in the differential diagnosis of a metastatic adenocarcinoma of unknown primary site. Of particular value in this differential diagnosis is the panel of CK7 and CK20, as the CK7/CK20 profiles of carcinomas of a variety of sites have been extensively studied. Endometrioid and serous ovarian carcinomas are typically CK7+/CK20−. This panel is most useful in distinguishing gastrointestinal primary carcinomas from ovarian mucinous carcinomas (see Mucinous Tumors, Differential Diagnosis later in this chapter). Breast carcinoma, which is usually CK7+/CK20−, is typically GCDFP-15 positive and WT1 negative, while ovarian carcinomas are GCDFP-15 negative and WT1 positive. However 30–40% of breast carcinomas are negative for GCDFP-15 [20, 355]. TTF1 is not of great value in distinguishing ovarian from lung and thyroid carcinoma because it is positive in a significant number of ovarian carcinomas.

Molecular Biology Because serous carcinomas comprise the majority of ovarian carcinomas, most published studies of generic "ovarian cancer" or "ovarian carcinoma" in the older literature, unless otherwise indicated, likely included mainly serous carcinomas. Although recent clinical and molecular studies of ovarian cancer are more likely to take histological type into account, they are also usually weighted toward serous carcinomas since these tumors comprise the majority of malignant epithelial tumors. As a consequence, molecular alterations in typical (high-grade) serous carcinomas as well as a spectrum of benign, borderline, and low-grade malignant ovarian serous neoplasms have been studied quite extensively. In keeping with the now well-recognized adenoma–carcinoma sequence in colorectal cancer pathogenesis, for many years it was widely assumed that ovarian serous tumors likely progress from benign serous cystadenoma to atypical proliferative (borderline) serous tumor (APST), to low-grade serous carcinoma, and ultimately to high-grade serous carcinoma. However, the correlation of clinicopathological observations with molecular genetic data has led to a paradigm shift, and we now recognize distinct pathways leading to the development of low-grade (Type I) versus high-grade (Type II) serous carcinomas.

Mutational Analyses Our understanding of gene mutations in serous carcinomas will undoubtedly become more refined in the near future by new technologies allowing large-scale sequencing of the genome in primary tumors. Unbiased genome sequencing of large numbers of primary serous carcinomas will almost certainly uncover as yet unsuspected gene mutations that occur frequently in these tumors. Indeed, ovarian serous carcinoma is one of three cancer types initially selected for analysis by *The Cancer Genome Atlas*, a comprehensive and coordinated effort jointly sponsored by the National Cancer Institute and National Human Genome Research Institute to accelerate our understanding of the molecular basis of cancer through the application of comprehensive genome analysis technologies [232]. These data are in the process of being collected and will be publicly released. Until then, investigators continue to evaluate primary tumors for mutations largely on a gene-by-gene basis. To date, relatively few genes have been found to be mutated in the majority of ovarian serous tumors. *TP53* is mutated in 50% or more of advanced stage, high-grade serous carcinomas [327, 328]. *TP53* mutation frequency was found to be even higher (~80%) in high-grade serous carcinoma when purified tumor samples were used for sequence analysis [286]. In their study of early (stage I) serous carcinomas Leitao and colleagues identified overexpression of p53 and mutation of *TP53* in well over half of the cases, suggesting that *TP53* mutation is an early event in the development of high-grade serous carcinomas [183]. On a related note, a small series of intraepithelial serous carcinomas in the fallopian tube and coexisting ovarian serous carcinomas were recently found to share identical *TP53* mutations, suggesting a common origin of tumors in the two sites and providing further evidence of a role for *TP53* mutations early in serous carcinoma pathogenesis [149]. Mutations in several other tumor suppressor genes and oncogenes such as *BRCA1/2*, *PTEN*, and *PIK3CA* have also been reported in ovarian serous carcinomas, but their mutation frequency is generally low (<10%) [220, 231, 376].

DNA Copy Number Changes Several studies have analyzed global DNA copy number alterations specifically in high-grade and low-grade serous carcinomas [164, 204, 215, 230] A general conclusion that can be drawn from these studies is that high-grade serous carcinomas are characterized by more diffuse and higher levels of subchromosomal gains and losses than low-grade serous carcinomas and APSTs, suggesting that chromosomal instability is more pronounced in high-grade serous carcinomas than in low-grade serous carcinomas and APSTs. Based on single nucleotide polymorphism (SNP) array analysis of DNA copy number alterations in purified ovarian serous carcinoma samples, Nakayama and colleagues found the most frequently amplified subchromosomal regions harbor the *CCNE1* (cyclin E1), *AKT2*, *NOTCH3*, *RSF1*, and *PIK3CA* loci [230]. Dual-color fluorescence in situ hybridization (FISH) was performed to validate the findings in a sizeable independent set of serous carcinomas. The results showed high-level DNA copy number gains/amplification of *CCNE1*, *NOTCH3*, *RSF1*, *AKT2*, and *PIK3CA* loci in 36%, 32%, 16%, 14%, and 11% of high-grade serous carcinomas, respectively. In contrast, low-grade serous tumors did not show high-level amplification at any of the above loci. These gene amplifications have both biological and clinical significance. For example, deregulation of the PI3K/Pten signaling pathway through amplification of *PIK3CA*, which encodes the catalytic subunit of PI3K, has been shown to play a causal role in invasion, metastasis, and chemoresistance in ovarian cancer [11, 218]. *CCNE1* gene amplification and overexpression contributes to oncogenesis and genetic instability, particularly in the presence of mutant p53, which is present in most high-grade serous carcinomas [23, 334]. Moreover, expression of low-molecular-weight cyclin E is associated with worse clinical outcome in ovarian cancer patients [69]. The functional consequences of other gene amplifications in ovarian serous carcinomas are just beginning to be elucidated. Notably, although early studies identified rather frequent *HER2/neu* (*ERBB2*) amplification/copy number gains in ovarian serous carcinomas, a recent analysis using comprehensive genome-wide digital karyotyping technologies failed to identify high levels of *ERBB2* gene amplification in 33 high-grade or 10 low-grade serous carcinomas [230].

Gene Expression Transcriptome-wide gene expression profiling using serial analysis of gene expression (SAGE) and oligonucleotide microarrays has been applied to ovarian serous tumors including high-grade carcinomas, low-grade carcinomas, and APSTs [28, 106, 128, 129, 215]. Several of these studies found that low-grade and high-grade serous carcinomas are distinguishable based on their gene expression profiles. In those studies that included APSTs, the APSTs always clustered with low-grade rather than high-grade serous carcinomas. This finding provides further evidence that APSTs and low-grade serous carcinomas are closely related and both tumors are distinct from high-grade serous carcinomas.

Although somatic mutations of *BRCA1* and *BRCA2* are known to be rather uncommon in sporadic ovarian carcinomas, accumulated studies suggest these genes may be inactivated, particularly in serous carcinomas, through mechanisms other than mutation [41]. Horiuchi and colleagues found reduced expression of *BRCA1* transcripts in serous carcinomas, often associated with loss of heterozygosity at the *BRCA1* locus [372]. Hypermethylation of the *BRCA1* promoter accompanied by loss of Brca1 protein expression has been observed in 15–31% of sporadic ovarian carcinomas [21]. Moreover, high-grade serous carcinomas with genetic versus epigenetic inactivation of *BRCA1* have recently been shown to have distinct molecular abnormalities involving the PI3K/Pten signaling pathway [265]. Specifically, tumors with *BRCA1* mutations typically had decreased *PTEN* mRNA levels, while those with epigenetic loss of BRCA1 had copy number gains of *PIK3CA*. Finally, *WT1* (Wilms' tumor 1) encodes a protein that plays important roles in genitourinary tract development. Several studies have noted preferential expression of WT1 in serous carcinomas (both low-grade and high-grade) compared to the other histologic types of ovarian carcinoma [1, 237]. Because *TP53* mutations in high-grade serous carcinomas are most often missense mutations that result in protein stabilization, strong and diffuse nuclear expression of p53 protein is also observed in many of these tumors.

Clinical Behavior and Treatment

The survival rates for ovarian carcinoma, of which the majority are serous, are shown in ➲ *Table 14.9*. As discussed above, stage I patients who have been carefully staged have a 5-year survival rate that exceeds 90%; however, comprehensively staged high-grade serous carcinomas are rarely stage I [182, 301] (1.1% of ovarian carcinomas in our series (➲ *Table 14.4*) and 0.5% of ovarian carcinomas in a population-based study from British Columbia (stages IA and IB only in the latter study [287])). In fact, serous histology may be a poor prognostic factor in stage I especially in patients who have not been comprehensively staged [313]. The vast majority of stage III and IV ovarian carcinomas are high-grade serous and overall survival is poor. However, these tumors are often very sensitive to PBC and the 5-year survival rate approaches 50% for optimally debulked patients; there are occasional 10-year survivors of advanced-stage high-grade serous carcinoma. Most studies show that survival for peritoneal serous carcinoma is the same as that for ovarian carcinoma when stratified by stage [19, 26, 134, 144]. Stage II tumors are uncommon (3% of serous carcinomas (➲ *Table 14.4*)) and represent an intermediate group, which, depending on other factors including completeness of surgical removal and substage, can have widely varying survival and cure rates [299]. Microscopic serous carcinoma, so-called early de novo carcinoma, despite its small size (less than 7 mm) is associated with recurrence and death in about a third of cases, usually with widespread peritoneal disease (➲ *Fig. 14.71*).

A recent study examining the histology of ovarian carcinoma after neoadjuvant chemotherapy (NAC) followed by interval debulking found that those patients with no residual tumor or only scattered solitary tumor cells had a significantly better survival than those with larger residual tumor, with median survival of 45 and 26 months, respectively [291]. A similar study showed that a moderate or marked degree of tumor necrosis, found in 49% of 73 patients treated with NAC, significantly correlated with a longer time to first recurrence independent of other established risk factors, but did not correlate with survival [173].

Serum levels of CA125 correlate with volume of disease but are not independent prognostic factors. Although high preoperative CA125 levels may predict unresectability and poor survival, postoperative CA125 levels appear to be more prognostic. CA125 levels are commonly used to monitor for recurrence.

Mucinous Tumors

At the outset, it must be noted that diagnosis of the mucinous cell type in ovarian epithelial tumors is based solely on hematoxylin and eosin-stained sections. Mucin stains do not play a role in classification as they can be positive in other cell types. Primary ovarian mucinous tumors include cystadenomas, atypical proliferative mucinous tumors (APMT; also referred to as borderline or low malignant potential tumors), and carcinomas (intraepithelial and invasive). The cystadenomas, followed by APMT, are the most commonly encountered, whereas primary ovarian mucinous carcinomas are much less common. Cystadenomas and APMT are noninvasive, and are distinguished from each other primarily by their degree of complexity and epithelial proliferation. The invasive carcinomas are distinguished from these two types by the presence of stromal invasion. There is a morphologic spectrum of epithelial proliferation in mucinous tumors which includes cystadenomas with focal epithelial proliferation and APMT with intraepithelial carcinoma and/or microinvasion, providing evidence that these tumors comprise a biologic spectrum with individual types representing steps in the sequence of ovarian mucinous carcinogenesis. Molecular studies support this view (see ➲ Molecular Biology below).

The other types of mucinous tumors encountered in the ovary include metastatic mucinous carcinomas, most commonly from the gastrointestinal tract, and low-grade mucinous tumors of appendiceal origin secondarily involving the ovary in association with the clinical syndrome of pseudomyxoma peritonei (PMP). Both metastatic mucinous carcinomas and low-grade mucinous tumors of appendiceal origin can simulate primary ovarian mucinous tumors, including both APMT and primary ovarian mucinous carcinoma. Refined criteria for diagnosis of ovarian mucinous tumors in recent years, with distinction of these non-ovarian tumors from true primary ovarian mucinous tumors, have been instrumental in clarifying the behavior of ovarian mucinous tumors and in providing more appropriate therapy.

Studies using refined diagnostic criteria for ovarian mucinous tumors, particularly those focused on recognition of metastatic mucinous carcinomas that simulate primary ovarian mucinous tumors, have established that primary ovarian mucinous carcinomas are much less common than previously believed [306]. However, despite improved recognition of metastases, the problem of distinguishing primary and metastatic mucinous carcinomas persists (see ➲ Chap. 18, Metastatic Tumors of the Ovary). The difficulty in recognizing metastases that morphologically simulate primary ovarian mucinous tumors is compounded by the fact that some metastases present first in the ovary without a clinically evident extraovarian primary. In addition, ancillary techniques such as immunohistochemistry, while useful in certain situations (see ➋ Differential Diagnosis below), are limited in their ability to distinguish some metastases from primary ovarian mucinous tumors. It is important to recognize this difficulty when evaluating the literature on behavior and therapeutic responses of ostensibly primary ovarian mucinous carcinomas, as older reports, particularly those prior to and even including the 1990s, likely include a subset of misclassified metastases. Even in expert hands, distinction of primary from metastatic mucinous carcinoma may be very difficult at times, and we estimate that the frequency of misclassification or genuine diagnostic uncertainty is at least 5%.

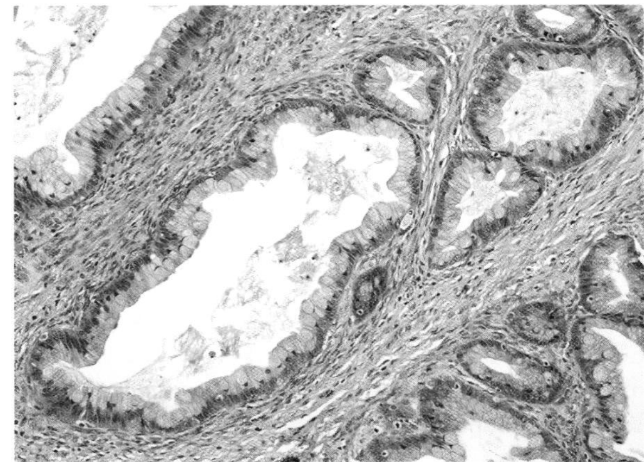

Fig. 14.72
Mucinous cystadenoma. **The nuclei are small, bland, and uniform. The cytoplasm contains abundant lightly basophilic mucin**

Benign Mucinous Tumors, Intestinal and Müllerian (Seromucinous, Endocervical-like) Types

Mucinous cystadenomas (including the müllerian type; see below) comprise 13% of benign ovarian epithelial neoplasms (➋ *Table 14.5*). Over 80% are of the intestinal type. The mean patient age is about 50 years. Intestinal-type mucinous cystadenomas are unilocular or multilocular tumors of variable size, ranging from a few centimeters to over 30 cm, with a mean of about 10 cm. They are typically unilateral (95%). The capsule is typically thick and white with a smooth outer surface. The cysts contain thick gelatinous material. The vast majority are composed of glands and cysts lined by simple non-stratified mucinous epithelium resembling gastric foveolar-type epithelium or intestinal epithelium containing goblet cells (➋ *Fig. 14.72*). The peripheral aspects of the cysts can form crypt-like structures where nuclei may appear reactive and exhibit mitotic activity, but the epithelium of the cysts generally lacks atypia or displays focal mild atypia. The epithelium can appear undulating but epithelial stratification and tufting are generally absent; when epithelial proliferation is present resembling APMT, this feature must be limited to <10% for the tumor to qualify as a cystadenoma (➋ *Fig. 14.73*). Tumors composed predominantly of cystadenoma with <10% of APMT are diagnosed as mucinous cystadenoma with focal proliferation [277] or focal atypia [310]. The majority of tumors contain calcification which is usually spiculated rather than psammomatous. Muciphages, pseudoxanthoma cells, and luteinized stromal cells are each present in 40–50%. Dissection of acellular mucin in the tumor stroma, referred to as "pseudomyxoma ovarii," is seen in 10%, and 10% also display multinucleated giant cells [302]. Rarely, benign mucinous neoplasms are solid and adenofibromatous; these are referred to as mucinous adenofibroma. Up to 18% of mucinous cystadenomas contain transitional cell nests, also referred to as a Brenner tumor component, often in a discrete nodule which is usually interpreted as a concurrent Brenner tumor [302]. When the Brenner component is prominent or intimately admixed with the mucinous component, the tumor can be classified as metaplastic Brenner tumor or mixed mucinous–Brenner tumor (see ➋ Brenner Tumors,

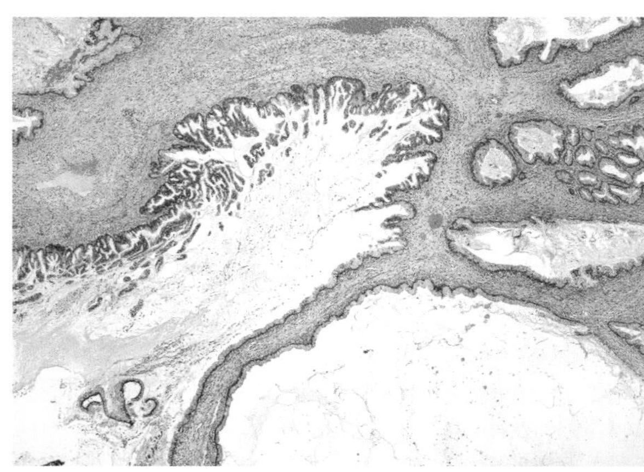

Fig. 14.73
Mucinous cystadenoma with focal proliferation. **The area of epithelial proliferation occupied less than 10% of the tumor**

and Mixed Epithelial Tumors, later in this chapter). In light of these findings and other observations, it has been suggested that the majority of intestinal type mucinous tumors arise from Brenner tumors or transitional cell nests.

Occasionally, cystadenomas have endocervical-type mucinous epithelium. These are referred to as müllerian-type mucinous, endocervical-like mucinous, or seromucinous cystadenoma. They are unilocular or multilocular cystic tumors, often with papillary architecture in contrast to the pure glandular pattern of the intestinal type. The epithelium closely resembles endocervical mucinous epithelium with columnar cells having apical mucin and basally situated bland nuclei. When stringent criteria are applied to avoid misclassification as gastrointestinal-type tumors, which can occasionally have very few goblet cells when lined by foveolar-type epithelium, this subtype is uncommon. Mucinous cystadenomas and adenofibromas are benign but can recur if incompletely excised. Tumor rupture has not been associated with recurrence.

Atypical Proliferative Mucinous Tumor (Mucinous Borderline Tumors), Intestinal Type

Although the borderline category was intended mainly for serous tumors (see Serous Tumors earlier in this chapter), the concept was also extended to mucinous tumors since they also appeared to have intermediate forms. These alleged intermediate forms were most often characterized by PMP and were felt to be analogous to serous borderline tumors with peritoneal implants, with the characteristic peritoneal mucin deposits of PMP representing the peritoneal implants of ovarian mucinous tumors. In the late 1970s, the term "atypical proliferative" or "atypically proliferating tumor" was introduced. Currently, three terms are used to refer to these tumors: "atypical proliferative mucinous tumor," "mucinous borderline tumor," and "mucinous tumor of low malignant potential." The 2003 Borderline Ovarian Tumor Conference established that the three terms are synonymous; "tumor of low malignant potential," was the least favored of the three [277, 310].

There are two types of APMT corresponding to the two types of mucinous cystadenomas: the gastrointestinal type and the endocervical-like (müllerian, or seromucinous) type. The gastrointestinal type of APMT is typically a large, multicystic tumor with a smooth capsule, and is usually unilateral (>95%) with mean and median sizes of about 20–22 cm [272, 391]. The locules of the tumor are usually filled with mucinous material and the lining appears smooth, without grossly evident papillations. Microscopically, the cysts are lined by stratified, proliferative gastrointestinal-type mucinous epithelium exhibiting tufted and villoglandular or papillary intraglandular growth and displaying variable (usually mild to moderate) nuclear atypia; by definition, stromal invasion is absent (*Figs. 14.74–14.79*).

The clinical behavior of mucinous tumors is summarized in *Table 14.16*. Review of the literature on tumors meeting the diagnostic criteria for APMT, gastrointestinal type, reveals an overwhelmingly benign behavior [148, 179, 235, 236, 272, 274]. More than 600 stage I tumors have been reported, and less than 1% of patients have died of disease. Parenthetically, most fatal tumors had inadequate or unknown degree of sampling and are reported in the older literature; most recent studies report 100% survival.

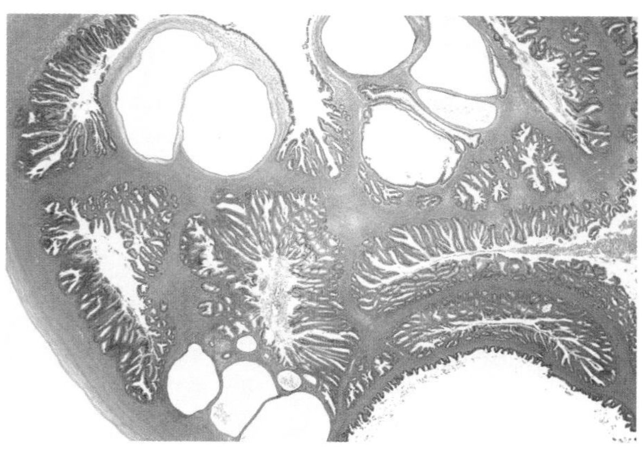

Fig. 14.74
Atypical proliferative (borderline) mucinous tumor (APMT). **An extensive but orderly epithelial proliferation lacking destructive infiltrative growth**

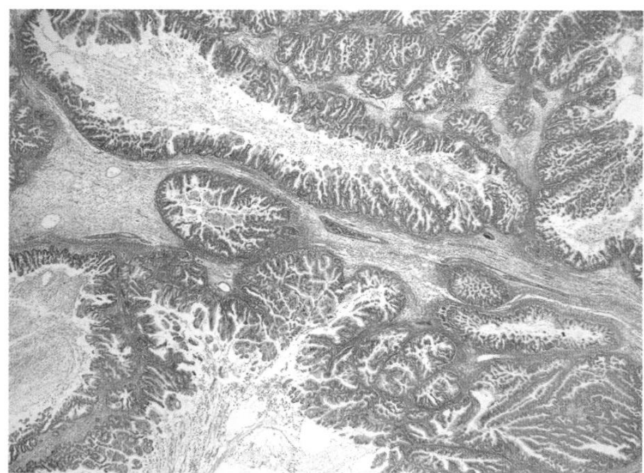

Fig. 14.75
Atypical proliferative (borderline) mucinous tumor. **Extensive epithelial proliferation with stratification and focal detachment of cell clusters**

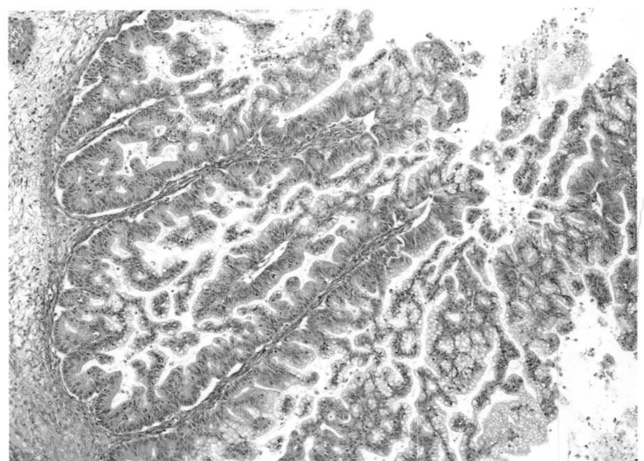

Fig. 14.76
Atypical proliferative (borderline) mucinous tumor. **Fusion of papillae focally creates small cribriform foci**

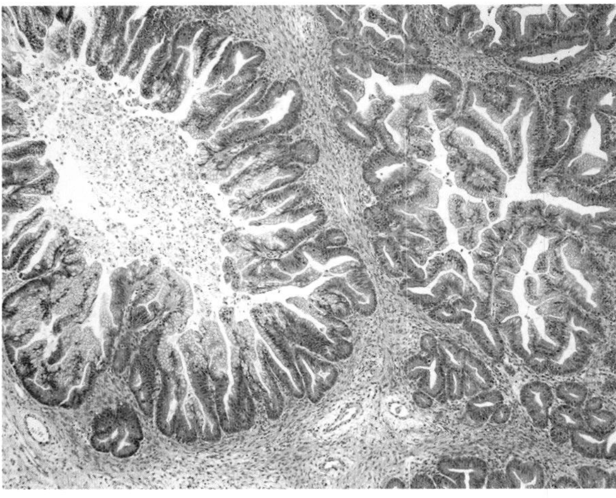

Fig. 14.77
Atypical proliferative (borderline) mucinous tumor. **Small neoplastic glands are in orderly clusters adjacent to the larger glands displaying proliferation**

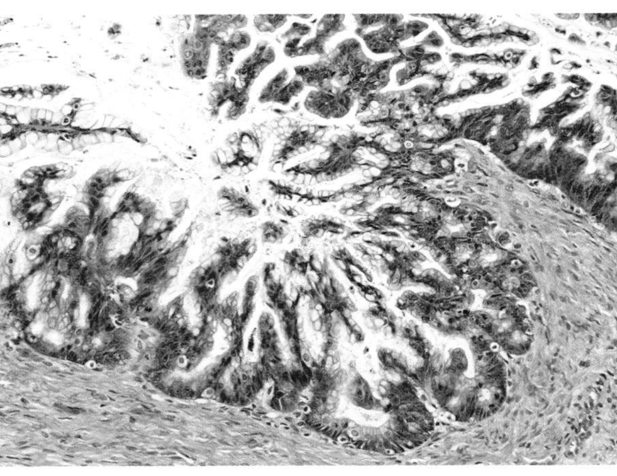

Fig. 14.78
Atypical proliferative (borderline) mucinous tumor. **Mild cytologic atypia and fusion of papillae**

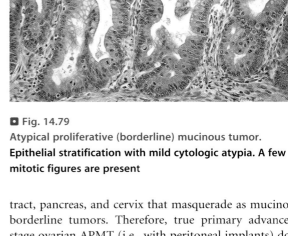

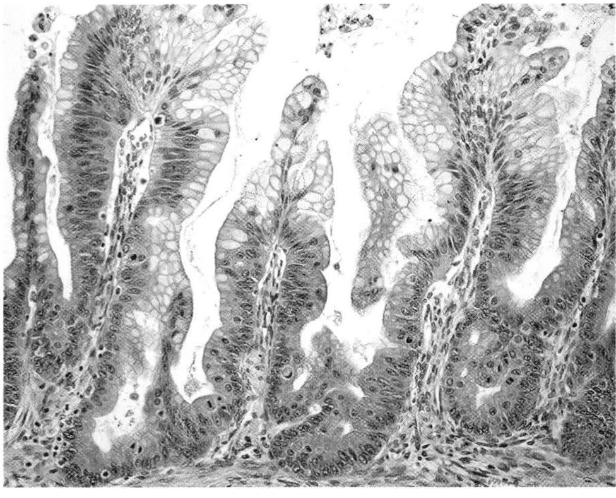

Fig. 14.79
Atypical proliferative (borderline) mucinous tumor. **Epithelial stratification with mild cytologic atypia. A few mitotic figures are present**

Approximately 100 of so-called advanced-stage borderline mucinous tumors have been reported, with nearly 50% mortality. Of these, about 85% have been associated with PMP. Recent studies have established that virtually all cases of PMP are of gastrointestinal (usually appendiceal), not ovarian, origin (see Mucinous Tumors Associated with Pseudomyxoma Peritonei (PMP) below) [278, 280, 362, 363, 365]. The remaining 15% of advanced-stage mucinous borderline tumors reported are, in all likelihood, metastatic mucinous carcinomas typically from the biliary tract, pancreas, and cervix that masquerade as mucinous borderline tumors. Therefore, true primary advanced-stage ovarian APMT (i.e., with peritoneal implants) does not exist. When these latter tumors are removed from the APMT category, the remainder consist of stage I tumors with benign behavior. Rarely, a mucinous cystadenoma or APMT is associated with a localized collection of mucin involving the pelvic peritoneum, and may even contain a few strips of benign mucinous epithelium. This is probably due to tumor rupture and should not be classified as PMP or APMT with peritoneal implants.

Table 14.16
Behavior of ovarian mucinous tumors

Tumor type	Survival rate[c]
Atypical proliferative mucinous tumors (APMTs), stage I	>99%
Atypical proliferative mucinous tumors, advanced stage[a]	(see PMP category)
Atypical proliferative mucinous tumors with intraepithelial carcinoma[a]	~95%
Atypical proliferative mucinous tumors with microinvasion	>99%
Primary ovarian mucinous carcinomas, confluent glandular type[a]	~90%
Primary ovarian mucinous carcinomas, infiltrative type[a]	<<50%
Ovarian mucinous tumors associated with pseudomyxoma peritonei (PMP)[b]	~50%
Metastatic mucinous carcinomas	<<50%

[a]May include some misclassified metastatic mucinous carcinomas.
[b]Virtually all tumors are derived from the gastrointestinal tract (usually appendix) and are thus not ovarian in origin.
[c]Data derived from review in [277].

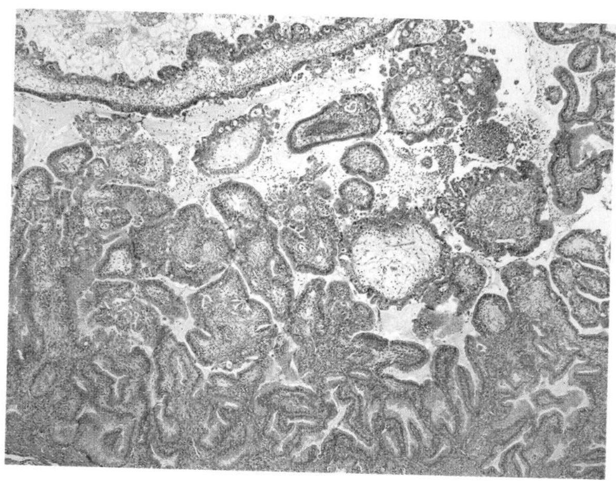

Fig. 14.80
Atypical proliferative (borderline) seromucinous tumor (APSMT). **Complex papillary proliferation at low magnification architecturally resembles atypical proliferative serous tumor**

Atypical Proliferative Mucinous Tumor, Seromucinous (Endocervical-like or Müllerian) Type

The seromucinous-type APMT (APSMT) is grossly, microscopically, and immunophenotypically distinct from the gastrointestinal-type tumor [361]. The seromucinous tumors are much less common, smaller, more frequently bilateral, architecturally resemble APST, and are much more often associated with endometriosis. In addition, they frequently display acute inflammation of the stroma, and a combination of endocervical mucinous and serous (ciliated)-type epithelium, often admixed with minor components (<10%) of other cell types (endometrioid, squamous, and eosinophilic "indifferent" cells) [228] (*Figs. 14.80–14.83*). The term "seromucinous" is more accurate than endocervical-type mucinous tumor for this group of tumors as it reflects the morphologic and behavioral features that are shared with the serous tumors, and that differ from the typical mucinous tumors of gastrointestinal type. Based on a small number of studies, these tumors, including very few with implants and intraepithelial and microinvasive carcinomas, have demonstrated a benign behavior [77, 273, 316].

Atypical Proliferative Mucinous Tumors with Intraepithelial (Noninvasive) Carcinoma

Based on the FIGO and WHO classifications of the early 1970s, the absence of stromal invasion distinguishes

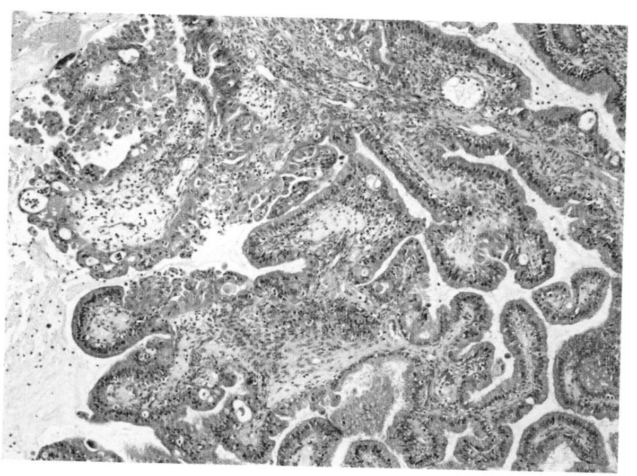

Fig. 14.81
Atypical proliferative (borderline) seromucinous tumor. **Areas of epithelial stratification and detachment of cell clusters. Many cells contain abundant eosinophilic cytoplasm. An acute inflammatory reaction and microabscesses in the epithelium are characteristic of this tumor**

APMT from mucinous carcinoma. Shortly thereafter, the criteria for mucinous carcinoma were expanded to include marked overgrowth of atypical epithelial cells manifested as stratification in excess of three layers, cribriform intraglandular proliferations, or fingerlike projections of solid cellular masses without connective tissue support; these patterns were often accompanied by marked nuclear

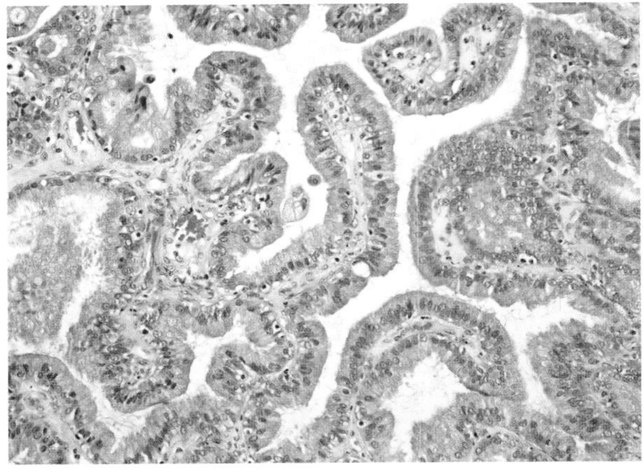

■ Fig. 14.82
Atypical proliferative (borderline) seromucinous tumor. **The epithelium displays minimal cytologic atypia and lightly basophilic cytoplasm resembling endocervical (müllerian) mucinous epithelium**

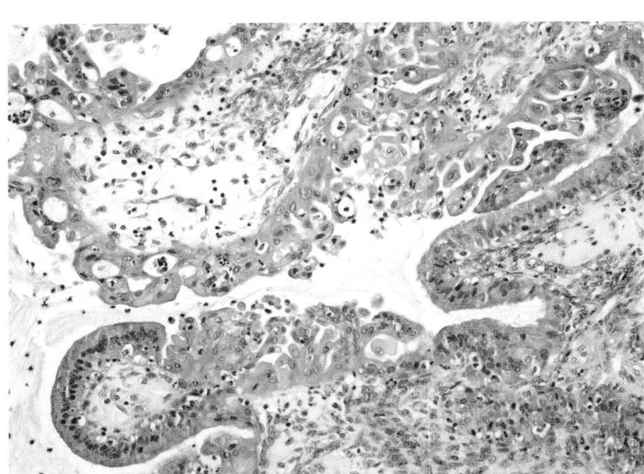

■ Fig. 14.83
Atypical proliferative (borderline) seromucinous tumor. **Mild cytologic atypia and cytoplasmic eosinophilia are present. Note acute inflammatory cells in the epithelium**

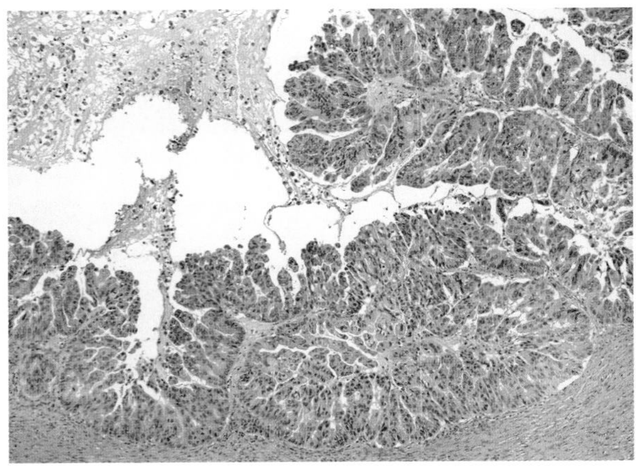

■ Fig. 14.84
Atypical proliferative (borderline) mucinous tumor with intraepithelial carcinoma. **Marked stratification of epithelium**

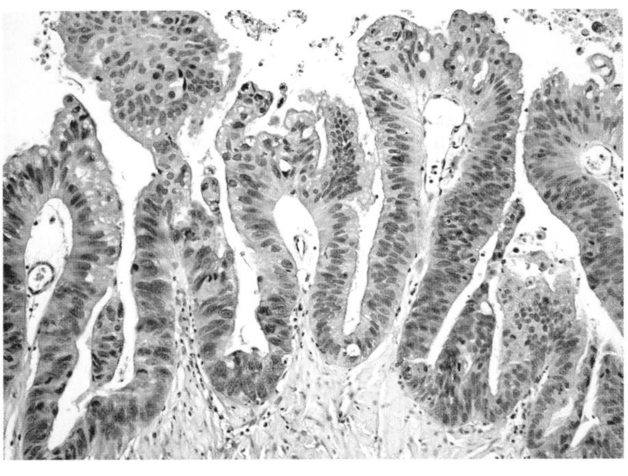

■ Fig. 14.85
Atypical proliferative (borderline) mucinous tumor with intraepithelial carcinoma. **Marked cytologic atypia is present**

atypia. In addition, the presence of marked nuclear atypia alone was added as a diagnostic feature of mucinous carcinoma. Since then, mucinous tumors lacking stromal invasion but displaying epithelial overgrowth and atypia have been referred to as "noninvasive," "intraglandular," or "intraepithelial" carcinomas. Proposed diagnostic criteria for intraepithelial carcinoma vary slightly among different studies [179, 236, 272, 273, 277]. All studies consider noninvasive tumors with marked nuclear atypia as intraepithelial carcinomas, and this is the preferred criterion (➲ *Figs. 14.84–14.86*). Excessive epithelial stratification and other complex intraglandular growth patterns can be seen in typical APMT and should not be used to diagnose intraepithelial carcinoma in the absence of severe atypia [277].

Intraepithelial carcinomas confined to the ovaries have an excellent prognosis (about 95% survival, with most recent studies reporting 100% survival) [148, 179, 236, 272, 273, 277]. A small number of so-called advanced stage intraepithelial mucinous carcinomas have been reported,

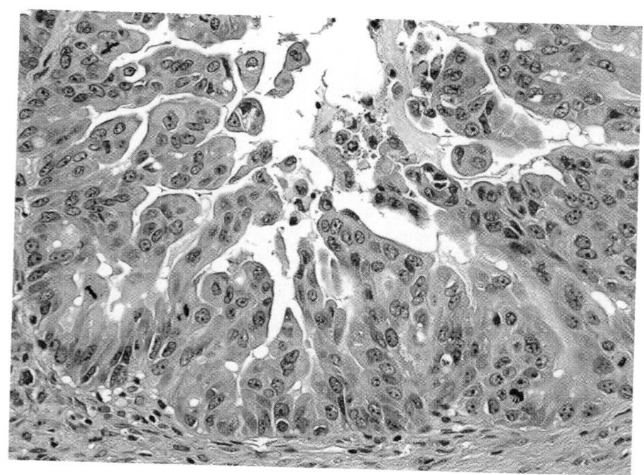

◘ Fig. 14.86
Atypical proliferative (borderline) mucinous tumor with intraepithelial carcinoma. **Marked cytologic atypia and mitotic figures are present**

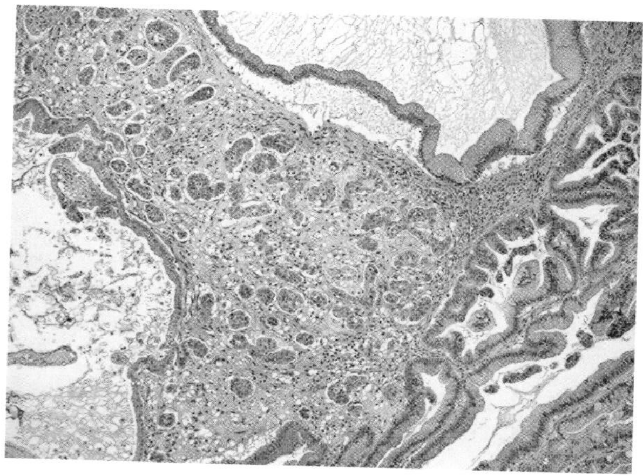

◘ Fig. 14.87
Atypical proliferative (borderline) mucinous tumor with microinvasion. **Haphazard infiltrative growth of small glands and nests measuring less than 5 mm in greatest dimension**

with a few tumor deaths. In view of the ability of metastatic mucinous carcinomas to simulate APMT with intraepithelial carcinoma (see below), it is likely that some of these apparent advanced-stage intraepithelial carcinomas with adverse outcome represent metastases from occult extraovarian primary tumors. It is also possible that some of these represent true primary ovarian mucinous carcinomas with foci of destructive invasion in unsampled tissue. Finally, these tumors may display patterns of invasion that are not recognizable as such using current criteria.

APMT with Microinvasion

Microinvasion in APMT has been defined as either small foci of stromal invasion characterized by single cells, glands, or small clusters or nests of mucinous epithelial cells within the stroma, or as small foci of confluent glandular or cribriform growth within the stroma (➲ *Figs. 14.87–14.91*). The size criterion for each focus has varied from 2 to 5 mm, with no requirement regarding the number of foci allowed [277]. Some tumors with microinvasion also have intraepithelial carcinoma. Based on the relatively small number of microinvasive tumors with follow-up that have been reported, no well-documented recurrences or deaths due to disease have been reported [148, 179, 235, 236, 272, 273, 277]. Although microinvasion in mucinous tumors often resembles the lesion designated "microinvasive carcinoma" in serous tumors, the metastatic potential of small foci of invasion in mucinous tumors is probably low but there are no published studies specifically addressing this issue. Accordingly, the behavior of tumors with these minute

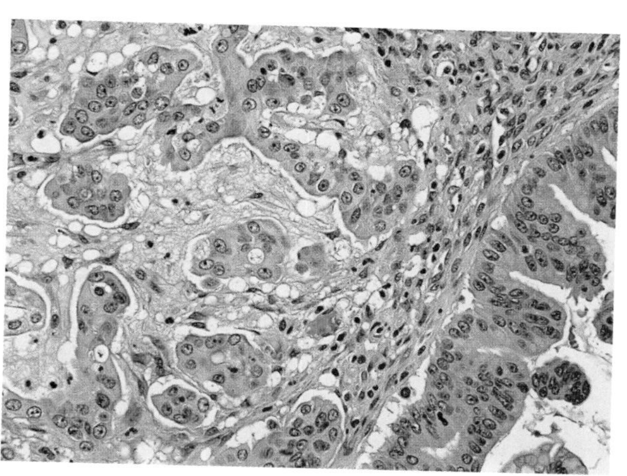

◘ Fig. 14.88
Atypical proliferative (borderline) mucinous tumor with microinvasion. **High magnification reveals cytologic atypia and extracellular mucin around infiltrative nests of cells (same case as ➲ *Fig. 14.87*)**

invasive foci is uncertain; the consensus among experts in the field is to use the term microinvasion [277].

Mucinous Tumors Associated with Pseudomyxoma Peritonei (PMP)

PMP has historically referred to the presence of mucinous ascites or mucoid nodules adherent to peritoneal surfaces and has not had a consistently applied histopathological

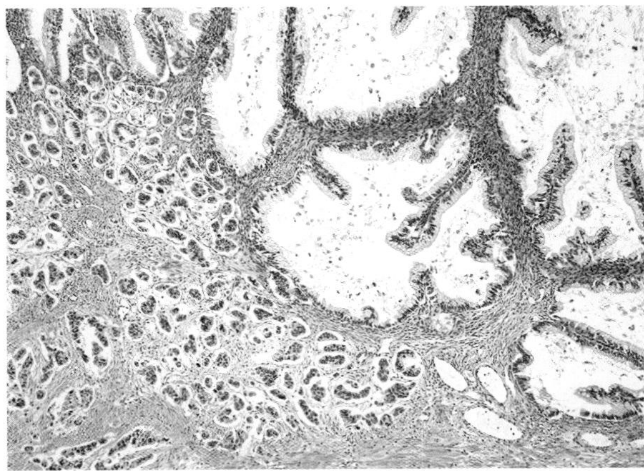

Fig. 14.89
Atypical proliferative (borderline) mucinous tumor with microinvasion. **Haphazard infiltrative growth of small nests adjacent to noninvasive neoplastic glands**

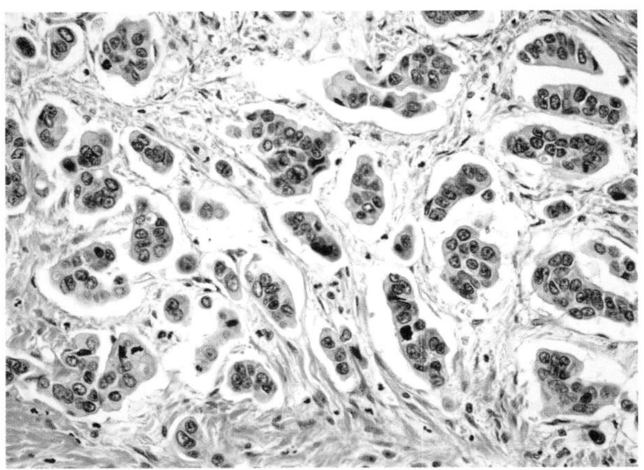

Fig. 14.90
Atypical proliferative (borderline) mucinous tumor with microinvasion. **High magnification reveals infiltrative small cords and nests surrounded by a space**

description. Recent studies have defined PMP as a clinicopathologic syndrome in which mucinous ascites is accompanied by low-grade neoplastic mucinous epithelium associated with pools of extracellular mucin and fibrosis [280]. Morphologic, immunohistochemical, and molecular genetic studies have provided compelling evidence that virtually all cases of PMP are derived from low-grade (adenomatous) mucinous tumors of the appendix, and that the ovarian involvement is secondary [278, 280, 281]. This concept is further supported by other studies showing that ruptured primary ovarian mucinous tumors have

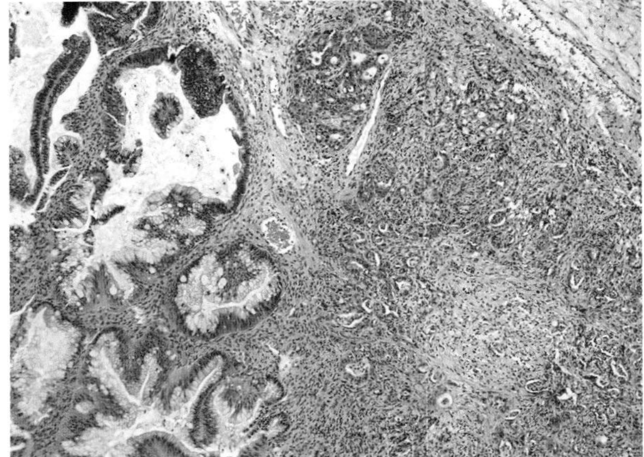

Fig. 14.91
Atypical proliferative (borderline) mucinous tumor with microinvasion. **The invasive area on the *right* is about 5 mm, and therefore is the boundary between APMT with microinvasion and mucinous carcinoma**

not been associated with the subsequent development of PMP [179]. Because the ovarian mucinous tumors associated with PMP are almost invariably derived from the gastrointestinal tract, usually the appendix, they are now reported as secondary involvement of the ovary by low-grade (adenomatous) mucinous tumor [277]. The term "metastatic mucinous carcinoma" should be avoided for the ovarian lesions (see Metastatic Mucinous Carcinoma). When intraoperative consultation with frozen section leads to a diagnosis of a mucinous ovarian tumor in the setting of PMP, the need for appendectomy as well as thorough examination of the gastrointestinal and pancreaticobiliary tracts should be conveyed to the surgeon. The pathologist should examine the entire appendix microscopically. The rare exception to the gastrointestinal origin of PMP is the occurrence of mucinous tumors arising in ovarian mature cystic teratomas associated with mucinous ascites [211, 279]. Accordingly these are classified as germ cell tumors (see Chap. 16, Germ Cell Tumors of the Ovary).

The terms "disseminated peritoneal adenomucinosis" (DPAM) and "involvement by low-grade appendiceal mucinous neoplasm" are now recommended as specific pathologic diagnostic terms for these low-grade peritoneal and ovarian mucinous tumors, respectively [278, 280, 281]. The term PMP is restricted to use as a clinical descriptor for the syndrome and is maintained as a general term for historical continuity. This recommendation is based on studies demonstrating that peritoneal mucinous tumors with the histologic features of the low-grade tumors are pathologically and prognostically distinct from mucinous carcinomas, with the latter having significantly worse survival [280, 388]. Some investigators have proposed the terms, "mucinous carcinoma peritonei, low grade" for DPAM, and "mucinous carcinoma peritonei, high grade" for the carcinomatous tumors [30]. The DPAM terminology is already in widespread use and has the added advantage of not changing the term for the high-grade variant, which has always been referred to as invasive mucinous carcinoma or mucinous carcinomatosis. The distinguishing morphologic features of DPAM and mucinous carcinomatosis are shown in *Table 14.17*, and those of ovarian involvement by DPAM and primary ovarian mucinous tumors in *Table 14.18* (*Figs. 14.92* and *14.93*).

Table 14.17

Distinguishing features of disseminated peritoneal adenomucinosis (DPAM) and peritoneal mucinous carcinomatosis (PMCA)

Feature	DPAM	PMCA
Primary site	Appendix	Appendix, colon, small intestine
Primary diagnosis	Mucinous adenoma; low grade mucinous neoplasm	Mucinous adenocarcinoma
Surgical appearance	Mucinous ascites with characteristic distribution[a]	Carcinomatosis with invasive implants
Peritoneal tumor		
Cellularity	Scant	Moderate to abundant
Morphology	Abundant extracellular mucin containing simple to focally proliferative mucinous epithelium	Moderate to abundant extracellular mucin containing extensively proliferative mucinous epithelium or mucinous glands, clusters of cells, or individual cells consistent with carcinoma
Cytologic atypia	Minimal	Moderate to marked
Mitotic activity	Rare	Infrequent to abundant
Lymph node involvement	Rare	Frequent
Parenchymal organ involvement	Rare (except ovary)	Frequent

[a]The distribution is characterized by superficial noninvasive involvement of the omentum, undersurface of the diaphragm, pelvis, right retrohepatic space, left abdominal gutter, and ligament of Treitz, with sparing of the peritoneal surfaces of the bowel.

Table 14.18

Distinction of ovarian mucinous tumors associated with pseudomyxoma peritonei (PMP) from primary ovarian mucinous tumors

Feature	Ovarian mucinous tumors in pseudomyxoma peritonei	Primary ovarian atypical proliferative mucinous tumors
Size	Variable (mean/median = 14 cm)[a]	Large (mean/median = 22 cm)[b]
Laterality	Bilateral (80%)[a]	Unilateral (100%)[b]
Location of tumor	Surface, superficial cortex, stroma	Within stroma (rarely on surface when ruptured)
Pseudomyxoma ovarii	Often prominent	Usually absent or limited
Amount and pattern of epithelium	Usually scant; haphazard when more abundant	Abundant; organized cysts with peripheral crypts
Associated appendiceal mucinous tumor	Virtually all cases	None

[a]Data derived from combination of data in [278, 391].
[b]Data derived from [391].

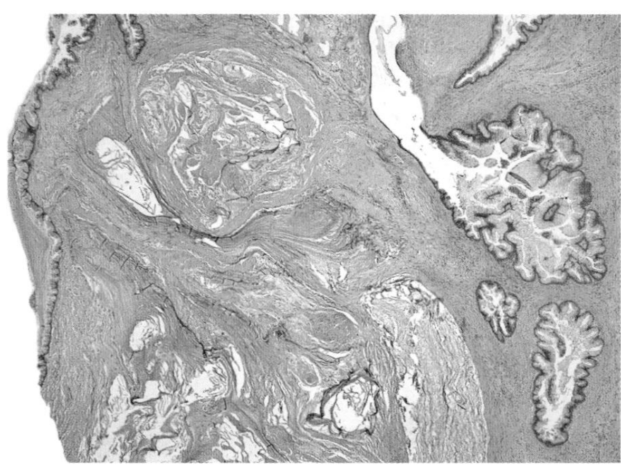

Fig. 14.92
Ovarian involvement by disseminated peritoneal adenomucinosis (DPAM). **Large lakes of mucin dissecting through the ovarian stroma**

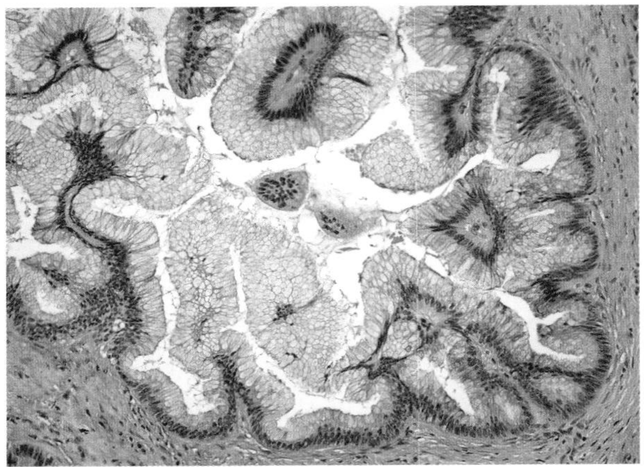

Fig. 14.93
Ovarian involvement by disseminated peritoneal adenomucinosis. **The neoplastic mucinous epithelium closely resembles that in a primary ovarian mucinous neoplasm**

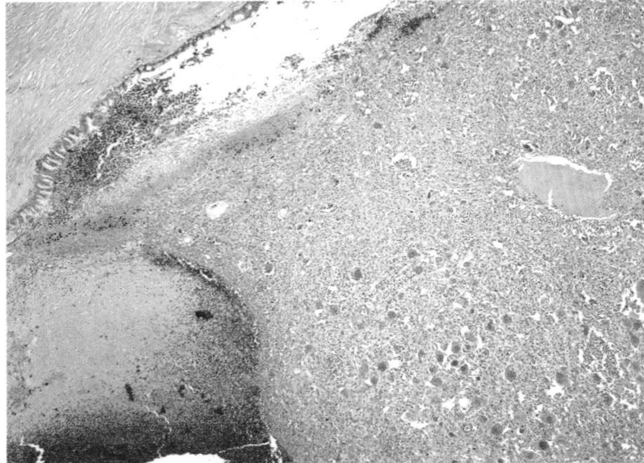

Fig. 14.94
Atypical proliferative mucinous tumor with sarcoma-like mural nodule. **Neoplastic mucinous epithelium on the *left* is adjacent to a solid proliferation of markedly atypical cells including multinucleated giant cells**

Mucinous Tumors with Mural Nodules

Ovarian mucinous cystic neoplasms of all types can occasionally contain mural nodules. Three varieties of mural nodules have been described, including true sarcomas, sarcoma-like mural nodules, and foci of anaplastic carcinoma. In general, the sarcomatous nodules and foci of anaplastic carcinoma tend to occur in older patients and are characterized by larger size, poor circumscription, a monotonous spindle cell population in the former, evidence of carcinomatous differentiation in the latter, and aggressive behavior. In contrast, sarcoma-like mural nodules tend to occur in younger women and are characterized by smaller size, sharp demarcation, a heterogeneous cell population, and no demonstrable impact on the prognosis. The sarcoma-like mural nodules can have various histologic appearances, including a pleomorphic and epulis-like type with multinucleated giant cells, a pleomorphic and spindle cell type, and a giant cell-histiocytic type (*Figs. 14.94* and *14.95*). The nodules can be solitary or multiple and mixtures of these histologic types can be encountered, with the pleomorphic and epulis-like type being the most common. Hemorrhage, necrosis, and a mixed inflammatory cell component are commonly seen. It is not clear whether sarcoma-like mural nodules are neoplastic or represent a reaction to hemorrhage within or rupture of a mucinous cyst. Sarcoma-like mural nodules usually coexpress vimentin (strong/diffuse) and cytokeratin (focal/weak), similar to true sarcomas yet distinct from anaplastic carcinomas that usually have strong/diffuse cytokeratin expression.

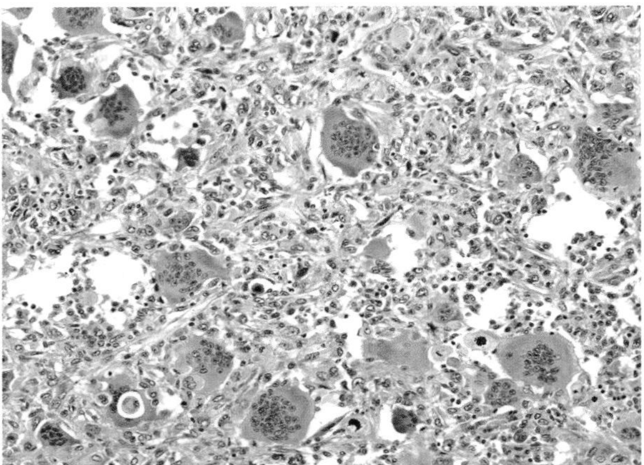

Fig. 14.95
Mucinous neoplasm with sarcoma-like mural nodule. **Epulis-like multinucleated giant cells are scattered in a background of ovoid and spindle cells with mild atypia and mitotic figures**

Mucinous tumors with malignant mural nodules are probably best classified as variants of mucinous carcinoma or carcinosarcoma. Malignant mural nodules are fatal in 50% of cases. Sarcoma-like mural nodules, though believed to be benign, should be regarded with caution as their histologic appearance is worrisome and clinical follow-up data are very limited.

Invasive Mucinous Carcinomas

Mucinous carcinomas of the intestinal type are rare, and comprise 2–3% of ovarian carcinomas (➲ *Tables 14.4* and ➲ *14.5*) [301, 342].

Clinical and Operative Findings

Primary ovarian mucinous carcinomas most often present as large unilateral ovarian masses, usually without evidence of ovarian surface involvement or extraovarian disease, similar to APMT.

Gross Findings

The gross findings are similar to APMT in that they are typically large, unilateral, multicystic mucus-containing tumors with smooth white capsules and have mean and median sizes of 18–22 cm. They may contain solid areas and foci of necrosis and hemorrhage.

Microscopic Findings

Mucinous carcinomas of intestinal type typically are architecturally well differentiated and display a variety of glandular patterns, with many tumors having areas of APMT adjacent to areas of carcinoma (➲ *Figs. 14.96–14.101*). The traditional definition of mucinous carcinoma required the presence of destructive stromal infiltration by malignant mucinous epithelium as the primary microscopic feature to establish a diagnosis of invasive carcinoma. Tumors exhibiting typical APMT-type growth patterns with excessive epithelial stratification and lacking significant nuclear atypia or stromal invasion have not been associated with adverse outcome and are accepted as APMT.

Recent studies have drawn attention to a second pattern of invasion, termed the "confluent glandular" or "expansile" pattern [52, 179, 272]. In this pattern, the glandular epithelium is markedly crowded, with little intervening stroma, and interconnected in a confluent or labyrinthine pattern (➲ *Figs. 14.96–14.98*). Primary ovarian mucinous carcinomas commonly exhibit this pattern

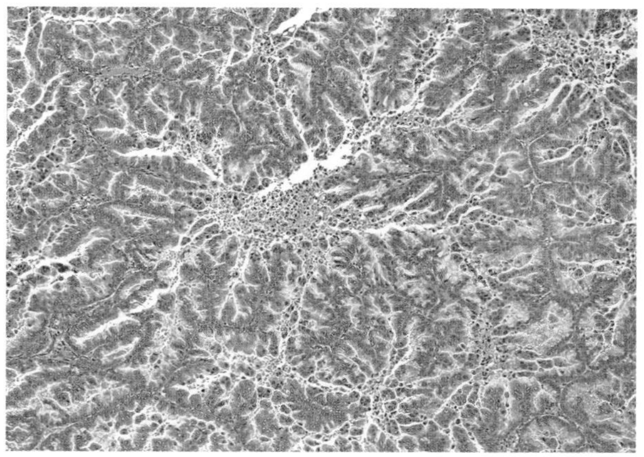

◘ Fig. 14.97
Mucinous carcinoma. **Confluent growth of complex interconnecting papillae**

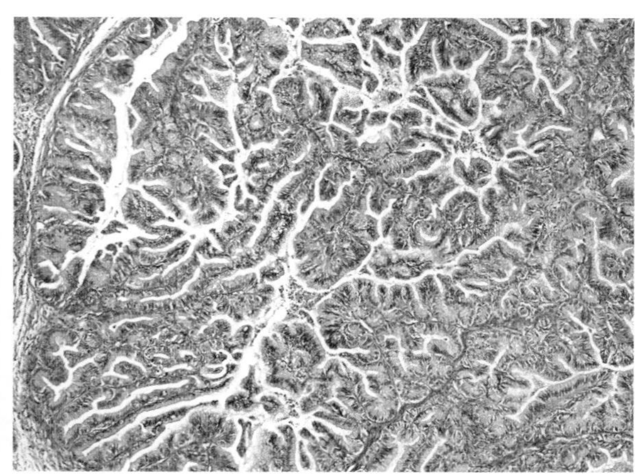

◘ Fig. 14.96
Mucinous carcinoma. **A confluent or "expansile" pattern of invasion**

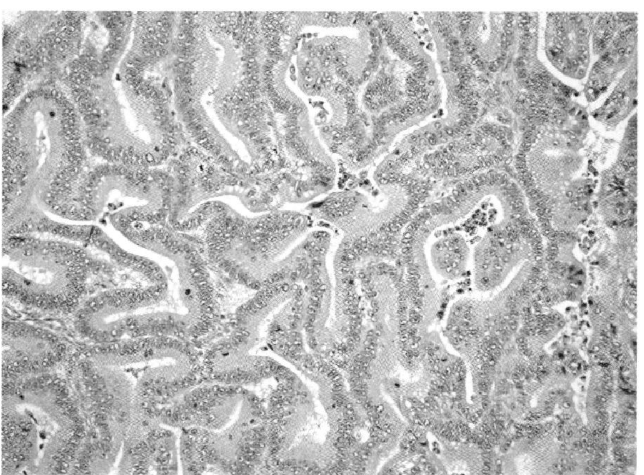

◘ Fig. 14.98
Mucinous carcinoma. **A confluent glandular pattern with complex interconnecting neoplastic glands**

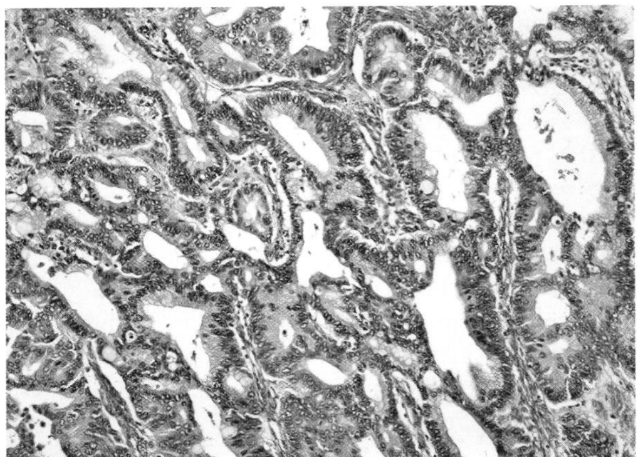

Fig. 14.99
Mucinous carcinoma. **Glands of varying shape and size with complex interconnections and marked cytologic atypia**

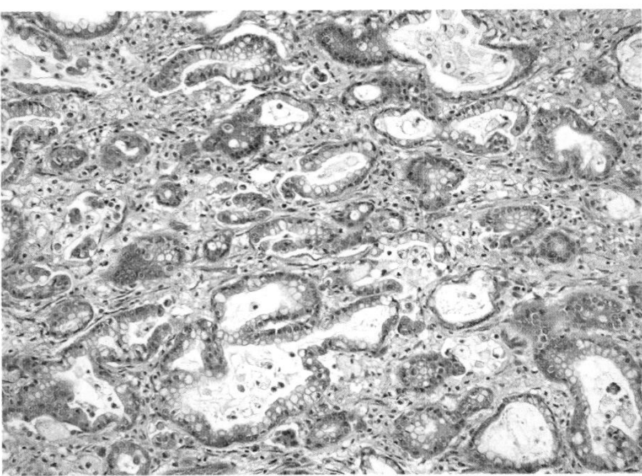

Fig. 14.101
Mucinous carcinoma. **Haphazard infiltrative pattern of small glands with marked cytologic atypia. Muciphages are present in the stroma**

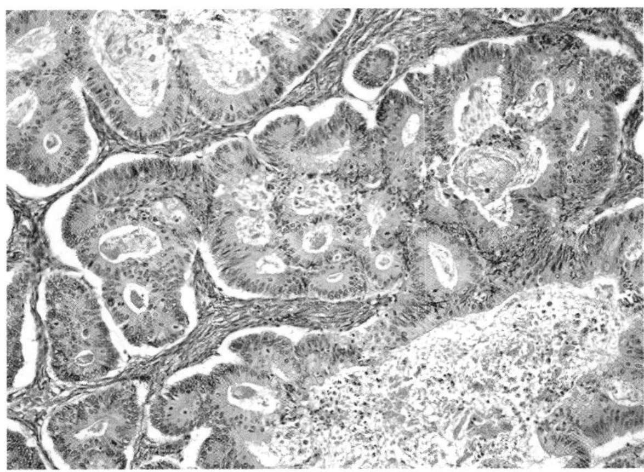

Fig. 14.100
Mucinous carcinoma. **Cribriform pattern. Necrotic debris is present in gland lumens**

of invasion, and the presence of an infiltrative pattern of stromal invasion should raise concern for metastatic mucinous carcinoma (see Differential Diagnosis below). The confluent glandular pattern reflects invasive mucinous carcinoma. High nuclear grade is significantly more common with the infiltrative pattern [342]. For tumors composed predominantly of APMT, the foci of confluent growth should measure more than the upper size limit allowed for microinvasion (5 mm) to qualify for the diagnosis of invasive carcinoma.

The grading of mucinous carcinoma has not been well-studied. Primary ovarian mucinous carcinomas are nearly always predominantly glandular and papillary and therefore architecturally low grade. The nuclear grade is therefore the best discriminator and we prefer the binary system described earlier (see High-Grade Serous Carcinoma; Microscopic Findings; Grade, earlier in this chapter).

Mucinous carcinomas of the seromucinous (müllerian or endocervical-like) type are quite uncommon. They are clinically and grossly similar to the atypical proliferative tumors of this type. Microscopically, they also resemble APSMT but exhibit destructive stromal invasion or sufficient complex papillary or confluent glandular growth to be classified as carcinoma [177, 316].

Immunohistochemistry

Ovarian mucinous tumors, including APMTs of gastrointestinal type and mucinous carcinomas, are characterized by generally diffuse expression of cytokeratin 7 (CK7) and variable expression of CK20, with the majority being positive for CK20 but virtually always with less-diffuse staining compared with CK7 expression [362]. They can express CDX2 (nuclear staining); exhibit generally patchy expression of p16; and are negative for ER, PR, and CA125 [363–365]. Mucinous tumors arising in association with mature cystic teratomas, some of which have architectural features of APMTs, are more heterogeneous in their CK7 and CK20 coordinate expression profiles [211, 366]. A subset with morphologic features of lower intestinal tract tumors, often accompanied by pseudomyxoma ovarii, is strongly associated with the CK7−/CK20+ immunoprofile [211]. The morphology and this profile can suggest a metastatic mucinous tumor of lower intestinal tract origin. APSMTs are CK7+/CK20− and express ER and PR [361].

Differential Diagnosis

It is critical when evaluating a mucinous carcinoma involving the ovary to consider the possibility of an extraovarian primary. Metastatic mucinous carcinomas are usually readily recognized as such when the ovarian tumors exhibit at least two of the following features: bilaterality, small size (typically less than 10–12 cm), ovarian surface involvement, a nodular pattern of ovarian involvement, and a haphazard infiltrative pattern of stromal invasion (➲ *Table 14.19*) [272, 306, 391]. Immunohistochemistry can be of great value in this distinction. (see ➲ Immunohistochemistry above, and ➲ Metastatic Mucinous Carcinoma" below.)

An algorithm has been proposed to assist in the distinction of primary versus metastatic mucinous carcinoma, particularly at the time of intraoperative evaluation when only limited histologic material can be examined. As originally proposed, bilateral mucinous carcinomas and unilateral ones smaller than 10 cm are metastatic, and unilateral ones larger than 10 cm are primary [306]. This algorithm correctly classified 90% of mucinous carcinomas. Subsequent studies have confirmed and refined the algorithm, also with close to 90% accuracy, and suggest that 13 cm is a better cutoff than 10 cm [391].

Molecular Biology

The molecular changes in ovarian mucinous tumors have not been as extensively studied as in serous and endometrioid tumors. This is probably due to the relative rarity of primary mucinous carcinomas, now that metastatic mucinous adenocarcinomas to the ovary are being more rigorously excluded. As a consequence, most studies in the published literature have analyzed only limited numbers of mucinous carcinomas, and therefore the true prevalence of many specific molecular alterations in these tumor types is unknown.

In primary ovarian mucinous carcinomas, *KRAS* mutation is a very common molecular alteration – occurring in upward of 75% of ovarian mucinous carcinomas [85, 102, 133]. Mucinous adenocarcinomas often contain areas indistinguishable from mucinous cystadenoma and mucinous borderline tumor and progression from benign to borderline and from borderline to malignant neoplasia has been proposed. Interestingly, identical *KRAS* mutations have been detected in mucinous carcinomas and adjacent mucinous cystadenoma and borderline tumor [67], a molecular finding supporting this morphological continuum of tumor progression in ovarian mucinous neoplasia, and in turn, their classification as Type I tumors in the dualistic model of ovarian cancer pathogenesis (see ➲ Morphologic and Molecular Pathogenesis earlier in this chapter).

Genome-wide analyses of DNA copy number changes in primary ovarian mucinous carcinomas have not yet been reported. Not unexpectedly, the pattern of gene

Table 14.19

Distinction of primary and metastatic mucinous carcinomas in the ovary

Feature	Primary ovarian mucinous tumors[a]	Metastatic mucinous tumors
Laterality	Unilateral (>>95%)[a]	Commonly bilateral (~65% overall; varies by site of origin)
Size	Large (mean/median = 22/21 cm)[a]	Typically smaller (mean/median = 13/12 cm; values vary by site of origin, from 2–18 cm)
Gross features	Multicystic (+/− solid foci), smooth capsule	Often nodular with surface involvement but can be multicystic with smooth capsule
Location of tumor	Within stroma	Surface, superficial cortex, stroma
Microscopic features	Well-differentiated mucinous epithelium forming organized cysts with peripheral crypts in atypical proliferative (borderline) tumors; well-differentiated mucinous epithelium most commonly with confluent glandular/cribriform pattern but occasionally infiltrative pattern in carcinomas	Typically infiltrative pattern of mucinous glands, often with nodules throughout or in superficial cortex; can have confluent glandular and borderline-like patterns without desmoplasia; nuclear atypia is often greater than expected relative to the low grade architecture
Extraovarian disease	Usually absent (stage I)	Often present (peritoneum, omentum)

[a]Atypical proliferative tumors and carcinomas.
[b]Data derived from [391].

expression of mucinous carcinomas is largely distinguishable from serous, endometrioid, and clear cell carcinomas based on comprehensive gene expression profiling [120, 296]. Using high-density oligonucleotide microarrays, Heinzelmann-Schwarz and colleagues identified a characteristic gene expression profile associated with mucinous ovarian tumors [120]. Ovarian mucinous tumors express several mucin genes (*MUC2*, *MUC3*, and *MUC17*) that are characteristic of mucinous carcinomas irrespective of their tissue origins. Because primary ovarian mucinous tumors often display intestinal-type differentiation, it is not surprising that additional genes with preferential expression in ovarian mucinous tumors encode markers of intestinal differentiation such as the caudal-type homeobox transcription factors *CDX1* and *CDX2*, and *LGALS4* (galectin 40), which encodes an intestinal cell surface adhesion molecule that is overexpressed in intestinal carcinomas. Immunohistochemical analysis of LGALS4 expression in a spectrum of ovarian mucinous neoplasms showed that LGALS4 is not detectable in normal ovarian surface epithelium, but is expressed at high levels in mucinous cystadenomas, borderline tumors, and carcinomas, indicating that increased LGALS4 expression occurs early during mucinous ovarian tumor progression [120].

Behavior and Treatment

Patients with stage I mucinous carcinomas displaying a confluent or expansile type of invasion have a survival of about 90%; despite a few exceptions, adverse prognosis is more commonly associated with the infiltrative rather than the confluent glandular pattern of invasion [52, 179, 272, 274]. For patients with APMT with microinvasion and/or intraepithelial carcinoma, a staging procedure is unlikely to yield positive findings, but no data are available to address the value of staging.

As with the other cell types of ovarian carcinomas, platinum–paclitaxel is standard treatment for mucinous carcinoma. However, because of classification problems discussed earlier, published data on the value of this regimen for those with true primary ovarian mucinous carcinoma are of uncertain validity.

Metastatic Mucinous Carcinomas

Metastatic mucinous carcinomas are typically bilateral, small (typically less than 10–12 cm), display ovarian surface and superficial cortical involvement, a nodular pattern of ovarian involvement, and a haphazard infiltrative pattern of stromal invasion (➋ *Table 14.19*) [272, 306, 391]. However, some metastatic mucinous carcinomas, especially those derived from the colorectum, pancreaticobiliary tract, appendix, and endocervix, can exhibit gross and microscopic features simulating a primary ovarian mucinous tumor. In particular, metastases can be large, unilateral (thus misclassified by the algorithm discussed earlier), and multicystic, and can display deceptive patterns of ovarian involvement. If these patterns are not recognized, these metastatic mucinous carcinomas can be misinterpreted as primary ovarian APMT with intraepithelial carcinoma or well-differentiated mucinous carcinoma [84, 391]. Not infrequently, some of these metastases display highly differentiated areas adjacent to carcinomatous areas, simulating benign and APMT precursor lesions. Recognizing such tumors as metastases is especially problematic when the ovarian tumor is the initial manifestation of disease and an extraovarian primary mucinous carcinoma is occult. When mucinous carcinomas in the ovaries are rigorously classified based on refined criteria and awareness of the deceptive patterns, metastatic mucinous carcinomas are much more commonly encountered than primary ovarian mucinous carcinomas, even if the obviously metastatic signet ring cell carcinomas are excluded [306, 391]. In general, the presence of a mucinous carcinoma in the ovary, particularly if extraovarian disease is present, should always prompt the pathologist to consider the possibility of metastatic mucinous carcinoma. Immunohistochemical analysis can be useful for identifying some metastatic mucinous carcinomas, especially those lacking characteristic features of metastases, which simulate primary ovarian mucinous tumors; however the utility of currently available markers is limited due to overlapping immunoprofiles of primary tumors and certain subsets of metastases (see ➋ Immunohistochemistry above) [139, 362–365]. Clinical evaluation is usually required to exclude metastatic mucinous carcinoma in the ovary derived from a clinically occult extraovarian source.

Endometrioid Tumors

The vast majority of endometrioid ovarian neoplasms are carcinomas. Endometrioid adenofibromas and atypical proliferative endometrioid tumors are uncommon (➋ *Table 14.5*). Molecular biological studies have shown that endometrioid ovarian carcinomas have similarities with, and differences from, their uterine counterparts. For example, mutations of *PTEN*, *PIK3CA*, and *CTNNB1* (β-catenin) are observed in subsets of both uterine and ovarian endometrioid adenocarcinomas, although the relative frequency of these alterations in carcinomas from the two sites are not identical. Comprehensive gene expression studies have shown differences in gene expression profile when comparing uterine and ovarian endometrioid adenocarcinomas [318, 398].

Ovarian endometriosis (including endometriomas and endometriotic cysts) is far more common than benign endometrioid neoplasms. Since the majority of ovarian endometriotic cysts are monoclonal and have a variety of molecular alterations, they are neoplastic [159, 374]. If endometriotic cysts were classified as benign endometrioid neoplasms, the relative proportions of ovarian epithelial tumors seen in *Table 14.5* would be significantly altered. As noted earlier, endometriosis would qualify as the most common ovarian neoplasm, and endometrioid carcinomas would be much less common than benign endometrioid neoplasms.

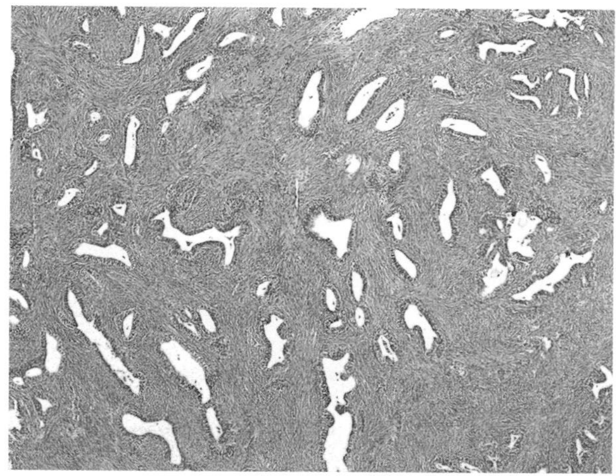

Fig. 14.102
Endometrioid adenofibroma. **Endometrioid-type glands are scattered in a densely fibrotic stroma**

Endometrioid Adenofibromas

Endometrioid adenofibromas are uncommon, comprise 1% of ovarian epithelial neoplasms, and 83% are unilateral. The median age is 57 years. The mean diameter is about 10 cm. The external surface is smooth and the cut surface is densely fibrous, often with intermixed cystic areas creating a honeycomb appearance. The cysts contain clear or yellowish fluid. Microscopically, the dominant pattern is that of an adenofibroma or cystadenofibroma. The epithelial elements are arranged in branching tubular glands and cysts, and usually resemble those of proliferative or mildly hyperplastic endometrium (*Figs. 14.102* and *14.103*). The epithelium lining the glands is tall and columnar with oval nuclei containing coarse chromatin and small nucleoli; the cytoplasm is basophilic to amphophilic. The epithelium is often ciliated and resembles tubal epithelium. Sometimes the nuclei resemble those of atrophic or inactive endometrium, with uniform, elongated dark nuclei and scanty cytoplasm. Mitoses are variable but usually rare. Secretory changes and focal squamous differentiation may be present. The stroma is usually densely fibrotic; focal areas often resemble ovarian cortical stroma. Endometrioid adenofibromas are frequently associated with endometriosis. The distinction of endometrioid adenofibroma from serous adenofibroma may be arbitrary at times, as both may have ciliated epithelium. Tubular glands and lack of the multiple cysts and fibrous papillae of serous adenofibroma favor endometrioid differentiation. These tumors are benign, although rarely they may recur.

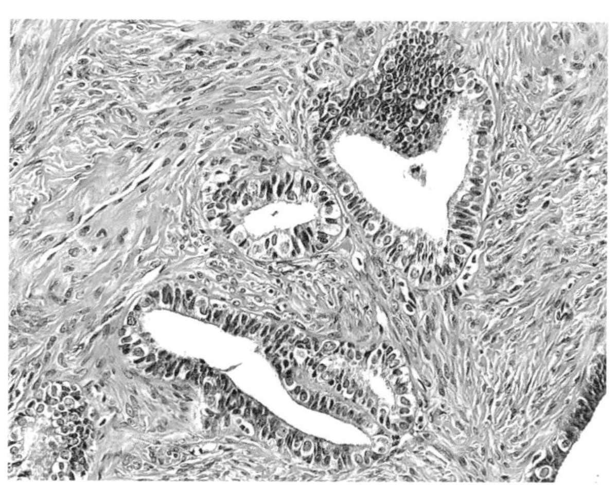

Fig. 14.103
Endometrioid adenofibroma. **The glandular epithelium resembles tubal epithelium in a fibrotic ovarian stroma**

Atypical Proliferative Endometrioid Tumors (APET)

There is a spectrum of epithelial proliferation, glandular crowding, and cytologic atypia in benign endometrioid neoplasms ranging from mild atypia, mild glandular crowding, and epithelial stratification slightly beyond what is seen in endometrioid adenofibromas to confluent epithelial proliferation lacking stromal support in areas up to 5 mm in diameter resembling atypical hyperplasia and well-differentiated adenocarcinoma of the endometrium. A variety of terms have been employed for these tumors, including proliferating or proliferative endometrioid tumor, atypical endometrioid adenofibroma, endometrioid tumor of low malignant potential, endometrioid borderline tumor, and atypical proliferative endometrioid tumor. APET with microinvasion (<5 mm), which is very rare, constitutes the upper end of this spectrum after which a diagnosis of low-grade endometrioid carcinoma is used. The criteria for these diagnoses have differed among several series. Since the behavior of all of the tumors up to and including those with microinvasion has been benign, we prefer to combine these groups and refer to them as "APET." The lower end of the spectrum characterized by slightly crowded glands lacking cytologic atypia is best classified as endometrioid adenofibroma.

APET comprise only 0.2% of ovarian epithelial neoplasms. Among five series [182, 282, 308], there were 134 patients with a mean age of about 51 years. Six patients (4%) had bilateral tumors, and all but two were confined to the ovaries; one had a colonic "implant" and one was stage IIC [282]. The mean tumor size was about 9 cm. The characteristic gross appearance is cystic in two thirds and solid and cystic in the rest; the cyst fluid is usually hemorrhagic, and brown or green. Many patients have had endometriosis and some have also had endometrial hyperplasia. In a recent series of 30 cases, 63% had endometriosis and 39% of those whose endometrium was examined had endometrial hyperplasia or carcinoma [282].

The two characteristic microscopic architectural appearances of APET are adenofibromatous and glandular/papillary. The glandular/papillary proliferation can show varying degrees of glandular complexity and crowding (➲ *Figs. 14.104–14.107*). An underlying adenofibroma is present in about half the cases [282]. When the glandular proliferation becomes confluent, this is considered evidence of invasion and is classified as microinvasion if the confluent area is less than 5 mm. Some investigators prefer to classify these as APET with intraepithelial carcinoma. A confluent epithelial proliferation or unequivocal invasion that exceeds 5 mm in diameter warrants a diagnosis of carcinoma. The glands show crowding, mild or moderate cytologic atypia, and epithelial stratification (➲ *Fig. 14.104–14.107*); tufting and bridging may be present. Severe cytologic atypia warrants a diagnosis of intraepithelial carcinoma, but this is rare. One third display a cribriform pattern [282]. Squamous metaplasia is present in nearly half of cases (➲ *Figs. 14.104–14.106*). The stroma may be cellular or fibrotic, and occasionally displays periglandular cuffing characterized by increased stromal cellularity around the glandular elements; however these areas lack the stromal mitoses and atypia of adenosarcoma. Necrosis is common and is often confined to gland lumens or cysts (➲ *Fig. 14.104*). The two reported cases with apparent extraovarian disease may represent independent lesions arising in endometriosis [282]. Among 134 reported APETs, all of those with clinical follow-up have had a benign behavior after a mean follow-up period of

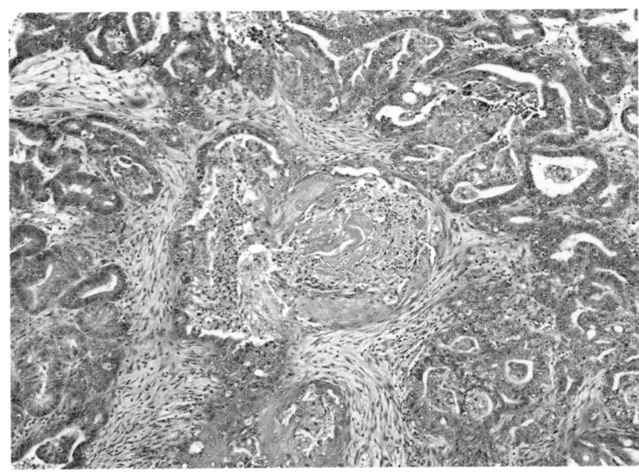

Fig. 14.104
Atypical proliferative (borderline) endometrioid tumor (APET). **Squamous differentiation is present. A stromal reaction is noted. The glands in the center contain necrotic debris**

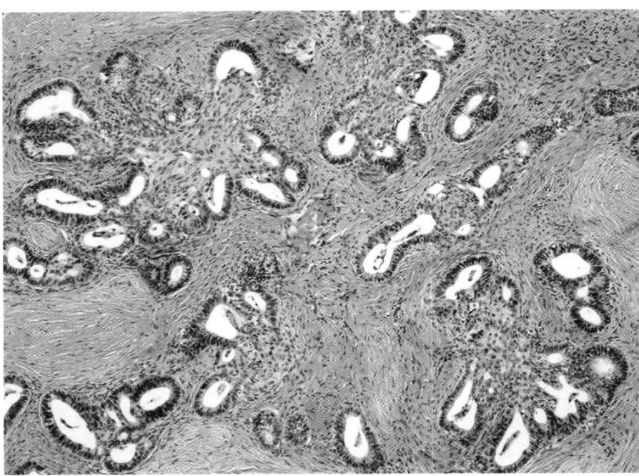

Fig. 14.105
Atypical proliferative (borderline) endometrioid tumor. **Clusters of endometrioid glands with squamous (morular) metaplasia**

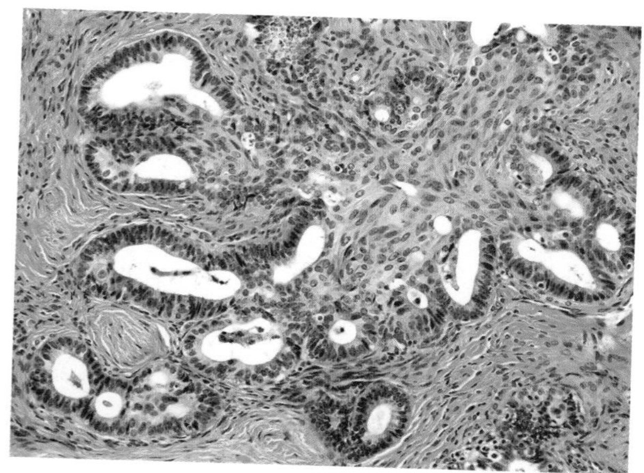

Fig. 14.106
Atypical proliferative (borderline) endometrioid tumor. **Mild cytologic atypia is present in both the endometrioid glands and the squamous morules**

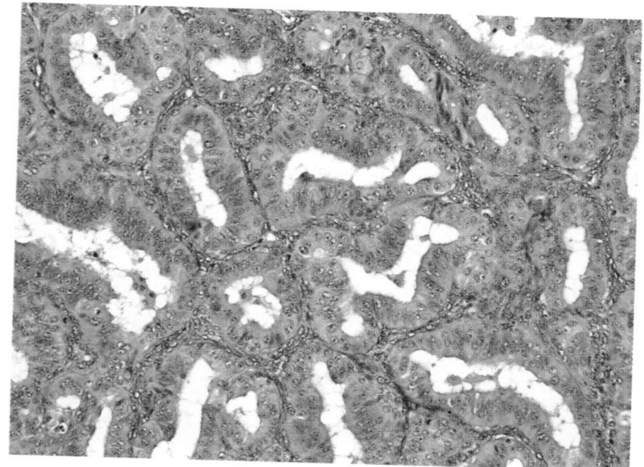

Fig. 14.107
Atypical proliferative (borderline) endometrioid tumor. **Moderate cytologic atypia in markedly crowded glands is seen**

approximately 5 years. Rarely, an endometriotic cyst is lined by markedly atypical epithelial cells that have cytologic features of malignancy (see Chap. 13, Diseases of the Peritoneum). If the lesion is well sampled and invasion is not found, a designation of APET with intraepithelial carcinoma should be used.

Criteria for microinvasion in APETs differ among investigators. In two series, microinvasion was characterized by a haphazard infiltrative pattern of single cells, glands, and nests with cytologically malignant features. Among the five APETs with microinvasion reported in these series, all patients were alive and well after a mean of 5.3 years. Different criteria employed by another group required one or more foci of confluent (expansile) glandular growth, each measuring less than 5 mm, for a designation of APET with microinvasion. The five cases in that series had limited follow-up; all were alive but only two were known to be free of disease at 2 years of follow-up. Others have used a combination of these criteria [282]. In summary, microinvasion (12 cases), intraepithelial carcinoma (7 cases), and confluence of glandular growth when limited in extent, are atypical morphologic features and appear to be biologically benign, but only a few cases have been reported and clinical follow-up data are limited.

The immunohistochemical features of this tumor are similar to those of endometrioid carcinoma (see below). EMA and many cytokeratins are positive. P16 can be positive in up to half of cases, but staining is usually focal [364].

Endometrioid Adenocarcinoma

In the older literature, about 15–20% of reported ovarian carcinomas are endometrioid, up to 25% in some reports [338], but when strict criteria are applied, the figure is lower and probably in the range of 10–15%. When very strict criteria are used, requiring a readily recognized resemblance to uterine endometrioid carcinoma and relegating nonspecific high-grade adenocarcinomas to the serous group, the figure is about 7.5% (*Table 14.4*; see Differential Diagnosis below).

Clinical Findings

These tumors are most common in the fifth and sixth decades, and the mean patient age is 55–58 years, slightly but significantly lower than that for serous carcinoma [338]. The most common symptoms are abdominal distention and pelvic or abdominal pain. Abnormal vaginal bleeding is also frequent. This is, in part, related to the association of endometrioid ovarian carcinoma with endometrial hyperplasia and carcinoma (see below). Most patients have an adnexal mass on pelvic examination.

Operative Findings

Tumor size ranges from 12 to 20 cm, with a mean of about 15 cm. The stage distribution differs significantly from serous carcinoma. A high proportion of endometrioid carcinomas are diagnosed in stage I: 43% in a review of 874 cases from 19 series, and 50% at the Washington Hospital Center (*Table 14.4*). In the FIGO database, 52% of patients are diagnosed in stage I or II. About 13% of early stage (FIGO I–II) cases are bilateral. Endometriosis, which may be extraovarian, in the ipsilateral or contralateral ovary or within the tumor itself, is found in at least 15–20% of patients.

Gross Findings

Endometrioid carcinomas have a smooth outer surface. On cut section, they are solid and cystic, with the cysts containing friable soft masses and bloody fluid. Cysts occasionally contain mucus or greenish fluid. Less commonly, the tumor is solid with extensive hemorrhage and necrosis. Tumors arising in endometriosis may display gross findings of an endometriotic cyst containing chocolate-colored fluid, with one or more solid nodules or papillary excrescences protruding from the wall and containing carcinoma.

Microscopic Findings

Destructive infiltrative growth characterizes one pattern of endometrioid carcinoma. This pattern is characterized by angulated glands with an infiltrative pattern, jagged irregularly spaced and unevenly shaped nests, often with an edematous or inflammatory stromal reaction, solid sheets with jagged edges, and single cell infiltration [52]. More commonly, a confluent glandular epithelial proliferation exceeding 5 mm (the limit for microinvasion) is present; this has also been termed "expansile invasion." This pattern typically excludes intervening stroma and is characterized by extensive glandular branching, budding, true cribriform architecture, and highly complex papillary proliferations (➲ *Figs. 14.108* and ➲ *14.109*). Confluent or expansile invasion is the predominant pattern in most endometrioid carcinomas [52] (➲ *Figs. 14.109–14.111*).

Architecturally well-differentiated endometrioid adenocarcinoma accounts for the majority of cases and is characterized by a confluent or cribriform proliferation of glands lined by tall, stratified columnar epithelium with sharp luminal margins (➲ *Figs. 14.109–14.111*). A villoglandular growth pattern also occurs. Despite the low-grade architecture, high-grade nuclear features, at least focally, can be observed [313]. Mitotic figures are commonly seen. Squamous differentiation is present in up to 50% of cases. Degeneration of squamous cells may induce a foreign body-type giant cell reaction in the stroma. Focal secretory changes are seen in up to a third of cases. In the majority of cases, a component of endometriosis, endometrioid adenofibroma, or APET can be identified and often occupies a significant proportion of the tumor volume [52, 389]. This corresponds to the Type I pathway of tumorigenesis in which a noninvasive precursor is identified (see ➲ Morphologic and Molecular Pathogenesis earlier in this chapter).

Luteinized stromal cells are seen in 12% of cases. Moderately and poorly differentiated endometrioid carcinomas show solid growth, complex glandular and microglandular patterns with marked nuclear pleomorphism, and mitotic activity (➲ *Figs. 14.110* and ➲ *14.111*); however the majority of high-grade carcinomas with these features are usually classified as serous (see ➲ Differential Diagnosis below). It has been suggested that solid areas in some endometrioid adenocarcinomas may reflect an undifferentiated component [325].

At present, clinicopathologic and molecular data indicate that it is important to be strict about classifying

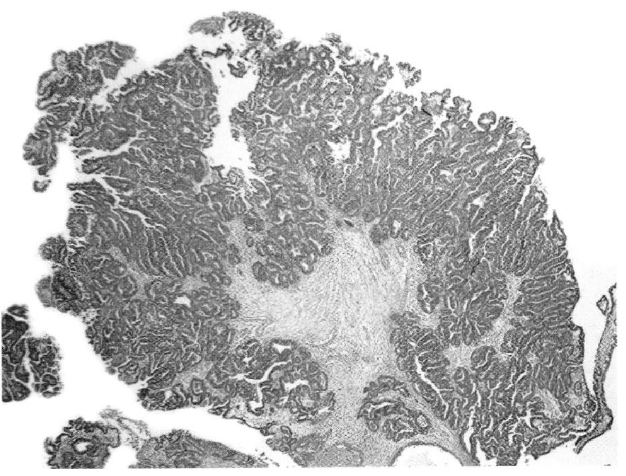

◘ Fig. 14.108
Well-differentiated endometrioid carcinoma arising in an atypical proliferative endometrioid tumor. **The confluent glandular/papillary proliferation reflects invasion in the absence of destructive infiltrative growth**

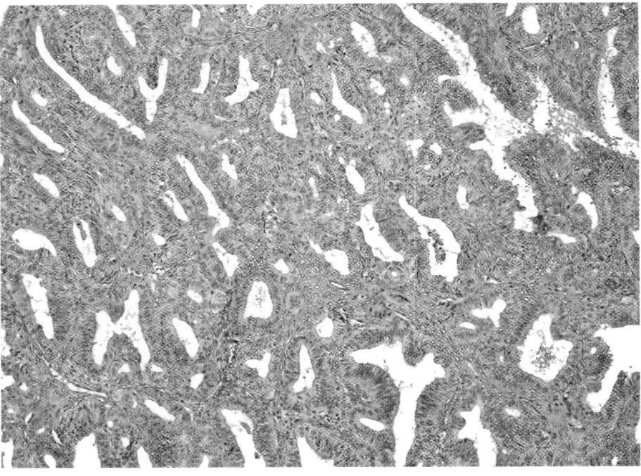

◘ Fig. 14.109
Well-differentiated endometrioid carcinoma. **Most of the glands are back-to-back, but confluent foci are present. The proliferation resembles endometrioid carcinoma of the uterine corpus**

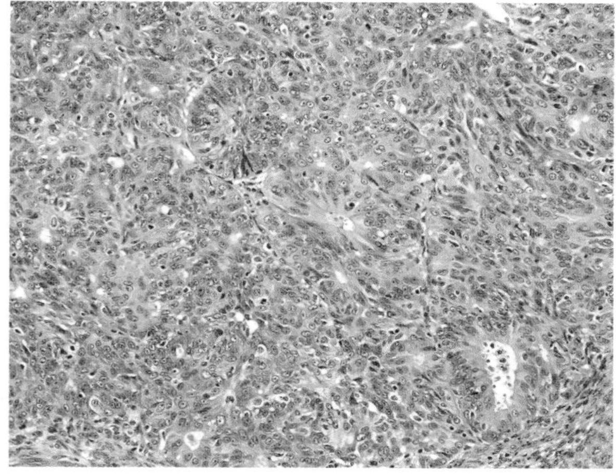

Fig. 14.110
Poorly differentiated endometrioid carcinoma. **The tumor displays almost entirely solid growth in this field**

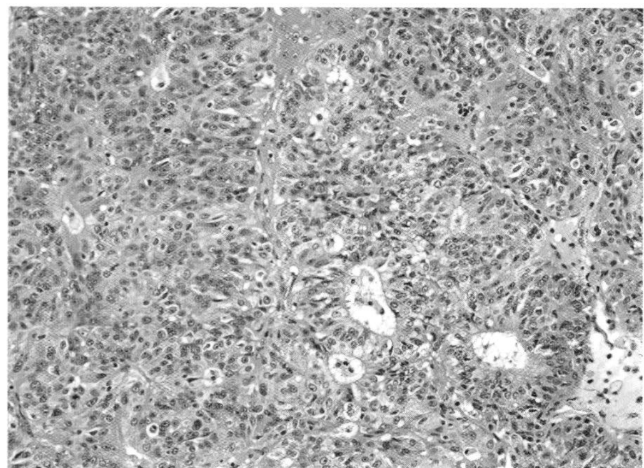

Fig. 14.111
Moderately differentiated endometrioid carcinoma. **Solid and glandular areas are present**

an adenocarcinoma as endometrioid type. Most predominantly glandular, non-clear cell, non-mucinous high-grade ovarian carcinomas should be classified as serous carcinoma [154]. Glandular, cribriform, and solid patterns are common in serous carcinoma (see Serous Tumors above). A bona fide endometrioid adenocarcinoma should resemble eutopic endometrial carcinomas (*Table 14.15*) [207]. When strict criteria are applied, only 7.5% of ovarian carcinomas are of endometrioid type (*Table 14.4*) and virtually all of these are well differentiated. Most tumors classified as poorly differentiated are more likely variants of high-grade serous carcinoma showing foci of gland formation. A diagnosis of mixed serous–endometrioid carcinoma can be made on occasion; we classified only 1.5% of ovarian carcinomas as mixed serous–endometrioid type.

There is no standard grading system for endometrioid carcinoma, although the WHO system for grading endometrial adenocarcinoma is often used (see Chap. 9, Endometrial Carcinoma). When strict criteria are used to separate high grade endometrioid carcinoma from high grade serous carcinoma (see above), most endometrioid carcinomas are architecturally well-differentiated as they are predominantly glandular or glandular and papillary. The nuclear grade is therefore the best discriminator and we prefer the binary system described earlier (see High-Grade Serous Carcinoma; Microscopic Findings; Grade earlier in this chapter). It is important to note that neither the WHO 3-grade system nor the binary system has been adequately tested for endometrioid carcinomas.

In addition to pure endometrioid carcinoma, which is the most common, several of the variants of endometrioid carcinoma of the uterine corpus also occur in the ovary. These include endometrioid carcinoma with squamous differentiation, and secretory and ciliated variants. Other variant microscopic patterns of endometrioid ovarian carcinoma have been described. One variant has been designated "sertoliform endometrioid carcinoma," or "endometrioid carcinoma resembling sex cord-stromal tumor." These tumors are characterized by a predominant pattern resembling a sex cord–stromal tumor, usually Sertoli–Leydig cell tumor (SLCT), characterized by small tubular glands lined by cuboidal or low columnar epithelium with a paired cell arrangement resembling well-differentiated Sertoli cell tumor. Anastomosing solid tubules are often present (*Figs. 14.112* and *14.113*). Moderately cellular fibrous stroma resembling the spindle cell component of stromal tumors may also be present. In a few cases, large islands of cells with round nuclei and scanty cytoplasm may mimic a granulosa cell tumor, but nuclear grooves are generally absent. In nearly all of these cases, foci of typical endometrioid carcinoma can be identified. Among 30 patients in three series, 87% were FIGO stage I.

Endometrioid carcinomas occasionally contain a prominent spindle cell component that usually reflects a spindled squamous component. These should not be classified as carcinosarcomas unless the stroma displays unequivocally sarcomatous features (see Sarcomas; Carcinosarcoma later in this chapter). Other very rare variants include those with an undifferentiated neuroendocrine component [368], adenoid cystic-like and basaloid types, oxyphilic endometrioid carcinoma, and a ciliated cell variant.

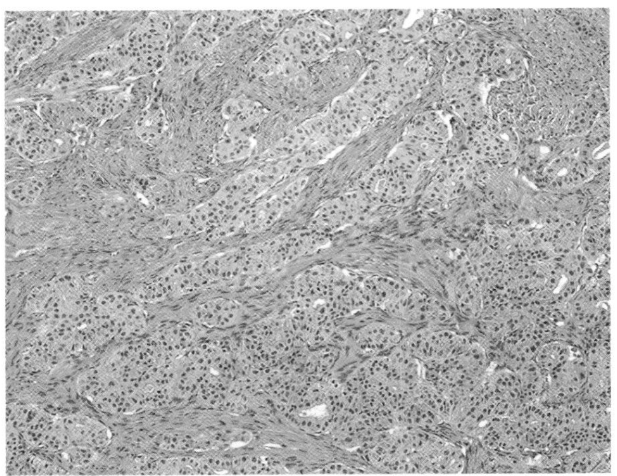

Fig. 14.112
Sertoliform endometrioid carcinoma. **Cords and tubules with a paired cell arrangement resemble a Sertoli cell tumor or a well-differentiated Sertoli–Leydig cell tumor (SLCT)**

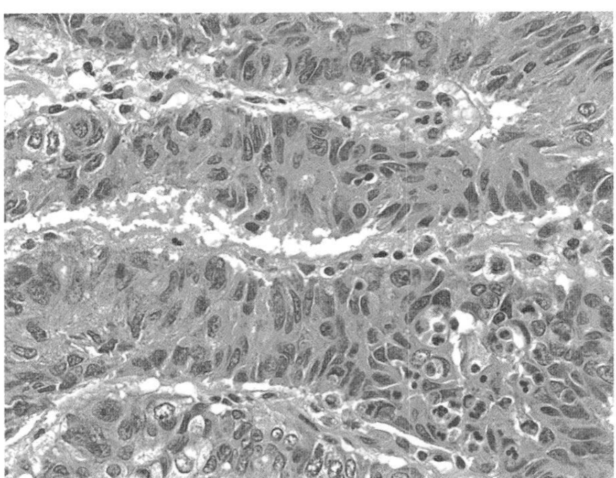

Fig. 14.113
Sertoliform endometrioid carcinoma. **The degree of cytologic atypia is high**

Peritoneal keratin granulomas may be found in women with endometrioid ovarian carcinomas, presumably as a result of rupture of the neoplasm or exfoliation of squamous cells. The keratin within the metaplastic squamous component of these tumors incites a foreign-body-type granulomatous reaction. Follow-up of a limited number of these patients reveals that these lesions have no prognostic significance and therefore should not be considered evidence of advanced-stage disease. Endometrioid carcinoma after chemotherapy can show extensive keratin granulomas due to necrosis of the squamous component, and therefore peritoneal keratin granulomas after chemotherapy probably reflect devitalized tumor.

Immunohistochemistry

Endometrioid carcinomas stain strongly with epithelial markers including cytoplasmic staining for keratins (CK7, 97%; CK20, 13% positive) and membranous staining for EMA. The frequency of positivity for other markers is as follows: vimentin, 31%; B72.3, 86%; CEA, 30%; and OC-125, 76%. The immunohistochemical profiles of typical endometrioid carcinoma and sertoliform endometrioid carcinoma appear to be identical. ER and PR are positive in the majority of cases [178]. WT1 and p16 are usually negative [1, 124, 205, 206, 237] but WT1 can be positive in 17–29% [47, 395, 396] and p16 can be positive in up to half but is usually focal [364]. Brca1 protein is usually positive (nuclear staining) [352]. Inhibin is rarely positive. Calretinin is strongly positive in 10%, and weakly positive in an additional 10–25% [47, 194]. TTF1 is usually negative [162]. CD99 is often positive. *PTEN* expression is negative in well-differentiated carcinomas; however *PTEN* immunostaining is not that reliable [109]. Loss of staining for hMLH1and hMSH2 proteins occurs in the majority of tumors with the microsatellite instability–high phenotype, which represent approximately 20% of ovarian endometrioid adenocarcinomas [186].

Differential Diagnosis

The sertoliform or sex cord-like variant of endometrioid carcinoma creates the most problems in the differential diagnosis. The age of the patient is helpful since the mean age of patients with SLCTs is 25 years, while women with endometrioid carcinoma are usually peri- or postmenopausal. In addition, hormonal manifestations such as virilization can be associated with sex cord–stromal tumors and generally not with endometrioid carcinomas. The retiform variant of SLCT, which occurs in adolescents, can rarely simulate endometrioid or serous carcinoma, but this pattern is usually only focal. In most cases of sertoliform endometrioid carcinoma, extensive sampling of the tumor will disclose areas of typical endometrioid carcinoma. Other helpful features include squamous metaplasia, which does not occur in sex cord–stromal tumors, an adenofibromatous component that is typical of endometrioid carcinoma, endometriosis, and prominent luminal mucin, which occur in endometrioid carcinomas.

Although sex cord–stromal tumors often stain with keratins, they are almost always negative for EMA. In addition, inhibin is a very useful marker that is positive in the vast majority of granulosa and SLCTs, and nearly always negative in ovarian epithelial tumors, although inhibin is nearly always positive in the non-neoplastic stromal cells within the tumor. Similarly, calretinin is nearly always positive in stromal tumors, but can stain endometrioid carcinomas, focally in 18–33% and strongly in up to 10% [364, 396]. Other epithelial markers including neuron-specific enolase, OM-1, and B72.3 are negative in granulosa and most SLCTs, and positive in the majority of endometrioid carcinomas. Positivity for CK7 and EMA together can help exclude yolk sac tumor (YST), which is negative for both; this may be a consideration when there is a clear cell component or to rule out the rare endometrioid variant of YST [267]. Occasionally, a prominent spindle cell component in an endometrioid carcinoma will create an appearance resembling a sex cord–stromal tumor, an adnexal tumor of wolffian origin, or a carcinosarcoma. The spindle cells are generally uniform and have nuclear features resembling the glandular component. In most cases, the spindle cells merge imperceptibly with the glands. The spindle cells in the spindle cell variant of endometrioid carcinoma are strongly positive for keratins and EMA.

Another common problem in the differential diagnosis of endometrioid carcinoma is metastatic adenocarcinoma, particularly from colonic carcinoma. Colonic metastases to the ovaries are often cystic and grossly mimic primary ovarian neoplasms. Useful features in the distinction are a characteristic "garland" pattern characterized by cysts lined by cytologically malignant tall columnar cells in which the epithelium displaying a cribriform pattern surrounds large areas of dirty necrosis. In addition, metastatic tumors are typically bilateral and display surface involvement. Although garlands and dirty necrosis are characteristic features of metastatic colonic carcinoma, they can also be seen in primary ovarian carcinomas, though usually only focally. The CK7/CK20 panel is of value in the distinction of primary ovarian versus metastatic colonic carcinoma, as ovarian endometrioid carcinoma is typically diffusely and strongly CK7 positive and CK20 negative, while most colon carcinomas are CK7 negative and are nearly always strongly and diffusely CK20 positive (see ➋ Metastatic Mucinous Carcinoma earlier in this chapter, and ➋ Chap. 18, Metastatic Tumors of the Ovary).

Molecular Biology

The association of ovarian endometrioid carcinoma with endometriosis is well established. The identification of genetic alterations in endometriotic lesions and the observation of a morphological transition from endometriosis to carcinoma in over one third of cases have led many to consider endometriosis a likely precursor of endometrioid carcinoma [285, 351]. Progression from endometriosis to benign endometrioid neoplasm to well-differentiated endometrioid carcinoma is analogous to that proposed for progression of low-grade serous carcinoma from serous borderline tumor. Hence, low-grade (well-differentiated) endometrioid carcinomas are classified as Type I tumors in the dualistic model of ovarian cancer pathogenesis. Classification of high-grade endometrioid carcinomas is less clear. Overlap of both morphological and molecular features between high-grade endometrioid and high-grade serous carcinomas has led some pathologists to default the vast majority of gland forming or near-solid cytologically high-grade ovarian carcinomas to the serous category, to the degree that "true" high-grade endometrioid carcinomas are considered by some to be very uncommon [207]. The molecular and morphological criteria for reliably distinguishing high-grade endometrioid from high-grade serous carcinomas have not yet been established, and for now, high-grade endometrioid carcinomas are classified as Type II tumors.

Mutational Analyses Well-differentiated ovarian endometrioid carcinomas share many molecular genetic features with their uterine counterparts. Indeed, mutations in several of the same tumor suppressor genes, oncogenes, and genes involved in DNA repair have been observed in both endometrial and ovarian endometrioid carcinomas. The molecular genetics of endometrial carcinomas have been recently reviewed by Di Cristofano and Ellenson [73].

The canonical Wnt (i.e., Wnt/β-catenin/Tcf, hereafter Wnt/β-cat) signaling pathway is involved in the regulation of several important cellular processes, including cell fate determination, proliferation, motility, and survival. In this pathway, β-catenin is a key effector that is stabilized as a consequence of selected Wnt ligands binding to their cell surface receptors. β-catenin-mediated signaling is deregulated in 16–38% of human ovarian endometrioid carcinomas, usually on the basis of activating mutations of *CTNNB1*, the gene that encodes β-catenin, and rarely because of inactivating mutations in genes encoding negative regulators of β-catenin such as *APC, AXIN1*, or *AXIN2* [383]. Notably, *CTNNB1* mutations are very uncommon in the other major types of ovarian carcinoma [98, 382]. Several studies have noted the association of *CTNNB1* mutation with squamous differentiation, low tumor grade, and favorable outcome [98, 383]. Inactivating mutations of the tumor suppressor gene *PTEN* have been reported in 14–21% of ovarian endometrioid carcinomas, and like *CTNNB1, PTEN* mutations are uncommon in the other major types of ovarian carcinomas [45, 238]. Inactivation of Pten, the lipid phosphatase that converts PIP3 to PIP2, is one mechanism by which activation of phosphotidylinositol 3-kinase (PI3K) signaling occurs in human tumors.

An alternative mechanism by which PI3K signaling is activated in endometrioid adenocarcinomas is through activating mutations of *PIK3CA*, which encodes the p110 catalytic subunit of PI3K. Most reported *PIK3CA* mutations are clustered in exons 9 and 20, and *PIK3CA* mutations in these exons have been identified in 20% of ovarian endometrioid and clear cell carcinomas but in only 2% of ovarian serous carcinomas [12, 40]. Oda and colleagues reported a high frequency of concomitant *PIK3CA* and *PTEN* mutations in uterine endometrioid adenocarcinomas, and functional studies suggested that mutation of both genes may have an additive effect on PI3K pathway activation [240]. *PIK3CA* and *PTEN* mutations also co-occur in a subset of ovarian endometrioid carcinomas. In both the ovary and the endometrium, *PIK3CA* mutations are associated with adverse prognostic indicators [46, 376]. In a recent mutational analysis of 72 primary ovarian endometrioid carcinomas, Wu and colleagues found that mutational defects in canonical Wnt signaling were significantly associated with mutations predicted to deregulate PI3K/Pten signaling [383]. Tumors with these mutations were typically low grade and low stage. Hence, defects in these two signaling pathways appear to be particularly characteristic of low-grade endometrioid adenocarcinoma, a finding with implications for future therapeutic strategies that include molecularly targeted agents. Activating mutations in *KRAS* and *BRAF* have been reported in ovarian endometrioid carcinomas, but the frequency of mutations in these genes is rather low at less than 7% [85, 203, 383]. *TP53* mutations are common in both uterine and ovarian endometrioid carcinomas. *TP53* mutations have been reported in upward of 60% of endometrioid carcinomas arising in the ovary overall, and in a greater percentage of high-grade tumors [157]. Wu and colleagues documented *TP53* mutations in approximately half of the aforementioned series of 72 endometrioid carcinomas, and mutations were significantly associated with high tumor grade, and were uncommon in tumors with documented Wnt/β-cat and/or PI3K/Pten signaling defects.

Akin to the serous carcinomas, the molecular findings support the division of ovarian endometrioid carcinomas into two subgroups. Low-grade tumors are characterized by mutations that deregulate the canonical Wnt/β-cat and PI3K/Pten signaling pathways and typically lack *TP53* mutations. High-grade tumors often harbor mutations of *TP53* and lack Wnt/β-cat or PI3K/Pten signaling pathway defects. Whether some of the high-grade tumors in this series would have been more appropriately considered high-grade serous carcinomas remains unresolved.

DNA Copy Number Changes Given their reduced abundance compared to the serous carcinomas, comprehensive studies of DNA copy number changes specifically in ovarian endometrioid carcinomas are rather few. Using conventional comparative genomic hybridization (CGH) methods, Tapper and colleagues identified gains of chromosome 1q in five of eight cases, but the genes presumably targeted by these gains were not identified [349]. These investigators also evaluated several serous and mucinous carcinomas and found divergence of DNA copy number changes between the three tumor types, providing additional molecular evidence for each type as a distinct disease entity. More recently, Mayr and associates used both conventional and array CGH to identify frequent gains at the *JUNB, KRAS2, MYCN, ESR*, and *CCND2* loci in six endometrioid carcinomas [204]. Clearly, comprehensive analysis of a larger number of cases is needed to help identify additional oncogenes and tumor suppressor genes that participate in the molecular pathogenesis of this group of ovarian cancers.

Gene Expression A number of investigators have used comprehensive high-throughput technologies to profile gene expression in ovarian cancers, including endometrioid carcinomas [200, 293, 296, 383, 398]. One of the more informative studies is that of Wu and colleagues, who used high-density oligonucleotide microarrays to analyze global gene expression in 41 serous, 37 endometrioid, 13 mucinous, and 8 clear cell ovarian carcinomas [383]. Notably, all of the endometrioid tumors were annotated with data on the mutational status of the *TP53, CTNNB1, PTEN, PIK3CA*, and *KRAS* genes. Although the gene expression profiles of both clear cell and mucinous carcinomas were found to be largely distinct from each other and from serous carcinomas, substantial overlap between the expression profiles of endometrioid and serous carcinomas was identified. When the mutational status of the above genes was taken into account, it was noted that endometrioid tumors with gene expression profiles similar to serous carcinomas were usually high grade and harbored *TP53* mutations, while the endometrioid tumors with expression patterns distinct from the serous carcinomas tended to be low grade and harbor mutations of *CTNNB1, PTEN*, and/or *PIK3CA*. Once again, the molecular data support the division of endometrioid carcinomas into two major groups based at least in part, on tumor grade. Shared genetic alterations such as *TP53* mutation may be responsible for similarities in global gene expression pattern between high-grade endometrioid carcinomas and high-grade serous carcinomas. Some of the overlap in gene expression between serous carcinomas and high-grade endometrioid carcinomas may be due to pathologists' inability to reliably distinguish between the two based solely on morphological criteria. Further studies are needed to address this issue and to determine whether moderately differentiated endometrioid carcinomas have molecular features more in keeping with high-grade versus low-grade tumors. Moreover, it is worth noting that the study of Wu and colleagues identified at least a few tumors with molecular features typical of both low-grade (i.e., Wnt/β-cat and/or PI3K/Pten pathway mutations) and high-grade (*TP53* mutations) tumors suggesting that "progression" from Type I to Type II endometrioid carcinoma may occur in a subset of cases.

Microsatellites are segments of DNA in which a short sequence motif, usually one to five nucleotides in length, is repeated several times. Microsatellite instability (MSI) refers to alterations in the DNA of tumor cells in which the number of sequence repeats within these microsatellites is different from the number of repeats at the same locus in DNA from the patient's non-neoplastic cells. MSI in tumor cells is associated with mutational or epigenetic inactivation of genes that encode proteins involved in DNA mismatch repair, such as *MSH2, MSH6*, and *MLH1.* A recent meta-analysis of ovarian carcinomas estimates the frequency of the microsatellite instability phenotype in unselected ovarian cancers at approximately 12%, with overrepresentation of non-serous histologic subtypes [251]. MSI has been observed in 13–20% of ovarian endometrioid carcinomas, and is usually associated with loss of expression of proteins involved in mismatch repair, particularly hMLH1 and less frequently, hMSH2 [45, 186]. Loss of expression is most often attributable to promoter hypermethylation rather than inactivating mutations in sporadic ovarian carcinomas with MSI [101].

Clinical Behavior and Treatment

Overall, endometrioid carcinomas of the ovary have a better prognosis than typical serous carcinomas due to the high proportion of stage I cases. The favorable prognosis may also be due, in part, to endometrioid carcinoma being low grade significantly more often than serous carcinoma, although data on the influence of grade on prognosis are less clear because grade and stage are mutually confounding factors (see ➲ Prognostic Factors, Grade above). One recent large prospective series found that in stages II and III, the prognosis was significantly better for endometrioid as compared to serous carcinoma. In that series, however, endometrioid carcinomas were significantly more likely to be optimally debulked as compared to serous carcinomas, and occurred in younger women. In addition, neither substage nor grade was considered in that analysis [338]. Treatment for endometrioid carcinoma is generally the same as that for other ovarian carcinomas. However, progestational agents, antiestrogens, tamoxifen, and other hormonal therapies have been used with limited success in previously treated endometrioid carcinomas; 10–15% response rates have been reported. There may be a correlation between the presence of steroid hormone receptors in tumor tissue and response rates, but data are limited. Hormonal therapy may be an option for the treatment of recurrence in patients who have failed or cannot tolerate chemotherapy or surgery.

Endometrioid Carcinoma Associated with Uterine Endometrial Carcinoma

Approximately 14% of women with endometrioid ovarian carcinoma also have endometrial cancer of the uterine corpus. Endometrial hyperplasia is also commonly present. As both tumors are often well-differentiated endometrioid adenocarcinomas, they resemble each other, and excluding the possibility that the ovarian tumor is metastatic can be a problem. Usually this can be determined based on a careful evaluation of the clinicopathologic features [201]. If the uterine endometrial tumor is low grade with no or only inner half myometrial invasion, its metastatic potential is very low, and the ovarian tumor can confidently be regarded as independent. If the endometrial tumor is high grade and/or deeply myoinvasive, the features of the ovarian tumors come into play. Bilaterality and a multinodular pattern, as well as other patterns characteristic of metastatic disease (See ➲ Chap. 18, Metastatic Tumors of the Ovary) indicate metastatic tumor. Close association of the ovarian tumors with either an underlying adenofibroma or endometriosis can also provide evidence that the ovarian tumor is independent.

The median age is about 50 years, significantly lower than high-grade serous carcinomas (about 60 years), but closer to that for women with endometrioid carcinomas (55–58 years). The median ovarian tumor size is about 9 cm. The majority of tumors in both sites are well differentiated. The 5-year survival is 70–92%, and the median survival is 10 years or longer [332, 338, 394]. Therefore, follow-up supports two independent tumors because most of these patients survive without recurrence, a finding more suggestive of stage I endometrial and ovarian carcinomas as compared to stage III endometrial cancer. It is conceivable, however, that an endometrioid carcinoma with an isolated ovarian metastasis may have a good prognosis. In one large series, 14% of patients had a relative with a gastrointestinal cancer and 18% had either a personal history of, or relative with, breast cancer [332]. In young women (<45 years) with endometrial cancer, 10–29% have synchronous ovarian cancer.

Over the last few years, investigators have employed several different molecular strategies to assess the likelihood that simultaneously detected endometrioid adenocarcinomas in the ovary and endometrium represent a single versus two independent primaries. Most of these have relied upon the presence or absence of shared genetic alterations in the ovarian and endometrial adenocarcinomas to identify single or dual primaries, respectively. Unfortunately, these approaches are rather labor-intensive and time-consuming, in part because investigators do not know, a priori, the specific genetic alterations present in a given tumor. Moreover, the certainty with which one can claim single versus dual primaries increases with the number of specific genetic alterations that can be compared in the ovarian and endometrial tumors. The difficulty of correctly classifying some of these cases is highlighted by the fact that virtually every published series of synchronous ovarian and uterine endometrioid adenocarcinomas includes cases that, after diagnosed using standard histologic criteria, would be reclassified based on molecular analysis [31, 91, 93, 270].

Endometrioid Carcinoma Arising in Endometriosis

On average, 15–20% of endometrioid carcinomas of the ovary are associated with endometriosis that may occur within the tumor, the ipsilateral or contralateral ovary, or elsewhere [392]. The frequency can be as high as 42%. It is likely that when strict criteria are applied to diagnose endometrioid carcinoma (see ➋ Differential Diagnosis above), some cases would be reclassified as high-grade serous carcinomas and therefore the percentage of endometrioid carcinomas associated with endometriosis would be higher. Accordingly, the majority of bona fide endometrioid carcinomas can be shown to be associated with endometriosis when extensive histologic sampling and meticulous searching for the histologic features of endometriosis are performed, and strict diagnostic criteria are used. In only a minority of cases, however, can direct continuity from endometriosis to atypical hyperplasia to carcinoma be demonstrated. This is most commonly seen in the lining of an endometriotic cyst that may display a thickening of the cyst wall, papillary excrescences, or a nodule protruding into the cyst. The mean age of women with endometrioid carcinoma associated with endometriosis is about 5–10 years younger than when unassociated with endometriosis. Tumors associated with endometriosis, and particularly those arising in an endometriotic cyst, are usually architecturally well differentiated and stage I, and therefore the prognosis is excellent. On rare occasions, a limited atypical epithelial proliferation in an endometriotic cyst will raise the differential diagnosis of atypical hyperplasia similar to the type seen in the uterine corpus, versus well-differentiated endometrioid adenocarcinoma. In such cases, criteria for this distinction used in the uterine corpus have been applied with minor modifications [298].

One study suggests that ovarian endometriosis has more chromosomal aberrations and may be more likely to undergo neoplastic transformation as compared to extraovarian endometriosis [159]. Another study suggests that expression of estrogen receptor alpha increases with transformation of endometriosis to endometrioid adenocarcinoma, the reverse of what is observed with transformation of endometriosis to clear cell carcinoma [3].

Clear Cell Tumors

The müllerian nature of clear cell tumors of the ovary, previously thought to be of mesonephric origin and referred to as "mesonephroma," is supported by the close association with endometriosis, their frequent admixture with endometrioid carcinoma, the occurrence of identical tumors in the endometrium, and their origin in vaginal adenosis in DES-exposed women. The vast majority of clear cell neoplasms of the ovaries are carcinomas, and comprise 8.5% of ovarian carcinomas (➋ *Table 14.4*). Clear cell adenofibromas and atypical proliferative clear cell neoplasms are vanishingly rare (➋ *Table 14.5*).

Clear Cell Adenofibromas

These are among the rarest of the ovarian epithelial tumors; we did not find a single example among 1,000 consecutive epithelial tumors (➋ *Table 14.5*). Among 12 reported cases of benign clear cell tumors, the mean age was 45 years. One tumor was bilateral. The median diameter was 12 cm. The tumors display a smooth lobulated external surface and the cut surfaces have a fine honeycomb appearance with minute cysts embedded in firm rubbery stroma ("parvilocular"). The cyst fluid is clear. Microscopically, the tumor is characterized by tubular glands lined by one or two layers of peg-like or hobnail cells that may bulge into the lumen or are flattened. The cytoplasm is either scanty, often in the hobnail cells, or abundant clear, granular, or eosinophilic in the large polyhedral cells. Nuclear atypia and mitotic activity are minimal. The stroma is compact and fibrocollagenous. The apical cell borders and lumens often contain mucin. The cytoplasm usually contains glycogen. The clinical behavior appears benign, although data are very limited.

Atypical Proliferative Clear Cell Tumors (APCCT)

APCCT comprise 0.2% of ovarian epithelial tumors (➋ *Table 14.5*). Among approximately 30 cases of APCCT (clear cell adenofibroma of borderline malignancy or low malignant potential) in the literature, the mean age is 60–70 years. The mean tumor diameter is about 15 cm. The gross appearance is similar to that of the clear cell adenofibroma, but in addition there are softer and fleshier areas. Microscopically, the architecture is similar to the clear cell adenofibroma, but glands are more crowded. The tumor has greater epithelial proliferation and atypia than the adenofibroma and lacks stromal invasion. The cell types lining the glands and cystic spaces are similar to those in benign tumors but display significant nuclear atypia with coarse chromatin clumping, prominent nucleoli, and mitotic activity up to 3 per 10 HPF. The epithelium may display stratification and budding; true papillary structures are uncommon. Small solid nests of clear cells, significant gland crowding, or papillary growth should raise the suspicion of stromal invasion. Distinction of an APCCT from clear cell carcinoma is one of the most difficult distinctions in gynecologic pathology. Some clear cell carcinomas lack an obviously infiltrative pattern and are characterized solely by crowded glands. The point at which gland crowding in a clear cell neoplasm reflects invasion is not well defined. The vast majority of tumors in which this differential is considered are usually classified as clear cell carcinoma. This practice helps ensure comprehensive staging where metastases might be found and thereby confirm a diagnosis of carcinoma. Furthermore, it gives the patient the potential benefit of chemotherapy if there is doubt about the diagnosis.

Occasionally, an endometriotic cyst is lined by atypical epithelial cells with clear cytoplasm. This has been designated "atypical endometriosis" (see ➋ Chap. 13, Diseases of the Peritoneum) [298]. Rarely, cytologic features of malignancy are present in this setting. If the lesion is well sampled and invasion is not found, the lesion is classified as APCCT with intraepithelial carcinoma. Microinvasion should be diagnosed if invasive areas measure less than 5 mm, but this finding should prompt additional sampling to look for diagnostic features of carcinoma. There are virtually no published data on clear cell tumors with microinvasion or intraepithelial carcinoma, both of which are exceedingly rare.

The rarity of clear cell adenofibroma and APCCT could reflect the fact that precursors of clear cell carcinoma most often have the morphology of endometriosis with atypia rather than a clear cell neoplasm. Peritoneal "implants" have not been described with APCCTs. Among the limited reported APCCTs, there is one alleged recurrence and no tumor deaths.

Clear Cell Carcinomas

Clinical Findings

The mean age of patients with clear cell carcinoma is 50–53 years. Symptoms usually relate to a pelvic or abdominal mass. Clear cell carcinoma is the most common epithelial ovarian neoplasm to be associated with vascular thrombotic events (18–46% of patients) and paraneoplastic hypercalcemia (2–10%)[254, 345] (see ➋ Chap. 15, Sex Cord-Stromal, Steroid Cell, and Other Ovarian Tumors with Endocrine, Paraendocrine, and Paraneoplastic Manifestations). In a large series from Australia, 27% of patients with clear cell carcinoma had a thromboembolic event as compared to 7% of those with other cell types of ovarian carcinoma [202].

Operative Findings

The relationship with endometriosis is strongest for clear cell carcinoma among all cell types of ovarian carcinoma. Accordingly, endometriotic implants are commonly present in close proximity to the tumor or elsewhere in the pelvis or abdomen. About 35–60% of clear cell carcinomas present in FIGO stage I, and 9–22% in stage II [255, 369]. Eight percent are bilateral; 4% of stage I cases are bilateral [353]. As noted earlier, several recent studies have shown that stage I clear cell carcinoma is more likely to be stage IC (55–74%) as compared to the other cell types [57, 224, 313, 341, 343, 353, 369]. The reason for this is not clear but it seems to be correlated with a higher risk of tumor rupture [224].

Gross Findings

Tumors range up to 30 cm in diameter with a mean of about 13–15 cm. Although they may be solid and fibrous with a honeycomb cut surface resembling benign and atypical proliferative clear cell tumors, more commonly the cut surfaces reveal a thick-walled unilocular cyst with multiple yellow-beige fleshy nodules protruding into the lumen, or a multiloculated cystic mass with cysts containing watery or mucinous fluid. Most tumors arise in endometriosis and display features of an endometriotic cyst, which typically contains chocolate-brown fluid, and a thickened, polypoid or nodular area in the wall, or a larger solid area reflecting the focus of malignant transformation. Less commonly, there is a prominent adenofibromatous component which is solid; this pattern is not as strongly associated with endometriosis [369].

Microscopic Findings

Clear cell carcinomas display several different patterns, which often occur together (➲ *Figs. 14.114–14.122*). These include papillary, tubulocystic, and solid. In a minority of cases, there is a prominent adenofibromatous component [369] (➲ *Figs. 14.121* and ➲ *14.122*). Recently, some investigators have subdivided clear cell carcinomas into those arising in a cyst and those that have an adenofibromatous background [369]. The cystic tumors are more frequently papillary, whereas the tubulocystic pattern tends to dominate in the adenofibromatous tumors. The cystic variant is more frequently associated with endometriosis. In addition, the behavior of the two types of tumors may be different although the data have been conflicting [369]. These findings suggest that the two variants arise along different pathways.

The solid pattern of clear cell carcinoma is characterized by sheets of polyhedral cells with abundant, clear cytoplasm separated by delicate fibrovascular septae or dense fibrotic stroma. The papillary pattern is characterized by papillae that are either fibrotic but more often are hyalinized (➲ *Figs. 14.116*, ➲ *14.117*, and ➲ *14.120*). In fact, the hyalinized papillary cores are a very characteristic feature of this tumor. The tubulocystic pattern is characterized by varying size tubules and cysts (➲ *Fig. 14.114*). The majority of tumors display combinations of all of these patterns [369]. Despite being designated clear cell carcinoma, many of the cells comprising clear cell carcinoma contain slightly granular eosinophilic cytoplasm.

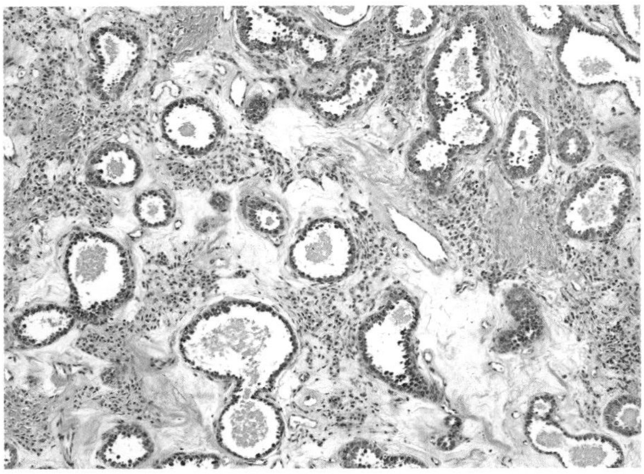

Fig. 14.115
Clear cell carcinoma. **The tumor is composed of tubules lined by a single layer of epithelium containing a large number of hobnail cells**

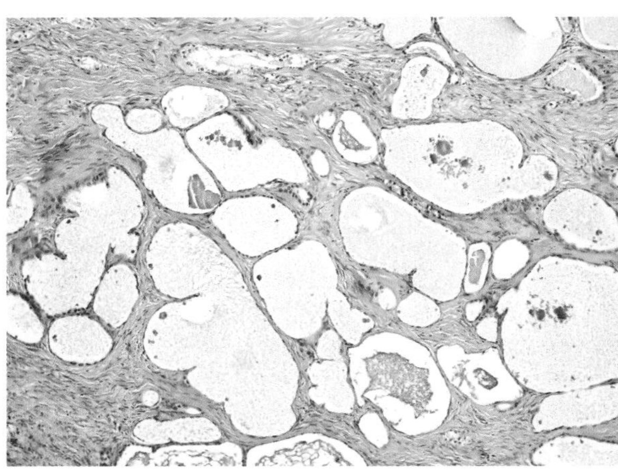

Fig. 14.114
Clear cell carcinoma. **Tubulocystic pattern. The glands are cystically dilated and the epithelium is flattened. As a consequence nuclear atypia can appear beguilingly innocuous**

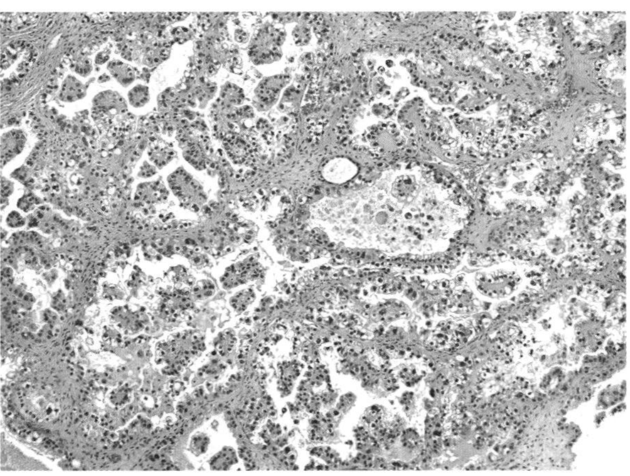

Fig. 14.116
Clear cell carcinoma. **Tubulopapillary architecture with hobnail and clear cells**

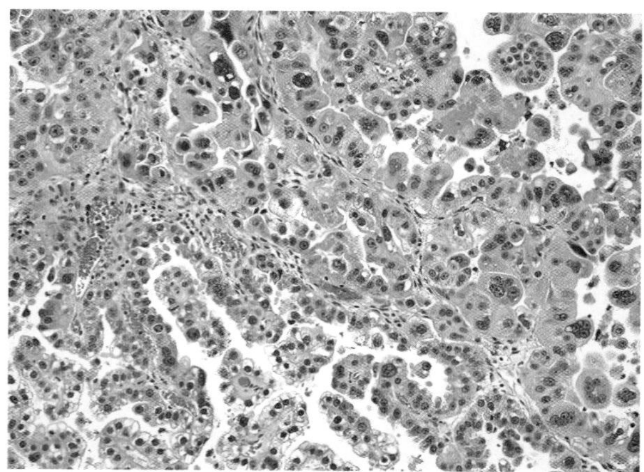

Fig. 14.117
Clear cell carcinoma. **Clear cells and cells with abundant eosinophilic cytoplasm (oxyphilic cells). Marked variation in nuclear atypia ranging from minimal to marked. This is not an unusual feature of clear cell carcinoma**

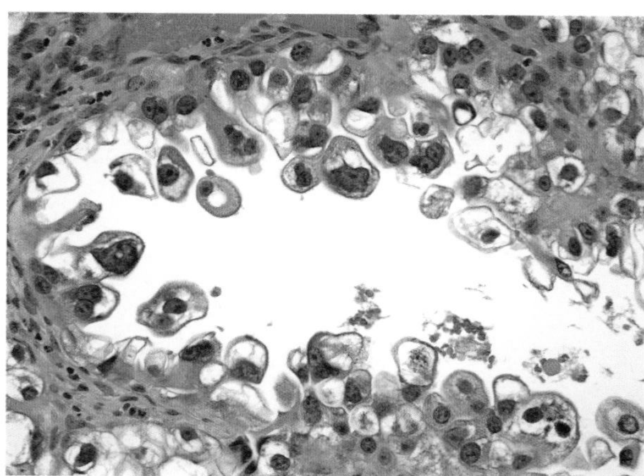

Fig. 14.119
Clear cell carcinoma. **Hobnail cells with marked nuclear atypia and clear cytoplasm**

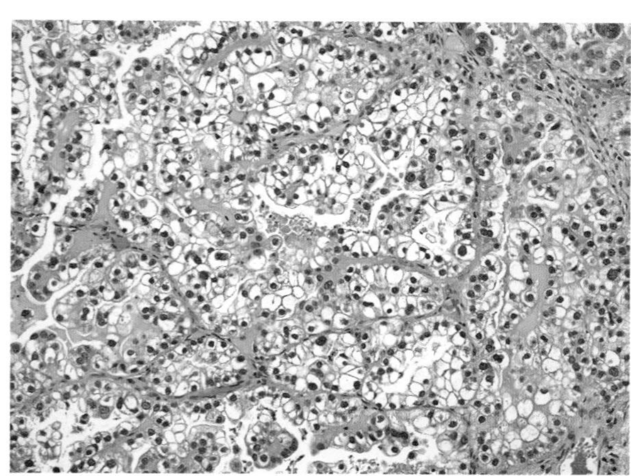

Fig. 14.118
Clear cell carcinoma. **Solid and glandular pattern composed exclusively of cells with clear cytoplasm. Note homogeneous eosinophilic stromal hyalinization**

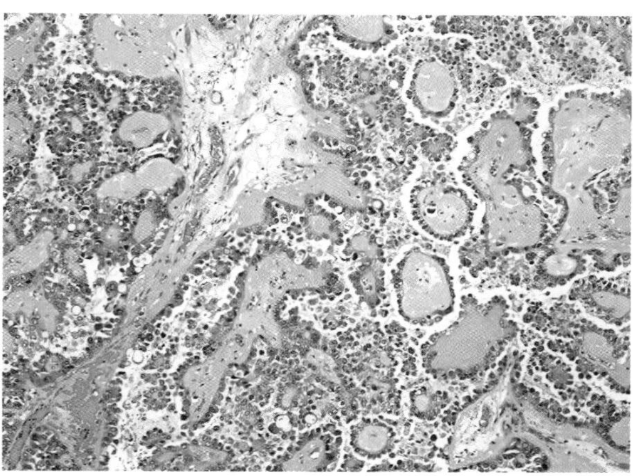

Fig. 14.120
Clear cell carcinoma. **Papillae lined by hobnail cells. Note hyalinized eosinophilic stroma, a characteristic feature of clear cell carcinoma**

When the majority of the cells have this appearance the term "oxyphilic clear cell carcinoma" has been used (*Fig. 14.117*). So-called hepatoid carcinoma may be a variant of oxyphilic clear cell carcinoma and can be mixed with serous and mucinous components [354]. The cells with clear cytoplasm contain glycogen and at times intracytoplasmic mucinous inclusions. The majority of clear cell carcinomas contain hyaline globules that are PAS positive. The nuclei vary from small and rounded and angular to large and pleomorphic with prominent nucleoli (*Figs. 14.117–14.119* and *14.122*). Often, the nuclear grade within a tumor varies from mild to markedly atypical. However, even when the majority of cells display only mild nuclear atypia, cells with marked atypia will be present. Accordingly, the nuclear grade is nearly always high regardless of the grading system used

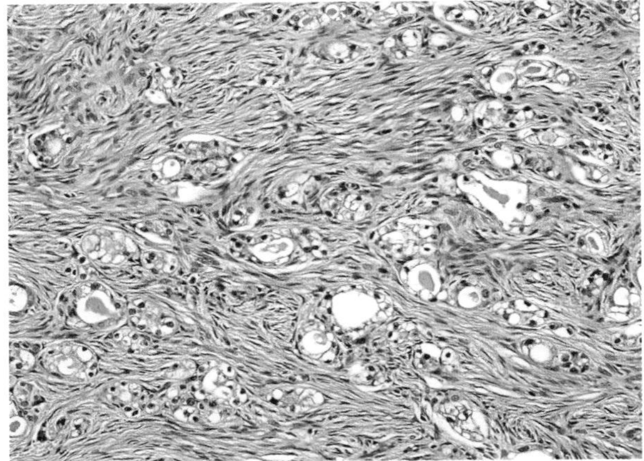

Fig. 14.121
Clear cell carcinoma. **Adenofibromatous pattern of clear cell carcinoma with small angulated glands**

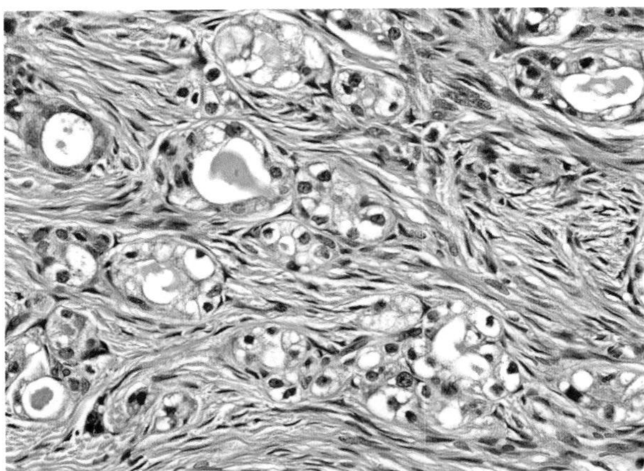

Fig. 14.122
Clear cell carcinoma. **Moderate cytologic atypia is present (same case as *Fig. 14.121*)**

and for that reason all clear cell carcinomas are considered high grade. Mitotic activity tends to be low, exceeding 10 per 10 HPF in only one fourth of cases [369]. In the tubulocystic and papillary patterns, the cells often have a hobnail appearance with the nucleus protruding from the papillae, tubule, or cyst into the lumen (*Figs. 14.115*, *14.116*, *14.119*, and *14.120*). Occasionally, the epithelium lining the tubules and cysts is flattened (*Fig. 14.114*), and the nuclear grade is low in these areas but careful scrutiny will reveal cells with high-grade nuclei elsewhere [387]. Necrosis, hemorrhage, and stromal lymphocytic infiltrates are variable. Luteinized stromal cells and psammomatous calcifications are occasionally present.

Clear cell carcinomas arising in endometriosis are usually cystic and may display atypia of the lining of an endometriotic cyst with either a gradual or abrupt transition to cytologic features of malignancy and invasive clear cell carcinoma. This can be seen in one third of clear cell carcinomas [369]. If cytologic atypia is marked and invasion is absent, a diagnosis of APCCT with intraepithelial carcinoma is warranted. Cystic clear cell carcinomas are significantly more likely to be associated with endometriosis and atypical endometriosis as compared to the adenofibromatous type [369].

About 30–35% of reported ovarian clear cell carcinomas are associated with endometriosis either in the involved ovary or elsewhere in the pelvis or abdomen. These figures vary widely and many recent studies have observed 50% or greater associated with endometriosis [369, 389]; one clinical study found that 88% of clear cell carcinomas were preceded by a sonographically detected endometriotic cyst [387]. One recent large study found endometriosis to be present in about 90% of cystic clear cell carcinomas, while the association of endometriosis with adenofibromatous clear cell carcinomas was only 44% [369]. When carefully sought, nearly all ovarian clear cell carcinomas are associated with endometriosis and at least one third of cases can be demonstrated to have arisen within endometriosis, usually an endometriotic cyst [336, 369].

Immunohistochemistry

Like other ovarian carcinomas, clear cell carcinomas stain strongly and diffusely for epithelial markers including keratins, particularly CK7, CAM5.2, EMA, Leu M1, and B72.3. Alpha fetoprotein, CK20, p53, and CD 10 are generally negative [20, 39, 116, 206], although CD10 can be positive in up to 20%, usually at the apical border [242]. CEA is negative in most cases [130], and vimentin is positive in about 50%. OC125 is usually positive [130, 206]. BRCA1 is usually positive [352]. WT1 is positive in 10–22% [1, 116, 124, 130]. TTF1 is positive in less than 20% [20, 130, 162]. Estrogen receptor [116, 290] and progesterone receptor are usually negative [92, 130, 178], and evidence suggests that expression of these receptors is lost during malignant transformation of endometriosis which is usually receptor positive [3]. 34β E12 (high-molecular-weight cytokeratin) is always positive [242]. The hyalinized stroma is immunoreactive for type IV collagen and laminin.

Several reports indicate that clear cell carcinoma expresses a variety of investigational markers significantly more frequently than the other cell types. These include hepatocyte nuclear factor 1β [384], ABCF2 [234], early mitotic inhibitor-1 protein [113], and GPX3 [128, 296].

Differential Diagnosis

Germ cell tumors including yolk sac (endodermal sinus) tumor, dysgerminoma, and rarely struma ovarii are important to consider in the differential diagnosis of a clear cell neoplasm in the ovary. Clinical information including young age for yolk sac tumors and dysgerminomas, and elevated serum AFP levels in women with yolk sac tumors, is helpful. Morphologically, the papillary structures of clear cell carcinomas are more complex and have hyalinized cores, thus differing from the festoon pattern of yolk sac tumors. In addition, yolk sac tumors display a variety of features not seen in clear cell carcinoma including the characteristic Schiller–Duvall bodies as well as other patterns (see Chap. 16, Germ Cell Tumors of the Ovary). Lack of staining for alpha fetoprotein (AFP) is an important feature in excluding yolk sac tumor, although rare clear cell carcinomas have been reported to secrete AFP. The combination of positive LeuM1 and negative AFP may help discriminate clear cell carcinoma from yolk sac tumor, but the sensitivity and specificity of AFP are not high. A more useful panel is CK7 and EMA, which, when both are positive, excludes YST, which is negative for these antibodies [267]. Glypican-3 can also be of value in this distinction [290]. Positivity for EMA and strong diffuse positivity for cytokeratins help exclude dysgerminoma. The solid pattern of clear cell carcinoma can resemble dysgerminoma, but dysgerminoma lacks the tubulocystic and papillary patterns of clear cell carcinoma and displays primitive-appearing nuclei. In addition, clear cell carcinoma lacks stromal chronic inflammation and granulomas frequently present in dysgerminomas. Extensive sampling may reveal other germ cell components or endometriosis that can assist in diagnosis.

A papillary pattern with low to moderate nuclear grade can mimic APST, particularly on frozen section when sampling is limited. "Pink cell" tufting in APST may cause confusion with the hobnail pattern. The characteristic detached cell clusters of APST can be seen in cyst lumens in clear cell carcinoma. Psammomatous calcification and low mitotic index are frequent in both tumors. Clear cell carcinomas are more frequently unilateral and occur in an older age group as compared to APST, but these features are not very helpful in an individual case. A useful panel is WT1 and ER. APST is positive for both, while clear cell carcinoma is usually negative [290].

The clear cytoplasm of these tumors has been overemphasized in differential diagnosis. The histologic patterns particularly the tubulocystic and papillary patterns are quite characteristic and warrant a diagnosis of clear cell carcinoma even in the absence of cells with clear cytoplasm. The papillae of clear cell carcinoma are thinner and delicate and the stroma is more frequently hyalinized as compared to serous carcinoma. Conversely, serous carcinomas not infrequently contain focal areas with clear cytoplasm (*Fig. 14.70*); these should not be diagnosed as clear cell carcinoma in the absence of the typical papillary and tubulocystic architecture of clear cell carcinoma [207, 333]. A useful panel for this distinction is ER, HNF-1β, and WT1. The most common profiles are WT1+, ER+, and HNF-1β- in high-grade serous carcinoma and WT1-, ER-, HNF-1β+ in clear cell carcinoma [155].

Although hyaline globules are commonly found in clear cell carcinomas, these are nonspecific. They are a characteristic feature of yolk sac tumor, but also occur in the majority of carcinosarcomas, and in a small minority of endometrioid, serous, and mucinous ovarian neoplasms.

Endometrioid carcinomas with secretory changes can mimic clear cell carcinoma. When the cells are tall columnar with sub- or supranuclear vacuoles resembling early secretory endometrium, the tumor is classified as the secretory variant of endometrioid carcinoma. When the clear cell changes are more extensive and the cells become more cuboidal, the distinction is more difficult. Rarely, a metaplastic squamous component of an endometrioid carcinoma, in which the squamous cells contain abundant glycogen, can be confused with clear cell carcinoma. Steroid cell tumors of the ovary can have prominent areas of clear cytoplasm. Benign or low-grade nuclear features, a delicate fibrovascular stroma, small size, well-circumscribed border, and confinement within the ovarian stroma are features of a steroid cell tumor that help to distinguish it from clear cell carcinoma.

Rarely, struma ovarii will mimic a clear cell tumor if the thyroid follicles become so cystic that the pattern resembles the tubulocystic pattern of clear cell carcinoma, and classic features of thyroid are not recognizable. Extensive sampling to identify other teratomatous elements can be of value, and staining for thyroglobulin is also useful. Metastatic clear cell neoplasms such as renal cell carcinoma are very rare (see Chap. 18, Metastatic Tumors of the Ovary). A useful panel for this distinction is CD10 and CK7; renal cell carcinomas are typically CK7 negative and CD10 positive [39, 242], the reverse of the pattern for ovarian clear cell carcinoma, but CK7 can be focally positive in up to 37.5% [242]. 34βE12 can also be helpful and is always negative in renal cell carcinoma [242].

Molecular Biology

The molecular changes in ovarian clear cell tumors have not been as extensively studied as in serous and endometrioid tumors. This is probably due to the relative rarity of clear cell tumors. As a consequence, most studies in the published literature have analyzed only limited numbers of clear cell carcinomas and therefore the true prevalence of many specific molecular alterations is unknown. In addition, the extent to which serous carcinomas containing clear cells have been misclassified as clear cell carcinomas and consequently affected these studies is unknown. Nevertheless, some important conclusions can be drawn regarding the role of a few molecular alterations in the pathogenesis of these tumors.

Mutation Analyses Mutations in *KRAS*, *BRAF*, and *TP53* are present in some clear cell carcinomas but their frequency is generally low [203, 376]. For example, *TP53* mutation and *BRAF* mutation were found in 8.3% and 6.3% of clear cell carcinomas, respectively. Mutations predicted to deregulate PI3K/Pten signaling are more common in clear cell carcinomas, with *PIK3CA* mutations reported in 20–25% and *PTEN* mutations in 8% of tumors in a few small series [40, 292, 376]. Kuo and colleagues recently analyzed 97 affinity-purified primary ovarian clear cell carcinomas for mutations in *PIK3CA, TP53, KRAS, PTEN, CTNNB1*, and *BRAF*. Mutations were identified in 33%, 15%, 7%, 5%, 3%, and 1% of cases, respectively [165]. Interestingly, Sato et al. demonstrated somatic mutations of *PTEN* in 21% of ovarian endometriotic cysts, indicative of shared molecular alterations between clear cell and endometrioid carcinomas of the ovary and their putative precursor lesion [292]. Among seven clear cell carcinomas with synchronous endometriosis, allelic deletions/loss of heterozygosity (LOH) at the *PTEN* locus in both the carcinoma and associated endometriosis was detected in three cases, and one case displayed LOH only in the carcinoma. In no cases were there LOH events involving *PTEN* in the endometriosis only. The findings suggest that inactivation of the *PTEN* tumor suppressor gene, when it occurs, is a relatively early event in the development of ovarian clear cell carcinoma. Although studies to date are rather limited, the clear cell carcinomas do not appear to share many other changes with endometrioid carcinomas, as canonical Wnt signaling pathway defects and microsatellite instability have not been observed with significant frequency in the clear cell tumors overall [94, 150, 376]. However, a recent study of microsatellite instability and mismatch repair protein defects in ovarian cancers affecting patients <50 years of age found evidence of mismatch repair defects in a significant proportion (17%) of ovarian clear cell carcinomas [138].

DNA Copy Number Changes At least two independent reports describe the use of classical CGH to study DNA copy number changes in clear cell carcinomas [72, 339]. In their analysis of 18 tumors, Dent and colleagues found that chromosome 9p21 deletion was the most common copy number alteration, followed by losses on chromosomes 1p, 11q, and 10q (including the *PTEN* locus at 10q23.3). DNA copy number gains were generally not detected [72]. In contrast, in their analysis of 12 ovarian clear cell carcinomas, Suehiro and colleagues identified increased DNA copy number at several chromosomal regions as well as frequent losses of chromosome 19p [339]. The discordant findings between the two studies suggest that clear cell carcinomas may be quite heterogeneous and analysis of large numbers of tumor samples using more advanced technologies with higher resolution may be needed to reliably identify common alterations of DNA copy number in clear cell carcinomas. Toward this end, Tsuda and colleagues employed a cDNA microarray platform to perform simultaneous genomic and expression array analyses on 30 ovarian clear cell carcinomas [357]. Using this approach, 12 and 5 genes showed significant increase and decrease, respectively, in both DNA copy number and mRNA levels compared to serous carcinomas. Although the clinical and biological significance of these molecular alterations remains unclear, overexpression of one gene, *ABCF2*, was associated with poor response to chemotherapy. In order to test the notion that some clear cell carcinomas might arise from clear cell adenofibromas and borderline tumors, Yamamoto and colleagues evaluated DNA isolated from clear cell adenofibromas/borderline tumors and adjacent clear cell carcinomas for LOH at 17 different polymorphic loci on 11 chromosomal arms [386]. The overall frequency of LOH was significantly higher in the clear cell carcinomas (49%) than in adjacent areas of borderline tumor (30%) or adenofibroma (22%). Furthermore, an identical LOH pattern involving the same alleles at one or more loci was found in 13 of 14 cases, a finding highly unlikely to have occurred at random. Allelic losses on chromosomes 5q, 10q, and 22q were frequent in clear cell carcinomas and their putative precursors, while LOH on 1p and 13q were frequent in the carcinomas but not in the adenofibromas. The data suggest that clear cell adenofibromas and borderline tumors can serve as clonal precursors for a subset of clear cell carcinomas [386].

Gene Expression Several comprehensive gene expression analyses of ovarian carcinomas have noted that clear cell carcinomas are readily distinguishable from the other histological types of ovarian carcinomas based on their global gene expression profiles [293, 296, 398]. A number of genes have been reported to be preferentially expressed in ovarian clear cell carcinomas and in some cases, in associated endometriosis. Among these overexpressed genes, HNF-1β appears to be a relatively specific marker of ovarian clear cell carcinoma [356]. HNF-1β is a nuclear homeodomain protein that participates in regulating gene expression in liver and several other tissues including secretory endometrium. Given that HNF-1β is essential in controlling multiple genes involved in glucose/glycogen metabolism, HNF-1β upregulation may be in part responsible for the characteristic cytological feature (i.e., the glycogen-rich, clear-appearing cytoplasm) of clear cell carcinoma. Furthermore, many genes relatively specific to clear cell carcinoma are also regulated by HNF-1β [315, 346]. Although not specific for clear cell differentiation, a recent study found that IGF2BP3 expression is a marker of unfavorable prognosis in ovarian clear cell carcinomas [156].

Clinical Behavior and Treatment

There are conflicting data on the behavior of clear cell carcinoma. In some studies, the prognosis appears similar to that for other ovarian carcinomas, but in others, the prognosis is said to be worse. Comprehensively staged ovarian carcinoma (of all histologic types) in FIGO stage I has a 90% or better 5-year survival, and several recent studies have shown comparable survival rates for clear cell carcinoma (see ➋ Prognostic Factors, earlier in this chapter). Evidence that clear cell histology is an adverse prognostic factor in advanced stage is somewhat more convincing [49, 50, 256]. The treatment is similar to that of other epithelial cell types of ovarian carcinoma.

Brenner (Transitional Cell) Tumors

Transitional cell tumors comprise 10% of ovarian epithelial tumors. Nearly all of these are benign Brenner tumors; atypical proliferative and malignant forms are very uncommon. The transitional epithelial cell type, characterized by a relatively uniform population of stratified cells with ovoid nuclei displaying nuclear grooves, is named because of its resemblance to urothelium. Evidence suggests that benign Brenner tumors have some true urothelial differentiation, while transitional cell carcinoma (unassociated with a benign Brenner component) is a variant of high-grade serous carcinoma [246, 271]. The same type of epithelium is characteristic of peritoneal Walthard cell nests (see ➋ Chap. 13, Diseases of the Peritoneum).

Brenner (Benign Transitional Cell) Tumors

The mean patient age is 56 years. These are common incidental findings and are often microscopic in size. Therefore, the presenting symptoms are often unrelated to the ovarian tumor. Most tumors are 2 cm or smaller, and although a 1 cm minimum size is used for the other cell types of ovarian epithelial tumors, this has not been applied to Brenner tumors that frequently measure only a few millimeters. Multiple microscopic tumors are seen in 17% of patients. Occasionally they are large and may exceed 10 cm. Most tumors are well circumscribed, firm, and rubbery, with a smooth or slightly bosselated serosal surface. The cut surfaces are typically solid and fibrous; usually gray, white, or yellow; and may be whorled or lobulated; occasionally a cystic component is present. Small tumors can usually be seen to be arising in the ovarian cortex or hilus.

Microscopically, the characteristic feature is sharply demarcated epithelial nests in a dense fibrous stroma (➋ *Figs. 14.123* and ➋ *14.124*). The epithelial cells are relatively uniform in size with prominent cell borders and pale to eosinophilic cytoplasm. The nuclei are oval, often with small nucleoli, and longitudinal grooves are usually present (➋ *Fig. 14.125*). Atypia and mitotic activity

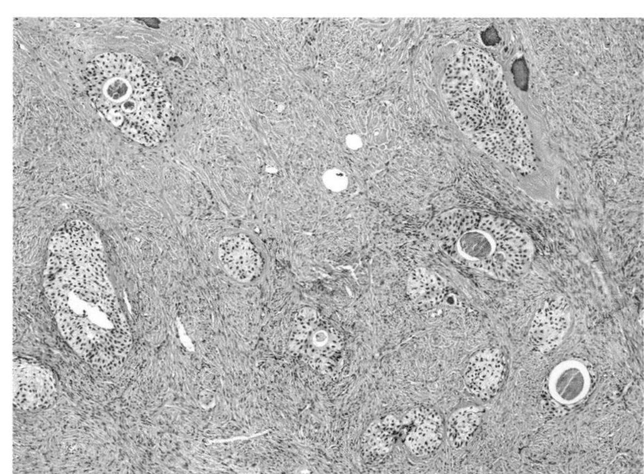

Fig. 14.123
Brenner tumor. **Rounded and ovoid nests of transitional cells are dispersed in a densely fibrotic stroma. Some nests are cystic and contain eosinophilic material. Spiculated calcification is seen at the *top right***

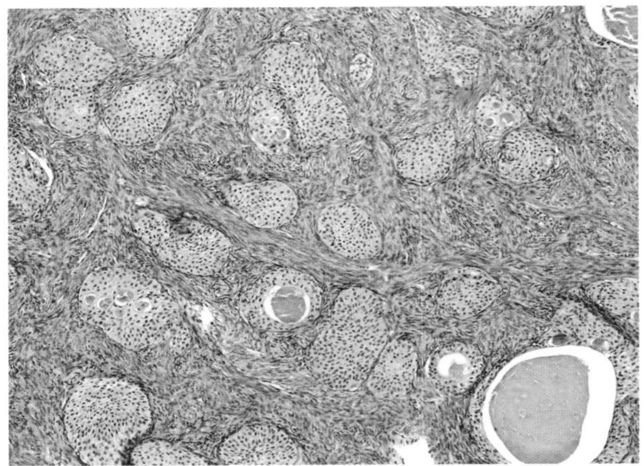

Fig. 14.124
Brenner tumor. **Transitional cell nests have smooth contours**

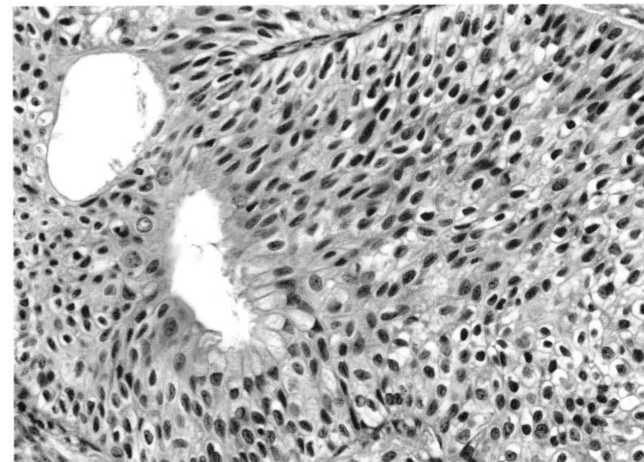

Fig. 14.125
Brenner tumor. **Cells with ovoid nuclei and longitudinal grooves create a resemblance to urothelial tumors. Metaplastic mucinous epithelium is present within a nest**

are generally not present. The nests often become cystic and contain eosinophilic debris or mucin. In 30%, metaplastic mucinous epithelium lines the cystic nests (*Fig. 14.125*); when extensive, some investigators have termed these tumors, "metaplastic Brenner tumor." The metaplastic mucinous component may occasionally form the dominant part of the tumor and accounts for the association of Brenner tumors with mucinous cystadenomas (*Fig. 14.126*). It has been suggested that the majority of nonteratomatous mucinous tumors arise in Brenner tumors as an overgrowth of the mucinous component [302] (see Mixed Brenner-Mucinous Tumors below). The stroma varies from closely resembling ovarian cortical stroma to densely fibrous. Hyalinized areas are common, and dystrophic, spiculated calcification is present in about half of cases (*Fig. 14.123*). Calcification is seen in 20% of tumors smaller than 1 cm and in over 80% of larger tumors [302]. Rare examples of "epidermoid cyst" of the ovary may represent cystic variants of Brenner tumor with squamous metaplasia (see Squamous Tumors later in this chapter) [146]. Walthard nests are seen in 50% of patients with Brenner tumors, significantly more often than those with serous, clear cell, or endometrioid tumors, but similar to those with mucinous tumors [302]. The clinical behavior is benign.

Histochemical stains indicate that the neoplastic cells contain glycogen, and mucin is present at the luminal borders and in the luminal contents. Immunoperoxidase stains reveal that the epithelial nests stain strongly for epithelial markers including keratins and EMA. CK7 is typically positive, and CK20 negative. Calretinin [194], inhibin, and WT1 are negative [47]. Uroplakin III, a urothelium-specific marker, is focally positive in a luminal pattern in a majority of cases. Thrombomodulin, a sensitive but less specific marker of urothelium, shows strong membranous staining in 82% [20, 187, 271]. CEA and CA 19-9 are positive in the majority of cases. The tumors are weakly reactive or negative for p16, cyclin D1, EGFR and Ras protein, and negative for p53 and Rb [66]. Stains for steroidogenic enzymes are usually negative.

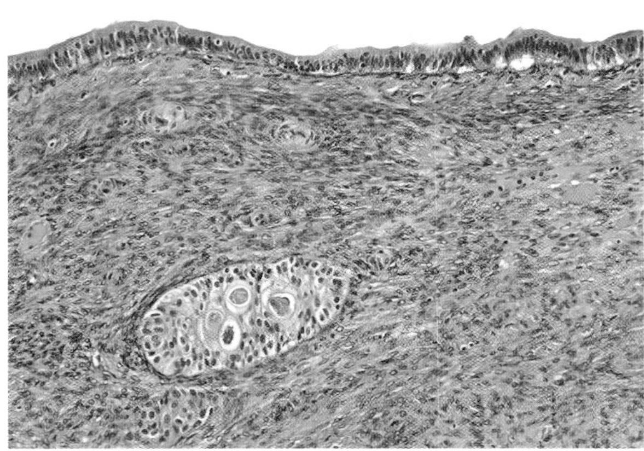

Fig. 14.126
Brenner tumor associated with mucinous cystadenoma. **A solitary Brenner nest is present beneath a layer of benign mucinous epithelium**

Mixed Brenner-Mucinous Tumors

Tumors containing both Brenner and mucinous components are more common than previously appreciated (◉ *Fig. 14.126*). These are believed to be variants of Brenner tumor and can be classified as metaplastic Brenner tumor (see above) or mixed Brenner–mucinous tumor (see ◉ Mixed Epithelial Tumors later in this chapter). One fourth of benign ovarian epithelial tumors that have a mucinous component also contain a Brenner component. Conversely, 16% of tumors with a Brenner component contain a mucinous component. These patients are significantly older than those with pure mucinous or pure Brenner tumor, with a mean age of 68 years. They are unilateral and most often have discrete Brenner and mucinous components, but in 30% the components are admixed. The other clinical and pathologic features are similar to their pure counterparts [302].

Atypical Proliferative Brenner (Transitional Cell) Tumors

These rare neoplasms, also termed "proliferating" or "borderline" transitional cell or Brenner tumor, or transitional cell or Brenner tumor "of low malignant potential," present in patients whose mean age is 59 years. They are always unilateral and confined to the ovary. They are larger than their benign counterparts, are usually cystic, and measure 10–28 cm with a mean diameter of 18 cm. Friable papillary or polypoid masses project into the cyst lumens, and there is usually a benign Brenner component present with a more solid and fibrous cut surface. Microscopically, the intracystic papillary component is composed of transitional-type epithelium resembling low-grade noninvasive papillary transitional cell neoplasms of the urinary tract (◉ *Figs. 14.127–14.130*). Mucinous metaplasia may be present in the epithelium lining the papillae (◉ *Fig. 14.130*). Underneath the papillae and within the wall there may be solid areas of transitional epithelium with little intervening stroma. Nearly all cases display areas of benign transitional cell neoplasm, and occasionally, the proliferating component can be seen to be arising directly from the benign component. The cytologic features are similar to those in benign transitional cell tumors, but occasionally significant atypia and mitotic activity are present. Some authors have separately classified "proliferative" and "low malignant potential" transitional cell tumors. The former are characterized by a resemblance to grade I–II urothelial papillary transitional cell carcinoma, whereas the latter display high-grade nuclear atypia resembling grade III urothelial papillary transitional cell carcinoma or in situ squamous cell carcinoma. In all cases, stromal invasion is absent; microinvasion has not been reported. EGFR, Ras, and CEA are usually positive. Rb, cyclin D1, p16, and p53 are usually weak or negative [66]. Among over 50 reported cases of atypical proliferative transitional cell tumors, there has been one local recurrence and no convincing evidence of malignant behavior. Accordingly, we prefer the term, "atypical proliferative transitional cell (Brenner) tumor."

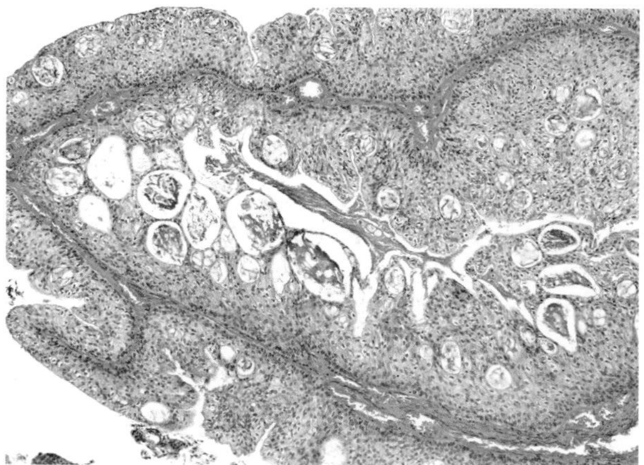

◘ Fig. 14.127
Atypical proliferative (borderline) Brenner tumor. **Large nest of proliferating transitional-type epithelium in center of field with extensive stratification and cystic change**

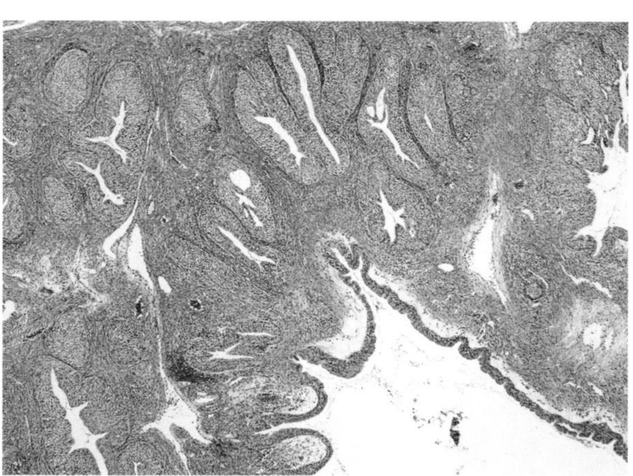

◘ Fig. 14.128
Atypical proliferative (borderline) Brenner tumor. **Transitional cell nests are larger and more densely packed than in a benign Brenner tumor**

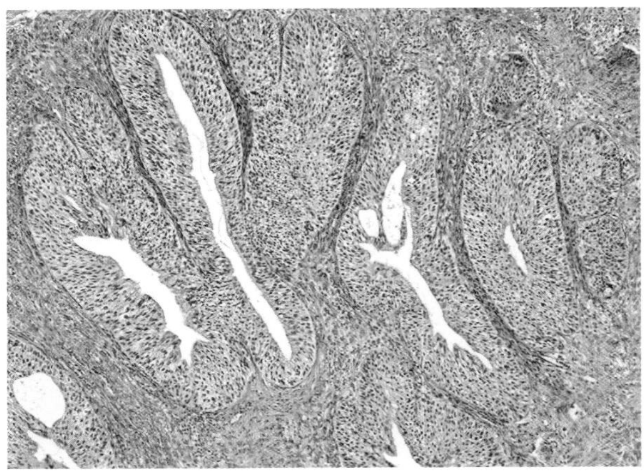

Fig. 14.129
Atypical proliferative (borderline) Brenner tumor. Proliferating transitional-type epithelium fills and expands the epithelial nests without invading the stroma

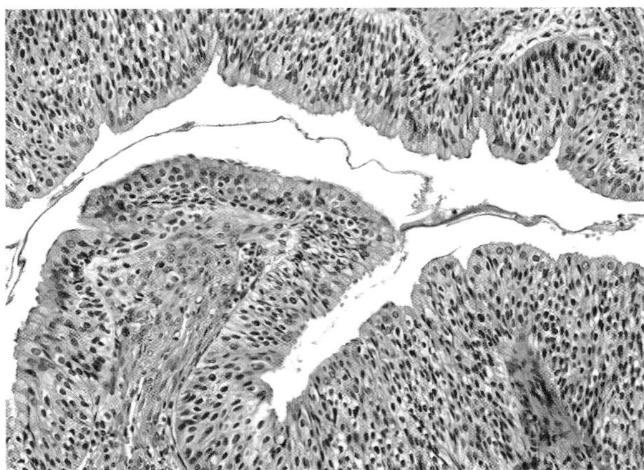

Fig. 14.130
Atypical proliferative (borderline) Brenner tumor. Transitional epithelium is highly stratified and has a surface layer of mucinous epithelium

Malignant Transitional Cell Tumors (Malignant Brenner Tumors and Transitional Cell Carcinomas)

Malignant transitional cell tumors are difficult to define clinicopathologically for several reasons. First, published data are very limited. Second, large databases including the FIGO annual report and the SEER database do not separately classify ovarian transitional cell carcinomas (TCC); in addition, malignant Brenner tumor is erroneously classified by SEER in a miscellaneous category for non-carcinomas. Third, serous carcinomas not infrequently have focal areas that display features resembling TCC. Nearly all tumors classified as ovarian transitional cell carcinomas are now regarded as high-grade serous carcinomas with transitional-like features.

Some investigators have found that approximately 10–15% of advanced-stage ovarian carcinomas contain a transitional cell component; others have found that a transitional cell pattern predominates in 22% of advanced-stage ovarian carcinomas. In contrast, we found only 3% of advanced-stage serous carcinoma were classifiable as TCC (*Table 14.4*), although we tend not to diagnose TCC unless the features are absolutely classic [301]. Some investigators have defined two clinicopathologic types of malignant transitional cell tumor: malignant Brenner tumor, in which a benign or atypical proliferative Brenner component is identified, and TCC, in which no benign or atypical proliferative Brenner component is identified.

Clinical Findings

The clinical presentation is nonspecific and is similar to those of the more common cell types of ovarian cancer; thus pelvic or abdominal pain and a mass are common. Malignant Brenner tumors occur at a mean age of 63 years, while TCCs present at a mean age of 56 years [81].

Operative Findings

The size of malignant Brenner tumors ranges up to 25 cm with a mean diameter of 14 cm. Among stage I tumors, 16% are bilateral. The stage distribution is as follows: stage I, 64%; stage II, 12%; stage III 18%; and stage IV, 6%. In contrast, 53% of transitional cell carcinomas present in advanced stage. The mean size is 10 cm [81].

Gross Findings

The gross appearance of TCC is similar to high-grade serous carcinoma, typically solid and cystic. The cysts may exhibit polypoid, friable mural nodules, and the cyst fluid is watery or mucinous. Hemorrhage and necrosis may be prominent, and half have foci of gritty calcification. In the malignant Brenner tumor, the benign Brenner component may be identifiable as a solid fibrous nodule within a cyst wall. Sometimes malignant Brenner tumor is completely solid. Serous carcinomas that have a transitional cell component have the gross features of serous carcinoma (see "Malignant serous tumors" above).

Microscopic Findings

The histologic patterns of TCC are often mixed with other types of carcinoma, most often serous. Approximately 10% of ovarian carcinomas containing the TCC pattern are said to be pure. More than 50% of the tumor should display the patterns of TCC for a diagnosis of TCC. A diagnosis of malignant Brenner tumor is warranted when a benign or atypical proliferative Brenner component is identified within or contiguous with the tumor.

The characteristic microscopic feature is thick, blunt, and often elongated papillary folds with fibrovascular cores, lined by transitional-type epithelium resembling urothelium (➲ *Fig. 14.131*). The papillae often appear to arise from a cyst wall with a similar lining of stratified and atypical transitional cells. A solid pattern is present in about half the cases. Microspaces, large cysts, and necrosis are seen in the majority of cases [81]. Foci of squamous or glandular differentiation are seen in less than 20%. Stromal invasion is present and characterized by haphazard infiltrative growth of epithelium at the base of the papillae into the cyst wall, or extensive areas of solid epithelial proliferation with scant or no fibrovascular support. Another architectural pattern of malignant Brenner tumor is characterized by a solid tumor resembling benign Brenner tumor, but the epithelial nests are more angulated and have a disorderly growth pattern that appears invasive. Stromal desmoplasia is occasionally present. Slit-like fenestrations are found in half of TCCs [81], highlighting the resemblance to serous carcinoma. Cytologic atypia is usually prominent and corresponds to grade II or III papillary transitional cell carcinoma of the urinary tract. High-grade pleomorphic nuclear features and bizarre giant cells occur in about one third, further supporting that these tumors are transitional-like variants of serous carcinoma. In the solid type of malignant Brenner tumor with angulated and disorderly nests, mild or moderate atypia may be present (➲ *Fig. 14.132*). Mitotic activity may be prominent. In addition, malignant Brenner tumors, like their benign counterparts, often have prominent stromal calcification that is usually spiculated, in contrast to TCCs in which calcification is less common and more often psammomatous.

Immunohistochemistry

Ovarian TCCs are positive for CK7 as well as WT1, p16, and p53 [66, 206]. They are negative for CK 20 in contrast to TCCs of the urinary tract, which are usually CK20 positive. EGFR, Ras, and cyclin D1 are usually weakly reactive or negative [66]. A minority of TCCs are positive for CEA and CA 19-9. Urothelial markers uroplakin III and thrombomodulin are positive in only a small minority [187, 246, 271]. Published data on the immunohistochemistry of malignant Brenner tumors are very limited.

Differential Diagnosis

On occasion, a predominantly solid serous carcinoma resembles TCC due to dropout of large areas of necrosis, which gives rise to an undulating or apparent

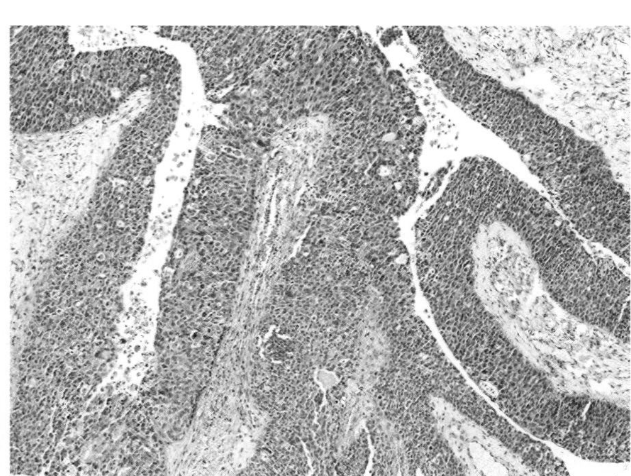

Fig. 14.131
Transitional cell carcinoma (TCC). **Thick papillae are lined by malignant epithelium resembling urothelium and mimicking papillary transitional cell carcinoma of the urinary tract**

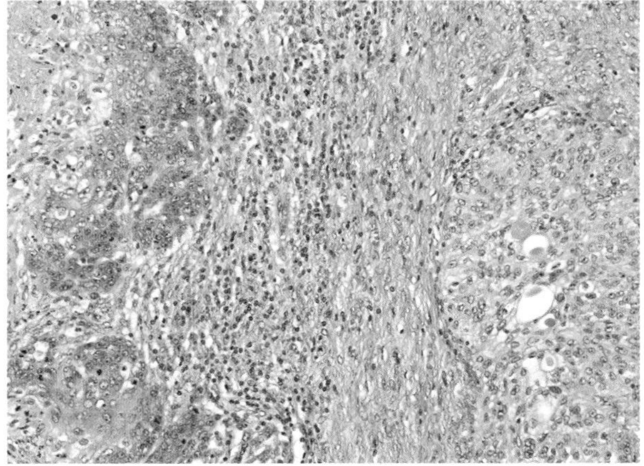

Fig. 14.132
Malignant Brenner tumor. **Infiltrating high-grade carcinoma on the *left*, and Brenner nest with only mild atypia on *right***

macropapillary pattern [81]. TCCs must be distinguished from metastatic TCC from the urinary tract. This is rarely a clinical problem as urothelial carcinomas that metastasize to the ovaries do so late in their evolution and are clinically evident.

Malignant Brenner tumor is diagnosed only in the presence of a benign or atypical proliferative Brenner component. Otherwise, a designation of TCC has been used. The appearance of thick, blunt papillae of transitional cell differentiation contrasts with the papillae of typical high-grade serous carcinoma, which are generally thinner.

Clinical Behavior and Treatment

Limited data suggesting that TCC is more chemosensitive than serous carcinoma have not shown a prognostic difference independent of stage and volume of residual disease [158]. Ovarian TCC is clinically different from malignant Brenner tumor. TCC presents in advanced stage, while most malignant Brenner tumors present in stage I. TCC is a variant of high-grade serous carcinoma and thus is a Type II tumor. This is supported by similar clinical and pathologic features between these two types of ovarian carcinoma, and an immunophenotype that more closely resembles serous carcinoma rather than TCC of the urinary tract. In contrast, malignant Brenner tumor has features of a Type I tumor (see ➋ Morphologic and Molecular Pathogenesis earlier in this chapter).

Squamous Tumors

Benign Squamous Tumors (Epidermoid Cyst)

Epidermoid cysts comprise 1.4% of ovarian epithelial tumors. They are lined by squamous epithelium and lack teratomatous elements. About half of these have either contralateral mature cystic teratomas suggesting that they are insufficiently sampled or monodermal teratomas, foci of Brenner tumor suggesting that they are Brenner tumors with squamous metaplasia, or features indicating a metaplastic change in endometriosis. Occasionally, other teratomatous elements are identified after extensive sampling of an apparent epidermoid cyst. Accordingly, pure epidermoid cyst is quite rare and comprises less than 1% of surface epithelial tumors [146].

Squamous Cell Carcinoma

Pure invasive squamous cell carcinoma is very rare, comprising 0.5% of ovarian carcinomas. In a series of 18 cases, endometriosis was found in 7 cases, and no underlying lesion was found in 11 cases. Invasive squamous cell carcinoma in the ovary is most commonly due to malignant transformation of a mature cystic teratoma; in such cases, the tumor is classified as a germ cell tumor with malignant transformation (see ➋ Chap. 16, Germ Cell Tumors of the Ovary). Rarely, metastatic disease from the uterine cervix is the source of squamous cell carcinoma in the ovary, and very rarely, in situ squamous cell carcinoma of the cervix spreads intraepithelially into the endometrium, fallopian tubes, and may involve the ovaries. Rare reports of nonteratomatous in situ squamous cell carcinoma of the ovary not extending from the cervix probably reflect atypical proliferative transitional cell tumors (see ➋ Atypical Proliferative Brenner (Transitional Cell) Tumors above). Rarely, an endometrioid carcinoma with a prominent metaplastic squamous component will mimic a pure squamous cell carcinoma.

The majority of patients with primary ovarian squamous cell carcinoma are in advanced stage and die within 1 year. Although data are limited, there appears to be a significantly worse prognosis compared to high-grade serous carcinoma as well as squamous cell carcinoma arising in a mature cystic teratoma.

Mixed Epithelial Tumors

The presence of two epithelial cell types in an ovarian epithelial neoplasm, each comprising at least 10% of the tumor, warrants a designation of a mixed epithelial tumor. Nonetheless, as mixed epithelial tumors are by necessity a heterogeneous group, it is more convenient and of no significant clinical import to ignore the minor components and classify tumors based solely on the predominant component, unless the minor component is malignant in an otherwise benign tumor, or is of a higher grade than the remainder of the tumor. As the prognosis for all cell types is essentially the same when stratified by stage, it is preferable to designate tumors based on the predominant component. We prefer to minimize the use of the mixed category, particularly for carcinomas, and accordingly require at least 25% of the minor component.

Serous and endometrioid differentiation may occur together. In particular, poorly differentiated serous and endometrioid carcinomas often display overlapping features, and at times, assignment to one or the other group is arbitrary and varies among observers. As discussed earlier, it has been suggested that there is no clinical or molecular basis for separating high-grade serous and endometrioid carcinomas. Many experts believe that most of these tumors are preferably classified as serous, reserving endometrioid for those tumors that display easily recognizable and characteristic features of eutopic endometrioid adenocarcinomas. Similarly, endometrioid and clear cell differentiation are not infrequently mixed. A mucinous component is often observed in benign transitional cell neoplasms (see "Mixed transitional cell–mucinous tumors"). Among atypical proliferative tumors, the most common mixed type is seromucinous, also called müllerian mucinous, or endocervical-like atypical proliferative ("borderline") mucinous tumor. Serous (papillary) architectural features and mucinous cytologic features in these tumors are often mixed with other cell types. However, APSMT is a unique variant of APST rather than simply a mixture of different cell types (see ➋ Atypical Proliferative Mucinous Tumor, Seromucinous (Endocervical-like or Müllerian) Type above).

Undifferentiated Carcinomas

Undifferentiated carcinomas show no readily identifiable features of any of the cell types of ovarian surface epithelial neoplasms. Therefore, any element of glands, papillae, or psammoma bodies removes a tumor from this category. Solid carcinomas with rare foci of glands or papillae are preferably classified as serous, although a few experts include such tumors in the undifferentiated category. There are four types of primary ovarian undifferentiated carcinoma, referred to as follows: undifferentiated carcinoma NOS, non-small-cell neuroendocrine carcinoma, the hypercalcemic type of small cell carcinoma, and the pulmonary type of small cell carcinoma. When strict pathologic criteria are employed for these diagnoses, all types are very uncommon, together comprising less than 1% of invasive carcinomas. In the Washington Hospital Center series of 435 carcinomas (➋ *Table 14.4*), there was a solitary case (0.23%) of undifferentiated small cell carcinoma (hypercalcemic type). In all cases when a diagnosis of undifferentiated carcinoma is considered, it is very important to exclude metastatic tumor, particularly from the lungs.

Although data are limited, undifferentiated carcinoma NOS appears to be more common than the other three types that are very rare. The small cell type of undifferentiated carcinoma associated with hypercalcemia is the most common type of undifferentiated carcinoma in women <40 years. The usual type of undifferentiated carcinoma shares many clinical and pathologic features with high-grade serous carcinoma. The mean age at presentation is 60 years. Seventy-eight percent present in stages III and IV. Tumors are composed of solid sheets of large pleomorphic cells with high-grade nuclear features, and usually with abundant cytoplasm that is often eosinophilic. Immunoperoxidase stains for epithelial markers (EMA, CAM 5.2, and B72.3) are positive. In nearly all cases, CK7 is positive and CK20 is negative; 21% stain for CEA, and 79% for OC-125. Overall, 22% survive 5 years, but only 14% of stage III and IV patients survive 5 years. Although overall survival appears worse than that for serous carcinoma, when stratified by stage, they do not have a significantly worse prognosis.

Non-small cell neuroendocrine carcinoma is usually associated with another cell type of surface epithelial carcinoma, most often mucinous carcinoma [241, 368], and therefore is best classified according to the better-differentiated component. Undifferentiated small cell carcinoma associated with hypercalcemia is a distinctive neoplasm, and is described in detail in ➋ Chap. 15, Sex Cord-Stromal, Steroid Cell, and Other Ovarian Tumors with Endocrine, Paraendocrine, Paraneoplastic Manifestations. Undifferentiated small cell carcinoma, pulmonary type, is extremely rare and is described in ➋ Chap. 17, Nonspecific Tumors of the Ovary Including Mesenchymal Tumors.

Malignant Mixed Mesodermal Tumor (Carcinosarcoma)

Previously thought to be rare, MMMTs comprise about 7.5% of ovarian carcinomas in the United States (➋ *Table 14.4*) and 2.5% in Thailand [147]. The mean age, 64–66 years, is higher than that for serous carcinoma [198]. These tumors are typically large, ranging from 15–20 cm in diameter. The stage distribution is identical to that of serous carcinoma [35]. The morphology is similar to its uterine counterpart (see ➋ Chap. 9, Endometrial Carcinoma). The characteristic microscopic feature is an intimate admixture of malignant epithelial and stromal elements. The malignant epithelial element is most commonly a high-grade serous or endometrioid carcinoma, but can be of any of the surface epithelial cell types of ovarian tumors. The stromal component usually contains sheets of hyperchromatic rounded to spindled cells with marked nuclear atypia and a high mitotic index. Heterologous elements, most commonly cartilage, osteoid, and rhabdomyoblasts, are commonly found and, as in the uterine counterpart, their frequency depends on the diligence with which they are sought. Occasionally, a tumor that is otherwise a typical carcinoma has a small focus of malignant stroma. Although there are few published data on such tumors, they are classified as MMMTs. Immunohistochemical stains for epithelial markers are often positive in the sarcomatous component, and their behavior and patterns of spread are similar to high-grade serous carcinomas. Like endometrial carcinosarcomas, the majority have been demonstrated to be monoclonal [140]. These observations suggest that these tumors should be classified as metaplastic carcinomas like their uterine counterparts [201], and accordingly represent a Type II tumor (see ➲ Morphologic and Molecular Pathogenesis earlier in this chapter). Immunohistochemistry for skeletal muscle markers such as desmin, MyoD1, and myogenin can be used to help identify heterologous rhabdomyoblasts. In the older literature, MMMTs were considered aggressive, rapidly fatal tumors with a median survival of ~1 year, but more recent data suggest that with cisplatin and either a taxane or ifosfamide therapy, survival rates approaching those for serous carcinoma can be achieved [181, 324]. When stratified by stage, however, limited data suggest that the prognosis is worse than that for serous carcinoma [35, 198]. Most but not all studies have shown that like their uterine counterpart the presence of heterologous elements does not influence prognosis [13].

Sarcomas

Though nonepithelial, these tumors are included in this chapter for convenience. Although primary pure or mixed sarcomas of the ovary are very uncommon, they constitute a heterogeneous group with four different types of neoplasms: endometrioid stromal sarcoma, adenosarcoma, sarcoma arising in a mature teratoma, and miscellaneous soft tissue sarcomas. Most carcinosarcomas are no longer considered sarcomas and are discussed above (see ➲ Malignant Mixed Mesodermal Tumor (Carcinosarcoma) above). All of these tumors are extremely rare. Sarcomas arising in teratomas are classified as germ cell tumors with secondary malignant transformation (see ➲ Chap. 16, Germ Cell Tumors of the Ovary). Miscellaneous soft tissue sarcomas rarely arise in the ovary. Their pathologic features do not appear to be significantly different from their soft tissue counterparts (see ➲ Chap. 22, Soft Tissue Lesions Involving Female Reproductive Organs).

Endometrioid Stromal Sarcoma (ESS)

ESS is an extremely rare primary ovarian neoplasm that is morphologically identical to its uterine counterpart (see ➲ Chap. 10, Mesenchymal Tumors of the Uterus). Among approximately 27 reported cases, 63% have been closely associated with endometriosis from which the tumor probably arises. The mean patient age is 52 years. The mean tumor size is 10 cm. Over 70% present in advanced stage (FIGO II–III). Since primary uterine ESS is often slow growing and prone to late recurrence, it is important to consider the possibility of metastatic tumor from a uterine primary, even if the patient has had a hysterectomy in the remote past. Ovarian sex cord–stromal tumors with a predominant spindle cell component, including cellular fibroma, thecoma, and poorly differentiated SLCT, are also important differential diagnostic considerations, and rarely an ovarian stromal tumor will have spindle cell patterns that are virtually identical to ESS. The behavior appears to parallel that of advanced-stage uterine ESS, although data are limited.

Müllerian Adenosarcoma and "Aggressive Endometriosis"

Müllerian adenosarcoma of the ovary is very rare. It is morphologically similar to its uterine counterpart (see ➲ Chap. 10, Mesenchymal Tumors of the Uterus). Nearly 60 cases have been reported [82]. The mean age is 54 and the mean tumor size is 14 cm; 65% present in FIGO stage I. Nearly all cases are unilateral. Grossly, the majority are predominantly solid with some cystic areas, and 10% are predominantly cystic. The characteristic microscopic feature is periglandular stromal condensation with atypia and mitotic activity in these hypercellular areas of stroma. Leaflike processes of stroma covered by a single layer of benign epithelium are another characteristic pattern. The mitotic index averages about 4 per 10 HPF. About 15% have sex cord-like elements and 30% have sarcomatous overgrowth. In the largest series [82], among 40 cases, 9 tumors were considered high grade (moderate or severe atypia and/or 10 or more mitoses per 10 HPF in the most active areas) and 31 were low grade; 63% of stage I tumors recurred. The 5-year recurrence-free survival was 45% for low grade and 25% for high grade. The overall 5-year survival is about 65%. Interestingly, among 40 patients, 2 had small synchronous adenosarcomas that appeared to be independent: one in the endometrium and one arising in appendiceal endometriosis.

Rarely, histologically benign endometriosis appears infiltrative to the surgeon and/or displays perineural and vascular invasion. The stroma can be cellular but there is no atypia and mitotic activity is very low. It can prove difficult to resect and consequently may display low-grade malignant behavior. This may be a form of low-grade adenosarcoma and has been referred to as "aggressive endometriosis." It has also been suggested that these are low-grade endometrial stromal sarcomas with endometrioid glandular differentiation [208]. There are no large series of this entity and it is therefore poorly understood (see Chap. 13, Diseases of the Peritoneum).

Acknowledgment

The authors thank Jonathan A. Cosin, M.D., for reviewing the clinical portions of the chapter, and Peter Russell, M.D., for his contributions in previous editions.

References

1. Acs G, Pasha T, Zhang PJ (2004) WT1 is differentially expressed in serous, endometrioid, clear cell, and mucinous carcinomas of the peritoneum, fallopian tube, ovary, and endometrium. Int J Gynecol Pathol 23:110–118
2. Agoff SN, Mendelin JE, Grieco VS et al (2002) Unexpected gynecologic neoplasms in patients with proven or suspected BRCA-1 or -2 mutations: implications for gross examination, cytology, and clinical follow-up. Am J Surg Pathol 26:171–178
3. Akahne T, Sekizawa A, Okuda T et al (2005) Disappearance of steroid hormone dependency during malignant transformation of ovarian clear cell cancer. Int J Gynecol Pathol 24:369–376
4. Akeson M, Jakobsen A-M, Zetterqvist BM et al (2009) A population-based 5-year cohort study including all cases of epithelial ovarian cancer in western Sweden: 10-year survival and prognostic factors. Int J Gynecol Cancer 19:116–123
5. Akeson M, Zetterqvist BM, Dahllof K et al (2008) Population-based cohort follow-up study of all patients operated for borderline ovarian tumor in western Sweden during an 11-year period. Int J Gynecol Cancer 18:453–459
6. Ali-Fehmi R, Khalifeh I, Bandyopadhyay S et al (2006) Patterns of loss of heterozygosity at 10q23.3 and microsatellite instability in endometriosis, atypical endometriosis, and ovarian carcinoma arising in association with endometriosis. Int J Gynecol Pathol 25: 223–229
7. Allison KH, Swisher EM, Kerkering KM et al (2008) Defining an appropriate threshold for the diagnosis of serous borderline tumor of the ovary: when is a full staging procedure unnecessary? Int J Gynecol Pathol 27:10–17
8. Alphs HH, Zahurak ML, Bristow RE et al (2006) Predictors of surgical outcome and survival among elderly women diagnosed with ovarian and primary peritoneal cancer. Gynecol Oncol 103:1048–1053
9. American Cancer Society (2008) Cancer facts and figures. American Cancer Society, Atlanta
10. Andersen MR, Goff BA, Lowe KA et al (2008) Combining a symptoms index with CA 125 to improve detection of ovarian cancer. Cancer 113:484–489
11. Arboleda MJ, Lyons JF, Kabbinavar FF et al (2003) Overexpression of AKT2/protein kinase beta leads to up-regulation of beta1 integrins, increased invasion, and metastasis of human breast and ovarian cancer cells. Cancer Res 63:196–206
12. Armes JE, Lourie R, de Silva M et al (2005) Abnormalities of the RB1 pathway in ovarian serous papillary carcinoma as determined by overexpression of the p16(INK4A) protein. Int J Gynecol Pathol 24:363–368
13. Athavale R, Thomakos N, Godfrey K et al (2007) The effect of epithelial and stromal tumor components on FIGO stages III and IV ovarian carcinosarcomas treated with primary surgery and chemotherapy. Int J Gynecol Cancer 17:1025–1030
14. Ayhan A, Al RA, Baykal C et al (2004) The influence of splenic metastases on survival in FIGO stage IIIC epithelial ovarian cancer. Int J Gynecol Cancer 14:51–56
15. Ayhan A, Gultekin M, Dorsun P et al (2008) Metastatic lymph node number in epithelial ovarian carcinoma: does it have any clinical significance? Gynecol Oncol 108:428–432
16. Ayhan A, Gultekin M, Taskiran C et al (2007) Ascites and epithelial ovarian cancers: a reappraisal with respect to different aspects. Int J Gynecol Cancer 17:68–75
17. Ayhan A, Guven ESG, Guven S et al (2005) Recurrence and prognostic factors in borderline ovarian tumors. Gynecol Oncol 98:439–445
18. Ayhan A, Kurman RJ, Vang R et al (2009) Defining the cut point between low grade and high grade ovarian serous carcinomas: a clinicopathologic and molecular genetic analysis. Am J Surg Pathol 33:1220–1224
19. Ayhan A, Taskiran C, Yigit-Celik N et al (2006) Long-term survival after paclitaxel plus platinum-based combination chemotherapy for extraovarian peritoneal serous papillary carcinoma: is it different from that for ovarian serous papillary cancer? Int J Gynecol Cancer 16:484–489
20. Baker PM, Oliva E (2005) Immunohistochemistry as a tool in the differential diagnosis of ovarian tumors: an update. Int J Gynecol Pathol 24:39–55
21. Baldwin RL, Nemeth E, Tran H et al (2000) BRCA1 promoter region hypermethylation in ovarian carcinoma: a population-based study. Cancer Res 60:5329–5333
22. Barda G, Menczer J, Chetrit A et al (2004) Comparison between primary peritoneal and epithelial ovarian carcinoma: a population-based study. Am J Obstet Gynecol 190:1039–1045
23. Bedrosian I, Lu KH, Verschraegen C et al (2004) Cyclin E deregulation alters the biologic properties of ovarian cancer cells. Oncogene 23:2648–2657
24. Bell DA, Longacre TA, Prat J et al (2004) Serous borderline (low malignant potential, atypical proliferative) ovarian tumors: workshop perspectives. Hum Pathol 35:934–948
25. Bell KA, Sehdev AES, Kurman RJ (2001) Refined diagnostic criteria for implants associated with ovarian atypical proliferative serous tumors (borderline) and micropapillary serous carcinomas. Am J Surg Pathol 25:419–432
26. Bloss JD, Brady MF, Liao SY et al (2003) Extraovarian peritoneal serous papillary carcinoma: a phase II trial of cisplatin and cyclophosphamide with comparison to a cohort with papillary serous ovarian carcinoma – A Gynecologic Oncology Group Study. Gynecol Oncol 89:148–154
27. Bommer GT, Gerin I, Feng Y et al (2007) p53-mediated activation of miRNA34 candidate tumor suppressor genes. Curr Biol 17: 1298–1307
28. Bonome T, Lee JY, Park DC et al (2005) Expression profiling of serous low malignant potential, low-grade, and high-grade tumors of the ovary. Cancer Res 65:10602–10612
29. Boyle P, Levin B (eds) (2008) World cancer report 2008. World Health Organization, Lyon

30. Bradley RF, Stewart JH, Russell GB et al (2006) Pseudomyxoma peritonei of appendiceal origin: a clinicopathologic analysis of 101 patients uniformly treated at a single institution, with literature review. Am J Surg Pathol 30:551–559
31. Brinkmann D, Ryan A, Ayhan A et al (2004) A molecular genetic and statistical approach for the diagnosis of dual-site cancers. J Natl Cancer Inst 96:1441–1446
32. Bristow RE, Chi DS (2006) Platinum-based neoadjuvant chemotherapy and interval surgical cytoreduction for advanced ovarian cancer: a meta-analysis. Gynecol Oncol 103:1070–1076
33. Bristow RE, Eisenhauer EL, Santillan A et al (2007) Delaying the primary surgical effort for advanced ovarian cancer: a systematic review of neoadjuvant chemotherapy and interval cytoreduction. Gynecol Oncol 104:480–490
34. Bristow RE, Gossett DR, Shook DR et al (2002) Recurrent micropapillary serous carcinoma: the role of secondary cytoreductive surgery. Cancer 95:791–800
35. Brown E, Stewart M, Rye T et al (2004) Carcinosarcoma of the ovary: 19 years of prospective data from a single center. Cancer 100: 2148–2153
36. Brustmann H (2007) Poly(adenosine diphosphate-ribose) polymerase expression in serous ovarian carcinoma: correlation with p53, MIB-1 and outcome. Int J Gynecol Pathol 26:147–153
37. Burks RT, Sherman ME, Kurman RJ (1996) Micropapillary serous carcinoma of the ovary. A distinctive low- grade carcinoma related to serous borderline tumors. Am J Surg Pathol 20:1319–1330
38. Buys SS, Partridge E, Greene MH et al (2005) Ovarian cancer screening in the Prostate, Lung, Colorectal and Ovarian (PLCO) cancer screening trial: findings from the initial screen of a randomized trial. Am J Obstet Gynecol 193:1630–1639
39. Cameron RI, Ashe P, O'Rourke DM et al (2003) A panel of immunohistochemical stains assists in the distinction between ovarian and renal clear cell carcinoma. Int J Gynecol Pathol 22:272–276
40. Campbell IG, Russell SE, Choong DY et al (2004) Mutation of the PIK3CA gene in ovarian and breast cancer. Cancer Res 64:7678–7681
41. Cannistra SA (2007) BRCA-1 in sporadic epithelial ovarian cancer: lessons learned from the genetics of hereditary disease. Clin Cancer Res 13:7225–7227
42. Carcangiu ML, Peissel B, Pasini B et al (2006) Incidental carcinomas in prophylactic specimens in BRCA1 and BRCA2 germ-line mutation carriers with emphasis on fallopian tube lesions: report of 6 cases and review of the literature. Am J Surg Pathol 30:1222–1230
43. Carcangiu ML, Radice P, Manoukian S et al (2004) Atypical epithelial proliferation in fallopian tubes in prophylactic salpingo-oophorectomy specimens from BRCA1 and BRCA2 germline mutation carriers. Int J Gynecol Pathol 23:35–40
44. Casey MJ, Synder C, Bewtra C et al (2005) Intra-abdominal carcinomatosis after prophylactic oophorectomy in women of hereditary breast ovarian cancer syndrome kindreds associated with BRCA1 and BRCA2 mutations. Gynecol Oncol 97:457–467
45. Catasus L, Bussaglia E, Rodriguez I et al (2004) Molecular genetic alterations in endometrioid carcinomas of the ovary: similar frequency of beta-catenin abnormalities but lower rate of microsatellite instability and PTEN alterations than in uterine endometrioid carcinomas. Hum Pathol 35:1360–1368
46. Catasus L, Gallardo A, Cuatrecasas M et al (2008) PIK3CA mutations in the kinase domain (exon 20) of uterine endometrial adenocarcinomas are associated with adverse prognostic parameters. Modern Pathol 21:131–139
47. Cathro HP, Stoler MH (2005) The utility of calretinin, inhibin and WT1 immunohistochemical staining in the differential diagnosis of ovarian tumors. Hum Pathol 36:195–201
48. Chambers SK (2005) Systematic lymphadenectomy in advanced epithelial ovarian cancer: two decades of uncertainty resolved. J Natl Cancer Inst 97:548–549
49. Chan JK, Teoh D, Hu JM et al (2008) Do clear cell ovarian carcinomas have poorer prognosis compared to other epithelial cell types? A study of 1411 clear cell ovarian cancers. Gynecol Oncol 109:370–376
50. Chan JK, Tian C, Monk B et al (2008) Prognostic factors for high-risk early-stage epithelial ovarian cancer: a Gynecologic Oncology Group study. Cancer 112:2202–2210
51. Chang SJ, Ryu HS, Chang KH et al (2008) Prognostic significance of the micropapillary pattern in patients with serous borderline ovarian tumors. Acta Obstet Gynecol Scand 87:476–481
52. Chen S, Leitao MM, Tornos C et al (2005) Invasion patterns in stage I endometrioid and mucinous ovarian carcinomas: a clinicopathologic analysis emphasizing favorable outcomes in carcinomas without destructive stromal invasion and the occasional malignant course of carcinomas with limited destructive stromal invasion. Modern Pathol 18:903–911
53. Chen S, Parmigiani G (2007) Meta-analysis of BRCA1 and BRCA2 penetrance. J Clin Oncol 25:1329–1333
54. Cheng EJ, Kurman RJ, Wang M et al (2004) Molecular genetic analysis of ovarian serous cystadenomas. Lab Invest 84:778–784
55. Chiesa-Vottero AG, Malpica A, Deavers MT et al (2007) Immunohistochemical overexpression of p16 and p53 in uterine serous carcinoma and ovarian high-grade serous carcinoma. Int J Gynecol Pathol 26:328–333
56. Cho KR, Shih IM (2009) Ovarian Cancer. Annu Rev Pathol Mech Dis 4:287–313
57. Chung HH, Hwang SY, Jung KW et al (2007) Ovarian cancer incidence and survival in Korea. Int J Gynecol Cancer 17:595–600
58. Cliby WA, Aletti GD, Wilson TO et al (2006) Is it justified to classify patients to stage IIIC epithelial ovarian cancer based on nodal involvement only? Gynecol Oncol 103:797–801
59. Colgan TJ (2003) Challenges in the early diagnosis and staging of fallopian-tube carcinomas associated with BRCA mutations. Int J Gynecol Pathol 22:109–120
60. Colgan TJ, Boerner SL, Murphy J et al (2002) Peritoneal lavage cytology: an assessment of its value during prophylactic oophorectomy. Gynecol Oncol 85:397–403
61. Colgan TJ, Murphy J, Cole DEC et al (2001) Occult carcinoma in prophylactic oophorectomy specimens: prevalence and association with BRCA germline mutation status. Am J Surg Pathol 25:1283–1289
62. Collaborative Group on Epidemiological Studies of Ovarian Cancer (2008) Ovarian cancer and oral contraceptives: collaborative reanalysis of data from 45 epidemiological studies including 23,257 women with ovarian cancer and 87,303 controls. Lancet 371:303–314
63. Comin CE, Saieva C, Messerini L (2007) h-caldesmon, calretinin, estrogen receptor, and Ber-EP4: a useful combination of immunohistochemical markers for differentiating epithelioid peritoneal mesothelioma from serous papillary carcinoma of the ovary. Am J Surg Pathol 31:1139–1148
64. Connolly DC, Bao R, Nikitin AY et al (2003) Female mice chimeric for expression of the simian virus 40 TAg under control of the MISIIR promoter develop epithelial ovarian cancer. Cancer Res 63:1389–1397
65. Cosary CL (2007) Chapter 16: Cancer of the ovary. In: Ries LAG et al (eds) SEER survival monograph. Cancer survival among adults. US SEER program, 1988-2001. Patient and tumors characteristics. National Cancer Institute, NIH publication no. 07-6215

66. Cuatrecasas M, Catasus L, Palacios J et al (2009) Transitional cell tumors of the ovary: a comparative clinicopathologic, immunohistochemical, and molecular genetic analysis of Brenner tumors and transitional cell carcinomas. Am J Surg Pathol 33:556–567
67. Cuatrecasas M, Villanueva A, Matias-Guiu X et al (1997) K-ras mutations in mucinous ovarian tumors: a clinicopathologic and molecular study of 95 cases. Cancer 79:1581–1586
68. Cusido M, Balaguero L, Hernandez G et al (2007) Results of the national survey of borderline ovarian tumors in Spain. Gynecol Oncol 104:617–622
69. Davidson B, Skrede M, Silins I et al (2007) Low-molecular weight forms of cyclin E differentiate ovarian carcinoma from cells of mesothelial origin and are associated with poor survival in ovarian carcinoma. Cancer 110:1264–1271
70. Deavers MT, Gershenson DM, Tortolero-Luna G et al (2002) Micropapillary and cribriform patterns in ovarian serous tumors of low malignant potential: a study of 99 advanced stage cases. Am J Surg Pathol 26:1129–1141
71. Demopoulos RI, Aronov R, Mesia A (2001) Clues to the pathogenesis of fallopian tube carcinoma: a morphological and immunohistochemical case control study. Int J Gynecol Pathol 20:128–132
72. Dent J, Hall GD, Wilkinson N et al (2003) Cytogenetic alterations in ovarian clear cell carcinoma detected by comparative genomic hybridisation. Br J Cancer 88:1578–1583
73. Di Cristofano A, Ellenson LH (2007) Endometrial carcinoma. Annu Rev Pathol 2:57–85
74. Diebold J, Seemuller F, Lohrs U (2003) K-RAS mutations in ovarian and extraovarian lesions of serous tumors of borderline malignancy. Lab Invest 83:251–258
75. Dinulescu DM, Ince TA, Quade BJ et al (2005) Role of K-ras and Pten in the development of mouse models of endometriosis and endometrioid ovarian cancer. Nat Med 11:63–67
76. Djordjevic B, Malpica A (2010) Lymph node involvement in ovarian serous tumors of low malignant potential: a clinicopathologic study of thirty-six cases. Am J Surg Pathol 34:1–9
77. Dube V, Roy M, Plante M et al (2005) Mucinous ovarian tumors of mullerian-type: an analysis of 17 cases including borderline tumors and intraepithelial, microinvasive, and invasive carcinomas. Int J Gynecol Pathol 24:138–146
78. Dusenbery KE, Bellairs EE, Potish RA et al (2005) Twenty-five year outcome of sequential abdominal radiotherapy and melphalan: implications for future management of epithelial carcinoma of the ovary. Gynecol Oncol 96:307–313
79. Earle CC, Schrag D, Neville BA et al (2006) Effect of surgeon specialty on processes of care and outcomes for ovarian cancer patients. J Nat Cancer Inst 98:172–180
80. Eichorn JH, Bell DA, Young RH et al (1999) Ovarian serous borderline tumors with micropapillary and cribriform patterns: a study of 40 cases and comparison with 44 cases without these patterns. Am J Surg Pathol 23:397–409
81. Eichorn JH, Young RH (2004) Transitional cell carcinoma of the ovary: a morphologic study of 100 cases with emphasis on differential diagnosis. Am J Surg Pathol 28:453–463
82. Eichorn JH, Young RH, Clement PB et al (2002) Mesodermal (mullerian) adenosarcoma of the ovary: a clinicopathologic analysis of 40 cases and a review of the literature. Am J Surg Pathol 26:1243–1258
83. Eisenkop SM, Spirtos NM, Lin W-CM (2006) "Optimal" cytoreduction for advanced epithelial ovarian cancer: a commentary. Gynecol Oncol 103:329–335
84. Elishaev E, Gilks CB, Miller D et al (2005) Synchronous and metachronous endocervical and ovarian neoplasms: evidence supporting interpretation of the ovarian neoplasms as metastatic endocervical adenocarcinomas simulating primary ovarian surface epithelial neoplasms. Am J Surg Pathol 29:281–294
85. Enomoto T, Weghorst CM, Inoue M et al (1991) K-ras activation occurs frequently in mucinous adenocarcinomas and rarely in other common epithelial tumors of the human ovary. Am J Pathol 139:777–785
86. Euscher ED, Malpica A, Deavers MT et al (2005) Differential expression of WT-1 in serous carcinomas in the peritoneum with or without associated serous carcinoma in endometrial polyps. Am J Surg Pathol 29:1074–1078
87. Euscher ED, Silva EG, Deavers MT et al (2004) Serous carcinoma of the ovary, fallopian tube, or peritoneum presenting as lymphadenopathy. Am J Surg Pathol 28:1217–1223
88. Finch A, Beiner B, Lubinski J et al (2006) Salpingo-oophorectomy and the risk of ovarian, fallopian tube, and peritoneal cancers in women with a BRCA1 or BRCA2 mutation. JAMA 296:185–192
89. Flesken-Nikitin A, Choi KC, Eng JP et al (2003) Induction of carcinogenesis by concurrent inactivation of p53 and Rb1 in the mouse ovarian surface epithelium. Cancer Res 63:3459–3463
90. Fritz A, Percy C, Jack A et al (2000) International classification of diseases for oncology, 3rd edn. WHO, Geneva
91. Fuji H, Matsumoto T, Yoshida M et al (2002) Genetics of synchronous uterine and ovarian endometrioid carcinoma: combined analyses of loss of heterozygosity, PTEN mutation, and microsatellite instability. Hum Pathol 33:421–428
92. Fujimara M, Hidaka T, Kataoka K et al (2001) Absence of estrogen receptor–[alpha] expression in human ovarian clear cell adenocarcinoma compared with ovarian serous, endometrioid, and mucinous adenocarcinoma. Am J Surg Pathol 25:667–672
93. Fujita M, Enomoto T, Wada H et al (1996) Application of clonal analysis-differential diagnosis for synchronous primary ovarian and endometrial cancers and metastatic cancer. Am J Clin Pathol 105:350–359
94. Fujita M, Enomoto T, Yoshino K et al (1995) Microsatellite instability and alterations in the hMSH2 gene in human ovarian cancer. Int J Cancer 64:361–366
95. Furuya M, Suyama T, Usui H et al (2007) Up-regulation of CXC chemokines and their receptors: implications for proinflammatory microenvironments of ovarian carcinomas and endometriosis. Hum Pathol 38:1676–1687
96. Gaarenstroom KN, van der Hiel B, Tollenaar RAEM et al (2006) Efficacy of screening women at high risk of hereditary ovarian cancer: results of an 11-year cohort study. Int J Gynecol Cancer 16 (suppl 1):54–59
97. Gadducci A, Conte PF (2008) Intraperitoneal chemotherapy in the management of patients with advanced epithelial ovarian cancer: a critical review of the literature. Int J Gynecol Cancer 18:943–953
98. Gamallo C, Palacios J, Moreno G et al (1999) beta-catenin expression pattern in stage I and II ovarian carcinomas: relationship with beta-catenin gene mutations, Clinicopathological features, and clinical outcome. Amer J Pathol 155:527–536
99. Garg R, Zahurak ML, Trimble EL et al (2005) Abdominal carcinomatosis in women with a history of breast cancer. Gynecol Oncol 99:65–70
100. Gayther SA, Mangion J, Russell P et al (1997) Variation of risks of breast and ovarian cancer associated with different germline mutations of the BRCA2 gene. Nat Genet 15:103–105
101. Geisler JP, Goodheart MJ, Sood AK et al (2003) Mismatch repair gene expression defects contribute to microsatellite instability in ovarian carcinoma. Cancer 98:2199–2206

102. Gemignani ML, Schlaerth AC, Bogomolniy F et al (2003) Role of KRAS and BRAF gene mutations in mucinous ovarian carcinoma. Gynecol Oncol 90:378–381
103. Gershenson DM, Sun CC, Lu KH et al (2006) Clinical behavior of stage II-IV low-grade serous carcinoma of the ovary. Obstet Gynecol 108:361–368
104. Gilks CB (2004) Subclassification of ovarian surface epithelial tumors based on correlation of histologic and molecular pathologic data. Int J Gynecol Pathol 23:200–205
105. Gilks CB, Alkushi A, Yue JJW et al (2003) Advanced-stage serous borderline tumors of the ovary: a clinicopathological study of 49 cases. Int J Gynecol Pathol 22:29–36
106. Gilks CB, Ionescu DN, Kalloger SE et al (2008) Tumor cell type can be reproducibly diagnosed and is of independent prognostic significance in patients with maximally debulked ovarian carcinoma. Hum Pathol 39:1239–1251
107. Gilks CB, Kobel M, Kalloger SE et al (2009) Significant differences in tumor cell type in early versus advanced stage ovarian carcinoma. Modern Pathol 22(S1):215A
108. Goldstein NS, Ceniza N (2000) Ovarian micropapillary serous borderline tumors: clinicopathologic features and outcome of seven surgically staged patients. Am J Clin Pathol 114:380–386
109. Gomes CP, Andrade LALA (2006) PTEN and p53 expression in primary ovarian carcinomas: immunohistochemical study and discussion of pathogenetic mechanisms. Int J Gynecol Cancer 16(suppl1):254–258
110. Goodman MT, Shvetzov YB (2009) Incidence of ovarian, peritoneal and fallopian tube carcinomas in the United States, 1995-2004. Cancer Epidemiol Biomarkers Prev 18:132–139
111. Granstrom C, Sundquist J, Hemminki K (2008) Population attributable fractions for ovarian cancer in Swedish women by morphological type. Br J Cancer 98:199–205
112. Gu J, Roth LM, Younger C et al (2001) Molecular evidence for the independent origin of extraovarian papillary serous tumors of low malignant potential. J Natl Cancer Inst 93:1122–1123
113. Gutgemann I, Lehman N, Jackson PK et al (2008) Emi1 protein accumulation implicates misregulation of the anaphase promoting complex/cyclosome pathway in ovarian clear cell carcinoma. Modern Pathol 21:445–454
114. Guth U, Huang DJ, Bauer G et al (2007) Metastatic patterns at autopsy in patients with ovarian carcinoma. Cancer 110: 1272–1280
115. Halperin R, Zehavi S, Langer R et al (2001) Primary peritoneal serous papillary carcinoma: a new epidemiologic trend? A matched-case comparison with ovarian serous papillary cancer. Int J Gynecol Cancer 11:403–408
116. Han G, Gilks CB, Leung S et al (2008) Mixed ovarian epithelial carcinomas with clear cell and serous components are variants of high-grade serous carcinoma: an interobserver correlative and immunohistochemical study of 32 cases. Am J Surg Pathol 32:955–964
117. Harter P, Gnauert K, Hils R et al (2007) Pattern and clinical predictors of lymph node metastases in epithelial ovarian cancer. Int J Gynecol Cancer 17:1238–1244
118. Hashi A, Yuminamochi T, Murata S-I et al (2003) Wilms tumor gene reactivity in primary serous carcinomas of the fallopian tube, ovary, endometrium, and peritoneum. Int J Gynecol Pathol 22:374–377
119. Heintz APM, Odicino F, Maisonneuve P et al (2006) Carcinoma of the ovary. In: 26th annual report on the results of treatment in gynecological cancer. Int J Gynecol Obstet 95(Suppl 1):S161–S192
120. Heinzelmann-Schwarz VA, Gardiner-Garden M, Henshall SM et al (2006) A distinct molecular profile associated with mucinous epithelial ovarian cancer. Br J Cancer 94:904–913
121. Heller DS, Murphy P, Westhoff C (2005) Are germinal inclusion cysts markers of ovulation? Gynecol Oncol 96:496–499
122. Hermsen BBJ, von Mensdorff-Pouilly S, Berkhof J et al (2007) Serum CA125 in relation to adnexal dysplasia and cancer in women at hereditary high risk of ovarian cancer. J Clin Oncol 25:1383–1389
123. Hess LM, Benham-Hutchins M, Herzog TJ et al (2007) A meta-analysis of the efficacy of intraperitoneal cisplatin for the front-line treatment of ovarian cancer. Int J Gynecol Cancer 17:561–570
124. Highlander B, Repasky E, Shrikant P et al (2006) Expression of Wilm's tumor gene (WT1) in epithelial ovarian cancer. Gynecol Oncol 101:12–17
125. Ho CL, Kurman RJ, Dehari R et al (2004) Mutations of BRAF and KRAS precede the development of ovarian serous borderline tumors. Cancer Res 64:6915–6918
126. Hogg R, Scurry J, Kim SN et al (2007) Microinvasion links ovarian serous borderline tumor and grade 1 invasive carcinoma. Gynecol Oncol 106:44–51
127. Holland WW, Stewart S, Masseria C (2006) Policy brief: screening in Europe. World Health Organization; European Observatory on Health Systems and Policies. http://www.euro.who.int/Document/E88698.pdf. Accessed 9 Feb 2008
128. Hough CD, Cho KR, Zonderman AB et al (2001) Coordinately up-regulated genes in ovarian cancer. Cancer Res 61:3869–3876
129. Hough CD, Sherman-Baust CA, Pizer ES et al (2000) Large-scale serial analysis of gene expression reveals genes differentially expressed in ovarian cancer. Cancer Res 60:6281–6287
130. Howell NR, Zheng W, Cheng L et al (2007) Carcinomas of ovary and lung with clear cell features: can immunohistochemistry help in differential diagnosis? Int J Gynecol Pathol 26:134–140
131. Hsu CY, Bristow R, Cha MS et al (2004) Characterization of active mitogen-activated protein kinase in ovarian serous carcinomas. Clin Cancer Res 10:6432–6436
132. Hsu C-Y, Kurman RJ, Vang R et al (2005) Nuclear size distinguishes low- from high-grade ovarian serous carcinoma and predicts outcome. Hum Pathol 36:1049–1054
133. Ichikawa Y, Nishida M, Suzuki H et al (1994) Mutation of K-ras protooncogene is associated with histological subtypes in human mucinous ovarian tumors. Cancer Res 54:33–35
134. Jaaback KS, Ludeman L, Clayton NL et al (2006) Primary peritoneal carcinoma in a UK cancer center: comparison with advanced ovarian carcinoma over a 5-year period. Int J Gynecol Cancer 16(suppl1):123–128
135. Jaeger W, Ackermann S, Kessler H et al (2001) The effect of bowel resection on survival in advanced epithelial ovarian cancer. Gynecol Oncol 83:286–291
136. Jemal A, Siegel R, Ward E et al (2008) Cancer statistics, 2008. CA Cancer J Clin 58:71–96
137. Jemal A, Siegel R, Xu J, Ward E (2010) Cancer statistics 2010. American Cancer Society, Inc. doi:10.1002/caac.20073. Accessed July 21 2010
138. Jensen KC, Mariappan MR, Putcha GV et al (2008) Microsatellite instability and mismatch repair protein defects in ovarian epithelial neoplasms in patients 50 years of age and younger. Am J Surg Pathol 32:1029–1037
139. Ji H, Isacson C, Seidman JD et al (2002) Cytokeratins 7 and 20, Dpc4, and MUC5AC in the distinction of metastatic mucinous carcinomas in the ovary from primary ovarian mucinous tumors:

Dpc4 assists in identifying metastatic pancreatic carcinomas. Int J Gynecol Pathol 21:391–400

140. Jin Z, Ogata S, Tamura G et al (2003) Carcinosarcomas (malignant mullerian mixed tumors) of the uterus and ovary: a genetic study with special reference to histogenesis. Int J Gynecol Pathol 22: 368–373
141. Jordan SJ, Green AC, Whiteman DC et al (2007) Risk factors for benign, borderline and invasive mucinous ovarian tumors: epidemiologic evidence of a neoplastic continuum? Gynecol Oncol 107:223–230
142. Karam AK, Stempel M, Barakat R et al (2009) Patients with a history of epithelial ovarian cancer presenting with a breast and/or axillary mass. Gynecol Oncol 112:490–495
143. Kauff ND, Satagopan JM, Robson ME et al (2002) Risk-reducing salpingo-oophorectomy in women with a BRCA1 or BRCA2 mutation. N Engl J Med 346:1609–1615
144. Khalifeh I, Munkarah AR, Lonardo F et al (2004) Expression of cox-2, CD34, Bcl-2, and p53 and survival in patients with primary peritoneal serous carcinoma and ovarian serous carcinoma. Int J Gynecol Pathol 23:162–169
145. Khalifeh I, Munkarah AR, Schimp V et al (2005) The impact of c-Kit and Ki-67 expression on patients prognosis in advanced ovarian serous carcinoma. Int J Gynecol Pathol 24:228–234
146. Khedmati F, Chirolas C, Seidman JD (2009) Ovarian and paraovarian squamous-lined cysts (epidermoid cysts): a clinicopathologic study of 18 cases with comparison to mature cystic teratomas. Int J Gynecol Pathol 28:193–196
147. Khunamornpong S, Suprasert P, Na Chiangmai W et al (2006) Metastatic tumors to the ovaries: a study of 170 cases in Northern Thailand. Int J Gynecol Cancer 16(suppl 1):132–138
148. Kim KR, Lee HI, Lee SK et al (2007) Is stromal microinvasion in primary mucinous ovarian tumors with "mucin granuloma" true invasion? Am J Surg Pathol 31:546–554
149. Kindelberger DW, Lee Y, Miron A et al (2007) Intraepithelial carcinoma of the fimbria and pelvic serous carcinoma: evidence for a causal relationship. Am J Surg Pathol 31:161–169
150. King BL, Carcangiu ML, Carter D et al (1995) Microsatellite instability in ovarian neoplasms. Br J Cancer 72:376–382
151. Klaren HM, van't Veer LJ, van Leeuwen FE et al (2003) Potential for bias in studies on efficacy of prophylactic surgery for BRCA1 and BRCA2 mutation. J Natl Cancer Inst 95:941–947
152. Kobayashi H, Sumimoto K, Moniwa N et al (2007) Risk of developing ovarian cancer among women with ovarian endometrioma: a cohort study in Shizuoka, Japan. Int J Gynecol Cancer 17:37–43
153. Kobayashi H, Yamada Y, Sado T et al (2008) A randomized study of screening for ovarian cancer: a multicenter study in Japan. Int J Gynecol Cancer 18:414–420
154. Kobel M, Kalloger SE, Baker PM et al (2010) Diagnosis of ovarian carcinoma cell type is highly reproducible: a transcanadian study. Am J Surg Pathol 34:984–993
155. Kobel M, Kalloger SE, Carrick J et al (2009) A limited panel of immunomarkers can reliably distinguish clear cell and high grade serous carcinoma of the ovary. Am J Surg Pathol 33:14–21
156. Kobel M, Xu H, Bourne PA et al (2009) IGF2BP3 (IMP3) expression is a marker of unfavorable prognosis in ovarian carcinoma of clear cell subtype. Modern Pathol 22:469–475
157. Kolasa IK, Rembiszewska A, Janiec-Jankowska A et al (2006) PTEN mutation, expression and LOH at its locus in ovarian carcinomas. Relation to TP53, K-RAS and BRCA1 mutations. Gynecol Oncol 103:692–697
158. Kommoss F, Kommoss S, Schmidt D et al (2005) Survival benefit for patients with advanced-stage transitional cell carcinomas vs. other subtypes of ovarian carcinoma after chemotherapy with platinum and paclitaxel. Gynecol Oncol 97:195–199
159. Korner M, Burckhardt E, Mazzucchelli L (2006) Higher frequency of chromosomal aberrations in ovarian endometriosis compared to extragonadal endometriosis: a possible link to endometrioid adenocarcinoma. Modern Pathol 19:1615–1623
160. Kraus JA, Seidman JD (2010) The relationship between papillary infarction and microinvasion in ovarian atypical proliferative ("borderline") serous and seromucinous tumors. Int J Gynecol Pathol 29:303–309
161. Krishnamurti U, Sasatomi E, Swalsky PA et al (2005) Microdissection-based mutational genotyping of serous borderline tumors of the ovary. Int J Gynecol Pathol 24:56–61
162. Kubba LA, McCluggage WG, Liu J et al (2008) Thyroid transcription factor-1 expression in ovarian epithelial neoplasms. Modern Pathol 21:485–490
163. Kumaran GC, Jayson GC, Clamp AR (2009) Antiangiogenic drugs in ovarian cancer. Br J Cancer 100:1–7
164. Kuo KT, Buan B, Feng Y et al (2009) Analysis of DNA copy number alterations in ovarian serous tumors identifies new molecular genetic changes in low-grade and high-grade carcinomas. Cancer Res 69:4036–4042
165. Kuo KT, Mao TL, Jones S et al (2009) Frequent activating mutations of PIK3CA in ovarian clear cell carcinoma. Am J Pathol 174: 1597–1601
166. Kurian AW, Balise RR, McGuire V et al (2005) Histologic types of epithelial ovarian cancer: have they different risk factors? Gynecol Oncol 96:520–530
167. Kurman RJ, Shih I-M (2008) Pathogenesis of ovarian cancer: lessons from morphology and molecular biology and their clinical implications. Int J Gynecol Pathol 27:151–160
168. Kurman RJ, Shih I-M (2010) The origin and pathogenesis of epithelial ovarian cancer: a proposed unifying theory. Am J Surg Pathol 34:433–443
169. Kurman RJ, Trimble CL (1993) The behavior of serous tumors of low malignant potential: are they ever malignant? Int J Gynecol Pathol 12:120–127
170. Kurman RJ, Visvanathan K, Roden R et al (2008) Early detection and treatment of ovarian cancer: shifting from early stage to minimal volume of disease based on a new model of carcinogenesis. Am J Obstet Gynecol 198:351–356
171. Laki F, Kirova YM, This P et al (2007) Prophylactic salpingo-oophorectomy in a series of 89 women carrying a BRCA1 or a BRCA2 mutation. Cancer 109:1784–1790
172. Lamb JD, Garcia RL, Goff BA et al (2006) Predictors of occultneoplasia in women undergoing risk-reducing salpingo-oophorectomy. Am J Obstet Gynecol 194:1702–1709
173. Le T, Shahriari P, Hopkins L et al (2006) Prognostic significance of tumor necrosis in ovarian cancer patients treated with neoadjuvant chemotherapy and interval surgical debulking. Int J Gynecol Cancer 16:986–990
174. Lee CH, Huntsman DG, Cheang MCU et al (2005) Assessment of Her-1, Her-2, and Her-3 expression and Her-2 amplification in advanced stage ovarian carcinoma. Int J Gynecol Pathol 24:147–152
175. Lee KW, Kang NJ, Heo YS et al (2008) Raf and MEK protein kinases are direct molecular targets for the chemopreventive effect of quercetin, a major flavonol in red wine. Cancer Res 68:946–955
176. Lee ES, Leong AS-Y, Kim Y-S et al (2006) Calretinin, CD34 and α–smooth muscle actin in the identification of peritoneal invasive

implants of serous borderline tumors of the ovary. Modern Pathol 19:364–372

177. Lee KR, Nucci MR (2003) Ovarian mucinous and mixed epithelial carcinomas of mullerian (endocervical-like) type: a clinicopathologic analysis of four cases of an uncommon variant associated with endometriosis. Int J Gynecol Pathol 22:42–51
178. Lee P, Rosen DG, Zhu C et al (2005) Expression of progesterone receptor is a favorable prognostic marker in ovarian cancer. Gynecol Oncol 96:671–677
179. Lee KR, Scully RE (2000) Mucinous tumors of the ovary: a clinicopathologic study of 196 borderline tumors (of intestinal type) and carcinomas, including an evaluation of 11 cases with "pseudomyxoma peritonei". Am J Surg Pathol 24:1447–1464
180. Leeper K, Garcia R, Swisher C et al (2002) Pathologic findings in prophylactic oophorectomy specimens in high-risk women. Gynecol Oncol 87:52–56
181. Leiser AL, Chi DS, Ishill NM et al (2007) Carcinosarcoma of the ovary treated with platinum and taxane: the memorial Sloan-Kettering Cancer Center experience. Gynecol Oncol 105:657–661
182. Leitao MM, Boyd J, Hummer A et al (2004) Clinicopathologic analysis of early-stage sporadic ovarian carcinoma. Am J Surg Pathol 28:147–159
183. Leitao MM, Soslow RA, Baergen RN et al (2004) Mutation and expression of the TP53 gene in early stage epithelial ovarian carcinoma. Gynecol Oncol 93:301–306
184. Levine DA, Argenta PA, Yee CJ et al (2003) Fallopian tube and primary peritoneal carcinomas associated with BRCA mutations. J Clin Oncol 21:4222–4227
185. Lewis MR, Deavers MT, Silva EG et al (2006) Ovarian involvement by metastatic colorectal adenocarcinoma: still a diagnostic challenge. Am J Surg Pathol 30:177–184
186. Liu J, Albarracin CT, Chang K-H et al (2004) Microsatellite instability and expression of hMLH1 and hMSH2 proteins in ovarian endometrioid cancer. Modern Pathol 17:75–80
187. Logani S, Oliva E, Amin MB et al (2003) Immunoprofile of ovarian tumors with putative transitional cell (urothelial) differentiation using novel urothelial markers: histogenetic and diagnostic implications. Am J Surg Pathol 27:1434–1441
188. Loizzi V, Cormio G, Resta L et al (2005) Neoadjuvant chemotherapy in advanced ovarian cancer: a case-control study. Int J Gynecol Cancer 15:217–223
189. Loizzi V, Rossi C, Cormio G et al (2005) Clinical features of hepatic metastasis in patients with ovarian cancer. Int J Gynecol Cancer 15:26–31
190. Longacre TA, McKenney JK, Tazelaar HD et al (2005) Ovarian serous tumors of low malignant potential (borderline tumors): outcome-based study of 276 patients with long-term (>5-year) follow-up. Am J Surg Pathol 29:707–723
191. Longacre TA, Oliva E, Soslow RA (2007) Recommendations for the reporting of fallopian tube neoplasms. Hum Pathol 338:1160–1163
192. Lu KH, Bell DA, Welch WR et al (1998) Evidence for the multifocal origin of bilateral and advanced human serous borderline ovarian tumors. Cancer Res 58:2328–2330
193. Lu KH, Garber JE, Cramer DW et al (2000) Occult ovarian tumors in women with BRCA1 or BRCA2 mutations undergoing prophylactic oophorectomy. J Clin Oncol 18:2728–2732
194. Lugli A, Forster Y, Haas P et al (2003) Calretinin expression in human normal and neoplastic tissues: a tissue microarray analysis on 5233 tissue samples. Hum Pathol 34:994–1000
195. Malander S, Rambech E, Kristoffersson U et al (2006) The contribution of the hereditary nonpolyposis colorectal cancer syndrome to the development of ovarian cancer. Gynecol Oncol 101:238–243
196. Malpica A, Deavers MT, Lu K et al (2004) Grading ovarian serous carcinoma using a two-tier system. Am J Surg Pathol 28:496–504
197. Malpica A, Deavers MT, Tornos C et al (2007) Introbserver and intraobserver variability of a two-tier system for grading ovarian serous carcinoma. Am J Surg Pathol 31:1168–1174
198. Mano MS, Rosa DD, Azambuja E et al (2007) Current management of ovarian carcinosarcoma. Int J Gynecol Cancer 17:316–324
199. Markman M (2009) Hyperthermic intraperitoneal chemotherapy in the management of ovarian cancer: a critical need for an evidence-based evaluation. Gynecol Oncol 113:4–5
200. Marquez RT, Baggerly KA, Patterson AP et al (2005) Patterns of gene expression in different histotypes of epithelial ovarian cancer correlate with those in normal fallopian tube, endometrium, and colon. Clin Cancer Res 11:6116–6126
201. Matias-Guiu X, Lagarda H, Catasus L et al (2002) Clonality analysis in synchronous or metachronous tumors of the female genital tract. Int J Gynecol Pathol 21:205–211
202. Matsuura Y, Robertson G, Marsden DE et al (2007) Thromboembolic complications in patients with clear cell carcinoma of the ovary. Gynecol Oncol 104:406–410
203. Mayr D, Hirschmann A, Lohrs U et al (2006) KRAS and BRAF mutations in ovarian tumors: a comprehensive study of invasive carcinomas, borderline tumors and extraovarian implants. Gynecol Oncol 103:883–887
204. Mayr D, Kanitz V, Anderegg B et al (2006) Analysis of gene amplification and prognostic markers in ovarian cancer using comparative genomic hybridization for microarrays and immunohistochemical analysis for tissue microarrays. Am J Clin Pathol 126:101–109
205. McCluggage WG (2004) WT1 is of value in ascertaining the site of origin of serous carcinomas within the female genital tract. Int J Gynecol Pathol 23:97–99, editorial
206. McCluggage WG (2006) Immunohistochemical and functional biomarkers of value in female genital tract lesions. Int J Gynecol Pathol 25:101–120
207. McCluggage WG (2008) My approach to and thoughts on the typing of ovarian carcinomas. J Clin Pathol 61:152–163
208. McCluggage WG, Ganesan R, Herrington CS (2009) Endometrial stromal sarcomas with extensive endometrioid glandular differentiation: report of a series with emphasis on the potential for misdiagnosis and discussion of the differential diagnosis. Histopathology 54:365–373
209. McKenney JK, Balzer BL, Longacre TA (2006) Lymph node involvement in ovarian serous tumors of low malignant potential (borderline tumors): pathology, prognosis, and proposed classification. Am J Surg Pathol 30:614–624
210. McKenney JK, Balzer BL, Longacre TA (2006) Patterns of stromal invasion in ovarian serous tumors of low malignant potential (borderline tumors): a reevaluation of the concept of stromal microinvasion. Am J Surg Pathol 30:1209–1221
211. McKenney JK, Soslow RA, Longacre TA (2008) Ovarian mature teratomas with mucinous epithelial neoplasms: morphologic heterogeneity and association with pseudomyxoma peritonei. Am J Surg Pathol 32:645–655
212. Medeiros F, Muto MG, Lee Y et al (2006) The tubal fimbria is a preferred site for early adenocarcinoma in women with familial ovarian cancer syndrome. Am J Surg Pathol 30:230–236
213. National Health and Medical Research Council, Australian Government. Clinical practice guidelines for the management of women

with ovarian cancer. http://www.nhmrc.gov.au/publications/synopses/_files/cp98_2.pdf. Accessed 6 Oct 2008
214. Meeuwissen PAM, Seynaeve C, Brekelmans CTM et al (2005) Outcome of surveillance and prophylactic salpingo-oophorectomy in asymptomatic women at high risk for ovarian cancer. Gynecol Oncol 97:476–482
215. Meinhold-Heerlein I, Bauerschlag D, Hilpert F et al (2005) Molecular and prognostic distinction between serous ovarian carcinomas of varying grade and malignant potential. Oncogene 24:1053–1065
216. Melichar B, Urminska H, Kohlova T et al (2004) Brain metastases of epithelial ovarian carcinoma responding to cisplatin and gemcitabine combination chemotherapy: a case report and review of the literature. Gynecol Oncol 94:267–276
217. Menczer J, Liphshitz I, Barchana M (2006) A decreasing incidence of ovarian carcinoma in Israel. Int J Gynecol Cancer 16:41–44
218. Meng Q, Xia C, Fang J et al (2006) Role of PI3K and AKT specific isoforms in ovarian cancer cell migration, invasion and proliferation through the p70S6K1 pathway. Cell Signal 18:2262–2271
219. Menon U, Gentry-Maharaj A, Hallett R et al (2009) Sensitivity and specificity of multimodal and ultrasound screening for ovarian cancer, and stage distribution of detected cancers: results of the prevalence screen of the UK Collaborative Trial of Ovarian Cancer Screening (UKCTOCS). Lancet Oncol 10:327–340
220. Merajver SD, Pham TM, Caduff RF et al (1995) Somatic mutations in the BRCA1 gene in sporadic ovarian tumours. Nature Genet 9:439–443
221. Miller K, Price JH, Dobbs SP et al (2008) An immunohistochemical and morphological analysis of post-chemotherapy ovarian carcinoma. J Clin Pathol 61:652–657
222. Mink PJ, Sherman ME, Devesa SS (2002) Incidence patterns of invasive and borderline ovarian tumors among white women and black women in the United States: results from the SEER program, 1978-1998. Cancer 95:2380–2389
223. Misdraji J, Vaidya A, Tambouret RH et al (2006) Psammoma bodies in cervicovaginal cytology specimens: a clinicopathological analysis of 31 cases. Gynecol Oncol 103:238–246
224. Mizuno M, Kikkawa F, Shibata K et al (2003) Long-term prognosis of stage I ovarian carcinoma: prognostic importance of intraoperative rupture. Oncology 65:29–36
225. Mok SC, Bell DA, Knapp RC et al (1993) Mutation of K-ras protooncogene in human ovarian epithelial tumors of borderline malignancy. Cancer Res 53:1489–1492
226. Morice P, Camatte S, Rey A et al (2003) Prognostic factors for patients with advanced stage serous borderline tumours of the ovary. Ann Oncol 14:592–598
227. Movahedi-Lankarani S, Kurman RJ (2002) Calretinin, a more sensitive but less specific marker than alpha-inhibin for ovarian sex cord-stromal neoplasms: an immunohistochemical study of 215 cases. Am J Surg Pathol 26:1477–1483
228. Nagai Y, Kishimoto T, Nikaido T et al (2003) Squamous predominance in mixed- epithelial papillary cystadenomas of borderline malignancy of mullerian type arising in endometriotic cysts: a study of four cases. Am J Surg Pathol 27:242–247
229. Nakatsuka S, Oji Y, Horiuchi T et al (2006) Immunohistochemical detection of WT1 protein in a variety of cancer cells. Modern Pathol 19:804–814
230. Nakayama K, Nakayama N, Jinawath N et al (2007) Amplicon profiles in ovarian serous carcinomas. Int J Cancer 120:2613–2617
231. Nakayama K, Nakayama N, Kurman RJ et al (2006) Sequence mutations and amplification of PIK3CA and AKT2 genes in purified ovarian serous neoplasms. Cancer Biol Ther 5:779–785
232. National Cancer Institute and National Human Genome Research Institute. The cancer genome atlas. http://cancergenome.nih.gov/. Accessed 11 July 2010
233. Ness RB, Modugno F (2006) Endometriosis as a model for inflammation-hormone interactions in ovarian and breast cancers. Eur J Cancer 42:691–703
234. Nishimura S, Tsuda H, Ito K et al (2007) Differential expression of ABCF2 protein among different histologic types of epithelial ovarian cancer and in clear cell adenocarcinomas of different organs. Hum Pathol 38:134–139
235. Nomura K, Aizawa S (2000) Noninvasive, microinvasive, and invasive mucinous carcinomas of the ovary: a clinicopathologic analysis of 40 cases. Cancer 89:1541–1546
236. Nomura K, Aizawa S, Hano H (2004) Ovarian mucinous borderline tumors of intestinal type without intraepithelial carcinoma: are they still tumors of low malignant potential? Pathol Int 54:420–424
237. O'Neill CJ, Deavers MT, Malpica A et al (2005) An immunohistochemical comparison between low-grade and high-grade ovarian serous carcinomas: significantly higher expression of p53, MIB1, BCL2, HER-2/neu, and C-KIT in high grade neoplasms. Am J Surg Pathol 29:1034–1041
238. Obata K, Morland SJ, Watson RH et al (1998) Frequent PTEN/MMAC mutations in endometrioid but not serous or mucinous epithelial ovarian tumors. Cancer Res 58:2095–2097
239. Obermair A, Fuller A, Lopez-Varela E et al (2007) A new prognostic model for FIGO stage I epithelial ovarian cancer. Gynecol Oncol 104:607–611
240. Oda K, Stokoe D, Taketani Y et al (2005) High frequency of coexistent mutations of PIK3CA and PTEN genes in endometrial carcinoma. Cancer Res 65:10669–10673
241. Ohira S, Itoh K, Shiozawa T et al (2004) Ovarian non-small cell neuroendocrine carcinoma with paraneoplastic parathyroid hormone-related hypercalcemia. Int J Gynecol Pathol 23:39–397
242. Ohta Y, Suzuki T, Shiokawa A et al (2005) Expression of CD10 and cytokeratins in ovarian and renal clear cell carcinoma. Int J Gynecol Pathol 24:239–245
243. Oliva E, Branton PA, Scully RE (2005) Ovary. College of American Pathologists. http://cap.org. Accessed 12 May 2009
244. Oliva E, Branton PA, Scully RE (2005) Peritoneum. College of American Pathologists. http://cap.org
245. Olivier RI, van Beurden M, Lubsen MA et al (2004) Clinical outcome of prophylactic oophorectomy in BRCA1/BRCA2 mutation carriers and events during follow-up. Br J Cancer 90:1492–1497
246. Ordonez NG (2000) Transitional cell carcinomas of the ovary and bladder are immunophenotypically different. Histopathology 36:433–438
247. Ordonez NG (2005) Value of estrogen and progesterone receptor immunostaining in distinguishing between peritoneal mesotheliomas and serous carcinomas. Hum Pathol 36:1163–1167
248. Ordonez NG (2007) What are the current best immunohistochemical markers for the diagnosis of epithelioid mesothelioma? A review and update. Hum Pathol 38:1–16
249. Orsulic S, Li Y, Soslow RA, Vitale-Cross LA et al (2002) Induction of ovarian cancer by defined multiple genetic changes in a mouse model system. Cancer Cell 1:53–62
250. Ozols RF, Rubin SC, Thomas GM et al (2005) Epithelial ovarian cancer. In: Hoskins WJ et al (eds) Principles and practice of gynecologic oncology, 4th edn. Lippincott, New York, pp 895–987
251. Pal T, Permuth-Wey J, Kumar A et al (2008) Systematic review and meta-analysis of ovarian cancers: estimation of microsatellite-high

frequency and characterization of mismatch repair deficient tumor histology. Clin Cancer Res 14:6847–6854

252. Park JY, Kim DY, Kim JH et al (2009) Surgical management of borderline ovarian tumors: the role of fertility sparing surgery. Gynecol Oncol 113:75–82
253. Partridge E, Kreimer AR, Greenlee RT et al (2009) Results from four rounds of ovarian cancer screening in a randomized trial. Obstet Gynecol 113:775–782
254. Pather S, Quinn MA (2004) Clear cell cancer of the ovary – is it chemosensitive? Int J Gynecol Cancer 15:432–437
255. Pectasides D, Fountzilas G, Aravantinos G et al (2006) Advanced stage clear-cell epithelial ovarian cancer: the Hellenic Cooperative Oncology Group experience. Gynecol Oncol 102:285–291
256. Pectasides D, Pectasides A, Psyrri A et al (2006) Treatment issues in clear cell carcinoma of the ovary: a different entity? Oncologist 11:1089–1094
257. Petit T, Velten M, d'Hombres A et al (2007) Long-term survival of 106 stage III ovarian cancer patients with minimal residual disease after second-look laparotomy and consolidation radiotherapy. Gynecol Oncol 104:104–108
258. Piek JMJ, Kenemans P, Verheijen RHM (2004) Intraperitoneal serous adenocarcinoma: a critical appraisal of three hypotheses on its cause. Am J Obstet Gynecol 191:718–732
259. Pohl G, Ho CL, Kurman RJ, Bristow R et al (2005) Inactivation of the mitogen-activated protein kinase pathway as a potential target-based therapy in ovarian serous tumors with KRAS or BRAF mutations. Cancer Res 65:1994–2000
260. Poli Neto OB, Candido Dos Reis FJ, Zambelli-Ramalho LN et al (2006) p63 expression in epithelial ovarian tumors. Int J Gynecol Cancer 16:152–155
261. Powell CB, Kenley E, Chen L et al (2005) Risk-reducing salpingo-oophorect omy in BRCA mutation carriers: role of serial sectioning in the detection of occult malignancy. J Clin Oncol 23:127–132
262. Prat J, de Nictolis M (2002) Serous borderline tumors of the ovary: a long-term follow-up study of 137 cases, including 18 with a micropapillary pattern and 20 with microinvasion. Am J Surg Pathol 26:1111–1128
263. Prat J, Ribe A, Gallardo A (2005) Hereditary ovarian cancer. Hum Pathol 36:861–870
264. Prentice RL, Thomson CA, Caan B et al (2007) Low-fat dietary pattern and cancer incidence in the Women's Health Initiative dietary modification randomized controlled trial. J Natl Cancer Inst 99:1534–1543
265. Press JZ, De Luca A, Boyd N et al (2008) Ovarian carcinomas with genetic and epigenetic BRCA1 loss have distinct molecular abnormalities. BMC Cancer 8:17
266. Pusiol T, Parolari A, Piscioli I et al (2008) Prevalence of and significance of psammoma bodies in cervicovaginal smears in a cervical cancer screening program with emphasis on a case of primary bilateral ovarian psammocarcinoma. Cytojournal 5:7
267. Ramalingam P, Malpica A, Silva EG et al (2004) The use of cytokeratin 7 and EMA in differentiating ovarian yolk sac tumors from endometrioid and clear cell carcinomas. Am J Surg Pathol 28:1499–1505
268. Ramus SJ, Harrington PA, Pye C et al (2007) Contribution of BRCA1 and BRCA2 mutations to inherited ovarian cancer. Hum Mutat 28:1207–1215
269. Rebbeck TR, Lynch HT, Neuhausen SL et al (2002) Prophylactic oophorectomy in carriers of BRCA1 or BRCA2 mutations. N Engl J Med 346:1616–1622
270. Ricci R, Komminoth P, Bannwart F et al (2003) PTEN as a molecular marker to distinguish metastatic from primary synchronous endometrioid carcinomas of the ovary and uterus. Diagn Mol Pathol 12:71–78
271. Riedel I, Czernobilsky B, Lifschitz-Mercer B et al (2001) Brenner tumors but not transitional cell carcinomas of the ovary show urothelial differentiation: immunohistochemical staining of urothelial markers including cytokeratins and uroplakins. Virchows Archiv 438:181–191
272. Riopel MA, Ronnett BM, Kurman RJ (1999) Evaluation of diagnostic criteria and behavior of ovarian intestinal-type mucinous tumors: atypical proliferative (borderline) tumors and intraepithelial, microinvasive, invasive, and metastatic carcinomas. Am J Surg Pathol 23:617–635
273. Rodriguez IM, Irving JA, Prat J (2004) Endocervical-like mucinous borderline tumors of the ovary: a clinicopathologic analysis of 31 cases. Am J Surg Pathol 28:1311–1318
274. Rodriguez IM, Prat J (2002) Mucinous tumors of the ovary: a clinicopathologic analysis of 75 borderline tumors (of intestinal type) and carcinomas. Am J Surg Pathol 26:139–152
275. Rollins SE, Young RH, Bell DA (2006) Autoimplants in serous borderline tumors of the ovary: a clinicopathologic study of 30 cases of a process to be distinguished from serous adenocarcinoma. Am J Surg Pathol 30:457–462
276. Roma AA, Malpica A, Deavers MT, Silva EG (2008). Ovarian serous borderline tumors with a predominant micropapillary pattern are aggressive neoplasms with an increased risk for low grade serous carcinoma. Modern Pathol 21:221A. Abstract
277. Ronnett BM, Kajdacsy-Balla A, Gilks CB et al (2004) Mucinous borderline ovarian tumors: points of general agreement and persistent controversies regarding nomenclature, diagnostic criteria, and behavior. Hum Pathol 35:949–960
278. Ronnett BM, Kurman RJ, Zahn CM et al (1995) Pseudomyxoma peritonei in women: A clinicopathologic analysis of 30 cases with emphasis on site of origin, prognosis, and relationship to ovarian mucinous tumors of low malignant potential. Hum Pathol 26:509–524
279. Ronnett BM, Seidman JD (2003) Mucinous tumors arising in ovarian mature cystic teratomas: relationship to the clinical syndrome of pseudomyxoma peritonei. Am J Surg Pathol 27:650–657
280. Ronnett BM, Yan H, Kurman RJ et al (2001) Patients with pseudomyxoma peritonei associated with disseminated peritoneal adenomucinosis have a significantly more favorable prognosis than patients with peritoneal mucinous carcinomatosis. Cancer 92:85–91
281. Ronnett BM, Zahn CM, Kurman RJ (1995) Disseminated peritoneal adenomucinosis and peritoneal mucinous carcinomatosis. A clinicopathologic analysis of 109 cases with emphasis on distinguishing pathologic features, site of origin, prognosis, and relationship to "pseudomyxoma peritonei". Am J Surg Pathol 19:1390–1408
282. Roth LM, Emerson RE, Ulbright TM (2003) Ovarian endometrioid tumors of low malignant potential: a clinicopathologic study of 30 cases with comparison to well-differentiated endometrioid adenocarcinoma. Am J Surg Pathol 27:1253–1259
283. Rufford B, Jacobs IJ (2004) Screening and diagnosis of ovarian cancer in the general population. In: Gershenson DM et al (eds) Gynecologic cancer: controversies in management. Elsevier, Philadelphia, pp 355–368
284. Russo A, Calo V, Bruno L et al (2009) Hereditary ovarian cancer. Crit Rev Oncol Hematol 69:28–44
285. Sainz de la Cuesta R, Eichhorn JH, Rice LW et al (1996) Histologic transformation of benign endometriosis to early epithelial ovarian cancer. Gynecol Oncol 60:238–244

286. Salani R, Kurman RJ, Giuntoli R 2nd et al (2008) Assessment of TP53 mutation using purified tissue samples of ovarian serous carcinomas reveals a higher mutation rate than previously reported and does not correlate with drug resistance. Int J Gynecol Cancer 18:487–491
287. Salvador S, Gilks B, Kobel M et al (2009) The fallopian tube: primary site of most pelvic high grade serous carcinomas. Int J Gynecol Cancer 19:58–64
288. Sangha N, Wu R, Kuick R et al (2008) Neurofibromin 1 (NF1) defects are common in human ovarian serous carcinomas and co-occur with TP53 mutations. Neoplasia 10:1362–1372
289. Sangoi AR, McKenney JK, Dadras SS et al (2008) Lymphatic vascular invasion in ovarian serous tumors of low malignant potential with stromal microinvasion: a case control study. Am J Surg Pathol 32:261–268
290. Sangoi AR, Soslow RA, Teng NN et al (2008) Ovarian clear cell carcinomas with papillary features: a potential mimic of serous tumor of low malignant potential. Am J Surg Pathol 32:269–274
291. Sassen S, Schmalfeldt B, Avril N et al (2007) Histopathologic assessment of tumor regression after neoadjuvant chemotherapy in advanced stage ovarian cancer. Hum Pathol 38:926–934
292. Sato N, Tsunoda H, Nishida M (2000) Loss of heterozygosity on 10q23.3 and mutation of the tumor suppressor gene PTEN in benign endometrial cyst of the ovary: possible sequence progression from benign endometrial cyst to endometrioid carcinoma and clear cell carcinoma of the ovary. Cancer Res 60:7052–7056
293. Schaner ME, Ross DT, Ciaravino G et al (2003) Gene expression patterns in ovarian carcinomas. Mol Biol Cell 14:4376–4386
294. Schmeler KM, Lynch HT, Chen L et al (2006) Prophylactic surgery to reduce the risk of gynecologic cancers in the Lynch syndrome. N Engl J Med 354:261–269
295. Schmeler KM, Sun CC, Bodurka DC et al (2008) Neoadjuvant chemotherapy for low-grade serous carcinoma of the ovary or peritoneum. Gynecol Oncol 108:510–514
296. Schwartz DR, Kardia SL, Shedden KA et al (2002) Gene expression in ovarian cancer reflects both morphology and biological behavior, distinguishing clear cell from other poor-prognosis ovarian carcinomas. Cancer Res 62:4722–4729
297. Scully RE, Sobin LH et al (1999) Histological typing of ovarian tumours, 2nd edn. Springer, New York
298. Seidman JD (1996) Prognostic importance of atypia and hyperplasia in endometriosis. Int J Gynecol Pathol 15:1–9
299. Seidman JD, Cosin JA, Wang B et al (2010) Upstaging pathologic stage I ovarian carcinoma based on dense adhesions is not warranted. A clinicopathologic study of 84 patients originally classified as FIGO stage II. Gynecol Oncol (2010), doi:10.1016/j.ygyno.2010.07.002. Accessed 15 July 2010
300. Seidman JD, Horkayne-Szakaly I, Cosin JA et al (2006) Testing of two binary grading systems for FIGO stage III serous carcinoma of the ovary and peritoneum. Gynecol Oncol 103:703–708
301. Seidman JD, Horkayne-Szakaly I, Haiba M et al (2004) The histologic type and stage distribution of ovarian carcinomas of surface epithelial origin. Int J Gynecol Pathol 23:41–44
302. Seidman JD, Khedmati F (2008) Exploring the histogenesis of ovarian mucinous and transitional cell (Brenner) tumors: a study of 120 tumors. Arch Pathol Lab Med 132:1753–1760
303. Seidman JD, Kraus JA, Yemelyanova A et al (2009) Ovarian low grade serous neoplasms: evaluation of sampling recommendations based on tumors expected to have invasion (those with peritoneal invasive low grade serous carcinoma (invasive implants)). Modern Pathol 22(Suppl 1):236A, Abstract
304. Seidman JD, Kurman RJ (1996) Subclassification of serous borderline tumors of the ovary into benign and malignant types: a clinicopathologic study of 65 advanced stage cases. Am J Surg Pathol 20:1331–1345
305. Seidman JD, Kurman RJ (2000) Ovarian serous borderline tumors: a critical review of the literature with emphasis on prognostic indicators. Hum Pathol 31:539–557
306. Seidman JD, Kurman RJ, Ronnett BM (2003) Primary and metastatic mucinous adenocarcinomas in the ovaries: incidence in routine practice with a new approach to improve intraoperative diagnosis. Am J Surg Pathol 27:985–993
307. Seidman JD, Mehrotra A (2005) Benign ovarian serous tumors: a re-evaluation and proposed reclassification of serous "cystadenomas" and "cystadenofibromas". Gynecol Oncol 96:395–401
308. Seidman JD, Russell P, Kurman RJ (2002) Surface epithelial tumors of the ovary. In: Kurman RJ (ed) Blaustein's pathology of the female genital tract, 5th edn. Springer, New York, pp 791–904
309. Seidman JD, Sherman ME, Bell KA et al (2002) Salpingitis, salpingoliths and serous tumors of the ovaries: is there a connection? Int J Gynecol Pathol 21:101–107
310. Seidman JD, Soslow RA, Vang R et al (2004) Borderline ovarian tumors: diverse contemporary viewpoints on terminology and diagnostic criteria with illustrative images. Hum Pathol 35:918–933
311. Seidman JD, Varallo MR (2007) Micropapillary serous carcinoma: the solution to the ovarian borderline tumor conundrum. Pathol Case Rev 12:136–142
312. Seidman JD, Wang B (2007) Evaluation of normal-sized ovaries associated with primary peritoneal serous carcinoma for possible precursors of ovarian serous carcinoma. Gynecol Oncol 106: 201–206
313. Seidman JD, Yemelyanova AV, Khedmati F et al (2010) Prognostic factors for stage I ovarian carcinoma. Int J Gynecol Pathol 29:1–7
314. Seidman JD, Yemelyanova A, Zaino RJ, Kurman RJ. The fallopian tube-peritoneal junction: a potential site of carcinogenesis. Int J Gynecol Pathol, in press
315. Senkel S, Lucas B, Klein-Hitpass L et al (2005) Identification of target genes of the transcription factor HNF1beta and HNF1alpha in a human embryonic kidney cell line. Biochim Biophys Acta 1731:179–190
316. Shappell HW, Riopel MA, Smith-Sehdev AE et al (2002) Diagnostic criteria and behavior of ovarian seromucinous (endocervical-type mucinous and mixed cell-type) tumors: atypical proliferative (borderline) tumors, intraepithelial, microinvasive, and invasive carcinoma. Am J Surg Pathol 26:1529–1541
317. Shaw P, McLaughlin JR, Zweemer RP et al (2002) Histopathologic features of genetically determined ovarian cancer. Int J Gynecol Pathol 21:407–411
318. Shedden KA, Kshirsagar MP, Schwartz DR et al (2005) Histologic type, organ of origin, and Wnt pathway status: effect on gene expression in ovarian and uterine carcinomas. Clin Cancer Res 11:2123–2131
319. Sherman ME, Berman J, Birrer MJ et al (2004) Current challenges and opportunities for research on borderline ovarian tumors. Human Pathol 35:961–970
320. Sherman ME, Mink PJ, Curtis R et al (2004) Survival among women with borderline ovarian tumors and ovarian carcinoma: a population-based analysis. Cancer 100:1045–1052
321. Shvartsman HS, Sun CC, Bodurka DC et al (2007) Comparison of the clinical behavior of newly diagnosed stages II-IV low-grade serous carcinoma of the ovary with that of serous ovarian tumors of low malignant potential that recur as low grade serous carcinoma. Gynecol Oncol 105:625–629

322. Sieben NL, Kolkman-Uljee SM et al (2003) Molecular genetic evidence for monoclonal origin of bilateral ovarian serous borderline tumors. Am J Pathol 162:1095–1101
323. Sieben NL, Macropoulos P, Roemen GM et al (2004) In ovarian neoplasms, BRAF, but not KRAS, mutations are restricted to low-grade serous tumours. J Pathol 202:336–340
324. Silasi DA, Illuzzi JL, Kelly MG et al (2008) Carcinosarcoma of the ovary. Int J Gynecol Cancer 18:22–29
325. Silva EG, Deavers MT, Bodurka DC et al (2006) Association of low grade endometrioid carcinoma of the uterus and ovary with undifferentiated carcinoma: a new type of dedifferentiated carcinoma? Int J Gynecol Pathol 25:52–58
326. Silva EG, Gershenson DM, Malpica A et al (2006) The recurrence and the overall survival rates of ovarian serous borderline neoplasms with noninvasive implants is time-dependent. Am J Surg Pathol 30:1367–1371
327. Singer G, Oldt R 3rd, Cohen Y et al (2003) Mutations in BRAF and KRAS characterize the development of low-grade ovarian serous carcinoma. J Natl Cancer Inst 95:484–486
328. Singer G, Stohr R, Cope L et al (2005) Patterns of p53 mutations separate ovarian serous borderline tumors and low- and high-grade carcinomas and provide support for a new model of ovarian carcinogenesis: a mutational analysis with immunohistochemical correlation. Am J Surg Pathol 29:218–224
329. Skirnisdottir I, Seidal T, Karlsson MG et al (2005) Clinical and biological characteristics of clear cell carcinomas of the ovary in FIGO stages I-II. Int J Oncol 26:177–183
330. Slomovitz BM, Caputo TA, Gretz HF et al (2002) A comparative analysis of 57 serous borderline tumors with and without a noninvasive micropapillary component. Am J Surg Pathol 26:592–600
331. Smith-Sehdev AE, Sehdev PS, Kurman RJ (2003) Noninvasive and invasive micropapillary (low grade) serous carcinoma of the ovary: a clinicopathologic analysis of 135 cases. Am J Surg Pathol 27:725–736
332. Soliman PT, Slomovitz BM, Broaddus RR et al (2004) Synchronous primary cancers of the endometrium and ovary: a single institution review of 84 cases. Gynecol Oncol 94:456–462
333. Soslow RA (2008) Histologic subtypes of ovarian carcinoma: an overview. Int J Gynecol Pathol 27:161–174
334. Spruck CH, Won KA, Reed SI (1999) Deregulated cyclin E induces chromosome instability. Nature 401:297–300
335. Stadlmann S, Gueth U, Reiser U et al (2006) Epithelial growth factor status in primary and recurrent ovarian cancer. Modern Pathol 19:607–610
336. Stern RC, Dash R, Bentley RC et al (2001) Malignancy in endometriosis: frequency and comparison of ovarian and extraovarian types. Int J Gynecol Pathol 20:133–139
337. Stewart BW, Kleihues P et al (eds) (2003) World cancer report. World Health Organization International Agency for Research on Cancer Press, Lyon, p 219
338. Storey DJ, Rush R, Stewart M et al (2008) Endometrioid epithelial ovarian cancer: 20 years of prospectively collected data from a single center. Cancer 112:2211–2220
339. Suehiro Y, Sakamoto M, Umayahara K et al (2000) Genetic aberrations detected by comparative genomic hybridization in ovarian clear cell adenocarcinomas. Oncology 59:50–56
340. Surveillance, Epidemiology, End Results (SEER). http://www.seer.cancer.gov/statfacts/html/ovary.html?statfacts_page=ovary.html&x=15&y=17. Accessed 9 Mar 2008
341. Suzuki S, Kajiyama H, Shibata K (2008) Is there any association between retroperitoneal lymphadenectomy and survival benefit in ovarian clear cell carcinoma patients? Ann Oncol 19:1284–1287
342. Tabrizi AD, Kalloger SE, Kobel M et al (2010) Primary ovarian mucinous carcinoma of intestinal type: significance of pattern of invasion and immunohistochemical expression profile in a series of 31 cases. Int J Gynecol Pathol 29:99–107
343. Takano M, Kikuchi Y, Yaegashi N et al (2006) Clear cell carcinoma of the ovary: a retrospective multicentre experience of 254 patients with complete surgical staging. Br J Cancer 94:1369–1374
344. Tam KF, Cheung ANY, Liu KL et al (2003) A retrospective review on atypical glandular cells of undetermined significance (AGUS) using the Bethesda 2001 classification. Gynecol Oncol 91:603–607
345. Tan DSP, Kaye S (2007) Ovarian clear cell adenocarcinoma: a continuing enigma. J Clin Pathol 60:355–360
346. Tanaka T, Tomaru Y, Nomura Y et al (2004) Comprehensive search for HNF-1beta-regulated genes in mouse hepatoma cells perturbed by transcription regulatory factor-targeted RNAi. Nucleic Acids Res 32:2740–2750
347. Tangjitgamol S, Levenback CF, Beller U et al (2004) Role of surgical resection for lung, liver, and central nervous system metastases in patients with gynecological cancer: a literature review. Int J Gynecol Cancer 14:399–422
348. Tanner EJ, Zahurak ML, Bristow RE et al (2008) Surgical care of young women diagnosed with ovarian cancer: a population-based perspective. Gynecol Oncol 111:221–225
349. Tapper J, Butzow R, Wahlstrom T et al (1997) Evidence for divergence of DNA copy number changes in serous, mucinous and endometrioid ovarian carcinomas. Br J Cancer 75:1782–1787
350. Tetsche MS, Dethlefsen C, Pedersen L, Sorenson HT, Norgaard M (2008) The impact of comorbidity and stage on ovarian cancer mortality: a nationwide Danish cohort study. BMC Cancer 8:31
351. Thomas EJ, Campbell IG (2000) Molecular genetic defects in endometriosis. Gynecol Obstet Invest 50(Suppl 1):44–50
352. Thrall M, Gallion HH, Kryscio R et al (2006) BRCA1 expression in a large series of sporadic ovarian carcinomas: a Gynecologic Oncology Group study. Int J Gynecol Cancer 16(suppl 1):166–171
353. Timmers PJ, Zwinderman AH, Teodorovic I et al (2009) Clear cell carcinoma compared to serous carcinoma in early ovarian cancer: same prognosis in a large randomized trial. Int J Gynecol Cancer 19:88–93
354. Tochigi N, Kishimoto T, Supriatna Y et al (2003) Hepatoid carcinoma of the ovary: a report of three cases admixed with a common surface epithelial carcinoma. Int J Gynecol Pathol 22:266–271
355. Tornos C, Soslow R, Chen S et al (2005) Expression of WT1, CA 125 and GCDFP-15 as useful markers in the differential diagnosis of primary ovarian carcinomas versus metastatic breast cancer to the ovary. Am J Surg Pathol 29:1482–1489
356. Tsuchiya A, Sakamoto M, Yasuda J et al (2003) Expression profiling in ovarian clear cell carcinoma: identification of hepatocyte nuclear factor-1 beta as a molecular marker and a possible molecular target for therapy of ovarian clear cell carcinoma. Am J Pathol 163:2503–2512
357. Tsuda H, Ito YM, Ohashi Y et al (2005) Identification of overexpression and amplification of ABCF2 in clear cell ovarian adenocarcinomas by cDNA microarray analyses. Clin Cancer Res 11:6880–6888
358. Tworoger SS, Gertig DM, Gates MA et al (2008) Caffeine, alcohol, smoking, and the risk of incident epithelial ovarian cancer. Cancer 112:1169–1177
359. van der Velde NM, Mourits MJ, Arts HJ et al (2009) Time to stop ovarian cancer screening in BRCA1/2 mutation carriers? Int J Cancer 124:919–923

360. Van Nagell JR jr, DePriest PD, Ueland FR et al (2007) Ovarian cancer screening with annual transvaginal sonography: findings of 25000 women screened. Cancer 109:1887–1896
361. Vang R, Gown AM, Barry TS et al (2006) Ovarian atypical proliferative (borderline) mucinous tumors: gastrointestinal and seromucinous (endocervical-like) types are immunophenotypically distinctive. Int J Gynecol Pathol 25:83–89
362. Vang R, Gown AM, Barry TS et al (2006) Cytokeratins 7 and 20 in primary and secondary mucinous tumors of the ovary: analysis of coordinate immunohistochemical expression profiles and staining distribution in 179 cases. Am J Surg Pathol 30:1130–1139
363. Vang R, Gown AM, Barry TS et al (2006) Immunohistochemistry for estrogen and progesterone receptors in the distinction of primary and metastatic mucinous tumors in the ovary: an analysis of 124 cases. Mod Pathol 19:97–105
364. Vang R, Gown AM, Farinola M et al (2007) p16 expression in primary ovarian mucinous and endometrioid tumors and metastatic adenocarcinomas in the ovary: utility for identification of metastatic HPV-related endocervical adenocarcinomas. Am J Surg Pathol 31:653–663
365. Vang R, Gown AM, Wu LS et al (2006) Immunohistochemical expression of CDX2 in primary ovarian mucinous tumors and metastatic mucinous carcinomas involving the ovary: comparison with CK20 and correlation with coordinate expression of CK7. Mod Pathol 19:1421–1428
366. Vang R, Gown AM, Zhao C et al (2007) Ovarian mucinous tumors associated with mature cystic teratomas: morphologic and immunohistochemical analysis identifies a subset of potential teratomatous origin that shares features of lower gastrointestinal tract mucinous tumors more commonly encountered as secondary tumors in the ovary. Am J Surg Pathol 31:854–869
367. Vang R, Shih I-M, Salani R et al (2008) Subdividing ovarian and peritoneal serous carcinoma into moderately differentiated and poorly differentiated does not have biologic validity based on molecular genetic and in vitro drug resistance data. Am J Surg Pathol 32:1667–1674
368. Veras E, Deavers MT, Silva EG et al (2007) Ovarian nonsmall cell neuroendocrine carcinoma: a clinicopathologic and immunohistochemical study of 11 cases. Am J Surg Pathol 31:774–782
369. Veras E, Mao T-L, Ayhan A et al (2009) Cystic and adenofibromatous clear cell carcinomas of the ovary: distinctive tumors that differ in their pathogenesis and behavior: a clinicopathologic analysis of 122 cases. Am J Surg Pathol 33:844–853
370. Vernooij F, Heintz APM, Witteveen PO et al (2008) Specialized care and survival of ovarian cancer patients in the Netherlands: nationwide cohort study. J Natl Cancer Inst 100:399–406
371. Vogelstein B, Kinzler KW (2004) Cancer genes and the pathways they control. Nat Med 10:789–799
372. Wang C, Horiuchi A, Imai T et al (2004) Expression of BRCA1 protein in benign, borderline, and malignant epithelial ovarian neoplasms and its relationship to methylation and allelic loss of the BRCA1 gene. J Pathol 202:215–223
373. Watson P, Butzow R, Lynch HT et al (2001) The clinical features of ovarian cancer in hereditary nonpolyposis colorectal cancer. Gynecol Oncol 82:223–228
374. Wells M (2004) Recent advances in endometriosis with emphasis on pathogenesis, molecular pathology, and neoplastic transformation. Int Gynecol Pathol 23:316–320
375. Werness BA, Ramus SJ, DiCioccio RA et al (2004) Histopathology, FIGO stage, and BRCA mutation status of ovarian cancers from the Gilda Radner Familial Ovarian Cancer Registry. Int J Gynecol Pathol 23:29–34
376. Willner J, Wurz K, Allison KH et al (2007) Alternate molecular genetic pathways in ovarian carcinomas of common histological types. Hum Pathol 38:607–613
377. Wimberger P, Lehmann N, Kimmig R et al (2006) Impact of age on outcome in patients with advanced ovarian cancer treated within a prospectively randomized phase III study of the Arbeitsgemeinschaft Gynaekologische Onkologie Ovarian Cancer Study Group (AGO-OVAR). Gynecol Oncol 100:300–307
378. Winter WE, Maxwell L, Tian C et al (2007) Prognostic factors for stage III epithelial ovarian cancer: a Gynecologic Oncology Group Study. J Clin Oncol 25:3621–3627
379. Wong KK (2009) Recent Developments in Anti-Cancer Agents Targeting the Ras/Raf/ MEK/ERK Pathway. Recent Patents Anticancer Drug Discov 4:28–35
380. Wong HF, Low JJH, Chua Y et al (2007) Ovarian tumors of borderline malignancy: a review of 247 patients from 1991–2004. Int J Gynecol Cancer 17:342–349
381. Wong K-K, Lu KH, Malpica A et al (2007) Significantly greater expression of ER, PR, and ECAD in advanced-stage low-grade ovarian serous carcinoma as revealed by immunohistochemical analysis. Int J Gynecol Pathol 26:404–409
382. Wright K, Wilson P, Morland S et al (1999) Beta-catenin mutation and expression analysis in ovarian cancer: exon 3 mutations and nuclear translocation in 16% of endometrioid tumours. Int J Cancer 82:625–629
383. Wu R, Hendrix-Lucas N, Kuick R et al (2007) Mouse model of human ovarian endometrioid adenocarcinoma based on somatic defects in the Wnt/B-catanin and PI3K/Pten signaling pathways. Cancer Cell 11:321–333
384. Yamamoto S, Tsuda H, Aida S et al (2007) Immunohistochemical detection of hepatocyte nuclear factor 1beta in ovarian and endometrial clear-cell adenocarcinomas and nonneoplastic endometrium. Hum Pathol 38:1074–1080
385. Yamamoto S, Tsuda H, Kita T et al (2007) Clinicopathological significance of WT1 expression in ovarian cancer: a possible accelerator of tumor progression in serous adenocarcinoma. Virch Arch 451:27–35
386. Yamamoto S, Tsuda H, Takano M et al (2008) Clear-cell adenofibroma can be a clonal precursor for clear-cell adenocarcinoma of the ovary: a possible alternative clear-cell carcinogenic pathway. J Pathol 216:103–110
387. Yamamoto S, Tsuda H, Yoshikawa T et al (2007) Clear cell adenocarcinoma associated with clear cell adenofibromatous components: a subgroup of ovarian clear cell adenocarcinoma with distinct clinicopathologic characteristics. Am J Surg Pathol 31:999–1006
388. Yan TD, Black D, Savady R et al (2007) A systematic review on the efficacy of cytoreductive surgery and perioperative intraperitoneal chemotherapy for pseudomyxoma peritonei. Ann Surg Oncol 14:484–492
389. Yemelyanova AV, Cosin JA, Bidus MA (2008) Pathology of stage I versus stage III ovarian carcinoma with implications for pathogenesis and screening. Int J Gynecol Cancer 18:465–469
390. Yemelyanova A, Mao T-L, Nakayama N (2008) Low grade serous carcinoma of the ovary displaying a macropapillary pattern. Am J Surg Pathol 32:1800–1806
391. Yemelyanova AV, Vang R, Judson K et al (2008) Distinction of primary and metastatic mucinous tumors involving the ovary: analysis of size and laterality data by primary site with reevaluation of an algorithm for tumor classification. Am J Surg Pathol 32:128–138
392. Yoshikawa H, Jimbo H, Okada S et al (2000) Prevalence of endometriosis in ovarian cancer. Gynecol Obstet Invest 50(Suppl 1):11–17

393. Young RC, Brady MF, Nieberg RK et al (2003) Adjuvant treatment for early ovarian cancer: a randomized phase III trial of intraperitoneal ^{32}P or intravenous cyclophosphamide and cisplatin- a Gynecologic Oncology Group study. J Clin Oncol 21:4350–4355
394. Zaino R, Whitney C, Brady MF et al (2001) Simultaneously detected endometrial and ovarian carcinomas: a prospective clinicopathologic study of 74 cases – a Gynecologic Oncology Group study. Gynecol Oncol 83:355–362
395. Zhao C, Bratthauer GL, Barner R et al (2007) Diagnostic utility of WT1 immunostaining in ovarian Sertoli cell tumor. Am J Surg Pathol 31:1378–1386
396. Zhao C, Bratthauer GL, Barner R et al (2007) Comparative analysis of alternative and traditional immunohistochemical markers for the distinction of ovarian Sertoli cell tumor from endometrioid tumors and carcinoid tumor: a study of 160 cases. Am J Surg Pathol 31:255–266
397. Zhou B, Sun Q, Cong R et al (2008) Hormone replacement therapy and ovarian cancer risk: a meta-analysis. Gynecol Oncol 108:641–651
398. Zorn KK, Bonome T, Gangi L et al (2005) Gene expression profiles of serous, endometrioid, and clear cell subtypes of ovarian and endometrial cancer. Clin Cancer Res 11:6422–6430

15 Sex Cord-Stromal, Steroid Cell, and Other Ovarian Tumors with Endocrine, Paraendocrine, and Paraneoplastic Manifestations

Robert H. Young

R. J. Kurman, L. Hedrick Ellenson, B. M. Ronnett (eds.), *Blaustein's Pathology of the Female Genital Tract (6th ed.)*, DOI 10.1007/978-1-4419-0489-8_15,

Sex Cord-Stromal Tumors

This category includes all ovarian neoplasms that contain granulosa cells, fibroblasts, theca cells (and their luteinized derivatives), Sertoli cells, Leydig cells, singly or in various combinations and in varying degrees of differentiation. Those who believe that all these cell types are derived from the "specialized stroma" of the genital ridge favor the term gonadal stromal tumors for these neoplasms [110]. Others, recognizing that many embryologists favor the participation of coelomic and mesonephric epithelium in the formation of sex cords, which are the proximal precursors of granulosa cells and Sertoli cells, favor the term sex cord-stromal tumors, and it is now the most widely accepted designation [144].

In the developing testis, the sex cords are clearly distinguishable by the fifth week of embryonic life as slender columns of primitive Sertoli cells, but similar cords, at least in the sense of thin columns, are not encountered in the developing ovary; instead, packets of small pregranulosa cells enveloping germ cells become evident later in embryonic life. For that reason, the term sex cords has been criticized as inaccurate to describe the progenitors of granulosa cells. Nevertheless, the long-established usage of this designation by embryologists and the lack of a better term justify its retention. The term sex cord-stromal tumors has the advantage of acknowledging the presence of neoplasms in this general category of derivatives of either or both the sex cords and the stroma. The components derived from the sex cords (granulosa and Sertoli cells) typically are arranged in epithelial configurations, whereas those derived from the stroma have the appearance of cellular gonadal stroma or its specialized derivatives, the theca and Leydig cells.

Most sex cord-stromal tumors (granulosa-stromal cell tumors) are composed of ovarian cell types but some (Sertoli-stromal cell tumors) contain cells that differentiate toward patterns more typical of the testis. Occasional tumors have significant components which in isolation would be in the granulosa-stromal or Sertoli-stromal categories and the term gynandroblastoma has been historically used for such cases. Although this heading is used in a section here, in accordance with the current World Health Organization classification, in our own practice, we prefer to categorize such neoplasms as mixed sex cord-stromal tumors and itemize the components present, and their quantity, roughly, in accord with the manner of dealing with mixed germ cell tumors of the gonads. This gives the clinician more cogent information than the gynandroblastoma terminology. When the neoplastic cells are immature and their appearance is intermediate between those of testicular and ovarian cell types, or when the architectural patterns of the tumor are not specific for either the testis or ovary, it may be impossible to determine whether the tumor belongs in the granulosa-stromal or Sertoli-stromal cell category; in such cases the term sex cord-stromal tumor, unclassified is used.

The classification of sex cord-stromal tumors used in this chapter is presented in *Table 15.1*. Sex cord-stromal tumors account for approximately 8% of all ovarian tumors, with fibromas accounting for approximately half the cases. The majority of clinically malignant tumors in the overall category are granulosa cell tumors and thus they are, practically, the most important neoplasm being considered here simply due to that and their frequency which exceeds significantly that of all other malignant tumors in the group. Accordingly, it and other neoplasms

Table 15.1
Classification of sex cord–stromal tumors

Granulosa–stromal cell tumors
Granulosa cell tumor
(i) Adult type
(ii) Juvenile type
Tumors in the thecoma–fibroma group
(i) Thecoma
(a) Typical
(b) Luteinized
(c) Of the type usually associated with sclerosing peritonitis
(d) Unclassified
(ii) Fibroma–fibrosarcoma
(a) Fibroma
(b) Cellular fibroma
(c) Fibrosarcoma
(iii) Stromal tumors with minor sex cord elements
(iv) Sclerosing stromal tumor
(v) Microcystic stromal tumor
(vi) Signet-ring stromal tumor
(vii) Unclassified
Sertoli–stromal cell tumors
Sertoli cell tumor
Leydig cell tumor
Sertoli–Leydig cell tumors
(i) Well differentiated
(ii) Of intermediate differentiation
(iii) Poorly differentiated
(iv) With heterologous elements
(v) Retiform
Gynandroblastoma (specify components)
Sex cord tumor with annular tubules
Unclassified

in the granulosa-stromal cell category are considered first after some comments on the overall aproach to evaluating these tumors, including a few remarks on immunohistochemistry.

Within the overall category of tumors considered in this chapter, one finds some of the most mundane diagnoses in ovarian tumor pathology, such as a typical fibroma, and on the other hand, a great array of other cases in which diverse patterns can bring almost any other ovarian tumor into the differential diagnosis. Fundamental to the approach to evaluating the more difficult cases is a broad knowledge of the great diversity of cell types and patterns seen in ovarian tumors, and the overlap that exists between various categories [184]. As difficult as some of these cases can be, it should also be noted that in many cases, one of the most crucial aspects of ovarian tumor evaluation, thorough sampling, will uncover foci that point firmly to the correct diagnosis. Accordingly, in an age when there is often a rush to apply immunohistochemistry, the importance of exceedingly thorough sampling of challenging cases cannot be overemphasized. The sampling must be based not only on the size of the tumor but also its overall gross characteristics and differing features thereof, and, of course, the differential diagnosis engendered when the initial sections are evaluated. Although in certain cirumstances these should point to judicious application of immunohistochemistry, they should also often cause reflection as to whether even further sections might give clues to the diagnosis. Although immunohistochemistry can be exceedingly helpful, the extent to which it is done in the current era is not matched by the aid actually provided from the viewpoint of arriving at the correct diagnosis. In some cases, it is also confusing, such as when a negative inhibin stain is obtained in a case of granulosa cell tumor, not a rare event.

Apart from thorough sampling, other fundamentals of ovarian tumor evaluation such as knowledge of the clinical background and awareness of the age of the patient should never be overlooked, albeit they are by no means always significant. The diagnostic formulation is impacted if the patient is known to have had a deeply invasive melanoma a few years ago; such tumors metastatic in the ovary can simulate a malignant steroid cell tumor or both adult and juvenile granulosa cell tumors quite closely. From the viewpoint of the age, clearly one approaches an ovarian tumor with a pattern of slit-like spaces and papillae differently in the first 10 years of life compared to in the seventh decade; in the first situation, a retiform pattern of Sertoli–Leydig cell tumor is high on the list, whereas of course in the older patient, one is most likely looking at another routine serous neoplasm.

The above emphasis on thorough sampling, awareness of age, and clinical history notwithstanding, there certainly is a role for immunohistochemistry in this area, although the extent to which it will be called upon will inevitably vary depending upon the experience of the evaluating pathologist with the spectrum of morphology of these tumors in general. Since Dr. Robert E. Scully first wrote an essay on the application of immunohistochemistry in ovarian tumor pathology in 1985 [142], there has been a vast literature on this topic. No attempt is made here to be complete from the viewpoint of citation and many excellent papers are not cited. Periodic reviews of this topic appear and three of those are cited here [11, 87, 93] as are a selected group of peer-reviewed contributions [24, 26, 34, 36, 39, 50, 57, 74, 85, 87–91, 104, 116, 131, 132, 158, 159, 197–201]. Some of these deal with now well-known applications such as that of inhibin and calretinin, but a few deal with more recently explored topics, whose benefit remains to be fully characterized with ongoing experience.

The most helpful triad that currently exists in evaluating sex cord-stromal tumors and their mimics is that of inhibin, calretinin, and epithelial membrane antigen (EMA). The first two are typically positive in sex cord tumors and the third, typically negative [2]. However, routine evaluation still dominates in arriving at the correct diagnosis and an appreciable minority of typical granulosa cell tumors in our experience are negative for inhibin and even occasionally for calretinin. Also, rare carcinomas are positive for inhibin [88]. If a tumor is negative for inhibin and calretinin and positive for EMA, that it is a granulosa, cell tumor is close to unheard of. If a tumor shows squamous differentiation, it rules out a sex cord-stromal tumor, irrespective of any immunohistochemical results. One of the most helpful findings in this area of differential diagnosis is the lack of squamous differentiation in sex cord-stromal tumors and its frequent presence, albeit often in abortive form, in one of the tumors that most often mimics a sex cord tumor, endometrioid carcinoma. Another area discussed here where immunohistochemistry may be important is in the realm of steroid cell tumors in which the broad differential of an oxyphilic neoplasm may pertain, particularly when the neoplasm is not one of the typical low-grade steroid cell tumors but one with atypical features. Staining for inhibin, calretinin, or melan-A may be very helpful positive results, as may certain negative results (such as those related to malignant melanoma), that would rule out other oxyphilic malignant tumors. It should be remembered that the luteinized stromal cells of many ovarian tumors may be inhibin-calretinin positive, and this occasionally causes confusion if the lack of staining of epithelial cells of the neoplasm is overlooked. Although immunohistochemistry has largely supplanted electromicroscopy as a diagnostic aid in ovarian tumor interpretation, there is still an occasional role for ultrastructural evaluation in showing, for example, dense core granules in tumors of neuroendocrine type and even Charcot–Bottcher filaments in some Sertoli cell tumors. From the converse viewpoint, ultrastructural evaluation may show, for example in malignant melanoma, distinctive features of that neoplasm ruling out a sex cord-stromal or steroid cell neoplasm.

Finally, the molecular pathogenesis of sex cord-stromal tumors is unknown as there have been very few molecular genetic studies of these neoplasms. Recently, it has been reported that mutation of FOXL2, a gene encoding a transcription factor critical for granulosa cell development, was present in 86 of 89 adult granulosa cell tumors (97%). Interestingly, the mutation was detected in only one of the ten juvenile granulosa cell tumors (10%), leading the authors to speculate that the juvenile granulosa cell tumor is a distinct disease from the adult type. Mutant FOXL2 was found in 3 of 14 thecomas (21%) and was absent in 49 sex cord tumors of other types, including Sertoli–Leydig tumors, fibromas, and steroid cell tumors, and in 329 unrelated ovarian and breast tumors. The findings suggest that mutant FOXL2 is a potential driver in the pathogenesis of adult-type granulosa tumors [150].

Granulosa-Stromal Cell Tumors

This category includes all ovarian tumors composed of granulosa cells, theca cells, and fibroblasts, singly or in any combination and in varying degrees of differentiation. Granulosa cell tumors that occur typically in middle-aged and older women differ in several important respects from those that usually arise in children and young adults and these two subtypes, which are referred to as adult and juvenile granulosa cell tumors, are discussed separately. It should be noted that the designations "adult" and "juvenile" are terms of convenience to capture the fact that the morphology seen under those headings is typically seen in adults and juveniles as the case may be. However, there are exceptions, some adult tumors being seen in young patients, even children, and some juvenile tumors being seen in the middle to later years of life. The adult and juvenile designations, however, are appropriate terms of convenience, as the many differences between adult and juvenile granulosa cell tumors would be difficult to encapsulate in other than extremely lengthy descriptive designations. Tumors in the thecoma–fibroma group are composed exclusively or almost exclusively of theca cells, fibroblasts of ovarian stromal origin, or both. The presence of occasional small nests of granulosa cells or occasional tubules lined by Sertoli cells does not exclude tumors from this category; such tumors have been referred to as fibromas or thecomas with minor sex cord elements [185]. A distinctive tumor in the thecoma–fibroma group is the sclerosing stromal tumor. It has its own unique constellation of features, described below, which set it apart from other neoplasms. It can be viewed as a variant of luteinized thecoma inasmuch as it is a stromal tumor with lutein cells, but its particular features, and their rather repetitive nature warrant its separate categorization. Another tumor that best belongs in the stromal category on the basis of current knowledge is the recently described microcystic stromal tumor.

Adult Granulosa Cell Tumor

Clinical Features

Adult granulosa cell tumors account for approximately 1% of all ovarian tumors and 95% of all granulosa cell tumors. They occur more often in postmenopausal than premenopausal women, with a peak incidence between 50 and 55 years of age [14, 16, 110, 152, 155]. They are the most common estrogenic ovarian tumors clinically, but the precise proportion of adult granulosa cell tumors that secrete hormones is difficult to establish because a specimen of endometrium to evaluate the effects of estrogenic stimulation often is unavailable. The typical endometrial alteration associated with functioning tumors in this category is simple hyperplasia, usually exhibiting some degree of precancerous atypicality. Carcinoma of the endometrium, which almost always is well differentiated, has been reported in from slightly less than 5% to slightly more than 25% of the cases; the wide variation in these figures is attributable, at least in part, to differing views of the dividing line between complex atypical hyperplasia and grade 1 adenocarcinoma. If strict criteria for the diagnosis of carcinoma are used, and if all patients with a granulosa cell tumor, not only those who have had an endometrial curettage or hysterectomy, are considered, the best estimate for the frequency of associated endometrial carcinoma is under 5%.

The endometrial changes associated with adult granulosa cell tumors are manifested clinically in women in the reproductive age group by irregular, excessive uterine bleeding, but amenorrhea, lasting from months to years, may precede the abnormal bleeding or may be the only hormonal manifestation. Postmenopausal bleeding is the most common endocrine symptom in older women, in whom carcinoma of the endometrium is encountered about twice as often as in younger patients. Occasionally, swelling and tenderness of the breasts are prominent symptoms. Elevated levels of estrogens have been reported in the blood and urine, and vaginal cytologic smears typically show increased maturation of squamous epithelial cells. Alterations resembling those seen in a secretory endometrium have been observed rarely in association with granulosa cell tumors, suggesting the possibility of a significant production of progesterone in these cases [180].

Rarely, androgenic changes are the sole endocrine manifestation of an adult granulosa cell tumor [105, 111]. Most of the patients have been frankly virilized, but some have been only hirsute. The tumors may be solid or solid and cystic. The cysts typically are thin walled and may be single or multiple, resembling serous cystadenomas. Because granulosa cell tumors in general are composed exclusively of thin-walled cysts in only about 3% of the cases, the almost 50% frequency of a cystic gross appearance of tumors associated with androgenic manifestations is of interest but remains an enigma [105].

Hemoperitoneum occurs in about 10% of cases of granulosa cell tumor, and an acute abdominal presentation is accordingly more typical of that tumor than other forms of ovarian cancer.

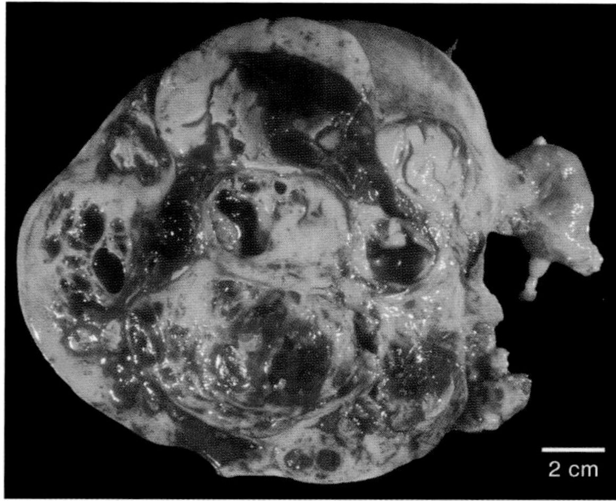

Fig. 15.1
Adult granulosa cell tumor. **The sectioned surface of the neoplasm is mostly solid and yellow but is focally cystic with abundant hemorrhage**

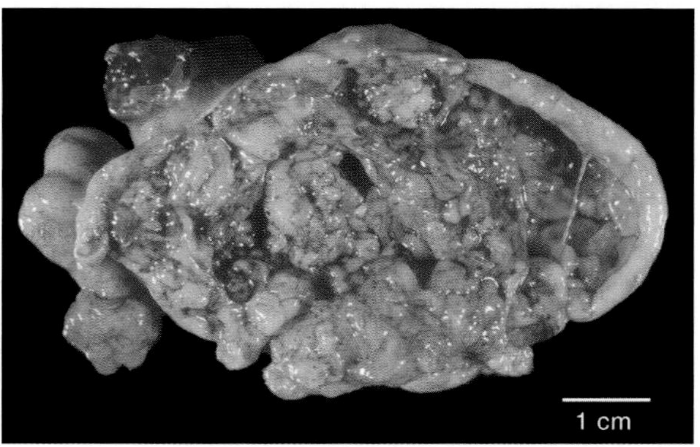

Fig. 15.2
Adult granulosa cell tumor. **The tumor has a friable appearance**

Gross Findings

Adult granulosa cell tumors (*Figs. 15.1–15.3*) vary in size from those that are too small to be felt on pelvic examination (10–15%) [46] to very large masses that distend the abdomen; the average diameter is approximately 12 cm. At operation, the tumor may appear predominantly solid or predominantly cystic and is unilateral in more than 95% of the cases.

The external surface may show a site of rupture with blood occasionally associated with it. In most cases, however, it is intact and mostly smooth. Sectioning a solid tumor reveals a gray-white or yellow color, depending on its lipid content, and a soft or firm consistency, depending on its relative content of neoplastic cells and fibrothecomatous stroma. Hemorrhage, which may be massive, is common as at least a focal finding. A friable nature may heighten the resemblance of some tumors to surface epithelial carcinomas (*Fig. 15.2*). Most characteristically, the tumor is solid and cystic, with numerous discrete compartments that are typically filled with fluid or clotted blood, or has ill-defined zones of hemorrhage, separated by solid tissue (*Fig. 15.1*). The occasional tumor that is

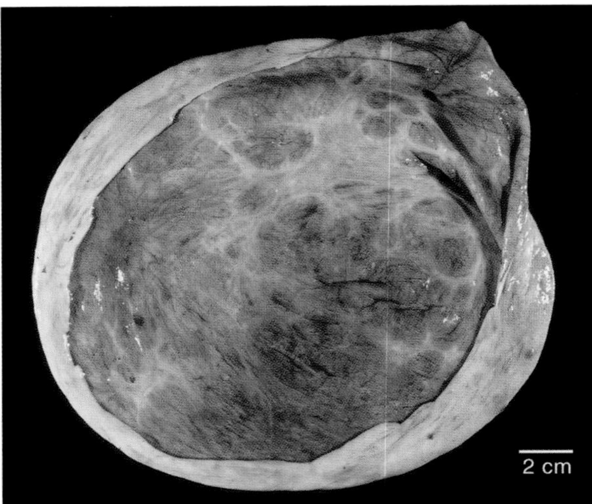

■ Fig. 15.3
Adult granulosa cell tumor. **The neoplasm is a unilocular cyst with a smooth inner lining**

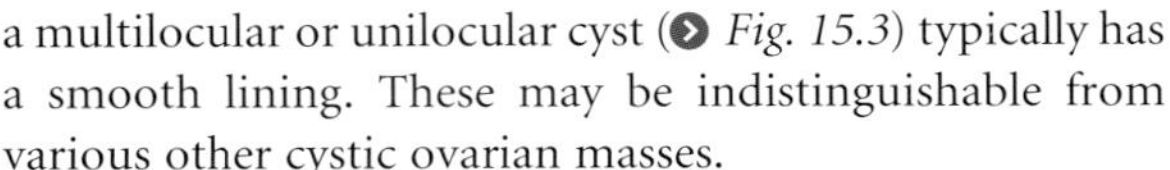
a multilocular or unilocular cyst (➲ *Fig. 15.3*) typically has a smooth lining. These may be indistinguishable from various other cystic ovarian masses.

Microscopic Findings

Microscopic examination of an adult granulosa cell tumor reveals only granulosa cells or, more often, an additional component of theca cells, fibroblasts, or both; in some cases, the latter cell types predominate. The granulosa cells grow in a wide variety of patterns, which are commonly admixed (➲ *Figs. 15.4–15.21*): diffuse, microfollicular, macrofollicular, insular, corded to trabecular, solid-tubular, rarely hollow-tubular, miscellaneous other epithelial formations (➲ *Fig. 15.16*), and sarcomatoid (➲ *Fig. 15.17*). Although the microfollicular pattern is the best known (➲ *Fig. 15.14*), it is less common, particularly as striking initial morphology, than a more or less diffuse

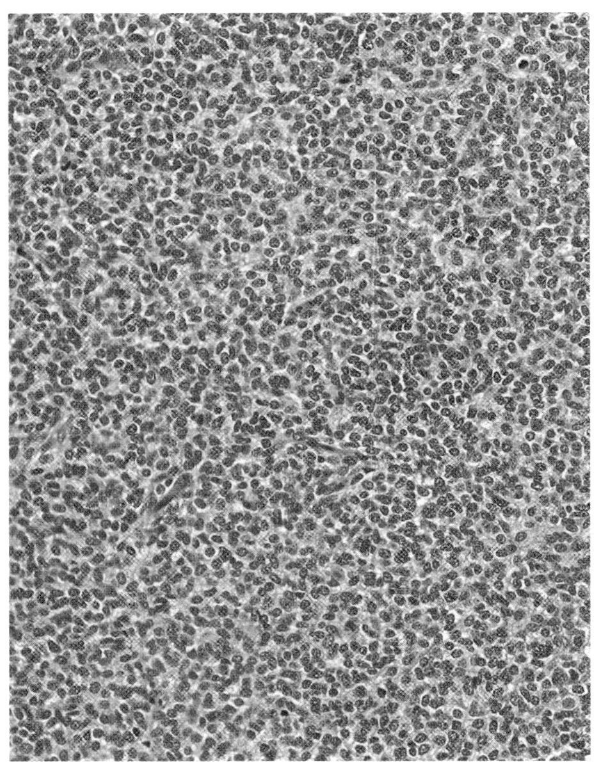

■ Fig. 15.4
Adult granulosa cell tumor, diffuse pattern

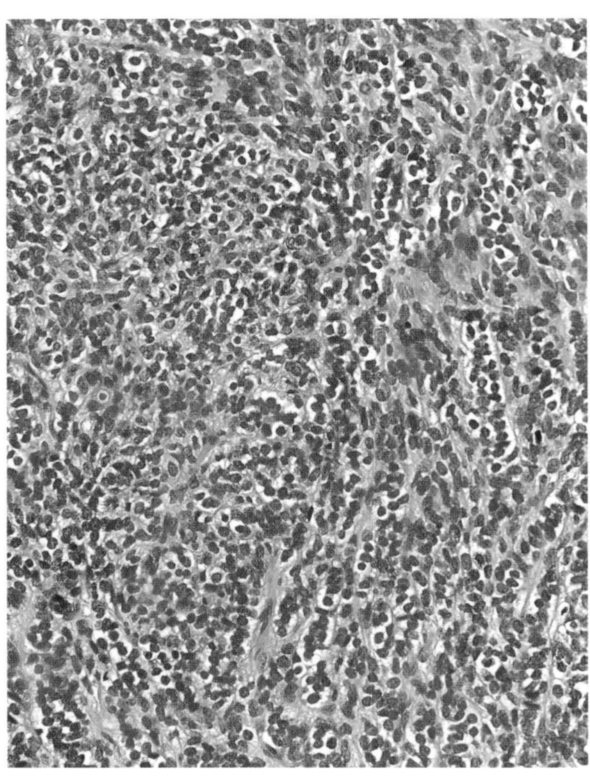

■ Fig. 15.5
Adult granulosa cell tumor. **Focal cords and clusters idicating an epithelial nature are seen in region close to that depicted in ➲ *Fig. 15.4***

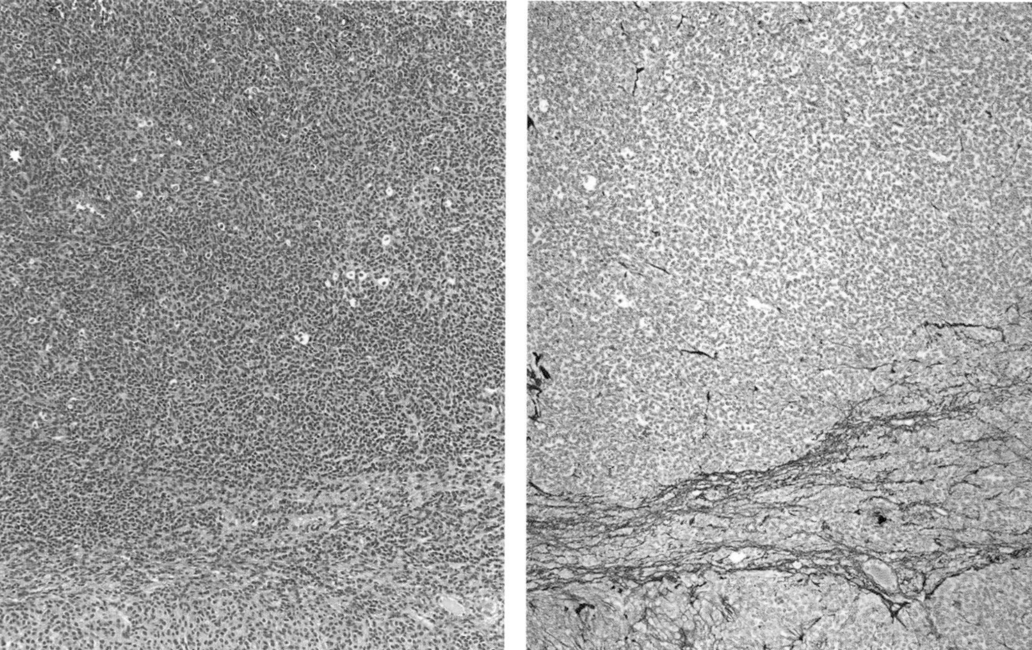

Fig. 15.6
Adult granulosa cell tumor. The tumor displays a diffuse pattern with focal subtle cords (*left*). A reticulum stain (*right*) shows a paucity of staining overall supporting the diagnosis

pattern. However, although regions of neoplasms that fall in the category of a "diffuse" granulosa cell tumor do have a mostly nonspecific sheet-like growth of cells, in the great majority of cases, sometimes most strikingly at the periphery, one sees various, admittedly often somewhat subtle, patterns of epithelial differentiation on medium- to high-power scrutiny (*Figs. 15.4–15.6*). Most typically, delicate cords are the initial clue to the diagnosis of a granulosa cell tumor and overall, cords are probably the commonest epithelial arrangement.

The trabecular (*Fig. 15.8*) and insular (*Fig. 15.11*) patterns are characterized by bands and islands of granulosa cells, separated by a fibromatous or thecomatous stroma. In the solid tubular pattern, the tubules may be uniformly cellular or contain peripheral nuclei and central masses of cytoplasm; occasionally, a few hollow tubules or gland-like structures are encountered. The various tubular patterns encountered in granulosa cell tumors are indistinguishable from those of well-differentiated Sertoli cell tumors; their presence is ignored as a diagnostic criterion unless they account for a significant portions of the tumor (10% or more); in such cases, a diagnosis of mixed granulosa cell and Sertoli cell tumor, or gynandroblastoma, is warranted. Other patterns of granulosa cell tumor are watered silk (moiré silk), gyriform (*Fig. 15.13*), and pseudopapillary [69]. The first two patterns are manifested by undulating or zigzag rows of granulosa cells, generally in single file. The third is likely a degenerative phenomenon.

The microfollicular pattern, which only rarely predominates, is characterized by the presence of numerous small cavities simulating the Call–Exner bodies of the developing graafian follicle (*Fig. 15.14*). These cavities may contain eosinophilic fluid and often one or a few degenerating nuclei, hyalinized basement membrane material, or rarely basophilic fluid. The microfollicles are separated typically by well-differentiated granulosa cells that contain scanty cytoplasm and pale, angular or oval, often grooved nuclei arranged haphazardly in relation to one another and to the follicles. The macrofollicular pattern of the granulosa cell tumor (*Fig. 15.15*) is uncommon and characterized by cysts lined by well-differentiated granulosa cells, beneath which theca cells often are present.

The neoplastic granulosa cells typically have scant cytoplasm and pale nuclei, some of which have nuclear grooves (*Fig. 15.18*). The pallor and frequency of nuclear grooves is variable from region to region and

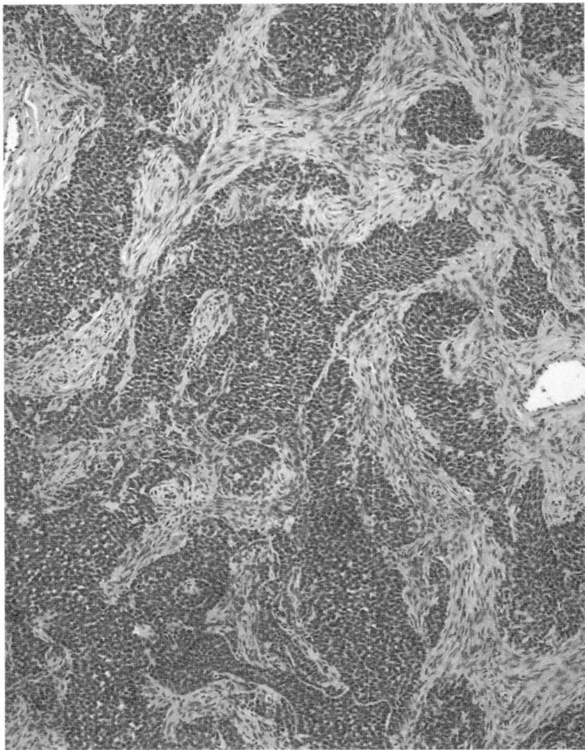

Fig. 15.7
Adult granulosa cell tumor. **Large irregular aggregates and smaller nests in a cellular fibrous stroma**

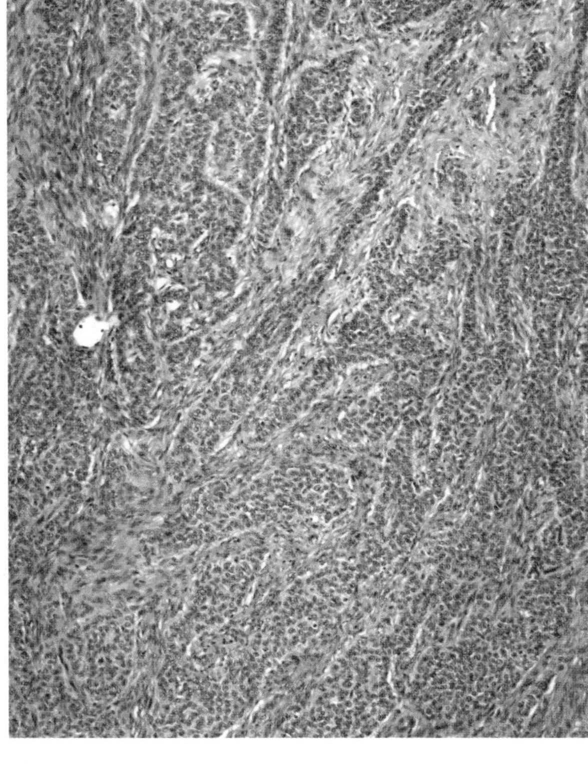

Fig. 15.8
Adult granulosa cell tumor. **A trabecular pattern is present**

case to case and can be impacted amongst other things by vagaries of fixation and staining. The mitotic rate in the tumors is also variable. It is generally not brisk, but there are exceptions; however, in cases with a brisk mitotic rate, particular care should be made to make sure one is not misinterpreting a mimic of a granulosa cell tumor as that neoplasm. In some granulosa cell tumors, the neoplastic cells contain abundant dense or vacuolated cytoplasm, approaching, to varying degrees, the appearance of the granulosa cells of the corpus luteum; in such cases, the term luteinized granulosa cell tumor is appropriate. Rarely, the neoplastic granulosa cells have a signet-ring cell morphology, more typical of the signet-ring cell stromal tumor considered later. Exceptionally, a granulosa cell tumor undergoes sarcomatous transformation [160] or transforms into an anaplastic carcinoma [144]. A handful of granulosa cell tumors have been intimately associated with a mucinous cystic tumor [95, 128].

An exception to the characteristic nuclear features described above is seen in approximately 2% of granulosa cell tumors that contain bizarre, enlarged hyperchromatic nuclei, including multinucleated forms [186] (*Figs. 15.19* and *15.20*). Cells with these nuclear features typically are a focal finding but rarely are conspicuous and may overshadow more characteristic foci, which can be overlooked if not carefully sought.

The prominence and nature of the stromal component in granulosa cell tumors vary considerably. In some cases, usually those with a diffuse pattern, it is essentially absent. In tumors in which the granulosa cells form nests or trabeculae, the stroma is usually conspicuous and composed of fibroblasts and theca cells that contain appreciable to abundant eosinophilic or vacuolated lipid-rich cytoplasm. The stroma is often quite vascular (*Fig. 15.9*), and this may be striking on low-power examination.

Rarely, crystals of Reinke are present in the lutein-type cells of a granulosa cell tumor, enabling them to be specifically identified as Leydig cells [4]. Another recently recognized rare component of the stromal compartment of granulosa cell tumors is hepatic-type cells [4, 109]

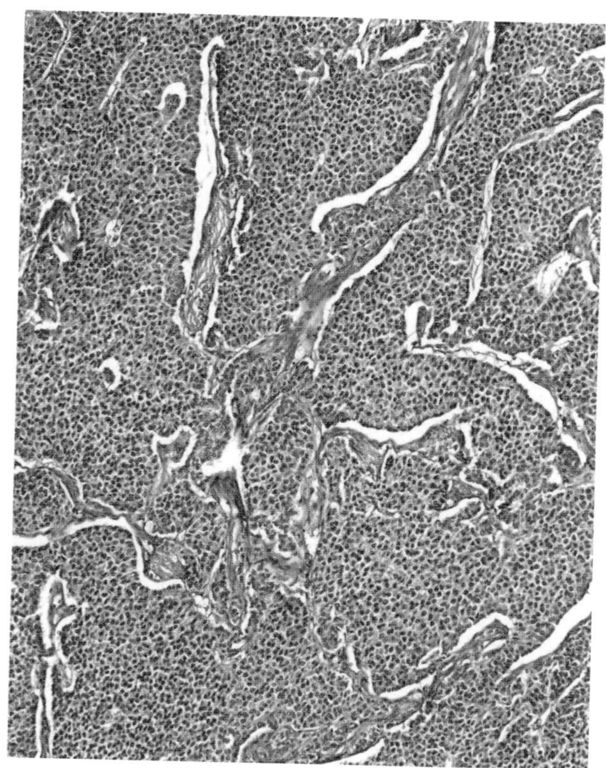

■ Fig. 15.9
Adult granulosa cell tumor. **Large islands of neoplastic granulosa cells separated by scant, but prominently vascular, stroma**

(➲ *Fig. 15.21*). These cells are typically larger and have denser eosinophilic cytoplasm than lutein or Leydig cells. Bile pigment has been detected in canaliculi between some of the hepatic-type cells in three cases. The hepatic-type cells have been immunoreactive for epithelial membrane antigen (EMA), carcinoembryonic antigen (CEA), which stained canaliculi between the cells, and CAM 5. In contrast to lutein or Leydig cells, the hepatic-type cells are negative for inhibin [4].

The presence of theca cells in varying quantities in most granulosa cell tumors has led to the occasional usage of the term granulosa–theca cell tumor. Although this designation accurately describes the cellular content of many of these neoplasms, the term granulosa cell tumor is more widely accepted for tumors containing both cell types. One reason for this preference is the probability that the presence of theca cells in some cases reflects a response of the ovarian stroma to the growth of granulosa cells rather than the coexistence of a second neoplastic cell component. Evidence favoring such an interpretation includes the nonspecific presence of theca-like cells in a variety of ovarian tumors, both benign and malignant and both primary and metastatic, and the observation that theca cells usually are absent in granulosa cell tumors that have extended beyond the ovary [47]. It is possible, however, that some tumors in which the theca cell element is prominent or even greatly preponderant are truly mixed neoplasms. The theca cells in granulosa cell tumors may resemble theca externa or theca interna cells and may be luteinized. In some tumors, particularly those with a diffuse pattern, differentiation of granulosa and theca cells with routine staining may be difficult or impossible. In such cases a reticulum stain may be helpful. Just as in a developing graafian follicle, so in a granulosa cell tumor, the fibrils typically invest theca cells individually. In contrast, the granulosa cell layer of a follicle contains no fibrils, and in a granulosa cell tumor, the reticulum usually is sparse, being typically confined to perivascular zones.

The presence of blood-filled cysts in many granulosa cell tumors results in the frequent presence in the tumors of related changes that are nonspecific, but in the context of other typical features of granulosa cell tumors are at the same time quite characteristic. For example, the cysts often are lined by fibrous tissue associated with evidence of old and recent hemorrhage that is sometimes conspicuous.

Several histochemical reactions that are characteristic of steroid hormone-producing cells, particularly those that demonstrate various types of lipid content or oxidative enzyme activity, usually are positive in the theca cells and negative or only weakly positive in the granulosa cells of a tumor containing both cell types [79–81, 146]. This finding, as well as ultrastructural observations, has led some observers to conclude that the theca cell component of granulosa cell tumors produces the hormones responsible for estrogenic manifestations. Additional evidence in favor of this conclusion is the observation that granulosa cell tumors that recur outside ovarian tissue and lack theca cells typically are not obviously estrogenic. In some cases, however, histochemical and other evidence has suggested a role for the granulosa cells in estrogen secretion [7, 42]. The above histochemical studies are rarely indicated other than for academic interest.

Differential Diagnosis

Misinterpretation of an undifferentiated carcinoma as an adult granulosa cell tumor (AGCT) with a diffuse pattern occasionally occurs. If the clinical course of the patient is

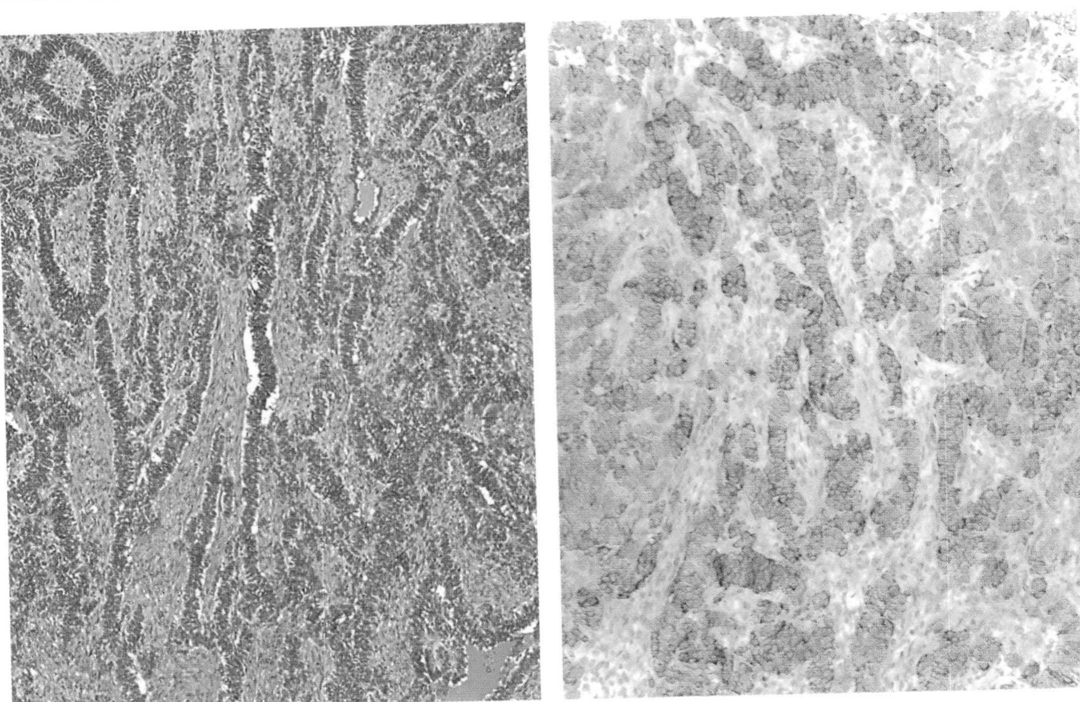

Fig. 15.10
Adult granulosa cell tumor. Long ribbons of cells (*left*). Positive staining for inhibin (*right*)

atypically malignant for an AGCT, the possibility of such a misdiagnosis must be considered. The single best criterion for distinguishing these two tumors is the appearance of the nuclei, which are typically uniform, pale, and often grooved in the AGCT (tumors with bizarre nuclei being a noteworthy exception) and are hyperchromatic, usually of unequal size and shape, and rarely grooved in undifferentiated carcinomas; atypical mitotic figures often are found in the latter as well. Other features helpful in the differential diagnosis are summarized in *Table 15.2*. The highly malignant small cell carcinoma, which usually is associated with hypercalcemia, also may be misdiagnosed as an AGCT. The differential features of these tumors are presented in *Table 15.3*. The most helpful features are the much higher mitotic rate of the small cell carcinoma and the lack in that tumor of the typical cytologic features of the AGCT. Immunohistochemical differences will also aid if this step is deemed indicated [3, 92]. A diffuse AGCT occasionally is confused with a primary endometrioid stromal sarcoma or metastatic endometrial stromal sarcoma of the ovary, but a variety of features, including the frequent high stage and bilaterality of the latter tumors, the characteristic pattern of growth in extraovarian sites of spread, their typical content of numerous arterioles, and their rich reticulum content aid in this differential diagnosis. In this, as in other problems in the diagnosis of granulosa cell and other sex cord-stromal tumors, extensive sampling of the specimen often is helpful as is an appreciation of the rarity of bilaterality and extraovarian spread at presentation in cases of sex cord-stromal tumors.

AGCTs may be difficult to distinguish from pure stromal tumors such as cellular thecomas, particularly those that are more cellular than is normal, fibromas, and fibrosarcomas. Reticulum stains may show abundant intercellular fibrils in these tumors, unlike the scant reticulum of AGCTs. In some cases, the pattern of fibrils is intermediate between an AGCT and a thecoma, and in such cases, the differential diagnosis may be difficult or impossible. The almost exclusive spindle cell nature of the cells in fibromas and fibrosarcomas is rarely seen in an AGCT.

Occasionally, the distinction of a unilocular or multilocular macrofollicular AGCT from one or more follicular cysts may be troublesome; this is particularly likely if the patient is pregnant, or in the puerperium, because a large solitary luteinized follicle cyst of pregnancy and the puerperium is indistinguishable grossly from a unilocular cystic AGCT. The large luteinized cells of the former, some of which contain large bizarre nuclei, differ

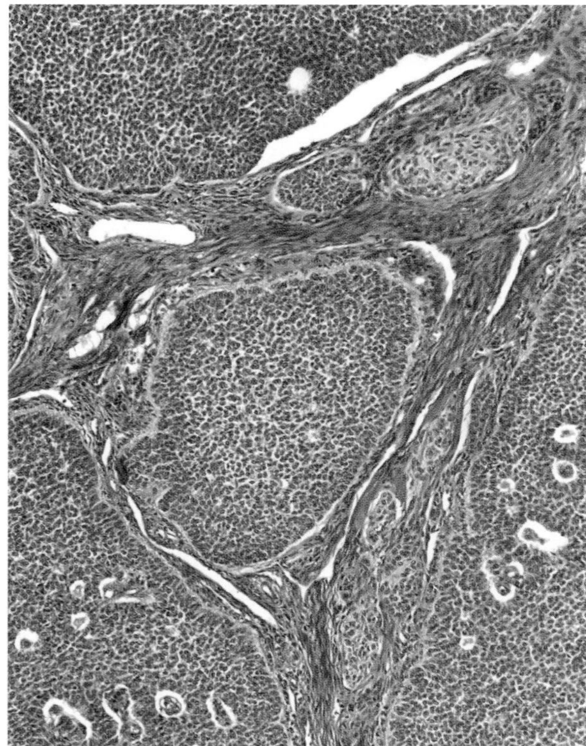

Fig. 15.11
Adult granulosa cell tumor, insular pattern

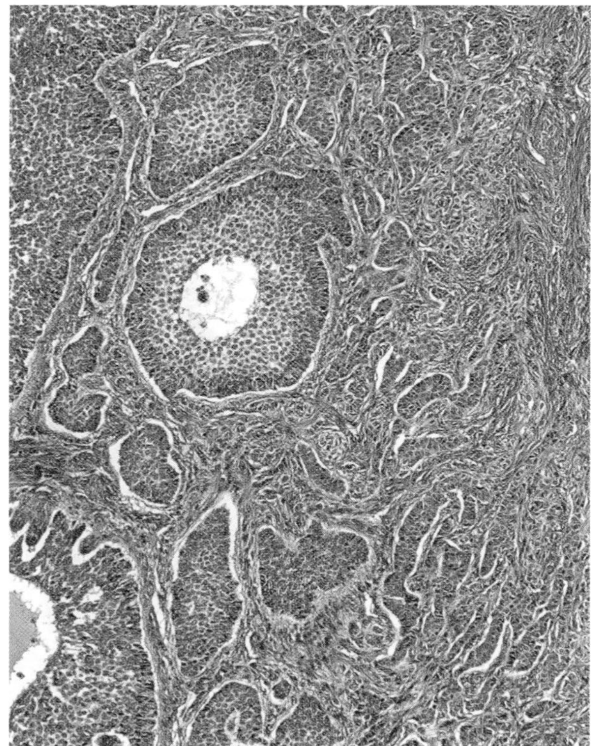

Fig. 15.12
Adult granulosa cell tumor, insular and trabecular patterns

from those of a unilocular AGCT, which are rarely uniformly luteinized and rarely contain bizarre nuclei lining the cysts.

Endometrioid carcinomas occasionally are misdiagnosed as AGCT when the former have small acini imparting a microfollicular pattern. Also, some endometrioid carcinomas have an insular pattern that on low power may suggest the diagnosis of an insular AGCT. Another source of confusion is the presence in some endometrioid carcinomas of a focal diffuse pattern that is occasionally difficult to distinguish from the diffuse pattern of an AGCT. In thoroughly sampled tumors, there will almost invariably be various patterns of one or the other tumor which will, however, establish the correct diagnosis. In the case of endometrioid tumors with a diffuse pattern, the focal presence of abortive squamous differentiation is a very major clue to the diagnosis. In most of these cases, the cytologic features in an endometrioid carcinoma differ from those of an AGCT, although there are rare cases in which the former tumors have pale nuclei that on cytologic grounds are consistent with a diagnosis of AGCT. In our experience, a combination of at least focal cytologic differences, and the presence in endometrioid tumors that are well sampled of other foci incompatible with the diagnosis of an AGCT, such as squamous foci, establish the diagnosis. Immunohistochemistry will aid if necessary, as noted in the introductory section of the chapter.

The rare AGCT in which the cells are extensively luteinized [180] may superficially resemble a steroid cell tumor. The focal presence of areas with the architectural and cytologic features of an AGCT usually facilitates the diagnosis in these cases. AGCTs should be distinguished from the small proliferations of granulosa cells within atretic follicles that are typically an incidental finding within the ovaries of pregnant women. Another rare problem in differential diagnosis is the distinction between a granulosa cell tumor, usually a luteinized one, and an epithelioid smooth muscle tumor. The latter diagnosis does not tend to be considered as quickly, not unreasonably, when examining an ovarian tumor as it does when evaluating a uterine one. This is an area in which immunohistochemistry, specifically strong desmin staining and negative staining for inhibin and calretinin, may play a major role.

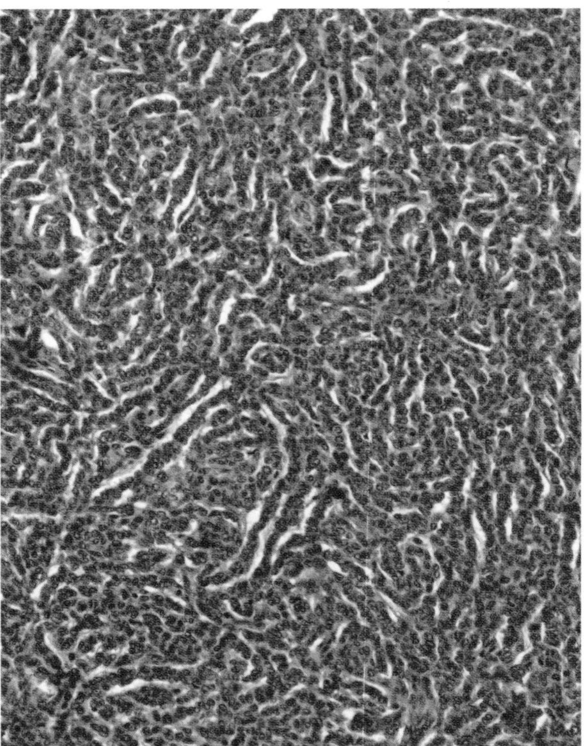

Fig. 15.13
Adult granulosa cell tumor, gyriform pattern

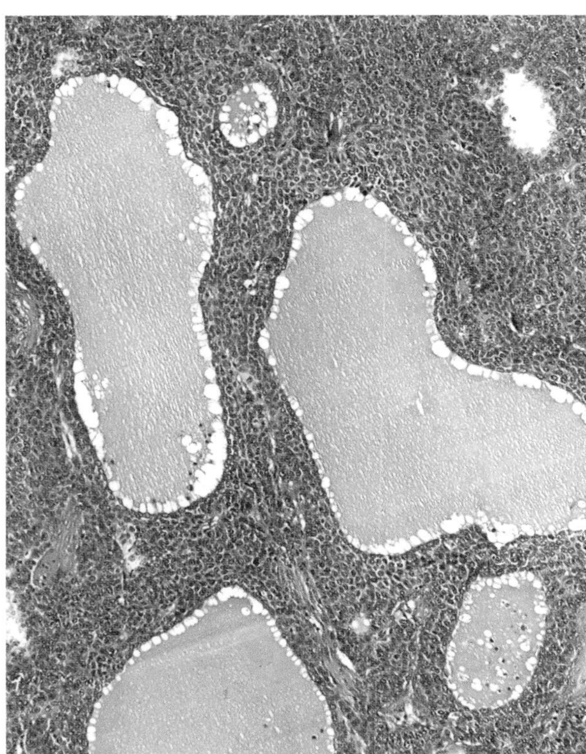

Fig. 15.15
Adult granulosa cell tumor, macrofollicular pattern

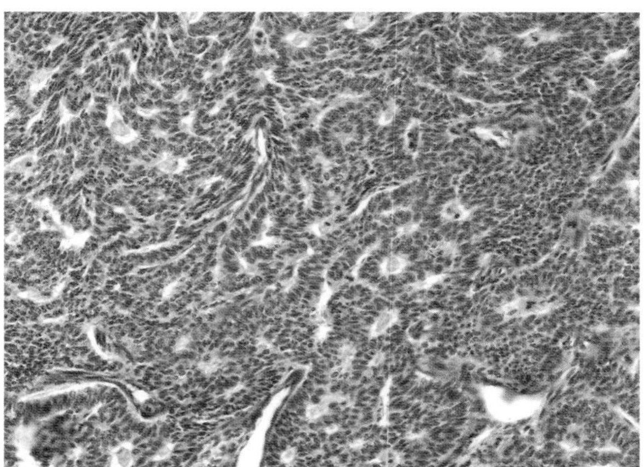

Fig. 15.14
Adult granulosa cell tumor, microfollicular pattern

It is important to distinguish the Call–Exner bodies of AGCTs from the acini of carcinoid (*Table 15.4*) and from the hyaline bodies that are seen in gonadoblastomas and sex cord tumors with annular tubules. The acini of carcinoids often contain dense eosinophilic secretion that is sometimes calcified; the latter is not a feature of the AGCT. The nuclei of carcinoids, which have coarse chromatin, contrast with the pale nuclei of the AGCT. The hyaline bodies of gonadoblastomas and sex cord tumors with annular tubules typically are larger than Call–Exner bodies. Sometimes, the hyaline bodies can be observed to be continuous with hyaline thickenings of the basement membrane along the periphery of the tumor cell nests; these bodies also undergo calcification.

The AGCT may be confused with two types of metastatic tumors, metastatic malignant melanoma and metastatic breast carcinoma. Metastatic melanomas may have cells with scant cytoplasm that grow diffusely, imparting a low-power appearance that may closely mimic that of an AGCT. Patterns of growth incompatible with a diagnosis of AGCT usually are found when a tumor is thoroughly sampled, and the finding of melanin pigment or immunohistochemical stains may be helpful in problematic cases. Metastatic breast carcinoma sometimes also has a diffuse growth of cells with scant cytoplasm, particularly in cases of lobular carcinoma. The history often is helpful

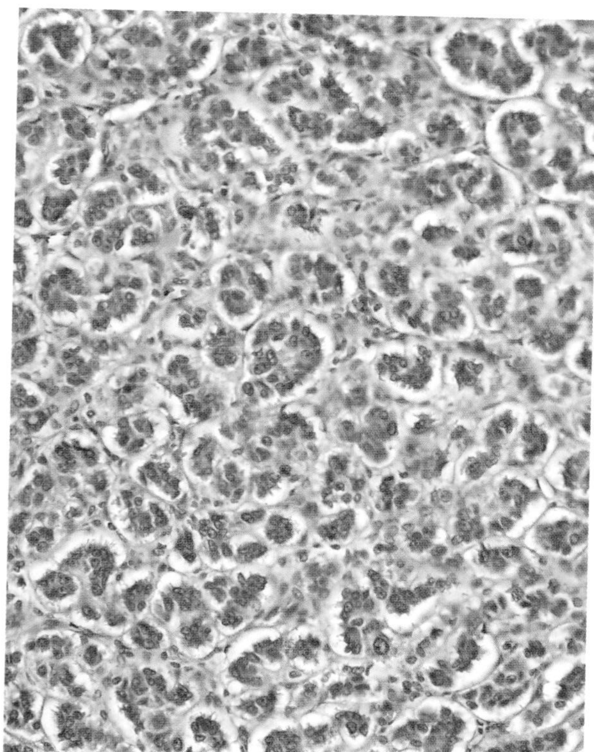

Fig. 15.16
Adult granulosa cell tumor. **A peculiar pattern of regular small clusters of cells**

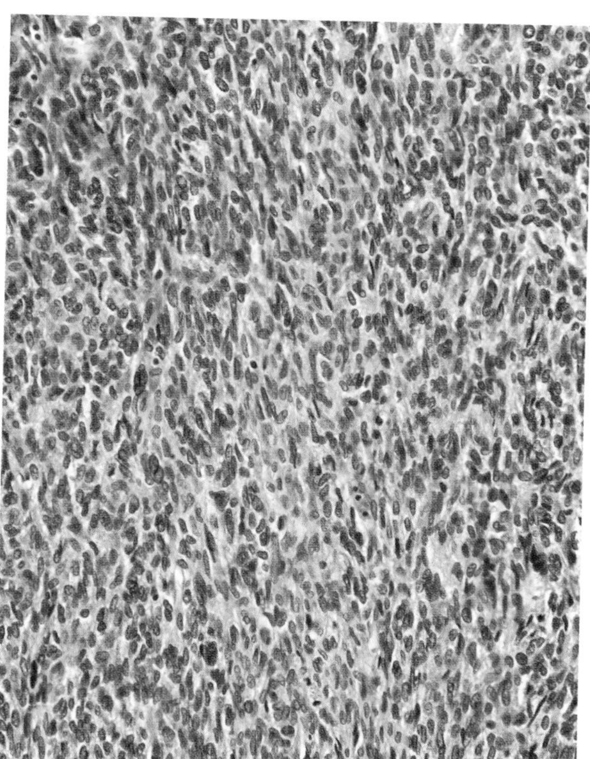

Fig. 15.17
Adult granulosa cell tumor, sarcomatoid pattern

in these cases because breast carcinoma rarely presents with an ovarian metastasis. In cases in which a breast cancer is not known in the patient, it is only the presence of focal patterns more suggestive of breast cancer than a granulosa cell tumor and a lack of the typical cytologic features of granulosa cell tumor that will alert the pathologist to the possible correct diagnosis. In both this situation and that of metastatic melanoma, the ovarian metastatic tumors are much more frequently bilateral than is the AGCT. Immunohistochemical staining for gross cystic disease fluid protein 15, S-100, and HMB45 can be helpful in the distinction of metastatic breast carcinoma and metastatic malignant melanoma from the adult granulosa cell tumor.

Clinical Behavior and Treatment

After the removal of a granulosa cell tumor, the manifestations of hyperestrinism typically regress. If the uterus has been conserved in a young woman, estrogen withdrawal bleeding usually occurs in 1 or 2 days, and regular menses ensue shortly thereafter. Granulosa cell tumors of all patterns have a malignant potential, with a capacity to extend beyond the ovary or recur after apparently successful removal. Spread is largely within the pelvis and lower abdomen; distant metastases are rare but have been reported in many sites. Although recurrences may appear within 5 years, they often are not evident until a much longer postoperative interval has elapsed, and numerous cases have been reported in which the tumor has reappeared two or even three or more decades after the initial therapy. The 10-year survival figures that have been recorded in the literature have varied widely from less than 60% to more than 90%, and progressive declines in survival have been documented after longer follow-up periods [14–16, 155]. Unfortunately, many old studies of granulosa cell tumor are suspect from the viewpoint of the impact of various features on prognosis, and survival figures overall, because of the almost certain inclusion in some of them of tumors that are not granulosa cell tumors, differential features between the granulosa cell tumor and its various mimics having been much more appreciated in the last several decades.

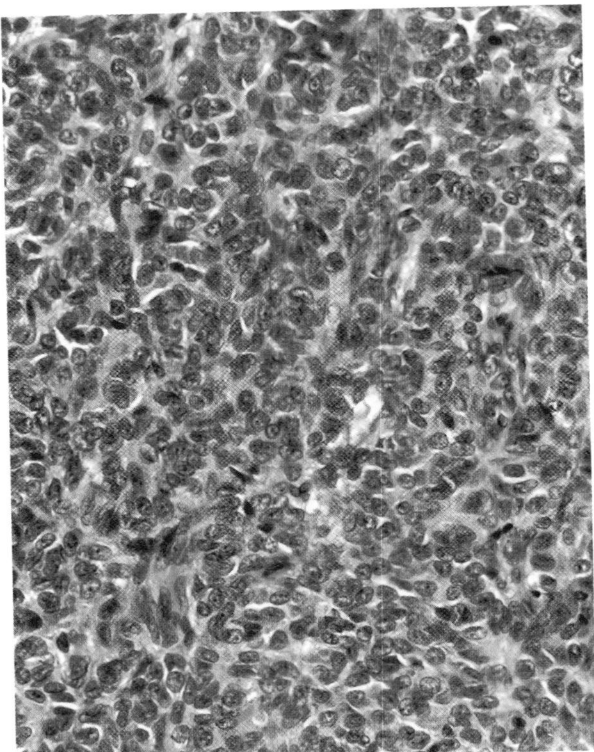

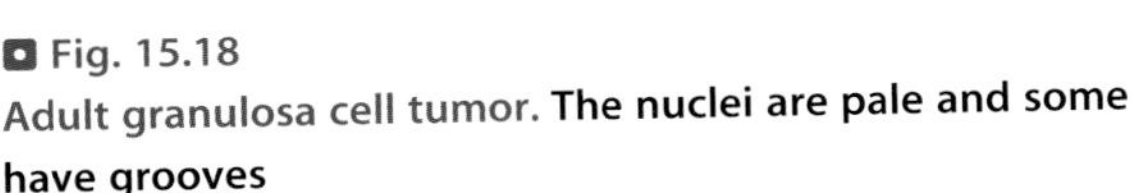

Fig. 15.18
Adult granulosa cell tumor. The nuclei are pale and some have grooves

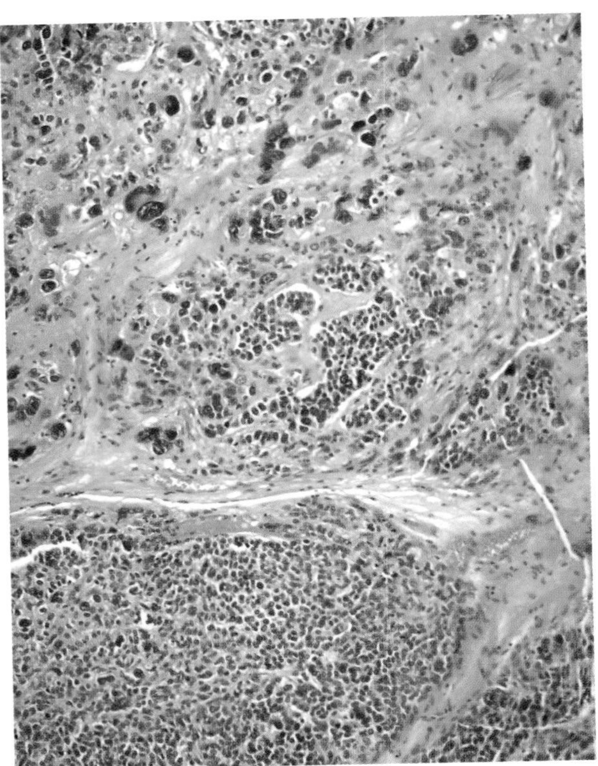

Fig. 15.19
Adult granulosa cell tumor with bizarre nucleil. Typical foci are also present (*bottom*) and a clue to the diagnosis

The optimal treatment of a granulosa cell tumor in menopausal or postmenopausal women is total hysterectomy with bilateral salpingo-oophorectomy. In younger women in whom the preservation of fertility is an important consideration, however, removal of only the ovary and the adjacent fallopian tube is justifiable if spread beyond the ovary is not demonstrable and examination of the contralateral ovary shows no suggestion of involvement. Some recurrent tumors have been treated successfully by reoperation, radiation therapy, or a combination of these.

At least 90% of granulosa cell tumors are stage I, and these tumors have a considerably better prognosis than the higher-stage tumors, as shown by an 86% versus a 49% relative survival at 10 years, respectively, in one large series and a 96% versus a 26% survival in another [16]. Rupture also adversely affects the outlook, with an 86% relative 25-year survival of patients with intact stage I tumors compared with only 60% survival of those with ruptured tumors that are otherwise in the same stage [16]. The impact of the stage has been confirmed in a recent study [9].

The size of granulosa cell tumors also has been related to their prognosis. In one series, all the patients with tumors 5 cm or less in diameter survived 10 years, but only 57% of those with tumors 6–15 cm in diameter and 53% of those with even larger tumors survived for that period of time [51]. Another investigation reported a 73% crude overall survival of patients with tumors less than 5 cm in diameter, a 63% survival of those with tumors between 5 and 15 cm, and a 34% survival of those with a tumor greater than 15 cm in diameter [155]. In a final series, stage I tumors 5 cm or less in diameter were associated with a 100% relative 10-year survival in contrast to a 92% survival of patients with larger stage I tumors [16]. The last series is the only one in which the survival rate was corrected for stage, and on that basis, the improvement in prognosis for the smaller stage I tumors was not statistically significant. Therefore, a relationship between tumor size and prognosis independent of stage has not been clearly established. Attempts to correlate the histologic pattern and the degrees of nuclear atypia and mitotic activity with prognosis have met with varying

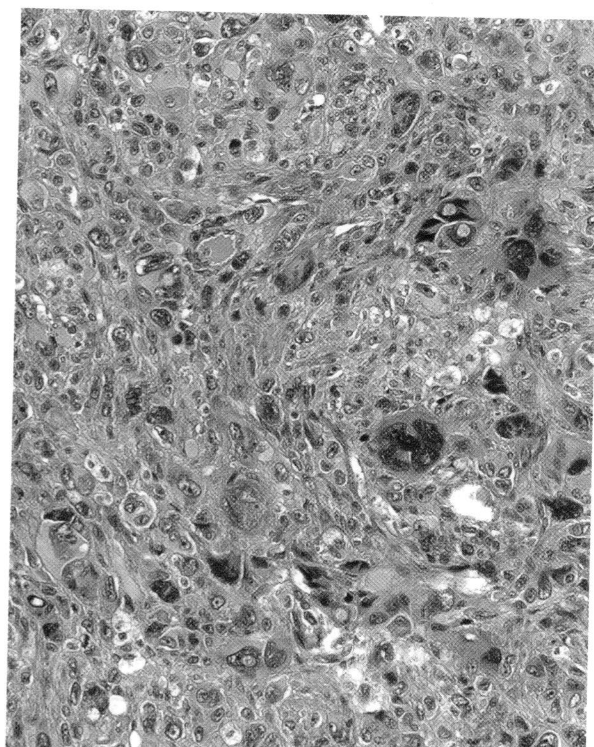

Fig. 15.20
Adult granulosa cell tumor with bizarre nuclei. In isolation the picture is alarming

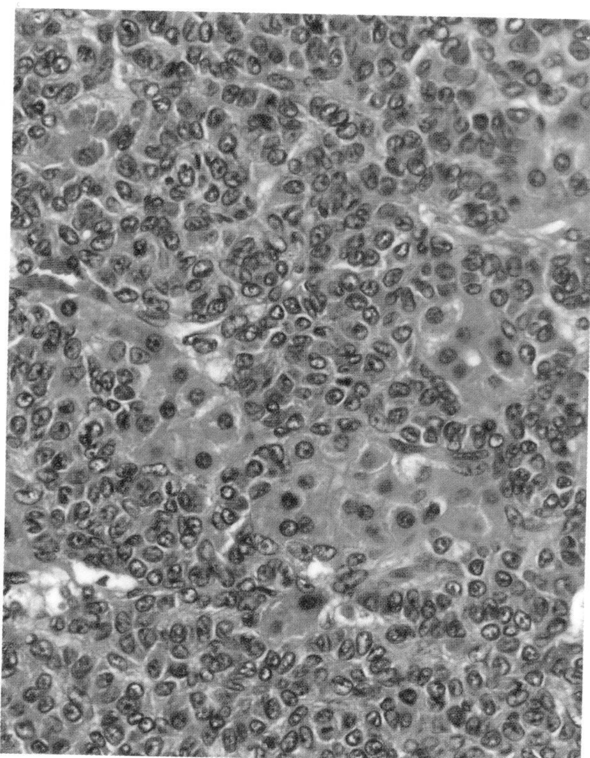

Fig. 15.21
Adult granulosa cell tumor with hepatic-like cells

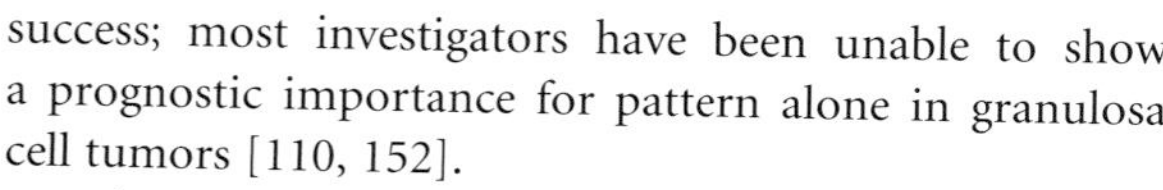

success; most investigators have been unable to show a prognostic importance for pattern alone in granulosa cell tumors [110, 152].

The degree of nuclear atypicality within granulosa cell tumors has been correlated with their prognosis. In one study, the 5-year survival of patients whose tumors showed no atypia was 92% compared with 80% for those with slight atypicality and 30% for those with moderate atypicality [155]. In another study, there was an 80% relative 25-year survival in cases with grade 1 nuclear atypicality in contrast to only a 60% survival in those with grade 2 atypia [16]. In both of these studies, nuclear atypicality was the most reliable prognostic index in cases of stage I tumors; for higher-stage tumors, nuclear atypicality and mitotic rate were of similar significance. With regard to the relation of nuclear atypicality to prognosis, it should be noted that assessment of its degree is somewhat subjective. Also, as noted earlier, approximately 2% of granulosa cell tumors contain mononucleate and multinucleate cells with large, bizarre, and hyperchromatic nuclei (*Figs. 15.19* and *15.20*), the

Table 15.2
Granulosa cell tumor versus undifferentiated carcinoma and poorly differentiated adenocarcinoma

Granulosa cell tumor	Carcinoma
Bilateral, less than 5%	Bilateral, more than 25%
Stage I in 90% of cases	Stage III or IV in most cases
Nuclei round to angular, pale and commonly grooved[a]	Nuclei hyperchromatic, often bizarre with atypical mitoses
Mucin occasionally in follicles (mainly in juvenile type)	Intracellular droplets or extracellular pools of mucin, psammoma bodies, or glands may be present
Good prognosis	Poor prognosis
Indolent course, when clinically malignant[b]	Rapid course

[a]Exception: dark, ungrooved nuclei of juvenile granulosa cell tumor.
[b]Exception: rare juvenile granulosa cell tumors.

Table 15.3
Granulosa cell tumors (GCTs) versus small cell carcinoma

Juvenile GCT	Adult GCT	Small cell carcinoma
Mostly before 30 years	All ages, but mostly postmenopausal	Always premenopausal
Rarely malignant	Occasionally malignant, often with protracted course	Highly malignant
No hypercalcemia	No hypercalcemia	Hypercalcemia common
Usually estrogenic	Usually estrogenic	Never estrogenic
Thecomatous component common	Fibrothecomatous component common	Stroma scanty and nonspecific
Mucinous epithelium absent	Mucinous epithelium rare	Mucinous epithelium 12% of cases
Cytoplasm usually abundant	Cytoplasm usually scanty	Cytoplasm usually scanty, but may be abundant
Nuclei dark, ungrooved, and pleomorphic 13% of cases	Nuclei pale and often grooved	Nuclei dark, uniform, and ungrooved
Mitoses usually numerous	Mitoses variable	Mitoses numerous

Table 15.4
Granulosa cell tumor versus carcinoid

Granulosa cell tumor	Insular carcinoid
Variety of patterns	Islands, round acini, solid tubules, and ribbons
Call–Exner bodies, ill-defined, with watery to dense eosniophilic content, occasionally pyknotic	Acini sharply outlined with dense content, nucleisometimes calcified
Nuclei round to angular, pale, often grooved, haphazardly oriented	Nuclei round with coarse chromatin and regular orientation
Thecomatous stroma common, at least focally	Fibromatous or hyalinized stroma, may be focally luteinized
Usually uninodular and almost always unilateral; no teratomatous elements	Often multinodular and almost always bilateral if metastatic; always unilateral and usually associated with other teratomatous elements if primary
Cells nonargentaffin; may contain fine argyrophilic granules	Cells usually argentaffin; almost always argyrophilic

presence of which has not been shown to worsen the prognosis. These nuclear changes, which resemble those seen in the uterine leiomyoma with bizarre nuclei, also are encountered in occasional Sertoli–Leydig cell tumors and thecomas and probably are degenerative. In a study of 8 granulosa cell tumors, 7 Sertoli–Leydig cell tumors and 2 thecomas with bizarre nuclei, follow-up was obtained on 11 patients, all of whom were alive without evidence of disease 3–21 years postoperatively [186].

The mitotic activity of granulosa cell tumors also has been correlated with their prognosis. In one study there was a 70% 10-year survival associated with tumors that had two or fewer mitotic figures (MF) per ten high-power fields (HPF) compared with only a 37% survival for those with three or more [155]. In another investigation [110], tumors with many mitotic figures were associated with a worse prognosis than those with few, but most of the tumors with high mitotic rates also were at a higher stage than those with low mitotic rates, and differences in mitotic rate did not have a statistically significant effect on the prognosis of stage I tumors.

Juvenile Granulosa Cell Tumor

Clinical Features

Somewhat less than 5% of granulosa cell tumors are diagnosed before the age of normal puberty [82]. The great majority of these tumors as well as many granulosa cell tumors in young adults differ histologically from adult granulosa cell tumors (*Table 15.5*), and the designation juvenile has been selected for such tumors because 97% of them occur in the first 3 decades [178]. Approximately,

Table 15.5
Adult versus juvenile granulosa cell tumor (GCT)

Adult GCT	Juvenile GCT
Less than 1% prepubertal	50% prepubertal
Usual after 30 years	Rare after 30 years
Mature follicles and Call–Exner bodies occasional	Immature follicles with mucin content Call–Exner bodies rare
Nuclei pale, angular, commonly grooved	Nuclei darker, round, rarely grooved
Luteinization infrequent	Luteinization frequent

80% of juvenile granulosa cell tumors (JGCTs) occurring in children result in isosexual precocity, accounting for 10% of cases of that syndrome in the female. More common forms of isosexual precocity are those of central origin, with premature release of gondadotropins from the anterior pituitary gland and those resulting from apparently autonomous formation of one or more follicle cysts. The precocity caused by granulosa cell tumors is more specifically designated pseudoprecocity because there is no associated ovulation or progesterone production, precluding the possibility of pregnancy, which exists, in contrast, in cases of true sexual precocity. Typically, pseudoprecocity is heralded by the development of the breasts, followed by the appearance of pubic and axillary hair, stimulation and enlargement of the external and internal secondary sex organs, irregular uterine bleeding, and a whitish vaginal discharge, believed to originate in the stimulated endocervical glands. Somatic and skeletal development typically are accelerated as well. Androgenic manifestations such as clitoromegaly occasionally occur [178].

When it occurs after puberty, the JGCT usually presents with abdominal pain or swelling, sometimes associated with menstrual irregularities or amenorrhea. Approximately, 6% of all the patients present with acute abdominal symptoms because of rupture of the tumor and hemoperitoneum. An interesting clinical association of the JGCT has been its association with Ollier's disease (enchondromatosis) in some patients and with Maffucci's syndrome (enchondromatosis and hemangiomatosis) in a few others. The JGCT is bilateral in only about 2% of the cases. It appears ruptured at operation in approximately 10% of the cases, and ascites is present in a similar percentage. Spread beyond the ovary is unusual; in our series only 2% of the tumors were stage II; rare tumors are stage III [178]. The diameter of the tumor has ranged from 3 to 32 cm, with an average of 12.5 cm. Because of a usual moderate to large size of the tumor, an adnexal mass is almost always detectable clinically. Rarely, however, a mass has not been palpable preoperatively even on bimanual rectal examination.

Gross Findings

The range of gross appearances of the JGCT is similar to that of the adult form. Like the latter, the single most common presentation is as a solid and cystic neoplasm in which the cysts may contain hemorrhagic fluid (*Fig. 15.22*). Uniformly solid and uniformly cystic neoplasms also are encountered; the latter may be multilocular or, rarely, unilocular. The solid component typically is yellow-tan or gray, and occasionally exhibits extensive necrosis, hemorrhage, or both.

Microscopic Findings

Microscopic examination (*Figs. 15.23–15.26*) typically reveals a solid cellular neoplasm, with focal follicle formation (*Fig. 15.23*), but the tumor also may be uniformly solid or uniformly follicular. In the solid areas, the neoplastic cells may be arranged diffusely or divided into nodules by fibrous septa; occasionally, small clusters of tumor cells are present in a fibrous stroma. In the solid foci the granulosa cells usually predominate, but often there is an admixture of theca cells, and in some areas the latter may predominate. Occasionally, the granulosa cells and theca cells are admixed in a haphazard fashion. Foci resembling typical thecoma with hyaline bands are encountered rarely but usually are minor in extent. Rarely, areas of sclerosis and calcification are seen. A pseudopapillary pattern (*Fig. 15.26*) analogous to that seen in the AGCT may be seen.

The follicles usually vary in size and shape but may be regular and round to oval. They generally do not reach the large size of the follicles in the rare macrofollicular form of AGCT. Their lumens contain eosinophilic or basophilic secretion, which stains with mucicarmine in approximately two thirds of the cases. Granulosa cells of varying layers of thickness line the follicles and occasionally are surrounded by mantles of theca cells. More often, however, the granulosa cells lining the follicles blend into the intervening diffusely cellular areas. Rarely, the lining cells resemble hobnail cells.

The two characteristic cytologic features of the neoplastic granulosa cells that distinguish them from those of

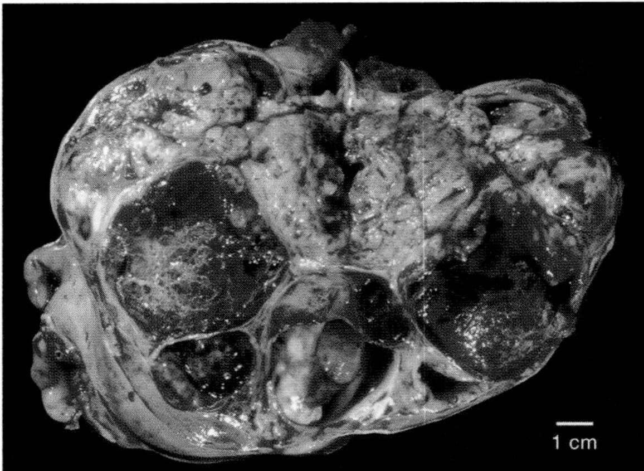

Fig. 15.22
Juvenile granulosa cell tumor. **The sectioned surface of the neoplasm is solid and cystic. Clotted blood is present in most of the cysts**

the AGCT are their generally rounded, hyperchromatic nuclei, which lack grooves in most cases, and their frequent abundant content of eosinophilic (luteinized) cytoplasm (*Fig. 15.24*). The theca cell element of the tumors usually is also luteinized, and lipid stains typically disclose moderate to large amounts of fat within the cytoplasm of both cellular components. The theca cells are more often spindle shaped than the granulosa cells and, like the latter, usually contain hyperchromatic nuclei. In rare JGCTs, small foci more characteristic of the AGCT are encountered.

Nuclear atypicality in JGCTs varies from minimal to marked. In approximately 13% of the cases severe degrees are present (*Fig. 15.25*) [178]. The mitotic rate also varies greatly but is generally higher than that seen in AGCTs.

There are very rare neoplasms that we designate anaplastic juvenile granulosa cell tumor. In contrast to conventional neoplasms with striking nuclear atypia but

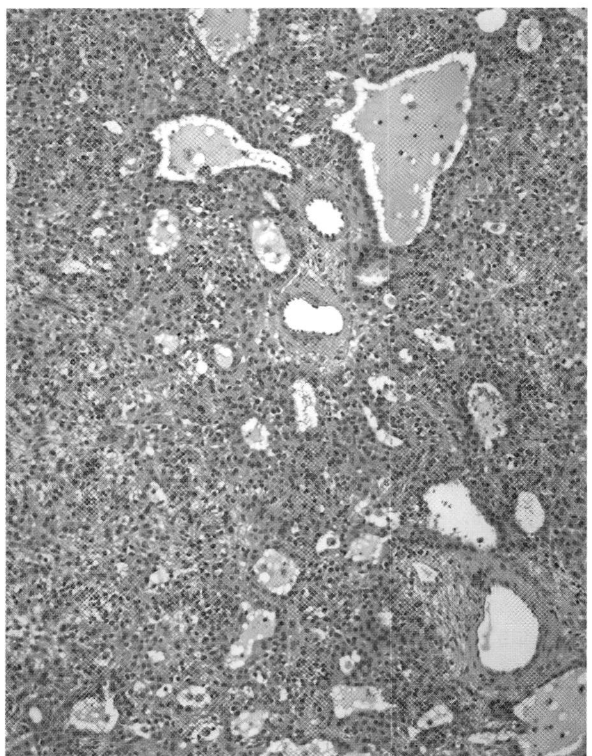

Fig. 15.23
Juvenile granulosa cell tumor. **Follicles of varying sizes and shapes are separated by cellular areas**

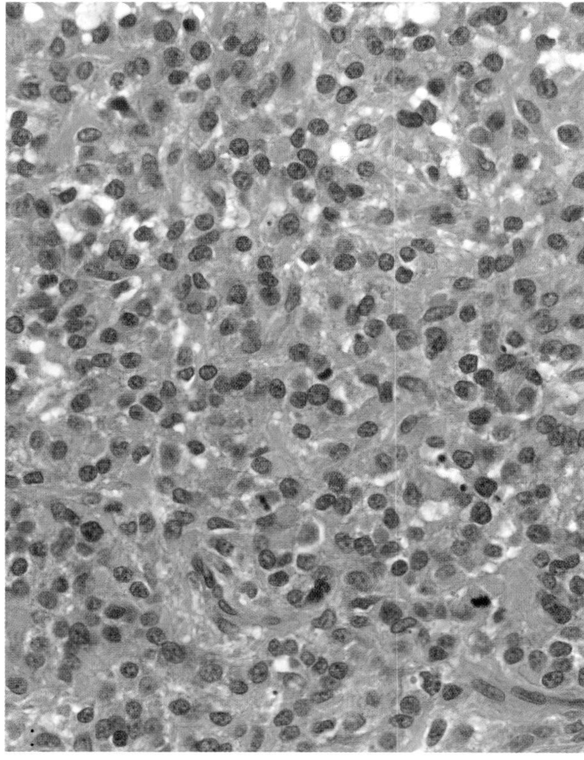

Fig. 15.24
Juvenile granulosa cell tumor. **The cells have abundant cytoplasm; their nuclei lack grooves and exhibit mitotic activity**

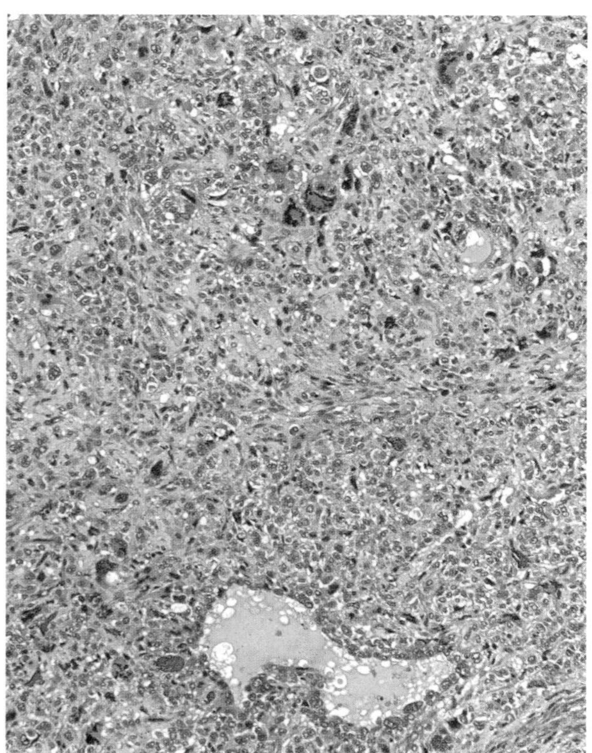

Fig. 15.25
Juvenile granulosa cell tumor. **Focally marked nuclear atypicality is present**

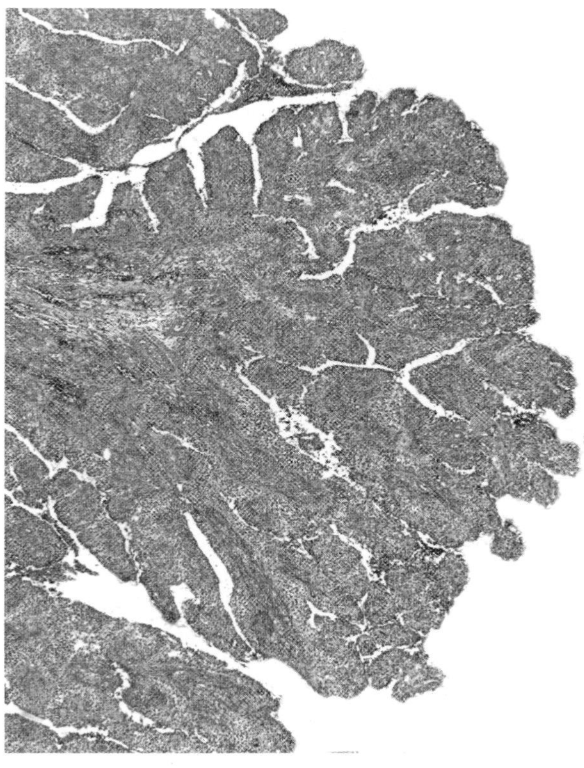

Fig. 15.26
Juvenile granulosa cell tumor, pseudopapillary pattern

which still have an orderly architecture, these neoplasms have zones with a sheet-like growth that when viewed in isolation are not recognizable as juvenile granulosa cell tumor and indeed, in some instances, resemble undifferentiated carcinoma. A diagnosis of anaplastic juvenile granulosa cell tumor can only be made when thorough sampling discloses characteristic features of that neoplasm in the form of the typical follicles.

Differential Diagnosis

The differential diagnosis of the JGCT includes the AGCT and a wide variety of other neoplasms. The follicles of the JGCT are more irregular in size and shape than those of an AGCT, and its cells are more extensively luteinized with nuclei that are typically round and more hyperchromatic and lack nuclear grooves (see *Table 15.5*). The mucicarminophilic, often basophilic follicular content in the JGCT, also differs from the eosinophilic fluid often accompanied by degenerating nuclei or basement membrane material that is usually present in the microfollicles of AGCTs.

The JGCT may be misdiagnosed as a malignant germ cell tumor. The latter may be associated with human chorionic gonadotropin (hCG)-induced isosexual pseudoprecocity. The nuclei of the JGCT are not as primitive appearing as those of either a yolk sac tumor or an embryonal carcinoma, and the follicular pattern of the JGCT is not a feature of either germ cell tumor, although the cysts of the polyvesicular variant of yolk sac tumor can superficially resemble the follicles of a JGCT in rare cases. Immunohistochemical demonstration of hCG in embryonal carcinomas and of alpha fetoprotein in yolk sac tumors may be helpful in difficult cases.

The JGCT is sometimes misinterpreted as a thecoma because of the occasional absence or rarity of follicles, the typically abundant cytoplasm of the neoplastic cells and the occasional predominance of theca cells. Thorough sampling to demonstrate follicles and the performance of reticulum stains to establish the granulosa cell nature of at least some of the tumor cells are important diagnostically. Also, thecomas rarely exhibit significant mitotic activity, uncommonly occur before 30 years of age and are exceptionally rare in children. A focally diffuse pattern in a luteinized JGCT may suggest the diagnosis of a steroid cell tumor, but the uniformity of the pattern and cytologic features of the latter tumor would be unusual for a JGCT, which almost always contains more diagnostic areas. The pregnancy luteoma rarely contains rounded follicle-like spaces and may suggest a luteinized JGCT but, like the steroid cell tumor, its cells are uniform in appearance, and it is multiple and bilateral in one half and one third of the cases, respectively.

The common epithelial tumors with which a JGCT may be confused are clear cell, undifferentiated, and transitional cell carcinomas. The tubulocystic variant of the clear cell carcinoma is rarely suggested when follicles in a JGCT are lined by cells resembling hobnail cells, and JGCTs with high-grade nuclear atypia may suggest an undifferentiated carcinoma. Transitional cell carcinoma is mimicked in rare cases in which a cystic JGCT contains pseudopapillae lined by uniform granulosa cells [69]. The young age of the patient and the presence of follicles and of other areas typical of a JGCT should help indicate the correct diagnosis in these cases.

The JGCT may be confused with a small cell carcinoma of hypercalcemic type (see ➋ *Table 15.3*) because both neoplasms contain follicles, and both are characteristically found in young patients. In the typical case of small cell carcinoma, the presence of cells with scanty cytoplasm is in marked contrast to the JGCT, in which the tumors almost without exception have cells with appreciable to abundant cytoplasm. The follicles in the small cell carcinoma rarely contain the basophilic secretion that is seen in many JGCTs. Although the JGCT characteristically has easily found mitotic figures, mitoses are in general much more numerous in the small cell carcinoma. Particular difficulty may be caused by cases of small cell carcinoma in which the tumor cells have abundant eosinophilic cytoplasm. The tumors usually can be distinguished even in these cases because the small cell carcinomas have a much more disorderly growth than seen in the JGCT. Additionally, the large cells seen in the cases of small cell carcinoma often have a rather distinctive dense, globular cytoplasm, a feature only occasionally seen in the JGCT.

The only metastatic tumor that we have seen confused with a JGCT is metastatic malignant melanoma, because some malignant melanomas, like many metastatic tumors, contain follicle-like spaces and this metastatic tumor frequently has cells with abundant eosinophilic cytoplasm. The result may be a striking simulation of the solid and follicular pattern of a JGCT. It is helpful clinically that metastatic malignant melanoma is very rare in the first 2 decades, when approximately 80% of JGCTs are encountered. The clinical history, of course, is helpful in many cases but as the history of malignant melanoma may be remote, or the primary tumor may have regressed, the possibility of malignant melanoma should be considered when entertaining the diagnosis of JGCT in a patient over 20 years of age. The likelihood of this diagnosis will be heightened if the ovarian tumor is bilateral. Other features of metastatic melanoma also may be helpful as will immunohistochemistry.

Clinical Behavior and Treatment

Although the JGCT usually appears less well differentiated than the adult type, follow-up to date indicates a high cure rate [82, 178, 193]. In contrast to AGCTs, which often recur late, all the clinically malignant juvenile tumors have reappeared within 3 years and several have had a rapid course.

In our series, the feature of greatest prognostic significance was the stage of the tumor [178]. Only 2 of the 80 stage I tumors for which follow-up information was available were clinically malignant. Rupture did not have an adverse effect on prognosis. Two of the ten stage IC tumors were malignant; in one of them, malignant cells were present on cytologic examination of the ascitic fluid. All three stage II tumors were fatal. Although both the mitotic rate and the degree of nuclear atypicality correlated with the prognosis when tumors of all stages were considered, no such correlation was evident when only stage I tumors were evaluated. In conclusion, despite the frequent presence of disquieting features such as severe nuclear atypicality and very high mitotic rates, a JGCT that is confined to the ovary appears to have an excellent prognosis with rare exceptions.

In view of the rarity of bilateral ovarian involvement, and their excellent prognosis, a stage IA JGCT can be treated by a unilateral salpingo-oophorectomy. Little experience has accumulated on the role of radiation therapy and chemotherapy in the management of persistent or recurrent tumor, but isolated examples of the efficacy of these modes of therapy have been recorded.

The comments just made on behavior, prognosis, and therapy do not apply to the rare cases that we designate anaplastic juvenile granulosa cell tumor, which are highly malignant in our experience.

Thecoma

Although different criteria for the microscopic separation of thecoma and fibroma have resulted in varying estimates of the frequency of these tumors, thecomas are approximately one third as common as granulosa cell tumors. The thecoma occurs at an older average age than the granulosa cell tumor, being very rare before puberty and uncommon before the age of 30 years. In one large series, 84% of the patients were postmenopausal, with a mean age of 59 years; only 10% of the patients were under 30 years of age [17]. In the same series, 60% of the postmenopausal women presented because of uterine bleeding, and 21% of the patients had endometrial carcinoma. Thecomas can be divided into typical and luteinized forms [12, 17, 55, 67, 136, 196].

Thecomas range in size from small, impalpable tumors to large, solid masses; most are medium size, 5–10 cm in diameter. Sectioning typically discloses a solid yellow mass (*Fig. 15.27*), but in some cases, the tumor is white with only focal tinges of yellow; cystic change and foci of hemorrhage and necrosis occur occasionally. Microscopic examination reveals masses of cells, often intersected by fibrous bands or hyaline plaques (*Fig. 15.28*). The tumor cells are ill defined and oval or rounded; the cytoplasm usually is moderate to abundant. It most often has a pale, almost dull grey appearance (*Fig. 15.29*) and its lipid-rich character has been overemphasized. However, in some cases, the cytoplasm is to a degree vacuolated, containing moderate to abundant amounts of lipid. Rarely it is strikingly vacuolated. In occasional cellular thecomas the cytoplasm is inconspicuous. The nuclei vary from round to spindle shaped, indicating the overlap between fibromas and thecomas (*Fig. 15.28*). There is usually little or no atypia, but bizarre nuclei are rarely seen; mitoses are absent or infrequent. In thecomas, in contrast to granulosa cell tumors, reticulum fibrils typically surround individual tumor cells although sometimes they surround small clusters of cells. The stroma is sometimes myxoid (*Fig. 15.30*) and rare tumors, particularly in the young, are calcified [176] (*Fig. 15.30*).

Typical thecomas are unilateral in 97% of the cases and are almost never malignant. A number of tumors have been reported as "malignant thecomas," but some of these tumors are better interpreted as endocrinologically inactive fibrosarcomas or diffuse granulosa cell tumors [175]. In cases in which the preservation of fertility is important, a thecoma can be treated adequately by oophorectomy. Total hysterectomy with bilateral salpingo-oophorectomy is indicated, however, in most patients who are menopausal or postmenopausal.

Tumors that are predominantly fibromatous or thecomatous but also contain collections of steroid-type

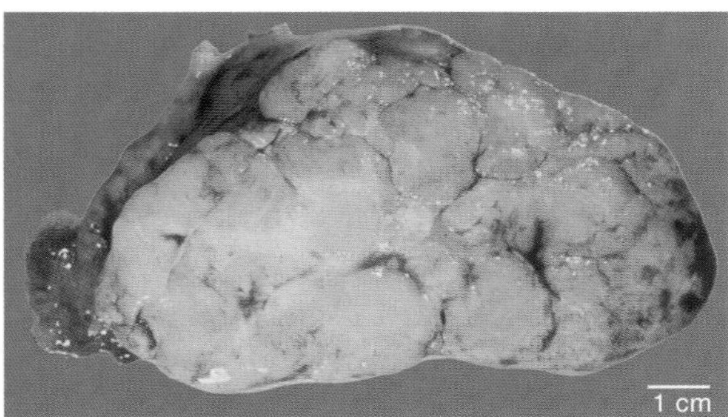

Fig. 15.27
Thecoma. **The sectioned surface of the neoplasm is uniformly solid, yellow, and lobulated**

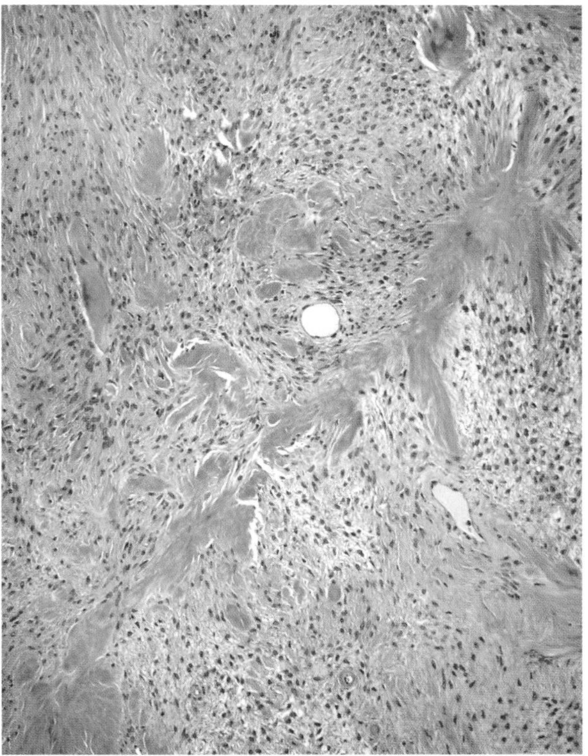

Fig. 15.28
Thecoma. **Hyaline plaques are conspicuous. This region of what was overall a thecoma had hybrid thecoma–fibroma features**

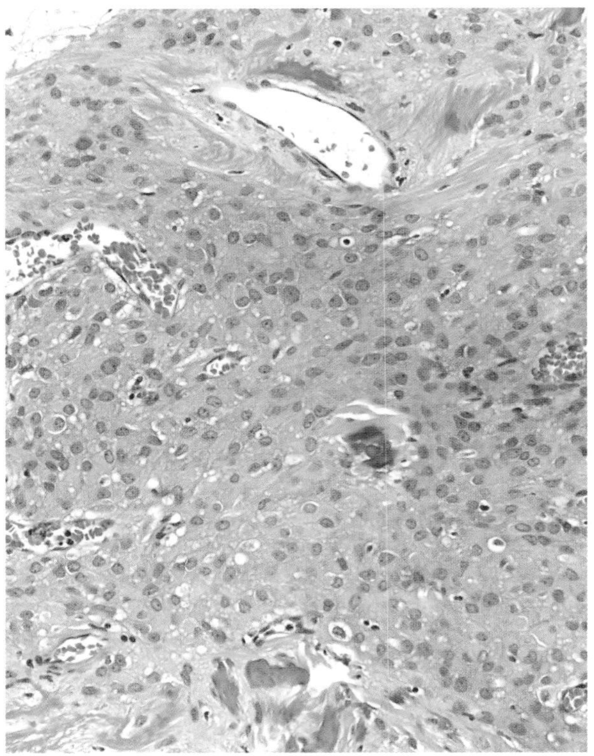

Fig. 15.29
Thecoma. **Typical appearance of cytoplasm in many cases**

cells, resembling luteinized theca and luteinized stromal cells have been called luteinized thecomas. In our series of 46 cases of these tumors, half of them were estrogenic, 39% were nonfunctioning, and 11% were androgenic [196]. Two of the four patients with tumors of this type described by Roth and Sternberg [136] also were virilized. This relatively high frequency of masculinization contrasts with its great rarity in association with nonluteinized thecomas. Luteinized thecomas also occur in a younger age group than typical thecomas; although they are most frequent in postmenopausal women, 30% of them have occurred in patients under 30 years of age. When, on rare occasions, crystals of Reinke are identified in the steroid-type cells [120], the term stromal-Leydig cell tumor is appropriate [18, 119, 141, 157, 196]. Approximately half of these tumors have been virilizing.

A rare subtype of luteinized thecoma with distinctive features (*Figs. 15.31–15.33*) is that usually associated with potentially fatal sclerosing peritonitis [31, 154]. In contrast to typical thecomas and luteinized thecomas of the usual type, this lesion is nearly always bilateral. In some cases, it enlarges the ovary irregularly, often resulting in a striking expansion of the cortex and an exaggerated cerebriform appearance, suggesting a nonneoplastic process in some cases (*Fig. 15.31*). In other cases it forms a discrete mass. Microscopic examination discloses a process with dense cellular areas and less cellular areas in which edema with microcystic change is often conspicuous (*Fig. 15.33*). Lutein cells are present but are smaller and less easy to recognize (*Fig. 15.32*) than those in the usual luteinized thecoma. The proliferation frequently incorporates preexisting ovarian structures such as follicles. Another unusual aspect of this neoplasm is the brisk mitotic activity present in many cases, despite the lack of evidence that the lesion has the potential to metastasize. While the luteinized cells stain with sex cord markers such as inhibin and calretinin, the spindle cell component typically does not. The associated sclerosing peritonitis (seen in nearly all cases although sometimes only histologically) may cause significant morbidity and has occasionally been fatal [154]. The pathogenesis of the sclerosing peritonitis in these cases remains a mystery.

Fibroma

This tumor, which is composed of spindle cells forming variable amounts of collagen, accounts for 4% of all ovarian tumors. Fibroma occurs at all ages, but is most frequent during middle age, with an average age of 48 years [41]; fewer than 10% of the cases are encountered under the age of 30 years. The fibroma is rarely associated with steroid hormone production but may be accompanied by two unusual clinical syndromes, Meigs' syndrome [98] and the basal cell nevus syndrome (Gorlin's syndrome) [56]. The former, which complicates about 1% of ovarian fibromas, is defined as ascites and pleural effusion accompanying a fibrous ovarian tumor, usually a fibroma, and disappearing after the removal of the tumor. Ascites alone is present in association with 10–15% of ovarian fibromas larger than 10 cm in diameter [139]. The most widely accepted explanation of Meigs' syndrome is seepage of fluid from the tumor through its serosal surface into the peritoneal cavity, with subsequent passage into one or both pleural cavities either via lymphatics or through a communication between the abdominal and pleural cavity such as the foramen of Bochdalek.

The hereditary basal cell nevus syndrome is characterized by one or more of the following findings: basal cell carcinomas appearing early in life, keratocysts of the jaw, calcification of the dura, mesenteric cysts, and other less common abnormalities [56] as well as ovarian fibromas, which typically are bilateral, multinodular, and calcified

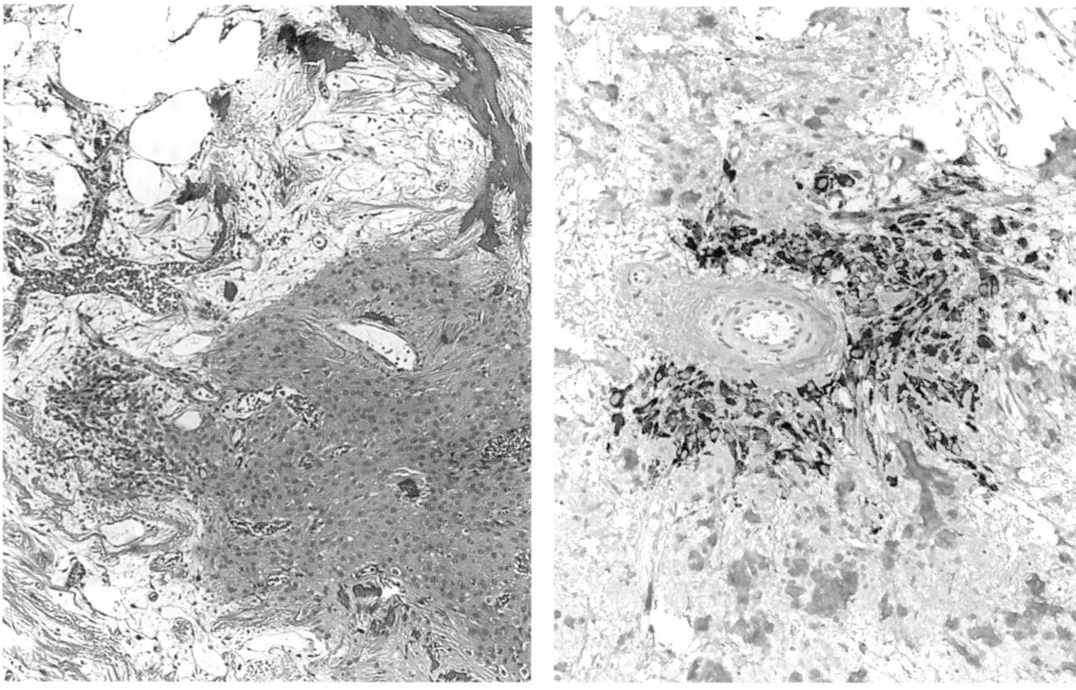

Fig. 15.30
Thecoma. **There is myxoid stroma and focal calcification (*left*). An inhibin stain is positive (*right*)**

(Fig. 19.28). A case of fibrosarcoma of the ovary in a child with the basal cell nevus syndrome has been reported [77].

Fibromas range in size from microscopic to very large. Sectioning typically reveals hard, flat, chalky-white surfaces that have a whorled appearance. Areas of edema, occasionally with cyst formation, are relatively common (*Fig. 15.34*). Focal or diffuse calcification and bilaterality are each observed in fewer than 10% of the cases but, as already mentioned, these features are characteristic of the fibromas associated with the basal cell nevus syndrome. Microscopic examination reveals intersecting bundles of spindle cells producing collagen; a storiform pattern may be encountered. The presence of bands of hyalinized fibrous tissue is not uncommon. Many tumors show varying degrees of intercellular edema. The cytoplasm of the neoplastic cells of fibromas may contain small quantities of lipid (*Fig. 15.35*). In rare tumors, the cytoplasm contains small red granules reminiscent of hyaline bodies, probably representing a degenerative phenomenon. As previously mentioned, an occasional fibroma contains a minor component of sex cord elements.

The fibroma must be distinguished from several nonneoplastic ovarian processes, specifically massive edema, fibromatosis, and stromal hyperplasia. The first two disorders usually are unilateral but may be bilateral and are characterized by proliferation of ovarian stromal cells with marked intercellular edema and the production of abundant dense collagen, respectively. Unlike fibromas, which almost always displace follicles, corpora lutea, and corpora albicantia, massive edema and fibromatosis encompass these structures. Stromal hyperplasia, in contrast to the ovarian fibroma, is bilateral and is characterized by a multinodular or diffuse proliferation of closely packed, small stromal cells with minimal collagen formation.

Occasional fibromas have varied cellularity (*Fig. 15.36*) and some vascularity, which may cause them to be misinterpreted as sclerosing stromal tumor. The distinct pseudolobulation, lutein cells, and ectatic vessels, in aggregate, set the sclerosing stromal tumor apart from fibromas that may mimic them to a limited degree. Some fibromas undergo prominent cystic degeneration and may be misconstrued as surface epithelial stromal tumors. However, the cysts (pseudocysts) do not have an epithelial lining.

A subset of ovarian fibromas are intensely cellular and merit the descriptive designation "cellular fibroma" [126]. Even when these have relatively brisk mitotic activity, over

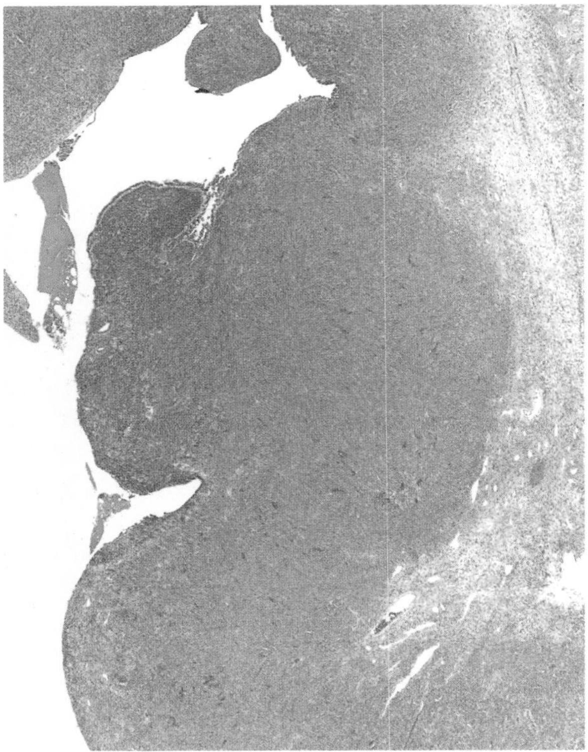

Fig. 15.31
Luteinized thecoma of type associated with sclerosing peritonitis. The ovarian cortex is strikingly cerebriform

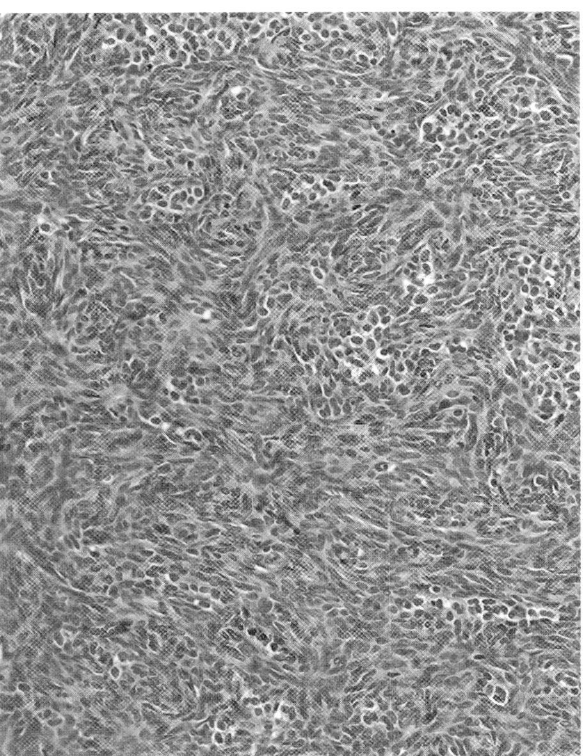

Fig. 15.32
Luteinized thecoma of type associated with sclerosing peritonitis. Ill-defined aggregates of lutein cells are seen

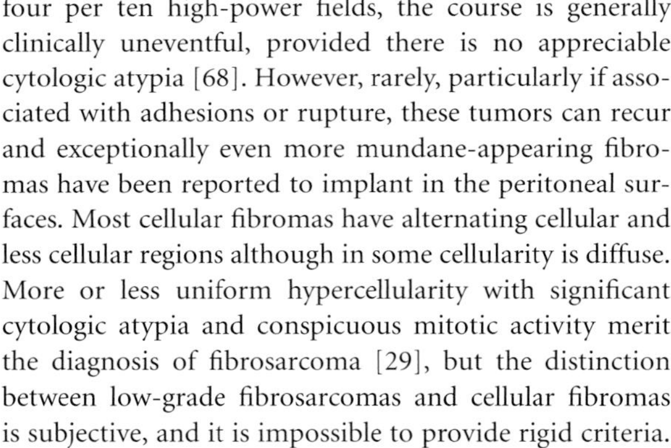

four per ten high-power fields, the course is generally clinically uneventful, provided there is no appreciable cytologic atypia [68]. However, rarely, particularly if associated with adhesions or rupture, these tumors can recur and exceptionally even more mundane-appearing fibromas have been reported to implant in the peritoneal surfaces. Most cellular fibromas have alternating cellular and less cellular regions although in some cellularity is diffuse. More or less uniform hypercellularity with significant cytologic atypia and conspicuous mitotic activity merit the diagnosis of fibrosarcoma [29], but the distinction between low-grade fibrosarcomas and cellular fibromas is subjective, and it is impossible to provide rigid criteria.

Sclerosing Stromal Tumor

This tumor differs from the fibroma and the thecoma both clinically and pathologically [28]. Although the latter tumors are uncommon in the first 3 decades, more than 80% of sclerosing stromal tumors have been encountered during the second and third decades, with an average age at diagnosis of 27 years. In contrast to the thecoma, the sclerosing stromal tumor has been associated with evidence of estrogen or androgen secretion, or both in only a few cases. All sclerosing stromal tumors encountered to date have been benign.

Gross examination typically reveals a unilateral, discrete, sharply demarcated mass; the neoplasm is rarely bilateral [71]. Its sectioned surface is solid and white but often shows areas of edema and cyst formation and foci of yellow discoloration (*Fig. 15.37*). A rare specimen presents as a unilocular cyst. Microscopic examination discloses a number of distinctive features: a pseudolobular pattern (*Fig. 15.38*), in which cellular nodules are separated by less cellular areas of dense collagenous or edematous connective tissue, sclerosis within the nodules, prominent thin-walled vessels in some of the nodules (*Fig. 15.39*), and a disorganized admixture of fibroblasts and rounded, vacuolated cells within the nodules (*Fig. 15.40*). Occasionally, the vacuolated cells have a signet cell appearance, creating some confusion with

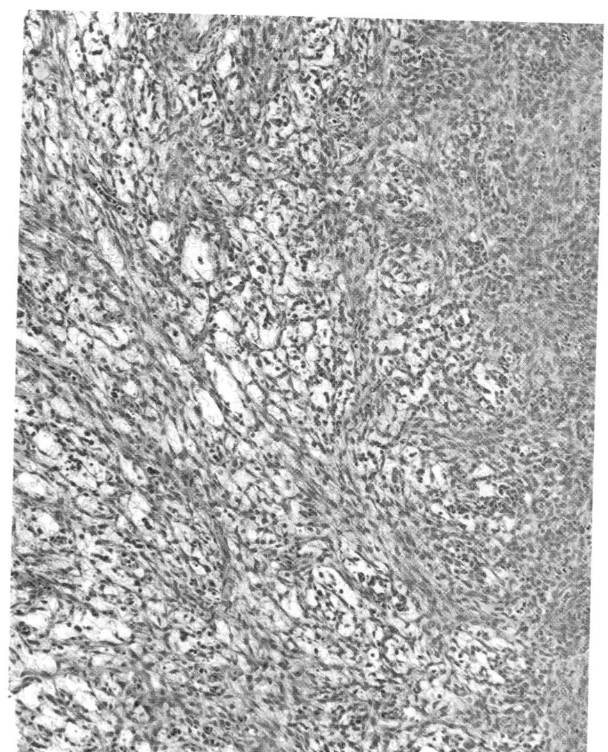

Fig. 15.33
Luteinized thecoma of type associated with sclerosing peritonitis. **Edema with microcystic change is conspicuous**

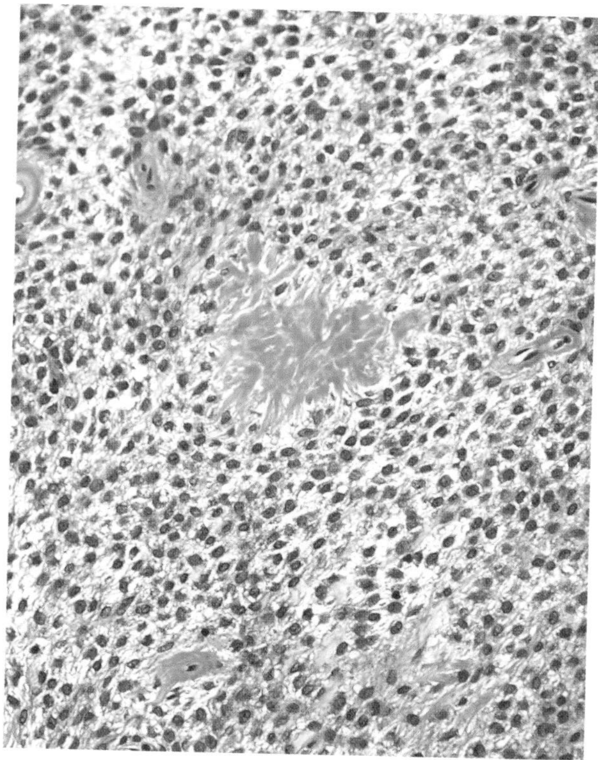

Fig. 15.35
Fibroma. **When cells are cut transversely and have pale cytoplasm due to a minor lipid content, an erroneous diagnosis of thecoma may result**

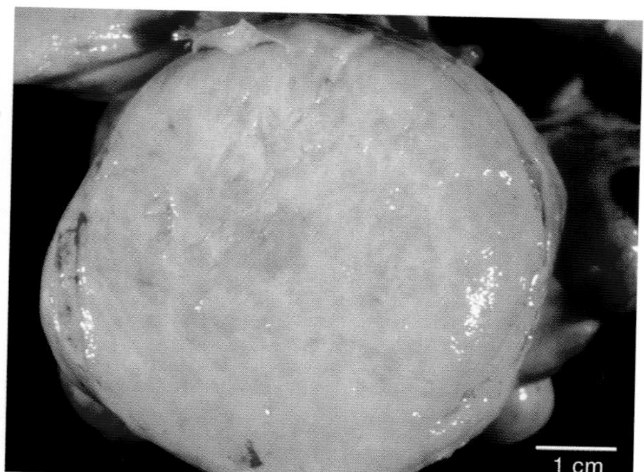

Fig. 15.34
Fibroma. **The sectioned surface of the neoplasm is solid, white, and slightly edematous**

the signet cells of a Krukenberg tumor, but the former cells contain lipid instead of mucin. The lipid-laden cells appear to be inactive or weakly active lutein cells; in the rare functioning tumors, the lutein cells resemble more closely those encountered in a luteinized thecoma. Rare sclerosing stromal tumors are prominently myxomatous, opening the possibility that there may be overlap in some cases with the rare ovarian myxoma [35]. Although overlap exists between fibromas, thecomas, sclerosing stromal tumors, and even steroid cell tumors, the presence of various distinctive features of these four tumors, which are presented in *Table 15.6*, almost always allows a specific diagnosis.

Microcystic Stromal Tumor

These rare tumors have recently been described as a distinctive variant within the stromal category [70]. All

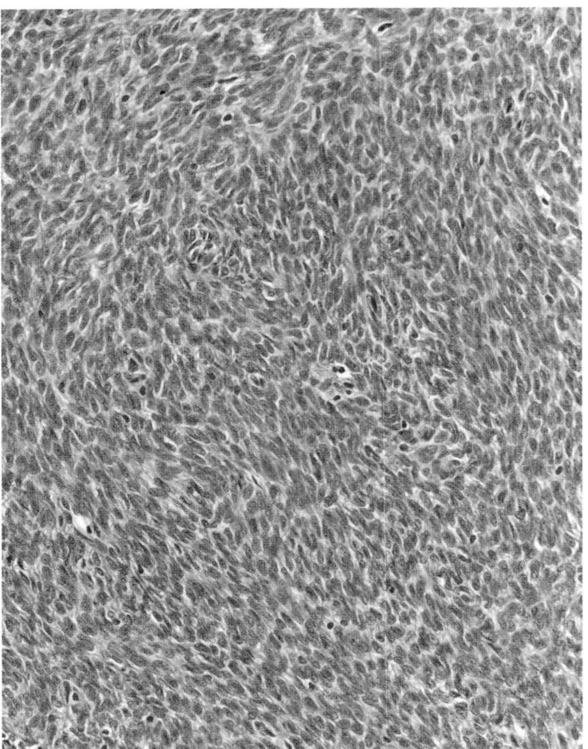

Fig. 15.36
Cellular fibroma

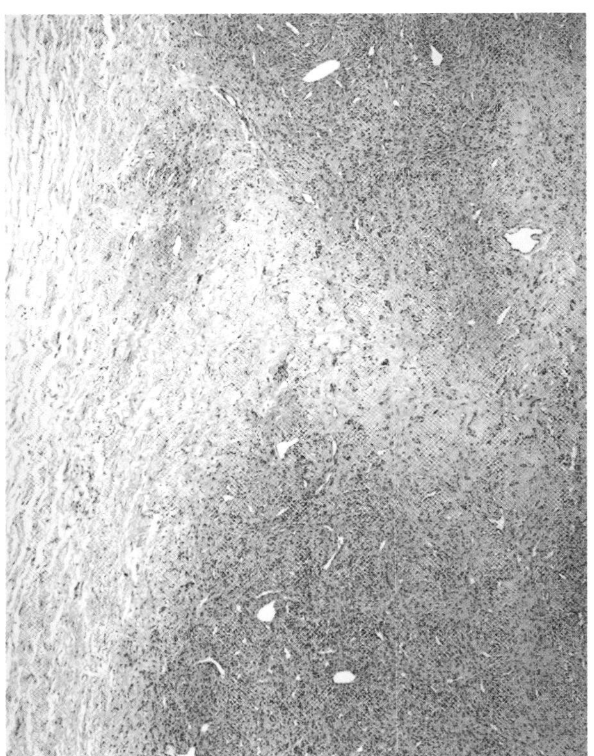

Fig. 15.38
Sclerosing stromal tumor. **Cellular pseudolobules are separated by edematous hypocellular tumor**

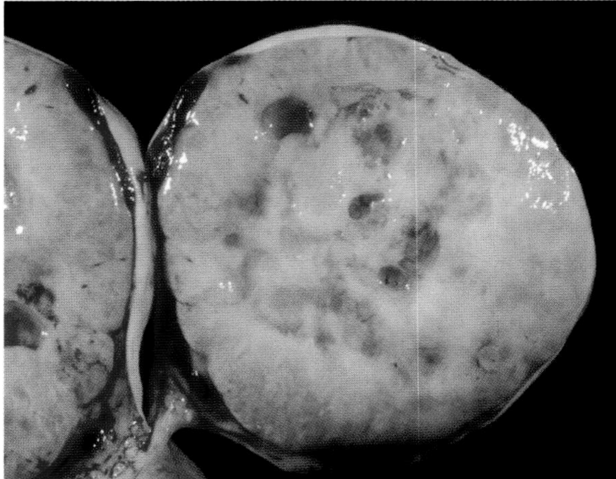

Fig. 15.37
Sclerosing stromal tumor. **The sectioned surface of the neoplasm is mostly solid with focal cystic degeneration particularly in the central region which was softer than the peripheral yellow component**

the 16 tumors encountered to date have been in adults, nonfunctioning, and stage I with a mean size of 10 cm. They may be cystic or solid and cystic. On microscopic examination, there are typically lobulated cellular regions separated by hyaline bands and fibrous plaques (*Fig. 15.41*). Definitionally, however, these regions are punctuated, oftentimes strikingly so, by small cysts (*Fig. 15.42*) that anastomose with each other, giving a distinctive appearance and resulting in the designation that has been given to this tumor. The neoplastic cells contain finely granular faintly eosinophilic cytoplasm and round to oval nuclei with small nucleoli. Mitotic figures are rare. Occasionally there is bizarre nuclear atypia of the degenerative type. The tumors are typically negative for inhibin but positive for CD10. About one third of the tumors examined to date have been cytokeratin positive but they have been EMA negative.

The differential diagnosis of this tumor is broad and has been recently presented in detail elsewhere [70] so will not be repeated here. As a great many other ovarian

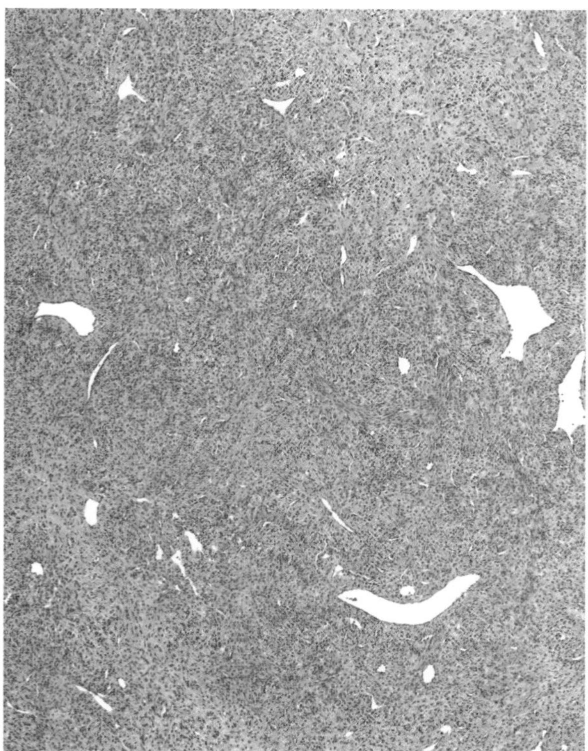

Fig. 15.39
Sclerosing stromal tumor. **Pseudolobule is richly vascularized**

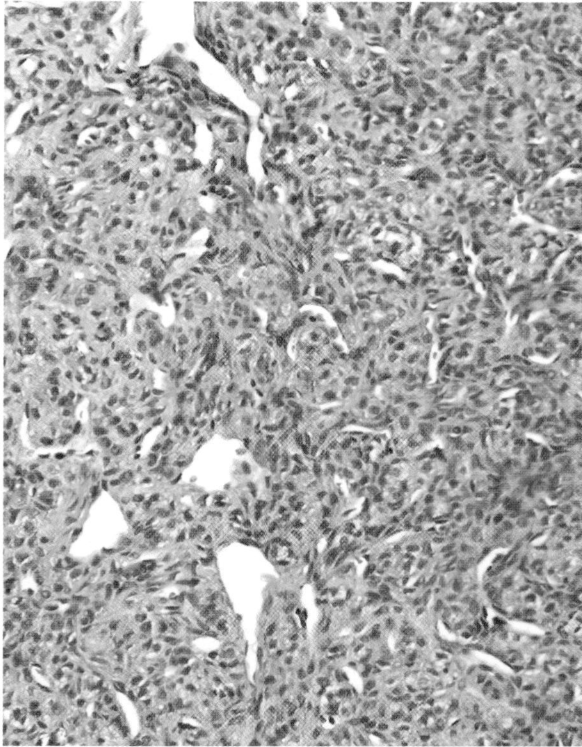

Fig. 15.40
Sclerosing stromal tumor. **Spindle cells are mixed with more rounded weak lutein cells**

tumors may have microcysts, the designation of microcystic stromal tumor should only be made after neoplasms have been thoroughly sampled to disclose other foci that may merit separate categorization.

Signet-Ring Stromal Tumor

In 1976, Ramzy [129] described an unusual ovarian tumor from a 28-year-old woman, which he designated signet-ring stromal tumor. These tumors are rare and only a small number of cases have been reported subsequently, all of them being in adults, nonfunctioning and benign [172]. There are no unique gross features. On microscopic examination, spindle cells are diffusely distributed and merge imperceptibly with rounded cells containing eccentric nuclei and single large vacuoles, resembling signet-ring cells (*Fig. 15.43*). These cells may be diffusely scattered or focally distributed. Stains for lipid and mucin are negative. Electron microscopic examination has shown that in some cases the vacuoles result from generalized edema of the cytoplasmic matrix, in others from swelling of mitochondria, and in still others from cytoplasmic pseudoinclusions of edematous extracellular matrix [40]. Negative staining for mucin excludes a Krukenberg tumor, the most important lesion in the differential diagnosis. There are many other differences between the two tumors. The signet-ring stromal tumor lacks the pseudolobulation, lipid-rich cells, and prominent vascularity of the sclerosing stromal tumor. Rarely a signet-ring change similar to that seen in this neoplasm may be encountered in granulosa cell tumors.

Unclassified Tumors

Rare tumors in the intermediate zone between fibromas and thecomas are impossible to classify more specifically. Such tumors are made up of cells having some but not all the features of theca cells, containing small to

Table 15.6
Sclerosing stromal tumor versus fibroma, thecoma, and steroid cell tumors

	Sclerosing stromal tumor	Fibroma	Thecoma	Steroid cell tumor
Age	80% under 30 years	10% under 30 years	Average age 63 years	25% under 30 years
Function	Almost always absent	Absent	Typically estrogenic[a]	Typically androgenic
Gross variegation	Yes	No	No	No
Pseudolobulation	Yes	Rare	Rare	No
Prominent ectatic vessels	Yes	Rare	Rare	Rare
Two cell types	Yes	No	Only in luteinized form	No
Hyaline plaques	No	Common	Common	No
Behavior	Benign	Almost always Benign	Almost always benign	Sometimes malignant

[a]Luteinized form androgenic in 11% of cases.

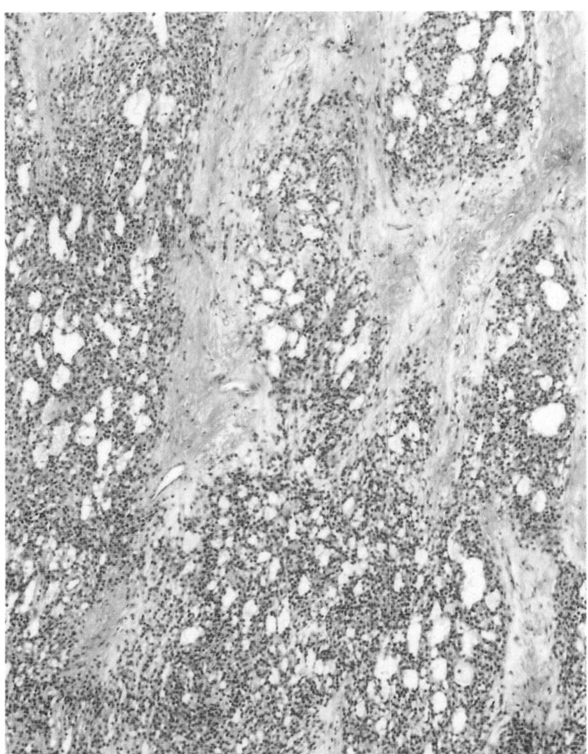

Fig. 15.41
Microcystic stromal tumor, typical low power

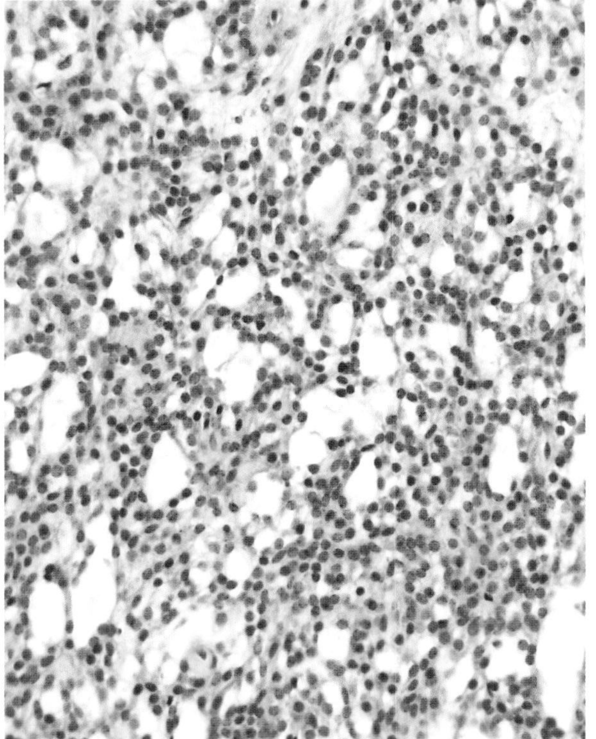

Fig. 15.42
Microcystic stromal tumor, high power showing microcysts

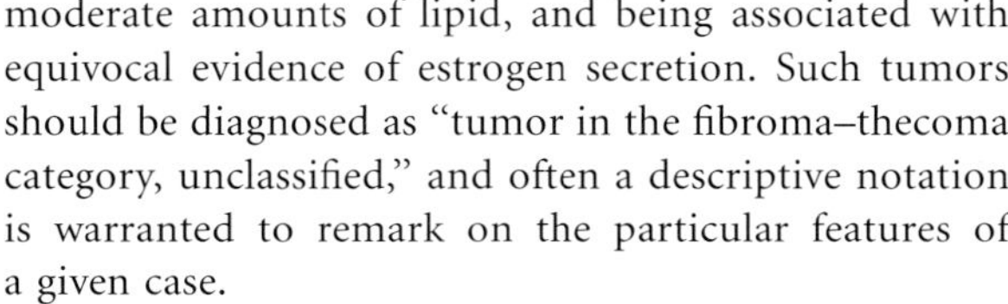

moderate amounts of lipid, and being associated with equivocal evidence of estrogen secretion. Such tumors should be diagnosed as "tumor in the fibroma–thecoma category, unclassified," and often a descriptive notation is warranted to remark on the particular features of a given case.

Sertoli-Stromal Cell Tumors

Sertoli-stromal cell tumors contain Sertoli cells, Leydig cells, fibroblasts, or all these cells, in varying proportions and varying degrees of differentiation. Most tumors in this family are Sertoli–Leydig cell tumors. Other tumors

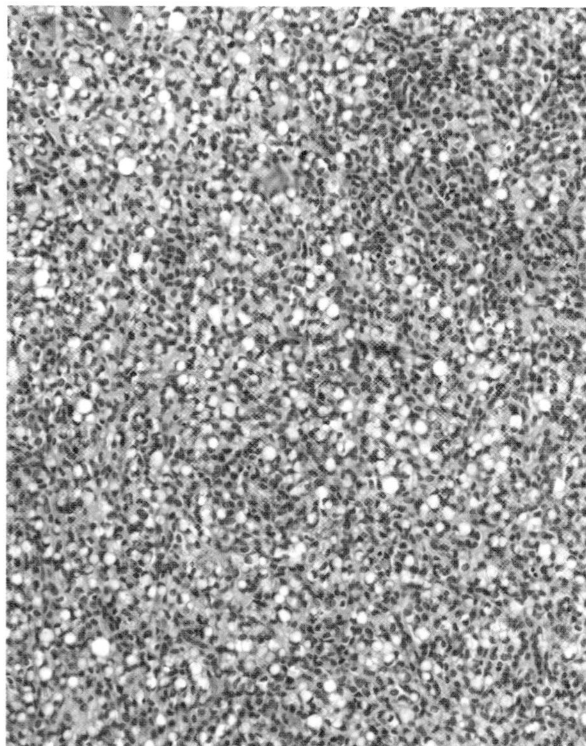

Fig. 15.43
Signet-ring stromal tumor

within this group are pure Sertoli cell tumors, pure Leydig cell tumors, and stromal-Leydig cell tumors; the latter already have been mentioned in the discussion of luteinized thecomas, and pure Leydig cell tumors are considered in the section on steroid cell tumors.

Sertoli Cell Tumors

Sertoli cell tumors account for approximately 4% of Sertoli-stromal cell tumors [114, 164, 166, 188]. The tumors are usually nonfunctioning but seven Sertoli cell tumors, most or all of which appear to have been of the lipid-rich type, have resulted in isosexual pseudoprecocity. Two of these tumors were from patients with Peutz–Jeghers syndrome [153, 188]. One Sertoli cell tumor was associated with progesterone as well as estrogen production [168]. All the Sertoli cell tumors reported to date have been unilateral and most have been stage I.

They have averaged approximately 9 cm in diameter and typically have formed lobulated, solid, yellow or brown masses. Microscopic examination usually shows a uniform tubular pattern or at least focal tubules, but a rare neoplasm is uniformly diffuse. The tubules may be hollow or solid. The hollow tubules are lined by bland columnar to cuboidal cells with moderate amounts of pale or slightly eosinophilic cytoplasm. Their lumens are usually empty but may contain an eosinophilic secretion and rarely even mucin. The solid tubules are typically elongated but may be round or oval. An apparent solid pattern results when tubules are closely packed, and in some cases, there is a true solid pattern, particularly when the tumors are less well differentiated than usual. In some of these cases, there is focally an interruption of a generally solid pattern by a fibrous stroma, which rarely can impart an alveolar to nested pattern (*Figs. 15.44–15.46*) akin to that occasionally seen with testicular Sertoli cell tumors. As in that situation, rarely a low-power picture vaguely reminiscent of the alveolar pattern of dysgerminoma may result but high-power scrutiny shows differing cytologic features (*Fig. 15.45*) and if indicated of course, immunohistochemical differences will be stark (*Fig. 15.46*). Other less common patterns of Sertoli-cell neoplasia include the presence of cords, and also trabecular pseudopapillary, retiform, and even spindled patterns. Tumors with the latter patterns can impart many problems in differential diagnosis as discussed in detail recently elsewhere [114]. When the Sertoli cells contain abundant cytoplasmic lipid, the term lipid-rich Sertoli cell tumor is appropriate. Occasional Sertoli cell tumors have cells with abundant eosinophilic cytoplasm [49]. There is usually little if any nuclear atypia or mitotic activity, and the prognosis is generally excellent. A few tumors exhibit moderate degrees of nuclear atypicality, and exceptionally there is a malignant appearance with metastases [114, 125].

The differential diagnosis of Sertoli cell tumors is broadly similar to that of Sertoli–Leydig cell tumors, considered below. Brief note should be made of the rare tumors with little or no tubules, one of which is illustrated (*Figs. 15.44–15.46*). Their distinction from granulosa cell tumor is aided by lack of typical patterns of that tumor and nuclei lacking the distinctive features of it also. Distinction of these rare tumors from other neoplasms reasonably in the differential is one of the best examples of aid of staining for inhibin (*Fig. 15.46*) but of course, it will only be obtained if the diagnosis is entertained.

Sertoli–Leydig Cell Tumors

Sertoli–Leydig cell tumors account for less than 0.5% of all ovarian tumors. They are divided into three main

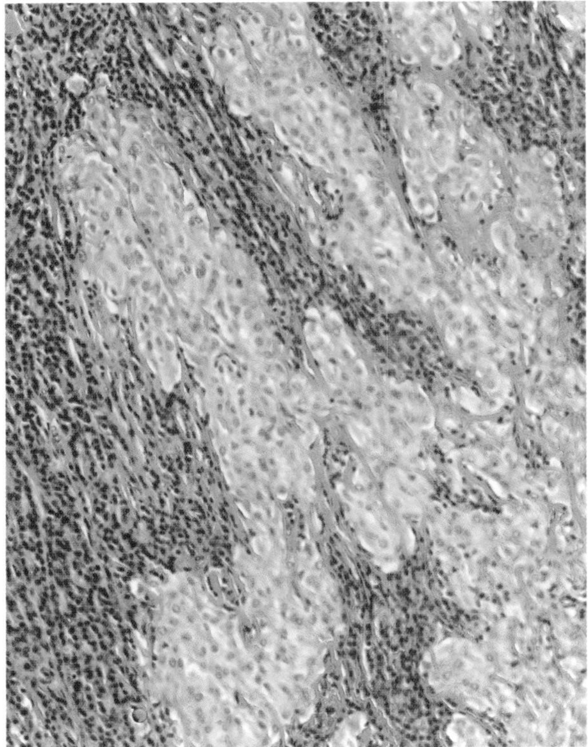

Fig. 15.44
Sertoli cell tumor. **Aggregates of cells with eosinophilic cytoplasm are separated by septa with an inflammatory cell infiltrate**

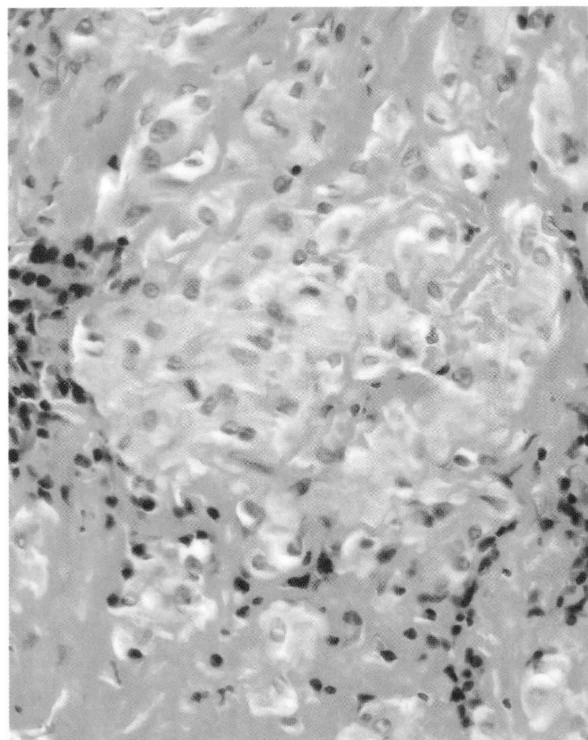

Fig. 15.45
Sertoli cell tumor. **High power showing typical cytology**

subtypes: well differentiated, of intermediate differentiation, and poorly differentiated. The latter two categories may additionally contain heterologous elements, a retiform component,or both, complicating an already often complex appearance. Sertoli–Leydig cell tumors occur in all age groups but are encountered most often in young women. The average age is 25 years; 75% of the patients are 30 years of age or younger and only about 10% are over 50 years [133, 191, 194]. The well-differentiated tumors [190] occur on an average a decade later, and retiform tumors [187] a decade earlier, than other Sertoli–Leydig cell tumors. Tumors with a retiform pattern are more common in the first decade than any other subtype. Recent molecular evidence [45] has indicated a true neoplastic nature for the Leydig cell component of these tumors. It should be emphasized that in some Sertoli–Leydig cell tumors, usually those that are poorly differentiated, recognizable Leydig cells are few, and in even some cases objectively cannot be appreciated. The tumor is still put in the Sertoli–Leydig category when the overall patterns fit best with that designation.

Clinical Features

Although the most striking mode of presentation of Sertoli–Leydig cell tumors is virilization, it develops in only about one third of the cases. In such cases, a patient who has been having normal menstrual periods typically begins to have oligomenorrhea, followed within a few months by amenorrhea. There is a concomitant loss of female secondary sex characteristics, with atrophy of the breasts and disappearance of normal bodily contours. Progressive masculinization is heralded by acne, with hirsutism, temporal balding, deepening of the voice, and enlargement of the clitoris following in its wake. Androgenic manifestations are lower in tumors containing heterologous elements and lower again in those having a prominent retiform component. The androgen secretion by the tumor also may result in erythrocytosis.

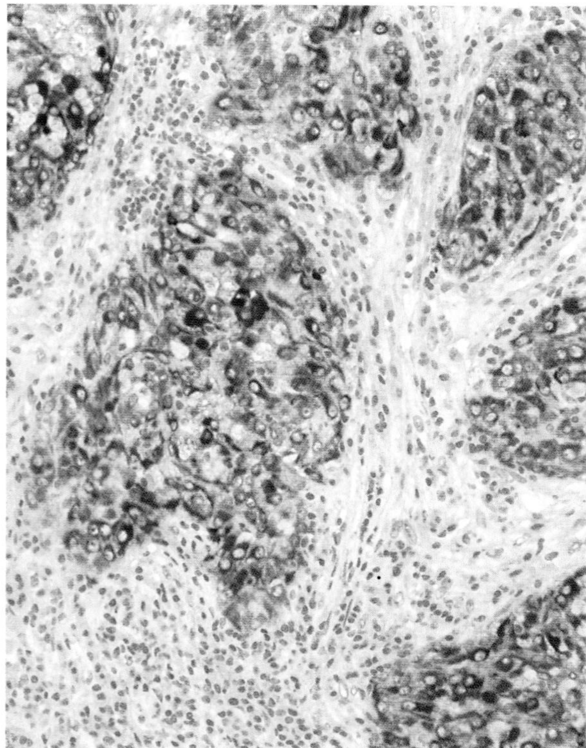

Fig. 15.46
Sertoli cell tumor. Positive inhibin stain of tumor seen in two prior figures

Plasma levels of testosterone, androstenedione, and other androgens, alone or in combination, may be elevated in patients with Sertoli–Leydig cell tumors. The urinary 17-ketosteroid values usually are normal or only slightly raised, although occasionally a high level has been recorded. These findings are in contrast to those associated with virilizing adrenal tumors, which often are accompanied by high urinary levels of 17-ketosteroids. The values for plasma androgens and urinary 17-ketosteroids are not reliable, however, in the differentiation of ovarian and adrenal virilizing tumors because the latter often are associated with elevated testosterone and normal urinary 17-ketosteroid levels [5]; also, tests involving attempted stimulation by tropic hormones and suppression by gonadal and adrenocortical steroids have not proved decisive in differentiating these tumors. Occasional Sertoli–Leydig cell tumors are associated with elevated plasma levels of alpha-fetoprotein but values as high as those accompanying yolk sac tumors are rare [13, 53].

Approximately, 50% of patients with Sertoli–Leydig cell tumors have no endocrine manifestations and usually complain of abdominal swelling or pain. Occasional tumors have been associated with various estrogenic syndromes similar to those of the granulosa cell tumor.

At laparotomy, almost all Sertoli–Leydig cell tumors are unilateral. The tumors are stage Ia in about 80% of the cases; in 12% the tumor has either ruptured or involved the external surface of the ovary, and in 4% ascites is present. Only about 2.5% of the tumors have spread beyond the ovary, usually within the pelvis and rarely into the upper abdomen. Poorly differentiated tumors more often are ruptured and present at a higher stage than tumors of intermediate differentiation. Well-differentiated tumors are essentially invariably state Ia.

Gross Findings

Sertoli–Leydig cell tumors vary greatly in their gross appearance (*Figs. 15.47–15.49*), like granulosa cell tumors, and these neoplasms usually cannot be distinguished on gross examination alone. There are, however, a few general differences. Sertoli–Leydig cell tumors contain blood-filled cysts less often than granulosa cell tumors and, unlike the latter, almost never have the appearance of a unilocular thin-walled cyst. Sertoli–Leydig cell tumors vary in size from microscopic to huge masses but most are between 5 and 15 (average, 13.5) cm in diameter. Poorly differentiated tumors including those with mesenchymal heterologous elements tend to be larger than those of better differentiation and contain areas of hemorrhage and necrosis more frequently. Tumors with heterologous or retiform components are cystic more often than tumors without these elements. The heterologous tumors occasionally simulate mucinous cystic tumors on gross examination, and retiform tumors may contain large, edematous papillae, resembling serous papillary tumors or be very soft (*Fig. 15.49*). The latter aspects are rare or absent features of granulosa cell tumor.

Well-Differentiated Tumors

These tumors are characterized by a predominantly tubular pattern (*Fig. 15.50*) [190]. On low-power examination, a nodular architecture often is conspicuous, with fibrous bands separating lobules composed of hollow or less often solid tubules; in some tumors tubules of

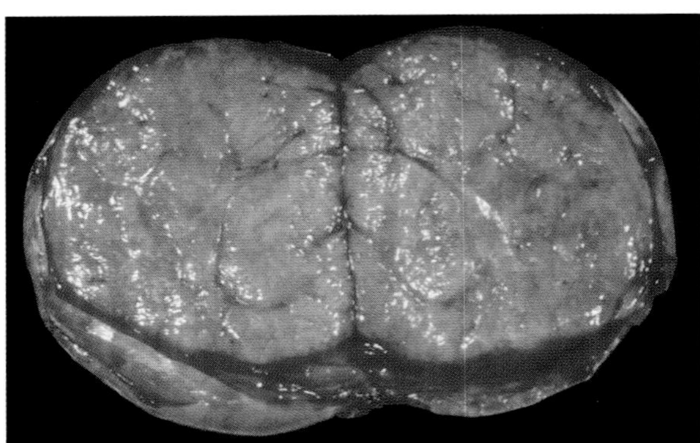

Fig. 15.47
Sertoli–Leydig cell tumor. **The sectioned surface of the neoplasm is solid yellow and lobulated**

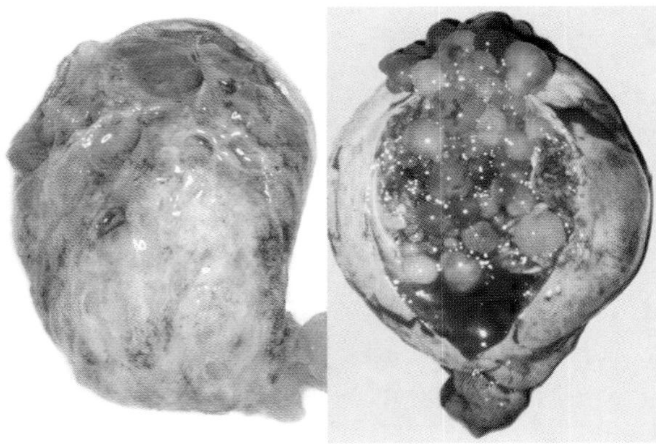

Fig. 15.49
Sertoli–Leydig cell tumor with retiform pattern. **The tumor on the left was soft and "spongy," a feature of many such tumors. Edematous polypoid structures project into the lumen of another neoplasm that was more cystic (*right*)**

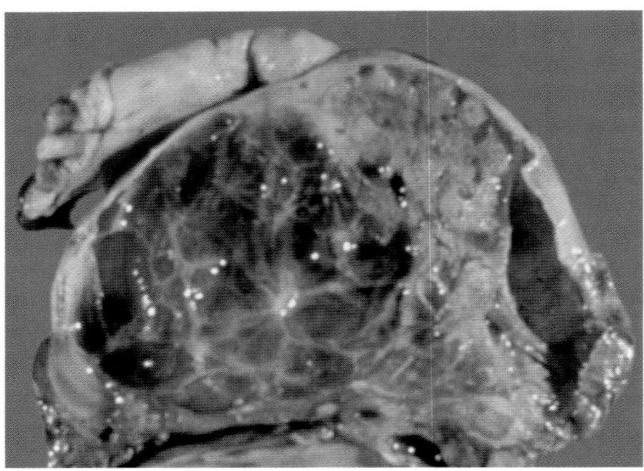

Fig. 15.48
Sertoli–Leydig cell tumor with mucinous heterologous elements. **The sectioned surface of the tumor is mostly mucoid with a minor solid yellow component**

both types are present. The hollow tubules typically are round to oval and small, but may be cystically dilated, and some of them resemble the tubular glands of a well-differentiated endometrioid adenocarcinoma (*Fig. 15.51*) [94]. The lumens usually are devoid of conspicuous secretion but in some cases eosinophilic fluid, which is occasionally mucicarminophilic, is present. The solid tubules typically are elongated but may be round or oval and occasionally resemble prepubertal or atrophic testicular tubules. The tubules contain cuboidal to columnar epithelial cells with round or oblong nuclei without

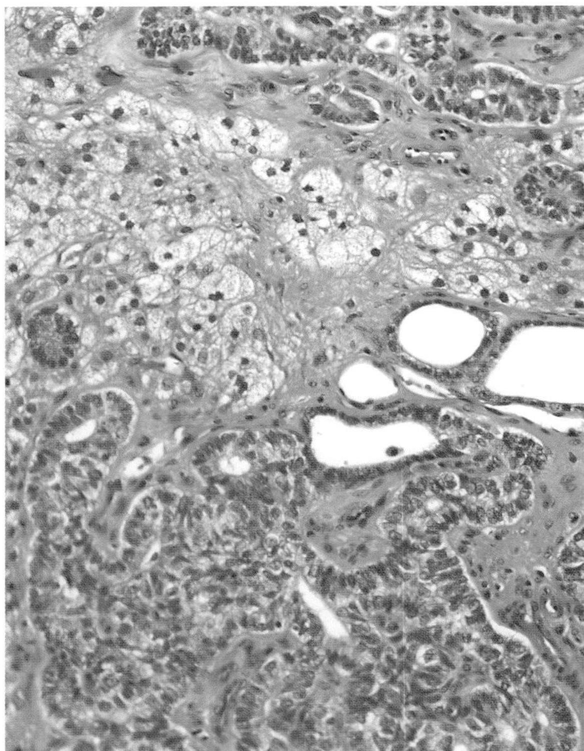

Fig. 15.50
Sertoli–Leydig cell tumor, well differentiated. **Hollow and solid tubules are separated by Leydig cells in intervening stroma**

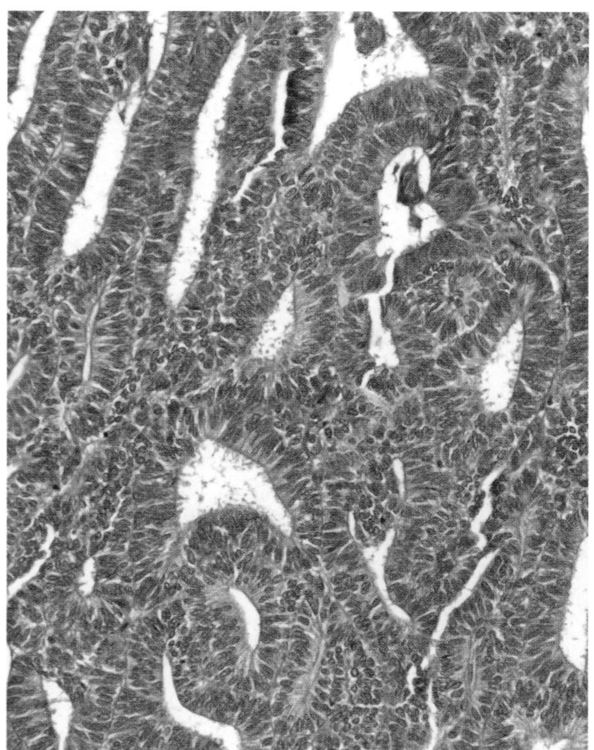

◘ Fig. 15.51
Sertoli–Leydig cell tumor, well differentiated.
Pseudoendometrioid tubules

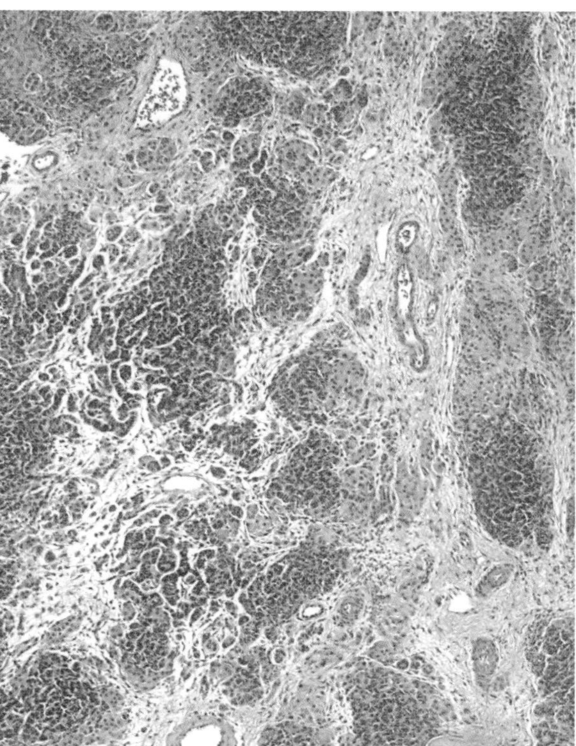

◘ Fig. 15.52
Sertoli–Leydig cell tumor of intermediate differentiation.
Cellular lobules are intersected by a slightly edematous stromal component containing Leydig cells

prominent nucleoli. Nuclear atypicality usually is absent or minimal, and mitotic figures are rare. The cells lining the hollow tubules and filling the solid tubules typically contain moderate amounts of dense cytoplasm, but in some cases, varying numbers of them have abundant pale cytoplasm rich in lipid. The stromal component consists of bands of mature fibrous tissue containing variable but usually conspicuous numbers of Leydig cells (➋ *Fig. 15.40*). These cells may contain abundant lipochrome pigment; crystals of Reinke are identified in some of the Leydig cells in approximately 20% of the cases. Ossification has been described in one case [101].

Tumors of Intermediate and Poor Differentiation

These tumors form a continuum characterized by a variety of patterns and combinations of cell types (➋ *Figs. 15.52–15.57*). Some tumors exhibit intermediate differentiation in some areas and poor differentiation in others and, less commonly, tumors of intermediate differentiation contain well-differentiated foci. Either the Sertoli cells or Leydig cells or both may exhibit varying degrees of immaturity. In the tumors of intermediate differentiation, immature Sertoli cells with small, round, oval, or angular nuclei are arranged typically in poorly defined masses, often creating a lobulated appearance on low power (➋ *Fig. 15.52*); solid and hollow tubules (➋ *Fig. 15.55*), nests, thin cords resembling the sex cords of the embryonic testis, and broad columns of Sertoli cells often are present. There is sometimes an alveolar pattern (➋ *Fig. 15.54*) and as with some well-differentiated tumors some tubules may be pseudoendometrioid. Cysts that range from small to large may be seen (➋ *Fig. 15.57*) and when they contain eosinophilic secretion, may create a thyroid-like appearance; follicle-like spaces are encountered rarely. The Sertoli cells, or the Leydig cells, may have bizarre nuclei similar to those seen in some granulosa cell

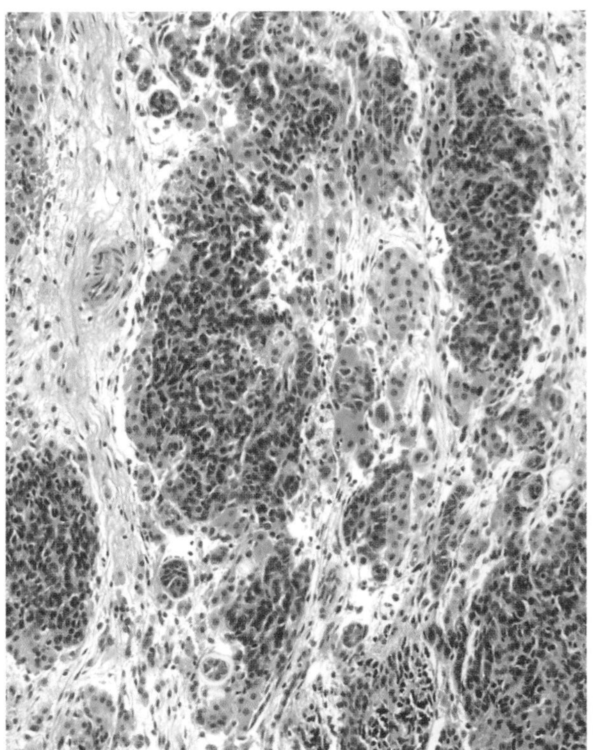

Fig. 15.53
Sertoli–Leydig cell tumor of intermediate differentiation. **Nests and cords of immature Sertoli cells and clusters of Leydig cells with abundant cytoplasm**

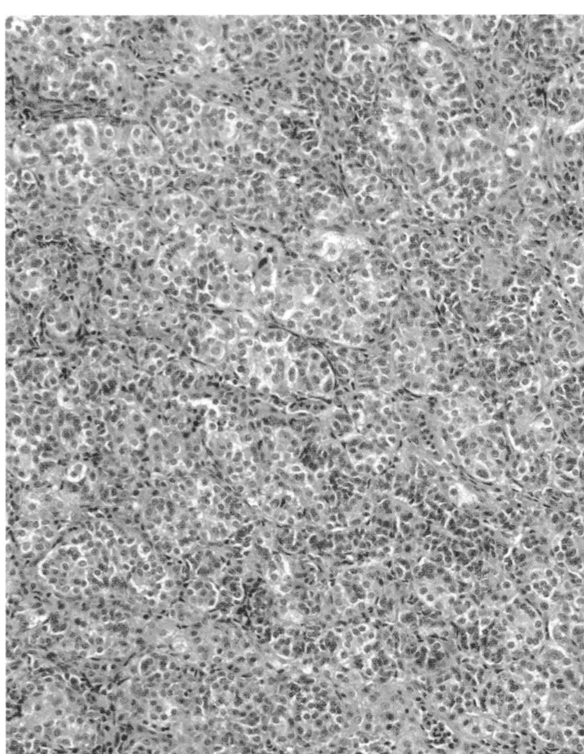

Fig. 15.54
Sertoli–Leydig cell tumor of intermediate differentiation, alveolar pattern

tumors [186]. The Sertoli cell aggregates are separated by a stromal component that ranges from fibromatous to densely cellular to edematous and typically contain clusters of well-differentiated Leydig cells. Occasionally, part or all of the stromal component is made up of immature, cellular mesenchymal tissue resembling a nonspecific sarcoma. The Sertoli and Leydig cell elements, singly or together, may contain varying and sometimes large amounts of lipid in the form of small or large droplets. Poorly differentiated Sertoli–Leydig cell tumors originally were classified as sarcomatoid because, aside from the presence of specifically diagnostic elements, they resemble fibrosarcomas; however, they often have a diffuse pattern that is not clearly recognizable as that of a fibrosarcoma. We reserve the designation "poorly differentiated" for Sertoli–Leydig cell tumors that lack in large areas, any recognizable patterns of the neoplasm, but definitionally there must be at least minor foci that enable categorization as Sertoli–Leydig cell tumor.

Retiform Sertoli–Leydig Cell Tumor

Fifteen percent of Sertoli–Leydig cell tumors are composed, usually partially but occasionally entirely, of tubular structures arranged in a pattern resembling that of the rete testis [99, 134, 161, 187]. So far a retiform pattern has been encountered only in tumors that are otherwise intermediate or poorly differentiated. Microscopic examination reveals a network of irregularly branching, elongated, narrow, often slit-like tubules and cysts into which papillae or polypoid structures may project (*Figs. 15.58* and *15.59*). The tubules and cysts may contain eosinophilic secretion; they are lined by epithelial cells that exhibit varying degrees of stratification and nuclear atypicality. The papillae and polyps are of three types: most commonly they are small and rounded or blunt, often containing hyalinized cores; sometimes they are large and bulbous, containing edematous cores. Finally, in some cases, they are delicate and branch extensively and may be lined by stratified cells, simulating the papillae of

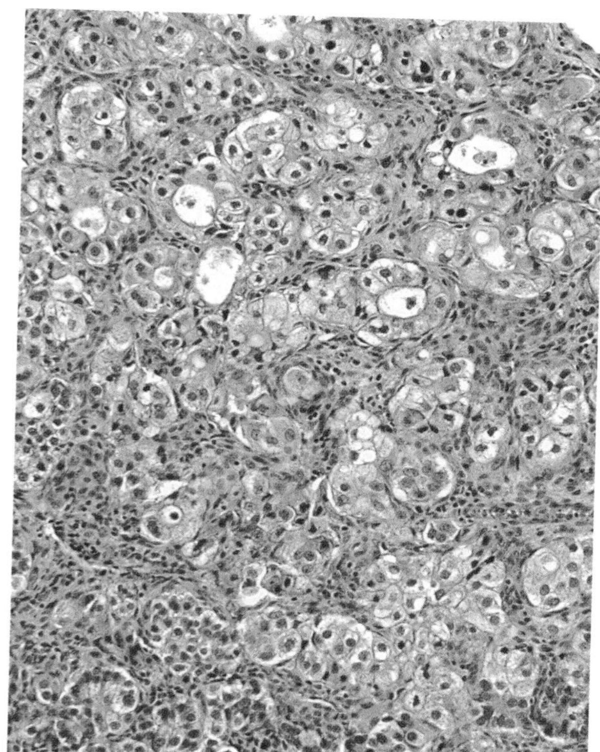

Fig. 15.55
Sertoli–Leydig cell tumor of differentiation. **Solid tubules and rare hollow tubules**

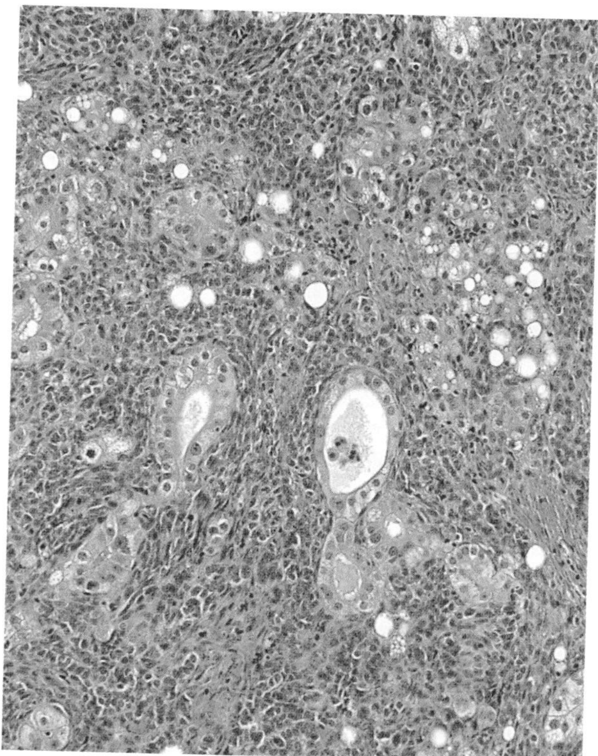

Fig. 15.56
Sertoli–Leydig cell tumor of intermediate differentiation. **Jumbled admixture of Sertoli and Leydig cells and focal tubules**

a serous tumor of borderline or invasive type. A common finding in the retiform Sertoli–Leydig cell tumor is the presence of columns or ribbons of immature Sertoli cells. The stroma within a retiform area may be hyalinized or edematous (*Fig. 15.60*), moderately cellular, or densely cellular and immature.

Heterologous Sertoli–Leydig Cell Tumor

Heterologous elements occur in approximately 20% of Sertoli–Leydig cell tumors, most of which are of intermediate differentiation but some are poorly differentiated [105, 156]. Glands and cysts lined by moderately to well-differentiated gastric-type or intestinal-type epithelium (*Fig. 15.61*) are most common. The intestinal-type epithelium at times may contain goblet cells, argentaffin cells, and rarely Paneth cells [183]. The argentaffin cells [1] rarely give rise to small foci of carcinoid [145], typically taking the form of tiny aggregates or cords of cells (*Fig. 15.62*) that may have admixed goblet cells, imparting a goblet-cell carcinoid morphology. Exceptionally, there is a more classic closely packed appearance of insular carcinoid that sometimes can even form a grossly evident nodule. Stromal heterologous elements are seen in 5% of all Sertoli–Leydig cell tumors [127]. Islands of fetal-type cartilage arising on a sarcomatous background, areas of embryonal rhabdomyosarcoma, or both (*Fig. 15.63*) are seen. Rarely, Sertoli–Leydig cell tumors of conventional or heterologous type contain cells resembling hepatocytes [100, 182], and one contained retinal tissue and another had neuroblastoma in recurrent tumor [127].

Differential Diagnosis

Because of their many patterns, Sertoli-stromal cell tumors often are difficult to differentiate from tumors outside the sex cord-stromal category as well as from granulosa cell tumors. The small hollow tubular structures, solid tubular aggregates, and cords that occasionally

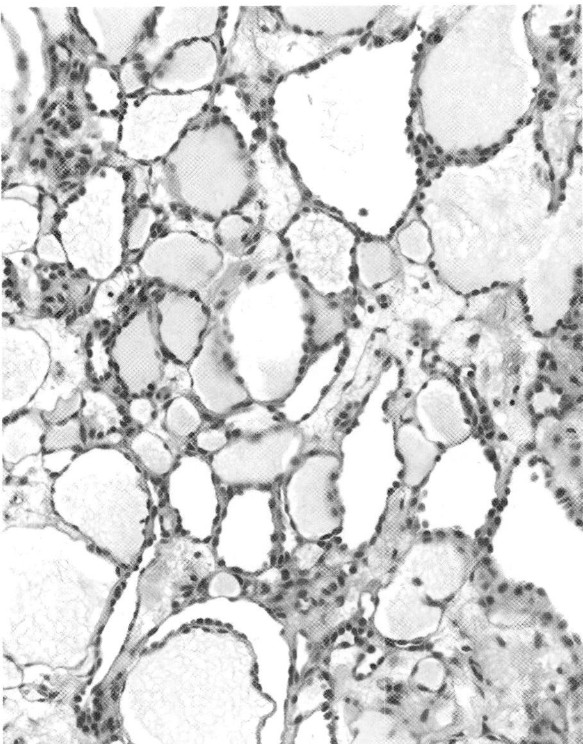

Fig. 15.57
Sertoli–Leydig cell tumor, of intermediate differentiated, microcystic pattern

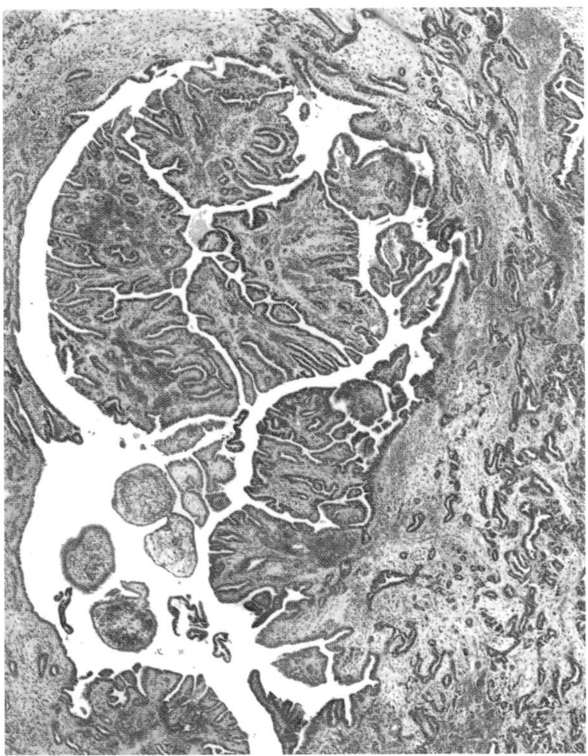

Fig. 15.58
Sertoli–Leydig cell tumor with retiform pattern. Prominent papillae

are seen in endometrioid carcinomas may closely mimic structures characteristically encountered in Sertoli and Sertoli–Leydig cell tumors. Endometrioid carcinomas also may contain luteinized stromal cells that resemble Leydig cells, creating an even greater problem in differentiation. Mucin secretion, areas of squamous differentiation that range from nests of uniform immature spindle-shaped epithelial cells to morules to keratinizing foci, and an adenofibromatous component of common epithelial type are present in most endometrioid carcinomas, facilitating their diagnosis. Clinical features, such as the usual older age of the patient and the absence of androgenic manifestations, support the diagnosis of endometrioid carcinoma, but it must be emphasized that endometrioid carcinomas occasionally have a functioning stroma, which sometimes is manifested clinically by estrogenic changes and rarely by virilization. Immunohistochemical staining for EMA may be helpful in difficult cases because it is almost always positive in cases of endometrioid carcinoma and only rarely focally positive in a few cells within a Sertoli–Leydig cell tumor. Sertoli–Leydig cell tumors may be simulated by primary or metastatic endometrioid stromal sarcomas. Criteria that are applicable in the differential diagnosis of these tumors with granulosa cell tumors also are helpful in this situation.

Rarely the alveolar pattern of a Sertoli–Leydig cell tumor, or Sertoli cell tumor, may suggest the diagnosis of dysgerminoma. There is not the typical scattering of lymphocytes of the germ cell tumor and on high-power scrutiny, there are marked differences in the cytologic features of the neoplastic cells. Should it be indicated, immunohistochemistry will have differing results.

The tubular Krukenberg tumor may mimic a Sertoli–Leydig cell tumor especially if luteinization of the stroma is present; further, confusion arises if the former tumor is associated with virilization. Tubular Krukenberg tumors are bilateral, however, in most cases and contain markedly atypical cells, including signet-ring cells that contain mucin, easily demonstrable by special stains. Other general features of metastatic tumors will aid in cases of Krukenberg tumor.

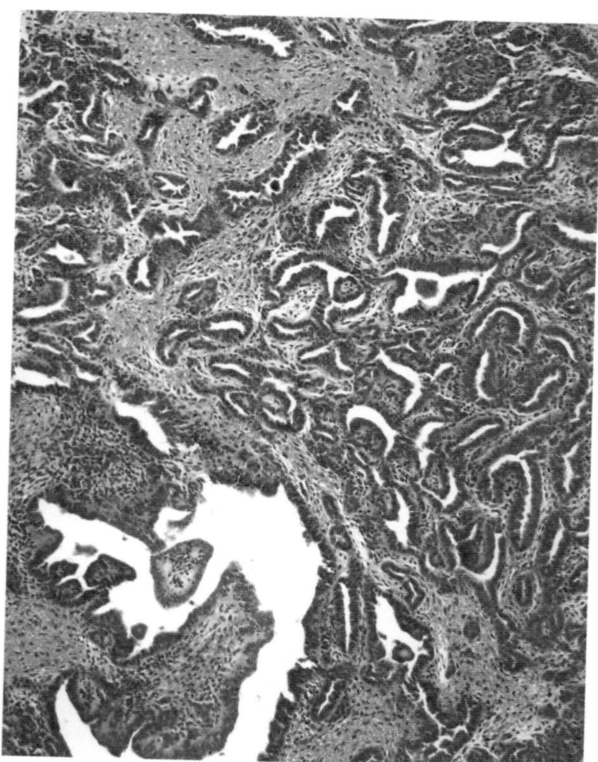

Fig. 15.59
Sertoli–Leydig cell tumor with retiform pattern. **Slit-like spaces are conspicuous**

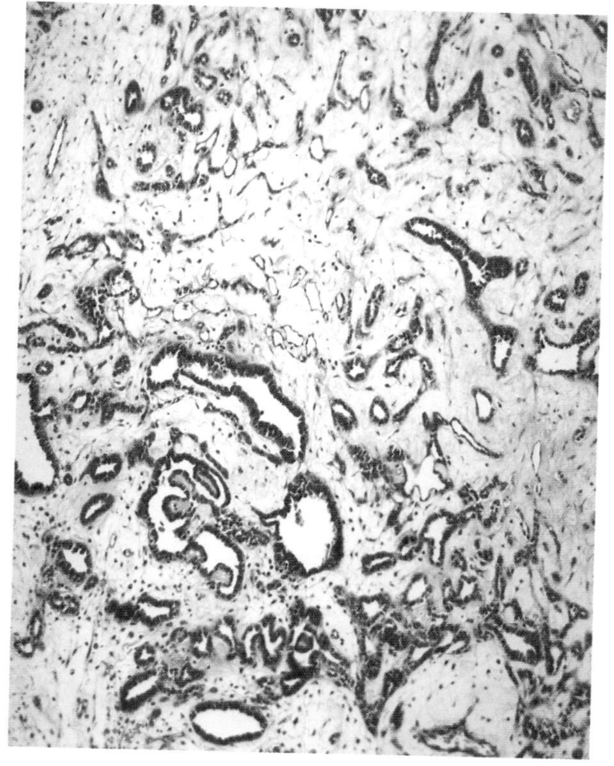

Fig. 15.60
Sertoli–Leydig cell tumor with retiform pattern. **Prominent edematous stroma**

Carcinoid tumors, especially those of the trabecular type, may be confused with Sertoli–Leydig cell tumors of intermediate differentiation. The ribbons of the former, however, are longer, thicker, and more uniformly distributed than the sex cord-like formations of the latter. Also, rare carcinoid tumors with a solid tubular pattern can be difficult to distinguish from well-differentiated Sertoli cell tumors. Examination of the stroma of carcinoid tumors may be helpful in the differential diagnosis. It is typically less cellular and more fibromatous than that of Sertoli–Leydig cell tumors and rarely contains Leydig cells, typically at the periphery. Primary carcinoid tumors are associated with teratomatous elements in 70% of the cases, and metastatic carcinoids are almost always bilateral and usually are associated with an obvious primary tumor of the intestine and metastases elsewhere in the abdomen. Immunohistochemistry should be definitive in the occasional case in which it is needed.

The tubules seen in ovarian wolffian tumors may be indistinguishable from those seen in Sertoli and Sertoli–Leydig cell tumors but are virtually always accompanied by other patterns that exclude the diagnosis of a sex cord-stromal tumor.

Although in the past, Sertoli–Leydig cell tumors with heterologous elements were sometimes considered "teratomatous" [130], there are marked differences in the overall constituents of Sertoli–Leydig cell tumors and teratomatous neoplasms such that distinction between the two should be straightforward in the great majority of cases. Rare heterologous neoplasms have a dominant mucinous cystic component and the diagnostic Sertoli–Leydig elements can be absent on certain slides, but judicious sampling will variably show them, by definition.

The retiform variant of Sertoli–Leydig cell tumor causes specific problems in differential diagnosis. A common misdiagnosis is yolk sac tumor, which is suggested clinically by the young age of the patient and pathologically by the presence of papillae within cystic spaces. The occurrence of androgenic manifestations with about 20% of cases of retiform Sertoli–Leydig cell

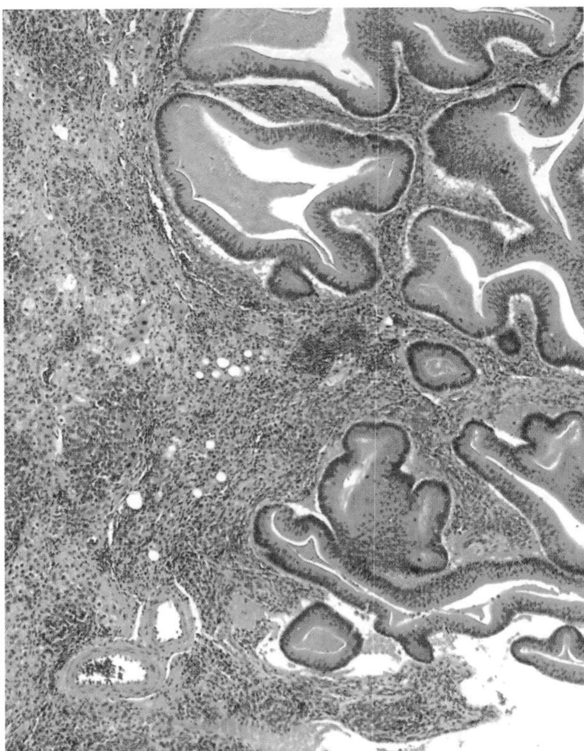

Fig. 15.61
Sertoli–Leydig cell tumor with heterologous elements. **Mucinous glands are separated by intermediate form of tumor**

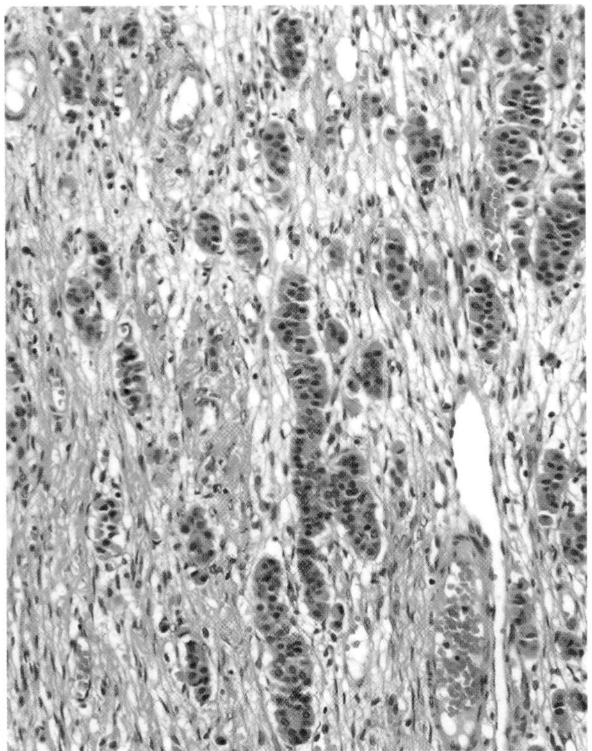

Fig. 15.62
Sertoli–Leydig cell tumor with heterologous elements. **Clusters and cords of carcinoid cells**

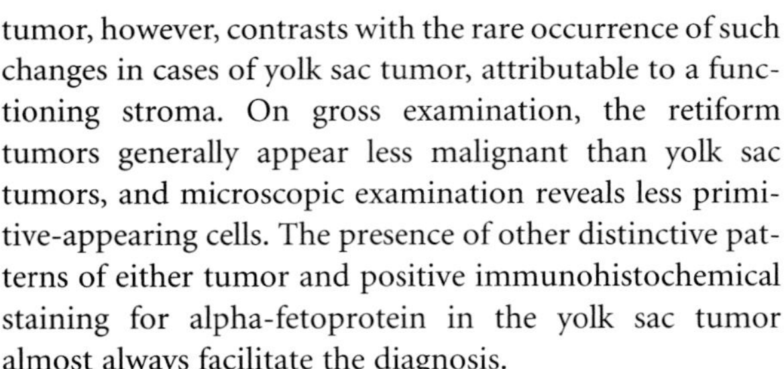

tumor, however, contrasts with the rare occurrence of such changes in cases of yolk sac tumor, attributable to a functioning stroma. On gross examination, the retiform tumors generally appear less malignant than yolk sac tumors, and microscopic examination reveals less primitive-appearing cells. The presence of other distinctive patterns of either tumor and positive immunohistochemical staining for alpha-fetoprotein in the yolk sac tumor almost always facilitate the diagnosis.

A greater problem in the differential diagnosis of retiform Sertoli–Leydig cell tumors arises because of their characteristic papillary patterns and the frequent presence of cellular stratification particularly if those features predominate. Under such circumstances, a misdiagnosis of a serous tumor of borderline malignancy or a serous or endometrioid carcinoma occasionally is made. A variety of clinical and pathologic features, including the young age of the patient, the association with virilization, and the presence of other more easily recognizable patterns of Sertoli–Leydig cell tumor, are helpful clues to the correct diagnosis. Finally, the juxtaposition of epithelial and immature mesenchymal elements in some retiform tumors, and in some cases additional mesenchymal heterologous elements, has caused confusion with a malignant mesodermal mixed tumor, but the features already outlined also serve to exclude the latter diagnosis.

Because occasional sex cord-stromal tumors have a morphologic appearance intermediate between granulosa cell tumors and Sertoli–Leydig cell tumors or exhibit features of both tumors, it is sometimes difficult to decide whether a given tumor should be placed in the granulosa, Sertoli–Leydig cell, or mixed category. Major criteria that help to differentiate granulosa cell tumors and Sertoli–Leydig cell tumors are listed in *Table 15.7.*

Clinical Behavior and Treatment

After the removal of a virilizing Sertoli–Leydig cell tumor, normal menses characteristically resume in about 4 weeks.

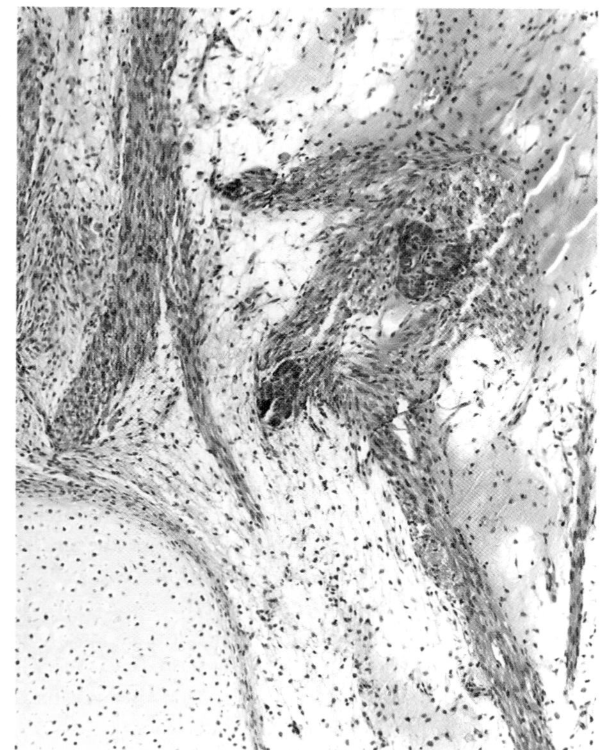

Fig. 15.63
Sertoli–Leydig cell tumor with heterologous elements. **Rare nests of darkly staining Sertoli cells with bands of skeletal muscle and focus of cartilage**

The excessive hair usually diminishes to some extent. Clitoromegaly and deepening of the voice are less apt to regress. The prognosis in cases of Sertoli–Leydig cell tumor is closely related to their stage and degree of differentiation. The rare tumors that present in an advanced stage have a poor prognosis, with a mortality rate of 100% in our series [191]. The survival rates of patients with stage I tumors correlate with the degree of differentiation. In our series, none of the well-differentiated tumors, 11% of those of intermediate differentiation, 59% of the poorly differentiated tumors, and 19% of those with heterologous elements were clinically malignant. The homologous component of the tumor was poorly differentiated in all eight clinically malignant tumors in the heterologous category, and in seven of these the heterologous elements included skeletal muscle, cartilage, or both.

Earlier studies in the literature failed to establish a relation between the degree of differentiation of Sertoli–Leydig cell tumors and their prognosis, but later investigations have supported the findings in our series. In our study, there also was evidence that the presence of a retiform pattern had an adverse effect on the prognosis; 25% of stage I tumors of intermediate differentiation with a retiform component were malignant as opposed to 10% of those with no retiform component [191]. It is noteworthy that the only stage III tumor of intermediate differentiation in our series had an almost completely retiform pattern, and we have seen an additional Sertoli–Leydig cell tumor with a predominantly retiform pattern that was stage III. Rupture also adversely affected the outcome of stage I tumors. Thirty percent of the tumors of intermediate differentiation that had ruptured were clinically malignant, in contrast to only 7% of those that were intact; in the poorly differentiated category, 86% of the ruptured tumors were malignant compared with 45% of those that had not ruptured.

In contrast to granulosa cell tumors, which often recur many years after primary therapy, Sertoli–Leydig cell tumors typically reappear relatively early. Sixty-six percent of the malignant tumors in our series recurred within 1 year and only 6.6% recurred after 5 years. The recurrent tumor usually is confined to the pelvis and abdomen, but distant metastases to the lung, scalp, and supraclavicular

Table 15.7
Adult granulosa cell tumor versus Sertoli–Leydig cell tumor

Granulosa cell tumor	Sertoli–Leydig cell tumor
All age groups, mostly postmenopausal	Mainly young women
Usually estrogenic, rarely androgenic	Usually androgenic, occasionally estrogenic
Microfollicular, macrofollicular, trabecular, insular and diffuse patterns	Hollow or solid tubules, cords, diffuse patterns
Granulosa cells usually mature with pale, often grooved nuclei	Sertoli cells often immature
Fibrothecomatous component common	Fibromatous component uncommon; mesenchyme often immature and cellular, or edematous
Steroid-type cells (lutein cells) usually not prominent and uncommonly clustered	Steroid-type cells (Leydig cells) tend to cluster; rarely contain crystals of Reinke
Heterologous elements rare	Heterologous elements in 20% of cases
Retiform elements absent	Retiform elements in 15% of cases

lymph nodes have been reported. Three of the patients in our series had parenchymal liver metastases.

The treatment of a patient with Sertoli–Leydig cell tumor depends on her age, the stage of her tumor, the presence or absence of rupture, and the degree of differentiation. In young women, the low frequency of bilaterality justifies the performance of a unilateral salpingo-oophorectomy if the tumor is stage IA and preservation of fertility is desired. More aggressive surgical therapy and adjuvant therapy are indicated for advanced-stage tumors. Adjuvant therapy also may be advisable for stage I tumors that are poorly differentiated, contain mesenchymal heterologous elements, or are ruptured tumors of intermediate differentiation.

Other Types of Sex Cord-Stromal Tumors

Gynandroblastoma

Gynandroblastoma, an extremely rare tumor [5], has been greatly overdiagnosed. Because small foci of ovarian cell types often are encountered in well-sampled, otherwise typical Sertoli–Leydig cell tumors and conversely, testicular cell types are demonstrable focally in occasional granulosa-stromal cell tumors, the diagnosis of gynandroblastoma should be restricted to the very rare tumors that contain significant components of both forms of neoplasia. According to our criteria, the minor component should account for at least 10% of a tumor in the sex cord-stromal category to warrant a diagnosis of gynandroblastoma. As indicated in the introductory remarks, we prefer to avoid the designation gynandroblastoma for reasons noted there. The nature of the hormones secreted by a sex cord-stromal tumor should not determine its morphologic diagnosis in view of the proven capacity of tumors of testicular cell types to secrete estrogens and of those of ovarian cell types to produce androgens.

Sex Cord Tumor with Annular Tubules

This neoplasm is characterized basically by the presence of simple and complex annular tubules (➋ *Figs. 15.64–15.66*) [143, 192]. The simple tubules have the shape of a ring, with the nucleus oriented peripherally and around a central hyalinized body composed of basement membrane material; an intervening anuclear cytoplasmic zone forms the major component of the ring. The much more numerous complex tubules are rounded structures made up of intercommunicating rings revolving around multiple hyaline bodies. Tumors containing annular tubules have been interpreted as Sertoli cell tumors by some observers [164] and granulosa cell tumors by others [59], but the pattern of growth has features intermediate between these two tumors, albeit focal differentiation into both typical Sertoli cell tumor with elongated tubules and typical granulosa cell tumor with Call–Exner bodies is seen in some of the cases. Sertoli-type cells have been identified ultrastructurally by the demonstration of Charcot–Bottcher filament bundles [164] which are considered specific cytoplasmic inclusions of Sertoli cells.

Sex cord tumors with annular tubules vary both clinically and pathologically, depending on whether the patient has Puetz–Jeghers syndrome or not (➋ *Table 15.8*). Almost all female patients with this syndrome whose ovaries have been examined microscopically have had sex cord tumorlets with annular tubules, which have been multifocal and bilateral in at least two thirds of the cases; the largest reported lesion in a patient with this syndrome was 3 cm in diameter. Focal calcification has been seen in more than half the cases. In almost all the patients, the lesions have been incidental findings in ovaries removed for other reasons. All the tumorlets associated with Peutz–Jeghers syndrome have been benign, warranting conservative treatment.

In patients without Peutz–Jeghers syndrome (➋ *Fig. 15.66*), in contrast, the tumors are almost always unilateral and usually form palpable masses. Transitions to typical granulosa cell tumor are much more common than in tumorlets associated with Peutz–Jeghers syndrome. A focal solid proliferation of cells with eosinophilic cytoplasm may be seen (➋ *Fig. 15.66*). Forty percent of the patients have had manifestations of estrogen secretion; progesterone secretion, as evidenced by a decidual change of the endometrium, is relatively common. At least one fifth of the tumors have been clinically malignant, with a characteristic spread via the lymphatic system. Recurrences often are late. In one remarkable case, multiple recurrences occurred, mostly within regional and distal lymph nodes, over a period of 24 years, with each recurrent tumor removed surgically. In that case, the tumor produced large amounts of müllerian-inhibiting substance as well as progesterone, both of which were found useful as tumor markers in the serum in monitoring the course of the patient [58].

Four other ovarian tumors from girls with Peutz–Jeghers syndrome have caused sexual precocity. Two of them, occurring in sisters, had the features of Sertoli cell tumors with lipid storage [153], whereas the other two had microscopic findings that were unique in our experience, including diffuse areas, tubular differentiation, microcysts, and papillae, and the presence of two distinctive cell types,

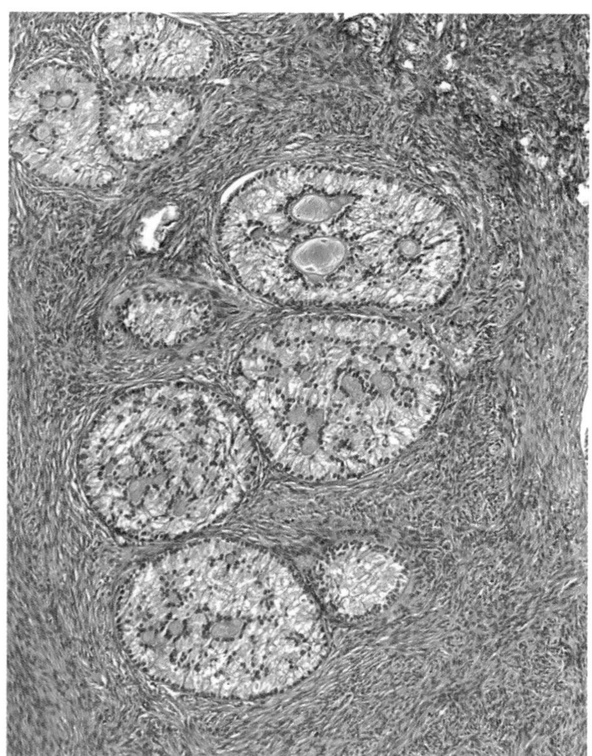

Fig. 15.64
Sex cord tumor with annular tubules. **Several foci are present within ovary from patient with Peutz–Jeghers syndrome**

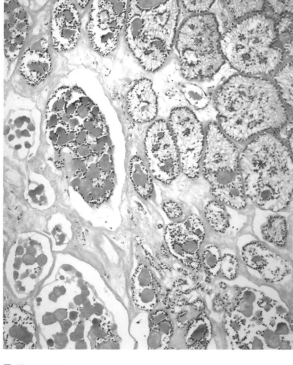

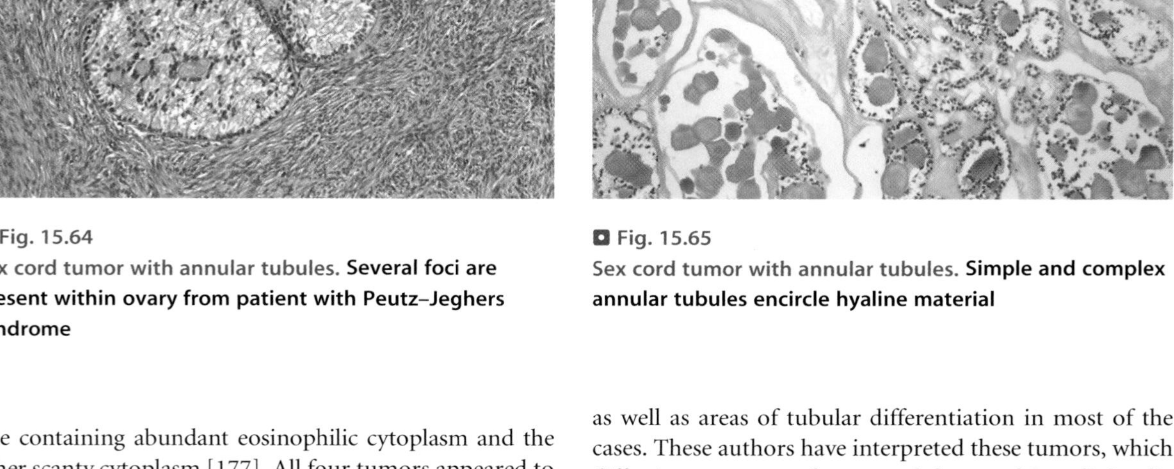

Fig. 15.65
Sex cord tumor with annular tubules. **Simple and complex annular tubules encircle hyaline material**

one containing abundant eosinophilic cytoplasm and the other scanty cytoplasm [177]. All four tumors appeared to be clinically benign.

Sex Cord-Stromal Tumors, Unclassified

Sex cord-stromal tumors, unclassified, is a poorly defined group of tumors that accounts for less than 10% of those in the sex cord-stromal category [148, 151]. This group includes neoplasms in which a predominant pattern of testicular or ovarian differentiation is not clearly recognizable. The boundary lines between these tumors and those of both ovarian and testicular cell types are vague because interpretations of intermediate patterns of growth and closely similar cell types inevitably are subjective.

Talerman and his associates [162] have described a group of sex cord-stromal tumors, containing diffuse fibrothecomatous and/or granulosa cell-like proliferation as well as areas of tubular differentiation in most of the cases. These authors have interpreted these tumors, which differ in appearance from usual forms of Sertoli–Leydig cell tumor, as diffuse nonlobular androblastomas, but in our opinion, it is more appropriate to place them in the unclassified sex cord-stromal category.

Sex Cord-Stromal Tumors During Pregnancy

Sex cord-stromal tumors may be particularly difficult to subclassify when they occur in pregnant patients because of alterations of their usual clinical and pathologic features. Their diagnosis is rarely suggested clinically because estrogenic manifestations are not recognizable during pregnancy, and androgenic manifestations are rare, possibly because of the ability of the placenta to aromatize androgens to estrogens. Indeed, virilization of a pregnant patient is much more likely to be caused by a nonneoplastic lesion such as the pregnancy luteoma or hyperreactio luteinalis or by a tumor with functioning stroma than a sex cord-stromal tumor. In one study, 17% of 36 sex cord-stromal tumors that were removed during pregnancy were placed in the unclassified group, and many of those which were classified in the granulosa cell or Sertoli–Leydig cell category had large areas with an indifferent appearance [179]. The features that led to difficulty in classification were the presence of prominent intercellular edema (Fig. 15.67), increased luteinization in the granulosa cell tumors, and marked degrees of Leydig cell maturation in one third of the Sertoli–Leydig cell tumors. All these changes, which were most common in tumors removed during the third trimester, tended to obscure the underlying architecture. The behavior of sex cord-stromal tumors during pregnancy appeared to be similar to that of tumors of similar type unassociated with pregnancy on the basis of limited follow-up of 36 cases.

Steroid Cell Tumors

The terms lipid cell tumor and lipoid cell tumor were applied for many years to ovarian neoplasms composed

Table 15.8
Sex cord tumor with annular tubules with and without Peutz–Jeghers syndrome

	With	Without
Bilateral	62%	5%
Grossly visible	27%	75%
Size	3 cm or less	Usually large
Multifocal	82%	6%
Calcification	62%	12%
Clinically malignant	0	20%[a]
Adenoma malignum	Occassional	Absent

[a]Only grossly visible tumors used in this evaluation.

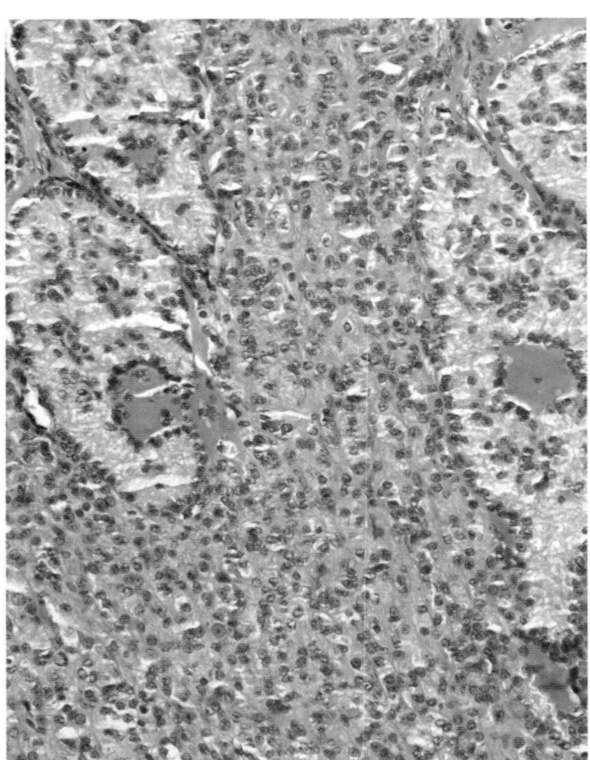

Fig. 15.66
Sex cord tumor with annular tubules. **There is a focal solid proliferation. There was no evidence of Peutz–Jeghers syndrome in the patient with this neoplasm**

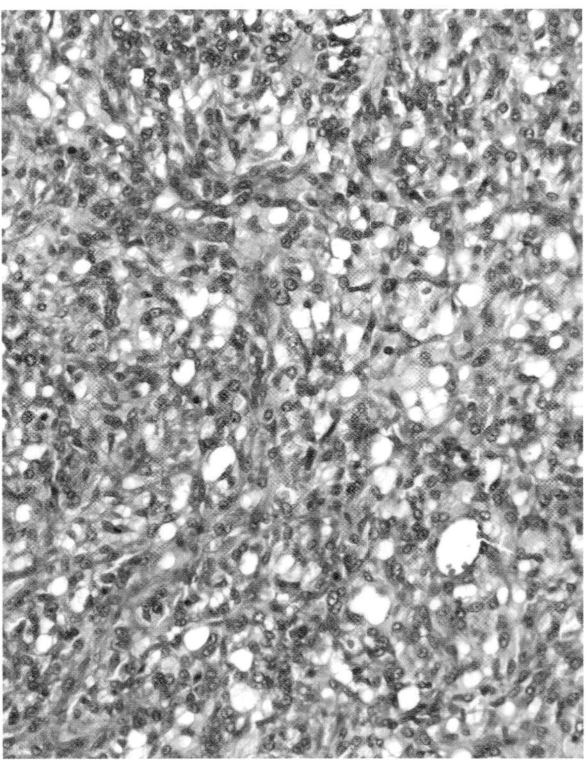

Fig. 15.67
Sex cord-stromal tumor with unclassified features. **The pateint was pregnant. There is prominent edema**

entirely of cells resembling typical steroid hormone-secreting cells, that is, lutein cells, Leydig cells, and adrenal cortical cells [165]. However, as many as 25% of tumors in this category contain little or no lipid, and several years ago, the term steroid cell tumors was introduced for these neoplasms, because it reflects both the morphologic features of the neoplastic cells and their propensity to secrete steroid hormones [144]. These tumors, which account for approximately 0.1% of ovarian tumors, have been subdivided into two subtypes according to their cell of origin and a third subtype whose specific cell lineage is unknown (*Table 15.9*). The features of the various subtypes of steroid cell tumors are contrasted in *Table 15.10*.

Stromal Luteoma

The stromal luteoma accounts for approximately 25% of steroid cell tumors [61]. This designation is applied to small steroid cell tumors that lie within the ovarian stroma (Fig. 19.69) and therefore are presumed to arise from it. Such an origin is supported by the capacity of the ovarian stroma to differentiate into lutein cells in the nonneoplastic disorder designated stromal hyperthecosis [157]. Adrenal rest cells and Leydig cells, the other possible sources of tumors of this type, on the other hand, have been identified within the ovarian stroma on only extremely rare occasions. The diagnosis of stromal luteoma is supported in approximately 90% of the cases by the finding of stromal hyperthecosis elsewhere in the same or contralateral ovary. In some cases of the latter disorders, the nests of lutein cells may form nodules (nodular hyperthecosis). The dividing line between a large hyperthecotic nodule and a stromal luteoma is arbitrary; we reserve the former designation for large nodular foci of microscopic size and the latter for nodules that are grossly visible.

Stromal luteomas are almost always less than 3 cm in diameter and, with rare exceptions, are unilateral. They are well circumscribed, solid, and usually gray-white or yellow, but one third of them have red or brown areas or are uniformly so (*Fig. 15.68*).

Table 15.9
Steroid cell tumors

Steroid cell tumors
Stromal luteoma
Leydig cell tumors
Hilus cell tumor
Leydig cell tumor, nonhilar type
Steroid cell tumor, not otherwise specified

Microscopic examination of a stromal luteoma reveals a more or less rounded nodule of cells of lutein type that generally contain relatively little lipid. Intracytoplasmic lipochrome pigment may be conspicuous. The nuclei are

Table 15.10
Clinical and pathologic features of steroid cell tumors

	Stromal luteoma	C+ hilus cell tumor	C− hilus cell tumor	Steroid cell tumor NOS
Age range, years (mean)	28–74 (58)	32–75 (57)	34–82 (61)	2–80 (43)
Virilization/ hirsutism	12%	83%	33%	52%
Estrogenic manifestations	60%	0	44%	8%
Duration of androgenic manifestations	1.5–5 years	2–20 years	1–24 years	0.5–30 years
Cushing's syndrome	0	0	0	6%
Diameter, cm (mean)	1.3	2.4	1.8	8.4
Stromal hyperthecosis	92%	42%	67%	23%

C, Reinke crystal; NOS, not otherwise specified.
Source: From [120].

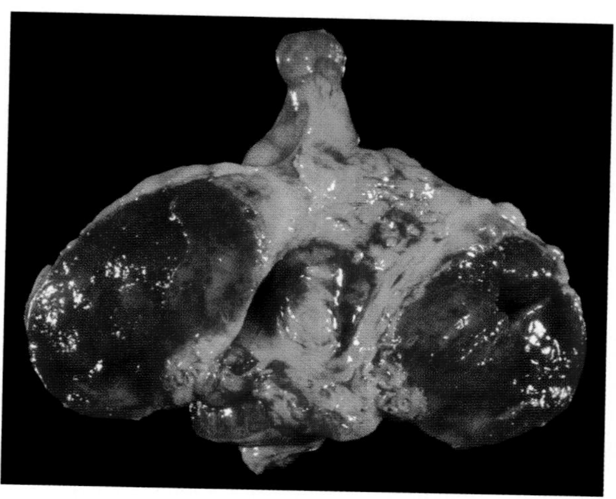

Fig. 15.68
Stromal luteoma. **The tumor is dark brown**

small and round with a single prominent nucleolus. Mitoses generally are rare. The cells may be arranged diffusely or in small nests or cords and are more or less completely surrounded by ovarian stroma. One confusing feature, seen in about 20% of the cases, is focal degeneration, with the formation of irregular spaces that may simulate glands or vessels. These spaces may contain, or be surrounded by, lipid-laden cells and chronic inflammatory cells and may be associated with fibrosis. In some cases they contain red blood cells. Some steroid cell tumors in the "not otherwise specified" category may be overgrown stromal luteomas, but the specific diagnosis cannot be made with certainty when the tumor is no longer confined to the ovarian stroma.

Eighty percent of stromal luteomas occur in postmenopausal women. The initial symptom in 60% of patients is abnormal vaginal bleeding probably related to hyperestrinism, although whether the tumor secretes estrogen directly or secretes an androgen that is converted peripherally to an estrogen is unknown. Androgenic manifestations are present in only 12% of the cases. This profile of hormonal function is the opposite of that associated with other categories of steroid cell tumor, which usually are androgenic and only occasionally estrogenic. Underlying stromal hyperthecosis may contribute to the clinical picture in some cases, particularly those in which there is a long history of hormonal disturbance. Stromal luteomas are benign.

Leydig Cell Tumors

A Leydig cell nature of a steroid cell tumor can be proved only by the identification of the more or less specific crystals of Reinke in the cytoplasm of the neoplastic cells on either light microscopic or electron microscopic examination [156]. Because only 35–40% of Leydig cell tumors of the testis contain crystals of Reinke on light microscopic examination and Leydig cells cannot be differentiated from lutein cells or adrenal cortical cells in the absence of these inclusions, it is probable that a number of unclassified steroid cell tumors are Leydig cell tumors that cannot be identified specifically as such.

Ovarian Leydig cell tumors have been divided into two subtypes by Roth and Sternberg [135], the hilus cell tumor and the Leydig cell tumor, nonhilar type. The former, which is much more common, originates in the ovarian hilus from hilar Leydig cells, which have been identified in 80–85% of adult ovaries, usually lying in relation to nonmedullated nerve fibers [156]. Hilus cell tumors, which account for approximately 20% of steroid cell tumors [120], occur at an average age of 58 years and cause hirsutism or virilization in three quarters of the cases; they are rarely associated with estrogenic manifestations. The androgenic changes typically have a less abrupt onset and are milder than those associated with Sertoli–Leydig cell tumors. They sometimes have been present for many years. The urinary 17-ketosteroid levels usually are normal or only slightly elevated because these tumors produce predominantly the potent androgen, testosterone, which is not a 17-ketosteroid, instead of the weaker androgens androstenedione and dehydroepiandrosterone, elevations of which are typically associated with high values of urinary 17-ketosteroids. Hilus cell tumors exceptionally are palpable preoperatively. They are rarely bilateral. There is no convincing example of malignant Leydig cell tumor in the literature.

Hilus cell tumors usually are reddish brown to yellow, are centered in the hilar region, and rarely are large (mean diameter, 2.4 cm). Microscopic examination typically reveals a circumscribed mass of steroid cells with abundant eosinophilic cytoplasm and little intracellular lipid; cytoplasmic lipochrome pigment may be abundant. The cells usually are distributed diffusely but occasionally their nuclei cluster and are separated by nucleus-free eosinophilic zones. This pattern (➋ *Fig. 15.69*) is highly suggestive of a hilus cell tumor even in the absence of crystals of Reinke. In some tumors, the presence of a prominent fibrous stroma imparts a nodular appearance. An unusual feature in one third of the cases is fibrinoid replacement of the walls of moderate-sized vessels (➋ *Fig. 15.69*), unaccompanied by inflammatory cell infiltration. Degenerative spaces similar to those seen in stromal luteomas may be present. The tumor cells typically contain abundant granular eosinophilic cytoplasm; occasional cells have spongy cytoplasm, indicating the presence of lipid. Cytoplasmic lipochrome pigment, which usually is sparse, is present in most cases. The typically round nuclei often are hyperchromatic and contain single small nucleoli; there may be slight to moderate variation in nuclear size and shape, and occasionally bizarre nuclei (➋ *Fig. 15.69*) and multinucleated cells are encountered. Rare mitotic figures occasionally are present. Pseudoinclusions of cytoplasm into the nucleus may be seen. Elongated eosinophilic Reinke crystals of varying sizes are present in varying numbers in the cytoplasm or sometimes in the nucleus, but often are found only after prolonged search.

The diagnosis of hilus cell tumor is favored if a crystal-free steroid cell tumor located in the hilus has a background of hilus cell hyperplasia, is associated with nonmedullated nerve fibers, has fibrinoid necrosis of blood vessel walls, or shows nuclear clustering with intervening nucleus-free

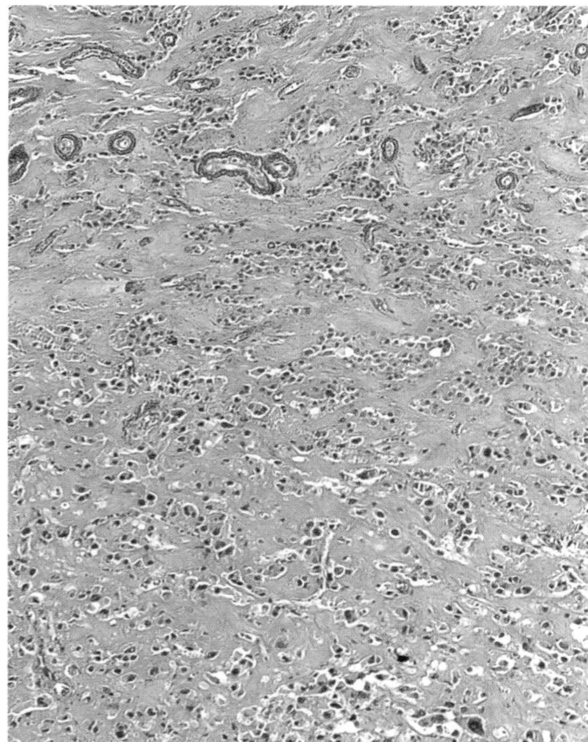

Fig. 15.69
Hilus cell tumor. **Several noteworthy features, all clues to this variant of steroid cell tumor, are seen – clusters of tumor cells, fibrinoid necrosis of vessel walls, and focal bizarre nuclei**

zones [120]. On electron microscopic examination, crystals of Reinke typically are needle shaped when cut longitudinally and hexagonal when cut in cross section. The interior of the crystal has a cross-hatched appearance. Intracytoplasmic eosinophilic spheres, which may be crystal precursors, also are typically present but are not specific for hilus cell tumors. Stromal hyperthecosis, hilus cell hyperplasia, or both are associated findings in occasional cases. The Leydig cell tumor of nonhilar type is thought to arise directly from ovarian stromal cells. Only four examples of this tumor have been reported [135] and, except for their location, their clinical and pathologic features have not differed from those of hilus cell tumors. An ovarian stromal cell derivation of these tumors is supported by the very rare finding of Leydig cells containing crystals in the steroid cell nests of ovaries that otherwise have the typical appearance of stromal hyperthecosis. In some cases in which a Leydig cell tumor is in equal contact with ovarian stroma and hilar stroma, it may be impossible to determine whether it is of the hilar or nonhilar type.

Steroid Cell Tumor, Not Otherwise Specified

These tumors occur at any age but typically at a younger age (mean, 43 years) than other types of steroid cell tumor, and in contrast to the latter, occasionally occur before puberty [60]. Steroid cell tumors not otherwise specified (NOS) are associated with androgenic changes, which may be of many years duration, in approximately half the cases, estrogenic changes, including rare examples of isosexual pseudoprecocity in approximately 10% of the cases, and occasionally progestagenic changes. A few tumors have secreted cortisol and caused Cushing's syndrome [189] and others have been accompanied by elevated cortisol levels in the absence of clinical manifestations of the syndrome; one secreted aldosterone. Rare tumors have been associated with hypercalcemia, erythrocytosis, or ascites. The remaining cases have not been accompanied by endocrine or paraendocrine manifestations. Hormone studies performed in patients with androgenic changes, Cushing's syndrome, or both typically show elevated urinary levels of 17-ketosteroids and 17-hydroxycorticosteroids as well as increased serum levels of testosterone and androstenedione. The tumors that resulted in Cushing's syndrome were associated with elevated levels of free cortisol in the blood or urine.

Gross Findings

The tumors typically are solid and well circumscribed, occasionally are lobulated, and have a mean diameter of 8.4 cm; only about 5% of them are bilateral. The sectioned surfaces typically are yellow or orange if large amounts of intracytoplasmic lipid are present, red to brown if the cells are lipid poor, or dark brown to black if large quantities of intracytoplasmic lipochrome pigment are present. Necrosis, hemorrhage, and cystic degeneration occasionally are observed.

Microscopic Findings

On microscopic examination, the cells typically are usually arranged diffusely, but occasionally they grow in large aggregates, small nests, irregular clusters, thin cords, or columns. The stroma is inconspicuous in most cases, but in approximately 15% of them it is relatively prominent

(➔ *Fig. 15.70*). A minor fibromatous component may be seen. Rarely the stroma is edematous or myxoid, with tumor cells loosely dispersed within it and, exceptionally, it exhibits calcification and even psammoma body formation. Necrosis and hemorrhage may be prominent, particularly in tumors that have significant cytologic atypia.

The polygonal to rounded tumor cells have distinct cell borders, central nuclei, and moderate to abundant amounts of cytoplasm that varies from eosinophilic and granular (lipid free or lipid poor) to vacuolated and spongy (lipid rich) (➔ *Figs. 15.70* and ➔ *15.71*); lipid was present in 75% of the tumors in one series [60]. Steroid cell tumors NOS have lipid-rich cytoplasm more often than other subtypes of steroid cell tumor. Rarely, cells with large fat droplets have a signet-ring appearance. Intracytoplasmic lipochrome pigment has been found in 40% of the cases. In 60% of the cases in the largest published series, nuclear atypia was absent or slight, and mitotic activity was low (less than 2 MF/10 HPFs) [60]. In the remaining cases, grades 1–3 nuclear atypia, usually associated with an increase in mitotic activity (up to 15 MFs/10 HPFs), was present.

Clinical Behavior and Treatment

Extraovarian spread of tumor is present at the time of operation in a small minority of cases; three of the patients with Cushing's disease had extensive intraabdominal spread of tumor [189]. In the two largest series in the literature, the proportion of tumors that were clinically malignant was 25% and 43% [60, 165]; rare tumors have recurred as many as 19 years postoperatively. Patients with clinically malignant tumors were on average 16 years older than patients with benign tumors in one series [60]; no malignant steroid cell tumors have been reported in patients in the first 2 decades.

The best pathologic correlates with malignant behavior in one series [60] were 2 or more MF/10 HPFs (92% malignant), necrosis (86% malignant), a diameter of 7 cm

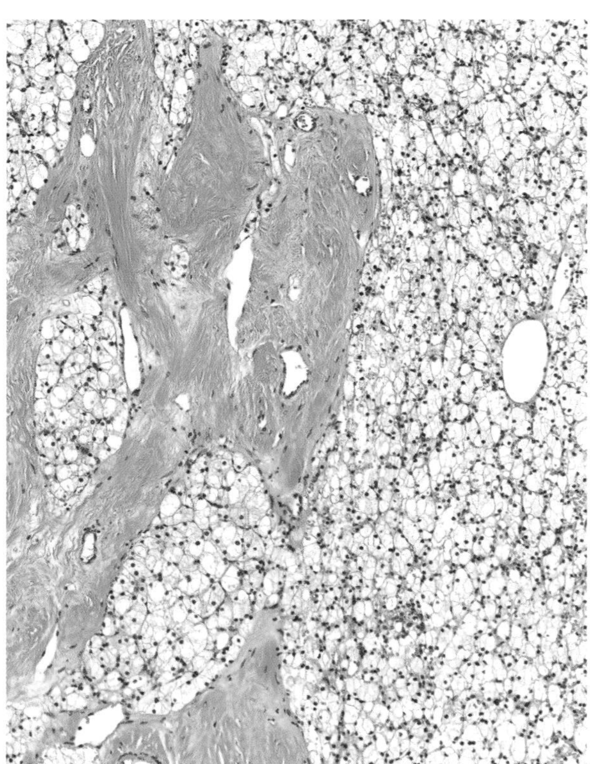

■ Fig. 15.70
Steroid cell tumor, not otherwise specified. **Cells with abundant pale cytoplasm focally separated by fibrous bands**

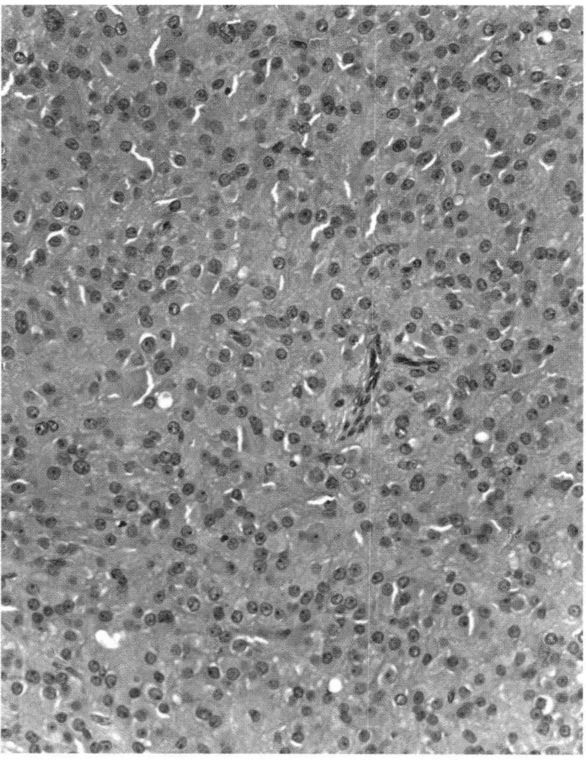

■ Fig. 15.71
Steroid cell tumor, not otherwise specified. **Typical oxyphil cells**

(78% malignant), hemorrhage (77% malignant), and grade 2 or 3 nuclear atypia (64% malignant), occasional tumors that appear cytologically benign, however, may be malignant. The metastatic tumor appears similar to the primary tumor in some cases but more poorly differentiated in others.

Differential Diagnosis of Steroid Cell Tumors

Stromal luteomas and Leydig cell tumors usually do not pose great diagnostic difficulty for the pathologist because of their characteristic locations and obvious composition of steroid-type cells, which contain crystals of Reinke in the Leydig cell tumor. The extensive formation of spaces in occasional tumors in these categories, however, may cause confusion with an adenocarcinoma and more often with a vascular tumor. Awareness of this degenerative phenomenon and its association with cellular debris, inflammatory cell infiltration, and fibrosis, as well as the finding of typical areas elsewhere in the specimen, particularly at the periphery, should facilitate the diagnosis.

Steroid cell tumors in the NOS category vary more widely in appearance than the stromal luteoma and Leydig cell tumor, both architecturally and cytologically and are accordingly the cause of greater diagnostic difficulty. The tumors that may enter the differential diagnosis include extensively luteinized granulosa cell tumors and thecomas, lipid-rich Sertoli cell tumors, clear cell carcinomas, particularly those of the oxyphilic type, rare oxyphilic endometrioid carcinomas, hepatoid yolk sac tumors and hepatoid carcinomas, endocrine tumors such as oxyphilic struma ovarii, pituitary-type tumors and paragangliomas (pheochromocytoma), metastatic renal cell carcinomas, adrenocortical carcinomas, hepatocellular carcinomas, other metastatic tumors with oxyphilic appearance, and primary and metastatic melanomas.

The presence of characteristic nonluteinized cells in both luteinized granulosa cell tumors and thecomas, as well as the typical cytologic features and patterns of these neoplasms, and the finding of abundant reticulum in thecomas are of help in the identification of these tumors. The recognition of areas with a solid tubular pattern helps distinguish a usually estrogenic lipid-rich Sertoli cell tumor with a predominant diffuse pattern from a typically androgenic steroid cell tumor. In contrast to steroid cell tumors, the clear cells of clear cell carcinomas and metastatic renal cell carcinomas have glycogen-rich cytoplasm and eccentric nuclei. Also, the presence of tubular, glandular, and papillary patterns, which are inconsistent with a steroid cell tumor, generally facilitate the differential diagnosis. Radiologic studies to rule out a renal cell carcinoma may be additionally helpful.

Oxyphilic clear cell carcinomas and endometrioid carcinomas and hepatoid yolk sac tumors and hepatoid carcinomas are all characterized by neoplastic cells with abundant eosinophilic cytoplasm. The first two tumors generally exhibit epithelial patterns, may contain glandular lumens, and are almost always accompanied by more easily recognized patterns. The oxyphilic clear cell carcinoma is almost always accompanied by a variable component of clear and hobnail cells not seen in steroid cell tumors. The hepatoid tumors also have epithelial patterns and may contain glandular lumens; they are characterized by immunohistochemical staining for alpha-fetoprotein. Primary and metastatic melanomas can simulate steroid cell tumors if amelanotic, and if they are pigmented, the pigment granules may be confused with the lipochrome granules of a steroid cell tumor. Melanomas generally have more malignant nuclear features than steroid cell tumors. Special staining, including staining for S-100 protein and HMB-45, may be helpful in difficult cases. An association with other teratomatous elements and the presence of colloid and immunohistochemical staining for thyroglobulin should enable one to distinguish an oxyphil struma from a steroid cell tumor NOS.

A rare pituitary-type tumor containing cells with abundant eosinophilic cytoplasm that arose in a wall of a dermoid cyst secreted ACTH and caused Cushing's syndrome [10]. Such a tumor might be confused with a steroid cell tumor. In that case, immunohistochemical staining for ACTH and several other pituitary hormones was positive. In one case, we have seen of pheochromocytoma of the ovary, immunohistochemical staining of the tumor cells for chromogranin, was helpful in establishing that diagnosis over steroid cell tumor. Electron microscopic examination of most of the neoplasms that simulate steroid cell tumors should disclose strikingly different features. Finally, the presence or absence of endocrine manifestations and their nature may be important clinical clues to the diagnosis.

Pregnancy luteomas, which are hyperplastic nodules composed of lutein cells that develop during pregnancy, may form large masses that resemble steroid cell tumors grossly and microscopically. As with the latter, they also may be virilizing (in about one quarter of the cases). Unlike steroid cell tumors, however, approximately one third of pregnancy luteomas are bilateral and approximately one half are multiple. Microscopic examination reveals masses of cells with abundant eosinophilic cytoplasm containing little or no lipid; mitotic figures may be numerous, sometimes up to 2 or 3/10 HPF. In contrast, a steroid cell tumor with minimal cytologic atypia that resembles a pregnancy luteoma usually contains only rare mitotic figures. Although it may be impossible to distinguish a lipid-poor or lipid-free steroid cell tumor from a solitary pregnancy luteoma, a lesion encountered during the third trimester of pregnancy is presumed to be a solitary pregnancy luteoma unless clear-cut evidence indicates otherwise.

Other Ovarian Tumors with Endocrine Function

Ovarian Tumors with Functioning Stroma

A wide variety of ovarian tumors other than those in the sex cord-stromal and steroid cell categories may be hormonally active as a result of steroid hormone production by stromal cells [66] within or adjacent to the tumor (➲ *Figs. 15.72* and ➲ *15.73*). These tumors, which have been designated ovarian tumors with functioning stroma, may be benign or malignant and, if in the latter category, primary or metastatic. Almost every ovarian tumor has been reported to be associated with steroid hormone production, but this phenomenon is seen much more often with some neoplasms than others.

Ovarian tumors with functioning stroma [86] are associated infrequently with overt endocrine manifestations but commonly accompanied by subclinical elevations of steroid hormone values. The stromal cells responsible for the hormone secretion in ovarian tumors with functioning stroma typically resemble lutein or Leydig cells and have been referred to as luteinized stromal cells. These cells almost always lie within the tumor singly, diffusely, or in clusters, but rarely they are mainly distributed just outside the tumor, sometimes forming a peripheral band (➲ *Fig. 15.73*) [137]. Exceptionally, crystals of Reinke can be identified in the lutein-like

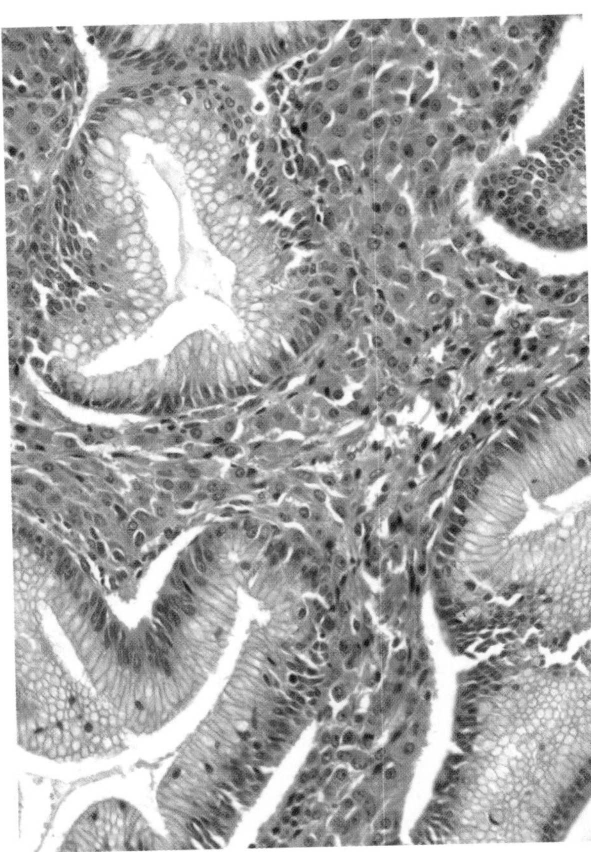

Fig. 15.72
Mucinous cystic tumor from virilized pregnant patient. **The neoplastic glands are separated by luteinized stromal cells**

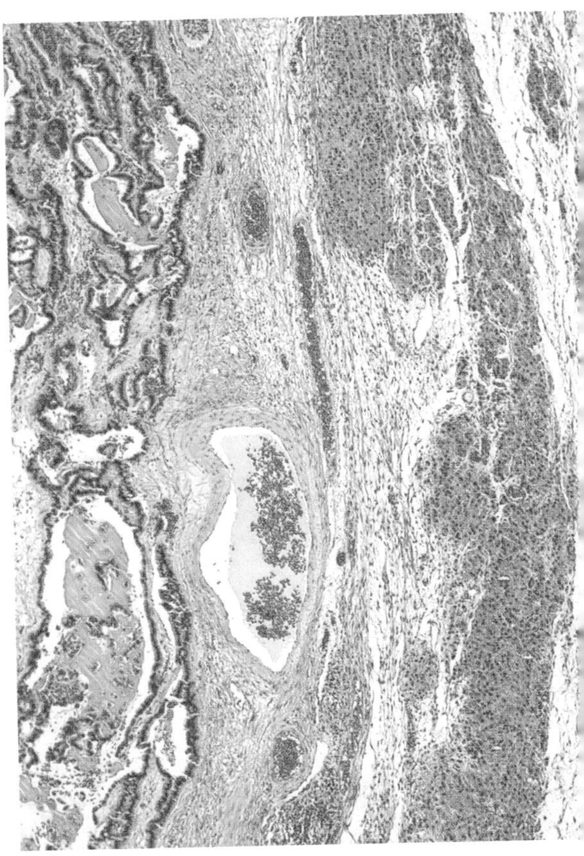

Fig. 15.73
Strumal carcinoid. **There is a peripheral band of steroid-ty cells**

cells, warranting their interpretation as Leydig cells [75]. It must be emphasized, however, that steroid-type cells may be prominent in the absence of clinical evidence of hormone overproduction and, conversely, evidence of function may exist in the absence of fully developed cells of steroid type. Ovarian tumors with functioning stroma can be divided into three major categories. In the first two categories, germ cell tumors that contain syncytiotrophoblast cells and tumors in pregnant patients, the luteinized stromal cells probably develop as a result of stimulation by hCG. The cause of the stromal alteration in the third (idiopathic) group, which accounts for most of the cases, is unclear, but ectopic production of hCG or some other stromal stimulant by the neoplastic cells may be responsible.

Germ Cell Tumors Containing Syncytiotrophoblast Cells

Two dysgerminomas with syncytiotrophoblast cells have been associated with luteinization of the stroma and endocrine manifestations; one was accompanied by isosexual precocity and the other by postpubertal virilization [171].

Germ cell tumors that produce hCG, including dysgerminomas with syncytiotrophoblast giant cells [195], choriocarcinomas, embryonal carcinomas, and polyembryomas and mixed primitive germ cell tumors, also may cause manifestations of steroid hormone secretion as a result of hCG stimulation of the ovary contralateral to the tumor to form luteinized follicles that secrete steroid hormones.

Tumors with Functioning Stroma Occurring During Pregnancy

Although it is logical to speculate that ovarian tumors with functioning stroma in pregnant patients may secrete estrogens, this possibility has not been investigated by hormone assay, and clinical manifestations of estrogen excess are not expected to be present during gestation. In contrast, more than 20 examples of virilization caused by ovarian tumors with functioning stroma during pregnancy have been reported. These tumors were mostly Krukenberg tumors or mucinous cystic tumors, but a few have been Brenner tumors or isolated other tumor types. The onset of the virilization in these patients has ranged from the third to the ninth month of gestation. Female offspring may be virilized.

Idiopathic Group

Although ovarian tumors with functioning stroma in the first two categories are encountered in young girls, patients with tumors in the idiopathic group usually are postmenopausal, reflecting the higher prevalence of ovarian tumors, both primary and metastatic, and possibly the higher levels of circulating luteinizing hormone in this age group. A wide variety of ovarian tumors has been associated with an idiopathic functioning stroma, but its frequency has varied from one type of neoplasm to another.

Mucinous tumors often contain functioning stroma, occasionally resulting in either estrogenic or androgenic manifestations (➲ *Fig. 15.74*). Brenner tumors have been accompanied by endometrial hyperplasia in 10–16% of

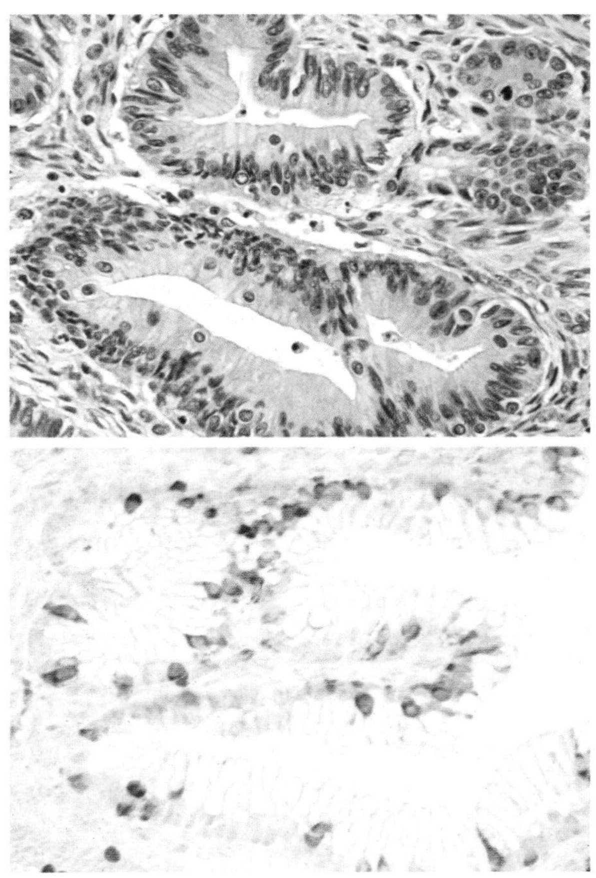

Fig. 15.74
Mucinous cystic tumor of borderline malignancy that was associated with the Zollinger–Ellison syndrome. In the bottom panel some of the neoplastic cells are immunoreactive for gastrin

the cases and occasionally are virilizing. Rare cases of endometrioid carcinoma have been reported to be associated with endometrial hyperplasia in postmenopausal women, and in one case, virilization and breast secretion developed. We have seen a well-differentiated endometrioid carcinoma from a patient with an elevated serum testosterone level and the recent development of hirsutism. Serous and clear cell tumors have been accompanied only exceptionally by hormone manifestations. Germ cell tumors of various types lacking trophoblastic cells have been associated rarely with stromal luteinization and evidence of steroid hormone secretion in the absence of pregnancy. The germ cell tumors within the idiopathic category that have been accompanied by androgenic or estrogenic manifestations have included a variety of subtypes such as dermoid cyst, struma ovarii, carcinoid tumors, embryonal carcinoma, and yolk sac tumor. The steroid cells that are stimulated in cases of germ cell tumor are peripheral rather than within the tumor in many, if not most, of the cases. The lesions associated with peripheral steroid cell formation in the series of Rutgers and Scully [137] describing this phenomenon were struma ovarii (nine cases), strumal or trabecular carcinoids (four cases), rete cysts (four cases), mucinous cystadenomas (three cases), dermoid cysts (two cases), and single examples of dysgerminoma with syncytiotrophoblast giant cells and metastatic carcinoid. In three of the cases, all strumas, a yellow color was appreciated grossly at the periphery or on the surface of the tumor.

The steroid cells that develop adjacent to ovarian tumors rather than within them are of three types: lutein cells within adjacent ovarian stroma, Leydig cells within ovarian stroma, and hilus cells, which are present only along the hilar border of the tumor. The number of cases in each of these three categories in the series of Rutgers and Scully [137] were 14, 2, and 8, respectively. The tumors with hilus cell hyperplasia were typically large with an average greatest diameter of 18 cm. The lutein cells and stromal Leydig cells were located predominantly or exclusively in the cortex or medulla peripheral to the tumor and were arranged singly and in nests, forming a discontinuous band up to 2 mm in thickness. The hilus cells were arranged singly and in small nests forming discontinuous bands in the walls of the cysts in which they arose. Lutein cell formation is accompanied most often by estrogenic manifestations, whereas stromal Leydig cell formation and hilar Leydig cell hyperplasia are associated most often with androgenic changes.

Metastatic carcinomas that contain mucinous cells, such as primary mucinous tumors of the ovary, frequently are associated with luteinization of the stroma and in a significant proportion of cases with clinical evidence of elevated steroid hormone levels. Scully and Richardson [147] found clinical evidence of excess estrogens as manifested by irregular premenopausal bleeding or postmenopausal bleeding in one quarter of patients with metastatic adenocarcinoma from the large intestine and stomach. Occasional Krukenberg tumors from nonpregnant patients have been associated with virilization. Other metastatic tumors are associated much less often with stromal luteinization. One postmenopausal woman was virilized as a result of luteinization caused by bilateral metastatic lobular carcinoma of the breast [25]. One metastatic colonic carcinoid was associated with peripheral stromal luteinization [137].

Ovarian Tumors with Thyroid Hyperfunction

Although strumas and strumal carcinoids of the ovary have been demonstrated by immunohistochemical staining to contain thyroglobulin, triiodothyronine, and thyroxine and, therefore, probably produce thyroid hormones at subclinical levels in many cases, clinical evidence suggestive of hyperthyroidism is present in only 25% of the cases, and florid thyrotoxicosis in only about 5%. Factors that make it difficult to determine accurately the frequency of hyperthyroidism in patients with struma ovarii include variable criteria for the amount of thyroid tissue required for a diagnosis of struma, the observation that approximately one sixth of patients with struma ovarii have concomitant enlargement of the thyroid gland, and a lack of confirmation of the hyperthyroidism by modern laboratory tests in most of the reported cases.

In some patients with clinical or laboratory evidence of hyperthyroidism, the preoperative diagnosis of hyperfunctioning struma ovarii has been established by high iodine uptake in the pelvis with low radioiodine uptake in the neck [21]. Other cases of struma-associated hyperthyroidism have not been recognized until the symptoms regressed after removal of an ovarian tumor. In some of these cases, a prior thyroidectomy had had no effect on the hyperthyroidism. Occasionally, oophorectomy for struma may precipitate compensatory enlargement of the thyroid gland, increased uptake of radioactive iodine by the thyroid gland, or an episode of thyrotoxicosis. Similarly, torsion of an ovary containing a struma precipitated striking hyperthyroxinemia in a pregnant patient. Occasional strumal carcinoids have been accompanied by evidence of hypersecretion of thyroid hormone in the form of postoperative thyroid storm or hypothyroidism, and thyroglobulin has been demonstrated in the colloid within tumors of this type.

Ovarian Tumors Associated with the Carcinoid Syndrome

Of the four major categories of primary carcinoid tumor of the ovary, insular, trabecular, strumal, and mucinous, one third of the insular tumors and a single example of strumal carcinoid have been associated with the carcinoid syndrome. One patient with the syndrome also had elevated serum levels of calcitonin [149]. Metastatic carcinoids involving the ovary are associated with the carcinoid syndrome in almost half the cases. The volume of the carcinoid is an important factor determining the presence or absence of the syndrome in cases of primary carcinoids. The syndrome is present in about two thirds of the cases when the tumor is large. One 74-year-old woman had the carcinoid syndrome attributable to an ovarian tumor that resembled an atypical carcinoid with areas of neuroendocrine (oat cell) carcinoma [20]. That patient also was virilized and had Cushing's syndrome. Although no immunohistochemical staining was performed, the authors concluded that the tumor was elaborating both serotonin and ACTH. The carcinoid syndrome typically occurs in the absence of hepatic or other metastases in cases of ovarian carcinoid, because the hormonal effluent of the tumor enters the systemic circulation directly, bypassing the portal venous system and avoiding inactivation in the liver. The carcinoid syndrome caused by a primary ovarian carcinoid, therefore, is usually curable if the tumor is confined to the ovary and irreversible damage to cardiac valves has not occurred.

Ovarian Tumors Associated with Zollinger–Ellison Syndrome

Eleven mucinous tumors (two cystadenomas, five borderline tumors, and four cystadenocarcinomas) have caused the Zollinger–Ellison syndrome with disappearance of the syndrome after removal of the tumor [19, 54]. Most of the tumors were large, with a mean diameter of 21.5 cm. Gastrin-containing cells were identified immunohistochemically within the cyst lining in all cases in which staining was performed (➋ *Fig. 15.74*), and gastrin was demonstrated within the cyst fluid in about half of them.

The association between ovarian mucinous tumors and Zollinger–Ellison syndrome is consistent with the frequent finding of neuroendocrine intestinal-type cells within mucinous tumors. A number of studies have shown that all categories of mucinous tumors (benign, borderline, and malignant) commonly contain argyrophil and hormone-immunoreactive cells, although in most of the studies, these cells have been found most frequently in mucinous borderline tumors. The argyrophilic cells often are immunoreactive for serotonin and a variety of polypeptide hormones. The most commonly identified of the latter have been corticotropin, gastrin, somatostatin, glucagon, secretion, and pancreatic polypeptide; in many cases, the tumors have been immunoreactive for multiple hormones.

Ovarian Tumors with Paraendocrine Disorders

A variety of paraendocrine disorders have been described in association with numerous types of ovarian tumor, some manifested by signs and symptoms of a well-known endocrine disease and others by subclinical laboratory abnormalities, indicating ectopic production of hormones or hormone-like substances by the tumor cells. In some of these cases, the hormone being produced has been identified whereas in others, such as in cases of hypercalcemia, the mechanism of the disorder remains unclear. In all the cases included within this category of neoplasms, successful therapy of the tumor has led to disappearance of the paraendocrine state.

Hypercalcemia, Including Small Cell Carcinoma

About 60% of these tumors have been a distinctive type of small cell carcinoma [181]; almost half the remainder have been clear cell carcinomas with serous carcinomas, squamous cell carcinoma arising in a dermoid cyst, dysgerminoma, and miscellaneous other neoplasms, each accounting for about one quarter of the remainder.

The mechanism of the hypercalcemia associated with ovarian cancers is unknown [113]. Attempts to demonstrate parathormone (PTH) within the tumor cells have been unsuccessful with rare exceptions, and in several cases in which PTH has been measured in the serum, the level was normal. Recent evidence has implicated PTH-related peptide (PTHRP) which has been elevated in the serum [62, 169] or detected by radioimmunoassay in some cases [52]; three tumors (one, a small cell carcinoma) were immunoreactive for PTHRP [22, 169]. Because of the binding of PTHRP to a receptor common for PTH and PTHRP, the secretion of PTHRP by a neoplasm may produce the biochemical features of hyperparathyroidism. In one case, the patient also had abnormally high serum concentrations of 1,25-dihydroxyvitamin D (1,25-DHD) and increased intestinal calcium absorption [62]. Tumor removal was followed by normalization of the serum calcium, PTHRP, and 1,25-DHD levels, suggesting an intestinal contribution to the maintenance of the hypercalcemia in this patient.

The small cell carcinoma of hypercalcemic type is the most common form of undifferentiated carcinoma of the ovary in females under 40 years of age and has been accompanied by elevated levels of calcium in 66% of the cases in which it has been measured [181]. The age of the patients has ranged from 14 months to 44 (average, 24) years. The presenting symptoms usually are abdominal pain and swelling.

At laparotomy almost all the tumors have been unilateral; spread beyond the ovary is usual. Gross examination reveals fleshy white to pale tan masses, often containing large areas of hemorrhage and necrosis (➲ *Fig. 15.75*). The most common microscopic appearance is a diffuse arrangement of closely packed epithelial cells interrupted focally in most cases by distinctive follicle-like structures containing eosinophilic fluid (➲ *Fig. 15.76*). The neoplastic cells typically have scanty cytoplasm and small nuclei (➲ *Fig. 15.77*) that typically contain single small nucleoli; mitotic figures are numerous. The tumor cells also grow in nests, cords, and irregular groups. In many tumors, large cells with abundant eosinophilic cytoplasm resembling lutein cells to varying extent have been present focally (➲ *Figs. 15.78* and ➲ *15.79*); rarely, these cells predominate. In about 10% of the cases, occasional glands lined by mature mucinous epithelium, signet cells, or highly atypical cells containing mucin are present. The stroma is generally relatively scanty and consists of nonspecific fibrous tissue.

Special staining and immunohistochemical [3] and ultrastructural [96] examination have not revealed any features that identify the specific cell type of this epithelial tumor; dense-core granules have been absent in most cases. Flow cytometry on paraffin-embedded material typically shows that the cells are diploid [44]. The age distribution and the characteristic presence of uniform small cells and follicle formation suggest a sex cord derivation, but transitions to recognizable forms of sex cord tumors have not been observed.

The small cell carcinoma often is confused with a granulosa cell tumor of either adult or juvenile type. The features of these three types of tumor are contrasted in ➲ *Table 15.3*. Diffuse small cell carcinomas also may resemble malignant lymphomas, particularly on low-power examination, but adequate sampling reveals patterns of

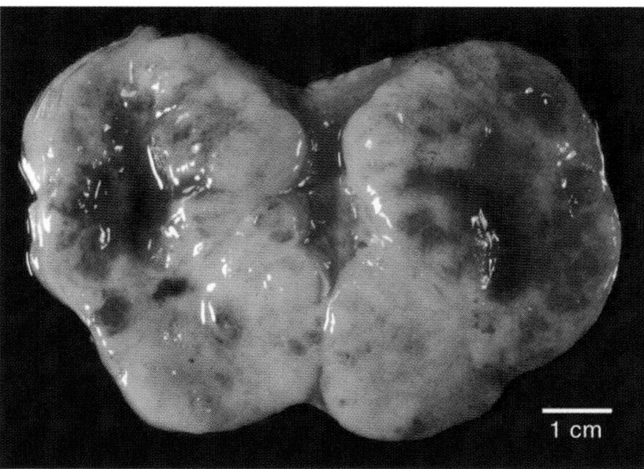

Fig. 15.75
Small cell carcinoma, hypercalcemic type. **The sectioned surface of the neoplasm is mostly creamy white with focal hemorrhage and necrosis**

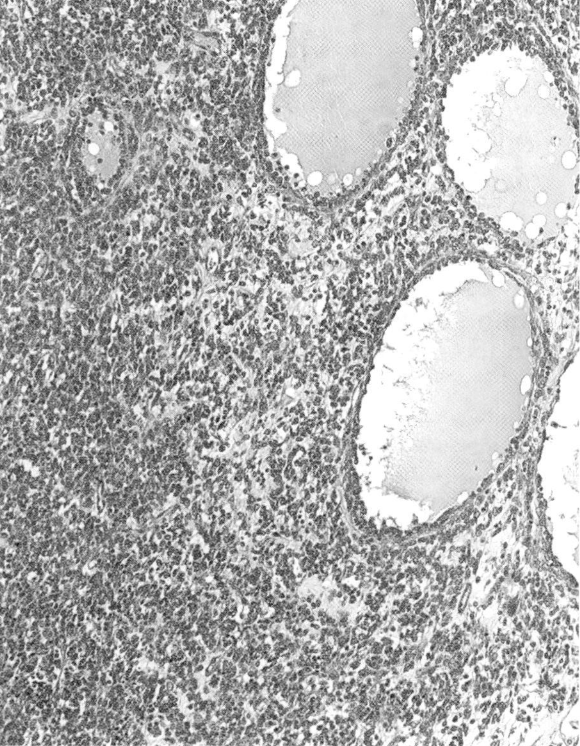

Fig. 15.76
Small cell carcinoma, hypercalcemic type. **Follicles are present within an otherwise densely cellular neoplasm**

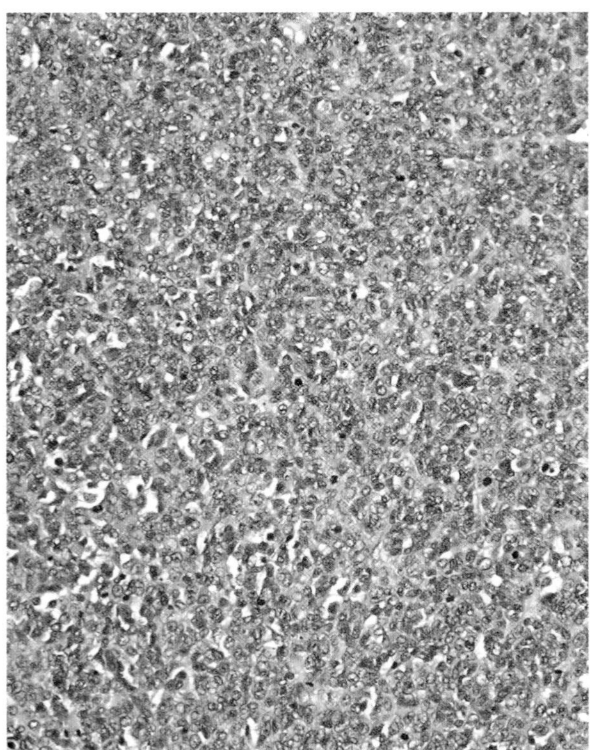

Fig. 15.77
Small cell carcinoma, hypercalcemic type. **Typical small cells**

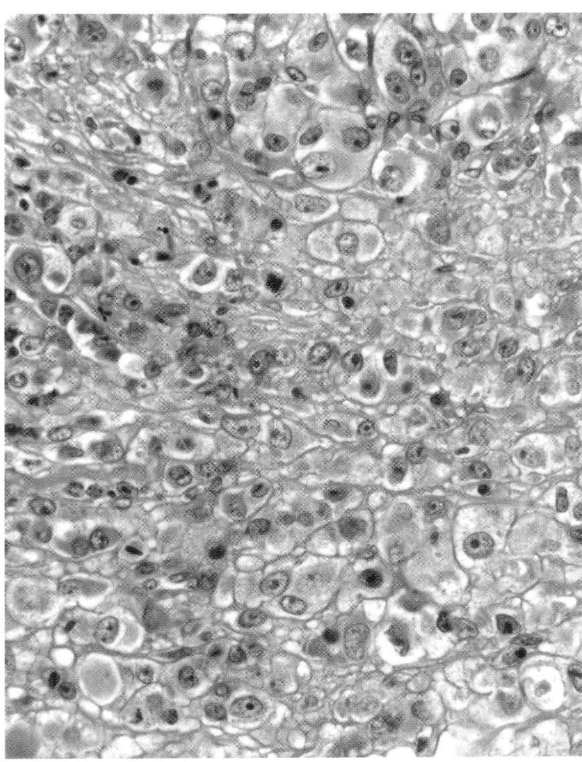

Fig. 15.78
Small cell carcinoma, hypercalcemic type. **Typical large cells**

growth that indicate the epithelial nature of the tumor; also, the cytologic features of the neoplastic cells are incompatible with any form of malignant lymphoma. Exceptionally, the differential diagnosis of a small cell carcinoma includes other small cell malignant tumors of the ovary, including several metastatic tumors such as metastatic melanoma and metastatic small cell sarcomas. The small cell carcinoma has a poor prognosis even when at stage I and no form of adjuvant therapy is of proven benefit.

Cushing's Syndrome

Five cases of clinically typical and biochemically documented Cushing's syndrome have been caused by cortisol production by a steroid cell tumor [189]. Most of the tumors occurred in adults and had metastasized within the abdomen at the time of presentation and had atypical cytologic features. Rarely, primary ovarian tumors other than those of steroid cell type have been associated with Cushing's syndrome, probably in most cases on the basis of ectopic production of corticotropin or corticotropin-releasing factor.

These cases have included bilateral endometrioid adenocarcinoma [38], a poorly differentiated adenocarcinoma [121], a malignant Sertoli cell tumor [108], a trabecular carcinoid (in which the tumor cells were immunoreactive for corticotropin) [144], and a tumor that resembled an atypical carcinoid and small cell carcinoma of the lung [20]. Finally, two cases have been described in which anterior pituitary tissue within a dermoid cyst caused Cushing's syndrome. In one of these cases, it was not clear whether the pituitary tissue was neoplastic or hyperplastic, but in the other case, there was a chromophobe adenoma in which the neoplastic cells were immunoreactive for corticotropin [32].

Human Chorionic Gonadotropin Secretion

Ectopic hCG production was reported by Civantos and Rywlin [30] in three women with serous papillary or

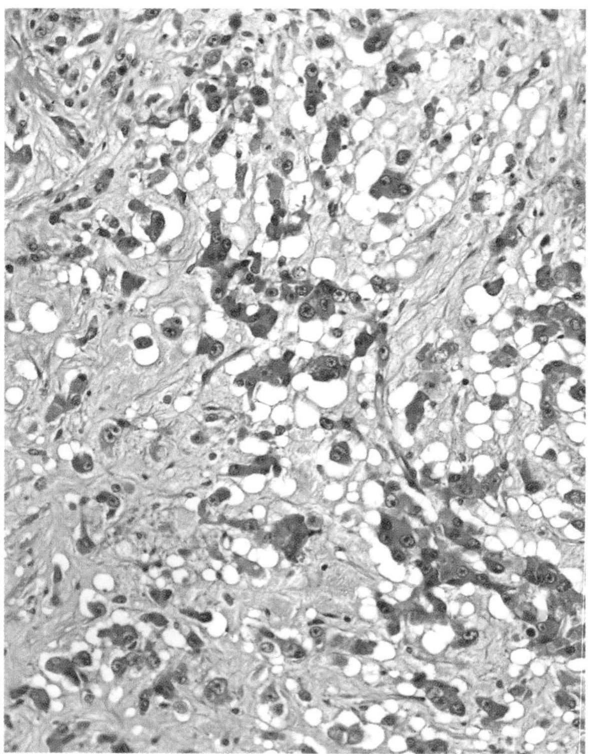

Fig. 15.79
Small cell carcinoma, hypercalcemic type. **The large cell variant pattern sometimes has a prominent myxoid background**

mucinous adenocarcinomas of the ovary. All the patients had elevated urinary hCG level. Each tumor contained poorly differentiated areas with cells resembling syncytiotrophoblast cells; these cells were positive for hCG on immunofluorescence. In one case, the contralateral ovary contained numerous lutein cells, and a decidual reaction was present in the endometrium; that patient had vaginal bleeding, but no endocrine effects were present in the others. Two poorly differentiated surface epithelial carcinomas with a choriocarcinomatous component had elevated serum hCG levels [115]. The choriocarcinoma appeared grossly as a necrotic, hemorrhagic, circumscribed, brown nodule. Matias-Guiu and Prat [86] conducted the most extensive immunohistochemical investigation of hCG in ovarian tumors, using single polyclonal antibodies to the whole hormone and its beta subunit and four monoclonal antibodies to the whole hormone, its beta subunit, and two regions of the carboxyl terminal of the beta subunit. Correlating positive staining results with the presence or absence of an "active" stroma of the tumor (luteinization and/or "condensation"), these authors found that the epithelial cells of 41% of the tumors with active stroma reacted with the polyclonal antibodies and 62% with the monoclonal antibodies; the corresponding figures for the epithelial cells of the tumor with an inactive stroma were 14% and 37%, respectively.

Hypoglycemia

Six ovarian neoplasms have been associated with hypoglycemia: a serous cystadenocarcinoma, a dysgerminoma, a fibroma, a malignant schwannoma, a strumal carcinoid, and a carcinoid tumor with a mixed insular and trabecular pattern [8, 103, 144]. In the case of the malignant schwannoma, insulin and proinsulin were recovered from the tumor tissue and the cells of the carcinoid tumor were immunoreactive for insulin. The patient with the insular-trabecular carcinoid tumor also had a parathyroid adenoma and pituitary hyperplasia.

Renin and Aldosterone Secretion

Three cases of hypertension related to hormone secretion by an ovarian tumor have been reported; two of the patients also had Gorlin's syndrome. In eight cases, the hypertension was associated with a renin-secreting tumor, hyperreninism, and secondary hyperaldosteronism [6, 76]. In three cases, an aldosterone-secreting ovarian tumor resulted in primary hyperaldosteronism associated with low or normal plasma renin levels [72, 78, 167]. Elevated aldosterone levels were present in the 12th case (but plasma renin levels were not measured) [144] and in the 13th case (neither renin nor aldosterone levels were determined) [144], reported in 1966. In four cases, the tumor also elaborated steroid hormones as manifested by isosexual pseudoprecocity in two cases and elevated serum levels of estradiol and testosterone in two. Eight of the ovarian tumors were interpreted as sex cord-stromal tumors and two as steroid cell tumors. Three tumors in the first category were well-differentiated Sertoli cell tumors, whereas the other four had an appearance that was too nonspecific or poorly differentiated to subclassify. One of these last four tumors occurred in a woman with Peutz–Jeghers syndrome and was benign, whereas the other three were clinically malignant and two were fatal. One of the "steroid cell" tumors occurred in a 7-year-old girl and had a prominent follicular pattern, more in keeping with a diagnosis of JGCT. The final two tumors were a leiomyosarcoma and a mucinous adenocarcinoma.

Immunohistochemical staining in five of the sex cord-stromal tumors and the leiomyosarcoma showed cells containing immunoreactive renin or prorenin.

Prolactin Secretion

Two ovarian dermoid cysts have been associated with the elaboration of prolactin [73, 118]. The patients were both in the reproductive age group. In one case, the dermoid cyst contained a 2.5-cm tumor composed of small rounded nests of epithelial cells, some of which surrounded lumens filled with colloid-like material (➋ *Fig. 15.80*). The cells had scanty cytoplasm and small, round, uniform, mitotically inactive nuclei. Most of the tumor cells were strongly immunoreactive for prolactin (➋ *Fig. 15.80*). In the other case, pathologic examination of an otherwise typical dermoid cyst disclosed a 1-mm focus of pituitary tissue composed of large polygonal cells with abundant eosinophilic cytoplasm that was immunoreactive for prolactin. In one patient with gonadoblastoma [63], a prolactin gradiant was present between the vein draining the tumor and peripheral veins, although the patient did not have hyperperlactonemia. Cells within the gonadoblastoma that resembled Sertoli cells were immunoreactive for prolactin.

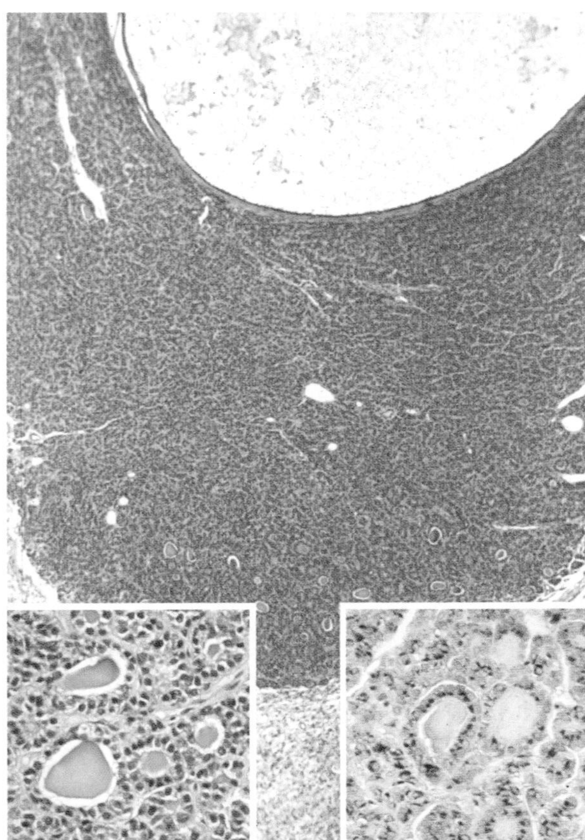

Fig. 15.80
Prolactinoma within ovarian dermoid cyst, partly seen at the top, with cellular proliferation of pituitary type cells beneath it. **The tumor was composed of epithelial cells with scanty cytoplasm and small round uniform nuclei; there were a few lumens filled with colloid-like material (*bottom left*). Most of the tumor cells were strongly immunoreactive for prolactin (*bottom right*)**

Ovarian Tumors Associated with Paraneoplastic Syndromes

Nervous System Disorders

Ovarian cancer of surface epithelial type is one of the malignant tumors most often associated with nervous system disorders. The tumor is occasionally occult [84]. A variety of lesions affecting both the gray matter and white matter of the cerebrum, cerebellum, spinal cord, the peripheral nerves, and the myoneural junction, accompanied by myasthenia gravis, may occur [170]. Paraneoplastic subacute cerebellar degeneration (SCD) is one of the most common lesions, with ovarian cancer accounting for from 16% to 47% of the cases [123]. The cerebellar manifestations usually antedate recognition of the cancer, and typically there is no improvement after the removal of the tumor. In one case, manifestations of the cerebellar degeneration partially regressed after plasmapheresis [32]. The pathogenesis of SCD in these cases appears to be related to the presence of circulating anti-Purkinje cell antibodies that have been shown to react with antigens in the tumor. The presence of such antibodies appears to be much more common in patients with SCD and gynecologic or breast cancer than in patients with SCD and other types of carcinoma. Inflammatory limbic encephalitis has been associated with dermoid cysts [138] and in these cases, N-Methyl-D asparate receptor antibodies have been found in the blood and cerebrospinal fluid.

Connective Tissue Disorders

The connective tissue disorder most commonly associated with ovarian cancer is dermatomyositis. In one study of ten patients with dermatomyositis or polymyositis and a malignant tumor of the female genital tract, five had ovarian cancer [173]. The tumors are most commonly high-grade, high-stage serous carcinomas [102], but there is one case of dysgerminoma and one of leiomyoma associated with dermatomyositis. The onset of the dermatomyositis generally precedes recognition of the tumor, which usually becomes evident within 2 years. Medsger and his associates [97] described six patients with ovarian carcinoma in whom polyarthritis and palmar fasciitis preceded the diagnosis of carcinoma by 5–25 months. The arthritic symptoms were similar to those of rheumatoid arthritis. Four of the ovarian tumors were endometrioid carcinomas, one a serous carcinoma, and one an undifferentiated carcinoma. Occasional patients have had hypertrophic pulmonary osteoarthropathy, rheumatoid arthritis, scleroderma, systemic lupus erythematosus, or the shoulder–hand syndrome.

Cutaneous Disorders

Acanthosis nigricans occurs in some, typically young, women in association with polycystic ovary disease (POD), stromal hyperthecosis, or combinations thereof [43], representing a component of the so-called HAIR-AN syndrome (hyperandrogenemia, insulin resistance, and acanthosis nigricans). Four cases of so-called malignant acanthosis nigricans have been cases of ovarian carcinoma. The sign of Leser–Trelat, the sudden onset and rapid increase in size of numerous seborrheic keratoses in association with an occult cancer, considered by some a variant of "malignant" acanthosis nigricans, has been associated with ovarian cancer in one case [64]. Rarely, ovarian carcinomas have occurred in patients with the Torre–Muir syndrome [33] or Sweet's syndrome [107]. Cutaneous melanosis has occurred with a strumal carcinoid [8]; the tumor cells were immunoreactive for alpha-melanocyte-stimulating hormone. Other uncommon associations of ovarian neoplasms and skin lesions are sporadically reported [48].

Nephrotic Syndrome

In cases of the nephrotic syndrome, 5–10% have a paraneoplastic background, although the causative tumors in such cases are located only rarely in the female genital tract. Hoyt and Hamilton [65] described a 65-year-old woman who was found to have the nephrotic syndrome 8 months before the detection of a stage IV poorly differentiated serous carcinoma of the ovary. A renal biopsy showed membranous glomerulopathy. The proteinuria markedly diminished after debulking of the tumor, and after 10 months of combination chemotherapy, the proteinuria had disappeared and there was no evidence of tumor at a second-look laparotomy.

Hematologic Disorders

Approximately 30 ovarian tumors have been reported to be associated with autoimmune hemolytic anemia, which is usually Coombs positive. Most of these tumors have been dermoid cysts [122], but occasional examples of carcinoma and a single case of granulosa cell tumor also have been reported [122]. In the latter case, the patient also had splenic angiomas. In many cases, corticosteroid therapy, splenectomy, or both have resulted in little or no improvement, but removal of the ovarian tumor has produced a rapid remission of the hemolytic disorder. Payne and coworkers [122] have listed several mechanisms proposed to explain the relation of the dermoid cyst to the anemia: (1) liberation by the tumor of a substance that alters the surface of red cells, making them antigenic to the host, (2) stimulation of production of an antibody that cross-reacts with the red cells by an antigen in the wall or lumen of the cyst, and (3) direct production of a red cell antibody by the tumor. Support for the last theory is provided by the finding of immunoglobulin in the cyst fluid in several cases.

Ovarian tumors are commonly associated with laboratory evidence of disseminated intravascular coagulation (DIC), but clinical manifestations of this disorder are uncommon. Ovarian tumors also have been associated with migratory thrombophlebitis (Trousseau's syndrome). Nonbacterial thrombotic endocarditis also has been recorded as a complication of ovarian cancer, as has microangiopathic hemolytic anemia. Excluding cases of mild erythrocytosis that may accompany androgenic ovarian tumors, paraneoplastic erythrocytosis, is associated only rarely with ovarian tumors [122]. Examples of erythropoetin-secreting ovarian tumors have included a dermoid cyst and a steroid cell tumor [122]. Other hematologic abnormalities that have been described rarely in association with ovarian tumors include nonthrombocytopenic purpura (mucinous cystadenoma), granulocytosis (clear cell carcinoma), thrombocytosis (serous carcinoma), thrombocytopenia (hemangioma and adenofibroma) [174], and pancytopenia (granulosa cell tumor).

Miscellaneous Rare Conditions

One ovarian example of inappropriate antidiuresis syndrome has been reported in association with a serous carcinoma that had a component of small cell carcinoma of pulmonary type [163]. Electron microscopic examination of the tumor disclosed neuroendocrine granules, and the neoplastic cells were also immunoreactive for antidiuretic hormone.

A small number of patients with ovarian tumors, usually with high-stage serous carcinomas but rarely with low-stage endometrioid carcinomas, have had hyperamylasemia [117]. Monitoring the serum amylase level may be a marker of tumor progression and response to therapy in such cases. Rarely, patients with ovarian cancer have had a clinical presentation that has mimicked that of acute pancreatitis [112]. In one unusual case, a patient with pseudo Meigs' syndrome had a pleural infusion rich in amylase that disappeared after removal of a serous tumor or borderline malignancy, which had ruptured preoperatively [37]. Six patients with poorly differentiated surface epithelial carcinomas [27] have had uveal melanocytic lesions as may be seen with other visceral cancers. Microscopic examination of the eyes of these patients who undergo progressive blurring and loss of vision shows bilateral diffuse proliferation of melanocytes throughout the uvueal tracts with the involvement of the sclerae in some instances [83]. Rarely, pyrexia is a presenting manifestation of a patient with ovarian carcinoma [140]. One of the two cases in this category was classified as a clear cell carcinoma, and the other was not subclassified.

Acknowledgment

When the late Dr. Ancel Blaustein prepared the first edition of this book in the mid-1970s, he asked Dr. Robert E. Scully to contribute the chapter on ovarian sex cord-stromal tumors and it duly appeared in 1977. In the 1980s, I had the pleasure and privilege of reviewing numerous sex cord-stromal tumors of the ovary in Dr. Scully's remarkable collection and a number of original publications with Dr. Scully and others came to pass. This resulted in Dr. Scully asking me if I would co-author the contribution on this topic for the third edition, expanded by the inclusion of consideration of steroid cell tumors and a variety of miscellaneous other neoplasms associated with various interesting clinical manifestations. This chapter appeared in the 1987 third edition. Dr. Scully, being retired, declined to participate in this most recent reedition of the chapter and although many of the words were initially written, or edited by him, given his customary awareness of the importance of ethics in medicine, he declined to have his name associated with a work which he did not actively participate in at this time. However, I would like to acknowledge my debt to Dr. Scully for the initial chapter, which laid the groundwork for everything to follow, the opportunity to learn from his cases, and most important of all, to be educated by him on the remarkable and fascinating microscopic spectrum encountered within the family of tumors reviewed in this chapter. Similar remarks pertain to ➲ Chap. 18, Metastatics Tumors of the Ovary.

References

1. Aguirre P, Scully RE, Delellis RA (1986) Ovarian heterologous Sertoli–Leydig cell tumors with gastrointestinal-type epithelium. An immunohistochemical analysis. Arch Pathol Lab Med 110: 528–533
2. Aguirre P, Thor AD, Scully RE (1989) Ovarian endometrioid carcinomas resembling sex cord-stromal tumors: an immunohistological study. Int J Gynecol Pathol 8:364–373
3. Aguirre P, Thor AD, Scully RE (1989) Ovarian small cell carcinoma: histogenetic considerations based on immunohistochemical and other findings. Am J Clin Pathol 92:140–149
4. Ahmed E, Young RH, Scully RE (1999) Adult granulosa cell tumor of the ovary with foci of hepatic cell differentiation. A report of four cases and comparison with two cases of granulosa cell tumor with Leydig cells. Am J Surg Pathol 23:1089–1093
5. Anderson MC, Rees DA (1975) Gynandroblastoma of the ovary. Br J Obstet Gynaecol 82:68–73
6. Anderson PW, Macaulay L, Do YS et al (1989) Extrarenal renin-secreting tumors: Insights into hypertension and ovarian renin production. Medicine (Baltim) 68:257–268
7. Armstrong DT, Papkoff H (1976) Stimulation of aromatization by endogenous and exogenous androgens in ovaries of hypophysectomized rats in vivo by FSH. Endocrinology 99:1144–1151
8. Ashton MA (1995) Strumal carcinoid of the ovary associated with hyperinsulinemic hypoglycemia and cutaneous melanosis. Histopathology (Oxf) 27:463–467
9. Auranen A, Sundstrom JI, Ijas J, Grenman S (2007) Prognostic factors of ovarian granulosa cell tumor: a study of 35 patients and review of the literature. Int J Gynecol Cancer 17:1011–1018
10. Axiotis CA, Lippes HA, Merino MJ, deLanerolle NC, Stewart AF, Kinder B (1987) Corticotroph cell pituitary adenoma within an ovarian teratoma. A new cause of Cushing's syndrome. Am J Surg Pathol 11:218–224
11. Baker PM, Oliva E (2004) Immunohistochemistry as a tool in the differential diagnosis of ovarian tumors: an update. Int J Gynecol Pathol 24:39–55
12. Banner EA, Dockerty MB (1945) Theca cell tumors of the ovary. A clinical and pathological study of twenty-three cases (including thirteen new cases) with a review. Surg Gynecol Obstet 81:234–242
13. Benfield GFA, Tapper-Jones L, Stout TV (1982) Androblastoma and raised serum alpha-fetoprotein with familial multinodular goitre. Case report. Br J Obstet Gynaecol 89:323–326
14. Bjorkholm E (1980) Granulosa cell tumors: a comparison of survival in patients and matched controls. Am J Obstet Gynecol 138:329–331
15. Bjorkholm E, Pettersson F (1980) Granulosa-cell and theca-cell tumors. The clinical picture and long term outcome for the Radiumhemmet series. Acta Obstet Gynecol Scand 59:361–365
16. Bjorkholm E, Silfversward C (1981) Prognostic factors in granulosa cell tumors. Gynecol Oncol 11:261–274

17. Bjorkholm E, Silfversward C (1980) Theca-cell tumors. Clinical features and prognosis. Acta Radiol Oncol Radiat Phys Biol 19:241–244
18. Bohm J, Roder-Weber M, Hofler H (1991) Bilateral stromal Leydig cell tumor of the ovary. Case report and literature review. Path Res Pract 187:348–352
19. Boixeda D, Roman AL, Pascasio JM et al (1990) Zollinger-Ellison syndrome due to gastrin-secreting ovarian cystadenocarcinoma. Case report. Acta Chir Scand 156:409–410
20. Brown H, Lane M (1965) Cushing's and malignant carcinoid syndromes from ovarian neoplasm. Arch Intern Med 115:490–494
21. Brown WW, Shetty KR, Rosenfeld PS (1973) Hyperthyroidism due to struma ovarii: demonstration by radioiodine scan. Acta Endocrinol 73:266–272
22. Burton PBJ, Knight DE, Quirke P et al (1990) Parathyroid hormone related peptide in ovarian carcinoma. J Clin Pathol 43:784
23. Callen JP (1986) Dermatomyositis and female malignancy. J Surg Oncol 32:121–124
24. Cao QJ, Jones JG, Li M (2001) Expression of calretinin in human ovary, testis and ovarian sex cord-stromal tumors. Int J Gynecol Pathol 20:346–352
25. Caron P, Roche H, Gorguet B, Martel P, Bennet A, Carton M (1990) Mammary ovarian metastases with stroma cell hyperplasia and postmenopausal virilization. Cancer (Phila) 66:1221–1224
26. Cathro HP, Stoler MH (2005) The utility of calretinin, inhibin and WT1 immunohistochemistry staining in the differential diagnosis of ovarian tumors. Hum Pathol 36:195–201
27. Chahud F, Young RH, Remulla JF et al (2001) Bilateral diffuse uveal melanocytic proliferation associated with extraocular cancers. Am J Surg Pathol 25:212–218
28. Chalvardjian A, Scully RE (1973) Sclerosing stromal tumors of the ovary. Cancer (Phila) 31:664–670
29. Christman JE, Ballon SC (1990) Ovarian fibrosarcoma associated with Maffucci's syndrome. Gynecol Oncol 37:290–291
30. Civantos F, Rywlin AM (1972) Carcinomas with trophoblastic differentiation and secretion of chroionic gonadotrophins. Cancer (Phila) 29:789–798
31. Clement PB, Young RH, Hanna W, Scully RE (1994) Sclerosing peritonitis associated with luteinized thecomas of the ovary. A clinicopathological analysis of six cases. Am J Surg Pathol 18:1–13
32. Cocconi G, Ceci G, Juvarra G et al (1985) Successful treatment of subacute cerebellar degeneration in ovarian carcinoma with plasmapheresis. A case report. Cancer (Phila) 56:2318–2320
33. Cohen PR, Kohn SR, Kurzrock R (1991) Association of sebaceous gland tumors and internal malignancy: the Muir-Torre syndrome. Am J Med 90:606–613
34. Costa MJ, Ames PF, Walls J, Roth LM (1997) Inhibin immunohistochemistry applied to ovarian neoplasms: a novel, effective, diagnostic tool. Hum Pathol 281:247–254
35. Costa MJ, Morris R, DeRose PB, Cohen C (1993) Histologic and immunohistochemical evidence for considering ovarian myxoma as a variant of the thecoma-fibroma group of ovarian stromal tumors. Arch Pathol Lab Med 117:802–808
36. Costa MJ, Morris RJ, Wilson R, Judd R (1992) Utility of immunohistochemistry in distinguishing ovarian Sertoli-stromal cell tumors from carcinosarcomas. Hum Pathol 23:787–797
37. Cramer SF, Bruns DE (1979) Amylase-producing ovarian neoplasm with pseudo-Meigs' syndrome and elevated pleural amylase. Cancer (Phila) 44:1715–1721
38. Crawford SM, Pyrah RD, Ismail SM (1994) Cushing's syndrome associated with recurrent endometrioid adenocarcinoma of the ovary. J Clin Pathol 47:766–768
39. Deavers MT, Malpica A, Liu J, Broaddus R, Silva E (2003) Ovarian sex cord-stromal tumors: An immunohistochenical study including a comparison of calretinin and inhibin. Mod Pathol 16:584–590
40. Dickersin GR, Young RH, Scully RE (1995) Signet-ring stromal and related tumors of the ovary. Ultrastruct Pathol 19:401–419
41. Dockerty MB, Masson JC (1944) Ovarian fibromas: a clinical and pathologic study of two hundred and eighty-three cases. Am J Obstet Gynecol 47:741–752
42. Dorrington JH, Moon YS, Armstrong DT (1975) Estradiol-17b biosynthesis in cultured granulosa cells from hypophysectomized immature rats: stimulation by FSH. Endocrinology 97:1328–1331
43. Dunaif A, Hoffman AR, Scully RE et al (1985) Clinical, biochemical, and ovarian morphologic features in women with acanthosis nigricans and masculinization. Obstet Gynecol 66:545–552
44. Eichhorn JH, Bell DA, Young RH et al (1992) DNA content and proliferative activity in ovarian small cell carcinomas of the hypercalcemic type. Implications for diagnosis, prognosis and histogenesis. Am J Clin Pathol 98:579–586
45. Emerson RE, Wang M, Roth L, Zheng W, Abdul-Karim FW, Liu F, Ulbright TM, Eble JN, Cheng L (2007) Int J Gynecol Pathol 26:368–374
46. Fathalla MF (1967) The occurrence of granulosa and theca tumors in clinically normal ovaries. A study of 25 cases. J Obstet Gynaecol Br Commonw 74:279–282
47. Fathalla MF (1968) The role of the ovarian stroma in hormone production by ovarian tumors. J Obstet Gynaecol Br Commonw 75:78–83
48. Fathizadeh A, Medenica MM, Soltani K et al (1982) Aggressive keratoacanthoma and internal malignant neoplasm. Arch Dermatol 118:112–114
49. Ferry JA, Young RH, Engel G, Scully RE (1994) Oxyphilic Sertoli cell tumor of the ovary: a report of three cases, two in patients with the Peutz-Jeghers syndrome. Int J Gynecol Pathol 13:259–266
50. Flemming P, Wellmann A, Maschek HJ et al (1995) Monoclonal antibodies against inhibin represents key markers of adult granulosa cell tumors of the ovary even in their metastases. Am J Surg Pathol 19:927–933
51. Fox H, Agrawal K, Langley FA (1975) A clinicopathological study of 92 cases of granulosa cell tumor of the ovary with special reference to the factors influencing prognosis. Cancer (Phila) 35:231–241
52. Fujino T, Watanabe T, Yamaguchi K et al (1992) The development of hypercalcemia in a patient with an ovarian tumor producing parathyroid hormone-related protein. Cancer (Phila) 70:2845–2850
53. Gagnon S, Tetu B, Silva EG, McCaughey WTE (1989) Frequency of a-fetoprotein production by Sertoli-Leydig cell tumors of the ovary: an immunohistochemical study of eight cases. Mod Pathol 2:63–67
54. Garcia-Villaneuva M, Figuerola NB, del Arbol LR, Ortiz MJH (1990) Zollinger–Ellison syndrome due to a borderline mucinous cystadenoma of the ovary. Obstet Gynecol 75:549–551
55. Geist SH, Gaines JA (1938) Theca cell tumors. Am J Obstet Gynecol 35:39–51
56. Gorlin RJ (1987) Nevoid basal-cell carcinoma syndrome. Medicine (Baltim) 66:98–113
57. Guerrieri C, Frånlund B, Malmström H, Boeryd B (1998) Ovarian endometrioid carcinomas simulating sex cord-stromal tumors: a study using inhibin and cytokeratin 7. Int J Gynecol Pathol 17:266–271
58. Gustafson ML, Lee MM, Scully RE et al (1992) Müllerian inhibiting substance as a marker for ovarian sex-cord tumor. N Engl J Med 326:466–471

59. Hart WR, Kumar N, Crissman JD (1980) Ovarian neoplasms resembling sex cord tumors with annular tubules. Cancer (Phila) 45:2352–2363
60. Hayes MC, Scully RE (1987) Ovarian steroid cell tumor (not otherwise specified): a clinicopathological analysis of 63 cases. Am J Surg Pathol 11:835–845
61. Hayes MC, Scully RE (1987) Stromal luteoma of the ovary: a clinicopathological analysis of 25 cases. Int J Gynecol Pathol 6:313–321
62. Hoekman K, Tjandra Y, Papapoulos SE (1991) The role of 1, 25–dihydroxyvitamin D in the maintenance of hypercalcemia in a patient with an ovarian carcinoma producing parathyroid hormone-related protein. Cancer (Phila) 68:642–647
63. Hoffman WH, Gala RR, Kovacs K, Subramanian MG (1987) Ectopic prolactin secretion from a gonadoblastoma. Cancer (Phila) 60: 2690–2695
64. Holguin T, Padilla RS, Ampuero F (1986) Ovarian adenocarcinoma presenting with the sign of Leser–Trelat. Gynecol Oncol 25:128–132
65. Hoyt RE, Hamilton JF (1987) Ovarian cancer associated with the nephrotic syndrome. Obstet Gynecol 70:513–514
66. Hughesdon PE (1958) Thecal and allied reactions in epithelial ovarian tumours. J Obstet Gynaecol Br Commonw 65:702–709
67. Hughesdon PE (1983) Lipid cell thecomas of the ovary. Histopathology (Oxf) 7:681–692
68. Irving JA, Alkushi A, Young RH, Clement PB (2006) Cellular Fibromas of the ovary: a study of 75 cases including 40 mitotically active tumors emphasizing their distinction from fibrosarcoma. Am J Surg Pathol 30:928–938
69. Irving JA, Young RH (2008) Granulosa cell tumors of the ovary with a pseudopapillary pattern: a study of 14 cases of an unusual morphologic variant emphasizing their distinction from transitional cell neoplasms and other papillary ovary tumors. Am J Surg Pathol 32:581–586
70. Irving JA, Young RH (2008) Microcystic stromal tumor of the ovary. Report of 16 cases of a hitherto uncharacterized distinctive ovarian neoplasm. Am J Surg Pathol 33:367–375
71. Ismail SM, Walker SM (1990) Bilateral virilizing sclerosing stromal tumours of the ovary in a pregnant woman with Gorlin's syndrome: implications for pathogenesis of ovarian stromal neoplasms. Histopathology (Oxf) 17:159–163
72. Jackson B, Valentine R, Wagner G (1986) Primary aldosteronism due to a malignant ovarian tumour. Aust NZ J Med 16:69–71
73. Kallenberg GA, Pesce CM, Norman B, Ratner RE, Silverberg SG (1990) Ectopic hyperprolactinemia resulting from an ovarian teratoma. JAMA 263:2472–2474
74. Kommoss F, Oliva E, Bhan AK, Young RH, Scully RE (1998) Inhibin expression in ovarian tumors and tumor-like lesions: an immunohistochemical study. Mod Pathol 11:656–664
75. Konishi I, Fujii S, Ishikawa Y, Suzuki A, Okamura H, Mori T (1986) Ovarian fibroma with Leydig cell hyperplasia of the adjacent stroma: a light and electron microscopic study. Int J Gynecol Pathol 5:170–178
76. Korzets A, Nouriel H, Steiner Z et al (1986) Resistant hypertension associated with a renin-producing ovarian Sertoli cell tumor. Am J Clin Pathol 85:242–247
77. Kraemer BB, Silva EG, Sneige N (1984) Fibrosarcoma of the ovary. A new component in the nevoid basal-cell carcinoma syndrome. Am J Surg Pathol 8:231–236
78. Kulkarni JN, Mistry RC, Kamat MR, Chinoy R, Lotlikar RG (1990) Autonomous aldosterone-secreting ovarian tumor. Gynecol Oncol 37:284–289
79. Kurman RJ, Andrade D, Goebelsmann U, Taylor CR (1978) An immunohistochemical study of steroid localization in Sertoli–Leydig tumors of the ovary and testis. Cancer (Phila) 42:1772–1783
80. Kurman RJ, Ganjei P, Nadjii M (1984) Contributions of immunocytochemistry to the diagnosis and study of ovarian neoplasms. Int J Gynecol Pathol 3:3–26
81. Kurman RJ, Goebelsmann U, Taylor CR (1979) Steroid localization in granulosa–theca tumors of the ovary. Cancer (Phila) 43:2377–2384
82. Lack EE, Perez-Atayde AR, Murthy ASK, Goldstein DP, Crigler JF, Vawter GF (1981) Granulosa theca cell tumors in premenarchal girls. A clinical and pathologic study of ten cases. Cancer (Phila) 48:1846–1854
83. Margo CE, Pavan PR, Gendelman D, Gragoudas E (1987) Bilateral melanocytic uveal tumors associated with systemic non-ocular malignancy. Malignant melanomas or benign paraneoplastic syndrome? Retina 7:137–141
84. Mason WP, Dalman J, Curtin MP, Posner JB (1997) Normalization of the tumor marker CA-125 after oophorectomy in a patient with paraneoplastic cerebellar degeneration without detectable cancer. Gynecol Oncol 65:1558–1563
85. Matias-Guiu X, Pons C, Prat J (1998) Müllerian inhibiting substance, alpha-inhibin, and CD99 expression in sex cord stromal tumors and endometrioid ovarian carcinomas resembling sex cord-stromal tumors. Hum Pathol 29:840–845
86. Matias-Guiu X, Prat J (1990) Ovarian tumors with functioning stroma. An immunohistochemical study of 100 cases with human chorionic gonadotropin monoclonal and polyclonal antibodies. Cancer (Phila) 65:2001–2005
87. McCluggage WG (2008) Immunohistochemical markers as a diagnostic aid in ovarian pathology. Diagn Histopathol 14:335–351
88. McCluggage WG, Maxwell P (1999) Adenocarcinomas of various sites may exhibit immunoreactivity with anti-inhibin antibodies. Histopathology 35:216–220
89. McCluggage WG, Maxwell P (2001) Immunohistochemical staining for calretinin is useful in the diagnosis of ovarian sex cord-stromal tumours. Int J Gynecol Pathol 20:346–352
90. McCluggage WG, Maxwell P, Sloan JM (1997) Immunohistochemical staining of ovarian granulosa cell tumors with monoclonal antibodies against inhibin. Hum Pathol 28:1034–1038
91. McCluggage WG, McKenna M, McBride HA (2007) CD56 is a sensitive and diagnostically useful immunohistochemical marker of ovarian sex cord-stromal tumors. Int J Gynecol Pathol 26: 322–327
92. McCluggage WG, Oliva E, Connolly LE, Young RH (2004) An immunohistochemical analysis of ovarian small cell carcinoma of hypercalcemic type. Int J Gynecol Pathol 23:330–336
93. McCluggage WG, Young RH (2005) Immunohistochemistry as a diagnostic aid in the evaluation of ovarian tumors Semin Diagin Pathol 22:3–32
94. McCluggage WG, Young RH (2007) Ovarian Sertoli-Leydig cell tumors with pseudoendometrioid tubules (pseudoendometrioid Sertoli-Leydig cell tumors). Am J Surg Pathol 31:592–596
95. McKenna M, Kenny B, Dorman G, McCluggage WG (2005) Combined adult granulosa cell tumor and mucinous cystadenoma of the ovary: Granulosa cell tumor with heterologous mucinous elements. Int J Gynecol Pathol 24:224–227
96. McMahon JT, Hart WR (1988) Ultrastructural analysis of small cell carcinomas of the ovary. Am J Clin Pathol 90:523–529
97. Medsger TA, Dixon JA, Garwood VF (1982) Palmar fasciitis and polyarthritis associated with ovarian carcinoma. Ann Intern Med 96:424–431
98. Meigs JV (1954) Fibroma of the ovary with ascites and hydrothorax. Meigs' syndrome. Am J Obstet Gynecol 67:962–987

99. Mooney EE, Nogales FF, Bergeron C, Tavassoli FA (2002) Retiform Sertoli-Leydig cell tumours: clinical, morphological and immunohistochemical findings. Histopathology 41:110–117
100. Mooney EE, Nogales FF, Tavassoli FA (1999) Hepatocytic differentiation in retiform Sertoli-Leydig cell tumors: distinguishing a heterologous element from Leydig cells. Hum Pathol 30:611–617
101. Mooney EE, Vaidya KP, Tavassoli FA (2000) Ossifying well-differentiated Sertoli-Leydig cell tumor of the ovary. Ann Diagn Pathol 4:34–38
102. Mordel N, Margalioth EJ, Harats N et al (1988) Concurrence of ovarian cancer and dermatomyositis. A report of two cases and literature review. J Reprod Med 33:649–655
103. Morgello S, Schwartz E, Horwith M et al (1988) Ectopic insulin production by a primary ovarian carcinoid. Cancer (Phila) 61: 800–805
104. Movahedi-Lankarani S, Kurman RJ (2002) Calretinin, a more sensitive but less specific marker than α-inhibin for ovarian sex cord-stromal neoplasms. An immunohistochemical study of 215 cases. Am J Surg Pathol 26:1477–1483
105. Nakashima N, Young RH, Scully RE (1984) Androgenic granulosa cell tumors of the ovary. A clinicopathological analysis of seventeen cases and review of the literature. Arch Pathol Lab Med 108:786–791
106. Napoli VM, Wallach H (1976) Pancytopenia associated with a granulosa-cell tumor of the ovary. Report of a case. Am J Clin Pathol 65:344–350
107. Nguyen KQ, Hurst CG, Pierson DL et al (1983) Sweet's syndrome and ovarian carcinoma. Cutis 32:152–154
108. Nichols J, Warren JC, Mantz FA (1962) ACTH-like excretion from carcinoma of the ovary. JAMA 182:713–718
109. Nogales FF, Concha A, Plata C, Ruiz-Avila I (1993) Granulosa cell tumor of the ovary with diffuse true hepatic differentiation simulating stromal luteinization. Am J Surg Pathol 17:85–90
110. Norris HJ, Taylor HB (1968) Prognosis of granulosa-theca tumors of the ovary. Cancer (Phila) 21:255–263
111. Norris HJ, Taylor HB (1969) Virilization associated with cystic granulosa tumors. Obstet Gynecol 34:629–635
112. Norwood SH, Torma MJ, Fontanelle LJ (1981) Hyperamylasemia due to poorly differentiated adenosquamous carcinoma of the ovary. Arch Surg 116:225–226
113. Nussbaum SR, Gas R, Arnold A (1990) Hypercalcemia and ectopic secretion of parathyroid hormone by an ovarian carcinoma with rearrangement of the gene for parathyroid hormone. N Engl J Med 323:1324–1328
114. Oliva EA, Alvarez T, Young RH (2005) Sertoli cell tumors of the ovary. A clinicopathological and immunohistochemical study of 54 cases. Am J Surg Pathol 29:143–156
115. Oliva E, Andrada E, Pezzica E, Prat J (1993) Ovarian carcinomas with choriocarcinomatous differentiation. Cancer (Phila) 72:2441–2446
116. Oliva E, Garcia-Miralles N, Vu Q, Young RH (2007) CD10 expression in pure stromal and sex cord-stromal tumors of the ovary: an immunohistochemical analysis of 101 cases. Int J Gynecol Pathol 26:359–367
117. O'Riordan T, Gaffney E, Tormey V, Daly P (1990) Hyperamylasemia associated with progression of a serous surface papillary carcinoma. Gynecol Oncol 36:432–434
118. Palmer PE, Bogojavlensky S, Bhan AK, Scully RE (1990) Prolactinoma in wall of ovarian dermoid cyst with hyperprolactinemia. Obstet Gynecol 75:540–543
119. Paoletti M, Pridjian G, Okagaki T, Talerman A (1987) A stromal Leydig cell tumor of the ovary occurring in a pregnant 15-year-old girl. Ultrastructural findings. Cancer (Phila) 60:2806–2810
120. Paraskevas M, Scully RE (1989) Hilus cell tumor of the ovary. A clinicopathological analysis of 12 Reinke crystal-positive and 9 crystal-negative cases. Int J Gynecol Pathol 8:299–310
121. Parsons V, Rigby R (1958) Cushing's syndrome associated with adenocarcinoma of the ovary. Lancet 2:992–994
122. Payne D, Muss HB, Homesley HD, Jobson VW, Baird FG (1981) Autoimmune hemolytic anemia and ovarian dermoid cysts: case report and review of the literature. Cancer (Phila) 48:721–724
123. Peterson K, Rosenblum MK, Kotanides H, Posner MP (1992) Paraneoplastic cerebellar degeneration. I. A clinical analysis of 55 anti-Yo antibody-positive patients. Neurology 42:1931–1937
124. Pelkey TJ, Frierson HF, Mills SE, Stoler MH (1998) The diagnostic utility of inhibin staining in ovarian neoplasms. Int J Gynecol Pathol 17:97–105
125. Phadke DM, Weisenberg E, Engel G, Rhone DP (1999) Malignant Sertoli cell tumor of the ovary metastatic of the lung mimicking neuroendocrine carcinoma: report of a case. Ann Diagn Pathol 3:213–219
126. Prat J, Scully RE (1981) Cellular fibromas and fibrosarcomas of the ovary: a comparative clinicopathologic analysis of seventeen cases. Cancer (Phila) 47:2663–2670
127. Prat J, Young RH, Scully RE (1982) Ovarian Sertoli-Leydig cell tumors with heterologous elements. (ii) cartilage and skeletal muscle: a clinicopathologic analysis of twelve cases. Cancer (Phila) 50:2465–2475
128. Price A, Russell P, Elliott P, Bannatyne P (1990) Composite mucinous and granulosa-cell tumor of ovary: case report of a unique neoplasm. Int J Gynecol Pathol 9:372–378
129. Ramzy I (1976) Signet-ring stromal tumor of ovary. Histochemical, light, and electron microscopic study. Cancer (Phila) 38:166–172
130. Reddick RL, Walton LA (1982) Sertoli-Leydig cell tumor of the ovary with teratomatous differentiation. Cancer (Phila) 50:1171–1176
131. Riopel MA, Perlman EJ, Seidman JD et al (1998) Inhibin and epithelial membrane antigen immunohistochemistry assist in the diagnosis of sex cord-stromal tumors and provide clues to the histogenesis of hypercalcemic small cell carcinomas. Int J Gynecol Pathol 17:46–53
132. Rishi M, Howard LN, Bratthauer GL, Tavassoli FA (1997) Use of monoclonal antibodies against human inhibin as a marker for sex cord-stromal tumors of the ovary. Am J Surg Pathol 19:927–933
133. Roth LM, Anderson MC, Govan ADT, Langley FA, Gowing NFC, Woodcock AS (1981) Sertoli-Leydig cell tumors. A clinicopathologic study of 34 cases. Cancer (Phila) 48:187
134. Roth LM, Slayton RE, Brady LW, Blesdsing JA, Johnson G (1985) Retiform differentiation in ovarian Sertoli–Leydig cell tumors. A clinicopathologic study of six cases from a gynecologic oncology study group. Cancer (Phila) 55:1093–1098
135. Roth LM, Sternberg WH (1973) Ovarian stromal tumors containing Leydig cells. II. Pure Leydig cell tumor, non-hilar type. Cancer (Phila) 32:952–960
136. Roth LM, Sternberg WH (1983) Partly luteinized theca cell tumor of the ovary. Cancer (Phila) 51:1697–1704
137. Rutgers J, Scully RE (1986) Functioning ovarian tumors with peripheral steroid cell proliferation: a report of twenty-four cases. Int J Gynecol Pathol 5:319–337
138. Sabin TD, Jednacz JA, Staats PN (2008) Case 26-2008: a 26-year-old woman with headache and behavioral changes. N Engl J Med 359:842–853

139. Samanth KK, Black WC (1970) Benign ovarian stromal tumors associated with free peritoneal fluid. Am J Obstet Gynecol 107:538–545
140. Schofield PM, Kirsop BA, Reginald P, Harington M (1985) Ovarian carcinoma presenting as pyrexia of unknown origin. Postgrad Med J61:177–178
141. Scully RE (1953) An unusual ovarian tumor containing Leydig cells but associated with endometrial hyperplasia, in a postmenopausal woman. J Clin Endocrinol Metab 13:1254–1263
142. Scully RE (1985) Immunohistochemistry of ovarian tumors. In: Russo J, Russo I (eds) Immunocytochemistry in tumor diagnosis. Martinus Nijhoff, Boston, MA, pp 293–320
143. Scully RE (1970) Sex cord tumor with annular tubules. A distinctive ovarian tumor of the Peutz–Jeghers syndrome. Cancer (Phila) 25:1107–1121
144. Scully RE, Young RE, Clement PB (1998) Tumors of the ovary, maldeveloped gonads, fallopian tube, and broad ligament. In: Atlas of tumor pathology, 3rd series, fasc 23. Armed Forces Institute of Pathology, Washington, DC
145. Scully RE, Aguirre P, DeLellis RA (1984) Argyrophilia, serotonin, and peptide hormones in the female genital tract and its tumors. Int J Gynecol Pathol 3:51–70
146. Scully RE, Cohen RB (1964) Oxidative-enzyme activity in normal and pathologic human ovaries. Obstet Gynecol 24:667–681
147. Scully RE, Richardson GS (1961) Luteinization of the stroma of metastatic cancer involving the ovary and its endocrine significance. Cancer (Phila) 14:827–840
148. Seidman JD (1996) Unclassified ovarian gonadal stromal tumors. A clinicopathologic study of 32 cases. Am J Surg Pathol 20:699–706
149. Sens MA, Levenson TB, Metcalf JS (1982) A case of metastatic carcinoid arising in an ovarian teratoma. Case report with autopsy findings and review of the literature. Cancer (Phila) 49:2541–2546
150. Shah SP, Kobel M, Senz J, Morin RD, Clarke BA et al (2009) Mutation of FOXL2 in granulosa-cell tumors of the ovary. N Eng J Med 360:2719–2729
151. Simpson JL, Michael H, Roth LM (1998) Unclassified sex cord-stromal tumors of the ovary. A report of eight cases. Arch Pathol Lab Med 122:52–55
152. Sjostedt S, Wahlen T (1961) Prognosis of granulosa cell tumors. Acta Obstet Gynecol Scand 40:1–26
153. Solh HM, Azoury RS, Najjar SS (1983) Peutz–Jeghers syndrome associated with precocious puberty. J Pediatr 103:593–595
154. Staats PN, McCluggage WG, Clement PB, Young RH (2008) Luteinized thecomas (thecomatosis) of the type typically associated with sclerosing peritonitis. Am J Surg Pathol 32:1273–1290
155. Stenwig JT, Hazekamp JT, Beecham JB (1979) Granulosa cell tumors of the ovary. A clinicopathological study of 118 cases with long-term follow-up. Gynecol Oncol 7:136–152
156. Sternberg WH (1949) The morphology, endocrine function, hyperplasia and tumors of the human ovarian hilus cells. Am J Pathol 25:493–511
157. Sternberg WH, Roth LM (1973) Ovarian stromal tumors containing Leydig cells. 1. Stromal-Leydig cell tumor and non-neoplastic transformation of ovarian stroma to Leydig cells. Cancer (Phila) 32:940–951
158. Stewart CJR, Jeffers MD, Kennedy A (1997) Diagnostic value of inhibin immunoreactivity in ovarian gonadal stromal tumours and their histological mimics. Histopathology (Oxf) 31:67–74
159. Stewart CJR, Nandini CL, Richmond JA (2000) Value of A103 (melan-A) immunostaining in the differential diagnosis of ovarian sex cord stromal tumours. J Clin Pathol 53:206–211
160. Susil BJ, Sumithran E (1987) Sarcomatous change in granulosa cell tumor. Hum Pathol 18:397–399
161. Talerman A (1987) Ovarian Sertoli-Leydig cell tumor (androblastoma) with retiform pattern: a clinicopathologic study. Cancer (Phila) 60: 3056–3064
162. Talerman A, Hughesdon PE, Anderson MC (1982) Diffuse nonlobular ovarian androblastoma usually associated with feminization. Int J Gynecol Pathol 1:155–171
163. Taskin M, Barker B, Calanog A, Jormark S (1996) Syndrome of inappropriate antidiuresis in ovarian serous carcinoma with neuroendocrine differentiation. Gynecol Oncol 62:400–404
164. Tavassoli FA, Norris HJ (1980) Sertoli tumors of the ovary. A clinicopathologic study of 28 cases with ultrastructural observations. Cancer (Phila) 46:2282–2297
165. Taylor HB, Norris HJ (1967) Lipid cell tumors of the ovary. Cancer (Phila) 20:1953–1962
166. Teilum G (1958) Classification of testicular and ovarian androblastoma and Sertoli cell tumors. Cancer (Phila) 11:769–782
167. Todesco S, Terribile V, Borsatti A et al (1975) Primary aldosteronism due to a malignant ovarian tumor. J Clin Endocrinol Metab 41:809–819
168. Tracy SL, Askin FB, Reddick RL, Jackson B, Kurman RJ (1985) Progesterone secreting Sertoli cell tumor of the ovary. Gynecol Oncol 22:85–96
169. Tsunematsu R, Saito T, Iguchi H, Fukuda T, Tsukamoto N (2000) Hypercalcemia due to parathyroid hormone-related protein produced by primary ovarian clear cell adenocarcinoma: case report. Gynecol Oncol 76:218–222
170. Tyler HR (1974) Paraneoplastic syndromes of nerve, muscle, and neuromuscular junction. Ann NY Acad Sci 230:348–357
171. Ueda G, Nobuaki H, Hayakawa K et al (1972) Clinical histochemical and biochemical studies of an ovarian dysgerminoma with trophoblasts and Leydig cells. Am J Obstet Gynecol 114: 748–754
172. Vang R, Vague S, Tavassoli F, Prat J (2003) Signet-ring stromal tumor of the ovary: clinicopathologic analysis and comparison with Krukenberg tumor. Int J Gynecol Pathol 23:45–51
173. Verducci MA, Malkasian GD, Friedman SJ, Winkelmann RK (1984) Gynecologic carcinoma associated with dermatomyositis-polymyositis. Obstet Gynecol 64:695–698
174. von dem Borne AEGK, van Oers RHJ, Wiersinga WM et al (1990) Complete remission of autoimmune thrombocytopenia after extirpation of a benign adenofibroma of the ovary. Br J Rheumatol 74:119–120
175. Waxman M, Vuletin JC, Urcuyo R, Belling CG (1979) Ovarian low-grade stromal sarcoma with thecomatous features. A critical reappraisal of the so-called "malignant thecoma. Cancer (Phila) 44:2206–2217
176. Young RH, Clement PB, Scully RE (1988) Calcified thecomas in young women. A report of four cases. Int J Gynecol Pathol 7:343–350
177. Young RH, Dickersin GR, Scully RE (1983) A distinctive ovarian sex cord–stromal tumor causing sexual precocity in the Peutz–Jeghers syndrome. Am J Surg Pathol 7:233–243
178. Young RH, Dickersin GR, Scully RE (1984) Juvenile granulosa cell tumor of the ovary. A clinicopathologic analysis of 125 cases. Am J Surg Pathol 8:575–596
179. Young RH, Dudley AG, Scully RE (1984) Granulosa cell. Sertoli-Leydig cell and unclassified sex cord-stromal tumors associated with pregnancy. A clinicopathological analysis of thirty-six cases. Gynecol Oncol 18:181–205

180. Young RH, Oliva E, Scully RE (1994) Lutenized adult granulosa cell tumors of the ovary: a report of four cases. Int J Gynecol Pathol 13:302–310
181. Young RH, Oliva E, Scully RE (1994) Small cell carcinoma of the ovary, hypercalcemia type. A clinicopathological analysis of 150 cases. Am J Surg Pathol 18:1102–1116
182. Young RH, Perez-Atayde AR, Scully RE (1984) Ovarian Sertoli-Leydig cell tumor with retiform and heterologous components. Report of a case with hepatocytic differentiation and elevated serum alpha-fetoprotein. Am J Surg Pathol 8:709–718
183. Young RH, Prat J, Scully RE (1982) Ovarian Sertoli-Leydig cell tumors with heterologous elements. (i) Gastrointestinal epithelium and carcinoid: a clinicopathologic analysis of thirty-six cases. Cancer (Phila) 50:2448–2456
184. Young RH, Scully RE (2001) Differential diagnosis of ovarian tumors based primarily on their patterns and cell types. Semin Diagn Pathol 18:161–235
185. Young RH, Scully RE (1983) Ovarian stromal tumors with minor sex cord elements: a report of seven cases. Int J Gynecol Pathol 2:227–234
186. Young RH, Scully RE (1983) Ovarian sex cord-stromal tumors with bizarre nuclei. A clinicopathologic analysis of seventeen cases. Int J Gynecol Pathol 1:325–335
187. Young RH, Scully RE (1983) Ovarian Sertoli-Leydig cell tumors with a retiform pattern: a problem in histopathologic diagnosis. A report of 25 cases. Am J Surg Pathol 7:755–771
188. Young RH, Scully RE (1984) Ovarian Sertoli cell tumors. A report of ten cases. Int J Gynecol Pathol 2:349–363
189. Young RH, Scully RE (1987) Ovarian steroid cell tumors associated with Cushing's syndrome. A report of three cases. Int J Gynecol Pathol 6:40–48
190. Young RH, Scully RE (1984) Well-differentiated ovarian Sertoli–Leydig cell tumors. A clinicopathological analysis of 23 cases. Int J Gynecol Pathol 3:277–290
191. Young RH, Scully RE (1985) Ovarian Sertoli-Leydig cell tumors. A clinicopathological analysis of 207 cases. Am J Surg Pathol 9:543–569
192. Young RH, Welch WR, Dickersin GR, Scully RE (1982) Ovarian sex cord tumor with annular tubules: review of 74 cases including 27 with Peutz–Jeghers syndrome and 4 with adenoma malignum of the cervix. Cancer (Phila) 50:1384–1402
193. Zaloudek C, Norris HJ (1982) Granulosa tumors of the ovary in children. A clinical and pathologic study of 32 cases. Am J Surg Pathol 6:503–512
194. Zaloudek C, Norris HJ (1984) Sertoli-Leydig tumors of the ovary. A clinicopathologic study of 64 intermediate and poorly differentiated neoplasms. Am J Surg Pathol 8:405–418
195. Zaloudek CJ, Tavassoli FA, Norris HJ (1981) Dysgerminoma with syncytiotrophoblastic giant cells. A histologically and clinically distinctive subtype of dysgerminoma. Am J Surg Pathol 5:361–367
196. Zhang J, Young RH, Arseneau J, Scully RE (1982) Ovarian stromal tumors containing lutein or Leydig cells (luteinized thecomas and stromal Leydig cell tumors). A clinicopathological analysis of fifty cases. Int J Gynecol Pathol 1:270–285
197. Zhao C, Bratthauer GL, Barner R, Vang R (2006) Immunohistochemical analysis of S*ox9* in ovarian Sertoli cell tumors and other tumors in the differential diagnosis. Int J Gynecol Pathol 26:1–9
198. Zhao C, Bratthauer GL, Barner R, Vang R (2007) Diagnostic Utility of WT1 immunostaining in ovarian Sertoli cell tumor. Am J Surg Pathol 31:1378–1386
199. Zhao C, Bratthauer GL, Barner R, Vang R (2007) Comparative analysis of alternative and traditional immunohistochemical markers for the distinction of ovarian Sertoli cell tumor from endometrioid tumors and carcinoid tumor: a study of 160 cases. Am J Surg Pathol 31:255–266
200. Zhao C, Barner R, Vinh TN, McManus K, Dabbs D, Vang R (2008) SF-1 is a diagnostically useful immunohistochemical marker and comparable to other sex cord-stromal tumor markers for the differential diagnosis of ovarian Sertoli cell tumor. Int J Gynecol Pathol 27:507–514
201. Zheng W, Sung CJ, Hanna I et al (1997) a and b subunits of inhibin/activin as sex cord-stromal differentiation markers. Int J Gynecol Pathol 16:263–271

16 Germ Cell Tumors of the Ovary

Aleksander Talerman · Russell Vang

R. J. Kurman, L. Hedrick Ellenson, B. M. Ronnett (eds.), *Blaustein's Pathology of the Female Genital Tract (6th ed.)*, DOI 10.1007/978-1-4419-0489-8_16,

Germ cell tumors are composed of a number of histologically different tumor types derived from the primitive germ cells of the embryonic gonad. The concept of germ cell tumors as a specific group of gonadal neoplasms has evolved over the last several decades. It is based on (1) the common histogenesis of these neoplasms, (2) the relatively frequent presence of histologically different neoplastic elements within the same tumor, (3) the presence of histologically similar neoplasms in extragonadal locations along the line of migration of the primitive germ cells from the wall of the yolk sac to the gonadal ridge [253], and (4) the remarkable homology between the various tumors in the male and the female. In no other group of gonadal neoplasms is this homology better illustrated. Although the strong morphologic resemblance between the testicular seminoma and its ovarian counterpart, the dysgerminoma was noted soon after these neoplasms were first described, for a long time there was no agreement as to their histogenesis. Nevertheless, these were the first neoplasms to become accepted as originating from germ cells. It was not until the studies by Teilum [231, 232] on the homology of ovarian and testicular neoplasms, the studies by Friedman and Moore [59] and Dixon and Moore [50] on testicular tumors, and those by Friedman [58] on related extragonadal neoplasms that the germ cell origin of other neoplasms belonging to this group was proposed. These views were supported by the embryologic studies of Witschi [253] and Gillman [66], and later by the experimental work of Stevens [200–202] and Pierce et al [149, 151] on germ cell tumors in rodents.

Although occasional unusual neoplasms composed of germ cells and sex cord derivatives had been noted previously, it was not until Scully's detailed description of gonadoblastoma [181] that these neoplasms were established as a distinct entity. More recently, another neoplasm composed of germ cells and sex cord derivatives, the mixed germ cell–sex cord–stromal tumor, has been described in detail [209, 210]. This chapter, therefore, is devoted not only to neoplasms of germ cell origin, but also to those composed of germ cells and sex cord derivatives.

Histogenesis

The histogenesis and interrelationships of the various types of germ cell neoplasms, as suggested by Teilum [235], are shown in ➋ *Fig. 16.1*. According to Teilum [235], dysgerminoma (seminoma) is a primitive germ cell neoplasm that has not acquired the potential for further differentiation. Embryonal carcinoma is regarded as a conceptual as well as a morphologic entity and represents a germ cell neoplasm composed of multipotential cells that are capable of further differentiation. This process can take place in an embryonal or somatic direction, resulting in teratomatous neoplasms showing various degrees of maturity, or in an extraembryonal direction along either of two pathways: vitelline, differentiating toward yolk sac (endodermal sinus) tumor, or trophoblastic, differentiating toward a choriocarcinoma. The process of differentiation is dynamic and, therefore, neoplasms may be composed of different elements showing various stages of development. According to this view [235], dysgerminoma was considered incapable of further differentiation, but immunohistochemical evidence indicates that some seminoma or dysgerminoma cells can differentiate into embryonal carcinoma and further [137]. The intimate admixture of dysgerminoma cells with other neoplastic germ cell elements seen in some germ cell tumors also supports this concept [82].

Classification

The World Health Organization (WHO) classification [186] divides germ cell tumors into a number of groups and also includes neoplasms composed of germ cells and sex cord–stromal derivatives. In the most recent version (➋ *Table 16.1*) [230], the yolk sac tumor category has been expanded to include the polyvesicular vitelline, hepatoid, and glandular subtypes, which unlike other patterns of differentiation in yolk sac tumors can occur in pure form and thus pose diagnostic problems. The new classification also expands the category of teratoma, dividing it into biphasic or triphasic teratoma and monodermal teratoma and somatic-type tumors associated with biphasic or triphasic teratoma [230]. The tumors composed of germ cells and the sex cord–stromal derivatives are divided into two categories: gonadoblastoma and mixed germ cell–sex cord–stromal tumor; each of these is subclassified to include those tumors associated with dysgerminoma or other germ cell tumors.

Clinical and Pathologic Features of Germ Cell Tumors

Germ cell tumors constitute the second largest group o ovarian neoplasms after the surface epithelial–strom tumors and comprise approximately 20% of all ovaria neoplasms observed in Europe and North America. I countries in Asia and Africa, where the prevalence surface epithelial–stromal tumors is much lower, ger

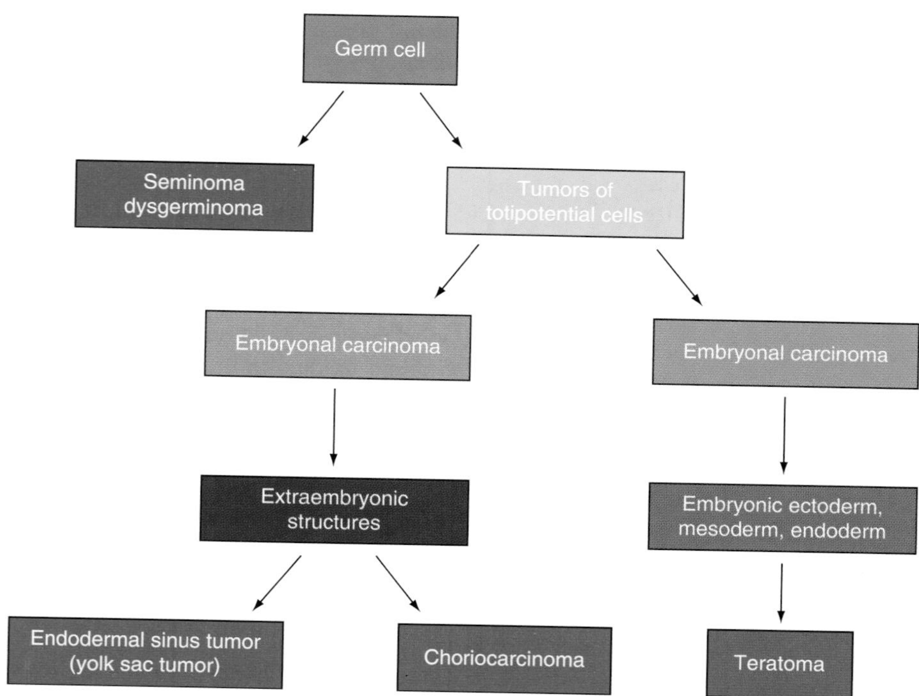

Fig. 16.1
Hypothetical model of histogenesis of germ cell tumors as proposed by Teilum (Modified from [232])

cell tumors constitute a much larger proportion of ovarian neoplasms. Germ cell tumors are encountered at all ages from infancy to old age but are seen most frequently from the first to the sixth decades. They also have been observed during fetal life. In children and adolescents, more than 60% of ovarian neoplasms are of germ cell origin, and one third are malignant [129]. In adults, the great majority of germ cell tumors (95%) are benign and consist of mature cystic teratomas (dermoid cysts). Malignant ovarian germ cell tumors occur in the first four decades and are rare thereafter.

Dysgerminoma

Histogenesis

Dysgerminoma is composed entirely of germ cells that show morphologic, ultrastructural [105], and histochemical [116] similarity to primordial germ cells. The cells of dysgerminoma are considered to be in an early and sexually indifferent stage of differentiation; they have been believed to be arrested at a developmental stage at which they have not yet gained the ability for further differentiation [232]. However, there is evidence that occasional cells may acquire this ability and differentiate to embryonal carcinoma and further [120, 137]. An origin from the primordial germ cells that migrate to the ovary during early embryogenesis from their site of origin in the wall of the yolk sac [253] is the most widely accepted view of the histogenesis of dysgerminoma. It is supported by the occurrence of homologous neoplasms in the testis (seminoma) and along the route of migration of the primordial germ cells from the wall of the yolk sac to the primitive gonad, in the mediastinum, retroperitoneum, posterior abdominal wall, and parapineal and sacrococcygeal regions.

Cytogenetic and Molecular Features

An increased amount of DNA, double the amount present in normal somatic cells, is present in the nuclei of dysgerminoma [9, 93]. The demonstration of a small isochromosome, i(12p), as a specific abnormality and therefore a possible chromosomal marker for testicular germ cell tumors, especially seminoma [11], has been noted in dysgerminomas [12, 43]. However, i(12p) has also been

Table 16.1
WHO classification of germ cell tumors of the ovary

Germ cell tumors
Dysgerminoma
Variant – with syncytiotrophoblastic cells
Yolk sac tumor (endodermal sinus tumor)
Variants
Polyvesicular vitelline tumor
Hepatoid
Glandular
Embryonal carcinoma
Polyembryoma
Choriocarcinoma
Teratomas
Immature
Mature
Solid
Cystic (dermoid cyst)
With secondary tumor formation (specify type)
Fetiform (homunculus)
Monodermal and highly specialized types
Struma ovarii
Variant – with thyroid tumor (specify type)
Carcinoid
Insular
Trabecular
Strumal carcinoid
Mucinous carcinoid
Neuroectodermal tumors
Sebaceous tumors
Others
Mixed (specify type)
Mixed forms (tumors composed of two or more of the above pure types)
Tumors composed of germ cells and sex cord–stromal derivatives
Gonadoblastoma
Variant – with dysgerminoma or other germ cell tumor
Germ cell–sex cord–stromal tumor
Variant – with dysgerminoma or other germ cell tumor

WHO, World Health Organization.

identified in non-dysgerminatous components of ovarian germ cell tumors [153].

Comparative genomic hybridization has revealed multiple DNA copy number changes in dysgerminoma [94, 159]. Common alterations include gains on chromosome arms 12p, 12q, 21q, and 22q and losses from 13q. A subset of tumors exhibits mutation of the *KIT* oncogene [77].

Prevalence

Dysgerminoma is an uncommon tumor, accounting for 1–2% of primary ovarian neoplasms and 3–5% of ovarian malignancies [121, 173]. It is the most common malignant ovarian germ cell neoplasm occurring in pure form. The exact prevalence of dysgerminoma in different parts of the world is not known because most cancer registry reports do not differentiate between the various types of ovarian neoplasms. Although most reports emanate from Europe and North America, dysgerminoma has been encountered in all parts of the world and in all races. In some countries, there are considerable regional variations.

Clinical Features

Dysgerminoma has been reported in infants from 7 months to women aged 70 years [121], but most cases occur in the second and third decades; nearly half the patients are under 20 years of age, and 80% are under 30 years [9, 24, 69, 121]. Dysgerminoma occurs not infrequently before puberty but is very rare after menopause. Therefore, dysgerminoma is one of the most common malignant ovarian neoplasms of childhood, adolescence, and early adult life [9, 24, 69, 121, 129].

Pure dysgerminoma has been reported in siblings [223] as well as in a mother and daughter. The symptomatology of dysgerminoma is not distinctive and is similar to that observed in patients with other solid ovarian neoplasms [9, 24, 69, 121]. The duration of symptoms is usually short; despite this, the tumor is often large, indicating rapid growth [24]. The most common presentation is abdominal enlargement and presence of a mass in the lower abdomen, which sometimes is associated with abdominal pain due to torsion. Loss of weight may also occur. In a number of cases, the tumor has been found incidentally; in these, the tumor is usually small. In pregnancy, the tumor may be discovered as an incidental finding or may obstruct labor.

The common association of dysgerminoma with gonadoblastoma, a tumor that nearly always occurs in patients with dysgenetic gonads [174, 175, 182], indicates that there is a relationship between dysgerminoma and genetic and somatosexual abnormalities. Several reports emphasize the occurrence of dysgerminoma in normal female patients [9, 24] and some have even cast doubt on the relationship with developmental and sexual abnormalities [9].

Dysgerminoma may also be discovered incidentally in patients investigated for primary amenorrhea; in these cases, it is usually associated with gonadoblastoma [174, 175, 182, 251]. Occasionally, menstrual and endocrine abnormalities may be the presenting symptoms, but this finding tends to be more common in patients with dysgerminoma containing syncytiotrophoblastic giant cells or when combined with other neoplastic germ cell elements, especially choriocarcinoma. The latter qualifies as a mixed germ cell tumor. In children, precocious sexual development may occur [171]. Dysgerminoma associated with evidence of virilization is found mostly in association with gonadoblastoma in patients with pure or mixed gonadal dysgenesis. A case of dysgerminoma associated with hypercalcemia has been reported and was found to be due to increased circulating levels of active form of vitamin D, 1,25-dihydroxyvitamin D3, rather than increased synthesis of parathyroid hormone-related peptide, as seen in other ovarian tumors with hypercalcemia [56]. Dysgerminoma has also been encountered in a patient with triple-X syndrome [86].

Gross Features

Dysgerminoma affects the right ovary in approximately 50% of cases and the left in 35%, and it is bilateral in 15% [9, 69, 121]. A much higher frequency of bilateral tumors is observed in patients with dysgerminoma associated with gonadoblastoma, the dysgerminoma arising from and overgrowing the gonadoblastoma [174, 175, 182]. Thus, inclusion of such cases tends to increase the prevalence of bilaterality.

Pure dysgerminomas are solid tumors that are round, oval, or lobulated, with a smooth, gray-white, slightly glistening fibrous capsule. They vary in size from a few centimeters in diameter to large masses measuring 50 cm across [9], which fill the pelvic and abdominal cavities. Tumors weighing more than 5 kg have been described [121]. The capsule is usually intact but may be ruptured, especially in large tumors, which may lead to the formation of adhesions between the tumor and surrounding structures. The consistency of dysgerminoma varies from firm and rubbery in small and medium-sized tumors to soft in large ones. On cut surface (*Fig. 16.2*), the tumor is solid and varies from gray-pink to light tan. Red, brown,

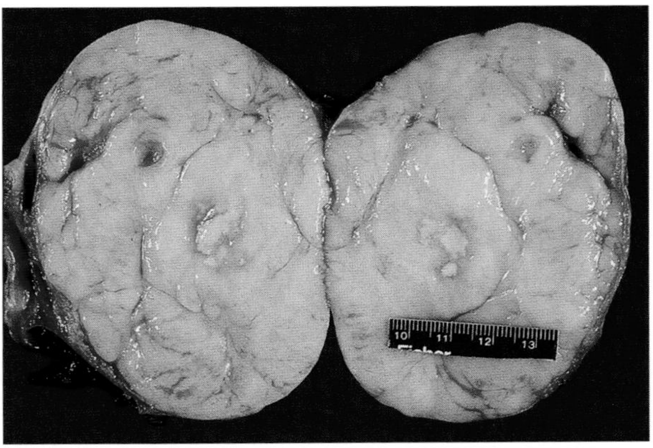

Fig. 16.2
Dysgerminoma. **The cut surface is solid. There is some lobulation. Focally, hemorrhage is present**

or yellow discoloration caused by hemorrhage or necrosis is also seen, especially in large tumors; this may sometimes lead to the formation of small cysts, but generally dysgerminomas are solid. The presence of cystic areas suggests the possibility that other neoplastic elements may be present, most likely teratoma. In view of the important therapeutic and prognostic implications concerning the presence of other neoplastic germ cell elements, extensive and judicious sampling of different parts of the tumor, especially of the less typical areas, is recommended.

Microscopic Features

Dysgerminoma is identical to seminoma of the testis. It is composed of aggregates, islands, or strands of large uniform cells surrounded by varying amounts of connective tissue stroma containing lymphocytes (*Figs. 16.3–16.5*). The cells are large and measure from 15 to 25 μm in diameter. They are oval or round and usually have distinguishable cytoplasmic borders. In well-fixed material, the cell boundaries are well defined. The cells contain an ample amount of pale, slightly granular eosinophilic or clear cytoplasm.

The centrally located vesicular nucleus is large, occupying nearly half the cell. The nucleus is oval or round, has a sharp nuclear membrane with unevenly dispersed finely granular chromatin, and contains usually one, but sometimes two, prominent eosinophilic nucleoli. Some variation in the size of the cells and nuclei and in the amount of nuclear chromatin is usually seen. Large or giant

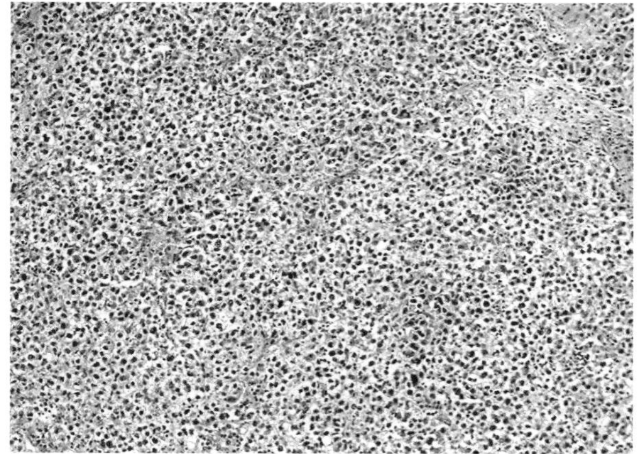

Fig. 16.3
Dysgerminoma. **The tumor is composed of large aggregates of uniform cells**

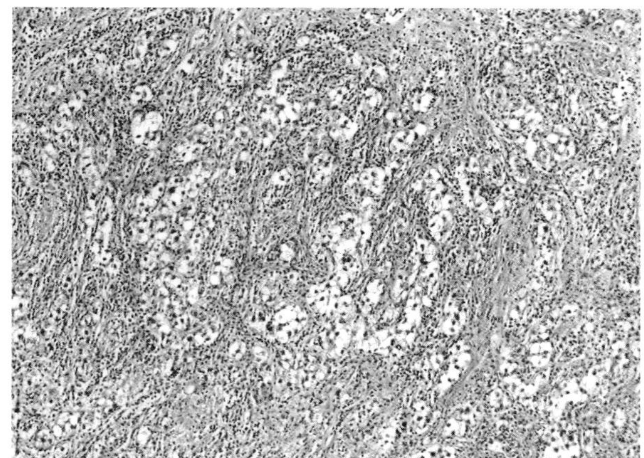

Fig. 16.5
Dysgerminoma. **Nests of tumor cells are present within fibrous stroma, which contains abundant lymphocytic component**

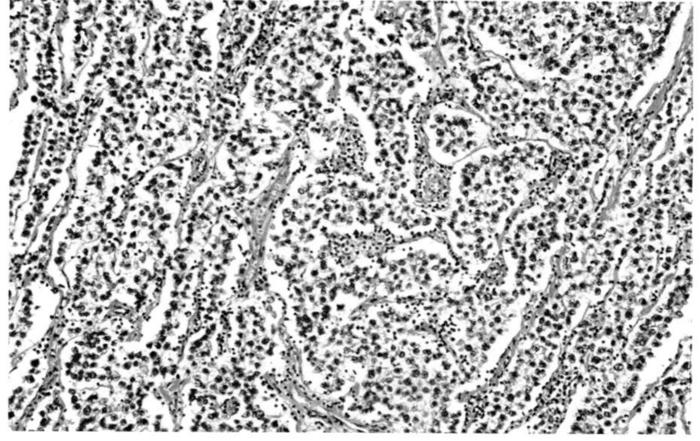

Fig. 16.4
Dysgerminoma. **The tumor is composed of trabeculae of tumor cells surrounded by connective tissue stroma containing lymphocytes**

mononucleate tumor cells, which in all other respects resemble typical dysgerminoma cells, may be seen. Mitotic activity is almost always detectable and may vary from slight to brisk. This difference in mitotic activity may be observed not only in different tumors but also in different parts of the same tumor.

The cytoplasm of the tumor cells contains glycogen, which can be demonstrated with the periodic acid–Schiff (PAS) reaction and is removed by diastase digestion. The amount of glycogen in tumor cells is variable, and glycogen is lost from the cytoplasm on prolonged fixation in formalin. In view of this, the PAS reaction may vary from strong to very weak. Lipid can be demonstrated in the cytoplasm of the tumor cells in frozen tissue.

The stroma that surrounds the tumor cells almost always displays lymphocytic infiltration, which can vary from slight to marked (*Fig. 16.5*). Occasionally, lymphoid follicles containing germinal centers may be seen. Plasma cells, eosinophils, and sometimes a granulomatous reaction are present in the connective tissue stroma. The lymphoreticular cell infiltrate has previously been studied immunohistochemically, and most of the cells are T cells and macrophages. There are relatively few B cells, natural killer cells, and other types of lymphoreticular cells [49].

The connective tissue stroma shows considerable variation ranging from a fine, delicate fibrovascular network that can be loose and edematous to densely hyalinized. Depending on the amount of stroma, the tumor cells form large aggregates, smaller nests, islands, cords, or strands. Occasionally, the amount of stroma may be very abundant leading to wide separation of the nests of tumor cells. In some cases hyalinization may be so marked that tumor cells are detected with difficulty. At the opposite end of the spectrum, there are tumors that are cellular and contain only an imperceptible amount of stroma. There may be considerable variation in the amount of stroma in various parts of the same tumor.

Foci of necrosis and hemorrhage are frequently found and may be extensive in large tumors or in tumors that have undergone torsion. Calcification is only occasionally seen in dysgerminoma. It occurs as small spots or flecks of calcified material that are found in association with necrosis, hemorrhage, fibrosis, or hyalinization. Occasionally,

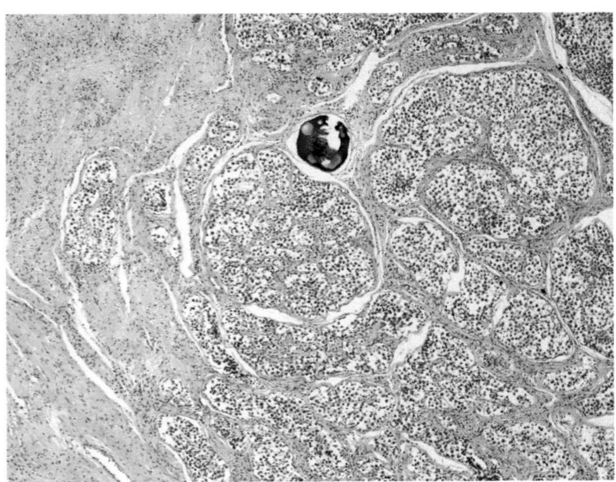

◘ Fig. 16.6
Dysgerminoma arising from gonadoblastoma. A large calcified concretion is present. Nests of gonadoblastoma were found in other parts of the tumor

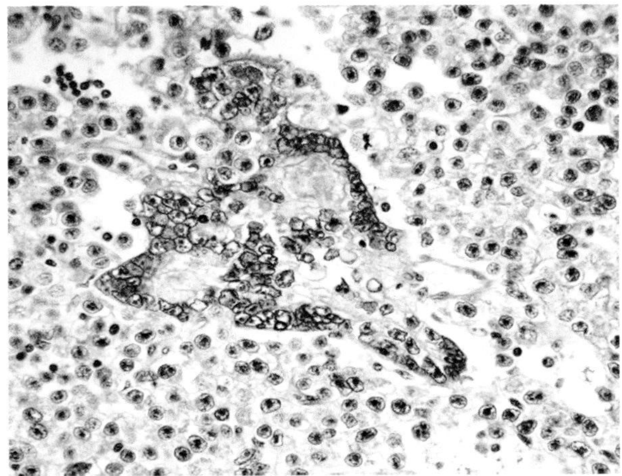

◘ Fig. 16.7
Dysgerminoma with a large syncytiotrophoblastic giant cell

relatively large, round, or ovoid calcified bodies are found, which may indicate the presence of a burnt-out gonadoblastoma [182] (➲ *Fig. 16.6*).

In 6–8% of dysgerminomas, there are individual or collections of syncytiotrophoblastic giant cells that produce human chorionic gonadotropin (hCG). The presence of these cells is associated with elevation of serum hCG levels; hCG can also be demonstrated in tissue sections by immunohistochemistry. This evidence provides another possible explanation, apart from the presence of true choriocarcinomatous elements, for the occasional presence of endocrine activity in cases of dysgerminoma. However, there remains a small group of cases in which, despite a careful search, trophoblastic elements have not been found. In some of these cases, the dysgerminoma has been associated with an increase in luteinized stromal cells and it is likely that they may be responsible for the feminizing side effects and occasionally virilization [171].

The syncytiotrophoblastic giant cells may form large syncytial masses resembling the syncytiotrophoblast of a choriocarcinoma, but they differ from the latter because there is no cytotrophoblast (➲ *Fig. 16.7*). The presence of choriocarcinoma in association with dysgerminoma is not frequent, but most of the reported series contain cases of this type [141, 173]. The syncytiotrophoblastic cells must also be differentiated from foreign body and Langhans' giant cells and from mononucleate and multinucleate tumor giant cells, which are seen in some dysgerminomas. There is no evidence that dysgerminomas containing syncytiotrophoblastic giant cells are associated with a worse prognosis [259]. The serum hCG level can be monitored as a tumor marker in the same way as in patients with gestational trophoblastic disease (see ➲ Chap. 20, Gestational Trophoblastic Tumors and Related Tumor-Like Lesions) or with mixed germ cell tumors containing choriocarcinoma. The serum hCG levels in these cases are much lower compared with dysgerminoma admixed with typical choriocarcinoma.

Pure dysgerminoma is not associated with elevated levels of serum alpha-fetoprotein (AFP) [227]. The presence of elevated levels of AFP is an indication of presence of other neoplastic germ cell elements, virtually always yolk sac tumor, either within the primary tumor or its metastases.

Immunohistochemical Features and Differential Diagnosis

SALL4 is highly sensitive and specific for primitive germ cell tumors, including dysgerminoma [32]. Immunohistochemical staining for placental alkaline phosphatase (PLAP) has been used less extensively in ovarian dysgerminoma as compared to testicular seminoma [82], but when applied PLAP stains dysgerminoma cells in the same way as testicular seminoma cells, showing membrane-bound staining in most cells [82]. As PLAP also stains the tumor cells in other malignant germ cell tumors, it cannot be used to differentiate dysgerminoma from other malignant germ cell neoplasms [82]. It may be useful in differentiating dysgerminoma from nongerm cell malignancies that occasionally may resemble it such as clear cell carcinoma, lymphoma, and granulosa cell tumor. Dysgerminoma shows expression of the c-kit

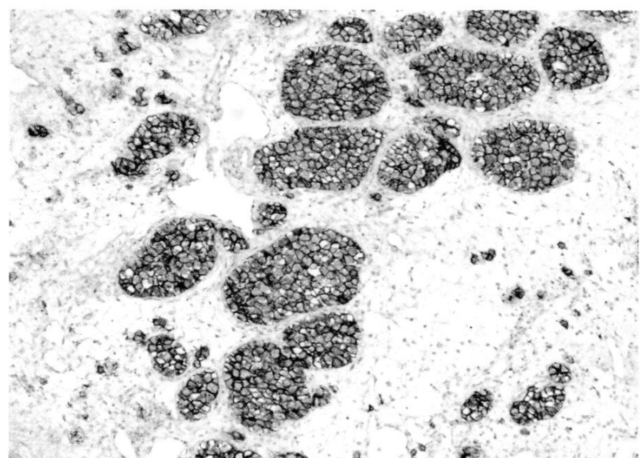

Fig. 16.8
Dysgerminoma. **Diffuse expression of CD117**

proto-oncogene product (CD117) (Fig. 16.8) [188, 242]. It has been suggested that this finding may have potential therapeutic value as the c-kit receptor may serve as a target for site-specific immunotherapy [188]. Recently, OCT-4 nuclear staining has been shown to be specific for dysgerminoma, seminoma, and embryonal carcinoma and was found to be negative in other germ cell tumors, thus providing another useful immunohistochemical marker for dysgerminoma [36]. Although D2-40 (podoplanin) is not specific for germ cell origin, it is expressed in dysgerminoma and negative in other ovarian germ cell tumors [35]. Most dysgerminoma cells do not show immunohistochemical staining for low molecular weight cytokeratin although occasional cells may show expression [42, 119, 120]. Thus, low molecular weight cytokeratin is useful for distinguishing dysgerminoma from embryonal carcinoma and yolk sac tumor, in which the latter two show diffuse expression [82, 119, 120].

The main tumors in the differential diagnosis of dysgerminoma include embryonal carcinoma, yolk sac tumor, clear cell carcinoma, and steroid cell tumor. Solid patterns of embryonal carcinoma, yolk sac tumor, and clear cell carcinoma can overlap with the histologic appearance of dysgerminoma, but (a) the admixture of glandular and papillary growth patterns in embryonal carcinoma, yolk sac tumor, and clear cell carcinoma; (b) lobulated architecture with lymphocytes in the interlobular fibrous septae seen in some dysgerminomas; and (c) immunohistochemical differences mentioned above usually allow for distinction. In addition, embryonal carcinoma typically shows a greater degree of nuclear pleomorphism than dysgerminoma. Histologically, dysgerminoma and steroid cell tumor can occasionally resemble one another because of sheets of clear cells. The younger age of patients with dysgerminoma, lobulated architecture with lymphocytes in the interlobular fibrous septae seen in some dysgerminomas, finely vacuolated cytoplasm of steroid cell tumor, and immunohistochemical expression of inhibin and calretinin in steroid cell tumor and CD117 and OCT-4 in dysgerminoma should facilitate the correct diagnosis.

Clinical Behavior and Treatment

Dysgerminoma is a malignant neoplasm capable of metastatic and local spread. Despite its less aggressive behavior compared with other malignant germ cell neoplasms, the malignant potential of dysgerminoma should not be underestimated. Dysgerminoma is a rapidly growing neoplasm, but metastatic spread does not occur early in the course of the disease (although it is not possible to predict this in individual cases). When the tumor is small and freely mobile, its capsule is usually intact, but large tumors may be adherent to surrounding structures or may rupture. Rupture may occur either spontaneously or at operation; this leads to spillage of the tumor contents and peritoneal implantation, causing serious consequences. Penetration of the ovarian surface by the tumor and formation of adhesions to surrounding structures may lead to direct extension by the tumor.

Metastatic spread occurs via the lymphatic system; the lymph nodes in the vicinity of the common iliac arteries and the terminal part of the abdominal aorta are first affected. Occasionally, there may be marked enlargement of these lymph nodes, with formation of large masses. Usually the enlargement is slight to moderate and can be detected by computerized tomography (CT) scanning or magnetic resonance imaging (MRI). From the abdominal lymph nodes, the tumor spreads to the mediastinal and supraclavicular lymph nodes. Hematogenous spread to distant organs occurs later, and any organ may be affected, although involvement of the liver, lungs, and bones tends to be most common [9, 24, 121]. In cases of pure dysgerminoma, the metastases usually present a similar histologic appearance to the primary tumor, but occasionally tumors composed of pure dysgerminoma may be associated with metastases composed of other neoplastic germ cell elements. This metastatic pattern is observed much more commonly in combined tumors. It has been suggested that cellular tumors with marked atypia and high mitotic activity and small amounts of stroma with only slight lymphocytic infiltration tend to be more aggressive [10]. However, there is at present no good evidence that the behavior of an individual tumor can be assessed by its histologic appearance [24]. The presence of other malignant germ cell elements, however, has an adverse effect on prognosis [9, 24, 98, 141].

Dysgerminoma, similar to its testicular counterpart seminoma, is associated with elevated levels of serum lactic dehydrogenase (LDH) and its isoenzyme-1 (LDH-1). These substances can be used as tumor markers [60, 180]. There is a good correlation between the volume of tumor tissue present and the serum levels of the enzymes.

The prognosis of patients with pure dysgerminoma is very favorable with a 5-year survival ranging from 75% to >90% [24, 64, 69, 104, 140, 237]. The 5-year survival of patients with unilateral encapsulated dysgerminoma has been reported as >90% [9, 24, 64, 104, 140, 237], although patients treated by unilateral salpingo-oophorectomy have recurrence rates ranging from 18% to 52%. Unfavorable prognostic features include presence of metastases at the time of diagnosis, presence of adhesions, spread into adjacent structures, bilaterality, and large size of the tumor [69, 141]. It should be noted that even when these features are present many patients have been cured with chemotherapy. Age does not appear to be an important prognostic factor [9, 24, 64, 140].

Like other malignant germ cell tumors, dysgerminoma responds very well to combination chemotherapy of cisplatin, etoposide (VP16), and bleomycin (BEP). In the cases studied, 80% of recurrences occur in the first 2 years after diagnosis [141], and it has been reported that more than 75% occur in the first year. In rare cases, recurrences occurred many years after excision of the original tumor.

For young women with unilateral encapsulated pure dysgerminoma, two different therapeutic approaches have been advocated. One consists of unilateral oophorectomy, or salpingo-oophorectomy, and careful follow-up. The second approach advocates similar surgical therapy, but to decrease and prevent metastases and recurrences, adjuvant chemotherapy is administered. The advantages of the first approach are that fertility is preserved and there are no genetic hazards associated with administration of chemotherapy. Although the second approach tends to decrease the risk of metastases and recurrences [24, 223], this risk is not very serious especially because metastases or recurrences can be treated successfully by combination chemotherapy [9, 24, 64, 140]. The conservative approach to the therapy of unilateral encapsulated dysgerminoma is recommended, but each individual case should be considered on its merits. It should be noted that before this mode of treatment can be considered, the opposite ovary must be normal, there should be no evidence of spread of the tumor in the abdominal cavity, and the abdominal and pelvic lymph nodes must be free from metastases on inspection, CT scanning, and MRI. In addition, the patient must have a normal female 46,XX karyotype.

In patients with widely disseminated metastases, administration of three to four cycles of combination chemotherapy composed of cisplatin, etoposide (VP16), and bleomycin combination (BEP) has been successful in eradicating the disease [64, 140]. The treatment of patients with dysgerminoma occurring in dysgenetic gonads must be hysterectomy and bilateral salpingo-gonadectomy in view of the high risk of development of bilateral neoplasms in these patients [61]. Furthermore, their gonads are hormonally and functionally inactive. Therefore, determination of the karyotype of all patients with dysgerminoma, especially those with evidence of virilization or developmental and menstrual abnormalities, is recommended. This is important in prepubertal patients, because these patients lack other signs of abnormal function, such as primary amenorrhea, virilization, and absence of normal sexual development. Following adnexectomy, patients are given hormone replacement therapy. Adequate treatment in these cases prevents development of a tumor in the opposite gonad [61]. Follow-up is advisable to prevent any deleterious effects of hormone replacement therapy.

Yolk Sac Tumor

Histogenesis

Yolk sac tumor is a malignant germ cell neoplasm that is thought to originate from the undifferentiated and multipotential embryonal carcinoma by selective differentiation toward yolk sac or vitelline structures, in the same way as nongestational choriocarcinoma differentiates trophoblastic structures. The recognition and classification of yolk sac (endodermal sinus) tumor as a specific entity stems from the studies of Teilum [232–234]. The concepts regarding the histogenesis of this neoplasm that Teilum proposed have been supported by the experimental studies of the neoplastic rodent yolk sac by Pierce et al [151]. The hyaline, PAS-positive material in yolk sac tumor has been found to be similar to the hyaline material produced by mouse teratocarcinoma during its conversion to the ascitic form, and this is considered to be a strong argument in favor of the yolk sac origin of the tumor [146, 147, 151]. When examined with the electron microscope, the cells of yolk sac tumor resemble those of the normal human yolk sac [68, 82, 124].

In 1939, Schiller [177] described an ovarian neoplasm composed of clear and hobnail cells with a pattern that he designated a mesonephroma because of the presence of structures resembling immature glomeruli. Other investigators [85] were unable to demonstrate the mesonephric origin of this tumor and considered it an endothelioma of the ovary [179]. In 1946, Teilum [232] demonstrated that the tumor described as mesonephroma [177] included two distinct neoplasms with different histogenesis, histologic pattern, age distribution, and clinical behavior. One of these tumors was highly malignant, occurred in young patients, was homologous with certain testicular neoplasms, and was of germ cell origin [232]. The other tumor was less aggressive, occurred in older women, and ultimately was shown by Scully to be of müllerian-type origin. He designated this neoplasm "clear cell carcinoma."

In addition to the terms mesonephroma and endothelioma, yolk sac tumors have been designated as embryonal carcinoma because of certain similarities to embryonal carcinoma of the testis [50]. Although embryonal carcinoma showing the histologic pattern resembling the typical embryonal carcinoma of the testis [50] is seen occasionally in ovarian tumors [97], most ovarian tumors of this type show a distinctive pattern with differentiation toward yolk sac or vitelline structures [234, 235] and should be termed yolk sac tumor.

The term yolk sac tumor is more inclusive than the original term endodermal sinus tumor. Ovarian yolk sac tumor differs from the undifferentiated embryonal carcinoma [50] and resembles closely the yolk sac tumor of both infantile and adult testes [212, 234, 235]. It is now generally accepted that the term embryonal carcinoma should be used only to designate ovarian neoplasms showing the typical histologic pattern of the embryonal carcinoma as described in testicular tumors [50, 97]. It is notable that most true ovarian embryonal carcinomas are combined with yolk sac tumor. The not infrequent combination of yolk sac tumor elements in ovarian tumors with other neoplastic germ cell elements [82, 98] is one of the arguments in favor of the germ cell origin of this neoplasm. Yolk sac tumor, either pure or combined with other neoplastic germ cell elements, has been encountered in extragonadal locations where germ cell tumors are known to occur, in the mediastinum, sacrococcygeal region, pineal gland, and vagina.

Alpha-fetoprotein (AFP) was first identified as a specific constituent of normal human fetal serum by Bergstrand and Czar [21] in 1956. In the human embryo, serum AFP peaks at approximately 3,000 mg/L at about 12–13 weeks of gestation. The level decreases slowly until birth, when it is approximately 55 mg/L. After birth, AFP disappears rapidly from the serum, and 3 weeks after full-term delivery, it can be detected only in very small amounts (0–15 ng/mL) by radioimmunoassay or sensitive enzyme immunoassays. In fetal development, AFP is produced by the yolk sac, liver, and upper gastrointestinal tract. Certain histologic components of germ cell neoplasms correlate with elevated serum AFP. It has been demonstrated that germ cell tumors in patients with elevated serum AFP are either composed entirely of, or contain, yolk sac tumor elements [128, 227]. Elevation of serum AFP has not been observed in patients with pure dysgerminoma [227], mature cystic teratoma of the ovary [227], or pure gonadoblastoma [227]. Slight elevations of serum AFP have been noted in occasional cases of immature teratoma of the ovary; this is most likely related to the presence of neuroepithelium.

Apart from yolk sac tumor, elevated levels of serum AFP are seen in patients with hepatoid carcinoma of the ovary and occasional Sertoli–Leydig cell tumors, especially those showing a retiform pattern [215, 219, 257]. Slightly elevated levels of serum AFP up to 60 ng/mL (upper limit of normal serum AFP, 20 ng/mL) have been observed in some cases of embryonal carcinoma of the testis [227]. Using immunohistochemical techniques, AFP has been identified in the cells of yolk sac tumor and embryonal carcinoma of the ovary [82, 97], and in the eosinophilic, PAS-positive, diastase-resistant globules present both inside and outside the tumor cells. Large amounts of AFP have been extracted from tumor tissue in yolk sac tumors of the ovary and testis [226].

In view of the fact that normal yolk sac in the human and other mammalian species has been shown to be associated with AFP synthesis [67], it is reasonable to assume that the selective synthesis of AFP by yolk sac tumors provides further support to the view that yolk sac tumor develops as a result of differentiation of primitive malignant germ cell elements in the direction of yolk sac or vitelline structures [82, 96, 218, 227]. The immunohistochemical localization of AFP in embryonal carcinoma and in areas of yolk sac tumor showing no morphologic evidence of yolk sac differentiation suggests that the biochemical manifestations of yolk sac differentiation, such as AFP synthesis, precede morphologic differentiation [82, 97].

Clinical Features

Yolk sac tumor is the second most common malignant ovarian germ cell neoplasm after dysgerminoma. It is one of the most common malignant ovarian neoplasms of childhood, adolescence, and early adult life [82].

Yolk sac tumor has been encountered in all races [65, 82, 96]. The reported age distribution of patients with yolk sac tumor ranges from 16 months to 46 years, but most patients have been under 30 years of age [65, 82, 96]. Yolk sac tumor is encountered most frequently in the second and third decades, followed by first and fourth, and is rare in women in the fifth decade. It has been encountered in occasional postmenopausal patients. Yolk sac tumor associated with an ovarian surface epithelial tumor has been rarely reported in elderly patients [113, 125, 172]. Although the histogenesis of these tumors is uncertain, the likely explanation is that it originates from the surface epithelium by a process of neoplastic differentiation and therefore the histogenesis is totally different from that of germ cell neoplasms [113, 172]. In some cases studied by one of the authors (AT), the yolk sac tumor component overgrew the surface epithelial–stromal element, and only extensive sectioning demonstrated focal presence of the latter. The serum AFP level was highly elevated, reflecting the presence of the yolk sac tumor component. A small series of similar cases has been reported [125].

Most patients with yolk sac tumor present with abdominal enlargement, pain, and a lower abdominal or pelvic mass [65, 82, 96]. Occasionally, symptoms are acute and severe and may lead to the diagnosis of acute appendicitis or a ruptured ectopic pregnancy; this usually is caused by torsion of the tumor. A number of cases have been encountered during pregnancy [82, 96]. The presence of yolk sac tumor is not associated with endocrine manifestations. On clinical examination, a tumor mass is usually palpable and is frequently of considerable size [65, 82, 96]. Increased levels of AFP are found in the sera [65, 128, 226], and this is a useful diagnostic test for the presence of yolk sac tumor elements in the primary tumor, its metastases, and recurrences [226, 227].

Gross Features

Yolk sac tumors are almost always unilateral [65, 82, 96, 226]. Bilaterality typically is a manifestation of metastatic spread. Yolk sac tumor shows a certain predilection for the right ovary [82, 96]. The tumor is usually large, varying in size from 3 to 30 cm in diameter, with most tumors measuring more than 10 cm [82, 96, 226]. It frequently weighs more than 500 g; tumors weighing 5 kg have been recorded. The tumor is usually encapsulated, round, oval, or globular; firm, smooth, or somewhat lobulated; and gray-yellow, with areas of hemorrhage and cystic or gelatinous changes. The tumor may form adhesions to the surrounding structures and invade them. On sectioning, yolk sac tumors are mainly solid, but cystic spaces containing gelatinous fluid frequently are present. Necrosis and hemorrhage and the presence of other neoplastic germ cell elements, especially teratoma, may alter the appearance of the tumor.

Microscopic Features

Yolk sac tumors exhibit a wide range of histologic patterns that differ considerably from each other and, although all the different patterns may be observed in the same tumor, one or two may predominate. The following histologic patterns may be observed in yolk sac tumor: (1) microcystic or reticular, (2) endodermal sinus, (3) solid, (4) alveolar–glandular, (5) polyvesicular vitelline, (6) myxomatous, (7) papillary, (8) macrocystic, (9) hepatoid, and (10) glandular or primitive endodermal (intestinal) (*Figs. 16.9–16.20*) [82].

The polyvesicular vitelline, the hepatoid, and the primitive endodermal (intestinal) patterns tend to occur in pure form, unassociated with other yolk sac tumor elements. Although such tumors are rare, they pose considerable diagnostic difficulties, and because of this they have been classified as specific subtypes of yolk sac tumor in the revised WHO classification of ovarian neoplasms [184, 186, 230] (see *Table 16.1*).

Endodermal sinuses or perivascular formations (Schiller–Duval bodies) are the hallmark of the tumor

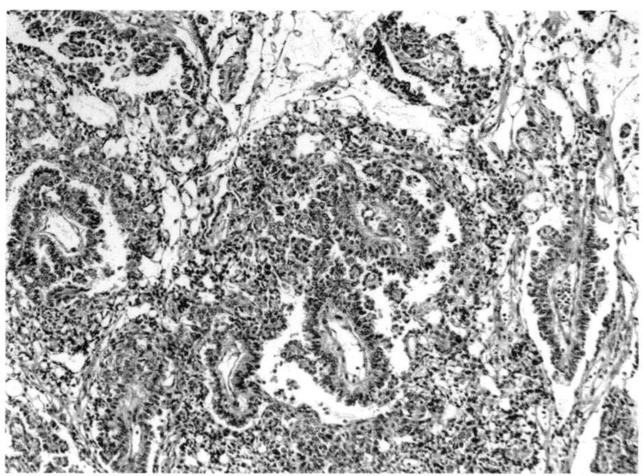

Fig. 16.9
Yolk sac tumor. **The tumor shows classical perivascular formations (Schiller–Duval bodies)**

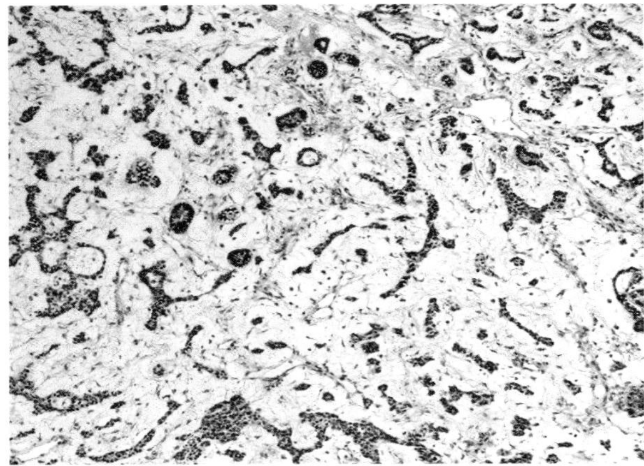

Fig. 16.10
Yolk sac tumor, myxomatous pattern. **Small collections of epithelial-like cells forming cords or gland-like structures are seen within myxoid stroma**

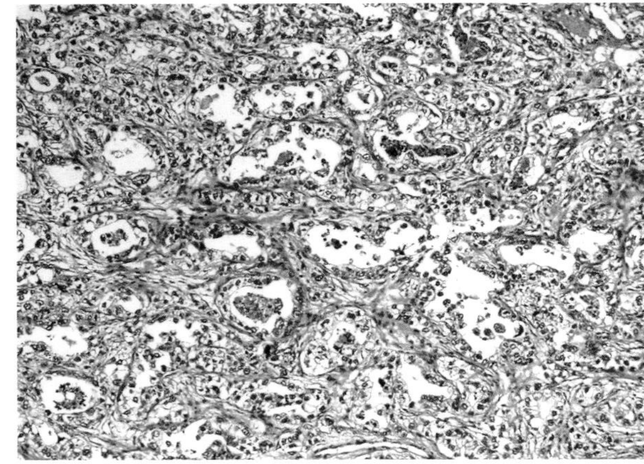

Fig. 16.12
Yolk sac tumor showing pronounced glandular pattern. **The glands are lined by large atypical cells with large hyperchromatic nuclei**

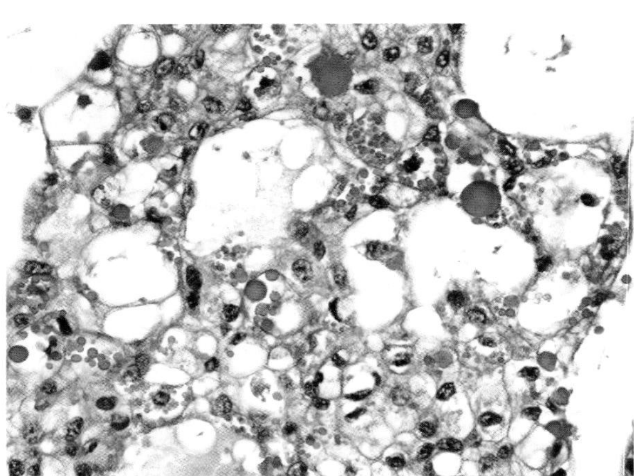

Fig. 16.11
Yolk sac tumor. **Numerous round hyaline globules are present inside the cells. Larger precipitates of this material are seen at the *top***

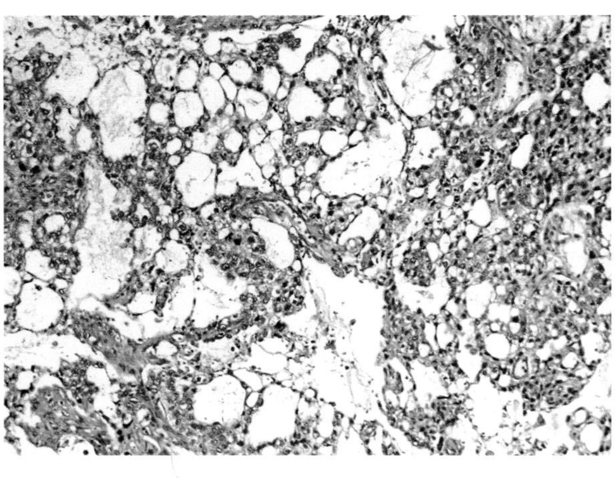

Fig. 16.13
Yolk sac tumor. **The tumor displays a macrocystic and microcystic patterns**

(*Fig. 16.9*). The microcystic or reticular pattern (*Fig. 16.13*) and myxomatous pattern (*Fig. 16.10*) are composed of a loose vacuolated network with small cystic spaces or microcysts forming a honeycomb pattern. The microcysts are lined by flat, pleomorphic, mesothelial-like cells with large hyperchromatic or vesicular nuclei that show brisk mitotic activity. There is usually some variation in the size of the cysts (*Fig. 16.13*). In the underlying capillary spaces, hematopoiesis may be seen. The vacuolated network may contain pale, PAS-positive, mucinous material forming small lakes or precipitates as well as small, round, brightly eosinophilic, PAS-positive, diastase-resistant globules or droplets. These globules are also found within the cytoplasm of the tumor cells (*Fig. 16.11*). Areas composed of fine, loose myxomatous tissue containing alveolar spaces, occasional gland-like structures lined by cuboidal epithelium, and small cellular aggregates, often merging with the microcystic or other patterns, are also present. The loose myxomatous pattern

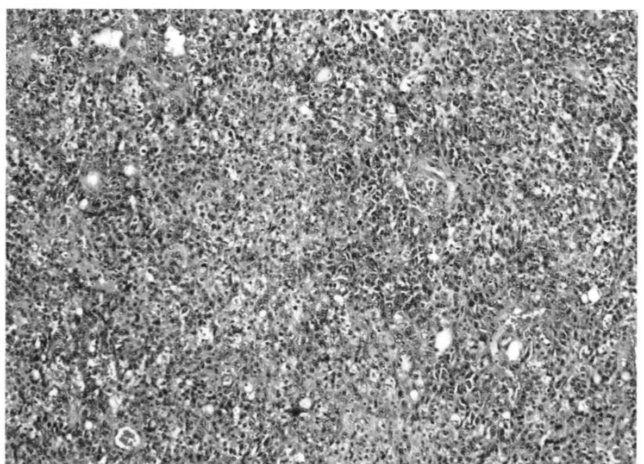

■ Fig. 16.14
Yolk sac tumor. **The tumor has a solid pattern**

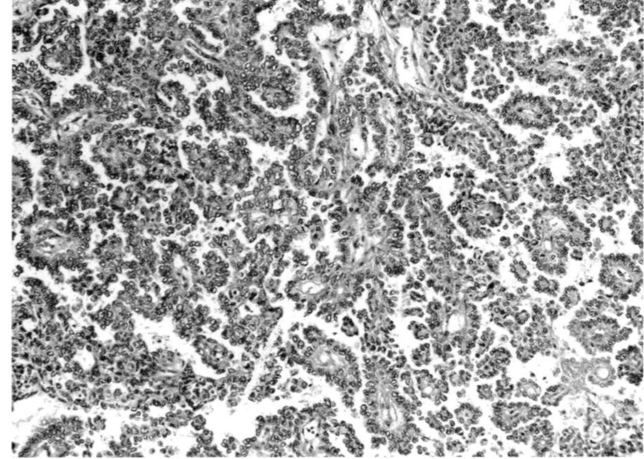

■ Fig. 16.15
Yolk sac tumor. **The tumor displays a pronounced papillary pattern**

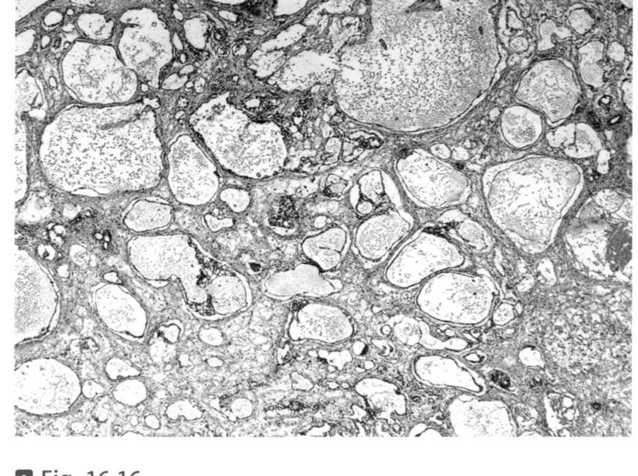

■ Fig. 16.16
Yolk sac tumor, polyvesicular vitelline pattern. **The tumor is composed of numerous small vesicles surrounded by connective tissue**

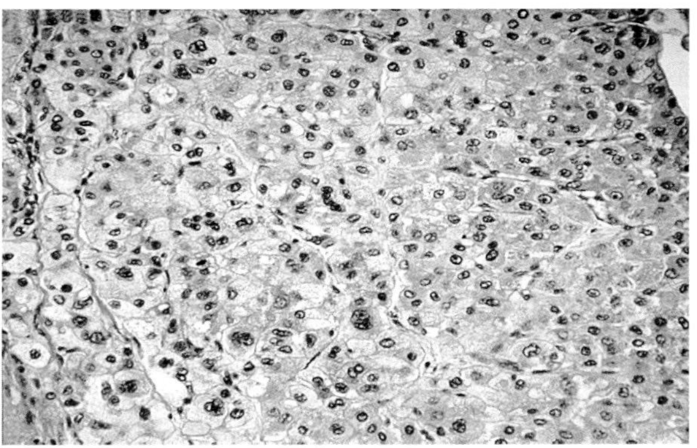

■ Fig. 16.17
Yolk sac tumor, hepatoid pattern. **The tumor is composed of solid aggregates or cords of polygonal cells with even or granular eosinophilic cytoplasm resembling hepatocytes**

was considered to be analogous to the *magma reticulare* or the extraembryonic mesoderm of the exocoelom, and the presence of this pattern led to the recognition of the mesoblastic nature of this tumor [233].

The endodermal sinus pattern (➋ *Fig. 16.9*) is composed of perivascular formations, consisting of a narrow band of connective tissue with a capillary blood vessel in the center and lined by a layer of cuboidal or low columnar embryonal epithelial-like cells. The cells have large, slightly vesicular nuclei, prominent nucleoli, and show mitotic activity. The surrounding capsular sinusoid space is lined by a single layer of flat cells with prominent hyperchromatic nuclei. These characteristic perivascular formations are said to recapitulate the so-called endodermal sinuses [234, 235] that, although not conspicuous in the human placenta, are well-defined embryologic structures in the rat placenta. These structures are also known as sinuses of Duval, Schiller–Duval bodies, or glomerulus-like structures and resemble superficially immature renal glomeruli. When sectioned longitudinally, the perivascular structures consist of a central connective tissue core containing a longitudinal vessel surrounded by epithelial-like cells that often form small papillary formations projecting into the surrounding capsular sinusoid space.

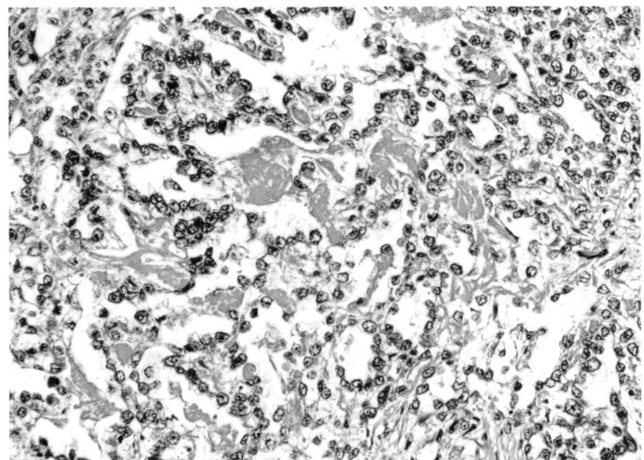

Fig. 16.18
Yolk sac tumor. **Basement membrane material is frequently observed in these tumors**

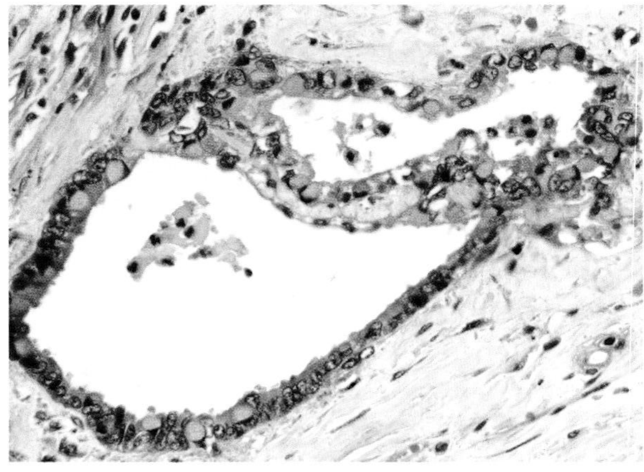

Fig. 16.19
Yolk sac tumor, endodermal (intestinal) pattern. **The cells show abundant goblet cells**

The presence of these perivascular formations or Schiller–Duval bodies can be considered diagnostic of yolk sac tumor, but in some tumors they may be poorly represented, somewhat atypical, or absent. Although the tumor should always be examined carefully and searched to identify these structures, their absence does not preclude the diagnosis, if the appearances of the tumor are typical in all other respects. Apart from the presence of the perivascular structures, this pattern consists of a complicated labyrinth of communicating cavities and channels. In addition, there are papillary processes and blood vessels surrounded by narrow connective tissue cores and epithelial-like cells radiating into the

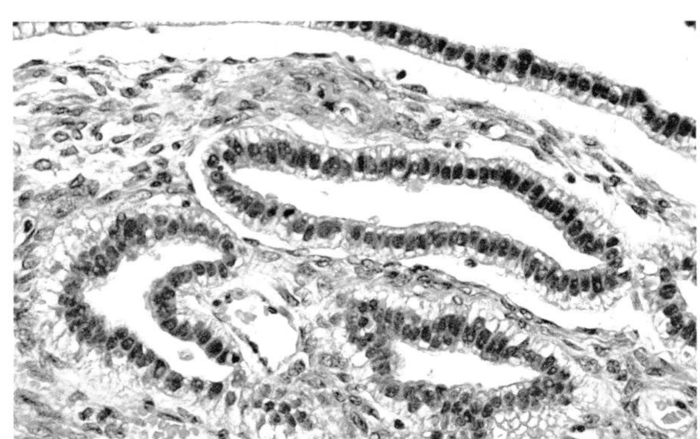

Fig. 16.20
Yolk sac tumor, endodermal pattern. **The so-called endometrioid variant resembles secretory endometrial adenocarcinoma**

surrounding stroma, resembling the typical perivascular formations but differing from them by the absence of the sinusoid space.

The solid pattern (*Fig. 16.14*) is composed of aggregates of small epithelial-like polygonal cells with clear cytoplasm and large vesicular or pyknotic nuclei with prominent nucleoli and exhibits brisk mitotic activity. The tumor cells in the solid aggregates may resemble dysgerminoma cells, but they usually show greater pleomorphism and presence of at least occasional microcysts. The presence of the latter helps differentiate between these two entities. The presence of other patterns of yolk sac tumor is also helpful in this respect, as is diffuse or focal staining for AFP and uniformly positive staining for low molecular weight cytokeratin, which are observed in yolk sac tumor and not in dysgerminoma.

The alveolar–glandular pattern (*Figs. 16.12*) is composed of alveolar, gland-like, or larger cystic spaces and cavities lined by flat or cuboidal epithelial-like cells with large, prominent nuclei and surrounded by myxomatous stroma or cellular aggregates. Some of these spaces may be lined by more than one layer of cells, and sometimes the lining cells form small papillary projections protruding into the lumen. The layer of cells lining these spaces may be continuous with the lining of the perivascular sinusoid spaces [234]. Gland-like formations lined by columnar or cuboidal epithelial-like cells may be seen and in some tumors may be prominent and may form bizarre patterns. The macrocystic pattern is observed when yolk sac tumor exhibits larger cysts in contrast to microcysts or alveolar spaces. In some tumors, this pattern may predominate.

The papillary pattern (➋ *Fig. 16.15*) is composed of papillary structures consisting of connective tissue cores lined by epithelial-like cells showing a considerable degree of cellular and nuclear pleomorphism and mitotic activity. The connective tissue may show variable hyalinization. This pattern may be the predominant pattern within a tumor.

The polyvesicular vitelline pattern [235] is composed of numerous cysts or vesicles surrounded by compact connective tissue stroma, which may vary from dense to loose (➋ *Fig. 16.16*). The vesicles are lined partly by columnar or cuboidal epithelial cells, frequently showing basal or paraluminal vacuolation, and partly by flat mesothelial-like cells. The individual vesicles or cysts vary in size and shape. The wall of the cyst may show a constriction dividing the part lined by the mesothelial cells from that lined by the columnar or cuboidal epithelium. This division was considered to reflect the embryologic conversion of the primary yolk sac into the secondary yolk sac [235]. Occasionally, the whole tumor may exhibit the polyvesicular vitelline pattern; such tumors have been designated as polyvesicular vitelline tumors [235].

The eosinophilic, hyaline droplets may be present either within the tumor cells or outside them; they may be numerous and prominent in some tumors (➋ *Fig. 16.11*). The droplets may be observed in tumors exhibiting all the histologic patterns described, and their identification is a helpful diagnostic feature. However, their presence is not diagnostic of yolk sac tumor because they are observed in many malignant, often poorly differentiated neoplasms, particularly clear cell carcinoma. The droplets are considered to be secreted by the tumor cells and accumulate within the cytoplasm. As the amount of secretion increases, the cell becomes distended and ruptures, discharging its contents into the surrounding tissue. Previously, these globules in yolk sac tumors have been shown by immunohistochemical techniques to contain AFP [82, 96, 191]. Other globules may contain alpha$_1$-antitrypsin and other plasma proteins such as transferrin [82, 191, 240].

The hepatoid pattern is composed of cells with eosinophilic, uniform, or granular cytoplasm, showing a solid pattern and considerable resemblance to hepatocytes. Such collections of hepatocyte-like cells are not infrequently observed in yolk sac tumors; however, if these cells are the dominant population, the neoplasm is designated "hepatoid yolk sac tumor" [154] (➋ *Fig. 16.17*). These tumors are infrequently admixed with other histologic patterns of yolk sac tumor or other neoplastic germ cell elements, and this, together with the rarity of the tumor, may cause diagnostic problems. The presence of a solid ovarian tumor composed of hepatocyte-like cells surrounded by connective tissue and forming solid aggregates, cords, or clusters and associated with elevated serum AFP in a young patient would strongly favor a diagnosis of yolk sac tumor with a hepatoid pattern. It should be noted that this variant also shows immunohistochemical expression of hepatocyte paraffin 1, similar to primary ovarian hepatoid carcinoma and metastatic hepatocellular carcinoma involving the ovary [152].

The presence of hyaline, PAS-positive material forming bands or connective tissue cores surrounded by tumor cells is not an infrequent finding in yolk sac tumor; in some tumors, it may be a prominent feature, with the tumor cells resting on and surrounding the bands of hyaline material (➋ *Fig. 16.18*). When this material is deposited in linear bands in stroma, other authors have designated this the "parietal pattern" of yolk sac tumor [185]. There may be an increased amount of the eosinophilic, PAS-positive globules described here in the vicinity of the hyaline bands, suggesting a relationship between them and a possibility of common origin [235].

Although scattered primitive endodermal glands are not uncommon in yolk sac tumors, the glandular or primitive endodermal (intestinal) pattern, in which the tumor is composed entirely of primitive endodermal glands, is encountered only occasionally [40] (➋ *Fig. 16.19*). This pattern has been designated as "glandular (intestinal) yolk sac tumor." The tumor in these cases is composed of nests or collections of primitive endodermal glands surrounded by connective tissue, which varies from loose and edematous to dense and hyalinized. The degree of differentiation varies from primitive to relatively well differentiated. The glands may contain inspissated secretion within the lumen, and the tumor may resemble a mucin-secreting adenocarcinoma. Ultrastructurally, the nuclei are large and show prominent nucleolonema, whereas the cytoplasm contains many ribosomes, rough endoplasmic reticulum, and mitochondria. Dense amorphous intracellular material is also present. Yolk sac tumors showing this pattern have been associated with very high serum levels of AFP [40]. It is of interest that the only tumor that was diploid in a series of 20 yolk sac tumors was a tumor of the pure glandular (primitive intestinal) type, whereas all the other tumors were aneuploid [93].

The presence of primitive endodermal glandular tissue, lobular or nest-like pattern, and high levels of serum AFP differentiate this type of yolk sac tumor from mucinous tumors of the ovary. A variant of this pattern composed of primitive glands of various sizes lined by tall columnar or cuboid cells with basophilic or clear cytoplasm containing subnuclear vacuoles resembling

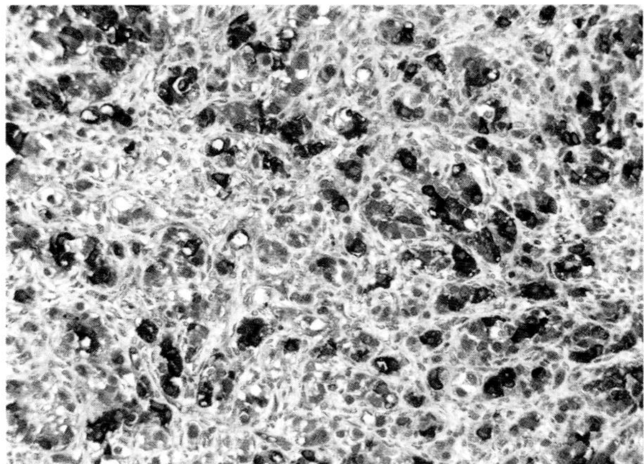

Fig. 16.21
Yolk sac tumor. **The tumor shows uniform strongly positive staining for AFP**

secretory endometrial carcinoma, so-called endometrioid variant (Fig. 16.20), has been described [39]. This variant may be seen in pure form, showing a pronounced glandular or villoglandular pattern, or may be composed of glands surrounded by fibrous or densely cellular stroma [39]. Elevated serum levels of AFP and immunohistochemical demonstration of AFP within the tumor cells confirm the diagnosis of yolk sac tumor (Fig. 16.21).

Occasionally, yolk sac tumor may exhibit a greater degree of cellular and nuclear pleomorphism with some giant cells, usually mononucleated, but sometimes multinucleated. This picture may be seen in association with the solid, papillary, and glandular–alveolar patterns. The pleomorphic cells show variable immunohistochemical staining for AFP, and the absence of hCG confirms that the giant cells are not trophoblastic in origin but are part of a yolk sac tumor.

Immunohistochemical Features and Differential Diagnosis

Yolk sac tumor may be confused with clear cell and endometrioid carcinomas, embryonal carcinoma, and dysgerminoma. Clear cell carcinoma shows more regular tubular patterns, lacks the honeycomb network composed of microcysts, and has papillary frond-like projections that are often lined by clear or hobnail cells. The typical perivascular formations, endodermal sinuses, or Schiller–Duval bodies present in yolk sac tumor are absent. The epithelial cells lining the tubules are cuboidal with clear cytoplasm or are hobnail with nuclei bulging into the lumen. Areas composed of large polygonal cells with clear cytoplasm and small, dark, uniform, centrally situated nuclei resembling those of renal carcinoma are present. When clear cell carcinoma is composed entirely of tubules or spaces, confusion may arise with the polyvesicular vitelline pattern of yolk sac tumor. However, the epithelial lining in clear cell carcinoma is usually composed of hobnail cells and not of the two types of epithelia in the vesicles comprising the polyvesicular vitelline pattern. The cystic spaces are more tubular and less vesicle-like. Clear cell carcinoma shows diffuse immunohistochemical expression of CK7 and EMA and is usually negative for AFP while yolk sac tumor typically shows the opposite immunoprofile [54, 157]. Glypican-3 is usually diffusely expressed in yolk sac tumor, whereas clear cell carcinoma is either negative or focally positive; [54] however, the extent of expression of this marker can overlap between both tumors [107]. SALL4 is highly sensitive and specific for primitive germ cell tumors, including yolk sac tumor [32].

The endometrioid-like glandular variant of yolk sac tumor can simulate endometrioid carcinomas with secretory differentiation. However, women with yolk sac tumor are typically younger and have an elevated serum AFP level while a subset of patients with endometrioid carcinoma has endometriosis in the ipsilateral ovary or elsewhere in the pelvic cavity. Other admixed classic patterns of yolk sac tumor and endometrioid carcinoma, as well as hyaline globules in the former and squamous differentiation in the latter, help support either diagnosis. Demonstrating immunohistochemical expression of AFP in yolk sac tumor and CK7 and EMA in endometrioid carcinoma is also useful [157]. Estrogen and progesterone receptors are not detected in yolk sac tumors [92], but diffuse expression of these markers is common in endometrioid carcinomas [261]. It should be noted, however, that rare cases of mixed yolk sac tumor and endometrioid carcinoma have been reported [125].

The embryonal carcinoma, which is uncommon in the ovary [82, 97, 234], lacks the specific patterns observed in the yolk sac tumor. In its undifferentiated form, it is composed of aggregates of primitive embryonal cells. The tumor cells are frequently larger than those seen in the solid cellular aggregates in yolk sac tumor. The cytoplasm is more granular, there is more marked cellular and nuclear pleomorphism, and the nucleoli are more prominent. Even when the tumor is better differentiated, with the embryonal cells forming cords, tubules, or papillae and lining clefts or spaces, it still lacks the typical patterns associated with yolk sac tumor.

Yolk sac tumor with a solid pattern may be confused with dysgerminoma. The cells of dysgerminoma are usually more uniform, lack microcysts, and are usually associated with lymphocytic and granulomatous reactions. The cells of yolk sac tumor are uniformly low molecular weight cytokeratin positive [119, 120]. The presence of this feature as well as positive staining for AFP and lack of expression of CD117 and OCT-4 differentiate between yolk sac tumor and dysgerminoma, in which the latter shows only occasional cytokeratin-positive cells.

Yolk sac tumor, because of its cystic pattern and the presence of numerous small blood vessels, has been confused with vascular tumors, but careful examination reveals that the pattern is more cystic, and a vascular tumor can be excluded with the use of appropriate immunohistochemical stains. It should be pointed out that yolk sac tumor elements may show hematopoiesis and are sometimes intimately associated with immature vascular tissue in some mixed germ cell tumors; this may also contribute to diagnostic problems. Confusion may arise occasionally, with some Sertoli–Leydig cell tumors showing a retiform pattern, especially when the latter are associated with elevated serum levels of AFP [215, 257]. The presence of more marked cellular and nuclear pleomorphism, brisk mitotic activity, and other histologic patterns observed in yolk sac tumor (as well as their absence in Sertoli–Leydig cell tumors) aid in the differential diagnosis. Immunohistochemical expression of inhibin further confirms the diagnosis of Sertoli–Leydig cell tumor.

Occasionally, confusion may arise with juvenile granulosa cell tumor when it presents with small vesicle-like collections of cells surrounded by connective tissue stroma that simulate the vesicles seen in polyvesicular vitelline yolk sac tumor. Presence of solid nests typical of juvenile granulosa cell tumor, absence of the various patterns of yolk sac tumor, absence of immunohistochemical staining for AFP, immunohistochemical expression of inhibin, and a lack of elevated serum levels of AFP indicate that the tumor is a juvenile granulosa cell tumor.

Clinical Behavior and Treatment

Yolk sac tumor is highly malignant, metastasizing early and invading surrounding structures and organs. Local invasion and intra-coelomic spread frequently lead to extensive involvement of the abdominal cavity. Yolk sac tumor metastasizes first via the lymphatic system to the para-aortic and common iliac lymph nodes and then to the mediastinal and supraclavicular lymph nodes. Hematogenous spread occurs later, with metastases found in the lungs, liver, and other organs. The tumor is locally aggressive, and spread beyond the ovary is observed in a number of patients at diagnosis [65, 82, 96]. Recurrences in the pelvis are frequent, even when the tumor and the affected adnexa have been excised completely [82, 96]. Such recurrences usually appear within a few weeks or months after excision of the primary tumor.

Until the advent of efficacious combination chemotherapy, the treatment of patients with yolk sac tumor was very disappointing. The treatment was primarily surgical [96, 234]. Extensive surgery did not improve prognosis [96, 234]. The few long-term survivors in the past had tumors confined to the ovary, and most were treated by unilateral adnexectomy [96, 234]. Since then, there has been marked improvement in prognosis with conservative surgery (unilateral salpingo-oophorectomy) and adjuvant multiagent combination chemotherapy [64, 140]. The combination chemotherapy originally used was dactinomycin, vincristine, and cyclophosphamide or dactinomycin, 5-fluorouracil, and cyclophosphamide. Although this therapy proved to be effective in many cases, recurrences were still frequent.

The introduction of a combination of cisplatin, bleomycin, and vinblastine, which has been superseded by less toxic cisplatin, etoposide (VP 16), and bleomycin (BEP) in combination, has been found to be much more effective and has produced remissions in patients with advanced-stage disease and in patients in whom other combinations of multiagent chemotherapy have failed [64, 140]. This combination chemotherapy has revolutionized the treatment of patients with yolk sac tumor. Complete cure for all stages is more than 80% [64, 140]. The occasional cases of pure hepatoid and glandular (primitive intestinal) yolk sac tumor show a less satisfactory response to combination chemotherapy and are therefore associated with poorer prognosis [39, 40, 154].

Serum AFP determination is useful diagnostically and in monitoring therapy. It should be noted, however, that a normal result may not always indicate the absence of active disease but only the absence of the tumor element associated with AFP synthesis. Preoperatively, if the tumor contains yolk sac tumor elements, considerable amounts of AFP can be detected in the serum. AFP levels fall postoperatively and, if there are no metastases, reach normal levels within 4–6 weeks, depending on the preoperative serum AFP level. Serum alpha$_1$-antitrypsin levels can also be used to monitor disease activity, but it is inferior to AFP [224].

Beta-hCG is normal in patients with yolk sac tumor. Carcinoembryonic antigen (CEA) has also been studied in patients with germ cell neoplasms and has been found to be of no value as a tumor marker in this group of patients [225].

Embryonal Carcinoma

The term embryonal carcinoma in this text includes only ovarian neoplasms showing histologic appearances resembling those observed in embryonal carcinomas occurring in the testis of adults. Dixon and Moore [50] consider embryonal carcinoma as both a morphologic and a conceptual entity, and this interpretation is being followed. Embryonal carcinoma is considered to be the least differentiated form of germ cell tumor, which may differentiate either to somatic (teratomatous tumors of various degrees of differentiation) or extraembryonal structures, forming yolk sac or vitelline (yolk sac tumor) or trophoblastic structures (choriocarcinoma) (➋ *Fig. 16.1*). Although ovarian embryonal carcinoma [82, 97] shows similar appearances and is considered to be homologous with its testicular counterpart, it is uncommon as a component of mixed germ cell tumors and rare as a pure entity. However, tumors showing this histologic pattern are relatively frequent in the testis. The reason for this difference is unknown. Ovarian embryonal carcinoma is usually combined with other neoplastic germ cell elements, most frequently yolk sac tumor, and forms a part of a mixed germ cell tumor [82, 98, 226]. Embryonal carcinoma occasionally has been observed in association with gonadoblastoma [182, 211, 216].

Clinical Features

The age, clinical presentation, and findings of embryonal carcinoma are similar to those observed in patients with other malignant germ cell neoplasms, with the tumor almost always occurring in children and young adults [82, 97, 226].

Embryonal carcinoma may produce AFP, even when it is not combined with yolk sac tumor, but the serum AFP levels in such cases are only slightly elevated. When embryonal carcinoma contains syncytiotrophoblastic giant cells, as is often the case, or is combined with choriocarcinoma, it produces hCG and is associated with endocrine manifestations, such as isosexual precocious puberty in children and abnormal vaginal bleeding in adults [97]. A positive pregnancy test is found in almost all such patients.

Gross Features

Because embryonal carcinoma usually is a component of mixed germ cell tumors, the appearances of the tumor vary according to the type and amount of the different components present. On sectioning, the embryonal carcinomatous component is solid, gray-white, and slightly granular, with foci of necrosis and hemorrhage in the larger tumors.

Microscopic Features

In its most primitive and undifferentiated form, embryonal carcinoma is composed of solid aggregates of epithelial-like, medium to large, polygonal or ovoid cells containing an ample amount of somewhat pale eosinophilic granular cytoplasm, with poorly defined cytoplasmic borders, frequently forming a syncytial arrangement (➋ *Figs. 16.22*–16.24). The cells have a large, prominent, centrally situated, and somewhat irregular vesicular or hyperchromatic nucleus with a fine nuclear membrane and frequently more than one nucleolus. Mitotic activity is usually brisk, and abnormal mitoses are frequently seen. Pleomorphism is usually marked. Giant cells and multinucleated cells may be seen.

In the better differentiated tumors, the cells, apart from forming solid areas, also tend to line clefts and spaces and form papillae. The cells appear more epithelial than those of the more undifferentiated type, being more cuboidal or columnar in shape. Although there is

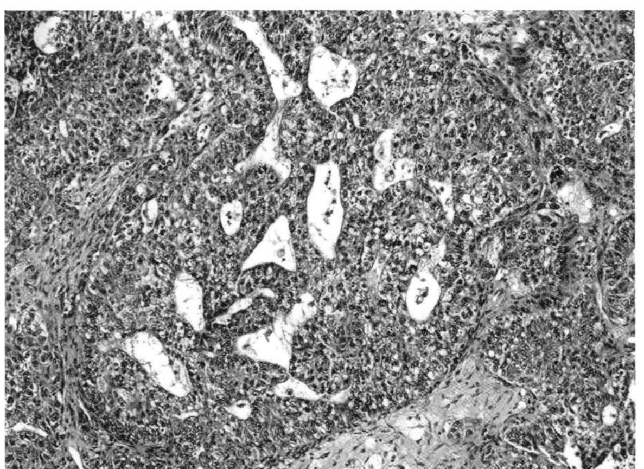

Fig. 16.22
Embryonal carcinoma. **The tumor shows pseudoglandular and solid patterns**

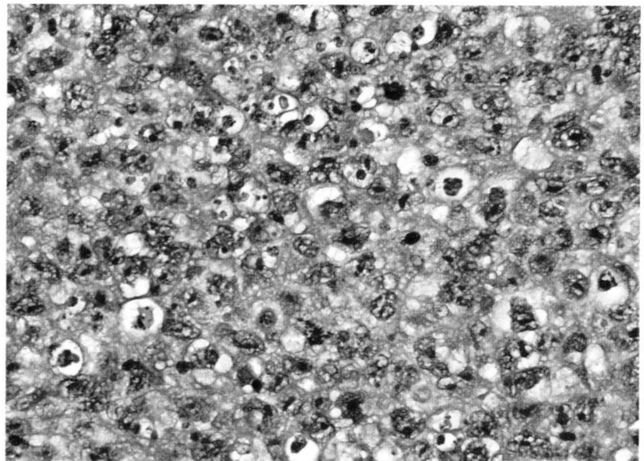

Fig. 16.23
Embryonal carcinoma. **The tumor cells display more nuclear pleomorphism and overlapping of nuclei compared with dysgerminoma**

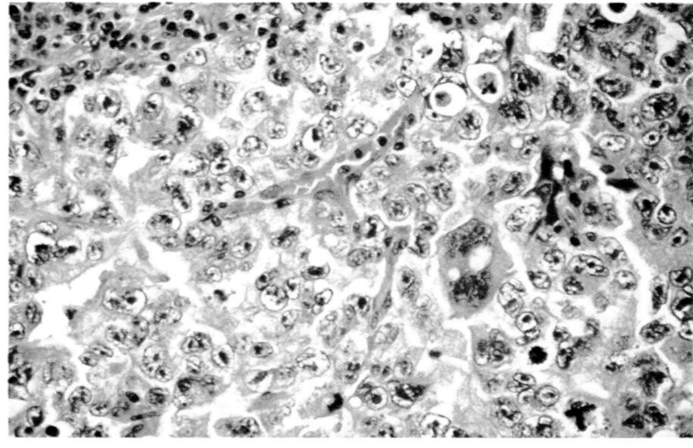

Fig. 16.24
Embryonal carcinoma. **The tumor shows a solid pattern and a syncytiotrophoblastic giant cell. Note the characteristic nuclei of embryonal carcinoma**

a suggestion of glandular differentiation, true gland formation is absent. The papillae are composed of solid collections of cells or may contain a cystic space or a small vessel surrounded by tumor cells. They must be differentiated from perivascular formations observed in yolk sac tumor. Very primitive mesenchymal tissue may be present in conjunction with the epithelial-like component. Syncytiotrophoblastic giant cells immediately adjacent to aggregates of embryonal carcinoma cells or lying isolated in the stroma are frequently found. Foci of necrosis and hemorrhage are also frequent.

Immunohistochemical Features and Differential Diagnosis

Embryonal carcinoma may be present in the form of small solid aggregates or pseudoglandular or cleft-like formations surrounded by better-differentiated malignant teratomatous elements showing somatic differentiation. It may coexist with other neoplastic germ cell elements, such as yolk sac tumor, immature or mature teratoma, choriocarcinoma, polyembryoma, or dysgerminoma. Differentiation from dysgerminoma is important because of a totally different prognosis and response to treatment. It is usually the solid primitive type of embryonal carcinoma that is more likely to be confused with dysgerminoma, but the presence of clefts, alveoli, or cell-lined spaces militates against the diagnosis of dysgerminoma.

The cells of embryonal carcinoma are usually larger and show much more pleomorphism. Mitotic activity is usually more prominent, and bizarre mitoses are more frequent. The nuclear membrane is less sharp and the nuclei are more irregular, larger, and usually contain more than one dark hyperchromatic nucleolus, in contrast with the rounded, prominent, usually single, and frequently eosinophilic nucleolus of dysgerminoma. The presence of connective tissue stroma infiltrated by lymphocytes and at times a granulomatous reaction is a prominent feature of dysgerminoma. These features usually are absent in embryonal carcinoma. Embryonal carcinoma shows immunohistochemical expression of cytokeratin, whereas most dysgerminomas are negative. In contrast, dysgerminoma expresses CD117, which is negative in embryonal carcinoma. In addition, some embryonal carcinomas stain for AFP, in contrast to dysgerminomas, which are invariably negative. Most embryonal carcinomas stain for CD30 (*Fig. 16.25*), whereas only occasional dysgerminomas are CD30-positive. Recently, OCT-4 has been found to be consistently positive in embryonal carcinoma, but this marker is also expressed in dysgerminoma. SALL4 is highly sensitive and specific for primitive germ cell tumors, including embryonal carcinoma [32].

Clinical Behavior and Treatment

Embryonal carcinoma of the ovary is a highly malignant neoplasm. It is aggressive locally, spreads extensively in the abdominal cavity, and metastasizes early. The metastatic spread is similar to that of other malignant germ cell neoplasms, taking place first via the lymphatics and later by hematogenous spread. The primary treatment of embryonal carcinoma is unilateral salpingo-oophorectomy and

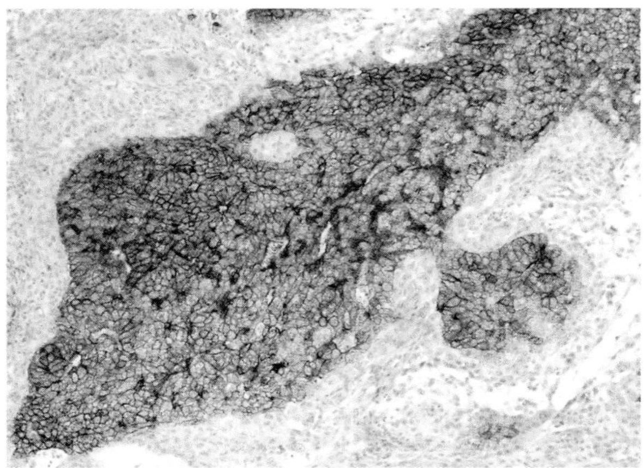

Fig. 16.25
Embryonal carcinoma. **Diffuse expression of CD30**

chemotherapy. The response to combination chemotherapy using bleomycin, vinblastine, and cisplatin or, preferably, cisplatin, etoposide (VP 16), and bleomycin [64, 140] is similar to that observed in patients with embryonal carcinoma of the testis.

Polyembryoma

General Features

Polyembryoma is a rare ovarian germ cell neoplasm composed of numerous embryoid bodies resembling morphologically normal presomite embryos [19, 89, 207]. Similar homologous neoplasms occur more frequently in the human testis [19, 55], although pure polyembryoma is very rare. In all ovarian cases, the polyembryoma was associated with other neoplastic germ cell elements, mainly immature or mature teratoma [19, 89, 192, 207]. All these tumors occurred in young patients or in patients in the reproductive age group [19, 89, 192, 207]; the oldest patient was 38 years old [192]. The clinical findings are similar to those observed in patients with other malignant germ cell neoplasms of the ovary. It should be noted that polyembryoma is not the same entity as "diffuse embryoma," which is a form of mixed germ cell tumor composed of yolk sac tumor and embryonal carcinoma with a unique admixture of both components [185].

Histogenesis

There are conflicting views of the origin of embryoid bodies. It has been suggested that they arise by parthenogenic development from primitive germ cells present in an immature (malignant) teratoma [111, 145, 192]. Other investigators question this view as well as the entire concept that embryoid bodies bear a close similarity to early human embryos because embryoid bodies never appear to develop beyond the 18-day stage [19]. They consider that embryoid bodies probably develop transiently by bizarre differentiation, possibly in response to local release of factors in malignant teratomas of the gonads.

Another view that has been advanced accepts the morphologic similarities between the early embryo and the embryoid bodies but disputes their parthenogenic origin [55, 147, 201]. It maintains that embryoid bodies are formed after initiation of teratogenesis, most likely from multipotential malignant embryonal cells present in a tumor and not directly from germ cells [202]. This concept is supported by the observations of the development of embryoid bodies from undifferentiated embryonal cells in strain 129 mice. The tumor, a teratoma that had been serially transplanted for many years, was considered to be devoid of germ cells [147, 201]. These findings are in accordance with the view that embryoid bodies probably persist only transiently within the tumor, and while new embryoid bodies are being formed others lose their identity and their multipotential cells undergo further differentiation [55]. Although the origin and development of embryoid bodies are still a matter of dispute, the view that they originate from multipotential malignant embryonal cells, which is supported by experimental observations [147, 201], is most favored at present.

Gross Features

Polyembryoma is usually unilateral. Macroscopically, the tumor resembles other malignant germ cell tumors, varying in size from 9.5 cm [19] to tumors filling almost the whole abdominal cavity and invading the surrounding structures [192]. The tumor is usually solid and contains hemorrhagic and necrotic areas.

Microscopic and Immunohistochemical Features

Polyembryoma is composed of numerous embryoid bodies, and the better-differentiated ones are composed of structures resembling an embryonic disk, amniotic cavity, and yolk sac surrounded by primitive extraembryonic mesenchyme (*Fig. 16.26*). Sometimes trophoblastic

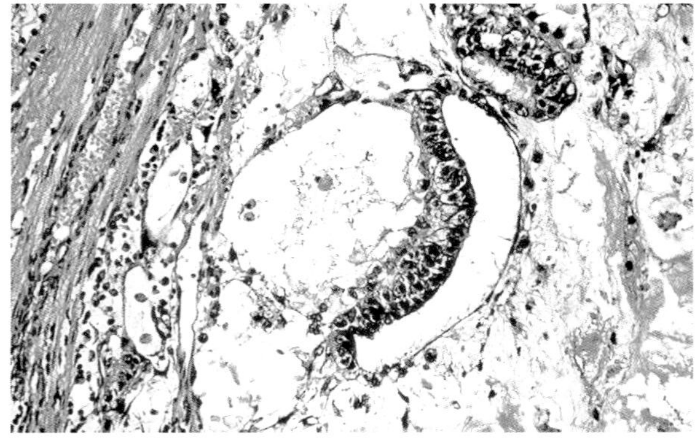

Fig. 16.26
Polyembryoma. **The embryoid body shows amniotic cavity (*right*), embryonic disk (*center*), and atypical yolk sac (*left*)**

differentiation may be seen in the vicinity of the embryoid body. When the embryoid bodies are less well formed, they are composed of a medullary plate and amnion associated with a blastocystic space or with extraembryonic mesenchyme. They may have two or more amniotic cavities and share a single yolk sac cavity or vice versa. There may be a considerable disproportion between the two cavities, and the cavities may be malformed. There also may be considerable variation in size between the different embryoid bodies; some may be more primitive and others appear to be better developed.

Some embryoid bodies may be malformed and show bizarre appearances. None of the embryoid bodies appear to have developed beyond the 18-day stage. The embryonic disk of a typical embryoid body is lined on one side by cuboidal epithelial cells of uniform size, resembling endoderm, and on the other by tall columnar epithelium, resembling ectoderm. The latter merges with low cuboidal epithelium lining the rest of the cavity, which resembles the amnion. The cavity resembling the yolk sac is on the opposite side of the embryonic disk from the amnion (*Fig. 16.26*). The embryoid bodies are surrounded by extraembryonic mesenchyme, which is composed of either closely or more loosely packed spindle-shaped cells of regular appearance and showing occasional mitotic figures. Loose myxomatous areas may be present.

Occasionally, embryoid bodies resemble earlier developmental stages, mainly the blastocyst and morula stage and form numerous round or oval structures. In some tumors this pattern may predominate, although occasional fully developed embryoid bodies may be seen [89]. Teratomatous structures in various stages of differentiation are frequently seen interspersed with the embryoid bodies. In one reported case [19], hCG and human placental lactogen were demonstrated within syncytiotrophoblastic cells that were present in the vicinity of the embryoid bodies. Cytotrophoblastic cells were not identified in this tumor. In another reported case, there was elevation of serum AFP and hCG. AFP was demonstrated by immunohistochemistry within the cells lining the yolk sac cavities and hCG within the syncytiotrophoblastic giant cells that were present in the vicinity of the embryoid bodies [207].

Clinical Behavior and Treatment

Polyembryoma is a highly malignant germ cell neoplasm. In most cases, it has been associated with invasion of adjacent structures and extensive metastases, which were mainly confined to the abdominal cavity [192].

The primary treatment of polyembryoma is surgical, and because the tumor is usually unilateral unless there is spread beyond the ovary, excision of the tumor and the adjoining adnexa is the treatment of choice. Polyembryoma responds to the combination chemotherapy used in treatment of malignant germ cell tumors [64, 207].

One patient with a relatively small mobile tumor, absence of capsular penetration, and no evidence of metastases survived more than 5 years [19]. Another patient was alive and free of disease for more than 12 years after excision of the affected adnexa and excision of intra-abdominal metastases composed of grade 1 immature teratoma [89]. A third patient was well and disease-free 6 months after diagnosis [207]. Before the introduction of effective combination chemotherapy, most patients with polyembryoma died of their disease.

Choriocarcinoma

General Features

Pure ovarian choriocarcinoma of germ cell origin is a rare neoplasm [81, 82, 185, 247], and even the presence of choriocarcinomatous elements admixed with other neoplastic germ cell elements is uncommon. In most cases, the tumor is admixed with other neoplastic germ cell elements, and their presence is diagnostic of non-gestational choriocarcinoma, except for the remote possibility of the tumor being a gestational choriocarcinoma metastatic to an ovarian germ cell tumor. The presence of other neoplastic germ cell elements is a particularly helpful diagnostic feature in postmenarchal patients in whom exclusion of gestational origin of the tumor may be difficult. In view of this, non-gestational choriocarcinoma may be diagnosed with confidence in postmenarchal patients and not only in young children, as had been considered earlier. A small number of ovarian germ cell tumors containing choriocarcinoma have been reported [81, 112, 247]. The tumor occurs in children and young adults. In some series, 50% of cases occurred in children who had not reached puberty [112]. This high frequency in children may stem from the reluctance of making the diagnosis in adults. Detection of paternal DNA has been successful in differentiating gestational and non-gestational choriocarcinoma. In two cases, DNA polymorphism analysis confirmed the non-gestational origin of the tumor [190, 241].

Histogenesis

Choriocarcinoma of the ovary may originate in three different ways: (1) as a primary gestational choriocarcinoma associated with ovarian pregnancy, (2) as metastatic choriocarcinoma from a primary gestational choriocarcinoma arising in other parts of the genital tract, mainly the uterus, and (3) as a germ cell tumor differentiating in the direction of trophoblastic structures, usually admixed with other neoplastic germ cell elements. In each case, it is important to ascertain the mode of origin of the tumor because this has important therapeutic and prognostic implications. Alternatively, choriocarcinoma of the ovary may be divided into two broad groups: (1) gestational choriocarcinoma encompassing the first two groups mentioned and (2) non-gestational choriocarcinoma, a germ cell tumor differentiation toward trophoblastic structures. As this chapter is concerned solely with germ cell tumors, only the non-gestational choriocarcinoma is discussed here.

Clinical Features

The clinical findings in patients with ovarian non-gestational choriocarcinoma are similar to those observed in patients with other malignant ovarian germ cell neoplasms, except that they may be modified by the endocrine activity of the tumor, which secretes hCG. This effect is particularly noticeable in prepubertal children who show evidence of isosexual precocious puberty, with mammary development, growth of pubic and axillary hair, and uterine bleeding. Adult patients may have signs of ectopic pregnancy. Very occasionally, the tumor may cause symptoms of thyrotoxicosis, including a severe acute form. Because the non-gestational choriocarcinoma, resembling its gestational counterpart, is associated with increased production of hCG, determination of urinary or plasma hCG is a useful diagnostic test. Serum hCG levels are useful in monitoring response to therapy. It should be noted that normal levels of hCG do not exclude the presence of metastases or recurrences composed of other neoplastic germ cell elements.

Gross Features

The tumor typically is large, unilateral, solid, gray-white, and hemorrhagic. Necrosis may be evident. Because most of these tumors are composed of a combination of neoplastic germ cell elements, the appearances tend to vary according to the elements present in the tumor.

Microscopic and Immunohistochemical Features

Choriocarcinoma is composed of two cell populations, mononucleate and multinucleate trophoblast (*Fig. 16.27*). The former is composed of cytotrophoblast and intermediate trophoblast and contains medium-sized polygonal, round, or oval cells with clear cytoplasm and sharp borders. Some cells have centrally situated, small, round, and hyperchromatic nuclei, whereas others have larger vesicular nuclei containing nucleoli and showing

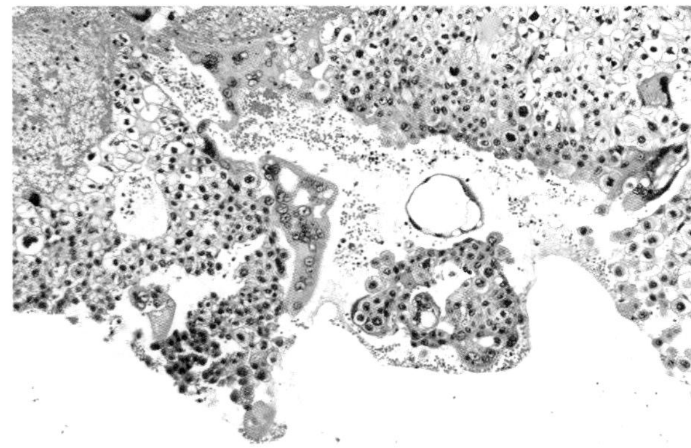

Fig. 16.27
Choriocarcinoma. **Cytotrophoblast composed of medium-sized cells are situated centrally; syncytiotrophoblast composed of very large multinucleated cells are situated peripherally**

brisk mitotic activity. The multinucleate population corresponds to syncytiotrophoblast, which is composed of large basophilic, vacuolated cells with irregular outlines, and although frequently elongated they may vary in shape. These cells contain multiple hyperchromatic nuclei, varying in shape and size. The cytotrophoblastic cells are usually disposed centrally within a tumor mass and are partly or completely surrounded by irregular collections or layers of the syncytiotrophoblastic cells.

There is a considerable variation in the pattern and in the ratio of the two components in different parts of the same tumor and in different tumors. The tumor cells form solid aggregates, nearly always associated with hemorrhage and necrosis. At times the tumor is limited to the periphery of the hemorrhagic mass. When the tumor is combined with other germ cell elements, the choriocarcinoma may form small nodules associated with hemorrhage and surrounded by other germ cell elements. The presence of other germ cell elements within the tumor is a frequent finding. As choriocarcinoma is often hemorrhagic, a careful search may be necessary to demonstrate the presence of choriocarcinomatous elements.

The cytotrophoblast is the more primitive element, and the syncytiotrophoblast is formed from it either directly or indirectly. The syncytiotrophoblast is the differentiated, nondividing, hormone-secreting component. These findings are supported by electron microscopic and immunohistochemical studies [148, 150]. Immunohistochemical staining for beta-hCG provides a useful confirmatory diagnostic method. Although intermediate trophoblastic cells may be seen occasionally in non-gestational choriocarcinomas, ovarian placental site trophoblastic tumors have been reported only rarely [8, 14, 41].

Clinical Behavior and Treatment

Non-gestational choriocarcinoma of the ovary is a highly malignant germ cell neoplasm. It invades adjacent structures, spreads widely throughout the abdominal cavity, and metastasizes via the lymphatics and the blood vessels. Although gestational choriocarcinoma tends to spread primarily via the bloodstream, non-gestational choriocarcinoma shows lymphatic and intra-abdominal spread as well as hematogenous spread. Sometimes the hematogenous spread may be less marked.

Until the introduction of effective combination chemotherapy, the prognosis of patients with choriocarcinoma was distinctly unfavorable but was somewhat better than of patients with yolk sac tumor. Treatment has been revolutionized by the introduction of combination chemotherapy containing cisplatin with marked improvement in prognosis and survival. Cisplatin, etoposide (VP 16), and bleomycin currently is the most favored combination [64, 140].

Teratoma

The origin of teratomas has been a matter of interest, speculation, and dispute for centuries. The parthenogenic theory, which suggests an origin from the primordial germ cell, is now the most widely accepted. Two other theories, one suggesting an origin from blastomeres segregated at an early stage of embryonic development and the second suggesting an origin from embryonal rests have few adherents currently. Support for the germ cell theory has come from the anatomic distribution of the tumors, which occur along the line of migration of the primordial germ cells from the yolk sac to the primitive gonad, and from the fact that the tumors occur most commonly during the years of reproductive activity. Support also comes from animal experiments in which cystic teratomas can be produced only during the period of reproductive activity of the gonad, as in roosters injected with zinc and copper salts [15, 33], and from the karyotyping of teratomas. The karyotype of mature ovarian teratomas is 46,XX [103, 158].

The histogenesis of mature cystic teratoma of the ovary has been studied using both cytogenetic techniques and the electrophoretic patterns of four enzymes in normal as well as in tumor cells. These studies demonstrated that teratomas are of germ cell origin and arise from a single germ cell after the first meiotic division [102, 103]. Subsequent studies using more advanced cytogenetic techniques further confirmed these observations. Although most mature cystic teratomas arise in this manner, some arise before the first meiotic division [126, 138]. This indicates that both modes of origin occur. The classification of ovarian teratomas is shown in ➋ *Table 16.1*. Briefly, they are divided into three main groups: (1) immature teratomas, (2) mature teratomas, and (3) monodermal and highly specialized teratomas. Most cases (99%) are mature cystic teratomas also known as dermoids or dermoid cysts.

Immature Teratoma

Immature teratomas are composed of tissues derived from the three germ layers – ectoderm, mesoderm, and endoderm – and, in contrast to the much more common mature teratoma, they contain immature or embryonal structures. Mature tissues are frequently present and sometimes may predominate. In these cases, the tumor should be differentiated from a mature teratoma with malignant transformation. The presence of immature or embryonal elements as opposed to the neoplastic transformation of mature tissues differentiates between these two types of neoplasm.

Clinical Features

The immature teratoma of the ovary is an uncommon tumor, comprising less than 1% of teratomas of the ovary [27, 34, 109, 168, 185, 255]. In contrast with the mature cystic teratoma, which is encountered most frequently during the reproductive years but occurs at all ages, the immature teratoma has a specific age incidence, occurring most commonly in the first 2 decades of life and being almost unknown after the menopause [27, 31, 109, 185, 255]. In view of this, teratomas occurring in childhood, adolescence, and early adult life should always be examined carefully and thoroughly sampled.

The tumor is usually asymptomatic until it reaches a considerable size. It tends to grow rapidly and may manifest itself as a pelvic or lower abdominal mass. It may cause pressure symptoms, abdominal heaviness, dull pain, or it may undergo torsion, causing acute abdominal pain.

Gross Features

The tumor is usually unilateral [27, 31, 34, 74, 255], but may coexist with a mature cystic teratoma in the opposite ovary [252], as is seen in at least 10–15% of cases. Immature teratomas are usually larger than their mature counterparts, with the reported range from 9 to 28 cm in the largest dimension [31]. They may form a round, oval, or lobulated, soft or firm solid mass, which frequently contains cystic structures with solid areas present in the cyst wall [27, 31, 34, 74, 109, 252]. The tumor is often prone to perforate its capsule, which is not always well defined [31, 252]. The cut surface is usually variegated, trabeculated, and lobulated, varying in color from gray to dark brown. Occasionally, foci of cartilage or bone may be recognizable and hair may be present. The cystic areas are usually filled with serous or mucinous fluid, colloid, or fatty material.

Microscopic Features

Immature teratomas are composed of a variety of immature and mature tissues derived from the three germ layers although usually derivatives of all the three germ layers are present. Occasionally, the tumor may be composed of a small number of tissues. Ectoderm is usually represented by neural tissue. Glia, ganglion cells, neuroblastic tissue, neuroepithelium, nerve trunks, and ocular structures are often represented (◉ *Figs. 16.28* and ◉ *16.29*). Skin elements, including pilosebaceous units, sweat eccrine glands, and hair, are frequently present. Mesodermal elements include fibrous connective tissue; cartilage; bone; muscle, usually smooth but sometimes striated (◉ *Fig. 16.30*); lymphoid tissue; and undifferentiated embryonic mesenchyme. Endodermal elements are usually represented by tubules lined by columnar, sometimes

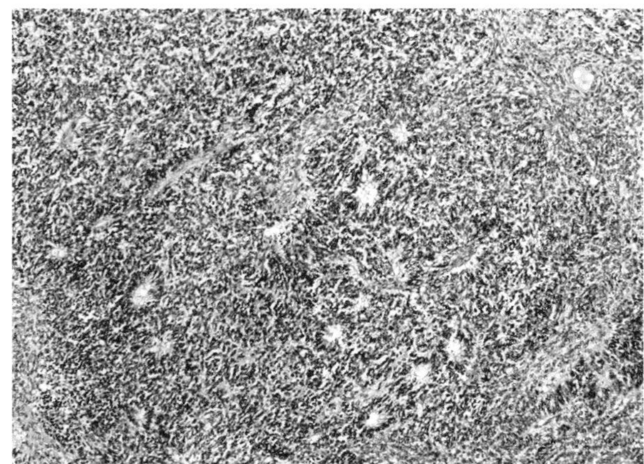

Fig. 16.28
Immature teratoma. **The immature neuroepithelium is composed of solid patterns punctuated by rosettes**

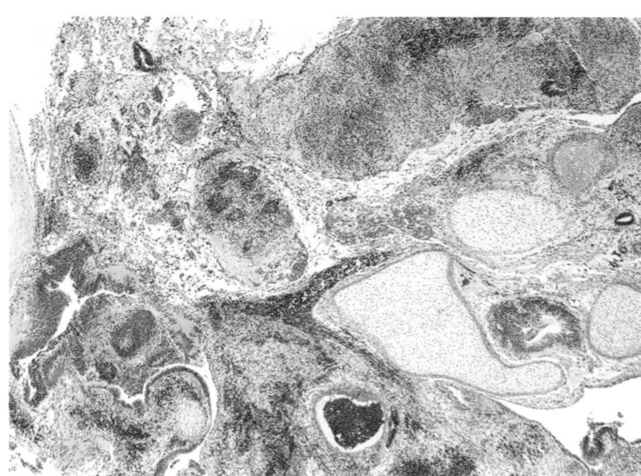

Fig. 16.29
Immature teratoma. **The tumor shows both immature neuroepithelial and mesenchymal elements**

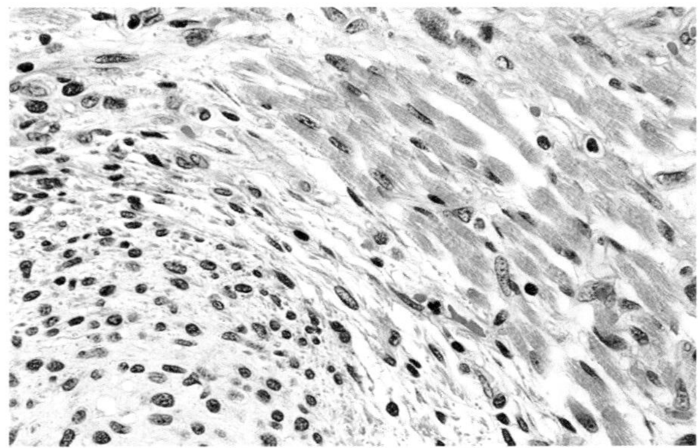

Fig. 16.30
Immature teratoma. **The tumor shows immature cartilage and rhabdomyoblastic components**

ciliated, epithelium. Occasionally, gastrointestinal or renal epithelium may be present. Endocrine elements may be present but, apart from thyroid tissue, are uncommon.

All these tissues, which may be in stages of maturity varying from embryonic to mature, are scattered haphazardly throughout the tumor and so differ from the orderly organoid arrangement seen in a mature teratoma. In cases in which the tumor is composed mainly of mature tissues, differentiation from mature teratoma may be difficult, and patients have been diagnosed as having a benign lesion only to return within a short time with recurrence. In a number of such cases, review of the material taken from the original tumor has revealed immature elements. Therefore, careful examination and thorough sampling of the tumor are strongly recommended. Immature teratoma may be combined with other neoplastic germ cell elements, such as yolk sac tumor, dysgerminoma, embryonal carcinoma, choriocarcinoma, and polyembryoma. It can therefore form a part of a malignant germ cell tumor composed of two or more neoplastic germ cell elements (mixed germ cell tumor). Immature teratoma has been reported to develop from the germ cell element of gonadoblastoma and mixed germ cell–sex cord–stromal tumor.

Differential Diagnosis

Immature teratoma must be differentiated from malignant mesodermal mixed tumor (MMMT), which although occurring most frequently in the uterus, also occurs in the ovary. MMMT is composed of tissue resembling derivatives of müllerian mesoderm, a primitive structure that gives rise to both the stroma and the epithelium of the endometrium. The characteristic histologic appearance of MMMT combined with the absence of other germ layer derivatives distinguish MMMT from teratoma; neuroectodermal derivatives, prominent in solid immature teratoma, are seen only exceptionally in MMMT. MMMT occurs most frequently in postmenopausal women between the ages of 50 and 70 years and, unlike immature teratoma, occurs only occasionally in younger patients. MMMTs are composed of sarcomatoid and carcinomatous tissue. The carcinoma is invariably an adenocarcinoma, squamous cell carcinoma, or adenosquamous carcinoma, and the sarcomatoid elements may be composed of a wide variety of tissues, including leiomyosarcoma, chondrosarcoma, rhabdomyosarcoma, fibrosarcoma, undifferentiated sarcomatous tissue, and myxomatous tissue. MMMT does not exhibit the great variety of tissues present in teratoma, and the tissues present in MMMT generally form more typical sarcomatous or carcinomatous patterns (see ❯ Chap. 10, Mesenchymal Tumors of the Uterus).

Clinical Behavior and Treatment

Immature teratoma is a malignant neoplasm that usually grows rapidly, penetrates its capsule, and forms adhesions to the surrounding structures. It spreads throughout the peritoneal cavity by implantation and metastasizes first to the retroperitoneal, para-aortic, and more distant lymph nodes and later to the lungs, liver, and other organs. Peritoneal implants and metastases are not infrequently present at operation for the removal of the primary tumor [31, 252]. Excision of the tumor is often followed by a local recurrence within a few weeks or months. Recurrences usually occur within the first year after the primary treatment [31]. Rupture of the tumor with spillage of the contents during operation is not infrequent, but because of the satisfactory response of the tumor to combination chemotherapy the favorable prognosis is not affected. The metastases and peritoneal implants may be composed of different tissues, and thus their teratomatous nature is readily apparent, but they may also be composed of a single tissue. The histologic appearances of the metastases and of the peritoneal implants may or may not reflect the appearances of the primary tumor. In two related conditions, the growing teratoma syndrome and chemotherapeutic retroconversion [51], the metastases of immature teratoma may consist of pure mature teratoma after chemotherapy.

It has been noted that there is a good correlation between the histologic appearances of the tumor and prognosis [27, 74, 130, 131]. Very immature and poorly differentiated tumors have been found to be associated with worse prognosis, whereas a more favorable outcome has been observed in patients with more mature and better differentiated tumors [74, 130, 252]. One study of immature teratoma in children showed that less mature tumors were more likely to be associated with yolk sac tumor [74].

Grading

O'Connor and Norris [131] proposed that immature teratomas should be divided into two grades, those with a slight degree of immaturity (grade 1; low grade), which are not treated with combination chemotherapy, and those with a more marked degree of immaturity (grades 2 and 3; high grade), which are treated. It was demonstrated that although there was considerable inter- and intraobserver disagreement when a large series of immature teratomas were being graded into three grades, this was markedly decreased when a two-grade system was used. The study further confirmed the good correlation between the grade of the tumor and behavior. Furthermore, it should be noted that rare and small microscopic foci of immature tissue within a mature cystic teratoma have been associated with an excellent outcome [256].

Ovarian immature teratomas and their metastases should be graded because the grade correlates with outcome and determines which patients receive chemotherapy. In order to ensure that the primary ovarian tumor has been adequately sampled, one block of tissue per centimeter of the greatest tumor dimension should be submitted. The currently used grading system is the Armed Forces Institute of Pathology (AFIP) system, which is endorsed by the WHO. In this system, it is the immature neuroepithelium that is graded. The grade is based on the *aggregate amount* of immature neuroepithelium on *any single slide* [130, 131] ❯ *Table 16.2*:

Metastases/implants are considered Grade 0 when no immature tissue is present, regardless of the grade of the ovarian tumor. In particular, a specific type of Grade 0 implant composed entirely of mature glial tissue ("gliomatosis peritonei") is associated with an excellent outcome.

Table 16.2
Grading of immature teratomas

Grade 1	Amount of immature neuroectoderm occupies ≤1 low-power (4× objective) magnification field
Grade 2	Amount of immature neuroectoderm occupies >1 but ≤3 low-power (4× objective) magnification fields
Grade 3	Amount of immature neuroectoderm occupies >3 low-power (4× objective) magnification fields

In the opinion of some authorities on the topic, when tissues other than neuroepithelium are present, their degree of immaturity must also be taken into consideration when grading; however, this is not the method specified by the WHO.

The recommended treatment for patients with grade 1 (low-grade) immature teratoma confined to one ovary is unilateral salpingo-oophorectomy and careful follow-up. This treatment is curative in nearly all cases [27, 140]. For grade 2 and 3 (high-grade) tumors, adjuvant chemotherapy is administered following unilateral salpingo-oophorectomy, resulting in complete cure in the majority of patients [27]. More extensive surgery is necessary if the tumor extends beyond the ovary. Current combination therapy is vincristine, dactinomycin, and cyclophosphamide (VAC); vinblastine, bleomycin, and cisplatin (VBP); or cisplatin, etoposide (VP 16), and bleomycin (BEP) regimens. Therapy with VAC had been the treatment of choice [130] because the results obtained were considered to be similar to those with VBP or BEP regimens and the latter are more toxic. There is evidence that the recurrence rate with BEP is less than with VAC regimen, and for patients with metastatic disease, the cisplatin-containing regimens are the treatment of choice, especially as the BEP regimen is less toxic than the VBP [27, 64, 140].

In a collaborative study of immature teratoma (ovarian, testicular, and extra-gondal) in children [74], it was demonstrated that pure immature teratomas in this population have a very good prognosis. The authors concluded that the presence of microscopic foci of yolk sac tumor rather than the grade of immature teratoma was the only valid predictor of recurrence; however, it should be noted that ovarian cases were not separately analyzed for correlation between grade and outcome.

Mature Solid Teratoma

General Features

Mature solid teratoma is an uncommon ovarian teratoma. The age at presentation is similar to that of immature solid teratoma, the tumor occurring mainly in children and young adults [142, 255]. Most solid ovarian teratomas are composed at least partly of immature tissues and therefore are considered to be malignant. The occasional cases of solid ovarian teratoma composed entirely of mature tissues have usually been included in this group and thus misinterpreted as malignant. As the presence of immature neural elements immediately excludes the tumor from this group, it is very important to recognize the mature tissue as such, as by definition only tumors composed entirely of mature tissues may be diagnosed as mature solid teratoma.

Gross Features

The tumors are usually large, do not exhibit any specific features, and show similar appearance to most solid teratomas, which are composed of immature tissues. They grow slowly in comparison with immature solid teratoma, but because they are usually discovered after they have reached a considerable size, this feature is of little help in diagnosis. In all reported cases of mature solid teratoma, the tumor has been unilateral [142, 252, 255].

Microscopic Features

Mature solid teratoma is composed entirely of mature tissues derived from the three germ layers. Rigid diagnostic criteria must be used, and the examination and sampling of the tumor must be thorough, because inclusion of cases with immature elements completely changes the prognosis of this neoplasm [142, 252, 255]. The tissues derived from the three germ layers are arranged in an orderly manner resembling the much more common mature cystic teratoma, except that the neoplasm is solid or at least predominantly solid. Neurogenic elements, which are among the most common tissues present in this tumor, often pose diagnostic problems because they may not be recognized as mature. Occasionally, mature solid teratoma may be associated with peritoneal implants composed entirely of mature glial tissue (gliomatosis) (➋ *Fig. 16.31*). Despite extensive peritoneal disease and irrespective of the mode of therapy employed, the prognosis is excellent [160, 168, 185]. Presence of peritoneal implants composed entirely of mature glial tissue occasionally may be observed in patients with immature solid teratoma and with mature cystic teratoma. The presence of these implants does not affect the prognosis [74, 123, 160, 168, 185].

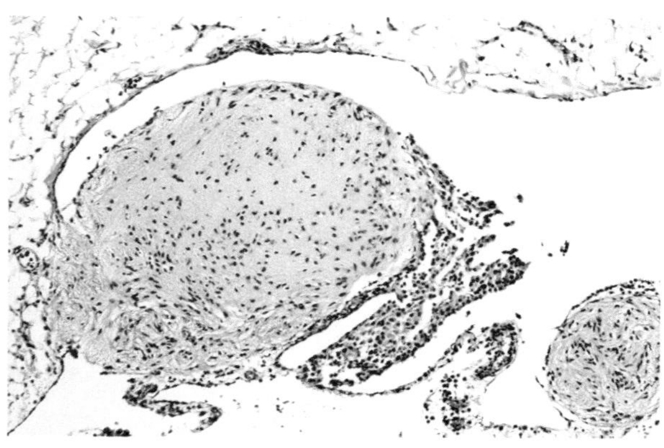

Fig. 16.31
Mature glial implant. **Mature glial implants on omentum ("*gliomatosis peritonei*")**

Clinical Behavior and Treatment

Because the tumor is unilateral, oophorectomy or unilateral adnexectomy is the treatment of choice, resulting in a complete cure [142, 252, 255].

Mature Cystic Teratoma

General Features

Mature cystic teratoma of the ovary, or dermoid cyst, has been known since antiquity. The tumor is composed of well-differentiated derivatives of the three germ layers – ectoderm, mesoderm, and endoderm – with ectodermal elements predominating. In its pure form, mature cystic teratoma is always benign, but occasionally it may undergo malignant change in one of its elements. It may also form a part of a germ cell neoplasm composed of a number of different neoplastic germ cell elements (mixed germ cell tumor).

Clinical Features

Mature cystic teratoma is the most common type of ovarian teratoma and the most common type of ovarian germ cell neoplasm. It occurs relatively frequently and comprises approximately 20% of all ovarian neoplasms [144, 168, 185]. Mature cystic teratoma occurs most commonly during the reproductive years, but, unlike other germ cell tumors of the ovary, it has a wider age distribution and may be encountered at any age from infancy to old age [13, 34, 144]. In some series, more than 25% of cases have been observed in postmenopausal women [110]. It has also been encountered in newborns. Mature cystic teratoma is often discovered as an incidental finding on physical examination, radiologic examination, or during abdominal surgery performed for other indications.

Patients present with abdominal pain (47.6%), abdominal mass or swelling (15.4%), and abnormal uterine bleeding (15.1%) [144]. The abdominal pain is usually constant, slight, or moderate but, in a number of cases, may be severe and acute because of torsion or rupture of the tumor. In children and young adults, the tumors tend to be more easily mobile and therefore are more frequently affected by torsion. Abnormal uterine bleeding and its cessation after excision of the tumor suggest hormone synthesis by the tumor, but histologic examination has failed to reveal any explanation for the endocrine function [110]. Slightly decreased fertility has been observed in patients with mature cystic teratoma, but in most cases there is no satisfactory explanation. In 10% of cases, the tumor is diagnosed during pregnancy [13, 34]. Mature cystic teratoma has been diagnosed radiologically because of the presence of teeth, bone, and cartilage [110, 144].

Cytogenetic Features

Mature cystic teratomas are diploid, have a normal 46,XX karyotype, and have been considered to originate from germ cells after the first meiotic division; thus, they are in contrast to mature teratomas of the postpubertal testis, which are malignant, are aneuploid, have complex cytogenetic abnormalities including 12p amplification, and are considered to originate from other forms of germ cell tumor [10, 102, 244]. Of note, ovarian mature cystic teratomas and prepubertal testicular mature teratomas are similar in that both are diploid, have normal karyotypes, and are benign [244]. Previous studies [126, 138] using banding techniques demonstrated diverse modes of origin of mature cystic teratoma. Although most ovarian mature cystic teratomas originate from germ cells after the first meiotic division, some originate before this event [126, 138]. This distinction also applies to immature ovarian teratomas, which tend to be aneuploid, resembling their testicular counterparts.

Gross Features

Mature cystic teratoma does not have a predilection for either ovary; 8–15% of cases are bilateral [144, 168, 185]. The tumor varies in size from very small (0.5 cm) to large (measuring more than 40 cm) and can weigh up to several kilograms. Approximately 60% of mature cystic teratomas measure from 5 to 10 cm, and more than 90% measure less than 15 cm [144]. The tumor is round, oval, or globular, with a smooth, gray-white, and glistening surface (◉ *Fig. 16.32*). It is usually freely mobile but occasionally may form adhesions to surrounding structures, especially if there has been leakage. On palpation, the tumor is soft and fluctuant, with firm or hard areas; this is usually observed immediately after its removal, because at room temperature the tumor tends to solidify. The contents of the tumor are liquid at temperatures above 34°C and become solid at temperatures below 25°C [25]. The cut surface of the tumor reveals a cavity filled with fatty material and hair surrounded by a firm capsule of varying thickness. The fatty material is similar to normal sebum. The tumor is usually unilocular but may be multilocular. Several tumors may be present in the same ovary.

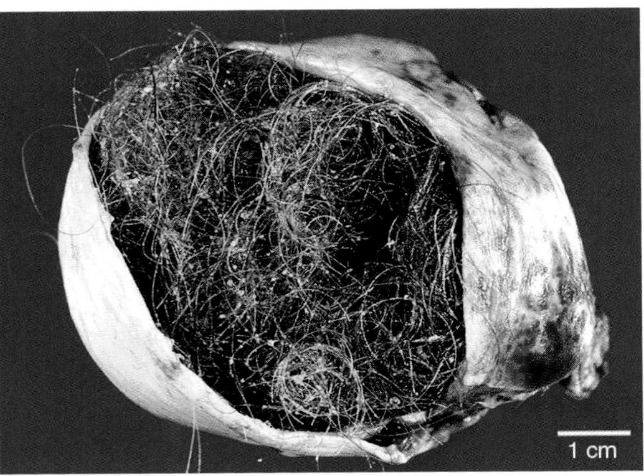

Fig. 16.32
Mature cystic teratoma. **Well-encapsulated tumor containing hair**

Arising from the cyst wall and projecting into the cavity is a protuberance that may vary in size from a small nodule to a rounded elevated mass. It is usually single but may be multiple and is frequently solid but may be partly cystic. This protuberance has been variously termed dermoid mamilla, dermoid protuberance, Rokitansky protuberance, embryonic node, or dermoid nipple. The hair present in the tumor arises from this protuberance, and when bone or teeth are present (◉ *Fig. 16.33*), they tend to be located within this area, which is composed of a variety of different tissues and is one of the sites that should always be carefully sampled. Mature cystic teratomas contain macroscopically recognizable and well-formed teeth in 31% of cases [25]. Phalanges, long and other bones, parts of the rib cage, loops of intestine, and even fetus-like structures are occasionally encountered [1, 250]. They have been classified as fetiform teratomas or homunculi [1, 250].

Microscopic Features

The outer side of the cyst wall is composed of ovarian stroma that may often be hyalinized, making its recognition difficult. The cavity of the cyst is lined mainly by skin, and in small tumors cutaneous structures may form the entire lining. The skin is composed of keratinized squamous epithelium and usually contains abundant sebaceous and eccrine glands associated with fat (◉ *Fig. 16.34*). In some tumors, a lipogranulomatous, fat necrosis-like, sieve-like, or pneumatosis cystoides-like pattern may be prominent. Hair and other dermal appendages are usually present. Occasionally, the cyst

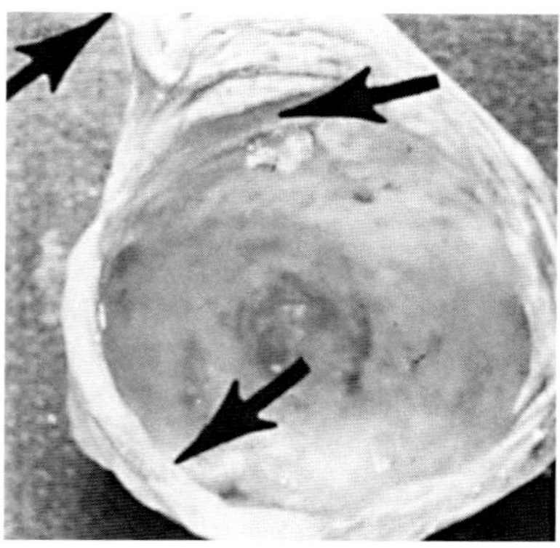

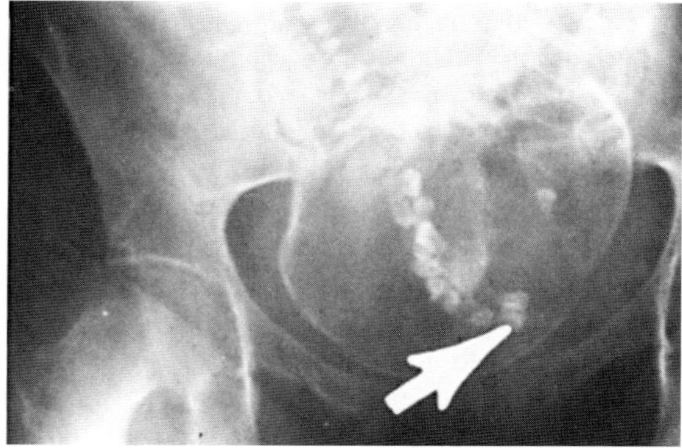

Fig. 16.33
Mature cystic teratoma. *Left*: Well-encapsulated spherical cystic mass. *Arrows* point to teeth. *Right*: The tumor was diagnosed via pelvic radiograph. A row of teeth is seen at *arrow* tip (Courtesy of A. Blaustein, M.D.)

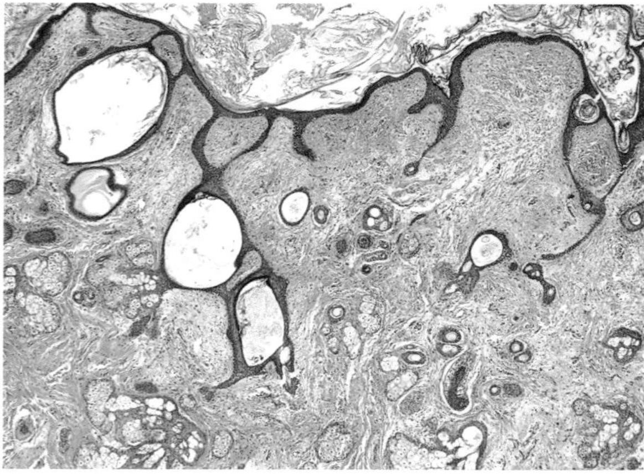

Fig. 16.34
Mature cystic teratoma. The lining of the cyst is composed of skin with its appendages

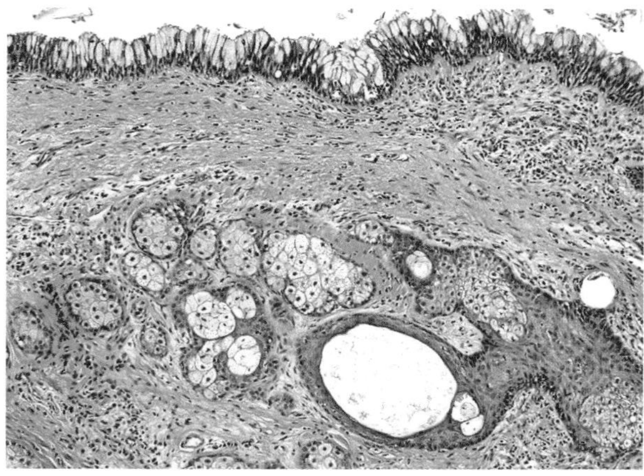

Fig. 16.35
Mature cystic teratoma. Mature cystic teratoma lined by well-differentiated mature respiratory epithelium. Mature adnexal structures are seen beneath the lining

wall may be lined by bronchial or gastrointestinal epithelium or epithelium of columnar or cuboidal type (*Fig. 16.35*). The squamous epithelium may be present only in the region of the dermoid protuberance. Sometimes there may be loss of the lining epithelium caused by desquamation, and this may be associated with a foreign body giant cell reaction. The latter may be seen in other parts of the tumor as a reaction to the contents of the tumor. Foreign body giant cell reactions may also be seen when the contents of the tumor are spilled, leading to the formation of adhesions.

The area around the dermoid protuberance may contain a large variety of tissues derived from the three germ layers. Ectodermal tissue, represented by squamous epithelium and other skin derivatives, is usually most abundant. Brain tissue, glia, neural tissue, retina, choroid plexus, and ganglia may also be encountered. In occasional cases, the glial tissue may be highly cellular, making the distinction between gliosis and a low-grade glial tumor, such as astrocytoma or oligodendroglioma, arising in a teratoma very difficult. Criteria have not been established for this distinction in the ovary. Furthermore, in view of the rarity of this problem in teratomas, the precise behavior of such lesions is not known, but in our experience (unpublished data), we are not aware of an adverse outcome.

Mesodermal tissue is represented by bone, cartilage, smooth muscle, and fibrous and fatty tissue. Endodermal tissue is represented by gastrointestinal and bronchial epithelium and glands, thyroid, and salivary gland tissue. In a careful study of 100 cases, ectodermal structures were found in 100%, mesodermal in 93%, and endodermal in 71% of cases [25]. Rare tissues, such as prostate, have been reported [71]. The various tissues present in mature cystic teratoma show an orderly organoid arrangement forming cutaneous, bronchial, and gastrointestinal tissues, as well as bone and other structures. Although these tissues may be scattered diffusely, they do not exhibit the disorderly haphazard arrangement that is observed in immature teratoma.

With the exception of thyroid tissue, the presence of endocrine tissue of other types is distinctly uncommon in mature cystic teratoma, but pituitary, adrenal, and parathyroid tissues have been documented. Occasionally functioning endocrine tissue, forming an adenoma, may be found in a mature cystic teratoma [168, 185]. Mature cystic teratoma must be differentiated from the rare cases of fetus in fetu, considered most likely to be caused by an inclusion of a monozygotic diamniotic twin [29]. Fetus in fetu can be distinguished from a teratoma by its location in the retroperitoneal space, presence of vertebral organization with formation of limb buds, and a well-developed organ system. Fetus in fetu shows better organization than the most differentiated teratomas. Like mature cystic teratoma, fetus in fetu is a benign lesion [29].

Clinical Behavior and Treatment

Mature cystic teratoma of the ovary may be associated with various complications. In view of the fact that in many of these cases the condition is amenable to cure, their recognition is of considerable importance. These complications include (1) torsion, (2) rupture, (3) infection, (4) hemolytic anemia, and (5) development of malignancy.

Torsion is the most frequent complication [13, 34, 133, 144], occurring in 16.1% of cases in one large series [144]. This complication tends to be more common during pregnancy and puerperium [110, 144]. Mature cystic teratoma is said to comprise from 22% to 40% of ovarian tumors in pregnancy, and from 0.8% to 12.8% of reported cases of mature cystic teratoma have occurred during pregnancy [34, 144]. The fact that these tumors, when they occur during pregnancy, are more liable to be associated with torsion is of considerable importance. Torsion is also more common in children and younger patients [133, 144]. The patients usually have severe acute abdominal pain, and the condition is an acute abdominal emergency. Excision of the affected ovary or salpingo-oophorectomy is the treatment of choice.

Torsion tends to predispose to rupture of the tumor. Rupture of mature cystic teratoma is an uncommon complication, occurring in approximately 1% of cases [110, 144]. The immediate result of the rupture may be shock or hemorrhage, especially during pregnancy or labor, but the prognosis even in these cases is usually favorable. Rupture of the tumor into the peritoneal cavity may be followed by chemical peritonitis caused by the spillage of the contents of the tumor. It produces a marked granulomatous reaction and leads to the formation of dense adhesions throughout the peritoneal cavity. Rupture of the tumor occasionally may be followed by the development of glial implants on the peritoneum. This condition occurs when the tumor contains mature neuroglial elements, and spillage leads to deposition of numerous small nodules composed of mature glia in the peritoneal cavity. Despite the wide dissemination of these deposits throughout the peritoneal cavity, the prognosis is favorable, and simple surgical excision of the primary tumor is considered to be adequate therapy [160]. Mature cystic teratoma may rupture not only into the peritoneal cavity but also into adjacent organs, usually the bladder or the rectum. Several such cases have been reported [44]. Infection is an uncommon complication and occurs in approximately 1% of cases [110]. The infecting organism is usually a coliform, but *Salmonella* infection causing typhoid fever has also been reported [75].

Autoimmune hemolytic anemia has been noted occasionally in patients with teratoma of the ovary, mainly mature cystic teratoma. Excision of the tumor in these cases resulted in the disappearance of the anemia and a complete cure [22, 46, 139]. A small number of mature cystic teratomas and other cystic ovarian tumors associated with this complication have been reported [22, 139]. The patients have symptoms and signs of progressive anemia, which may be moderate or severe; it is accompanied by reticulocytosis, spherocytosis, and increased osmotic fragility. Normoblasts may be present in the peripheral blood. The indirect serum bilirubin is elevated, and the direct antiglobulin test (Coombs' test) is positive, indicating the presence of autoantibodies that react with the patient's red blood cells. The platelets are normal in number. The spleen may be palpable but is only slightly enlarged. Steroids are only transiently effective in treating the disease, and splenectomy has no effect on the progress of the disease [22, 139]. Excision of the ovarian tumor leads to the permanent disappearance of the anemia [22, 46, 139]. The following possible pathogenetic mechanisms have been suggested [22]:

(1) Presence in the tumor of substances that are antigenically different from the host and that stimulate the

production of antibodies by the host, which cross-react with the patient's own red blood cells; (2) Antibody production by the tumor directed specifically against the host's red blood cells resembling the graft-versus-host reaction; and (3) Coating of red blood cells with products secreted by the tumor, resulting in changed red blood cell antigenicity.

In view of this, pelvic and radiologic examination is indicated in a young woman with autoimmune hemolytic anemia that does not respond to steroid treatment, as it may help detect an ovarian teratoma and prevent an unnecessary splenectomy [139].

The treatment of choice for an uncomplicated mature cystic teratoma in young patients is excision of the cyst with conservation of part of the ovary if possible. This treatment usually results in a complete cure. Local recurrences after conservative treatment for mature cystic teratoma are uncommon and occur in less than 1% of cases.

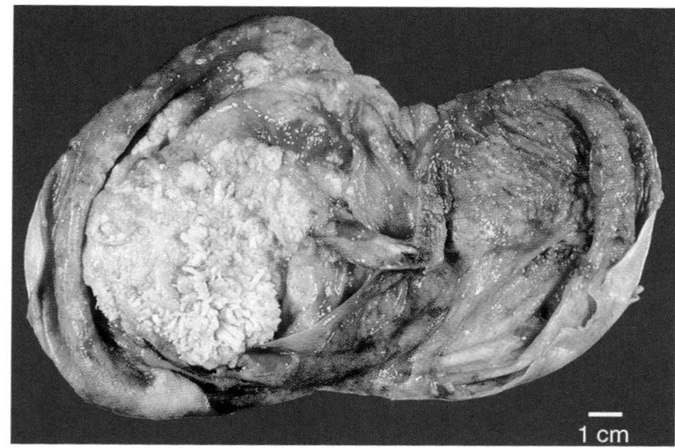

Fig. 16.36
Squamous cell carcinoma (*left*) arising in and overgrowing mature cystic teratoma

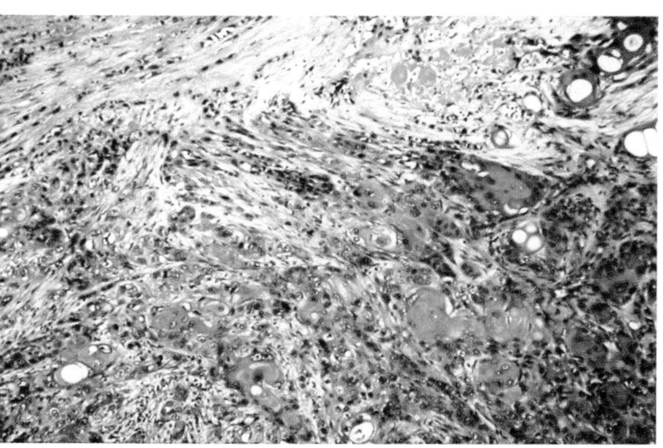

Fig. 16.37
Squamous cell carcinoma arising in mature cystic teratoma. The tumor has an infiltrating pattern showing numerous keratin pearls

Mature Cystic Teratoma (Dermoid Cyst) with Malignant Transformation

General Features

Malignant transformation is an uncommon complication of mature cystic teratoma. It occurs in approximately 2% of cases [13, 95, 110, 136, 143, 168, 185, 199], although in one report the frequency was almost 4% [134]. The age of patients with this complication as reported in the literature ranges from 19 to 88 years [143], but this tumor usually is observed in postmenopausal patients [95, 110, 134, 143, 199].

Clinically, this tumor cannot be readily differentiated from an uncomplicated mature cystic teratoma or other ovarian tumor although evidence of its rapid growth, pain, loss of weight, and other systemic signs and symptoms suggest the presence of a malignant tumor. Sometimes, the tumor may be an incidental finding.

Gross Features

The tumor is frequently larger than the average mature cystic teratoma [34, 95, 185, 199]; it may exhibit a more solid appearance (Fig. *16.36*), but differentiation usually cannot be made on gross examination. Malignant transformation in mature cystic teratoma tends to occur in patients with unilateral tumors [143, 144].

Microscopic Features

The most common tumor component to undergo malignant transformation is squamous epithelium, with formation of a typical squamous cell carcinoma (*Figs. 16.37* and *16.38*) [34, 76, 95, 134, 143, 199]. Any of the tissues present in a mature cystic teratoma may undergo malignant transformation, and a variety of malignant tumors have been reported, including mucinous carcinoma, carcinoid tumor, thyroid carcinoma, basal cell carcinoma, malignant melanoma, leiomyosarcoma, chondrosarcoma, and angiosarcoma (*Figs. 16.39* and *16.40*) [70, 114, 117, 143, 243, 248]. The malignant element invades other parts of the tumor and its wall, which may perforate. The malignant component may overgrow the remaining part of the mature cystic teratoma and pose diagnostic problems.

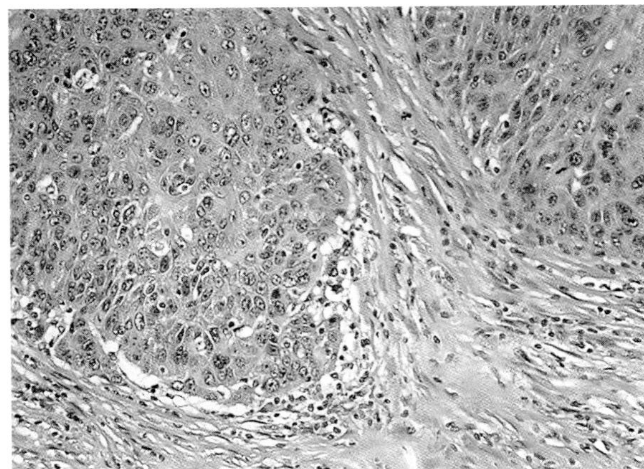

Fig. 16.38
Squamous cell carcinoma arising in a mature cystic teratoma. **The tumor displays a pushing pattern**

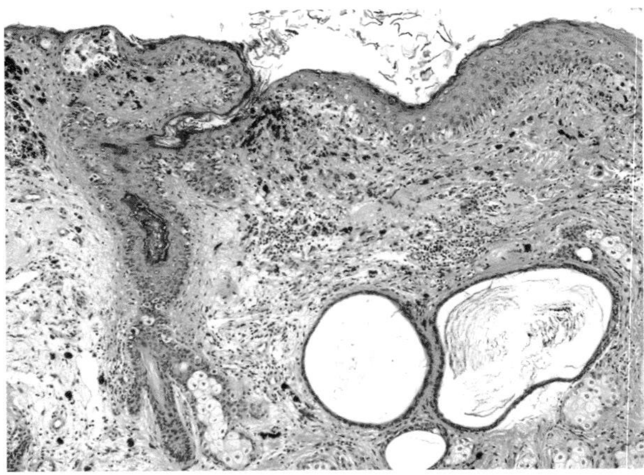

Fig. 16.39
Melanoma arising in mature cystic teratoma. **Note nested pattern within squamous epithelium**

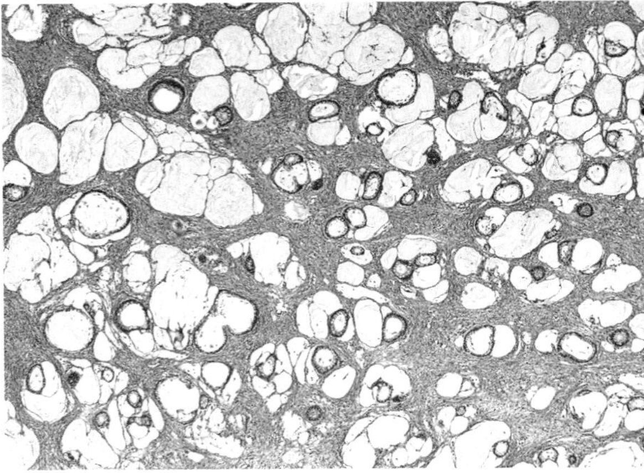

Fig. 16.40
Invasive mucinous carcinoma arising within mature cystic teratoma. **Note extensive glandular component, slightly haphazard glandular arrangements, and prominent pseudomyxoma ovarii. The diagnosis of invasion in examples such as this can be very difficult, particularly with regard to distinction from non-carcinomatous tumors that have pseudomyxoma ovarii coupled with a slightly less extensive glandular proliferation and density of glands**

Clinical Behavior and Treatment

The mode of spread of the malignant tumor differs from that observed in other tumors of germ cell origin. The tumor spreads by direct invasion and peritoneal implantation and generally does not metastasize to the lymph nodes [95, 143]. Extensive local invasion and absence of lymph node involvement usually is observed at laparotomy [134, 199]. Hematogenous dissemination is uncommon.

The prognosis of patients with mature cystic teratoma with malignant transformation is unfavorable [95, 134, 143, 199]; only 15–30.8% of patients survive 5 years [95, 143]. Better prognosis has been reported when the malignant element is a squamous cell carcinoma confined to the ovary and is excised without spillage of the contents. In such cases, the reported 5-year survival is 63% [143].

Treatment is hysterectomy and bilateral adnexectomy [95, 199]. Because the tumors are usually unilateral, in cases where there is no penetration of the capsule and no involvement of the adjacent structures, a more conservative surgical procedure may be just as effective. However, because malignant transformation of a mature cystic teratoma usually occurs in postmenopausal women, total abdominal hysterectomy and bilateral salpingo-oophorectomy is performed. If the tumor has spread beyond the confines of the ovary and there is involvement of the adjacent structures, a more radical procedure with resection of the tumor and the involved structures or viscera is advocated [134]. Response to chemotherapy is unsatisfactory [95, 134].

Mucinous Tumors Arising in Mature Cystic Teratoma

General Features

In general, the vast majority of primary ovarian mucinous tumors are of surface epithelial origin, but a subset is of germ cell origin. In the cases studied, 2–11% of ovarian mature cystic teratomas are associated with a mucinous tumor, and many of the latter in this setting are likely of germ cell origin.

Microscopic Features

Primary ovarian mucinous tumors associated with a mature cystic teratoma show a spectrum of histologic appearances [117, 248]. At the lower end of the spectrum, tumors display a cystadenomatous pattern. Proliferative tumors with architectural complexity and epithelial stratification resemble atypical proliferative (borderline) mucinous tumor of ovarian surface epithelial origin or low-grade adenomatous mucinous neoplasm of the appendix. Pseudomyxoma ovarii can be seen with some cystadenomatous and proliferative neoplasms. Compared to tumors without pseudomyxoma ovarii, neoplasms with pseudomyxoma ovarii more closely resemble lower gastrointestinal tract adenomatous tumors and tend to have hypermucinous columnar epithelium and abundant goblet cells. Other tumors may show goblet cell carcinoid-like morphology. At the upper end of the spectrum, the carcinomatous neoplasms may be of glandular (➋ *Fig. 16.40*) or signet-ring cell type. Pseudomyxoma ovarii can also be associated with goblet cell carcinoid-like tumors or carcinoma.

Immunohistochemical Features and Differential Diagnosis

Immunohistochemical stains for CK7 and CK20 show variable coordinate expression profiles [248]. Tumors *without* pseudomyxoma ovarii and having cystadenomatous or proliferative patterns show a variety of CK7/CK20 profiles, including a CK7 diffuse/CK20 variable pattern (a pattern frequently seen in ovarian surface epithelial tumors). Those *with* pseudomyxoma ovarii and having cystadenomatous, proliferative, or goblet cell carcinoid-like patterns characteristically display a CK7(−)/CK20 diffuse or CK7 focal/CK20 diffuse profile (patterns typical of lower gastrointestinal tract tumors). A minority of these tumors histologically and immunohistochemically resembling lower gastrointestinal tract adenomatous tumors can have the clinical syndrome of pseudomyxoma peritonei without a tumor in the appendix. Parenthetically, it should be emphasized that although nearly all cases of pseudomyxoma peritonei are of appendiceal origin, rare cases are of primary ovarian origin due to an appendiceal-type mucinous tumor arising within a mature cystic teratoma. The carcinomas can have variable CK7/CK20 profiles, but some will show a CK7(−)/CK20 diffuse or CK7 focal/CK20 diffuse pattern.

Ovarian mucinous tumors of germ cell origin with histologic and immunohistochemical features typical of primary lower gastrointestinal tract tumors can be misclassified as metastatic or secondary tumors involving the ovary. Thus, it is important to search for focal teratomatous components in such ovarian mucinous tumors in order to suggest a possible primary ovarian origin. Nonetheless, when problematic mucinous neoplasms in ovarian mature cystic teratomas histologically and immunohistochemically resemble lower gastrointestinal tract tumors, extensive sampling of the gross specimen and further clinical evaluation to exclude the rare possibility of a similar primary mucinous tumor in the appendix or colorectal region as part of a tumor-to-tumor metastasis (e.g., a primary lower gastrointestinal tract tumor with a metastasis to a coexisting ovarian teratoma) are recommended.

Primary ovarian mucinous tumors arising in a teratoma, which histologically and immunohistochemically resemble lower gastrointestinal tumors, are considered to be of germ cell origin. Tumors that are histologically and immunohistochemically analogous to ovarian surface epithelial mucinous cystadenoma or atypical proliferative (borderline) mucinous tumor may have developed in the same ovary containing a teratoma as an independent tumor; however, it should also be considered that some of those mucinous tumors could be of germ cell origin as it is possible that they arose from upper gastrointestinal/pancreaticobiliary or sinonasal tissue in a teratoma, which would have histologic and immunohistochemical features similar to mucinous tumors of ovarian surface epithelial origin.

Nomenclature

For primary ovarian mucinous tumors histologically and immunohistochemically resembling lower gastrointestinal tract tumors, descriptive terminology that parallels the nomenclature for tumors in lower gastrointestinal sites (e.g., low-grade adenomatous mucinous neoplasm for ovarian tumors histologically and immunohistochemically analogous to those of the appendix) is preferred, considering that (a) terms such as borderline tumor or atypical proliferative tumor are used for surface epithelial tumors of the ovary, (b) these mucinous tumors are of germ cell rather than surface epithelial origin, and (c) they resemble their counterparts in the lower gastrointestinal tract.

Clinical Behavior and Treatment

Data on the behavior of mucinous ovarian tumors of germ cell origin are limited, but in the series of McKenney et al.

and Vang et al., patients with cystadenomatous and proliferative/low malignant potential tumors on follow-up remained well and disease-free [117, 248]. In the same series, mucinous carcinomas showed variable outcome but exhibited the potential for aggressive behavior. However, Ueda et al [243] reported a case of a patient with an adenocarcinoma arising in a mature cystic teratoma who has survived for more than 15 years. Furthermore, the present authors have seen a case of a patient with an intestinal-type adenocarcinoma arising in a mature cystic teratoma who has survived for more than 5 years.

Struma Ovarii

General Features

Thyroid tissue is a relatively frequent constituent of mature cystic teratoma and has been demonstrated in 5–20% of cases. Struma ovarii is considered a one-sided development of a teratoma in which the thyroid tissue has overgrown all other tissues, or one in which only the thyroid tissue has developed. The term struma ovarii should be reserved for tumors composed either entirely or predominantly of thyroid tissue [168, 169, 185].

Clinical Features

Struma ovarii is uncommon; it comprises nearly 3% of ovarian teratomas. The age distribution of patients with struma ovarii is generally the same as that of patients with mature cystic teratoma and ranges from 6 to 74 years. Most patients are in the reproductive years [168, 169, 254]. There are usually no specific symptoms; the clinical findings are similar to those observed in patients with mature cystic teratoma. The only differences are that in some cases struma ovarii is associated with enlargement of the thyroid gland, and in other cases there is clinical evidence that the struma ovarii is responsible for the development of thyrotoxicosis although this has not been confirmed preoperatively by laboratory tests [193, 254]. The ectopic thyroid tissue present within struma ovarii, therefore, may be the subject of the same physiologic and pathologic changes as the thyroid gland [193].

Gross Features

Struma ovarii is usually unilateral but is often associated with mature cystic teratoma and rarely with a cystadenoma in the contralateral ovary [168, 169, 185, 254]. In some cases, the teratoma present in the contralateral ovary contained thyroid tissue.

Struma ovarii varies in size, but usually measures less than 10 cm. The surface is usually smooth and, before sectioning, the tumor resembles a mature cystic teratoma. Occasionally, adhesions may be present. The cut surface of the tumor may be composed entirely of light tan, glistening thyroid tissue. Hemorrhage, necrosis, and foci of fibrosis may be present. Solid tumors with small amounts of colloid appear less glistening and more fleshy. Some tumors may be cystic [205].

Microscopic and Immunohistochemical Features

The tumor is composed of mature thyroid tissue consisting of acini of various sizes, lined by a single layer of columnar or flattened epithelium (*Fig. 16.41*). The acini contain eosinophilic, PAS-positive colloid. The intensity of the staining may vary. There may be a considerable variation in the size of the acini, which may be large, containing a large amount of colloid, or may be small. Thyroglobulin and TTF-1 can be identified in the epithelial cells by immunohistochemistry (*Fig. 16.42*). Occasionally, the lining of the acini may be columnar, containing small papillary projections not unlike those seen in hyperactive thyroid gland. Sometimes the appearances may resemble a nodular adenomatous goiter. Adenoma-like lesions may also be observed. When the tumor exhibits markedly crowded follicles without features of malignancy, the designation "proliferative struma ovarii" has been suggested (*Fig. 16.43*) [48]. Struma ovarii showing appearances suggestive of Hashimoto's thyroiditis has also been reported [52]. Rarely, the tumor may show clear cell or cystic patterns [205, 206].

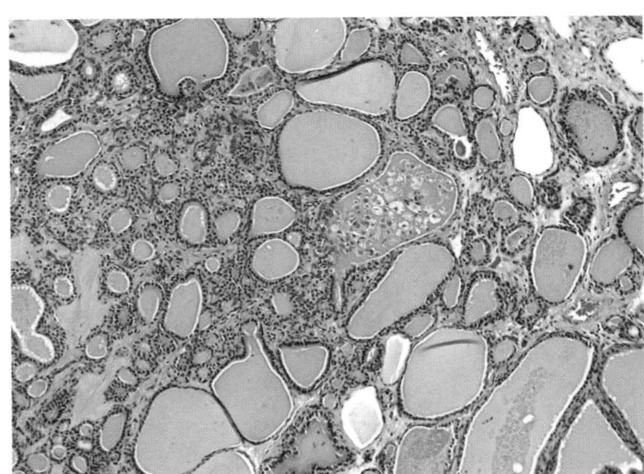

Fig. 16.41
Struma ovarii. **The tumor is composed of normal thyroid tissue**

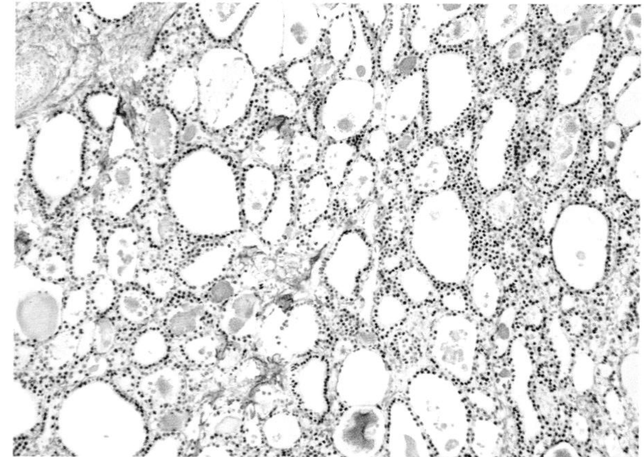

Fig. 16.42
Struma ovarii showing diffuse expression of TTF-1

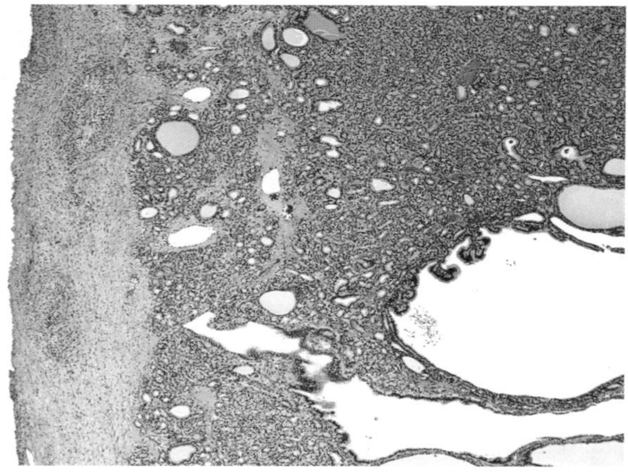

Fig. 16.43
Proliferative struma ovarii. **The follicles are markedly crowded, but features diagnostic of follicular thyroid carcinoma are not seen**

Clinical Behavior and Treatment

Most cases of struma ovarii are benign and can be treated by excision of the ovary or by unilateral salpingo-oophorectomy. In a small number of cases, there are complications, the most important being the development of malignancy [48, 62, 165, 168, 170]. In one series [48], proliferative struma ovarii was benign; however, in another series 26% of cases were clinically malignant, but the entire cohort of proliferative struma ovarii had good overall survival (98% survival at 10 years, 92% at 25 years) [165]. Another complication is the presence of ascites or ascites associated with pleural effusion producing a pseudo-Meigs' syndrome [84]. Ascites may be found in 17% of cases of struma ovarii, and its presence does not indicate that the tumor is malignant [193]. The cause of the ascites and pleural effusion has not been fully elucidated. In most reported cases, excision of the tumor led to complete remission.

Occasionally, struma ovarii may be associated with extra-ovarian extension caused either by rupture of the tumor or by local spread. In such cases, the peritoneal cavity contains tumor deposits, which may be numerous and are composed of mature thyroid tissue. The condition is thought by some to be benign and is termed benign strumosis [87], although some authorities believe that it represents a very well-differentiated follicular carcinoma [165, 167]. This condition is only rarely associated with untoward side effects, which are mainly caused by the formation of adhesions. As most patients with this rare condition have been treated by excision of the tumor deposits and by administration of radioactive iodine (^{131}I) with successful outcome, or have been lost to follow-up after varying periods of time with no ill effects, it is not possible to resolve this controversy. However, rare patients with strumosis have died of disease [165].

Malignancy Arising in Struma Ovarii

Clinical Features

Malignant change in struma ovarii, in which the tumor shows histologic/cytologic features of thyroid carcinoma ("malignant struma ovarii"), is uncommon (3% of all cases of struma ovarii in one study [165]). A number of reported cases of malignant struma ovarii were actually examples of strumal carcinoid. Patients with malignant struma ovarii are relatively young. The mean ages of women with the different types of thyroid carcinoma arising in struma ovarii range from 38 to 46 years [170]. Most patients with papillary thyroid carcinoma and typical follicular carcinoma present with stage I disease.

Microscopic Features

More than a hundred well-documented cases have been reported [62, 165, 170]. Microscopically, most of the tumors were of the papillary type (Fig. 16.44), including its follicular variant, followed by follicular carcinoma. A few tumors showed features of poorly differentiated carcinoma. *BRAF* mutations and *RET/PTC* rearrangements, as seen in papillary thyroid carcinoma of the eutopic thyroid gland, have been identified in papillary thyroid carcinoma arising in struma ovarii [28, 178].

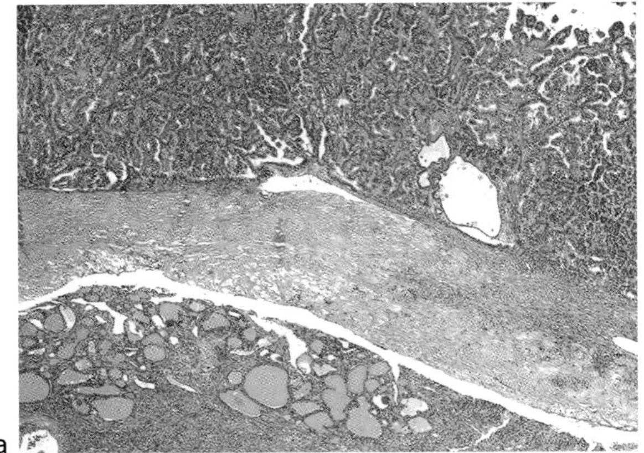

a

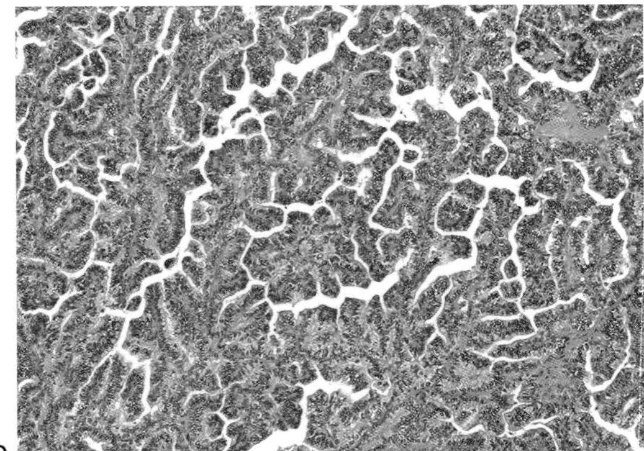

b

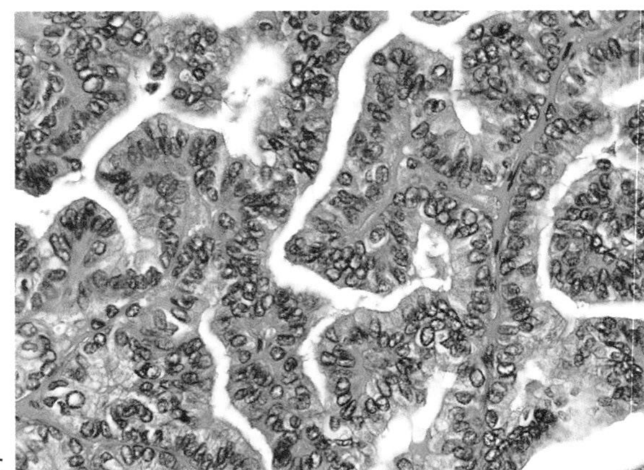

c

Fig. 16.44
Papillary thyroid carcinoma arising in struma ovarii. (a) Low power. Struma ovarii is present at the bottom, and carcinoma is present at the *top*. (b) Prominent papillary architecture. (c) Nuclear features characteristic of papillary thyroid carcinoma

In a number of reported cases, the diagnosis was based on the histology of the tumor, and there were no metastases or other features of malignancy [48, 169, 170]. Whether malignant struma ovarii should be diagnosed based on the same criteria used for tumors in the eutopic thyroid gland is unclear. Application of the eutopic thyroid diagnostic criteria for the follicular variant of papillary thyroid carcinoma (FVPTC) in struma ovarii (optically clear nuclei, overlapping nuclei, nuclear pseudoinclusions, nuclear grooves [165]) may be difficult given the recognized interobserver variability in diagnosis for tumors in eutopic thyroid locations. It should be noted that even ovarian tumors with subtle atypical nuclear features, which are suggestive of but not fully diagnostic for the FVPTC still have the ability to metastasize [62]. Therefore, it has been recommended that whenever an ovarian follicular thyroid-type tumor with cytologic features borderline for the FVPTC is encountered, it should be reviewed by at least two surgical pathologists with experience in thyroid pathology in order to prevent under- or overdiagnosis [62]. Application of eutopic thyroid criteria for the diagnosis of follicular carcinoma in struma ovarii (tumor invasion of cortex with growth on ovarian serosa and vascular invasion [165]) is also problematic, particularly because the ovary lacks a true capsule. Furthermore, ovarian tumors that histologically qualify as struma ovarii but which have an extra-ovarian metastasis or recurrence that histologically resembles non-neoplastic thyroid tissue have been designated "highly differentiated follicular carcinoma." [167] Thus, this form of follicular carcinoma can only be diagnosed when an extra-ovarian lesion is identified. It should be noted, however, that this entity is controversial and considered "peritoneal strumosis" by others. However, tumor deposits of obviously malignant papillary thyroid carcinoma and typical follicular carcinoma should be diagnosed as such.

For any ovarian tumor featuring a problematic proliferation of thyroid tissue, extensive sampling is strongly suggested. In rare and unusual cases (especially those with bilateral tumors), it may be necessary to recommend further clinical evaluation in order to exclude the possibility of a metastasis from the thyroid gland with secondary involvement of the ovary.

Clinical Behavior and Treatment

See above section on Malignancy Arising in Struma Ovarii for behavior of proliferative struma ovarii. In addition to peritoneal involvement by malignant struma ovarii, other routes of spread are via the lymphatics to the para-aortic and other lymph nodes and via the bloodstream to the lungs and bones [170]. Metastases are uncommon [62, 170]. The disease is treatable with good outcome in most cases, including those with metastatic disease. Only 7%, 14%, and 0% of patients with papillary thyroid carcinoma, typical follicular carcinoma, and "highly differentiated follicular carcinoma," respectively, in struma ovarii died of disease [170]. In a recent study by Robboy et al of all histologically malignant thyroid-type tumors in struma ovarii, 81% and 60% of patients were alive at 10 years and 25 years, respectively [165]. In that study, malignant struma ovarii was assessed for pathologic features that might predict aggressive behavior, and the size of the strumal component correlated with malignant outcome. It was also demonstrated that abundant peritoneal fluid, numerous adhesions, or ovarian serosal defects were more common in clinically malignant tumors. In general, however, it is not possible to reliably determine which cases will develop progressive disease.

Treatment of malignant struma ovarii should consist of at least oophorectomy but may also include thyroidectomy, radioactive iodine (^{131}I), and follow-up with serum thyroglobulin measurement. Long-term follow-up is important as metastases can occur decades later.

Carcinoid

Carcinoid tumors of the ovary may be primary or metastatic. Primary carcinoids are subdivided into four categories: (1) insular, (2) trabecular, (3) strumal, and (4) mucinous. Mixed types also occur (composed of any combination of the pure types). The latter are uncommon and often associated with a mature cystic teratoma. Of the metastatic carcinoids, the insular carcinoid tumor is the most common, followed by the trabecular and mucinous types. Metastatic carcinoid tumors of the ovary are discussed in ➲ Chap. 18, Metastatic Tumors of the Ovary.

Insular Carcinoid

General Features Insular carcinoid tumor, considered to be of midgut derivation, is the most common type of primary ovarian carcinoid tumor. It usually arises in association with gastrointestinal or respiratory epithelium present in a mature cystic teratoma. It may also be observed within a solid teratoma, a mucinous tumor, in association with a Sertoli–Leydig cell tumor [258], or may occur in a pure form [163, 195, 214]. The latter is considered to arise either as a one-sided development of a teratoma or from enterochromaffin cells present within the ovary. The former is much more likely. Approximately 40% of ovarian insular carcinoids occur in pure form; the remaining 60% are combined [185, 195, 214].

Clinical Features More than 200 cases of primary ovarian insular carcinoid tumors have been reported [45, 163, 185, 214]. The age of patients ranges from 31 to 83 years, but most patients are either postmenopausal or perimenopausal [45, 163, 195]. One third of the reported cases have been associated with the typical carcinoid syndrome, despite the absence of metastases [45, 163, 195]. This is in contrast to intestinal carcinoids, which are associated with the syndrome only when there is metastatic spread to the liver. The reason for this difference is that the blood flow from the ovary goes directly into the systemic circulation and does not pass through the liver, which inactivates the serotonin produced by the tumor. The presence or absence of symptoms of carcinoid syndrome is also dependent on the number of secreting tumor cells.

Functioning ovarian carcinoid tumors, with only one exception, have all measured approximately 10 cm in greatest dimension, whereas intestinal carcinoids are usually smaller. Thus, there is a good correlation between the size of the tumor and the presence of carcinoid syndrome. The excision of the tumor is associated with rapid remission of the symptoms, disappearance of 5-hydroxyindole acetic acid (5-HIAA) from the urine [163], and marked decrease of serum serotonin. Determination of serum serotonin and urinary 5-HIAA may be used to monitor disease activity and response to therapy. If the tumor is nonfunctioning, there is no specific presentation.

Gross Features The tumor shows similar appearances to those of mature cystic teratoma within which it is usually found. The same applies if the tumor is associated with a solid teratoma or a mucinous tumor. If the carcinoid is not associated with other tissue elements, the tumor is solid. The carcinoid may vary in size from microscopic to 20 cm in greatest dimension and is solid and homogeneous. Its color may vary from light brown to yellow or pale gray. Primary ovarian carcinoids practically always are unilateral, although they may be associated with a mature cystic teratoma in the contralateral ovary.

Microscopic Features Primary ovarian insular carcinoid usually shows the typical appearance associated with midgut carcinoids [163]. The tumor is composed of collections of small acini and solid nests of uniform polygonal cells with ample amounts of cytoplasm and round or oval, centrally located hyperchromatic nuclei (➲ *Fig. 16.45*). Mitotic activity is low. The cytoplasm is basophilic or amphophilic and may contain red, brown, or orange argentaffin or argyrophil granules, which are demonstrated in the majority of cases of primary ovarian carcinoids [163]. Ultrastructurally, the cells of the ovarian

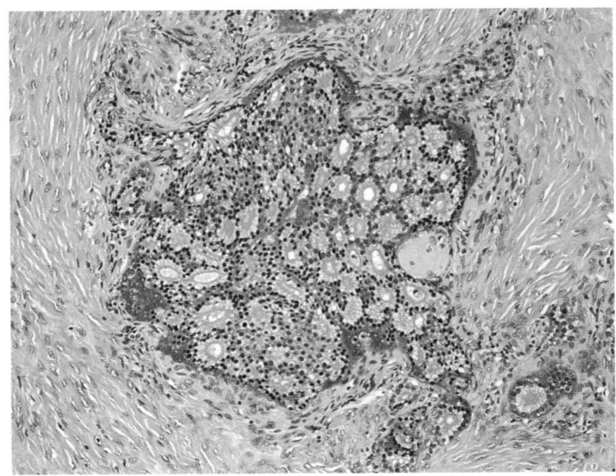

Fig. 16.45
Primary insular carcinoid tumor of the ovary. **Note the bright pink staining of the tumor cells due to the presence of neurosecretory granules**

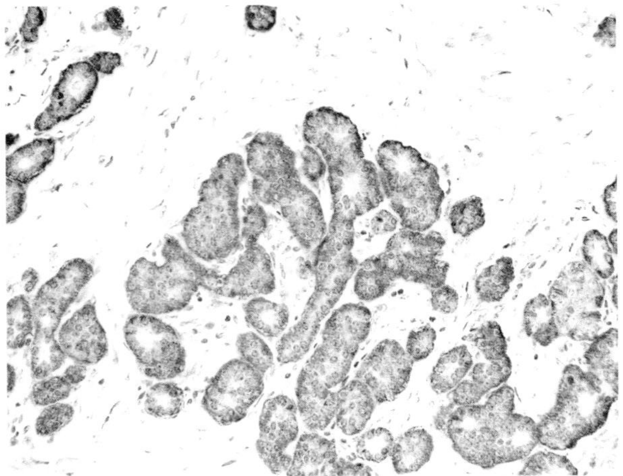

Fig. 16.46
Primary insular carcinoid tumor of the ovary. **The tumor shows diffuse expression of chromogranin. Note that the compartments of the cells showing chromogranin expression are the same compartments containing bright pink cytoplasmic granules in *Fig. 16.45***

insular carcinoid show similar appearances to those of insular carcinoid tumors from other locations [214] and show abundant neurosecretory granules, which exhibit marked variation in size and shape, being round, oval, or elongated.

Immunohistochemical Features and Differential Diagnosis

Demonstration of immunohistochemical expression of chromogranin and synaptophysin (*Fig. 16.46*) further supports the diagnosis and has become the method of choice to confirm the diagnosis. These two markers frequently show diffuse and strong staining [261]. Serotonin may be demonstrated within the cytoplasm of the tumor cells by immunohistochemical techniques [197]. Occasionally, other neurohormonal polypeptides may also be demonstrated within the cytoplasm of the tumor cells, but their finding is much less frequent than in trabecular or strumal carcinoids [197]. The connective tissue surrounding the tumor nests is frequently dense and hyalinized as a result of the fibrogenic effect of the serotonin produced by the tumor. If immunohistochemistry is needed because a carcinoma is in the differential diagnosis, one should be aware that carcinoid frequently expresses pan-cytokeratin and low molecular weight cytokeratin (CK8/18), which occasionally may be diffuse. CK7 and EMA are more specific in that they are frequently expressed in carcinoma and expressed uncommonly in carcinoid [261]. In carcinoids positive for CK7 and EMA, expression tends to be of limited extent. Also, ER and PR are usually negative in carcinoid and positive in endometrioid carcinomas and can be added to an immunohistochemical panel [261].

Primary insular carcinoid of the ovary must be differentiated from metastatic insular carcinoid of the ovary, which is usually of gastrointestinal origin. Metastatic carcinoid nearly always affects both ovaries [162], unlike primary ovarian carcinoid, which is unilateral [163]. Macroscopically, the metastatic carcinoid is composed of tumor nodules, whereas primary ovarian carcinoid forms a single homogeneous mass. Presence of other teratomatous elements associated with an ovarian carcinoid confirms that it is primary [163, 214].

Primary ovarian carcinoid sometimes may be confused with Brenner tumor, but the appearances of the cell nests and the grooved coffee-bean nuclei of the cells of Brenner tumor are against the diagnosis of a carcinoid, whereas the typical small acinar pattern and expression of chromogranin A are in favor of a carcinoid. Confusion with granulosa cell tumor may also arise because Call–Exner bodies may be mistaken for carcinoid acini, but the cells of the carcinoid tumor usually show an acinar pattern and contain more cytoplasm and argentaffin granules [163]. Cystic areas that may be present in a granulosa cell tumor are nearly always absent in a carcinoid. Presence of nuclear grooves typical of adult granulosa cell tumor further supports this diagnosis. Inhibin and calretinin are typically negative in carcinoid [261].

Occasionally, ovarian carcinoid may be confused with a Krukenberg tumor, but the latter is usually bilateral and larger. The cells of Krukenberg tumor tend to merge with the stroma, are larger, and show greater pleomorphism, at least focal signet-ring appearance, and more brisk mitotic activity. An acinar pattern is less evident. Demonstration of chromogranin and synaptophysin expression supports a diagnosis of carcinoid.

Clinical Behavior and Treatment Although insular carcinoid tumors of the ovary are considered to be malignant, they are slow growing and only occasionally are associated with metastases. Metastases have been observed in 11 patients, 7 of whom died with metastatic disease [45, 163]; this includes 6 patients with metastatic disease from a series of 9 cases of insular carcinoid tumors of the ovary collected over 40 years by Davis et al [45]. This series suggested that metastatic disease may be more frequent than generally reported. Although the malignant potential of insular carcinoid should not be minimized, it is considered that the series of Davis et al [45]. was somewhat selective as regards its content of metastasizing tumors and lethal outcome.

In occasional patients, features of carcinoid syndrome, such as tricuspid incompetence resulting in right-sided heart failure, may progress after the excision of the tumor and lead to the death of the patient, as has been observed in two cases [163]. In most patients with the carcinoid syndrome, the symptoms and signs of the syndrome observed preoperatively disappear or regress during the postoperative period [163]. Because nearly all patients with this tumor are postmenopausal or perimenopausal, bilateral salpingo-oophorectomy and hysterectomy is the treatment of choice. Surgical excision of foci of extra-ovarian spread or of metastases if present is indicated. There is little experience with chemotherapy. Estimation of serum serotonin and 5-HIAA in the urine may be used to monitor the progress of the disease.

Trabecular Carcinoid

General Features Trabecular carcinoid includes carcinoid tumors of hindgut or foregut derivation. Primary trabecular or ribbon carcinoid usually arises in association with teratomatous elements [164, 195], but in a later study of four cases of trabecular carcinoid, two tumors were pure and not associated with teratomatous elements [217].

Clinical Features Trabecular carcinoid is rare. Patient age varies from 24 to 74 years, with most patients being postmenopausal [45, 164, 195, 217]. Trabecular carcinoid is a slowly growing neoplasm that can reach a large size.

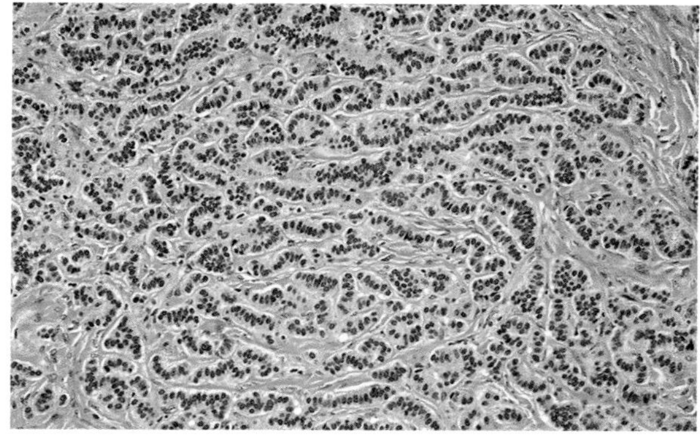

Fig. 16.47
Primary trabecular carcinoid tumor of the ovary. **The tumor is composed of long ramifying cords of tumor cells surrounded by dense fibrous stroma**

None of the known cases have been associated with the carcinoid syndrome. In three patients whose urine was examined immediately after the operation, 5-HIAA was normal [164].

Gross Features The appearance of trabecular carcinoid depends on whether the tumor is associated with teratomatous elements. When associated with teratoma, the appearance is similar to that of a mature cystic teratoma. When the tumor is pure, it is a solid, firm to hard, round or oval mass with a smooth outline and tan to yellow on cross section. The tumors have always been unilateral [164, 195, 217], but occasionally have been associated with mature cystic teratoma in the opposite ovary [164, 195]. In the reported cases, the tumors measured from 4 to 25 cm in greatest dimension [164, 195, 217].

Microscopic Features The tumor is composed of long, usually wavy ribbons, cords, or parallel trabeculae surrounded by fibromatous connective tissue stroma that is usually dense (*Fig. 16.47*). The ribbons, cords, or trabeculae are composed of cells that form usually one but sometimes two cell layers. The nuclei are elongated or ovoid and contain finely dispersed chromatin. The cytoplasm is abundant and often contains orange to red-brown granules, which usually stain with argyrophil and argentaffin stains. Ultrastructurally, the neurosecretory granules are round or oval and show slight variation in size [187, 220], thus differing from those seen in insular carcinoids.

Immunohistochemical Features and Differential Diagnosis See section on Insular Carcinoid for details of immunohistochemistry. Immunohistochemical staining demonstrates a much wider range of neurohormonal polypeptides than insular carcinoids; these include serotonin, pancreatic polypeptide, glucagon, enkephalin, gastrin, vasoactive intestinal polypeptide, and calcitonin [197].

Primary trabecular carcinoid must be distinguished from metastatic trabecular carcinoid, which is usually bilateral and frequently associated with metastases elsewhere. The presence of teratomatous elements, which are found frequently in the primary lesion, helps distinguish the primary from a metastatic lesion. Trabecular carcinoid sometimes may exhibit an insular pattern in foci, but unless this is a major component the tumor need not be classified as a mixed carcinoid.

The presence of thyroid follicles indicates that the tumor is a struma ovarii and carcinoid (strumal carcinoid), and their presence must be excluded before a diagnosis of trabecular carcinoid is made. Occasionally, trabecular carcinoid must be distinguished from a Sertoli–Leydig cell tumor showing a cord-like pattern. In contrast to a Sertoli–Leydig tumor, trabecular carcinoid lacks tubules. Immunohistochemical expression of chromogranin and synaptophysin and lack of staining for inhibin and calretinin confirm the diagnosis of carcinoid.

Clinical Behavior and Treatment The prognosis of patients with trabecular carcinoid of the ovary is favorable because these tumors are not associated with metastases [45, 164, 217]. In one case, a peritoneal implant was found 2 years after bilateral salpingo-oophorectomy and hysterectomy [164]. The optimal treatment is the excision of the affected adnexa, which results in a complete cure, but follow-up of the patient is advisable.

Mucinous Carcinoid (Goblet Cell Carcinoid)

General Features Mucinous carcinoid is a variant of carcinoid tumor that has been encountered mainly in the vermiform appendix [90, 203, 249] and occasionally has been observed in the ovary [2, 16, 214]. However, it should be noted that at least some of the tumors described as primary Krukenberg tumors of the ovary may have been examples of this entity. Also, it should be emphasized that before establishing a diagnosis of primary ovarian mucinous carcinoid, a metastatic appendiceal carcinoma with goblet cell carcinoid-like features must be excluded. A number of the latter have been reported [78], and several more are known to the authors. It is likely that a proportion of "primary ovarian" mucinous carcinoids reported in the literature really represent metastases from an occult appendiceal primary.

Clinical Features The age of patients ranges from 14 to 74 years. Mucinous carcinoid is usually observed in pure form but may be seen in association with mature cystic teratoma. The tumor is unilateral but may be associated with metastases in the contralateral ovary [2, 16, 214].

Gross Features Macroscopically, the tumor is usually of considerable size, ranging from 4 to 30 cm, and most of the tumors have been more than 8 cm in greatest dimension. The tumor is gray-yellow, firm, and usually solid but may contain cystic areas [2, 16, 214]. Similar appearances are encountered when the tumor forms part of a mature cystic teratoma.

Microscopic Features Microscopically, mucinous carcinoid is composed of numerous small glands or acini with very small lumens lined by uniform columnar or cuboid epithelium. The cells contain small round or oval nuclei or appear as goblet cells distended with mucin (*Fig. 16.48*). Some cells may be disrupted by excessive distension with mucin, which may result in the formation of small pools of mucin within the glands or even in the obliteration of the gland with pools of mucinous material within the connective tissue. The glands are surrounded by connective tissue, which may vary from loose and edematous to dense fibrous or hyalinized. Some of the glands or acini may be larger and occasionally may be cystic; this represents the typical or classical pattern of mucinous carcinoid. In some areas, the tumor cells tend to invade the surrounding connective tissue, often assuming signet-ring appearance. The tumor cells may form large solid aggregates and show a less uniform appearance

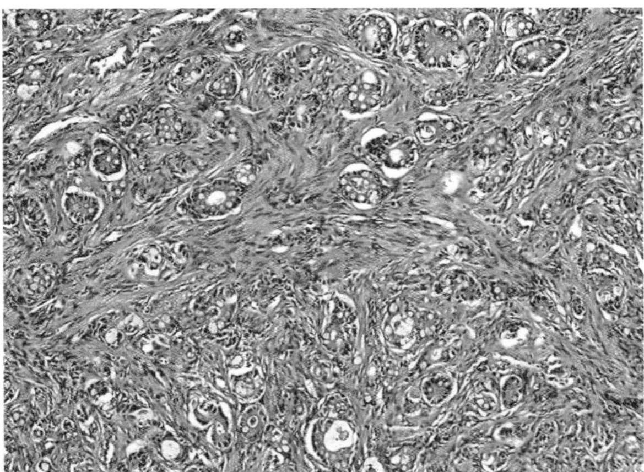

Fig. 16.48
Primary mucinous carcinoid tumor. **The tumor is composed of numerous small glands and acini with imperceptible or very small lumens. Numerous goblet cells distended with mucin are present**

and more atypical features, with large hyperchromatic nuclei and brisk mitotic activity.

In some tumors, such appearances may predominate. This second pattern resembles Krukenberg tumor and is described as atypical or Krukenberg tumor-like pattern. Sometimes mucinous carcinoid showing either the typical or atypical pattern or both merges with intestinal-like adenocarcinoma showing numerous neuroendocrine cells; this is regarded as a third pattern present in this tumor. Some mucinous carcinoids may be admixed with other types of carcinoid tumor, such as insular or trabecular, forming a mixed carcinoid tumor. Thus, primary ovarian mucinous carcinoid tumors can be divided into these four histologic types. In a study of 17 mucinous carcinoid tumors, 6 were of the typical type, 4 of the atypical or Krukenberg tumor-like type, 5 were admixed with intestinal-like adenocarcinoma, and 2 were of the mixed type [16]. The cytoplasm of the tumor cells may exhibit orange-red granules and may even be bright red. Argyrophil and argentaffin granules are always present and, in some tumors, may be abundant [2, 16, 214].

Ultrastructurally, neurosecretory granules are present in some cells and absent in others. The tumor cells may contain both neurosecretory granules and mucinous material. The neuroendocrine nature of the tumor cells is further confirmed using immunohistochemical stains.

Immunohistochemical Features and Differential Diagnosis The tumor cells react positively with chromogranin A. Using immunohistochemical techniques, some of the tumor cells have been shown to contain serotonin and gastrin, and these substances may be present within the same tumor cell. Other neurohormonal polypeptides such as pancreatic polypeptide and prolactin also have been detected in the tumor cells, but the range is narrower than that observed in trabecular carcinoids. CEA and low molecular weight cytokeratin also can be demonstrated within the cytoplasm of the tumor cells. These tumors are expected to show a CK7(−)/CK20 diffuse profile [248] (➲ *Fig. 16.49*).

Primary mucinous carcinoid tumor of the ovary must be differentiated from its metastatic counterpart although a number of the latter probably are appendiceal carcinomas with goblet cell carcinoid-like features [78, 214]. The latter, in common with other types of carcinoid metastatic to the ovary, is nearly always bilateral and instead of forming a single tumor mass shows scattered tumor deposits involving ovarian tissue. Depending on their size, these deposits may form tumor nodules observed macroscopically or may be detectable only microscopically. Histologically, they may have appearances indistinguishable from the primary tumor. The presence of teratomatous elements supports primary ovarian origin.

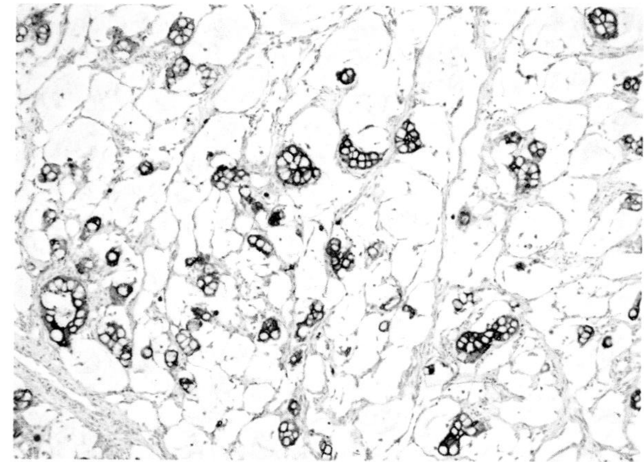

◘ Fig. 16.49
Primary mucinous carcinoid tumor

Mucinous carcinoid must be distinguished from mucinous tumors of the ovary, particularly, a mucinous carcinoma with goblet cell carcinoid-like features arising in a teratoma. That is especially so when the carcinoid tumor is composed of large acini, shows increased mucin production, and exhibits a pleomorphic pattern. Occasionally, confusion may arise with well-differentiated endometrioid tumors of the ovary, which may resemble mucinous tumors.

Mucinous carcinoid must be distinguished from a Krukenberg tumor. The differentiation between these two entities may be difficult, especially if the mucinous carcinoid assumes a predominantly Krukenberg-like pattern or if the Krukenberg tumor contains numerous argentaffin and argyrophil granules. The presence of these granules as well as of the neurosecretory granules observed ultrastructurally cannot be used for differentiation between these two entities. Involvement of both ovaries and the presence of primary extra-ovarian signet-ring or mucinous adenocarcinoma are indicative of Krukenberg tumor.

Clinical Behavior and Treatment Primary mucinous carcinoid of the ovary behaves in a somewhat more aggressive manner than other types of primary ovarian carcinoid tumors [2, 16, 214], similar to the behavior of mucinous carcinoid tumors of the vermiform appendix [90, 203, 249]. The tumor tends to spread mainly via the lymphatics, and metastases may be present at the time of initial laparotomy. Patients who do not exhibit metastatic disease at the time of diagnosis have a much better prognosis compared to those who have metastases, however small, at the time of diagnosis [2, 16, 214]. A series of 17 patients has been reported [16]. Six patients with mucinous carcinoid of the typical or classical type had tumors confined to the ovary, and all five with available follow-up (27–147 months) were well and disease-free after excision of the tumor. Three patients with mucinous carcinoid of the atypical type had tumors confined to the ovary and were well and disease-free after excision of the tumor (follow-up, 36–168 months). Of the eight women with carcinoma arising in mucinous carcinoid, six were stage I, one was stage II, and one was stage III. Seven had available follow-up. Two patients died of disease at 9 and 12 months, respectively. Four were alive and well with 48–120 months of follow-up, and a fifth patient died of other causes at 36 months.

The treatment is surgical, depending on the extent of the disease, but in postmenopausal women, patients with involvement of the contralateral ovary, and patients who do not want children, hysterectomy, bilateral salpingo-oophorectomy, and omentectomy, as well as excision of all the tumor deposits, are indicated. Para-aortic lymph node dissection may be necessary because metastatic tumor deposits may be present. Surgery may be followed by combination chemotherapy, including 5-fluorouracil, although the efficacy of this mode of therapy is not proven. Premenopausal patients with tumors localized to the ovary may be treated by unilateral salpingo-oophorectomy with careful follow-up.

Strumal Carcinoid

General Features Strumal carcinoid is an uncommon ovarian tumor composed of thyroid tissue intimately admixed with carcinoid tumor, showing a ribbon-like or cordlike pattern. Other teratomatous elements are also present in most of the tumors [161]. Tumors showing the histologic pattern of struma ovarii, merging imperceptibly with carcinoid tumor exhibiting the ribbon-like pattern observed in hindgut carcinoids, were usually interpreted as a carcinoma developing in a struma ovarii, although the resemblance to a carcinoid tumor has been noted in some cases.

Clinical Features More than 60 cases have been reported [161, 194, 195], and there are probably as many unreported cases. The age distribution is similar to struma ovarii, ranging from 21 to 77 years. The tumor is usually not associated with any specific clinical findings. In one reported case, it was associated with virilization. Like hindgut carcinoids and unlike the primary ovarian insular carcinoid, strumal carcinoid is not, as a rule, associated with the carcinoid syndrome [161, 194, 195] although this association has been described in a single case [244].

Gross Features Macroscopically, this tumor, if pure, may be similar to struma ovarii or carcinoid. If the tumor is a part of a teratoma, it manifests as a yellow nodule within the teratoma [161, 194].

Microscopic and Immunohistochemical Features Microscopically, strumal carcinoid is composed of thyroid follicles containing colloid that merge with ribbons of neoplastic cells usually set in dense fibrous tissue stroma similar to trabecular carcinoid (*Fig. 16.50*). The thyroid follicles are often small in size at the junction between the two types of tissue. The carcinoid is usually composed of long, winding or straight ribbons of columnar cells with elongated hyperchromatic nuclei. It may also be composed of small islands of tumor cells surrounded by dense fibrous tissue stroma. Slight mitotic activity is present in the carcinoid part of the lesion.

Argyrophil and argentaffin granules are identified in the carcinoid cells [161, 194, 198], as well as in some cells lining the thyroid follicles both histochemically and immunohistochemically. Chromogranin and synaptophysin are expressed in the carcinoid component. TTF-1 and CK7 are usually expressed in the strumal component with no expression in the carcinoid component [156]; however,

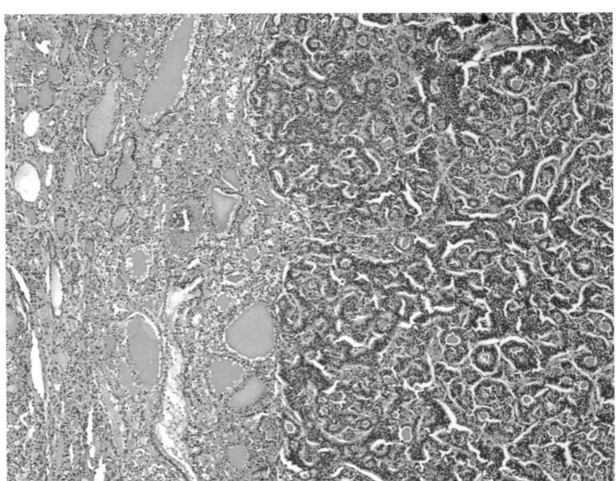

Fig. 16.50
Strumal carcinoid. **The carcinoid forms long narrow cords and ribbons (*right*) merging with thyroid follicles (*left*)**

we have seen cases with focal TTF-1 expression in the carcinoid component. Ultrastructural examination demonstrates neurosecretory granules in the carcinoid component and in some of the thyroid follicular cells [194, 198]. In two tumors, amyloid deposits were identified and were verified both immunohistochemically and ultrastructurally [6, 47].

Some investigators consider that strumal carcinoid is a carcinoid tumor and that the thyroid tissue only resembles thyroid [73]. Other investigators have conclusively demonstrated thyroglobulin and TTF-1 within the thyroid component of the tumor, thus indicating its thyroid nature [156, 161, 194]. It is, therefore, considered that in verified cases of strumal carcinoid, the tumor consists of thyroid tissue intimately admixed with a carcinoid. Strumal carcinoid should be distinguished from carcinoma of the thyroid arising in struma ovarii, with which it has often been confused. The carcinoma has the typical appearances observed in the eutopic thyroid and usually exhibits the follicular or papillary pattern.

Clinical Behavior and Treatment Strumal carcinoid only once has been associated with metastases, and even in this case the patient was apparently cured by a combination of surgery and radiation therapy [161]. All other cases have followed a benign course [161, 194].

Monodermal Teratomas with Neuroectodermal Differentiation

Cysts lined entirely by mature glial [246] or ependymal tissue [238] have been described in the ovary. More importantly, however, neuroectodermal tumors may also develop in the ovary and are considered monodermal teratomas with neuroectodermal differentiation. Kleinman et al. have reported a series of 25 cases of primary neuroectodermal tumors of the ovary [91]. The average age was 23 years (range 6–69 years). The tumors were cystic and/or solid with an average size of 14 cm (range 4–20 cm). They consisted of three histologic types: differentiated (ependymoma (*Fig. 16.51*)), primitive (medulloepithelioma, ependymoblastoma, neuroblastoma, and medulloblastoma), and anaplastic (glioblastoma). Some were associated with a mature cystic teratoma. Occasional patients may present with advanced stage disease. It is noteworthy that ependymomas may contain papillary areas mimicking serous tumors or gland-like structures resembling endometrioid tumors. In the small number of neoplasms tested, immunohistochemical expression of glial fibrillary acidic protein (GFAP) was seen in the differentiated and anaplastic tumors but not the primitive tumors. Survival was dependent on stage; however, the differentiated group showed superior outcome compared with the other two categories of tumors, and deaths with stage I tumors were seen in the anaplastic group.

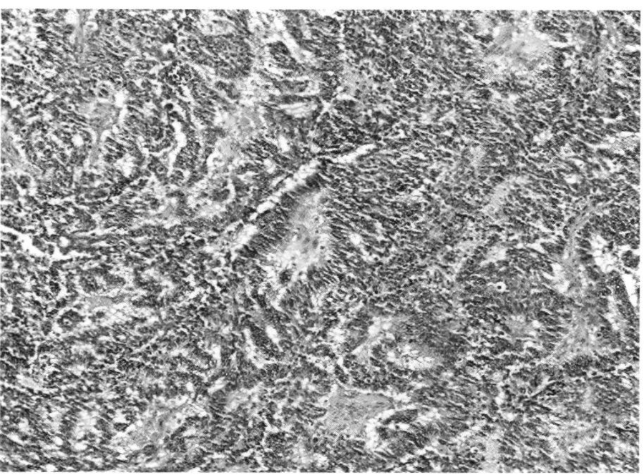

Fig. 16.51
Monodermal teratoma with ependymona. **Perivascular pseudorosettes are present**

Monodermal Teratoma Composed of Vascular Tissue

Another type of monodermal teratoma is represented by neoplasms composed entirely or predominantly of immature vascular tissue. These occur in children and young adults, and the patients present with symptoms and signs suggestive of an ovarian tumor. The tumors may vary in size and are smooth, soft, solid, and gray-pink but may be hemorrhagic. Microscopically, they consist of collections of small vascular spaces lined by immature endothelial cells and surrounded by connective tissue, which varies from loose and edematous to dense and fibrous. The lining of the vascular spaces may be multilayered and the endothelial cells may form small projections bulging into the lumen. Small collections of endothelial cells, some forming abortive lumina and some devoid of a lumen, are also seen within the connective tissue and may predominate.

The endothelial cells show a considerable degree of cellular and nuclear pleomorphism, and mitotic activity is usually evident. Occasionally, hematopoietic activity may be seen within some of the vascular spaces. When these tumors contain small teratomatous foci, their nature is more readily apparent, but when they occur in pure form, especially when the endothelial cells form a more solid pattern with fewer obvious vascular spaces, the nature of the lesion is more difficult to recognize. Occasionally, these tumors may be composed of immature pericytes and resemble a hemangiopericytoma. Further sectioning of the tumor, which may reveal a more typical vascular pattern, and immunohistochemical stains for CD31 and CD34 as well as for factor VIII may be helpful in reaching the correct diagnosis. This distinction is important because monodermal teratomas composed of immature vascular tissue or with a predominant vascular component behave on the whole in a less aggressive manner compared with high-grade immature teratomas and angiosarcomas of the ovary, with which they tend to be confused. As in most immature teratomas, the grade of the tumor is an important prognostic feature.

Baker et al. have reported a series of teratomas containing prominent benign vascular proliferations associated with neural tissue [17]. The underlying tumors were either mature cystic teratoma, immature teratoma, or a mixed germ cell tumor. The vascular proliferations consisted of long, thin-walled, and curved vessels or rounded cellular aggregates with glomeruloid patterns. Small vessels could be seen arranged in whorls, and focally, a trabecular pattern was present.

Monodermal Teratoma with Sebaceous Differentiation

Sebaceous tumors showing one-sided development of a teratoma or arising in mature cystic teratomas are rare [38]. The reported cases showed an age range from 31 to 79 years at presentation, but the majority of patients were older than 49 years. All presented with lower abdominal enlargement. The ovarian tumors found at laparotomy were large, ranging from 10 to 35 cm. Some of the patients were found to have a mature cystic teratoma in the contralateral ovary. The tumors were mainly cystic. Partly solid yellow and tan masses protruded into the cysts. The latter contained necrotic or cheesy material [38]. Similar findings were also noted in a case of sebaceous carcinoma recently seen by the authors.

Microscopically, the tumors consisted of sebaceous adenoma, basal cell carcinoma with sebaceous differentiation, and sebaceous carcinoma [38]. The adenomas were all composed of nodules or lobules of proliferating normal sebaceous cells showing various degrees of maturity, with mature cells predominating. The basal cell carcinomas with sebaceous differentiation were composed of masses or nests of malignant basal cells containing collections of mature sebaceous cells. The sebaceous carcinoma was composed of sebaceous cells showing marked cellular and nuclear pleomorphism growing in an infiltrative pattern. The tumor cells had the typical appearance of sebaceous cells. Lipid stains were strongly positive in all the tumors, confirming the diagnosis [38].

The patients were treated either by excision of the affected adnexa or by hysterectomy and bilateral salpingo-oophorectomy [38]. The outcome was favorable; only one tumor was known to have recurred. The tumor, a basal cell carcinoma with sebaceous differentiation, recurred in the pelvis; further follow-up was not available. All the other patients were well and disease-free for periods ranging from 1.5 to 6 years postoperatively. One patient had, in addition to the sebaceous adenoma, a squamous cell carcinoma arising in the same ovary and died as a result of disseminated disease 1 year after the diagnosis. The patient with sebaceous carcinoma was well and disease-free 6 years after diagnosis [38]. In the case of sebaceous carcinoma recently seen by the authors, the patient was well after complete excision of the tumor. There were no adhesions or metastases. Chemotherapy was also administered. Whether this additional treatment was necessary is debatable.

Other Types of Monodermal Teratoma

Some mucinous tumors of germ cell origin arising in mature cystic teratomas may overgrow the background teratomatous component and appear to be entirely composed of a mucinous tumor (see section on Mucinous Tumors Arising in Mature Cystic Teratoma) [248]. This phenomenon is similar to the situation in which thyroid tissue in a pure struma ovarii or carcinoid has developed in a pure form or has overgrown all the other tissues. The presence of occasional teratomatous tumors composed mainly of mucinous (intestinal-type) epithelium of endodermal derivation and only a small amount of other teratomatous elements, as well as a 5% association of mature cystic teratoma with mucinous cystadenoma, lends strong support to this mode of origin for at least some mucinous tumors.

Mucinous epithelium resembling intestinal epithelium has been observed in association with struma ovarii and with strumal carcinoid. In these cases, it was the only other tissue element present. The mucinous epithelium frequently contains goblet cells resembling intestinal rather than endocervical epithelium. In 21% of cases, the epithelium lining mucinous tumors of the ovary contains argyrophil and argentaffin granules. In a considerable number of cases, Paneth cells are also present. These findings are considered to be a strong argument in favor of the derivation of at least some mucinous ovarian tumors from intestinal-type epithelium and their teratomatous (germ cell) origin. Molecular studies will help clarify the origin of pure mucinous tumors of the ovary and confirm that some of these are of germ cell origin [108].

Other rare examples of monodermal teratomatous neoplasms observed in the ovary include the epidermoid cyst, which is lined by epidermis without appendages, the melanotic tumor, resembling the retinal anlage tumor [88], and the possible benign cystic counterpart of the latter [5]. Monodermal teratomatous origin of some malignant connective tissue tumors is difficult to prove because of the occurrence of connective tissue neoplasms derived from normal ovarian tissue. Monodermal teratomatous origin of tumors derived from ectodermal or endodermal tissues is more easily acceptable, and there may be as yet undescribed tumors of this type.

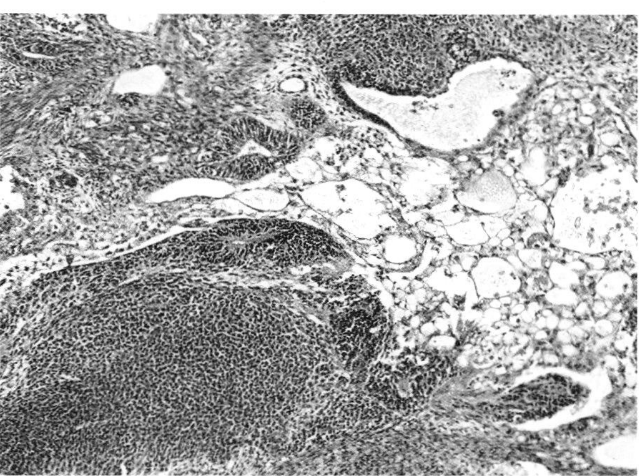

Fig. 16.52
Malignant mixed germ cell tumor. **The tumor is composed of poorly differentiated neuroepithelial elements and yolk sac tumor (*right*)**

Mixed Germ Cell Tumors

Mixed germ cell tumors are tumors composed of more than one neoplastic germ cell element, such as dysgerminoma combined with teratoma, yolk sac tumor, choriocarcinoma, embryonal carcinoma, or polyembryoma, as well as any other possible combination of these tumor types (*Fig. 16.52*). Some tumors may contain all these neoplastic germ cell elements. Histologically, the different neoplastic germ cell elements may be intimately admixed or found separated from one another. Some studies indicate a greater frequency of mixed germ cell tumors [98, 141] as compared with earlier reports [121]. This finding is a result of a more detailed examination of the tumors and a better recognition of the fact that germ cell tumors may be composed of histologically different neoplastic elements occurring in combination. This group includes only neoplasms composed entirely of neoplastic germ cell elements and does not include gonadoblastoma and mixed germ cell–sex cord–stromal tumor, which in addition to germ cells contain sex cord–stromal derivatives as an integral component. The relatively frequent finding of different neoplastic germ cell elements in gonadal tumors of germ cell origin is considered to be a strong argument in favor of the common histogenesis of this group of neoplasms. The various tumor elements present in these tumors may be intimately admixed or may form separate areas adjacent to each other and separated by fibrous septa.

Although many ovarian tumors belonging to this group are classified according to the predominant element present, it is emphasized that when these tumors are examined, all areas of varying appearance should be sampled carefully. All the neoplastic germ cell elements observed within the tumor, however small, should be reported and described and, if possible, their relative size estimated. This is important because the behavior and treatment of these neoplasms vary considerably, and the presence of a small area composed of a more malignant element may alter the therapeutic approach and prognosis. This is especially true in children [74] where most immature teratomas behave in a nonaggressive manner; however, the presence of small foci of yolk sac tumor (YST) in an immature teratoma is associated with aggressive behavior.

Even though the presence of very small foci of YST or high-grade immature teratoma may not alter the behavior of a mixed germ cell tumor largely composed of less-aggressive components, the presence of larger amounts of more malignant elements within a tumor is usually associated with a more aggressive behavior. Before the introduction of effective combination chemotherapy, the presence of YST or other more aggressive elements was associated with an unsatisfactory response to therapy and poor prognosis [9, 98, 223]. However, it should be noted that the clinical course in most patients with tumors composed of yolk sac tumor associated with dysgerminoma or other germ cell elements usually does not differ materially from that observed in patients with pure yolk sac tumor [64, 140]. The different response to treatment and the different behavior of some cases of dysgerminoma described in the past may have been a result of the presence of other germ cell elements that were not identified. Although in the past mixed germ cell tumors were considered to be uncommon, they tend to figure quite frequently in subsequent reports, probably because of more careful and extensive examination of the tumors.

Clinical and Pathologic Features of Tumors Composed of Germ Cells and Sex Cord–Stromal Derivatives

Gonadoblastoma

General Features

In 1953, Scully [181] described two patients with a distinctive gonadal tumor, which he designated gonadoblastoma. The tumor was composed of germ cells and sex cord–stromal derivatives, resembling immature granulosa and Sertoli cells. One of the tumors also contained stromal elements indistinguishable from lutein or Leydig cells. Both tumors occurred in phenotypic females who showed abnormal sexual development. The older patient, who was postpubertal, showed virilization, and it was considered that the tumor was capable of steroid hormone secretion. The tumors were located at the site of normal ovaries, but normal ovarian tissue was not discernible and the exact nature of the gonads in which the tumors had originated could not be determined. Both patients had bilateral tumors that were partly overgrown by dysgerminoma. The tumor was designated gonadoblastoma because it appeared to recapitulate the development of the gonads and because it occurred in individuals with abnormal sexual development and in gonads, the nature of which could not be determined [182]. It was subsequently demonstrated that both patients were sex chromatin negative.

The neoplastic nature of gonadoblastoma has been questioned because some lesions are very small and may undergo complete regression by hyalinization and calcification. Furthermore, when malignancy supervenes, it manifests itself as germ cell neoplasia despite the fact that gonadoblastoma is composed of two or three different cell types. When the tumor has metastasized, gonadoblastoma as such has never been observed in the metastases. Nevertheless, gonadoblastoma shows exactly the same pattern in the very small lesions as in the large ones, including mitotic activity in the germ cell element and early overgrowth by dysgerminoma. The association with dysgerminoma is seen in 50% of cases and with other more malignant germ cell neoplasms in an additional 10% [182]. In view of this, the concept that gonadoblastoma represents an in situ germ cell malignancy is considered to be fully justified.

Genetic and Molecular Features

Gonadoblastoma occurs almost entirely in patients with pure or mixed gonadal dysgenesis or in male pseudohermaphrodites. Occasional patients are of short stature and may have other stigmata of Turner syndrome [30, 174, 189]. Nearly all patients with gonadoblastoma whose karyotype was recorded (96%) were found to have a Y chromosome [174]. Eight patients had 46,XX karyotype [20, 53, 122, 132, 228, 260], and four of these were fertile [20, 53, 122, 228, 260]. One patient had a 45,X/46,XX mosaicism [181]. The most frequently encountered karyotype was 46,XY, which was seen in half the cases; this was followed by 45,X/46,XY mosaicism, which was seen in a quarter of the cases. The remainder showed many different forms of mosaicism [174]. Six patients had morphologic abnormalities of the Y chromosome. Of 25 patients with gonadal dysgenesis and dysgerminoma, 24 had a Y chromosome. The karyotype was 46,XY in 60%, followed by 45,X/46,XY in 24%. The remainder showed various forms of mosaicism [174]. One patient had 45,X monosomy and Turner syndrome. All other patients with features of Turner syndrome had various forms of mosaicism containing a Y chromosome.

The similarity between the distribution of the karyotypes in the gonadoblastoma group and the patients with dysgerminoma and gonadal dysgenesis is striking, and 62% of the former group and 45% of the latter had clitoral hypertrophy [174]. Gonadal dysgenesis and dysgerminoma has been reported in a female with a 46,XX karyotype who had no evidence of Y chromosomal DNA [101]. Gonadoblastoma was not detected in the affected gonad, but the authors [101] suggested that it was probably overgrown by the dysgerminoma. This finding indicates that gonadoblastoma and gonadal dysgenesis may occur in patients who do not have Y chromosomal DNA.

Family history of gonadal dysgenesis has been noted in at least 10 reports of patients with gonadoblastoma [3, 4, 26, 208]. Evidence of gonadal dysgenesis affecting three generations of the family of a patient with gonadoblastoma was obtained in two instances [3, 18]. Gonadoblastoma has been reported in one pair of twins [56] and in four pairs of siblings [3, 4, 26, 208]. All these patients had 46,XY karyotype. It has been postulated that the mode of inheritance is either an X-linked recessive gene or an autosomal sex-linked mutant gene [18, 174, 175]. The *TSPY* gene has been suggested as playing a role in the pathogenesis of gonadoblastoma [100].

Endocrine Features

The association of gonadoblastoma with certain endocrine abnormalities was noted in one of the two cases first reported [181]. In view of the fact that gonadoblastoma occurs almost entirely in patients with gonadal dysgenesis, the defective gonadal development present in these patients should not be confused with the presence of endocrine effects that are associated with the tumor and are not a result of the abnormal gonadal development. Although the virilization produced by the tumor may regress after the excision of the tumor, there is no further gonadal development and the gonadal abnormalities remain. Although the exact source of the steroid hormone production was not originally known, the interstitial cells resembling Leydig or lutein cells were considered to be the most likely source of the androgens [181]. Further observations have shown that the presence of Leydig or lutein-like cells is not always associated with the presence of virilization, although they are encountered more frequently in tumors from virilized phenotypic female patients than in those from non-virilized patients. The possibility that the tumor may secrete estrogens, as evidenced by complaints of hot flushes and other menopausal symptoms after the excision of the tumor, has also been noted [182]. Originally the evidence of hormone secretion was mainly clinical, usually evidenced by virilization occurring after puberty and manifesting itself as masculine body contour, hirsutism, and clitoromegaly. Slight elevation of the urinary 17-ketosteroid excretion was noted in some cases. The gonadotropins, when estimated, were usually elevated.

Subsequently, it has been shown that gonadoblastoma is capable of producing testosterone and estrogens from progesterone in vitro [4, 166]. Evidence of testosterone secretion in vivo in patients with gonadal dysgenesis has been presented [83]. Androgen and estrogen formation from progesterone in vitro has been demonstrated in a streak gonad that did not contain any Leydig and lutein cells microscopically, but from the description, it may have contained a small burned-out gonadoblastoma [106]. Although in vitro testosterone formation has been ascribed to the Leydig or lutein-like cells present in gonadoblastoma [166], the demonstration of steroid production by a streak gonad that did not contain Leydig or lutein cells indicates that the nondescript stromal tissue also has the capability of steroid synthesis [106].

Despite the advances in the understanding of the hormonal aspects of gonadoblastoma and dysgenetic gonads, a number of questions remain, the most important being why some patients become virilized and others do not. Although there is an approximate relationship between virilization and the presence of Leydig or lutein-like cells in the tumor, this relationship is not constant. It may be that the amount of steroid secretion is inadequate to produce virilization because of a small cell mass. Another possible explanation is that the steroid metabolic pathways may be different and that some gonadoblastomas may produce hormones that are metabolically nonfunctioning whereas other gonadoblastomas produce metabolically active steroids.

Clinical Features

The exact prevalence of gonadoblastoma is not known, but it is certainly uncommon. Gonadoblastoma is usually seen in young patients, occurring most frequently in the second decade and somewhat less frequently in the third and first decades, in that order. With a few exceptions, all the reported cases occurred in patients under 30 years of age. Patients with gonadoblastoma usually have primary amenorrhea, virilization, or developmental abnormalities of the genitalia. The discovery of gonadoblastoma is made in the course of investigations of these conditions. Another mode of presentation is the presence of a gonadal tumor. The gonadoblastoma forms part of the tumor in these cases and is discovered on histologic examination. Most patients with gonadoblastoma (80%) are phenotypic females, and the remainder are phenotypic males with cryptorchidism, hypospadias, and female internal secondary sex organs. Among the phenotypic females, 60% are virilized and the remainder are normal in appearance [182].

Most of the phenotypic female patients exhibit abnormal genital development, and breast development is often diminished even among the non-virilized females. Although primary amenorrhea is a common presenting symptom among phenotypic females with gonadoblastoma, a few patients have episodes of spontaneous cyclical bleeding, but in most of these patients the episodes are sporadic and the bleeding scanty; occasional patients menstruate normally [182]. The virilization present in phenotypic female patients with gonadoblastoma usually does not regress after excision of the tumor, although this has been seen in occasional cases, and in a few additional cases there was partial regression.

Although most patients have gonadal dysgenesis, gonadoblastoma has been described in patients who have had normal pregnancies. These include patients with a 46,XX karyotype [20, 53, 122, 260] and true hermaphrodites [228].

In seven true hermaphrodites with gonadoblastoma, four had a 46,XX karyotype [115, 228] and the other three had 46,XY [135, 204]. Gonadoblastoma has also been diagnosed in five males with normally descended testes [79, 216], some of whom fathered children subsequent to the excision of the testis bearing the lesion.

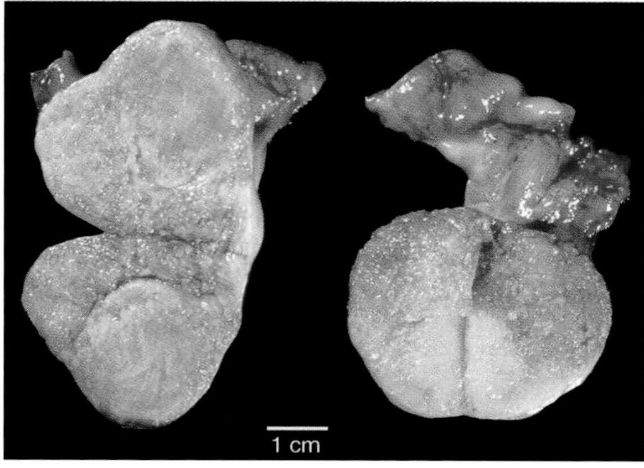

Fig. 16.53
Bilateral gonadoblastomas with dysgerminoma. **The outer surface is smooth, and the cut surface is solid, granular, and yellow-brown. The white nodule in the lower pole of the tumor on the *right* is a dysgerminoma (Published with kind permission of Dr. Robert E. Scully, Boston, MA)**

Gross Features

Gonadoblastoma has been found more often in the right gonad than in the left and has been bilateral in 40% of cases or higher [182, 221]. Although some tumors are recognized on gross examination, in a number of cases the lesion is detected only on histologic examination; this may be the case with bilateral tumors, only one of which may be recognized macroscopically. In most cases, the gonad of origin is indeterminate because it is overgrown by the tumor. When the nature of the gonad can be identified, it is usually a streak or a testis. The contralateral gonad in these cases may be a streak or a testis, and the former is more likely to harbor a gonadoblastoma [182, 221]. Occasionally gonadoblastoma has been found in otherwise normal ovaries [122, 127, 155].

Pure gonadoblastoma varies in size from a microscopic lesion to 8 cm, with most tumors measuring a few centimeters. When gonadoblastoma becomes overgrown by dysgerminoma or other malignant germ cell elements, much larger tumors may be observed [182, 211, 221]. The macroscopic appearance of the tumor varies to some extent according to the presence of hyalinization and calcification, as well as overgrowth by dysgerminoma.

Gonadoblastoma is a solid tumor and presents a smooth or slightly lobulated surface. It varies from soft and fleshy to firm and hard. It is speckled with calcific granules and may be almost completely calcified. Calcification has been recognized on gross examination in 45% of cases, and in more than 20% it has been detected radiologically [182]. The tumor varies in color from gray or yellow to brown, and on cross section it appears to be somewhat granular (➲ *Fig. 16.53*).

Although the external sex organs in patients with gonadoblastoma present a wide variety of appearances ranging from normal to completely ambiguous, the secondary internal sex organs consist almost always of a uterus, which is hypoplastic in most cases, and two or occasionally one normal fallopian tube; this is also seen in the phenotypic males. Male secondary internal sex organs, such as the epididymis, vas deferens, and prostate, are found occasionally in the virilized phenotypic females and are always found in the phenotypic male pseudohermaphrodites [182].

Microscopic and Immunohistochemical Features

Gonadoblastoma is composed of collections of cellular nests surrounded by connective tissue stroma (➲ *Figs. 16.54–16.56*). The nests are solid, usually small, and oval or round but occasionally may be larger and elongated. The cellular nests contain a mixture of germ cells and sex cord derivatives resembling immature Sertoli and granulosa cells (➲ *Fig. 16.55*). The germ cells are large

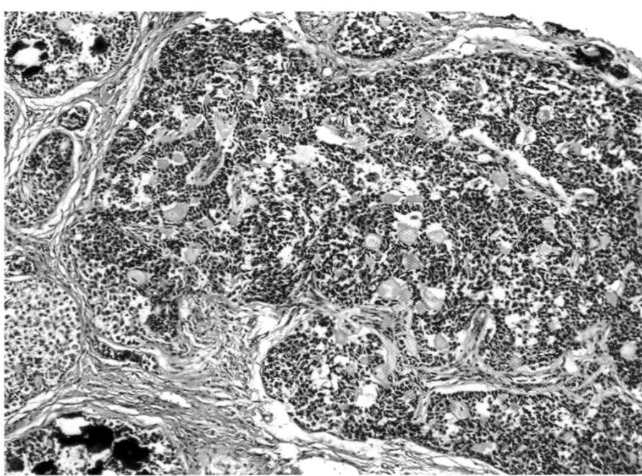

Fig. 16.54
Gonadoblastoma. **Cellular nests surrounded by connective tissue stroma. Note foci of calcification**

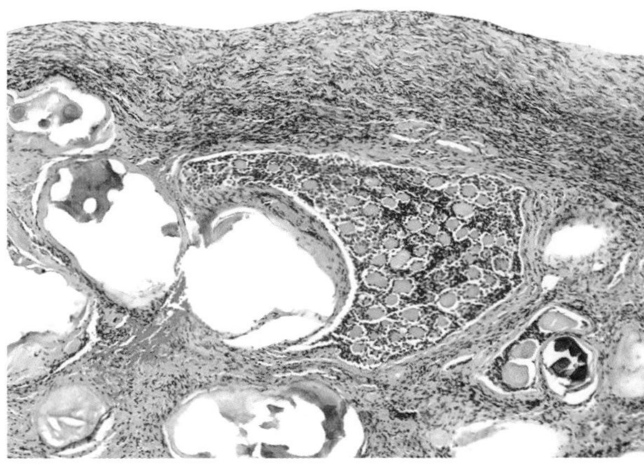

Fig. 16.56
Microscopic gonadoblastoma arising in a normal ovary. **It should be noted that microscopic gonadoblastoma-like foci can also be found in a subset of normal fetuses and newborns [185]**

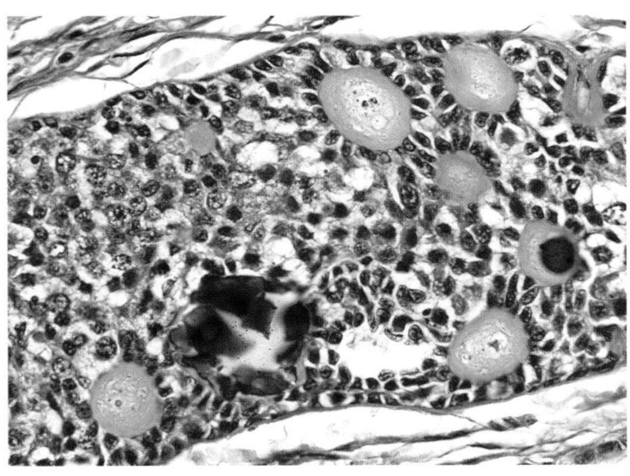

Fig. 16.55
Gonadoblastoma. **A nest composed of large germ cells is intimately admixed with smaller sex cord derivatives. Hyaline Call–Exner-like bodies also are seen**

and round, with pale or slightly granular cytoplasm and large round vesicular nuclei, often with prominent nucleoli showing histologic and ultrastructural appearances and histochemical and immunohistochemical (CD117[+], OCT-4[+], and SALL4[+] [32]) staining patterns similar to the germ cells of dysgerminoma or seminoma. The sex cord cells will show immunohistochemical expression of inhibin.

The germ cells show mitotic activity, which may be marked in some cases. They are intimately admixed with immature Sertoli and granulosa cells, which are smaller and epithelial-like. The latter are round or oval and have dark, oval or slightly elongated carrot-shaped nuclei. Mitotic activity is not seen in these cells. The immature Sertoli and granulosa cells are arranged within the cell nests in three typical patterns: (1) along the periphery of the nests in a coronal pattern, (2) surrounding individual or collections of germ cells in the same way as the follicular epithelium surrounds the ovum of the primary follicle, or (3) surrounding small round spaces containing amorphous hyaline, eosinophilic, and PAS-positive material that resemble Call–Exner bodies.

The connective tissue stroma surrounding the cellular nests frequently contains collections of cells indistinguishable from Leydig cells or luteinized stromal cells. There is considerable variation in the number of these cells from case to case; in some cases they are numerous, in others they are identified with difficulty, or they may be absent.

Although in many cases the cells are indistinguishable from Leydig cells and may contain lipochrome granules, Reinke crystals, which are specifically diagnostic of Leydig cells, have never been identified in their cytoplasm. The Leydig or lutein-like cells are identified in 66% of cases, and they are present nearly twice as frequently in older patients as in those 15 years of age or younger [182]. The presence of Leydig or lutein-like cells is not necessary for the diagnosis of gonadoblastoma. The connective tissue stroma surrounding the cellular nests may be scanty or abundant, and may vary from dense and hyalinized to cellular, resembling ovarian stroma. These latter appearances are more common in tumors that either have arisen in, or are suspected to originate in, a gonadal streak [182]. Occasionally, the stroma may be loose and edematous.

The basic composition of gonadoblastoma, consisting of the two cell types present within the cellular nests and with the Leydig or lutein-like cells present in the stroma, has been confirmed by electron microscopy [63, 80, 106]. Although there is agreement concerning the nature of the germ cells, the nature of the sex cord–stromal cells is in dispute. They are considered by some to be Sertoli cells or granulosa cells or their precursors [106], whereas others consider them to be primitive sex cord–stromal cells and are unable to differentiate them further [182, 213]. The latter view is more widely accepted. The nature of the amorphous, hyaline, and eosinophilic material forming Call–Exner-like bodies also was a matter of dispute. It was considered to be either of basement membrane origin [80, 106] or composed of fibrillar material formed by the stromal cells before they undergo fragmentation and cell death. The former view is supported by most investigators.

The basic histologic appearance of gonadoblastoma may be altered by three processes: hyalinization, calcification, and overgrowth by dysgerminoma [182, 213, 221]. Hyalinization takes place by coalescence of the hyaline Call–Exner-like bodies within the nests and of the basement membrane-like band of similar material present around the nests. The hyaline material replaces the tumor cells, and the whole nest may be replaced. Calcification is a common feature (➋ *Fig. 16.54*) and is seen microscopically in 81% of cases; it usually begins in the Call–Exner-like bodies with formation of small calcific spherules that are frequently laminated, resembling psammoma bodies. The process continues with enlargement and fusion of the calcified bodies and calcification of the hyalinized material, resulting in formation of a calcified mass embracing the whole nest. The process may extend to the stroma, which may also undergo hyalinization and calcification. In such cases, tumor cells become very scarce or absent, and the presence of smooth, rounded, and calcified masses may be the only evidence that gonadoblastoma was present (➋ *Fig. 16.6*). Although this finding is not considered to be diagnostic of gonadoblastoma, and has been called a burned-out gonadoblastoma [182, 213, 221], it is a strong argument in favor of the diagnosis and indicates that a careful search should be made for more viable areas of the tumor.

Gonadoblastoma is frequently overgrown by dysgerminoma, as is seen in 50% of cases [182, 213, 221]. The overgrowth may vary from the presence of a small collection of malignant germ cells in the stroma outside the gonadoblastoma nests to massive overgrowth of the whole tumor, in which occasional nests of gonadoblastoma may be seen. The dysgerminoma in these cases shows the typical appearances of pure dysgerminoma or seminoma – histologically, histochemically, immunohistochemically, and ultrastructurally. It should be noted that when gonadoblastoma becomes overgrown by dysgerminoma, the germ cell component present within the gonadoblastoma nests shows marked proliferative activity and overgrows the sex cord elements. When gonadoblastoma undergoes regressive changes, they manifest first as a decrease in germ cells. Gonadoblastoma may also be associated with, and overgrown by, other more malignant germ cell neoplasms, such as immature teratoma, yolk sac tumor, embryonal carcinoma, and choriocarcinoma, as occurs in 10% of cases [182, 213, 221]. A gonadoblastoma overgrown by dysgerminoma and containing a proliferation of sex cord element resembling a Sertoli cell tumor and occurring in a dysgenetic gonad of a 19-year-old phenotypic female with 46,XY karyotype has been reported [127]. Although it has been postulated that gonadoblastoma may coexist with mixed germ cell–sex cord–stromal tumor, the two cases describing such an association [23, 37] were in reality typical gonadoblastomas and not combined tumors.

Differential Diagnosis

Gonadoblastoma, because of its distinctive histologic appearance and its cellular composition, cannot be easily confused with any of the well-recognized gonadal neoplasms. Gonadoblastoma may be confused with the mixed germ cell–sex cord–stromal tumor [208, 209], which shares with gonadoblastoma the unique distinction of being composed of germ cells and sex cord–stromal derivatives. The mixed germ cell–sex cord–stromal tumor shows less uniform appearance, absence of nest-like pattern, absence of calcification and hyalinization, a more pronounced proliferative activity involving also the sex cord–stromal derivatives, the tendency to occur in normal gonads, and other genetic, endocrine, and somatic differences. The other lesion resembling gonadoblastoma is the ovarian sex cord tumor with annular tubules [183], which is frequently found in patients with Peutz–Jeghers syndrome. This lesion, which is also frequently bilateral, is composed of tubules lined by Sertoli and granulosa-like cells, contains similar round, eosinophilic, and hyaline Call–Exner-like bodies, and tends to calcify in the same manner as gonadoblastoma. The basic difference from gonadoblastoma is the absence of germ cells (see ➋ Chap. 15, Sex Cord-Stromal, Steroid Cell, and Other Ovarian Tumors with Endocrine, Paraendocrine, and Paraneoplastic Manifestations).

Clinical Behavior and Treatment

The prognosis of patients with pure gonadoblastoma is excellent, provided the tumor and the contralateral gonad, which may be harboring an undetectable gonadoblastoma, are excised. When gonadoblastoma is associated with dysgerminoma, the prognosis is still very good. Metastases tend to occur later and more infrequently than in dysgerminoma that is not associated with a gonadoblastoma. All patients with gonadoblastoma and dysgerminoma with known follow-up, including the occasional cases with metastases [72, 176, 182], are alive and well after treatment, with the exception of two patients who died of disseminated dysgerminoma [72, 236]. The prognosis is different when gonadoblastoma is associated with more malignant germ cell neoplasms, such as embryonal carcinoma, yolk sac tumor, choriocarcinoma, and immature teratoma. In the past, none of these patients survived longer than 18 months [211]. Subsequently, the administration of combination chemotherapy used successfully in the treatment of malignant germ cell tumors has markedly improved the prognosis, which with adequate treatment is now favorable.

Because gonadoblastoma occurs almost entirely in patients with dysgenetic gonads, which are not capable of normal function, and that the gonadoblastoma may act as a source from which malignant germ cell neoplasms may originate [174], there is general agreement that excision of the gonads is the treatment of choice [175, 182, 213, 221]. This consensus applies not only to a contralateral gonad that appears to be abnormal but also, in most cases, to a normal-appearing gonad. There is no complete agreement regarding whether the uterus should be excised together with the gonads. It has been considered that for psychological reasons it should not be removed so that periodic bleeding simulating menstruation can take place on estrogen–progesterone substitution therapy. However, because estrogen administration is associated with a risk of development of endometrial carcinoma, excision of the uterus together with the gonads has been advocated by some [175].

Mixed Germ Cell–Sex Cord–Stromal Tumor

General Features

The descriptive term mixed germ cell–sex cord–stromal tumor originally was intended to embrace all the tumors composed of these cell types, including the gonadoblastoma. In view of the fact that the latter term is now so well established, the term mixed germ cell–sex cord–stromal tumor should be reserved for tumors composed of these cell types that exhibit distinctive histologic appearances differing from those of gonadoblastoma [209, 210]. This is the term used in the WHO classification.

Genetic and Molecular Features

Nearly all female patients with this neoplasm have had genotype and karyotype determinations and have been found to have the normal female chromosome complement of 46,XX. All the patients with this tumor showed normal somatosexual development. There is no evidence that patients with this tumor have chromosomal abnormalities or gonadal dysgenesis, except for a single patient reported to have monosomy 22 [196]. In a small number of tumors studied, a subset of neoplasms showed amplification of chromosome 12p, and no mutations of the *c-kit* or *PDGFRA* genes were identified [118].

Endocrine Features

Most patients with mixed germ cell–sex cord–stromal tumor do not exhibit any endocrine abnormalities as observed clinically. In most cases, tests of hormonal function have not been performed preoperatively. In cases in which tests have been performed postoperatively, function has been found to be normal. In one case, the patient, an 8-year-old girl, exhibited signs of precocious pseudopuberty manifesting as mammary development and menstrual bleeding for 3 years before the discovery of a large ovarian tumor [222]. There was an increased urinary estrogen excretion. After excision of the ovarian tumor, the uterine bleeding ceased and the urinary estrogens became normal [222].

Isosexual precocious pseudopuberty has been seen in nine other patients in the first decade, including four infants less than 1 year of age, who exhibited mammary development and vaginal bleeding. The urinary estrogens were elevated, and vaginal smears showed estrogen effect. After the excision of the tumor, there was a complete return to normality. There was no evidence of virilization in any of the patients. These findings indicate that female patients with this neoplasm either do not have any associated endocrine abnormalities or, if these are present, that they are manifested as feminization. One of the patients, who had a mixed germ cell–sex cord–stromal tumor excised at the age of 10 years [209], has developed normally and commenced menstruating at the age of 15 years. She was well and disease-free 12 years after excision of the tumor.

Clinical Features

These neoplasms are rare. A number of adequately documented cases have been reported [7, 99, 118], but it is likely that some cases may not have been recognized and have been included with tumors of germ cell origin or with sex cord–stromal tumors. This concept is supported by the fact that because this neoplasm has been recognized as a specific entity, additional well-documented and so far unreported cases have been encountered. Tumors of this type have been observed more frequently in normal phenotypic female patients but have also been encountered in normal adult males. Most of the known cases in females were encountered in children in the first decade. More than a dozen cases occurred in infants less than 1 year of age [210, 213]. In three cases, the tumor occurred in women aged 26, 31, and 43 years, respectively, who had normal pregnancies. In the ovary, the tumor is most common in the first decade, followed by the second and third, and is uncommon thereafter. Therefore, the age distribution of patients with this neoplasm differs from that of patients with gonadoblastoma [213].

Gross Features

The tumors encountered have been relatively large, varying from 7.5 to 18 cm and weighing from 100 to 1,050 g. The tumor was found to be unilateral in all except two patients, and the contralateral gonad has always been described as a normal ovary. In some cases in which excision or biopsy was performed, this was confirmed on microscopic examination.

The tumor is usually round or oval, firm in consistency, and surrounded by a smooth, slightly glistening gray or gray-yellow capsule. In most cases the tumor is solid [118, 209, 210, 221], but in some cases it is partly cystic [222]. The cut surface of the tumor is uniformly gray, pink, or yellow to pale brown. Neither calcified areas nor foci of necrosis have been observed on gross examination. The fallopian tubes and the uterus have always been found to be normal. There have been no abnormalities affecting the external genitalia.

Microscopic and Immunohistochemical Features

The tumor is composed of germ cells and sex cord derivatives, intimately admixed with each other. The tumor cells form four different histologic patterns [7, 118, 209, 210, 213, 222]. One is composed of long, narrow ramifying cords or trabeculae (*Figs. 16.57* and *16.58*), which in places expand to form wider columns and larger round

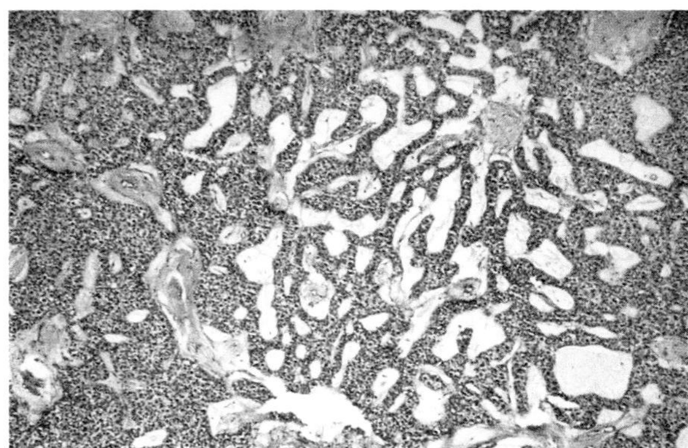

Fig. 16.57
Mixed germ cell–sex cord–stromal tumor. **The neoplasm is composed of large cellular aggregates and more slender cords**

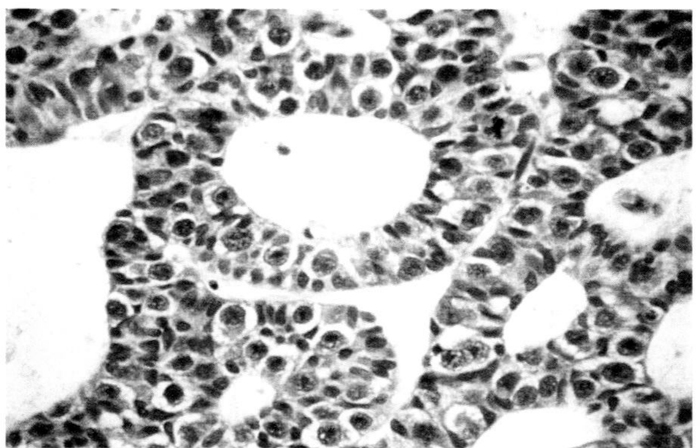

Fig. 16.58
Mixed germ cell–sex cord–stromal tumor. **Note large germ cells surrounded by sex cord–stromal cells**

or oval cellular aggregates surrounded by connective tissue stroma. The second consists of tubular structures devoid of a lumen and surrounded by a fine connective tissue network. In some places, the tubular pattern is less obvious, and the tumor forms small clusters or larger round or oval cellular masses surrounded by connective tissue stroma. The latter varies in amount and appearance and tends to be more abundant in tumors showing mainly the cord-like or trabecular pattern, whereas the tubular variety tends to be more cellular and contains less connective tissue. The stroma may vary from loose and edematous to dense fibrous and hyalinized. The former is seen more often where the cordlike pattern is most prominent, whereas the latter surrounds the larger cellular aggregates.

The third pattern consists of scattered collections of germ cells surrounded by sex cord elements that may be very abundant. The germ cells admixed with sex cord derivatives may also be scattered individually and in small groups within connective tissue stroma. Sometimes there may be a suggestion of an insular pattern with islands of various sizes surrounded by fine fibrovascular stroma coalescing and forming aggregates, or occasionally being separated by large amounts of connective tissue and forming a more pronounced insular pattern. Admixture with all these patterns is often seen. The typical nest-like pattern present in gonadoblastoma is not observed. In only one case were a few small collections of Leydig or lutein-like cells observed [209], but in all the remaining cases these cells were not identified.

The fourth more recently encountered pattern [7, 118] shows similar appearances to the sex cord tumor with annular tubules (SCTAT) [183, 185], but differs from the latter by the presence of germ cells as an additional cellular element within the tumor (➲ *Figs. 16.59* and ➲ *16.60*). The germ cells show similar appearances seen in the tumors showing the other three patterns, including mitotic activity. The sex cord elements are similar to those observed in typical sex cord tumors with annular tubules.

The two cellular elements present in the tumor, the germ cells and the sex cord derivatives, are intimately admixed. The sex cord derivatives are arranged peripherally in a single file, forming long rows at the periphery of the cords, or peripherally lining the tubular structures as well as surrounding individual or groups of germ cells within the small clusters or larger aggregates. The germ cells resemble those observed in dysgerminoma and gonadoblastoma in all respects, including ultrastructural, histochemical, and immunohistochemical (CD117[+] and OCT-4[+]) reactions. In some cases, a number of the germ cells present in this tumor appear more mature than the germ cells observed in gonadoblastoma or dysgerminoma and tend to resemble primordial germ cells. In view of this, it is possible that they may represent a later stage in the maturation of the germ cell than that seen in gonadoblastoma or dysgerminoma. The germ cells show brisk mitotic activity. The sex cord derivatives generally tend to resemble Sertoli cells more than granulosa cells. They show variable degrees of mitotic activity.

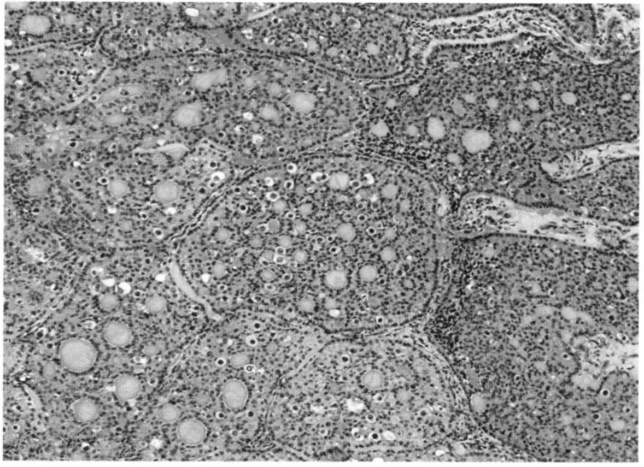

◻ Fig. 16.59
Mixed germ cell–sex cord–stromal tumor with SCTAT-like pattern. **Note the marked similarity to the sex cord tumor with annular tubules (SCTAT) but differing from it by the presence of germ cells**

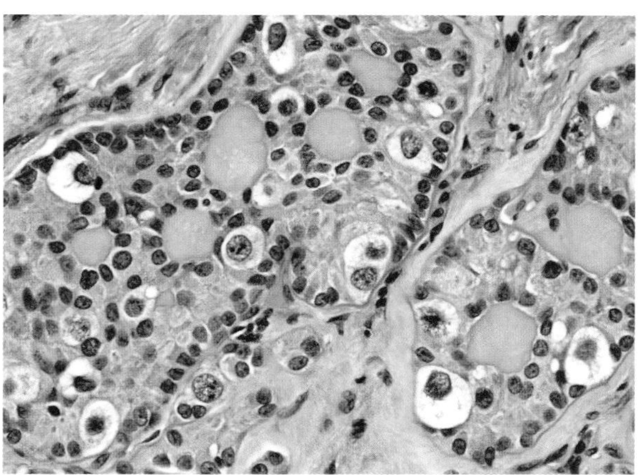

◻ Fig. 16.60
Mixed germ cell–sex cord–stromal tumor with SCTAT-like pattern. **Typical cytologic features. Compare with ➲ *Figs. 16.55* and ➲ *16.58***

The tumor does not show hyalinization, calcification, or the regressive changes observed in gonadoblastoma and appears to be actively proliferative. There is some variation in the cellular content in some parts of the tumor; in some areas there is a preponderance of germ cells, whereas in others the sex cord derivatives predominate. However, the intimate admixture of these two cell types is seen everywhere. Most tumors show a solid pattern, although occasional small clefts lined by sex cord elements may be present. In some tumors, cystic spaces of varying size either lined by sex cord derivatives or flattened epithelial-like cells or devoid of lining may be observed [222, 229, 239]; they closely resemble the cystic spaces observed in some retiform Sertoli–Leydig cell tumors [215, 219, 257] or cystic sex cord–stromal tumors. In occasional tumors, this pattern may be pronounced and may suggest that the tumor contains epithelial cells in addition to germ cells and sex cord derivatives [229]. It is considered that these cells are in fact sex cord derivatives and that the tumor in common with some sex cord tumors exhibits a retiform or cystic pattern or both.

Normal ovarian tissue as evidenced by the presence of normal ovarian stroma and at least some primordial follicles has been identified in all cases, including a case in which it could not be identified in the original sections available [209]. In a number of cases, graafian follicles also are present [210, 222]. In other cases, tumor deposits are found very close to the surface of the ovary, obliterating primordial and graafian follicles.

Differential Diagnosis

Histologically, this tumor is most likely to be confused with gonadoblastoma. In contrast to gonadoblastoma, this tumor lacks the typical nest-like pattern, has greater proliferative activity of both the germ cell and sex cord component, and lacks calcification, hyalinization, and in most cases Leydig or lutein-like cells. Macroscopically, the tumors are larger. The gonad of origin is a normal ovary, and there is no evidence of gonadal dysgenesis or any somatosexual abnormalities. The patients have a normal female 46,XX karyotype. There is no evidence of virilization, and if there are signs of abnormal endocrine activity, they manifest themselves as feminization.

Occasionally, if the germ cells are relatively scanty, the tumor may be confused with the sex cord–stromal tumors of the ovary, but the presence of germ cells should alert the observer to the true identity of the tumor. If the sex cord derivatives are few in number, are missed, or are disregarded, the tumor may be misclassified as a germ cell tumor, but the presence of sex cord elements intimately admixed with the germ cells should indicate its true identity. The presence of prominent clefts and cystic spaces, especially when the latter contain papillary projections, may cause confusion with Sertoli–Leydig cell tumors showing the retiform pattern or even with serous papillary tumors. The presence of germ cells admixed with sex cord derivatives indicates that the tumor is a mixed germ cell–sex cord–stromal tumor, irrespective of its pattern.

Clinical Behavior and Treatment

The prognosis of patients with mixed germ cell–sex cord–stromal tumor of the ovary occurring in pure form is favorable. In the great majority of known cases when the tumor was confined to the ovary and not associated with other malignant neoplastic germ cell elements, there has been no recurrence or metastases after excision of the affected adnexa. The patients are well and disease-free for periods varying from 1 to 15 years [118, 213, 221]. Accordingly, after a unilateral salpingo-oophorectomy, careful examination of the abdominal cavity is recommended. If the contralateral ovary shows signs of abnormality, biopsy is advisable. After this procedure, the patient should have chromosome studies. If the karyotype is 46,XX and if no other abnormalities are detected, further therapy is not necessary, although careful long-term follow-up is essential.

One well-documented case of metastasizing mixed germ cell–sex cord–stromal tumor occurring in an 8-year-old girl has been reported [99]. The metastases were found in the para-aortic lymph nodes and in the peritoneal cavity. The patient was well and disease-free 2 years after excision of the affected adnexa, para-aortic lymphadenectomy, excision of peritoneal metastases, and a course of cisplatin-based combination chemotherapy [99]. Another case of metastasizing mixed germ cell–sex cord–stromal tumor showing an unusual pattern resembling the SCTAT occurring in a 30-year-old woman has been reported [7]. Three years after excision of a right-sided ovarian tumor, a large tumor mass was noted in the region of the uterine fundus. The mass and a number of peritoneal implants were excised together with the uterus and the left ovary. The primary and the metastatic tumors showed identical appearances. The left ovary was normal. The patient was well and disease-free 1 year after excision of the metastases and administration of combination chemotherapy.

In three patients in their 20s, one in her early 30s, and one in her early 40s, the mixed germ cell–sex cord–stromal tumor was associated with dysgerminoma. There was no evidence of metastases. The patients are well and disease-free from 2 to 7 years after unilateral adnexectomy and radiation therapy.

In four children, aged 5–16 years, the tumor was overgrown by other malignant germ cell elements, including choriocarcinoma and yolk sac tumor. In three of these cases, the tumor metastasized and resulted in the death of the patient. The metastases were composed of the malignant germ cell elements. One patient treated with cisplatin-based chemotherapy was alive and well 5 years later. When the tumor is associated with malignant germ cell elements, the patient should be treated with the appropriate combination chemotherapy used in treatment of non-dysgerminomatous malignant germ cell tumors.

When the tumor is encountered in postmenarchal women, there is an increased possibility that the tumor may not present in pure form but be associated with other neoplastic germ cell elements. In such cases, in addition to excision of the affected adnexa appropriate therapy to treat the neoplastic germ cell elements present is recommended. This can be exemplified by a case of a 26-year-old woman with mixed germ cell sex cord stromal tumor associated with yolk sac tumor and immature teratoma. The patient was well and disease-free 3 years following excision of the tumor and a course of cisplatin-based combination chemotherapy.

References

1. Abbot TM, Herman WJ Jr, Scully RE (1984) Ovarian fetiform teratoma (homunculus) in a 9-year-old girl. Int J Gynecol Pathol 2:392
2. Alenghat E, Okagaki T, Talerman A (1986) Primary mucinous carcinoid tumor of the ovary. Cancer (Phila) 58:777
3. Allard S, Cadotte M, Boivin Y (1972) Dysgenesie gonadique pure familiale et gonadoblastome. Union Med Can 101:448–452
4. Anderson CT Jr, Carlson IH (1975) Elevated plasma testosterone and gonadal tumors in two 46XY "sisters". Arch Pathol 99:360
5. Anderson MC, McDicken IW (1971) Melanotic cyst of the ovary. J Obstet Gynaecol Br Commonw 78:1047
6. Arhelger RB, Kelly B (1974) Strumal carcinoid. Report of a case with electron microscopical observations. Arch Pathol 97:323
7. Arroyo JG, Harris W, Laden SA (1998) Recurrent mixed germ cell-sex cord-stromal tumor of the ovary in an adult. Int J Gynecol Pathol 17:281
8. Arroyo MR, Podda A, Cao D et al (2009) Placental site trophoblastic tumor in the ovary of a young child with isosexual precocious puberty. Pediatr Dev Pathol 12:73
9. Asadourian LA, Taylor HB (1969) Dysgerminoma. An analysis of 105 cases. Obstet Gynecol 33:370
10. Atkin NB (1973) High chromosome numbers of seminomata and malignant teratomata of the testis: a review of data on 103 tumors. Br J Cancer 28:275
11. Atkin NB, Baker MC (1983) i(12p): specific chromosomal marker in seminoma and malignant teratoma of the testis? Cancer Genet Cytogenet 10:199
12. Atkin NB, Baker MC (1987) Abnormal chromosomes including small metacentrics in 14 ovarian cancers. Cancer Genet Cytogenet 26:355
13. Ayhan A, Bukulmez O, Genc C, Kuramursel BS, Ayhan A (2000) Mature cystic teratomas of the ovary. A case series from one institution over 34 years. Eur J Obstet Gynecol 88:153
14. Baergen RN, Rutgers J, Young RH (2003) Extrauterine lesions of intermediate trophoblast. Int J Gynecol Pathol 22:362
15. Bagg HJ (1936) Experimental production of teratoma testis in a fowl. Am J Cancer 26:69
16. Baker PM, Oliva E, Young RH et al (2001) Ovarian mucinous carcinoids including some with carcinomatous component: a report of 17 cases. Am J Surg Pathol 25:557
17. Baker PM, Rosai J, Young RH (2002) Ovarian teratomas with florid benign vascular proliferation: a distinctive finding associated with the neural component of teratomas that may be confused with a vascular neoplasm. Int J Gynecol Pathol 21:16
18. Bartlett DJ, Grant JK, Pugh MA, Aherne W (1968) A familial feminizing syndrome. A family showing intersex characteristics with XY chromosomes in three female members. J Obstet Gynaecol Br Commonw 75:199
19. Beck JS, Fulmer HF, Lee ST (1969) Solid malignant ovarian teratoma with "embryoid bodies" and trophoblastic differentiation. J Pathol 99:67
20. Bergher de Bacalao E, Dominguez I (1969) Unilateral gonadoblastoma in a pregnant woman. Am J Obstet Gynecol 105:1279
21. Bergstrand CG, Czar B (1956) Demonstration of a new protein fraction in serum from human fetus. Scand J Lab Invest 8:174
22. Bernstein D, Naor S, Rikover M, Manahem H (1974) Hemolytic anemia related to ovarian tumor. Obstet Gynecol 43:276
23. Bhatena D, Haning RV Jr, Shapiro S, Hafez GR (1985) Coexistence of a gonadoblastoma and mixed germ cell–sex cord stroma tumor. Pathol Res Pract 180:203
24. Bjorkholm E, Lundell M, Gyftodimos A, Silversward C (1990) Dysgerminoma. The Radiumhemmet series 1927–1984. Cancer (Phila) 65:38
25. Blackwell WJ, Dockerty MB, Masson JC, Mussey RD (1946) Dermoid cysts of the ovary: clinical and pathological significance. Am J Obstet Gynecol 51:151
26. Boczkowski K, Teter J, Sternadel Z (1972) Sibship occurrence of XY gonadal dysgenesis with dysgerminoma. Am J Obstet Gynecol 113:952
27. Bonazzi C, Peccatori F, Colombo N, Lucchini V, Cantu MG, Mangioni C (1994) Pure ovarian immature teratoma, a unique and curable disease: 10 years experience of 32 prospectively treated patients. Obstet Gynecol 84:598
28. Boutross-Tadross O, Saleh R, Asa SL (2007) Follicular variant papillary thyroid carcinoma arising in struma ovarii. Endocr Pathol 18:182
29. Brand A, Alves MC, Saraiva C et al (2004) Fetus in fetu – diagnostic criteria and differential diagnosis – a case report and literature review. J Pediatr Surg 39:616
30. Brant WO, Rajinvale A, Lovell MA et al (2006) Gonadoblastoma and Turner syndrome. J Urol 175:1858
31. Breen JL, Neubecker RD (1967) Ovarian malignancy in children with special reference to the germ cell tumors. Ann NY Acad Sci 142:658
32. Cao D, Guo S, Allan RW et al (2009) SALL4 is a novel sensitive and specific marker of ovarian primitive germ cell tumors and is

particularly useful in distinguishing yolk sac tumor from clear cell. Am J Surg Pathol 33:894
33. Carleton RL, Friedman NB, Bomze EJ (1953) Experimental teratomas of testis. Cancer (Phila) 6:464
34. Caruso PA, Marsh MR, Minkowitz S, Karten G (1971) An intense clinicopathologic study of 305 teratomas of the ovary. Cancer (Phila) 27:343
35. Chang MC, Vargas SO, Hornick JL et al (2009) Embryonic stem cell transcription factors and D2-40 (podoplanin) as diagnostic immunohistochemical markers in ovarian germ cell tumors. Int J Gynecol Pathol 28:347
36. Cheng L, Thomas A, Roth LM et al (2004) OCT4: a novel biomarker for dysgerminoma of the ovary. Am J Surg Pathol 28:1341
37. Cholafranceschi M, Massi D (1995) Gonadoblastoma with coexistent features of mixed germ cell-sex cord-stromal tumor: a case report. Tumori 81:215
38. Chumas JC, Scully RE (1991) Sebaceous tumors arising in ovarian dermoid cysts. Int J Gynecol Pathol 10:356
39. Clement PB, Young RH, Scully RE (1987) Endometrioid-like variant of ovarian yolk sac tumor. A clinicopathological analysis of eight cases. Am J Surg Pathol 11:767
40. Cohen MB, Friend DS, Molnar JJ, Talerman A (1987) Gonadal endodermal sinus (yolk sac) tumor with pure intestinal differentiation; a new histologic type. Pathol Res Pract 182:609
41. Condous G, Thomas J, Okaro E (2003) Placental site trophoblastic tumor masquerading as an ovarian ectopic pregnancy. Ultrasound Obstet Gynecol 21:504
42. Cossu-Rocca P, Jones TD, Roth LM et al (2006) Cytokeratin and CD30 expression in dysgerminoma. Hum Pathol 37:1015
43. Cossu-Rocca P, Zhang S, Roth LM et al (2006) Chromosome 12p abnormalities in dysgerminoma of the ovary: a FISH analysis. Mod Pathol 19:611
44. Dandia SD (1967) Rectovesical fistula following an ovarian dermoid with recurrent vesical calculus. A case report. J Urol 97:85
45. Davis KP, Hartmann LK, Keeney GL, Shapiro H (1996) Primary ovarian carcinoid tumors. Gynecol Oncol 61:259
46. Dawson MA, Wilimer T, Yarbro JW (1971) Hemolytic anemia associated with an ovarian tumor. Am J Med 50:552
47. Dayal Y, Tashjian AH Jr, Wolfe HJ (1979) Immunocytochemical localization of calcitonin-producing cells in a strumal carcinoid with amyloid stroma. Cancer (Phila) 43:1331
48. Devaney K, Snyder R, Norris HJ et al (1993) Proliferative and histologically malignant struma ovarii: a clinicopathologic study of 54 cases. Int J Gynecol Pathol 12:333
49. Dietl J, Horny HP, Ruck P, Kaiserling E (1993) Dysgerminoma of the ovary. An immunohistochemical study of tumor-infiltrating lymphoreticular cells and tumor cells. Cancer (Phila) 71:2562
50. Dixon FJ, Moore RA (1952) Tumors of the male sex organs. Atlas of tumor pathology, sect VIII, fasc 31b, 32. Armed Forces Institute of Pathology, Washington, DC
51. Djordjevic B, Euscher ED, Malpica A (2007) Growing teratoma syndrome of the ovary: review of literature and first report of a carcinoid tumor arising in a growing teratoma of the ovary. Am J Surg Pathol 31:1913
52. Erez SE, Richart RM, Shettles LB (1965) Hashimoto's disease in a benign cystic teratoma of the ovary. Am J Obstet Gynecol 92:273
53. Erhan Y, Toprak AS, Ozdemir N, Tiras B (1992) Gonadoblastoma and fertility. J Clin Pathol 45:828
54. Esheba GE, Pate LL, Longacre TA (2008) Oncofetal protein glypican-3 distinguishes yolk sac tumor from clear cell carcinoma of the ovary. Am J Surg Pathol 32:600
55. Evans RW (1957) Developmental stages of embryo-like bodies in teratoma testis. J Clin Pathol 10:321
56. Evans KN, Taylor H, Zehnder D et al (2004) Increased expression of 25-hydroxyvitamin D-1alpha-hydroxylase in dysgerminoma: a novel form of hypercalcemia of malignancy. Am J Pathol 165:807
57. Frazier SD, Bashore RA, Mosier HD (1964) Gonadoblastoma associated with pure gonadal dysgenesis in monozygous twins. J Pediatr 64:740
58. Friedman NB (1951) The comparative morphogenesis of extragenital and gonadal teratoid tumors. Cancer (Phila) 4:265
59. Friedman NB, Moore RA (1946) Tumors of the testis. A report of 922 cases. Mil Surg 99:573
60. Fujii S, Konishi I, Suzuki A, Okamura H, Okazaki T, Mori T (1985) Analysis of serum lactic dehydrogenase levels and its isoenzymes in ovarian dysgerminoma. Gynecol Oncol 22:65
61. Galager HS, Lewis RP (1973) Sequential gonadoblastoma and choriocarcinoma. Obstet Gynecol 41:123
62. Garg K, Soslow RA, Rivera M et al (2009) Histologically bland "extremely well differentiated" thyroid carcinomas arising in struma ovarii recur and metastasize. Int J Gynecol Pathol 28:222
63. Garvin AJ, Pratt-Thomas HR, Spector M, Spicer SS, Williamson HO (1976) Gonadoblastoma: histologic ultrastructural and histochemical observations in five cases. Am J Obstet Gynecol 125:459
64. Gershenson DM (1993) Update on malignant ovarian germ cell tumors. Cancer (Phila) 71:1581
65. Gershenson DM, Del Junco G, Herson J, Rutledge FN (1983) Endodermal sinus tumor of the ovary. The M.D. Anderson experience. Obstet Gynecol 61:194
66. Gillman J (1948) The development of the gonads in man with consideration of the role of fetal endocrines and the histogenesis of ovarian tumors. Contrib Embryol 32:83
67. Gitlin D, Pericelli A, Gitlin G (1972) Synthesis of alpha-fetoprotein by liver, yolk sac and gastrointestinal tract of the human conceptus. Cancer Res 32:979
68. Gonzalez-Crussi F, Roth LM (1976) The human yolk sac and yolk sac carcinoma. Hum Pathol 7:675
69. Gordon A, Lipton D, Woodruff JD (1981) Dysgerminoma: a review of 158 cases from the Emil Novak Ovarian Tumor Registry. Obstet Gynecol 58:497
70. Gupta D, Deavers MT, Silva EG et al (2004) Malignant melanoma involving the ovary: a clinicopathologic and immunohistochemical study of 23 cases. Am J Surg Pathol 28:771
71. Halabi M, Oliva E, Mazal PR et al (2002) Prostatic tissue in mature cystic teratomas of the ovary: a report of four cases, including one with features of prostatic adenocarcinoma, and cytogenetic studies. Int J Gynecol Pathol 21:261
72. Hart WR, Burkons DM (1979) Germ cell neoplasms arising in gonadoblastomas. Cancer (Phila) 34:669
73. Hart WR, Regezi JA (1978) Strumal carcinoid of the ovary. Ultrastructural observations and long-term follow-up study. Am J Clin Pathol 69:356
74. Heifetz SA, Cushing B, Giller R et al (1998) Immature teratomas in children: Pathologic considerations. A report from the combined Pediatric Oncology Group/Children's Cancer Group. Am J Surg Pathol 22:1115
75. Hingorani V, Narula RK, Bhalla S (1963) Salmonella typhi infection in an ovarian dermoid. Report of a case. Obstet Gynecol 22:118
76. Hirakawa T, Tsuneyoshi M, Enjoji M (1989) Squamous cell carcinoma arising in mature cystic teratoma of the ovary. Clinicopathologic and topographic analysis. Am J Surg Pathol 13:397

77. Hoei-Hansen CE, Kraggerud SM, Abeler VM et al (2007) Ovarian dysgerminomas are characterised by frequent KIT mutations and abundant expression of pluripotency markers. Mol Cancer 6:12
78. Hristov AC, Young RH, Vang R et al (2007) Ovarian metastases of appendiceal tumors with goblet cell carcinoidlike and signet ring cell patterns: a report of 30 cases. Am J Surg Pathol 31:1502
79. Hughesdon PE, Kumarasamy T (1970) Mixed germ cell tumors (gonadoblastomas) in normal and dysgenetic gonads. Virch Arch (Pathol Anat) 349:258
80. Ishida T, Tagatz GE, Okagaki T (1976) Gonadoblastoma. Ultrastructural evidence of testicular origin. Cancer (Phila) 37:1770
81. Jacobs AJ, Newland JR, Green RK (1982) Pure choriocarcinoma of the ovary. Obstet Gynecol Surv 37:603
82. Jacobsen GK, Talerman A (1989) Atlas of germ cell tumors. Munksgaard, Copenhagen
83. Judd HL, Scully RE, Atkins L, Neer RM, Kliman B (1970) Pure gonadal dysgenesis with progressive hirsutism. N Engl J Med 282:881
84. Kawahara H (1963) Struma ovarii with ascites and hydrothorax. Am J Obstet Gynecol 85:85
85. Kazancigil TR, Laquer W, Ladewig P (1940) Papilloendothelioma of the ovary; report of three cases and discussion of Schiller's "mesonephroma ovarii". Am J Cancer 40:199
86. Kemp B, Hauptmann S, Schroder W, Amo-Takyi B, Leeners B, Rath W (1995) Dysgerminoma of the ovary in a patient with triple-X syndrome. Int J Obstet Gynecol 50:51
87. Kerseladze AI, Kulinich SI (1994) Peritoneal strumosis. Pathol Res Pract 190:1082
88. King ME, Mouradian JA, Micha JP, Chaganti RSK, Allen SL (1985) Immature teratoma of the ovary with predominant malignant retinal anlage tumor. A parthenogenetically derived tumor. Am J Surg Pathol 9:221
89. King ME, Hubbell MJ, Talerman A (1991) Mixed germ cell tumor of the ovary with prominent polyembryoma component. Int J Gynecol Pathol 10:88
90. Klein HZ (1974) Mucinous carcinoid tumor of the vermiform appendix. Cancer (Phila) 33:770
91. Kleinman GM, Young RH, Scully RE (1993) Primary neuroectodermal tumors of the ovary. A report of 25 cases. Am J Surg Pathol 17:764
92. Kommoss F, Franklin WA, Talerman A (1989) Estrogen and progesterone receptors in endodermal sinus (yolk sac) tumor. Evaluation of immunocytochemical and biochemical methods. J Reprod Med 34:943
93. Kommoss F, Bibbo M, Talerman A (1990) Nuclear deoxyribonucleic acid content (ploidy) of endodermal sinus (yolk sac) tumor. Lab Invest 62:223
94. Kraggerud SM, Szymanska J, Abeler VM et al (2000) DNA copy number changes in malignant ovarian germ cell tumors. Cancer Res 60:3025
95. Krumerman MS, Chung A (1977) Squamous carcinoma arising in benign cystic teratoma of the ovary. Cancer (Phila) 39:1237
96. Kurman RJ, Norris HJ (1976) Endodermal sinus tumor of the ovary. A clinical and pathological analysis of 71 cases. Cancer (Phila) 38:2404
97. Kurman RJ, Norris HJ (1976) Embryonal carcinoma of the ovary. A clinicopathologic entity distinct from endodermal sinus tumor resembling embryonal carcinoma of the adult testis. Cancer (Phila) 38:2420
98. Kurman RJ, Norris HJ (1976) Malignant mixed germ cell tumors of the ovary. A clinical and pathological analysis of 30 cases. Obstet Gynecol 48:579
99. Lacson AG, Gillis DA, Shawwa A (1988) Malignant mixed germ cell–sex cord stromal tumors of the ovary associated with isosexual precocious puberty. Cancer (Phila) 61:2122
100. Lau YF, Li Y, Kido T (2009) Gonadoblastoma locus and the TSPY gene on the human Y chromosome. Birth Defects Res C Embryo Today 87:114
101. Letterie GS, Page DC (1995) Dysgerminoma and gonadal dysgenesis in 46,XX female with no evidence of Y chromosomal DNA. Gynecol Oncol 57:423
102. Linder D, Power J (1970) Further evidence for postmeiotic origin of teratomas in the human female. Ann Hum Genet 34:21
103. Linder D, McCaw BK, Hecht F (1975) Parthenogenic origin of benign ovarian teratoma. N Engl J Med 292:63
104. Lu KH, Gershenson MD (2005) Update on the management of ovarian germ cell tumors. J Reprod Med 50:417
105. Lynn JA, Varon HH, Kingsley WB, Martin JH (1967) Ultrastructure and biochemical studies of estrogen-secreting capacity of a "nonfunctional" ovarian neoplasm (dysgerminoma). Am J Pathol 51:639
106. Mackay AM, Pattigrew N, Symington T, Neville AM (1974) Tumors of dysgenetic gonads (gonadoblastoma). Ultrastructural and steroidogenic aspects. Cancer (Phila) 34:1108
107. Maeda D, Ota S, Takazawa Y et al (2009) Glypican-3 expression in clear cell adenocarcinoma of the ovary. Mod Pathol 22:824
108. Magi-Galluzi C, O'Connell JT, Neffen E et al (2001) Are mucinous cystadenomas of the ovary derived from germ cells? A genetic analysis (Abstract). Mod Pathol 14:140A (abstract # 818)
109. Malkasian GD Jr, Symmonds RE, Dockerty MB (1965) Malignant ovarian teratomas. Report of 31 cases. Obstet Gynecol 25:810
110. Malkasian GD Jr, Dockerty MB, Symmonds RE (1967) Benign cystic teratomas. Obstet Gynecol 29:719
111. Marin-Padilla M (1965) Origin, nature and significance of the "embryoids" of human teratomas. Virchows Arch (Pathol Anat) 340:105
112. Marrubini G (1949) Primary chorionepithelioma of the ovary. Report of two cases. Acta Obstet Gynecol Scand 28:251
113. Mazur MT, Talbot WH Jr, Talerman A (1988) Endodermal sinus tumor and mucinous cystadenofibroma of the ovary. Occurrence in an 82-year-old woman. Cancer (Phila) 62:2011
114. McCluggage WG, Bissonnette JP, Young RH (2006) Primary malignant melanoma of the ovary: a report of 9 definite or probable cases with emphasis on their morphologic diversity and mimicry of other primary and secondary ovarian neoplasms. Int J Gynecol Pathol 25:321
115. McDonough PG, Byrd JR, Tho PT, Otken L (1976) Gonadoblastoma in a true hermaphrodite with 46XX karyotype. Obstet Gynecol 47:355
116. McKay DG, Hertig AT, Adams EC, Danziger S (1953) Histochemical observations on the germ cells of human embryos. Anat Rec 117:201
117. McKenney JK, Soslow RA, Longacre TA (2008) Ovarian mature teratomas with mucinous epithelial neoplasms: morphologic heterogeneity and association with pseudomyxoma peritonei. Am J Surg Pathol 32:645
118. Michal M, Vanecek T, Sima R et al (2006) Mixed germ cell sex cord-stromal tumors of the testis and ovary. Morphological, immunohistochemical and molecular genetic study of seven cases. Virchows Archs 448:612
119. Miettinen M, Talerman A, Wahlstrom T, Astengo-Osuna C, Virtanen I (1985) Cellular differentiation in ovarian sex cord-stromal and germ-cell tumors studied with antibodies to intermediate-filament proteins. Am J Surg Pathol 9:640

120. Miettinen M, Virtanen I, Talerman A (1985) Intermediate filament proteins in human testis and testicular germ-cell tumors. Am J Pathol 120:402
121. Mueller CW, Topkins P, Lapp WA (1950) Dysgerminoma of the ovary. An analysis of 427 cases. Am J Obstet Gynecol 60:153
122. Nakashima M, Nagasaka T, Fukata S, Oiwa N, Nara Y, Fukatsu T, Takeuchi J (1989) Ovarian gonadoblastoma with dysgerminoma in a woman with two normal children. Hum Pathol 20:814
123. Nielsen SNJ, Scheithauer BW, Gaffey TA (1985) Gliomatosis peritonei. Cancer (Phila) 56:2499
124. Nogales FF Jr, Silverberg SG, Bloustein PA, Martinez-Hernandez A, Pierce GB (1977) Yolk sac carcinoma (endodermal sinus tumor). Ultrastructure and histogenesis of gonadal and extragonadal tumors in comparison with normal human yolk sac. Cancer (Phila) 39:1462
125. Nogales FF, Bergeron C, Carvia RE, Alvaro T, Fulwood HR (1996) Ovarian endometrioid tumors with yolk sac tumor component, an unusual form of ovarian neoplasm. Analysis of six cases. Am J Surg Pathol 20:1056
126. Nomura K, Ohama K, Okamoto E, Fujiwara A (1983) Cytogenetic studies of multiple ovarian dermoid cysts in a single host. Acta Obstet Gynecol Jpn 35:1938
127. Nomura K, Matsui T, Aizawa S (1999) Gonadoblastoma with proliferation resembling Sertoli cell tumor. Int J Gynecol Pathol 18:91
128. Norgaard-Pedersen B, Albrechtsen R, Teilum G (1975) Serum alpha-fetoprotein as a marker for endodermal sinus tumor (yolk sac tumor), or a vitelline component of teratocarcinoma. Acta Pathol Microbiol Scand A 83:573
129. Norris HJ, Jensen RD (1972) Relative frequency of ovarian neoplasms in children and adolescents. Cancer (Phila) 30:713
130. Norris HJ, Zirkin HJ, Benson WL (1976) Immature (malignant) teratoma of the ovary. A clinical and pathologic study of 58 cases. Cancer (Phila) 37:2359
131. O'Connor DM, Norris HJ (1994) The influence of grade on the outcome of stage I ovarian immature (malignant) teratomas and the reproducibility of grading. Int J Gynecol Pathol 13:283
132. Obata NH, Nakashima N, Kawai M, Kikkawa F, Mamba S, Tomoda Y (1995) Gonadoblastoma with dysgerminoma in one ovary and gonadoblastoma with dysgerminoma and yolk sac tumor in the contralateral ovary in a girl with 46,XX karyotype. Gynecol Oncol 58:124
133. Pantoja E, Noy MA, Axtmayer RW, Colon FE, Pelegrina I (1975) Ovarian dermoids and their complications. Comprehensive historical review. Obstet Gynecol Surv 30:1
134. Pantoja E, Rodriguez-Ibanez I, Axtmayer RW, Noy MA, Pelegrina I (1975) Complications of dermoid tumors of the ovary. Obstet Gynecol 45:89
135. Park IJ, Pyeatte JC, Jones HW, Woodruff JD (1972) Gonadoblastoma in a true hermaphrodite with 46XY genotype. Obstet Gynecol 40:466
136. Park JY, Kim DY, Kim JH et al (2008) Malignant transformation of mature cystic teratoma of the ovary: experience at a single institution. Eur J Obstet Gynecol Reprod Biol 141:173
137. Parkash V, Carcangiu ML (1995) Transformation of ovarian dysgerminoma to yolk sac tumor: evidence for a histogenetic continuum. Mod Pathol 8:881
138. Parrington JM, West LF, Povey S (1984) The origin of ovarian teratomas. J Med Genet 21:4
139. Payne D, Muss HB, Homesley HD, Jobson VM, Baird FG (1981) Autoimmune hemolytic anemia and ovarian dermoid cysts. Case report and review of the literature. Cancer (Phila) 48:721
140. Peccatori F, Bonazzi C, Chiari F, Landoni F, Colombo N, Mangioni C (1995) Surgical management of malignant ovarian germ cell tumors: 10 years' experience with 129 patients. Obstet Gynecol 86:367
141. Pedowitz P, Felmus LB, Grayzel DM (1955) Dysgerminoma of the ovary. Prognosis and treatment. Am J Obstet Gynecol 70:1284
142. Peterson WF (1956) Solid histologically benign teratomas of the ovary. A report of four cases and review of the literature. Am J Obstet Gynecol 72:1094
143. Peterson WF (1957) Malignant degeneration of benign cystic teratomas of the ovary: a collective review of the literature. Obstet Gynecol Surv 12:793
144. Peterson WF, Prevost EC, Edmunds FT, Huntley JM Jr, Morris FK (1955) Benign cystic teratomas of the ovary. A clinicostatistical study of 1007 cases with review of the literature. Am J Obstet Gynecol 70:368
145. Peyron A (1939) Faits nouveaux relatifs l'origine et l'histogenese des embryomes. Bull Assoc Fr Cancer 28:658
146. Pierce GB Jr, Dixon FJ (1959) Testicular teratomas. 1. Demonstration of teratogenesis by metamorphosis of multipotential cells. Cancer (Phila) 12:573
147. Pierce GB Jr, Dixon FJ (1959) Testicular teratomas. 2. Teratocarcinoma as ascitic tumor. Cancer (Phila) 12:584
148. Pierce GB Jr, Midgley AR (1963) The origin and function of human syncytiotrophoblastic giant cells. Am J Pathol 43:153
149. Pierce GB Jr, Verney EL (1961) An in vitro and in vivo study of differentiation in teratocarcinomas. Cancer (Phila) 14:1017
150. Pierce GB Jr, Midgley AR, Beals TF (1962) An ultrastructural study of differentiation and maturation of trophoblast of the monkey. Lab Invest 13:451
151. Pierce GB Jr, Midgley AR, Sri Ram J, Feldman JD (1964) Parietal yolk sac carcinoma. Clue to the histogenesis of Reichert's membrane of the mouse embryo. Am J Pathol 41:549
152. Pitman MB, Triratanachat S, Young RH et al (2004) Hepatocyte paraffin 1 antibody does not distinguish primary ovarian tumors with hepatoid differentiation from metastatic hepatocellular carcinoma. Int J Gynecol Pathol 23:58
153. Poulos C, Cheng L, Zhang S et al (2006) Analysis of ovarian teratomas for isochromosome 12p: evidence supporting a dual histogenetic pathway for teratomatous elements. Mod Pathol 19:766
154. Prat J, Bhan AK, Dickersin GR, Robboy SJ, Scully RE (1982) Hepatoid yolk sac tumor of the ovary (endodermal sinus tumor with hepatoid differentiation). A light microscopic ultrastructural and immunohistochemical study of seven cases. Cancer (Phila) 50:2355
155. Pratt-Thomas HR, Cooper JM (1976) Gonadoblastoma with tubal pregnancy. Am J Clin Pathol 65:121
156. Rabban JT, Lerwill MF, McCluggage WG et al (2009) Primary ovarian carcinoid tumors may express CDX-2: a potential pitfall in distinction from metastatic intestinal carcinoid tumors involving the ovary. Int J Gynecol Pathol 28:41
157. Ramalingam P, Malpica A, Silva EG et al (2004) The use of cytokeratin 7 and EMA in differentiating ovarian yolk sac tumors from endometrioid and clear cell carcinomas. Am J Surg Pathol 28:1499
158. Rashad MH, Fathalla MF, Kerr MC (1966) Sex chromatin and chromosome analysis in ovarian teratomas. Am J Obstet Gynecol 96:461
159. Riopel MA, Spellerberg A, Griffin CA et al (1998) Genetic analysis of ovarian germ cell tumors by comparative genomic hybridization. Cancer Res 58:3105

160. Robboy SJ, Scully RE (1970) Ovarian teratoma with glial implants on the peritoneum. An analysis of 12 cases. Hum Pathol 1:643
161. Robboy SJ, Scully RE (1980) Strumal carcinoid of the ovary. An analysis of 50 cases of a distinctive tumor composed of thyroid tissue and carcinoid. Cancer (Phila) 46:2019
162. Robboy SJ, Scully RE, Norris HJ (1974) Carcinoid metastatic to the ovary. A clinicopathologic analysis of 35 cases. Cancer (Phila) 33:798
163. Robboy SJ, Norris HJ, Scully RE (1975) Insular carcinoid primary in the ovary: a clinicopathologic analysis of 48 cases. Cancer (Phila) 36:404
164. Robboy SJ, Scully RE, Norris HJ (1977) Primary trabecular carcinoid of the ovary. Obstet Gynecol 49:202
165. Robboy SJ, Shaco-Levy R, Peng RY et al (2009) Malignant struma ovarii: an analysis of 88 cases, including 27 with extraovarian spread. Int J Gynecol Pathol 28:405
166. Rose LI, Underwood RH, Williams GH, Pincus GS (1974) Pure gonadal dysgenesis. Studies of in vitro androgen metabolism. Am J Med 57:957
167. Roth LM, Kerseladze AI (2008) Highly differentiated follicular carcinoma arising from struma ovarii: a report of three cases, a review of the literature and reasessement of the so-called peritoneal strumosis. Int J Gynecol Pathol 27:213
168. Roth LM, Talerman A (2006) Recent advances in the pathology and classification of ovarian germ cell tumors. Int J Gynecol Pathol 25:305
169. Roth LM, Talerman A (2007) The enigma of struma ovarii. Pathology 39:139
170. Roth LM, Miller AWIII, Talerman A (2007) Typical thyroid-type carcinoma arising in struma ovarii: a report of 4 cases and review of the literature. Int J Gynecol Pathol 27:496
171. Rutgers JL, Scully RE (1986) Functioning ovarian tumors with peripheral steroid cell proliferation. A report of 24 cases. Int J Gynecol Pathol 5:319
172. Rutgers JL, Young RH, Scully RE (1987) Ovarian yolk sac tumor arising from endometrioid carcinoma. Hum Pathol 18:1296
173. Santesson L (1947) Clinical and pathological survey of ovarian tumours treated at the Radiumhemmet. 1. Dysgerminoma. Acta Radiol (Stockh) 28:643
174. Schellhas HF (1974) Malignant potential of the dysgenetic gonad. Part 1. Obstet Gynecol 44:298
175. Schellhas HF (1974) Malignant potential of the dysgenetic gonad. Part 2. Obstet Gynecol 44:455
176. Schellhas HF, Trujillo JM, Rutledge FN, Cork A (1971) Germ cell tumors associated with XY gonadal dysgenesis. Am J Obstet Gynecol 109:1197
177. Schiller W (1939) Mesonephroma ovarii. Am J Cancer 35:1
178. Schmidt J, Derr V, Heinrich MC et al (2007) BRAF in papillary thyroid carcinoma of ovary (struma ovarii). Am J Surg Pathol 31:1337
179. Schmitz EF (1925) Malignant endothelioma of perithelioma type in the ovary. Am J Obstet Gynecol 9:247
180. Schwartz PE, Morris JM (1988) Serum lactic dehydrogenase. A tumor marker for dysgerminoma. Obstet Gynecol 72:511
181. Scully RE (1953) Gonadoblastoma. A gonadal tumor related to dysgerminoma (seminoma) and capable of sex hormone production. Cancer (Phila) 6:455
182. Scully RE (1970) Gonadoblastoma. Cancer (Phila) 25:1340
183. Scully RE (1970) Sex cord tumor with annular tubules. A distinctive ovarian tumor of the Peutz–Jeghers syndrome. Cancer (Phila) 25:1107
184. Scully RE (1999) Histological typing of ovarian tumours, World Health Organization histological classification of tumours, 2nd edn. Springer, Heidelberg
185. Scully RE, Young RH, Clement PB (1998) Tumors of the ovary, maldeveloped gonads and broad ligament. Atlas of tumor pathology. Fascicle 23, 3rd series. Armed Forces Institute of Pathology, Washingon, DC
186. Serov SF, Scully RE, Sobin LH (1973) Histological typing of ovarian tumors. International histological classification of tumors, no 9. World Health Organization, Geneva
187. Serratoni FT, Robboy SJ (1975) Ultrastructure of primary and metastatic ovarian carcinoids: analysis of 11 cases. Cancer (Phila) 36:157
188. Sever M, Jones TD, Roth LM et al (2005) Expression of CD117 (c-kit) receptor in dysgerminoma of the ovary: diagnostic and therapeutic implications. Mod Pathol 18:1411
189. Shah KD, Kaffe S, Gilbert F, Dolgin S, Gertner M (1988) Unilateral microscopic gonadoblastoma in a prepubertal Turner mosaic with Y chromosome material identified by restriction fragment analysis. Am J Clin Pathol 90:622
190. Shigematsu T, Kamura T, Airnia T et al (2000) DNA polymorphism analysis of a pure nongestational choriocarcinoma of the ovary: case report. Eur J Gynecol Oncol 21:153
191. Shirai T, Itoh T, Yoshiki T, Noro T, Tomino Y, Hayasaka T (1976) Immunofluorescent demonstration of alpha-fetoprotein, and other plasma proteins in yolk sac tumor. Cancer (Phila) 38:1661
192. Simard LC (1957) Polyembryonic embryoma of the ovary of parthenogenetic origin. Cancer (Phila) 10:215
193. Smith FG (1946) Pathology and physiology of struma ovarii. Arch Surg 53:603
194. Snyder RR, Tavassoli FA (1986) Ovarian strumal carcinoid: Immunohistochemical, ultrastructural, and clinicopathologic observations. Int J Gynecol Pathol 5:187
195. Soga J, Osaka M, Yakawa Y (2000) Carcinoids of the ovary: an analysis of 329 reported cases. J Exp Clin Cancer Res 19:271
196. Speleman F, Dermaut B, DePotter CR et al (1997) Monosomy 22 in a mixed germ cell-sex cord-stromal tumor of the ovary. Genes Chromosomes Cancer 19:192
197. Sporrong B, Falkmer S, Robboy SJ et al (1982) Neurohormonal peptides in ovarian carcinoids. An immunohistochemical study of 81 primary carcinoids and of intraovarian metastases from six midgut carcinoids. Cancer (Phila) 49:68
198. Stagno PA, Petras RE, Hart WR (1987) Strumal carcinoids of the ovary. An immunohistologic and ultrastructural study. Arch Pathol Lab Med 111:440
199. Stamp GWH, McConnell EM (1983) Malignancy arising in cystic ovarian teratomas. Br J Obstet Gynecol 90:671
200. Stevens LC (1959) Embryology of testicular teratomas in strain 129 mice. J Natl Cancer Inst 23:1249
201. Stevens LC (1960) Embryonic potency of embryoid bodies derived from a transplantable testicular teratoma of the mouse. Dev Biol 2:285
202. Stevens LC (1962) The biology of teratomas including evidence indicating their origin from primordial germ cells. Ann Biol 1:585
203. Subbuswamy SG, Gibbs NM, Ross CF, Morson BC (1974) Goblet cell carcinoid of the appendix. Cancer (Phila) 34:338
204. Szokol M, Kondrai G, Papp Z (1977) Gonadal malignancy and 46 XY karyotype in a true hermaphrodite. Obstet Gynecol 49:358
205. Szyfelbein WM, Young RH, Scully RE (1994) Cystic struma ovarii: a frequently unrecognized tumor. A report of 20 cases. Am J Surg Pathol 18:785

206. Szyfelbein WM, Young RH, Scully RE (1995) Struma ovarii simulating ovarian tumors of other types. A report of 30 cases. Am J Surg Pathol 19:21
207. Takeda A, Ishizuka T, Goto T et al (1982) Polyembryoma of ovary producing alpha-fetoprotein and HCG. Immunoperoxidase and electron microscopic study. Cancer (Phila) 49:1878
208. Talerman A (1971) Gonadoblastoma and dysgerminoma in two siblings with dysgenetic gonads. Obstet Gynecol 38:416
209. Talerman A (1972) A distinctive gonadal neoplasm related to gonadoblastoma. Cancer (Phila) 30:1219
210. Talerman A (1972) A mixed germ cell-sex cord stroma tumor in a normal female infant. Obstet Gynecol 40:473
211. Talerman A (1974) Gonadoblastoma associated with embryonal carcinoma. Obstet Gynecol 43:138
212. Talerman A (1975) The incidence of yolk sac tumor (endodermal sinus tumor) elements in germ cell tumors of the testis in adults. Cancer (Phila) 36:211
213. Talerman A (1980) The pathology of gonadal neoplasms composed of germ cells and sex cord stroma derivatives. Pathol Res Pract 170:24
214. Talerman A (1984) Carcinoid tumors of the ovary. J Cancer Res Clin Oncol 107:125
215. Talerman A (1987) Ovarian Sertoli–Leydig cell tumor (androblastoma) with retiform pattern: A clinicopathologic study. Cancer (Phila) 60:3056
216. Talerman A, Delemarre JFM (1975) Gonadoblastoma associated with embryonal carcinoma in an anatomically normal male. J Urol 113:355
217. Talerman A, Evans MI (1982) Primary trabecular carcinoid tumor of the ovary. Cancer (Phila) 50:1407
218. Talerman A, Haije WG (1974) Alpha-fetoprotein and germ cell tumors. A possible role of yolk sac tumor in production of alpha-fetoprotein. Cancer (Phila) 34:1722
219. Talerman A, Haije WG (1985) Ovarian Sertoli cell tumor with retiform and heterologous elements. Am J Surg Pathol 9:459
220. Talerman A, Okagaki T (1985) Ultrastructural features of primary trabecular carcinoid tumor of the ovary. Int J Gynecol Pathol 4:153
221. Talerman A, Roth LM (2007) Recent advances in the pathology and classification of gonadal neoplasms composed of germ cells and sex cord derivatives. Int J Gynecol Pathol 26:313
222. Talerman A, van der Harten JJ (1977) A mixed germ cell-sex cord stroma tumor of the ovary associated with isosexual precocious puberty in a normal female child. Cancer (Phila) 40:889
223. Talerman A, Huyzinga WT, Kuipers T (1973) Dysgerminoma. Clinicopathologic study of 22 cases. Obstet Gynecol 41:137
224. Talerman A, Haije WG, Baggerman L (1977) Alpha-1-antitrypsin (AAT) and alpha-foetoprotein (AFP) in sera of patients with germ cell neoplasms. Value as tumor markers in patients with endodermal sinus tumour (yolk sac tumour). Int J Cancer 19:741
225. Talerman A, van der Pompe WB, Haije WG, Baggerman L, Boekestein-Tjahjadi HM (1977) Alpha-fetoprotein and carcinoembryonic antigen in germ cell neoplasms. Br J Cancer 35:288
226. Talerman A, Haije WG, Baggerman L (1978) Serum alpha-fetoprotein in diagnosis and management of endodermal sinus (yolk sac) tumor and mixed germ cell tumor of the ovary. Cancer (Phila) 41:272
227. Talerman A, Haije WG, Baggerman L (1980) Serum alpha-fetoprotein (AFP) in patients with germ cell tumors of the gonads and extragonadal sites. Correlation between endodermal sinus (yolk sac) tumor and raised serum AFP. Cancer (Phila) 46:340
228. Talerman A, Verp M, Senekjian E, Gilewski T, Vogelzang N (1990) True hermaphrodite with normal female 46, XX karyotype, bilateral gonadoblastomas and dysgerminomas and normal pregnancy. Cancer (Phila) 66:2668
229. Tavassoli FA (1983) A combined germ cell-gonadal stromal-epithelial tumor of the ovary. Am J Surg Pathol 7:73
230. Tavassoli FA, Devilee P (2003) Pathology and genetics of tumors of the breast and female genital organs, World Health Organization classification of tumors. IARC, Lyon
231. Teilum G (1944) Homologous tumours in ovary and testis: contribution to classification of gonadal tumours. Acta Obstet Gynecol Scand 24:480
232. Teilum G (1946) Gonocytoma; homologous ovarian and testicular tumours. 1. With discussion of "mesonephroma ovarii" (Schiller: Am J Cancer 1939). Acta Pathol Microbiol Scand 23:242
233. Teilum G (1950) "mesonephroma ovarii" (Schiller) extraembryonic mesoblastoma of germ cell origin in ovary and testis. Acta Pathol Microbiol Scand 27:249
234. Teilum G (1959) Endodermal sinus tumors of the ovary and testis. Comparative morphogenesis of the so-called mesonephroma ovarii (Schiller) and extraembryonic (yolk sac-allantoic) structures of the rat's placenta. Cancer (Phila) 12:1092
235. Teilum G (1965) Classification of endodermal sinus tumour (mesoblastoma vitellinum) and so-called embryonal carcinoma of the ovary. Acta Pathol Microbiol Scand 64:407
236. Teter J (1970) Prognosis, malignancy and curability of the germ cell tumor occurring in dysgenetic gonads. Am J Obstet Gynecol 108:894
237. Thomas GM, Dembo AJ, Hacker NE, DePetrillo AD (1987) Current therapy for dysgerminoma of the ovary. Obstet Gynecol 70:268
238. Tiltman AJ (1985) Ependymal cyst of the ovary. South Afr Med J 68:424
239. Tokuoka S, Aoki Y, Yokoyama T, Ishii T (1985) A mixed germ cell-sex cord stromal tumor of the ovary with retiform tubular structure. A case report. Int J Gynecol Pathol 4:161
240. Tsuchida Y, Kaneko M, Yokomori K et al (1978) Alpha-fetoprotein, prealbumin, albumin, alpha-1-antitrypsin, and transferrin as diagnostic and therapeutic markers for endodermal sinus tumors. J Pediatr Surg 13:25
241. Tsujioka H, Hamada T, Miyakawa H (2003) A pure nongestational choriocarcinoma of the ovary diagnosed with DNA polymorphism analysis. Gynecol Oncol 89:540
242. Tsuura Y, Hiraki H, Watanabe K et al (1996) Preferential localization of C-kit product in tissue mast cells, basal cells of skin, epithelial cells of breast, small cell lung carcinoma and seminoma/dysgerminoma in the human. Immunohistochemical study on formalin-fixed paraffin-embedded tissues. Virchows Arch 424:135
243. Ueda G, Fujita M, Ogawa H, Sawada M, Inoue M, Tanizawa O (1993) Adenocarcinoma in a benign cystic teratoma of the ovary. Report of a case with a long survival period. Gynecol Oncol 48:259
244. Ulbright TM (2005) Germ cell tumors of the gonads: a selective review emphasizing problems in differential diagnosis, newly appreciated, and controversial issues. Mod Pathol 18(Suppl 2):S61
245. Ulbright TM, Roth LM, Erlich CE (1982) Ovarian strumal carcinoid. An immunocytochemical and ultrastructural study of two cases. Am J Clin Pathol 77:622
246. Ulirsch RC, Goldman RL (1982) An unusual teratoma of the ovary: neurogenic cyst with lactating breast tissue. Obstet Gynecol 60:400
247. Vance RP, Geisinger KR (1985) Pure nongestational choriocarcinoma of the ovary. Report of a case. Cancer (Phila) 56:2321

248. Vang R, Gown AM, Zhao C et al (2007) Ovarian mucinous tumors associated with mature cystic teratoma. Morphologic and immunohistochemical analysis identifies a subset of potential teratomatous origin that shares features of lower gastrointestinal tract mucinous tumors more commonly encountered as secondary tumors of the ovary. Am J Surg Pathol 31:854
249. Warkel RL, Cooper PH, Helwig EB (1978) Adenocarcinoid, a mucin-producing carcinoid of the appendix. Cancer (Phila) 42:2781
250. Weldon-Linne CM, Rushovich AM (1983) Benign ovarian cystic teratomas with homunculi. Obstet Gynecol 61:88S
251. Williamson HO, Underwood PB Jr, Kreutner A Jr, Rogers JF, Mathur RS, Pratt-Thomas HR (1976) Gonadoblastoma: clinicopathologic correlation in six patients. Am J Obstet Gynecol 126:579
252. Wisniewski M, Deppisch LM (1973) Solid teratomas of the ovary. Cancer (Phila) 32:440
253. Witschi E (1948) Migration of the germ cells of human embryos from the yolk sac to the primitive gonadal folds. Contrib Embryol 32:69
254. Woodruff JD, Rauh JT, Markley RL (1966) Ovarian struma. Obstet Gynecol 27:194
255. Woodruff JD, Protos P, Peterson WF (1968) Ovarian teratomas. Relationship of histologic and ontogenic factors to prognosis. Am J Obstet Gynecol 102:702
256. Yanai-Inbar I, Scully RE (1987) Relation of ovarian dermoid cysts and immature teratomas: an analysis of 350 cases of immature teratoma and 10 cases of dermoid cyst with microscopic foci of immature tissue. Int J Gynecol Pathol 6:203
257. Young RH, Scully RE (1983) Ovarian Sertoli–Leydig cell tumors with a retiform pattern. A problem in histopathologic diagnosis. A report of 25 cases. Am J Surg Pathol 7:755
258. Young RH, Prat J, Scully RE (1982) Ovarian Sertoli–Leydig cell tumors with heterologous elements (1) gastrointestinal epithelium and carcinoid: a clinicopathologic analysis of thirty six cases. Cancer (Phila) 50:2448
259. Zaloudek C, Tavassoli FA, Norris HJ (1981) Dysgerminoma with syncytiotrophoblastic giant cells. A histologically and clinically distinctive subtype of dysgerminoma. Am J Surg Pathol 5:361
260. Zhao S, Kato N, Endoh Y et al (2000) Ovarian gonadoblastoma with mixed germ cell tumor in a woman with 46,XX karyotype and successful pregnancies. Pathol Int 50:332
261. Zhao C, Bratthauer GL, Barner R et al (2007) Comparative analysis of alternative and traditional immunohistochemical markers for the distinction of ovarian Sertoli cell tumor from endometrioid tumors and carcinoid tumor: a study of 160 cases. Am J Surg Pathol 31:255

17 Nonspecific Tumors of the Ovary, Including Mesenchymal Tumors

Aleksander Talerman · Russell Vang

R. J. Kurman, L. Hedrick Ellenson, B. M. Ronnett (eds.), *Blaustein's Pathology of the Female Genital Tract (6th ed.)*, DOI 10.1007/978-1-4419-0489-8_17,

The tumors discussed in this chapter comprise a heterogeneous group of neoplasms that are not specific to the ovary. They are uncommon in this location, occurring much more frequently in other parts of the body. Consequently, whenever they are encountered in the ovary, these tumors pose difficult problems in diagnosis, histogenesis, behavior, and therapy for the pathologist and clinician. These neoplasms must be differentiated from primary ovarian neoplasms containing mesenchymal tissue, as well as from metastatic and disseminated neoplasms affecting the ovary. Thus, mesenchymal neoplasms nonspecific to the ovary must be differentiated primarily from teratomatous neoplasms containing large amounts of mature or immature mesenchymal elements and from the malignant mesodermal mixed müllerian (mesodermal) tumors (MMMT), which are composed of different malignant connective tissue elements in addition to their malignant epithelial components. Tumors of teratomatous origin containing mesenchymal tissue are described in ➲ Chap. 16, Germ Cell Tumors of the Ovary, and MMMTs/carcinosarcomas, endometrioid stromal sarcomas, and adenosarcoma are discussed in ➲ Chap. 14, Surface Epithelial Tumors of the Ovary.

In addition to the connective tissue neoplasms nonspecific to the ovary, the adenomatoid tumor, which is of mesothelial origin, the ovarian tumor of probable wolffian origin, ovarian neoplasms of neural origin, hepatoid carcinoma of the ovary, small cell carcinoma of the ovary with pulmonary differentiation, and tumors of salivary gland type are included.

Mesenchymal Tumors Nonspecific to the Ovary

Mesenchymal neoplasms nonspecific to the ovary include all primary ovarian neoplasms of connective tissue origin found in the ovary that are nonspecific to it but are considered to originate from ovarian tissue, and are not of teratomatous or surface epithelial–stromal (müllerian) origin. However, this mode of origin cannot be excluded in a number of cases. The neoplasms discussed here are composed of a single neoplastic mesenchymal element, either benign or malignant, in contrast to teratomatous tumors or MMMTs, which usually are composed of a number of tissue elements.

Some issues of classification and histogenesis may not be reconcilable in view of the possibility of one-sided differentiation of a teratoma or of a malignant mixed müllerian tumor of the ovary. Thus, although some of these neoplasms can be shown to originate directly from ovarian tissue, a considerable number of cases are of indeterminate histogenesis and origin. Mesenchymal neoplasms nonspecific to the ovary can be benign or malignant, and are classified on the basis of the tissue of origin.

Myxoma

Primary myxoma of the ovary is a very rare neoplasm: only a very small number of cases have been reported in the literature [3, 13, 61]. The patients were aged 14–45 years, and in each case had an adnexal mass while the other adnexa was normal [3, 13, 61]. Macroscopically, the tumors measured from 5 to 22 cm in the greatest dimension [13, 61]. They were encapsulated, gray-white, and soft; on cut section, they were found to be partly cystic. Solid areas were slimy and mucinous, whereas the cystic spaces contained a viscous, glassy, gelatinous material.

Microscopically, the tumors showed typical appearances of myxoma as seen in other locations. They were composed of loose myxomatous stroma within which there were scattered stellate or spindle-shaped cells, some of which contained hyperchromatic nuclei. There was no nuclear pleomorphism, and mitotic activity was absent. The tumors varied from poorly vascularized, containing only a few capillary blood vessels and showing absence of plexiform vessels, to tumors with prominent capillary vessels within the tumor, and larger vessels with muscular walls at its periphery. The myxomatous stroma stained positively with alcian-blue stain and contained a network of fine reticulum fibers. Stains for fat were negative. In some areas, fibrosis was present. There were no other connective tissue elements, and the tumors had a homogeneous appearance.

Myxoma is immunoreactive for vimentin and focally for actin, but negative for desmin, cytokeratins, vascular markers, S-100, and neurofilaments [8, 13]. Most myxomas originate within connective tissue, and the origin of the tumor is still a matter of dispute. The histogenesis of ovarian myxomas is unknown; however, a gonadal stromal origin has been proposed [8].

Although myxoma is a benign neoplasm, because of its viscous nature it is difficult to excise it completely, and recurrences are not uncommon unless the entire adnexa bearing the tumor are excised. All the patients treated by unilateral adnexectomy and for whom there is follow-up information are free of disease after 1–13 years [13].

Myxoma must be differentiated from fibroma with myxoid degeneration, which contains normal fibrous tissue in some areas. Ovarian myxoma must be distinguished from massive edema of the ovary (see ➲ Chap. 12,

Nonneoplastic Lesions of the Ovary) [29, 78]. The patients with massive edema usually are younger, and the lesion shows entrapment of follicular derivatives, which is not observed in ovarian myxoma. More importantly, myxoma must be differentiated from myxomatous liposarcoma, which contains fat, is more vascularized, and shows lipoblasts at least in some areas. It also must be differentiated from mucinous cystadenomas and carcinomas, either primary or metastatic, which contain epithelial cells, show absence of stellate and spindle-shaped cells, and may show glandular differentiation. The epithelial tumor cells are cytokeratin-positive.

Myxoma also should be distinguished from embryonal rhabdomyosarcoma. The latter tumor shows less of a uniform appearance, displays greater cellular and nuclear pleomorphism, and contains rhabdomyoblasts. In addition, embryonal rhabdomyosarcoma shows immunohistochemical staining for muscle-specific actin, desmin, and myogenin. Ultrastructurally, Z-band formation, glycogen granules, and thick filament ribosomal complexes are observed.

Giant Cell Tumor of the Ovary

Giant cell tumor of the ovary, histologically indistinguishable from a giant cell tumor of bone, is very rare, and only a few cases have been reported [17, 36]. Most of the tumors were either associated with an epithelial component of surface epithelial stromal origin or were seen as part of mural nodules, but in two cases the tumor was composed entirely of multinucleated giant cells and small ovoid or spindle-shaped stromal cells [17, 36]. In the latter cases, the tumors were larger, showed hemorrhage, necrosis, and brisk mitotic activity in the smaller mononuclear component of the tumor. There was no evidence of metastases. One patient, a 31-year-old woman, was well and disease-free 4.5 years following surgery, while the other, a 76-year-old woman, died a few months following surgery and chemotherapy. Due to limited data it is not possible to draw any conclusions regarding the behavior of this tumor.

Undifferentiated Sarcoma

Some ovarian tumors are poorly differentiated, and although a diagnosis of sarcoma can be made, the tumor does not exhibit further differentiation beyond showing its mesenchymal origin. Careful and extensive gross sampling and histologic examination in such cases are helpful and may result in finding better-differentiated areas, which will yield a more accurate diagnosis. Immunohistochemical investigations may be very helpful in detecting accurately the tissue of origin and should be undertaken in all such cases. In some cases, a more precise diagnosis cannot be made despite very extensive investigations.

Tumors of Muscle Differentiation

Leiomyoma

Primary leiomyoma of the ovary is uncommon [10, 30, 34, 53, 61]. A small number of cases are on record, but it is likely that many cases are not reported, especially when the tumor is small and is discovered incidentally. More than a dozen unreported cases are known to the authors.

Primary ovarian leiomyoma probably originates from smooth muscle present in the walls of blood vessels in the cortical stroma, in the corpus luteum, and in the ovarian ligaments at their point of attachment to the ovary; its precise histogenesis is uncertain, however. This tumor usually is found in menopausal and postmenopausal women, but sometimes occurs in young women. The age of patients ranged from 3 to 65 years. Clinically, many patients are asymptomatic, and the tumor is discovered incidentally. When symptoms are present, they are related to the presence of an adnexal mass, often accompanied by abdominal swelling and pain. The latter may be acute because of torsion. Ascites is rare, and hydrothorax has not been reported. The uterus usually contains leiomyomas.

Ovarian leiomyoma is unilateral, although a single case of large bilateral ovarian leiomyomas occurring in a 21-year-old woman has been reported [30]. Macroscopically the tumors are solid, firm, and round or oval masses having a smooth surface. On cut section they have a white or gray-white solid whorled surface. Hemorrhage and necrosis may be evident, altering the appearance. Cyst formation caused by necrosis may occur, and calcification also may be present.

Microscopically, the tumor shows typical appearances of a leiomyoma, as observed in the uterus, the tumor being composed of smooth muscle cells that are uniformly spindle-shaped or elongated and contain elongated blunt-ended or cigar-shaped nuclei (➲ *Fig. 17.1*). Palisading of the nuclei may be present and may be prominent. Mitotic activity is absent or very low, and cellular and nuclear pleomorphism is not a feature. Most leiomyomas are of the typical type, but cellular, mitotically active, atypical, myxoid, and epithelioid types can be seen. The tumor cells form bundles intersected by fibrous septa that may be wide and show marked hyalinization. Other degenerative

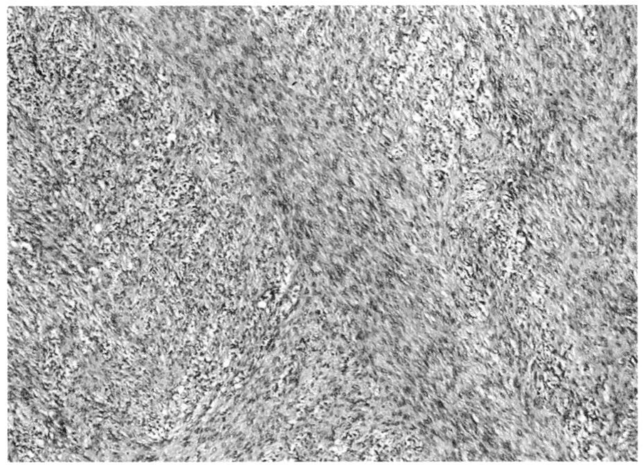

Fig. 17.1
Primary leiomyoma of the ovary. **The tumor shows an appearance similar to the much more common uterine leiomyoma**

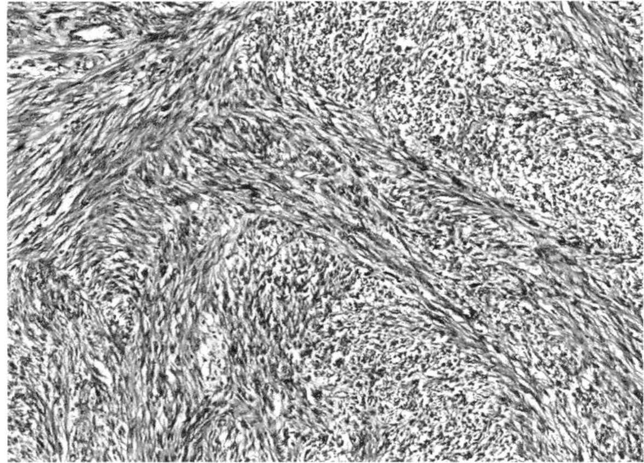

Fig. 17.2
Primary leiomyosarcoma of the ovary. **Low magnification. Note the similarity to the leiomyoma seen in** ***Fig. 17.1***

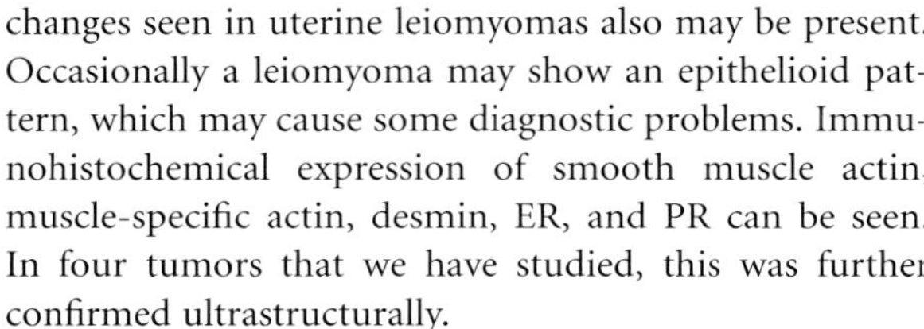

changes seen in uterine leiomyomas also may be present. Occasionally a leiomyoma may show an epithelioid pattern, which may cause some diagnostic problems. Immunohistochemical expression of smooth muscle actin, muscle-specific actin, desmin, ER, and PR can be seen. In four tumors that we have studied, this was further confirmed ultrastructurally.

A well-documented case of a large ovarian lipoleiomyoma occurring in a 63-year-old woman has been reported [41]. The tumor replaced nearly the entire ovary. The adipose tissue was found replacing and dissecting the smooth muscle within the tumor. There was no associated uterine leiomyomatosis.

Primary ovarian leiomyoma must be differentiated from pedunculated subserosal (parasitic) uterine leiomyoma, which has lost its attachment and instead has become attached to the ovary, from which it draws its blood supply. Leiomyoma also must be differentiated from ovarian fibroma as the latter is much more common. There is a tendency to diagnose leiomyoma as a fibroma, but use of immunohistochemical stains for this distinction should be used with caution since fibromas can also show expression of muscle markers [8, 70]. The treatment is excision of the affected adnexa.

Leiomyosarcoma

Primary leiomyosarcoma of the ovary is very rare. These tumors usually are found in postmenopausal women, but sometimes may be seen in younger women [1, 34]. The tumors usually are large and solid, and patients have symptoms and signs related to the presence of an abdominal or pelvic mass. The tumors are gray-yellow, soft, fleshy, and frequently associated with hemorrhage and necrosis.

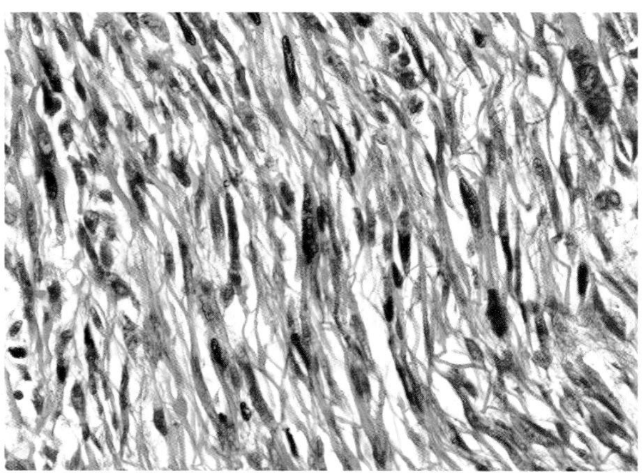

Fig. 17.3
Primary leiomyosarcoma of the ovary. **High magnification. Note the marked cellular and nuclear pleomorphism**

Microscopically, they differ from a leiomyoma by the presence of a variable combination of mitotic activity, cellular and nuclear pleomorphism, and necrosis (*Figs. 17.2* and *17.3*). It has been proposed that leiomyosarcoma should be diagnosed when ≥2 of the following histologic features are present: significant nuclear atypia, mitotic index ≥10 mitotic figures/10 high-power fields, and tumor cell necrosis; it has also been suggested that a smooth muscle tumor with nuclear atypia can qualify as a leiomyosarcoma if the mitotic index is ≥5 mitotic figures/10 high-power fields, even if tumor cell necrosis is not present [34]. The diagnosis of "smooth muscle tumor of uncertain malignant potential" can be used for tumors with histologic features intermediate between leiomyoma and leiomyosarcoma.

Most leiomyosarcomas are of the conventional type, but occasional ovarian leiomyosarcomas may be of the myxoid or epithelioid type. It is important to recognize these unusual variants, which are similar to their counterparts in the uterus. Primary leiomyosarcoma of the ovary metastasizes via the bloodstream; the prognosis is generally unfavorable. Primary leiomyosarcoma of the ovary must be distinguished from MMMTs containing a prominent leiomyosarcomatous component. Primary leiomyosarcoma also should be distinguished from immature teratoma with a prominent leiomymatous tissue component. It also must be distinguished from metastatic leiomyosarcoma of uterine or other origin, as well as from poorly differentiated sarcomas and carcinosarcomas, both primary and metastatic to the ovary.

Rhabdomyoma

No well-documented case of pure ovarian rhabdomyoma has been recorded. A case of mural nodules of rhabdomyoma within a serous cystadenoma in a 48 year old has been reported [25].

Rhabdomyosarcoma

Primary rhabdomyosarcoma of the ovary is uncommon. A small number of cases have been reported in the literature, and nine unreported cases are known to the authors. A careful review of the literature shows that some cases, such as the frequently quoted case reported by Sandison [58], were not pure rhabdomyosarcomas but rather examples of MMMT or teratomas with a marked rhabdomyoblastic component. Therefore, before a diagnosis of primary ovarian rhabdomyosarcoma can be made, the tumor must be sampled carefully and extensively to exclude the presence of other neoplastic elements, the presence of which would preclude a diagnosis of a pure rhabdomyosarcoma of the ovary.

The histogenesis of primary rhabdomyosarcoma of the ovary is uncertain. These tumors may originate from the connective tissue of the ovary, as a one-sided development of a teratoma, as a result of malignant transformation of a mature cystic teratoma with the malignant element overgrowing the tumor, or as a one-sided development of a MMMT.

The age of patients with ovarian rhabdomyosarcoma ranged from 2.5 to 84 years. The small number of cases makes it impossible to state whether there is a predilection for any particular age group, but, as with rhabdomyosarcomas occurring in other locations, the pleomorphic type occurs in older patients, whereas the embryonal and alveolar types occur in young women and children [5]. Patients with ovarian rhabdomyosarcoma usually have symptoms associated with the presence of a large, usually rapidly growing, abdominal mass, often associated with hemorrhagic ascites. Metastases frequently are seen at presentation.

Macroscopically, the tumors are unilateral, but metastatic involvement of the contralateral ovary may be present and should be differentiated from bilateral involvement. The tumors usually are large, exceeding 10 cm in diameter. They are solid, soft, fleshy, and gray-pink to yellow-tan, with areas of hemorrhage and necrosis that may be prominent.

Microscopically, the tumors may be of the embryonal (including the botryoid type), alveolar, or pleomorphic type and contain variable numbers of rhabdomyoblasts (*Figs. 17.4–17.6*). Tumors composed of the former types occur in children and young adults, whereas those of the

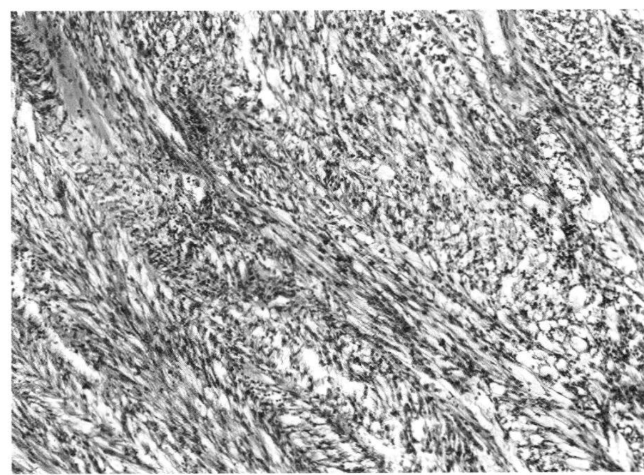

Fig. 17.4
Primary rhabdomyosarcoma of the ovary. **This portion of the tumor contains a significant spindle cell component**

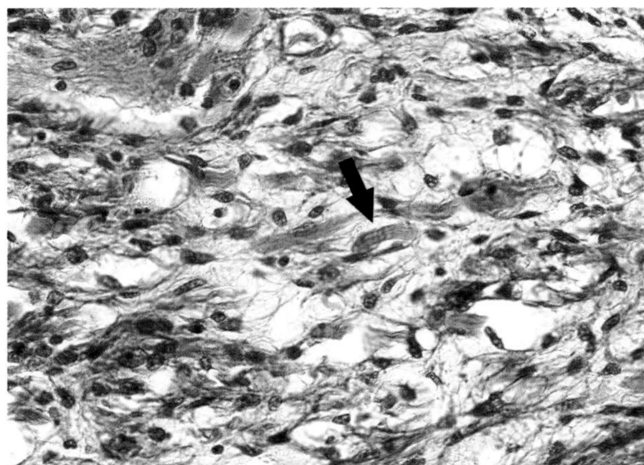

Fig. 17.5
Primary rhabdomyosarcoma of the ovary. **Distinctive cross-striations are seen (*arrow*)**

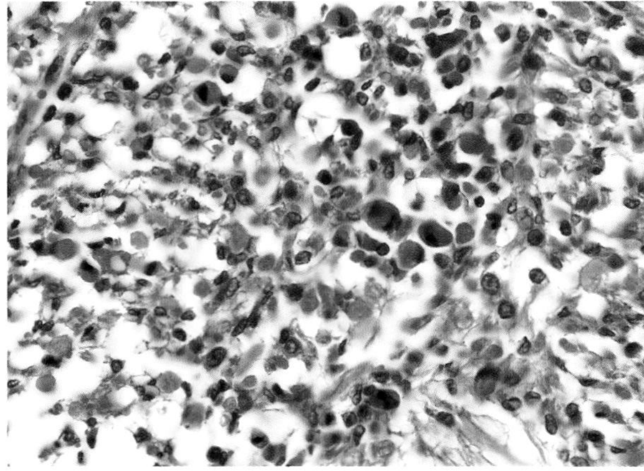

Fig. 17.6
Primary rhabdomyosarcoma of the ovary. **The tumor contains abundant rhabdomyoblasts, each of which have an ample amount of bright eosinophilic cytoplasm and eccentric nuclei**

pleomorphic type are observed in older women. The diagnosis of pleomorphic rhabdomyosarcoma should not present undue difficulty, because of the presence of at least some typical rhabdomyoblasts showing cross-striations. In cases of embryonal rhabdomyosarcoma, the diagnosis is much more difficult because the tumor cells are poorly differentiated, making rhabdomyoblastic differentiation discernible only with difficulty. Furthermore, it is necessary to recognize the distinctive alveolar or botryoid patterns, which also may not be easy.

The embryonal rhabdomyosarcoma is composed of small round primitive cells having a narrow rim of cytoplasm. They are poorly differentiated rhabdomyoblasts in various stages of differentiation. Therefore, the lesion is difficult to distinguish from poorly differentiated small cell carcinoma, lymphoma/leukemia, or even neuroblastoma [44, 48, 61]. Among the small round cells are scattered occasional rhabdomyoblasts, which are better-differentiated large cells with bright eosinophilic cytoplasm and eccentric nuclei (*Fig. 17.6*). Presence of these cells and their recognition may provide a diagnostic clue. Occasionally, large, more typical rhabdomyoblasts may be seen. The presence of cross-striations is not necessary for diagnosis, but the cells comprising the tumor may be well-enough differentiated to exhibit cross-striations (*Fig. 17.5*). Demonstration of Z bands or their precursors by electron microscopy is helpful in making the diagnosis. Immunohistochemical demonstration of myoglobin, desmin, muscle-specific actin, and myogenin are helpful in this respect (*Fig. 17.7*). The tumor is frequently affected by edema, hemorrhage, and necrosis, making the diagnosis even more difficult. Therefore,

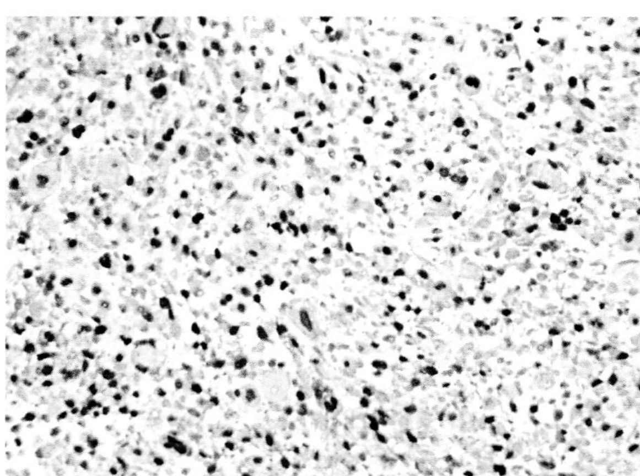

Fig. 17.7
Primary rhabdomyosarcoma of the ovary showing diffuse expression of myogenin.

thorough examination and sampling of the tumor are essential to make the correct diagnosis. The tumor may be more common than has been hitherto believed, but because of its poor differentiation, it may have been either assigned to the group of undifferentiated ovarian tumors or misdiagnosed. In some cases, the tumor infiltrated the bone marrow and was originally diagnosed as leukemia [48]. It is therefore emphasized that embryonal rhabdomyosarcoma must be considered in the differential diagnosis of undifferentiated small round cell tumor of the ovary in a young patient. The presence of other neoplastic elements always must be excluded when making this diagnosis.

The importance of making the correct diagnosis is not only academic but practical, in view of the advances that have been made in the therapy of embryonal rhabdomyosarcoma during the past few decades. In the past, the prognosis was poor, and in most reported cases, the patients died of extensive metastatic disease within 1 year of diagnosis. Recently, patients with embryonal rhabdomyosarcoma, some of whom had metastases, are well and disease-free after surgery, chemotherapy, and radiotherapy. The combination chemotherapy advocated for such patients consists of dactinomycin, vincristine, and cyclophosphamide. The addition of methotrexate with folinic acid rescue and doxorubicin to this combination also may be of value.

Myofibroblastoma

A well-documented case of an ovarian myofibroblastoma has been reported recently [54]. A 22-year-old woman who was involved in an automobile accident was found to have an enlarged right ovary but refused laparotomy. Over the next 3 years the mass gradually increased in size, and laparotomy was performed. A $9 \times 8.5 \times 6$ cm, right-sided ovarian tumor weighing 215 g and adherent to the right fallopian tube and omentum was found and excised. The tumor was solid, white-tan, and on sectioning revealed whorled areas and focal calcification. Microscopically, it was composed of uniform bland-looking spindle cells arranged haphazardly in fascicles separated by bands of hyalinized collagen. In some areas there was increased vascularity. There was no atypia or mitotic activity. The tumor cells showed vimentin, smooth muscle actin, and muscle-specific actin positivity. There was no immunoreactivity with desmin and cytokeratin. The patient was well and disease-free 21 months after treatment. Myofibroblastoma is a benign lesion, and complete excision results in cure.

Tumors of Vascular and Lymphatic Differentiation

Hemangioma

Hemangioma is found only occasionally in the ovary. Only a small number of well-documented cases have been reported. Although some cases may not have been recognized or recorded, all investigators consider ovarian hemangioma uncommon [33, 67]. This is somewhat surprising as the ovary has a very rich and complex vasculature.

The origin of ovarian hemangioma in common with hemangioma in general is a matter of controversy; it is considered either a hamartomatous malformation or a true neoplasm. It is likely that both modes of origin are responsible for their formation. The reported age of patients with ovarian hemangioma ranges from 4 months to 63 years [20, 33, 67], and does not show a predominance in any decade. In most patients, ovarian hemangioma has been noted as an incidental finding at operation or autopsy [67]. In a few cases, the lesion was large and the patient had abdominal enlargement because of the presence of an ovarian mass [19, 37, 38] or had acute abdominal pain associated with torsion of the tumor [37, 63]. In some cases, there was ascites [19, 38, 59]. The lesions usually are unilateral, although in four patients they were bilateral [67]. Ovarian hemangiomas have been noted in patients with generalized hemangiomatosis [33] and in patients with hemangiomas in other parts of the genital tract [33, 67]. One patient with bilateral ovarian hemangiomas and diffuse abdominopelvic hemangiomatosis had thrombocytopenia. The platelet count returned to normal after excision of the affected ovaries [33].

Macroscopically, the lesions are small, red or purple, round or oval nodules, measuring from a few millimeters to 1.5 cm in diameter. Larger lesions also have been encountered measuring up to 11.5 cm in the longest diameter [19, 37]. On cut section, they usually are spongy and show a honeycomb appearance. Although they have been found in different parts of the ovary, the medulla and the hilar region appear to be the most common sites [67].

Microscopically, ovarian hemangioma is of the cavernous or mixed capillary-cavernous type. It consists of collections of vascular spaces, which may vary in size but usually are small, lined by a single layer of endothelial cells, and usually contain red blood cells in their lumens (➲ *Fig. 17.8*). Occasionally, thrombosis may be seen. A small amount of connective tissue may be present within the lesion. In a few reported cases, the hemangioma was associated with the presence of luteinized cells in the stroma of the lesion. In one such case, there was evidence of hormonal function [59]. In a recent case, a patient with capillary hemangioma presenting as an adnexal mass had elevated serum CA-125 and massive ascites [19]. Excision of the affected adnexa resulted in a complete cure.

Hemangioma must be differentiated from proliferations of dilated blood vessels, frequently seen in the hilar region of the ovary. Although a very small hemangioma may not be easily distinguished from such vascular proliferations, the hemangioma usually forms a nodule or a small mass. The presence of a circumscribed nodule composed of vascular spaces tends to distinguish hemangioma from vascular proliferations, which usually are smaller and more diffuse. The presence of numerous blood cells within the vascular spaces and the absence of pale eosinophilic homogeneous material usually distinguish hemangioma from the less common lymphangioma. Hemangioma also must be distinguished from teratoma with a prominent vascular component. In such cases, careful sampling will detect other teratomatous elements, the presence of which distinguishes the lesion from a hemangioma.

The treatment of choice is oophorectomy, which results in a complete cure.

Angiosarcoma (Previously Referred to as Hemangiosarcoma, Hemangioendothelial Sarcoma, Hemangioendothelioma, and Lymphangiosarcoma in the Ovary)

Angiosarcoma is a very rare ovarian neoplasm [43, 47, 61]. Six unreported cases have been seen by the authors. In some reported cases, the angiosarcoma had arisen within a mature cystic teratoma or may have been associated with an immature teratoma. Such cases are considered as germ cell tumors and are excluded from consideration here. The age of the patients with angiosarcoma varied from 19 to 77 years. The tumor usually is unilateral, but bilateral tumors have been recorded. Bilaterality must be differentiated from metastatic spread to the contralateral ovary. The histogenesis of primary ovarian angiosarcoma is uncertain. It may originate from the vascular tissue present in the ovary, as a one-sided development of a teratoma, or from a teratoma in which the vascular component has overgrown the other parts of the tumor. Patients usually have symptoms related to the presence of a lower abdominal mass, which may be associated with torsion and rupture of the tumor and hemorrhage.

Macroscopically, the tumors usually are large, blue-brown, hemorrhagic, soft, and friable. They may be confined to the ovary, but often are associated with invasion of the surrounding structures.

Microscopically, they are composed of vascular spaces of varying size and appearance, lined by endothelial cells that usually are large, showing atypical appearance, bizarre nuclei, and mitotic activity (*Figs. 17.9* and *17.10*). In some areas, the tumor may contain a considerable amount of connective tissue interspersed between the vascular spaces. Fine papillary projections lined by atypical endothelial cells may be seen and are prominent. Some tumors are composed of small closely packed spaces lined by atypical cells with a suggestion of a solid pattern [47].

Angiosarcoma of the ovary must be distinguished from immature teratomatous neoplasms with a prominent

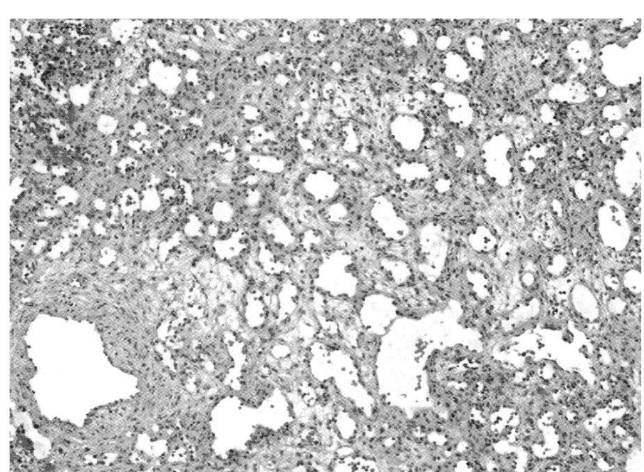

Fig. 17.8
Hemangioma of the ovary. **The tumor is composed of numerous small blood vessels, some of which contain red blood cells in their lumens**

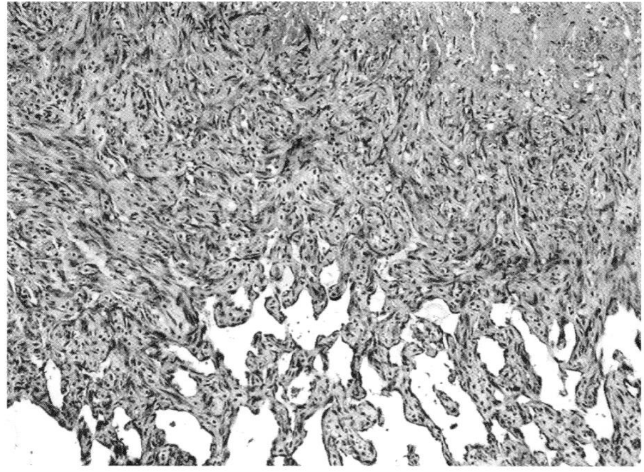

Fig. 17.9
Primary angiosarcoma of ovary. **The tumor contains closely packed vessels forming a solid spindle cell pattern (*top*). More typical vascular pattern is seen below**

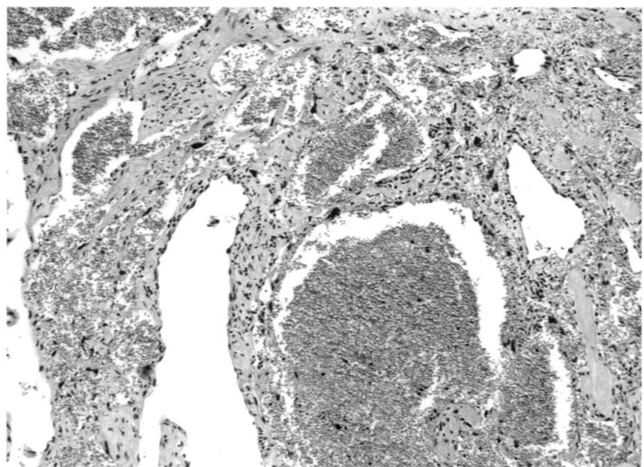

Fig. 17.10
Primary angiosarcoma of ovary. **The tumor is composed of dilated vascular spaces lined by enlarged hyperchromatic cells**

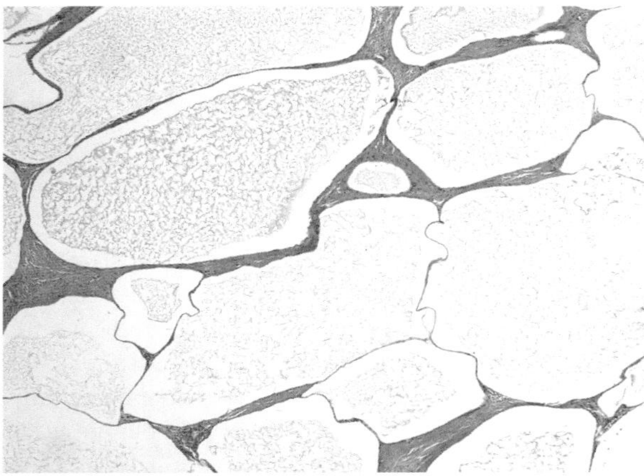

Fig. 17.11
Primary ovarian lymphangioma. **The tumor is composed of large and closely packed thin-walled lymphatic spaces lined by flattened endothelial cells and contains pale eosinophilic fluid**

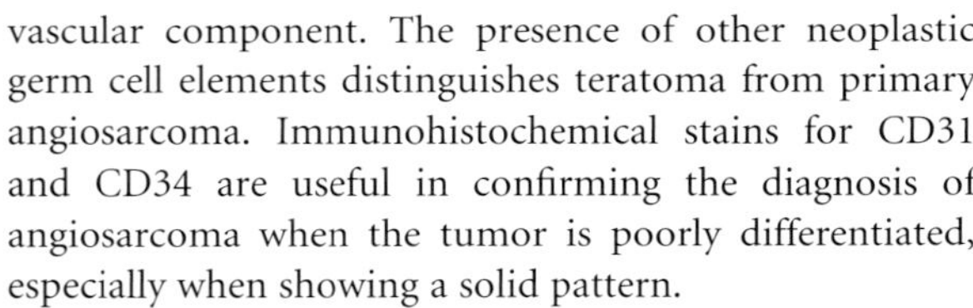

vascular component. The presence of other neoplastic germ cell elements distinguishes teratoma from primary angiosarcoma. Immunohistochemical stains for CD31 and CD34 are useful in confirming the diagnosis of angiosarcoma when the tumor is poorly differentiated, especially when showing a solid pattern.

The tumor invades locally and metastasizes via the bloodstream. Prognosis is poor, especially in patients who have metastases at the time of presentation. When the tumor is confined to the ovary, the prognosis is better and a few survivors have been reported. The tumor has not responded to combination chemotherapy regimens.

Lymphangioma

Lymphangioma of the ovary is very rare. We have seen two cases. In both cases, the tumor was small and was found incidentally. The tumor is usually unilateral but bilateral lesions have been reported. In the latter cases, it is possible that the lesions were malformations and neoplasms. Macroscopically, the tumor is small with a smooth, gray surface. On cut section, it is yellow, honeycombed, and composed of numerous small cystic spaces exuding clear yellow fluid.

Microscopically, lymphangioma of the ovary is composed of closely packed, thin-walled vascular spaces lined by flattened endothelial cells and containing pale, homogeneous eosinophilic fluid (*Fig. 17.11*). Lymphocytes may be seen within the vascular spaces. The histogenesis is a matter of controversy. Some investigators consider these lesions as malformations and some as neoplasms. Both modes of histogenesis are likely.

Lymphangioma is differentiated from a teratoma with a prominent vascular component by the absence of other germ cell elements. Lymphangioma also must be distinguished from hemangioma and an adenomatoid tumor that contains thin-walled, vessel-like spaces. In contrast to hemangioma, lymphangioma does not contain blood cells in the vascular spaces, and immunohistochemical expression of D2-40 is expected in the latter. The adenomatoid tumor has solid areas, and the cells lining the vessel-like spaces show immunohistochemical expression of cytokeratin and calretinin.

Tumors of Cartilage Differentiation

Chondroma

Only a few reports of ovarian chondroma are available, and documentation in most cases is unsatisfactory. One well-documented case considered to originate from the ovarian stroma has been reported [45]. The tumor, which measured 4 × 3 × 3 cm and was composed entirely of mature cartilage, was found incidentally. Although chondroma may originate from the connective tissue of the ovary by a process of metaplasia, it is more likely that most ovarian tumors described as chondroma were either fibromas showing cartilaginous metaplasia or teratomas having a prominent cartilaginous component.

Chondrosarcoma

A single example of pure chondrosarcoma of the ovary (*Figs. 17.12* and *17.13*) has been reported [68]. A 61-year-old woman had an abdominal mass that on extensive microscopic examination proved to be a pure, well-differentiated chondrosarcoma. The patient was well and disease-free 6 years after one-sided oophorectomy. The histogenesis of this tumor is uncertain, but the age of the patient and the histologic appearances of the tumor point to an origin in a dermoid cyst with malignant transformation and overgrowth by the malignant cartilaginous component [68]. A well-documented case of mature cystic teratoma (dermoid cyst) with malignant transformation of the cartilaginous element has been reported; the patient died of extensive metastatic disease [7]. In malignant ovarian tumors with cartilaginous differentiation, additional sampling is recommended in order to exclude an MMMT.

Tumors of Bone Differentiation

Osteoma

Few documented examples of osteoma occurring in the ovary exist. Although an origin from ovarian stroma is possible, most such lesions probably were examples of osseous metaplasia occurring in fibromas or leiomyomas, or possibly examples of metaplasia or heterotopia and not neoplasia occurring in the connective tissue of the ovary. Teratomatous origin is also possible. The lesions usually are small, but may be large, and are histologically composed of dense cortical bone.

Osteosarcoma

Few cases of pure osteosarcoma of the ovary have been reported [16, 23, 24, 74]. Patients range in age from 24 to 76 years. The tumor is frequently associated with extensive metastatic disease. Survival is poor. In one case metastatic tumor deposits affecting the abdominal cavity were excised at operation, and the patient was treated with triple chemotherapy consisting of cyclophosphamide, mitomycin C, and bleomycin [24]. The tumor recurred, and cisplatin and doxorubicin were added to the chemotherapeutic regimen. In spite of this, the tumor progressed and the patient died 8 months after diagnosis.

Histologically, the tumors show typical appearances of osteosarcoma occurring in the skeleton. Although it was believed that the tumors originated directly from ovarian stroma, their histogenesis is uncertain. Occasional cases of osteosarcoma originating in ovarian teratoma have been recorded [66], but such cases should not be confused with pure ovarian osteosarcoma or with cases of MMMT with a prominent osteosarcomatous component.

Tumors of Neural Differentiation

Ovarian tumors originating from neural tissue are rare. The presenting symptoms usually are related to the

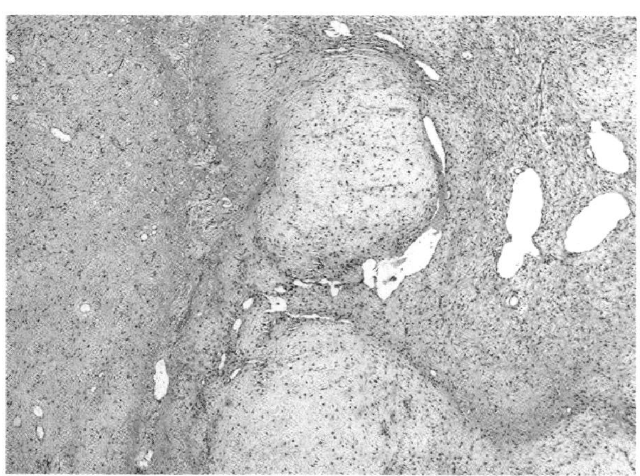

Fig. 17.12
Primary ovarian chondrosarcoma. **Low magnification**

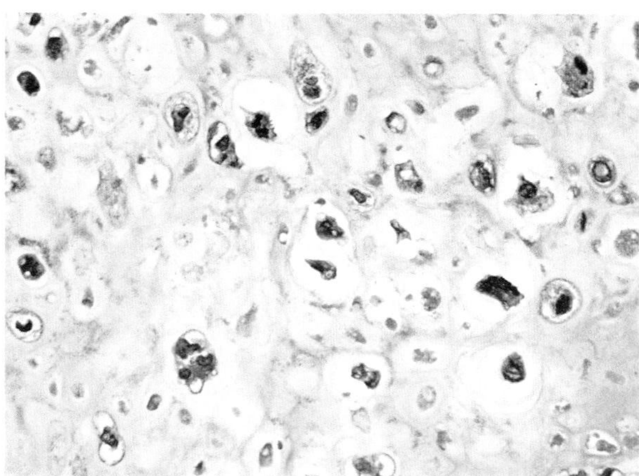

Fig. 17.13
Primary ovarian chondrosarcoma. **Marked nuclear atypia**

presence of an intraabdominal mass. The tumors are solid and usually are small. The histogenesis is uncertain and probably is similar to that of other mesenchymal tumors of the ovary.

Neurofibroma

Two cases of neurofibroma of the ovary have been reported in patients with generalized neurofibromatosis (von Recklinghausen's disease) [22, 64], one as an incidental finding [64]. Histologically, the tumors resembled neurofibroma occurring elsewhere.

Schwannoma (Neurilemmoma)

Three cases of ovarian schwannoma have been reported [40, 42]. In one case, the tumor was large [42]. The tumors were solid, and the patients were well and disease-free after the excision of the tumor. Histologically, the tumors resembled schwannoma occurring in other locations.

Malignant Peripheral Nerve Sheath Tumor

One case of "malignant neurilemmoma" (malignant schwannoma) of the ovary has been reported [65]. The affected patient, a 71-year-old nulliparous woman, was admitted for evaluation of lower abdominal enlargement and pain. There were no stigmata of generalized neurofibromatosis. At laparotomy, a 15 cm, firm, somewhat hemorrhagic tumor was found arising from the left ovary. There were numerous tumor deposits involving the peritoneal cavity. A debulking procedure was performed, and the ovarian tumor was excised together with the omentum. Histologic and ultrastructural examinations revealed that the tumor was a malignant neurilemmoma. After surgery, the patient was treated with combination chemotherapy consisting of doxorubicin and cyclophosphamide, but the disease progressed and she died 5 months after surgery of extensive intraabdominal metastatic disease [65]. One case of "neurofibrosarcoma" occurring in a 38-year-old woman with generalized neurofibromatosis (von Recklinghausen's disease) has been described [11]. The tumor was an incidental finding and had replaced the ovary. It was solid, and histologically showed the typical appearance of a neurofibrosarcoma with a moderate degree of nuclear pleomorphism and mitotic activity. There was no evidence of metastases, and the patient was well and disease-free 1 year after diagnosis [11]. A malignant epithelioid schwannoma of the ovary has been reported [32].

Paraganglioma/Pheochromocytoma

Paraganglioma of the ovary is rare. In a report of three cases, patients ranged in age from 22 to 68 years [39]. Two patients had hypertension. Some cases may have extra-ovarian spread of tumor. Tumors are characterized by the "zellballen" growth pattern seen in primary non-ovarian paragangliomas. With immunohistochemical stains, tumors are positive for neuroendocrine markers and negative for cytokeratin. Sustentacular cells can show expression of S-100. It should be noted that inhibin expression has been observed, which may create diagnostic confusion if a sex cord–stromal tumor is in the differential diagnosis.

A case of ovarian "pheochromocytoma" has been reported in a 15-year-old girl [18]. The patient had hypertension, convulsions, and a large, left-sided abdominal tumor mass. The tumor had undergone torsion and weighed 970 g. It was solid, and microscopic examination showed typical appearances of pheochromocytoma. Epinephrine and norepinephrine were extracted from tumor tissue. The symptoms disappeared after excision of the tumor, and the patient was well and disease-free 15 months after the operation [18]. Two additional cases were mentioned by Scully et al [61], but no further details were provided.

Ganglioneuroma

A single case of ovarian ganglioneuroma occurring in a 4-year-old girl has been reported [60]. The child had abdominal enlargement. The tumor was solid, weighing 200 g, and replaced nearly the whole ovary. Histologically, the tumor was composed of well-differentiated ganglion cells. There was a recurrence after the excision of the tumor. True ganglioneuroma must be differentiated from teratomas showing prominence of ganglion cells and from proliferations of ganglion cells occasionally seen in the hilar region of the ovary; the latter are nonneoplastic and probably hamartomatous in nature.

Tumors of Adipose Tissue Differentiation

Collections of adipose cells forming islands of fatty tissue that are not encapsulated are seen occasionally within ovarian tissue and are attributed to metaplasia of connective tissue of the ovary. These collections have been described as adipose prosoplasia. Benign adipose tissue seen in the ovary may be part of a teratoma with a prominent adipose tissue component. Pure benign fatty tumors in the ovary are very rare. A single case of a pure lipoma has been reported [81]. Malignant adipose tissue may be part of a MMMT with a prominent liposarcomatous component, or it may represent metastases from a liposarcoma occurring at another location. Well-characterized cases of pure malignant fatty tumors of the ovary have not been reported.

Tumors of Mesothelial Differentiation

Adenomatoid Tumor

The adenomatoid tumor, which in females is found most frequently in the fallopian tubes and broad ligament and occasionally in the uterus near the serosal surface, is found only rarely in the ovary (see Chap. 10, Mesenchymal Tumors of the Uterus and Chap. 11, Diseases of the Fallopian Tube and Paratubal Region). Although its histogenesis was long disputed, it is now considered to be of mesothelial origin, as is supported by morphologic, histochemical, immunohistochemical, and ultrastructural observations. Adenomatoid tumor is benign and, therefore, is considered a benign mesothelioma.

Few cases of ovarian adenomatoid tumor have been recorded, most of which occurred in patients in the third and fourth decades [61, 80]. The lesions, which are small, round or oval, and 0.5–3 cm in diameter, usually are found in the hilus of the ovary as incidental findings. In two cases the tumors were larger, measuring 6 and 8 cm in the longest diameter, respectively, and were symptomatic.

Histologically, the tumors show similar appearances to adenomatoid tumors occurring in other locations and are composed of clefts and spaces lined by cuboidal, low columnar, or flattened epithelial-like cells (*Fig. 17.14*) and of solid aggregates of similar cells surrounded by connective tissue that varies from loose and edematous to dense and hyalinized. The epithelial-like cells may exhibit marked vacuolation. An oxyphilic variant has been described [51]. They exhibit positive staining with alcian blue, which is digestible with hyaluronidase, and similarly staining material is present in the clefts and spaces. Occasionally, the cells may show weak PAS staining. The tumor cells show strong positive immunohistochemical staining for low molecular weight cytokeratin, WT-1, calretinin, and D2-40. ER, PR, and Ber-EP4 are

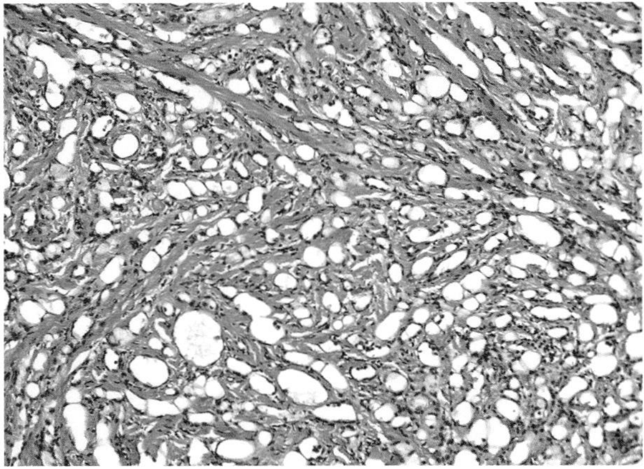

Fig. 17.14
Adenomatoid tumor. **The tumor has numerous clefts and small round spaces lined by a single layer of flattened cells**

negative. Ultrastructural observations support the mesothelial origin of this lesion and show an abundance of microvilli, bundles of cytoplasmic filaments, tight junctional complexes, and intercellular spaces. The lesion is benign, and its excision results in a complete cure.

Adenomatoid tumor may be confused with yolk sac tumor (YST) because the clefts and spaces may resemble the microcystic pattern of YST, but the nuclear appearances are totally different. The nuclei of adenomatoid tumor are bland and generally small and flattened, differing from the larger round and ovoid vesicular nuclei of YST, which exhibit brisk mitotic activity. The absence of other patterns associated with YST helps to distinguish adenomatoid tumor from YST. Confusion with lymphangioma may arise, and we have seen an adenomatoid tumor diagnosed as lymphangioma and vice versa. Immunohistochemical studies can be helpful in differentiating between these two entities. Lymphangioma is low molecular weight cytokeratin negative, whereas adenomatoid tumor is strongly positive. Vascular markers such as factor VIII, CD34, and CD31 show negative reactions with adenomatoid tumor and positive staining with lymphangioma. Calretinin and WT-1 are also expressed in adenomatoid tumor but negative in lymph-vascular tumors.

Peritoneal Malignant Mesothelioma

Occasionally, peritoneal mesothelioma may involve the surface of the ovary (see Chap. 13, Diseases of the

Peritoneum). When the tumor affects the ovary, confusion with primary ovarian neoplasms or benign conditions may occur [69]. The involvement of the ovary may be very extensive, and the presentation is that of a primary ovarian neoplasm. In one series of nine malignant peritoneal mesotheliomas presenting as ovarian masses, two tumors were considered as primary ovarian malignant mesotheliomas because the tumors were confined to the ovary [6, 61]. The histologic pattern, immunohistochemical and ultrastructural observations, and behavior and distribution of the lesion are helpful in making the correct diagnosis [2, 6, 50, 61, 69, 72]. Most patients with malignant peritoneal mesothelioma are middle-aged or elderly adults, and the tumor shows a considerable male predominance, and association with asbestos exposure. Very rarely, it may occur in children [69].

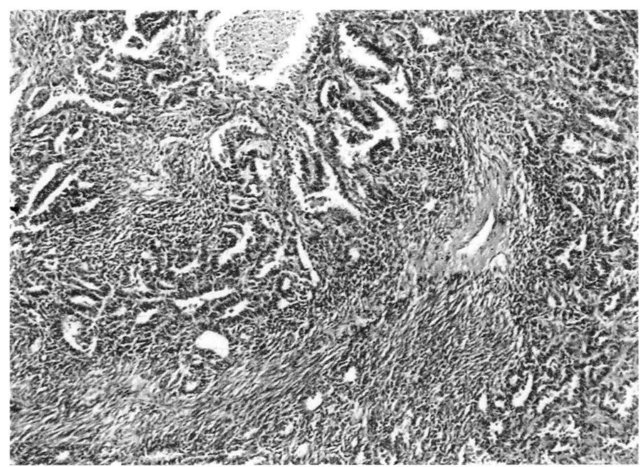

Fig. 17.15
Ovarian tumor of probable wolffian origin. **The tumor is composed of closely packed tubules and clefts with adjacent solid patterns containing spindle cells**

Ovarian Tumor of Probable Wolffian Origin (FATWO)

In the original report describing tumors of this type [31], all the tumors were located within the leaves of the broad ligament or were attached to it or to the fallopian tube; this also applied to subsequent reports dealing with this entity. Subsequently, a small number of ovarian tumors of probable wolffian origin were reported [9, 26, 77], indicating that tumors of this type also occur in the ovary. The age of most patients ranged from 28 to 79 years. Some patients had abdominal enlargement, and in other patients, the tumor was found on physical examination [26, 77]. All the tumors were unilateral. In most cases, they were confined to the ovary, but in one case metastatic deposits in the abdominal cavity were reported. In the latter case, the tumor contained foci of undifferentiated carcinoma [77]. Most tumors ranged in size from 2 to 20 cm in the largest diameter. They are smooth and often lobulated and are either solid or solid and cystic. The cysts vary in size and may range up to 11 cm [77].

Microscopically, the tumor is composed of relatively uniform epithelial cells that line cysts and tubules, sometimes forming a sieve-like pattern. The tumor cells also may form closely packed tubules, grow in a diffuse pattern, or fill tubules or tubular spaces (*Fig. 17.15*). They have uniform round or oval nuclei, and there is low mitotic activity. The tumor cells do not contain mucin but occasionally may contain glycogen. The amount of intervening connective tissue varies from imperceptible to considerable, forming fibrous bands separating the islands of tumor cells and producing a lobular pattern [77]. In two patients in whom the tumors were associated with aggressive behavior, there was brisk mitotic activity with 10 or more mitoses (MF)/10 high-power fields (HPF), and in one of the these patients, there was nuclear pleomorphism. Details of immunohistochemistry can be found in Chap. 11, Diseases of the Fallopian Tube and Paratubal Region.

Two patients have subsequently developed metastases [77]. Eight patients were known to be alive and disease-free from 1 to 15 years postoperatively, and one was lost to follow-up [77], indicating that in most cases the tumor is not associated with an aggressive course. It is also of note that there is a good correlation between the mitotic activity and the behavior of this neoplasm.

Ovarian tumor of probable wolffian origin may be confused with sex cord–stromal tumors, especially various types of Sertoli–Leydig cell tumors and surface epithelial–stromal tumors (see Chap. 15, Sex Cord-Stromal, Steroid Cell, and Other Ovarian Tumors with Endocrine, Paraendocrine, and Paraneoplastic Manifestations). The presence of the typical features of this tumor described here and the absence of the various patterns observed in Sertoli–Leydig cell tumors differentiate it from the latter. Female adnexal tumors of probable wolffian origin (FATWO) with a prominent spindle cell component may mimic cellular fibroma [35]. The tumor of probable wolffian origin is distinguished from the various surface epithelial–stromal tumors of the ovary by the absence of cellular and nuclear pleomorphism, papillary pattern, and intraluminal and intracellular mucin.

Lesions of the Rete Ovarii

Rete cysts/cystadenomas are uncommon, although probably more common than realized. The average age of patients with tumors of the rete ovarii is 59 years (range, 23–80 years). Patients can present with abdominal discomfort, pelvic pressure, virilization, postmenopausal bleeding, and/or hirsutism [56]. Most tumors are unilateral, and the average size is 9 cm. They may be uni- or multicystic, and the internal lining is usually smooth.

The rete lesions range in histologic type and include cyst, cystadenoma, adenoma, adenomatous hyperplasia, and adenocarcinoma [21, 46, 56]. Most are cysts/cystadenomas. Rete lesions are either found within the ovarian hilus or are anatomically related to the rete ovarii. The distinction between cyst and cystadenoma is arbitrary, but an upper limit of 1 cm for cysts has been proposed. The epithelial lining of the rete cyst/cystadenoma is simple, non-ciliated, and bland and characterized by irregular crevices. The periphery of rete adenoma is well circumscribed, and the tumor contains crowded tubules and papillae. The tubules and papillae have a simple layer of bland epithelial cells. Adenomatous hyperplasia is histologically similar to adenoma; however, the former is not well circumscribed.

Rete adenocarcinoma is rare. Only one well-documented case of adenocarcinoma of rete ovarii occurring in a 52-year-old woman with abdominal enlargement and ascites has been reported [56]. The patient had bilateral, partly solid and partly cystic tumors without specific macroscopic features. The tumor showed a predominant pattern of branching tubules and cysts containing simple papillae with fibrovascular or hyalinized cores. Some cysts contained eosinophilic material. Focally the tumor showed a solid tubular pattern. The cells lining the tubules and papillae were cuboidal, nonciliated, and atypical. Focally, they were multilayered and stratified. There was brisk mitotic activity. Adenocarcinoma of rete ovarii can only be diagnosed if the tumor has hilar location and is composed of collections of slit-like retiform tubules and cysts containing papillae lined by cells similar to those of normal rete ovarii [56, 61].

Rete cysts/cystadenomas are benign. The data on adenoma and adenocarcinoma is limited; thus, the behavior of these lesions is uncertain.

The most common lesion to histologically mimic rete cystadenoma is serous cystadenoma, but this is not a clinically important distinction. Rete cystadenoma is favored based on location in the hilus or anatomic connection with the rete ovarii, cyst lining with crevice-like contours, absence of ciliated cells, and smooth muscle and hilus cells within the cyst wall. Confusion may occur with retiform Sertoli–Leydig cell tumor, but the latter is likely to show other patterns of Sertoli–Leydig cell tumor and stain positively for inhibin. The role of immunohistochemistry in this setting is uncertain as immunohistochemical data on rete lesions is limited. Some serous carcinomas may also resemble adenocarcinoma of the rete ovarii, but they tend to be found in cortical location, generally do not show the fine slit-like papillae, and exhibit much greater nuclear pleomorphism.

Primary Ovarian Tumors of Uncertain Histogenesis

Hepatoid Carcinoma

In 1987, Ishikura and Scully [28] described five cases of ovarian carcinoma with hepatoid features, three of them primary and two probably primary. The age of the patients ranged from 42 to 78 years, and thus differed considerably from patients with YST with a hepatoid pattern, which is invariably seen in children, adolescents, and young women. The age range as well as the histologic appearances of the tumors showed considerable similarity to gastric carcinomas with hepatic features described some years earlier [27].

Unlike YST with a hepatoid pattern, which may be pure, mixed with other YST patterns, or combined with other germ cell tumors, hepatoid carcinoma of the ovary occurs in pure form, although occasionally it is associated with serous adenocarcinoma or other types of ovarian surface epithelial–stromal tumors [52, 61, 62, 71]. Hepatoid carcinoma of the ovary [28, 52, 71], like YST with hepatoid pattern and gastric adenocarcinoma with hepatoid features [27], is associated with alpha-fetoprotein (AFP) secretion, and AFP can be demonstrated within the tumor cells by immunohistochemical techniques. In three cases known to the authors, high levels of serum AFP were noted, and serum AFP was used to monitor the disease activity.

Clinically, patients present with symptoms and signs related to the presence of an adnexal mass. Abdominal enlargement, which may be associated with pain, malaise, and weight loss, is the main presenting sign [28].

Hepatoid carcinomas of the ovary are large and are associated with metastatic tumor deposits within the abdominal cavity (stage III) in most cases [28]. Histologically, the tumor shows a close resemblance to hepatocellular carcinoma (➊ *Fig. 17.16*), and is composed of solid sheets or aggregates of uniform cells with moderate or

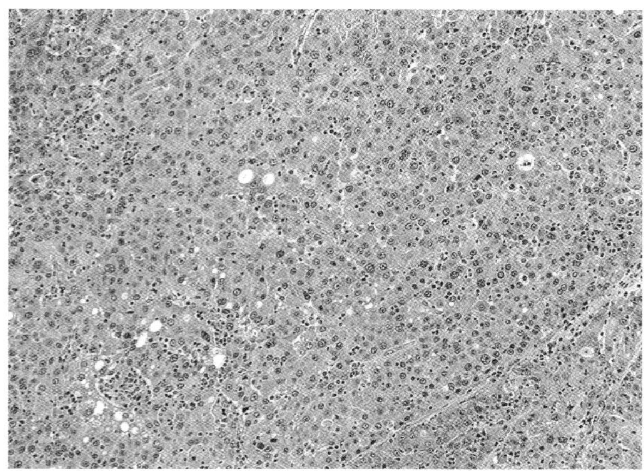

Fig. 17.16
Hepatoid carcinoma of the ovary. **Note the close resemblance to hepatocellular carcinoma**

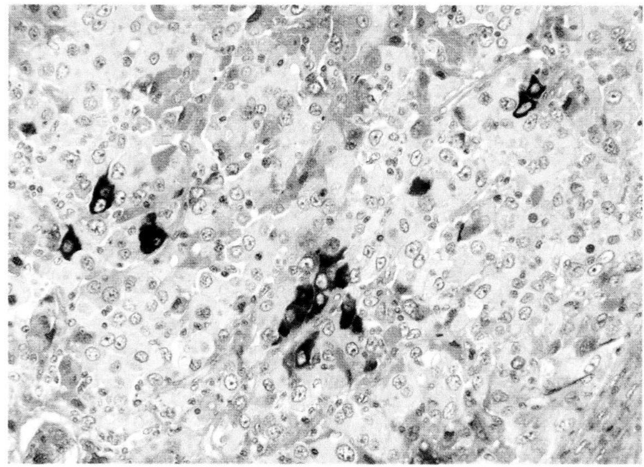

Fig. 17.17
Hepatoid carcinoma of the ovary showing expression of alpha-fetoprotein (AFP)

abundant eosinophilic cytoplasm, distinct cell borders, and centrally located nuclei with prominent nucleoli [28, 52, 71]. Mitotic activity generally is brisk, and abnormal forms are seen. In some parts of the tumor there may be a considerable degree of nuclear pleomorphism, and multinucleated giant cells may be seen [28]. PAS-positive diastase-resistant hyaline globules may be seen, and glycogen can be demonstrated within the cytoplasm of the tumor cells. Histologic patterns seen in germ cell tumors or surface epithelial–stromal tumors are not detectable when the tumor is seen in pure form [28, 61].

Immunohistochemical studies demonstrate the presence of AFP and hepatocyte paraffin 1 [52] in a considerable number of tumor cells (*Fig. 17.17*). In addition, the tumor cells are immunoreactive for albumin, alpha$_1$-antitrypsin, and alpha$_1$-antichymotrypsin. Focal positive immunostaining for carcinoembryonic antigen (CEA) also is seen [28].

Hepatoid carcinoma of the ovary is a highly malignant neoplasm [28, 61]. Most patients present with disseminated disease and die of the disease within a few years of diagnosis. One patient was well and disease free for 2 years after pelvic irradiation [28]. One patient was alive with evidence of disease 2 years after surgery and combination chemotherapy. She was treated with Taxol and for some time responded to treatment, as evidenced by some decrease in the highly elevated serum AFP level. She then relapsed and died of extensive disease.

The histogenesis of hepatoid carcinoma of the ovary has not been established. Unlike YST with hepatoid pattern, it is not of germ cell origin, as it occurs in older patients, is not associated with other neoplastic germ cell elements, and is not found in patients with gonadal dysgenesis. Because of the age distribution and the occasional association with ovarian surface epithelial–stromal tumors, it is likely that it is a metaplastic tumor and represents a variant of a surface epithelial–stromal tumor [28, 52, 61, 62, 71].

Hepatoid carcinoma of the ovary must be distinguished from YST with hepatoid pattern. It can be distinguished clinically by its occurrence in older, usually postmenopausal patients, and by its presentation in a more advanced clinical stage, usually in stage III. Histologically, hepatoid carcinoma shows a greater degree of cellular and nuclear pleomorphism, and tumor giant cells are much more frequently seen.

Demonstration of positive immunocytochemical staining for AFP in the tumor cells and elevated levels of serum AFP differentiate hepatoid carcinoma from other ovarian tumors such as undifferentiated adenocarcinomas, endometrioid adenocarcinomas with marked squamous differentiation, and steroid cell tumors [28]. Primary hepatoid carcinoma of the ovary also must be differentiated from hepatocellular carcinoma metastatic to the ovary [75]. Although the latter is uncommon, this possibility must be carefully excluded before the diagnosis of primary hepatoid carcinoma of the ovary is made.

Small Cell Carcinoma, Pulmonary Type

Eichhorn et al [15]. have reported 11 primary ovarian tumors that resembled small cell carcinoma of the lung and differed both clinically and histologically from primary small cell carcinoma of the ovary of hypercalcemic type [76]. The age of the patients ranged from 28 to 85 years [15]. Most patients presented with abdominal enlargement. Six of the tumors were unilateral, and five were bilateral. Spread beyond the ovary was noted in seven tumors. None of the patients had distant metastases at presentation [15]. The tumors measured from 4.5 to 26 cm in the greatest dimension; they were mostly solid with a variable minor cystic component [15].

Histologically, the tumor is composed of small to medium-sized round to spindle-shaped cells with scanty cytoplasm, hyperchromatic nuclei, and inconspicuous nucleoli forming sheets, large aggregates, and closely packed nests (➲ *Fig. 17.18*). Sometimes an insular or a trabecular pattern was seen [15]. In four tumors a component of endometrioid carcinoma was present, one tumor showed focal squamous differentiation, two tumors were associated with Brenner tumor, and one contained a cyst lined by atypical mucinous cells [15]. In two of six tumors, argyrophil granules were demonstrated. In nine cases, immunohistochemical studies were performed that demonstrated positive staining for cytokeratin in six cases, epithelial membrane antigen (EMA) in five, and chromogranin in two. All nine tumors were vimentin-negative. In a small number of cases evaluated, perinuclear dot-like staining for CK20 and variable TTF-1 expression have been observed [4, 55]. Flow cytometric studies performed on eight tumors showed that five tumors were aneuploid and three were diploid [15].

The tumors were aggressive, and of the nine patients with known follow-up, five died of the disease 1–13 months after diagnosis, one died after an unknown interval, and two had recurrent disease 6 and 8 months after surgery. Five of the patients with stage III tumors and two with stage I tumors were treated with combination chemotherapy, which included cisplatin in all cases and doxorubicin in most cases; one of these treated patients was alive at 7.5 years [15].

Aggressive treatment with agents effective in treating small cell pulmonary carcinoma appears to be the treatment of choice.

Primary ovarian small cell carcinoma with pulmonary differentiation must be distinguished from pulmonary small cell carcinoma metastatic to the ovary, which shows both clinical and pathologic differences [79]. It also must be differentiated from primary ovarian small cell carcinoma, usually associated with hypercalcemia [61, 76] (see ➲ Chap. 15, Sex Cord-Stromal, Steroid Cell, and Other Ovarian Tumors with Endocrine, Paraendocrine, and Paraneoplastic Manifestations). The patients with primary ovarian small cell carcinoma with pulmonary differentiation are older. The tumor is seen either in perimenopausal or postmenopausal women [15, 61]. Hypercalcemia is absent. The tumors are bilateral in 45% of cases, whereas in the hypercalcemic type, bilaterality is seen only rarely (1% of cases) [15].

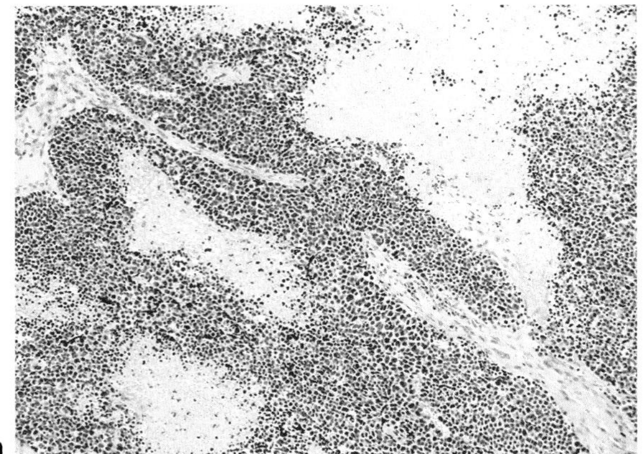

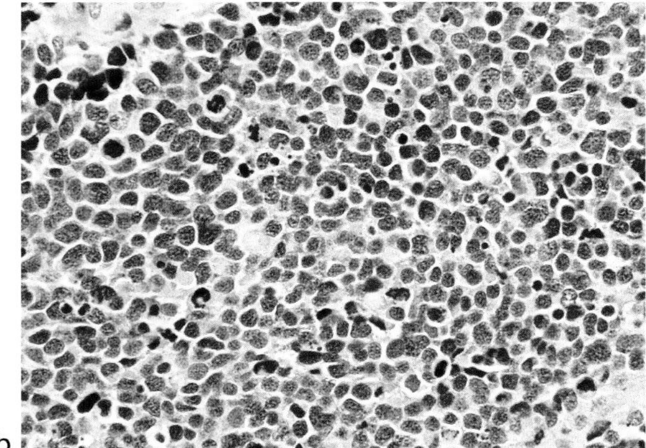

Fig. 17.18
Small cell carcinoma, pulmonary type. **(a) Solid growth pattern containing abundant geographic necrosis. (b) Small to medium-sized round cells with hyperchromatic nuclei, absence of nucleoli, scant cytoplasm, and numerous apoptotic bodies and mitotic figures (Case courtesy of Dr. Robert H. Young, Boston, MA)**

Histologically, the cells of primary ovarian small cell carcinoma with pulmonary differentiation differ from those of the hypercalcemic type in having finely dispersed chromatin and inconspicuous nucleoli, whereas the latter is composed of cells with nuclei showing clumped chromatin and prominent nucleoli, as well as showing the presence of larger cells with abundant eosinophilic cytoplasm in 40% of cases [15]. Follicle-like spaces are frequently seen in the hypercalcemic type and are virtually absent in the pulmonary type of small cell carcinoma [15]. Endometrioid and Brenner tumor components are present in more than half the small cell carcinomas with pulmonary differentiation and are absent in the hypercalcemic type. The former also tend to be more frequently aneuploid [15].

Although the histogenesis of the primary ovarian small cell carcinoma with pulmonary differentiation has not been established, the frequent association with endometrioid and Brenner tumors points toward a surface epithelial–stromal origin, as is supported further by the age range of the patients [15].

Neuroendocrine Carcinoma, Non-Small Cell Type

A small number of ovarian tumors composed of solid sheets, nests, cords, trabeculae, or solid islands of cells showing neuroendocrine differentiation have been reported [12, 61, 73]. These tumors were associated with either a surface epithelial-stromal or possibly germ cell component. The age of the patients ranged from 22 to 77 years. Some tumors were stage I, but in spite of this the prognosis was poor. Several cases presented with advanced stage disease, and the tumors demonstrated aggressive behavior, in common with neuroendocrine tumors occurring in other sites.

Histologically, the neuroendocrine component of the tumor consisted of solid islands or cords of medium to large epithelial cells with variable amount of cytoplasm and large nuclei, some of which had prominent nucleoli. Mitotic activity was variable but frequently high. The cellular islands and cords were surrounded only by a small amount of connective tissue. Immunohistochemical stains were frequently positive for pan-cytokeratin, CK7, CK20, chromogranin, and synaptophysin [73]. Other neurohormonal polypeptides were also detected in some of the tumors [12].

The neuroendocrine component of the tumor may resemble insular carcinoid tumor of the ovary, but the cells are usually larger and show much greater degree of cellular and nuclear pleomorphism. The presence of the surface epithelial–stromal component also helps to differentiate between these two entities. The distinction between them is very important because the prognosis of patients with neuroendocrine carcinoma is by far worse than that of patients with carcinoid tumors. The size of the tumor cells and the strong positive immunohistochemical reactions distinguish this tumor from the ovarian carcinoma of the small cell pulmonary type. The presence of the surface epithelial–stromal component confirming the ovarian origin differentiates this tumor from metastatic small cell tumors to the ovary [12].

Salivary Gland-like Carcinomas

Ovarian tumors resembling salivary gland carcinomas are rare, but a series of 12 tumors has been reported [14]. The tumors in six cases resembled adenoid cystic carcinoma. Most of the tumors also exhibited a minor component of surface epithelial–stromal neoplasia. The latter were of various histologic types and included serous, endometrioid, and clear cell carcinomas. The affected patients were elderly; nearly all were in the seventh or eighth decade. Most of the tumors were associated with extensive metastatic disease and the prognosis was poor, except for one case where the tumor was in pure form and another in which the associated surface epithelial–stromal component was of the serous borderline type. Histologically, the tumors showed architectural patterns seen in adenoid cystic carcinoma of the salivary glands (➲ *Fig. 17.19*). The tumor cells resemble myoepithelial cells, although this has not been confirmed immunohistochemically because in the majority of cases the cells did not stain positively for actin and S-100 protein [14, 61]. Histogenetically, these tumors are probably of surface epithelial–stromal origin because they are usually associated with a surface epithelial–stromal component or recurred as an adenoid cystic carcinoma in a patient for whom the original tumor was an endometrioid carcinoma.

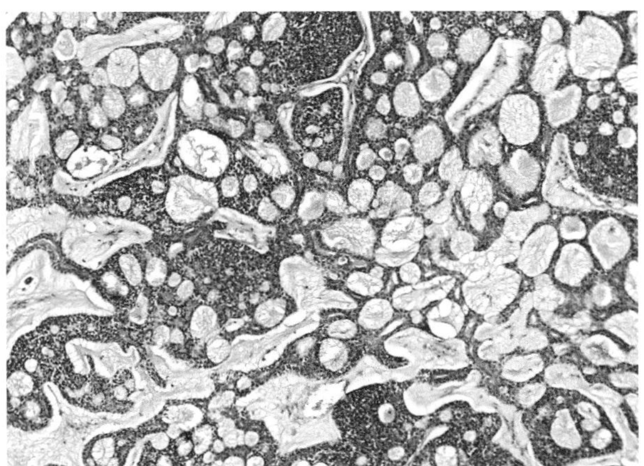

Fig. 17.19
Ovarian carcinoma resembling adenoid cystic carcinoma. (Case courtesy of Dr. Robert H. Young, Boston, MA)

The ovarian tumors in the remaining six cases from the study mentioned above showed basaloid or ameloblastomatous features [14, 61]. The age distribution was wide, ranging from 19 to 65 years. Most of the tumors were confined to the ovary (stage IA), and the prognosis was excellent after excision of the tumor although some of the follow-up periods were relatively short, varying from 16 to 71 months. Histologically, the tumors showed either a basaloid or ameloblastomatous pattern (➋ *Fig. 17.20*). Several of them showed focal squamous and glandular differentiation, and one showed a minor component of endometrioid adenocarcinoma [14, 61]. The histogenesis of this neoplasm is uncertain, but surface epithelial–stromal origin, particularly endometrioid carcinoma, appears to be most likely.

Nephroblastoma (Wilms' Tumor)

One case of ovarian nephroblastoma occurring in a 56-year-old woman has been reported [57]. The patient was treated by excision of the affected adnexa followed by radiotherapy and chemotherapy. She was well and disease-free 9 years after diagnosis. The tumor showed typical features of well-differentiated nephroblastoma with glomeruloid formations, small tubules, and prominent blastema. There were no other neoplastic elements [57]. A second case of a 3.5-year-old girl has also been reported. A left salpingo-oophorectomy was performed, and there was no evidence of metastasis [49].

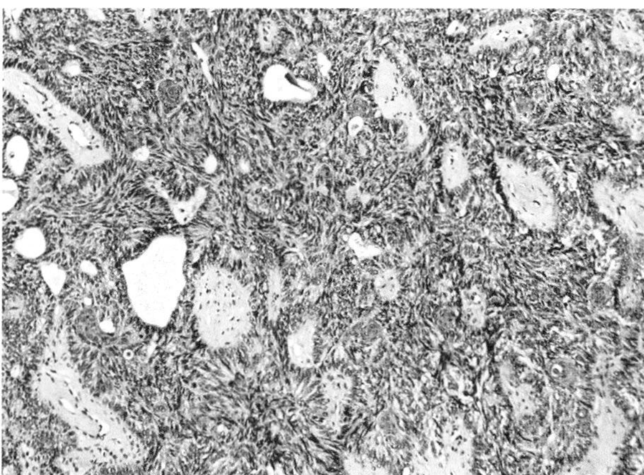

Fig. 17.20
Ovarian carcinoma with basaloid appearance. **Note peripheral palisading at interface between neoplastic epithelium and fibrovascular cores (Case courtesy of Dr. Robert H. Young, Boston, MA)**

Although the tumors were described as primary ovarian nephroblastomas, their histogenetic origin is uncertain. It is considered that one-sided development of a teratoma, or a teratoma overgrown by its nephroblastomatous component, is the likely origin of this tumor. Nephroblastomatous differentiation is seen in a number of ovarian teratomas and has not been seen in association with other ovarian neoplasms, providing support for this contention. Occasionally, retiform Sertoli–Leydig cell tumors, because of the presence of tubules and papillary pattern resembling glomeruloid formations, have been misdiagnosed as ovarian nephroblastomas. Careful sectioning and examination of the tumor for the presence of other patterns associated with Sertoli–Leydig cell tumors and absence of renal blastema are helpful in differentiating between these two entities. Demonstration of positive inhibin staining using immunohistochemistry further supports the diagnosis of Sertoli–Leydig cell tumor.

References

1. Balaton A, Vaury P, Imbert MC et al (1987) Primary leiomyosarcoma of the ovary. A histological and immunocytochemical study. Gynecol Oncol 28:116–120
2. Bollinger DJ, Wick MR, Dehner LP et al (1989) Peritoneal malignant mesothelioma versus serous papillary adenocarcinoma. A histochemical and immunohistochemical comparison. Am J Surg Pathol 13:659–670
3. Brady K, Page DV, Benn LE et al (1987) Ovarian myxoma. Am J Obstet Gynecol 156:1240–1242
4. Carlson JW, Nucci MR, Brodsky J et al (2007) Biomarker-assisted diagnosis of ovarian, cervical and pulmonary small cell carcinomas: the role of TTF-1, WT-1 and HPV analysis. Histopathology 51:305–312
5. Chan YF, Leung CS, Ma L (1989) Primary embryonal rhabdomyosarcoma of the ovary in a 4-year-old girl. Histopathology 15:309–311
6. Clement PB, Young RH, Scully RE (1996) Malignant mesotheliomas presenting as ovarian masses: a report of nine cases, including two primary ovarian mesotheliomas. Am J Surg Pathol 20:1067–1080
7. Climie AR, Heath LP (1968) Malignant degeneration of benign cystic teratoma of the ovary. Review of the literature and report of a chondrosarcoma and a carcinoid tumor. Cancer 22:824–832
8. Costa MJ, Morris R, DeRose PB et al (1993) Histologic and immunohistochemical evidence for considering ovarian myxoma as a variant of the thecoma-fibroma group of ovarian stromal tumors. Arch Pathol Lab Med 117:802–808
9. Devouassoux-Shisheboran M, Silver SA, Tavassoli FA (1999) Wolffian adnexal tumor, so-called female adnexal tumor of probable Wolffian origin (FATWO): immunohistochemical evidence in support of a Wolffian origin. Hum Pathol 30:856–863
10. Doss BJ, Wanek SM, Jacques SM et al (1999) Ovarian leiomyomas: clinicopathologic features in fifteen cases. Int J Gynecol Pathol 18:63–68

11. Dover H (1950) Neurofibrosarcoma of the ovary, associated with neurofibromatosis. Can Med Assoc J 63:488–490
12. Eichhorn JH, Lawrence WD, Young RH et al (1996) Ovarian neuroendocrine carcinomas of non-small cell type associated with surface epithelial adenocarcinomas. A study of five cases and review of the literature. Int J Gynecol Pathol 15:303–314
13. Eichhorn JH, Scully RE (1991) Ovarian myxoma. Clinicopathologic and immunocytologic analysis of five cases and a review of the literature. Int J Gynecol Pathol 10:156–169
14. Eichhorn JH, Scully RE (1995) "Adenoid cystic" and basaloid carcinomas of the ovary: evidence for a surface epithelial lineage. A report of 12 cases. Mod Pathol 8:731–740
15. Eichhorn JH, Young RH, Scully RE (1992) Primary ovarian small cell carcinoma of pulmonary type. A clinicopathologic, immunohistologic and flow cytometric analysis of 11 cases. Am J Surg Pathol 16:926–938
16. Fadare O, Bossuyt V, Martel M et al (2007) Primary osteosarcoma of the ovary: a case report and literature review. Int J Gynecol Pathol 26:21–25
17. Fadare O, Mariappan MR, Ocal IT et al (2003) A malignant ovarian tumor with osteoclast-like giant cells. Am J Surg Pathol 27:854–860
18. Fawcett FJ, Kimbell NKB (1971) Phaeochromocytoma of the ovary. J Obset Gynaecol Br Commonw 78:458–459
19. Gehrig PA, Fowler WC Jr, Liniger RA (2000) Ovarian capillary hemangioma presenting as adnexal mass with massive ascites and elevated CA-125. Gynecol Oncol 76:130–132
20. Gupta R, Singh S, Nigam S et al (2006) Benign vascular tumors of female genital tract. Int J Gynecol Cancer 16:1195–1200
21. Heatley MK (2000) Adenomatous hyperplasia of the rete ovarii. Histopathology 36:383–384
22. Hegg CA, Flint A (1990) Neurofibroma of the ovary. Gynecol Oncol 37:437–438
23. Hines JF, Compton DM, Stacy CC et al (1990) Pure primary osteosarcoma of the ovary presenting as an extensively calcified adnexal mass: a case report and review of the literature. Gynecol Oncol 39:259–263
24. Hirakawa T, Tsuneyoshi M, Enjoji M et al (1988) Ovarian sarcoma with histologic features of telangiectatic osteosarcoma of bone. Am J Surg Pathol 12:567–572
25. Huang TY, Chen JT, Ho WL (2005) Ovarian serous cystadenoma with mural nodules of genital rhabdomyoma. Hum Pathol 36:433–435
26. Hughesdon PE (1982) Ovarian tumors of wolffian or allied nature. Their place in ovarian oncology. J Clin Pathol 35:526–535
27. Ishikura H, Kirimoto K, Shamoto M et al (1986) Hepatoid adenocarcinomas of the stomach. An analysis of seven cases. Cancer 58:119–126
28. Ishikura H, Scully RE (1987) Hepatoid carcinoma of the ovary. A newly described tumor. Cancer 60:2775–2784
29. Kalstone CE, Jaffe RB, Abell MR (1969) Massive edema of the ovary simulating fibroma. Obstet Gynecol 34:564–571
30. Kandalaft PL, Esteban JM (1992) Bilateral massive ovarian leiomyomata in a young woman. A case report with review of the literature. Mod Pathol 5:586–589
31. Kariminejad MH, Scully RE (1973) Female adnexal tumor of probable wolffian origin. Cancer 31:671–677
32. László A, Ivaskevics K, Sápi Z (2006) Malignant epithelioid ovarian schwannoma: a case report. Int J Gynecol Cancer 16:360–362
33. Lawhead RA, Copeland LJ, Edwards CL (1985) Bilateral ovarian hemangiomas associated with diffuse abdominopelvic hemangiomatosis. Obstet Gynecol 65:597–599
34. Lerwill MF, Sung R, Oliva E et al (2004) Smooth muscle tumors of the ovary: a clinicopathologic study of 54 cases emphasizing prognostic criteria, histologic variants, and differential diagnosis. Am J Surg Pathol 28:1436–1451
35. Li F, Szallasi A, Young RH (2008) Wolffian tumor of the ovary with a prominent spindle cell component: report of a case with brief discussion of unusual problems in differential diagnosis, and literature review. Int J Surg Pathol 16:222–225
36. Lorentzen M (1980) Giant cell tumor of the ovary. Virchows Arch A Pathol Anat Histol 388:113–122
37. Mann LS, Metrick S (1961) Hemangioma of the ovary. Report of a case. J Int Coll Surg 36:500–502
38. McBurney RP, Trumbull M (1955) Hemangioma of the ovary with ascites. Miss Doct 32:271–274
39. McCluggage WG, Young RH (2006) Paraganglioma of the ovary: report of three cases of a rare ovarian neoplasm, including two exhibiting inhibin positivity. Am J Surg Pathol 30:600–605
40. Meyer R (1943) Nerve tumors of the female genitals and pelvis. Arch Pathol 36:437–464
41. Mira JL (1991) Lipoleiomyoma of the ovary. Report of a case and review of the English literature. Int J Gynecol Pathol 10:198–202
42. Mishura VI (1963) Report of large benign tumor – report of three cases. Vopr Onkol 9:103
43. Nielsen GP, Young RH, Prat J et al (1997) Primary angiosarcoma of the ovary. A report of seven cases and review of the literature. Int J Gynecol Pathol 16:378–382
44. Nielsen GP, Young RH, Rosenberg AE et al (1998) Primary ovarian rhabdomyosarcoma. A report of 13 cases. Int J Gynecol Pathol 17:113–119
45. Nogales FF (1982) Primary chondroma of the ovary. Histopathology 6:376
46. Nogales FF, Carvia RE, Donne C et al (1997) Adenomas of the rete ovarii. Hum Pathol 28:1428–1433
47. Nucci MR, Krausz T, Lifschitz-Mercer B et al (1998) Angiosarcoma of the ovary. Clinicopathologic and immunohistochemical analysis of 4 cases with a broad morphologic spectrum. Am J Surg Pathol 22:620–630
48. Nunez C, Abboud SL, Lemon NC et al (1983) Ovarian rhabdomyosarcoma presenting as leukemia. Case report. Cancer 52:297–300
49. Oner U, Tokar B, Açikalin MF et al (2002) Wilms' tumor of the ovary: a case report. J Pediatr Surg 37:127–129
50. Ordóñez NG (1998) Role of immunohistochemistry in distinguishing epithelial peritoneal mesotheliomas from peritoneal and ovarian serous carcinomas. Am J Surg Pathol 22:1203–1214
51. Phillips V, McCluggage WG, Young RH (2007) Oxyphilic adenomatoid tumor of the ovary: a case report with discussion of the differential diagnosis of ovarian tumors with vacuoles and related spaces. Int J Gynecol Pathol 26:16–20
52. Pitman MB, Triratanachat S, Young RH et al (2004) Hepatocyte paraffin 1 antibody does not distinguish primary ovarian tumors with hepatoid differentiation from metastatic hepatocellular carcinoma. Int J Gynecol Pathol 23:58–64
53. Prayson RA, Hart WR (1992) Primary smooth muscle tumors of the ovary. A clinicopathologic study of four leiomyomas and two mitotically active leiomyomas. Arch Pathol Lab Med 116:1068–1071
54. Rhoades CP, McMahon JT, Goldblum JR (1999) Myofibroblastoma of the ovary. Mod Pathol 12:907–911
55. Rund CR, Fischer EG (2006) Perinuclear dot-like cytokeratin 20 staining in small cell neuroendocrine carcinoma of the ovary (pulmonary-type). Appl Immunohistochem Mol Mophol 14:244–248

56. Rutgers JL, Scully RE (1988) Cysts (cystadenomas) and tumors of the rete ovarii. Int J Gynecol Pathol 7:330–342
57. Sahin A, Benda JA (1988) Primary ovarian Wilms' tumor. Cancer 61:1460–1463
58. Sandison AT (1955) Rhabdomyosarcoma of the ovary. J Pathol Bacteriol 70:433–438
59. Savargaonkar PR, Wells S, Graham I et al (1994) Ovarian hemangiomas and stromal luteinization. Histopathology 25:185–188
60. Schmeisser HC, Anderson WAD (1938) Ganglioneuroma of the ovary. J Am Med Assoc 111:2005–2007
61. Scully RE, Young RH, Clement PB (1998) Tumors of the ovary, maldeveloped gonads, Fallopian tube, and broad ligament, vol 23, 3rd ser. Armed Forces Institute of Pathology, Washington, DC
62. Scurry JP, Brown RW, Jobling T (1996) Combined ovarian serous papillary and hepatoid carcinoma. Gynecol Oncol 63:138–142
63. Shaeffer MD, Cancelmo JJ (1939) Cavernous hemangioma of the ovary in a girl twelve years of age. Am J Obstet Gynecol 38:722–723
64. Smith FR (1931) Neurofibroma of the ovary associated with Recklinghausen's disease. Am J Cancer 15:859–862
65. Stone GC, Bell DA, Fuller A et al (1986) Malignant schwannoma of the ovary. Report of a case. Cancer 58:1575–1582
66. Stowe LM, Watt JY (1952) Osteogenic sarcoma of the ovary. Am J Obstet Gynecol 64:422–426
67. Talerman A (1967) Hemangiomas of the ovary and the uterine cervix. Obstet Gynecol 30:108–113
68. Talerman A, Auerbach WM, Van Meurs AJ (1981) Primary chondrosarcoma of the ovary. Histopathology 5:319–324
69. Talerman A, Montero JR, Chilcote RR et al (1985) Diffuse malignant peritoneal mesothelioma in a 13-year-old girl. Am J Surg Pathol 9:73–80
70. Tiltman AJ, Haffajee Z (1999) Sclerosing stromal tumors, thecomas, and fibromas of the ovary: an immunohistochemical profile. Int J Gynecol Pathol 18:254–258
71. Tochigi N, Kishimoto T, Supriatna Y et al (2003) Hepatoid carcinoma of the ovary: a report of three cases admixed with a common surface epithelial carcinoma. Int J Gynecol Pathol 22:266–271
72. Vang R, Ronnett BM (2009) Metastatic and miscellaneous primary tumors of the ovary. In: Nucci MR, Oliva E (eds) Gynecologic pathology. Elsevier, Philadelphia, pp 539–613
73. Veras E, Deavers MT, Silva EG et al (2007) Ovarian nonsmall cell neuroendocrine carcinoma: a clinicopathologic and immunohistochemical study of 11 cases. Am J Surg Pathol 31:774–782
74. Yeasmin S, Nakayama K, Ishibashi M et al (2009) Primary osteosarcoma of ovary. Int J Clin Oncol 14:163–166
75. Young RH, Gersell DJ, Clement PB et al (1992) Hepatocellular carcinoma metastatic to the ovary: a report of three cases discovered during life with discussion of the differential diagnosis of hepatoid tumors of the ovary. Hum Pathol 23:574–580
76. Young RH, Oliva E, Scully RE (1994) Small cell carcinoma of the ovary, hypercalcemic type. A clinicopathologic analysis of 150 cases. Am J Surg Pathol 18:1102–1116
77. Young RH, Scully RE (1983) Ovarian tumors of probable wolffian origin. A report of 11 cases. Am J Surg Pathol 7:125–135
78. Young RH, Scully RE (1984) Fibromatosis and massive edema of the ovary, possibly related entities. A report of 14 cases of fibromatosis and 11 cases of massive edema. Int J Gynecol Pathol 3:153–178
79. Young RH, Scully RE (1985) Ovarian metastases from cancer of the lung. Problems in interpretation. A report of seven cases. Gynecol Oncol 21:337–350
80. Young RH, Silva EG, Scully RE (1991) Ovarian and juxtaovarian adenomatoid tumors: a report of six cases. Int J Gynecol Pathol 10:364–371
81. Zwiesler D, Lewis SR, Choo YC et al (2008) A case report of an ovarian lipoma. South Med J 101:205–207

18 Metastatic Tumors of the Ovary

Melinda F. Lerwill · Robert H. Young

R. J. Kurman, L. Hedrick Ellenson, B. M. Ronnett (eds.), *Blaustein's Pathology of the Female Genital Tract (6th ed.)*, DOI 10.1007/978-1-4419-0489-8_18,

Tumors that spread to the ovary from elsewhere are an important group of ovarian neoplasms because the misinterpretation of cases encountered as surgical pathology specimens may have significant adverse consequences for the patient. The spread may be from adjacent sites by direct local extension or from distant extragenital sites [27, 44, 61, 66, 90, 94, 111, 145, 152, 155, 161, 162]. The latter tumors are truly metastatic, whereas the designation "metastatic" is sometimes not used for those that are secondary from local sites. However, for simplicity, this discussion includes spread to the ovary from all sites.

We first review general principles of clinical, gross, and microscopic evaluation that aid the pathologist in arriving at the correct diagnosis of a metastatic tumor, also highlighting some general pitfalls that are encountered. The subsequent discussion is site- or organ-specific, with the exception that a few tumors that may originate at more than one site (Krukenberg tumors, carcinoids, or gastrointestinal stromal tumors) are considered under those headings. We divide our consideration into three basic categories: (1) spread from extragenital sites (the most significant practical issue), (2) spread from other sites in the genital tract, and (3) involvement by peritoneal tumors. Hematopoietic tumors are covered in a separate chapter.

General Principles

Confident recognition of the metastatic nature of an ovarian tumor depends on several factors: (1) an awareness of the frequency with which metastases occur and simulate a variety of primary tumors; (2) a thorough clinical history, which in some cases may require the pathologist to prompt the clinician to explore it in greater detail than first done; (3) when indicated, a thorough clinical and operative search by the surgeon for a primary tumor outside the ovary; (4) a careful evaluation of the gross and routine microscopic features of the ovarian tumor by the pathologist, including in some cases reinspection of the gross specimen and submission of additional sections; and (5) judicious use of conventional special stains and immunohistochemistry.

The diagnosis of a metastatic tumor is often missed by the pathologist because the existence of a concurrent or prior tumor in another organ is either not known or disregarded. The surgical and pathologic findings from previous operations should be reviewed if there is any possibility that they could be related to the ovarian tumor being evaluated. In some cases a search for an extraovarian primary tumor must be conducted postoperatively, based on the pathologist's suspicion that the ovarian tumor is metastatic. Even if an extraovarian primary tumor is not detected, a diagnosis of a metastasis to the ovary must be strongly considered if the distribution of disease is atypical for primary ovarian cancer or if pathologic examination is highly suggestive of metastasis. For example, the presence of pulmonary or hepatic metastases in the absence of extensive peritoneal disease would be an unusual pattern of spread for an ovarian cancer, but not for certain other tumors that are prone to metastasize to the ovary. The mere presence of tumor outside the ovaries should lead to the serious consideration of a metastasis in certain situations. For example, if a well-differentiated ovarian mucinous tumor is associated with extensive mucinous adenocarcinoma in the omentum and on the peritoneal surfaces, the possibility of spread to the ovary, particularly from the pancreas or biliary tract, should be entertained. Additionally, certain tumors, such as Sertoli cell tumors or primary carcinoid tumors, which are most often benign, should be diagnosed with caution in cases in which there is also extraovarian tumor. In cases of these types, the putative Sertoli cell tumor may prove to be a metastatic tumor that is mimicking it, such as tubular Krukenberg tumor [14], and the carcinoid tumor probably is metastatic rather than primary in the ovary. It also must be emphasized that an association of an ovarian tumor with clinical or pathologic evidence of excess estrogens, androgens, or progesterone does not exclude the diagnosis of a metastatic tumor, which may have a functioning stroma [128] (see ➋ Chap. 15, Sex Cord-Stromal, Steroid Cell, and Other Ovarian Tumors with Endocrine, Paraendocrine, and Paraneoplastic Manifestations).

For a variety of reasons, it is difficult to establish accurately the frequency of metastatic tumors among all ovarian tumors from the available literature. Some studies have been based on autopsy findings, others on surgical specimens, and still others on both. In addition, some series have included clinically silent metastases such as breast carcinoma found in prophylactic or therapeutic oophorectomy specimens and small metastases detected incidentally during operations for gastric or intestinal carcinoma. In contrast, other series have been restricted to metastatic tumors that presented clinically as pelvic or abdominal masses. Finally, some investigations have included as metastases ovarian carcinomas associated with uterine cancers of similar histologic type, but in many cases the ovarian tumors likely represent independent primary tumors [143, 184].

The frequency of metastases to the ovary also varies from one country to another because of wide differences in the prevalence of the various cancers that are associated with high rates of ovarian spread. For example, metastatic carcinoma accounts for approximately 40% of ovarian cancers in Japan where gastric carcinoma is common, but is far less common in Africa where this form of cancer is relatively rare. The frequency of metastases also has varied greatly in series in which differences in the prevalence of the primary tumors do not adequately explain the discrepant results. Such variations may be related, in part, to the frequency and thoroughness of microscopic examination of the ovaries, because gross inspection may not reveal evidence of involvement in one third to one half the cases. The figure for the frequency of ovarian metastases that is most meaningful is one that expresses the probability that an ovarian neoplasm found on exploration of a pelvic or abdominal mass is metastatic; this figure is on the order of 5–10%.

The age distribution of patients with ovarian metastases depends to a great extent on that of the corresponding primary tumors, but for each of the most common types (intestinal, gastric, and breast) the average age of patients with ovarian involvement is significantly lower than that of those without ovarian spread, suggesting that the richly vascularized ovaries of young women are more receptive to metastases than those of older patients.

Tumors spread to the ovary by several routes. Spread from distant sites is mainly via blood vessels and lymphatics. The frequent association of ovarian metastases with other blood-borne metastases, the common finding of tumor within ovarian blood vessels on microscopic examination in cases of metastasis, and the higher frequency of ovarian metastases in young patients support the important role of hematogenous spread.

Transcoelomic dissemination with surface implantation is an important route by which intraabdominal cancers spread to the ovary, as is supported by the common association of ovarian involvement with generalized peritoneal spread. The pathologist often encounters foci of metastatic carcinoma on the surface of the ovary or superficially located within the cortex, supporting implantation as the mechanism. It is possible that ovulation, by creating a defect in the ovarian surface, provides a portal of entry for cancer cells floating in the peritoneal cavity in premenopausal patients.

Direct spread is an important pathway for carcinomas of the fallopian tube and uterus, for mesotheliomas, and for occasional colonic carcinomas and retroperitoneal sarcomas. Another mechanism of spread of genital tract carcinomas is through the lumen of the fallopian tube and onto the surface of the ovary; this route is taken most often by carcinomas of the uterine corpus [23], but may also account for some cases of spread from the uterine cervix [113, 124].

The gross features of tumors metastatic to the ovary vary greatly and may resemble those of a variety of primary ovarian tumors [119]. Because of the relatively high frequency with which metastases are bilateral (two-thirds to three-quarters of the cases), the possibility of metastasis should especially be considered when evaluating bilateral tumors (*Fig. 18.1*) other than serous and undifferentiated carcinomas, which also are commonly bilateral. Endometrioid and mucinous carcinomas, in contrast, are bilateral in less than 15% of cases, and bilateral tumors with endometrioid-like or mucinous features merit more serious consideration for possibly being metastatic [181]. Still, many metastatic tumors are unilateral and, if the microscopic features of a tumor suggest metastasis, unilaterality should not be considered a significant argument against it. In general, almost 10% of bilateral ovarian cancers presenting as adnexal masses prove to be metastatic on careful evaluation. It has recently been suggested that a simple assessment of size and laterality can distinguish primary from metastatic mucinous neoplasms: bilateral tumors of any size or unilateral tumors under 10 cm have a strong likelihood of being metastatic, compared to unilateral tumors over 10 cm, which are usually primary [130].This is an appropriate general guideline and may be helpful, particularly in the intraoperative setting; however, there are unfortunately many exceptions [67, 134], especially in cases of colorectal and endocervical primaries [157]. It is also of note that metastatic tumors involving

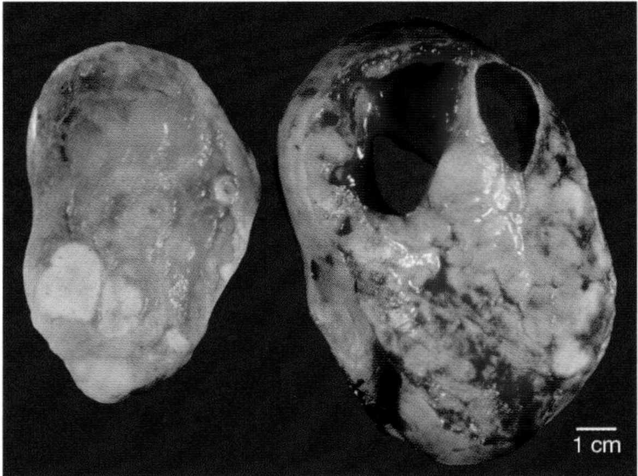

Fig. 18.1
Metastatic appendiceal adenocarcinoma. **The tumor is bilateral, and the smaller ovary shows several discrete nodules, mainly in the lower half. In the other ovary, the nodules have become confluent, but ill-defined nodularity is still evident**

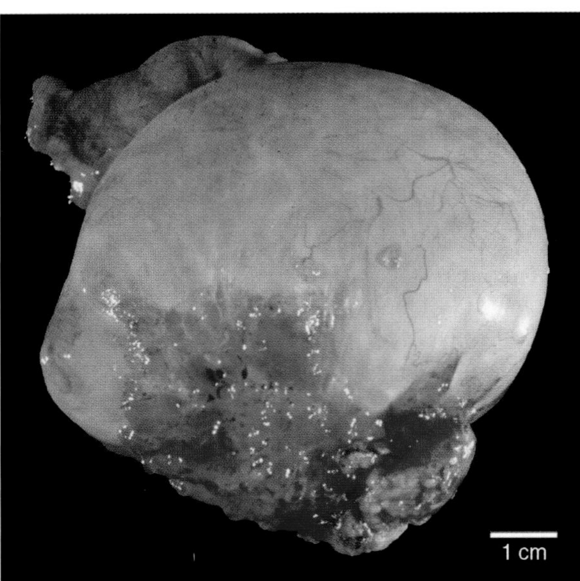

Fig. 18.2
Metastatic cecal adenocarcinoma. **Foci of mucoid tumor are seen on the ovarian surface**

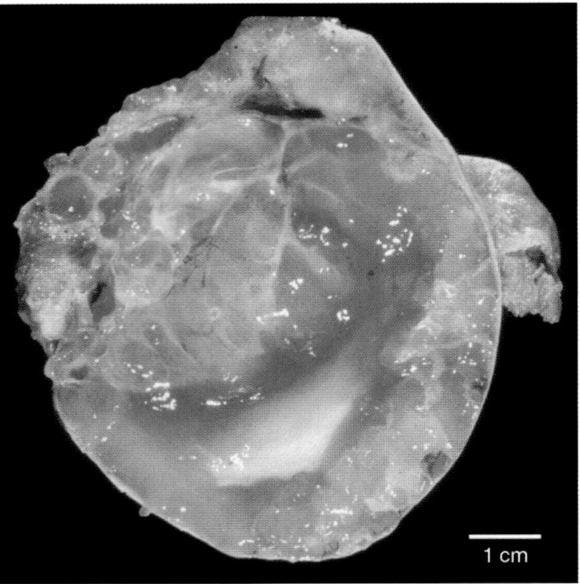

Fig. 18.3
Metastatic cecal adenocarcinoma. **Sectioned surface of tumor in prior figure showing a mainly cystic neoplasm grossly consistent with a primary neoplasm**

the ovary are often large and may dwarf their primary tumors.

Two other gross findings that are suggestive, but not pathognomonic, of metastasis are the presence of multiple tumor nodules (*Fig. 18.1*) and tumor on the surface of the ovary (*Fig. 18.2*), sometimes without significant involvement of the underlying parenchyma. As examples of the only suggestive nature of these findings, we note the well-known surface location of some serous carcinomas and in other cases, the multinodularity of some serous and undifferentiated carcinomas. The microscopic features of these carcinomas generally are not problematic, however. It should also be noted that some endometrioid carcinomas arise from foci of endometriosis in the superficial cortex or on the ovarian surface, and accordingly may project off the ovary. An association with endometriosis, which is easily overlooked, can be crucial in supporting an ovarian origin for such a tumor. A gross feature of some metastastic tumors that should not be regarded as establishing the primary nature of the tumor is the presence of cysts (*Fig. 18.3*). These are often large and occasionally thin-walled, and they can occur even when there is an absence of cysts in the primary neoplasm.

The microscopic appearance of a metastatic tumor obviously varies with the appearance of the primary neoplasm. In addition to the specific features of various primary tumors, the microscopic correlates of the findings

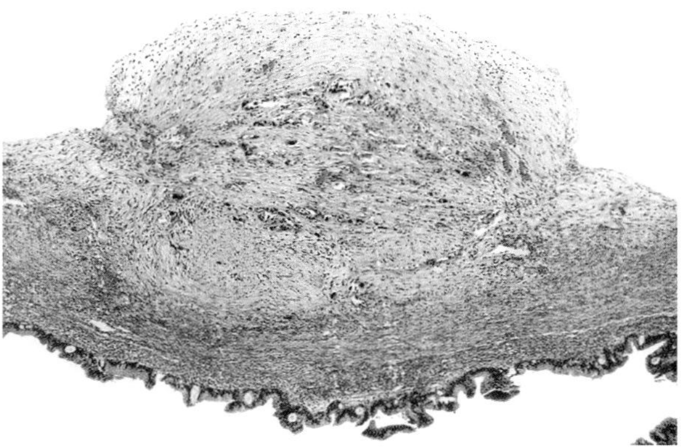

Fig. 18.4
Metastatic pancreatic adenocarcinoma. **Typical surface implant in the form of a nodular protrusion composed of infiltrating small glands and prominent stroma. Note maturation of the underlying cystic component (Reproduced with permission from Ref. [161])**

noted in the prior paragraph, namely implants on the surface of the ovary (*Fig. 18.4*) and multinodularity (*Fig. 18.5*), suggest metastasis in many cases, but with the same caveats as above. These findings have particular weight in cases with mucinous or endometrioid-like morphologies, as well as in those with any of a diverse number of unusual microscopic appearances. Surface implants typically are focal, often projecting above the surface of the adjacent cortex, and the tumor is frequently embedded in desmoplastic or sometimes hyalinized fibrous tissue (➋ *Fig. 18.4*). A conspicuous stromal reaction of the type just noted is also often seen in more central regions of metastatic tumors (➋ *Fig. 18.6*) and, particularly if multifocal, is on average much more common in metastatic tumors than in primary neoplasia. Metastatic tumors more often envelop preexisting normal ovarian structures than primary tumors (➋ *Fig. 18.7*).

Another feature more typical of metastasis is what has been referred to as heterogeneous or nodular invasive growth (➋ *Fig. 18.6*). This terminology is intended to reflect the varied appearance that results when scattered foci of obviously invasive growth, often in a desmoplastic stroma, are present within a background neoplasm that has a more leisurely growth and sometimes even deceptively benign features. Infiltrating moderate- to high-grade cancer with destructive invasion in a primary mucinous tumor may have a similar appearance, but it is generally not as multifocal nor as striking as in many cases of metastasis. Although certainly not diagnostic on its

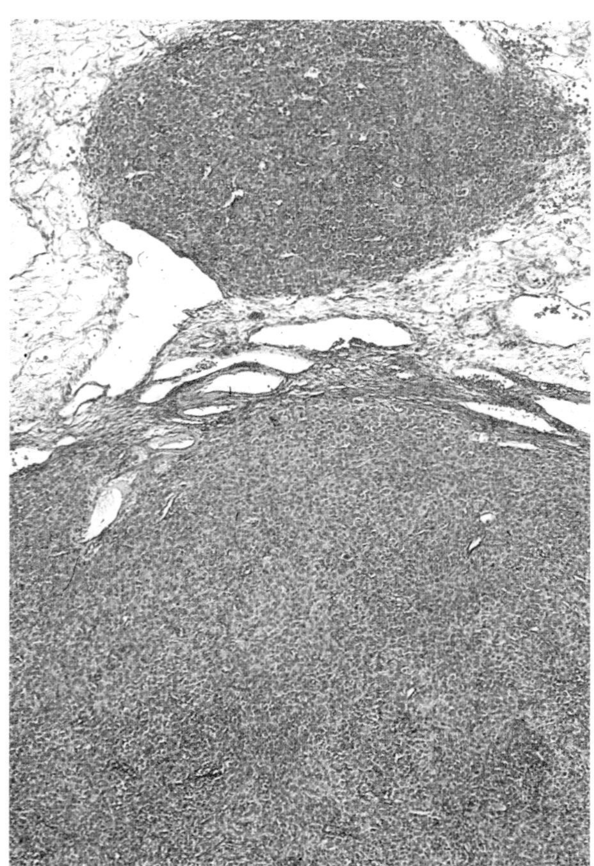

Fig. 18.5
Metastatic malignant melanoma. **Two discrete nodules of tumor are seen**

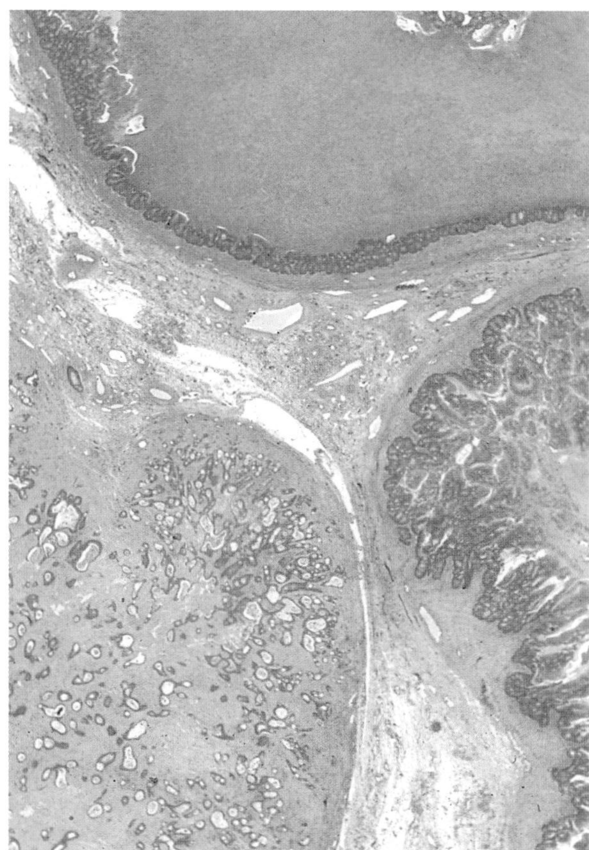

Fig. 18.6
Heterogeneous nodular growth. **Three separate distinct patterns of growth are evident in this case of metastatic colon cancer: a dilated gland at the *top*, conventional adenocarcinoma at the *right*, and small gland adenocarcinoma in a prominent desmoplastic stroma at the *bottom left* (Courtesy of Dr. Kenneth R. Lee; Reproduced with permission from Ref. [161])**

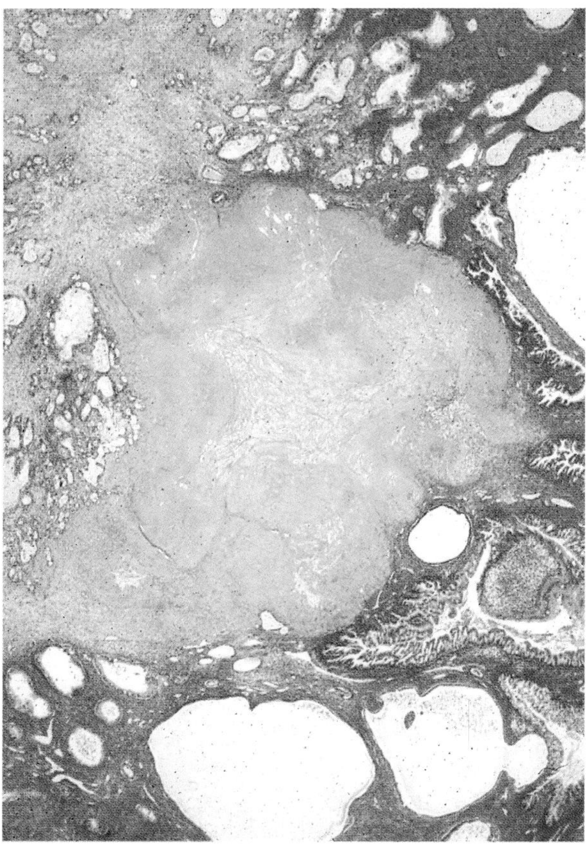

■ Fig. 18.7
Metastatic colon carcinoma surrounding a corpus albicans

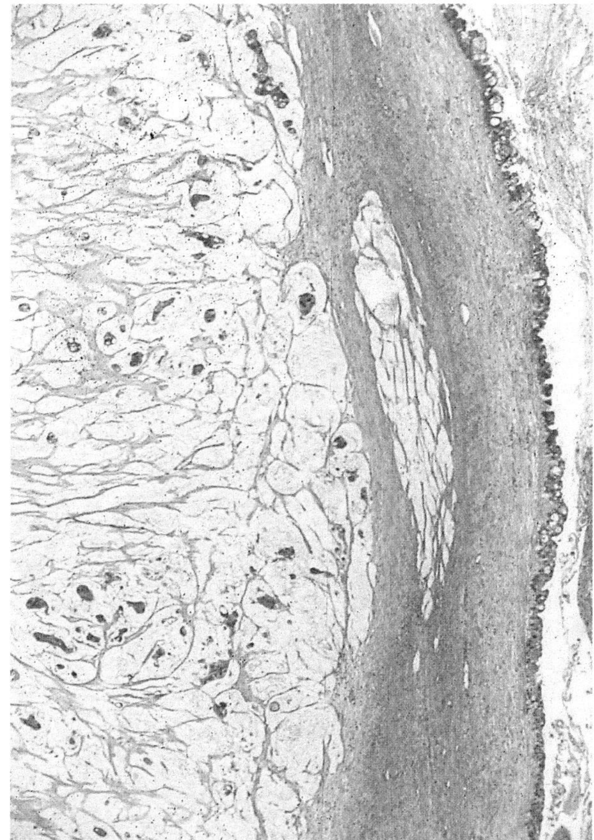

■ Fig. 18.8
Metastatic colloid adenocarcinoma. **This pattern of mucinous carcinoma is uncommonly primary in the ovary and accordingly such a picture should cause concern for a metastasis (Reproduced with permission from Ref. [161])**

own, this pattern should cause metastasis to be entertained and should be evaluated in context. A similar comment pertains to all features overall more typical of metastasis. The mere nature of the neoplasia may be important. For example, primary mucinous carcinomas of the ovary only rarely have a colloid morphology, whereas this is a well-known pattern of colonic carcinoma; when this morphology is seen in the ovary (➋ *Fig. 18.8*), metastasis should enter consideration and certainly be excluded before the tumor is accepted as a primary neoplasm.

The epithelium of most metastatic carcinomas in the ovary is clearly malignant, but a treacherous aspect is the propensity of some tumors, particularly those that are mucinous, to differentiate and result in a borderline-like or even cystadenoma-like appearance. This so-called maturation phenomenon [182] may even result in flattened epithelium that appears benign, and if separated by bland stroma, an adenofibroma or cystadenofibroma may be mimicked (➋ *Fig. 18.9*). Another confusing microscopic feature of some metastatic tumors is the presence of cysts, some of which simulate follicles. These follicle-like spaces (➋ *Fig. 18.10*) may be encountered in a variety of metastatic tumors including gastric and intestinal carcinomas, carcinoids, small cell carcinomas from various sites, and malignant melanomas. A wide variety of other patterns and cell types in metastatic tumors suggest diverse possible primary sites, as discussed in detail and presented in tabular form elsewhere [182]. Lymphatic or blood vessel invasion, sometimes particularly striking in the hilus, strongly suggests metastasis (➋ *Fig. 18.11*).

Immunohistochemistry, selectively applied based on a differential diagnosis generated by routine microscopic features, may aid in certain cases [7, 21, 91, 93, 94], but is uncommonly diagnostic on its own. Even after the most thorough evaluation, it is sometimes impossible for the pathologist to be definitive whether a neoplasm is primary or metastatic, but on the basis of the morphology one may

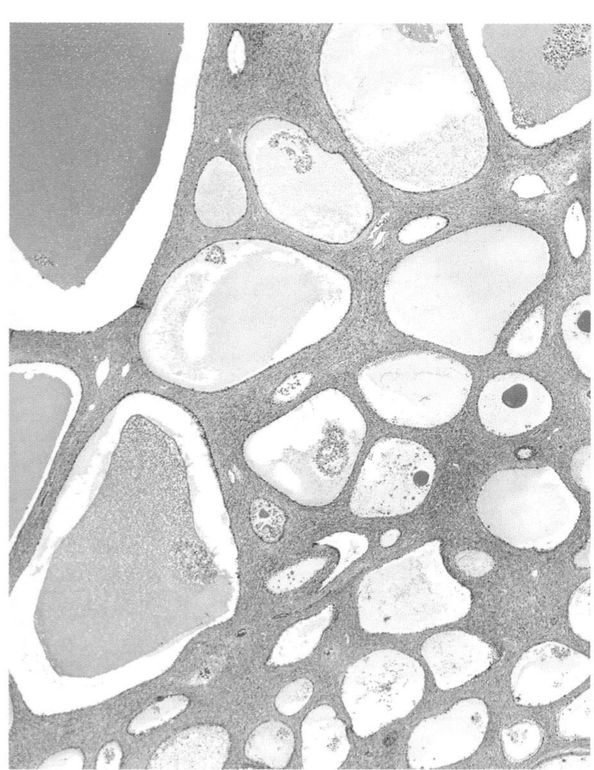

Fig. 18.9
Metastatic cholangiocarcinoma. **The epithelium has undergone marked maturation. The presence of a background cellular stroma results in mimickry of a cystadenofibroma**

suggest the most likely possible extra-ovarian primary sites to direct clinical evaluation. *Table 18.1* presents a comparison of various features of primary and metastatic mucinous tumors in the ovary, but is also broadly applicable, in great part, to the overall topic being considered here.

Extragenital Tumors

In this category, we begin with tumors of the gastrointestinal tract (except sarcomas, considered later) and associated structures, which cause in aggregate the majority of diagnostic problems. We first discuss the Krukenberg tumor, arguably one of the most well-known cancers involving the ovary [14, 28, 42, 49, 55, 71, 161].

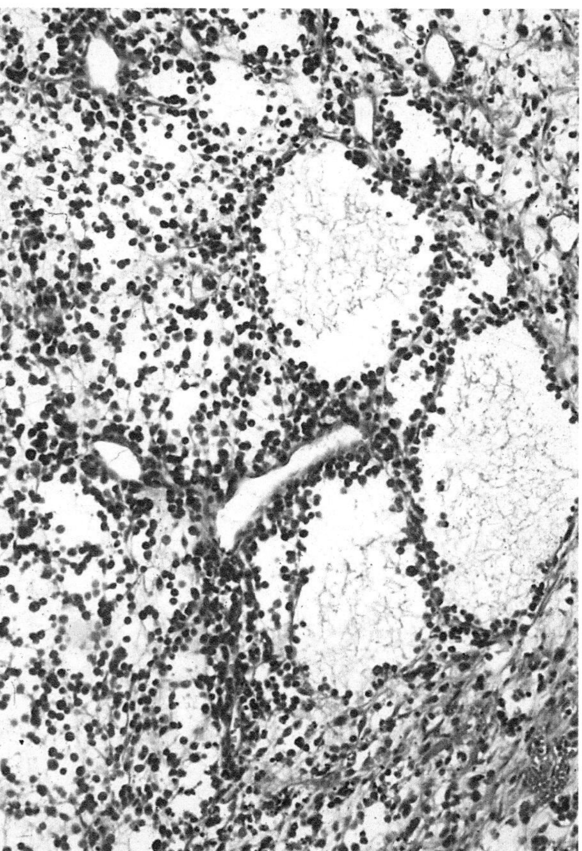

Fig. 18.10
Metastatic malignant melanoma. **Follicle-like spaces are clearly evident (Reproduced with permission from Ref. [161])**

Carcinoma of the Stomach

Metastatic Tumors with Signet Ring Cells (Krukenberg Tumor)

The great majority of metastatic gastric carcinomas to the ovary are Krukenberg tumors, which are defined by us as metastatic tumors characterized by the presence of mucin-filled signet-ring cells accounting for at least 10% of the tumor. The source of Krukenberg tumors in the great majority of reported cases is a gastric carcinoma, usually arising in the pylorus. Carcinomas of the large intestine, appendix, and breast are the next most common primary sites; the gallbladder, biliary tract, pancreas, cervix, and urinary bladder are rare sources of these tumors. Saphir [126] demonstrated in an autopsy study that signet-ring cell carcinomas of various organs are associated more

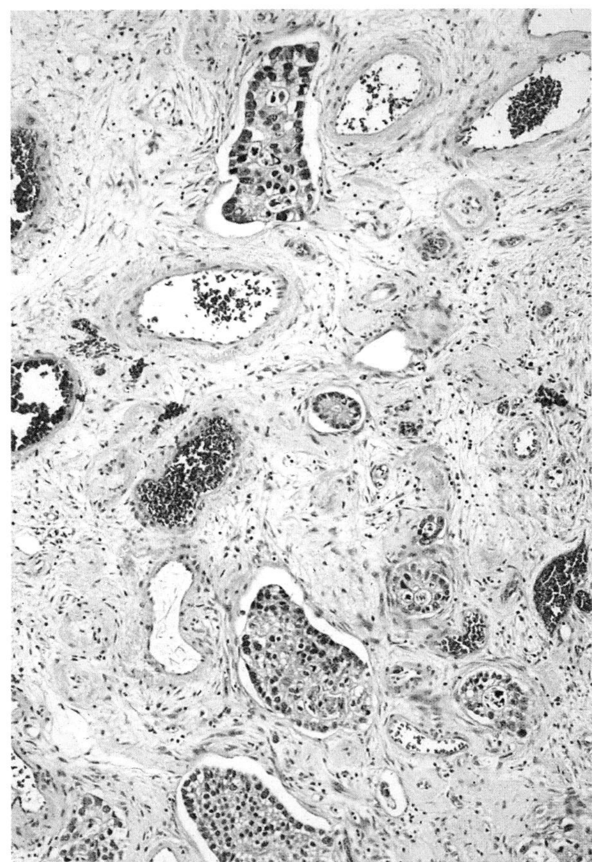

Fig. 18.11
Metastatic carcinoma. **Prominent lymphatic involvement (Reproduced with permission from Ref. [161])**

often with ovarian metastasis than carcinomas of other histologic types by a ratio of about 4:1. More recent studies have supported his observation: gastric signet-ring cell carcinomas metastasize to the ovary much more often than intestinal-type carcinomas of the stomach do [81], and signet-ring cell carcinomas of the colon also metastasize to the ovaries more frequently than conventional colonic adenocarcinomas [5].

The frequency of the Krukenberg tumor varies with that of gastric carcinoma in the population analyzed. In countries such as Japan, with a high prevalence of gastric carcinoma and a low prevalence of primary ovarian carcinoma, the Krukenberg tumor accounts for a large proportion of all ovarian cancers [156].

The average age of patients with Krukenberg tumors is about 45 years. One quarter to almost one half the patients are under 40 years, and only slightly more than 10% of them are over 60 years of age. This age distribution is related in part to the disproportionate frequency of gastric signet-ring cell carcinomas in young women as well as the greater vascularity of the ovary in young women. In one study, 10% of women 35 years or younger with this tumor had ovarian metastases at presentation [142].

Almost 90% of patients with Krukenberg tumors have symptoms related to ovarian involvement, the most common of which are abdominal pain and swelling; occasionally, there is abnormal uterine bleeding and rarely, particularly during pregnancy, overt signs of excess hormone production such as virilization. The remainder of the patients have gastrointestinal or miscellaneous

Table 18.1
Comparison of helpful clinicopathologic features in distinguishing metastatic from primary mucinous cystic tumors

Feature	Metastatic	Primary
History of, or clinical evidence of, extraovarian primary	Usual[a]	Rare[b]
Extraovarian disease	Common	Rare
Bilaterality	Common	Rare
Size >15 cm	Uncommon	Common
Gross tumor on surface of ovary	Occasional	Rare
Microscopic surface implants or surface mucin	Common	Rare
Heterogeneous nodular invasive growth	Common	Rare
Colloid pattern	Occasional	Rare
Mucin granulomas	Uncommon	Common
Vascular invasion	Occasional	Rare
Single cell growth	Occasional	Uncommon
Müllerian nature of epithelium	Rare	Occasional
Association with teratoma, endometriosis, adenofibroma, Brenner tumor[c]	Rare	Occasional
So-called mural nodules	Absent	Occasional

[a] In some cases the primary tumor may initially be occult and require clinical evaluation to detect.
[b] The possibility that a patient may have independent primary tumors always exists, particularly as primary mucinous tumors of the ovary and certain tumors that may mimic them when they spread to the ovary are common.
[c] As the four listed lesions are common, by happenstance they might be present in an ovary involved by metastasis. Also, it should be noted that maturation in some metastatic tumors may impart a focal adenofibroma-like appearance.
Modified from Lee and Young [78].

symptoms related to spread of the signet-ring cell cancer to other sites such as lungs or bone, or are asymptomatic. A history of prior carcinoma of the stomach or, less often, another organ can be obtained in 20–30% of the cases. The interval between the diagnosis of a gastric carcinoma and the subsequent discovery of ovarian involvement usually is 6 months or less, but periods as long as 12 years have been reported [42]. In most cases, the diagnosis of the gastric carcinoma is made preoperatively, during the operation for the ovarian metastasis, or within a few months thereafter. Not infrequently, the primary tumor is too small to be detected at operation, and radiographic examination of the upper gastrointestinal tract also may fail to reveal evidence of a tumor even after the diagnosis of Krukenberg tumor has been established. Rarely, the gastric carcinoma may not be detected until 5 or more years after discovery of the ovarian metastatic tumor. Primary carcinomas, particularly those arising in the breast and stomach, may be very small, requiring exhaustive sectioning to detect them, despite the presence of metastases in some cases. It is possible that tiny primary tumors were missed in these or other organs in the reported autopsied cases of "primary" Krukenberg tumors. Ulbright and Roth [144] cited a case observed by Kraus in which a primary tumor in the stomach was detected only after microscopic sections prepared from 200 blocks had been examined.

Almost all the patients die within a year of the diagnosis of ovarian metastasis, but a rare patient has survived, apparently free of tumor, for as long as 6 years after gastrectomy and bilateral oophorectomy [49]. Such a result, even though exceptional, justifies removal of both the stomach and the ovarian metastases for possible cure in cases in which the tumor appears limited to those organs. It also is prudent for the surgeon to remove the ovaries routinely in menopausal and postmenopausal women who have a gastric resection for carcinoma so as to prevent the later complication of ovarian metastasis and avoid another operation.

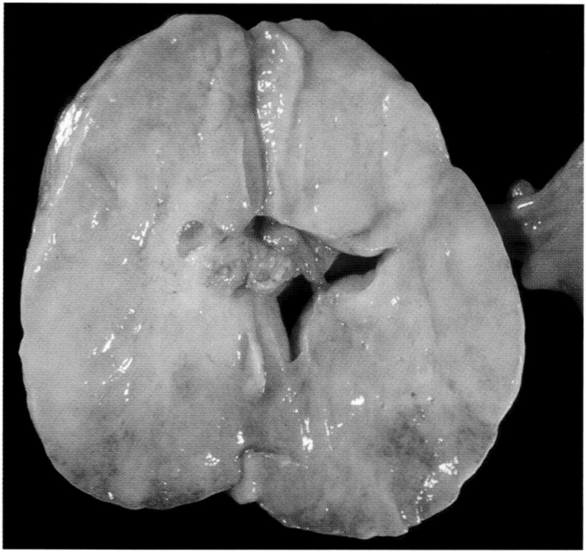

Fig. 18.12
Krukenberg tumor. **The sectioned surface is more or less uniform and tan**

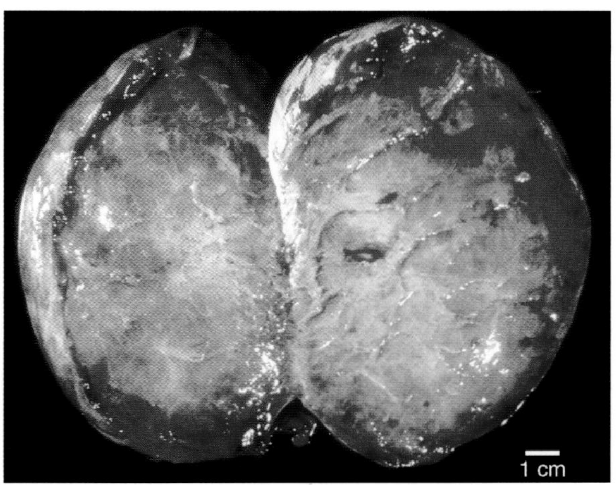

Fig. 18.13
Krukenberg tumor. **The central region in this case differed in appearance from the periphery, a feature occasionally seen**

Gross Findings

Krukenberg tumors typically form rounded or reniform, firm, white masses that may be bosselated and may attain a large size. The surfaces are generally devoid of appreciable adhesions. The sectioned surfaces usually are tan or white (*Fig. 18.12*), but areas of purple, red, or brown discoloration and extensive hemorrhage also are encountered. The appearance may be relatively uniform or, in other cases, ill-defined nodularity or even discrete nodules may be seen. The consistency is characteristically firm, but fleshy, gelatinous, or spongy areas are common. Sometimes the periphery is distinctly different in appearance from the central region, the latter often being softer than the periphery (*Fig. 18.13*). Occasionally, the gross presentation is atypical with large, thin-walled cysts containing mucinous or watery fluid, separated by relatively small amounts of solid tissue. Both ovaries are involved in 80% or more of the cases.

Microscopic Findings

The histologic appearance of these tumors is much more varied than the most emphasized morphology in the literature, namely that of signet-ring cells in a cellular stroma (➋ *Fig. 18.14*). This picture, which is of historical interest because it resulted in the initial confusion with fibrosarcoma, is present in only a minority of cases as a finding of any prominence. We first consider the low-power features of the Krukenberg tumor and then aspects related to signet-ring cells (and other cell types), other epithelial elements, and stroma in turn.

Like many metastatic tumors, growth as distinct nodules, or at least as vague nodules, is typically conspicuous on low-power examination (➋ *Fig. 18.15*), but the nodules and intervening stroma may be quite variable in appearance, particularly when the other features noted below are present (➋ *Figs. 18.16–18.32*). The tumor nodules are often separated by edematous stroma, and a picture of densely cellular pseudolobules is often seen (➋ *Fig. 18.16*). The nodules themselves are generally composed of jumbled admixtures of signet-ring cells, indifferent cells, glands, cysts, and background stroma. Similar admixtures of epithelial and stromal elements are seen in tumors that have a more diffuse arrangement. Sometimes a striking low-power feature is a greater cellularity at the periphery, with aggregates of tumor cells, stroma, or both ramifying from the periphery into central, more edematous regions (➋ *Fig. 18.17*). Residual ovarian structures may be present in the midst of the tumor (➋ *Fig. 18.18*).

The signet-ring cells vary greatly in amount and, accordingly, prominence. Occasionally vast numbers are

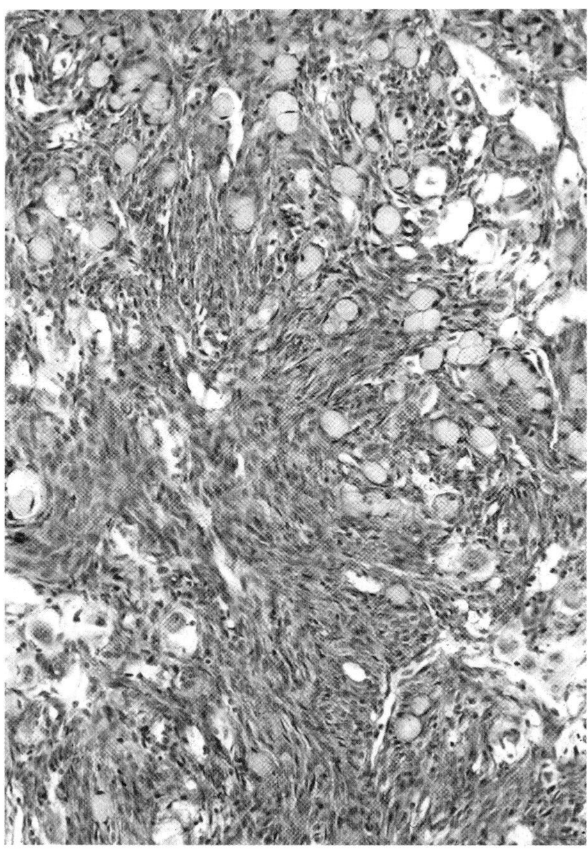

Fig. 18.14
Krukenberg tumor. **Numerous signet-ring cells are present within a cellular stroma**

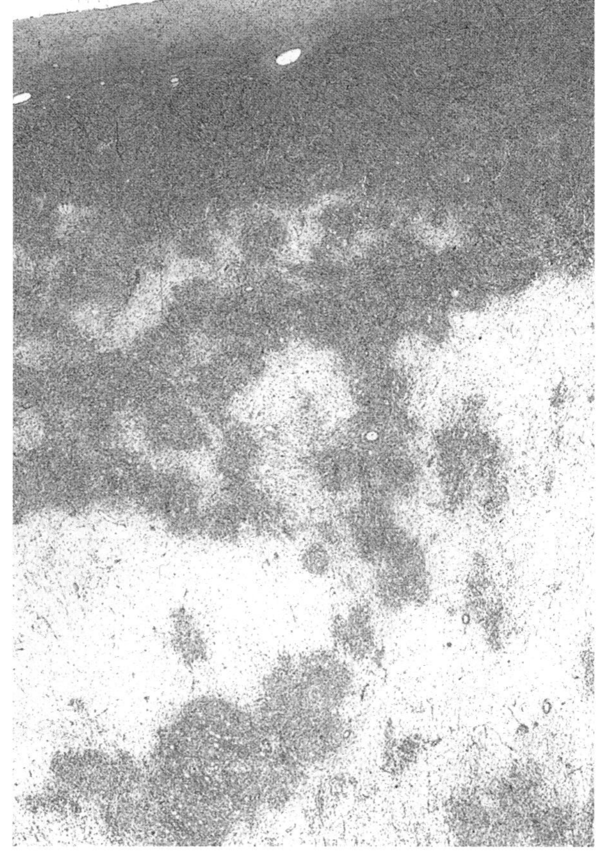

Fig. 18.15
Krukenberg tumor. **Typical alternating hypercellular and hypocellular regions**

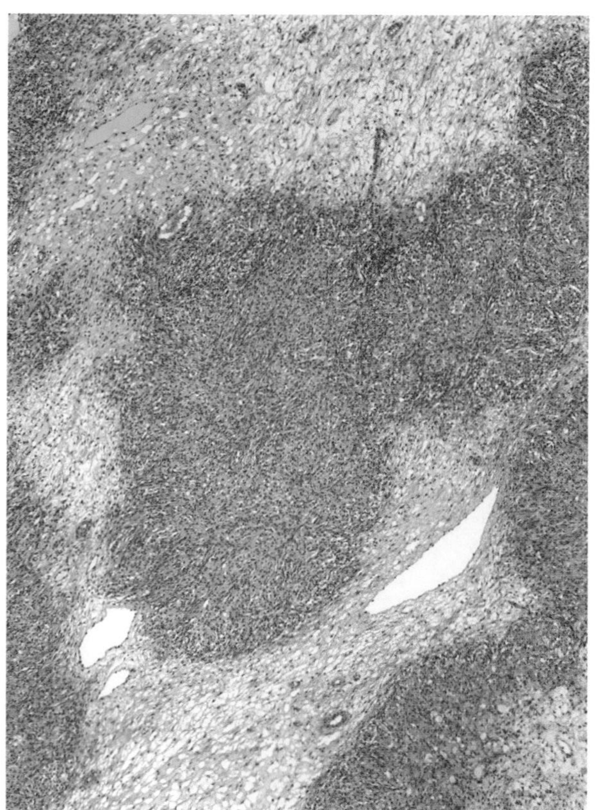

Fig. 18.16
Krukenberg tumor. **Pseudolobular pattern**

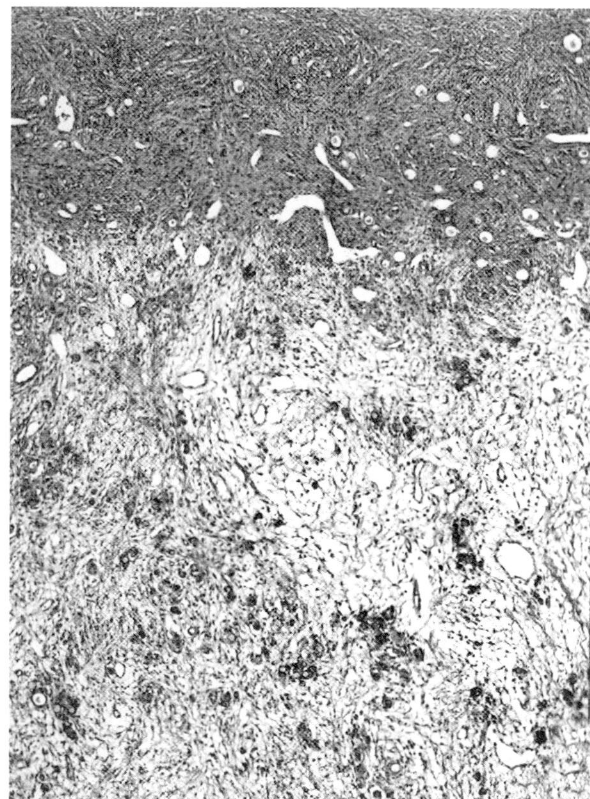

Fig. 18.17
Krukenberg tumor. **The outer region of the tumor (*top*) contrasts with the more central region that shows marked edema and clusters of tumor cells**

present, and a "sea" of signet-ring cells is immediately striking (*Fig. 18.19*). Conversely, it is not rare for these cells to be relatively inconspicuous, at least on initial low-power evaluation and even sometimes on high-power scrutiny. The arrangement of the signet-ring cells (*Fig. 18.20*) to one another and to other epithelial elements is equally variable. They may grow diffusely, in somewhat orderly clusters (*Fig. 18.21*), in pseudotubular formations, or in a totally random fashion within the stroma or between glands and cysts. The individual signet-ring cells are generally of relatively similar size and usually have pale to basophilic cytoplasm, which compresses the nucleus to the periphery in the well-known manner. This results in the nuclei often having rather deceptively bland cytologic characteristics. Occasionally the cytoplasm is eosinophilic, and sometimes densely so (*Fig. 18.22*). The cytoplasm may have a bull's-eye appearance, containing a large vacuole with a central eosinophilic body. Other neoplastic cells may be present that are mucinous but not of signet-ring cell morphology, and it is not rare for a component of the tumor to have nondescript mucin-free cells; such regions may be prominent (*Fig. 18.23*). Rarely, cells with clear cytoplasm are present (*Fig. 18.24*), and exceptionally, one can even see squamous or transitional-like cells.

It has recently been reemphasized that other epithelial elements, specifically glands and cysts, are present in most Krukenberg tumors [71, 161] (*Fig. 18.25*). In many cases, these can be as striking a finding as the signet-ring cells. The glands are usually small and often impart a microcystic appearance (*Fig. 18.26*), but a spectrum is encountered up through medium-sized glands to large cysts. The glands can appear indifferent or have a striking intestinal-type appearance, but the pseudoendometrioid morphology typical of non-signet-ring cell intestinal carcinoma (see below) is rarely present, and dirty necrosis is likewise uncommon. The glands and cysts may have

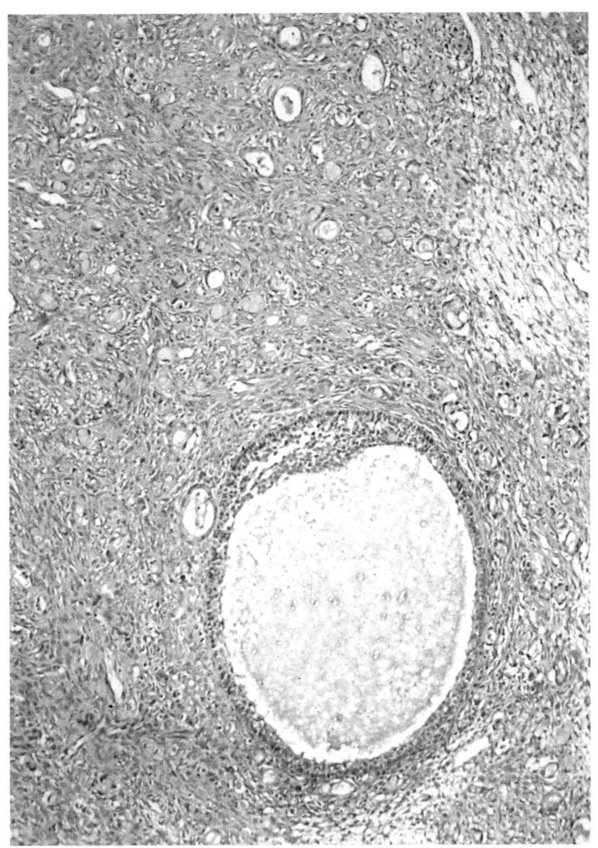

Fig. 18.18
Krukenberg tumor. **An entrapped follicle is evident**

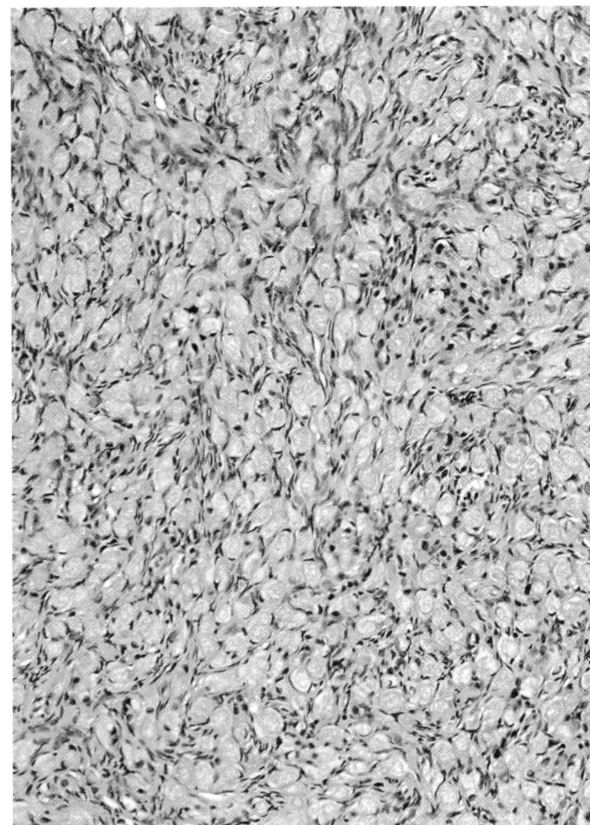

Fig. 18.19
Krukenberg tumor. **Numerous signet-ring cells**

attenuated lining cells or, uncommonly, columnar mucinous cells. Small round tubules, larger hollow tubules, and solid pseudotubular formations with or without signet-ring cells may all be seen (*Fig. 18.27*) and when prominent, account for the description "tubular Krukenberg tumor." Mucin stains may highlight signet-ring cells in these and other cases (*Fig. 18.28*). Many tumors have nondescript patterns of carcinoma, such as masses, nests, cords (*Fig. 18.29*), and individual cells, at least focally. Follicle-like spaces may be prominent (*Fig. 18.30*).

In our experience, the stroma is more often edematous than cellular, and a highly cellular "sarcoma-like" picture is distinctly uncommon. Indeed, densely cellular regions are more often due to a conspicuous content of small hyperchromatic epithelial cells with scant cytoplasm than to a cellular stromal proliferation. Mucin in the stroma is sometimes prominent and may contain signet-ring cells, form acellular mucin pools, or be separated by wispy collagen producing a pattern that has been referred to as feathery degeneration (*Fig. 18.31*). When glands are set in a relatively regular fashion on the background stroma, there may be a deceptively orderly architecture, albeit usually only focally. If the stroma is cellular in such instances, a superficial resemblance to an adenofibroma may result; this can be particularly treacherous at the time of frozen-section examination. If only a bland "fibroma-like" appearance of the stroma is captured for frozen section, a misdiagnosis of fibroma may result (*Fig. 18.32*). Occasionally, these fibromatous regions have a storiform appearance. The Krukenberg tumor is one of the ovarian tumors most often associated with stromal lutein cells (*Fig. 18.20*). They are often present in at least small numbers and may be prominent, particularly if the patient is pregnant as is sometimes the case given the relative youth of many patients. As with metastases in general, blood vessel and lymphatic invasion are common, generally identified at the periphery or in the hilar aspect of the neoplasm. In one unique case of a gastric primary,

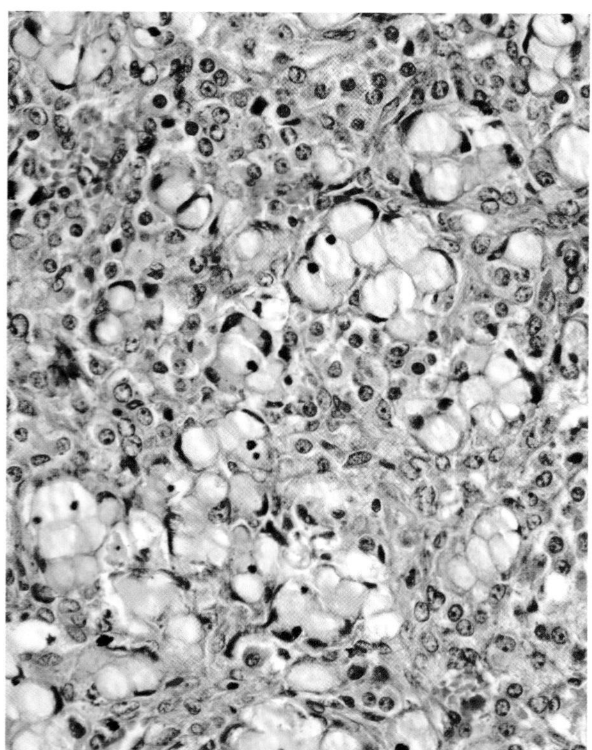

■ Fig. 18.20
Krukenberg tumor. **Typical signet-ring cells are intermingled with luteinized stromal cells**

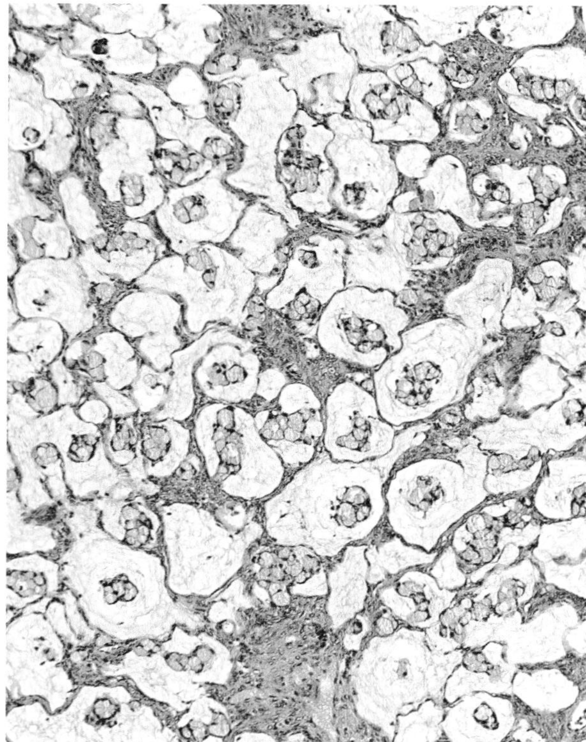

■ Fig. 18.21
Krukenberg tumor. **Signet-ring cells aggregate together in a rather orderly manner within uniform spaces**

the ovarian metastases showed yolk sac differentiation, none being identified in the primary tumor [186]. In two other unusual cases, metastatic signet-ring cell carcinoma in the ovaries originated in the cervix, a judgment based significantly on identification of human papilloma virus by in situ hybridization [151].

Differential Diagnosis

The Krukenberg tumor may resemble a fibroma or any other type of solid ovarian tumor on gross examination. Its appearance also occasionally may be deceptive on frozen section, as noted above, or low-power examination, but it should be readily diagnosable on high-power microscopic examination, especially with the aid of mucin stains. A frequent misdiagnosis is a Sertoli–Leydig cell tumor, particularly when a prominent tubular component and luteinization of the stroma are encountered [14]; signet-ring cells, however, are not a feature of Sertoli–Leydig cell tumors except for occasional tumors of heterologous type (see ➋ Chap. 15, Sex Cord-Stromal, Steroid Cell, and Other Ovarian Tumors with Endocrine, Paraendocrine, and Paraneoplastic Manifestations). The sclerosing stromal tumor may contain cells resembling signet-ring cells as well as a proliferating fibroblastic component, but such cells contain lipid rather than mucin. The rare signet-ring stromal tumor also may enter the differential diagnosis, but the signet-ring cells in that tumor also fail to react with mucin stains.

Surface epithelial tumors generally cause fewer problems in differential diagnosis than sex cord–stromal tumors. Cells with clear cytoplasm may raise the issue of clear cell carcinoma, but the clear cells in the latter contain glycogen; mucin, when present, is typically luminal and extracellular. In rare cases, clear cell carcinomas may have focal signet-ring cells, but the presence of other characteristic features, such as a typical tubulocystic pattern or papillae, permit their identification. Primary mucinous tumors are rarely difficult to distinguish from Krukenberg tumors, as the latter have so many features pointing to a metastatic process. It should be noted that rare mucinous tumors can contain signet-ring cells, but as recently emphasized, their similarity to Krukenberg tumors is otherwise minimal [95]. Occasional serous and even some endometrioid and undifferentiated carcinomas can have signet-ring cells [19], but the many

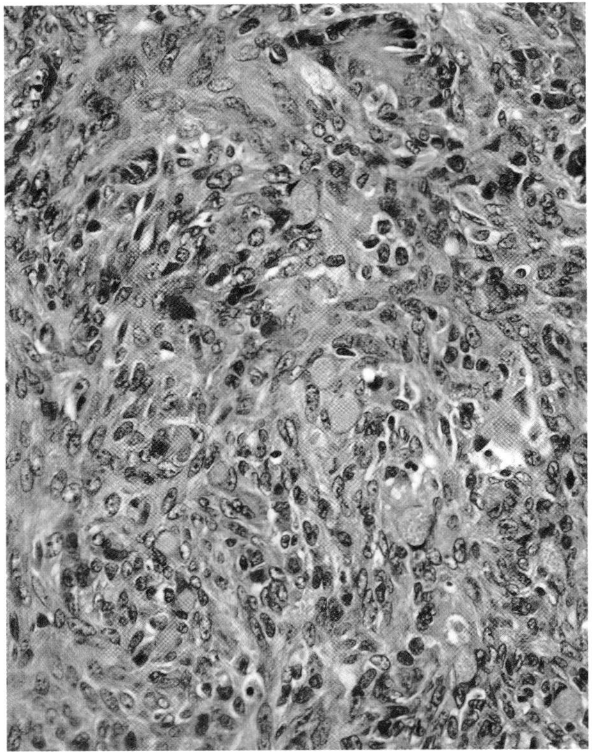

Fig. 18.22
Krukenberg tumor. **Many signet-ring cells in this illustration have dense eosinophilic cytoplasm**

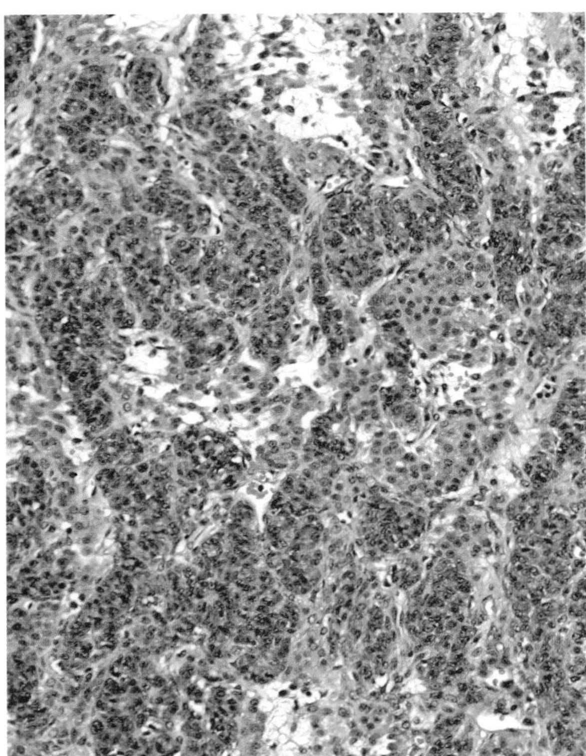

Fig. 18.23
Krukenberg tumor. **Epithelial cells without conspicuous mucin grow as cords and clusters separated by luteinized stromal cells, imparting a superficial resemblance to Sertoli–Leydig cell tumor**

differences between these tumors and Krukenberg tumors are such that resolving any issue in differential diagnosis should be straightforward.

Mucinous carcinoid tumors that contain large numbers of signet-ring cells are distinguished from Krukenberg tumors by their additional component of carcinoid, the presence of which can be confirmed by special stains. Infrequently, a mesothelial neoplasm may be a diagnostic consideration. The vacuoles of the rare adenomatoid tumor that involves the ovary may be misconstrued as signet-ring cells, but many differences, including even the much less ominous gross appearance of the adenomatoid tumor, should help one avoid misdiagnosis [112]. Adenomatoid-like foci may be seen in some malignant mesotheliomas [6], such that one involving the ovary could cause a Krukenberg tumor to be entertained in the differential diagnosis; however, the tubulo-papillary patterns of mesothelioma are generally distinctive, and these tumors lack the many above-described features seen in most Krukenberg tumors.

Finally, the rare nonneoplastic lesion, mucicarminophilic histiocytosis [73], which is caused by injection of substances containing polyvinylpyrrolidine, is characterized by signet-ring-like cells and may involve numerous tissues and organs including the ovaries. Although these cells are stained by mucicarmine, they are periodic acid–Schiff negative.

Metastatic Intestinal-Type Adenocarcinoma of the Stomach

Only a small number of cases of this type are documented [81]. This precludes firm conclusions on differing clinical features from the Krukenberg tumor, but the limited information available suggests that these patients are somewhat older than the usual patient with a Krukenberg tumor. To date, the endocrine manifestations seen with some cases of the latter have not been a feature of the intestinal-type cancers.

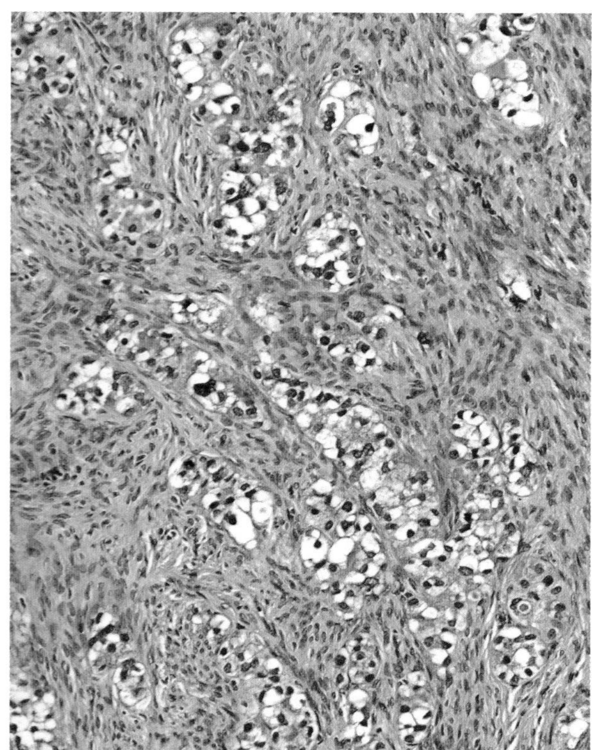

Fig. 18.24
Krukenberg tumor. **Cords and clusters of cells with appreciable clear cytoplasm are present in a moderately cellular fibrous stroma. The appearance in this field is non-specific**

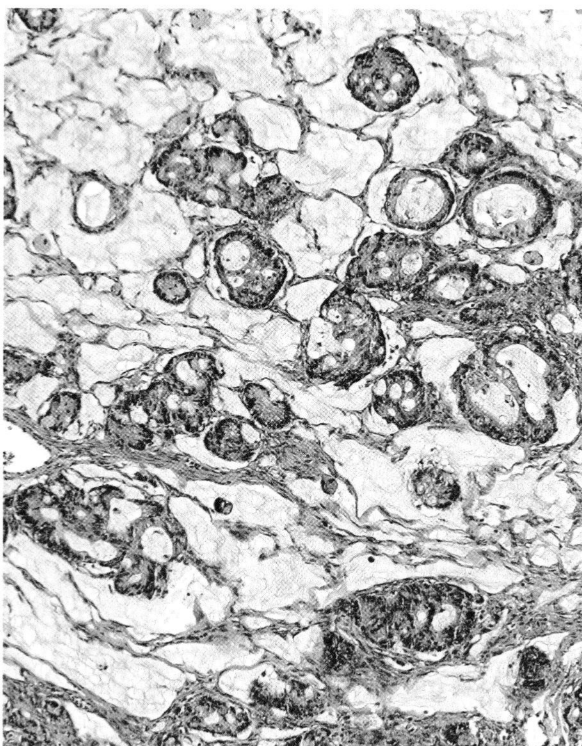

Fig. 18.25
Krukenberg tumor. **Glandular differentiation**

Gross Findings

The tumors are typically solid, cystic, and large, resembling metastatic colon cancer rather than the usual Krukenberg tumor. They may be bilateral or unilateral.

Microscopic Findings

The tumors are typically formed of medium-sized tubular glands, resulting in a pseudoendometrioid pattern (*Fig. 18.33*) as seen with metastatic colon cancer. Other familiar features of the latter such as dirty necrosis may also be encountered. Findings common to many cases of metastatic disease in the ovary, such as prominent stromal edema (*Fig. 18.34*) and notable morphologic variability within a small zone of tumor (*Fig. 18.35*), are seen, as are nonspecific patterns of growth such as cords. Less often the picture is that of a mucinous neoplasm. A very minor component (definitionally <10%) of signet-ring cells is present in some metastatic intestinal-type tumors.

Differential Diagnosis

The differential diagnosis is with other metastatic tumors that may have pseudoendometrioid or mucinous features, such as metastatic colorectal carcinoma, and with primary endometrioid and mucinous neoplasia. Clinical evaluation is paramount in the distinction from other metastatic tumors, and features elaborated elsewhere in this chapter are applicable in the distinction from primary neoplasms. Immunohistochemistry is of limited value, as the immunoprofile of gastric carcinoma overlaps with both primary and metastatic tumors in the differential diagnosis. Many, but not all, gastric carcinomas express cytokeratin 7 (CK7), whereas cytokeratin 20 (CK20) expression is variable [7]; this is essentially identical to the immunoprofile of primary ovarian mucinous neoplasms. Immunohistochemistry may provide more helpful information if the tumor has an endometrioid-like morphology. A CK7+ tumor is most likely non-colorectal in origin, as those tumors are characteristically CK7−/CK20+. Reactivity for CK20 points away from a primary endometrioid neoplasm (typically CK7+/CK20−). CDX2 positivity may

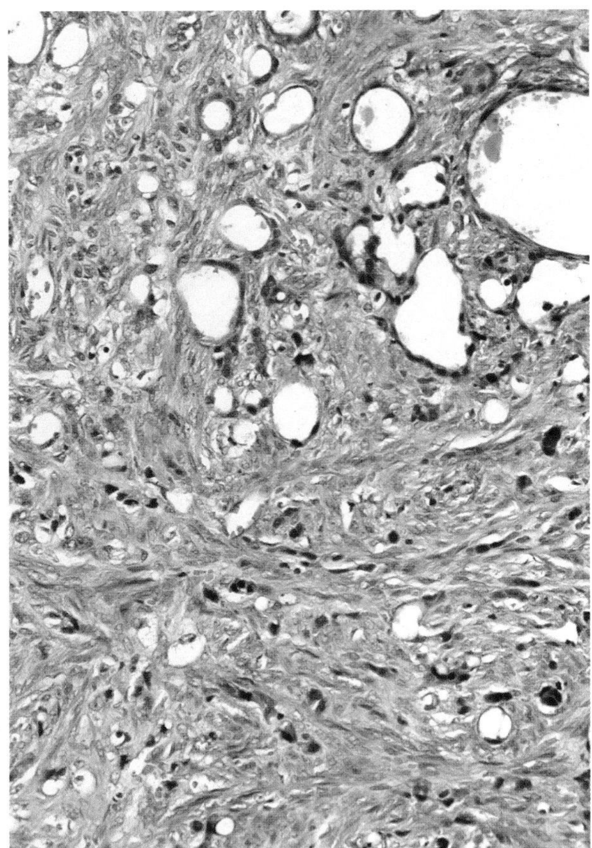

Fig. 18.26
Krukenberg tumor. **Small microcysts of the type seen in many cases**

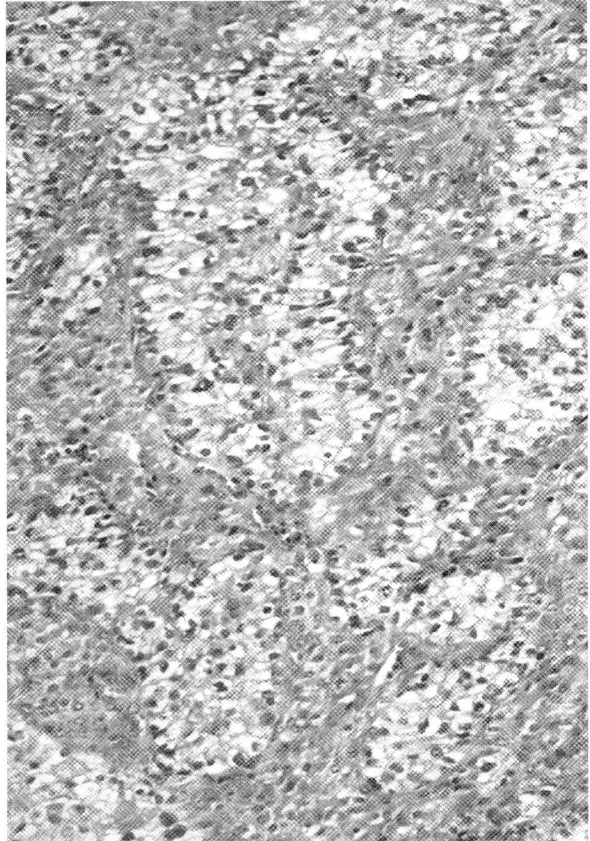

Fig. 18.27
Krukenberg tumor. **There is a prominent tubular pattern ("tubular Krukenberg tumor"). The cells have clear cytoplasm and could be misconstrued as the lipid-rich cells of a Sertoli cell tumor**

be seen in all the aforementioned tumors, but is usually strong and diffuse in colorectal carcinomas [7].

Intestinal Carcinoma

Most metastatic ovarian tumors of intestinal origin are from the large intestine, with occasional examples of small intestinal derivation. Ovarian metastases from intestinal carcinomas have been reported to be less common than those from gastric carcinomas at autopsy, 14% versus 38% respectively [126], but when malignant ovarian tumors encountered at the time of operation are evaluated, metastases from intestinal carcinomas are almost five times as frequent as those from gastric carcinomas [2, 11, 153]. Lash and Hart [75] have estimated that up to 45% of large intestinal metastases to the ovary are clinically thought to be primary ovarian tumors, and many are misinterpreted as such on pathologic examination even when there is a known intestinal cancer.

Approximately 4% of women with intestinal cancer have ovarian metastases at some time during the course of their disease [11], but in one study this figure was as high as 10% when the ovaries were sectioned into 2 mm slices [38]. Four of the six metastatic ovarian tumors in that series of 58 cases were not recognized on gross examination. Metastasis from the large intestine to the ovary is seen relatively more frequently when this cancer occurs in women under 40 years of age (in 18–27% of the patients in this age group) [114]. In one large series, one quarter of the patients were less than 40 years old [82] and in another about 43% were under 50 years [58]. In the latter study, it was noted that patients initially presenting with an ovarian mass were significantly younger than those having ovarian

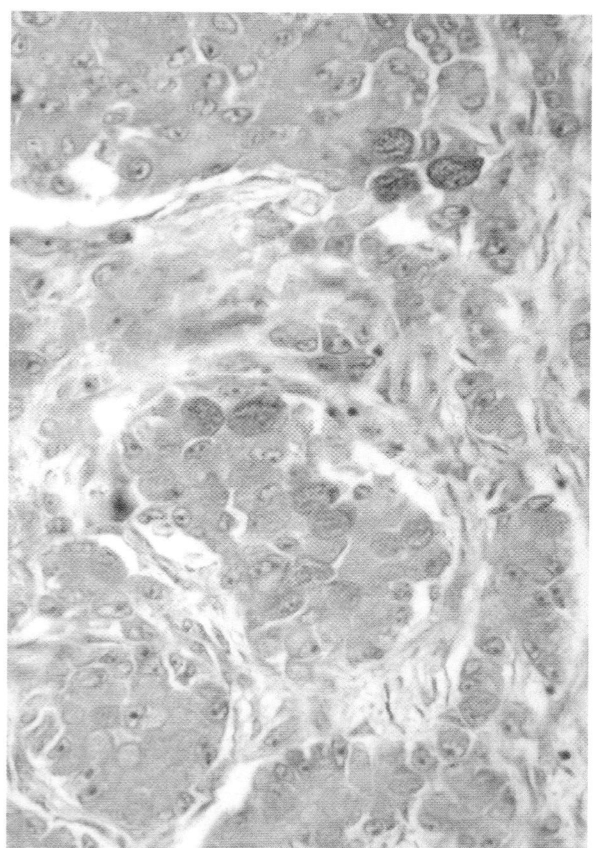

Fig. 18.28
Krukenberg tumor. **A mucicarmine stain highlights signet-ring cells in a tumor with a tubular pattern**

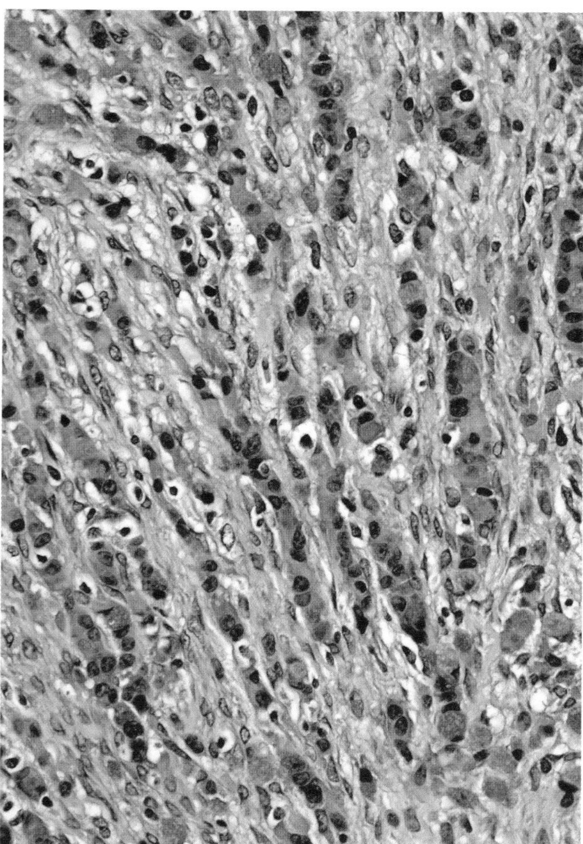

Fig. 18.29
Krukenberg tumor. **Indifferent tumor cells are growing as cords with only scattered signet-ring cells**

spread in the setting of a known colorectal primary (average 48 versus 61 years). We have seen ovarian spread in a 12-year-old girl. The serum CA-125 level may be elevated contributing to potential confusion with primary neoplasia.

From a clinical point of view, patients with this type of metastatic carcinoma fall into three categories: (1) patients with a known intestinal carcinoma (50–75% of the cases) that antedates diagnosis of the ovarian tumor by as much as 3 years in 90% of the cases, (2) patients in whom ovarian involvement is found unexpectedly during an operation for resection of an intestinal carcinoma, and (3) patients whose initial manifestations are those of an ovarian tumor (3–20% of the cases). Ovarian metastases have been found in up to 8% of patients who have bilateral prophylactic oophorectomy because of intestinal carcinoma [89]. In one study, 77% of the large intestinal primary tumors were in the rectum or sigmoid colon, 5% in the descending colon, 9% in the ascending colon, and 9% in the cecum [75] Three of the small number of clear cell adenocarcinomas of the intestine that spread to the ovaries were primary in the small intestine [170]. Occasional patients have luteinized stromal cells in the ovarian tumor with resultant hormone production and endocrine symptoms.

Gross Findings

These neoplasms, which are bilateral in approximately 60% of the cases, may form solid masses with a nonspecific appearance but are more often at least focally cystic (*Fig. 18.36*), and in many cysts predominate. Frequently the tumors are large, with a median largest dimension in one series of 11 cm [75], and they may closely simulate primary carcinomas of the ovary. Sectioning typically reveals friable or mushy yellow, red, or gray tissue with

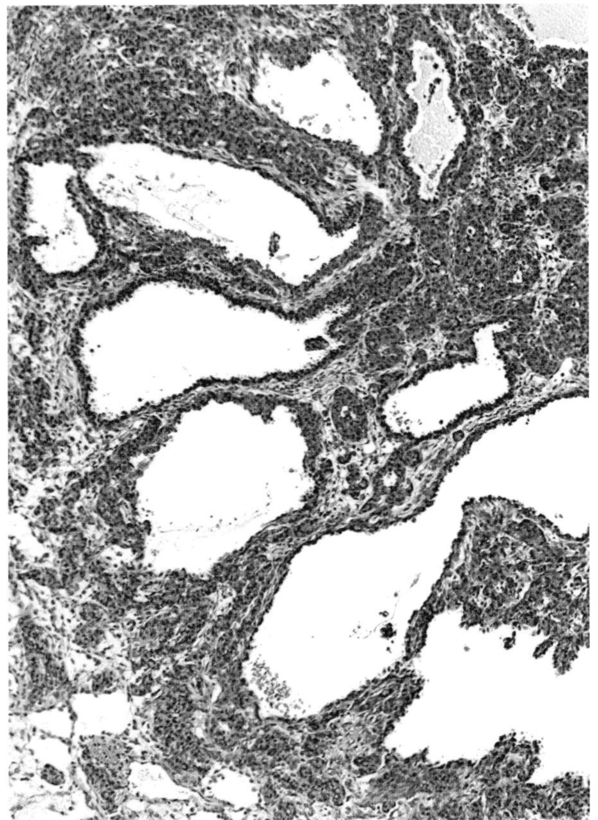

■ Fig. 18.30
Krukenberg tumor. **Prominent follicle-like spaces**

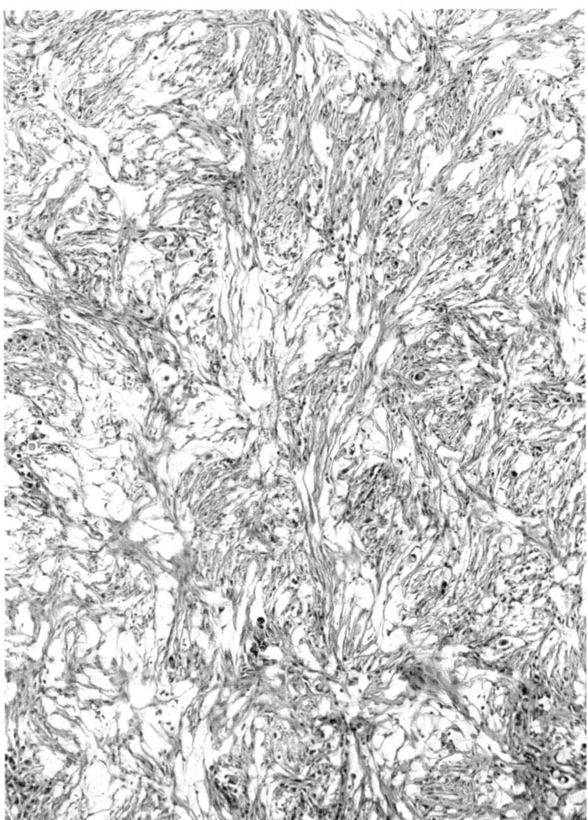

■ Fig. 18.31
Krukenberg tumor. **Mucin is separated by wispy collagen, imparting an appearance that has been referred to as "feathery degeneration"**

cystic compartments that contain necrotic tumor, mucinous or clear fluid, or fresh or old blood. Approximately 10% of the tumors rupture spontaneously during pelvic examination or removal. An occasional example is composed of multiple, thin-walled cysts filled with mucinous or clear fluid.

Microscopic Findings

The neoplastic cells grow in patterns similar to those of primary intestinal carcinomas of usual type, typically forming small or large glands with a frequent cribriform pattern [25] (➲ *Figs. 18.37* and ➲ *18.38*). Necrosis is common and often extensive, forming striking eosinophilic masses containing nuclear debris within the lumens; this feature, referred to as dirty necrosis (➲ *Fig. 18.37*), was present in all the cases in one series [75]. Two other features of the tumor, the frequent disposition of glands in a ring at the edge of the necrotic material (likened to a garland) (➲ *Fig. 18.37*) and focal segmental necrosis of the glandular epithelium (➲ *Fig. 18.39*), were emphasized by Lash and Hart [75]. Cysts may be prominent and contain central necrotic debris, clusters of tumor cells (➲ *Fig. 18.40*), or appear empty. A papillary pattern is seen occasionally. Mucin-containing cells (➲ *Fig. 18.41*), including goblet cells, may be scattered among mucin-free cells, the latter usually predominating or being the exclusive cell type. The epithelial cells are usually strikingly atypical (➲ *Fig. 18.42*). Glands and cysts lined by well-differentiated mucin-rich cells may be a prominent component of the tumor, and rarely the tumor has the pattern of colloid carcinoma. Signet-ring cells may be present in minor amounts, being present in 10% of cases in one series [82]. The stroma varies from negligible to abundant (➲ *Fig. 18.43*); it may be desmoplastic, edematous, or mucoid, and often contains luteinized stromal cells.

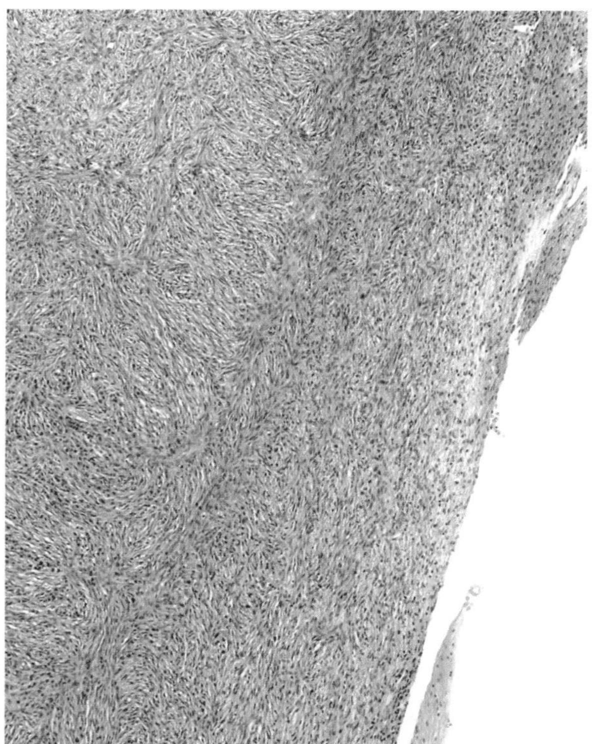

■ Fig. 18.32
Krukenberg tumor. **Fibroma-like stromal proliferation with paucity of signet-ring cells**

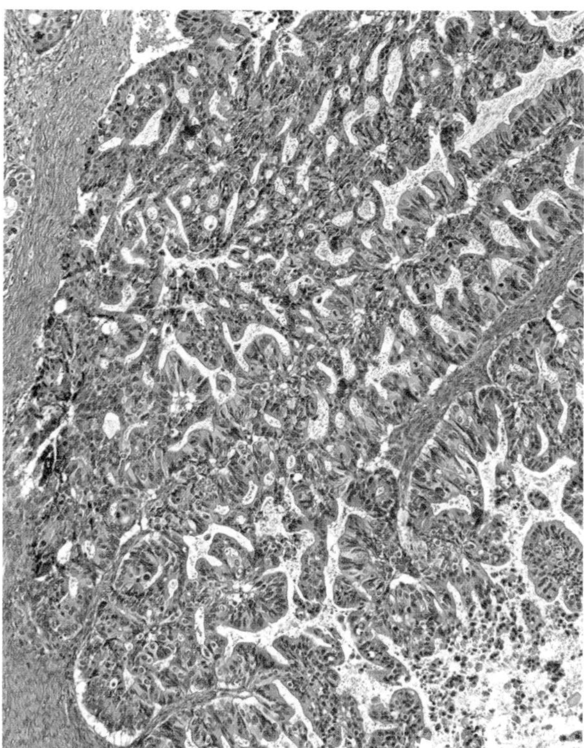

■ Fig. 18.33
Metastatic intestinal-type carcinoma from the stomach. **Glands of varying sizes and shapes impart a pseudoendometrioid appearance**

The tumors metastatic from intestinal clear cell adenocarcinomas have a glandular pattern architecturally similar to that of the usual intestinal adenocarcinoma metastatic in the ovary, including dirty necrosis. These tumors, however, differ in the conspicuous clear cytoplasm of the tumor cells (➲ *Fig. 18.44*). In some instances the clarity is subnuclear (➲ *Fig. 18.45*) imparting a resemblance to the secretory variant of endometrioid carcinoma, but in most the closest resemblance is to clear cell adenocarcinoma. In a few tumors, a colloid-like secretion has been conspicuous.

Signet-ring cell carcinomas of the colon may form typical Krukenberg tumors; 5.4% of the latter originated in the sigmoid colon in one large series [156]. Three cases of intestinal small cell carcinoma with ovarian metastases have been reported [30].

Differential Diagnosis

In one series, more than two thirds of the cases of metastatic intestinal carcinoma were initially misinterpreted as primary ovarian adenocarcinomas [145]. The most difficult tumors to exclude on microscopic examination are primary endometrioid and mucinous adenocarcinomas. In the series of 22 metastatic intestinal cancers described by Lash and Hart [75], 19 mimicked endometrioid carcinoma, 2 mucinous carcinoma, and 1 a mixed endometrioid and mucinous carcinoma. Aside from clinical clues, gross features may be helpful in the differential diagnosis. The usual bilaterality of metastatic intestinal carcinomas contrasts with the less than 15% frequency of bilateral involvement in cases of primary endometrioid and mucinous carcinomas. Endometrioid adenocarcinomas often are cystic, like many metastatic colonic cancers, but the cysts are sometimes filled with chocolate material. The presence of the latter is generally related to a background of endometriosis. A more homogeneous, less often necrotic, solid component is usually present.

With regard to the microscopic differential diagnosis of metastatic intestinal adenocarcinoma and endometrioid adenocarcinoma, the glands of the former typically are

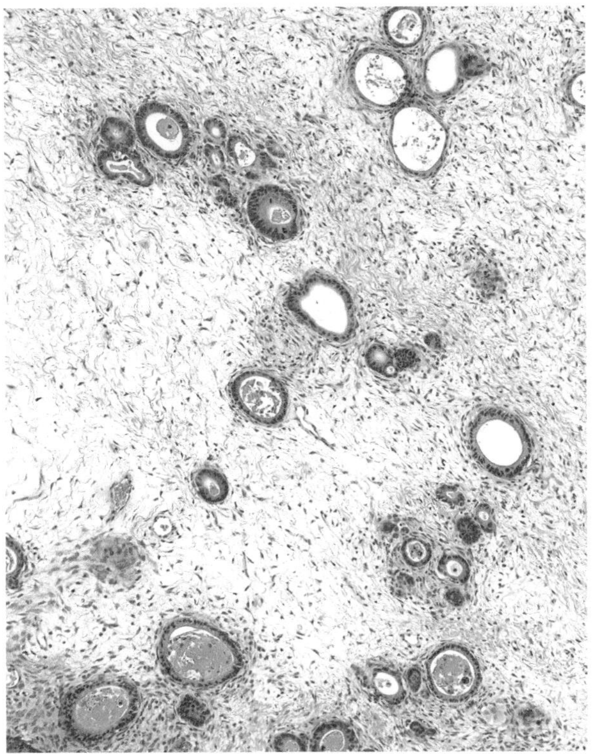

Fig. 18.34
Metastatic intestinal-type carcinoma from the stomach. **Small glands are separated by conspicuous edematous stroma**

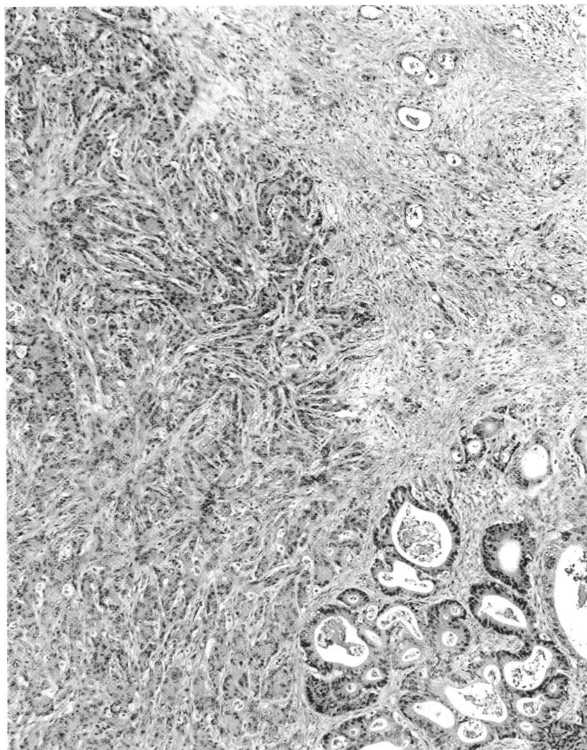

Fig. 18.35
Metastatic intestinal-type carcinoma from the stomach. **Markedly varied morphology within a small zone of tumor is a feature of many tumors metastatic to the ovary**

lined by more poorly differentiated cells with greater nuclear hyperchromatism and loss of polarity than those of endometrioid adenocarcinomas with a similar degree of glandular differentiation. In addition, extensive confluent necrosis is common in metastatic intestinal carcinomas, but uncommon in gland-forming endometrioid carcinomas. A similar comment pertains to so-called dirty necrosis within gland lumens, but it should be emphasized that this and the other features typical of metastatic intestinal carcinoma, such as focal segmental necrosis of glandular-lining epithelium, may be seen in some cases of endometrioid carcinoma [26]. Foci of squamous differentiation are frequent in endometrioid carcinomas but rare in intestinal carcinomas, and an adjacent or background adenofibromatous component or endometriosis strongly favors endometrioid carcinoma. The features just summarized, in conjunction with the general features of metastatic tumors to the ovaries and the clinical findings, also aid in the uncommon problem of differentiating a metastatic clear cell adenocarcinoma from the intestines

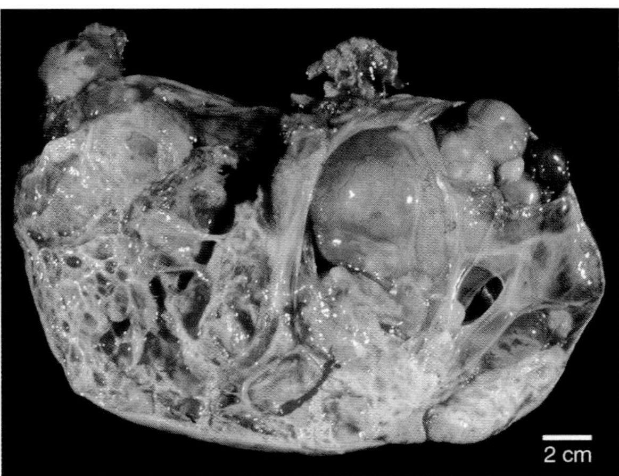

Fig. 18.36
Metastatic carcinoma from the colon. **The tumor is solid and cystic**

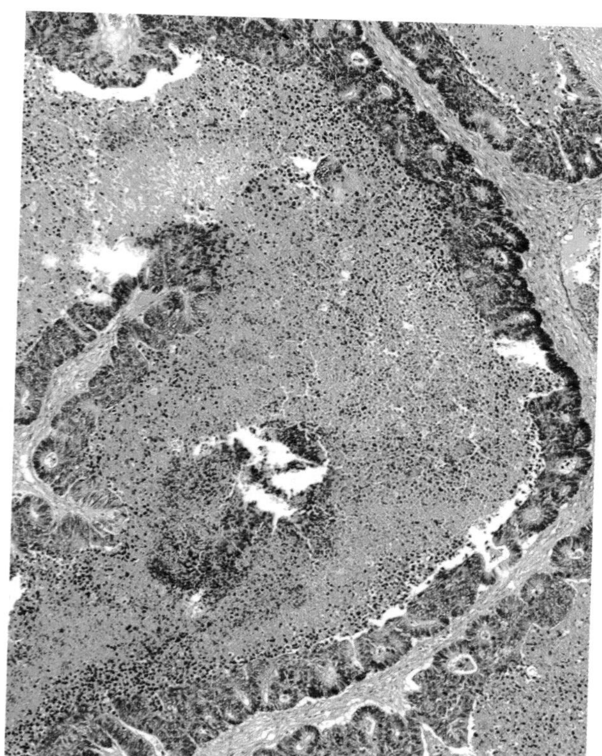

Fig. 18.37
Metastatic carcinoma from the colon. **There is extensive so-called dirty necrosis**

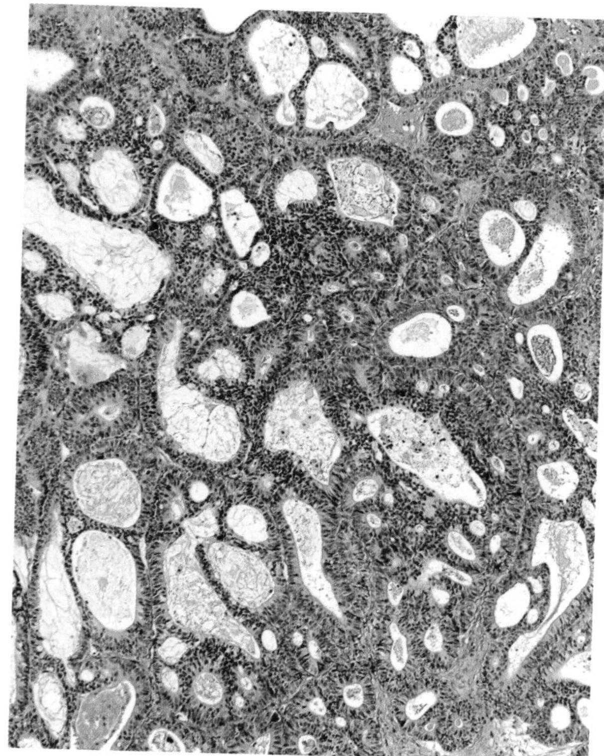

Fig. 18.38
Metastatic carcinoma from the colon. **Closely packed glands with focal cribriform pattern**

from a primary secretory endometrioid adenocarcinoma or clear cell adenocarcinoma.

In cases in which the differential is between a metastatic intestinal adenocarcinoma and primary mucinous adenocarcinoma, the frequent presence of glands and cysts lined by endocervical-type mucinous cells with basal nuclei favors a primary ovarian mucinous carcinoma over a metastasis, although differentiated glands and cysts are encountered in some metastatic intestinal carcinomas. Goblet cells are encountered more commonly in primary mucinous carcinomas, but they also may be seen in metastatic mucinous tumors. The other typical features of metastatic disease in the ovary already discussed are helpful in many cases, but occasionally it may be impossible to differentiate between a metastatic and primary mucinous adenocarcinoma on the basis of examination of the ovarian tumor alone. Metastatic mucinous carcinomas are more characteristically from the pancreas (discussed in more detail later), although they can derive from diverse sites. In one series eight metastatic mucinous adenocarcinomas were from the pancreas, six from the colon and rectum, three from the endocervix, two from the stomach, one possibly from the appendix, and one from the esophagus [119]. Other primary sites of metastatic mucinous carcinomas include the gall bladder and intra- and extrahepatic bile ducts, and even, exceptionally, urachus and lung.

Immunohistochemistry can be helpful in differentiating a typical metastatic large intestinal carcinoma from a primary endometrioid adenocarcinoma. Colorectal carcinomas are characteristically CK7−/CK20+, CEA+, and CA125−, whereas most endometrioid adenocarcinomas have the opposite immunoprofile [9, 91]. It should be noted, however, that right-sided colon carcinomas appear to be more frequently CK20− [76]. Cytokeratin stains are less helpful for the distinction of metastatic mucinous colorectal carcinomas from primary ovarian mucinous carcinomas. The former may be focally CK7+ and are usually CK20+, and the latter are usually CK7+ and may be focally CK20+, resulting in significant immunohistochemical overlap [93]. Furthermore, those mucinous carcinomas arising in teratomas may show a similar

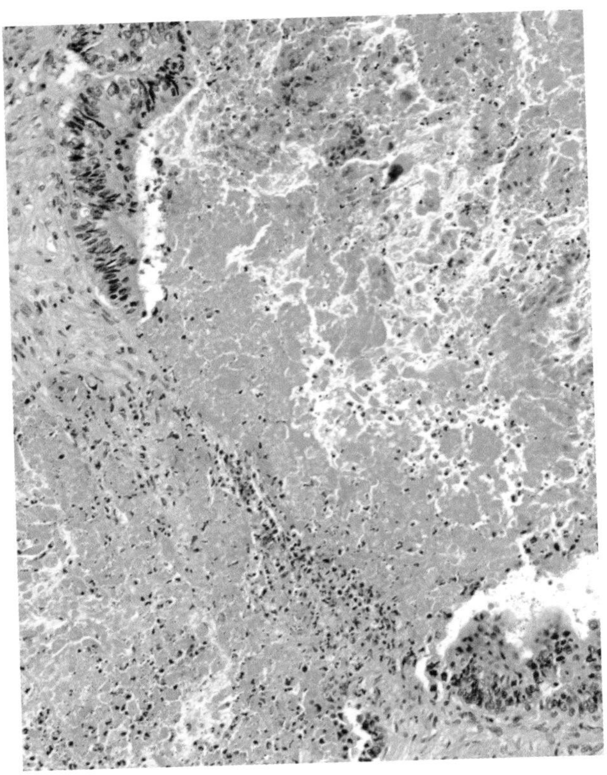

Fig. 18.39
Metastatic carcinoma from the colon. **Segmental necrosis of epithelium**

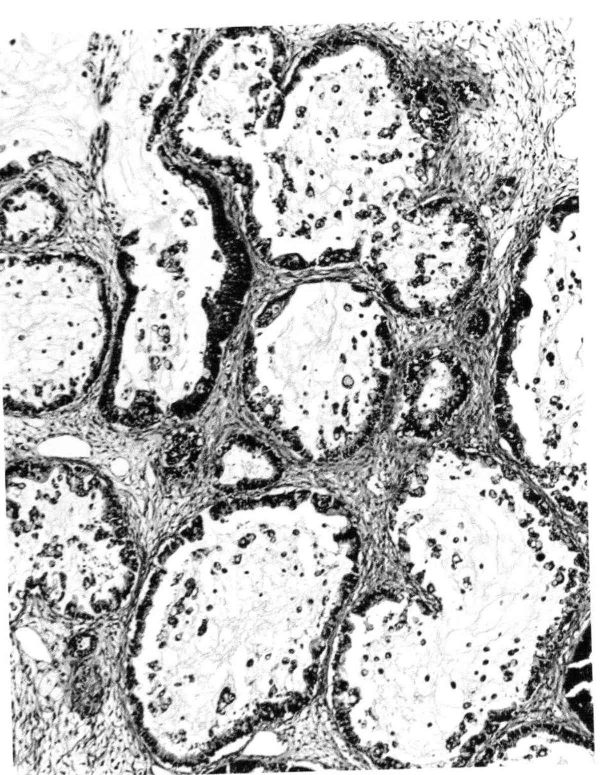

Fig. 18.40
Metastatic carcinoma from the colon. **Cysts contain clusters of tumor cells**

CK7−/CK20+ immunoprofile to many large intestinal carcinomas, reflective of their likely origin from intestinal elements [96, 147]. Small intestinal carcinomas are often CK7+ and are not infrequently CK20− [20, 76], and therefore in many cases they have a similar cytokeratin profile to primary ovarian carcinomas.

As mentioned previously, CDX2 is often strongly and diffusely positive in colorectal carcinomas, but it can also be positive in ovarian mucinous and endometrioid tumors [86, 148]. Colon carcinomas and mucinous ovarian carcinomas tend to show an inverse staining pattern for MUC2 and MUC5AC, with the former tumors usually positive for MUC2 and uncommonly positive for MUC5AC, and the latter showing MUC5AC positivity and limited MUC2 staining of goblet cells [7]. Estrogen receptor may be helpful for differentiating endometrioid adenocarcinomas from metastatic intestinal carcinomas, as the former are usually positive and the latter are negative [91]. In general, these immunohistochemical markers are most informative when the differential diagnosis is between a pseudoendometrioid metastasis and a primary endometrioid adenocarcinoma. Because most mucinous carcinomas and mucinous borderline tumors of the ovary are of intestinal type, they not surprisingly show a similar immunoprofile to tumors arising from the intestinal tract. It is important to remember that there are exceptions to all of the above "typical" immunoprofiles, and careful consideration of the clinical, gross, and standard morphologic features is critical and oftentimes most informative.

Tumors of the Appendix

Ovarian involvement is most common in cases of low-grade mucinous tumors of the appendix that often have the gross features of a so-called mucocele. Ovarian spread may also be seen in cases of frankly invasive adenocarcinomas of the usual intestinal and typical mucinous types

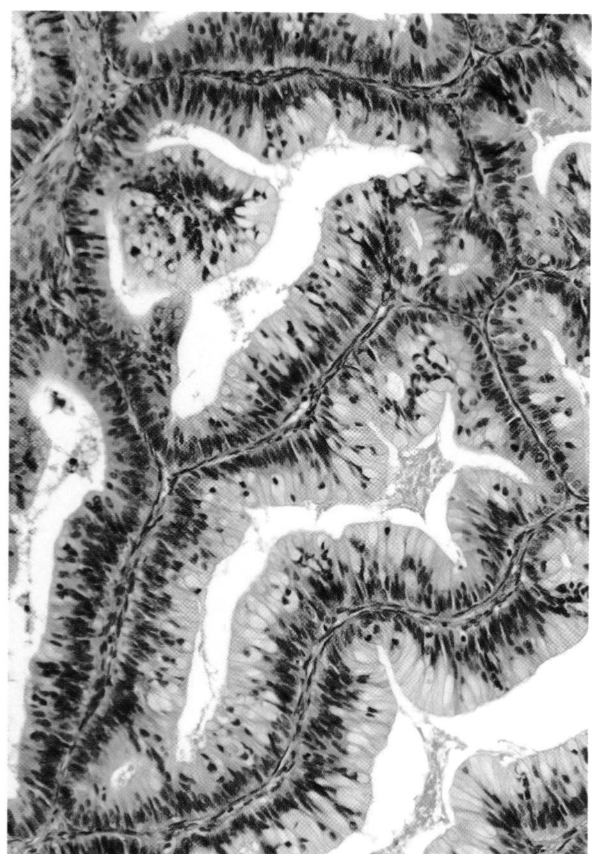

Fig. 18.41
Metastatic carcinoma from the colon. **In this tumor, many neoplastic cells were mucinous**

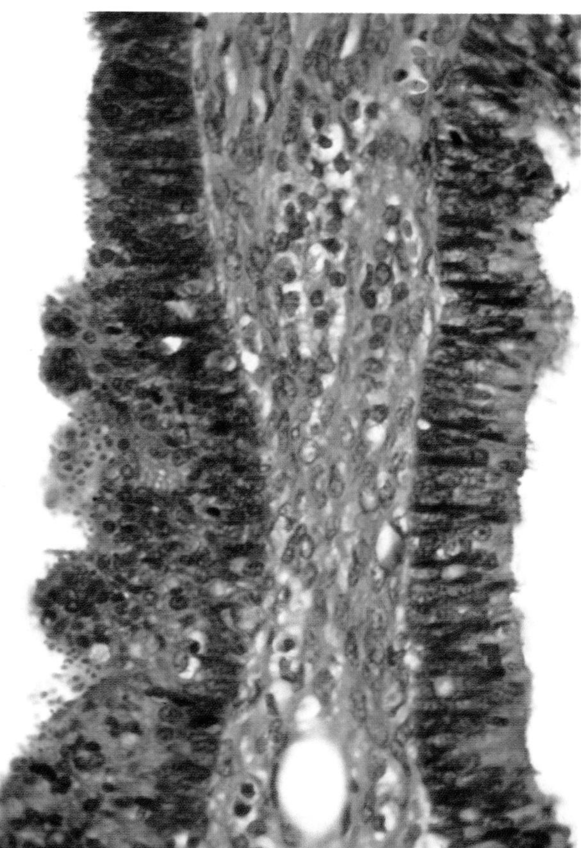

Fig. 18.42
Metastatic carcinoma from the colon. **Typical moderate- to high-grade cytology of the epithelial cells**

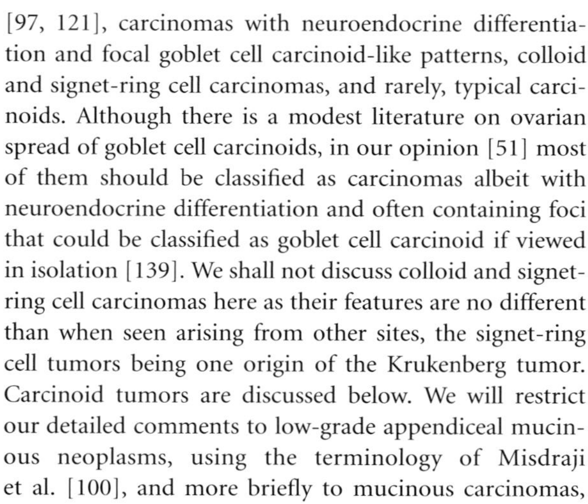

[97, 121], carcinomas with neuroendocrine differentiation and focal goblet cell carcinoid-like patterns, colloid and signet-ring cell carcinomas, and rarely, typical carcinoids. Although there is a modest literature on ovarian spread of goblet cell carcinoids, in our opinion [51] most of them should be classified as carcinomas albeit with neuroendocrine differentiation and often containing foci that could be classified as goblet cell carcinoid if viewed in isolation [139]. We shall not discuss colloid and signet-ring cell carcinomas here as their features are no different than when seen arising from other sites, the signet-ring cell tumors being one origin of the Krukenberg tumor. Carcinoid tumors are discussed below. We will restrict our detailed comments to low-grade appendiceal mucinous neoplasms, using the terminology of Misdraji et al. [100], and more briefly to mucinous carcinomas, intestinal-type carcinomas, and those with neuroendocrine differentiation.

Spread from Low-Grade Appendiceal Mucinous Neoplasms

The patients are usually middle aged to elderly, and typically present with symptoms referable to an adnexal mass. In many cases, this is the first evidence of an appendiceal neoplasm, although in some cases the ovarian manifestations follow some time after the patient is known to have had a primary appendiceal neoplasm. The appendix, if not previously removed, is usually dilated and often covered with mucus. In some cases, however, the right iliac fossa is so obscured by mucoid material that identification of the appendix is difficult or impossible.

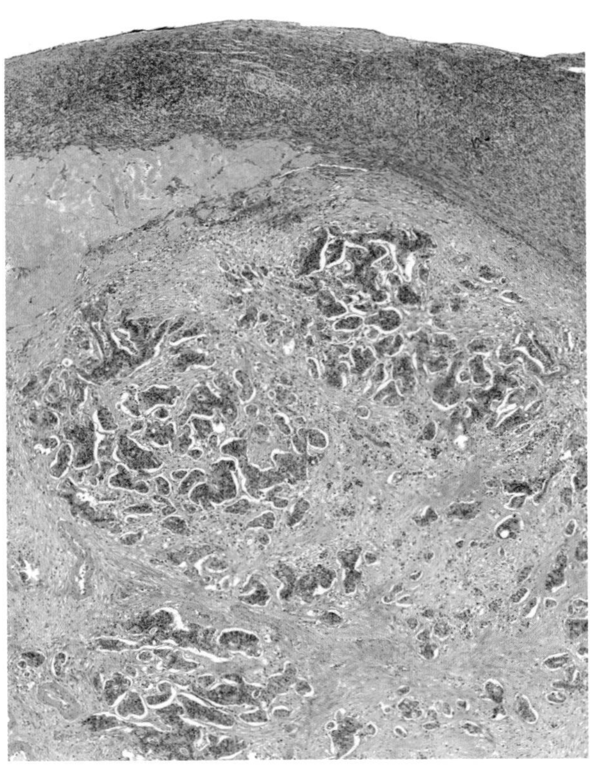

Fig. 18.43
Metastatic carcinoma from the colon. **There is a prominent stromal reaction surrounding small aggregates of neoplastic cells**

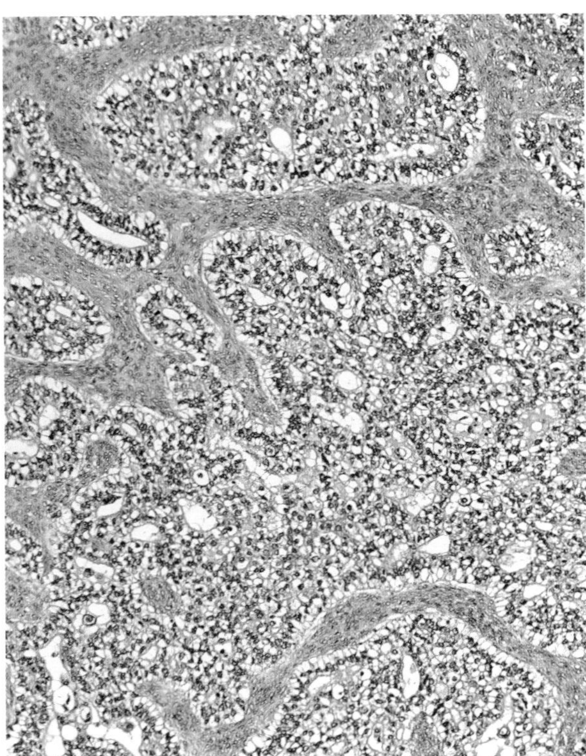

Fig. 18.44
Metastatic carcinoma from the intestine, clear cell type. **The clear cell morphology may cause confusion with clear cell carcinoma**

Gross Findings

Laparotomy typically discloses cystic ovarian tumors that are often bilateral (*Fig. 18.46*), average about 16 cm in diameter, and usually are multilocular. There is often generalized pseudomyoma peritonei [160], and the mucinous material may conspicuously coat the surfaces of one or both ovaries. Sectioning the ovaries typically reveals abundant jelly-like mucoid material (*Fig. 18.47*), although in some cases it has a firmer consistency. A multicystic appearance is most common, but organized mucin with fibrosis can impart a solid aspect in areas.

Microscopic Findings

Low-power examination shows glands and cysts growing in a leisurely fashion, often between residual recognizable ovarian elements. Mucin, with or without epithelial cells, may be prominent on the surface, or mucinous cells alone may line the surface (*Fig. 18.48*). Glands and cysts spread into the underlying stroma in a generally somewhat indolent-appearing manner (*Fig. 18.49*) The glands and cysts are lined by columnar mucinous epithelial cells (*Fig. 18.50*) that are typically taller than those seen in primary ovarian mucinous tumors and in other types of metastatic mucinous neoplasia. Mucin often appears to exude from the apical portion of the cytoplasm (*Fig. 18.51*). Although mild to moderate nuclear atypia is often seen, overall there is a remarkably banal appearance to the mucinous cells throughout most of these neoplasms in the majority of cases. The epithelium often lifts off its basement membrane, a likely artifact, but nonetheless one that has struck us as being a somewhat distinctive feature of these particular metastatic neoplasms (*Fig. 18.50*). In many cases, mucin dissects into the ovarian stroma (pseudomyxoma ovarii) (*Fig. 18.48*).

Differential Diagnosis

The first issue to briefly address is whether these are indeed cases of metastatic neoplasia, a point of some controversy in the past but now largely settled in favor of metastatic disease [116, 122, 123, 129, 137, 167]. The typical synchronous

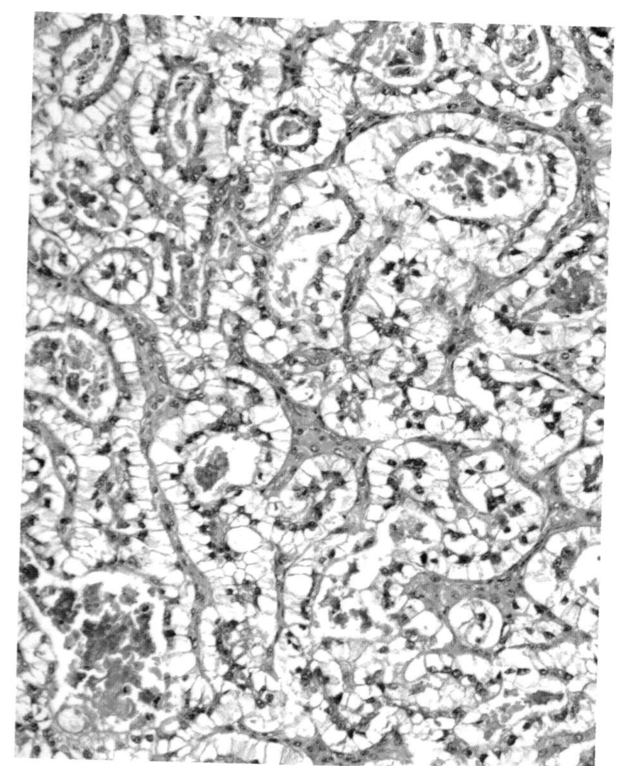

Fig. 18.45
Metastatic carcinoma from the intestine, clear cell type. **There is a prominent secretory-like appearance**

presentation of the ovarian and appendiceal tumors, their histologic similarity, the frequent bilaterality of the ovarian tumors, and the predominance of right-sided ovarian involvement in unilateral cases favors spread to the ovary. The lack of identification of appendiceal rupture has been used as an argument against the appendix being the primary site in these cases. Ongoing experience, however, has indicated that the site of rupture may be very small and require extensive sectioning to demonstrate it; such examinations have not been performed in most of the cases in which a site of rupture has not been identified. Additionally, in some cases a rupture site heals over, and is represented only by fibrosis in the appendiceal wall.

The association of the ovarian tumors with pseudomyxoma peritonei and, in most cases, known appendiceal pathology generally facilitate recognition of these tumors as metastatic. The rare primary mucinous tumors that are associated with pseudomyxoma peritonei usually have an additional teratomatous component; like primary appendiceal neoplasms, these are frequently CK7–/CK20+/CDX-2+, limiting the diagnostic utility of immunohistochemistry for determining site of origin in such cases [96, 149].

Mucinous Carcinoma and Intestinal-Type Carcinoma

These appendiceal tumors resemble those of similar type arising from elsewhere in the intestinal tract. Their features when they spread to the ovary have no unique characteristics, other than operative or other clinical findings drawing attention to the appendix as the likely primary site. A remarkable diversity of morphology is present in some cases.

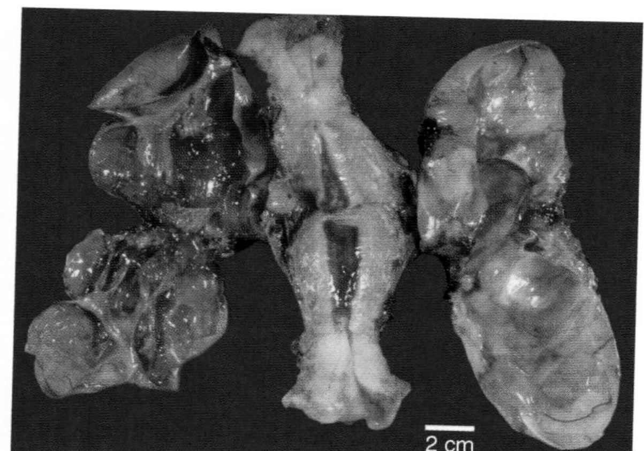

Fig. 18.46
Metastatic low-grade appendiceal mucinous neoplasm. **The ovarian tumors are cystic**

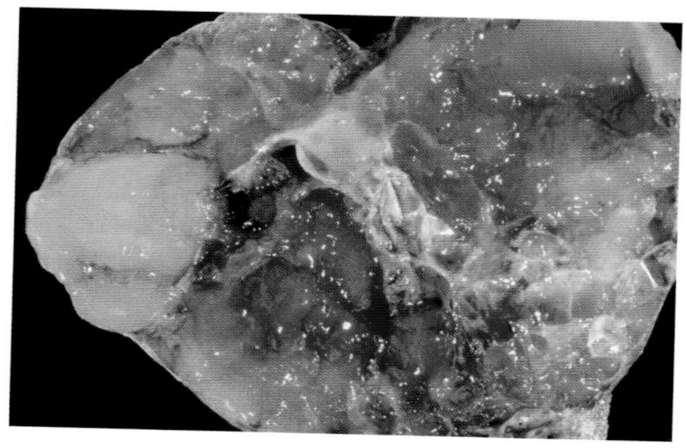

Fig. 18.47
Metastatic low-grade appendiceal mucinous neoplasm. **The tumor is strikingly mucoid**

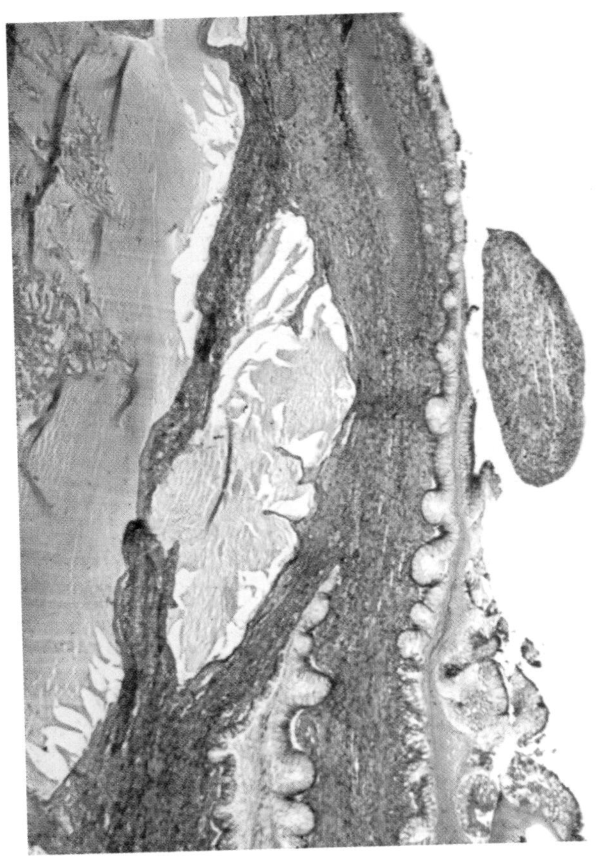

■ Fig. 18.48
Metastatic low-grade appendiceal mucinous neoplasm. **Columnar cells line the ovarian surface and mucin dissects into the ovarian stroma ("pseudomyxoma ovarii")**

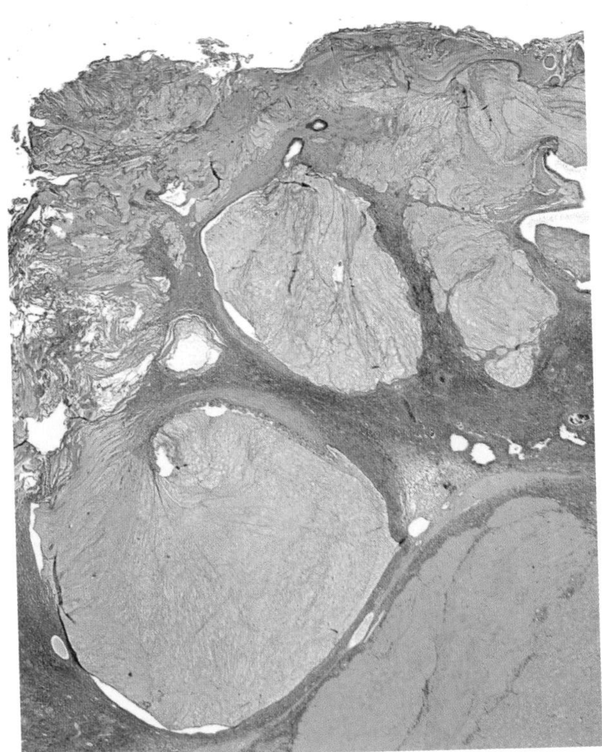

■ Fig. 18.49
Metastatic low-grade appendiceal mucinous neoplasm. **Mucin is on the surface and cystic glands invaginate in a leisurely fashion into the cortical stroma**

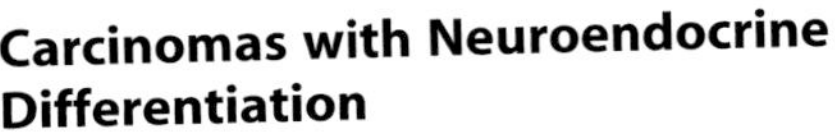

Carcinomas with Neuroendocrine Differentiation

Hristov and colleagues [51] recently reported a series of ovarian metastases of carcinomas of this type and emphasized that the overall clinical features and morphologic findings support classification of the appendiceal tumors as carcinomas rather than goblet cell carcinoids. They may have foci of the latter nature, but the presence of clearly infiltrative and destructive growth merits designation as frank carcinoma (● *Fig. 18.52*). Signet-ring cells are often a conspicuous feature, and metastases of such tumors constitute one form of the Krukenberg tumor. Although neuroendocrine stains may be done for academic interest, in our opinion they are not necessary for routine diagnostic purposes. The broad principles of evaluating metastatic tumors in the ovary assist in these cases. The prominent tubular component and neuroendocrine differentiation may place suspicion on the appendix if an appendiceal neoplasm is initially not evident.

Carcinoid Tumors and Neuroendocrine Carcinomas

Carcinoid tumors account for approximately 2% of metastases that form ovarian masses, and a similar percentage of small intestinal carcinoids greater than 1 cm in diameter spread to the ovary. Although most metastatic carcinoids are of small intestinal origin [120, 135], rarely the primary tumor originates in the appendix, colon, stomach, pancreas, or lung [13, 50, 145, 174]. In the largest series of carcinoids metastatic to the ovary, the age of the 35 patients ranged from 21 to 82 years, with a median of

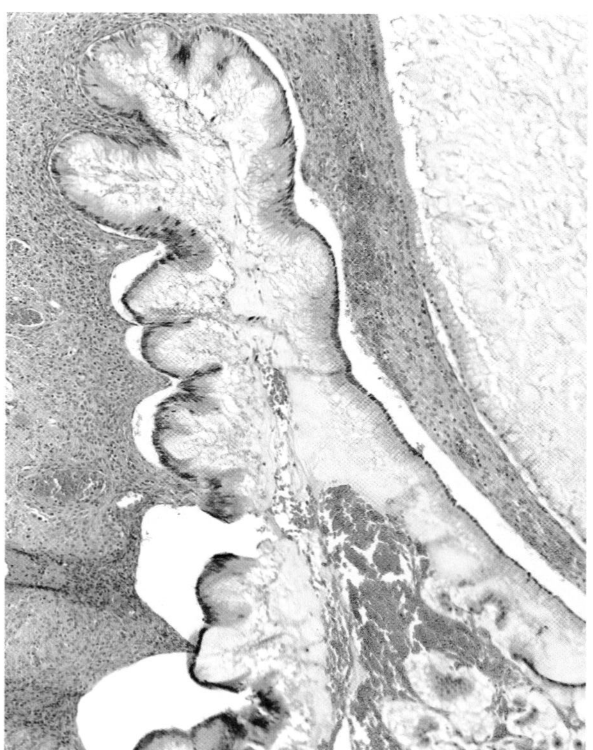

◘ Fig. 18.50
Metastatic low-grade appendiceal mucinous neoplasm. **The mucinous cells are tall and exhibit minimal atypia. There is retraction of the epithelium off its supporting basement membrane**

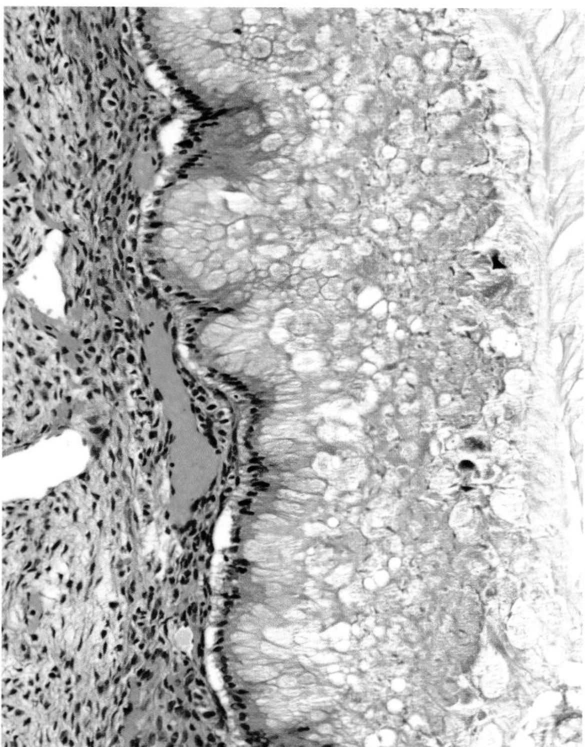

◘ Fig. 18.51
Metastatic low-grade appendiceal mucinous neoplasm. **Mucin appears to exude from the apical portion of the columnar cells**

57 years; almost all were older than 40 years [120]. Ten of the tumors in that series were not diagnosed until autopsy. Forty percent of the women whose metastases were discovered at operation had preoperative manifestations of carcinoid syndrome. Some of them also had signs and symptoms referable to intestinal or ovarian involvement. Extraovarian metastases were found in at least 90% of the cases, a figure that contrasts with the rarity of similar spread of primary ovarian carcinoids. The primary site usually was in the ileum, but cecum, jejunum, appendix, and pancreas were sources in occasional cases. One third of the patients died within 1 year and three fourths of them within 5 years after unilateral or bilateral salpingo-oophorectomy, which was accompanied by a hysterectomy and an intestinal operation in some of the cases. Six of the 25 patients, however, were asymptomatic for a median period of 5 years postoperatively. The symptoms of carcinoid syndrome generally abate after removal of the ovarian tumors.

In view of the occasional complication of ovarian metastasis, menopausal or postmenopausal patients with gastrointestinal carcinoids should have a bilateral oophorectomy even in the absence of obvious ovarian involvement to prevent the subsequent growth of occult metastases or the development of new metastases. Whenever bilateral ovarian carcinoids are detected, a careful search for an extraovarian primary tumor should be instituted. Both the metastases and the primary tumor, if found, should be excised whenever feasible. In a young woman with a unilateral neoplasm, careful examination of the intestine and its mesentery and other organs for a primary tumor, biopsy of the opposite ovary if enlarged, a thorough search for teratomatous elements in the tumor, postoperative radiologic studies, and measurement of 5-hydroxyindole acetic acid in the urine may be necessary before a determination of the primary or metastatic nature of the tumor can be made. Because the primary tumor in the intestine may be very small, it may not be detected by radiologic studies for a year or more after the diagnosis of the ovarian metastasis.

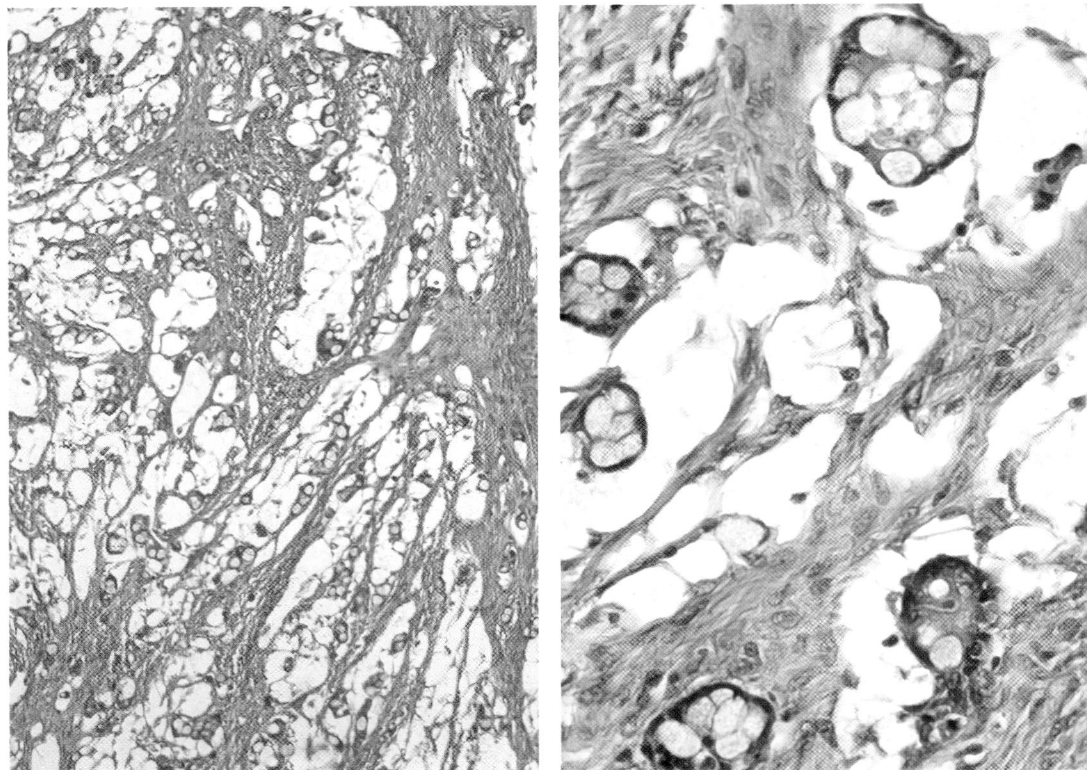

Fig. 18.52
Metastatic appendiceal carcinoma with neuroendocrine differentiation. **On the *left*, there is overt infiltration of an aggressive type. On the *right*, small clusters have an appearance consistent with goblet cell carcinoid**

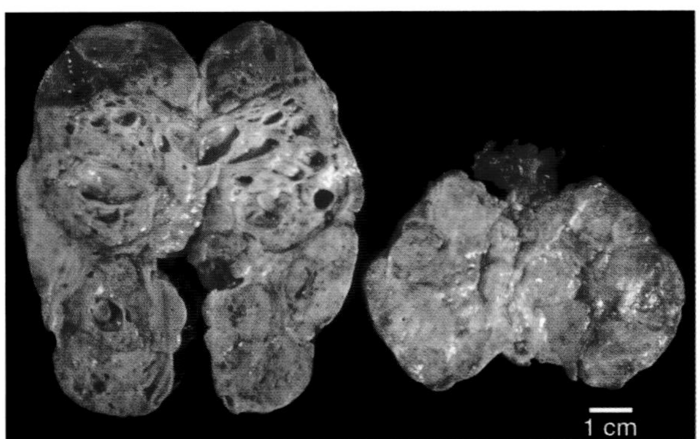

Fig. 18.53
Metastatic carcinoid. **The larger tumor contains multiple cysts simulating a cystadenofibroma**

Gross Findings

Most of these tumors are bilateral (Fig. 18.53) in contrast to primary ovarian carcinoids, which are almost always unilateral. The tumors are most often only of modest size but may be large and typically are predominantly solid, with smooth or bosselated surfaces. Sectioning reveals single or confluent, firm, white to yellow nodules, which may resemble ovarian fibromas or thecomas. Cysts of varying size occasionally are present (*Fig. 18.53*) and are often filled with clear, watery fluid, resulting in a gross appearance similar to that of a cystadenofibroma. Focal necrosis and hemorrhage may occur (*Fig. 18.54*).

Microscopic Findings

The microscopic features of metastatic carcinoids are generally similar to those of primary ovarian carcinoids except that teratomatous elements are not encountered, multinodularity is often prominent, and vascular invasion is occasionally observed. An insular pattern is most common (*Fig. 18.55*), but trabecular (*Fig. 18.56*), mixed, and rarely solid tubular patterns are also encountered. Acini, which typically are uniformly small and round,

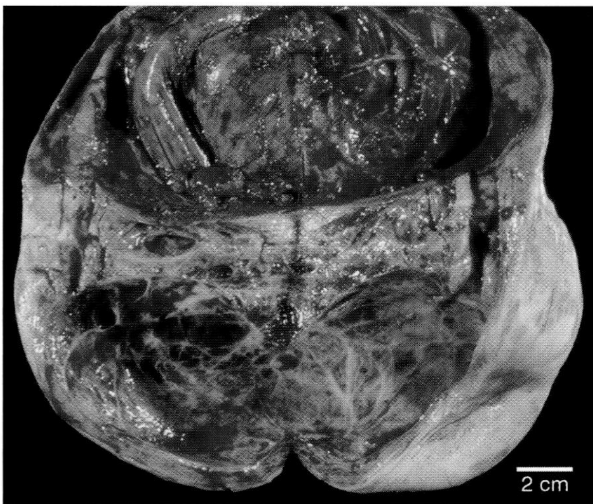

■ Fig. 18.54
Metastatic carcinoid. **The tumor is predominantly cystic with extensive hemorrhage**

are common (➋ *Fig. 18.57*); they often contain homogeneous eosinophilic secretions that may undergo calcification, sometimes in the form of psammoma bodies. The acini sometimes punctuate otherwise solid nests or, in some instances, are arrayed at the periphery in an orderly manner. Follicle-like spaces are frequently quite striking (➋ *Fig. 18.58*). They may appear empty, but in other cases neoplastic cells slough into the spaces in a conspicuous manner. Metastatic carcinoid often has an extensive paucicellular fibrous stroma (➋ *Fig. 18.59*); occasionally this stroma is extensively hyalinized. Indeed, this tumor is the metastatic neoplasm most often associated with a very quiescent yet prominent fibromatous stroma.

Differential Diagnosis

In addition to the absence of teratomatous elements and frequent bilaterality, which are the dominant findings that aid in distinction from a primary carcinoid in most cases, the metastatic tumors less often have a trabecular pattern and may show vascular invasion. Mucinous glands that are

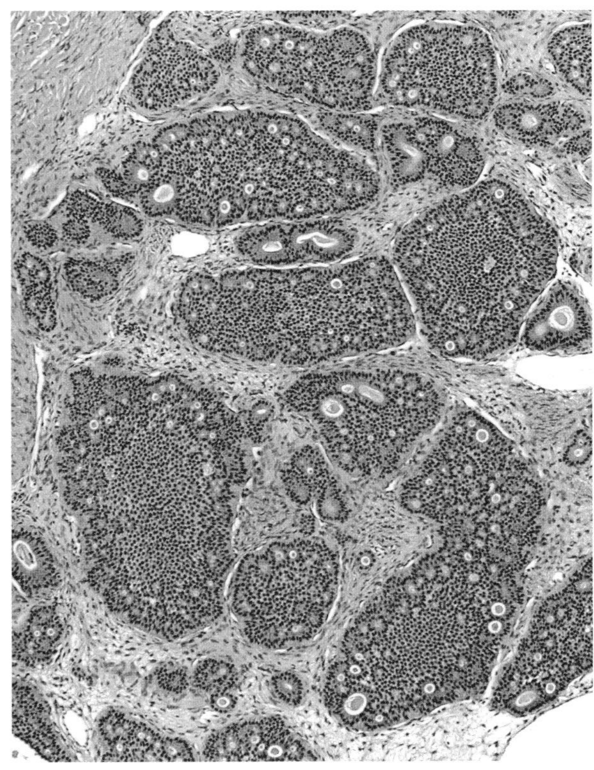

■ Fig. 18.55
Metastatic carcinoid. **Striking insular pattern**

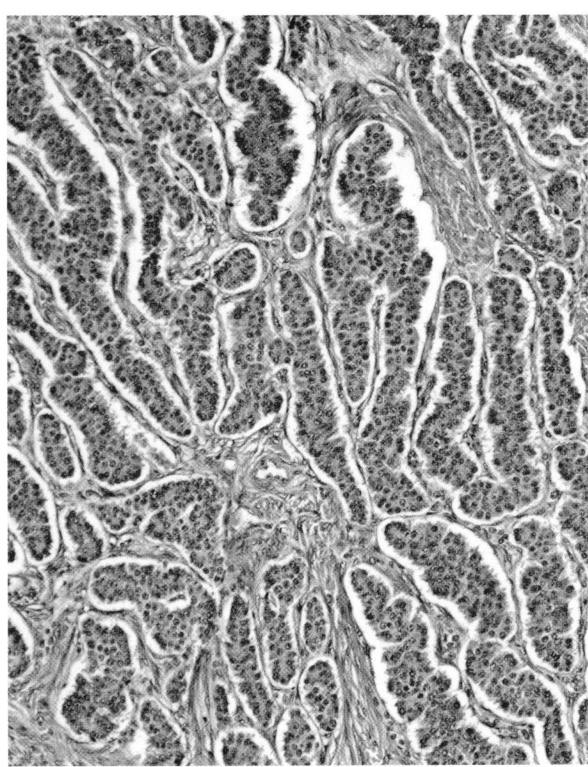

■ Fig. 18.56
Metastatic carcinoid. **Trabecular pattern**

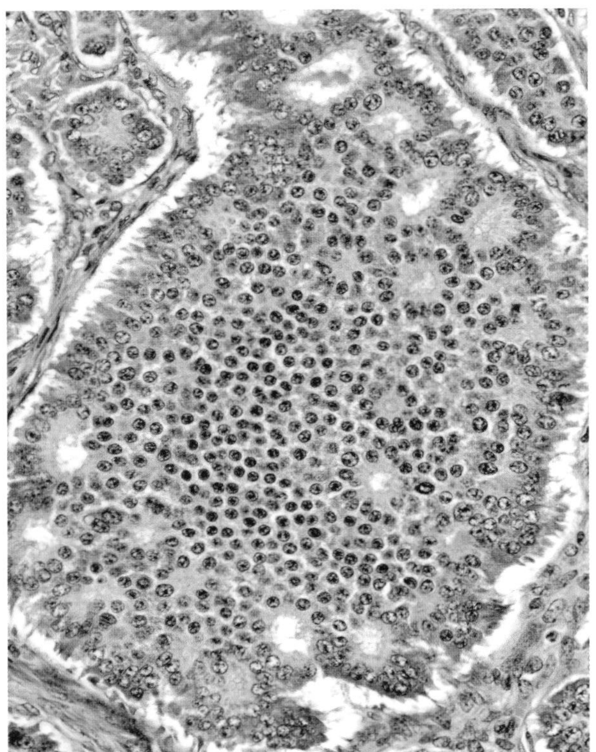

Fig. 18.57
Metastatic carcinoid. **Typical acini**

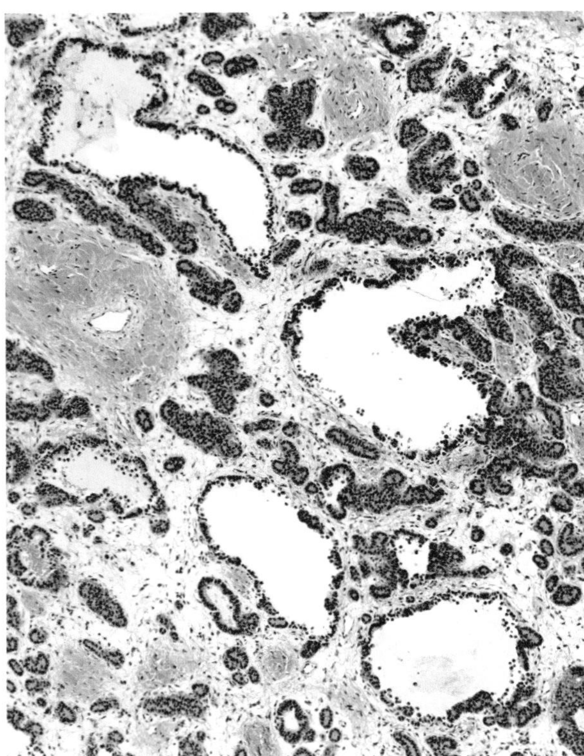

Fig. 18.58
Metastatic carcinoid. **Prominent follicle-like spaces**

common in the primary strumal carcinoid in particular are not a feature of metastatic carcinoid. The presence of foci of carcinoid outside the ovary strongly favors that the ovarian tumor is a metastasis. CDX-2 does not distinguish between tumors of intestinal origin and primary ovarian carcinoids [117].

Metastatic carcinoids may be confused with a number of tumors other than primary carcinoid tumors, including granulosa cell tumors, Sertoli or Sertoli–Leydig cell tumors, Brenner tumors, benign or borderline adenofibromas and cystadenofibromas, and adenocarcinomas of various types. The Call–Exner body of the granulosa cell tumor may resemble the acinus of the carcinoid when the latter is filled with dense eosinophilic basement membrane material, but the former differs by containing watery, eosinophilic fluid and shrunken nuclei in its lumen. The examination of the neoplastic cells is the most helpful clue to the correct diagnosis. The cells of a microfollicular granulosa cell tumor usually have scanty cytoplasm and ovoid, angular, or round nuclei that typically are pale and grooved. The cells are generally haphazardly oriented with respect to one another and the cavities of the Call–Exner bodies. In contrast, the cells of carcinoid tumors characteristically have round nuclei with coarse chromatin, and their cytoplasm often contains prominent red or red-brown argentaffin granules. The cells tend to have an orderly distribution and are polarized around the acinar spaces.

The sex cord-like formations of Sertoli–Leydig cell tumors may resemble the ribbons of the trabecular carcinoid, but the latter are usually longer and thicker and have a more orderly architecture. The tubules of Sertoli or Sertoli–Leydig cell tumors may simulate the acini of insular carcinoids. Further confusion may be caused by the presence of a carcinoid component, which typically is minor in extent, in a Sertoli–Leydig cell tumor with heterologous elements. The presence of other distinctive patterns of Sertoli–Leydig cell tumor and attention to the characteristic cytologic features of carcinoid cells, however, should enable one to differentiate the two.

The fibromatous stroma of a Brenner tumor is often indistinguishable from that of a carcinoid, but the epithelial nests of the former contain cells of urothelial type with oval, pale, and grooved nuclei rather than cells with the characteristic cytologic features of carcinoid tumors. Benign and malignant adenofibromatous tumors and

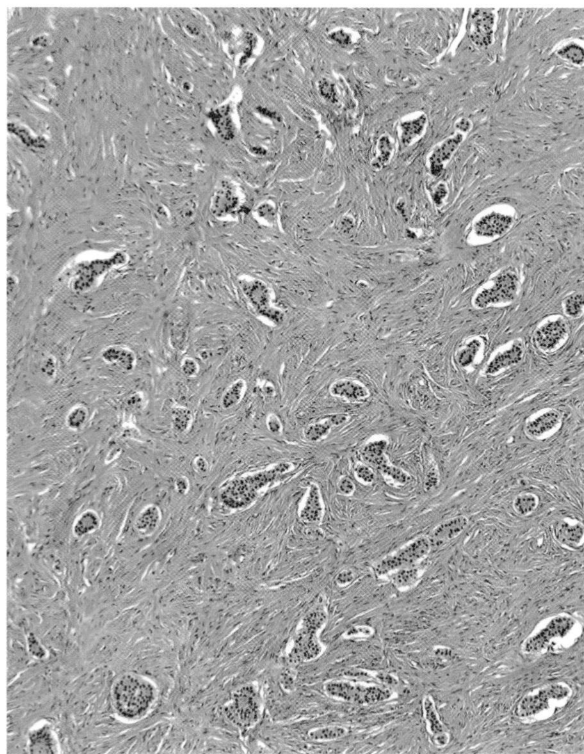

■ Fig. 18.59
Metastatic carcinoid. **Abundant stroma**

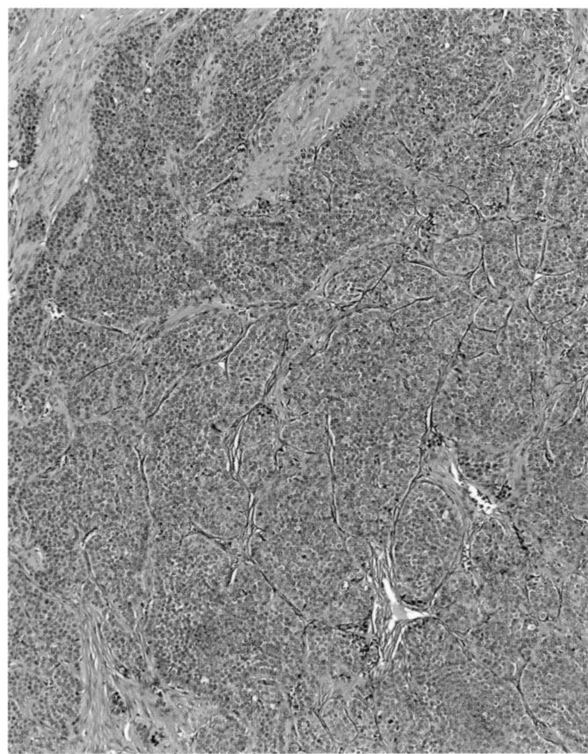

■ Fig. 18.60
Metastatic neuroendocrine carcinoma from small bowel. **There is an insular pattern, albeit less discrete than in the better-differentiated carcinoid tumor**

endometrioid adenocarcinomas containing small tubules and acini are generally readily distinguished from carcinoid tumors by recognition of the differing patterns and cytologic features of these tumors. Metastatic breast carcinoma with a prominent insular pattern may simulate a carcinoid tumor. Rarely, an acinar cell carcinoma of the pancreas metastasizes to the ovary and, in the absence of a known pancreatic primary tumor, may be misdiagnosed as a metastatic carcinoid (see below).

If the diagnosis of a carcinoid tumor is difficult in any of the above situations, more thorough sampling, immunohistochemical staining for neuroendocrine markers, and in rare situations in which those studies are not definitive, electron microscopy for dense-core granules should resolve the differential diagnosis.

It is our opinion, as stated earlier, that if strict criteria are used, mucinous carcinoids rarely spread to the ovary. However, we have already noted that carcinomas of the appendix with neuroendocrine differentiation may do so, and so may the spectrum of neoplasms ranging from neuroendocrine carcinoma (➋ *Fig. 18.60–18.62*) to small cell carcinoma of neuroendocrine type.

Tumors of the Pancreas

Usual Ductal Adenocarcinoma and Mucinous Cystadenocarcinoma

Spread of pancreatic carcinoma to the ovary was considered uncommon until relatively recently [125, 168], but current experience indicates that it is more common than was previously thought and has almost certainly been responsible for the miscategorization of some metastatic tumors in the ovary as primary mucinous carcinomas and even mucinous borderline tumors. Pancreatic primaries accounted for 7 of 82 nongenital cancers that spread to the ovary in one large series [111], and in another recent series of metastatic mucinous carcinomas, the single greatest number of cases, 8, originated in the pancreas [119]. The patients are usually in the mid to late years of life. Ovarian spread is often part of disseminated pre-terminal disease (or an autopsy finding in some cases), but in a sizeable subset of cases the ovarian manifestations have been

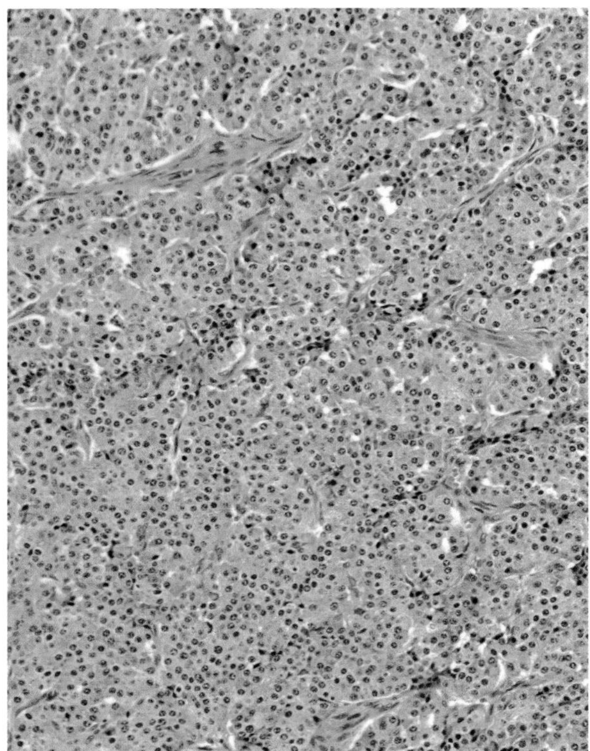

Fig. 18.61
Metastatic neuroendocrine carcinoma. **Striking oxyphil cells**

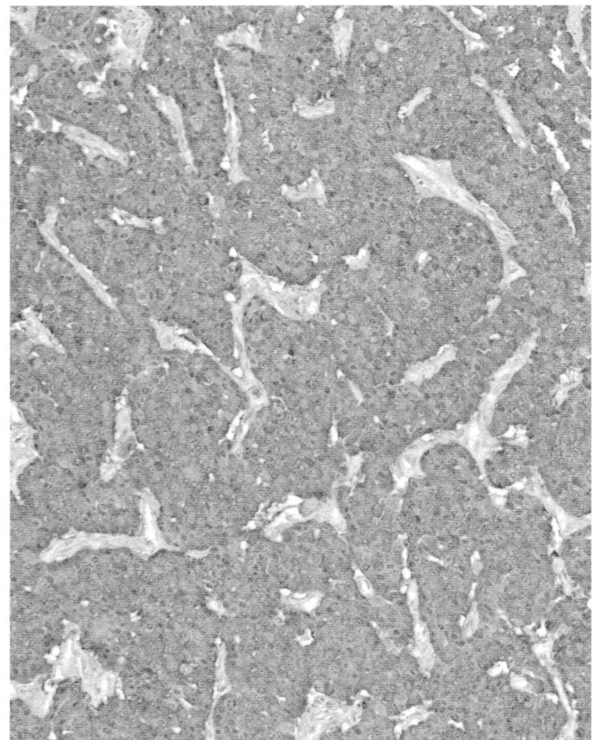

Fig. 18.62
Metastatic neuroendocrine carcinoma. **Positive chromogranin stain of tumor depicted in prior two illustrations**

a dominant clinical finding and in some instances have even accounted for the clinical presentation [125, 168].

Gross Findings

The ovarian disease is typically bilateral and often takes the form of solid nodules, characteristic of many examples of metastatic spread to the ovaries. However, the ovarian tumors can also be large, cystic, and multiloculated and sometimes unilateral, mimicking primary tumors (*Fig. 18.63*). Sectioning shows an appearance that may be indistinguishable from primary mucinous neoplasia, although in some cases surface nodules may be noted and raise suspicion for metastasis.

Microscopic Findings

In cases grossly represented by solid nodules, small glands randomly infiltrating in a desmoplastic stroma comprise the typical histologic appearance. In tumors that are grossly cystic, foci resembling mucinous cystadenoma, mucinous cystic tumor of borderline malignancy, and moderately or well-differentiated mucinous cystadenocarcinoma may be present (*Fig. 18.64*). However, foci of more obvious carcinoma, typical of the grossly solid tumors, are also often present (*Fig. 18.65*) but may be very minor in amount, and identification is very dependent on thorough sampling. In some cases, multifocal high-grade carcinoma randomly scattered among, and contrasting markedly with, much more indolent low-grade cystic neoplasia is a clue to the diagnosis. In both gross forms of disease, surface implants may be seen (*Fig. 18.66*). The maturation of epithelium in some of these cases is remarkable (*Fig. 18.67*), but high-power scrutiny of areas initially thought to represent benign neoplasia may show a degree of cytologic atypia disproportionate to the degree of architectural differentiation. Vascular invasion may be seen. The pancreatic tumors are usually typical ductal adenocarcinomas but are rarely mucinous cystadenocarcinomas.

Differential Diagnosis

A number of features are helpful in distinguishing between a primary and metastatic mucinous tumor in these cases and in other cases of metastatic mucinous carcinoma,

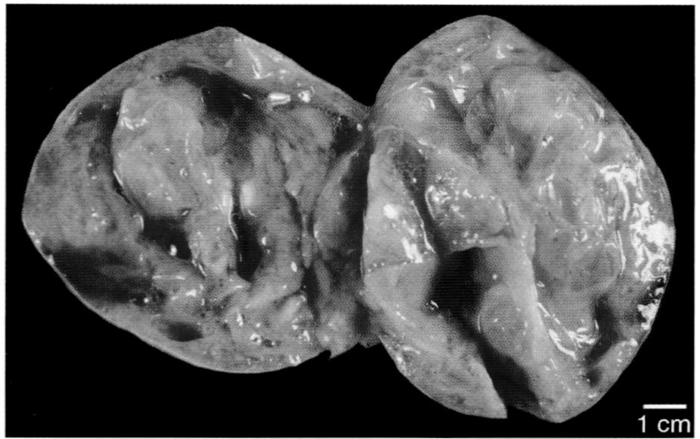

■ Fig. 18.63
Metastatic carcinoma from the pancreas. **The cystic tumor mimics a primary mucinous tumor**

irrespective of the primary site. Bilaterality of the ovarian tumors strongly favors metastasis. A helpful finding is the presence of desmoplastic implants of carcinoma on the ovarian surface and in the superficial ovarian cortex. The clinical findings often aid, and the frequent presence of intraabdominal spread is most consistent with secondary involvement of the ovary in cases of bilateral mucinous carcinomas. The heterogeneous picture noted in our microscopic description above may also be helpful. The reader is again referred to ➋ *Table 18.1.* We have recently added to it so-called mucin granulomas [68], which we feel are considerably more common in primary, compared to metastatic, mucinous tumors.

Immunohistochemistry is of limited utility for distinguishing metastatic pancreatic adenocarcinoma from a primary ovarian mucinous neoplasm. Both are usually CK7+ and show variable reactivity for CK20 (➋ *Fig. 18.68*) [91]. A lack of reactivity for Dpc4 suggests a pancreatic primary, since almost half of pancreatic adenocarcinomas

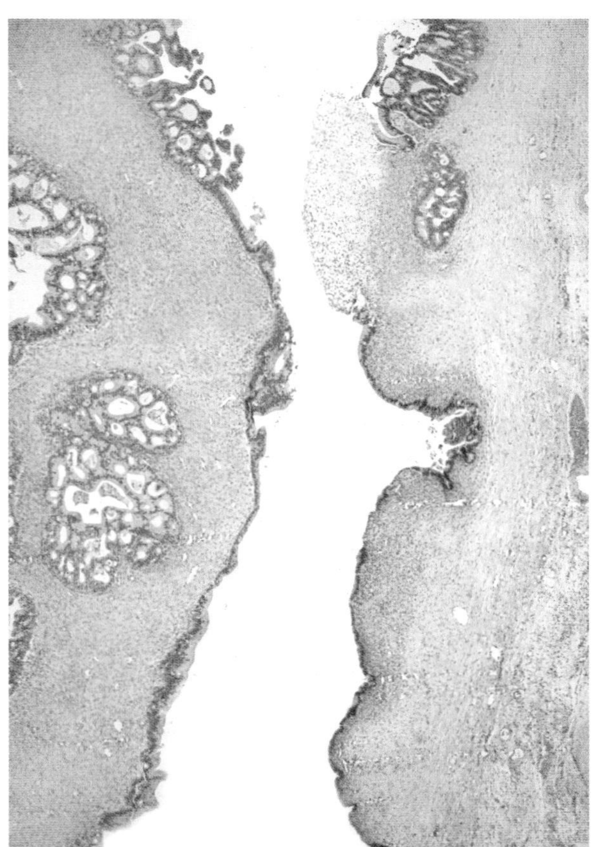

■ Fig. 18.64
Metastatic carcinoma from the pancreas. **The cystic nature and varied degree of differentiation are evident**

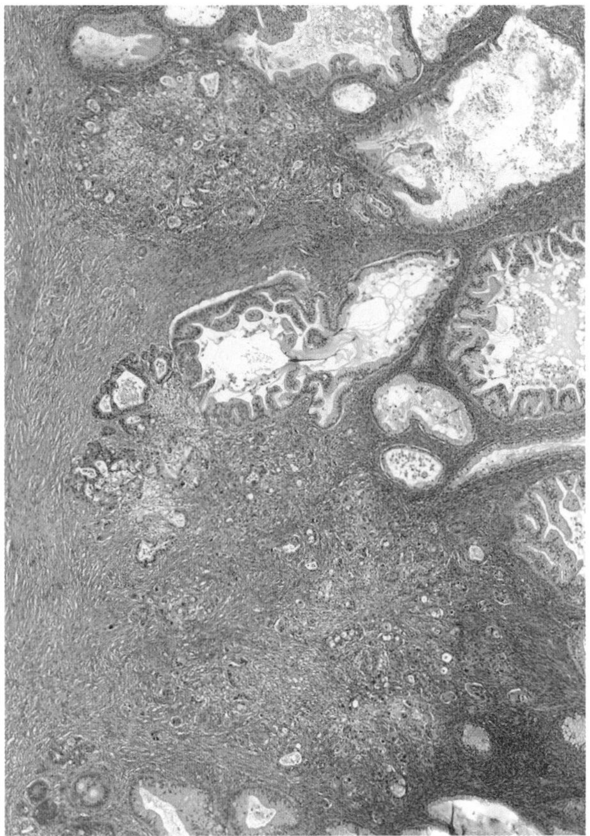

■ Fig. 18.65
Metastatic carcinoma from the pancreas. **Foci of high-grade carcinoma on background of more indolent morphology**

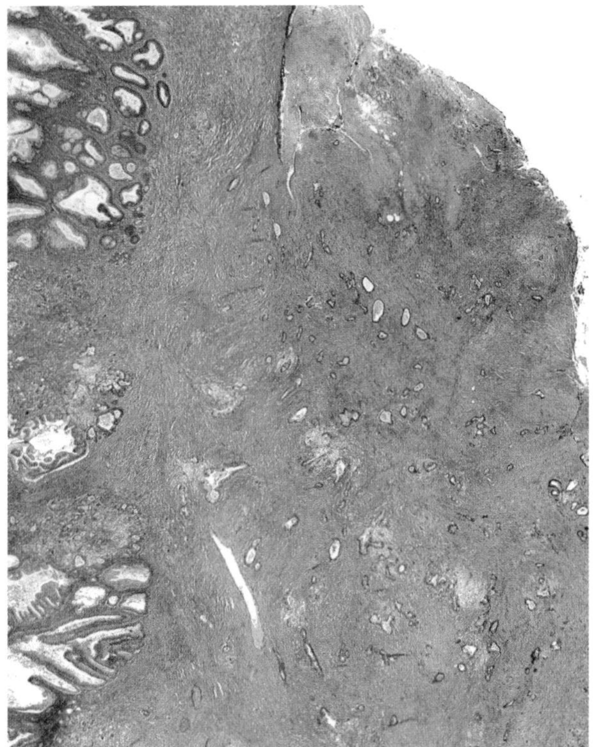

Fig. 18.66
Metastatic carcinoma from the pancreas. **Surface implant**

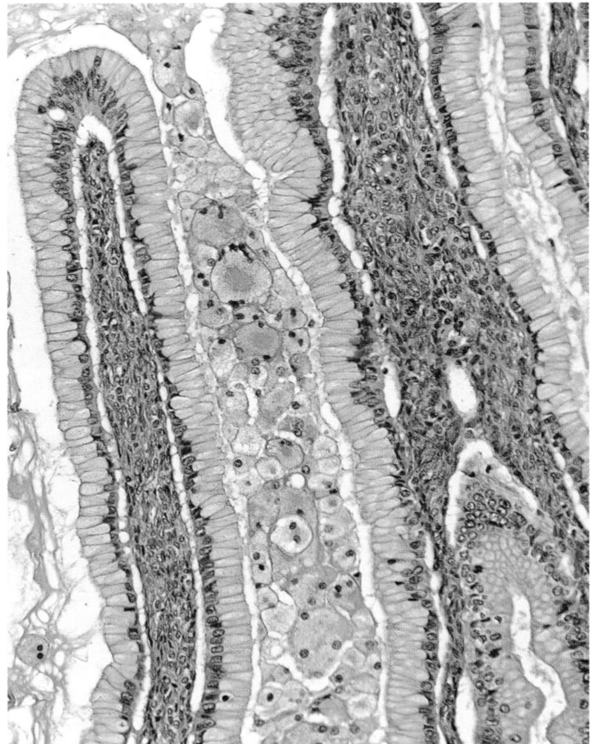

Fig. 18.67
Metastatic carcinoma from the pancreas. **Marked maturation of the neoplastic epithelium resulting in morphology indistinguishable from benign primary neoplasia**

show loss of this marker, whereas ovarian mucinous tumors express it [57]. However, a positive reaction for Dpc4 is obviously of no discriminatory value.

Acinar Cell Carcinoma

Four cases of ovarian spread of this carcinoma have been only recently reported, indicative of its rarity [146]. The patients were all adults, and in three of them the ovarian tumors were detected prior to the pancreatic neoplasm. In these three patients, however, the primary tumor became evident within a short period of time. Three patients also had involvement of sites other than the ovary or pancreas.

Gross Findings

The ovarian tumors, three of which were bilateral, had an average maximum dimension of about 7 cm, and were solid and firm for the most part, with only one showing "myxoid" degeneration.

Microscopic Findings

The neoplasms were characterized by solid nests and formations with lumina (*Fig. 18.69*), the latter ranging from small acini (*Fig. 18.70*) to larger tubules to even larger gland-like formations that were sometimes cystic (*Fig. 18.71*). There was little intervening stroma. Comedo-like necrosis was conspicuous in some cases. The tumor cells had abundant pale to eosinophilic, finely granular cytoplasm. Their nuclei were round with stippled chromatin and prominent nucleoli. The mitotic rate was typically brisk. Vascular invasion was seen in all cases. Immunostains showed positivity for chymotrypsin and trypsin in all cases (*Fig. 18.72*). Neuroendocrine stains were negative.

Differential Diagnosis

Because of the striking acinar differentiation, these tumors can be misdiagnosed as carcinoids or other forms of neuroendocrine neoplasia. Indeed, this initially happened in some of the reported cases. The at least focally brightly eosinophilic granular cytoplasm, reflecting the presence of zymogen granules, contrasts with the typical appearance of

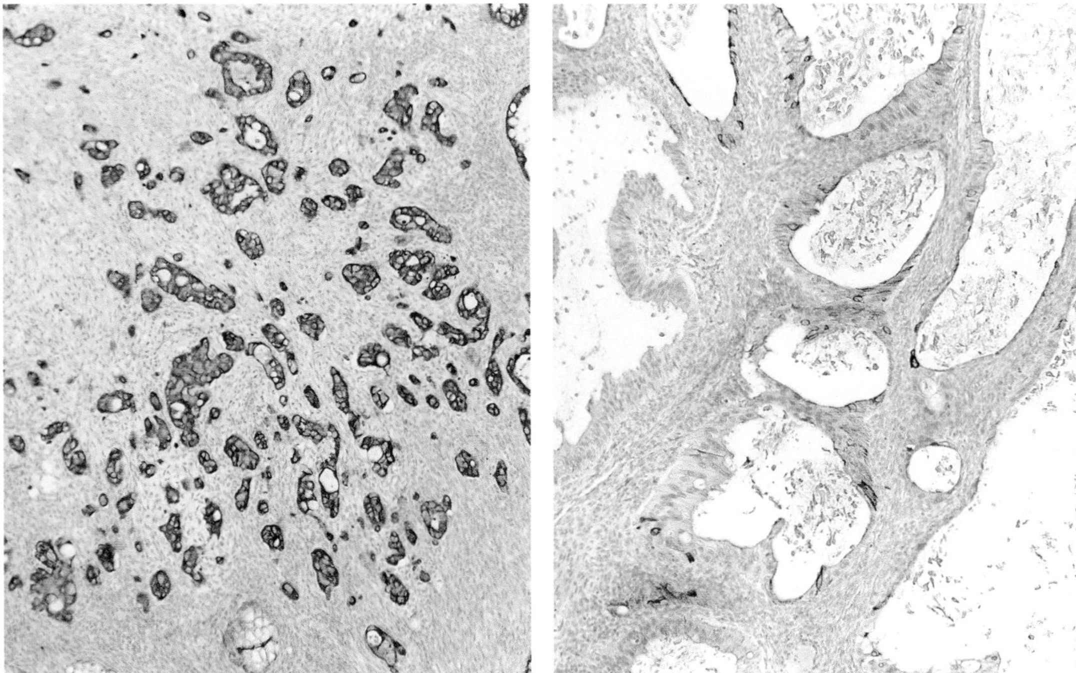

Fig. 18.68
Metastatic carcinoma from the pancreas. **Immunohistochemical stains show prominent CK7 staining (*left*) and more focal CK20 staining (*right*), as seen in many cases of this type**

the cytoplasm of neuroendocrine neoplasms. Acinar carcinoma cells also lack the typical "salt and pepper" chromatin of the latter. The large prominent single nucleolus typifying most of the acinar carcinoma cells is also a noteworthy difference. These contrasting features notwithstanding, the immunohistochemical differences noted above may play an important role in diagnosis. Other rare issues in differential diagnosis, such as consideration of Sertoli cell tumor, may also be aided by immunohistochemistry, and this and other aspects have elaborated in detail recently by Vakiani et al. [146].

Other Pancreatic Neoplasms

Rare islet cell carcinomas have spread to the ovaries [105, 113]. In the most recent case reported, a 41-year-old woman presented with hirsutism, Cushing's syndrome, and a pelvic mass. Work-up disclosed a primary pancreatic neuroendocrine neoplasm with bilateral solid and cystic metastatic tumors in the ovary [105].

Tumors of the Gall Bladder and Extrahepatic Bile Ducts

Sporadic examples of this phenomenon have been reported over the years [178], usually as isolated case reports, but Khunamornpong and colleagues [63] have recently reported the largest series whose features reflect the overall experience.

Their 16 cases occurred in patients from 21 to 87 (mean 59) years. Almost half the patients presented with gynecologic manifestations. The remaining patients had the usual symptoms attributable to biliary neoplasia.

Gross Findings

All but one ovarian tumor was bilateral. Most ovaries showed grossly evident disease with a mean size of 9.4 cm. The cut surfaces were variable, most often solid and cystic but sometimes uniformly solid and in five instances, multicystic.

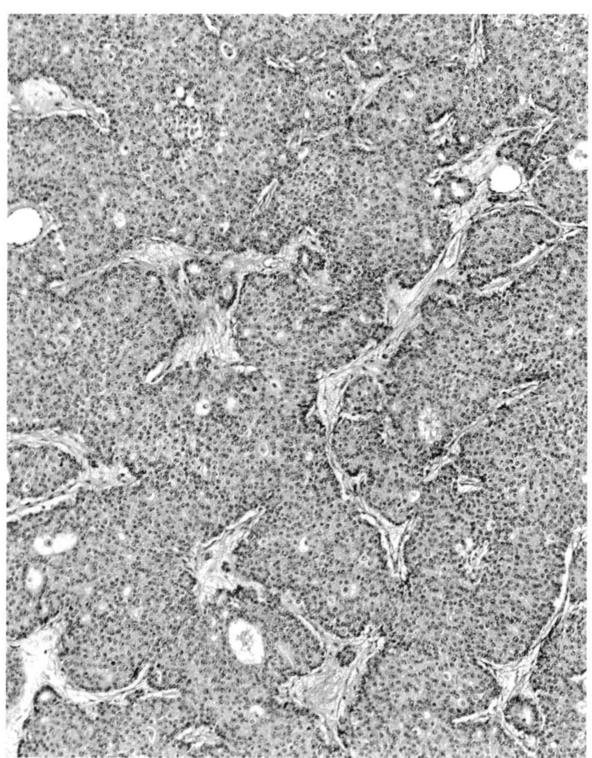

Fig. 18.69
Metastatic acinar cell carcinoma of the pancreas. **Islands of tumor cells contain numerous small acini. The tumor mimics a carcinoid tumor**

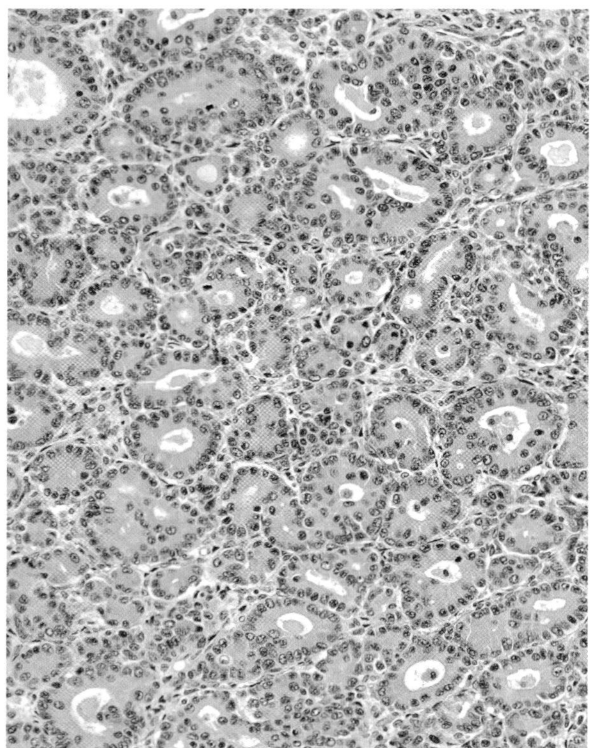

Fig. 18.70
Metastatic acinar cell carcinoma of the pancreas. **High-power view of typical small acini**

Microscopic Findings

The multinodular growth that typifies many examples of metastasis was seen in about 60% of the cases, and surface implants were seen in two thirds (*Fig. 18.73*). The overall features were similar to other cases of metastatic adenocarcinoma from various abdominal sites, including pancreas and colon. For example, a differentiated mucinous morphology as seen with pancreatic primaries was observed in some cases, whereas others showed a colloid (*Fig. 18.74*) or pseudoendometrioid morphology more typical of colonic metastases. Signet-ring cells justified the diagnosis of Krukenberg tumor in four cases.

Differential Diagnosis

This is broadly similar to that of other metastases from abdominal sites, with no unique features being evident other than the clinical determination of the primary site. Three tumors in the above series were hilar cholangiocarcinomas, five common bile duct carcinomas, and eight gallbladder carcinomas. Like primary ovarian mucinous neoplasms and other adenocarcinomas of the pancreatobiliary tract, these tumors tend to be CK7+ and show variable expression for CK20+ [63], so the cytokeratin profile does not provide discriminatory information.

Tumors of the Liver

Hepatocellular Carcinoma

The spread of hepatocellular carcinoma to the ovary is even rarer than that of pancreatic and biliary tumors, but five clinically important cases have been reported [64, 165]. The patients have all been adults. In two patients, bilateral ovarian tumors were discovered at the same time as the liver primary. In another patient, the liver tumor was discovered by radiologic investigation after bilateral

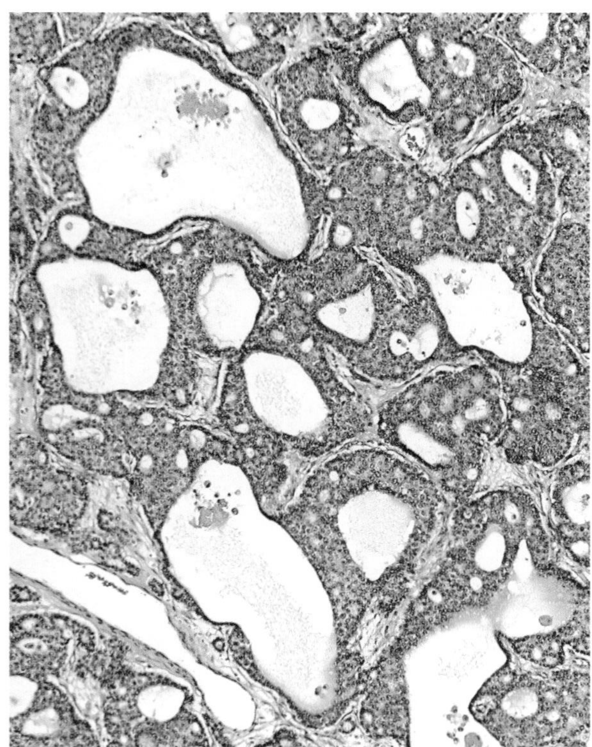

Fig. 18.71
Metastatic acinar cell carcinoma of the pancreas. **Cysts are conspicuous**

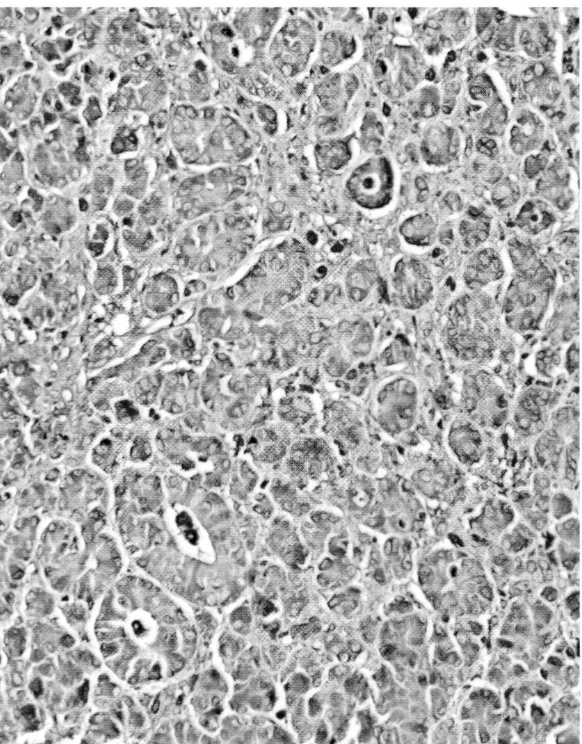

Fig. 18.72
Metastatic acinar cell carcinoma of the pancreas. **Immunoreactivity for chymotrypsin**

ovarian tumors had been removed. In the other two cases, unilateral ovarian tumors were discovered 3 and 7 months, respectively, after the liver tumors had been detected.

Pathologic Findings

The ovarian neoplasms ranged from 4 to 11 cm in diameter and three of them were solid. A green color may be a clue to the diagnosis (*Fig. 18.75*). Microscopic examination revealed features typical of metastatic disease, such as striking surface involvement in some cases (*Fig. 18.76*), and overall findings characteristic of hepatocellular carcinoma, except in one case in which cysts were prominent. A trabecular pattern is sometimes conspicuous, and the neoplastic cells almost invariably have moderate to abundant eosinophilic cytoplasm (*Figs. 18.77* and *18.78*).

Differential Diagnosis

The major differential diagnosis in these cases involves both primary and metastatic hepatoid tumors of the ovary. In most cases of hepatoid yolk sac tumor, the finding of foci of more typical yolk sac neoplasia or other germ cell elements excludes the diagnosis of metastatic hepatocellular carcinoma, and the young age of the patient will argue against the latter diagnosis. In a postmenopausal patient, the differential diagnosis involves hepatoid carcinoma rather than hepatoid yolk sac tumor. Hepatoid carcinomas usually contain foci of more typical surface epithelial carcinoma, typically serous. Bilaterality and other characteristic patterns of metastatic spread to the ovary may be helpful in indicating the metastatic nature of a tumor. Hepatoid carcinomas may also arise outside the ovary, for example in the stomach and lung, and may potentially metastasize to the ovary, although we are not aware of documented examples. HepPAR1 is not useful in distinguishing among metastatic hepatocellular carcinoma, hepatoid yolk sac tumor, and hepatoid ovarian carcinoma as it is expressed in all [115].

Intrahepatic Cholangiocarcinoma

Particularly in the Far East, spread of intrahepatic cholangiocarcinoma to the ovary is seen with some

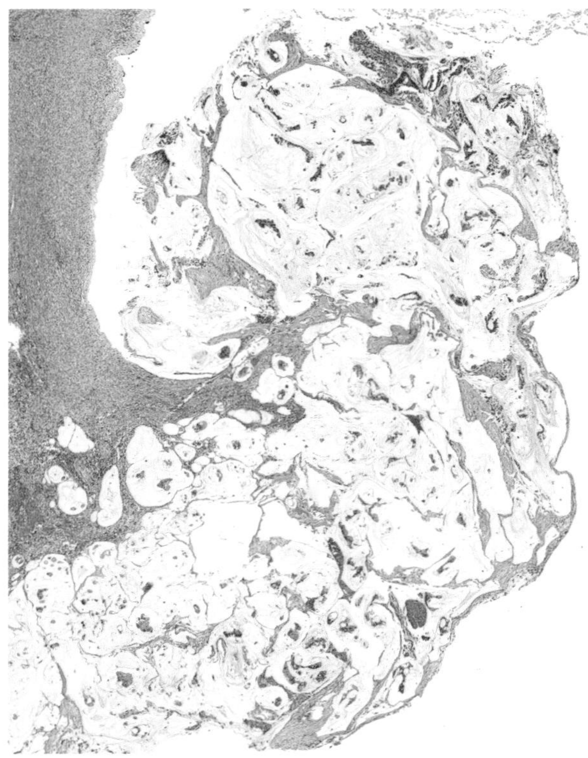

Fig. 18.73
Metastatic biliary tract carcinoma. **Surface involvement by colloid carcinoma**

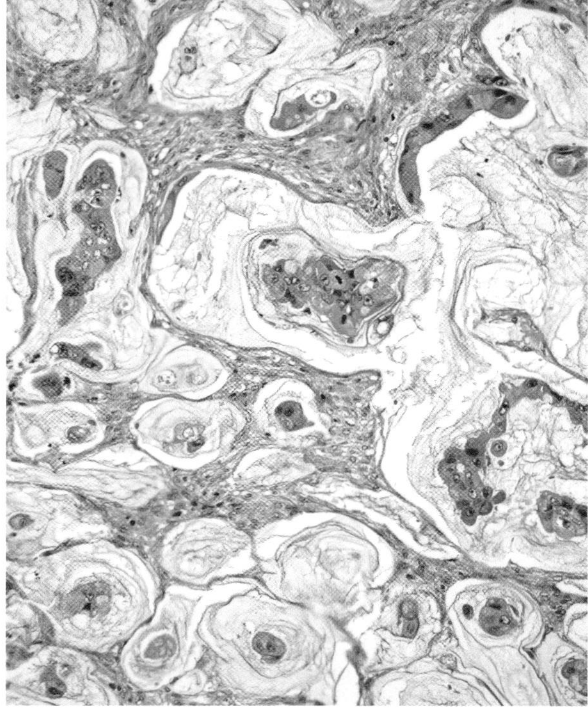

Fig. 18.74
Metastatic biliary tract carcinoma. **This tumor has a striking colloid morphology**

frequency because of the high incidence of that form of cancer due to endemic infestation with the trematode *Opisthorchis viverrini.* Only rarely has this tumor been documented to spread to the ovary in other parts of the world. A series of 16 cases has significantly expanded information on this topic [65].

Pathologic Findings

About two-thirds of these cases have been bilateral in the ovaries, and they have had a mean size of about 12 cm. The majority of tumors have been solid and cystic, but almost half have been cystic and the remainder uniformly solid. Microscopic examination showed a quite varied morphology, but typical features of metastatic disease were generally present, including prominent nodules, or at least a vague multinodular pattern (*Fig. 18.79*). In some cases striking maturation with a cystic pattern was seen (*Fig. 18.80*). Occasionally small micropapillae were encountered (*Fig. 18.81*). In many cases there was a degree of cytologic atypia that was discordant with the degree of glandular differentiation, a finding that can be

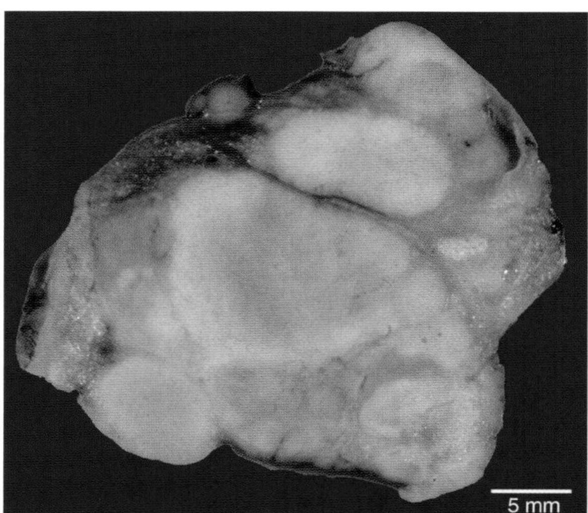

Fig. 18.75
Metastatic hepatocellular carcinoma. **Multiple nodules are visible on the sectioned surface of a yellow-green tumor**

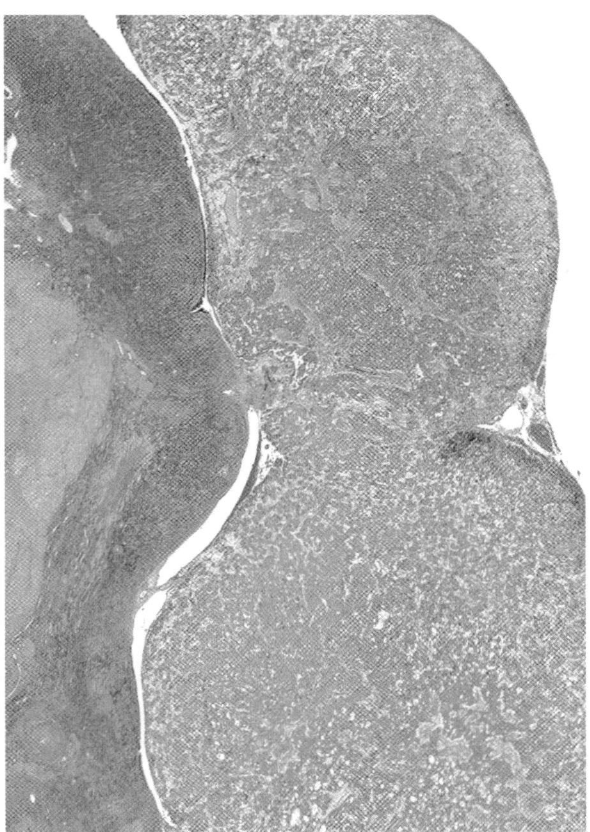

Fig. 18.76
Metastatic hepatocellular carcinoma. **Prominent surface involvement**

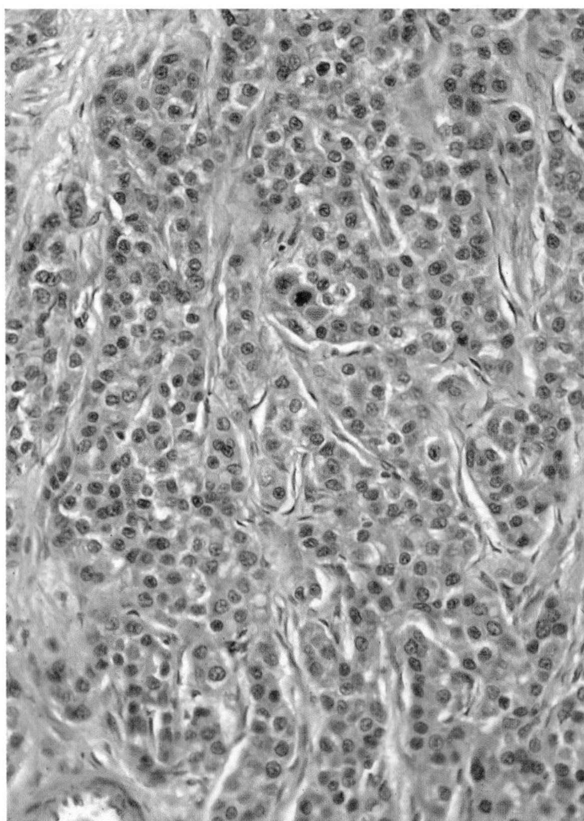

Fig. 18.77
Metastatic hepatocellular carcinoma. **Tumor cells with eosinophilic cytoplasm are arranged in trabeculae. Note the presence of bile (Reproduced with permission from Ref. [162])**

a subtle clue to the diagnosis of metastatic adenocarcinoma (*Fig. 18.82*).

Other Rare Neoplasms

A hepatoblastoma that occurred in a 19-year-old woman and was associated with bilateral ovarian metastases at presentation has been reported [40].

Breast Carcinoma

Ovarian involvement is seen at autopsy in about 10% of cases of breast cancer. The metastases are bilateral in approximately 80% of those cases and in approximately two thirds of all cases, autopsy and surgical combined. Most surgical pathology experience with ovarian metastases of mammary carcinoma has resulted from examination of ovaries removed to decrease the estrogen level in patients with known spread of the tumor [88]. In such cases, ovarian involvement has been reported in up to half the cases but is often only a microscopic finding.

It is unusual for metastatic carcinoma of the breast to produce signs or symptoms of an ovarian tumor, and only rarely is the ovarian metastasis evident before the primary tumor is detected [35, 163]. In one large series, breast carcinoma accounted for almost 40% of all metastases to the ovary, being slightly more common than gastrointestinal tract metastases [35]. However, 22 of the 59 breast metastases were autopsy findings, and 28 were incidental findings in therapeutic oophorectomy specimens. In four of the remaining nine cases, the ovarian metastases were incidental findings during an operation for another indication; in the remaining five patients, however, the ovarian

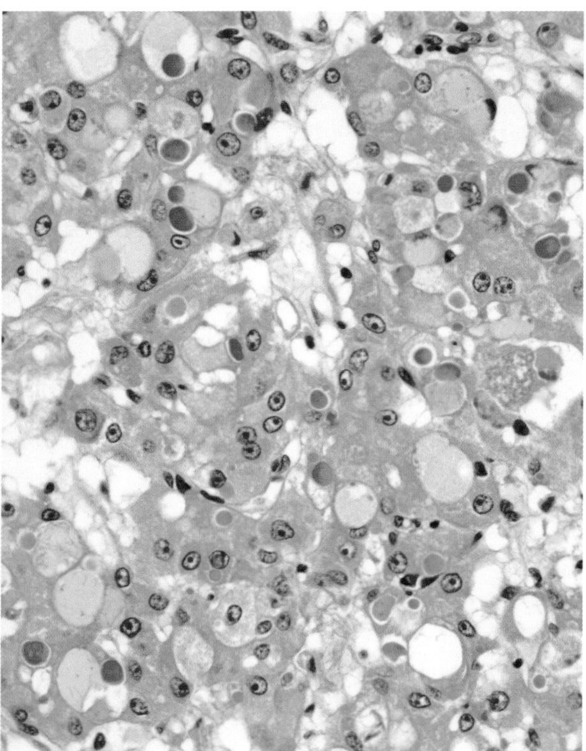

Fig. 18.78
Metastatic hepatocellular carcinoma. **The neoplastic cells have abundant eosinophilic cytoplasm. There are scattered hyaline droplets**

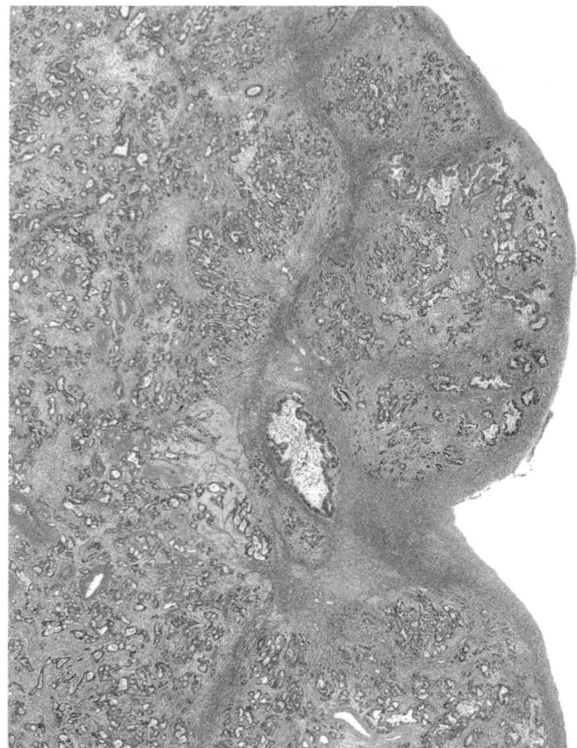

Fig. 18.79
Metastatic intrahepatic cholangiocarcinoma. **There is a vague multinodular pattern**

metastases caused a mass of sufficient size to be the clinical indication for operation. The ovarian metastatic tumor was detected before the breast cancer in only one case. This patient presented with hepatic and ovarian tumors, and her primary breast cancer was not identified until 15 months later. The median interval between the diagnosis of breast cancer and the ovarian metastasis was 11.5 months and was related to the stage of the breast cancer. The median survival after the diagnosis of ovarian metastasis was 16 months. One patient with metastatic breast carcinoma in the ovaries presented 10 years after initial treatment of the breast cancer, as a result of virilization caused by stromal luteinization associated with the ovarian metastasis [18]. Although ovarian metastases of breast cancer are usually accompanied by other foci of abdominal spread, isolated ovarian metastases occasionally are encountered. Lobular carcinomas, including those of signet-ring cell type, spread to the ovary more frequently than those of ductal type; in an autopsy study 36% of the former metastasized to the ovaries in contrast to only 2.6% of the latter [43].

Gross Findings

On gross examination, the visibly involved ovaries often have irregular, nodular surfaces and typically contain firm or gritty, white to yellow nodules of various sizes (*Fig. 18.83*). When the organ is replaced by tumor, it is transformed into a smooth-surfaced or bosselated mass; exceptionally, it contains cysts and very rarely it is entirely cystic. When all cases are considered, tumors larger than 5 cm are uncommon, accounting for only 15% of the cases in one large study [35].

Microscopic Findings

Microscopic examination reveals the same variety of patterns and cell types that are observed in primary breast carcinomas. In early examples, small cords and clusters of cells may be found in the ovarian cortex. In premenopausal women, small deposits often are situated in the highly vascular theca interna of a graafian follicle or in the

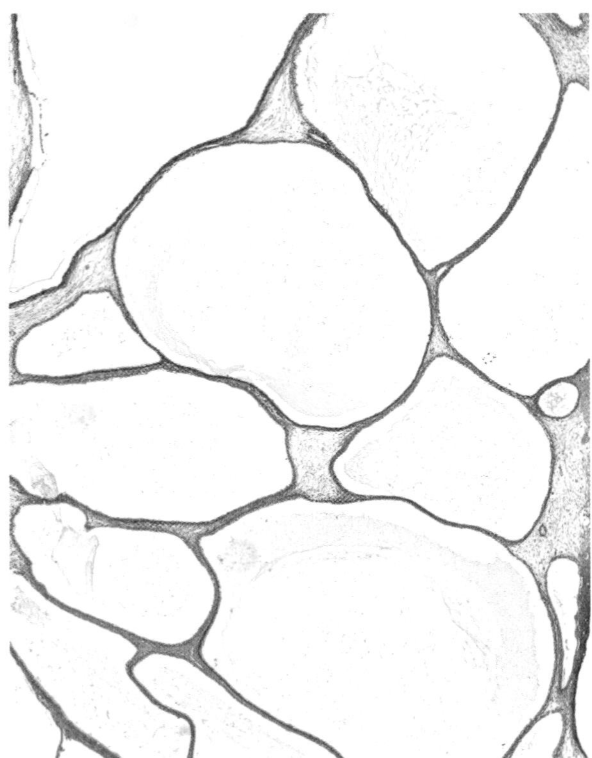

■ Fig. 18.80
Metastatic intrahepatic cholangiocarcinoma. **There is striking maturation with a resultant deceptively benign cystic pattern**

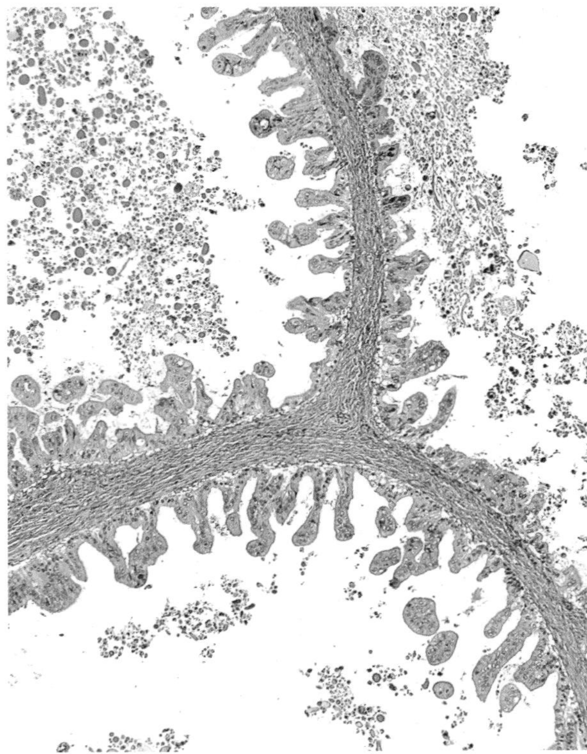

■ Fig. 18.81
Metastatic intrahepatic cholangiocarcinoma. **Micropapillary pattern**

granulosa or theca layer of a corpus luteum. Surface tumor may be seen (➋ *Fig. 18.84*) but is generally not as conspicuous as in metastatic tumors from the abdominal viscera. Multinodular growth may be striking (➋ *Fig. 18.85*). A pattern of tubular glands and nests similar to that of ductal carcinoma is common (➋ *Figs. 18.86* and ➋ *18.87*), as is the single-file pattern of lobular carcinoma (➋ *Fig. 18.88*); such patterns were seen in 42 and 32% of the cases, respectively, in one series [35]. A pure cribriform pattern is infrequent but focal cribriform areas are relatively common. In approximately 10% of the cases, there is a diffuse pattern, and occasionally the tumor cells grow as single cells or in clusters. Rarely, papillae are seen and equally uncommonly there is a striking oxyphilic appearance. Admixtures of these various patterns may occur. Signet-ring cells usually are not a conspicuous feature of metastatic breast carcinoma unless the primary tumor is of the relatively uncommon signet-ring type but, rarely, the features of a metastatic breast cancer are those of a Krukenberg tumor (➋ *Fig. 18.89*). The stroma of the tumor varies from sparse to abundant; it rarely shows luteinization in contrast to the stroma of metastatic carcinomas of intestinal origin. Lymphatic invasion was seen in 15% of the cases in one series [35].

Differential Diagnosis

The differential diagnosis of metastatic breast carcinoma may be difficult, particularly if the primary tumor is remote, not apparent, or its existence is not known by the pathologist. Rare, predominantly glandular tumors may resemble surface epithelial tumors, particularly those of endometrioid type, and the insular pattern may mimic a carcinoid tumor. Exceptionally, a tumor with a diffuse pattern or one with a single-file arrangement of the cells simulates a lymphoma or granulocytic sarcoma. Metastatic breast carcinomas also have been misinterpreted as granulosa cell tumors. The growth patterns and characteristics of the neoplastic cells and the clinical features, however, almost always permit their distinction from these and other tumors, but this is

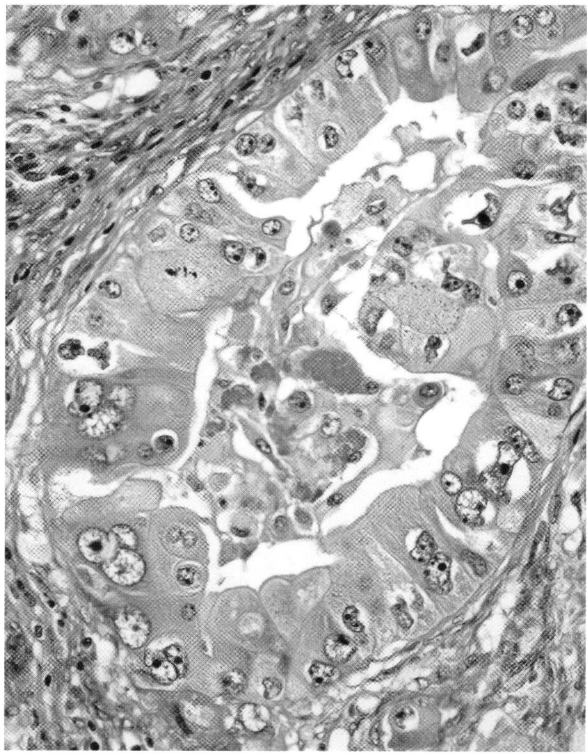

Fig. 18.82
Metastatic intrahepatic cholangiocarcinoma. **Striking atypia of cells lining a gland**

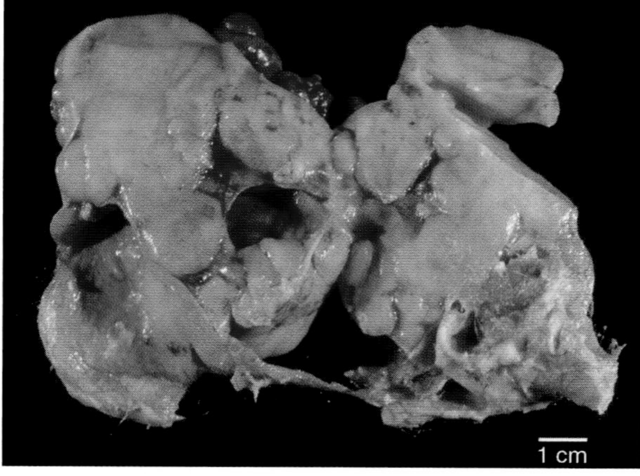

Fig. 18.83
Metastatic breast cancer. **The sectioned surface shows a lobulated yellow-white neoplasm. This tumor spread to an ovary involved by a dermoid cyst, which is evident in the picture**

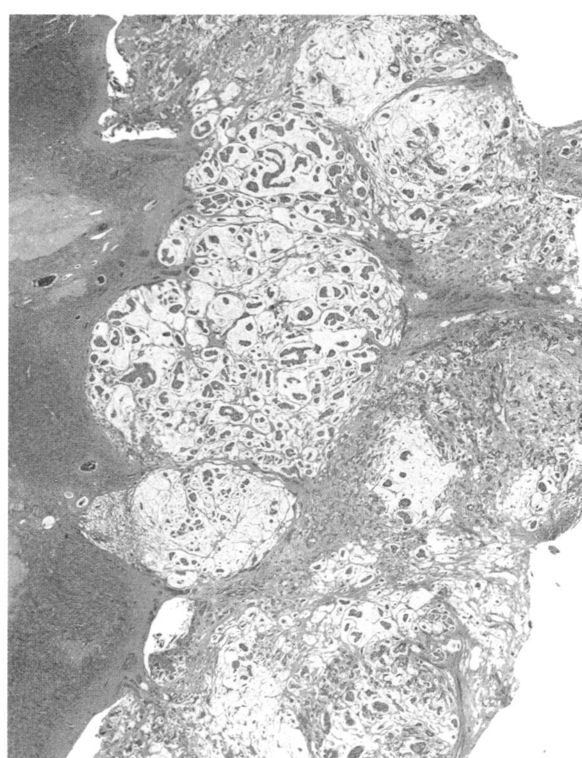

Fig. 18.84
Metastatic breast cancer. **Prominent surface involvement by a metastatic mucinous adenocarcinoma**

occasionally difficult on the evaluation of routinely stained sections alone. It should be remembered that patients with breast cancer have an increased frequency of ovarian carcinoma [24], especially those patients harboring BRCA mutations, and rarely ovarian carcinoma metastasizes to the breast.

Staining of an ovarian neoplasm immunohistochemically for gross cystic disease fluid protein-15 (GCDFP-15) (*Fig. 18.90*) may be helpful in distinguishing a metastasis from the breast from a primary ovarian carcinoma [101]. Between 40 and 70% of breast carcinomas metastatic to the ovary have been reported to be positive for GCDFP-15, whereas primary ovarian carcinomas are almost always negative [80, 141, 154]. GCDFP-15 expression in breast carcinoma is usually strong but focal. Mammoglobin is another marker of breast origin that is expressed in about 50% of breast carcinomas (*Fig. 18.91*) [10, 127]. It appears to show greater sensitivity but less specificity for breast origin than GCDFP-15. Mammoglobin expression has been demonstrated in rare ovarian serous carcinomas; its expression in other subtypes of ovarian carcinoma has not been

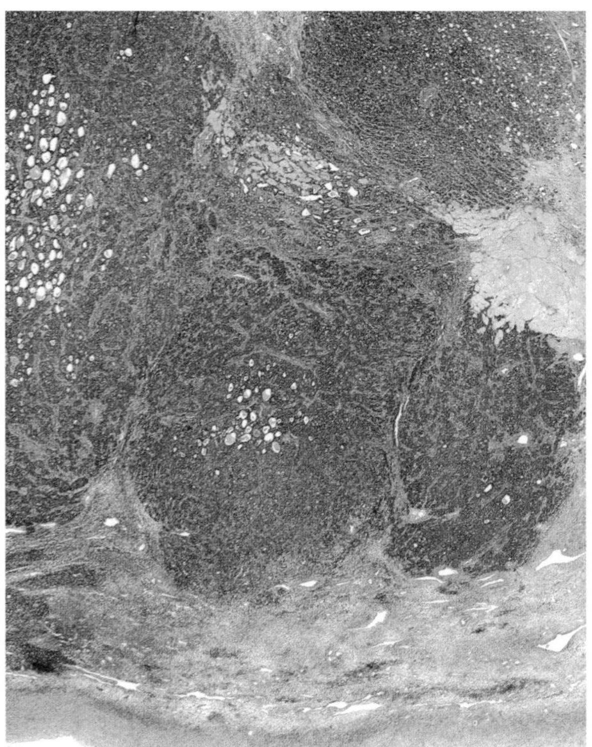

■ Fig. 18.85
Metastatic breast carcinoma. **Multinodular pattern**

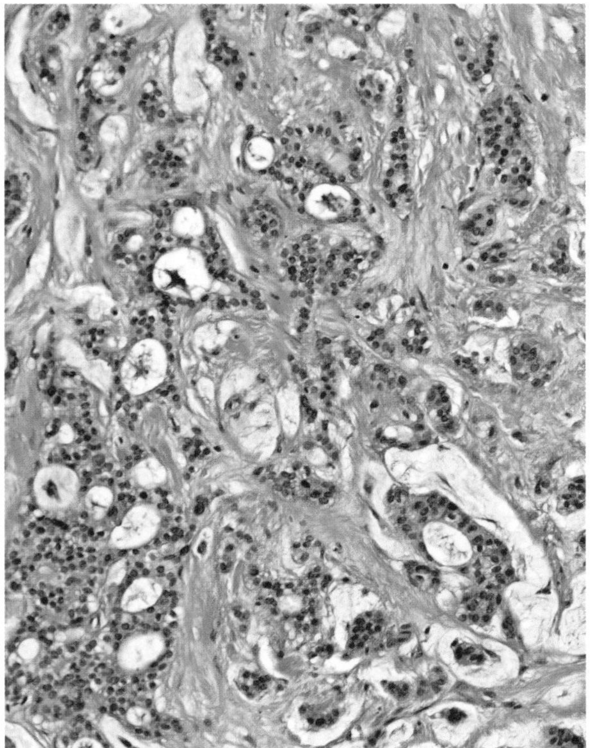

■ Fig. 18.86
Metastatic breast carcinoma. **Small glands typical of ductal carcinoma**

extensively studied, but it is noteworthy that mammoglobin is frequently positive in endometrioid carcinomas of the uterine corpus [10, 109].

Other markers are commonly expressed in primary ovarian carcinomas but not breast carcinomas. WT-1 is positive in >80% of serous and transitional cell carcinomas of the ovary, but it is only very exceptionally positive in breast carcinomas [77, 80, 102, 104, 141]. Similarly, mesothelin is frequently expressed in ovarian carcinomas but not breast carcinomas; its expression in the former, however, may be focal [45, 60]. In a tissue microarray study, nonmucinous ovarian carcinomas were immunoreactive for PAX-8 in greater than 88% of cases; 243 breast carcinoma samples were negative [104]. CA-125 reactivity may occur in either ovarian or breast carcinomas, but the latter express this antigen much less frequently [80, 102, 141]. As in other settings, when necessary, a panel of immunohistochemical stains is recommended as no currently available individual marker is entirely specific for breast or ovarian origin.

Finally, in cases of ovarian involvement by the intraabdominal desmoplastic small round cell tumor [164], the diagnosis of metastatic breast cancer may be suggested in areas. However, these patients usually are in their teens, when breast cancer is rare, and other more characteristic foci of the tumor and its typical immunohistochemical profile facilitate the interpretation. We have seen one case in which this tumor involved the breast, confusing the picture, but the breast involvement suggested metastasis and the tumor exhibited the characteristic immunohistochemical staining of the desmoplastic small round cell tumor.

Renal Tumors

Renal cell carcinoma rarely spreads to the ovary, with only 15 cases of clinically detectable ovarian metastatic tumors reported in detail [53, 133, 150, 169]. In seven of the cases, the ovarian tumor was discovered first, leading to the initial misdiagnosis of primary ovarian clear cell carcinoma in three cases. The renal tumors were usually detected within a short period of time in these patients, but in one the renal primary was not detected until 8 years

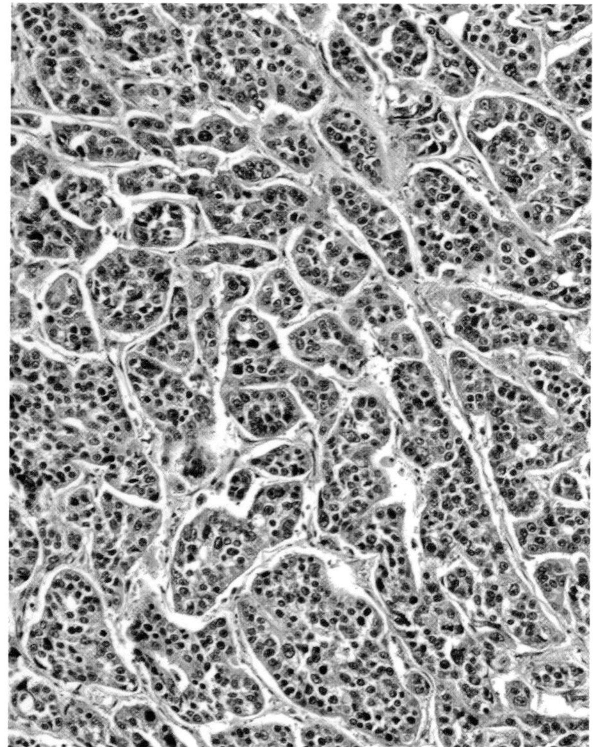

Fig. 18.87
Metastatic breast carcinoma. **Insular pattern**

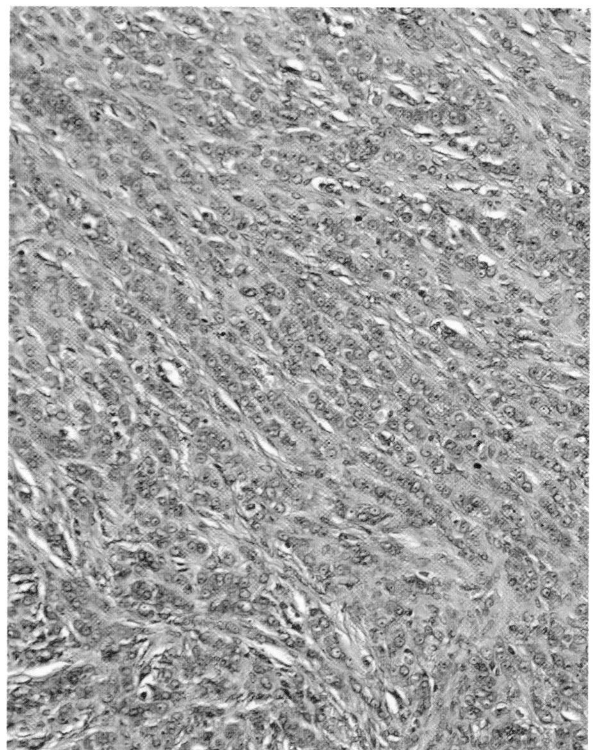

Fig. 18.88
Metastatic breast carcinoma. **Growth in cords typical of metastatic lobular carcinoma**

later. In the other cases the ovarian tumor was usually detected within 2 years after the renal tumors had been removed, but in one case the interval was 14 years.

Gross Findings

The ovarian tumors, only a minority of which were bilateral, were often large (average 12.5 cm in greatest dimension), and were either solid or solid and cystic, with one cystic tumor being unilocular and containing a 2.5 cm solid nodule in one area. The solid components of the tumors were either uniformly or focally yellow to orange (*Fig. 18.92*).

Microscopic Findings

With one possible exception the reported renal tumors were well-differentiated clear cell adenocarcinomas; microscopic examination showed a relatively uniform picture of diffuse sheets of clear cells or tubules lined by similar cells and containing eosinophilic material or blood; a prominent sinusoidal vascular pattern was almost always present (*Fig. 18.93*).

Differential Diagnosis

It is helpful in differential diagnosis that primary clear cell carcinoma of the ovary has a tubulocystic and papillary component, hobnail cells, and intraluminal mucin in the great majority of cases. Hobnail cells and conspicuous mucin production, in contrast, are exceptional in renal cell carcinomas. In addition, the typical sinusoidal vascular framework of renal cell carcinoma is not a feature of ovarian clear cell carcinoma. In cases of pure clear cell carcinoma of the ovary without hobnail cells or mucin secretion, radiologic evaluation of the kidney may rarely be necessary to exclude a renal cell carcinoma. A panel of antibodies may aid in evaluation: ovarian clear cell carcinomas are usually positive for CK7 and mesothelin and negative for CD10 and renal cell carcinoma marker (RCCma), whereas renal clear cell carcinomas often demonstrate the opposite immunoprofile

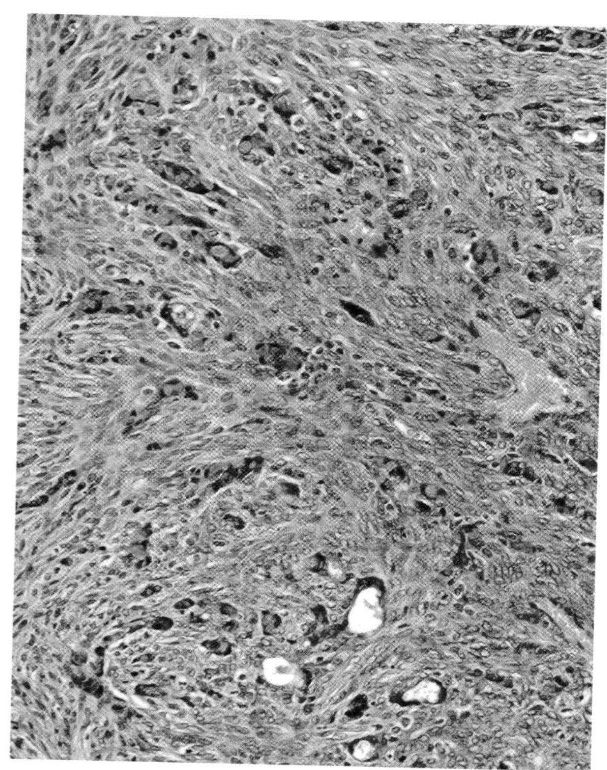

Fig. 18.89
Metastatic breast carcinoma. **This tumor had a signet-ring cell component qualifying it as a Krukenberg tumor**

(CK7-/mesothelin-/CD10+/RCCma+) (Fig. 18.94) [16, 79, 107]. Although PAX-2 may be a somewhat more sensitive marker than RCCma for metastatic renal cell carcinoma, it should be noted that about 40% of ovarian clear cell carcinomas also express this protein [36].

Renal transitional cell tumors rarely spread to the ovary, but exceptionally a patient with a renal pelvic tumor of this type has an ovarian metastasis at the time of presentation [52, 108]. Ovarian metastases from Wilms' tumor of the kidney are rare and no examples are present in several large series of this neoplasm. In one remarkable case, a patient with a rhabdoid tumor of the kidney presented with an ovarian metastasis, initially misinterpreted as a granulosa cell tumor, the primary renal tumor being undiscovered until autopsy [172].

Tumors of the Urinary Bladder, Ureter, and Urethra

Tumors from these sites uncommonly metastasize to the ovaries. Three signet-ring cell carcinomas metastatic from the bladder have had the appearance of a Krukenberg tumor [176]. In one of them the ovarian tumor was an autopsy finding and in another the ovarian involvement was an incidental finding on microscopic examination. In the third case, the ovarian metastatic tumor, which was symptomatic, was not discovered until 7 years after the primary bladder tumor had been resected. A small number of urachal adenocarcinomas have formed metastatic mucinous cystic tumors in the ovary [106, 159]. Only isolated examples of ovarian metastasis of ureteral or urethral cancer have been reported in the literature.

In many cases of possible transitional cell carcinoma metastatic to the ovary, it is difficult to distinguish between a metastatic tumor and a borderline or malignant Brenner tumor or independent primary transitional cell carcinoma of the ovary [132, 176]. In almost all borderline or malignant Brenner tumors, however, foci of typical benign Brenner tumor also can be found and the presence of associated benign mucinous elements also favors the diagnosis of a Brenner tumor. The extent of invasion of the primary extraovarian tumor, and the general features of metastatic involvement of the ovary, all have to be considered in the evaluation of these cases. The metastatic transitional cell carcinoma in the series of Ulbright et al. [145] was cystic, exemplifying the great propensity of ovarian metastases from various sites to undergo cystic change.

Transitional cell carcinomas of the bladder are often positive for CK20, uroplakin III, and thrombomodulin; they are typically negative for WT-1 [85]. Primary ovarian transitional cell carcinomas, on the other hand, are usually negative for CK20, uncommonly express uroplakin III and thrombomodulin, and are frequently positive for WT-1. This difference in immunoprofile supports that the shared histologic features of the two tumors do not indicate a shared histogenesis, and that primary ovarian transitional cell carcinomas are variants of surface epithelial neoplasia. Interestingly, Brenner tumors show a high frequency of uroplakin III and thrombomodulin expression, suggesting true urothelial differentiation in these tumors [85].

Adrenal Gland Tumors

Neuroblastoma spreads to the ovary more frequently than other tumors of the adrenal gland. From 25 to 50% females with neuroblastoma have ovarian involvement at autopsy [98]. Clinically significant metastases during life are rare but documented [136, 172]. Rarely, neuroblastoma is primary in the ovary, and such tumors must be distinguished from metastatic neuroblastomas.

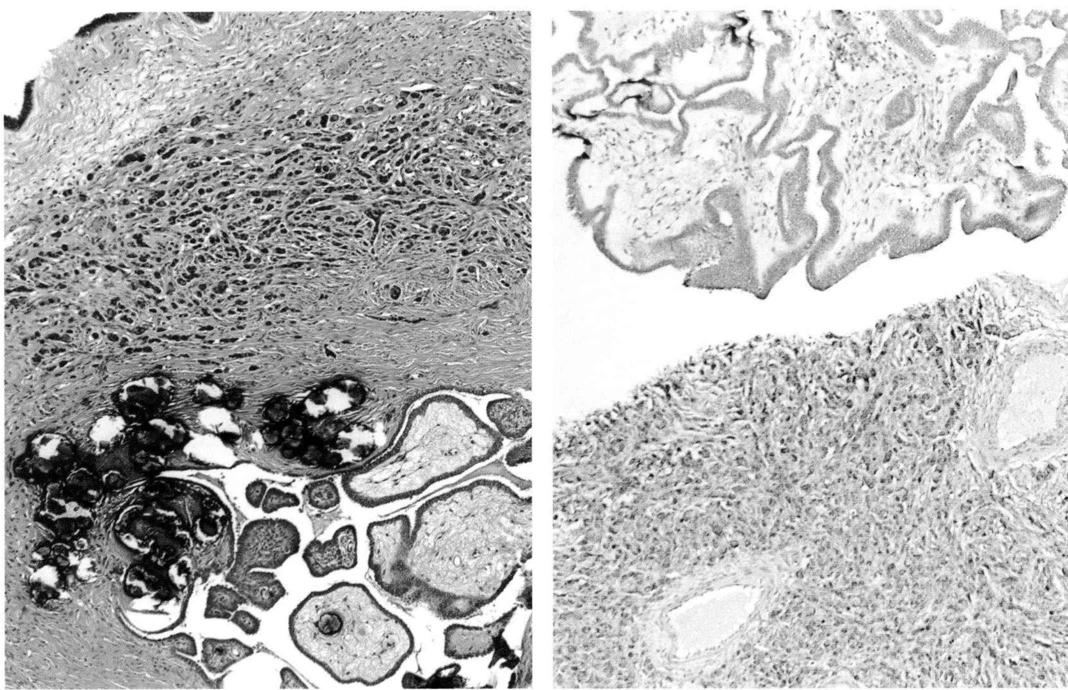

Fig. 18.90
Metastatic carcinoma to a serous neoplasm. **Confirmation that the infiltrating carcinoma was metastatic carcinoma from the breast rather than a component of the primary serous neoplasm was aided by positive immunohistochemical staining of the breast cancer for gross cystic disease fluid protein-15 (*right*)**

The unilaterality of the primary tumors, their occasional association with a teratoma, and the absence of a known primary tumor elsewhere are helpful in the differential diagnosis in individual cases. The prominent fibrillary background of neuroblastoma and the presence of pseudorosettes should aid in the distinction of metastatic neuroblastoma from other metastatic small cell tumors; immunohistochemical staining also may help in a case in which routine stains are not diagnostic.

Metastases of adrenal cortical carcinomas to the ovary are rarely found even at autopsy. One non-autopsy case resulted in the broad differential of a malignant oxyphilic ovarian tumor [74]. Pheochromocytomas spread to the ovary even less commonly; a review of the literature has failed to disclose a documented case.

Malignant Melanoma

Autopsies of patients who died of malignant melanoma have revealed ovarian involvement in about 20% of the cases. Most of the tumors have originated in the skin, but occasional examples have arisen in the choroid or elsewhere. Occasionally ovarian involvement is clinically symptomatic, as exemplified by many of the 52 cases in three relatively large series of melanomas metastatic to the ovary [34, 41, 180]. The patients in these reports had an average age of 38 years and two were teenagers. The usual presentation is abdominal swelling or pain, but a history of melanoma is usually existent, albeit not always immediately made known to the pathologist. Approximately 80% of the patients have metastatic tumor outside the ovary, usually within the pelvis and upper abdomen.

Gross Findings

The ovarian tumors average 10 cm in diameter; about 30% are noted to be black (➲ *Fig. 18.95*) or brown. About 80% have a minor cystic component. Rarely, a tumor is mostly cystic.

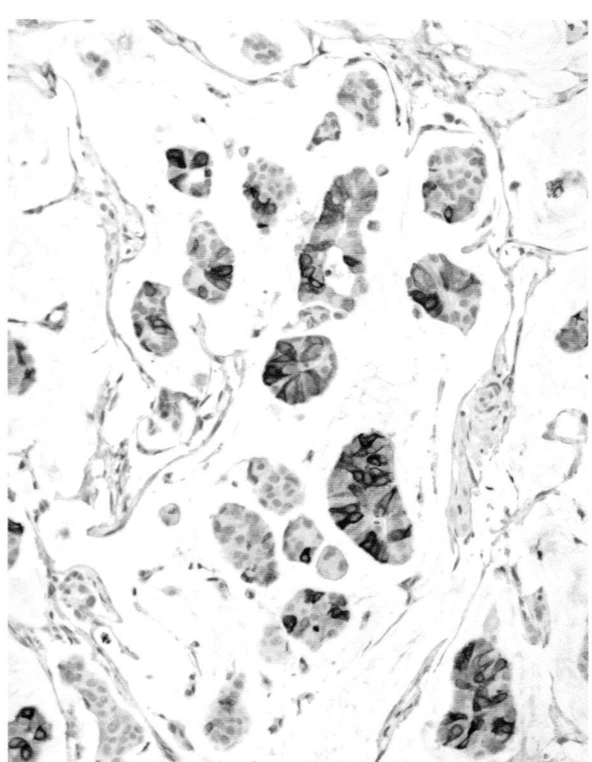

◘ Fig. 18.91
Metastatic breast carcinoma. **Immunohistochemical reactivity for mammoglobin**

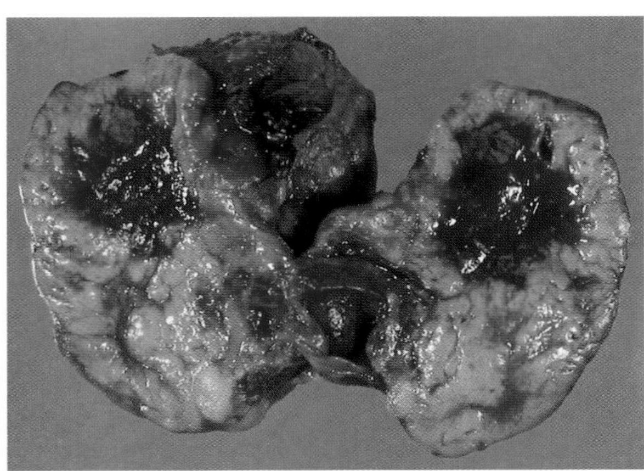

◘ Fig. 18.92
Metastatic renal cell carcinoma. **The tumor is orange (Courtesy of Dr. Mahul B. Amin)**

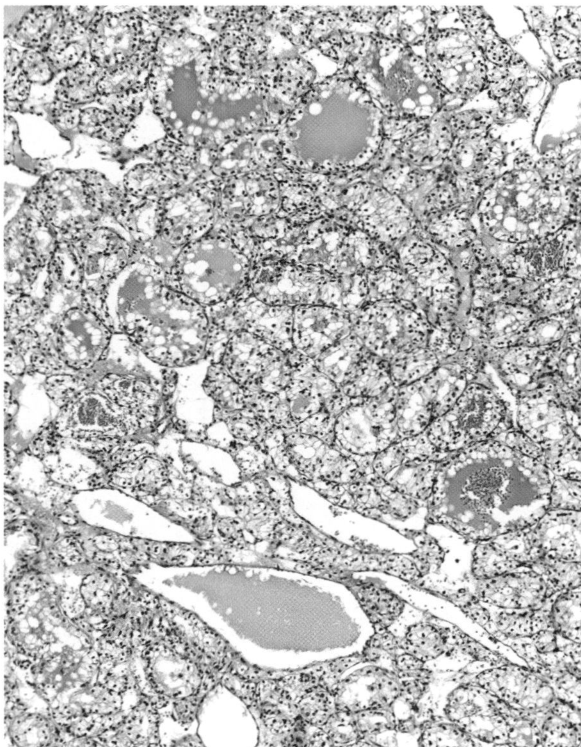

◘ Fig. 18.93
Metastatic renal cell carcinoma, clear cell type. **The primary tumor in this case was not diagnosed until 8 years after the removal of the metastasis. Note the sinusoidal vascular pattern**

Microscopic Findings

On low-power examination, a feature suggesting the metastatic nature in a number of the cases is growth of the tumor in the form of multiple nodules. The most common microscopic appearance is that of large cells with abundant eosinophilic cytoplasm (➲ *Fig. 18.96*). Occasional tumors are characterized by small cells with scanty cytoplasm (➲ *Fig. 18.97*), and a minority by spindle cells; admixtures of these cells types may be encountered. Follicle-like spaces are seen in approximately 40% of the cases (➲ *Fig. 18.10*). A helpful diagnostic feature of many metastatic melanomas is the presence of discrete rounded aggregates with a nevoid appearance (➲ *Fig. 18.98*). Prominent nucleoli are seen in many cases, and cytoplasmic pseudoinclusions are present in many nuclei in about 25%. The presence of melanin pigment is an obvious clue to the nature of the tumor in these cases, but melanin

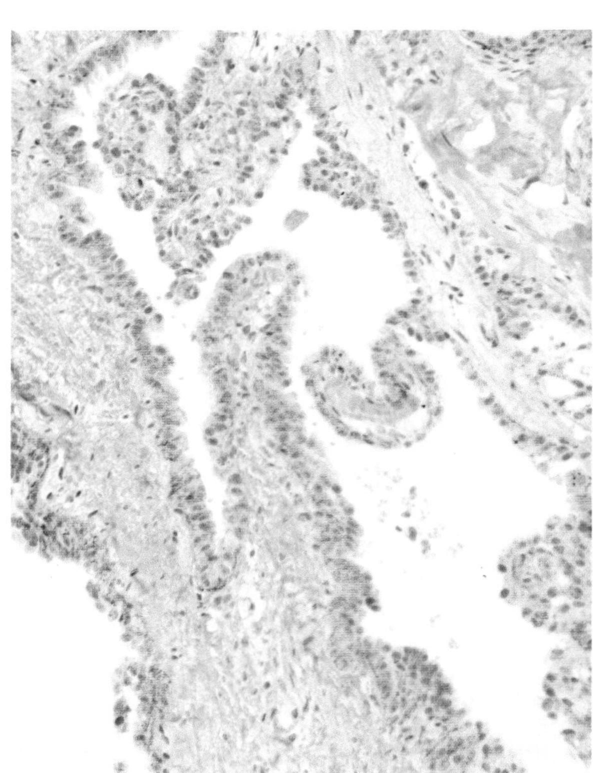

■ Fig. 18.94
Metastatic renal cell carcinoma. **This tumor, which had an unusual oxyphilic morphology, was immunoreactive for CD10**

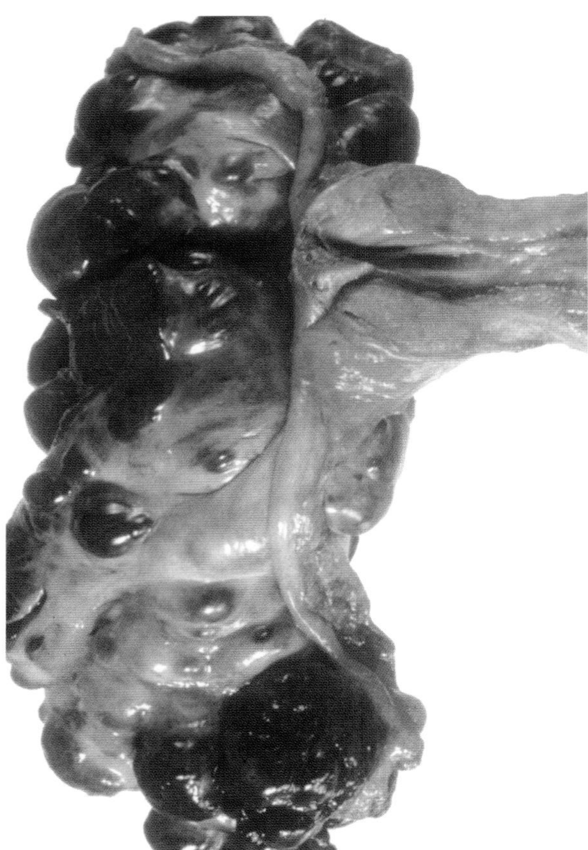

■ Fig. 18.95
Metastatic malignant melanoma. **The tumor has a bosselated external surface and is black**

was inconspicuous or absent in approximately half the cases in the reported series. Miscellaneous potentially confusing findings have been clear cells, rhabdoid cells, growth as cords, and myxoid stroma.

Differential Diagnosis

Metastatic melanoma must be distinguished from the rare primary melanoma [92] that usually arises in the wall of a dermoid cyst, which is sometimes accompanied by junctional activity beneath the squamous lining of the cyst or is associated with another teratomatous component such as struma ovarii. Because recognition of teratomatous elements is important in establishing the primary nature of a melanoma, the pathologist should sample the specimen extensively. In cases of apparently pure ovarian melanoma without obvious evidence of a primary tumor elsewhere, a meticulous search for an occult primary tumor should be conducted. If there is no evidence of a primary tumor elsewhere, it is possible that a primary cutaneous melanoma that has regressed was the source of the ovarian tumor. In these cases, bilaterality or growth of the ovarian tumor in the form of multiple nodules strongly suggests metastasis even in the absence of a known primary tumor. In some cases, removal of a primary melanoma may be remote and possibly not considered relevant by the patient or known by the clinician.

Metastatic melanoma, particularly if it is amelanotic, may resemble closely a lipid-poor steroid cell tumor or, if it is found during pregnancy, a pregnancy luteoma. Melanin can be misinterpreted as lipochrome pigment, the presence of which may be a feature of steroid cell tumors and impart a dark green-brown or almost black color to the neoplastic tissue. The presence of follicle-like spaces in metastatic melanomas has resulted in their confusion with small cell carcinomas of the hypercalcemic type (when the

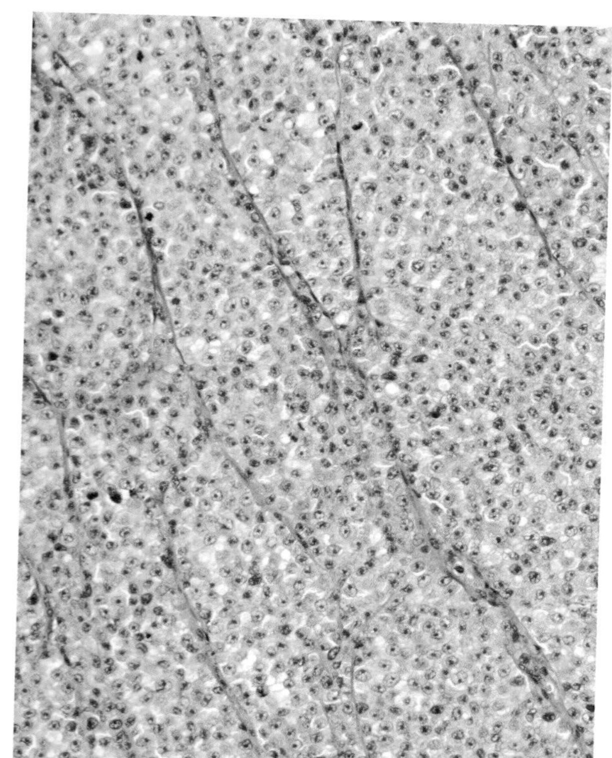

Fig. 18.96
Metastatic malignant melanoma. **The tumor cells have appreciable eosinophilic cytoplasm**

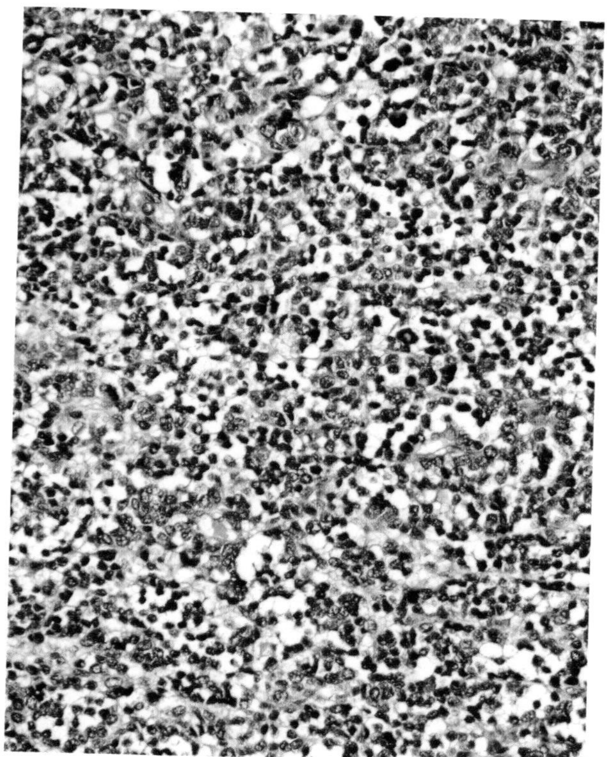

Fig. 18.97
Metastatic malignant melanoma. **The picture is that of a small cell malignant tumor**

cells are small) as well as juvenile granulosa cell tumors (when the cells have conspicuous eosinophilic cytoplasm). Rarely, surface epithelial neoplasms, particularly undifferentiated carcinoma and transitional cell carcinoma, may be reasonable considerations in the differential diagnosis, but surface epithelial neoplasms will often have at least minor obvious epithelial characteristics that rule out melanoma. In a young person, dysgerminoma is rarely entertained, but a variety of architectural and cytologic differences should resolve this issue. In all the aforementioned situations, the diagnosis of metastatic melanoma to the ovary may be confirmed by the immunohistochemical demonstration of S-100, HMB-45, and MART-1 positivity and negative staining for keratin and other antigens characteristic of other neoplasms that may be in the differential diagnosis.

Pulmonary and Mediastinal Tumors

Only approximately 5% of women with lung cancer have ovarian metastases at autopsy, and the surgical pathologist uncommonly encounters an ovarian tumor of this type. Exceptionally, an ovarian metastasis either precedes the discovery of a pulmonary tumor or is found simultaneously. Salient features of this phenomenon based on a relatively recent series, by far the largest on the topic, are summarized [56].

These tumors have occurred at an average age of 47 years. A history of lung cancer is known at presentation in slightly more than half the cases. In most of the remainder, the two tumors are discovered essentially synchronously, but in almost 20% the ovarian manifestations antedate recognition of the pulmonary primary, sometimes by as much as 2 years.

Gross Findings

The tumors have been bilateral in only about one third of the cases, and they average about 10 cm in maximum dimension. No unique gross characteristics have been evident in the cases encountered to date, but some have

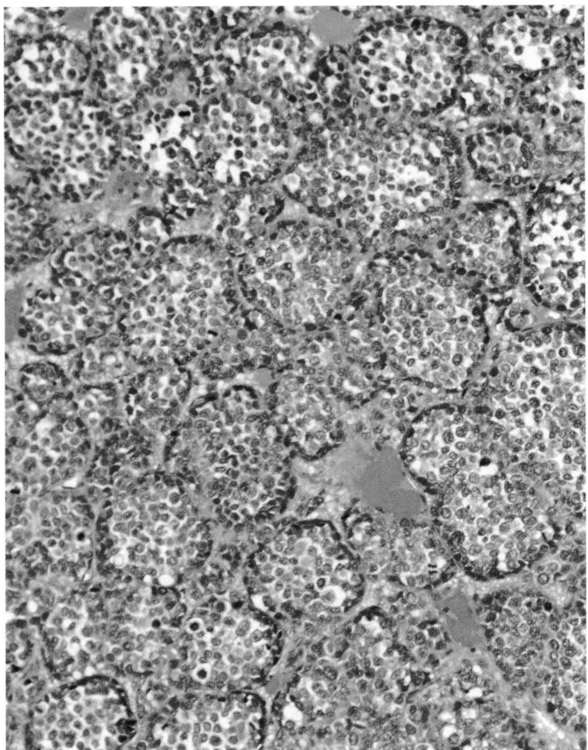

Fig. 18.98
Metastatic malignant melanoma. **Nests of cells have a nevoid appearance**

features, such as striking multinodularity (Fig. 18.99), in keeping with a metastatic neoplasm. Rarely a primary surface epithelial neoplasm is mimicked (Fig. 18.100).

Microscopic Findings

The greatest number of cases, about 44%, are small cell carcinomas (*Figs. 18.101* and *18.102*), the remaining neoplasms being largely split between adenocarcinoma and large cell carcinoma with a ratio of about 2:1. Rare more differentiated neuroendocrine neoplasms falling in the atypical carcinoid–neuroendocrine carcinoma group have spread to the ovary (*Fig. 18.103*). Perhaps surprisingly, spread of squamous cell carcinoma, although documented, is exceptionally uncommon. The morphologic features of the tumors in the ovary are similar to those encountered in the lung except for features relevant to metastatic ovarian disease, specifically surface involvement, nodularity, and vessel space invasion.

Differential Diagnosis

When a patient has pulmonary and ovarian neoplasms, it can be difficult to decide which tumor is primary. When the histologic features are typical of a lung carcinoma, a pulmonary origin can be assumed with rare exceptions. Small cell carcinomas of pulmonary type may be primary in the ovary, but there is typically no pulmonary

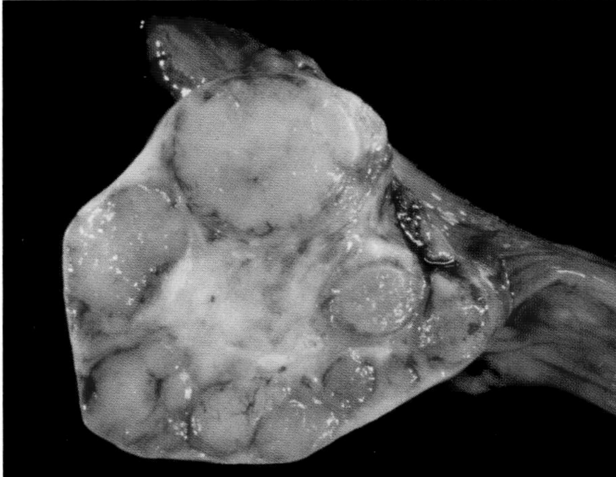

Fig. 18.99
Metastatic bronchioloalveolar carcinoma of the lung. **Note the multiple nodules (Courtesy of Dr. Jaime Prat)**

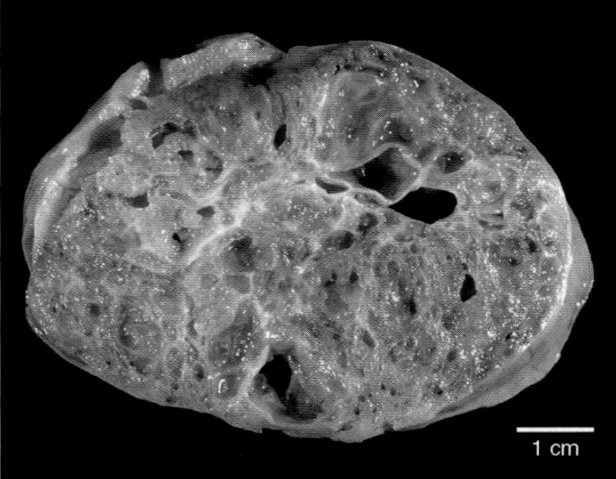

Fig. 18.100
Metastatic small cell carcinoma from the lung. **The solid and cystic sectioned surface mimics a surface epithelial neoplasm**

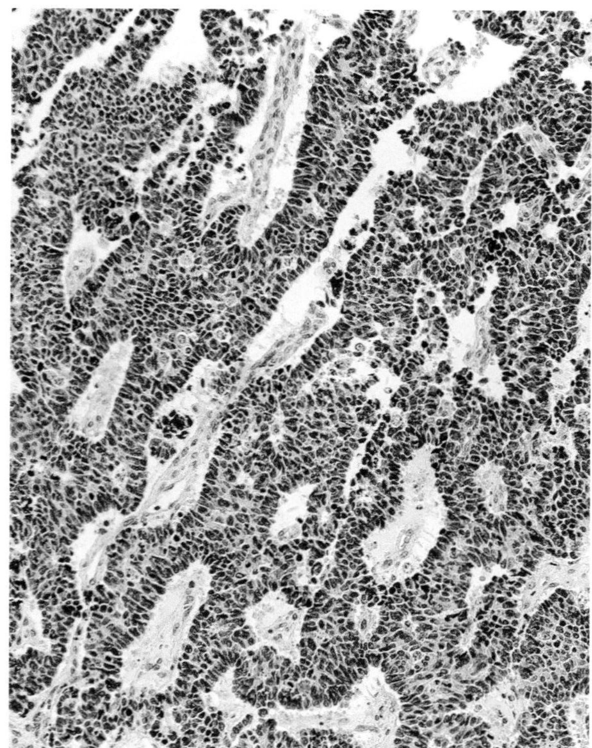

Fig. 18.101
Metastatic small cell carcinoma from the lung. **Trabecular pattern**

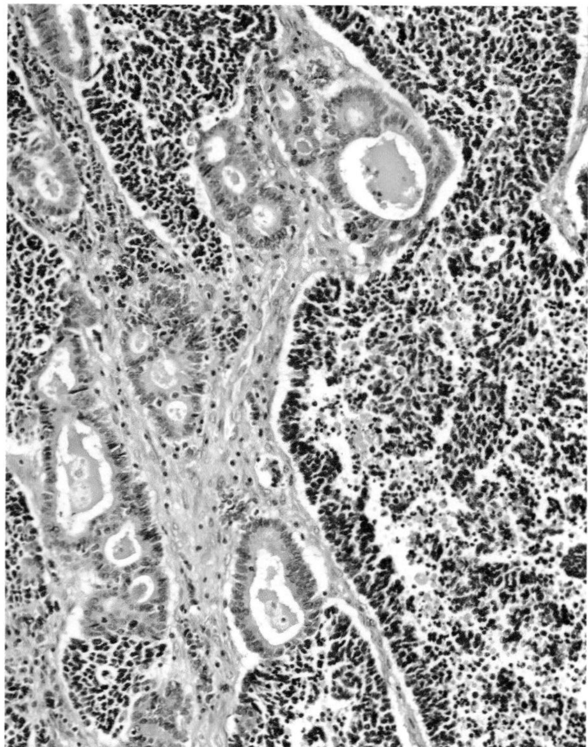

Fig. 18.102
Metastatic small cell carcinoma from the lung. **There is focal gland differentiation**

involvement in such cases, facilitating the diagnosis of an ovarian primary. The focal presence of a surface epithelial tumor is also sometimes helpful in excluding a metastasis. In the absence of such a finding and in the presence of tumor in the lung, it may be impossible to decide whether an ovarian small cell carcinoma of pulmonary type is primary or metastatic. Gland differentiation may be seen in some cases of metastatic small cell carcinoma (*Fig. 18.102*). This should be borne in mind in the differential diagnosis with a primary ovarian small cell carcinoma of pulmonary type, which is sometimes associated with endometrioid carcinoma; the latter may be suggested by the glands of what in fact is a metastatic small cell carcinoma. This exemplifies the diagnostic problems that can be hard to resolve in rare cases.

The metastatic adenocarcinomas generally have nonspecific glandular features, which, should a pulmonary neoplasm be known to exist, will aid in distinction from independent primary ovarian adenocarcinoma. Unfortunately, given the spectrum of primary ovarian neoplasia, particularly of endometrioid type, recognizing a tumor as metastatic in the absence of known pulmonary neoplasia may be difficult or impossible. The large cell carcinomas may have a broad differential diagnosis of oxyphilic tumors of the ovary.

The utility of TTF-1 in the recognition of metastatic lung carcinoma depends on the morphologic subtype under consideration. Approximately 75% of pulmonary adenocarcinomas are positive for TTF-1, whereas only 40% of large cell carcinomas are positive and the majority of squamous cell carcinomas are negative [29, 47, 62, 118]. TTF-1 may be also expressed in a subset of ovarian carcinomas [72, 187], including notably up to 37% of serous carcinomas in one study [72]. Its expression in primary ovarian tumors is usually focal but is occasionally diffuse. A negative reaction for TTF-1 does not exclude a lung primary, and although diffuse positivity may suggest a pulmonary origin, it is not independently diagnostic of such. Cytokeratin 7/20 profiles do not aid in the distinction of metastatic pulmonary from primary ovarian adenocarcinoma, as both are typically CK7+/CK20– [91].

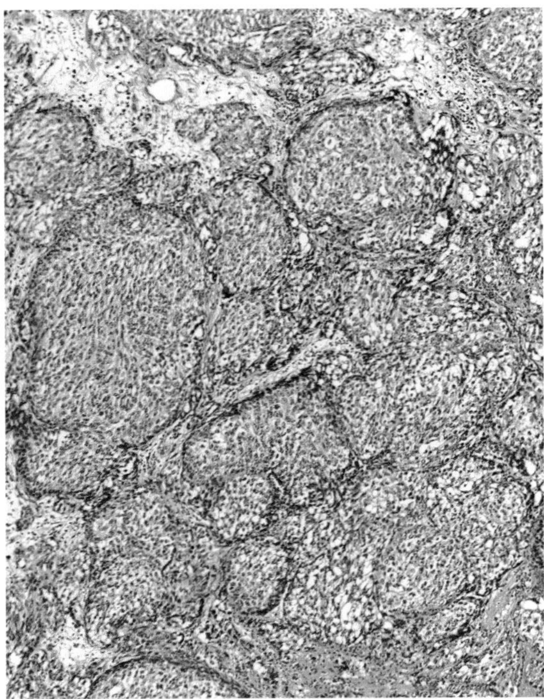
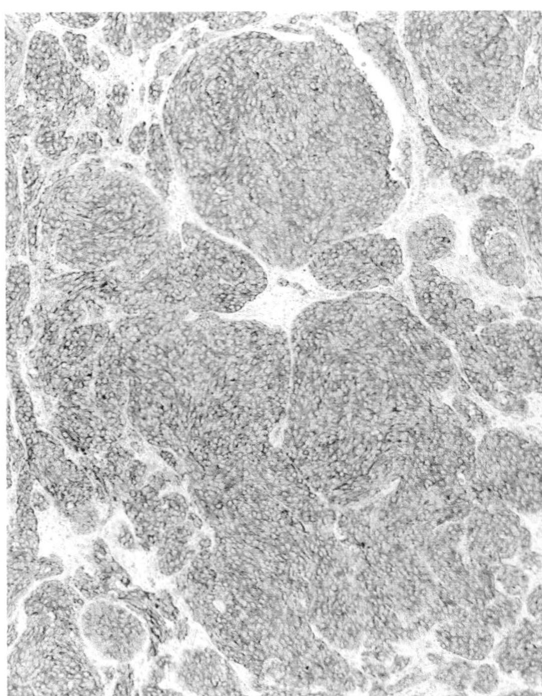

Fig. 18.103
Metastatic neuroendocrine carcinoma from the lung (*left*) with immunoreactivity for chromogranin (*right*)

Metastatic small cell carcinomas in the ovary may originate in sites other than the lung. Three such tumors were primary in the mediastinum, apparently of thymic origin, and had ovarian metastases at the time of presentation [30]. Small cell carcinomas from various sites express TTF-1, and thus TTF-1 positivity is not specific for pulmonary origin among tumors of this type [4]. One of two ovarian small cell carcinomas of pulmonary type was found to be positive for TTF-1 in a recent study [17].

One neuroblastoma primary in the posterior mediastinum metastasized to the ovary [172]. Thymomas have involved the ovary rarely [158].

Extragenital Sarcomas

Extragenital sarcomas, whether from the viscera or the soft tissues, uncommonly metastasize to the ovary except in late stages of the disease. An exception to this is the recently characterized gastrointestinal stromal tumor, a small series of which metastatic to the ovary pointed out some appreciable diagnostic problems [54].

The five patients described were all adults. In three, the primary (two small bowel and one its mesentery) and metastatic tumors were discovered synchronously. In one, however, ovarian masses were discovered 18 months before the gastric primary, and in the fifth case, ovarian spread was found 27 years after a primary small bowel tumor had been resected.

The ovarian tumors had no specific gross features but were often sizeable. Microscopic examination, as expected given the known morphology of this tumor, typically showed a low-grade spindle cell neoplasm (*Fig. 18.104*), but a number of features such as the presence of signet-ring-like cells and palisading (*Fig. 18.105*) complicated the appearance. The differential diagnosis may be broad and include cellular and typical fibromas, smooth muscle tumors, and other primary soft-tissue-type tumors. In cases in which any of these is a consideration but there is an atypical feature, such as bilaterality or extraovarian disease, immunohistochemistry for c-kit (*Fig. 18.106*) is appropriate to rule out the possibility of a gastrointestinal stromal neoplasm.

Eleven rhabdomyosarcomas metastatic to the ovary have been reported in patients 6 to 27 years of age [177]. Six tumors were alveolar rhabdomyosarcomas, three embryonal, one mixed embryonal and alveolar rhabdomyosarcoma, and one of unstated subtype. In most of the

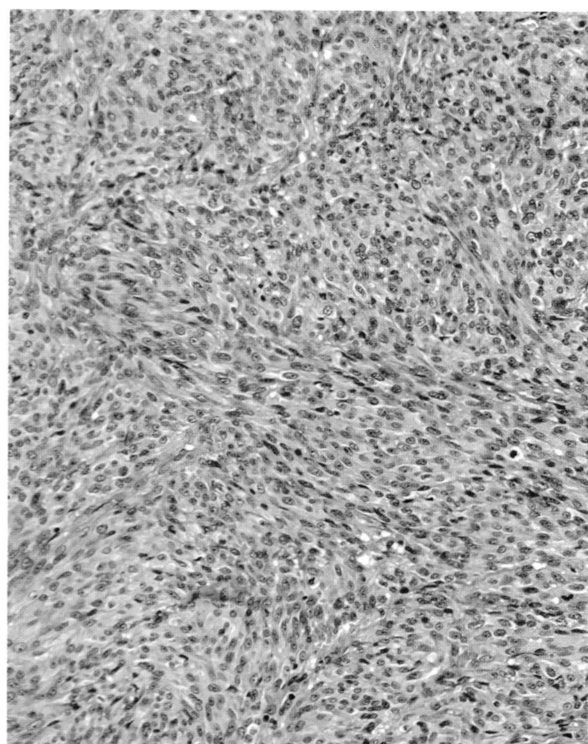

Fig. 18.104
Metastatic gastrointestinal stromal tumor. **The picture may be confused with cellular fibroma**

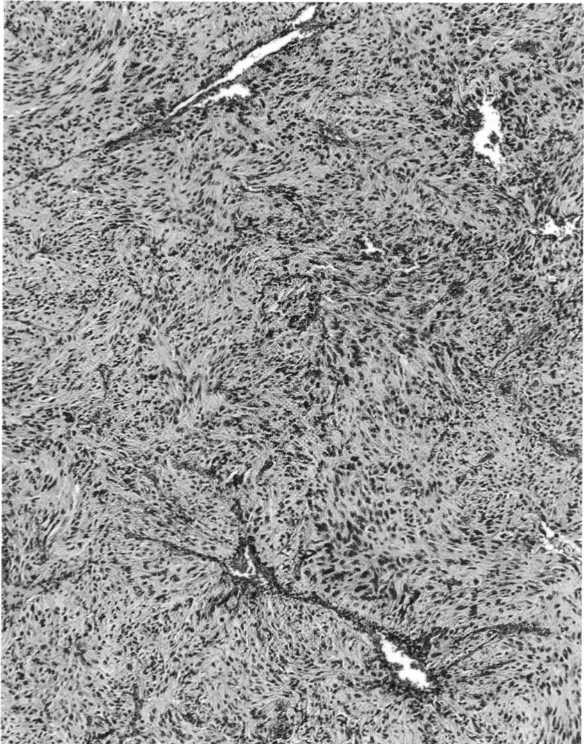

Fig. 18.105
Metastatic gastrointestinal stromal tumor. **Palisading is seen**

cases, the ovarian spread was a late manifestation of disease. The ovarian tumors were symptomatic in only two patients, in whom the ovarian involvement was detected within a few weeks of discovery of a soft tissue mass by the patient. The ovarian tumors were bilateral in two cases. In cases of embryonal rhabdomyosarcoma metastatic to the ovary, the diagnosis of rhabdomyosarcoma usually is evident because of the presence of strap cells, and the tumor must be distinguished from a primary embryonal rhabdomyosarcoma, which is the most common subtype of primary malignant striated muscle tumor of the ovary. Because a primary alveolar rhabdomyosarcoma of the ovary has not, to the best of our knowledge, been reported, metastatic alveolar rhabdomyosarcoma more commonly raises the question of other primary and metastatic small cell tumors of the ovary in young women. A combination of clinical findings, thorough sampling, and immunohistochemistry to varying degrees in individual cases will help resolve what can be a very challenging area. Two other cases in which the ovary was involved by rhabdomyosarcoma have occurred in patients with a clinical picture that simulated acute leukemia [46].

In one study of 21 metastatic sarcomas to the ovary other than rhabdomyosarcoma, 10 were extragenital in origin and all were clinically significant [179]. These tumors have included a miscellaneous group of soft tissue sarcomas primary at a variety of sites. Rare cases of hemangiosarcoma that metastasized to the ovaries have been documented as have a few cases of Ewing's sarcoma. The latter are noteworthy as they may be part of the broad differential diagnosis of a small cell malignant tumor of the ovary.

Miscellaneous Rare Ovarian Metastases

Metastases to the ovary other than those already discussed are of great rarity and generally only of relevance to autopsy pathology. Carcinomas of the thyroid only exceptionally spread to the ovary even in autopsy series, but a few cases documented during life exist. In one case [171], a 29-year-old woman had a 17 cm right ovarian tumor

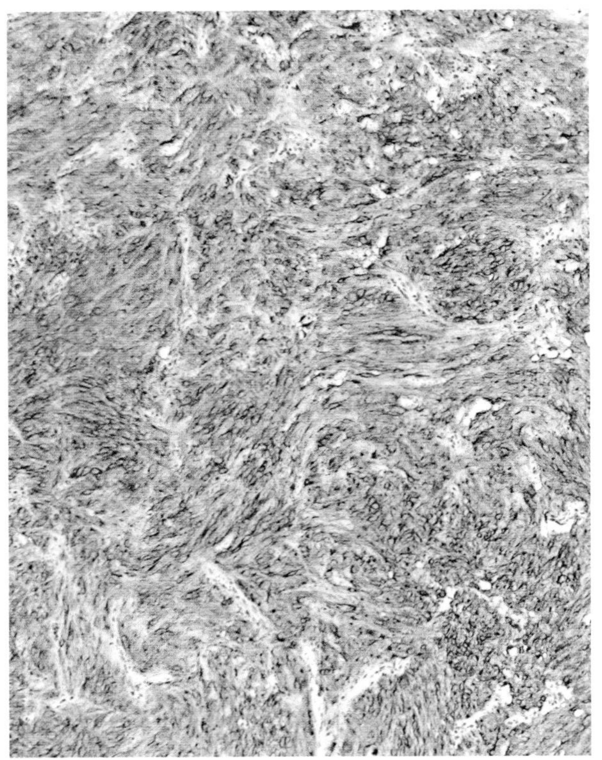

Fig. 18.106
Metastatic gastrointestinal stromal tumor. Immunoreactivity for c-kit

12 years after undergoing a partial thyroidectomy for follicular carcinoma. The tumor also had spread to the brain and one adrenal gland by the time the ovarian tumor was discovered. Initial consideration was given to the diagnosis of a malignant struma ovarii in this case because of the interval since the thyroid tumor, and also because it was only the existence of the ovarian tumor that prompted review of the thyroid neoplasm and its reinterpretation as carcinoma, a diagnosis not made initially. In another case [12], a 38-year-old woman with papillary carcinoma and local lymph node spread returned 7 years later with bilateral cystic ovarian metastases. In another case of papillary carcinoma, ovarian metastasis was uncovered after 10 years [84].

A review of the literature on parathyroid carcinoma has not disclosed any examples of ovarian metastasis. Rare examples of head and neck carcinoma metastatic to the ovary are documented and we have seen one case in which the primary tumor was an undifferentiated carcinoma of the ethmoid sinus. Salivary gland tumors also spread to the ovary with extreme rarity. We have seen a case of a young woman who had an adenoid cystic carcinoma of the parotid gland excised at the age of 12 years followed by local recurrence, lung metastasis, and bilateral symptomatic ovarian metastases 11 years after presentation. Longacre and colleagues [87] described a case of a 30-year-old woman with an adenoid cystic carcinoma of the submandibular gland who had a 10 cm left ovarian metastasis, followed by a smaller tumor in the opposite ovary 10 years later. These cases emphasize that a history of neoplasia of any type, even relatively remote, may be relevant in the evaluation of an unusual ovarian tumor. Esophageal cancer rarely spreads to the ovary. A case of metastatic esophageal adenocarcinoma to the ovary is briefly mentioned in one series [119].

There are only two reports to our knowledge in which ovarian spread of tumors of the central nervous system and cranium is mentioned. One was a case of metastatic meningioma and the other was a metastatic medulloblastoma in a 4-year-old girl, in whose ovary "a cleft near the hilum was full of tumor cells" [172]. Tumors of the skin, other than malignant melanoma, rarely spread to the ovary; clinically significant spread of Merkel cell tumor is documented [30]. One chordoma has metastasized to the ovary [188]. There are sporadic reports of a metastatic tumor involving an ovary that contains a primary ovarian neoplasm [48, 131], and there seem to be no unique features of these happenstance events, a few examples of which we have seen (*Fig. 18.90*).

Female Genital Tract Tumors

Tubal Carcinoma

The ovary is involved secondarily in 10–15% of tubal carcinomas, usually by direct extension, sometimes via tuboovarian inflammatory adhesions, and at other times by surface implantation on the ipsilateral or contralateral ovary. In some cases, there is clinical or pathologic evidence of salpingitis and salpingo-oophoritis, but often it is unclear whether the inflammatory process preceded or followed the development of the carcinoma. If the involvement of the tube and the ovary is extensive, the primary site of the tumor may not be established with certainty; the term tuboovarian carcinoma has been suggested for these cases. Green and Scully [39] encountered six such tumors in an investigation of 24 carcinomas initially considered to be of tubal origin. The tuboovarian carcinomas formed solid or cystic masses; at least one of the cystic tumors appeared to have developed in a postinflammatory tuboovarian cyst.

Because most tubal carcinomas closely resemble serous, endometrioid, or undifferentiated carcinomas of the ovary, microscopic examination often fails to establish whether a carcinoma involving both organs is primary in one or the other unless the tumor is grossly clearly centered in one of them. Because of the great rarity of primary mucinous and clear cell carcinomas of the fallopian tube, a tumor of either of these cell types involving both organs usually is considered primary in the ovary. It should be emphasized that surface growth within the tube may be seen as a result of implantation from an ovarian carcinoma and does not necessarily indicate a tubal primary.

Recent studies from one group have raised the possibility that a greater number of serous carcinomas of the ovary than hitherto thought may actually represent spread of fallopian tube cancers, especially those of the fimbria [70].

Endometrial Carcinoma

Ovarian involvement in cases in which a diagnosis of endometrial carcinoma has been made has been reported in 34–40% of autopsy cases [8, 15] and 5–15% of hysterectomy and bilateral salpingo-oophorectomy specimens. Conversely, in approximately one third of the cases in which a diagnosis of endometrioid carcinoma of the ovary has been made, an endometrial carcinoma also has been found. When the uterine corpus and the ovary are both involved by carcinomas, the question arises whether both cancers are primary or one is metastatic from the other [31, 143, 184]. If the endometrial carcinoma extends deeply into the myometrium with lymphatic or vascular invasion; if tumor is present in the lumen of the fallopian tube; or if tumor is on the ovarian surface, within its lymphatics, or in blood vessels, it is usually reasonable to conclude that the ovarian involvement is secondary. On the other hand, if lymphatic or hematogenous spread is absent, if the corpus carcinoma is small and limited to the endometrium or superficial myometrium, if it arises on a background of atypical hyperplasia, and if the ovarian tumor arises on a background of endometriosis, the tumors probably are independent primaries. Criteria that are helpful in the determination of primary versus metastatic concomitant ovarian and endometrial carcinomas are presented in ➋ *Table 18.2.* Although synchronous ovarian and uterine tumors are of endometrioid type in most cases, occasionally they are of similar but other cell types, and rarely the histologic type of tumor is different in the two organs [31].

In some cases of combined involvement it is impossible to establish the site of origin even after consideration of the features just described. In our experience and that of most series, most synchronous ovarian and corpus carcinomas are independent primary tumors; in one study, however, the ovarian tumors were interpreted as metastatic from the corpus in most of the cases [143], and other valid cases of metastasis are reported in the literature. An independent primary explanation for most concomitant ovarian and corpus carcinomas is supported by the survival rates associated with this combination of tumors, which have generally been high. These results would be surprising if either the ovarian or corpus carcinoma was metastatic in most of the cases.

Rarely, spread to the ovary from an adenocarcinoma of the uterine corpus with squamous differentiation takes the form of deposits of keratin or degenerated mature squamous cells associated with a foreign body giant cell response on the serosal surface of one or both ovaries [69]. If no viable-appearing tumor cells can be identified in these deposits on careful sampling, this finding does not appear to worsen the prognosis even when the granulomas are also found elsewhere on the peritoneum.

Cervical Carcinoma

Ovarian spread of cervical carcinomas of all types generally has been considered rare. There has been considerable recent interest in this topic [33, 59, 83, 175], however, simulated in part by observations suggesting that it is more common in cases of adenocarcinoma than in cases of squamous cell carcinoma, and raising the question of whether ovarian conservation is justified in patients with cervical adenocarcinoma. In addition, occasional patients with cervical carcinomas of diverse types have had clinically significant ovarian metastases [166].

One of the most detailed studies of ovarian spread of cervical carcinoma is that of Tabata et al. [138] In their autopsy series, ovarian metastases were detected in 104 of 597 (17%) cases of squamous cell carcinoma and in 22 of 77 (28.6%) cases of adenocarcinoma. The frequency of ovarian metastases of squamous cell carcinoma at autopsy in their series is much higher than the 3% frequency in the prior literature. Ovarian metastases discovered during life are much rarer. In their series of 318 patients with stage IA cervical carcinoma treated by hysterectomy with ovarian preservation, Tabata et al. [138] found no examples of subsequent ovarian metastasis during follow-up periods that exceeded 5 years in more than half the cases. In cases of stage IB, II, and III carcinoma in their series, there were no ovarian metastases in 278 cases of squamous cell carcinoma in contrast to 6 ovarian metastases of 48 (12.5%) cases of adenocarcinoma. In another series there were

Table 18.2
Criteria for interpretation of nature of concomitant uterine corpus and ovarian carcinomas

Corpus primary Ovarian metastasis	Ovarian primary Corpus metastasis	Ovarian primary Corpus primary	Ovarian metastasis Corpus metastasis	Uncertain primary
Direct extension to ovary from large corpus tumor	Direct extension to corpus from large ovarian primary	No direct extension of either tumor	Usually no direct extension of tumors	Massive involvement of both organs or conflicting findings listed in first four columns
Deep myometrial invasion from endometrium	Myometrial invasion from serosal surface	Myometrial invasion usually absent or superficial	Tumor characteristically in endometrial stroma	Myometrial invasion may be present
Lymphatic or blood vessel invasion in corpus, ovary, or both	Lymphatic or blood vessel invasion in corpus, ovary, or both	No lymphatic or blood vessel invasion	Lymphatic or blood vessel invasion frequent in ovary and corpus	
Atypical hyperplasia of endometrium frequent	Atypical hyperplasia of endometrium usually absent	Atypical hyperplasia of endometrium frequent	Atypical hyperplasia of endometrium absent	
Tumor present in fallopian tube	Tumor present on peritoneal surfaces and sometimes in fallopian tube	Usually both tumors confined to primary sites or have spread minimally	Tumor usually evident outside female genital tract	
Tumor predominant on surface of ovary	Tumor predominant within ovary	Tumor predominant within ovary and endometrium	Ovarian tumor usually bilateral, ovarian surface involvement frequent	
Usually no endometriosis in ovary	Endometriosis sometimes present in ovary	Endometriosis sometimes present in ovary	Endometriosis absent	
Histological types uniform and consistent with corpus primary	Histological types uniform and consistent with ovarian primary	Histological types uniform or dissimilar	Type of tumor inconsistent with or unusual for either organ	

3 cases of microscopic ovarian metastasis in 185 cases of stage IIB cervical carcinoma [140]; in the same series, there were no metastases in 335 cases of stage IB disease, 71 cases of stage IIA disease, and 6 cases of stage IIIB disease. One of the ovarian metastases was from a squamous cell carcinoma (0.2% of all squamous cell carcinomas), whereas two were from adenocarcinomas (5.5% of these tumors). The cervical carcinomas in these three cases had invaded the uterine corpus and vascular spaces. Tabata et al. [138] also found that ovarian metastasis was much more common when a cervical carcinoma had invaded the uterine corpus.

Adenocarcinomas

The commonest cervical carcinoma to exhibit ovarian spread is what we refer to as endocervical adenocarcinoma of the usual type. We have seen many unpublished examples and a series of 29 cases has recently been reported [124]. These experiences enable the following observations. We shall only comment in detail on the ovarian aspects, but it is pertinent to briefly note that the primary cervical tumors may only be microinvasive or even have features that objectively make recognition of definite invasion questionable. It has been suggested that contiguous spread to the corpus may contribute to the development of metastases by heightening the chance of transtubal spread to the ovarian surface [124].

The ovarian tumors are bilateral in only about one third of the cases and are often over 10 cm. Given that usual endocervical adenocarcinoma has a somewhat distinctive histologic appearance, it is not surprising that this morphology is also seen in the ovaries (*Figs. 18.107–18.109*).

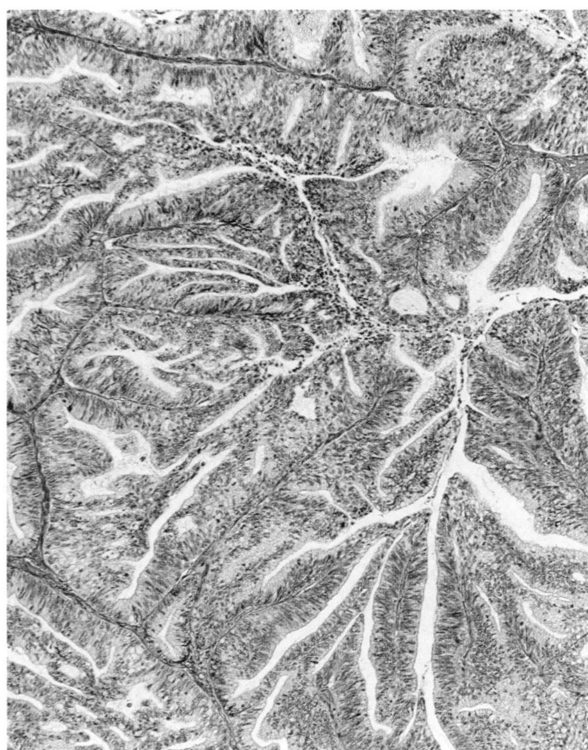

Fig. 18.107
Metastatic endocervical adenocarcinoma of the usual type. There is a pseudoendometrioid picture

Approaching the topic from the ovarian perspective, the picture is more often pseudoendometrioid than truly mucinous in nature, and yet the morphology is not typical of classic endometrioid glandular neoplasia. As summarized elegantly by Ronnett et al. [124], the tumors often have a hybrid appearance with low-power endometrioid-like features but with apical mucin appreciable on higher power. The nuclei are typically hyperchromatic and elongated (*Fig. 18.109*), more atypical than seen in true endometrioid carcinomas with a similar degree of gland differentiation. Apically located mitotic figures are usually prominent, and apoptotic cells are often numerous. With increasing experience, it is possible to suspect a cervical origin when confronted with cases with this morphology, but it is a difficult area given the inherent subjectivity. As recently emphasized, help may be garnered by p16 immunohistochemical staining (*Fig. 18.108*), which supports a secondary nature but is not specific. Should p16 be positive, more definitive evidence can be obtained by evaluating the ovarian tumor for human papilloma virus using in situ hybridization or polymerase chain reaction. Cases have been documented in which these results have prompted evaluation of a clinically non-suspicious cervix and subsequent identification of the occult primary neoplasm [124].

Less often, the rarer primary mucinous adenocarcinoma of the cervix with ovarian spread is encountered (*Fig. 18.110*). In a series from the Armed Forces Institute of Pathology, as many as 10% of mucinous adenocarcinomas of the cervix were reported to metastasize to the ovary [59], although the referral nature of that material may have introduced some bias in the frequency of the phenomenon; occasional other examples have been reported in detail [175] or included in series of metastatic mucinous carcinomas in the ovary [119]. When a cervical mucinous adenocarcinoma and an ovarian mucinous adenocarcinoma coexist, the general features of metastatic spread to the ovary usually help in diagnosis.

Squamous Cell Carcinomas

There are only eight well-documented examples of clinically significant ovarian metastases from invasive squamous cell carcinomas of the cervix [103, 166]. The youngest patient was 30 years old and the oldest 59 years. The ovarian and cervical tumors were discovered at essentially the same time in three of the patients. In four others, the ovarian metastases occurred 18 months to 10 years after the cervical primary tumor had been treated. In the eighth case the cervical tumor was not discovered until autopsy 7 months after the patient had been treated for a squamous cell carcinoma involving the left ovary. The cervical tumor in that case was invasive only to 3.8 mm, whereas in the other cases there appears to have been deep infiltration of the cervical wall with frequent extrauterine extension of the neoplasm [166]. The ovarian tumors, two of which were bilateral, ranged from 5 to 17 cm in greatest dimension. Four of the 10 tumors in these patients were solid, 3 solid and cystic, and 3 cystic. Microscopic examination has shown the typical features of squamous cell carcinoma except that many of the tumors had striking cystification within the squamous nests. In one case, a cervical squamous cell carcinoma that was invasive to only 1.2 mm extended in an in situ manner to involve the endometrium and the surface and inclusion glands and cysts within one ovary, tumor cells presumably having spread there via the tubal lumen. In a final remarkable case, a cervical squamous cell carcinoma in situ was associated with contiguous spread to the endometrium, fallopian tubes, and ovaries, extensively replacing the endometrial and tubal epithelium and focally invading the wall of the tubes and parenchyma of both ovaries [113].

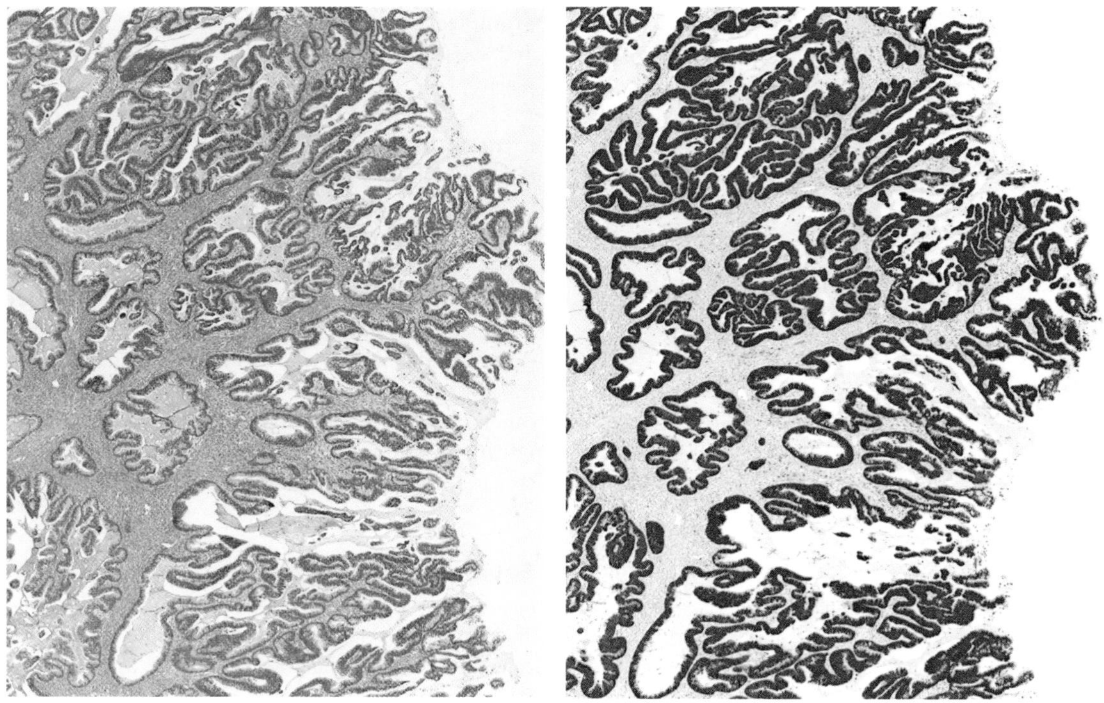

Fig. 18.108
Metastatic endocervical adenocarcinoma of the usual type. Companion staining with hematoxylin and eosin (*left*) and for p16 (*right*)

The differentiation of metastatic squamous cell carcinoma from the cervix from primary squamous cell carcinoma of the ovary usually has been aided by the knowledge of the presence of a cervical tumor, but in the one case in which the cervical tumor was not detected until autopsy and some of the others, there were major problems in diagnosis [166]. Before the diagnosis of primary squamous cell carcinoma of the ovary is made, the possibility of spread from a cervical tumor, even one that is occult, should be considered unless overt features of primary neoplasia are immediately obvious. As most squamous cell carcinomas of the ovary arise on the background of a preexistent neoplasm such as a dermoid or endometriotic cyst, thorough sampling to identify such a component may be crucial in determining the primary nature of the neoplasm. Although the evidence strongly points to the ovarian tumors being metastatic when both organs have been involved by squamous cell carcinoma, the rare association of squamous cell carcinoma of the ovary with squamous cell carcinoma in situ of the cervix leaves open the possibility of independent primary neoplasms in some cases. Although the differential in these cases is generally between primary and metastatic squamous cell carcinoma, in some cases metastatic squamous cell carcinoma undergoes cystic degeneration and as squamous and transitional cell types are closely related, a resemblance to primary transitional cell carcinoma may result (*Fig. 18.111*).

Other Carcinomas

Two adenosquamous carcinomas and two glassy cell carcinomas with ovarian metastases have been reported [166]. Both metastatic adenosquamous carcinomas were discovered at the same time as the cervical primary tumors. The ovarian tumors were bilateral in both cases, and the cervical tumors were deeply invasive with extracervical extension, findings facilitating the diagnosis in these cases. In one of the cases of glassy cell carcinoma the ovarian involvement was a microscopic finding; in the other the ovarian involvement was grossly evident but the ovary was not enlarged.

Four cases have been reported in detail in which cervical small cell carcinomas or mixed tumors with a component of adenocarcinoma and small cell carcinoma or poorly

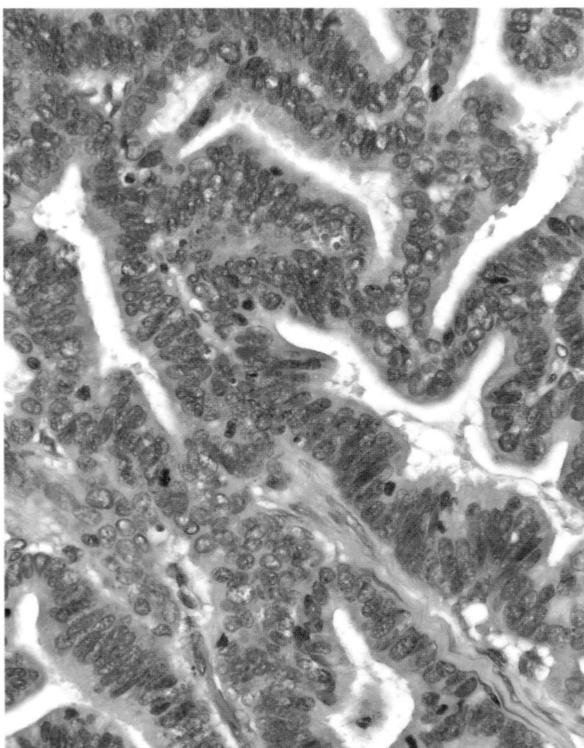

Fig. 18.109
Metastatic endocervical adenocarcinoma of the usual type. **Typical cytologic features**

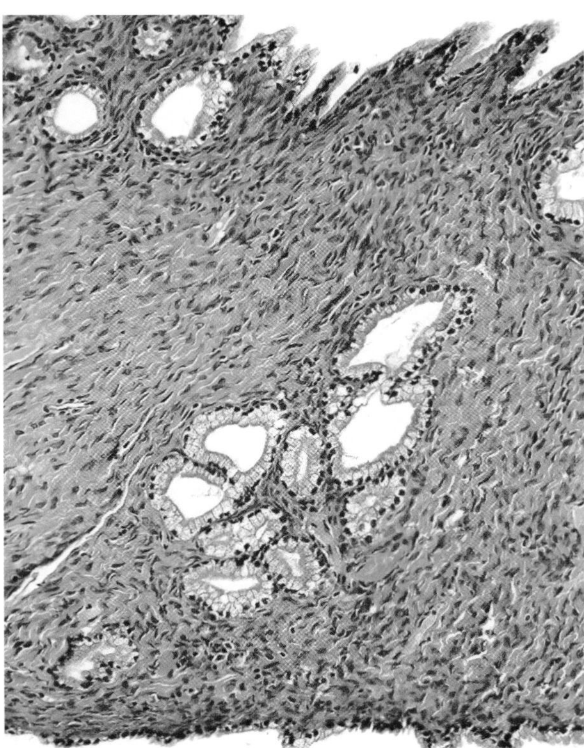

Fig. 18.110
Metastatic endocervical adenocarcinoma, mucinous type. **Highly differentiated glands of the type seen in adenoma malignum**

differentiated carcinoid have been associated with ovarian metastases. In each of these four cases, the ovarian spread was manifest clinically [166]. In one, the patient had evidence of the carcinoid syndrome. The four patients were from 23 to 34 years of age. The cervical tumors and ovarian tumors were synchronous findings in two of them. In the other two, the ovarian tumors were discovered 10 months and 3 years after the cervical tumors. In one final case, a cervical transitional cell carcinoma metastasized to the ovary and was detected before the cervical tumor, which was not discovered until pathologic examination. The ovarian metastatic tumor in this case was a large cystic mass that was indistinguishable microscopically from a primary transitional cell carcinoma of the ovary but was associated with prominent vascular space invasion, suggesting its metastatic nature.

Other Uterine Tumors

The most important of these by far is metastatic endometrial stromal sarcoma because it has some proclivity for ovarian spread and can cause a wide array of problems in differential diagnosis. This sarcoma metastasizes to the ovary more frequently than leiomyosarcoma. In a series of 11 uterine sarcomas that metastasized to the ovary (none of which were autopsy findings), 8 were endometrial stromal sarcomas and 3 leiomyosarcomas [179]. The patients with endometrial stromal sarcomas ranged from 33 to 79 (average 50) years of age; 5 of them were less than 50 years old. The ovarian metastases accounted for the clinical presentation in three of the patients. In two patients, the primary uterine tumors were not discovered until 7 months and 10 months after bilateral ovarian tumors had been resected. In four of the other cases the ovarian and uterine tumors were found synchronously, and in the remaining two the ovarian metastases occurred 4 to 9 years after the uterine neoplasms had been discovered. The ovarian tumors were bilateral in six cases, and ranged up to 17 cm in greatest dimension. These tumors usually are solid (*Fig. 18.112*) or solid and cystic, but rarely are cystic.

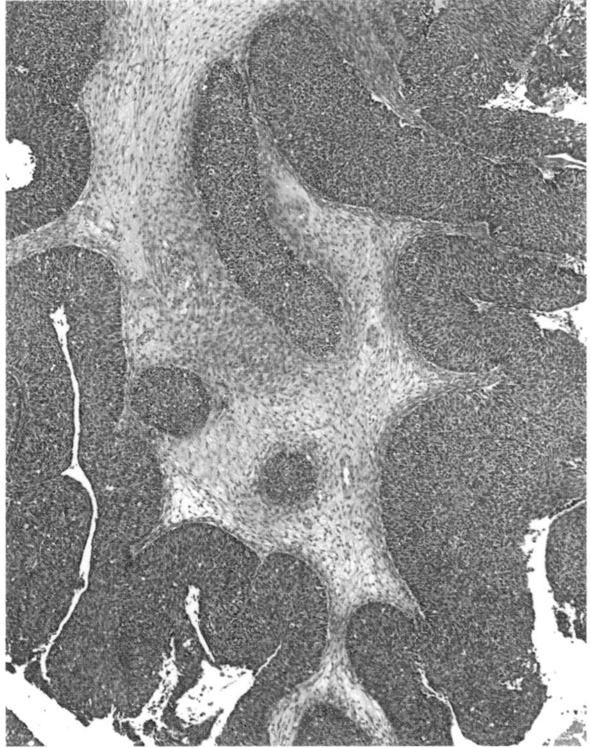

◘ Fig. 18.111
Metastatic squamous cell carcinoma from cervix. **The lining of cysts by thick undulating bands of neoplastic cells without overt squamous differentiation imparts a resemblance to a primary transitional cell carcinoma of the ovary**

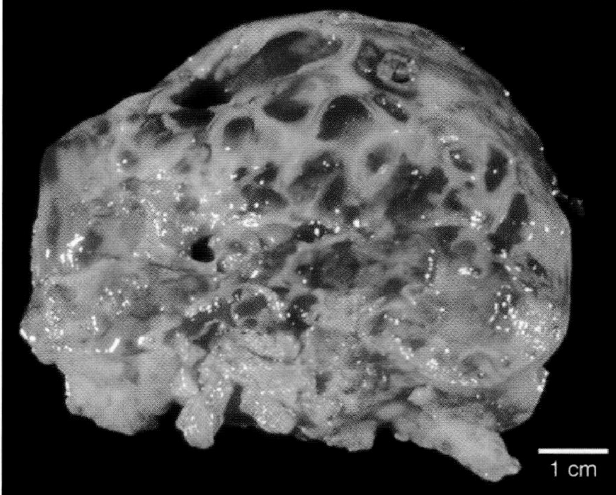

◘ Fig. 18.112
Metastatic endometrial stromal sarcoma. **Peculiar nodular growth**

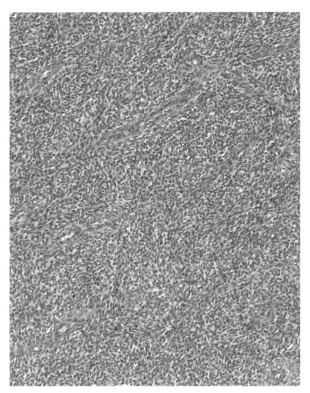

◘ Fig. 18.113
Metastatic endometrial stromal sarcoma. **The tumor has a diffuse pattern**

The major problem with the interpretation of these tumors on microscopic examination is that, in the ovary, the tongue-like pattern of infiltration characteristic of this neoplasm often is inconspicuous. A diffuse pattern is common (➋ *Fig. 18.113*). Other diagnostic problems result from the presence in some of the tumors of large fibromatous areas (➋ *Fig. 18.114*) and hyaline plaques (➋ *Fig. 18.115*). Yu et al. [183] described the case of a 24-year-old woman with a metastatic endometrial stromal sarcoma that was misinterpreted initially as a thecoma for this reason. In other cases with a diffuse pattern, the characteristic small arteries resembling the spiral arteries of the endometrium are inconspicuous, resulting in a resemblance to a diffuse granulosa cell tumor. Confusion with sex cord–stromal tumors may be heightened by the occasional presence of areas of sex-cord-like differentiation in metastatic endometrial stromal sarcomas. However, high-power examination does not show the typical nuclear features of granulosa cell tumors and careful examination usually demonstrates, at least focally, the typical vascular pattern of endometrial stromal tumors

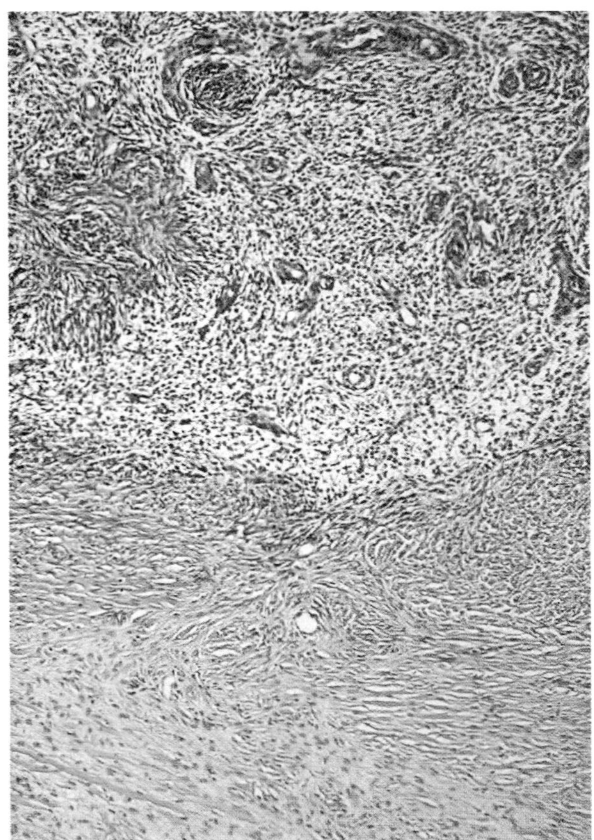

◘ Fig. 18.114
Metastatic endometrial stromal sarcoma. **Typical pattern at the *top* and unusual fibroma-like morphology at the *bottom***

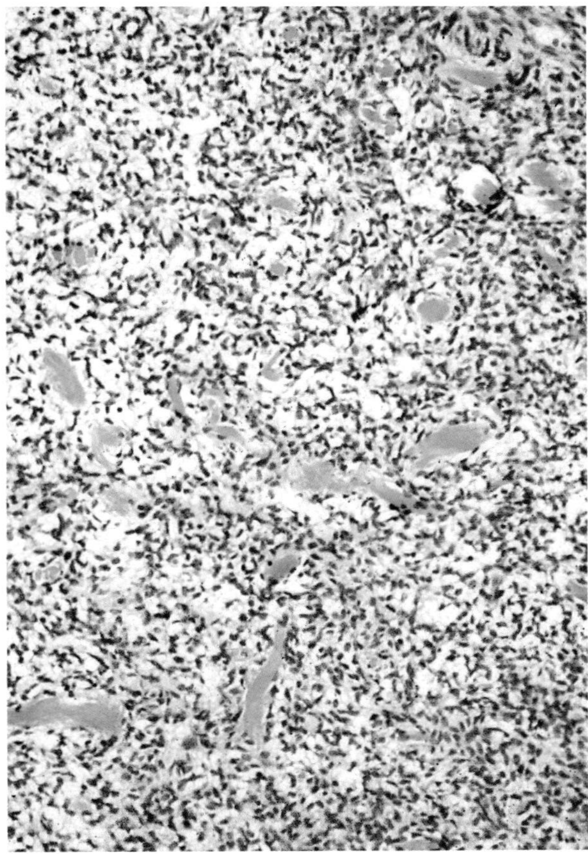

◘ Fig. 18.115
Metastatic endometrial stromal sarcoma. **Hyaline plaques are conspicuous and may cause the diagnosis of thecoma to be entertained**

(➲ *Fig. 18.116*). Reticulum stains may be helpful in the differential diagnosis by showing individual cell investment by fibrils in endometrial stromal sarcoma and only small amounts, mainly perivascular, in granulosa cell tumor. Bilaterality also is far more common in the former than the latter, as is the presence of extraovarian tumor, examination of which often shows the distinctive growth pattern of endometrial stromal sarcoma.

Metastatic endometrial stromal sarcomas in the ovary must be distinguished from primary endometrioid stromal sarcomas [173]. An association of the tumor with endometriosis is evidence for an ovarian origin. Bilaterality favors metastasis, although it is possible that some bilateral tumors may represent independent primaries.

Leiomyosarcomas of the uterus with ovarian metastases are probably more common than the rare reports in the literature suggest, particularly in patients with widespread disease. The three leiomyosarcomas with ovarian metastases in our series occurred in patients 35, 44, and 49 years of age [179] In the first patient, a large ovarian metastatic tumor became symptomatic 14 months after hysterectomy. In the second patient, the ovarian metastatic tumor occurred in the setting of widespread disease. In the third case, the ovarian involvement was only microscopic. Ovarian spread of malignant mixed müllerian tumors is common but not usually a diagnostic problem. Ovarian involvement in cases of müllerian adenosarcoma of the uterus is uncommon and in some cases may be an independent primary, particularly if it is associated with endometriosis.

Gestational choriocarcinoma of the uterus may spread to the ovary, but in the light of known uterine disease is not a diagnostic problem [3]. If such an ovarian tumor in

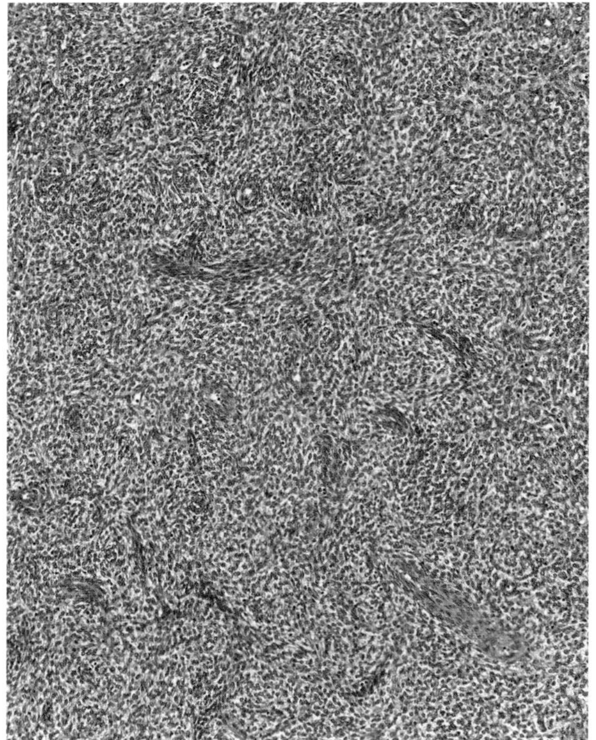

Fig. 18.116
Metastatic endometrial stromal sarcoma. **Typical arterioles are present (same tumor as in** *Fig. 18.113***)**

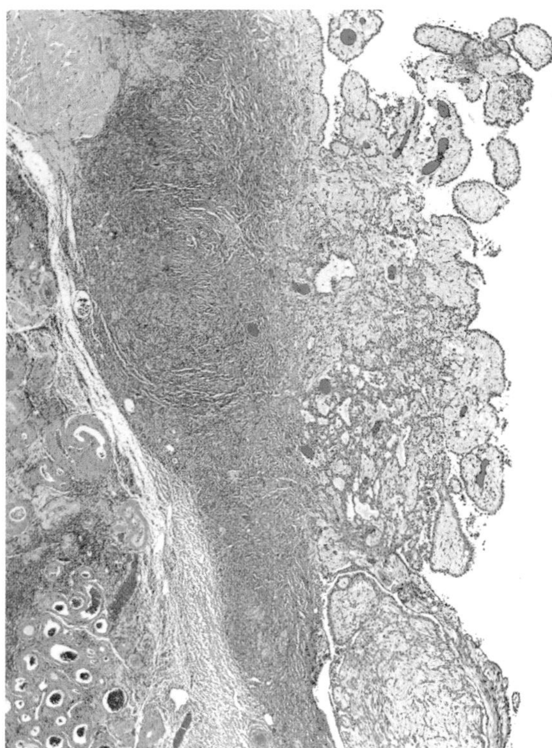

Fig. 18.117
Ovarian involvement by malignant mesothelioma of peritoneum. **Note typical tubulopapillary pattern**

a woman of childbearing age is not clearly metastatic from a uterine or tubal choriocarcinoma, thorough sampling may be needed to demonstrate the presence or absence of teratomatous elements. If such elements are not found, it may be difficult or impossible to differentiate between a primary choriocarcinoma of the ovary of either gestational or germ cell origin and a metastatic tumor from a choriocarcinoma of the uterus that has regressed. Invasive hydatidiform mole has also been documented to spread to the ovary, and in rare cases the placental site trophoblastic tumor has spread through the uterine wall to involve an ovary [1, 99].

Vulvar and Vaginal Tumors

Vulvar and vaginal carcinomas rarely exhibit ovarian spread. Occasional vaginal clear cell adenocarcinomas have metastasized to the ovary, in most cases associated with extensive pelvic spread.

Ovarian Involvement by Peritoneal Tumors

Although ovarian involvement in cases of peritoneal serous carcinoma may be secondary in most of the cases, this subject is generally not included in discussions of secondary tumors of the ovary because the ovarian involvement is only one part of widespread peritoneal disease. More pertinent to our interest here are cases of significant ovarian involvement in cases of malignant mesothelioma that may engender a broader array of problems in differential diagnosis [6].

In one series of peritoneal mesotheliomas, ovarian involvement was common [37], and this phenomenon was the focus of another report that included seven cases of peritoneal malignant mesothelioma that presented clinically as "ovarian cancer" [22]. The differential diagnosis in these cases is primarily with an ovarian surface epithelial carcinoma, particularly serous carcinoma. Although there is some overlap, in typical cases the tubulopapillary (*Fig. 18.117*) and diffuse patterns of mesothelioma, and

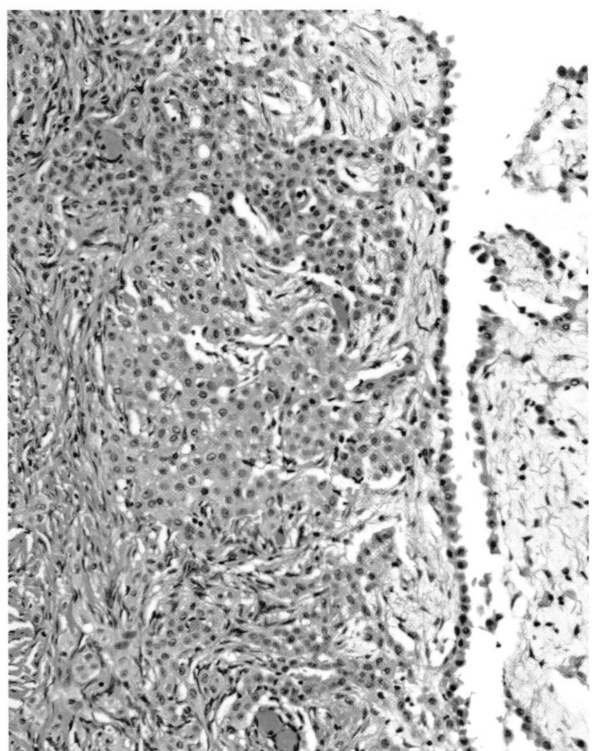

◘ Fig. 18.118
Ovarian involvement by malignant mesothelioma of peritoneum. **Note typical eosinophilic cytoplasm and relatively bland cytology**

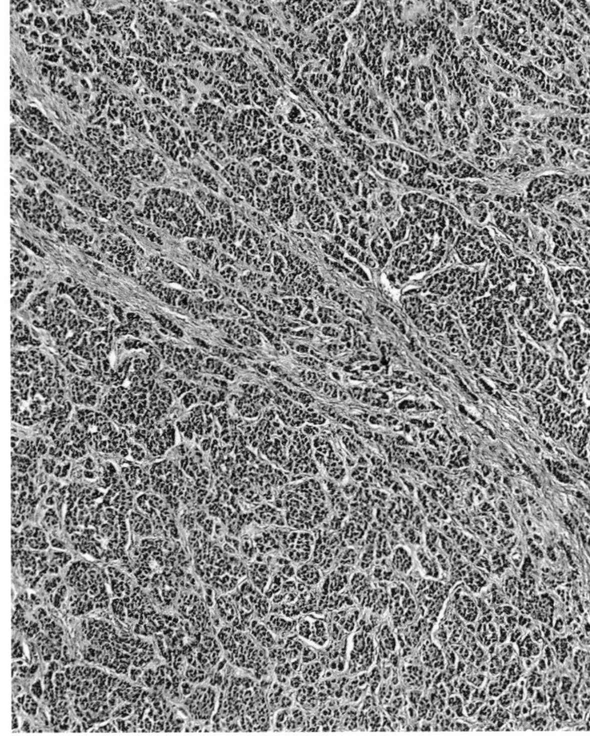

◘ Fig. 18.119
Ovarian involvement by intraabdominal desmoplastic small round cell tumor. **Nested pattern**

the characteristic cuboidal to rounded cells with abundant eosinophilic cytoplasm (➋ *Fig. 18.118*), produce a picture that is distinctly different from that of serous carcinoma. Psammoma bodies, although occasionally seen in mesotheliomas, are rarely numerous and if present in significant number, they favor a serous neoplasm. Histochemical and immunohistochemical stains may aid in this differential. Special stains in serous tumors frequently reveal apical or luminal neutral mucin and one or more antigens that are usually absent in mesothelioma including TAG-72, S-100, Leu-M1, PLAP, CEA, and Ber-EP4 [22].

The broad spectrum of morphology of peritoneal mesothelioma may result in other diverse but generally rare issues in differential diagnosis, should a case be dominated by ovarian involvement. This topic has been reviewed in detail by Baker et al. [6] and only two issues that have struck us as being perhaps more realistic than most are briefly noted here. A superficial resemblance to clear cell carcinoma may be imparted in some cases by the tubular and papillary patterns of mesothelioma, but the latter is generally less cytologically atypical and when the spectrum of morphology is evaluated, the two neoplasms should be distinguishable. A malignant mixed mesodermal tumor may be entertained when a mesothelioma has a spindle cell morphology or a prominent myxoid stroma, but the mesothelial cells are almost always less pleomorphic than the high-grade carcinomatous component of a malignant mixed mesodermal tumor.

Another peritoneal tumor that may have ovarian manifestations as a major component of the clinical presentation and present as "ovarian cancer" is the intraabdominal desmoplastic small round cell tumor with divergent differentiation. A small number (circa 10) of these tumors with ovarian involvement at presentation have been described in patients in the second and third decades, the oldest patient being 27 years old [32, 110, 164, 185]. In some cases the ovarian tumor initially was thought to be the primary neoplasm. In all the cases there was extensive extraovarian tumor at the time of presentation.

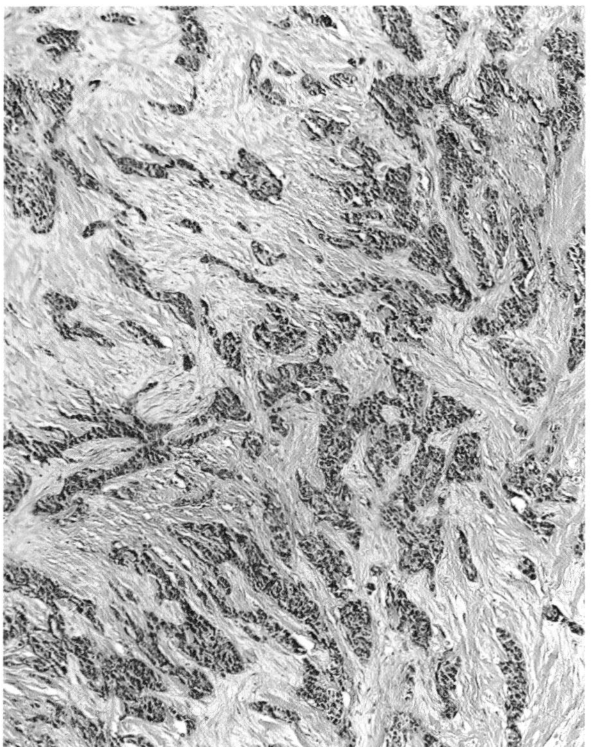

Fig. 18.120
Ovarian involvement by intraabdominal desmoplastic small round cell tumor. In this illustration, desmoplastic stroma is conspicuous and, in the setting of widespread abdominal disease, is a strong clue to the diagnosis, particularly in a young female

The ovarian involvement is usually bilateral. Microscopic examination of the ovarian tumors shows large nodules, smaller nests, and clusters composed predominantly of small cells with hyperchromatic nuclei and scanty cytoplasm surrounded by a prominent desmoplastic stroma (*Figs. 18.119* and *18.120*). The neoplasms exhibit the characteristic immunohistochemical staining profile, with many of the tumor cells staining for cytokeratin, epithelial membrane antigen, desmin, and vimentin.

The differential diagnosis in these cases is extensive and is primarily related to a number of small cell tumors that may involve the ovary, either primarily or secondarily in young females, as presented in detail elsewhere [177]. Rarely other problems in diagnosis may be encountered related to unusual findings such as focal tubular differentiation or cells with more appreciable eosinophilic cytoplasm than is typical. Generally these are only focal findings in neoplasms dominated by more distinctive morphology.

References

1. Abdul-Hafeez M, Akhtar M, Aqeel HSB, Kidess EA (1987) Placental site trophoblastic tumor: report of a case with review of literature. Ann Saudi Med 7:340–344
2. Abu-Rustum NR, Barakat RR, Curtin JP (1997) Ovarian and uterine disease in women with colorectal cancer. Gynecol Oncol 89:85–87
3. Acosta-Sison H (1958) The relative frequency of various anatomic sites as the point of first metastasis in 32 cases of chorionepithelioma. Am J Obstet Gynecol 75:1149–1152
4. Agoff SN, Lamps LW, Philip AT, Amin MB, Schmidt RA, True LD, Folpe AL (2000) Thyroid transcription factor-1 is expressed in extrapulmonary small cell carcinomas but not in other extrapulmonary neuroendocrine tumors. Mod Pathol 13:238–242
5. Amorn Y, Knight WA (1978) Primary linitis plastica of the colon: report of two cases and review of the literature. Cancer (Phila) 41:2420–2425
6. Baker PM, Clement PB, Young RH (2005) Malignant peritoneal mesothelioma in women. A study of 75 cases with emphasis on their morphologic spectrum and differential diagnosis. Am J Clin Pathol 123:724–737
7. Baker PM, Oliva E (2004) Immunohistochemistry as a tool in the differential diagnosis of ovarian tumors: an update. Int J Gynecol Pathol 24:39–55
8. Beck RP, Latour JPA (1963) Necropsy reports on 36 cases of endometrial carcinoma. Am J Obstet Gynecol 85:307–311
9. Berezowski K, Stastny JF, Kornstein MJ (1996) Cytokeratins 7 and 20 and carcinoembryonic antigen in ovarian and colonic carcinoma. Mod Pathol 9:426–429
10. Bhargava R, Beriwal S, Dabbs DJ (2007) Mammaglobin vs GCDFP-15. An immunohistologic validation survey for sensitivity and specificity. Am J Clin Pathol 127:103–113
11. Birnkrant A, Sampson J, Sugarbaker PH (1986) Ovarian metastasis from colorectal cancer. Dis Colon Rectum 29:767–771
12. Brogioni S, Viacava P, Tomisti L, Martino E, Macchia E (2007) A special case of bilateral metastases in a woman with papillary carcinoma of the thyroid. Exp Clin Endocrinol Diabetes 115:397–400
13. Brown BL, Scharifker DA, Gordon R, Deppe GG, Cohen CJ (1980) Bronchial carcinoid tumor with ovarian metastasis. A light microscopic and ultrastructural study. Cancer 46:543–546
14. Bullon A, Arseneau J, Prat J, Young RH, Scully RE (1981) Tubular Krukenberg tumor. A problem in histopathologic diagnosis. Am J Surg Pathol 5:225–232
15. Bunker ML (1959) The terminal findings in endometrial carcinoma. Am J Obstet Gynecol 77:530–538
16. Cameron RI, Ashe P, O'Rourke DM, Foster H, McCluggage WG (2003) A panel of immunohistochemical stains assists in the distinction between ovarian and renal clear cell carcinoma. Int J Gynecol Pathol 22:272–276
17. Carlson JW, Nucci MR, Brodsky J, Crum CP, Hirsch MS (2007) Biomarker-assisted diagnosis of ovarian, cervical and pulmonary small cell carcinomas: the role of TTF-1, WT-1 and HPV analysis. Histopathology 51:305–312
18. Caron P, Roche H, Gorguet B, Martel P, Bennet A, Carton M (1990) Mammary ovarian metastases with stromal cell hyperplasia and postmenopausal virilization. Cancer (Phila) 66:1221–1224
19. Che M, Tornos C, Deavers MT (2001) Ovarian mixed-epithelial carcinomas with a microcystic pattern and signet-ring cells. Int J Gynecol Pathol 20:323–328

20. Chen ZME, Wang HL (2004) Alteration of cytokeratin 7 and cytokeratin 20 expression profile is uniquely associated with tumorigenesis of primary adenocarcinoma of the small intestine. Am J Surg Pathol 28:1352–1359
21. Chu PG, Weiss LM (2004) Immunohistochemical characterization of signet-ring cell carcinomas of the stomach, breast, and colon. Am J Clin Pathol 121:884–892
22. Clement PB, Young RH, Scully RE (1996) Malignant mesotheliomas presenting as ovarian masses. A report of nine cases, including two primary ovarian mesotheliomas. Am J Surg Pathol 20:1067–1080
23. Creasman WT, Lukeman J (1972) Role of the fallopian tube in dissemination of malignant cells in corpus cancer. Cancer (Phila) 20:456–457
24. Curtin JP, Barakat RR, Hoskins WJ (1994) Ovarian disease in women with breast cancer. Obstet Gynecol 84:449–452
25. Daya D, Nazerali L, Frank GL (1992) Metastatic ovarian carcinoma of large intestinal origin simulating primary ovarian carcinoma. A clinicopathologic study of 25 cases. Am J Clin Pathol 97:751–758
26. DeCostanzo DC, Elias JM, Chumas JC (1997) Necrosis in 84 ovarian carcinomas: a morphologic study of primary versus metastatic colonic cancer with a selective immunohistochemical analysis of cytokeratin subtypes and carcinoembryonic antigen. Int J Gynecol Pathol 16:245–249
27. Demopoulos RI, Touger L, Dubin N (1987) Secondary ovarian carcinoma: a clinical and pathological evaluation. Int J Gynecol Pathol 6:166–175
28. Diddle AW (1955) Krukenberg tumors: diagnostic problem. Cancer (Phila) 8:1026–1034
29. DiLoreto C, Di Lauro V, Puglisi F et al (1997) Immunocytochemical expression of tissue specific transcription factor-1 in lung carcinoma. J Clin Pathol 50:30–32
30. Eichhorn JH, Young RH, Scully RE (1993) Non-pulmonary small cell carcinomas of extragenital origin metastatic to the ovary: a report of seven cases. Cancer (Phila) 71:177–186
31. Eifel P, Hendrickson M, Ross J, Ballon S, Martinez A, Kempson R (1982) Simultaneous presentation of carcinoma involving the ovary and the uterine corpus. Cancer (Phila) 50:163–170
32. Elhajj M, Mazurka J, Daya D (2002) Desmoplastic small round cell tumor presenting in the ovaries: report of a case and review of the literature. Int J Gynecol Cancer 12:760–763
33. Elishaev E, Gilks CB, Miller D, Srodon M, Kurman RJ, Ronnett BM (2005) Synchronous and metachronous endocervical and ovarian neoplasms. Evidence supporting interpretation of the ovarian neoplasms as metastatic endocervical adenocarcinomas simulating primary ovarian surface epithelial neoplasms. Am J Surg Pathol 29:281–294
34. Fitzgibbons PL, Martin SE, Simmons TJ (1987) Malignant melanoma metastatic to the ovary. Am J Surg Pathol 11:959–964
35. Gagnon Y, Tetu B (1989) Ovarian metastases of breast carcinoma. A clinicopathologic study of 59 cases. Cancer (Phila) 64:892–898
36. Gokden N, Gokden M, Phan DC, McKenney JK (2008) The utility of PAX-2 in distinguishing metastatic clear cell renal cell carcinoma from its morphologic mimics. An immunohistochemical study with comparison to renal cell carcinoma marker. Am J Surg Pathol 32:1462–1467
37. Goldblum J, Hart WR (1995) Localized and diffuse mesotheliomas of the genital tract and peritoneum in women. A clinicopathological study of nineteen true mesothelial neoplasms, other than adenomatoid tumors, multicystic mesotheliomas and localized fibrous tumors. Am J Surg Pathol 19:1124–1137
38. Graffner HOL, Alm POA, Oscarson JEA (1983) Prophylactic oophorectomy in colorectal carcinoma. Am J Surg 146:233–235
39. Green TH Jr, Scully RE (1962) Tumors of the fallopian tube. Clin Obstet Gynecol 5:886–906
40. Green LK, Silva EG (1989) Hepatoblastoma in an adult with metastasis to the ovaries. Am J Clin Pathol 92:110–115
41. Gupta D, Deavers MT, Silva EG et al (2004) Malignant melanoma involving the ovary. A clinicopathologic and immunohistochemical study of 23 cases. Am J Surg Pathol 28:771–780
42. Hale RW (1968) Krukenberg tumor of the ovaries. A review of 81 records. Obstet Gynecol 32:221–225
43. Harris M, Howell A, Chrissohou M, Swindell RIC, Hudson M, Sellwood RA (1984) A comparison of the metastatic pattern of infiltrating lobular carcinoma and infiltrating duct carcinoma of the breast. Br J Cancer 50:23–30
44. Hart WR (2005) Diagnostic challenge of secondary (metastatic) ovarian tumors simulating primary endometrioid and mucinous neoplasms. Pathol Int 55:321–343
45. Hassan R, Kreitman RJ, Pastan I, Willingham MC (2005) Localization of mesothelin in epithelial ovarian cancer. Mol Morphol 13:243–247
46. Hayashi Y, Kikuchi F, Oka T et al (1988) Rhabdomyosarcoma with bone marrow metastasis simulating acute leukemia. Report of two cases. Acta Pathol Jpn 38:789–798
47. Hecht JL, Pinkus JL, Weinstein LJ et al (2001) The value of thyroid transcription factor-1 in cytologic preparations as a marker for metastatic adenocarcinoma of lung origin. Am J Clin Pathol 116:483–488
48. Hines JR, Gordon RT, Widger C et al (1976) Cystosarcoma phyllodes metastatic to a Brenner tumor of the ovary. Arch Surg 111:299–300
49. Holtz F, Hart WR (1982) Krukenberg tumors of the ovary. A clinicopathologic analysis of 27 cases. Cancer (Phila) 50:2438–2447
50. Hopping RA, Dockerty MB, Masson JC (1942) Carcinoid tumor of the appendix. Report of a case in which extensive intra-abdominal metastases occurred, including involvement of the right ovary. Arch Surg 45:613–622
51. Hristov AC, Young RH, Vang R, Yemelyanova AV, Seidman JD, Ronnett BM (2007) Ovarian metastases of appendiceal tumors with goblet cell carcinoid-like and signet ring cell patterns: A report of 30 cases. Am J Surg Pathol 31:1502–1511
52. Hsiu J-G, Kemp GM, Singer GA, Rawls WH, Siddiky MA (1991) Transitional cell carcinoma of the renal pelvis with ovarian metastasis. Gynecol Oncol 41:178–181
53. Insabato L, DeRosa G, Franco R et al (2003) Ovarian metastasis from renal cell carcinoma: a report of three cases. Int J Surg Pathol 11:309–312
54. Irving JA, Lerwill MF, Young RH (2005) Gastrointestinal stromal tumors metastatic to the ovary. A report of five cases. Am J Surg Pathol 29:920–926
55. Irving JA, Vasques DR, McGuinness TB, Young RH (2006) Krukenberg tumor of renal pelvic origin: report of a case with selected comments on ovarian tumors metastatic from the urinary tract. Int J Gynecol Pathol 25:147–150
56. Irving JA, Young RH (2005) Lung carcinoma metastatic of the ovary. A clinicopathologic study of 32 cases emphasizing their morphologic spectrum and problems in differential diagnosis. Am J Surg Pathol 29:997–1006
57. Ji H, Isacson C, Seidman JD, Kurman RJ, Ronnett BM (2002) Cytokeratins 7 and 20, Dpc4, and MUC5AC in the distinction of metastatic mucinous carcinomas in the ovary from primary ovarian mucinous tumors: Dpc4 assists in identifying metastatic pancreatic carcinomas. Int J Gynecol Pathol 21:391–400

58. Judson K, McCormick C, Vang R, Yemelyanova AV, Wu LSF, Bristow RE, Ronnett BM (2008) Women with undiagnosed colorectal adenocarcinomas presenting with ovarian metastases: Clinicopathologic features and comparison with women having known colorectal adenocarcinomas and ovarian involvement. Int J Gynecol Pathol 27:182–190
59. Kaminski PF, Norris HJ (1984) Coexistence of ovarian neoplasms and endocervical adenocarcinoma. Obstet Gynecol 64:553–556
60. Kanner WA, Galgano MT, Stoler MH, Mills SE, Atkins KA (2008) Distinguishing breast carcinoma from mullerian serous carcinoma with mammaglobin and mesothelin. Int J Gynecol Pathol 27:491–495
61. Karsh J (1951) Secondary malignant disease of the ovaries. A study of 72 autopsies. Am J Obstet Gynecol 61:154–160
62. Kaufmann O, Dietel M (2000) Thyroid transcription factor-1 is the superior immunohistochemical marker for pulmonary adenocarcinomas and large cell carcinomas compared to surfactant proteins A and B. Histopathology 36:8–16
63. Khunamornpong S, Lerwill MF, Siriaunkgul S, Suprasert P, Pojchamarnwiputh S, Chiangmai WN, Young RH (2008) Carcinoma of extrahepatic bile ducts and gallbladder metastatic to the ovary: a report of 16 cases. Int J Gynecol Pathol 27:366–379
64. Khunamornpong S, Siriaunkgul S, Chunduan A (1999) Metastatic hepatocellular carcinoma of the ovary. Int J Gynecol Obstet 64:189–191
65. Khunamornpong S, Siriaunkgul S, Suprasert P, Pojchamarnwiputh S, Chiangmai WN, Young RH (2007) Intrahepatic cholangiocarcinoma metastatic to the ovary: A report of 16 cases of an underemphasized form of secondary tumor of the ovary that may mimic primary neoplasia. Am J Surg Pathol 31:1788–1799
66. Khunamornpong S, Suprasert P, Chiangmai WN, Siriaunkgul S (2006) Metastatic tumors to the ovaries: a study of 170 cases in Northern Thailand. Int J Gynecol Cancer 16:132–138
67. Khunamornpong S, Suprasert PS, Pojchamarnwiputh S, Chiangmai WN, Settakorn J, Siriaunkgul S (2006) Primary and metastatic mucinous adenocarcinomas of the ovary: evaluation of the diagnostic approach using tumor size and laterality. Gynecol Oncol 101:152–157
68. Kim KR, Lee HI, Lee SK, Ro JY, Robboy SJ (2007) Is stromal microinvasion in primary mucinous ovarian tumors with "mucin granuloma" true invasion? Am J Surg Pathol 31:546–554
69. Kim K-R, Scully RE (1990) Peritoneal keratin granulomas with carcinomas of endometrium and ovary and atypical polypoid adenomyoma of endometrium. A clinicopathological analysis of 22 cases. Am J Surg Pathol 14:925–932
70. Kindelberger DW, Lee Y, Miron A, Hirsch MS, Feltmate C, Medeiros F, Callahan MJ, Garner EO, Gordon RW, Birch C, Berkowitz RS, Muto MG, Crum CP (2007) Intraepithelial carcinoma of the fimbria and pelvic serous carcinoma: evidence for a causal relationship. Am J Surg Pathol 31:161–169
71. Kiyokawa T, Young RH, Scully RE (2006) Krukenberg tumors of the ovary. A clinicopathologic analysis of 120 cases with emphasis on their variable pathologic manifestations. Am J Surg Pathol 31:277–299
72. Kubba LA, McCluggage WG, Liu J, Malpica A, Euscher ED, Silva EG, Deavers MT (2008) Thyroid transcription factor-1 expression in ovarian epithelial neoplasms. Mod Pathol 21:485–490
73. Kuo T-T, Hsueh S (1984) Mucicarminophilic histiocytosis. A polyvinylpyrrolidone (PVP) storage disease simulating signet-ring cell carcinoma. Am J Surg Pathol 8:419–428
74. Kurek R, Von Knoblock R, Feek U, Heidenreich A, Hofmann R (2001) Local recurrence of an oncocytic adrenocortical carcinoma with ovary metastasis. J Urol 166:985
75. Lash RH, Hart WR (1987) Intestinal adenocarcinomas metastatic to the ovaries. A clinicopathological evaluation of 22 cases. Am J Surg Pathol 11:114–121
76. Lee MJ, Lee HS, Kim WH, Choi Y, Yang M (2003) Expressions of mucins and cytokeratins in primary carcinomas of the digestive system. Mod Pathol 16:403–410
77. Lee AHS, Paish EC, Marchio C, Sapino A, Schmitt FC, Ellis IO, Reis-Filho JS (2007) The expression of Wilms' tumour-1 and Ca125 in invasive micropapillary carcinoma of the breast. Histopathology 51:824–828
78. Lee KR, Young RH (2003) The distinction between primary and metastatic mucinous carcinomas of the ovary. Am J Surg Pathol 2:281–292
79. Leroy X, Farine MO, Buob D, Wacrenier A, Copin MC (2007) Diagnostic value of cytokeratin 7, CD10 and mesothelin in distinguishing ovarian clear cell carcinoma from metastasis of renal clear cell carcinoma. Histopathology 51:846–876
80. Lerwill MF (2004) Current practical applications of diagnostic immunohistochemistry in breast pathology. Am J Surg Pathol 28:1076–1091
81. Lerwill MF, Young RH (2006) Ovarian metastases of intestinal-type gastric carcinoma. A clinicopathologic study of 4 cases with contrasting features to those of the Krukenberg tumor. Am J Surg Pathol 31:1382–1388
82. Lewis MR, Deavers MT, Silva EG, Malpica A (2006) Ovarian involvement by metastatic colorectal adenocarcinoma. Still a diagnostic challenge. Am J Surg Pathol 30:177–184
83. LiVolsi VA, Merino MJ, Schwartz PE (1983) Coexistent endocervical adenocarcinoma and mucinous adenocarcinoma of ovary: a clinicopathological study of four cases. Int J Gynecol Pathol 1:391–402
84. Logani S, Baloch ZW, Snyder PJ, Weinstein R, LiVolvi VA (2001) Cystic ovarian metastasis from papillary thyroid carcinoma: a case report. Thyroid 11:1073–1075
85. Logani S, Oliva E, Amin MB, Folpe AL, Cohen C, Young RH (2003) Immunoprofile of ovarian tumors with putative transitional cell (urothelial) differentiation using novel urothelial markers. Histogenic and diagnostic implications. Am J Surg Pathol 27:1434–1441
86. Logani S, Oliva E, Arnell PM, Amin MB, Young RH (2005) Use of novel immunohistochemical markers expressed in colonic adenocarcinoma to distinguish primary ovarian tumors from metastatic colorectal carcinoma. Mod Pathol 18:19–25
87. Longacre TA, O'Hanlan K, Hendrickson MR (1996) Adenoid cystic carcinoma of the submandibular gland with symptomatic ovarian metastases. Int J Gynecol Pathol 15:349–355
88. Lumb G, Mackenzie DH (1959) The incidence of metastases in adrenal glands and ovaries removed for carcinoma of the breast. Cancer (Phila) 12:521–526
89. MacKeigan JM, Ferguson JA (1979) Prophylactic oophorectomy and colorectal cancer in premenopausal patients. Dis Colon Rectum 22:401–405
90. Mazur MT, Hsueh S, Gersell DJ (1984) Metastases to the female genital tract. Analysis of 325 cases. Cancer (Phila) 53: 1978–1984
91. McCluggage WG (2008) Immunohistochemical markers as a diagnostic aid in ovarian pathology. Diagn Histopathol 14:335–351

92. McCluggage WG, Bissonnette JP, Young RH (2006) Primary malignant melanoma of the ovary: A report of 9 definite or probable cases with emphasis on their morphologic diversity and mimicry of other primary and secondary ovarian neoplasms. Int J Gynecol Pathol 25:321–329
93. McCluggage WG, Wilkinson N (2005) Metastatic neoplasms involving the ovary: a review with an emphasis on morphological and immunohistochemical features. Histopathology 47:231–247
94. McCluggage WG, Young RH (2005) Immunohistochemistry as a diagnostic aid in the evaluation of ovarian tumors. Semin Diagn Pathol 22:3–32
95. McCluggage WG, Young RH (2008) Primary ovarian mucinous tumors with signet ring cells: report of three cases with discussion of so-called primary Krukenberg tumor. Am J Surg Pathol 32:1373–1379
96. McKenney JK, Soslow RA, Longacre TA (2008) Ovarian mature teratomas with mucinous epithelial neoplasms: Morphologic heterogeneity and association with pseudomyxoma peritonei. Am J Surg Pathol 32:645–655
97. Merino MJ, Edmonds P, LiVolsi V (1985) Appendiceal carcinoma metastatic to the ovaries and mimicking primary ovarian tumors. Int J Gynecol Pathol 4:110–120
98. Meyer WH, Yu GW, Milvenan ES, Jeffs RD, Kaizer H, Leventhal BG (1979) Ovarian involvement in neuroblastoma. Med Pediatr Oncol 7:49–54
99. Milingos D, Doumplis D, Savage P, Seckl M, Lindsay I, Smith JR (2007) Placental site trophoblastic tumor with an ovarian metastasis. Int J Gynecol Cancer 17:925–927
100. Misdraji J, Yantiss RK, Graeme-Cook FM, Balis UJ, Young RH (2003) Appendiceal mucinous neoplasms. A clinicopathologic analysis of 107 cases. Am J Surg Pathol 27:1089–1103
101. Monteagudo C, Merino MJ, Laporte N, Neumann RD (1991) Value of gross cystic disease fluid protein-15 in distinguishing metastatic breast carcinomas among poorly differentiated neoplasms involving the ovary. Hum Pathol 22:368–372
102. Moritani S, Ichihara S, Hasegawa M, Endo T, Oiwa M, Yoshikawa K, Sato Y, Aoyama H, Hayashi T, Kushima R (2008) Serous papillary adenocarcinoma of the female genital organs and invasive micropapillary carcinoma of the breast. Are WT1, CA125, and GCDFP-15 useful in differential diagnosis? Hum Pathol 39:666–671
103. Nguyen L, Brewer CA, DiSaia PJ (1998) Ovarian metastasis of Stage 1B1 squamous cell cancer of the cervix after radical parametrectomy and oophoropexy. Gynecol Oncol 68:198–200
104. Nonaka D, Chiriboga L, Soslow RA (2008) Expression of Pax8 as a useful marker in distinguishing ovarian carcinomas from mammary carcinomas. Am J Surg Pathol 32:1566–1571
105. Oberg KC, Wells K, Seraj IM et al (2002) ACTH-secreting islet cell tumor of the pancreas presenting as bilateral ovarian tumors and Cushing's syndrome. Int J Gynecol Pathol 21:276–280
106. Ohira S, Shiohara S, Itoh K et al (2003) Urachal adenocarcinoma metastatic to the ovaries: case report and literature review. Int J Gynecol Pathol 22:189–193
107. Ohta Y, Suzuki T, Shiokawa A, Mitsuya T, Ota H (2005) Expression of CD10 and cytokeratins in ovarian and renal clear cell carcinoma. Int J Gynecol Pathol 24:239–245
108. Oliva E, Musulen E, Prat J, Young RH (1993) Transitional cell carcinoma of the renal pelvis with symptomatic ovarian metastases. Int J Surg Pathol 2:231–236
109. Onuma K, Dabbs DJ, Bhargava R (2008) Mammaglobin expression in the female genital tract: immunohistochemical analysis in benign and neoplastic endocervix and endometrium. Int J Gynecol Pathol 27:418–425
110. Parker LP, Duong JL, Wharton JT, Malpica A, Silva EG, Deavers MT (2002) Desmoplastic small round cell tumor: report of a case presenting as a primary ovarian neoplasm. Eur J Gynaec Oncol 23:199–202
111. Petru E, Pickel H, Heydarfadai M, Lahousen M, Haas J, Schaider H, Tamussino K (1992) Nongenital cancers metastatic to the ovary. Gynecol Oncol 44:83–86
112. Phillips V, McCluggage WG, Young RH (2006) Oxyphilic adenomatoid tumor of the ovary: a case report with discussion of the differential diagnosis of ovarian tumors with vacuoles and related spaces. Int J Gynecol Pathol 26:16–20
113. Pins MR, Young RH, Crum CP, Leach IH, Scully RE (1997) Cervical squamous carcinoma in situ with superficial extension to corpus and tubes and invasion of tubes and ovaries. Int J Gynecol Pathol 16:272–278
114. Pitluk H, Poticha SM (1983) Carcinoma of the colon and rectum in patients less than 40 years of age. Surg Gynecol Obstet 157:335–337
115. Pitman MB, Triratanachat S, Young RH, Oliva E (2003) Hepatocyte paraffin 1 antibody does not distinguish primary ovarian tumors with hepatoid differentiation from metastatic hepatocellular carcinoma. Int J Gynecol Pathol 23:58–64
116. Prayson RA, Hart WR, Petras RE (1994) Pseudo-myxoma peritonei. A clinicopathologic study of 19 cases with emphasis on site of origin and nature of associated ovarian tumors. Am J Surg Pathol 18:591–603
117. Rabban JT, Lerwill MF, McCluggage WG, Grenert JP, Zaloudek CJ (2009) Primary ovarian carcinoid tumors may express CDX-2: a potential pitfall in distinction from metastatic intestinal carcinoid tumors involving the ovary. Int J Gynecol Pathol 28:41–48
118. Reis-Filho JS, Carrilho C, Valenti C et al (2000) Is TTF1 a good immunohistochemical marker to distinguish primary from metastatic lung adenocarcinomas? Pathol Res Pract 196:835–840
119. Riopel MA, Ronnett BM, Kurman RJ (1999) Evaluation of diagnostic criteria and behavior of ovarian intestinal-type mucinous tumors. Atypical proliferative (borderline) tumors and intraepithelial, microinvasive, invasive, and metastatic carcinomas. Am J Surg Pathol 23:617–635
120. Robboy SJ, Scully RE, Norris HJ (1974) Carcinoid metastatic to the ovary. A clinicopathologic analysis of 35 cases. Cancer (Phila) 33:798–811
121. Ronnett BM, Kurman RJ, Shmookler BM, Sugarbaker PH, Young RH (1997) The morphologic spectrum of ovarian metastases of appendical adenocarcinomas. A clinicopathologic and immunohistochemical analysis of tumors often misinterpreted as primary ovarian tumors or metastatic tumors from other gastrointestinal sites. Am J Surg Pathol 2:1144–1155
122. Ronnett BM, Kurman RJ, Zahn CM, Shmookler BM, Jablonski KA, Kass ME (1995) Pseudomyxoma peritonei in women. A clinicopathologic analysis of 30 cases with emphasis on site of origin, prognosis, and relationship to ovarian mucinous tumors of low malignant potential. Hum Pathol 26:509–524
123. Ronnett BM, Shmookler BM, Diener-West M, Sugarbaker PH, Kurman RJ (1997) Immunohistochemical evidence supporting the appendiceal origin of pseudomyxoma peritonei in women. Int J Gynecol Pathol 16:1–9
124. Ronnett BM, Yemelyanova AV, Vang R, Gilks CB, Miller D, Gravitt PE, Kurman RJ (2008) Endocervical adenocarcinomas with ovarian metastases. Analysis of 29 cases with emphasis on minimally

invasive cervical tumors and the ability of the metastases to simulate primary ovarian neoplasms. Am J Surg Pathol 32:1835–1853

125. Ronnett BM, Zahn CM, Kurman RJ, Kass ME, Sugarbaker PH, Shmookler BM (1995) Disseminated peritoneal adenomucinosis and peritoneal mucinous carcinomatosis: a clinicopathologic analysis of 109 cases with emphasis on distinguishing pathologic features, site of origin, prognosis, and relationship to "pseudomyxoma peritonei". Am J Surg Pathol 19:1390–1408
126. Saphir O (1951) Signet-ring cell carcinoma. Mil Surg 109:360–369
127. Sasaki E, Tsunoda N, Hatanaka Y, Mori N, Iwata H, Yatabe Y (2007) Breast-specific expression of MGB1/mammaglobin: an examination of 480 tumors from various organs and clinicopathological analysis of MGB1-positive breast cancers. Mod Pathol 20:208–214
128. Scully RE, Richardson GS (1961) Luteinization of the stroma of metastatic cancer involving the ovary and its endocrine significance. Cancer (Phila) 14:827–840
129. Seidman JD, Elsayed AM, Sobin LH, Tavassoli FA (1993) Association of mucinous tumors of the ovary and appendix. A clinicopathologic study of 25 cases. Am J Surg Pathol 17:22–34
130. Seidman JD, Kurman RJ, Ronnett BM (2003) Incidence in routine practice with a new approach to improve intraoperative diagnosis. Primary and metastatic mucinous adenocarcinomas in the ovaries. Am J Surg Pathol 27:985–993
131. Smale L (1980) Metastatic breast adenocarcinoma to Brenner tumors. Gynecol Oncol 9:251–253
132. Soslow RA, Rouse RV, Hendrickson MR, Silva EG, Longacre TA (1996) Transitional cell neoplasms of the ovary and urinary bladder: a comparative immunohistochemical analysis. Int J Gynecol Pathol 15:257–265
133. Spencer JR, Eriksen B, Garnett JE (1993) Metastatic renal tumor presenting as ovarian clear cell carcinoma. Urology 41:582–584
134. Stewart CJR, Brennan BA, Hammond IG et al (2005) Accuracy of frozen section in distinguishing primary ovarian neoplasia from tumors metastatic to the ovary. Int J Gynecol Pathol 24:356–362
135. Strosberg J, Nasir A, Cragun J, Gardner N, Kvols L (2007) Metastatic carcinoid tumor to the ovary: a clinicopathologic analysis of seventeen cases. Gynecol Oncol 106:65–68
136. Sty JR, Kun LE, Casper JT (1980) Bone scintigraphy in neuroblastoma with ovarian metastasis. Wis Med J 79:28–29
137. Szych C, Staebler A, Connolly DC, Wu R, Cho KR, Ronnett BM (1999) Molecular genetic evidence supporting the clonality and appendiceal origin of pseudomyxoma peritonei in women. Am J Pathol 154:1849–1855
138. Tabata M, Ichinoe K, Sakuragi N, Shina Y, Yamaguchi T, Mabuchi Y (1987) Incidence of ovarian metastasis in patients with cancer of the uterine cervix. Gynecol Oncol 28:255–261
139. Tang LH, Shia J, Soslow RA, Dhall D, Wong WD, O'Reilly E, Qin J, Paty P, Weiser MR, Guillem J, Temple L, Sobin LH, Klimstra DS (2008) Pathologic classification and clinical behavior of the spectrum of goblet cell carcinoid tumors of the appendix. Am J Surg Pathol 32:1429–1443
140. Toki N, Tsukamoto N, Kaku T et al (1991) Microscopic ovarian metastasis of the uterine cervical cancer. Gynecol Oncol 41:46–51
141. Tornos C, Soslow R, Chen S et al (2005) Expression of WT1, CA 125, and GCDFP-15 as useful markers in the differential diagnosis of primary ovarian carcinomas versus metastatic breast cancer to the ovary. Am J Surg Pathol 29:1482–1489
142. Tso PL, Bringaze WL III, Dauterive AH, Correa P, Cohn I Jr (1987) Gastric carcinoma in the young. Cancer (Phila) 59:1362–1365
143. Ulbright TM, Roth LM (1985) Metastatic and independent cancers of the endometrium and ovary: a clinicopathologic study of 34 cases. Hum Pathol 16:28–34
144. Ulbright TM, Roth LM (1985) Secondary tumors of the ovary. In: Roth LM, Czernobilsky B (eds) Tumors and tumor-like conditions of the ovary, vol 6, Contemporary issues in surgical pathology. Churchill-Livingstone, New York, pp 129–152
145. Ulbright TM, Roth LM, Stehman FB (1984) Secondary ovarian neoplasia. A clinicopathologic study of 35 cases. Cancer (Phila) 53:1164–1174
146. Vakiani E, Young RH, Carcangiu ML, Klimstra DS (2008) Acinar cell carcinoma of the pancreas metastatic to the ovary. A report of 4 cases. Am J Surg Pathol 32:1540–1545
147. Vang R, Gown AM, Barry TS, Wheeler DT, Yemelyanova A, Seidman JD, Ronnett BM (2006) Cytokeratins 7 and 20 in primary and secondary mucinous tumors of the ovary: analysis of coordinate immunohistochemical expression profiles and staining distribution in 179 cases. Am J Surg Pathol 30:1130–1139
148. Vang R, Gown AM, Wu LSF, Barry TS, Wheeler DT, Yemelyanova A, Seidman JD, Ronnett BM (2006) Immunohistochemical expression of CDX2 in primary ovarian mucinous tumors and metastatic mucinous carcinomas involving the ovary: comparison with CK20 and correlation with coordinate expression of CK7. Mod Pathol 19:1421–1428
149. Vang R, Gown AM, Zhao C, Barry TS, Isacson C, Richardson MS, Ronnett BM (2007) Ovarian mucinous tumors associated with mature cystic teratomas. Morphologic and immunohistochemical analysis identifies a subset of potential teratomatous origin that shares features of lower gastrointestinal tract mucinous tumors more commonly encountered as secondary tumors in the ovary. Am J Surg Pathol 31:854–869
150. Vara A, Madrigal B, Veiga M, Diaz A, Garcia J, Calvo J (1998) Bilateral ovarian metastases from renal clear cell carcinoma. Acta Oncol (Stockh) 37:379–380
151. Veras E, Srodon M, Neijstrom ES, Ronnett BM (2009) Metastatic HPV-related cervical adenocarcinomas presenting with thromboembolic events (Trousseau syndrome): clinicopathologic characteristics of two cases. Int J Gynecol Pathol 28:134–139
152. Webb MJ, Decker DG, Mussey E (1975) Factors influencing survival. Cancer metastatic to the ovary. Obstet Gynecol 45:391–396
153. Wheelock MC, Putong P (1959) Ovarian metastases from adenocarcinomas of colon and rectum. Obstet Gynecol 14:291–295
154. Wick MR, Lillemoe TJ, Copland GT, Swanson PE, Manivel JC, Kiang DT (1989) Gross cystic disease fluid protein-15 as a marker for breast cancer: immunohistochemical analysis of 690 human neoplasms and comparison with alpha-lactalbumin. Hum Pathol 20:281–287
155. Woodruff JD, Murthy YS, Bhaskar TN, Bordbar F, Tseng S-S (1970) Metastatic ovarian tumors. Am J Obstet Gynecol 107:202–209
156. Yakushiji M, Tazaki T, Nishimura H, Kato T (1987) Krukenberg tumors of the ovary: a clinicopathologic analysis of 112 cases. Acta Obstet Gynaecol Jpn 39:479–485
157. Yemelyanova AV, Vang R, Judson K, Wu LSF, Ronnett BM (2008) Distinction of primary and metastatic mucinous tumors involving the ovary: analysis of size and laterality data by primary site with reevaluation of an algorithm for tumor classification. Am J Surg Pathol 32:128–138
158. Yoshida A, Shigematsu T, Mori H, Yoshida H, Fukunishi R (1981) Non-invasive thymoma with widespread blood-borne metastasis. Virchows Arch (Path Anat) 390:121–126

159. Young RH (1995) Urachal adenocarcinoma metastatic to the ovary simulating primary mucinous cystadenocarcinoma of the ovary: report of a case. Virchows Arch 426:529–532
160. Young RH (2004) Pseudomyxoma peritonei and selected other aspects of the spread of appendiceal neoplasms. Semin Diagn Pathol 21:134–150
161. Young RH (2006) From Krukenberg to today: The ever present problems posed by metastatic tumors in the ovary. Part I. Historical perspective, general principles, mucinous tumors including the Krukenberg tumor. Adv Anat Pathol 13:205–227
162. Young RH (2007) From Krukenberg to today: the ever present problems posed by metastatic tumors in the ovary. Part II. Adv Anat Pathol 14:149–177
163. Young RH, Carey RW, Robboy SJ (1981) Breast carcinoma masquerading as a primary ovarian neoplasm. Cancer (Phila) 48:210–212
164. Young RH, Eichhorn JH, Dickersin GR, Scully RE (1992) Ovarian involvement by the intra-abdominal desmoplastic small round cell tumor with divergent differentiation. A report of three cases. Hum Pathol 23:454–464
165. Young RH, Gersell DJ, Clement PB, Scully RE (1992) Hepatocellular carcinoma metastatic to the ovary: a report of three cases discovered during life with discussion of the differential diagnosis of hepatoid tumors of the ovary. Hum Pathol 23:574–580
166. Young RH, Gersell DJ, Roth LM, Scully RE (1993) Ovarian metastases from cervical carcinomas other than pure adenocarcinomas: a report of 12 cases. Cancer (Phila) 71:407–418
167. Young RH, Gilks CB, Scully RE (1991) Mucinous tumors of the appendix associated with mucinous tumors of the ovary and pseudomyxoma peritonei: a clinicopathological analysis of 22 cases supporting an origin in the appendix. Am J Surg Pathol 15:415–429
168. Young RH, Hart WR (1989) Metastases from carcinomas of the pancreas simulating primary mucinous tumors of the ovary: a report of seven cases. Am J Surg Pathol 13:748–756
169. Young RH, Hart WR (1992) Renal cell carcinoma metastatic to the ovary: a report of three cases emphasizing possible confusion with ovarian clear cell adenocarcinoma. Int J Gynecol Pathol 11:96–104
170. Young RH, Hart WR (1998) Metastatic intestinal carcinomas simulating primary ovarian clear cell carcinoma and secretory endometrioid carcinoma. A clinicopathologic and immunohistochemical study of five cases. Am J Surg Pathol 22:805–815
171. Young RH, Jackson A, Wells M (1994) Ovarian metastasis from thyroid carcinoma twelve years after partial thyroidectomy mimicking struma ovarii. Report of a case. Int J Gynecol Pathol 13:181–185
172. Young RH, Kozakewich HPW, Scully RE (1993) Metastatic ovarian tumors in children: a report of 14 cases and review of the literature. Int J Gynecol Pathol 12:8–19
173. Young RH, Prat J, Scully RE (1984) Endometrial stromal sarcomas of the ovary. A clinicopathologic analysis of 23 cases. Cancer (Phila) 53:1143–1155
174. Young RH, Scully RE (1985) Ovarian metastases from cancer of the lung: problems in interpretation – a report of seven cases. Gynecol Oncol 21:337–350
175. Young RH, Scully RE (1988) Mucinous tumors of the ovary associated with mucinous adenocarcinomas of the cervix. A clinicopathological analysis of 16 cases. Int J Gynecol Pathol 7:99–111
176. Young RH, Scully RE (1988) Urothelial and ovarian carcinomas of identical cell types: problems in interpretation. A report of three cases and review of the literature. Int J Gynecol Pathol 7:197–211
177. Young RH, Scully RE (1989) Alveolar rhabdomyosarcoma metastatic to the ovary. A report of two cases and discussion of the differential diagnosis of small cell malignant tumors of the ovary. Cancer (Phila) 64:899–904
178. Young RH, Scully RE (1990) Ovarian metastases from carcinoma of the gallbladder and extrahepatic bile ducts simulating primary tumors of the ovary: a report of six cases. Int J Gynecol Pathol 9:60–72
179. Young RH, Scully RE (1990) Sarcomas metastatic to the ovary. A report of 21 cases. Int J Gynecol Pathol 9:231–252
180. Young RH, Scully RE (1991) Malignant melanoma metastatic to the ovary: a clinicopathologic analysis of 20 cases. Am J Surg Pathol 15:849–860
181. Young RH, Scully RE (1991) Metastatic tumors in the ovary: a problem-oriented approach and review of the recent literature. Semin Diagn Pathol 8:250–276
182. Young RH, Scully RE (2001) Differential diagnosis of ovarian tumors based primarily on their patterns and cell types. Semin Diagn Pathol 18:161–235
183. Yu TJ, Iwasaki I, Horie H, Tamaru J, Takahashi A (1986) Endolymphatic stromal myosis of the uterus with metastasis to ovary and recurrence in vagina. Acta Pathol Jpn 36:301–308
184. Zaino RJ, Unger ER, Whitney C (1984) Synchronous carcinomas of the uterine corpus and ovary. Gynecol Oncol 19:329–335
185. Zaloudek C, Miller TR, Stern JL (1995) Desmoplastic small cell tumor of the ovary: a unique polyphenotypic tumor with an unfavorable prognosis. Int J Gynecol Oncol 14:260–265
186. Zamecnik M, Voltr L, Stuk J, Chlumska A (2008) Krukenberg tumor with yolk sac tumor differentiation. Int J Gynecol Pathol 27:223–228
187. Zhang PJ, Gao HG, Pasha TL, Litzky L, LiVolsi V (2009) TTF-1 expression in ovarian and uterine epithelial neoplasia and its potential significance, an immunohistochemical assessment with multiple monoclonal antibodies and different secondary detection systems. Int J Gynecol Pathol 28:10–18
188. Zukerberg LR, Young RH (1990) Chordoma metastatic to the ovary: report of a case. Arch Path Lab Med 114:208–210

19 Diseases of the Placenta

Deborah J. Gersell · Frederick T. Kraus

R. J. Kurman, L. Hedrick Ellenson, B. M. Ronnett (eds.), *Blaustein's Pathology of the Female Genital Tract (6th ed.)*, DOI 10.1007/978-1-4419-0489-8_19,

The placenta is crucial for fetal growth and survival, performing the most important functions of many somatic organs before birth. Thus, pathologic processes interfering with placental function may result in abnormalities of fetal growth or development, malformation, or stillbirth, and there is increasing recognition that some long-term (especially neurologic) disabilities can be traced to injury occurring before birth. The purpose of this chapter is to describe clinically important placental lesions and to emphasize the context in which these lesions are directly or indirectly important to the fetus, the mother, or both.

Normal Anatomy and Development

The monograph by Boyd and Hamilton [23] provides a detailed description and exquisite illustrations of the various stages of human implantation. The ovum is fertilized in the fallopian tube and develops rapidly, reaching the endometrial cavity as a blastocyst. At this stage, the outer cell layer of the blastocyst has differentiated into trophoblast, and there are only a few cells in the inner cell mass from which the embryo will develop. The trophoblast attaches to and penetrates the endometrium on the 6th to 7th postovulatory day, and by the 10th to 11th postovulatory day, the blastocyst is totally embedded in endometrial stroma that has reestablished continuity over the penetration defect. The trophoblast grows rapidly and circumferentially, invading maternal blood vessels. Blood-filled spaces (lacunae) separate the trophoblast into trabecular columns (*Fig. 19.1*), with an outer syncytiotrophoblastic layer oriented radially around central solid cores of cytotrophoblast. As the extraembryonic mesenchyme penetrates the cytotrophoblastic cores, small blood vessels form within it, and these eventually connect with each other and with those forming independently in the allantois of the body stalk (chorioallantoic placentation), establishing the fetoplacental circulation by the 5th–6th week. A shell of solid trophoblast remains at the periphery of the stem villi, anchoring them to the basal plate and continuing to grow and expand the intervillous space (*Fig. 19.2*).

Successful implantation requires a series of complex, coordinated interactions between maternal tissue and trophoblast. The trophoblast consists of several morphologically and functionally distinct cell types, each with characteristic anatomic distribution. The great majority of cytotrophoblastic and syncytiotrophoblastic cells are located on the villi (villous trophoblast). Cytotrophoblast (CT), the germinative, mitotically active component of trophoblast, is present as a layer of uniform cells with single, round–oval nuclei, clear cytoplasm, and distinct cell borders directly overlying the stromal core of the villus. The syncytiotrophoblast (ST) overlies the CT and is the terminally differentiated component of trophoblast responsible for transport functions, protection, and pregnancy-specific protein and hormone production. Its abundant, often vacuolated cytoplasm is amphophilic with multiple small dark nuclei and a distinct brush border. Intermediate trophoblast (IT) is a constituent of villous trophoblast, primarily in the anchoring cell columns, but is most prevalent in extravillous sites. IT developing from the trophoblastic shell invades the endometrium and myometrium at the implantation site. Subpopulations of IT in the villi (villous IT), implantation site,

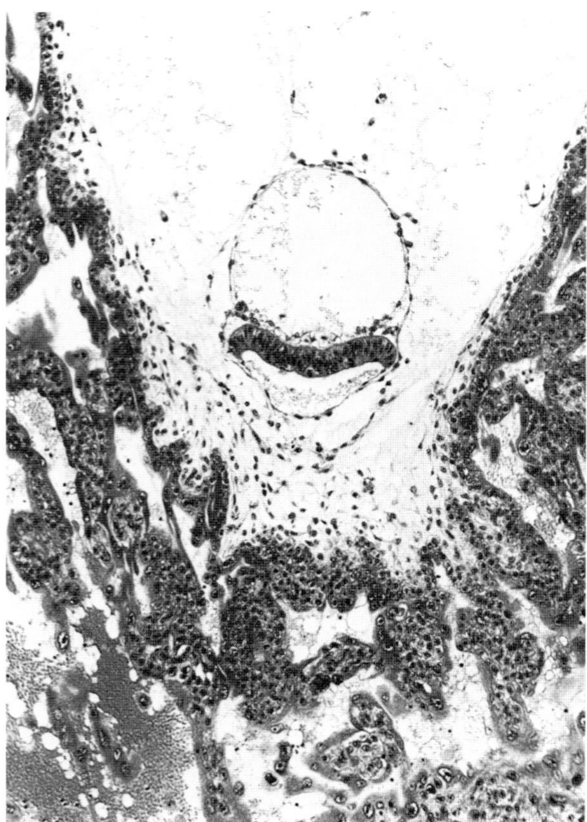

Fig. 19.1
Implantation at 13 days. **Trophoblast has differentiated into inner (cytotrophoblast) and outer (syncytiotrophoblast) layers. Focally, the cytotrophoblast has proliferated to form projections, the forerunners of the primary villi. The germ disk is located near the center (Reprinted courtesy of Department of Embryology, Davis Division, Carnegie Institute of Washington)**

and membranes (chorionic IT) are morphologically and immunohistochemically distinct [172]. IT nuclei are irregular and hyperchromatic with coarsely granular chromatin. Most cells are mononucleate, although multinucleate forms occur. IT may be round, polyhedral, or spindle shaped depending on location with abundant eosinophilic, amphophilic, or clear cytoplasm. The cytologic features are generally sufficiently distinctive to identify IT, but their intermingling with decidua at the implantation site is so intimate that it may be difficult to characterize any particular cell as maternal or fetal by conventional light microscopy. When findings are equivocal (as in some abortion specimens), immunohistochemical stains for keratin help distinguish IT (keratin positive) from decidua (keratin negative).

■ Fig. 19.2
Secondary villi. **Mesenchyme has penetrated the trophoblastic cores. The trophoblastic shell is peripheral**

The IT that infiltrates the decidua and myometrium at the implantation site is responsible for remarkable physiologic structural modifications in the spiral arteries. In the early weeks of pregnancy, IT invades the decidual segments of the spiral arteries, forming intraluminal plugs. Later, between the 12th and 20th weeks of pregnancy, endovascular IT extends from the decidual into the myometrial segments of the spiral arteries. Eventually, IT and fibrinoid completely replace the endothelium and the muscular and elastic tissue of the media (➲ *Fig. 19.3*). Altered by this process, the spiral arteries undergo progressive distension, eventuating in large funnel-shaped channels that augment blood flow to the implantation site. Dissolution of the muscular media results in fixed vascular dilatation unresponsive to vasculospastic influences.

As it grows and enlarges, the chorion undergoes gross structural modifications. Initially, villi surround the entire chorionic cavity, but as the chorion prolapses into the endometrial cavity, the villi oriented toward the uterine cavity undergo progressive atrophy to form the smooth chorion (chorion laeve) or fetal membranes (➲ *Fig. 19.4*). These atrophic villi are still apparent in sections of membranes in the mature placenta (➲ *Fig. 19.5*). The villi on the embryonic aspect of the chorion continue to proliferate, forming the definitive placenta (chorion frondosum). Differential villous atrophy and proliferation reflect maternal blood flow. Departure from the usual pattern of villous growth and atrophy is thought to result in some of the aberrant placental shapes described below. Continued growth and enlargement of the chorion results in eventual obliteration of the uterine cavity through fusion

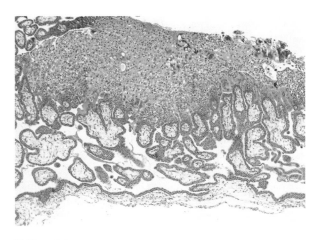

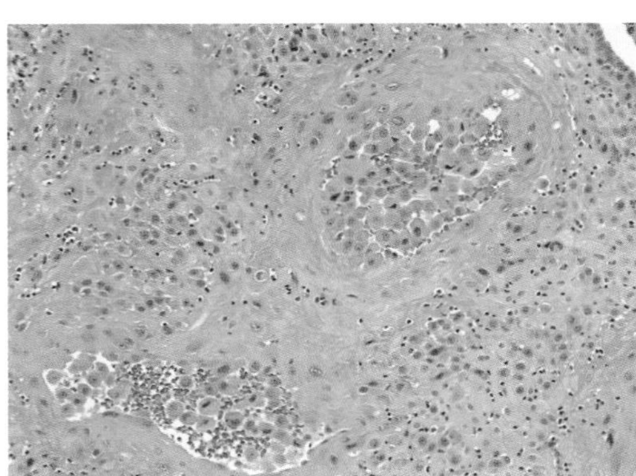

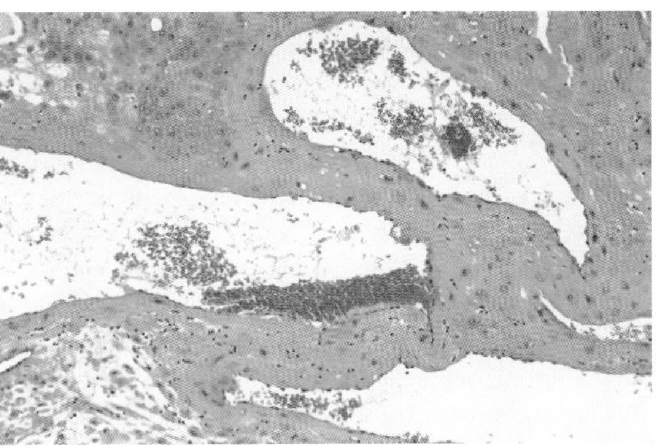

■ Fig. 19.3
Normal spiral artery remodeling. **Intraluminal IT (*left*) later invades and replaces the vascular media along with fibrinoid matrix (*right*)**

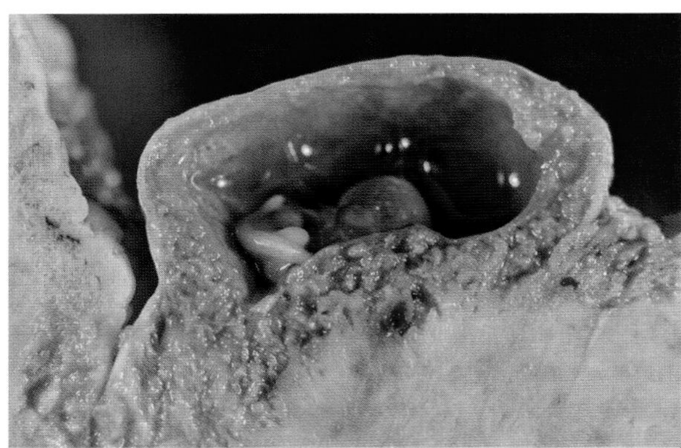

Fig. 19.4
Formation of chorion laeve. **As the chorion prolapses into the endometrial cavity, the villi on the intracavitary aspect atrophy to form the fetal membranes**

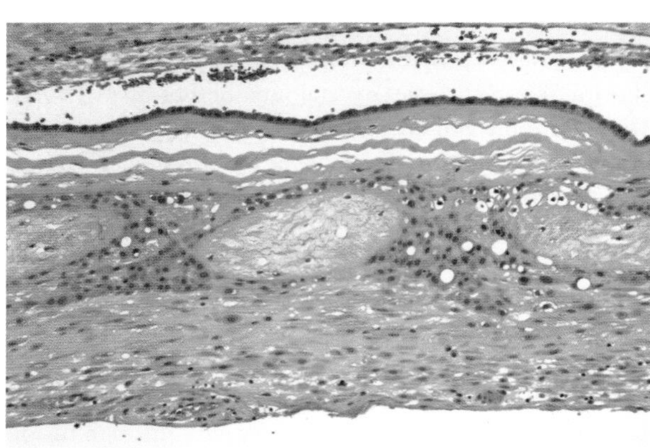

Fig. 19.5
Chorion laeve. **Atrophied villous remnants remain in the membranes at term**

of the decidua capsularis and the decidua vera of the opposite uterine wall, usually around 20 weeks. In time, the chorionic cavity is obliterated by progressive expansion of the amnion. Irregular folds of the basal plate drawn into the intervillous space by the relatively slow growth of anchoring villi form septae, appearing at about 3 months. IT islands are prominent in the septae. The septae partition the maternal surface incompletely and irregularly into 15 to 20 divisions that have no physiologic significance.

Villous structure changes dramatically over the course of a normal gestation reflecting placental growth, development,

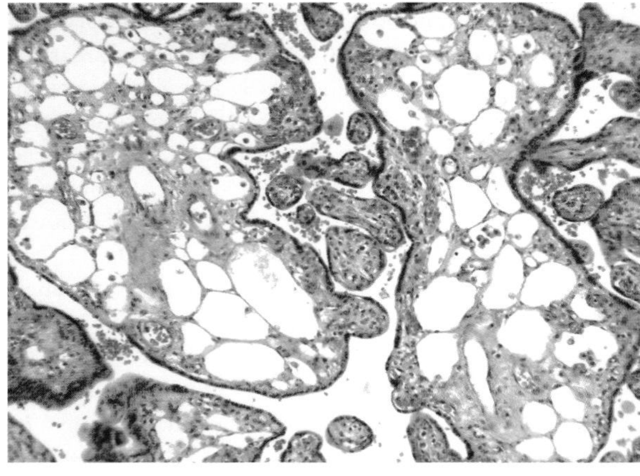

Fig. 19.6
Immature intermediate villi. **These are characterized by reticular stroma and channels containing Hofbauer cells**

and maturation. Five villous types have been detailed in the work of Kaufmann and others [17]. Mesenchymal villi are a primitive, transient stage in villous development. The loose stroma of mesenchymal villi is abundant with numerous Hofbauer cells, central small vessels, and an orderly surface bilayer of CT and ST. Mesenchymal villi predominate in early pregnancy but may be found in small numbers even at term. According to Kaufmann, mesenchymal villi begin to develop into immature intermediate villi around 7–8 weeks. Immature intermediate villi are defined by abundant loose reticular stroma with empty channels containing Hofbauer cells, features that may lead to erroneous interpretation as villous edema (*Fig. 19.6*). Immature intermediate villi predominate through the second trimester, but small clusters persist in the center of lobules at term (normally 0–5% volumetrically). Immature intermediate villi are gradually transformed into stem villi as their vessels acquire a distinct muscular media and progressively prominent adventitia and fibrous stroma. The stem villi divide progressively, and some insert into the basal plate, anchoring the placenta to the uterus. Stem villi support the villous tree and transport blood but do not participate significantly in oxygen or nutrient exchange. Stem villi comprise 20–25% of villi in a normal term placenta, with highest concentration centrally beneath the chorionic plate.

Beginning in the last trimester, newly formed mesenchymal villi transform into mature intermediate villi. Mature intermediate villi are long and slender with roughly the same diameter as terminal villi and numerous small vessels and capillaries, comprising less than 50% of the villus. Roughly one fourth of the villous volume at term is made up of mature intermediate villi. Terminal villi are the final ramifications of the villous tree produced along the surfaces of mature intermediate villi during the third trimester. Terminal villi have sinusoidally dilated capillaries (occupying more than 50% of the villous stroma) that bulge beneath overlying attenuated syncytiotrophoblast. Fusion of endothelial and trophoblastic basement membranes results in the formation of vasculosyncytial membranes (➋ *Fig. 19.7*). In these areas, where the maternal and fetal circulations are most closely approximated, gas and nutrient exchange occur. Normally, terminal villi make up more than 40% of the villous volume at term.

With villous maturation, the barrier between maternal and fetal circulations is reduced by thinning of syncytiotrophoblast, diminution in cytotrophoblast, decrease in mean villous diameter, and apposition of fetal capillaries to the villous surface. The factors that normally control villous maturation are not understood, but considerable evidence suggests that the maturational rate is altered in pathologic states. The villi in any placenta are not completely homogeneous. The peripheral villi and those beneath the chorionic plate tend to be smaller with more collagenous stroma and a thicker trophoblastic basement membrane than the less mature villi located centrally in the fetal lobule. These regional differences, probably related to maternal blood flow, should always be considered when judging placental maturity, which is best assessed in standardized sections from central placental zones.

The placenta has two circulations – maternal and fetal. Maternal blood is delivered to the intervillous space through spiral arterial inlets in the basal plate. Maternal blood flows toward the chorionic plate, disperses laterally, percolates around the villi, and exits through venous outlets concentrated peripherally in the placental floor. Deoxygenated fetal blood reaches the placenta through the two umbilical arteries that branch and divide in stem villi until they ultimately terminate in the complex capillary network of the terminal villi. Oxygenated and fortified fetal blood returns via venous tributaries to the umbilical vein. The placental circulation normally receives about 55% of the fetal cardiac output. Lacking autonomic innervation, it responds only to local factors such as pressure and flow.

Abnormal Placentation and Villous Development

Anomalous Shapes

The pattern of villous atrophy and proliferation that occurs during placental development resulting in ultimate placental shape and configuration is thought to be determined by maternal blood flow. The *accessory* or *succenturiate lobe* is a common shape variation (3–6% of placentas) in which usually one but occasionally multiple discrete masses of placental tissue are separated from the main placenta by fetal membranes (➋ *Fig. 19.8*). The umbilical cord usually

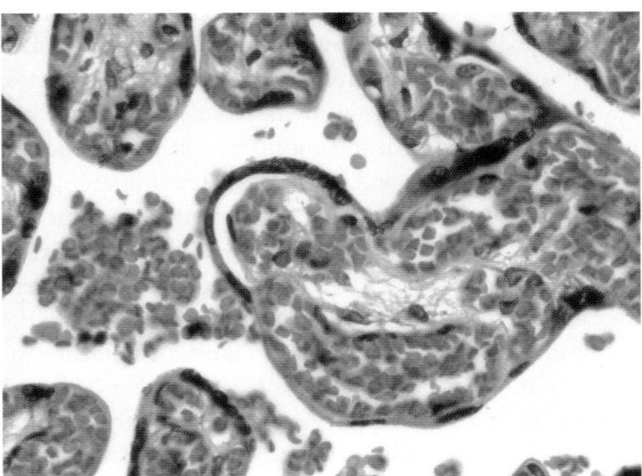

Fig. 19.7
Third-trimester terminal villi, vasculosyncytial membranes. **Fetal capillaries protrude beneath thinned syncytiotrophoblast cytoplasm between knots. The endothelial and syncytiotrophoblastic basement membranes fuse forming vasculosyncytial membranes**

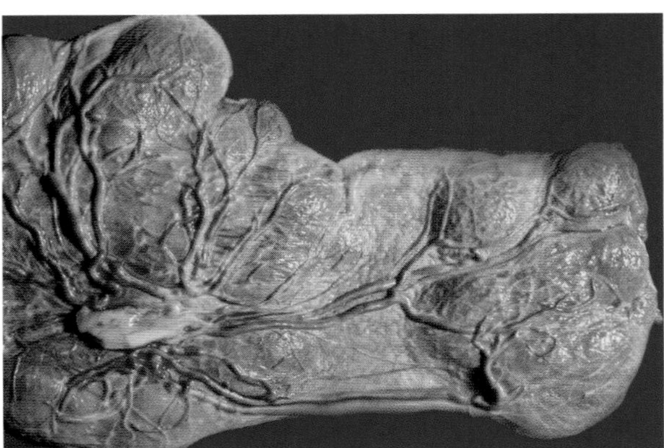

Fig. 19.8
Accessory (succenturiate) lobe. **A discrete mass of placental tissue is separated from the main disk by fetal membranes containing unsupported fetal vessels**

inserts into the main placental mass, and the fetal vessels supplying the accessory lobe traverse membranes unsupported by underlying villous parenchyma. If these membranous vessels are traumatized during delivery, severe fetal hemorrhage may result. Thrombosis of membranous vessels may be associated with fetal thromboembolic events. Occasionally, an accessory lobe presents as placenta previa or is retained in utero after delivery resulting in postpartum bleeding or infection. Succenturiate lobes have a tendency to atrophy or infarct but otherwise show no specific histologic changes. The *bilobate* or *bipartite placenta* is a variant in which two equally sized placental lobes are separated by fetal membranes or connected by a narrow isthmus of placental tissue. The umbilical cord often inserts centrally between the lobes.

Other anomalous shapes are uncommon. *Multilobate placentas* have multiple lobes defined by indentations measuring >50% of the disc diameter. *Placenta membranacea* is a large, thin placenta with functional chorionic villi covering the entire gestational sac. In this condition, differential atrophy of the chorion laeve and proliferation of the chorion frondosum do not occur. The placental parenchyma may vary in thickness, but only exceptionally is there a dominant area resembling a placental disk. Placenta membranacea occurs commonly in animal species but is extremely rare in humans. The few reported cases have been complicated by antepartum bleeding and abnormal placental adherence relating to the obligate placenta previa that accompanies this form of placentation. Nearly all cases are associated with preterm delivery and high fetal mortality. The annular or cylindrical *ring-shaped placenta* is very rare. In *fenestrate placentas*, focal absence of the villous parenchyma may result in a through-and-through hole or the chorionic plate may remain intact over the parenchymal defect.

Extrachorial Placenta

Extrachorial placentation is a common gross structural deviation in which the chorionic plate of the placenta is smaller than the basal plate. The chorionic plate does not extend to the placental margin as in a normal placenta, but undergoes transition to fetal membranes central to the disk edge, leaving a rim of bare placental tissue (extrachorial portion) extending beyond the limits of the chorionic plate (➲ *Fig. 19.9*). Fetal vessels appear to terminate at the margin of the chorionic plate but actually continue their course peripherally in the deeper villous tissue.

Etiology and pathogenesis. There have been many theories attempting to explain the etiology and pathogenesis

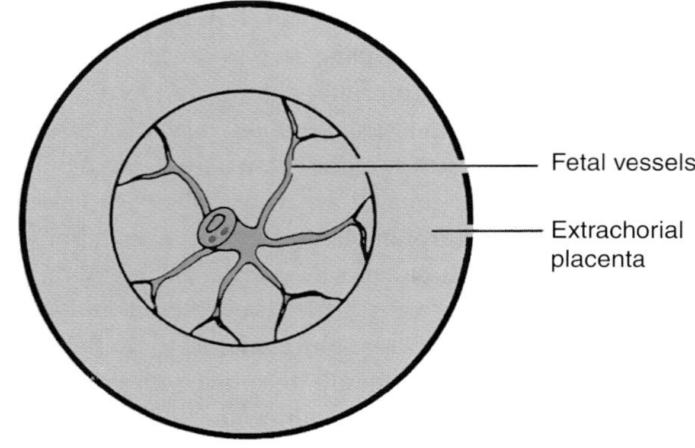

Fig. 19.9
Diagram of an extrachorial placenta, fetal side. **Vessels appear to terminate at the margin of the chorionic plate but continue peripherally in the extrachorial portion (After [44])**

of extrachorial placentation including abnormally deep implantation and premature fixation of the disc-membrane boundary. Recently, recurrent marginal hemorrhage resulting in circumvallation has been documented on serial ultrasound images, providing evidence that recurrent hemorrhage at the disk margin elevates and displaces the membrane insertion site centrally [151]. This may represent the pathologic correlate of recurrent and persistent maternal bleeding throughout pregnancy (chronic abruption). Amnionic fluid loss also contributes and is thought to be the primary mechanism in the circumvallation invariably associated with extramembranous pregnancy.

Pathology. Historically, extrachorial placentas have been subdivided into circummarginate and circumvallate types based on the nature of the transition from the chorionic plate to the fetal membranes. In circumvallate placentas, the marginal membrane ring is often reflected centrally, folded, and rolled back upon itself (➲ *Fig. 19.10*). Variable amounts of fibrin and recent and old blood clot are often found in the reflected membrane fold, with focal, or in severe cases, diffuse hemosiderin deposits in the chorionic plate. A flat transition from the chorionic plate to the membranes without reflection or prominent fibrin accumulation has been termed a circummarginate placenta (➲ *Fig. 19.11*). Either finding may be partial or complete, and they frequently merge imperceptibly with one another. Multiple authors have suggested that the term circummarginate should be abandoned and that all extrachorial placentas should be considered part of the spectrum of circumvallation [84].

Clinical behavior. Estimates of the frequency of extrachorial placentation vary widely presumably because the terms are not used uniformly. It is more common in

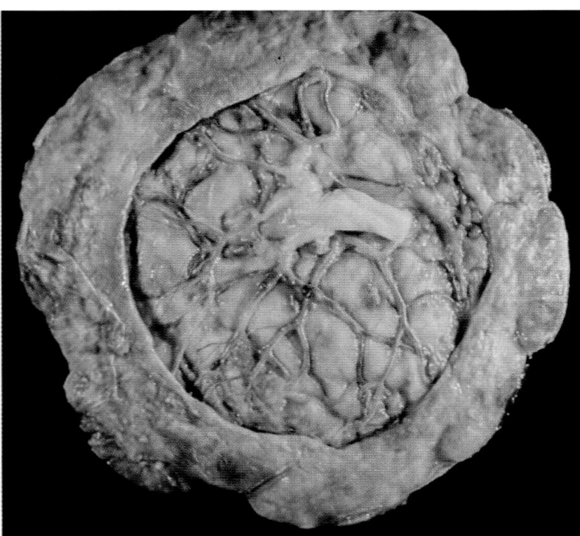

Fig. 19.10
Extrachorial placenta. **The fetal membranes do not extend to the peripheral margin of the disk, leaving a ring of placental tissue extending beyond the chorionic plate. This membrane ring is rolled and reflected centrally**

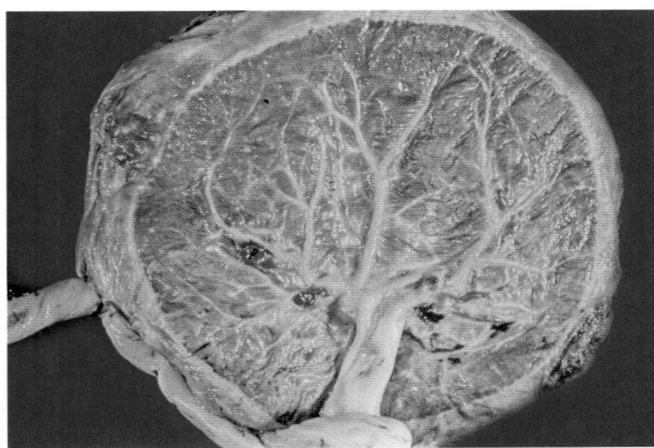

Fig. 19.11
Extrachorial placenta. **The membrane transition in this extrachorial placenta is flat**

multigravidas. The clinical sequellae seem to parallel the amount of associated hemorrhage. Mild or focal circumvallation without hemorrhage is clinically insignificant. More severe cases with chronic marginal abruption and oligohydramnios are associated with antepartum bleeding, preterm labor (PTL), intrauterine growth restriction (IUGR), and long-term neurologic impairment [145]. Circumvallate placentation may recur in successive pregnancies.

Placenta Accreta, Increta, and Percreta

Placenta accreta, increta, and percreta are defined as abnormal adherence of the placenta to the uterine wall so that placental separation does not occur after delivery of the newborn. The degree of abnormal adherence/invasion is variable; placental villi may adhere to (*placenta accreta*) or invade the myometrium (*placenta increta*), sometimes penetrating through the serosa (*placenta percreta.*) The condition may be total (involving the entire placenta), partial (involving one or more cotyledons), or focal (involving isolated foci).

Etiology. The pathologic basis of this condition is partial or complete absence of the decidua. Decidua normally regulates trophoblastic invasion during gestation and allows the placenta to separate from the myometrium after delivery. Lack of decidua explains the abnormal placental adherence that occurs in ectopic (cornual, tubal, or cervical) implantation or in scarred endometrium over leiomyomas or cesarean section scars.

Clinical features. The frequency of placenta accreta is difficult to determine. Reported figures have varied widely from 1 in 540 to 1 in 70,000 pregnancies. Fox emphasized the particular tendency of placenta accreta to occur in multigravid and obstetrically elderly women [45]. A number of predisposing factors have been linked to this condition, the two most significant being *placenta previa* (placental implantation in the lower uterine segment near or overlying the cervical os) and previous cesarean section. In some reports, as many as 64% of placentas accreta have been associated with placenta previa, many occurring in cesarean section scars. Often only the portion of the placenta implanted in the lower uterine segment or over a cesarean section scar is abnormally adherent. Other risk factors include prior uterine instrumentation or intrauterine infection, previous manual removal of the placenta, uterine structural defects (leiomyomas, septae), and nonfundic implantation. The common endpoint in all these conditions is a deficiency in, or absence of, the decidua. In less than 10% of cases, no risk factors are identified.

Pathology. The diagnosis is usually obvious in a hysterectomy performed at the time of delivery. The placenta is almost invariably implanted in the lower uterine segment or cervix, often anteriorly in the region of prior cesarean section (*Fig. 19.12*). The myometrium is variably but often markedly thinned. The uterus and placenta may be disrupted by attempts to remove the adherent placenta at the time of delivery. Microscopically, the cardinal feature is partial or complete absence of the decidua basalis. Placental villi adhere directly to, or invade

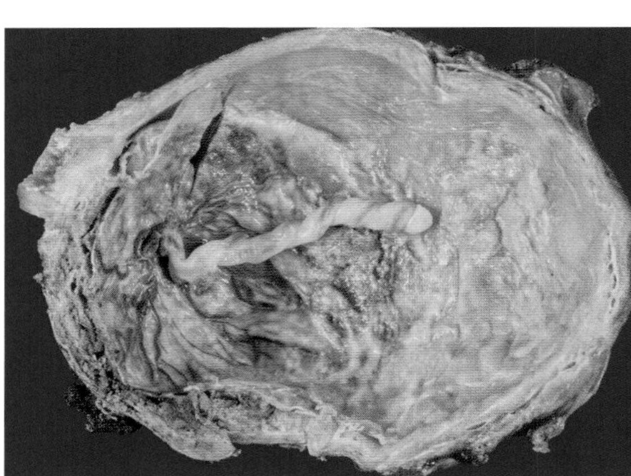
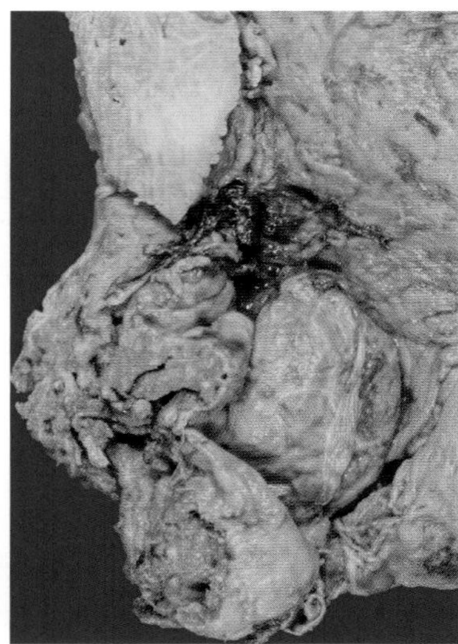

Fig. 19.12
Placenta percreta. **The placenta at left implanted over the cervical os (*upper left*) and penetrated the serosa. The placenta at right also penetrated the serosa in the anterior lower uterine segment at the site of three prior cesarean sections**

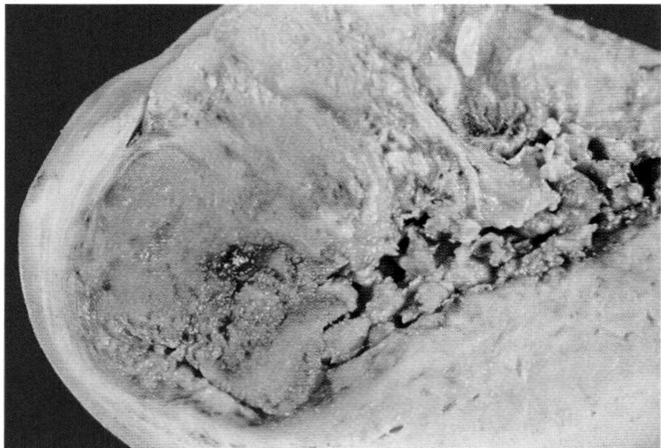
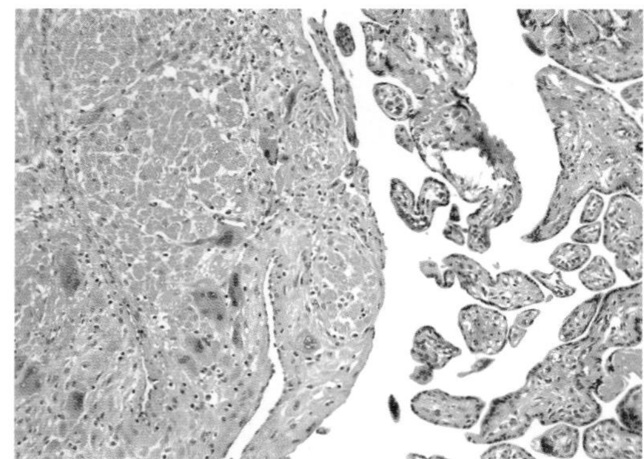

Fig. 19.13
Placenta increta. **The placenta has invaded the myometrium almost to the serosa. Villi invade the myometrium without intervening decidua**

into, the myometrium (*Fig. 19.13*), penetrating through the uterine serosa in some instances. The diagnosis can also be established on placental exam. Microscopic sections of grossly fragmented, low-lying, or manually removed placentas may show a thin layer of myometrial fibers adherent to the placenta without intervening decidua. Occasional smooth muscle cells in a basal plate containing decidua is not diagnostic of accreta. The diagnosis in a postpartum curettage calls attention to the potential for further bleeding or infection if all the placental tissue is not removed.

Clinical behavior and treatment. Placenta accreta is compatible with normal fetal growth and development. Although usually anticipated, it may not be suspected until the placenta fails to separate in the third stage of labor. Postpartum bleeding may be life threatening, requiring immediate hysterectomy, or bleeding may be delayed. Antepartum bleeding and premature labor are common due to the high frequency of associated placenta previa. Uterine rupture may occur at any stage of pregnancy or during labor. Maternal and fetal mortality are now uncommon.

Mesenchymal Dysplasia

Placentas with mesenchymal dysplasia are usually very large, often over 1,000 g. The chorionic vessels are aneurysmally dilated and often thrombosed. Enlarged cystic stem villi are recognizable grossly (➔ *Fig. 19.14*). Microscopically, the stem villi are large and edematous with cyst formation and prominent thick-walled muscular stem vessels (➔ *Fig. 19.15*). Terminal villi are usually normal but may show distal villous immaturity and chorangiosis. Chorangiomas are common. There is no trophoblastic hyperplasia. This rare lesion is often identified as partial hydatidiform mole on ultrasound. Over one half of reported cases have been associated with Beckwith Wiedemann syndrome. Mesenchymal dysplasia is associated with IUGR, intrauterine fetal demise (IUFD), and neonatal death [71, 101, 116]. Females are disproportionally affected.

Multiple Pregnancy

Multiple gestations are common and becoming more so with assisted reproductive techniques (ART). In the United States in 2000, ART accounted for 14% of all twin births, and 45% of ART births were twins [153]. Multiples are associated with a disproportionate share of complications including higher rates of morbidity, mortality, low birth weight, anomalous development, and malformation than singletons. Careful pathologic examination of the placenta(s) can provide important insight into problems peculiar to multiples, and pathologists must be aware of the special considerations required in the examination of placentas from multiple births.

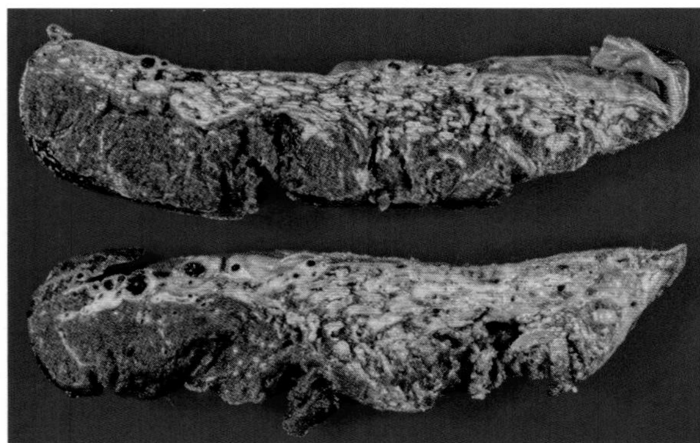

Fig. 19.14
Mesenchymal dysplasia. **The gross abnormalities in this placenta with mesenchymal dysplasia were identified on antenatal ultrasound. The infant was normal**

Twin Gestation

Zygosity

Definition. Twins may arise from the fertilization of two separate ova (dizygous or fraternal twins) or from the division of a single fertilized ovum (monozygous or identical twins). Monozygous twins are genetically and usually phenotypically identical, but dizygous twins are genetically dissimilar like singleton siblings. Rare variants of dizygous twinning result when ova are fertilized by sperm from different sources (*superfecundation*) or when ova are ovulated and fertilized at different times resulting in twins of disparate developmental ages (*superfetation*). A rare variant of monozygous twins, monozygous heterokaryotic twins, have different karyotypes and sometimes even different sex [14]. These twins are thought to result from chromosome non-disjunction, most commonly involving the sex chromosomes, but on occasion the autosomes as well. A third type of twinning, polar body or dispermic monovular twinning, presumably results from fertilization of an oocyte and a polar body. Bieber described a triploid acardiac/diploid twin gestation resulting from fertilization of an oocyte and its first polar body [20]. Theoretically, fertilization of the oocyte and second polar body could also occur. The frequency of this phenomenon is unknown. It has been hypothesized that dispermic monovular twins are monochorionic due to the proximity of the oocyte and the polar body and because cytoplasmic imbalance equips only the oocyte with its more abundant cytoplasm to implant.

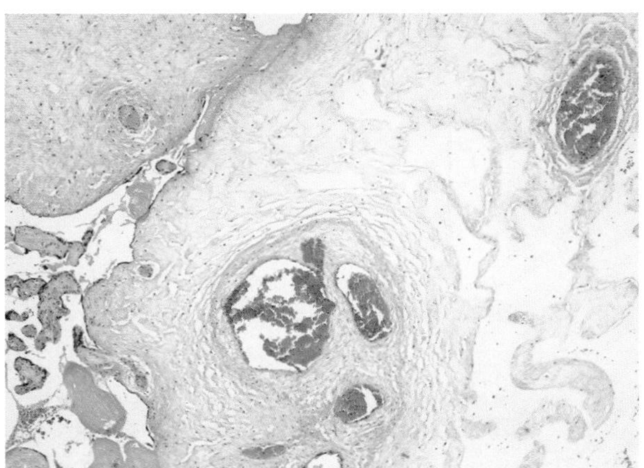

Fig. 19.15
Mesenchymal dysplasia. **The stem villi are greatly enlarged with abundant, focally degenerated cystic stroma and large thick muscular vessels**

Frequency and etiology. Twins occur in about 1 in 80 Caucasian pregnancies in the United States, and approximately 30% of these are monozygous. The frequency of monozygous twinning is relatively constant worldwide (about 3.5 in 1,000 pregnancies), but there are marked geographic differences in total twinning rate reflecting excess dizygous twinning in certain populations and families who have a genetic predisposition for high FSH and polyovulation. Dizygous twinning is also age-related, increasing with maternal age until 35 years, again probably reflecting a role for increasing FSH levels with age. The cause of monozygous twinning is unknown. Monozygous twinning is increased in pregnancies following ART [98]. ART has changed the epidemiology of multiple pregnancy. It is as yet unclear if or how this technology may affect developmental events [26]. So far, pathologic placental lesions do not appear to be increased in ART multiples [163].

Placentation

The object of placental exam in multiple gestation is the same as in singleton gestation – to identify pathologic processes affecting placental function. The gross and microscopic manifestations of these processes are identical in the placentas of singletons and multiples, although some lesions are particularly pertinent to the problems experienced by multiples. Comparison of the relative distribution of lesions in the placental territories and correlation with the size and condition of the fetuses is an important aspect of placental assessment in multiple gestation. Features unique to multiples include (1) the relationships of the disks and fetal membranes and (2) the pattern and degree of vascular anastomoses.

Chorionicity, Amnionicity, and Placental Mass

Placentas in twin gestation are either monochorionic or dichorionic. Virtually all dizygous twins have dichorionic placentas (diamnionic dichorionic – DiDi). In double ovulation, each blastocyst generates a placenta. If these implant in close proximity, varying degrees of fusion may result (DiDi fused); otherwise they are entirely separate. Monozygous twins may show any type of placentation depending on when division occurs (Fig. 19.16). If the single fertilized ovum divides very early, before differentiation of the chorion (first 5–6 days), the situation is analogous to dizygous twinning; two placentas develop that may be separate or fused (25% of monozygous

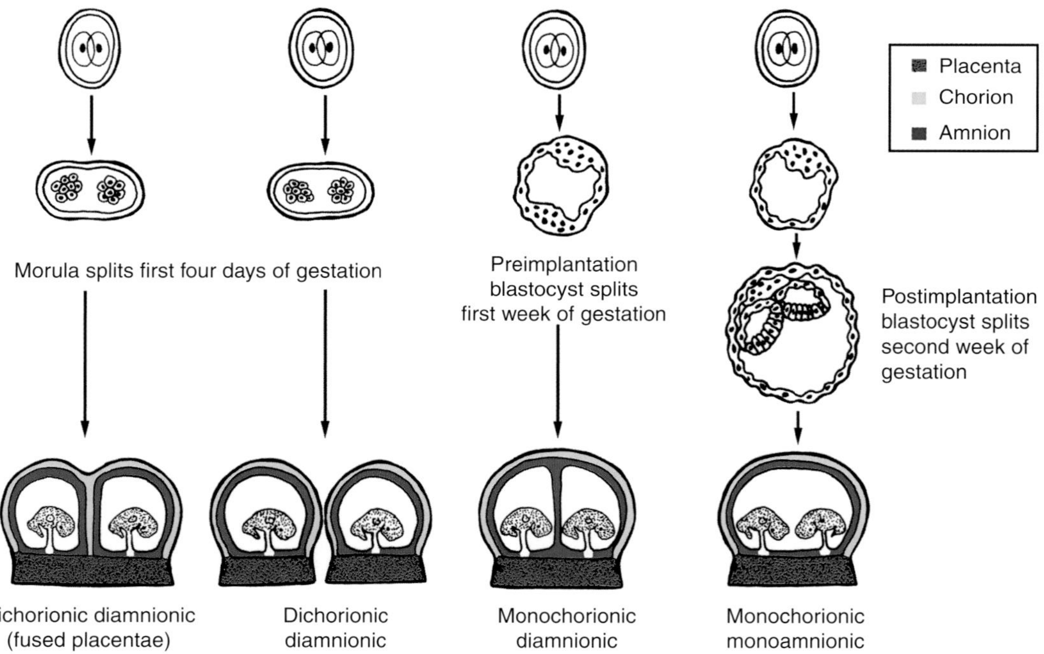

Fig. 19.16
Diagrammatic representation of twin placentation. (After [44] used with permission of the American Registry of Pathology/Armed Forces Institute of Pathology)

twins). If splitting occurs after formation of the chorion but before formation of the amnion (8th day after fertilization), there will be a single placenta with two amnionic sacs (diamnionic monochorionic – DiMo), occurring in about 75% of monozygous twins. A split after formation of the amnion (between the 8th and 15th days), will result in one placenta with one amnionic cavity (monoamnionic monochorionic – MoMo), and still later splitting, in conjoined twins (➋ *Fig. 19.17*). Practically speaking, twins with monochorionic placentas are monozygous with very rare exceptions (monovular dispermic and one case of dizygous monochorionic twins) [178]. Twins with dichorionic placentas, whether separate or fused, may be either dizygous or monozygous. Obviously, different fetal sex establishes a dizygous relation, but further investigation (blood group analysis, HLA typing, and DNA analysis) is required to determine zygosity in like-sex dichorionic twins.

Establishment of placentation type is important, not only as an initial step in determining zygosity, but primarily because it has an important relationship to the increased morbidity and mortality that occur in multiple gestations. Many factors contribute, importantly the premature onset of labor and delivery, but placentation is also a very significant risk factor. Twins with monochorionic placentas have much higher mortality rates than those with dichorionic placentas, and monoamnionic placentation is associated with a fetal mortality rate as high as 50%.

Placentation type is usually reliably established on gross examination. Two entirely separate placentas are obviously dichorionic (DiDi separate), each requiring routine examination. Frequently the disks are separate but the membranes are fused. The membranes of one twin may overlap the disk of the co-twin (irregular chorionic fusion) when there is differential expansion of the membranous sacs. When the blastocysts implant close to one another, the two placental disks fuse to form an apparently single disk with a dividing septum (DiDi fused).

The principal task for the pathologist is to distinguish between monochorionic and dichorionic fused placentas. The nature of the membranous septum and the pattern of chorionic vascularization are critical in this distinction. The septum in dichorionic fused placentas is relatively thick and opaque due to the presence of chorionic tissue between the two amnionic layers (➋ *Fig. 19.18*). Because each embryo is developing within its own chorion, any fusion between them will contain chorionic tissue. The chorionic tissue in the septum is continuous with the underlying placenta remaining firmly attached to the fetal surface. If the amnions are separated, chorionic tissue will remain as a ridge at the base of the septum. In contrast, the

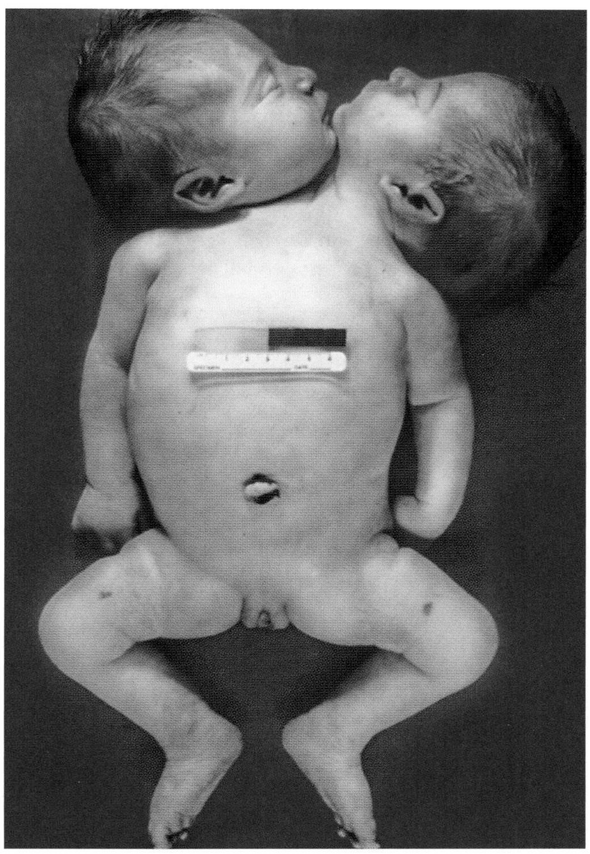

Fig. 19.17
Conjoined twins. **(Used with permission of the American Registry of Pathology/Armed Forces Institute of Pathology)**

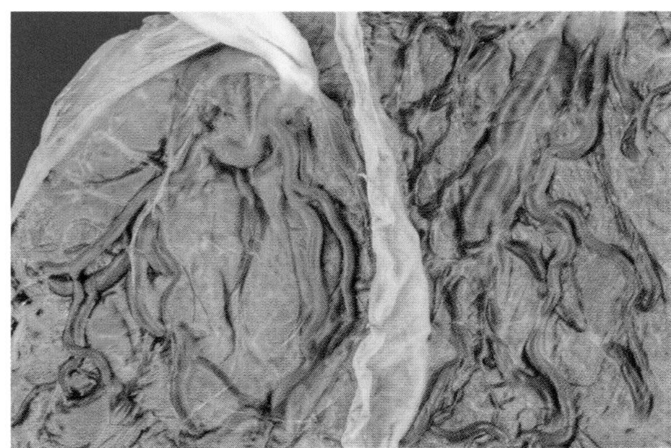

Fig. 19.18
DiDi fused placentas. **The two placentas are fused but discrete. The septal membrane is thick and the fetal vessels do not cross the line of fusion (Used with permission of the American Registry of Pathology/Armed Forces Institute of Pathology)**

septum in a diamnionic monochorionic placenta is thin and translucent, composed of two directly apposed layers of amnion (➲ *Fig. 19.19*). This septum, devoid of chorion, is easily detached from the placental surface. Some pathologists peel the dividing membranes in order to identify monochorionic placentas that require injection studies. Histologic examination of the membranous septum confirms the gross impression. This is most easily accomplished in a section of rolled septal membranes (➲ *Figs. 19.20* and ➲ *19.21*), although identical information may be obtained from a section of the T zone where the septum meets the fetal surface. The latter method is particularly useful when the septal membrane has been torn or otherwise distorted and cannot be rolled.

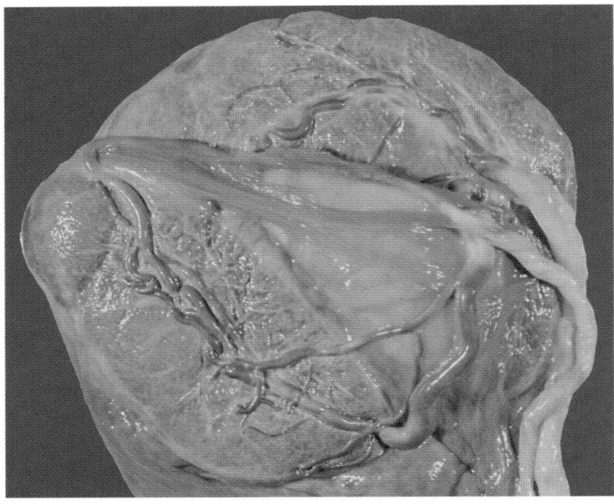

Fig. 19.19
DiMo twin placenta. **The septal membranes are thin and filmy. Note velamentous insertion of the cord into the septal membranes (Used with permission of the American Registry of Pathology/Armed Forces Institute of Pathology)**

The distribution of the fetal vessels on the chorionic plate is equally helpful in distinguishing DiDi fused from DiMo placentas. In dichorionic placentas, the septum represents the apposed borders of the two fused placentas and as such defines the vascular equator of the two placentas. In DiDi fused placentas, fetal chorionic vessels approach, but do not cross the area of fusion (➲ *Fig. 19.18*). In diamnionic monochorionic placentas, portions of the same placenta are shared by both fetuses, and the two vascular districts are intimately intermingled (➲ *Fig. 19.22*). The position of the membranous septum in the DiMo placenta is independent of, and does not necessarily conform to, the fetal vascular districts.

Rarely, a monochorionic placenta presents as two apparently distinct disks, superficially resembling dichorionic separate placentas. The nature of the septum and the intermingling of the vascular districts with anastomosis identify these as monochorionic. The appearance of two separate "disks" is due to involution or atrophy of intervening villous tissue related to factors at the implantation site affecting maternal blood supply.

Monoamnionic monochorionic placentas (MoMo) are very uncommon, accounting for less than 1% of twin gestations. In MoMo gestations, both twins develop within a single amnionic sac. Before considering a monochorionic placenta to be monoamnionic, the amnion between the cord insertions should be complete and continuous.

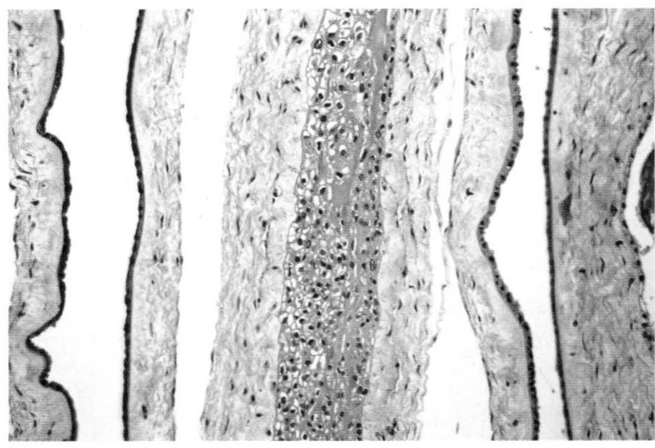

Fig. 19.20
DiDi septum. **A central layer of fused chorion intervenes between amnions**

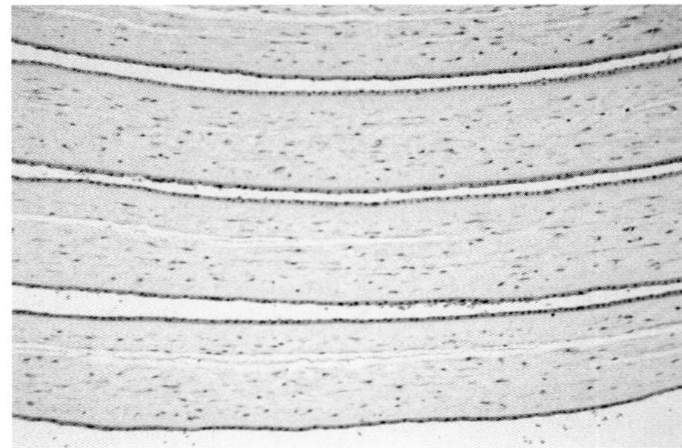

Fig. 19.21
DiMo Septum. **The septum is composed of two directly apposed amnions**

Because the amnion commonly separates from the underlying chorion and is often nearly completely detached at delivery, more apparently single sacs are artifactual than truly monoamnionic. Remnants of detached amnion and septum may be found encircling the cords or attached to the free membranes when carefully sought. Although membrane patterns are established early and persist throughout pregnancy, intragestational disruption of diamnionic septae has been reported. This suggests that at least some monoamnionic placentas may have been diamnionic originally. The umbilical cords in monoamnionic gestations are typically closely inserted, usually within 6 cm of each other (➲ *Fig. 19.23*). Rarely there is partial cord fusion. Large vessel anastomoses are frequent but not invariable between the closely inserted cords. Cord entanglement is common and a significant cause of morbidity and mortality (➲ *Fig. 19.24*).

The pattern and adequacy of chorionic vascularization, the relative proportion of the chorionic surface populated by vessels from each twin, and the relative placental mass serving each twin are pertinent observations in multiple gestations. Dichorionic fused placentas can be divided and weighed. Estimates of the placental mass serving monochorionic twins are based on the chorionic vasculature. The pattern of venous return is a good indicator of placental supply. Not all discordantly grown twins have asymmetric placentas, and not all twins with asymmetric placentas are discordantly grown, but these associations are not uncommon. In twins with discordant placental mass, the smaller placenta is frequently associated with a lesser number of chorionic vessels. Whether the smaller placenta impairs the growth of the fetus, or both fetus and placenta are small secondary to other influences is not always clear.

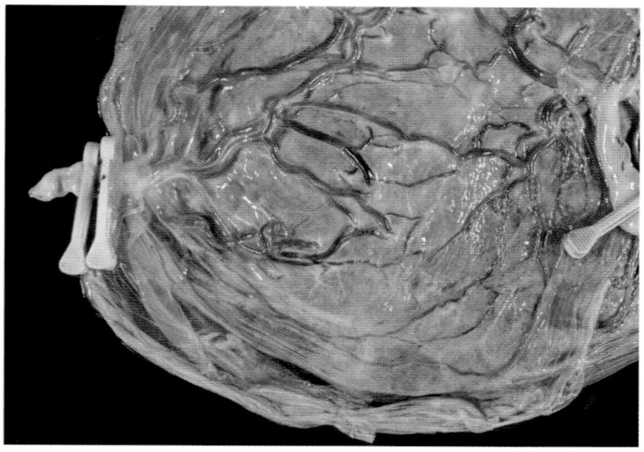

■ Fig. 19.22
DiMo twin placenta. **The fetal vessels are intimately intermingled, and some are anastomosed (Used with permission of the American Registry of Pathology/Armed Forces Institute of Pathology)**

Vascular Anastomoses

An important feature of monochorionic placentas is the presence of vascular communications between the two fetal circulations. The fetal circulation is established when small vessels developing independently within the villous mesenchyme connect with larger vessels in the chorionic plate and body stalk. When twins share the same placenta, the potential exists for the two developing circulations to merge in a number of different ways.

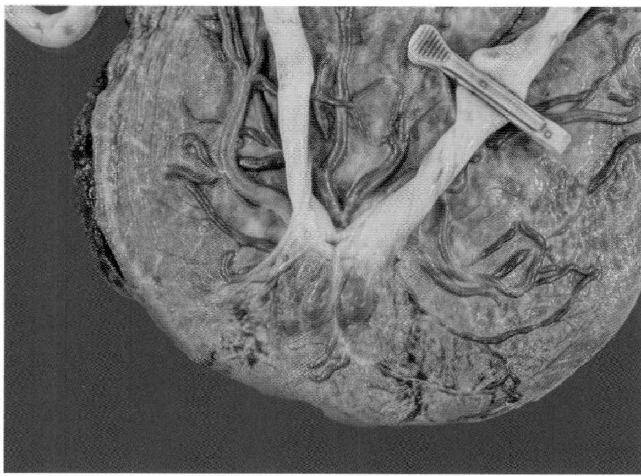

■ Fig. 19.23
Cord insertion, MoMo. **Close cord insertion is typical of MoMo placentation**

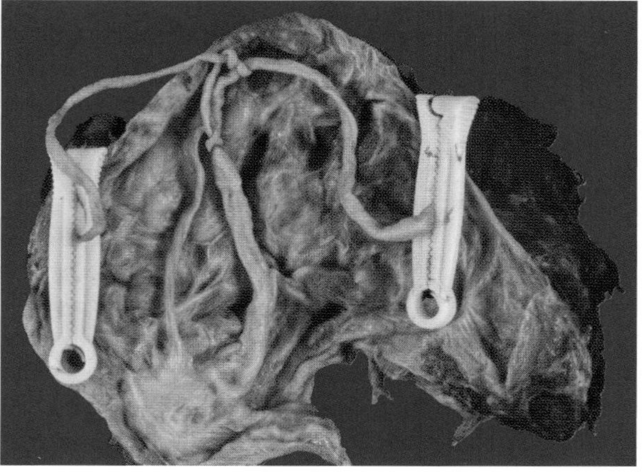

■ Fig. 19.24
Cord entanglement in MoMo. **This cord entanglement resulted in IUFD at 25 weeks**

For example, the capillary bed supplied by an artery from one twin might establish continuity with a vein returning to its co-twin resulting in a parenchymal arteriovenous (A–V) anastomosis. In contrast, the two circulations in dichorionic twins are established independently explaining why vascular communications in DiDi-fused placentas are absent with rare exception.

It is generally agreed that vascular communication is invariable in monochorionic placentas although the number, size, and type of anastomoses are highly variable. Anastomoses between large chorionic plate vessels are very common. The majority of large vessel anastomoses are between arteries (A–A); vein to vein (V–V) anastomoses are less common. Of greater physiologic significance are the arteriovenous (A–V) anastomoses that occur between capillaries deep within shared villous parenchyma. Vascular anastomoses may be compound with surface (large vessel) and parenchymal (villous capillary) connections involving the same vessels (➋ *Fig. 19.25*). A–A anastomoses alone (20–28%) and A–A with A–V anastomoses (25–40%) are most common. A–V anastomoses alone, unmodified by concomitant large vessel anastomoses, are estimated to occur in 11–20% of cases.

Large vessel anastomoses are easily identified grossly (➋ *Fig. 19.22*) and can be confirmed by moving blood back and forth between the contributing vessels or highlighted by the injection of dye or air (➋ *Fig. 19.26*). The size, diameter, location (central or peripheral), type (arteries cross over veins), and number of anastomoses should be recorded. A–V anastomoses are more important physiologically but are more difficult to identify as they occur between capillaries deep in the villous parenchyma and cannot be directly visualized. Potential sites of A–V anastomosis can be suspected when an unpaired artery from one twin penetrates the chorionic plate in close proximity to an unpaired vein from the co-twin (➋ *Fig. 19.27*). This configuration is highly suggestive of an underlying anastomosis as arteries and veins are normally paired. A simple method to confirm the presence of arteriovenous anastomoses is to inject air into the arterial branch supplying a suspected anastomosis and document its return to the venous district of the co-twin. This has the advantage of displacing blood from the shared placental district. The resulting pallor allows estimation of the volume of shared parenchyma. Air injection can be repeated at multiple sites in an attempt to document the extent of anastomoses. All injection studies are qualitative. They do not necessarily reflect the physiologic significance of an anastomosis, or the overall balance of blood flow in vivo. Nevertheless, their documentation is essential if vascular anastomosis is to be invoked as a cause of, or contributor to, discordant fetal

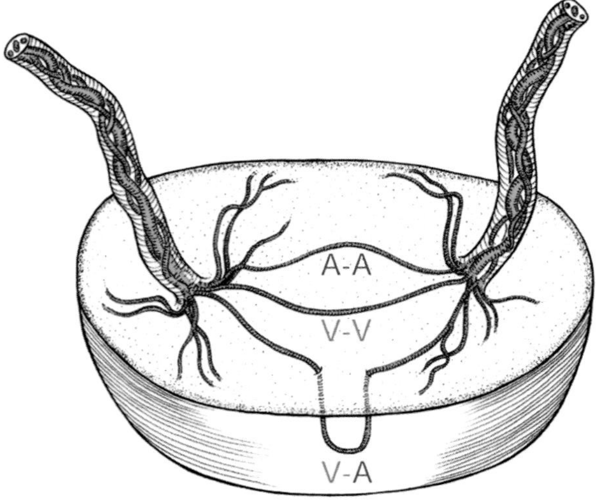

Fig. 19.25
Types of vascular anastomoses in monochorionic placentas. **Large vessel anastomoses (artery-artery and vein-vein) are easily identifiable on the chorionic plate. Arteriovenous anastomoses occur between capillaries in shared placental lobules. The presence of an unpaired artery penetrating the chorionic plate in the vicinity of an unpaired vein from its co-twin suggests this possibility. Superficial (large vessel) and capillary anastomoses may involve the same vessels (Used with permission of the American Registry of Pathology/Armed Forces Institute of Pathology)**

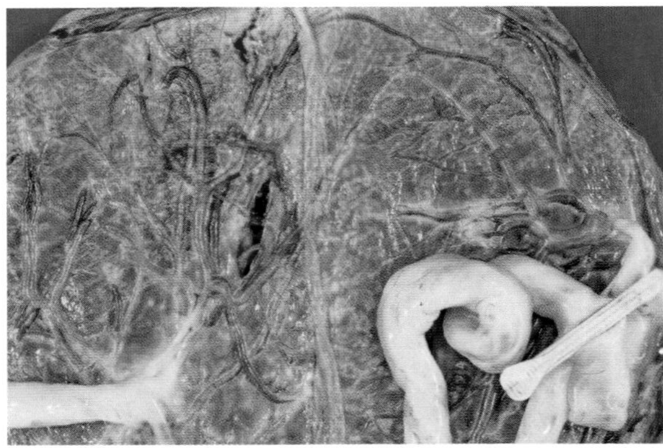

Fig. 19.26
Vascular anastomosis. **This large anastomosis has been highlighted by air injection (Used with permission of the American Registry of Pathology/Armed Forces Institute of Pathology)**

growth. Injection studies are precluded by fixation and may be compromised by villous disruption.

Umbilical Cord

Anomalies of the umbilical cord are much more common in multiple than in singleton gestations. The incidence of velamentous cord insertion in twins has been reported to be up to nine times higher than in singletons. The frequency of anomalous insertion (marginal and velamentous) increases with proximity of the twins (dichorionic separate < dichorionic fused < monochorionic). Anomalous cord insertion in multiples has the same significance as in singletons. In addition, there is some evidence that velamentous cord insertion is a factor that influences twin–twin transfusion and associated early delivery.

Single artery cords are also more frequent in multiple gestations, occurring in approximately 3% as compared to 0.53% of singletons. Most twins are discordant for single umbilical artery, although concordance is greater in monozygous than dizygous twins. The length of the umbilical cord is on average 7.6 cm shorter in twins than singletons, and the incidence of hypocoiled cords is also increased.

Twins that share an amnionic cavity (monoamnionic) are at increased risk for cord entanglements. Cord entanglements of all types occur in monochorionic twins with a reported frequency between 53 and 71%, and they may be remarkably complex (*Fig. 19.28*). Such entanglements may result not only in cord compression but in mistaken cord transection when one twin's cord is looped around its co-twin at delivery. Cord entanglement as a factor in fetal mortality is most common prior to 24 weeks while there is still sufficient room for fetal movement. After 30–32 weeks and in higher multiples, cord entanglement is less common as opportunity for movement decreases. Cord entanglements may result in chronic vascular compromise or they may not become a problem until the forces of labor result in acute vascular obstruction.

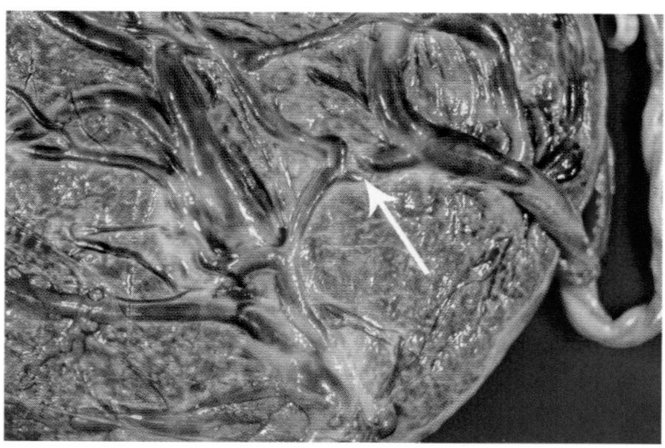

Fig. 19.27
Arteriovenous anastomosis. **An unpaired artery from the umbilical cord barely visible at bottom penetrates the chorionic plate adjacent to an unpaired dilated vein from the co-twin at right (Used with permission of the American Registry of Pathology/Armed Forces Institute of Pathology)**

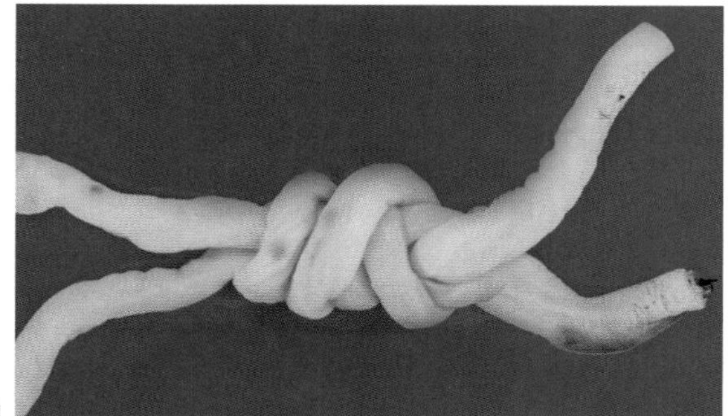

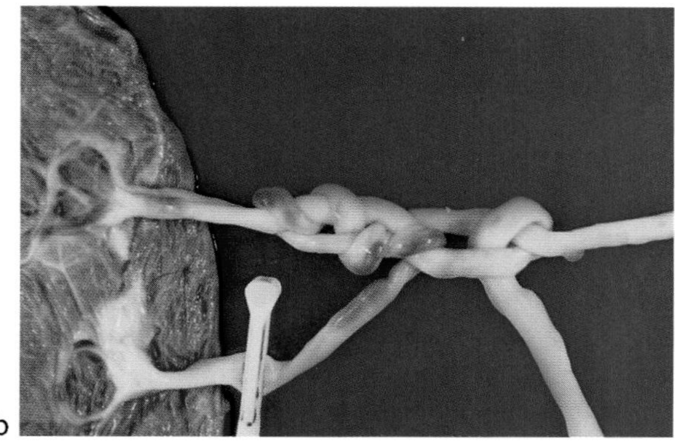

Fig. 19.28
Complex cord entanglements in MoMo twins (a and b)

Complications of Multiple Pregnancy

Twin–Twin Transfusion Syndrome (TTTS)

Vascular communications in monochorionic placentas create the potential for blood flow between the twins. When there is a net flow of blood from one twin to the other, the clinical manifestations depend on the size, number, and type of vascular communications. Capillary-sized arteriovenous (A–V) anastomoses involve the transfusion of small amounts of blood over long periods of time (chronic transfusion). A large volume of blood can be transferred rapidly through large caliber chorionic plate vessels often at the time of labor and delivery (acute transfusion). Not infrequently, both occur – an acute transfusion is superimposed on a chronic long-term process (acute on chronic transfusion). Large vessel anastomoses are likely to be bidirectional and A–V connections are likely to be unidirectional.

Chronic Transfusion

Definition and etiology. Chronic TTTS is the most common form of twin–twin transfusion, and is an important cause of perinatal mortality in monochorionic twins. Schatz proposed the view that the chronic TTTS results when there is unbalanced flow of blood from one twin (the donor) to its co-twin (the recipient) through A–V anastomoses deep within shared placental lobules (the "third circulation") [17]. Chronic unidirectional diversion of blood results in anemia, relative deprivation, and growth retardation of the donor as compared to the larger, polycythemic recipient. Hypervolemia and hypertension in the recipient result in increased urine output and polyhydramnios, while hypotension and hypovolemia in the donor lead to oliguria, oligohydramnios, and decreased movement (the "stuck" twin.) Either twin may be hydropic, reflecting cardiac dysfunction and congestive heart failure in the recipient and profound anemia in the donor.

Although vascular anastomoses are a necessary precondition for the development of the TTTS, additional factors beyond shifts of blood (differential protein, atriopeptin, growth factor concentration, or colloid osmotic pressure) may contribute. Velamentous cord insertion is significantly more common in monochorionic gestations with the TTTS. It has been proposed that velamentous cords are more easily compressed, resulting in decreased umbilical vein flow and enhanced flow through A–V anastomoses. Others have speculated that polyhydramnios may contribute to umbilical and chorionic vessel compression providing the therapeutic rationale for amniocentesis.

The clinical definition of the TTTS is complicated because twins commonly show asymmetric growth for reasons other than a chronic twin–twin transfusion (maternal, fetal, umbilical cord, or placental factors). A hemoglobin concentration difference >5 g/100 mL and twin weight difference of 15–20% are considered definitive criteria by some, although similar weight and hemoglobin discrepancies are just as common in dichorionic twins without an anatomic basis for transfusion [140]. Conversely, hemoglobin concentration in twins with the chronic twin–twin transfusion may be similar if the donor's compensatory hematopoiesis has been sufficient. A relatively selective criterion is a recipient heart weight that is two to four times that of the donor. This feature is generally not present in any other process resulting in twin weight–growth discordance. The disparity in heart size is due not only to a generalized growth differential but also to the increased cardiac work load associated with the hypervolemia, hypertension, and hyperviscosity experienced by the recipient twin. Heart size discrepancy may be the first manifestation of the chronic TTTS, evident on ultrasound as early as 10 weeks. Difference in overall fetal size is usually apparent only later in gestation. Discrepant amnionic fluid volumes, hydrops, and a "stuck twin" are other ultrasound findings very suggestive of the TTTS.

Frequency. Recent studies indicate close correspondence between the number of cases with well-documented twin–twin transfusion and the number of monochorionic twin placentas with A–V anastomoses without concomitant large-vessel anastomoses [18]. This occurs in 9–20% of monochorionic gestations. Superficial vascular anastomoses appear to mitigate against the effects of A–V transfusion probably by allowing transfer of blood back to the donor from the recipient. In the absence of superficial anastomoses, arteriovenous transfusions are uncompensated, resulting in marked growth discordance, hydramnios, early delivery, and high perinatal mortality. The TTTS is not a significant cause of fetal mortality in monoamnionic twins presumably because the majority of MoMo twins have large-vessel anastomoses that modify parenchymal connections. In addition, any intra-amnionic pressure differences that potentially could affect blood flow in diamnionic twins are equalized in monoamnionic twins. For unexplained reasons, the twin–twin transfusion syndrome is more common in females.

Gross and microscopic pathology. After delivery, there is a marked discrepancy in the size and appearance of the infants and their corresponding placental territories. The donor twin is smaller, pale, and anemic; the recipient is heavier, edematous, plethoric, and polycythemic (➲ *Fig. 19.29*). Either twin may be hydropic. The organs of the recipient are larger and heavier than those of the donor (➲ *Fig. 19.30*). The recipient's heart especially is comparatively enlarged, with myocardial hypertrophy involving all chambers. Smooth muscle mass is increased in the media of pulmonary and systemic arteries and arterioles. Pulmonary arterial calcification has been described in the recipient twin. The donor heart is usually small, and arterial muscle mass is decreased. Glomeruli are enlarged, up to twice normal size in the recipient twin, and they are either normal or small in the donor.

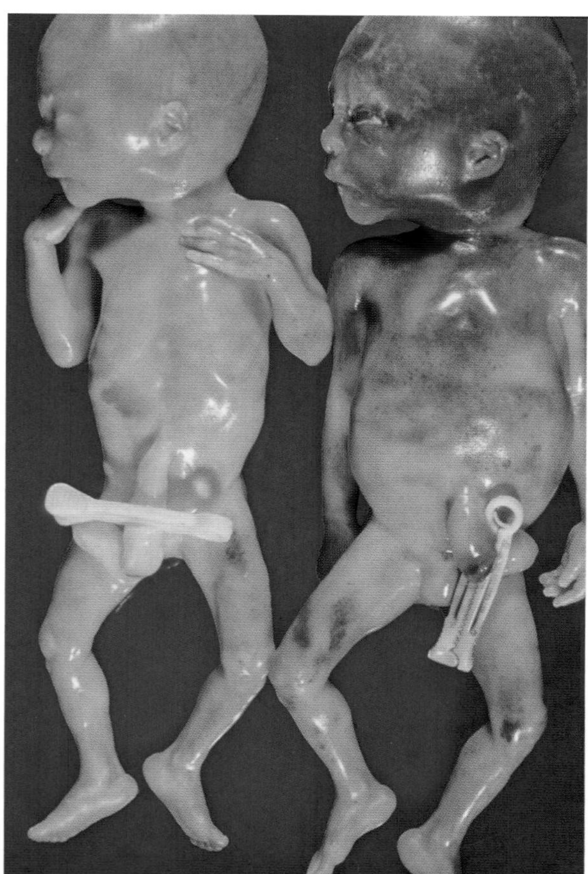

■ Fig. 19.29
Twin–twin transfusion syndrome (TTTS). **The donor twin (*left*) is smaller and pale. The recipient twin (*right*) is larger and plethoric (Used with permission of the American Registry of Pathology/Armed Forces Institute of Pathology)**

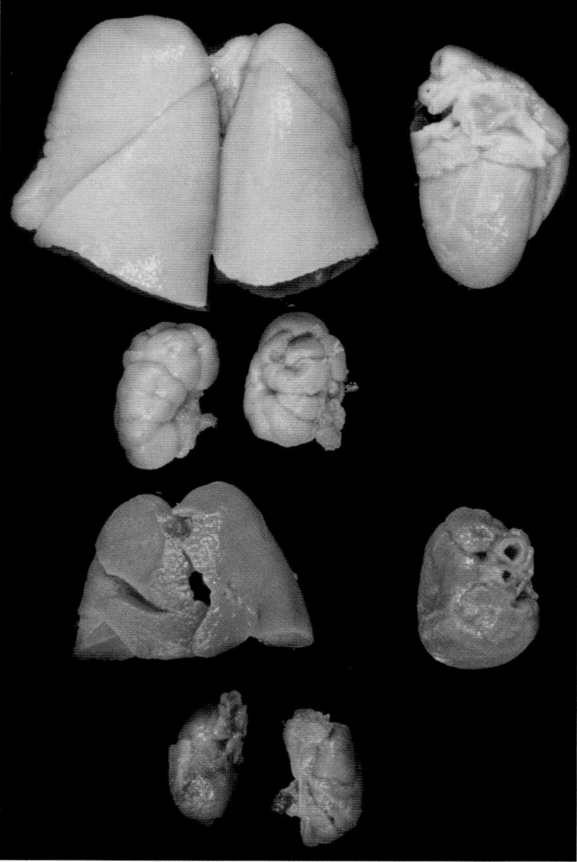

■ Fig. 19.30
Twin–twin transfusion syndrome (TTTS). **The organs of the recipient twin are larger and heavier. Congestion of the smaller (donor) organs and pallor of the larger (recipient) organs is a reversal of the expected pattern, suggesting that the recipient twin exsanguinated into the donor (Used with permission of the American Registry of Pathology/Armed Forces Institute of Pathology)**

The donor's placental territory may be large, bulky, and pale reflecting fetal anemia (➋ *Fig 19.31*). The villi are large and edematous with numerous Hofbauer cells and capillaries containing nucleated red blood cells (➋ *Fig. 19.32*). In other cases, the donor's placenta has been described as pale and atrophied. Amnion nodosum may be found when there is associated oligohydramnios. The recipient's placental territory is generally smaller, firm, and deep red. The villi are appropriately mature with dilated and intensely congested vessels (➋ *Fig. 19.33*).

Clinical features. Typically, the chronic TTTS is clinically manifest in the second trimester with acute hydramnios and growth discrepancy between the twins, but it may be suspected earlier based on the ultrasound demonstration of different amnionic fluid volumes. The consequences of the twin–twin transfusion syndrome are grave. Mortality rates are as high as 70–100% depending on the gestational age at diagnosis and delivery. The earlier the syndrome is manifest, the more likely the outcome will be fatal. When the condition develops in the second trimester, it is often associated with pre-term labor and death of one or both fetuses or significant morbidity if the neonates survive. Both twins are at great risk. The recipient twin is subject to cardiac failure, hemolytic jaundice, kernicterus, and thrombosis due to hemoconcentration. The donor twin may be severely anemic or hypoglycemic. Both twins are likely to suffer from

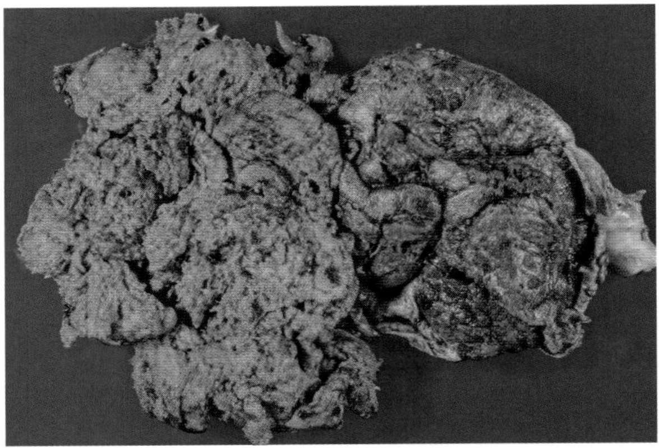

Fig. 19.31
Twin–twin transfusion syndrome (TTTS). **The donor's placental territory (*left*) is larger and pale reflecting anemia. The recipient's territory is smaller and congested (Used with permission of the American Registry of Pathology/Armed Forces Institute of Pathology)**

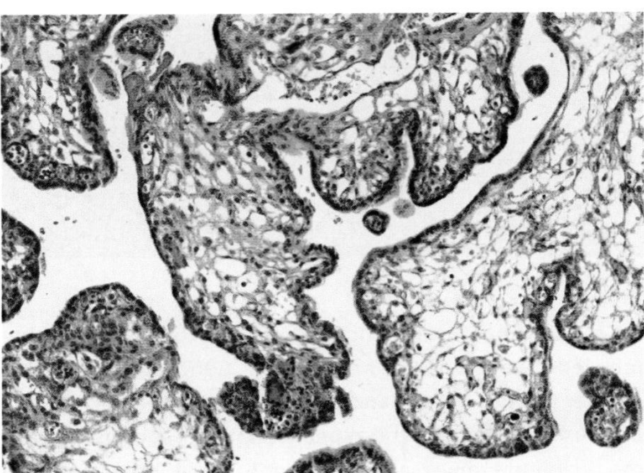

Fig. 19.32
Twin–twin transfusion syndrome (TTTS). **The donor's villi are large, relatively immature and edematous with numerous immature erythroid precursors**

complications of prematurity. Multiorgan necrotic lesions including white matter infarcts, leukoencephalopathy, hydranencephaly, porencephaly, intestinal atresia, renal cortical necrosis, and aplasia cutis (*Fig. 19.34*) may occur in either or both twins. These lesions are attributed to the altered hemodynamics, transitory cardiovascular compromise, and hypoperfusion associated with complex fluctuating placental vascular connections.

Although most chronic transfusions progress, some may fluctuate or even reverse. If one twin dies in utero and the transfusion ceases, the situation may resolve itself. Alternatively, the surviving twin (usually the recipient) may exsanguinate into the suddenly relaxed circulatory system of the dead co-twin (usually the donor) (*Fig. 19.30*). Acute hypotension and/or blood loss after co-twin death is considered a likely explanation for necrotic lesions in the surviving twin, a view supported by Doppler studies showing dramatic umbilical flow velocity changes in the surviving twin. It has been estimated that neurologic sequelae occur in as many as 27% of surviving twins. Cerebral lesions have been demonstrated sonographically in twins at birth and in utero, developing rapidly in some cases. These observations are important in attempting to explain the high incidence of cerebral palsy in twins, reportedly five times the incidence in singletons and affecting primarily monozygous twins. Recognition that lesions predictive of cerebral palsy are of prenatal onset is important not only in medicolegal considerations, but also when contemplating the possible consequences of intentional fetal reduction for the surviving twin.

Attempts to alter TTTS have included treatment with indomethacin to reduce fetal urine output and polyhydramnios, digoxin to treat congestive heart failure, decompressive amniocentesis to prolong pregnancy and affect fetal blood flow, division of intervening membranes, selective feticide, and laser ablation of anastomoses. The latter approach requires accurate prenatal mapping of physiologically significant arteriovenous anastomoses and their successful ablation in vivo. Increasingly sophisticated Doppler studies are used to tailor treatment strategies to individual vascular patterns and to assess the results of intervention. Pathologic evaluation of laser sites and mapping of residual anastomoses play an important part in this treatment strategy. The enthusiasm for intervention must be tempered by the knowledge that the two fetal circulations are connected and that any manipulation will potentially affect both fetuses. Given the complexity and uniqueness of the vascular anatomy, it is difficult to predict the consequences.

Acute Transfusion

Plethora of one twin and pallor of the other do not always signify a chronic transfusion, but may reflect acute shifts of blood through large superficial vascular anastomoses. A large blood volume may shift rapidly through large-vessel connections. Simple acute transfusions are usually diagnosed at birth. The donor is pale and the recipient plethoric, but there is no growth differential and hemoglobin and hematocrit levels are equal in initial assessments. Acute transfusions may occur when one twin experiences circulatory collapse for whatever reason or

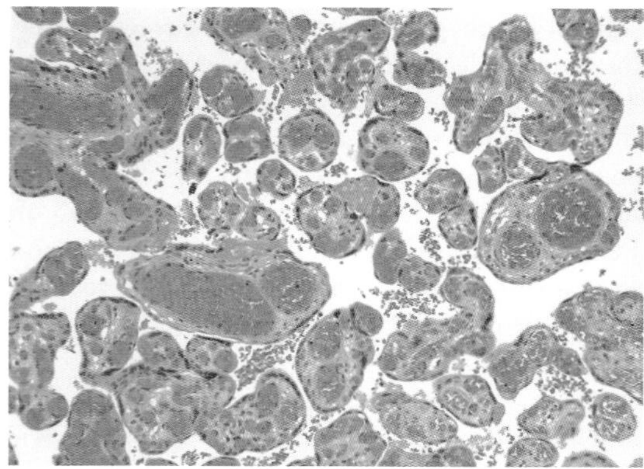

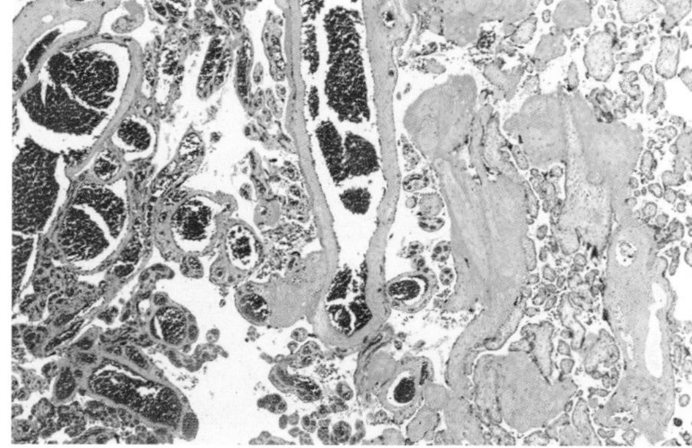

Fig. 19.33
Twin–twin transfusion syndrome (TTTS). **The recipient's villi are appropriately mature but congested (*left*). The contrast between the donor and recipient placental territories is dramatic (*right*)**

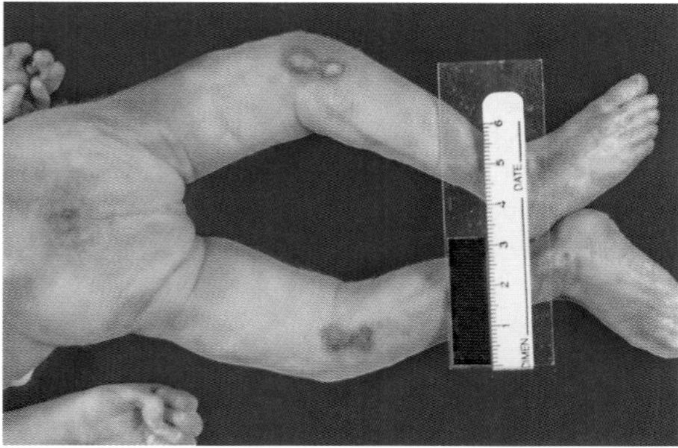

Fig. 19.34
Twin–twin transfusion syndrome (TTTS). **Both twins may have necrotic lesions including aplasia cutis as seen here in the donor twin (Used with permission of the American Registry of Pathology/Armed Forces Institute of Pathology)**

when a twin exsanguinates through the unclamped cord of its delivered co-twin. Although clinically documented simple acute transfusion is rare, silent cases occurring in utero may account for the dramatic increase in cerebral palsy in like-sex twins.

Acute on Chronic Transfusion

Superimposition of acute transfusion on established chronic transfusion is more common than simple acute transfusion, and when this occurs, there is reversal in the expected pattern with plethora of the smaller, original donor twin and pallor of the larger, recipient twin (*Fig. 19.30*). Whether this pattern develops after the donor dies and the recipient's blood drains into the donor's flaccid vascular tree, or the acute transfusion occurs first, overwhelming the capacity of the donor's heart causing death is unknown. Both mechanisms may be operative. On occasion, an acute transfusion and/or fetomaternal hemorrhage may occur in twins with discordant growth for reasons unrelated to chronic transfusion. While this scenario may mimic an acute on chronic transfusion, lack of evidence for adaptation to chronic transfusion (no heart-size discrepancy, polyhydramnios, or oligohydramnios) may help exclude chronic transfusion as a relevant contributing factor.

Asymmetric Growth

Established growth standards indicate that the growth curves for dichorionic and monochorionic twins approximate those of singletons prior to 30–34 weeks [7, 84]. Twins weigh progressively less than singletons as pregnancy advances. When twin growth is discordant, the larger twin approximates the growth of an age-matched singleton, and the growth rate of the smaller twin slows and may gradually decline into the range of small for gestational age (SGA). In dichorionic twins, growth discordancy is usually manifest around 25 weeks, but in monochorionic twins, the onset is more variable, commencing in some cases as early as 18–20 weeks.

Twin birth weight discordance is strongly associated with pre-term birth, perinatal death, and postnatal morbidity [28]. The majority of twins with discordant growth are dichorionic, and even among monochorionic twins, TTTS is not the most common cause of growth discrepancy. Even when chronic transfusion occurs, other factors may contribute as much or more to discordant growth. Cord anomalies including velamentous insertion and single umbilical artery are associated with decreased fetal weight, and both are much more frequent in twin gestations. In one recent study, peripheral cord insertion (velamentous, marginal, and markedly eccentric) was the strongest predictor of discordant growth and SGA in dichorionic and monochorionic twins [140]. Velamentous and marginal cord insertion may be accompanied by differences in placental vascularization; higher Doppler S–D ratios, and lower numbers of small muscular arteries in tertiary villi have been demonstrated in the smaller of discordant twins with peripheral cord insertion. Discordant birth weight is also associated with placental mass; smaller babies have smaller placentas. Since the fetal–placental weight ratio in smaller twins is normal to decreased, maternal vascular insufficiency is unlikely to be a major cause of impaired growth. Rather, poor placentation with asymmetrical trophotropism and abnormal cord insertion, asymmetric placental volume, and decreased placental vascularization are major causative factors in IUGR and twin growth discordance. These factors may also explain the coexistence of oligohydramnic, growth-restricted, and polyhydramnic larger twins (twin oligohydramnios–polyhydramnios sequence – TOPS) in dichorionic gestations and in monochorionic gestations in which twin–twin transfusion has been carefully excluded by marker erythrocyte studies [24]. Whether placental and fetal growth asymmetries reflect a generalized problem in the conceptus or result from a primary placental problem is unclear.

While discordant parenchymal lesions present a possible explanation for growth asymmetry, most placental disease processes involve twin placentas to similar degree; concordance for most findings is higher than might be expected based on their prevalence in singleton placentas. In one recent study, the only lesion significantly associated with discordant SGA twins was the finding of fibrotic avascular villi (FAV) [140]. This lesion, indicative of fetal vascular occlusion (fetal thrombotic vasculopathy) and associated with neurologic impairment in term infants, might contribute to the increased morbidity and mortality in twins. The incidence of fetal vessel thrombosis is higher in monochorionic than dichorionic placentas, correlating with peripheral cord insertion, vascular cushions, and IUGR [163].

Intragestational Fetal Loss

Multiples have higher mortality rates at all stages of gestation and after birth. The causes of intrauterine twin death vary with gestational age but are essentially the same as in singletons with the important addition of the specific complications of monochorionic placentation. Monochorionic twins are greatly over-represented among twin deaths at all gestational ages. The pathologic findings in intragestational fetal loss also depend on the time of fetal death and duration of retention in utero. One or both twins may die, concordantly or discordantly, and they may be delivered at intervals or retained and delivered together.

Vanishing Twin

Twin gestations are commonly converted to singletons with the embryonic/early fetal death of one twin (*vanishing twin*). Of twins diagnosed before 10 weeks, about 70% are born as singletons. When a twin dies spontaneously early in the first trimester, it is often difficult or impossible to identify any residue. A flattened mass of sclerotic placenta may remain as a vaguely thickened area in the membranes of the surviving co-twin. Microscopic examination may identify the membranous septum and establish chorionicity. Rarely there is an embryonic remnant, invariably severely degenerated (*Fig. 19.35*). Electively reduced embryonic remnants are more easily identified (*Fig. 19.36*).

Fetus Papyraceus

A twin dying in the second trimester may be retained, progressively compressed, and flattened by the growth of

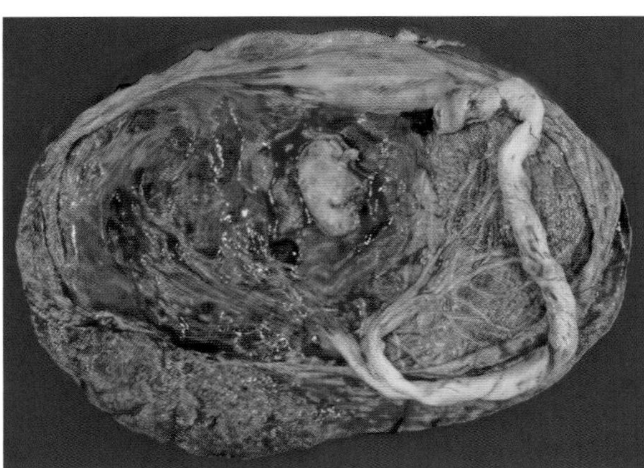

Fig. 19.35
Early twin demise. **This growth disorganized tiny twin was delivered at term with its normal co-twin. The abnormal morphology suggests that this early twin death was the result of an abnormal karyotype**

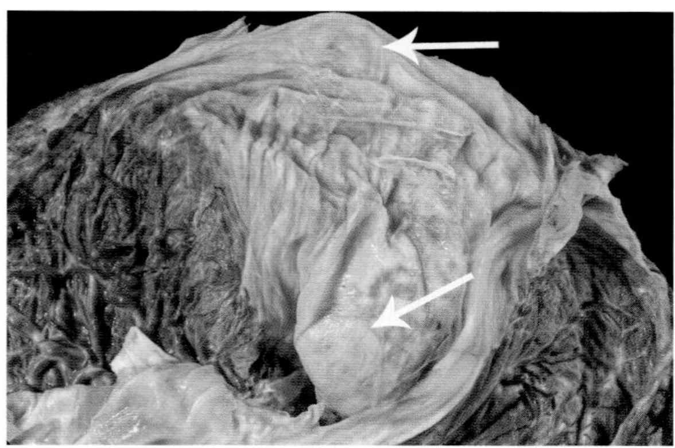

Fig. 19.36
Multiple pregnancy with elective reduction. **Reduced fetuses are usually about the same size and relatively easily identified in the membranes (Used with permission of the American Registry of Pathology/Armed Forces Institute of Pathology)**

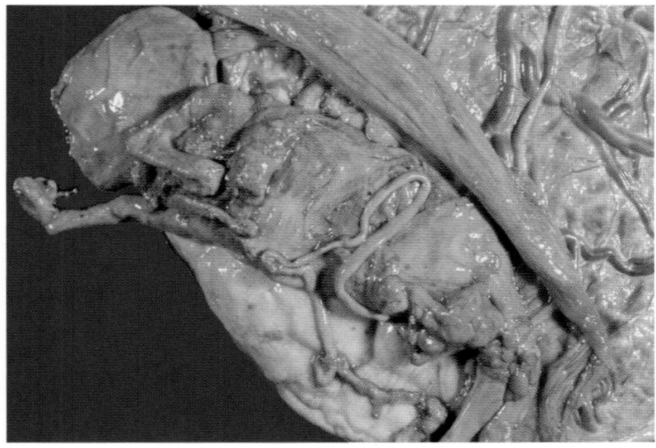

Fig. 19.37
Fetus papyraceus

the co-twin. Depending on the length of retention, this flattened dead twin, a *fetus papyraceus*, is variably altered (*Fig. 19.37*). Some are still easily recognizable and others resemble amorphous necrotic material. Specimen radiographs may reveal skeletal remnants. It has been estimated that the creation of a fetus papyraceus takes about 10 weeks. The degree of maceration generally precludes establishment of the cause of death, although anomalous cord insertion and TTTS have been implicated in many cases. Fetus papyraceus may occur in both monochorionic and dichorionic gestations. The amnionic cavity of the fetus papyraceus is gradually compressed as the amnionic fluid is resorbed. The corresponding placenta is generally pale, thinned, and sclerotic with avascular, fibrotic villi enmeshed in fibrin.

Survivors of Co-Twin Demise

Abnormalities including intestinal atresia, skin defects, amputations, gastroschisis, and especially brain damage have been reported in twins surviving the in utero death of a co-twin. The risk of serious cerebral damage in surviving twins is reportedly around 20% and may be even higher in certain subsets. Monochorionic twins appear to be at greatest risk [117]. At all gestational ages, the risk of cerebral palsy is higher in like-sex surviving co-twins. Lesions occurring in surviving co-twins are similar to those in monochorionic twins with complex vascular anastomoses, suggesting a similar pathogenesis. Survivors of co-twin death also have a higher postnatal mortality rate.

Duplication Abnormalities

Occasional monozygous twins show marked discrepancies in size and configuration or varying degrees of incomplete separation. These asymmetric and incomplete duplications include acardiac and parasitic twins and conjoined fetuses. A parasitic twin is a variably developed fetiform mass attached to its co-twin either internally or externally (*Fig. 19.38*). Conjoined twins retain their overall symmetry but are either incompletely separated or possibly secondarily fused during development. Neither parasitic nor conjoined twins show specific placental abnormalities.

Acardiac Twin (*Chorangiopagus Parasiticus*)

Acardiac twinning is the commonest form of asymmetric duplication anomaly, occurring in 1% of monochorionic twins. The acardius is a grossly malformed, often bizarre fetus of variable size, appearance, and degree of organogenesis. No two are alike. Some are amorphous, shapeless masses resembling teratomas (*Fig. 19.39*) and others are remarkably well developed. Commonly, acardiac fetuses have relatively well-developed legs and perineal structures, a trunk into which the umbilical cord inserts and a rounded, dome-like upper body (*Fig. 19.40*). A single body cavity may contain abdominal viscera, but thoracic structures and the heart are typically absent. Cardiac remnants or a deformed heart may be identified on occasion. Organ development is highly variable; some acardiacs may demonstrate absence of most organs, while in others, the organs may be well developed. Acardiacs may be hydropic, and some are larger than the co-twin.

The essential feature common to all acardiac fetuses is their circulation, which is maintained entirely by the co-twin (the "pump" twin). Blood from the normal "pump" twin reaches the acardiac through an artery to artery anastomosis, flows through the acardiac in reverse course, then returns to the normal twin through a vein to vein anastomosis (*twin reversed arterial perfusion – TRAP*). The majority of acardiacs have a single umbilical artery. The specific vascular communications between the acardiac and pump twins are large, occurring at the level of the umbilical cord or chorionic plate. There are no placental parenchymal vascular connections, and therefore the acardiac is analogous to a conjoined twin and not to the TTTS. The histologic features of the placenta in acardiac twinning have not been described in detail. Villous immaturity and recent and remote thrombosis of umbilical and chorionic plate veins have been reported [179]. Acardiacs may occur in diamnionic or monoamnionic monochorionic placentas, although monoamnionic placentation is especially prevalent. Acardiacs are greatly over-represented in triplet and higher multiple gestations.

The pump twin is at risk for cardiovascular overload. The extra work involved in circulating blood through the acardiac may result in cardiomegaly and high output failure associated with hydrops and hydramnios. Pump twins also tend to be growth impaired perhaps because the blood diverted away from the placenta to the acardiac returns deoxygenated. Many pump twins have congenital

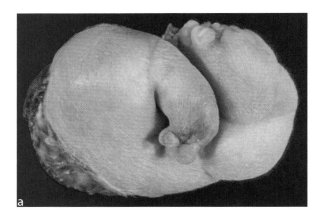

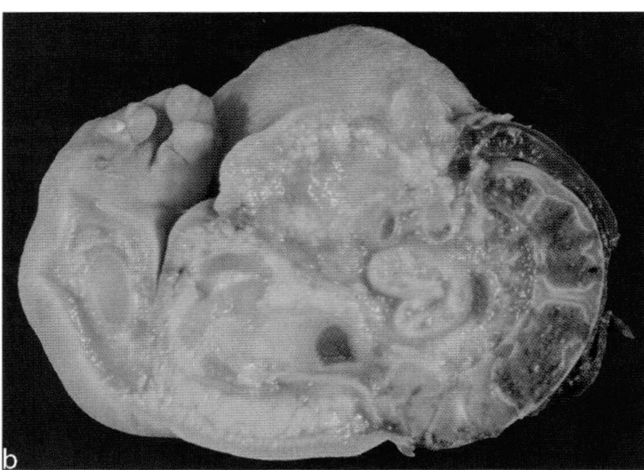

Fig. 19.38
Parasitic twin. **This parasitic twin (a and b) was removed from the abdominal cavity of its co-twin (Used with permission of the American Registry of Pathology/Armed Forces Institute of Pathology)**

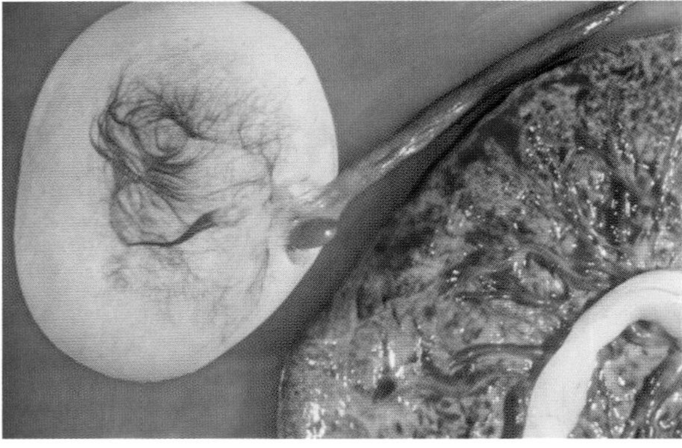

Fig. 19.39
Acardiac fetus. **This amorphous acardiac fetus had a single umbilical artery (Used with permission of the American Registry of Pathology/Armed Forces Institute of Pathology)**

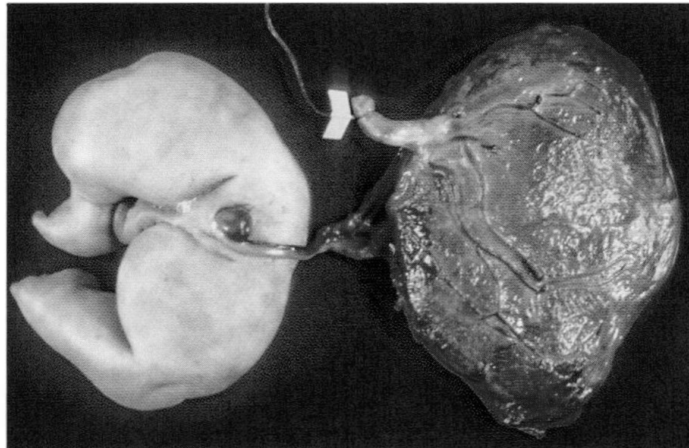

Fig. 19.40
Acardiac fetus. **A dome shaped upper body with lower extremities is a relatively common configuration in acardiac fetuses (Used with permission of the American Registry of Pathology/Armed Forces Institute of Pathology)**

anomalies. Classification of the acardiac anomaly based on prognostic factors including the cardiovascular condition of the pump twin and the size of the acardiac twin has been proposed [191]. Strategies similar to those employed in management of the twin–twin transfusion syndrome have been successful in ameliorating the effects of cardiac overload in the pump twin [180].

Higher Multiple Births

Examination of placentas from higher multiple births extend the observations applied to twins. Chorionicity, membrane relationships, cord insertion, chorionic vascularity, potential vascular anastomoses, and relative placental volumes are assessed as in twins. Patterns of placentation vary depending on zygosity. Triplets, for example, may be monochorionic, dichorionic, or trichorionic with variable amnionicity (➲ *Figs. 19.41* and ➲ *19.42*). Multichorionic placentas are usually fused as space in the uterus is limited. Combinations of monozygous and polyzygous multiples are common. With increasing use of assisted reproductive techniques, triplets and even quadruplets or quintuplets are no longer unusual in many institutions (➲ *Fig. 19.43*). Higher multiples experience the same complications as twins – prematurity, low birth weight, congenital anomalies, increased perinatal morbidity/mortality – all progressively problematic with increasing numbers. Acardiacs are much more frequent in higher multiples as compared to twins. Cord entanglement is less common in

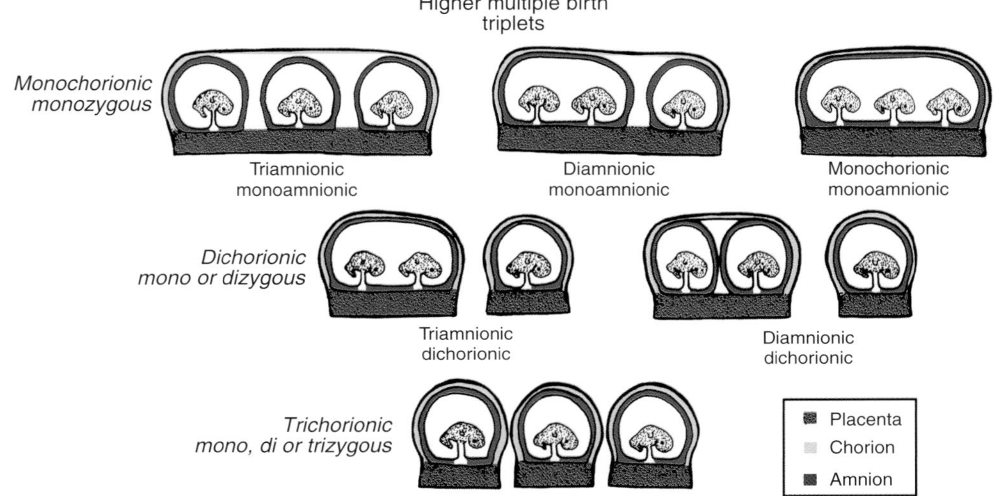

Fig. 19.41
Triplet placentation (After [44])

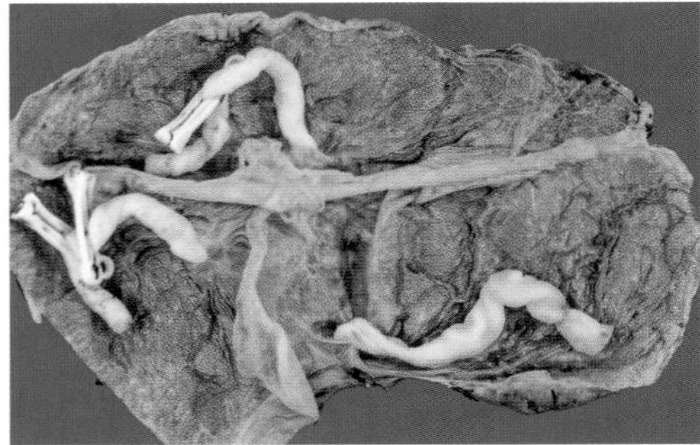

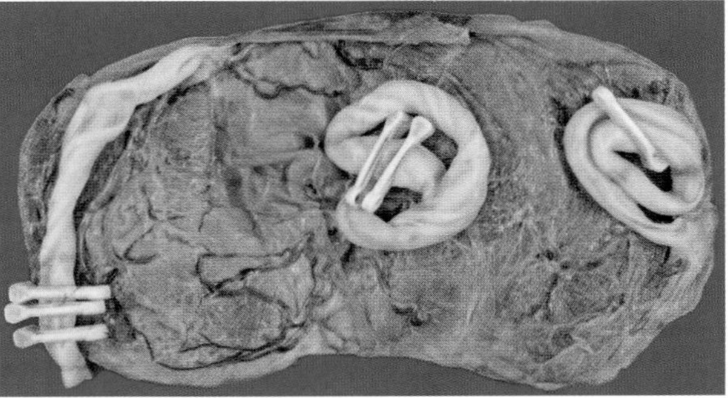

Fig. 19.42
Triplet placentation. **Tri-Tri triplets (*left*). DiMo triplets (*right*). Although the placental territory at left is discrete, the fetal vascular pattern confirms monochorionicity. The middle and right triplets are monoamnionic**

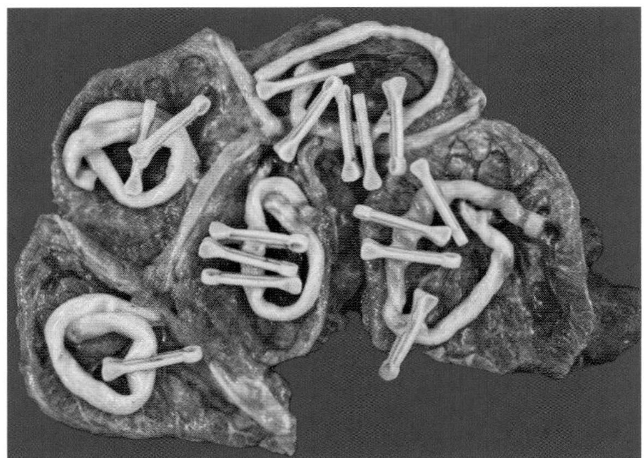

Fig. 19.43
Quintuplet placentas

monoamnionic higher-order multiples presumably due to limited opportunity for movement in the increasingly crowded uterus. While the outlook in higher multiple births has improved, complications are common and the outcome is often poor. Consequently, selective fetal reduction has been advocated, and there is now a substantial body of accumulated experience. Remnants of reduced fetuses are regularly identified when carefully sought.

Placental Inflammation and Intrauterine Infection

Placental inflammation is a common and important histologic finding. The character of a given inflammatory infiltrate and its pattern of involvement reflect, in general, its etiology and determine its clinical significance [127]. Placental inflammatory infiltrates can be divided into two major categories: (1) acute chorioamnionitis (ACA), an acute inflammatory reaction in the fetal membranes and umbilical cord; and (2) villitis – inflammation, usually chronic, of the villous parenchyma. ACA is invariably infectious due to microorganisms, usually bacteria, that ascend from the vagina or cervix (*ascending infection*). Villitis is almost invariably idiopathic, although rarely, it may be infectious, caused by microorganisms (viruses, some bacteria, or protozoa) that reach the placenta through the maternal blood (*hematogenous infection*). Passage through an infected birth canal is an important mode of fetal infection, but the placenta is not involved in this circumstance.

The consequences of intrauterine infection and inflammation include abortion, stillbirth, preterm birth (PTB), fetal malformation, active postnatal infection, and long-term sequelae, frequently neurologic. At worst, affected children may be severely handicapped, retarded, blind, or deaf. The social, financial, and emotional burden posed by the support of these children is enormous.

Ascending Infection and Acute Chorioamnionitis

Frequency, etiology, and pathogenesis. ACA is the most common form of placental infection and inflammation in humans [134]. Histologic ACA is found in approximately 10–15% of term and in up to 50–70% of preterm placentas. This striking inverse relationship between ACA and gestational age emphasizes the strong association between ACA and PTB. The term “chorioamnionitis” when used by clinicians to describe a symptom complex suggestive of intrauterine infection (maternal fever, uterine tenderness, or elevated white blood cell count) correlates poorly with histologic chorioamnionitis.

While historically controversial, it is now clear that ACA is a maternal and fetal acute inflammatory response to infectious agents that have gained access to the gestational sac. Microorganisms, usually bacteria, have been cultured from fetal membranes, amnionic fluid, cord blood, and fetal tissues in a high percentage of cases [194], and have been demonstrated by PCR in culture negative cases [48]. ACA can be produced experimentally in animals by the intraamnionic injection of bacteria but not by sterile exogenous irritants. Most cases of ACA result from the ascent of vaginal or cervical bacteria into the uterus. Other potential sources of intrauterine infection include endometritis or contiguous spread of organisms from the fallopian tubes, bladder, appendix, or intestines. Recent epidemiologic and experimental data have linked periodontal disease due to *Fusobacterium nucleatum* to PTL and have suggested that these microorganisms may reach the decidua hematogenously in some cases [57, 65].

ACA may either preceed or follow membrane rupture. There is a consistent and well-documented relationship between chorioamnionitis and membrane rupture; the longer membranes have been ruptured, the greater the likelihood that ACA will occur. Ascending infection and ACA, however, frequently precede membrane rupture, initiating premature rupture of membranes (PROM) and/or PTL, rather than following it, explaining the strong association between ACA and PTB. Outcome studies would suggest that ACA with intact membranes is a distinct entity with a greater risk to the developing fetus than ACA following membrane rupture, although the histologic changes are identical [129]. The bacteria most commonly identified in women with spontaneous

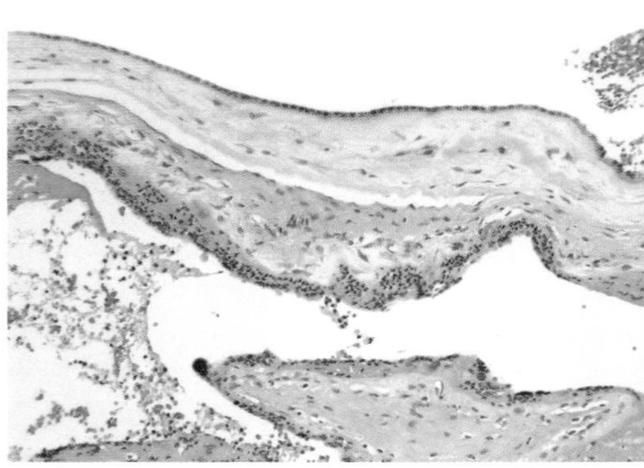
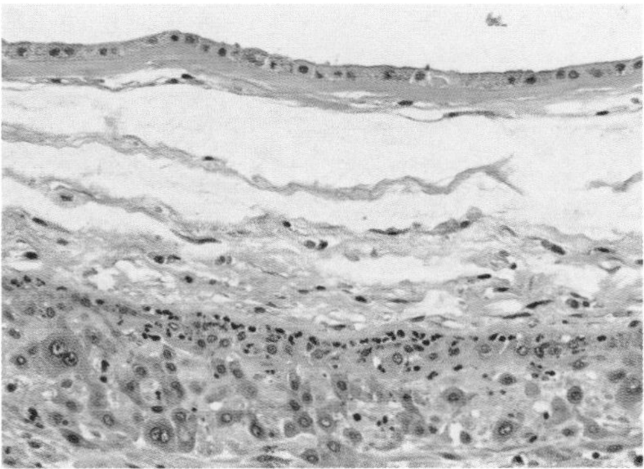

Fig. 19.44
ACA, maternal response (early, stage 1). **Maternal neutrophils migrate out of the intervillous space aggregating in the subchorionic fibrin (*left*) and from decidual vessels infiltrating the membranous chorionic trophoblast (*right*)**

PTL and intact membranes are low-virulence vaginal and enteric organisms – *Fusobacterium*, *Ureaplasma urealyticum*, *Mycoplasma hominis*, *Gardnerella vaginalis*, *Bacterioides* and *Peptostreptococcus* species. Whether susceptibility to ACA is more related to factors that facilitate access of microorganisms to the intrauterine environment or to the virulence of, and host response to, a given infectious agent is unclear. To some extent, the maternal response to intrauterine infection is blunted by adaptations in the immune system that prevent rejection of the fetus [129].

Pathology. Maternal response: In most cases of ACA, the fetal membranes are macroscopically normal. In cases of particularly severe, long-standing infection, they may be opaque, friable, or foul smelling. Histologically there is a maternal and often a fetal inflammatory response to amnionic infection that progress sequentially and predictably as originally described by Blanc [21]. The initial response is maternal, manifested by the migration of maternal neutrophils from the intervillous space and from vessels in the membranous decidua. Neutrophils accumulate first in the subchorionic fibrin (acute subchorionitis) and membranous chorionic trophoblast (early acute chorionitis) (*Fig. 19.44*), migrating progressively through the connective tissue layer of the chorion (acute chorionitis) and amnion (acute chorioamnionitis) (*Fig. 19.45*) and into the amnionic fluid in response to chemotactic factors released by the infecting agent and/or inflammatory reaction. With time, the neutrophils undergo apoptosis and karyorrhexis followed by amnionic epithelial necrosis (necrotizing chorioamnionitis) (*Fig. 19.46*).

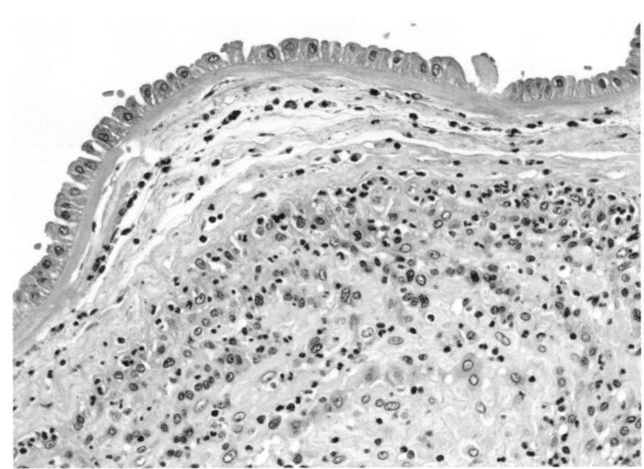

Fig. 19.45
ACA, maternal response (intermediate, stage 2). **Maternal neutrophils migrate into the connective tissue of the chorion and amnion**

The sequential changes and disease progression (stage) in the maternal inflammatory response are constant. A clinically relevant scheme for staging and grading the maternal inflammatory response has been proposed by the Perinatal Section of the Society for Pediatric Pathology (*Table 19.1*) [141]. The time course of progression in the maternal inflammatory response has been estimated based on personal observation and clinical correlation as well as experimental data. According to Redline, the initial maternal inflammatory response (acute subchorionitis) occurs within 6–12 h of infection. Involvement of amnionic connective tissue (ACA) most probably develops over 12–36 h after which the initial wave of neutrophils undergoes apoptosis and karryorhexis (36–48 h) [131]. Whether and how the timing of the maternal response may be altered by maternal factors such as preexisting

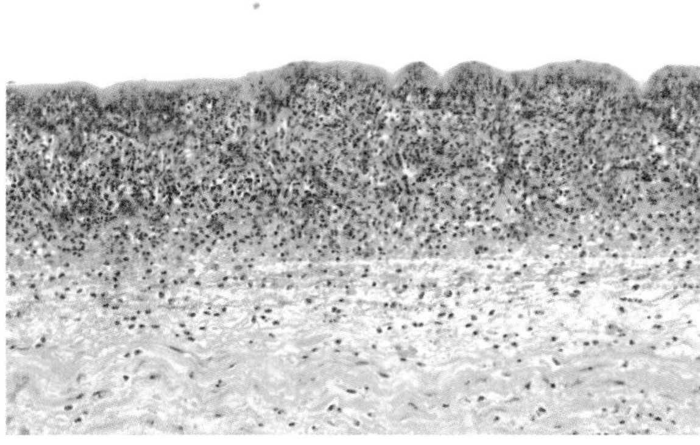

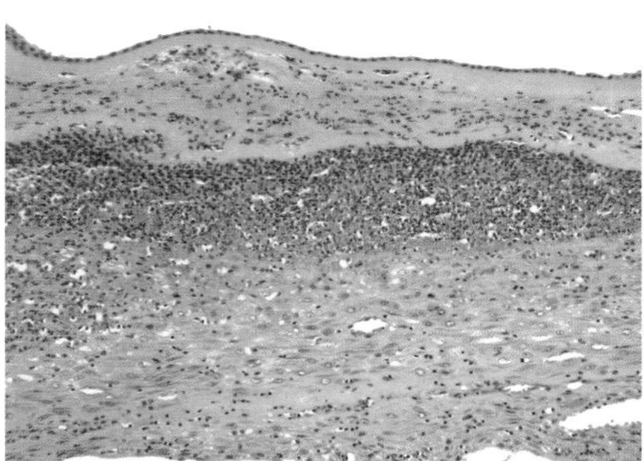

Fig. 19.46
ACA, maternal response (advanced stage 3, severe). **Diffuse intense inflammation with karyorrhexis of neutrophils and amnionic epithelial necrosis (*left*) and chorionic microabscesses (*right*)**

Table 19.1
Ascending infection

Maternal response	
Stage 1 early:	Acute subchorionitis/early chorionitis
Stage 2 intermediate:	Chorionitis/chorioamnionitis
Stage 3 late:	Necrotizing chorioamnionitis
	Subacute chorioamnionitis
Grade severe:	Subchorionic microabscesses
Fetal response	
Stage 1 early:	Umbilical phlebitis/chorionic vasculitis
Stage 2 intermediate:	Umbilical arteritis
Stage 3 late:	Necrotizing funisitis
Grade severe:	Intense chorionic vasculitis

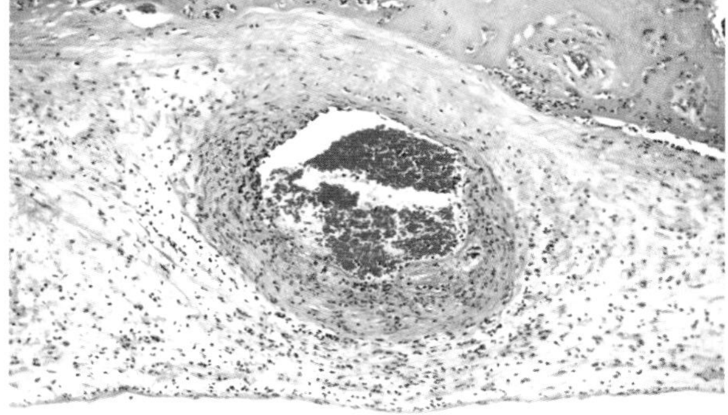

Fig. 19.47
ACA, fetal response (early, stage 1). **Fetal neutrophils migrate into the chorionic plate vessels (chorionic vasculitis)**

maternal antibodies or the characteristics of the specific causative organism is not understood. The intensity (grade) of the maternal inflammatory response is more difficult to quantify. Grading based on the number of neutrophils in the most inflamed area of the chorionic plate has been suggested. The formation of subchorionic microabscesses has long been recognized as an indicator of severity since associated with fetal sepsis by Keenan (*Table 19.1*) [78, 141].

Fetal inflammatory response: Depending on the gestational age and status of the fetal immune system, the fetus may also respond to amnionic infection. A fetal leukocytic response is often absent in gestations less than 19–20 weeks and in fetuses less than 500 g. The first manifestation of a fetal inflammatory reaction is the migration of fetal neutrophils into the umbilical vein (umbilical phlebitis) and/or chorionic plate vessels (chorionic vasculitis). The migration of inflammatory cells is crescent-shaped, oriented toward the source of infection in the amnionic cavity (*Fig. 19.47*). In later stages, fetal neutrophils migrate from the umbilical arteries (umbilical arteritis) and into Wharton's jelly. With increasing duration, the neutrophils undergo necrosis forming necrotic bands around the umbilical vessels (necrotizing/subacute necrotizing funisitis) that may undergo calcification or vascularization (*Fig. 19.48*). Umbilical cord inflammation is often segmental, sometimes identified in only one of multiple sections, often from the fetal end.

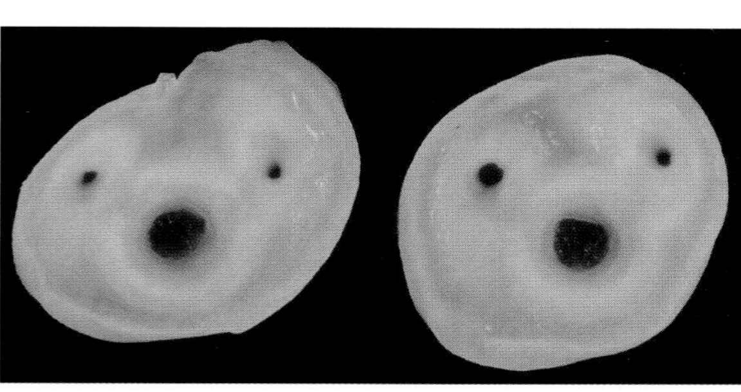

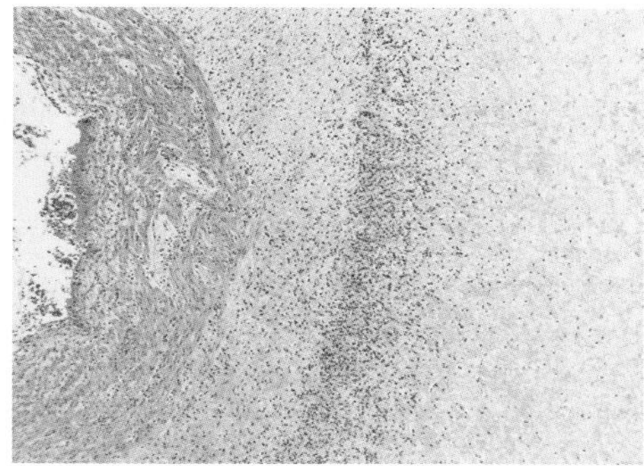

Fig. 19.48
ACA, fetal response (late, stage 3). **Necrotizing funisitis. Prominent crescentic band of necrotic leukocytes around umbilical vessels can be appreciated grossly**

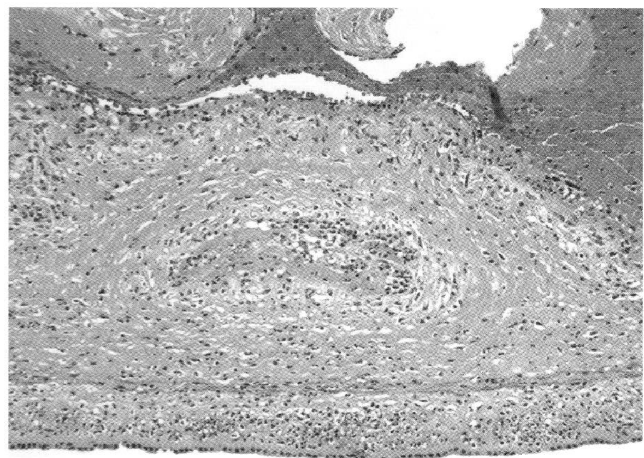

Fig. 19.49
ACA, fetal response (severe). **Fetal neutrophilic infiltration of chorionic vessels with medial disarray and in this case thrombosis**

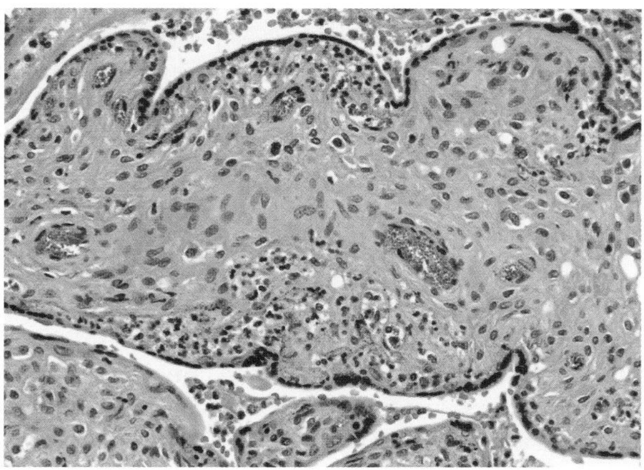

Fig. 19.50
Acute villitis. **Bacterial colonies are prominent in villous capillaries and neutrophils have accumulated beneath the trophoblast in the peripheral villous stroma**

Progression of the fetal inflammatory response has also been staged (*Table 19.1*), although the rate of progression of the fetal inflammatory response is more variable than the maternal response, depending significantly on gestational age. The intensity (grade) of the fetal inflammatory response has important associations with adverse fetal outcome. Scattered neutrophils in the chorionic plate or umbilical vessels are considered to be mild to moderate (grade 1). Intense chorionic vasculitis (severe/grade 2) is characterized by near confluent neutrophilic infiltration of vessels accompanied by attenuation or disarray of the vascular smooth muscle media (*Fig. 19.49*). Inflamed vessels may be thrombosed.

Amnionic infection, then, is a unique situation in which two individuals, mother and fetus, respond to the same infectious insult. The acute inflammatory infiltrate in chorioamnionitis is characteristically confined to the fetal membranes and umbilical cord. The villous parenchyma is not involved unless fetal septicemia results secondarily in villitis. In this event, bacteria (usually *Escherichia coli*, group B streptococci) are present in villous capillaries, often with accumulation of neutrophils beneath the trophoblastic basement membrane (*Fig. 19.50*). Although the majority of leukocytes in the fetal membranes are maternal, fluorescence in situ hybridization studies have demonstrated that the majority of neutrophils in amnionic fluid and fetal lung are fetal, emphasizing the important contributions of both maternal and fetal immune systems. The character of the inflammatory infiltrate is usually not specific enough to identify a particular offending agent. In fact, it is relatively unusual to find bacteria in histologic sections even when they have been demonstrated on smears of the amnion. Notable exceptions to this include infections with group B β-hemolytic streptococci in which colonies of the organism are frequently found without difficulty even in the absence of histologic evidence of chorioamnionitis. Fusobacterium species may also be visible on conventional H&E stains as long (at least 15 μm), faintly basophilic wavy organisms often associated with very severe inflammation and necrosis in the membranes. Fusobacteria may be demonstrated with silver stains but are only faintly gram-negative on Brown and Hopps stain. In rare instances of *Candida* infection, tiny white fungal colonies 2–3 mm in size may be seen grossly on the amnionic surface of the umbilical cord. Yeast and hyphal forms *Candida* may also be identified on conventional H&E stains, characteristically in small, superficial, crescentic microabscesses under the amnionic surface of the umbilical cord (peripheral funisitis) (➲ *Fig. 19.51*).

Clinical significance. Although there are maternal hazards associated with chorioamnionitis (maternal sepsis), the principal clinical impact of chorioamnionitis is its potential adverse affect on the fetus.

Preterm birth (PTB). It is estimated that approximately 70% of perinatal mortality and nearly half of long-term neurologic morbidity can be attributed to PTB [40]. Multiple factors contribute to PTB, but chorioamnionitis is implicated in a high percentage of cases. Intrauterine infection as a cause of PTB is usually asymptomatic until labor begins or the membranes rupture prematurely, and therefore, early diagnosis is difficult. Many recent strategies have been aimed at the identification of women at risk and the development of therapeutic interventions targeting infection and the inflammatory response to reduce spontaneous PTB and its associated mortality and long-term morbidity.

Data accumulating from experimental and human studies are clarifying how bacterial infection and chorioamnionitis result in spontaneous PTB. The inflammatory response to bacterial invasion results in the production of cytokines that initiate prostaglandin synthesis, resulting in uterine contractions. Certain bacterial species commonly associated with chorioamnionitis are high in phospholipase A2, which releases the prostaglandin precursor arachidonic acid from membrane phospholipids. The inflammatory response also results in increased synthesis of metalloproteases that are thought to remodel and soften cervical collagen and to degrade the extracellular matrix of the fetal membranes, leading to membrane rupture [85].

Placental villous edema in the context of ACA, most often in preterms, has been correlated with increased morbidity, mortality, and neurologic impairment [105, 144, 150].

Approximately 30% of cases of ACA at less than 25 weeks are associated with retroplacental hematoma eventuating in death and delivery in many [129].

Fetal inflammatory response syndrome (FIRS). Traditional thinking has attributed many of the neonatal complications of chorioamnionitis-induced PTB to prematurity, not to infection per se. Evidence is accumulating that pathologic lesions predictive of long-term morbidity (periventricular leucomalacia, intraventricular hemorrhage) are initiated in utero by the fetal response to placental infection (*fetal inflammatory response syndrome – FIRS*). Most data would not implicate infectious organisms as a direct cause of tissue damage but rather mediators of the fetal inflammatory reaction, principally cytokines (IL1, IL6, IL8, TNF-α) in the genesis of fetal lesions, especially white matter damage predictive of

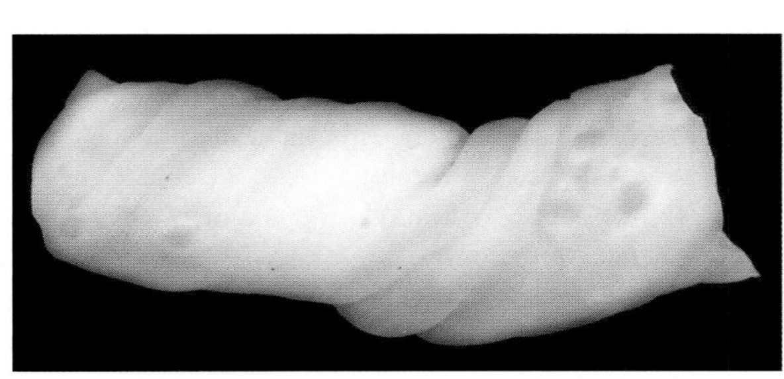

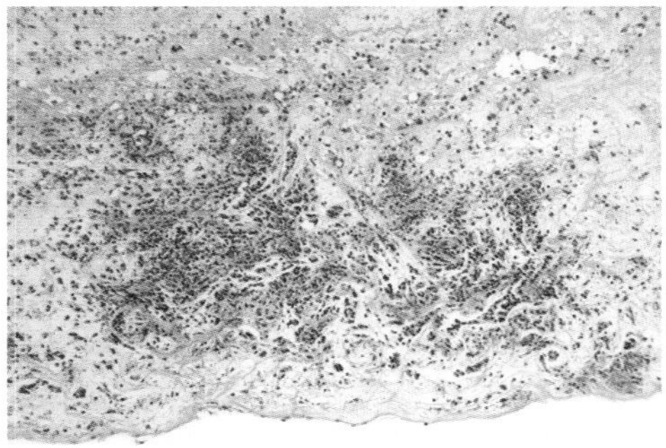

Fig. 19.51
Candida peripheral funisitis. **Small yellow foci on the umbilical cord correspond to superficial microabscesses**

cerebral palsy [54, 88]. Cytokines may cause white matter damage directly via a toxic effect or indirectly by activating endothelium and microglia resulting in thrombosis or increased vascular permeability. Whether endotoxins or exotoxins cross the placenta or blood–brain barrier to directly injure the central nervous system is unknown.

The only histologic finding directly correlated with CNS injury in ACA is the severity of the fetal inflammatory response. Umbilical arteritis is associated with higher levels of circulating fetal cytokines than inflammation of the umbilical vein alone [81, 157]. Intense chorionic vasculitis has been associated with increased risk of cerebral palsy in term and preterm infants [130, 150]. The concomitant presence of mural thrombi in inflamed chorionic plate vessels is an additional risk factor for neurologic impairment in very low birth weight (VLBW) infants [150].

Neonatal infection. ACA implies that the fetus has been exposed to infection but not necessarily that the fetus is infected. The exposed fetus may be infected through the fetal skin, eyes, nose, or ear canals or by inspiring or swallowing infected amnionic fluid. Infants whose placentas show ACA are at increased risk to develop sepsis and die in the neonatal period. Although neither mother nor neonate is overtly ill in most cases, neonatal infection is an important cause of perinatal death, and most serious neonatal infections are associated with ACA. Fetal outcome is determined by a number of factors including gestational age and causative organism. Group B β-hemolytic streptococcus, *E. coli*, and *Haemophilus influenzae* are the most common causes of significant neonatal infection. Placental features associated with increased risk of neonatal infection include severe maternal and fetal inflammatory responses [78, 194].

Subacute Chorioamnionitis

Subacute chorioamnionitis is characterized by a mixed inflammatory infiltrate of mononuclear cells and degenerating neutrophils, usually concentrated in the upper chorion. This pattern may result from ongoing low-grade or repetitive infection, and has been associated with chronic lung disease in a subgroup of VLBW infants with concomitant amnionic necrosis. The maternal history may include repetitive bouts of vaginal bleeding [111].

Villitis and Hematogenous Infection

Etiology. Villitis, inflammation of the villous parenchyma, is almost never due to documented infection. No causative organism has been identified despite intensive study, and no maternal symptoms, seasonal or geographic pattern of occurrence, neonatal inflammatory response, or congenital infections have been associated. Such cases have been termed *villitis of unknown etiology* (*VUE*). Recent investigations have identified the villous inflammatory cells as CD8 positive maternal T lymphocytes, supporting the theory that VUE represents a maternal immune response in fetal tissue (host versus graft reaction) [103, 135, 147].

Very rarely, villitis may result from a hematogenous infection in which infectious agents, usually viruses but also some bacteria and protozoa, reach the placenta through the maternal blood (*hematogenous infection*). In contrast to chorioamnionitis, a local infection, placental involvement in hematogenous infection is just one manifestation of maternal systemic disease. Although catastrophic fetoplacental infections caused by hematogenously acquired agents have been well documented, they are very infrequent.

Pathology. Villitis is almost always discovered incidentally on microscopic examination. Typically, there is neither clinical suspicion of nor gross pathologic clue to the underlying inflammatory process. There may be nonspecific findings – the placenta may be small or large and edematous – but only rarely are inflammatory foci identified grossly. The essential feature common to all villitides is an inflammatory infiltrate in the villi, but its character and the nature of associated changes are variable from case to case. The inflammatory infiltrate is usually chronic, composed of lymphocytes, histiocytes, and plasma cells in variable proportion (Fig. 19.52), but occasionally it may be granulomatous, and rarely neutrophils are prominent. Usually the inflammatory infiltrate is associated with appreciable alterations in villous landmarks, but rarely it may infiltrate

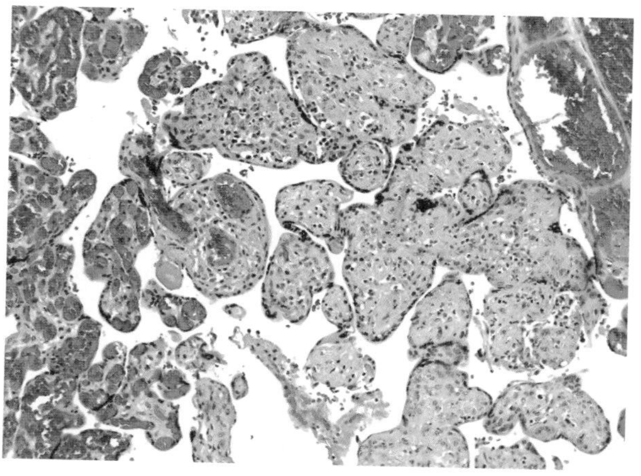

Fig. 19.52
Villitis of unknown etiology (VUE). **Villi infiltrated by lymphocytes and histiocytes**

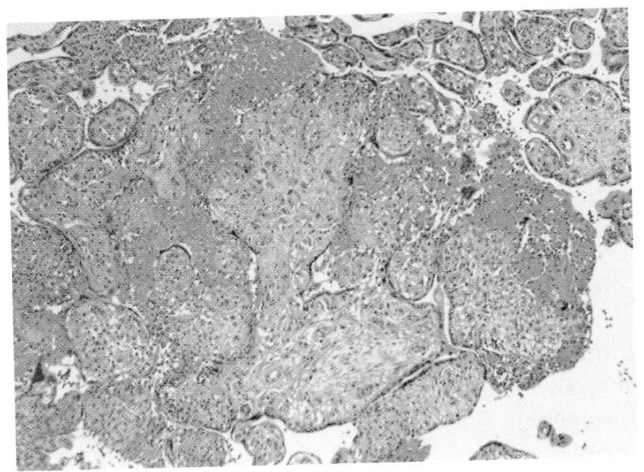

Fig. 19.53
Villitis of unknown etiology (VUE). **Inflammation involving the perivillous space with agglutination of adjacent inflamed villi**

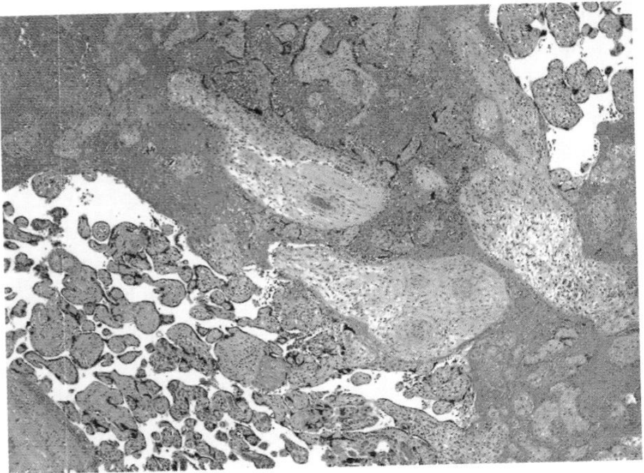

Fig. 19.54
Active chronic villitis with intervillositis and villous necrosis. **The villous stroma and intervillous space are infiltrated by neutrophils and chronic inflammatory cells. Fetal stem villous vasculitis, villous necrosis, and diffuse perivillous fibrin deposition result in grossly visible necrotic foci. Obliteration of stem vessels results in distal villous changes, here FAV**

passively. Necrosis, dystrophic calcification, and stromal hemosiderin deposition may be present in some cases. The inflammatory cells are generally concentrated within the villi, but may also extend into the surrounding intervillous space, a feature commonly associated with syncytiotrophoblastic necrosis, intervillous fibrin deposition, and agglutination of contiguous inflamed villi (*Fig. 19.53*). Occasionally an intervillous component (*intervillositis*) may predominate. Inflamed villi are usually randomly distributed, but in some cases may be concentrated in the basal regions of the placenta or juxtaposed to the septa. The degree of villous involvement varies greatly from case to case and may be graded semiquantitatively as outlined by Fox and Sebire (grades 1–4) [45] or Redline (focal, multifocal, patchy, and diffuse) [84] *Table 19.2.*

Table 19.2
Villous inflammation graded by extent

Grade 1:	Only one or two foci of villous inflammation, and in each focus only a very few villi are involved
Grade 2:	Up to six foci of villous inflammation, each focus containing up to twenty villi
Grade 3:	Multiple inflammatory foci, each occupying up to half a low power microscopic field
Grade 4:	Large areas of villous inflammation in most or all of the four sections
Focal:	Small clusters of five-ten villi in a single slide
Multifocal:	Small clusters of five-ten villi in multiple slides
Patchy:	Larger foci (more than ten villi)
Diffuse:	Diffuse involvement of all sections by groups of more than ten inflamed villi

Villitis of Unknown Etiology (VUE)

More than 95% of villitides are of unknown etiology. Although the extent and severity of VUE vary, it is very mild/mild or focal/multifocal in the majority of cases (60–75%). The villous inflammatory infiltrate is typically composed of macrophages and lymphocytes, but giant cells are common and are not indicative of infection. An active component with perivillous neutrophils may be present and when fulminant may be accompanied by intervillositis and fibrin deposition with villous necrosis (*active chronic villitis*) (*Fig. 19.54*). Since this pattern may be seen in some infectious villitides (gram-negative bacteria, nonsyphilitic spirochetes), special stains (gram, silver stains) should be considered. The inflammatory infiltrate is often confined to terminal villi but may also involve stem villi. Inflammatory obliteration of stem villous vessels with downstream fibrotic avascular villi (*VUE with fetal obliterative vasculopathy*) has been associated with neurologic impairment (*Fig. 19.55*) [84]. Chronic deciduitis and chronic chorioamnionitis may accompany VUE in some cases. Villitis involving basal/periseptal villi

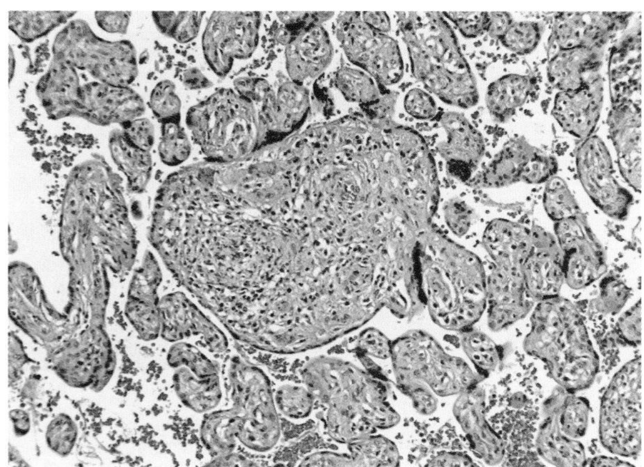

Fig. 19.55
Villitis of unknown etiology (VUE) with obliterative fetal vasculopathy. Vasculitis and obliteration of stem vessels result in avascular villi

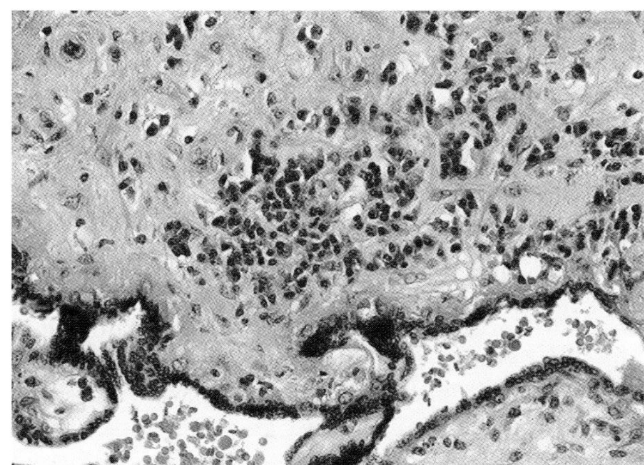

Fig. 19.56
CMV placentitis. Plasmacytic villous infiltrate

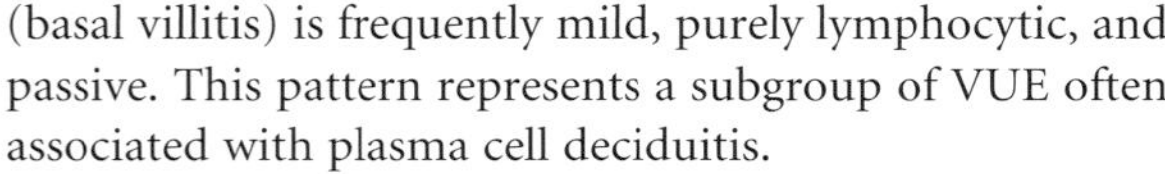

(basal villitis) is frequently mild, purely lymphocytic, and passive. This pattern represents a subgroup of VUE often associated with plasma cell deciduitis.

Clinical significance. VUE is a common lesion involving 5–15% of third-trimester placentas [135]. When mild, VUE is usually clinically silent and the infant unaffected. More severe, extensive VUE is associated with IUGR, IUFD, cerebral palsy, and other forms of neurologic impairment [145]. These complications correlate directly with the severity of the villitis. In VUE, maternal cells enter not only the villi but the fetus itself [135]. Whether this contributes to perinatal morbidity or mortality is unclear. When fatal, VUE is generally massive, suggesting that impaired placental function may be a mechanism of injury. VUE may recur (10–25% when diffuse), and is associated with total reproductive failure. IUGR, IUFD, and preterm delivery are especially likely in cases of recurrent VUE.

Specific Infectious Villitides

Rarely the morphologic features of a villitis suggest an infectious cause, although differences between the infectious villitides and VUE may be quite subtle. In general, infectious villitides tend to be more severe with more villous fibrosis, necrosis, calcification, and inflammation of fetal membranes and umbilical cord.

Cytomegalovirus (CMV)

Pathology. The placenta may be normal, small (in cases of IUGR) or large and edematous. Histologically the villi may exhibit any or all of a wide spectrum of changes

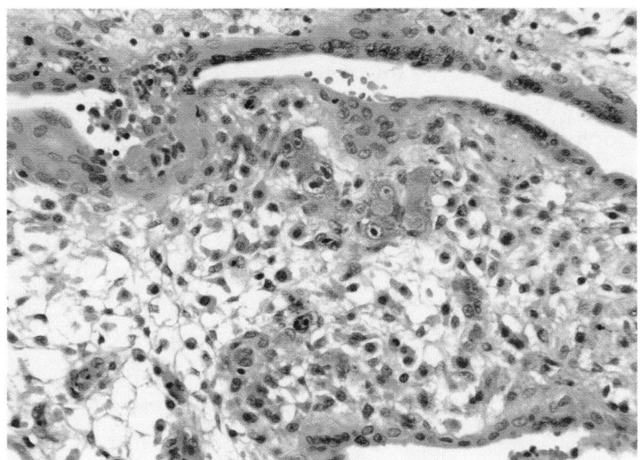

Fig. 19.57
CMV inclusions

related in part to gestational age. A plasmacytic villous infiltrate and stromal hemosiderin, often deposited around the remnants of occluded vessels, are characteristic (*Fig. 19.56*). Foci of stromal necrosis, calcification, and fibrosis may be found. The diagnostic cytopathic viral changes, large eosinophilic intranuclear and smaller basophilic cytoplasmic inclusions, may be present in endothelial cells, Hofbauer cells, or trophoblast (*Fig. 19.57*). They are most numerous and easily found in early, severe infections; as gestation proceeds, viral inclusions are typically scarce. When inclusions are not visualized on conventional H&E stains, CMV infection may be confirmed by immunohistochemistry, polymerase chain reaction (PCR), or in situ hybridization.

Clinical significance. CMV is the commonest identified infectious cause of villitis. The prevalence of congenital infection ranges from 0.2 to 2.2% of all live births. Transmission to the fetus may occur in utero, at birth, or postnatally. Intrauterine infection may result from either primary or recurrent maternal infection. Congenital infections resulting from reactivation of latent virus are less likely to produce fetal damage and late sequelae than those resulting from primary maternal infection. At the present time, CMV is the most commonly recognized infectious cause of developmental impairments. Late complications including mental retardation, chorioretinitis, seizures, and especially neurosensory hearing loss are most common among survivors of symptomatic congenital infection but may also occur later in children with no manifestations at birth.

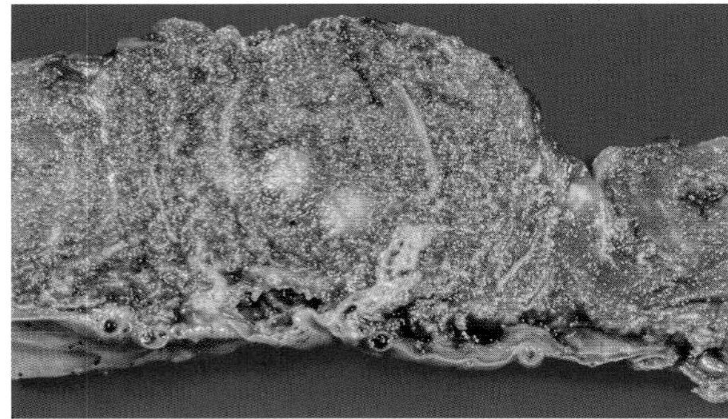

Fig. 19.58
Listeria placentitis. **Yellow white necrotic areas may be grossly apparent in some cases**

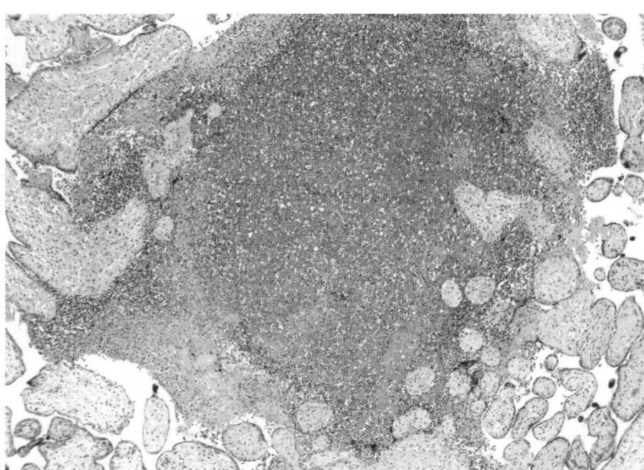

Fig. 19.59
Listeria placentitis. **Neutrophils aggregate in the intervillous space. Entrapped villi undergo necrosis forming abscesses. Neutrophils accumulate peripherally in the villous stroma beneath the trophoblast**

Treponema pallidum

Pathology. Infected placentas tend to be large and bulky. Histologically, the villi are large and relatively immature but not markedly edematous. The villous stroma is cellular as a result of the prominence of Hofbaur cells, and a lymphoplasmacytic infiltrate with subtrophoblastic neutrophils and microabscesses may be seen focally. Rarely, the inflammatory reaction has granulomatous features. Subendothelial and perivascular fibrosis resulting in luminal narrowing, recanalization, or occlusion of villous vessels is particularly characteristic. Marked decidual plasmacytic vasculitis and a chronic inflammatory infiltrate in the fetal membranes and umbilical cord have been noted in some cases. Necrotizing funisitis is a frequent finding but is not universal in, or specific for, congenital syphilis. The histologic changes in the placenta and umbilical cord are characteristic but not diagnostic. Definitive diagnosis depends on identification of spirochetes, most easily demonstrated in the umbilical cord whether inflamed or not.

Listeria monocytogenes

Pathology. The placenta is usually grossly normal but may contain minute yellow-white necrotic foci or rarely larger abscesses or infarcts (*Fig. 19.58*). The amnionic fluid is frequently meconium-stained. Unlike most other villitides, neutrophils predominate in Listeria villitis. Villi are commonly enmeshed in intervillous acute inflammation and fibrin, which, when extensive, may result in villous necrosis and abscesses. Neutrophils in the villi are often localized to a rim, often between the trophoblast and villous stroma (*Fig. 19.59*). Listeria villitis is usually accompanied by chorioamnionitis and often funisitis. *Listeria monocytogenes* is a small gram-positive motile bacillus with rounded ends that may be demonstrated with Brown–Hopps, Warthin–Starry, or Dieterle stains. Immunohistochemical stains have been utilized to establish the diagnosis and to exclude other infections (*Campylobacter* species, *E. coli*, *H. influenzae*, *Francisella tularensis*, *Streptococcus* species, *Brucella abortus*, *Chlamydia psittaci*, *Coccidioides immitis*) that have similar histologic findings.

Clinical significance. L. monocytogenes is a significant cause of intrauterine infection, spontaneous abortion, prematurity, and neonatal sepsis, morbidity, and death. Perinatal listeriosis takes one of two forms. In the "early type," congenital infection results in devastating neonatal sepsis (granulomatosis infantisepticum) in which microabscesses similar to those in the placenta are disseminated in fetal organs. The "late type" of perinatal listeriosis, presumably acquired during birth, presents as meningitis in the second or third week of life. *L. monocytogenes* usually does not cause serious disease in adults, although gravidas may experience a flu-like syndrome and fever. The most common mode of infection is the ingestion of contaminated food, often a milk product. A brief hematogenous phase is followed by fecal shedding until immunity is established. Placental infection can result from hematogenous dissemination or via the ascending route. The particular predisposition for significant listerial infection in pregnant women and the fetus appears to be related to local factors at the maternofetal interface that compromise an effective immune response [125, 126].

Toxoplasma gondii

Pathology. The placenta infected with *Toxoplasma gondii* may be grossly normal but is commonly large and edematous. Microscopically, the changes are highly variable, ranging from a subtle low-grade lymphocytic villous infiltrate to a destructive process associated with necrosis or fibrosis. True granulomas with central necrosis, palisaded histiocytes, and Langerhans giant cells may predominate. Nodular accumulations of histiocytes beneath the trophoblast or extending into the intervillous space, decidual plasmacytic infiltrates and vasculitis, and chronic inflammatory infiltrates in the fetal membranes and umbilical cord have been described. The encysted form of the organism may be found in the fetal membranes, chorionic plate, umbilical cord, or villi (*Fig. 19.60*). Toxoplasma cysts are typically unassociated with inflammation, but once ruptured, the tachyzoites incite an intense inflammatory reaction and necrosis. Identification of tachyzoites, very difficult on H&E stains, is aided by immunohistochemistry, immunofluorescence, or PCR.

Clinical significance. Congenital infection appears to result mainly from primary maternal infection acquired early in pregnancy, usually by the ingestion of oocytes in undercooked meat or by contact with cat feces. During the parasitemic stage of maternal infection, the organism is transmitted to the placenta and fetus. The risk of fetal infection in these circumstances is about 50%. The likelihood of fetal transmission increases with gestational age, although the severity of infection is greatest when the infection is acquired in the first trimester. The clinical spectrum of fetal involvement ranges from severe damage to the central nervous system and eyes to completely asymptomatic infection, recognized only by the development of chorioretinitis after months or years of follow-up. Prenatal diagnosis (via fetal blood sampling or culture) and antibiotic treatment seem to reduce the frequency of congenital infection. In the presence of maternal antibodies from past infections, fetal lesions, with rare exception, do not occur.

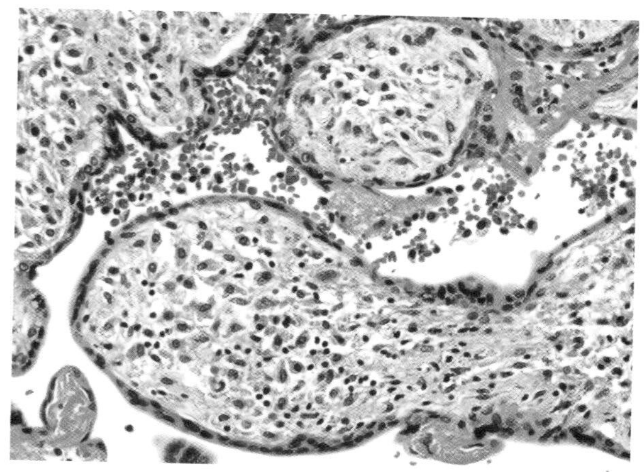

Fig. 19.60
Toxoplasma villitis. **A toxoplasma cyst is present in this chronically inflamed villus**

Parvovirus B19

Pathology. Pathologic changes in the placenta reflect fetal anemia. Parvovirus B19 preferentially infects actively replicating cells, especially erythroblasts, which are then destroyed. Grossly, the placentas are large, pale, and friable. Microscopically, there is a uniform pattern of relative villous immaturity and edema. Diagnostic intranuclear eosinophilic inclusions with peripheral chromatin condensation are present in erythroblasts in the villous vessels (*Fig. 19.61*). In situ hybridization and immunohistochemistry are somewhat more sensitive than conventional microscopy in identifying infected cells or PCR may be used to confirm the diagnosis. Unlike most other congenital hematogenous infections, there is no villous inflammation.

Clinical Significance. Human parvovirus B19 is the agent of "fifth disease," or erythema infectiosum, a mild, acute exanthematous disease of children. In adults, most infections are asymptomatic, although self-limited polyarthropathy is common especially in women, and aplastic crises occur in individuals with chronic hemolytic anemias. To date, the most commonly recognized consequences of fetal parvovirus infection are non-immune hydrops (which may resolve spontaneously) and abortion. Most abortions occur between the 10th and 28th weeks of pregnancy, but the risk of fetal loss is low, estimated to be

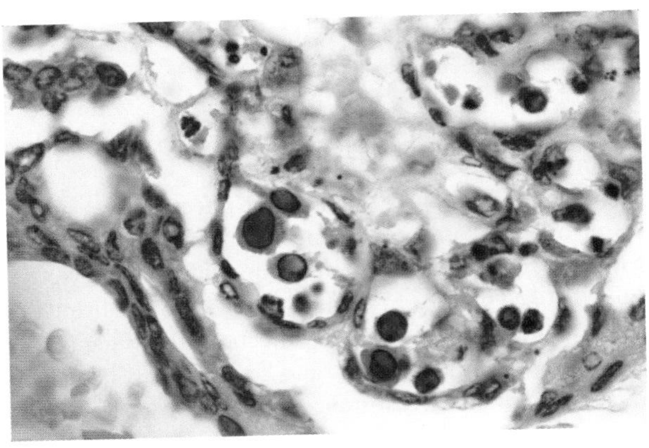

Fig. 19.61
Parvovirus infection. **Erythrocytes in the villous capillaries show central nuclear eosinophilic inclusions with peripheral chromatin condensation**

less than 10%. Neonatal anemia has been observed in a few infants infected in the third trimester, and malformations reminiscent of ocular rubella embryopathy have been reported very rarely.

Herpes Simplex Virus

Disseminated herpes simplex virus infection is an important cause of devastating disease and death in the newborn. Intrapartum infection of the fetus is the most common, although ascending and transplacental dissemination have been described. Villous necrosis and agglutination, lymphocytic villitis, and fibrinoid necrosis of villous vessels have been documented in cases of hematogenous infection. Acute necrotizing and chronic lymphoplasmacytic chorioamnionitis, amnionic viral inclusions, and funisitis have been described in cases of ascending infection. An increased frequency of spontaneous abortion and congenital malformations have been reported in patients with primary infection in the first 20 weeks of pregnancy.

Varicella Zoster

Varicella infection in pregnancy is uncommon in the United States because the majority of women of childbearing age (95%) are immune. In congenital infection, the placenta may show small, grossly visible necrotic foci and villous necrosis, vascular occlusion, lymphoplasmacytic infiltrates, and granulomas with giant cells. Viral inclusions have been reported in villi and decidua. The spectrum of fetal manifestations is wide, ranging from completely asymptomatic babies to those with perinatal varicella/zoster or full-blown embryopathy, the latter occurring in less than 5% of fetuses infected in the first trimester. Reactivation of maternal zoster during pregnancy does not appear to be associated with severe fetal sequelae.

Rubella

Congenital rubella infection is now rare due to the effectiveness of immunization programs. The placental findings have been well documented during previous rubella epidemics, mainly in first- and second-trimester abortions but in a few term placentas as well.

Human Immunodeficiency Virus

Human immunodeficiency virus (HIV) may be transmitted to the fetus transplacentally, at the time of delivery, or after birth (through breastfeeding). In utero transmission can be confirmed by the detection of virus in infants by PCR or coculture within 48 h of birth. Several factors (maternal, fetal, obstetric, and virologic) affect maternal–infant viral transmission, and timing of transmission may determine the subsequent course of infection in the infant. Antiretroviral therapy given to the mother before and during delivery and to the infant after delivery has reduced vertical transmission substantially. No histopathologic lesions directly attributable to HIV have been described in the placenta. Specifically, there have been no reports of villitis. Placentas from seropositive mothers have demonstrated an increased incidence of ACA.

Other Organisms

Massive chronic histiocytic intervillositis may occur in malaria [112]. Recurrent villitis has been described in association with nonsyphilitic spirochetes [1]. The placental lesions associated with hematogenous spread of other organisms are detailed elsewhere [45].

Other Patterns of Placental Inflammation

Chronic Histiocytic Intervillositis

Chronic histiocytic intervillositis is the diffuse uniform infiltration of the intervillous space by monocyte–macrophages accompanied by variable perivillous fibrin deposition (*Fig. 19.62*). Excluded from this category are cases with concomitant villitis or polymorphous intervillous inflammation. Placentas are often small for gestational age. The histologic features are very similar to those in placental malaria, distinguished from it by the absence of malarial pigment. Chronic histiocytic intervillositis is idiopathic, encountered most often in

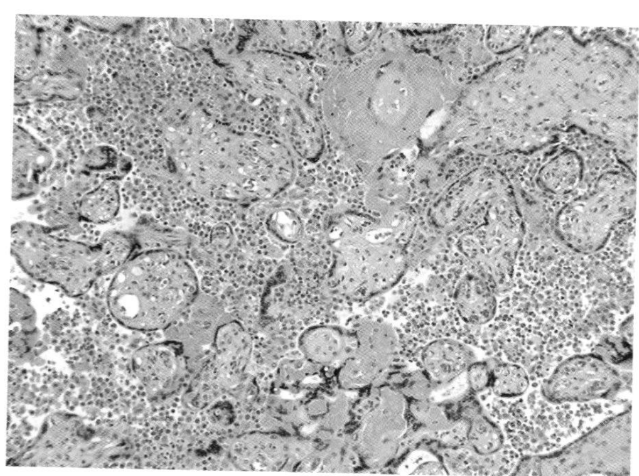

Fig. 19.62
Chronic histiocytic intervillositis. **There is diffuse infiltration of the intervillous space by monocyte-macrophages**

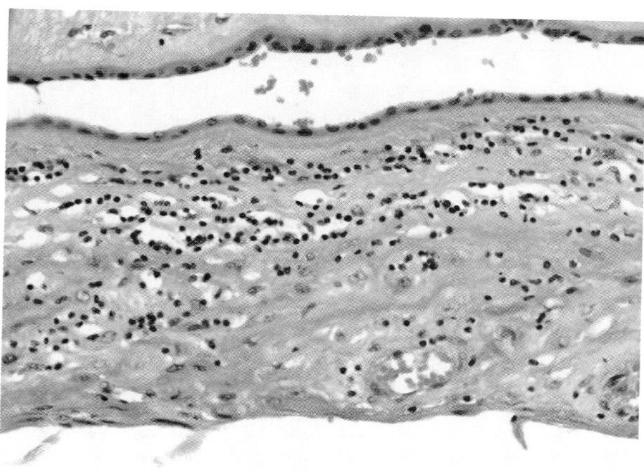

Fig. 19.63
Chronic chorioamnionitis. **Small lymphocytes infiltrate the amnion and chorion**

first-trimester spontaneous abortions. It is associated with recurrent spontaneous abortion, IUGR, IUFD, and a high overall perinatality mortality rate.

Chronic Deciduitis

Chronic deciduitis has been defined as either the presence of plasma cells or diffuse chronic inflammation (with or without plasma cells) in the decidua basalis. The chronic inflammatory response may be directed against maternal or fetal antigens or microorganisms. Chronic deciduitis is often associated with VUE at term and with ACA in preterm placentas, but it may also occur as an isolated finding.

Chronic Chorioamnionitis

Rarely, an inflammatory infiltrate occurring in the same distribution as ACA is composed of chronic inflammatory cells (*Fig. 19.63*). Typically, small mature lymphocytes predominate, but plasma cells, histiocytes, and rarely large lymphoid cells and immunoblasts are admixed [69]. In some cases, the chronic inflammatory cells may be accompanied by a minor component of neutrophils, which may be either entirely distinct from, or intimately admixed with, the chronic inflammatory component. The inflammatory infiltrate in chronic chorioamnionitis is commonly focal and typically mild. It is generally confined to the membranes, although involvement of the chorionic plate may occur. Rarely, the large fetal vessels of the chorionic plate and umbilical cord are also chronically inflamed. Chronic chorioamnionitis is often accompanied by villitis and occasionally by chronic or subacute necrotizing funisitis. A specific infectious etiology is not identified in the great majority of cases, although rarely chronic chorioamnionitis may occur in association with rubella, herpes simplex, *T. pallidum*, or *T. gondii* infection.

Eosinophilic/T Cell Vasculitis

Eosinophilic/T cell vasculitis is a chronic inflammatory infiltrate composed of fetal eosinophils and lymphocytes involving chorionic plate and large stem villous vessels (*Fig. 19.64*). There are no specific clinical associations, although in most reported cases there have been maternal or fetal abnormalities [47].

Circulatory Disorders

The placenta is a vascular organ with separate fetal and maternal circulations. The integrity of both circulations is essential to placental function. Clots, hematomas, and other pathologic processes affecting the vessels and spaces in and around the placenta may cause both fetal and maternal injury depending on their size, location, and extent. Measurement of size and evaluation of extent is important in assessing the significance of individual lesions. There is, however, no absolute "cutoff" beyond which a bad

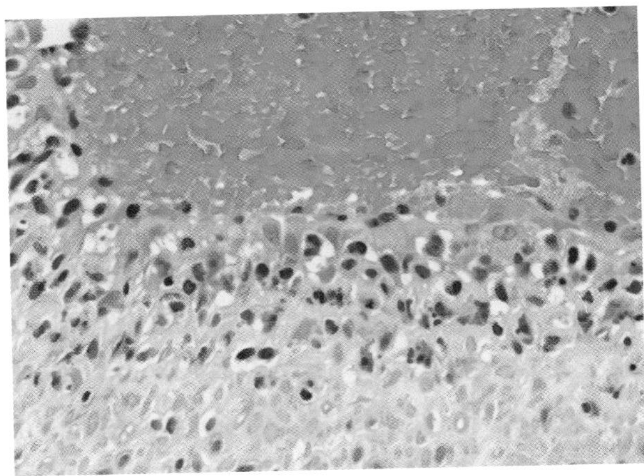

Fig. 19.64
Eosinophilic T-cell vasculitis. **Eosinophils and small lymphocytes invade the muscular wall of this chorionic plate vessel**

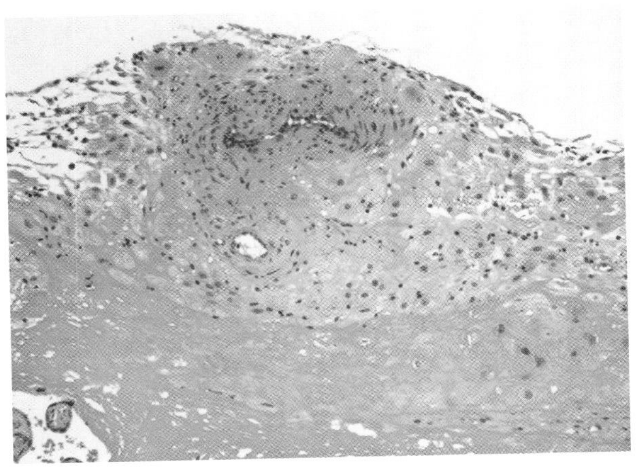

Fig. 19.65
Incomplete vascular remodeling. **This basal plate artery retains its muscular wall**

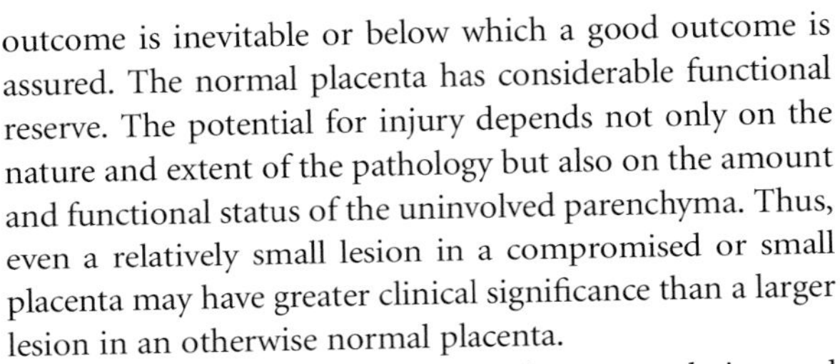

outcome is inevitable or below which a good outcome is assured. The normal placenta has considerable functional reserve. The potential for injury depends not only on the nature and extent of the pathology but also on the amount and functional status of the uninvolved parenchyma. Thus, even a relatively small lesion in a compromised or small placenta may have greater clinical significance than a larger lesion in an otherwise normal placenta.

A balance between factors that favor coagulation and fibrinolysis is necessary for homeostasis; pregnancy itself shifts that balance toward thrombosis. Within the maternal intervillous space, clotting inhibitors such as annexin V at the syncytiotrophoblastic surface normally inhibit clotting. Thrombogenic factors may overcome this, resulting in thrombi and infarcts [123, 124]. Within the fetal circulation, stasis, local injury from inflammation or compression, or thrombophilic factors may result in clotting. The existence of an intravascular clot, regardless of cause, confirms that the balance has been broken at least locally, and may also promote or be associated with clotting elsewhere in the circulation.

Maternal Circulation

In relation to placental pathophysiology, the maternal circulation includes the uterine arteries and their branches, the spiral arteries, the maternal intervillous space, and the venous drainage of the uterus. Many pathologic processes affecting the maternal circulation can be traced to abnormal implantation and vascular remodeling [136].

Decidual Vasculopathy, Incomplete Physiologic Change, Acute Atherosis, and Maternal Vascular Underperfusion

Etiology. When normal physiologic trophoblastic remodeling of the spiral arteries does not evolve properly, arterial smooth muscle persists, the lumina fail to expand, and uteroplacental blood flow is reduced. The maternal blood pressure rises, the maternal vascular endothelium is injured, and the maternal syndrome of preeclampsia develops.

Pathology. Non-remodeled spiral arteries with persistent musculoelastic media (*absence of physiologic change*) may be identified in the basal plate (*Fig. 19.65*). Non-remodeled spiral arteries are predisposed to develop a distinctive lesion, *acute atherosis*, characterized by necrosis and dense eosinophilia of the vessel wall with large foamy macrophages and inflammation (*Fig. 19.66*). The lumens may be partly or completely occluded by thrombus. Acute atherosis involves muscularized maternal arteries in the basal plate and membranous decidua. The latter is often the best place to find acute atherosis (*Fig. 19.67*). Immature IT in the superficial basal plate and trophoblastic giant cells in the deep basal plate are increased [149]. These changes together with the characteristic vascular alterations have been referred to as *superficial implantation* [84].

Mural hypertrophy of membrane arterioles is a less common pattern of decidual vasculopathy that occurs especially in women whose preeclampsia is complicated by diabetes mellitus [15]. The muscular walls of the affected vessels in the decidua parietalis are thickened, and there is marked luminal narrowing (Fig. 19.67). Mural hypertrophy is diagnosed when the mean wall diameter is greater than 30% of the overall vessel diameter [139].

The most direct adverse effect of decidual vasculopathy is the reduction of maternal blood flow into the intervillous space (*maternal vascular underperfusion*) leading to reduced placental growth and weight. Microscopic changes include increased and prominent syncytiotrophoblastic knots (Fig. 19.68). The nuclei in the small knots of a normal placenta undergo apoptosis and break away into the maternal circulation as membrane bound packets. In preeclampsia, the nuclei of the pathologic knots undergo ischemic necrosis ("aponecrosis") [67], releasing membrane fragments, DNA, and proteins into the maternal circulation. This circulating cellular debris may contribute to maternal endothelial injury in preeclampsia [67]. Adhesions between syncytial knots undergoing aponecrosis may result in the agglutination of small villous clusters (>2 <20) that commonly show karyorrhexis and stromal fibrosis (*villous agglutination*) (Fig. 19.69). With more severe underperfusion, intervillous fibrin is increased, first around stem villi, and then around distal villi, accumulating as small nodules at sites of trophoblastic necrosis. Ultimately, large aggregates of villi may be enmeshed in fibrin [139]. Fibrin accumulation in the intervillous space may be the result of decreased maternal perfusion and stasis or to abnormal coagulation or both.

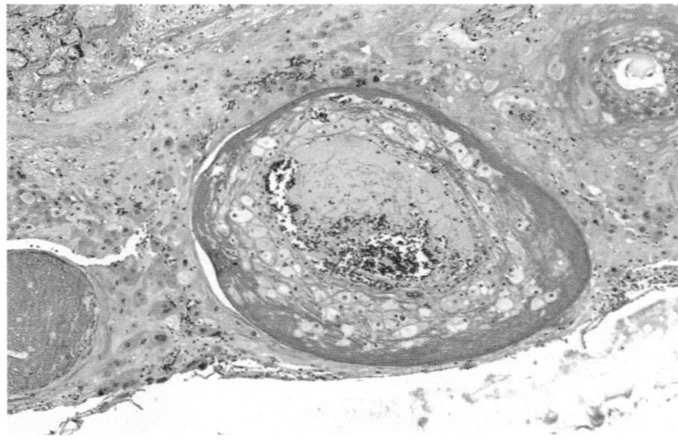

Fig. 19.66
Acute atherosis. **The spiral arteries show fibrinoid necrosis and accumulation of foamy macrophages. The largest artery is thrombosed, and there is infarction of the overlying placenta**

When reduced maternal blood flow is severe and longstanding, the villi develop abnormally. The distal villi are decreased in number and slender with reduced branching, and terminal villi are very small with increased syncytial knots. This constellation of features is referred to as *distal villous hypoplasia* (synonyms: *accelerated maturation, peripheral villous hypoplasia*) (Fig. 19.70). To be significant, these changes must be demonstrated centrally in the mid and basal zones of the placenta because similar changes occur normally in the less perfused peripheral and subchorionic regions [192]. Hypoxia-related gene expression in trophoblast occurs in these areas even in the normal placenta [192] Localized areas of severe ischemia result in infarcts that may be large and numerous in cases of severe preeclampsia (Fig. 19.71). Long-standing

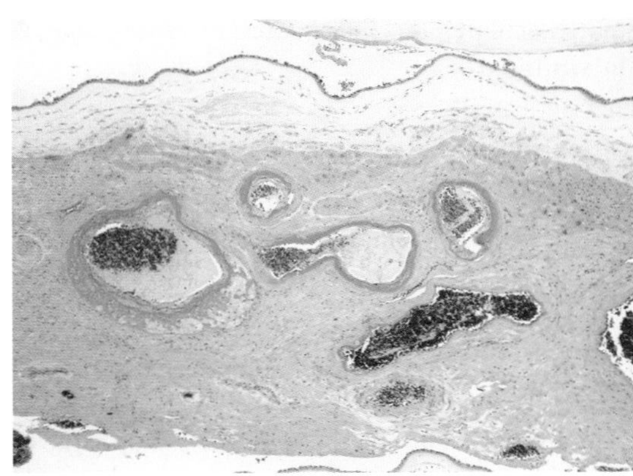

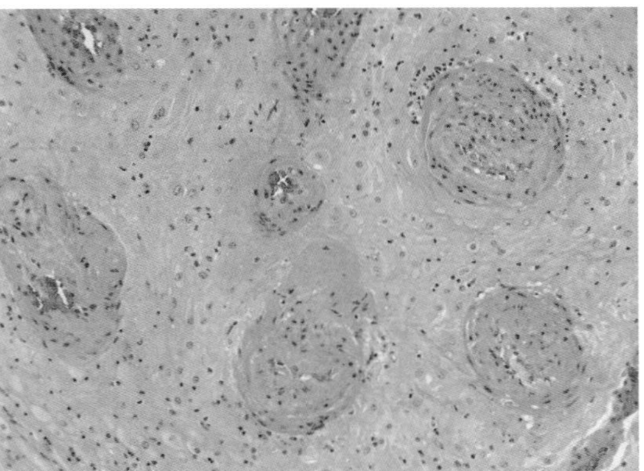

Fig. 19.67
Acute atherosis (*left*) and mural hypertrophy of membrane arterioles (*right*). **In mural hypertrophy, the vessel wall is greater than one third of the total vessel diameter**

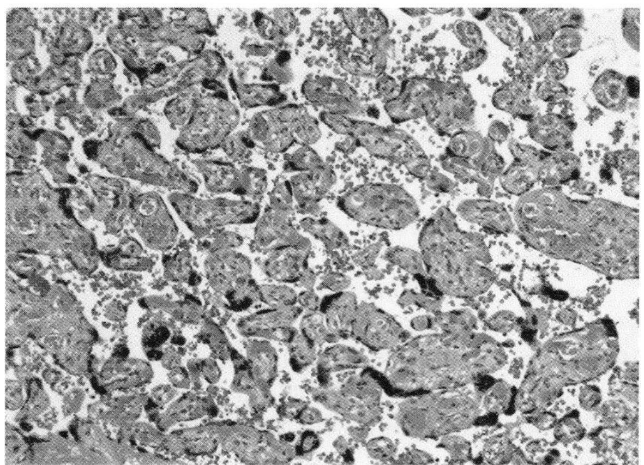

Fig. 19.68
Maternal underperfusion. **Increased syncytial knots. Syncytiotrophoblastic nuclei clustered in the distal villi**

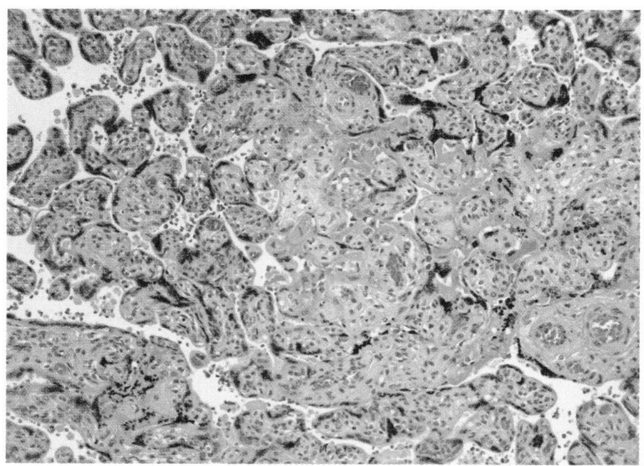

Fig. 19.69
Maternal underperfusion. **Villous agglutination. Clusters of degenerating distal villi are adherent to one another**

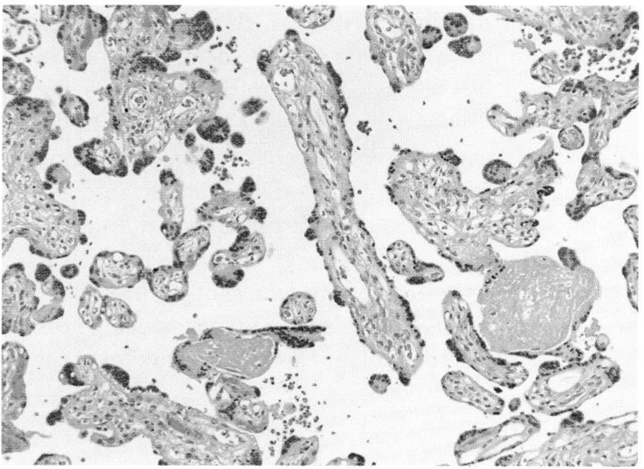

Fig. 19.70
Maternal underperfusion. **Distal villous hypoplasia. Chronic severe maternal underperfusion results in distal villi that are thin and non-branched when cut longitudinally and very small when cut in cross section. Syncytial knots are prominent**

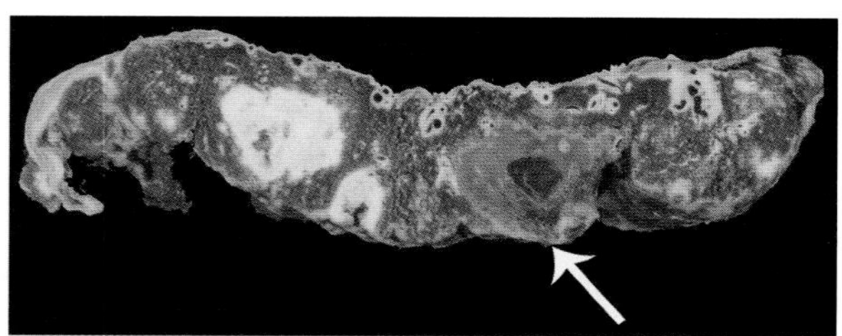

Fig. 19.71
Maternal underperfusion. **Infarcts of varying ages. Recent infarct is red**

maternal vascular underperfusion may cause fetal volume depletion, decreased extracellular fluid, and an abnormally thin cord.

Clinical significance. Maternal vascular compromise with placental underperfusion is one of the major causes of IUGR. Severe maternal vascular underperfusion may result in IUFD and is associated with cerebral palsy (CP) in VLBW infants [144]. Identical pathologic changes occur in the placentas of patients with systemic lupus erythematosus [93], scleroderma [38], the antiphospholipid antibody syndrome [159], and occasionally in the absence of hypertension. Similar changes in the spiral arteries with constrictions, dilations, hyalinization, and thrombi occur in the placenta when thrombotic thrombocytopenic purpura develops in pregnancy [70].

Infarct

Etiology. An infarct in the placenta, as in any other organ, is an area of ischemic necrosis resulting from obstruction of blood supply. The spiral arteries that supply the placenta may be narrowed by acute atherosis, occluded by thrombi, or disrupted by a retroplacental hematoma. Extensive placental infarcts have been reported in association with thrombophilic states [9, 37, 80].

Pathology. Infarcts are wedge-shaped areas of induration often located at the placental margin. Fresh infarcts are difficult to see; they differ little in color, but are firmer and drier than the surrounding placenta. Older infarcts grow progressively firmer and change from red to brown, then tan, yellow, or white (➲ *Fig. 19.71*). Microscopically, the earliest change is collapse of the intervillous space. The villi are crowded, separated by only a thin layer of fibrin, and trophoblastic nuclei cluster together forming knots. The syncytiotrophoblast, vascular endothelium, and villous stroma undergo progressive necrosis until eventually only crowded, ghostlike villous outlines remain (➲ *Fig. 19.72*). The mummified infarcted villi are not removed by macrophages or replaced by fibrous tissue as occurs in other organs. A mild acute inflammatory response may occur at the margin of an infarct.

Clinical behavior. Infarcts occur in about 25% of otherwise normal term placentas. The finding of a small peripheral infarct in an otherwise normal placenta is of no clinical significance. Multiple or large (>3 cm) infarcts, central infarcts, or infarcts in the first or second trimester are indicative of significant, underlying maternal vascular disease, most often preeclampsia. Extensive placental infarction is associated with fetal hypoxia, IUGR, and IUFD. These ill effects on the fetus are not simply the result of the destruction of villous tissue but reflect the superimposition of infarction on a placenta already compromised by low maternal blood flow.

Retroplacental Hematoma

Definition. A retroplacental hematoma is a clot located in the decidua between the placental floor and the myometrium. It represents the pathologic lesion responsible for the clinical diagnosis of placental abruption that is made by the obstetrician based on the presenting signs and symptoms manifested by the mother. These two terms should not be used interchangeably, a practice which leads to confusion between a clinical diagnosis with grave implications and a pathologically demonstrated clot whose impact depends primarily on size.

Frequency. Retroplacental hematomas are found in approximately 4.5% of placentas examined pathologically [45]. Based on data from the National Hospital Discharge Summary, symptomatic abruption occurs in 1% of singleton deliveries. The incidence appears to be increasing [6].

Etiology. The pathogenesis of retroplacental hematoma is not known, but bleeding from a decidual artery followed by dissection of the enlarging clot is the presumed sequence in most cases. An occluded ischemic artery that undergoes reperfusion may rupture, leading to a retroplacental hematoma. Retroplacental hematomas are increased threefold in women with preeclampsia, presumably due to the related vascular pathology. Other associations include PTL, chorioamnionitis, anemia, smoking, cocaine abuse, trauma, diabetes mellitus, and short umbilical cord. Traumatic separation of the attached placenta followed by bleeding from a disrupted vessel probably occurs, for instance, following an automobile accident.

Pathology. When confined by peripherally attached placenta, a retroplacental hematoma distorts and indents the overlying placental parenchyma (➲ *Fig. 19.73*). Separated from its blood supply, the overlying placenta infarcts. The characteristic depression and overlying infarct are easily recognized even when the clot itself has become detached during delivery. Larger clots may dissect

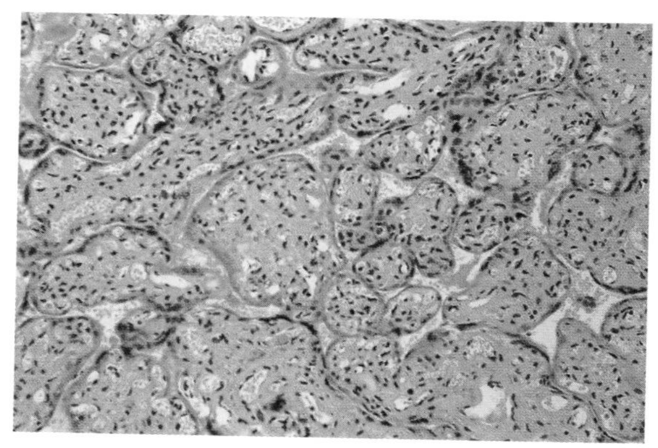

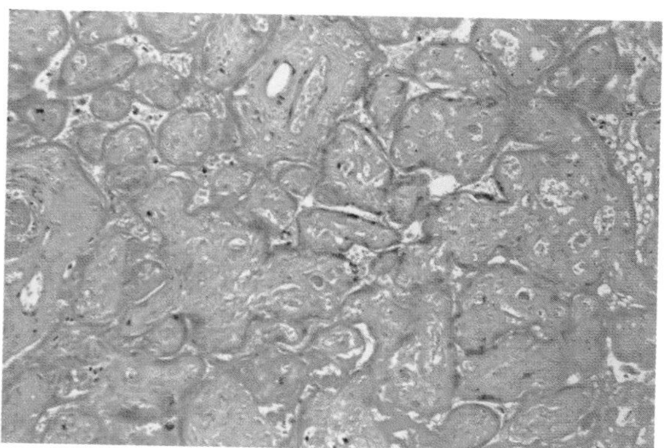

Fig. 19.72
Maternal underperfusion. **Infarcts. The intervillous space is collapsed with necrotic villi undergoing progressive necrosis eventuating in ghost like villous remnants**

into the basal region of the placenta. Older retroplacental hematomas may be much more subtle, forming only a thin, inconspicuous layer of red-brown clot beneath an infarct. When retroplacental hematomas extend to the placental margin, the blood may be evacuated without causing any indentation. Very recent extensive placental separation is typically associated with little, if any, gross or histologic change in the placenta. These large hematomas generally result in immediate fetal distress, necessitating emergent delivery. A large fresh clot behind a "floating" detached placenta observed at the time of cesarean section may be the only objective sign of an acute retroplacental hemorrhage. Obstetricians should document this observation and submit the clot along with the placenta. Microscopic examination of the clot may offer supportive evidence when clumps of decidua associated with strands of fibrin are demonstrated.

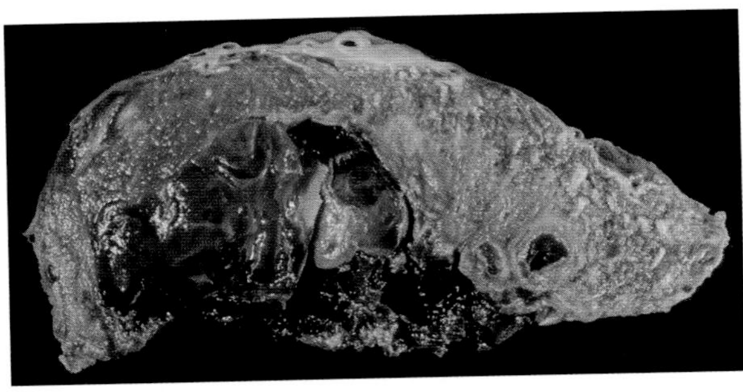

Fig. 19.73
Retroplacental hematoma. **The placenta is compressed and infarcted over this large retroplacental hematoma**

Retroplacental hematomas consist of stratified red cells and fibrin, the proportion of fibrin increasing as the lesion ages and the red cells degenerate. The time course of these evolutionary changes is unknown. The adjacent decidua may be necrotic. Macrophages containing hemosiderin are often present around older clots and sometimes involve the membranes. Organization may occur where the clot interfaces with the uterus, but not where it interfaces with the placenta. The placenta overlying the hematoma is often infarcted. Villous edema and villous stromal hemorrhage are secondary placental abnormalities indicating that the retroplacental hematoma has adversely affected the fetus. Nucleated fetal erythrocytes are often increased (*Fig 19.74*).

Clinical significance. The clinical significance of a retroplacental hematoma is related primarily to its size. Retroplacental clots block the passage of blood from the spiral artery into the intervillous space. Small clots may have little effect, since adjacent spiral arteries may suffice to keep the overlying placental villi functional. The larger the clot and infarct, the more likely it will exceed the functional reserve capacity of the placenta, which may be already marginal in a background of chronic uteroplacental ischemia. Older chronic lesions associated with hemosiderosis in the membranes indicate the possibility of chronic reduction of placental function. Extensive accumulations of blood lead to the full clinical picture of abruption – pain, and shock in the mother and severe acute hypoxia in the fetus.

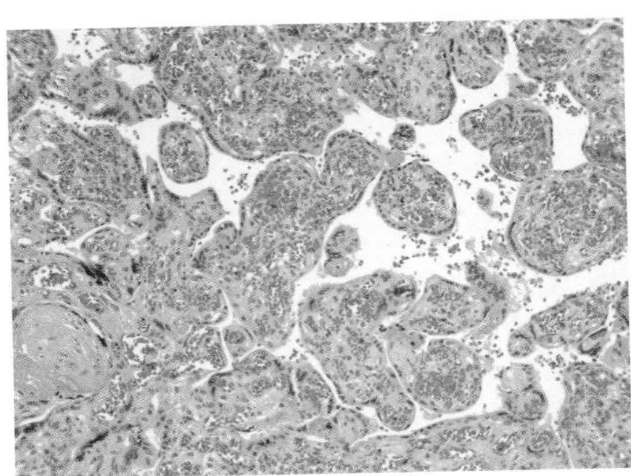

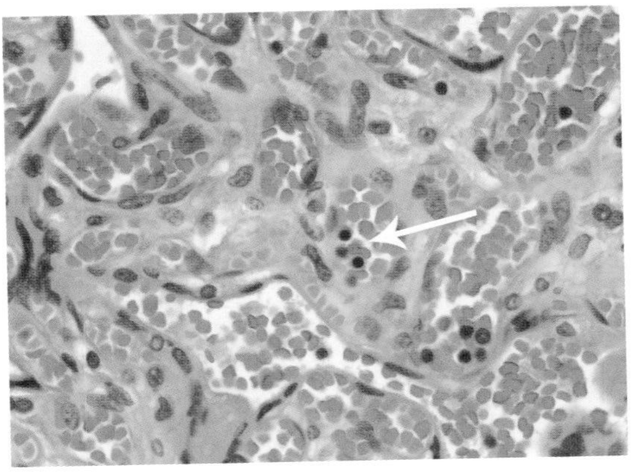

Fig. 19.74
Villous stromal hemorrhage. **Villous stromal hemorrhage is associated with acute retroplacental hematoma (*left*). nRBC are often increased (*right*)**

Marginal Hematoma

Definition. A marginal hematoma occurs where the lateral margin of the placental disk joins the fetal membranes.

Etiology. Acute marginal hematomas are thought to result from rupture of uteroplacental veins at the margin of a low-lying placenta. Chronic recurrent venous hemorrhage at the disk margin (*chronic marginal hematoma, chronic abruption*) elevates and centrally displaces the membrane insertion site, resulting in circumvallation.

Pathology. Grossly, an acute marginal hematoma forms a crescent-shaped clot at the lateral margin of the placenta. On cut section, the clot is triangular with the apex at the junction of the membranous and villous chorion. Microscopically, a recent marginal clot usually lies entirely outside the placental disk but may occasionally involve the intervillous space. With this exception, the presence of an acute marginal hematoma has no effect on the adjacent villi. Chronic marginal hematomas are tan-brown clots usually occurring in the region of circumvallate membrane insertion and associated with membrane hemosiderin deposition (*Fig. 19.75*).

Clinical significance. An acute marginal hematoma may be associated with antepartum bleeding, in some cases followed by onset of labor, but it does not have any untoward effect on the fetus. Chronic marginal hematomas and circumvallation are often associated with antenatal bleeding. In this context, retroplacental hematomas and abruption are also more frequent.

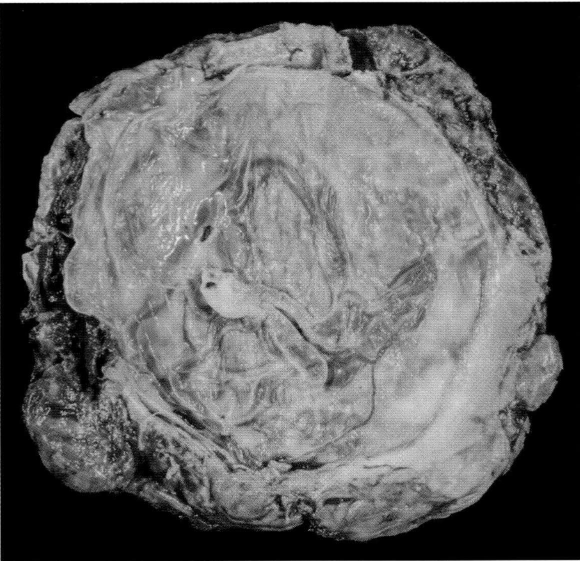

Fig. 19.75
Chronic marginal hematoma. **Old brown clot is prominent at the margin of this circumvallate placenta**

Intervillous (Intraplacental) Hematoma

Definition, frequency, and etiology. Intervillous hematomas are clots in the intervillous space. They are common, found in 36–48% of placentas. Intervillous hematomas are thought to be initiated by fetal bleeding into the intervillous space through ruptured vasculosyncytial membranes. Small amounts of fetal blood can be demonstrated, although most of the clot is composed of maternal blood [75]. Factors cited as potential causes of villous damage resulting in fetomaternal hemorrhage include trauma, amniocentesis, and external version. Basilar intervillous hematomas may have a different etiology.

Pathology. Intervillous hematomas are round or oval blood clots that may occur anywhere in the intervillous space but are most common midway between the chorionic and basal plates. They begin as red, fluid, or semifluid blood and become progressively laminated and depigmented with age. They may be single, although multiple lesions are common. Most are 1–3 cm in diameter. Microscopically, the thrombi consist of layered red cells and fibrin, the proportion of fibrin increasing as the lesion ages (*Fig. 19.76*). Villi displaced to the margins of the clot may be infarcted or fibrotic and avascular.

Clinical significance. An intervillous hematoma is significant in that it marks a site of hemorrhage from the fetal into the maternal circulation. Intervillous hematomas occur at the bleeding site. These are common and usually

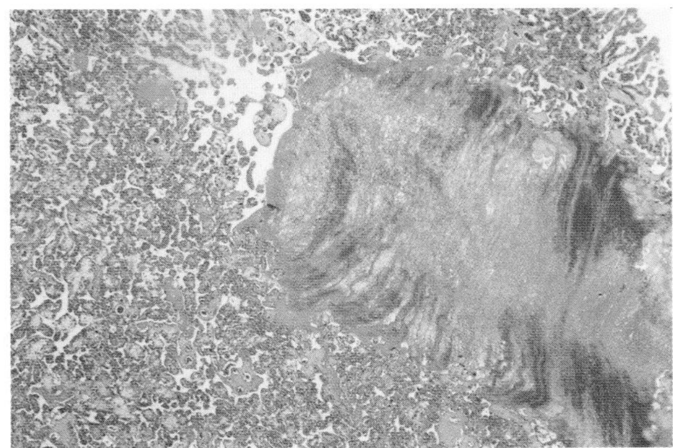

Fig. 19.76
Intervillous (intraplacental) hematoma. **A typical lesion composed of laminated fibrin and red cells**

do not indicate that a significant fetal blood loss has occurred. Occasionally, a larger fetomaternal hemorrhage results in fetal anemia and fetoplacental hydrops if it occurs slowly and chronically, or sudden unexpected death if severe and acute. Severe fetal morbidity and mortality result from hemorrhages of 150 mL or more, but lesser amounts can be significant if chronic bleeding has occurred episodically. It has been suggested that the risk is greater when the mother and fetus have compatible ABO blood types, perhaps because of deficient clot formation at the site of bleeding [195]. There is often no clinical evidence of fetal distress or injury, even in cases resulting in IUFD. The amount of fetomaternal hemorrhage can be quantitated using the Kleihauer–Betke test. Flow cytometry may be more sensitive [31, 41]. Correlation between the severity of fetomaternal hemorrhage and size and number of intervillous hematomas is variable. In some cases of severe fetomaternal hemorrhage, there may be no hematoma and a site of bleeding may not be identified.

Small amounts of fetal blood leak into the maternal circulation in virtually every pregnancy. Fetomaternal hemorrhage may lead to isoimmunization of Rh negative mothers resulting in hemolytic anemia and immune hydrops in the fetus.

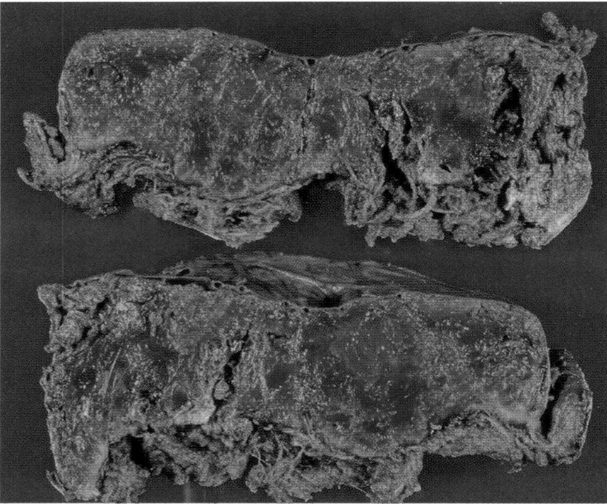

Fig. 19.77
Massive subchorial hematoma. **Thick fresh clot separates the chorionic plate from the underlying placental parenchyma**

Massive Subchorial Hematoma (Breus' Mole)

The massive subchorial hematoma has been defined as coagulated blood, at least 1 cm in thickness, separating the chorionic plate from the underlying placenta over much of its area (*Fig. 19.77*). These are generally relatively fresh, red hematomas that distort the chorionic plate and protrude as nodular masses into the amnionic cavity. They may dissect into the chorionic plate or extend into the intervillous space, sometimes as far as the basal plate. This is a rare lesion, the incidence estimated to be 0.53 per 1,000 deliveries in one large study [170]. The etiology and pathogenesis are unknown. Most authors agree that the hematomas are maternal.

Massive subchorial hematomas are usually acute because catastrophic reduction in placental function results in abortion or IUFD. Rarely babies are liveborn.

Maternal Floor Infarct (MFI) and Massive Perivillous Fibrin Deposition (MPF)

Definition. These two lesions have many similar features, differing mainly in the extent and distribution of abnormal fibrin(oid) in the placenta. *Massive perivillous fibrin* (*MPF*) deposits occur extensively throughout the placenta. In *maternal floor infarct* (*MFI*), the same type of fibrin-like material is concentrated in the basal plate.

Etiology. Currently two types of fibrinoid or fibrin-like material are identified in the placenta [46, 186]. Matrix-type fibrinoid is composed of oncofetal fibronectin, collagen IV, laminin, and tenascin and usually does not include fibrin. It is consistently associated with, and apparently produced by, extravillous trophoblast. This type of fibrinoid and associated trophoblast surrounds the villi in both MPF and MFI. Fibrin-type fibrinoid has immunohistochemical features of blood clot product and lacks the cellular trophoblast component. This form of fibrin accumulates in maternal vascular underperfusion associated with decidual vasculopathy and the syndrome of preeclampsia.

The fact that the intervillous space is involved would seem to implicate a maternal circulatory abnormality. Isolated reports have identified a group of associations including antiphospholipid antibody syndrome [166], polymyositis [3, 66], long-chain L-3-hydroxyacyl-coA dehydrogenase deficiency [96, 122], chronic intervillositis [189], and thrombophilias [9, 76]. Two separate reports, however, document involvement of only one of dichorionic twins, suggesting a role for the fetus [56, 143]. Whether the fibrinoid material that encases the terminal villi in these disorders reflects coagulation

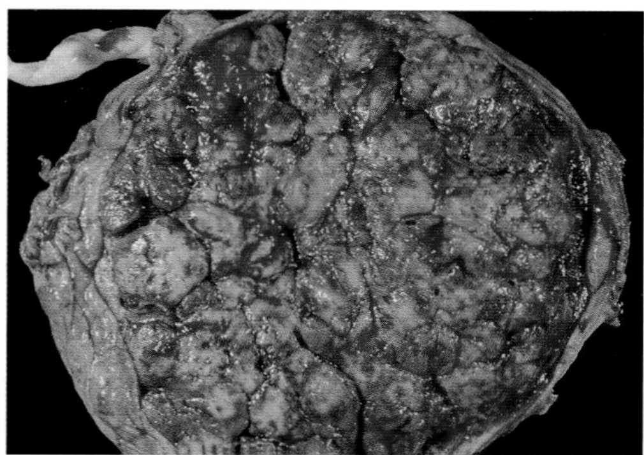

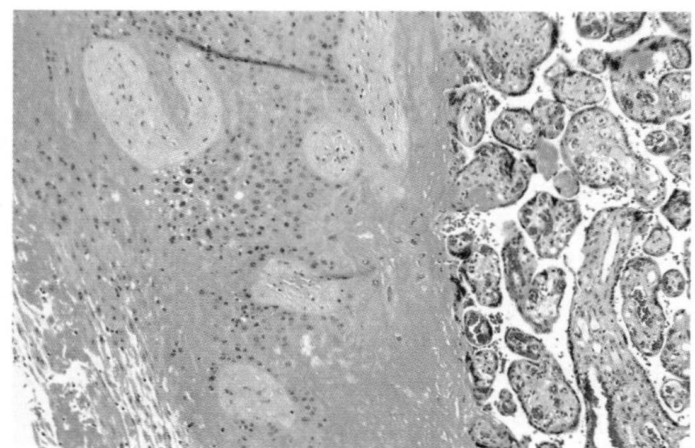

Fig. 19.78
Maternal floor infarct (MFI). **The maternal surface is diffusely discolored and firm (*left*). The basal villi are entrapped in fibrinoid (*right*)**

secondary to stasis of maternal blood in the intervillous space or aberrant secretion of matrix by villous trophoblast is unknown.

Pathology. Wide strands and interlacing clumps of hard waxy pale tan or gray material accumulate as a thickened rind in the basal portion and ramify throughout the placenta. When most of the material is concentrated basally, the term MFI best applies, even though other parts of the placenta may also be involved (*Fig. 19.78*). In MPF, the deposition of fibrinoid is diffuse without preferential basal concentration, although there may be patchy, sometimes extensive involvement of the maternal floor as part of the process (*Fig 19.79*). Classification based on fibrin distribution is subjective. When classified by criteria proposed by Katzman and Genest, 44% of lesions did not conform to any of the categories [77]. Microscopically, the villi are widely separated by pink amorphous matrix-type fibrinoid containing numerous mononuclear trophoblast cells (*Fig. 19.80*). The syncytiotrophoblast and capillary endothelium disappear from entrapped villi, but the villous stroma and villous outlines persist.

Clinical significance. The reported incidence ranges from 0.5 to 5 per 1,000 deliveries [143]. First-trimester spontaneous abortions, sometimes recurrent, and mid- and late-trimester IUFD are common when the process is massive. Survivors are often delivered preterm with IUGR or develop long-term neurologic impairment [2]. MFI may recur in successive pregnancies. Villi entrapped in fibrinoid are isolated and non-functional. MFI and MPF represent the most severe end of a continuum. Redline and Patterson observed that perivillous fibrin deposits that entrapped more than 20% of villi in the central basal portion of the placenta (thought to be the primary region

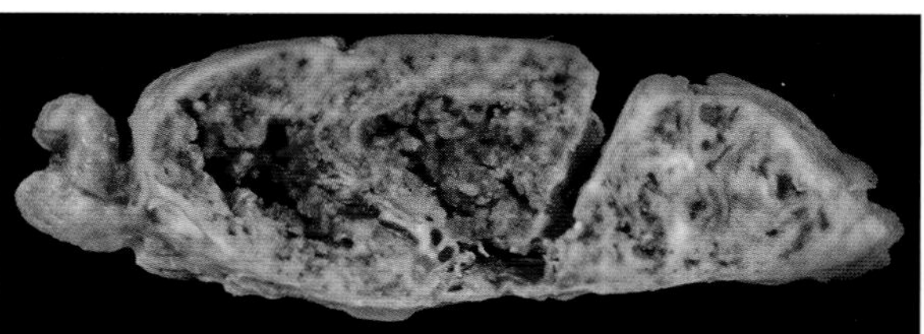

Fig. 19.79
Massive perivillous fibrin deposits. **Hard waxy material is distributed throughout the placenta including the maternal surface**

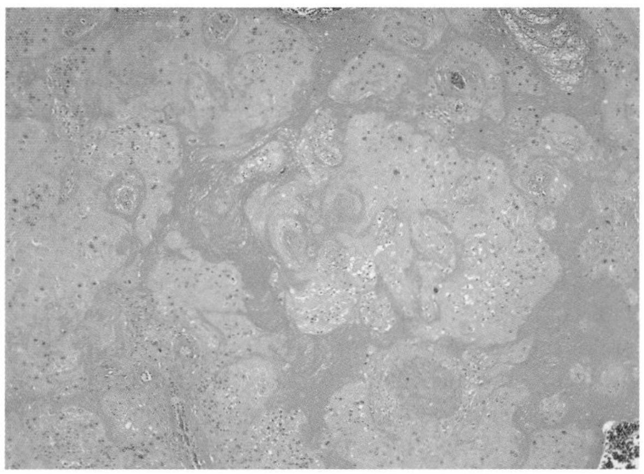

Fig. 19.80
Massive perivillous fibrin deposition (MFD). **Villi are separated by and enmeshed in dense perivillous fibrinoid containing IT**

of gas and nutrient exchange) were significantly associated with an IUGR and low placental weight [148]. Milder cases of perivillous fibrin deposition enveloping 5–20% of terminal villi showed a lesser degree of similar complications. Fibrin deposits at the placental margin or beneath the chorionic plate do not appear to have any adverse affect on the fetus.

Fetal Circulation

The fetal circulation of the placenta begins with the paired umbilical arteries, branches of the fetal iliac arteries. The umbilical arteries pass through the umbilical cord to the placenta where they branch on the chorionic plate and progressively rebranch in smaller stem villi ultimately reaching the villous capillaries where oxygen and nutrient exchange occur across vasculosyncytial membranes. The fortified blood flows through progressively larger veins in the stem villi and chorionic plate, reaching the umbilical vein, which passes back through the umbilical cord to drain into the sinus venosus of the fetus.

Fetal Thrombotic Vasculopathy (FTV) and Fetal Stem Vessel Thrombi

Definition. Clots that form in the fetal circulation obstruct blood flow to the villi, rendering them nonfunctional for the transfer of oxygen and nutrients from the mother to the fetus. *Fetal thrombotic vasculopathy* (*FTV*) refers to the changes in stem vessels and villi that follow occlusion and cessation of blood flow. Related lesions or terms with similar connotations include fetal stem artery thrombosis [43], fibrinous vasculosis [165], intimal fibrin cushion [35], avascular terminal villi [158, 160], and hemorrhagic endovasculitis [161, 162].

Etiology. The rules of Virchow's triad apply to thromboses in the placenta. Stasis, vascular injury, and a hypercoagulable state, especially in combination, may result in clots in the fetal circulation. The most common cause of stasis is chronic partial or recurrent intermittent umbilical cord compression resulting from cord entanglements or anatomic factors (excessive length, hypercoiling, etc.). Stasis may also result from compression of velamentous vessels or in the meandering vascular spaces of chorangiomas or mesenchymal dysplasia. Vascular injury may be due to a fetal inflammatory response to infection, exposure to cytokines or meconium, or vascular inflammation in VUE (*VUE with obliterative vasculopathy*). Hypercoagulable states occur in inherited (factor V Leiden, protein S or C deficiency, etc.) and acquired thrombophilias (antiphospholipidemias, lupus erythematosus). The occurrence of a thrombophilic state in the mother or newborn does not by itself predict vascular lesions in the placenta or fetus, but it may represent a risk factor in association with other conditions [10].

Pathology. Thrombi in large vessels of the chorionic plate or umbilical cord are often visible on gross inspection (➋ *Fig. 19.81*). Villi in the distribution of a large thrombosed vessel form a pale triangular area often with the same consistency as the surrounding parenchyma (➋ *Fig. 19.82*). Older lesions may be firmer, gray-white, and better delimited. Both thrombi and villous lesions are subtle, sometimes better estimated after formalin fixation. In the majority of cases, the occluded vessels are small,

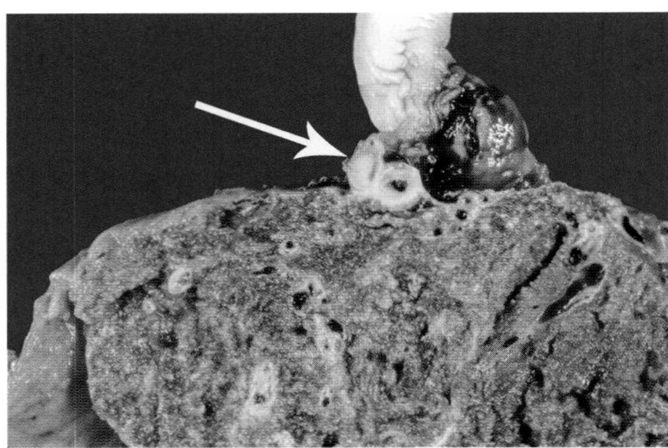

Fig. 19.81
Chorionic vessel thrombus. **This large chorionic plate vessel is occluded by a hard white thrombus**

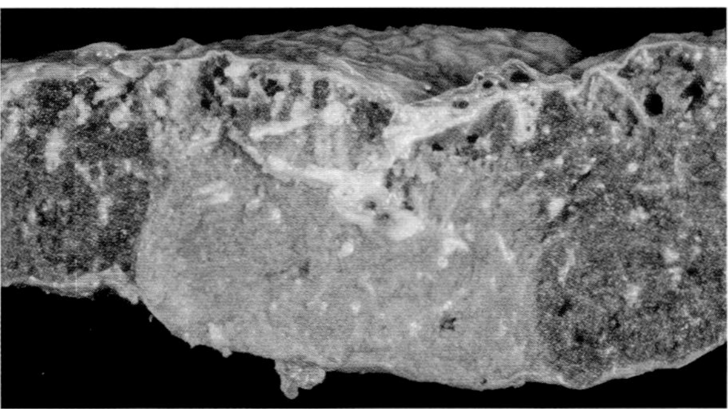

Fig. 19.82
Fetal vascular obstruction. **When a large fetal vessel is occluded, the downstream villous changes are visible as a pale wedge shaped area**

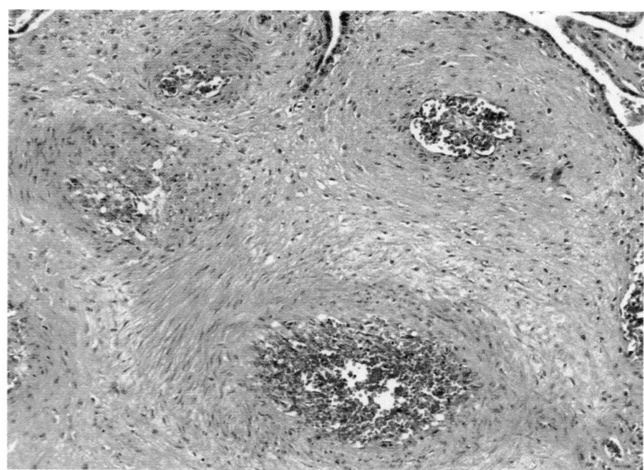

Fig. 19.83
Fetal vascular obstruction. **Red cell extravasation and septation in fetal stem vessels**

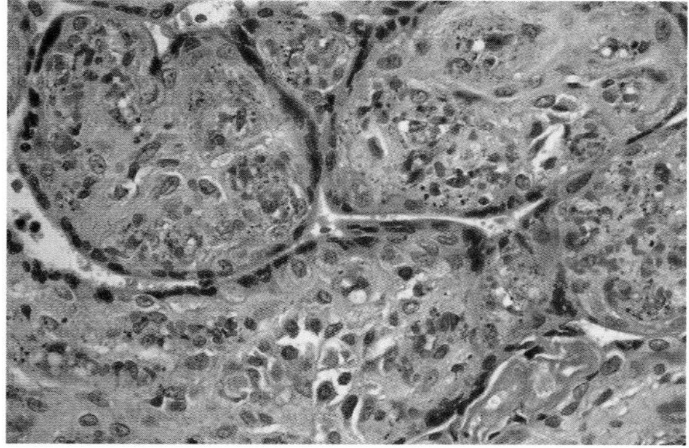

Fig. 19.84
Fetal vascular obstruction, villous stromal-vascular karyorrhexis. **Fragmented red cells are extravasated and there is nuclear debris in and around terminal villous capillaries. These represent early changes in villi downstream from an occluded vessel**

associated with small clusters of distal fibrotic avascular villi that are identifiable only microscopically.

The evolution of large vessel thrombi is similar to that in other sites except organization does not occur. Recent thrombi expand the vessel, are attached, and may have a layered appearance. The endothelium disappears and spindle-shaped cells invade the thrombus producing a multilocular pattern (*septation*) (*Fig. 19.83*). The erythrocytes fragment and blend into adjacent connective tissue. Smooth muscle may disappear and the wall may calcify.

The villi distal to an occluded vessel show a sequence of distinctive alterations. Early changes include karyorrhexis of intravascular, endothelial, and villous stromal cells with destruction of capillaries and extravasation of red cells (*Fig. 19.84*). The stroma is mineralized and may be hypercellular. This constellation of alterations, currently termed *villous stromal vascular karyorrhexis*, is identical to *hemorrhagic endovasculitis* as originally described by Sander [161]. Eventually, the villi become fibrotic with bland, densely collagenized, hyalinized stroma (*fibrotic avascular villi – FAV*) (*Fig. 19.85*). The surrounding syncytiotrophoblast is preserved and often knotted. Larger stem vessels distal to the occlusion show fibromuscular sclerosis. The thrombosed vessel resulting in these distal villous alterations may or may not be apparent depending on the plane of sectioning. The same sequence of changes occurs diffusely throughout the entire placenta after IUFD. The diffuse versus focal nature helps distinguish involutional from pathologic vascular alterations.

Clinical significance. A committee of the Perinatal Section of the Society for Pediatric Pathology has suggested terminology and criteria for the reproducible diagnosis of fetal vascular obstructive lesions. They emphasized that the prognostic importance of fetal vascular obstructive lesions is related to their severity, recommending that the diagnostic term *fetal thrombotic vasculopathy* (*FTV*) be reserved for cases with severe involvement defined as an average of >15 affected villi per slide [138]. FTV is associated with neonatal

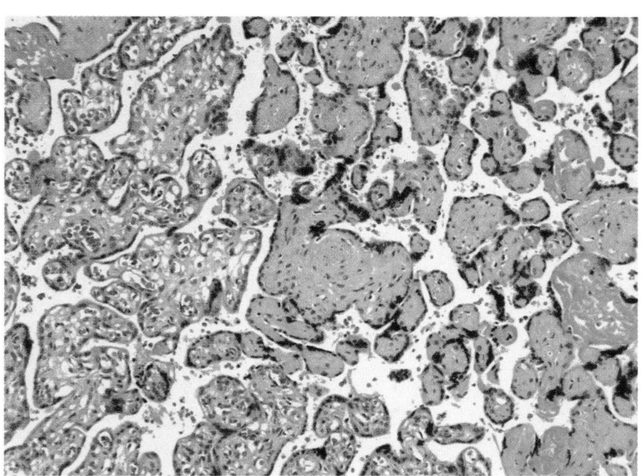

Fig. 19.85
Fetal vascular obstruction, fibrotic avascular villi. **Fibrotic avascular villi reflect fetal vessel occlusion, contrasting with the functional villi in this placenta from a liveborn baby**

encephalopathy [97], cerebral palsy [130], IUFD, and fetal and neonatal thromboocclusive disease [83, 146]. FTV represents a major placental pathologic finding in IUGR and discordant twin growth [140].

The negative effects of FTV occur in at least two ways. First, the presence of thrombi in fetal circulation of the placenta indicates the potential for thrombi to occur elsewhere either as a result of generalized activation of the fetal coagulation system or direct embolism. Thrombi or emboli and infarcts in the fetal brain, kidney, lung, and liver causing severe perinatal liver disease have been reported [25, 30, 83]. While there is definite connection when clots in the placenta and fetus occur together, the finding of FTV in the placenta alone is not predictive. The prevalence of systemic thrombi or infarcts among newborns with placental FTV is low [87]. A second form of injury results from reduction of placental reserve caused by loss of a significant fraction of the placental circulatory bed. The occurrence of multiple lesions in the same placenta compounds the prospects for injury [138, 145, 187].

Intimal Fibrin Cushions and Fibrinous Vasculosis

DeSa described *intimal fibrin cushions* composed of intramural fibrin deposits and proliferating fibroblasts forming non-occlusive intraluminal protrusions, some calcified, in chorionic veins (➋ *Fig. 19.86*) [35]. The finding was attributed to local injury from elevated venous pressure. Clinical associations included low birth weight, abruption, maternal hypertension, and intrapartem hypoxia. Emphasizing associated wall edema, Scott et al. described a similar lesion, *fibrinous vasculosis*, associated with stillbirth and other adverse outcomes [165]. Currently these large vessel lesions are classified as intimal fibrin cushions and are thought to be pressure-related changes affecting vessels between the actual site of fetal vascular obstruction and the terminal villi [138]. They are often associated with other evidence of fetal vascular occlusion in distal villi including fibrotic avascular villi and villous stromal vascular karyorrhexis.

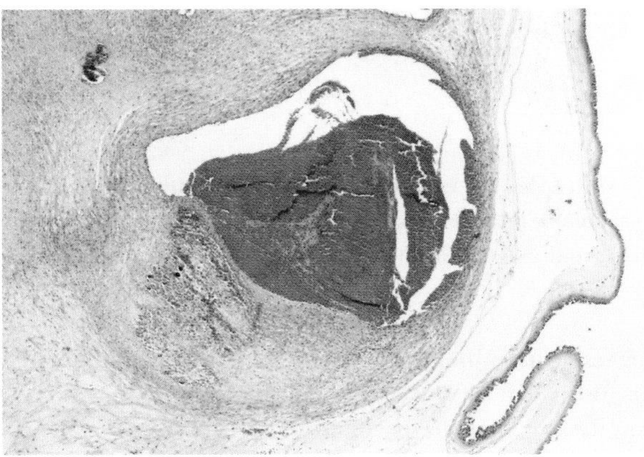

Fig. 19.86
Intimal fibrin cushion. **Fibrin(oid) is deposited in the wall of large chorionic plate vessel. Mural calcification is consistent with a long-standing process**

Fetal Vascular Narrowing and Increased Umbilical Vascular Resistance

Doppler velocimetry studies have identified a group of growth-restricted fetuses with increased resistance to fetal blood flow. In general, these placentas are small with distal villous hypoplasia. Small fetal stem arteries in such cases have been described as narrowed with thickened walls [53], an observation supported by morphometric studies [42, 100]. When severe and in the setting of a strong supporting clinical history, these changes may be noted, but they overlap significantly with post-delivery arterial vasospasm.

Villous Edema and Villous Stromal Hemorrhage

Abnormal accumulations of fluid in the villous stroma occur in three different contexts, each with distinct pathologic features. The first and most obvious form is the gross villous swelling of hydatidiform mole and certain other abnormal karyotypes (triploidy, monosomy X). A second pattern occurs in intermediate and terminal villi that are expanded by fluid in small discrete stromal lacunar spaces. Normal immature intermediate villi have a similar appearance but lack the expanded outlines caused by edema. This pattern of edema is associated with more severe grades and stages of ACA, most often in premature and VLBW newborns. In this context, severe edema is predictive of neurologic impairment [105, 138, 145]. Occasionally villous edema may occur with ACA at or near term or with abruption. The third category of villous edema occurs in fetoplacental hydrops in which all villi, terminal and stem, are diffusely edematous and relatively immature.

Hemorrhage into the villous stroma (*villous stromal hemorrhage*) is thought to result from capillary rupture due to acute ischemia. It is most common in preterm placentas with clinically suspected abruption (➋ *Fig. 19.74*).

Chorangiosis

Villous chorangiosis is a form of villous hypervascularity in which villi have expanded outlines and contain numerous capillaries. Groups of more than 10 terminal villi with more than 10 capillaries (actually more than 15 are usually present) involving several areas per microscopic section is definitional [4] (➲ *Fig. 19.87*). The capillaries are centrally located with a thin basement membrane, and pericytes are absent. This condition is distinguished from congestion in which capillaries are prominent but normally distributed and not numerically increased.

Chorangiosis occurs in approximately 7% of placentas, usually at or near term, and often large with delayed villous maturation. The changes are common in diabetics. The occurrence of chorangiosis in pregnancies at high altitude suggests that it is an adaptive response to hypoxia [177]. While frequent in cases with abnormal outcome, chorangiosis has not yet been shown to be an independent causative factor [110].

In *diffuse, multifocal chorangiomatosis*, villous capillaries are also numerically increased, but unlike chorangiosis, they are accompanied by pericytes, involve stem villi, and usually occur in immature placentas of less than 32 weeks. The clinical significance of this recently described and uncommon lesion has not been fully defined [110].

Subamnionic Hematoma

A subamnionic hematoma lies between the amnion and chorion on the fetal surface of the placenta. It most often results from trauma to the chorionic vessels during delivery, especially after excessive traction on the umbilical cord. Occasionally, particularly if the umbilical cord is short or entangled, sufficient traction may develop during labor to cause vessel rupture and significant fetal blood loss. This is virtually impossible to distinguish from the common third-stage hemorrhage. Laceration of chorionic plate vessels during amniocentesis may also lead to subamnionic hemorrhage, sometimes severe. Older subamnionic fibrin clots form dome-shaped blisters containing a mixture of brown-tinged fluid and fibrin. Lesions diagnosed by ultrasound between the 18th and 30th weeks of gestation have been associated with elevated maternal alpha-fetoprotein levels, vaginal bleeding, polyhydramnios, and IUGR [33].

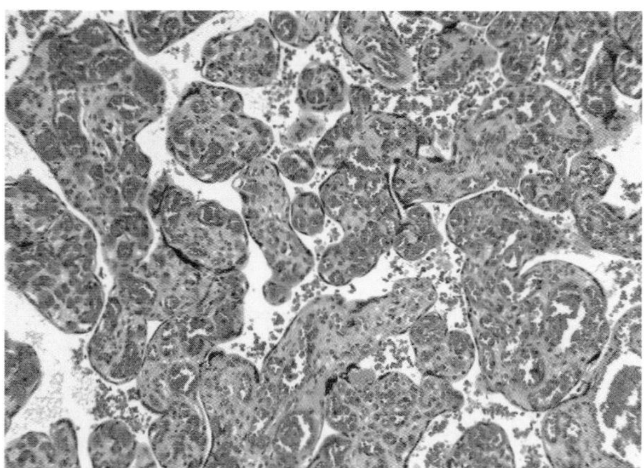

■ Fig. 19.87
Chorangiosis. **Small, central villous capillaries are greatly increased**

Fetal Membranes

The fetal membranes and contiguous placenta form a sac containing amnionic fluid in which the fetus grows and develops. The fetal membranes provide a crucial barrier against infection, contain the amnionic fluid, and have metabolic functions including the modulation of events related to the onset of labor. The fetal membranes examined in their natural anatomic configuration after reconstructing the gestational sac as it exists in utero permits assessment of size, completeness, membrane insertion, and point of rupture. The distance from the point of membrane rupture to the edge of the placental disk reflects the site of uterine implantation; the lower the implantation, the closer the membrane rupture site is to the disk. A configuration indicative of low implantation should prompt consideration of associated conditions such as marginal hematoma or placenta accreta. Microscopic sections of the fetal membranes include fetal amnion and chorion and maternal decidua. The amnion is composed of amnionic epithelium and a connective tissue layer separated from the surrounding chorion by a loose spongy layer. The chorion is also composed of a connective tissue layer and a cellular layer containing chorionic type IT and atrophied villi. The most peripheral layer is maternal decidua (➲ *Fig. 19.5*).

Squamous Metaplasia

Foci of squamous metaplasia are slightly elevated, sometimes targetoid, pearly-white macules that tend to be most numerous at the site of cord insertion (➲ *Fig. 19.88*). Although they are generally no more than a few millimeters, rarely they may form larger plaques. Histologically, foci of squamous epithelium, with or without keratinization, have a sharp transition with the surrounding amnionic epithelium. Squamous metaplasia has no clinical significance, but it is important to distinguish from amnion nodosum, which it superficially resembles grossly.

Amnion Nodosum

Definition and pathology. Amnion nodosum is a rare condition in which the amnionic surface is studded with small (1–5 mm), irregular, yellowish elevated nodules (➲ *Fig. 19.89*). These nodules are generally concentrated on the chorionic plate, particularly around the insertion of the umbilical cord, although they may occur anywhere on the amnionic surface. The nodules are composed of amorphous, eosinophilic material containing cells and hair fragments (➲ *Fig. 19.89*). The amnionic epithelium may be totally or partially preserved or absent beneath the nodules, and a layer of amnionic epithelium is commonly present over their surfaces.

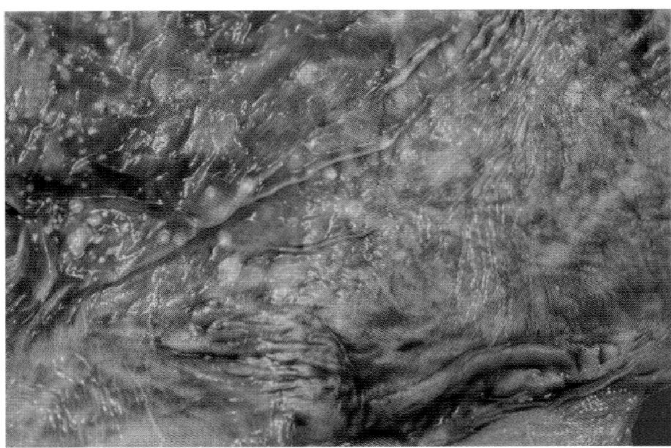

Fig. 19.88
Squamous metaplasia. **Squamous metaplasia is visible as elevated white macules**

Etiology and clinical features. Amnion nodosum is associated with oligohydramnios. The particulate debris and cellular elements from the fetal epidermis, oral cavity, urinary and gastrointestinal tracts, and the amnion itself are abnormally concentrated when amnionic fluid is scant and are deposited on the amnionic surface. The cause of the oligohydramnios varies. In many cases, a fetal urinary tract abnormality (renal agenesis or urinary tract obstruction) is responsible for diminished fetal urine resulting in decreased amnionic fluid. Oligohydramnios may occur in association with IUGR or in the donor twin in the twin–twin transfusion syndrome. Long-standing amniorrhea is less likely to result in amnion nodosum than decreased amnionic fluid production, presumably because in the former, the cellular and particulate debris are lost along with the amnionic fluid. Amnion nodosum is a reliable indicator of oligohydramnios that should prompt an investigation for fetal abnormalities known to accompany it, including urinary tract anomalies and pulmonary hypoplasia.

Amnionic Bands

Definition. Separation of the amnion and chorion results in amnionic fragmentation, shredding, and exposure of mesoblastic tissue, leading to the formation of thin fibrous strands. These encircle fetal limbs, digits, neck, and umbilical cord, causing characteristic constriction, amputation, and syndactyly (➲ *Fig. 19.90*). Some babies with characteristic amnionic band defects have additional structural

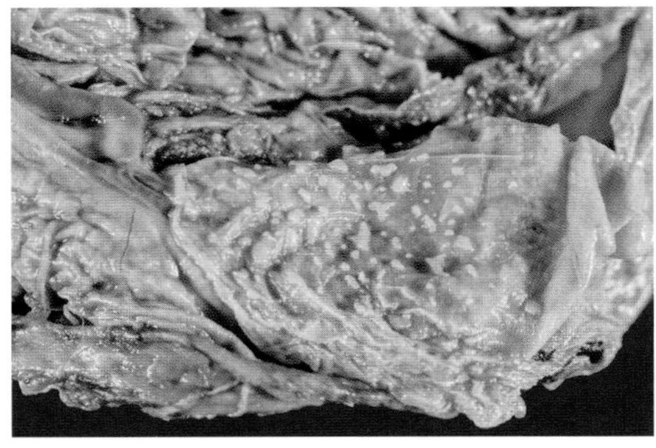

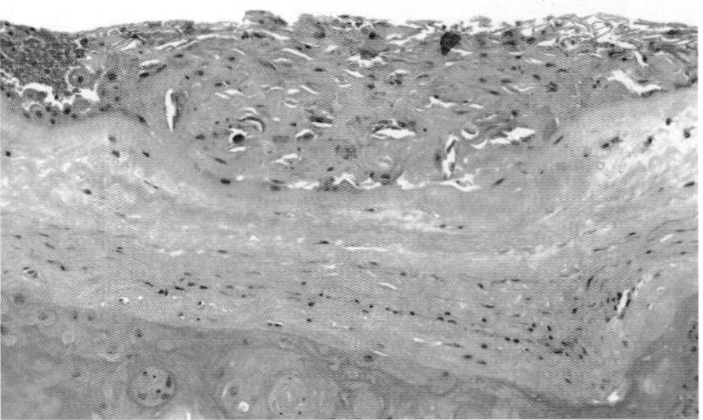

Fig. 19.89
Amnion nodosum. **Irregular elevated amnionic nodules (*left*) correspond to nodular deposits composed of degenerating cell fragments and hair embedded in amorphous granular material (*right*)**

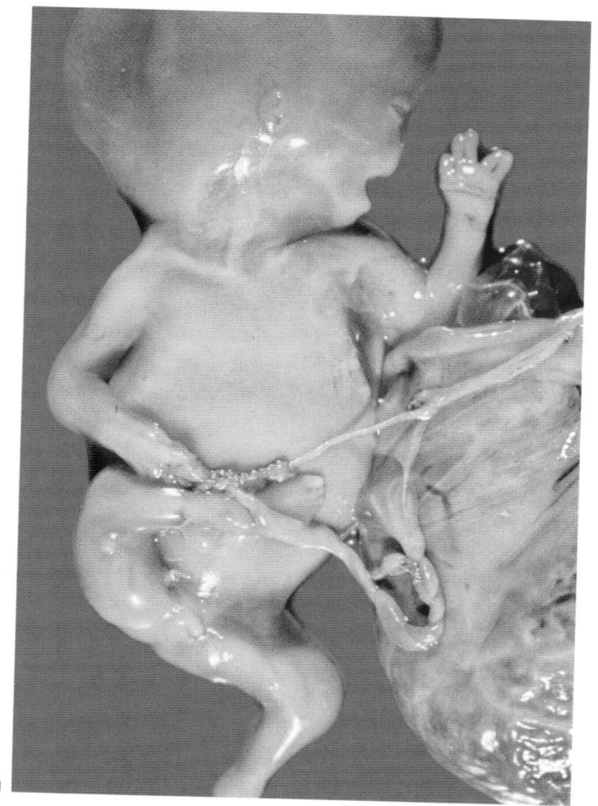

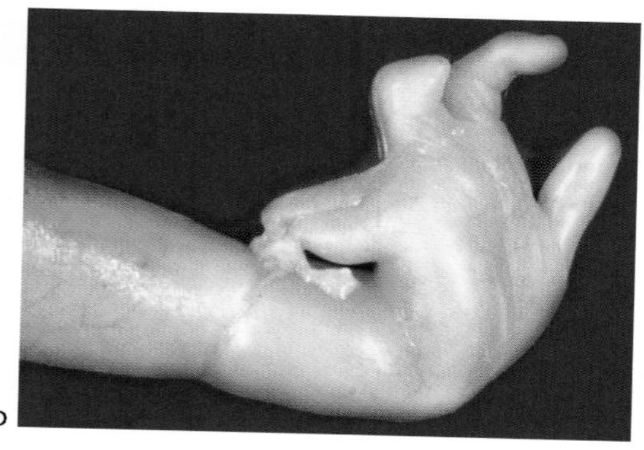

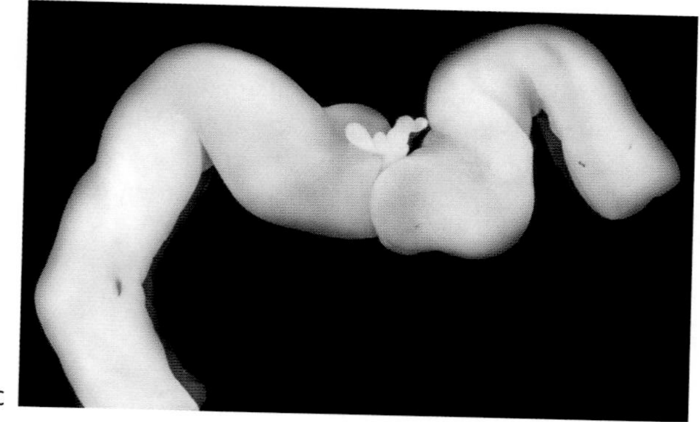

Fig. 19.90
Amnionic bands. **Amnionic bands entangle limbs (a), digits (b), and the umbilical cord (c)**

anomalies, usually severe, including major limb deficiencies, body wall or open cranial defects, short umbilical cord, club feet, or internal abnormalities. The wide spectrum of anomalies in this condition has been variously referred to as the *amnionic band syndrome*, *amnionic band disruption complex*, *early amnion rupture sequence*, *limb–body wall complex*, and *amnion adhesion malformation syndrome*.

Pathology. Gross identification of the bands and strings may be difficult, sometimes facilitated by submersion of the placenta in water. The surface of the placenta may be dull and slightly roughened, also subtle findings. Microscopically, the bands usually consist of fibrous tissue, but occasionally amnionic epithelium is recognizable. Amnion is absent from the placental surface and the chorion is fibrotic. In cases associated with body wall or open cranial defects, the amnion may be continuous with the fetal skin at the site of the defect. Broad adhesions may occur between the placenta and fetus.

Etiology. Multiple theories have been proposed to explain the abnormalities in this syndrome. Torpin strongly espoused the concept that amnionic bands cause the structural defects [182]. The widely variable nature of the defects has been attributed to the timing of amnionic rupture; early rupture is thought to result in fetal compression, tethering, or swallowing of bands, resulting in severe multisystem defects, whereas constriction and amputation defects in limbs and digits have been attributed to amnionic rupture later in pregnancy. Malformations are thought to result when a band interferes with the normal sequence of embryonic development. Kalousek maintains that the extent of amnionic bands is as important as the developmental stage at which they occur in determining of the pattern of fetal involvement [72]. The etiology of amnionic rupture is unknown. Amnionic bands have been noted rarely after trauma, amniocentesis, and in women with connective tissue disorders. Others have postulated that the amnionic bands are secondary and that the more severe fetal abnormalities are the result of vascular disruption or a primary embryologic defect.

Clinical significance. The recognition of amnion rupture and its consequences are important in counseling parents because the risk of recurrence is negligible. Unless accompanied by typical constriction/amputation lesions, major craniofacial or body wall defects may be difficult to diagnose. An important clue is the variety and asymmetry of the fetal defects, which are unlike the pattern of any heritable syndrome. No two cases are alike.

Meconium Stain

Definition and frequency. Meconium, the intestinal contents of the fetus, is commonly passed into the amnionic fluid. The reported prevalence ranges from 7 to 25%. Meconium passage is especially common in post-term placentas, present in up to 31%. It is unlikely to be present before 30 weeks.

Pathology. Meconium can often be identified on gross examination, its appearance correlating roughly with the chronicity of meconium passage. Meconium passed shortly before delivery may be recognizable as such. The membranes become progressively green-stained and slimy, with longer exposure, dark and edematous, and eventually dull, muddy brown (➋ *Fig. 19.91*).

Microscopically, free meconium consists of amorphous green-brown material and anucleate squames. The amnionic epithelium exposed to meconium shows degenerative changes including heaping, stratification, and eventually nuclear pyknosis and necrosis. There may be marked edema of the spongy layer. With time, meconium is engulfed by macrophages in the amnion, chorion, and decidua (➋ *Fig. 19.92*). In vitro studies indicate that meconium appears in amnionic macrophages in 1 h and in deeper chorionic macrophages within 3 h [99]. How closely these observations approximate events in vivo is unknown. Meconium is usually scant in the umbilical cord due to the paucity of macrophages. As meconium

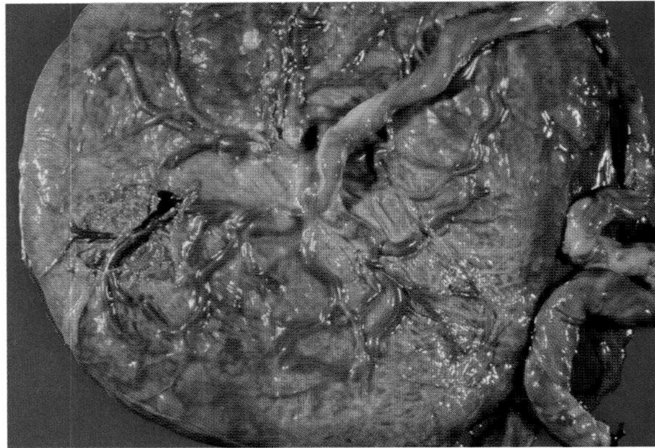

Fig. 19.91
Meconium stained placenta

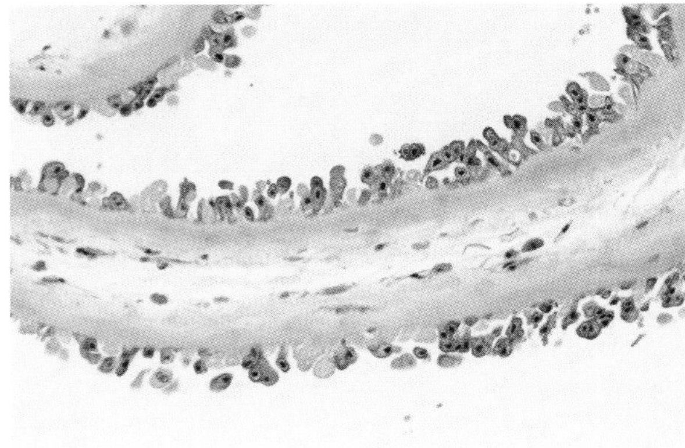

Fig. 19.92
Meconium reaction. **Amnionic epithelium is heaped and stratified with macrophages containing meconium in the subjacent stroma**

passes through the membranes and cord, it eventually reaches the large fetal vessels where the toxic effect of its constituents can lead to apoptotic cell death of medial smooth muscle cells at the periphery of umbilical or chorionic plate vessels (➲ *Fig. 19.93*).

Meconium must be distinguished from hemosiderin, generally a larger, more refractile, and yellowish crystalline granule. Iron stain is helpful when an ambiguous pigment is encountered. Lipochrome and nonhemosiderin, nonmeconium pigments of unknown composition, have been identified in a variety of diverse clinical situations. It has been hypothesized that these pigments may represent metabolites of remotely passed meconium.

Clinical significance. Meconium staining has long been perceived as an indicator of perinatal morbidity. Meconium passage has been significantly associated with parameters of fetal distress including low Apgar scores, umbilical artery pH of 7.0 or less, respiratory distress, seizures in the first 24 h, and need for delivery room resuscitation. Neonatal morbidity of all kinds has been significantly associated with meconium stained as compared to clear amnionic fluid [84]. Equally clear is that many infants, especially at term or post-term, pass meconium as a reflection of physiologic maturity, usually unassociated with significant problems. The role of meconium as the primary factor in perinatal injury is, therefore, controversial. The most important consideration is the circumstance under which meconium is passed. Meconium staining is often superimposed on other significant pathologies, especially chorioamnionitis, that may represent the major injurious factors. Meconium may, however, potentiate the effects of these underlying pathologies. For example, the growth of group B streptococcus is enhanced by the presence of meconium, and meconium has been shown to inhibit neutrophil function in vitro.

Meconium may induce injury directly (in amnionic epithelium and umbilical and chorionic plate vessels) and has also been demonstrated to cause vasoconstriction, a potential cause of ischemia [5, 173]. There is some evidence that meconium may interfere with surfactant function and, in high enough concentrations, have a direct toxic effect on type II pneumocytes, possibly contributing to the meconium aspiration syndrome [27]. The role of meconium as the primary factor in the meconium aspiration syndrome is controversial. Autopsy studies indicate that in most cases, meconium aspiration syndrome is of prenatal origin, especially in relation to intrauterine infection and chronic hypoxia [52].

Gastroschisis

Gastroschisis is a defect in the paraumbilical abdominal wall through which bowel protrudes. This is distinguished from the more common omphalocele in which bowel protrudes into a saccular defect at the cord insertion but remains enclosed in peritoneum and amnion. Gastroschisis is characterized by extensive fine, uniform vacuolization of amnionic epithelial cells (➲ *Fig. 19.94*).

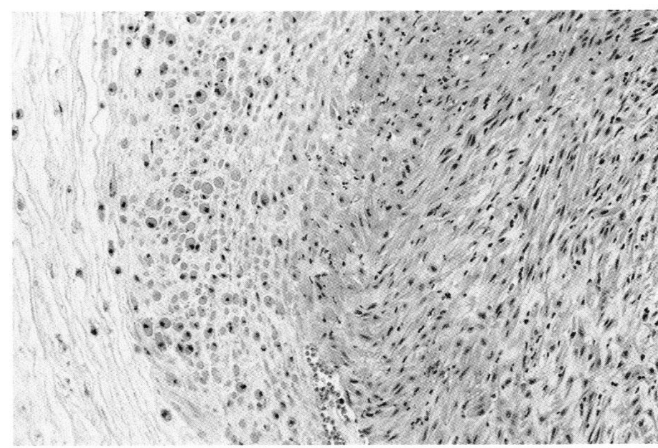

◘ Fig. 19.93
Meconium induced vascular changes. **The outer smooth muscle in the wall of this umbilical artery has undergone apoptosis in response to prolonged meconium exposure. The nuclei are pyknotic and the cytoplasm is dense and eosinophilic**

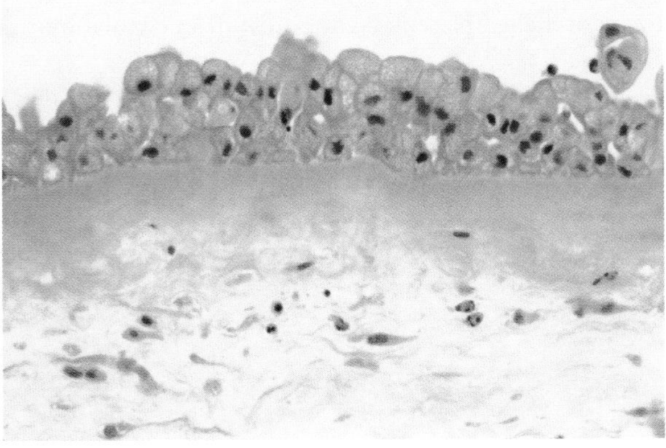

◘ Fig. 19.94
Gastroschisis. **The amnionic epithelium in gastroschisis shows fine vacuolation. The epithelial stratification in this case is the result of meconium passage**

Ultrastructural studies confirm that the vacuoles contain lipid, but the origin of the lipid is obscure. These amnionic changes are not present in omphalocele.

Extramembranous Pregnancy

Rarely the amnion and chorion rupture completely leaving the fetus to develop outside the membranes. The placenta is invariably circumvallate and the umbilical cord is short. Amnion nodosum and membrane hemosiderin deposits are common. Pulmonary hypoplasia is common and often fatal. Compression deformities may occur. There is often a maternal history of amniorrhea and vaginal bleeding.

Umbilical Cord

Normal Anatomy and Embryonic Development

Early in gestation, the blastocyst is filled with a loose meshwork of extraembryonic mesoderm that cavitates centrally to form the chorionic cavity. The embryonic structures are connected to the trophoblastic shell by a bridge of extraembryonic mesoderm, the connecting stalk, and forerunner of the umbilical cord. The yolk sac and the allantois protrude into the connecting stalk. As the amnion enlarges, the embryo prolapses into the amnionic cavity, progressively lengthening the connecting stalk. The allantoic vessels connect with vessels developing independently in the villi to establish the fetoplacental (chorio*allantoic*) circulation.

The normal umbilical cord contains two arteries and one vein suspended in Wharton's jelly, a loosely structured myxoid tissue covered by firmly attached amnion. Wharton's jelly is derived from the extraembryonic mesenchyme and consists of myofibroblasts and abundant ground substance. The combination of loose gel and contractile cells helps maintain turgor and protect the vessels against compression. The umbilical cord is supplied by oxygen and nutrients from the umbilical vessels. No other vessels or lymphatics are found in the normal umbilical cord. Most umbilical arteries are either fused or connected via an anastomosis (Hyrtl's anastomosis) generally within 1.5 cm of the placental insertion site. This connection is important to equalize flow and distribute blood uniformly to the placenta. The normal umbilical cord is spiraled, usually counterclockwise (counterclockwise/clockwise = 7:1), and the average number of coils is ~0.2 coil/cm. The spiral is established early in the first trimester as demonstrated sonographically.

Vestigial Remnants

Vestigial remnants dating back to formation of the connecting stalk and umbilical cord are common microscopic findings. The presence of vestigial remnants has not been correlated with congenital anomalies, maternal age, race, gravidity, or gestational age at delivery. Remnants of the allantoic duct are frequent (about 15%) in the proximal portion of the cord. They are lined by flat or cuboidal cells reminiscent of transitional epithelium, with or without a lumen (Fig. 19.95). *Allantoic remnants* are located between the umbilical arteries. Rarely, they are large

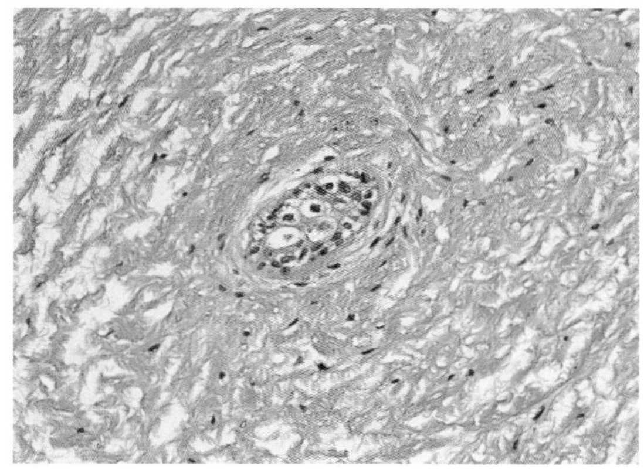
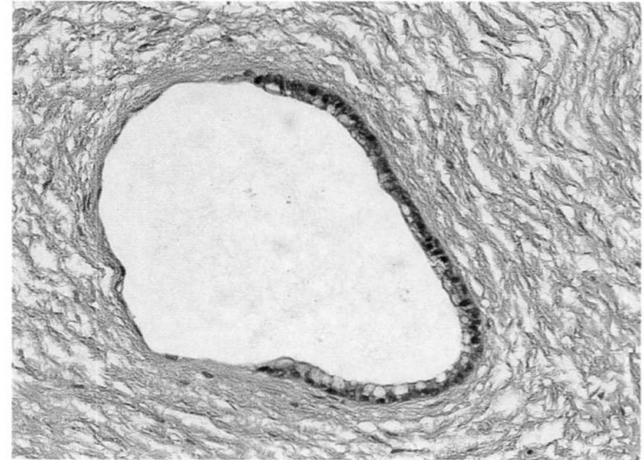
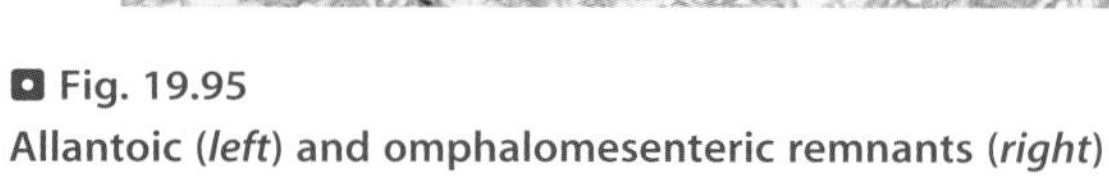

Fig. 19.95
Allantoic (*left*) and omphalomesenteric remnants (*right*)

enough to expand the cord or they may remain patent predisposing to urinary leakage from the cord stump.

Traces of the omphalomesenteric duct, which connects the fetal ileum and the yolk sac in the early embryo, are infrequent, occurring in 1.5% of umbilical cords. These remnants are usually discontinuous, located peripherally, and lined by columnar cells resembling intestinal epithelium (➋ *Fig. 19.95*). *Omphalomesenteric remnants* sometimes have a muscular wall, occasionally containing ganglion cells, liver, pancreas, gastric, or small intestinal mucosa. Vitelline vessels may accompany omphalomesenteric remnants or they may occur in isolation. These are usually paired but sometimes clustered, lined by endothelium lacking a muscular coat. Omphalomesenteric remnants are of little clinical significance. They are rarely associated with Meckel's diverticulum, small intestinal atresia, or intestinal protrusion into the cord that may be inadvertently clamped or cut. Cystic omphalomesenteric remnants are rare, more common in males (M:F = 4:1). The yolk sac remnant is commonly visible as a small white nodule between the amnion and chorion composed of amorphous basophilic material histologically.

Stasis Problems and "Cord Accidents"

The umbilical cord is a crucial lifeline between the fetus and placenta. Cessation of or diminished umbilical blood flow can result in severe fetal compromise or death. Umbilical flow may be compromised by mechanical factors (compression), vessel damage (trauma, inflammation, or meconium), or thrombosis. Cord abnormalities with the potential for obstruction of blood flow – abnormal coiling, stricture, abnormal length, true knots, entanglements, prolapse, and velamentous insertion – have been associated with increased risk of IUFD, IUGR, and neurologic injury [12, 13]. Many of these conditions are related; true knots and excessive coiling commonly occur in long cords, and stricture almost always occurs in a hypercoiled cord. Chronic partial or intermittent flow obstruction may be evidenced by umbilical, chorionic, or stem vessel dilatation and thrombosis, intimal fibrin cushions, and/or villous alterations reflecting fetal vascular occlusion (FAV/villous stromal–vascular karyorrhexis) [113]. Based on these findings, non-acute cord compression has been implicated in over half of unexplained fetal deaths. Acute flow obstruction may supervene when a knot or entanglement tightens during delivery or there is cord prolapse. Doppler studies have confirmed that cord obstruction and compression impede venous return. Increasingly sophisticated imaging techniques provide opportunities for better assessment of the relationship between pathologic findings and significant alterations in blood flow.

Cord Length

Umbilical cord length is an important parameter most accurately documented in the delivery room before the cord shrinks or cord segments are removed for other studies. Cord length declines by as much as 7 cm during the first few hours after delivery. Standards for cord length relative to gestational age have been established [84]. The mean cord length at term is about 55–60 cm.

Cord length reflects factors that influence its growth – mainly tensile forces related to fetal activity and intrauterine conditions affecting fetal movement. Umbilical cord growth slows during the last trimester as room for fetal movement declines, although some cord growth occurs normally until term. Conditions restricting fetal mobility – amnionic bands, oligohydramnios, and crowding (multiple pregnancy) – are often associated with relatively short cords. Infants with Down's syndrome have short cords. Naeye has correlated short cord with subsequent motor and mental impairment [104]. Whether cord length as an indirect indicator of fetal movement can be correlated ultimately with antenatal neurologic development deserves further study.

Extremes of cord length are associated with potentially adverse outcomes. Some consideration of relative as well as absolute cord length is appropriate. For example, a long cord with extensive looping may function as a relatively short cord.

Short Cord

Definition and frequency: Gardiner's calculation that a normal vertex delivery requires a minimum cord length of 32 cm provides a common definition of an abnormally short cord [49]. Using this definition, between 0.4 and 0.9% of umbilical cords are abnormally short. Berg and Rayburn found that 2% of cords are less than 35 cm [19].

Clinical significance: Unduly short cords have been linked to fetal distress in some cases, although blood pH and base deficit values in short cords are reportedly the same as in cords of normal length [19]. In the absence of fetal anomalies, short cords have been associated with low Apgar scores, neonatal hypotonia, and need for resuscitation. Short cords may be associated with rupture or hemorrhage, delayed second stage of labor, abruption, subamnionic hemorrhage, and uterine inversion. At the extreme, there may be complete or near-complete cord absence (acordia) characteristically associated with fetal anterior abdominal wall defects that are directly attached to the placenta.

Long Cord/Entanglements/Prolapse

Definition and frequency. Excessively long cords have been variously defined as greater than 70 [13], 80 [19], or 100 cm [84]. Cord entanglements encircling the fetal neck, body, and extremities are common, occurring in about 23% of deliveries, but they are much more common in excessively long cords. Umbilical cord prolapse is an obstetric emergency defined as presentation of the cord in advance of the presenting part, occurring in 0.25–0.5% of deliveries.

Clinical significance. Long cords have been associated with IUGR, IUFD, brain imaging abnormalities, and poor neurologic outcomes [12, 13]. Histological evidence consistent with venous obstruction has been described in the placenta. Abnormally long cords are also associated with excess knotting, hypercoiling, entanglements, and prolapse. Most cord entanglements do not have adverse outcomes, but some may result in cord compression. Tight entanglements have been associated with low Apgar scores and stillbirths. Babies with sonographically documented nuchal cords have higher rates of cesarean section and NICU admission. Nuchal cords have been demonstrated as a cause of IUGR, indicating that the deleterious effect is long term in some cases [175]. Tight nuchal cords restricting venous return may result in neonatal anemia or even hypovolemic shock. Cerebral palsy has been linked to tight nuchal cords at delivery [109]. Cord prolapse has a perinatal mortality rate of 20% [91].

Pathologic changes. Constriction of the umbilical cord and the encircled fetal part may be dramatic in some cord entanglements. Cord compression may be associated with edema, venous congestion, hemorrhage, and thrombosis of umbilical or large chorionic plate vessels and/or villous abnormalities reflecting fetal vascular occlusion.

Knots

Frequency and etiology. Between 0.35% and 0.5% of umbilical cords contain true knots. True knots (➲ *Fig. 19.96*) should be distinguished from false knots, which are focal accentuations of the vascular spiral, a varicosity, or excess Wharton's jelly (➲ *Fig. 19.97*). True knots are thought to be related to fetal movement and are increased in long cords, male fetuses, monoamnionic twins, multigravidae, and in association with excess amniotic fluid. They occur with equal frequency in abortions and term deliveries indicating that they probably develop early in pregnancy when there is ample opportunity for movement.

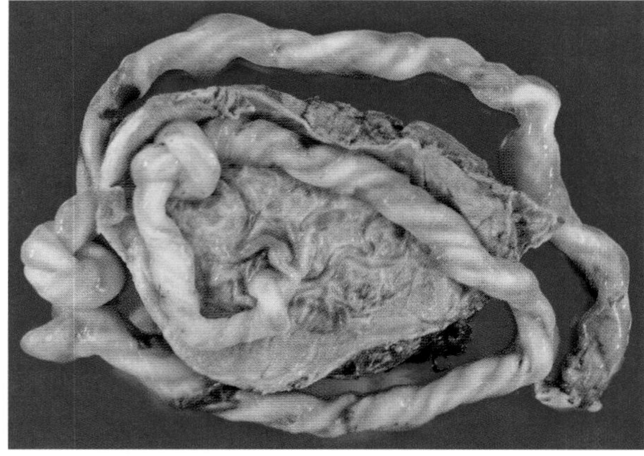

Fig. 19.96
True knots. **Long cord with two true knots (Used with permission of the American Registry of Pathology/Armed Forces Institute of Pathology)**

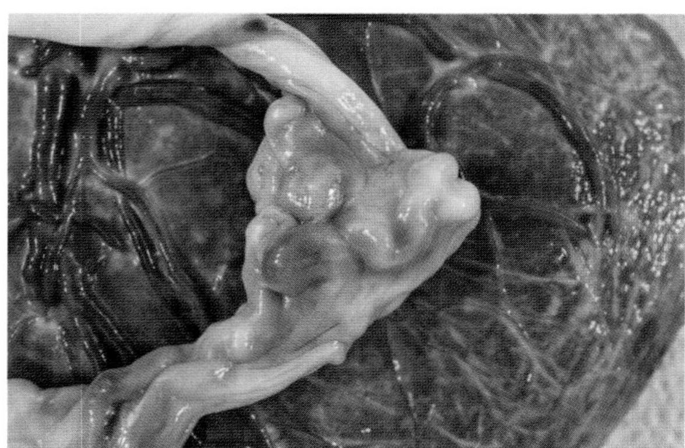

Fig. 19.97
False knot

Pathology. Umbilical cord knots should be assessed for evidence of chronicity, tightness, and circulatory compromise. In long-standing tight knots, there is grooving and loss of Wharton's jelly with constriction of blood vessels, changes that persist when the knot is untied. Thrombosis of umbilical or chorionic plate vessels, sometimes calcified, and villous alterations reflecting fetal vascular occlusion indicate chronic vascular obstruction. Acutely tightened knots may be associated with venous distention distal to the knot, edema, and villous vascular congestion.

Clinical significance. True knots are associated with an overall perinatal mortality rate of 8–11%, attributable to their potential for fetal circulatory obstruction (➋ *Fig. 19.98*). Either an acutely tightened or longstanding knot may be responsible for intrauterine or intrapartum fetal death [64]. False knots are generally of no clinical significance with only rare instances of thrombosis.

Torsion

Definition and frequency. The normal umbilical cord averages about 0.2 coils/cm (coiling index = no. of coils per cord length). Hypercoiled cords are generally considered to be those in which the coiling index is >0.3 coils/cm, and hypocoiled cords are those in which the coiling index is <0.1 coils/cm [84]. In one study, 7.5% of 120 unselected placentas had hypocoiled cords and 20% had hypercoiled cords [92]. About 4–5% of cords are noncoiled. Umbilical cord coiling is thought to reflect fetal movement; it is decreased in association with uterine constriction or fetal abnormalities that affect movement. Hypocoiled cords have been reported to occur more commonly in twins and in babies with chromosomal abnormalities. Hypercoiling is more common in long cords, male fetuses, multigravidae (presumably due to more room for fetal movement), and in association with maternal cocaine use.

Pathology. Hypercoiling may be localized or affect the entire cord (➋ *Fig. 19.99*) or be associated with stricture (➋ *Fig. 19.100*). Thrombosis of umbilical and chorionic plate vessels, intimal fibrin cushions, and vascular calcification suggest a chronic process in some cases. Hypocoiled cords are often thin with decreased Wharton's jelly.

Clinical significance. Hypercoiled cords have the potential for blood flow obstruction. Hypercoiling has been associated with adverse fetal outcome, including fetal IUGR, intolerance of labor, and IUFD [32]. Absent or minimal coiling is associated with fetal anomalies, chromosomal errors, fetal distress, and increased fetal and neonatal morbidity and mortality.

Stricture

Definition and etiology. An umbilical cord stricture is a sharply defined, usually short narrowed segment with decreased Wharton's jelly and vascular constriction

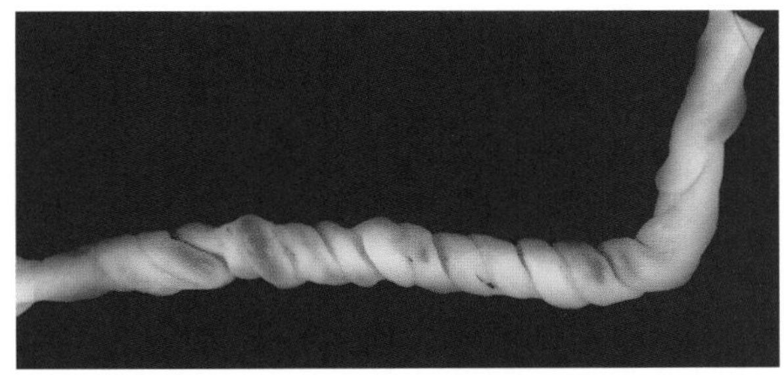

Fig. 19.99
Hypercoiled cord

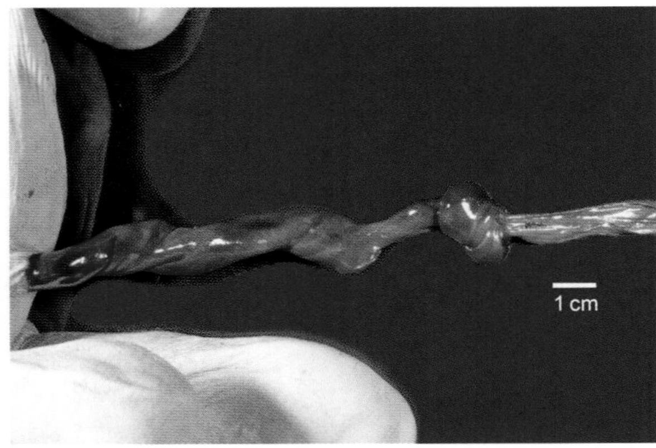

Fig. 19.98
Tight knot resulting in intrauterine fetal demise (IUFD). **(Used with permission of the American Registry of Pathology/Armed Forces Institute of Pathology)**

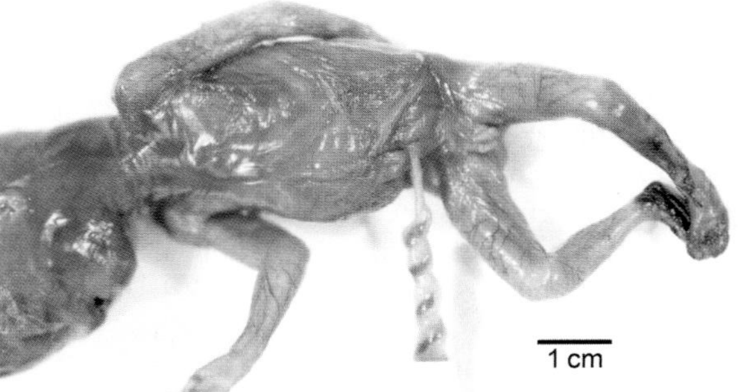

Fig. 19.100
Hypercoiled cord with stricture and intrauterine fetal demise (IUFD). **(Used with permission of the American Registry of Pathology/Armed Forces Institute of Pathology)**

(➲ *Fig. 19.100*). The etiology is unknown, but it rarely occurs outside the setting of excess torsion. Alternatively, it has been hypothesized to be the result of a primary deficiency of Wharton's jelly, perhaps an exaggeration of the normal gradual loss of Wharton's jelly at the fetal end of the umbilical cord.

Pathology. Strictures are most common at the fetal end of the cord, although occasionally they may occur at the placental end or elsewhere. They are usually associated with excessively long and hypercoiled cords. Many are seen in association with macerated fetuses, although the abnormality is not confined to abortions. The strictured segment shows decreased Wharton's jelly and vascular, especially venous, compression. Placental surface vessels may be thrombosed.

Clinical significance. Umbilical cord strictures are often associated with abortion [115]. Strictures have recurred in successive pregnancies and have been proposed as a cause of non-immune hydrops.

Cord Diameter

Umbilical cord diameter is affected by the number of vessels and the amount and fluid content of Wharton's jelly. Nomograms generated from uncomplicated pregnancies indicate a progressive increase in sonographic cord diameter and cross-sectional area until 32 weeks gestation with a decline thereafter presumably due to a reduction in fluid content of Wharton's jelly. Patel and colleagues established the normal cord circumference to be 37.7 ± 7.73 mm [114]. Silver and colleagues determined that cord diameter ranged from 1.25 to 2.00 cm and circumference from 2.4 to 4.4 cm [174]. The factors that determine the amount of Wharton's jelly and its water content are poorly understood. More cord jelly and vascular spiraling have been associated with better fetal outcome, while compression patterns on fetal heart tracings occur more often in cords with decreased fluid content [174]. A thin ("lean") cord with decreased or absent Wharton's jelly may be associated with IUGR. At present, a lean cord is defined as one with a cross-sectional area less than the tenth percentile as assessed sonographically or 8 mm or less along its entire length [121, 139]. Diminished size appears to be due to a reduction in Wharton's jelly. Lean cords tend to have a lower coiling index and reduced umbilical vein flow normalized for fetal weight [36].

Cord edema, focal or diffuse, occurs inconsistently in a variety of clinical situations, especially diabetes, but often the cause is unknown. Edema is more common in prematures.

Rupture

Complete cord rupture is very rare. Most cord ruptures complicate precipitous delivery, but rarely rupture may occur in the early stages of labor or before labor begins. Short and velamentously inserted cords, trauma, or inflammation are proposed etiologic factors.

Insertion

Velamentous Insertion and Membranous Vessels

Definition and frequency. In velamentous insertion, the cord inserts into the fetal membranes.

Velamentous insertion is a common anomaly, occurring in about 1% of placentas. It is greatly increased in multiple pregnancies, extrachorial placentas, and in single-artery cords. Velamentous insertion is also reportedly increased in association with cigarette smoking and advanced maternal age. An associated condition, *vasa previa*, occurs when membranous vessels in the fetal membranes present in advance of a fetal part.

Pathology. After insertion, the umbilical vessels usually branch in the fetal membranes (➲ *Fig. 19.101*). Having lost their protective covering of Wharton's jelly and unsupported by underlying villous tissue, membranous vessels are vulnerable to injury – traumatic rupture, hemorrhage (➲ *Fig. 19.102*), compression, and thrombosis, especially when they traverse the cervical os in advance of the fetus. The length of membranous vessels provides

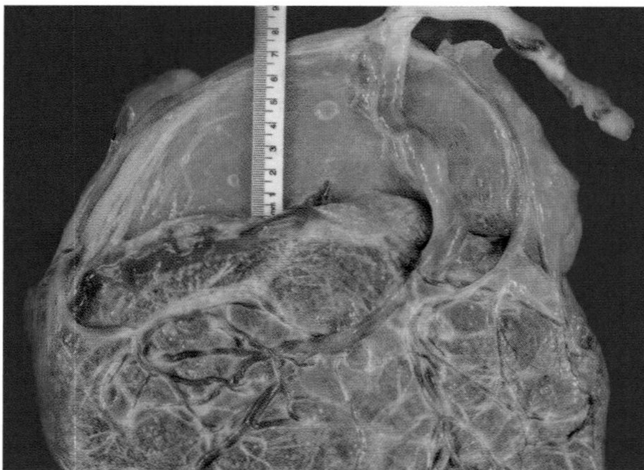

Fig. 19.101
Velamentous insertion

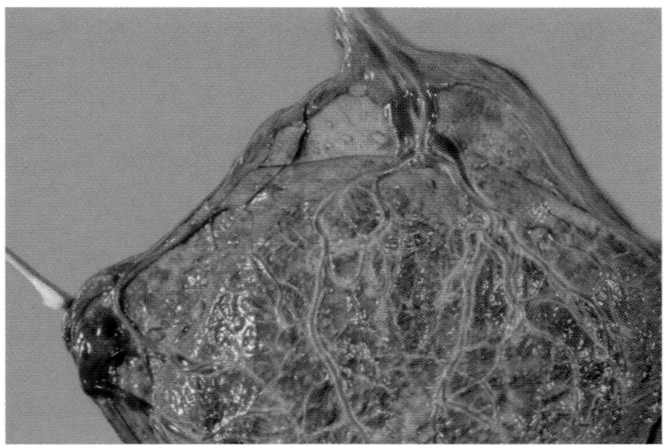

Fig. 19.102
Velamentous insertion. **A ruptured membranous vessel is associated with surrounding hemorrhage (Used with permission of the American Registry of Pathology/Armed Forces Institute of Pathology)**

one measure of the degree of their vulnerability. Membranous vessels are not limited to velamentously inserted cords but may arise aberrantly from marginally or even centrally inserted cords, and they regularly supply succenturiate lobes. As a site of significant pathologic alterations, all membranous vessels should be inspected carefully and included in sections for microscopic exam. Rarely a velamentously inserted cord retains its Wharton's jelly, running in the membranes before its vessels branch (*interposito velamentosa*).

Etiology. Velamentous cord insertion may be due to malpositioning of the blastocyst at implantation with consequent aberrant body stalk – placental disk orientation (polarity theory). Alternatively, velamentous insertion may result when the placenta "moves" from its initial implantation site, leaving the cord insertion behind (trophotropism theory). This placental remodeling, probably in response to uterine crowding and/or maternal vascular supply, involves simultaneous atrophy on one aspect and growth/expansion on the other. The increased frequency of velamentous cord insertion in multiples, in uteri with structural defects and foreign bodies and the sonographic documentation of eccentric placental expansion with conversion of placenta previa to a higher uterine position support the trophotropism theory.

Clinical features. Velamentous cord insertion has several important clinical associations. The best-documented complications are related to the vulnerability of membranous vessels. Vessel compression with severe fetal distress or laceration with blood loss, even exsanguination, may occur suddenly during labor. Although bleeding is most common from membranous vessels near the os at the time of labor, bleeding may also occur antepartum and from vessels located higher in the uterus. Thrombosis of membranous arteries and veins has been associated with major fetal thromboembolic events and fetal death.

Velamentous cord insertion also provides a marker for poor placentation with decreased placental vascularization. This may explain its reported association with low birth weight, low Apgar scores, and abnormal fetal heart-rate patterns. Velamentous cord insertion has also been associated with congenital anomalies, occurring in 8.5% of infants and in as many as 25% of spontaneous abortions with velamentous cords. The structural anomalies associated with velamentous cord insertion are deformations not malformations or disruptions indicating that they and the velamentous insertion are both the result of competition for intrauterine space. Velamentous cord insertion is significantly more common in monochorionic gestations with the twin–twin transfusion syndrome than in those without it.

Marginal Insertion

Definition and frequency. Umbilical cord insertion at the edge of the placental disk is termed a marginal or *Battledore* insertion. Marginal insertion occurs in about 7% of placentas and is hypothesized to develop via the same mechanism as velamentous insertion (abnormal primary implantation versus trophotropism).

Clinical associations. The clinical significance of marginal insertion is debated. Marginal insertion has been reported to occur with increased frequency in abortions and malformed infants and in association with neonatal asphyxia and PTL, although these associations have not been confirmed by others. Peripheral cord insertion (velamentous, marginal, and markedly eccentric) has been associated with discordant growth and SGA in twins [140].

Furcate Insertion

In furcate insertion, the cord loses Wharton's jelly before insertion, leaving the umbilical vessels unsupported (*Fig. 19.103*). Furcate cords may insert velamentously or into the placental disk.

The unsupported vessels are subject to the same complications as membranous vessels.

Tethered Insertion ("Amnionic Web")

Amnionic webs or chorda are amnionic folds that encase the cord at the insertion site (➋ *Fig. 19.104*).

Large tight amnionic webs may limit mobility of the cord, potentially compromising blood flow.

Umbilical Vessels

Numerical Variation

Single Umbilical Artery

Definition and frequency. The presence of a single umbilical artery (SUA) is a common and important cord abnormality. In prospective studies of consecutive deliveries, the frequency of single umbilical artery is consistently somewhat less than 1%, although the frequency is considerably higher in perinatal autopsy studies (2.7–12%) and in spontaneous abortions (1.5–2.7%). The frequency of single umbilical artery is higher in white women, diabetic mothers, multiples, and chromosome abnormalities especially trisomies.

The likelihood of diagnosing single umbilical artery is increased when fixed versus fresh cords are examined, and histologic exam provides the most accurate means of establishing the diagnosis. Cord vascularity should be assessed at least 3–5 cm from the placental insertion site because the umbilical arteries frequently fuse close to the placenta.

Etiology. Whether single umbilical artery is due to primary aplasia or secondary atrophy has long been debated. When specifically sought, histologic evidence of vascular remnants is demonstrable in some single artery cords. The higher incidence of single umbilical artery in fetuses as compared to early embryos provides circumstantial evidence that single umbilical artery may be an acquired defect.

Pathology. Muscular or elastic remnants of an atrophied vessel are identified in some cases. Single artery cords are commonly associated with velamentous insertion (as high as 12%), circumvallation, and a magistral pattern of chorionic blood vessels. On occasion, two umbilical arteries are present but are of markedly different size. A difference of at least 1 mm in umbilical artery diameter as established sonographically is considered discordance [120] (➋ *Fig. 19.105*). Marked umbilical

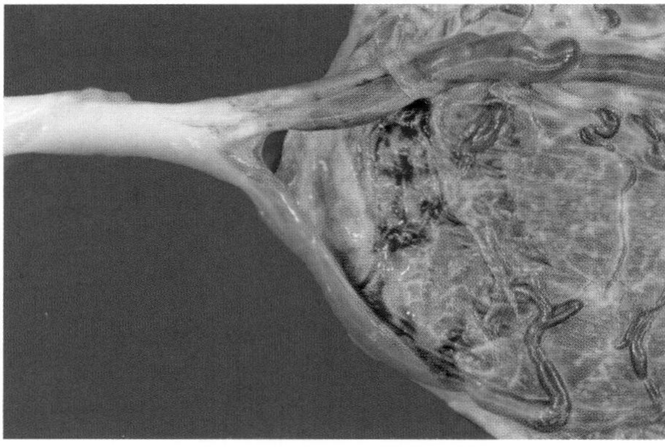

Fig. 19.103
Furcate insertion

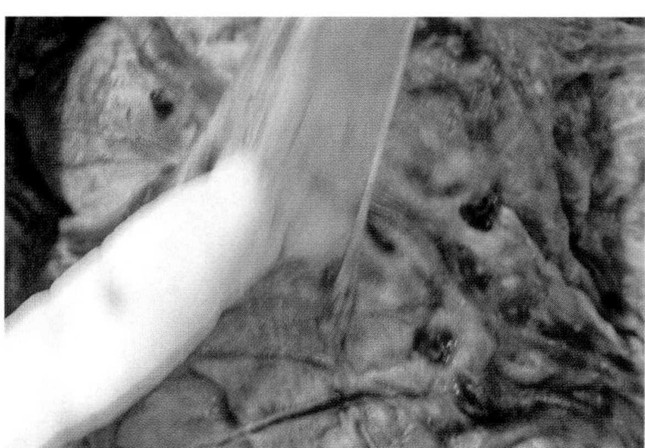

Fig. 19.104
Tethered insertion

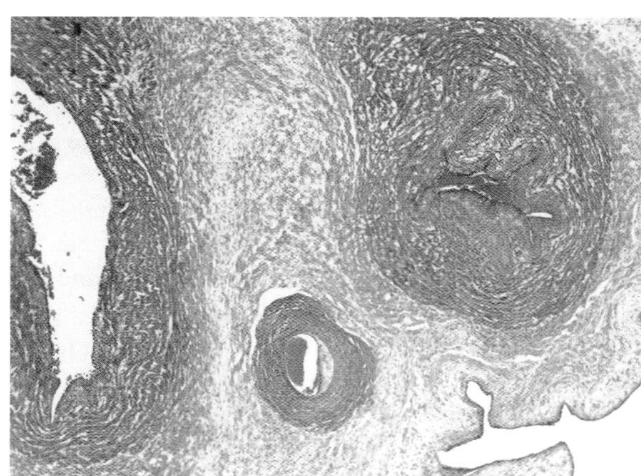

Fig. 19.105
Discordant umbilical arteries

artery discordance may be associated with fetal anomalies similar to those encountered with single umbilical artery.

Clinical Significance *Congenital malformations.* There is a well-documented association between single umbilical artery and fetal malformations, but there is no particular organ or specific abnormality characterizing this association. Any organ system may be affected, and malformations are frequently multiple. Congenital malformations are most numerous and most severe in stillborn and aborted babies and those dying in the neonatal period. Infants with single artery cords but no detectable abnormalities at birth who survive the neonatal period are unlikely to have other significant abnormalities detected subsequently. Single umbilical artery is almost invariable in sirenomelia and acardiac fetuses. Whether single umbilical artery plays a role in the development of congenital malformations or is just another manifestation of them is unclear.

Perinatal mortality. The perinatal mortality rate of infants with single umbilical artery is greatly increased (11–41%). This is attributable to associated major malformations in most instances, although otherwise normal infants with single umbilical artery have an increased perinatal mortality rate as well. The sonographic demonstration of decreased Wharton's jelly in single artery cords may contribute to cord vulnerability.

Low birth weight. Single umbilical artery is associated with low birth weight even when infants with malformations are excluded from analysis.

Vascular Abnormalities

Segmental Thinning

Quereshi and Jacques reported segmental thinning of umbilical vessels with virtual absence of the media in 1.5% of consecutively examined placentas [119]. The umbilical vein was involved in the majority of cases, although on occasion, one or both arteries exhibited identical changes. Both superficial and medial aspects of the vessels exhibited wall deficiencies. Segmental vascular thinning was accompanied by fetal malformations in a significant number of cases, and there was a high incidence of fetal distress.

Meconium-Induced Necrosis

Long-standing meconium exposure may induce muscle necrosis in umbilical and chorionic plate vessels. Myonecrosis usually involves the superficial aspects of the arteries closest to the surface. The necrotic cells are rounded with dense eosinophilic-smudged cytoplasm and pyknotic nuclei (*Fig. 19.93*) [82]. Meconium-associated vascular necrosis has been linked to cerebral palsy [145]. In addition to vascular damage, meconium has been shown to cause vasoconstriction of umbilical vessels in vitro [5].

Ulceration

Linear ulceration of Wharton's jelly with vascular necrosis, aneurysmal dilatation, and rupture may result in intraamnionic hemorrhage, profound fetal anemia, and fetal death in utero (*Fig. 19.106*). These cord anomalies

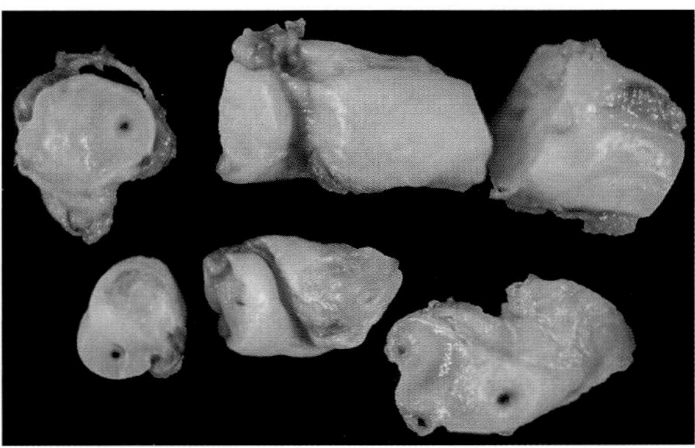

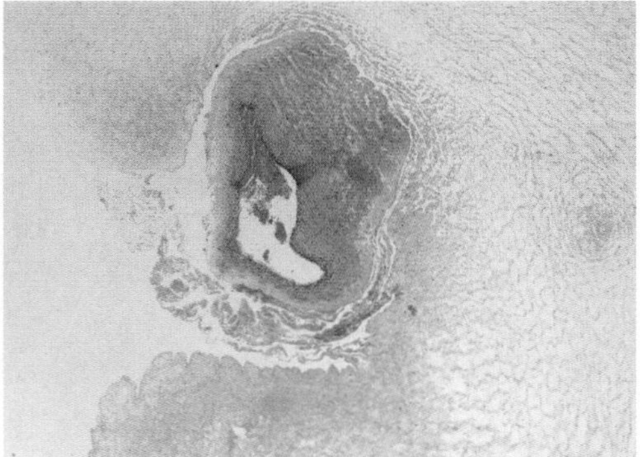

Fig. 19.106
Ulceration of Wharton's jelly. **Necrosis of Wharton's jelly with thinning and rupture of umbilical vessels resulted in IUFD in this baby with duodenal atresia (Used with permission of the American Registry of Pathology/Armed Forces Institute of Pathology)**

have been described in association with fetal intestinal atresia.

Thrombosis

Definition and frequency. Thrombosis of umbilical vessels may be occlusive or non-occlusive, and is often associated with similar changes in chorionic plate or stem villous vessels. Thrombosis of umbilical cord vessels is uncommon, occurring in 1 in 1,300 deliveries, 1 in 938 perinatal autopsies, and 1 in 250 high-risk pregnancies [164].

Etiology. Thrombi may be associated with cord compression, abnormal coiling, knots, stricture, hematoma, inflammation, anomalous insertion, amnionic bands, or entanglements. Other factors such as thrombophilic states could act synergistically to precipitate thrombosis. In many instances, the etiology is obscure.

Pathology. Thrombi more commonly involve the umbilical vein alone (71%) with a lesser frequency of combined vein and artery thrombosis (18%) or arterial thrombosis alone (11%). Thrombi may be associated with vessel calcification and necrosis (➋ *Fig. 19.107*). The chorionic plate and stem villous vessels may be similarly affected.

Clinical significance. Fetal morbidity and mortality is high, particularly with occlusion of both umbilical arteries. Thrombi may embolize to the fetus causing infarcts in fetal organs or they may result in the loss of a significant fraction of the fetoplacental circulatory bed. Thrombi have also been associated with cerebral palsy, massive fetomaternal hemorrhage, IUGR, and IUFD.

Hematoma

Definition and frequency. Umbilical cord hematomas are accumulations of blood in Wharton's jelly. They are uncommon.

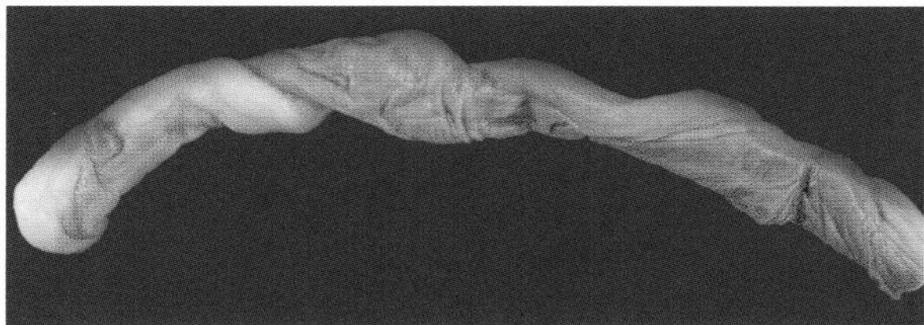

Fig. 19.107
Thrombosed umbilical artery. **This thrombosed umbilical artery, cause undetermined, is visible as a dark spiral and was completely necrotic (Used with permission of the American Registry of Pathology/Armed Forces Institute of Pathology)**

Etiology. In the great majority of cases, an obvious etiology is not apparent. Rarely, hemorrhage has a demonstrable origin from an umbilical vein or artery, and origin from omphalomesenteric vessels has been proposed. Rupture of a varix, traumatic damage at the time of amniocentesis or percutaneous umbilical cord sampling, or inflammation or structural anomalies of a vessel wall have been suggested as possible mechanisms.

Pathology. Most umbilical cord hematomas present as red-purple fusiform swellings (➋ *Fig. 19.108*). They are usually single, but may be multiple or even involve the full length of the umbilical cord. They are generally confined to the cord, but on occasion, they may rupture into the amnionic cavity. Small collections of fresh blood usually reflect cord blood sampling or traction at the time of delivery.

Clinical significance. A perinatal mortality rate in the range of 40–50% has been reported in association with umbilical cord hematoma. Fetal death may be due to blood loss or umbilical vascular compression with circulatory compromise.

Hemangioma

Definition. Hemangiomas are benign lesions composed of proliferating vessels sometimes associated with marked myxoid degeneration of Wharton's jelly (angiomyxoma).

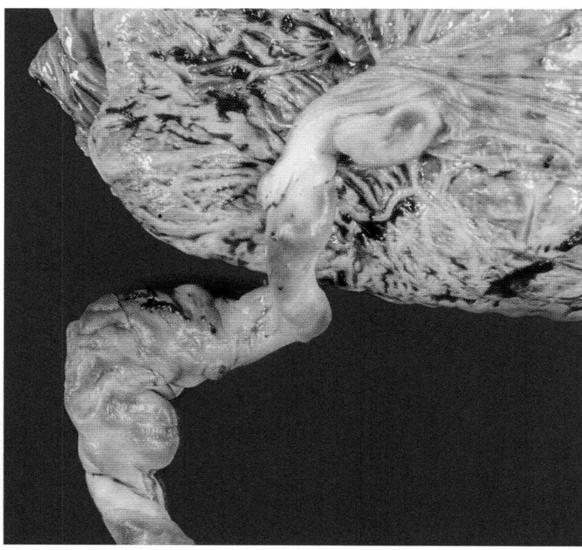

Fig. 19.108
Localized cord hematoma. **(Used with permission of the American Registry of Pathology/Armed Forces Institute of Pathology)**

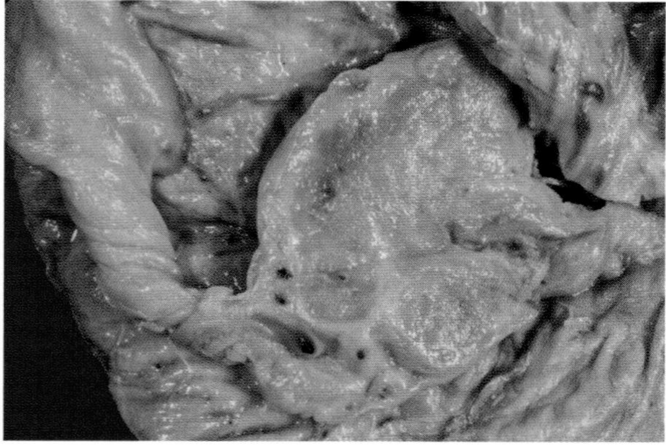

Fig. 19.109
Umbilical cord hemangioma. **(Used with permission of the American Registry of Pathology/Armed Forces Institute of Pathology)**

Pathology. Hemangiomas present as fusiform swelling of the umbilical cord usually at the placental end. They can attain substantial size (up to 900 g in one report) (*Fig. 19.109*). Microscopically, these benign tumors show features similar to benign hemangiomas at other body sites.

Clinical significance. Hemangiomas with myxoid degeneration (angiomyxoma) can be associated with hemorrhage, increased alpha fetoprotein levels, and rarely nonimmune fetal hydrops, presumably due to high output cardiac failure.

Aneurysm

Umbilical cord aneurysms are rare. They may be so large as to compress adjacent vessels resulting in fetal death. Umbilical artery aneurysm has been reported in trisomy 18 [168].

Clinical Syndromes and Their Pathologic Correlates in the Placenta

Placentas come to the pathologist with limited clinical data supplied by the obstetrician. The diagnoses or problems listed do not necessarily provide insight into the nature of the pathologic abnormalities that the pathologist should look for. Here follow definitions of common clinical conditions that lead to submission of a placenta for pathologic examination together with the relevant pathologic lesions.

Preeclampsia

Definition. A previously normotensive pregnant woman whose blood pressure reaches 140/90 mm Hg or greater after 20 weeks gestation on at least two occasions has *pregnancy-induced hypertension.* The addition of proteinuria (1+ or greater on urine dipstick confirmed by a 24 h collection containing ≥300 mg of protein) means that *preeclampsia* has occurred. *Severe preeclampsia* indicates the addition of one or more of the following: blood pressure over 160 mm Hg systolic or 110 mm Hg diastolic; proteinuria greater than 5 g/24 h or 3+ or greater on two dipstick evaluations at least 4 h apart; headache; visual disturbances, epigastric, or right upper quadrant pain; oliguria; thrombocytopenia or liver enzyme elevation; fetal growth restriction; and/or pulmonary edema. The *HELLP syndrome* is a form of severe preeclampsia with a specific triad of findings including hemolysis, elevated liver enzymes, and low platelet count. Seizures signify the onset of eclampsia. Delivery of the placenta, often premature, is the only effective medical intervention.

Etiology. The spiral arteries that supply maternal blood to the placenta must expand to accommodate the growing placentofetal unit. This is normally accomplished by trophoblastic remodeling of spiral arteries. A failure of this process results in decidual vasculopathy, reduced maternal flow, placental ischemia, and the maternal syndrome of preeclampsia [90].

In preeclampsia, there is generalized maternal endothelial dysfunction thought to be caused by soluble factors produced by ischemic trophoblast. Endoglin and sFlt-1 are two factors that have been implicated. Both appear prior to disease onset and cause endothelial dysfunction and hypertension in the mother. These factors act by neutralizing the angiogenic and vasodilatory effects of vascular endothelial growth factor and placental growth factor produced by the placenta [102]. When endoglin and sFlt-1 are overexpressed in an experimental rat model, the result is severe proteinuria, hypertension, and growth restriction as well as thrombocytopenia and liver dysfunction [185].

Pathology. Correlation between placental lesions and severity of maternal symptoms is poor. Two types of abnormal placentas are associated with preeclampsia. The first and most common is the small placenta with decidual vasculopathy, especially acute atherosis, the pathologic changes characteristic of maternal vascular underperfusion, and thin umbilical cord. Less common is the large placenta associated with a heterogenous group of conditions including diabetes mellitus, placental hydrops, multiple gestation, and hydatidiform mole.

Essential Hypertension

Patients with preexisting hypertension not complicated by superimposed preeclampsia may have similar but less pronounced abnormalities in the villi. Arteriosclerotic changes in the uterine or intramyometrial arteries may be sufficient to produce some degree of placental ischemia.

Diabetes Mellitus

Placentas associated with uncomplicated maternal diabetes mellitus vary. In about half of cases they appear normal, grossly, and microscopically. Correlation between placental findings, metabolic control, and clinical severity are poor. When they are abnormal, diabetic placentas tend to be large and heavy, with large and edematous umbilical cords. Villi in the larger placentas often show chorangiosis and *distal villous immaturity*, large distal villi with increased central capillaries, macrophages, and interstitial fluid (➋ *Fig. 19.110*). Placental, fetal, and neonatal thrombi are more frequent, a manifestation of the thrombophilia associated with diabetes. When complicated by hypertension or preeclampsia, the placenta may be small with evidence of low maternal flow.

Preterm Birth, Preterm Labor, and Preterm Rupture of Membranes

A term birth takes place between 37 and 42 weeks of gestation. The most severe sequelae for the newborn occur before the 34th week. The category of "VLBW" infants refers to live-born infants weighing between 500 and 1,500 g. These are at greatest risk of neonatal death, neurologic injury, and pulmonary immaturity. PTB occurs in 12–13% of all pregnancies in the United States. The result is a 40-fold increase in perinatal morbidity and mortality.

Most PTBs are due to ACA or preeclampsia. The two pathologic subgroups show very little overlap [8, 59]. ACA is most common, occurring in 61% of premature placentas delivered within 1 h of membrane rupture [58, 59]. ACA is more common in earlier PTB. Lesions resulting from impaired blood flow are more common in later PTB [61]. Premature labor and delivery also have a significant correlation with decidual hemorrhage, which may directly initiate prostaglandin release and labor.

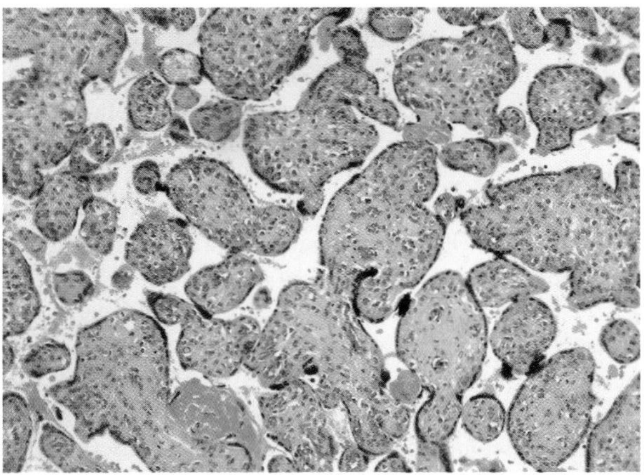

Fig. 19.110
Distal villous immaturity. **Increased numbers of large distal villi with increased capillaries and evenly distributed interstitial fluid**

Post-Term Pregnancy

A gestation longer than 42 completed weeks (294 days) is considered post-term. Perinatal mortality is increased. The postmature newborn has a characteristically slender, elongated body and limbs, dried, wrinkled, often meconium-stained skin, long fingernails, and an apprehensive expression. Meconium staining is more common in post-term placentas, but otherwise there are no distinctive or definitive pathologic changes in the placenta [17].

Fetal Growth Restriction, Intrauterine Growth Restriction (IUGR)

Prenatal evaluation of fetal growth is based on ultrasound measurements of abdominal circumference, head circumference, biparietal diameter, and femur length (among others), which may also be used to estimate fetal weight [152]. IUGR is a significant risk factor for poor outcome and stillbirth [184]. IUGR is symmetric when head and abdominal measurements are decreased proportionately, and asymmetric when there is a greater decrease in abdominal girth. When IUGR is identified, Doppler studies of blood flow through the umbilical cord, middle cerebral artery, or other sites may be obtained. Absent or reduced umbilical artery blood flow is a significant adverse finding, which may begin early and persist for weeks until delivery [154]. Infants whose birth weight lies below an expected percentile for gestational age (which may be arbitrarily set at the third, fifth, or tenth percentile) are classified as small for gestational age (SGA) and qualify as growth-restricted.

Maternal factors that contribute to IUGR include pre-eclampsia, hypertension, diabetes mellitus, thrombophilias, extreme malnutrition, chronic renal disease, tobacco and other drug abuse, and poor obstetric history in general. Fetal factors include chromosomal anomalies (including confined placental mosaicism), congenital malformations, and multiple gestation [190]. Placental lesions associated with IUGR include: (1) vascular lesions that reduce maternal blood flow (decidual vasculopathy or chronic abruption), (2) vascular lesions that reduce fetal blood flow, (FTV, large chorangiomas, or umbilical cord abnormalities), and (3) lesions that greatly reduce the amount of functional placenta (extensive chronic villitis, MPF, MFI, or multiple infarcts.) [167]

Neonatal Encephalopathy (NE), Cerebral Palsy (CP), and "Birth Asphyxia"

Historically, the occurrence of abnormal neurologic findings in the first week of life was assumed to have followed a period of asphyxia (severe hypoxia with metabolic acidosis) during labor and delivery. This concept led to such clinical terms as "birth asphyxia" and "hypoxic-ischemic encephalopathy." While episodes of pure hypoxia do occur (acute abruption is a good example), other factors – intrauterine infection and other acute and chronic placental lesions – are much more common. The transient clinical state, characterized by hypotonia, apnea, coma, and seizures, is now called *neonatal encephalopathy.* The incidence varies from 6 to 8 per 1,000 births.

Cerebral palsy, by contrast, is a chronic, non-progressive neurologic disorder, most often a form of spastic diplegia, hemiplegia, or quadriplegia, with an incidence of 2 per 1,000 births. It is usually not diagnosed much before age 2 years, certainly not at the time of delivery. Approximately 50% of cases develop after full-term birth following an apparently normal gestation. The remainder are divided between VLBW infants (<1.5 kg) and a heterogeneous group of low-birth-weight and near-term infants, some with IUGR [133]. Extreme prematurity is a risk factor for both NE and CP [108]. In a large population-based study of term infants with neonatal encephalopathy, 13% subsequently developed cerebral palsy, while 24% of CP patients had a prior history of NE [11]. The overall incidence of CP has not changed much over the past 50 years despite advances in intrapartum monitoring and antenatal diagnosis.

Clearly, the placenta from every newborn with NE deserves careful attention from the pathologist [79]. Acute lesions associated with NE include large retroplacental hematomas, meconium-associated vascular necrosis, and severe chorioamnionitis, especially with intense chorionic vessel inflammation [145, 150]. Chronic lesions include chorionic vessel thrombi, fetal thrombotic vasculopathy [97, 107], especially with cord abnormalities [128], placental or fetal hydrops, diffuse chronic villitis, especially with obliterative fetal vasculopathy, diffuse chorioamnionic hemosiderosis, and massive perivillous fibrin deposits [130].

Fetal and Placental Hydrops

Hydrops is a state of marked generalized edema, with accumulation of fluid in subcutaneous tissue, body cavities, placenta, and umbilical cord. Most cases are now detected by prenatal ultrasound. Prenatal investigation to assign a specific cause is urgent because many cases are potentially treatable. In fatal cases, determination of the cause is still important for parental counseling and for appropriate management of future pregnancies. Even in the absence of specific changes in the placenta, the pathologist has a primary role in coordinating other forms of laboratory testing, including cytogenetics, immunologic and microbiologic studies, immunohistochemistry, and fluorescence in situ hybridization.

Immune hydrops, caused by maternal isoimmunization to the Rh (mainly D) antigen expressed by the fetal red blood cells, still occurs, but is now rare due to anti-D gammaglobulin (Rhogam) prophyllaxis. *Nonimmune hydrops* is now more common, but still infrequent, with incidence figures from 1 in 1,400 to 1.34 per 1,000 live births [183]. There are numerous causes of non-immune placental or fetal hydrops. The main pathophysiologic categories are cardiac failure, anemia, and hypoproteinemia. Among the most important lesions are cardiac malformations, chromosomal anomalies (45XO, trisomies 21 and 18), thoracic lesions (congenital cystic adenomatoid malformation, pulmonary sequestration, or tumors), anemias (parvovirus infection or fetomaternal hemorrhage), fetal infections (TORCH group or syphilis), large tumors (sacrococcygeal teratoma or angiomas), and urinary tract anomalies [156]. Chromosomal anomalies are more common prior to 24 weeks; cardiac and pulmonary lesions are more common after 24 weeks [176]. Hydrops caused by parvovirus anemia, cardiac arrhythmias, and hydrothorax respond more favorably to prenatal treatment [176].

A hydropic placenta is often massively enlarged (exceeding 1,000 g), soft, friable, and pale (➋ *Fig. 19.31*). Histologically, the villi appear enlarged, cytotrophoblast

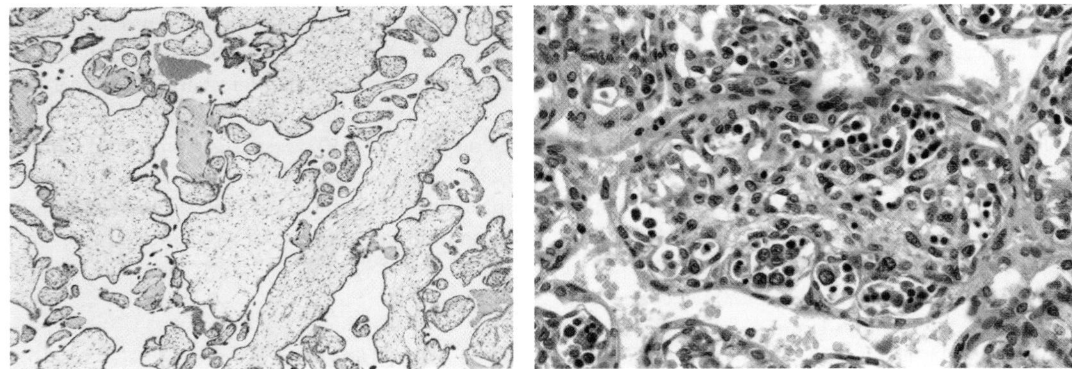

Fig. 19.111
Fetoplacental hydrops. **The villi are immature and edematous (*left*). When due to fetal anemia, nucleated red blood cells and erythroblasts expand the villous capillaries as in this case of Rh incompatibility**

cells are increased with occasional mitoses, villous capillaries are reduced or inconspicuous, and the stroma is edematous (Fig. 19.111). In cases of anemia, nucleated red blood cells (nRBC – erythroblasts and normoblasts) are very prominent, often in clusters that expand the capillary outlines.

Nucleated Red Blood Cells in the Fetal Circulation

nRBC are rare in sections of a normal term placenta or in the blood of normal newborns. Absolute counts in the range of 500–1,000 nRBC/mm^3 or 1–10 nRBC/100 white blood cells in fetal or neonatal blood are normal; counts in excess of these figures are abnormal [63]. An increased number of nRBC in the circulation of newborns is a well-recognized parameter of potential neonatal injury [63]. nRBC elevation is believed to be caused by acute or chronic fetal hypoxia resulting in erythropoetin release. The most dramatic nRBC elevations occur in the severe anemias associated with immune or non-immune hydrops and congenital infections (especially parvovirus). Anemia caused by fetomaternal hemorrhage, either acute or chronic, may elicit a marked nRBC elevation. nRBC elevation occurs in a number of other clinical settings including maternal diabetes, acidosis [89], IUGR, maternal smoking [193], and other infections [63].

Erythropoetin can be measured in amniotic fluid as well as in fetal blood. Elevations occur in maternal diabetes, fetal growth restriction, maternal smoking, fetal anemia, acidosis, prolonged heart rate deceleration (demonstrable prior to deceleration), and after acute or repeated fetal hemorrhages [181]. Amniotic fluid levels are lower but persist longer. Episodic periods of hypoxia in cord entanglement may be reflected in this way even when blood levels have returned to normal [60].

The time interval between an acute event and nRBC elevation is not established. Elevated lymphocyte and platelet counts (as well as increased nRBC) may correlate with the timing of prenatal neurologic injury; counts tend to be higher and last longer in newborns with long-standing hypoxic injury [106, 118].

Clinically significant nRBC elevations are usually evident on microscopic examination of the placenta (Fig. 19.74) [29, 137]. Redline found a highly significant correlation between cord blood counts and the number of nRBC observed in ten high-power fields (40× objective) in the placenta; 10 nRBC/10 HPF corresponded to an absolute count of 2,500 nRBC/mm^3 with 90% sensitivity and 82% specificity [137]. In this study of placentas from babies with cerebral palsy, an elevated nRBC count was significantly associated with placental lesions – multifocal avascular villi (FTV) or chronic villitis. Meconium-associated necrosis in vessels of the chorionic plate or umbilical cord showed a borderline association. Increased nRBC, with or without placental lesions, were unassociated with acidosis or birth asphyxia indicating that the underlying causes of nRBC elevation in this context antedated immediate peripartum events [137]. Persistent nRBC elevation in the first week of life of a preterm growth-restricted newborn has serious implications for additional complications, including bronchopulmonary dysplasia, necrotizing enterocolitis, and intraventricular hemorrhage [16].

Thrombophilias

Inherited and acquired coagulation disorders are risk factors for adverse pregnancy outcomes (early spontaneous abortion, IUFD, abruption, IUGR, and preeclampsia) [37, 55, 94, 95, 132, 155].

The most widely studied thrombophilias include the *G1691A* mutation in the factor V gene (factor V Leiden), the *G20210A* mutation in the prothrombin gene, the *C677T* mutation in the methylene tetrahydrofolate reductase gene, deficiencies in protein S, protein C, antithrombin III, hyperhomocysteinemia, and acquired thrombophilic states such as antiphospholipid antibody syndrome. Coagulopathies also occur in patients with diabetes mellitus. The mere identification of an inherited thrombophilia is not predictive for pregnancy complications. Estimates of the risk for different outcomes in mothers with specific thrombophilic conditions have been summarized recently [132].

There is no specific placental lesion unique to or specific for maternal thrombophilia. The placental pathology linking thrombophilia to adverse pregnancy outcome is essentially identical to other disorders associated with chronic maternal vascular underperfusion (increased syncytial knots, increased intervillous fibrin, infarcts, retroplacental hematoma, distal villous hypoplasia, decreased placental weight, and thin cord) [9, 83, 95]. Maternal thrombophilia has been associated with MPF/MFI and subchorionic hematomas in some reports [62, 132]. Whether coagulation abnormalities are underlying causes of abnormal placentation or exacerbate preexisting placental compromise is unknown. Acquired thrombophilic states such as the antiphospholipid antibody syndrome may promote intraplacental clotting, possibly by blocking the normal antithrombotic annexin V phospholipid-binding protein and by activating complement [123, 169]. A similar predisposition to placental clotting occurs in patients with lupus erythematosus [93] and scleroderma [38]. IgG antiphospholipid antibodies may cross the interhemal membrane to enter the fetal circulation.

Fetal thrombophilic mutations studied to date are by themselves not associated with fetal vascular thrombosis. The frequency of fetal thromboocclusive placental lesions in babies with fetal thrombophilias is not increased, and there is no increase in the prevalence of thrombophilic mutations in infants whose placentas have fetal thromboocclusive lesions. At most, fetal coagulation abnormalities may act in concert with other factors affecting fetal blood flow. FTV does have a clear and strong relationship with umbilical cord entanglement and cord abnormalities.

Placental pathology has poor predictive value in identifying patients with thrombophilia. Coagulation studies are probably best focused on patients with specific clinical scenarios such as severe early onset or recurrent pregnancy loss in association with typical placental lesions [132].

Acute Fatty Liver of Pregnancy and HELLP Syndrome

Both the HELLP syndrome (hemolysis, elevated liver enzyme levels, low platelet count) and acute fatty liver of pregnancy (AFLP) present as preeclampsia complicated by liver malfunction. The HELLP syndrome is more common and usually has a reasonably good prognosis under appropriate management. AFLP, although rare, has a significant mortality rate. Liver biopsy in AFLP shows characteristic changes including microvesicular steatosis.

Although recognized by maternal diseases, one very important cause is an inherited gene mutation in the fetus that causes a deficiency of long-chain 3-hydroxyl-CoA dehydrogenase, resulting in abnormal fatty acid metabolism [68]. The mother's acute problem is usually relieved by delivery. The infant has severe liver dysfunction, hypoglycemia, cardiomyopathy, and neuromuscular abnormalities. Appropriate early dietary management may reduce morbidity and mortality.

Fatty acids are an important source of energy for the fetus. More than 20 different genetically determined disorders of fatty acid metabolism have been recognized [171]. Although rare, together they represent the most common metabolic disorder with severe consequences for the mother and fetus. Retrospective studies have identified these disorders in a significant number of unexplained stillbirths and sudden infant deaths.

Placental lesions in the context of the HELLP syndrome include all of the features of decidual vasculopathy found in severe preeclampsia. There is little information on the placenta associated with AFLP. In one instance, a maternal floor infarct was found [96].

Sickle-Cell Trait/Disease and Other Hemoglobinopathies

Sickled maternal cells in the intervillous space may identify sickle cell disease, although low oxygen tension in the placenta may result in sickling of maternal erythrocytes in sickle trait as well [22]. Clinical problems and placental lesions are unlikely in uncomplicated sickle trait. Sickle cell disease has been associated with spontaneous abortion, stillbirth, premature delivery, and IUGR, although regular obstetric care and close hematologic surveillance have significantly reduced maternal and fetal morbidity. Placentas in sickle disease may be normal (with the exception of sickled maternal erythrocytes) or small and infarcted. We have seen an occasional instance of extensive placental infarction and postnatal morbidity in instances of sickle cell trait complicated by other hemoglobinopathies or maternal coagulopathies. Ultrastructural abnormalities in the umbilical vein have been attributed to hypoxia [34].

Storage Disorders

Metabolic storage disorders are rare and placental findings are incompletely documented. Placental abnormalities in some inherited metabolic storage diseases include vacuolar changes in trophoblastic, stromal, and Hofbauer cells. Placentas from two infants with Gaucher's disease causing nonimmune fetal hydrops and stillbirth were found to have circulating Gaucher cells. Genetic analysis and/or enzymatic and biochemical studies may aid in the identification of specific enzymatic defects.

Abortion, Stillbirth, and Intrauterine Fetal Death

Products of conception are commonly submitted for pathologic examination to confirm the presence of an intrauterine gestation, to exclude trophoblastic disease and, if possible, to explain why the pregnancy failed. The identification of embryonic or placental tissue – chorionic villi, implantation site infiltrated by IT, or isolated clumps of trophoblast – essentially confirms intrauterine pregnancy. Immunostaining for keratin highlights IT when findings are equivocal. When embryonic or placental tissue is not found, the possibility of an ectopic gestation cannot be excluded. It should be recognized that no combination of findings, including chorionic villi, can completely exclude an ectopic pregnancy because rarely intrauterine and tubal pregnancies occur simultaneously.

Approximately one half of all human gestations abort, of which about half are recognized by the mother or her physician. Of clinically recognized pregnancies, those that abort can be divided into two significantly different groups, early (up to 12 weeks) and late (>12 weeks). In general, embryonic/fetal factors, primarily chromosomal abnormalities, are responsible for most early abortions. Late spontaneous abortion/stillbirth is more likely to be associated with placental and maternal factors.

Early Abortion

The embryonic stage of development extends to the 8th gestational week. Early abortion includes losses up to the 12th week. More than half of early spontaneous abortions have demonstrable chromosomal anomalies, and most of these are eliminated in the embryonic period. Trisomies, triploidy, and monosomy X are most common [86].

In spontaneously passed tissue, the chorionic cavity, intact or disrupted, may be identified. The chorionic cavity is frequently empty but may contain remnants of cord or embryo. The amnionic sac, when present, is often abnormally large and prematurely fused to the chorion. Embryos frequently exhibit generalized abnormal development (growth disorganization), pointing to a high probability of a chromosomal anomaly (*Fig. 19.112*). Localized developmental defects (facial fusion defects, ocular anomalies, limb bud deformities, neural tube defects, and cervical edema) are also commonly genetically determined, although specific morphologic defects are often difficult to identify in the early embryo. These are more easily evaluated in the larger previable fetus. The finding of a well-developed, normal embryo suggests the possibility of a maternal causative factor (infection, inflammation, immune rejection, or coagulopathy), although 20–25% of morphologically normal embryos are also karyotypically abnormal, usually triploid. Accurate assessment of embryo morphology requires

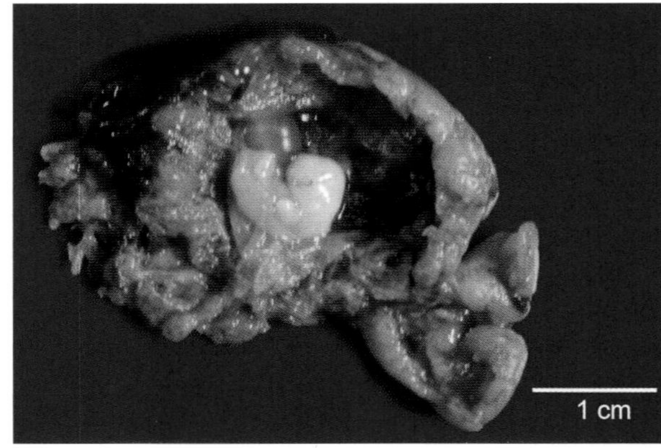

Fig. 19.112
Spontaneous abortion. **The abnormal embryo in this early abortion is closely correlated with an abnormal karyotype**

familiarity with normal developmental stages, which are well illustrated in the comprehensive work of Kalousek et al [74]. Gross assessment of the embryo and/or placenta is, at best, suboptimal in the dissociated tissues of curetted specimens.

The placenta is commonly retained in the uterus for a variable period after fetal death, and villi in abortion specimens often show alterations reflecting fetal death. Regardless of cause, fetal death leads to progressive involution of fetal vessels diffusely throughout the placenta. Involution begins with intravascular karyorrhexis (6 h), followed by septation of stem vessels (48 h) and ends with fibrous obliteration of vessels and villous stromal fibrosis (when extensive >2 weeks) [39, 50, 51]. This sequence of changes is identical to that which occurs locally in villi distal to an occluded fetal vessel.

The villi of abortions with abnormal karyotypes often appear abnormal, but the patterns are variable and nonspecific. Dysmorphic features suggestive of a chromosomal abnormality – villous enlargement with myxoid stroma, irregular villous outlines, multiple trophoblastic invaginations, and individual trophoblastic cells in the villous stroma – are common and may be more marked in karyotypically abnormal abortions, but are found in abortions with normal karyotypes as well. Complete and partial moles are the only morphologic entities with defined karyotypic abnormalities that can be diagnosed with any degree of confidence, although their distinction is becoming more difficult with earlier evacuation. Rarely, significant trophoblastic hyperplasia without molar change may occur in association with chromosomal abnormalities, (especially trisomies 7, 15, 21, and 22.) [142] These cases are best managed with a follow-up serum HCG titer to assure return to baseline.

Karyotyping may be clinically very useful in the evaluation of couples distressed by repeated spontaneous abortion. Trisomies can be identified by FISH in formalin fixed tissue. Occasionally, karyotypic abnormalities are confined to the placenta. In *confined placental mosaicism*, mosaicism is expressed in the placenta but not the fetus [73]. These placentas show no histologic abnormalities; their identification requires genetic evaluation of villous stroma and trophoblast and the fetus.

Late Abortion, Stillbirth, and Intrauterine Fetal Death

Chromosomal abnormalities still occur but are uncommon after 20 weeks. Important considerations in explaining late abortion, stillbirth, and IUFD include intrauterine infections and inflammatory processes, maternal and/or fetal circulatory compromise, destructive placental lesions, cord accidents, and fetal malformations. The gross and microscopic features of these conditions have been described throughout this chapter. Involutional changes that invariably occur following fetal death will be superimposed to greater or lesser extent. Fetomaternal hemorrhage is often overlooked as a cause of unexpected stillbirth. A Kleihauer–Betke test should be performed in all such cases. When the fetus is normally formed and the placental findings seem trivial, confined placental mosaicism is a consideration.

Recurrent pregnancy loss may be associated with thrombophilias, maternal vascular obstructive lesions, and VUE when these conditions are severe and of early onset. Massive perivillous fibrin deposition and chronic histiocytic intervillositis are rare lesions, but they almost always lead to recurrent reproductive loss in affected individuals [135, 188].

Nontrophoblastic and Metastatic Tumors

Hemangioma (Chorangioma)

Placental hemangiomas (chorangiomas) occur in about 0.5–1% of carefully examined placentas. They are usually small, entirely intraplacental, and may be difficult to appreciate, especially in the unfixed specimen. Large tumors distorting either the chorionic or basal plate are rare. Exceptionally a chorangioma is attached to the placenta by a thin pedicle. Chorangiomas are usually solitary (➲ *Fig. 19.113*), but they may be multiple or, rarely,

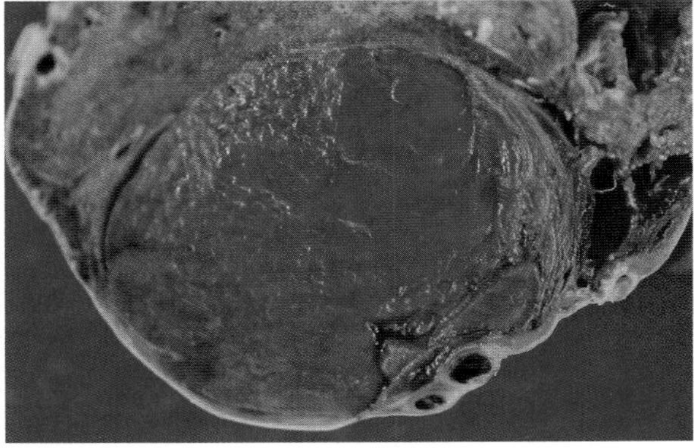

Fig. 19.113
Placental hemangioma

involve the placenta diffusely (➔ *Fig. 19.114*). They may be brown, yellow, tan, red, or white and are usually firm and well demarcated from the surrounding parenchyma. Most chorangiomas are composed of capillary-sized blood vessels supported by inconspicuous, loose stroma. Occasionally, they may be more cellular or show prominent myxoid change, hyalinization, necrosis, or calcification. Mitotic figures and nuclear atypicality have been reported in some chorangiomas, but these have not behaved aggressively. Trophoblastic hyperplasia may be prominent [110]. Localized groups of large stem villi with similar alterations but without nodular expansion have been termed localized chorangiomatosis [110].

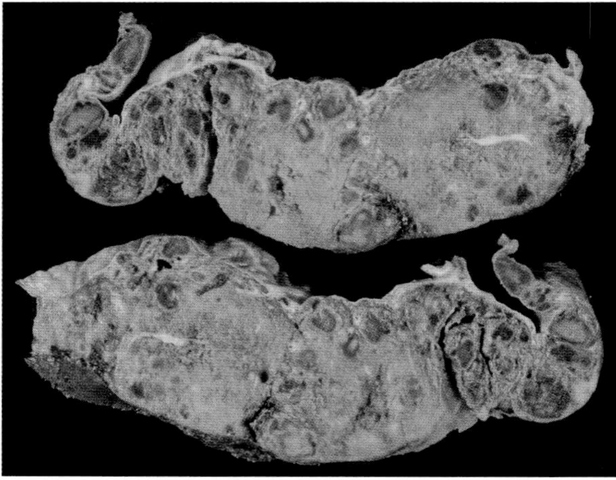

Fig. 19.114
Diffuse placental hemangioma

The tendency for chorangiomas to be found beneath the chorionic plate and at the placental margin in addition to their association with preeclampsia and high-altitude pregnancy suggest that decreased oxygen tension may play a role in their development. Although the majority of chorangiomas are of no clinical significance, various complications have been reported, usually in association with large lesions. Hydramnios and premature delivery are the most significant. Fetal cardiomegaly, congestive heart failure, and hydrops have been attributed the increased workload in shunting blood through a large chorangioma. When significant amounts of blood are directed through the chorangioma away from functional villi, chronic hypoxia may lead to intrauterine growth retardation. Complications including fetal anemia and thrombocytopenia reflect sequestration or destruction of cellular elements as they traverse the chorangioma. Skin angiomas have been reported in a few babies with placental hemangiomas.

Hepatocellular Adenoma and Adrenocortical Nodules

Rarely small nodules of hepatocytes occur in the placenta. Termed *hepatocellular adenoma*, these nodules may contain hematopoetic foci but lack bile ducts and central veins (➔ *Fig. 19.115*). Their immunoprofile is typical of hepatocytes. Tiny nodules of adrenal cortical cells have been considered heterotopias. The pathogenesis of these unusual findings is not understood.

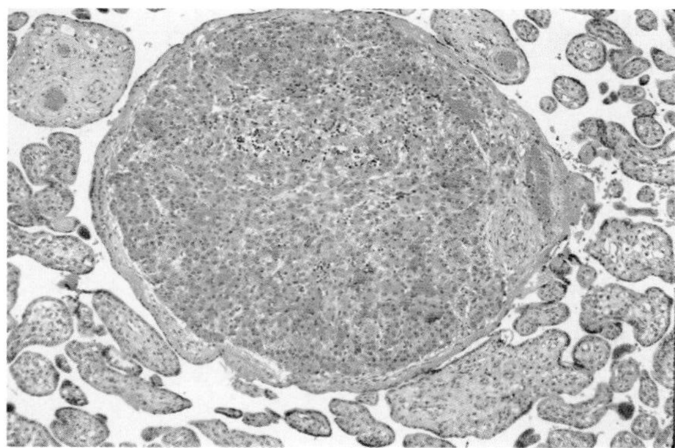

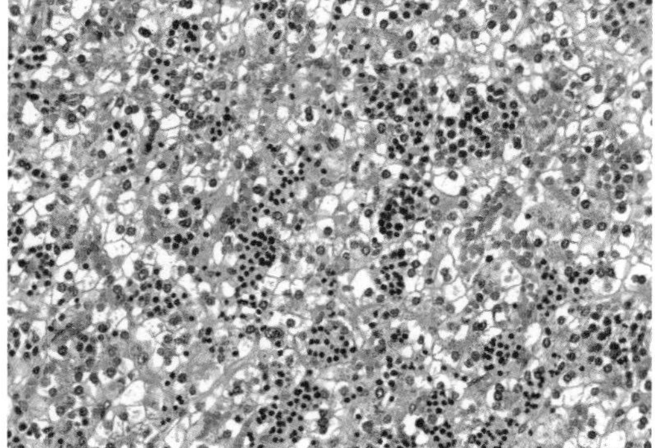

Fig. 19.115
Hepatic adenoma. This discrete collection of hepatocytes showed extramedullary hematopoiesis

Other Placental "Tumors"

Despite intraplacental location and infiltrative border, careful molecular analysis of one intraplacental leiomyoma documented its maternal origin. Teratomas have been reported to occur rarely between the amnion and chorion on the chorionic plate and in the umbilical cord. Although teratomas have been distinguished from acardiac fetuses by lack of an umbilical cord and disorganization of the component tissues, this distinction is a matter of dispute.

Placental Metastases

Either maternal or fetal neoplasms may metastasize to the placenta but they are very rare. Malignant melanoma is the most common maternal tumor to metastasize to the placenta despite the fact that other tumors are more common in this age group. Other maternal neoplasms metastasizing to the placenta have included leukemia, lymphoma, breast carcinoma, and lung carcinoma. Malignant melanoma, leukemia, and lymphoma have been reported to metastasize to the fetus transplacentally [84].

Placentas harboring maternal metastases are often normal on gross inspection, although metastatic tumor deposits may be apparent grossly (➋ *Fig. 19.116*). Tumor cells are usually confined to the intervillous space (➋ *Fig. 19.117*). Villous or fetal vascular invasion is very uncommon, and even when present, does not correlate well with fetal spread.

Dissemination of a congenital fetal tumor to the placenta is also very rare. Neuroblastoma is most common, but rare cases of fetal leukemia, lymphoma, hepatoblastoma, sarcoma, and sacrococcygeal teratoma have metastasized to the placenta (➋ *Fig. 19.118*). Disseminated histiocytosis involving the vessels of the umbilical cord has been documented. The placenta involved by a metastatic fetal tumor is consistently hydropic, pale, and bulky with tumor cells distending fetal vessels. Pigmented nevus cells may involve the villi in association with giant nevi, but these are not considered to be malignant or metastatic.

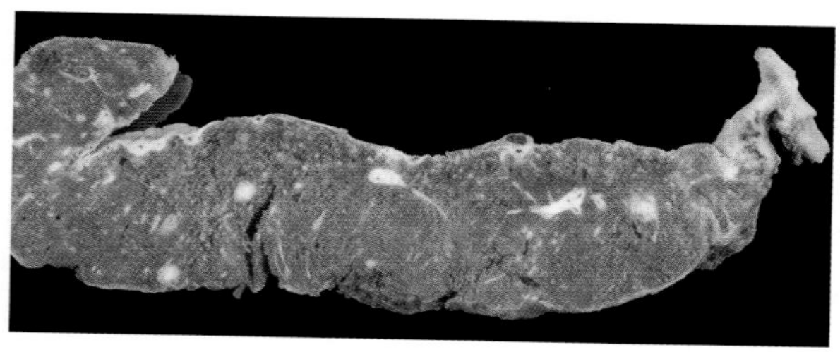

Fig. 19.116
Metastatic breast cancer. **The metastatic tumor is visible as small nodules (Used with permission of the American Registry of Pathology/Armed Forces Institute of Pathology)**

Examination of the Placenta

A gross examination of all placentas should be performed and recorded at the time of delivery by the clinician. Some

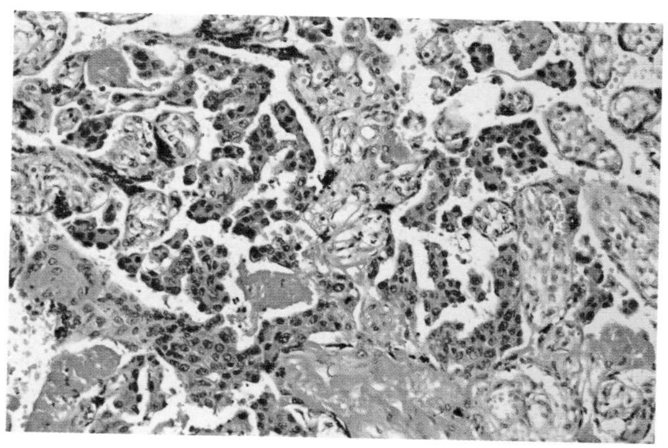

Fig. 19.117
Metastatic breast carcinoma. **Metastatic tumor cells are confined to the intervillous space**

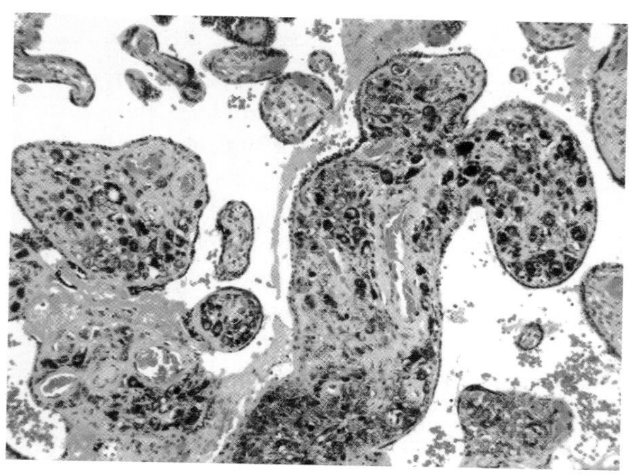

Fig. 19.118
Metastatic fetal melanoma. **This congenital scalp melanoma metastasized to the placenta**

information – length of umbilical cord, location of placenta in utero, retroplacental hematoma, ruptured membranous vessels, completeness of membranes or maternal surface – may be of immediate relevance and is best documented by the practitioner. Cultures for microorganisms and tissue for cytogenetics are best obtained at this time. Placentas are most commonly submitted to the pathologist when either the mother or infant is abnormal, the course of pregnancy, labor or delivery is complicated, a gross placental abnormality is noted, or for the evaluation of multiple pregnancy. Guidelines for submission of placentas for pathologic exam have been established [84]. A request for pathologic examination of the placenta should include the reason for submission with specific questions as well as a summary of the clinical history pertinent to that evaluation – the mother's gravidity, parity, details concerning previous pregnancies, underlying maternal disease, antepartum course, labor and deliver, and the infant's gestational age, weight, and Apgar scores. Placentas not submitted to pathology can be retained in the event that a complete placental exam should become necessary.

A good placental exam can be performed on a fresh or fixed placenta. In our institutions, the placenta is examined fresh to establish weight and pertinent measurements, perform vascular injection when indicated, and roll the membranes. After overnight fixation, the cut surfaces are examined and sections are submitted. Important abnormalities are unlikely to be overlooked when the placenta is approached systematically as follows.

Fetal membranes

Point of rupture: Measure the distance between the point of rupture and the closest placental margin. This provides information relating to the site of implantation (low-lying or placenta previa.)

Completeness: By attempting to reconstruct the amnionic sac, an estimation may be made as to whether membranes have been retained in utero.

Insertion: The membranes may insert at the margin of the placenta or central to the placental margin (circumvallate). Note extent (complete, partial) and associated changes.

Color and opacity: Opaque or cloudy membranes suggest infection. Green/brown staining suggests meconium or hemosiderin deposition.

Roll the membranes to include the point of rupture and the placental margin. Remove the membranes.

Umbilical cord

Length: Measure all pieces. The most accurate assessment of cord length is obtained in the delivery room. Umbilical cord length decreases by as much as 7 cm within a few hours of delivery.

Diameter: Measure greatest and least.

Insertion: Measure the distance between the insertion of the umbilical cord and closest placental margin. Note the mode and site of insertion and the condition of all membranous vessels.

Vessels: Normally 3.

Torsion: Degree of twist can be expressed as number of coils per 10 cm.

Other: Strictures, edema, thrombosis, hematomas, ulceration, knots.

Remove the cord flush with the placental surface.

Placenta

Measure: Measure the diameter and thickness.

Weigh: Weigh after fetal membranes, umbilical cord and large clots have been removed. Formalin fixation adds about 10% to placental weight.

Shape: Note anomalous shapes.

Fetal surface: Evaluate color (blue, green, brown) and chorionic vessels. Arteries cross over veins.

Maternal surface: The maternal surface should be complete. Missing fragments suggest retained placental tissue. Evaluate all clots for site, size, and related placental alterations. Breadloaf the placenta at 1 cm intervals.

Cut surface: Placental color reflects fetal blood content. Describe, measure, and locate focal abnormalities. Assess percentage when large lesions or significant proportions of the placenta are altered.

Sections

Two sections of umbilical cord and two sections of the membrane roll can be included in one block. Do not section the cord within 2 cm of the insertion site – this may give a false impression of SUA. We routinely submit at least three sections of placenta including two sections from grossly normal central placental parenchyma. Additional sections to demonstrate pathologic alterations are submitted as appropriate. Selection of microscopic sections should be tailored to the specific clinical scenario. For example, additional sections of the membrane roll or basal plate optimizes evaluation of maternal vessels when there is a history of preeclampsia.

Special aspects of Multiple Pregnancy

The delivering physician should identify the umbilical cords, but if not, they can be arbitrarily identified or by distinguishing characteristics (cord length, insertion site, etc.). Maintain the separate identity of each placenta grossly and microscopically.

Placentation type: Two entirely separate placentas are obviously dichorionic, requiring routine examination. To distinguish between DiMo and DiDi fused placentas, assess the dividing membranes and fetal vascular pattern. In DiDi fused placentas, the septum is opaque and the fetal vessels do not cross the line of fusion. In DiMo placentas, the septum is thin and the two vascular districts are intermingled.

Placental mass: Quantify the placental mass belonging to each infant. DiDi fused placentas can be separated along the line of fusion and weighed separately. The placental territories of monochorionic infants correspond best with their chorionic venous distribution.

Vascular anastomoses: Assess monochorionic placentas for vascular anastomoses. Large chorionic vessel anastomoses are easily identified grossly. Deep arteriovenous anastomoses cannot be seen but can be screened for with air injection. After clamping the arteries proximally, inject them with air using a plastic syringe. Anastomoses will allow air to pass from an artery into a vein of the co-twin. Repeat to establish the extent of anastomoses. Placental injection studies require fresh placentas and may be compromised by villous disruption.

Special Techniques

Cytogenetics: Placental tissue may be easier to grow and karyotype than other fetal tissue. Chorionic villous sampling early in pregnancy is being used for prenatal diagnosis. Flow cytometry may be useful in the evaluation of molar pregnancies. Genetic questions regarding specific chromosomes may be addressed by FISH.

Culture: This is usually done by the obstetrician. Cultures may be accomplished by swabs of the amnionic surface or subchorionic fibrin after searing the amnion.

Immunoperoxidase stains: This technique may be useful in the identification of infectious agents and the delineation of cell types (i.e., CD68 in chronic histiocytic intervillositis.)

References

1. Abramowsky C, Beyer-Patterson P et al (1991) Nonsyphilitic spirochetosis in second-trimester fetuses. Pediatr Pathol 11:827–838
2. Adams-Chapman I, Vaucher YE et al (2002) Maternal floor infarction of the placenta: association with central nervous system injury and adverse neurodevelopmental outcome. J Perinatol 22:236–241
3. Al-Adnani M, Kiho L et al (2008) Recurrent massive perivillous fibrin deposition associated with polymyositis: a case report and review of the literature. Pediatr Dev Pathol 11:226–229
4. Altshuler G (1984) Chorangiosis. An important placental sign of neonatal morbidity and mortality. Arch Pathol Lab Med 108:71–74
5. Altshuler G, Hyde S (1989) Meconium-induced vasocontraction: a potential cause of cerebral and other fetal hypoperfusion and of poor pregnancy outcome. J Child Neurol 4:137–142
6. Ananth CV, Oyelese Y et al (2005) Placental abruption in the United States, 1979 through 2001: temporal trends and potential determinants. Am J Obstet Gynecol 192:191–198
7. Ananth CV, Vintzileos AM et al (1998) Standards of birth weight in twin gestations stratified by placental chorionicity. Obstet Gynecol 91:917–924
8. Arias F, Rodriguez L et al (1993) Maternal placental vasculopathy and infection: two distinct subgroups among patients with preterm labor and preterm ruptured membranes. Am J Obstet Gynecol 168:585–591
9. Arias F, Romero R et al (1998) Thrombophilia: A mechanism of disease in women with adverse pregnancy outcome and thrombotic lesions in the placenta. J Matern Fetal Med 7:277–286
10. Ariel IB, Anteby E et al (2004) Placental pathology in fetal thrombophilia. Hum Pathol 35:729–733
11. Badawi N, Felix JF et al (2005) Cerebral palsy following term newborn encephalopathy. Devel Med Child Neurol 47:293–298
12. Baergen RN (2007) Cord abnormalities, structural lesions, and cord accidents. Semin Diag Pathol 24:23–32
13. Baergen RN, Malicki D et al (2001) Morbidity. mortality, and placental pathology in excessively long umbilical cords; retrospective study. Pediatr Devel Pathol 4:144–153
14. Baldwin VJ (1994) Pathology of multiple pregnancy. Springer, New York
15. Barth WH Jr, Genest DR et al (1996) Uterine arcuate artery Doppler and decidual microvascular pathology in pregnancies complicated by type I diabetes mellitus. Ultrasound Obstet Gynecol 8:98–103
16. Baschat AA, Gungor S et al (2007) Nucleated red blood cell counts in the first week of life: a critical appraisal of relationships with perinatal outcome in preterm growth restricted neonates. Am J Obstet Gynecol 197(3):286.e1–286.e8
17. Benirschke K, Kaufmann P et al (2006) Pathology of the human placenta, 5th edn. Springer, New York
18. Benirschke K, Masliah E (2001) The placenta in multiple pregnancy: outstanding issues. Reprod Fertil Dev 13(7–8):615–622
19. Berg TG, Rayburn WF (1995) Umbilical cord length and acid-base balance at delivery. J Reprod Med 40:1–12
20. Bieber FR, Nance WE et al (1981) Genetic studies of an acardiac monster: evidence of polar body twinning in man. Science 213:775–777
21. Blanc WA (1959) Amnionic infection syndrome. Pathogenesis, morphology, and significance in circumnatal mortality. Clin Obstet Gynaecol 2:705–734
22. Bloomfield RD, Suarez JR et al (1978) The placenta: a diagnostic tool in sickle cell disorders. J Natl Med Assoc 70:87–88

23. Boyd JD, Hamilton WJ (1970) The human placenta. Heffer, Cambridge
24. Bruner JP, Anderson TL et al (1998) Placental pathophysiology of the twin: oligohydramnios-polyhydramnios sequence and the twin-twin transfusion syndrome. Placenta 19:81–86
25. Burke CJ, Tannenberg AE (1995) Prenatal brain damage and placental infarction-An autopsy study. Devel Med Child Neurol 37:555–562
26. Chan OT, Mannino FL et al (2007) A retrospective analysis of placentas from twin pregnancies derived from assisted reproductive technology. Twin Res Hum Genet 10(2):385–393
27. Cleary GM, Wiswell TE (1998) Meconium-stained amnionic fluid and the meconium aspiration syndrome. An update. Pediatr Clin North Amer 45:511–529
28. Cooperstock MS, Tummara R et al (2000) Twin birth weight discordance and risk of preterm birth. Am J Obstet Gynecol 183:63–67
29. Curtin WM, Shehata BM et al (2002) The feasibility of using histologic placental sections to predict newborn nucleated red blood cell counts. Obstet Gynecol 110:305–310
30. Dahms B, Boyd T et al (2002) Severe perinatal liver disease associated with fetal thrombotic vasculopathy in the placenta. Pediatr Devel Pathol 5:80–85
31. Davis BH, Olsen S et al (1998) Detection of fetal red cells in fetomaternal hemorrhage using a fetal hemoglobin monoclonal antibody by flow cytometry. Transfusion 38:749–756
32. De Laat MWM, van Alderen ED et al (2007) The umbilical coiling index in complicated pregnancy. Eur J Obstet Gynecol Reprod Biol 130:66–72
33. Deans A, Jauniaux E (1998) Prenatal diagnosis and outcome of subamniotic hematomas. Ultrasound Obstet Gynecol 11:319–323
34. Decastel M, Leborgne-Samuel Y (1999) Morphological features of the human umbilical vein in normal, sickle cell trait, and sickle cell disease pregnancies. Hum Pathol 30(1):13–20
35. DeSa DJ (1973) Intimal cushions of foetal placental veins. J Pathol 110:347–352
36. Di Naro E, Ghezzi F et al (2001) Umbilical vein blood flow in fetuses with normal and lean umbilical cord. Ultrasound Obstet Gynecol 17:224–228
37. Dizon-Townson DS, Meline L et al (1997) Fetal carriers of the factor V Leiden mutation are prone to miscarriage and placental infarction. Am J Obstet Gynecol 177:402–405
38. Doss BJ, Jacques SM et al (1998) Maternal scleroderma: placenta findings and perinatal outcome. Hum Pathol 28:1524–1530
39. Dr G, Singer DB (1992) Estimating the time of death in stillborn fetuses: III. External fetal examination; a study of 86 stillborns. Obstet Gynecol 80:593–600
40. Esplin MS (2006) Preterm birth: a review of genetic factors and future directions for genetic study. Obstet Gynecol Survey 61:800–806
41. Fernandes BJ, von Dadelszen P et al (2007) Flow cytometric assessment of feto-maternal hemorrhage; a comparison with Bettke-Kleihauer. Prenat Diagn 27:641–643
42. Fok RY, Pavlova Z et al (1990) The correlation of arterial lesions with umbilical artery Doppler velocimetry in the placentas of small-for-dates pregnancies. Obstet Gynecol 75:578–583
43. Fox H (1966) Thrombosis of the foetal stem arteries in the human placenta. J Obstet Gynaecol Br Commonwealth 73:961–965
44. Fox H (1997) Pathology of the placenta, 2nd edn. Saunders, Philadelphia
45. Fox H, Sebire NJ (2007) Pathology of the placenta, 3rd edn. Saunders, Philadelphia
46. Frank HG, Malekzadeh F et al (1994) Immunohistochemistry of two different types of placental fibrinoid. Acta Anat 150:55–68
47. Fraser RB, Wright JR (2002) Eosinophilic/T-cell chorionic vasculitis. Pedatri Dev Pathol 5:350–355
48. Gardella C, Riley DE et al (2004) Identification and sequencing of bacterial rDNAs in culture-negative amniotic fluid from women in premature labor. Am J Perinatol 21:319–323
49. Gardiner JP (1922) The umbilical cord: normal length; length in cord complications; etiology and frequency of coiling. Surg Gynecol Obstet 34:252–256
50. Genest DR (1992) Estimating the time of death in stillborn fetuses: II. Histologic evaluation of the placenta; a study of 71 stillborns. Obstet Gynecol 80:585–592
51. Genest DR, Williams MA et al (1992) Estimating the time of death in stillborn fetuses: I. Histologic evaluation of fetal organs; an autopsy study of 150 stillborns. Obstet Gynecol 80:575–584
52. Ghidini A, Spong CY (2001) Severe meconium aspiration syndrome is not caused by aspiration of meconium. Am J Obstet Gynecol 185:931–938
53. Giles WB, Trudinger BJ et al (1985) Fetal umbilical artery flow velocity waveforms and placental resistance: pathological correlation. Brit J Obstet Gynaecol 92:31–38
54. Gomez R, Romero R et al (1998) The fetal inflammatory response syndrome. Am J Obstet Gynecol 179:194–202
55. Greer IA (1999) Thrombosis in pregnancy: maternal and fetal issues. Lancet 353:1258–1265
56. Gupta N, Sebire NJ et al (2004) Massive perivillous fibrin deposition associated with discordant fetal growth in a dichorionic twin pregnancy. J Obstet Gynaecol 24:579–580
57. Han YW, Redline RW et al (2004) *Fusobacterium nucleatum* induces premature and term stillbirths in pregnant mice: implication of oral bacteria in preterm birth. Infect Immun 72:2272–2279
58. Hansen AR, Collins MH et al (2000) Very low birthweight infant's placenta and its relation to pregnancy and fetal characteristics. Pediatr Devel Pathol 3:419–430
59. Hansen AR, Collins MH et al (2000) Very low birthweight placenta; clustering of morphologic characteristics. Pediatr Devel Pathol 3:431–438
60. Hashimoto K, Clapp JF (2003) The effect of nuchal cord on amniotic fluid and cord blood erythropoetin at delivery. J Soc Gynecol Investig 10:406–411
61. Hecht JL, Allred EN et al (2008) Histologic characteristics of singleton placentas delivered before the 28th week of gestation. Pathology 40:372–376
62. Heller DS, Rush D et al (2003) Subchorionic hematoma associated with thrombophilia: report of three cases. Pediatr Dev Pathol 6:261–264
63. Hermansen MC (2001) Nucleated red blood cells in the fetus and newborn. Arch Dis Child Fetal Neonatal Ed 84:F211–F215
64. Hershkovitz R, Silberstein T et al (2001) Risk factors associated with true knots of the umbilical cord. Eur J Obstet Gyneco Biol 93:36–39
65. Hill GB (1998) Preterm birth: associations with genital and possibly oral microflora. Ann Periodontal 3:222–232
66. Hung NA, Jackson C et al (2005) Pregnancy-related polymyositis and massive perivillous fibrin deposition in the placenta: are they pathogenetically related? Arthr Rhematism 55:154–156
67. Huppertz B, Kadyrov M et al (2006) Apoptosis and its role in the trophoblast. Am J Obstet Gynecol 195:29–39
68. Ibdah JA, Bennett MJ et al (1999) A fetal fatty acid oxidation disorder as a cause of liver disease in pregnant women. N Engl J Med 340:1723–1731

69. Jacques SM, Qureshi F (1998) Chronic chorioamnionitis: a clinicopathologic and immunohistochemical study. Hum Pathol 29:1457–1461
70. Jamshed S, Kouides P et al (2007) Pathology of thrombotic thrombocytopenic purpura in the placenta, with emphasis on the "snowman sign.". Pediatr Dev Pathol 10:455–462
71. Jauniaux E, Nicolaides KH et al (1997) Perinatal features associated with placental mesenchymal dysplasia. Placenta 18:701–706
72. Kalousek DK, Bamforth S (1988) Amnion rupture sequence in previable fetuses. Am J Med Genet 31:63–73
73. Kalousek DK, Barrett I (1994) Confined placental mosaicism and stillbirth. Pediatr Pathol 14:151–159
74. Kalousek DK, Fitch N et al (1990) Pathology of the human embryo and previable fetus. An atlas. Springer, New York
75. Kaplan C, Blanc WA et al (1982) Identification of erythrocytes in intervillous thrombi. A study using immunoperoxidase identification of hemoglobins. Hum Pathol 13:554–557
76. Katz VL, DiTomasso J et al (2002) Activated protein C resistance associated with maternal floor infarction treated with low-molecular-weight heparin. Am J Perinatol 19:273–277
77. Katzman PJ, Genest DR (2002) Maternal floor infarction and massive perivillous fibrin deposition: histological definitions, association with intrauterine fetal growth restriction, and risk of recurrence. Pediatr Devel Pathol 5:159–164
78. Keenan WJ, Steichen JJ et al (1977) Placental pathology compared with clinical outcome. Am J Dis Child 131:1224–1227
79. Keogh JM, Badawi N (2006) The origins of cerebral palsy. Curr Opin Neurol 19:129–134
80. Khong TY (1999) The placenta in maternal hyperhomocysteinaemia. Br J Obstet Gynaecol 106:2733–2738
81. Kim CJ, Yoon BH et al (2001) Umbilical arteritis and phlebitis mark different stages of the fetal inflammatory response. Am J Obstet Gynecol 185(2):496–500
82. King EL, Redline RW et al (2004) Myocytes of chorionic vessels from placentas with meconium-associated vascular necrosis exhibit apoptotic markers. Hum Pathol 35(4):412–417
83. Kraus FT, Acheen VI (1999) Fetal thrombotic vasculopathy in the placenta: cerebral thrombi and infarcts, coagulopathies, and cerebral palsy. Hum Pathol 30:759–769
84. Kraus FT, Redline RW et al (2004) Placental pathology. ARP/AFIP, Washington DC
85. Kumar D, Fung W et al (2006) Proinflammatory cytokines found in amniotic fluid induce collagen remodeling, apoptosis, and biophysical weakening of cultured human fetal membranes. Biol Report 74(1):29–34
86. Lash GB, Quenby S et al (2008) Gestational diseases – a workshop report. Placenta 22:S92–S94
87. Leistra-Leistra MJ, Timmer A et al (2004) Fetal thrombotic vasculopathy in the placenta: a thrombophilic connection between pregnancy complications and neonatal thrombosis? Placenta 25(Suppl A):S102–S105
88. Leviton A, Paneth N et al (1999) Maternal infection, fetal inflammatory response, and brain damage in very low birth weight infants. Developmental Epidemiology Network Investigators. Pediatr Res 46(5):566–575
89. Lim FT, Scherjon SA et al (2000) Association of stress during delivery with increased numbers of nucleated cells and hematologic progenitor cells in umbilical cord blood. Am J Obstet Gynecol 183:1144–1151
90. Lim LK, Zhou Y et al (1997) Human cytotrophoblast differentiation/invasion is abnormal in pre-eclampsia. Am J Pathol 151:1809–1818
91. Lin MG (2006) Umbilical cord prolapse. Obstet Gynecol Surv 61(4):269–277
92. Machin GA, Ackerman J et al (2000) Abnormal umbilical cord coiling is associated with adverse perinatal outcomes. Pediatr Devel Pathol 3:462–471
93. Magid MS, Kaplan C et al (1998) Placental pathology in systemic lupus erythematosus: a prospective study. Am J Obstet Gynecol 179:226–236
94. Many A, Elad R et al (2002) Third trimester unexplained intrauterine fetal death is associated with inherited thrombophilia. Obstet Gynecol 99:684–687
95. Many A, Schreiber L et al (2001) Pathologic features of the placenta in women with severe pregnancy complications and thrombophilia. Obstet Gynecol 98:1041–1044
96. Matern D, Shehata BM et al (2001) Placental floor infarction complicating the pregnancy of a fetus with long-chain 3-hydroxyacyl-CoA dehydrogenase (LCHAD) deficiency. Mol Genet Metab 72:265–268
97. McDonald DG, Kelehan P et al (2004) Placental fetal thrombotic vasculopathy is associated with neonatal encephalopathy. Hum Pathol 35:875–880
98. Menezo YJ, Sakkas D (2002) Monozygotic twining: is it related to apoptosis in the embryo? Hum Reprod 17:247–248
99. Miller PW, Coen RW et al (1985) Dating the time interval from meconium passage to birth. Obstet Gynecol 66:459–462
100. Mitra SC, Seshan SV et al (2000) Placental vessel morphometry in growth retardation and increased resistance of the umbilical artery Doppler flow. J Matern Fetal Med 9:282–286
101. Moscoso G, Jauniaux E et al (1991) Placental vascular anomaly with diffuse mesenchymal stem villous hyperplasia. A new clinico-pathological entity? Path Res Pract 187:324–328
102. Mutter WP, Karumanchi SA (2008) Molecular mechanisms of pre-eclampsia. Microvasc Res 75:1–8
103. Myerson D, Parkin RK (2006) The pathogenesis of villitis of unknown etiology: analysis with a new conjoint immunohistochemistry-in situ hybridization procedure to identify specific maternal and fetal cells. Pediatr Dev Pathol 9(4):257–265
104. Naeye RL (1985) Umbilical cord length: clinical significance. J Pediatr 107:278–281
105. Naeye RL, Maisels J et al (1983) The clinical significance of placental villous edema. Pediatrics 71:588–594
106. Naeye RL, Shaffer ML (2005) Postnatal laboratory timers of antenatal hypoxic-ischemic brain damage. J Perinatol 25:664–668
107. Nelson KB, Dambrosia JM et al (1998) Neonatal cytokines and coagulation factors in children with cerebral palsy. Ann Neurol 44:665–675
108. Nelson KB, Dambrosia JM et al (2005) Genetic polymorphisms and cerebral palsy in very preterm infants. Pediatr Res 57:494–499
109. Nelson KB, Grether KJ (1998) Potentially asphyxiating conditions and spastic cerebral palsy in infants of normal birth weight. Am J Obstet Gynecol 179:507–513
110. Ogino S, Redline RW (2000) Villous capillary lesions of the placenta: Distinctions between chorangioma, chorangiomatosis, and chorangiosis. Hum Pathol 31:945–954
111. Ohyama M, Itani Y et al (2002) Re-evaluation of chorioamnionitis and funisitis with a special reference to subacute chorioamnionitis. Hum Pathol 33:183–190
112. Ordi J, Ismail MR et al (1998) Massive chronic intervillositis of the placenta associated with malaria infection. Am J Surg Pathol 22:1006–1011

113. Parast MM, Crum CP et al (2008) Placental histological criteria for umbilical flow restriction in unexplained stillbirth. Hum Pathol 39:948–953
114. Patel D, Dawson M et al (1989) Umbilical cord circumference at birth. Am J Dis Child 143:638–639
115. Peng HW, Levitin-Smith M et al (2006) Umbilical cord stricture and overcoiling are common causes of fetal demise. Pediatr Dev Pathol 9:14–19
116. Pham T, Steele J et al (2006) Placental mesenchymal dysplasia is associated with high rates of intrauterine growth restriction and fetal demise. A report of 11 new cases and review of the literature. AOLP 126:67–78
117. Pharaoh P, Adi Y (2000) Consequences of in-utero death in twin pregnancy. Lancet 355:1597–1602
118. Phelan JP, Korst LM et al (1998) Neonatal nucleated red blood cell and lymphocyte counts in fetal brain injury. Obstet Gynecol 91:485–489
119. Qureshi F, Jacques SM (1994) Marked segmental thinning of the umbilical cord vessels. Arch Pathol Lab Med 118:826–830
120. Raio L, Ghezzi F (1998) The clinical significance of antenatal detection of discordant umbilical arteries. Obstet Gynecol 91:86–91
121. Raio L, Ghezzi F et al (1999) Prenatal diagnosis of a lean umbilical cord: A simple marker for the fetus at risk of being small for gestational age at birth. Ultrasound Obstet Gynecol 13:176–180
122. Rakheja D, Bennett MJ et al (2002) Long-chain L-3-hydroxyacyl-coenzyme A dehydrogenase deficiency: a molecular and biochemical review. Lab Invest 82:815–824
123. Rand JH (2000) Antiphospholipid antibody-mediated disruption of the annexin-V antithrombotic shield: a thrombogenic mechanism for the antiphospholipid syndrome. J Autoimmun 15:107–111
124. Rayne SC, Kraus FT (1993) Placental thrombi and other vascular lesions. Classification, morphology, and clinical correlations. Pathol Res Pract 189:2–17
125. Redline RW (1988) Role of local immunosuppression in murine fetoplacental listeriosis. J Clin Invest 79:1234–1241
126. Redline RW (1988) Specific defects in the anti-listerial immune response in discrete regions of the murine uterus and placenta account for susceptibility to infection. J Immunol 140:3947–3955
127. Redline RW (2002) Clinically and biologically relevant patterns of placental inflammation. Pediatr Dev Pathol 5:326–328
128. Redline RW (2004) Clinical and pathological umbilical cord abnormalities in fetal thrombotic vasculopathy. Hum Pathol 35:1494–1498
129. Redline RW (2004) Placental inflammation. Seminars Neonat 9:265–274
130. Redline RW (2005) Severe fetal placental vascular lesions in term infants with neurologic impairment. Am J Obstet Gynecol 192:452–457
131. Redline RW (2006) Inflammatory responses in the placenta and umbilical cord. Sem Fetal and Neonat Med 11:296–301
132. Redline RW (2006) Thrombophilia and placental pathology. Clin Obstet and Gynecol 49(4):885–894
133. Redline RW (2006) Placental pathology and cerebral palsy. Clin Perinat 33:503–516
134. Redline RW (2007) Infections and other inflammatory conditions. Sem Diag Pathol 24:5–13
135. Redline RW (2007) Villitis of unknown etiology: noninfectious chronic villitis in the placenta. Hum Pathol 38(10):1439–1446
136. Redline RW (2008) Placental pathology: a systematic approach with clinical correlations. Placenta 29:S86–S89
137. Redline RW (2008) Elevated circulating fetal nucleated red blood cells and placental pathology in term infants who develop cerebral palsy. Hum Pathol 39:1378–1384
138. Redline RW, Ariel IB et al (2004) Fetal vascular obstructive lesions: Nosology and reproducibility of placental reaction patterns. Pediatr Devel Pathol 7:443–452
139. Redline RW, Boyd T et al (2004) Maternal vascular underperfusion: nosology and reproducibility of placental reaction patterns. Pediatr Devel Pathol 7:237–249
140. Redline RW, Dinesh S et al (2001) Placental lesions associated with abnormal growth in twins. Pediatr Dev Pathol 4:473–481
141. Redline RW, Faye-Petersen O et al (2003) Amniotic infection syndrome: nosology and reproducibility of placental reaction patterns. Pediatr Dev Pathol 6:435–448
142. Redline RW, Hassold T et al (1998) Determinants of villous trophoblastic hyperplasia in spontaneous abortions. Mod Pathol 11(8):762–768
143. Redline RW, Jiang JG et al (2003) Discordancy for maternal floor infarction in dizygotic twin placentas. Hum Pathol 34:822–824
144. Redline RW, Minich N et al (2007) Placental lesions as predictors of cerebral palsy and abnormal neurocognitive function in extremely low birth weight infants (<1kg). Pediatr Dev Pathol 10:282–292
145. Redline RW, O' Riordan MA (2000) Placental lesions associated with cerebral palsy and neurologic impairment following term birth. Arch Pathol Lab Med 124:1785–1791
146. Redline RW, Pappin A (1995) Fetal thrombotic vasculopathy: the clinical significance of extensive avascular villi. Hum Pathol 26:80–85
147. Redline R, Patterson R (1993) Villitis of unknown etiology is associated with major infiltration of fetal tissues by maternal cells. Am J Pathol 143:332–336
148. Redline RW, Patterson P (1994) Patterns of placental injury: correlation with gestational age, placental weight, and clinical diagnosis. Arch Pathol Lab Med 118:698–701
149. Redline RW, Patterson P (1995) Preeclampsia is associated with an excess of proliferative immature intermediate trophoblast. Hum Pathol 26:594–600
150. Redline RW, Wilson-Costello D et al (1998) Placental lesions associated with neurologic impairment and cerebral palsy in very low birth weight infants. Arch Pathol Lab Med 122:1091–1098
151. Redline RW, Wilson-Costello D et al (1999) Chronic peripheral separation of placenta. The significance of diffuse chorioamniotic hemosiderosis. Am J Clin Pathol 111:804–810
152. Resnik R (2002) Intrauterine growth restriction. Obstet Gynecol 99:490–496
153. Reynolds MA, Schieve LA et al (2003) Trends in multiple births conceived using assisted reproductive technology, United States, 1997–2000. Pediatrics 111:1159–1162
154. Rigano S, Bozzo M et al (2001) Early and persistent reduction in umbilical vein flow in the growth restricted fetus: A longitudinal study. Am J Obstet Gynecol 185:834–838
155. Rodger MA, Paidas M et al (2008) Inherited thrombophilia and pregnancy complications revisited. Obstet Gynecol 112:320–324
156. Rodriguez MM, Chaves F et al (2002) Value of autopsy in nonimmune hydrops fetalis: Series of 51 stillborn fetuses. Pediatr Devel Pathol 5:365–374
157. Rogers BB, Alexander JM et al (2002) Umbilical vein interleukin-6 levels correlate with the severity of placental inflammation and gestational age. Hum Pathol 33:335–340
158. Salafia CM (1997) Placental pathology of fetal growth restriction. Clin Obstet Gynaecol 40:740–749

159. Salafia CM, Cowchock FS (1997) Placental pathology and antiphospholipid antibodies: a descriptive study. Am J Perinatol 14(8):435–441
160. Salafia CM, Pezzullo JC et al (1997) Placental pathology of absent and reversed end-diastolic flow in growth-restricted fetuses. Obstet Gynecol 90:830–836
161. Sander CH (1980) Hemorrhagic endovasculitis and hemorrhagic villitis of the placenta. Arch Pathol Lab Med 104:371–373
162. Sander CM, Gilliland D et al (2002) Livebirths with placental hemorrhagic vasculitis. Interlesional relationships and perinatal outcomes. Arch Pathol Lab Med 126:157–164
163. Sato Y, Benirschke K (2006) Increased prevalence of fetal thrombi in monochorionic-twin placentas. Pediatrics 117(1):e113–e117
164. Sato Y, Benirschke K (2006) Umbilical arterial thrombosis with vascular wall necrosis: clinicopathologic findings of 11 cases. Placenta 27:715–718
165. Scott JM (1983) Fibrinous vasculosis in the human placenta. Placenta 4:87–100
166. Sebire NJ, Backos M et al (2002) Placental massive perivillous fibrin deposition associated with antiphospholipid antibody syndrome. Br J Obstet Gynaecol 109:570–573
167. Sebire NJ, Sepulveda W (2008) Correlating placental pathology with ultrasound findings. J Clin Pathol 61:1276–1284
168. Sepulveda W, Corral E et al (2003) Umbilical artery aneurysm: prenatal identification in three fetuses with trisomy 18. Ultra Obstet Gynecol 21:292–296
169. Shamonki JM, Salmon JE et al (2007) Excessive complement is associated with placental injury in patients with antiphospholipid antibodies. Am J Obstet Gynecol 196(2):167.e1–167.e5
170. Shanklin DR, Scott JS (1975) Massive subchorial thrombohaematoma. (Breus' mole). Br J Obstet Gynaecol 82:476–487
171. Shekhawat P, Matern D et al (2005) Fetal fatty acid oxidation disorders, their effect on maternal health and neonatal outcome: Impact of expanded newborn screening on their diagnosis and management. Pediatr Res 57:78R–86R
172. Shih I-M, Seidman JD et al (1999) Placental site nodule and characterization of distinctive types of intermediate trophoblast. Hum Pathol 30:687–694
173. Sienko A, Altshuler G (1999) Meconium-induced umbilical vascular necrosis in abortuses and fetuses: a histopathologic study for cytokines. Obstet Gynecol 94:415–420
174. Silver RK, Dooley SL et al (1987) Umbilical cord size and amniotic fluid volume in prolonged pregnancy. Am J Obstet Gynecol 157:716–720
175. Soernes T (1995) Umbilical cord encirclements and fetal growth restriction. Obstet Gynecol 86:725–728
176. Sohan K, Carroll SG et al (2001) Analysis of outcome in hydrops fetalis in relation to gestational age at diagnosis, cause and treatment. Acta Obstet Gynecol Scand 80:726–730
177. Soma H, Watanabe Y et al (1996) Chorangiosis and chorangioma in three cohorts of placentas from Nepal, Tibet, and Japan. Reprod Fertil Devel 7:1533–1538
178. Souter VL, Kapur RP et al (2003) A report of dizygous monochorionic twins. NEJM 349:154–158
179. Steffensen T, Gilbert-Barness E et al (2008) Placental pathology in TRAP sequence: clinical and pathogenetic implication. Fetal Pediatr Path 27:13–29
180. Tan TYT, Sepulveda W (2003) Acardiac twin: a systematic review of minimally invasive treatment modalities. Ultrasound Obstet Gynaecol II 22:409–419
181. Teramo KA, Widness JA (2008) Increased fetal plasma and amniotic fluid erythropoetin concentrations: markers of intrauterine hypoxia. Neonatology 95(2):105–116
182. Torpin R (1965) Amniochorionic mesoblastic fibrous strings and amnionic bands: associated contricting fetal malformations of fetal death. Am J Obstet Gynecol 91:65–75
183. Trainor B, Tubman R (2006) The emerging pattern of hydrops fetalis-incidence, etiology, and management. Ulster Med J 75:185–186
184. Turan S, Miller J et al (2008) Integrated testing and management in fetal growth restriction. Semin Perinatol 32:194–200
185. Venkatesha S, Toporsian M et al (2006) Soluble endoglin contributes to the pathogenesis of preeclampsia. Nat Med 12:642–649
186. Vernof K, Benirschke K et al (1992) Maternal floor infarction: Relation to X cells, major basic protein, and adverse perinatal outcome. Am J Obstet Gynecol 167:1355–1363
187. Viscardi RM, Sun CC CC (2001) Placental lesion multiplicity: risk factor for IUGR and neonatal cranial ultrasound abnormalities. Early Hum Devel 62:1–10
188. Waters BL, Ashikaga T (2006) Significance of perivillous fibrin/oid deposition in uterine evacuation specimens. Am J Surg Pathol 30:760–765
189. Weber MA, Nikkels PGJ et al (2006) Co-occurrence of massive perivillous fibrin deposition and chronic intervillositis: case report. Pediatr Dev Pathol 9:234–238
190. Wilkins-Haug L, Quade B et al (2006) Confined placental mosaicism as a risk factor among newborns with fetal growth restriction. Prenat Diagn 26:428–432
191. Wong AE, Sepulveda W (2005) Acardiac anomaly: current issues in prenatal assessment and treatment. Prenat Diagn 25:796–806
192. Wyatt S, Kraus FT et al (2005) The correlation between sampling site and gene expression in the term human placenta. Placenta 26:372–379
193. Yeruchimovich M, Dollberg S et al (1999) Nucleated red blood cells in infants of smoking mothers. Obstet Gynecol 93:403–406
194. Zhang J, Kraus FT et al (1985) Chorioamnionitis: a comparative histologic, bacteriologic, and clinical study. Int J Gynecol Pathol 4:1–10
195. Ziska Z, Fait T et al (2008) ABO fetomaternal compatibility poses a risk for massive fetomaternal transplacental hemorrhage. Acta Obstet Gynecol Scand 87:1011–1014

20 Gestational Trophoblastic Tumors and Related Tumor-Like Lesions

Ie-Ming Shih · Michael T. Mazur · Robert J. Kurman

R. J. Kurman, L. Hedrick Ellenson, B. M. Ronnett (eds.), *Blaustein's Pathology of the Female Genital Tract (6th ed.)*, DOI 10.1007/978-1-4419-0489-8_20,

Introduction

Gestational trophoblastic disease (GTD) encompasses a heterogeneous group of lesions with specific clinical features, morphological characteristics, and pathogenesis. The World Health Organization classification of GTD includes complete and partial hydatidiform mole, invasive mole, choriocarcinoma, placental site trophoblastic tumor (PSTT), epithelioid trophoblastic tumor, exaggerated placental site, and placental site nodule (➔ *Table 20.1*) [145]. Some of these lesions are true neoplasms, whereas others represent abnormally formed placentas with a predisposition for neoplastic transformation of the trophoblast. Two benign entities, the exaggerated placental site and the placental site nodule, are included because they are trophoblastic lesions that must be distinguished from other entities with malignant potential. The literature on GTD is extensive and at times confusing because of inconsistencies in classification and terminology. In fact, the necessity of a morphologic classification has been questioned, because current management is largely medical and in the case of trophoblastic disease following a mole, treatment is often conducted in the absence of a histological diagnosis. Thus, all trophoblastic lesions are frequently combined under the rubric of GTD without applying specific pathological terms. However, recent studies demonstrate profound differences in the etiology, morphology, and clinical behavior of various forms of the disease. These studies underscore the importance of a uniform histological classification to facilitate standardized reporting of data and to ensure appropriate clinical management. Nonetheless, the term GTD has clinical utility, as the principles of human chorionic gonadotropin (hCG) monitoring in follow-up and the chemotherapy of metastatic or persistent disease are similar for all these entities.

This chapter discusses the clinical and pathological features of each specific form of GTD as well as their clinical behavior, management, and treatment. In addition, the morphologic and immunohistochemical features of the distinct subtypes of trophoblastic cells are reviewed since these have important implications for diagnosis. Recent studies have shed light on the molecular mechanisms of trophoblastic function, especially as it relates to trophoblastic disease and this material is reviewed since it enhances our understanding of the biology of these entities.

Table 20.1
World Health Organization classification of gestational trophoblastic disease

Hydatidiform moles (abnormally formed placentas)
Complete mole
Partial mole
Invasive mole
Trophoblastic tumor-like lesions (benign lesions)
Exaggerated placental site/reaction
Placental site nodule
Trophoblastic tumors (neoplastic diseases)
Choriocarcinoma
Placental site trophoblastic tumor (PSTT)
Epithelioid trophoblastic tumor (ETT)

Overview of Morphology, Development, and Biology of Trophoblast

The abnormal trophoblastic tissue in GTD recapitulates the trophoblast present in the early developing placenta and the implantation site. In normal placentation, the trophoblast growing in association with chorionic villi is referred to as villous trophoblast, whereas the trophoblast in all other locations is termed extravillous trophoblast. Three distinct types of trophoblastic cells have been recognized: cytotrophoblast (CT), syncytiotrophoblast (ST), and intermediate trophoblast (IT). Villous trophoblast is composed, for the most part, of CT and ST with small amounts of IT. In contrast, extravillous trophoblast that infiltrates the decidua, myometrium, and spiral arteries of the placental site is composed of IT.

CT (Langhans cells) is the germinative component of trophoblast, whereas ST is the differentiated component that interfaces with the maternal circulation and produces most of the placental hormones. IT is a distinct form of trophoblast that shares some of the morphologic and functional features of CT and ST. IT has been referred to X-cells, interstitial (cyto)trophoblast, extravillous (cyto) trophoblast, and "cytotrophoblast." The term "intermediate trophoblast" is preferred by pathologists since it more clearly reflects the morphological and functional features including hormone secretion of this unique cell population which is "intermediate" between cytotrophoblast and syncytiotrophoblast. Recent morphological and immunohistochemical studies have shown that intermediate trophoblast is a heterogeneous cell population that can be further categorized according to its anatomic location (➔ *Fig. 20.1*). Accordingly, we have proposed that intermediate trophoblast extending from the trophoblastic column at the anchoring villi be designated "villous

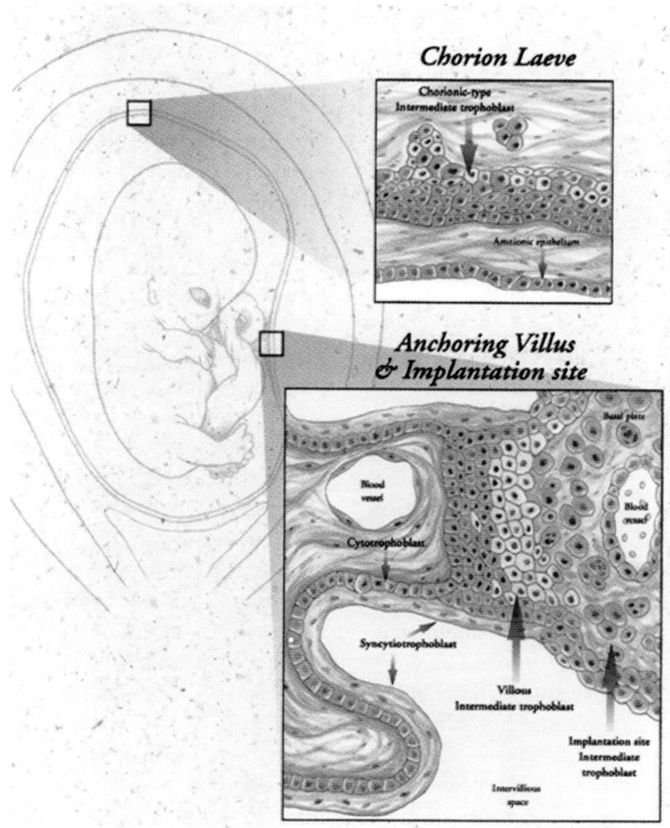

Fig. 20.1
Schematic representation of trophoblastic subpopulations in the placenta and fetal membranes (Reprinted by permission from reference [158])

intermediate trophoblast," in the placental site (or basal plate) "implantation site intermediate trophoblast," and in the chorion laeve of the fetal membranes "chorionic-type intermediate trophoblast" (Fig. *20.1*). The intermediate trophoblastic cells in the trophoblastic islands and placental septae appear to be equivalent to the implantation site intermediate trophoblastic cells.

Human trophoblast is derived from the trophoectoderm, the outermost layer of the blastocyst. Shortly after implantation (day 7–8), the trophoectoderm differentiates into a syncytiotrophoblastic mass at the implantation pole. Small intrasyncytial vacuoles then appear in the syncytiotrophoblastic mass and expand, becoming confluent and forming a system of lacunae that are separated by syncytiotrophoblastic trabeculae. On approximately day 12, the previllous mononucleate trophoblast from the primary chorionic plate invades the syncytiotrophoblastic trabeculae wherein the peripheral ends of the trabeculae join together and form the outermost layer of the trophoblast, the trophoblastic shell. After 2 weeks of gestation, the extraembryonic mesenchyme grows into the trabeculae, transforming them into the primary chorionic villi. The lacunae coalesce to form the intervillous space.

After the development of the chorionic villi, distinctive trophoblastic subpopulations can be recognized (Fig. *20.1*). The chorionic villus surface is lined by a continuous inner layer of cytotrophoblast and an outer layer of syncytiotrophoblast. Cytotrophoblast is the trophoblastic stem cell on the villous surface, demonstrating proliferative activity with a Ki-67 nuclear labeling index of approximately 30% in the first trimester. Cytotrophoblast, in early gestation, differentiates along two main pathways – villous and extravillous [145, 154]. On the villous surface, cytotrophoblast fuses directly to form syncytiotrophoblast. The differentiation of cytotrophoblast into syncytiotrophoblast is accompanied by complete loss of proliferation activity [151]. As gestation progresses, the proliferative activity of cytotrophoblast decreases with an increase in the relative number of syncytiotrophoblast to cytotrophoblast. The nuclei of syncytiotrophoblast gradually become apoptotic, forming so-called syncytial knots, clusters of pyknotic nuclei with a small amount of cytoplasm, which are eventually extruded into the intervillous space. The second pathway of differentiation of cytotrophoblast occurs at the pole of the villi that make contact with the placental bed. These villi, the so-called anchoring villi, display a morphologic spectrum of differentiation where cytotrophoblast merges imperceptibly into intermediate trophoblast within these trophoblastic columns (➲ *Fig. 20.1*). These intermediate trophoblastic cells in the trophoblastic columns are termed "villous intermediate trophoblast." The proliferative activity of villous intermediate trophoblast gradually decreases as the cells move away from the villi [151]. At the base of trophoblastic column at the junction with the endometrium, intermediate trophoblast infiltrates the decidua and myometrium and invades and replaces the spiral arteries of the implantation site (basal plate) to establish the maternal/fetal circulation. This subpopulation of intermediate trophoblast in the implantation site is designated "implantation site intermediate trophoblast." Although these trophoblastic cells extensively infiltrate the placental bed, they do not demonstrate proliferative activity. Some mononucleate implantation site intermediate trophoblastic cells fuse into multinucleated cells that are terminally differentiated. In contrast to anchoring villi, floating villi are not in contact with the placental bed. The trophoblast at the tips of these villi appears to be analogous to implantation site intermediate trophoblast. This cell population of trophoblast is associated with extensive deposition of extracellular matrix protein and fibrin forming "balloon-like" structures that have been designated "trophoblastic islands." Like implantation site intermediate trophoblast, the trophoblastic cells in the trophoblastic islands are not proliferative. In contrast, the intermediate trophoblast away from implantation site (i.e., the chorion frondosum) differentiates into "chorionic-type intermediate trophoblast." At around 20 weeks of gestation, the expanding gestational sac obliterates the endometrial cavity and the chorion frondosum fuses with the decidua parietalis to form the chorion laeve (➲ *Fig. 20.2*). As the surface area of the chorionic laeve increases towards term, the chorionic-type intermediate trophoblast continues to proliferate throughout gestation, albeit at a low level.

Morphology of Trophoblast

Previllous trophoblast. By light microscopy, the previllous trophoblast is composed of mononucleate trophoblast and primitive syncytiotrophoblast that invade the endometrium. The dimorphic pattern of previllous trophoblast is reminiscent of the dimorphic pattern of trophoblast in choriocarcinoma and it has been hypothesized that the morphologic appearance of choriocarcinoma is a recapitulation of the appearance of previllous trophoblast (➲ *Fig. 20.3*). Unlike choriocarcinoma, previllous trophoblastic cells are less pleomorphic and do not exhibit cellular necrosis.

Cytotrophoblast. Following the development of villi, cytotrophoblastic cells appear as small primitive epithelial cells, uniform, and polygonal to oval in shape (➲ *Fig. 20.4a*). Cytotrophoblastic cells have a single nucleus, clear to granular cytoplasm, and well-defined cell borders. Mitotic activity is evident.

Syncytiotrophoblast. Syncytiotrophoblast is composed of a large, multinucleate cellular mass with dense amphophilic cytoplasm often containing multiple vacuoles that vary in size (➲ *Fig. 20.4a*). A distinct brush border often lines the cell membrane. The syncytiotrophoblastic nuclei are dark and often appear pyknotic. They do not show mitotic activity.

Villous intermediate trophoblast. Villous intermediate trophoblastic cells are mononucleate and larger than cytotrophoblast with pale to clear cytoplasm and uniform round nuclei.

Implantation site intermediate trophoblast. Implantation site intermediate trophoblastic cells have a variable appearance, which to some extent is dependent on their anatomic location (➲ *Figs. 20.4b* and *c*). For example, implantation site intermediate trophoblastic cells in the endometrium are polygonal or round and contain abundant amphophilic cytoplasm closely resembling the decidualized stromal cells with which they are admixed. In contrast, implantation site intermediate trophoblastic cells in the myometrium are frequently spindle-shaped and resemble the smooth muscle cells of the myometrium. Generally, the cytoplasm of implantation site intermediate trophoblastic cells is abundant and is eosinophilic to amphophilic. Scattered small vacuoles may be present in the cytoplasm of implantation site intermediate trophoblastic cells. The nuclei of implantation site intermediate trophoblastic cells have highly irregular outlines and hyperchromatic, coarsely granular chromatin. Often the nuclei are lobulated or show multiple deep nuclear clefts. Nucleoli are smaller and less prominent than those

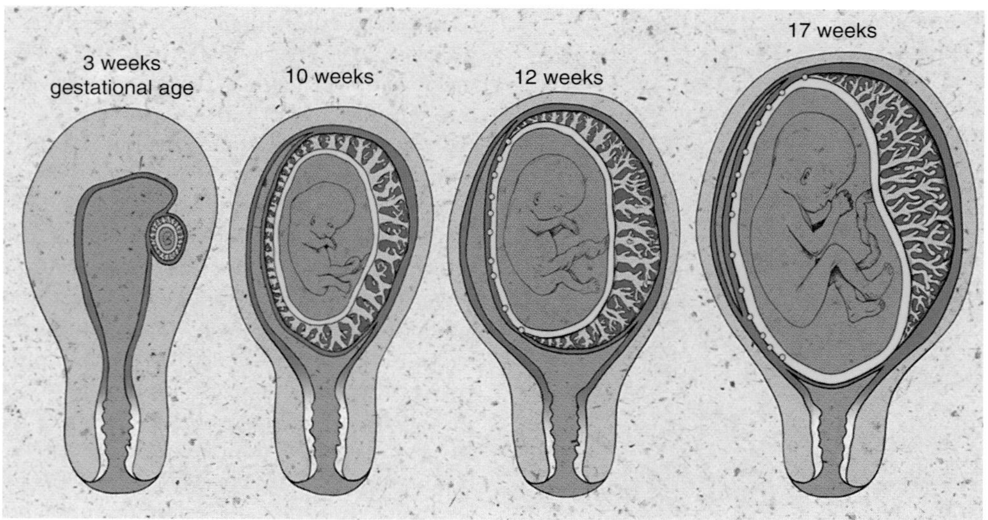

Fig. 20.2
Schematic representation of the formation of the chorion laeve (yellow). **At 3 weeks of gestation, the entire blastocyst is embedded in the endometrium at the implantation site and is surrounded by the trophoblastic shell. At 10 weeks, the definitive placenta is established at the implantation site and the chorionic villi at the opposite pole begin to degenerate. At approximately 12 weeks, the amnion (yellow)/chorion (blue) at the opposite end of the placental site fuses with the decidua capsularis. The intervillous space is obliterated and the chorionic villi (the small, round pale-gray structures) degenerate. This process continues and at approximately 17 weeks of gestation the uterine cavity is largely obliterated as the amnion and chorion laeve become apposed to the endometrium on the opposite side of the uterine cavity. The chorion laeve, amnion, and underlying decidua constitute the fetal membranes (Reprinted by permission from [158])**

in cytotrophoblast. Cytoplasmic nuclear invaginations may be seen. Mononucleate implantation site intermediate trophoblastic cells occasionally fuse into multinucleated cells.

Implantation site intermediate trophoblastic cells infiltrate the decidua, surround glands, and invade the myometrium, dissecting between smooth muscle fibers without destroying them. These cells characteristically invade spiral arteries replacing the smooth muscle of the vessel wall but leaving the overall structure intact. Eosinophilic fibrinoid material is often deposited around implantation site intermediate trophoblast. The material contains a variety of extracellular matrix proteins including adult-type and oncofetal fibronectin, type IV collagen, laminin, and a small amount of fibrin. Implantation site intermediate trophoblastic cells are the predominant cellular population of the exaggerated placental site and the PSTT.

The intermediate trophoblastic cells in the trophoblastic islands are mononucleate, round, and uniform in size and contain rounded nuclei. They are embedded in an abundant, homogeneous, and eosinophilic fibrinoid matrix. In vitro studies suggest that the cell islands are derived from the floating cell columns, which are not anchored to the endometrium. As a result, abundant extracellular matrix accumulates among the cells replacing those in the center of the islands.

Chorionic-type intermediate trophoblast. Chorionic-type intermediate trophoblast is composed for the most part of relatively uniform cells with either eosinophilic or clear (glycogen-rich) cytoplasm arranged in a cohesive layer in the chorion laeve (*Figs. 20.1* and *20.5*). Most of the cells are smaller than implantation site intermediate trophoblast but larger than cytotrophoblast. Occasionally, the cells form nests or cords that extend into the underlying decidua. As with implantation site intermediate trophoblastic cells, some chorionic-type intermediate trophoblastic cells are multinucleated. Chorionic-type intermediate trophoblast is the cellular population found in placental site nodules and epithelioid trophoblastic tumors [158].

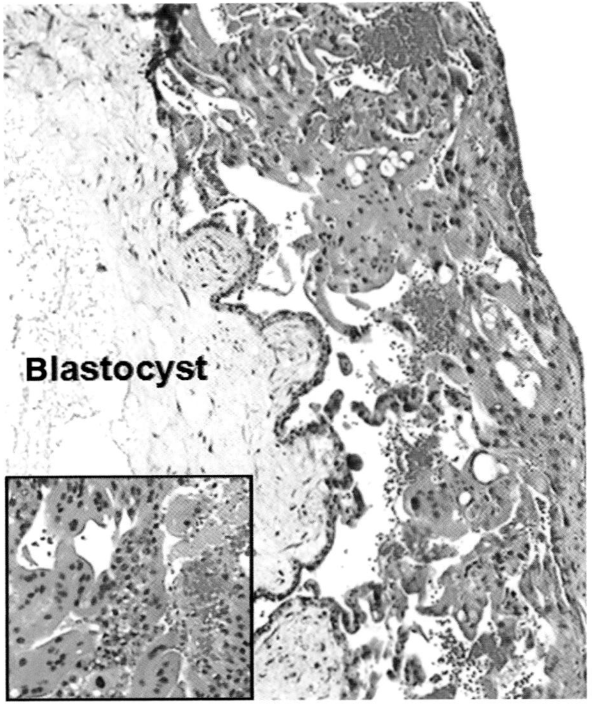

Fig. 20.3
Primitive trophoblast. **The previllous trophoblast surrounding the blastocyst demonstrates a dimorphic pattern composed of mononucleate trophoblastic cells and syncytiotrophoblastic cells that resemble choriocarcinoma. The mononucleate trophoblastic cells, in contrast to those in choriocarcinoma, are smaller, more uniform, and not atypical (*inset*). Unlike choriocarcinoma, the trophoblast does not invade and destroy adjacent tissue**

Gene Expression and Immunohistochemical Features of Trophoblastic Subpopulations

Trophoblast-associated gene expression as detected by immunohistochemistry has great value in the diagnosis of GTD as well as in the study of the biology of trophoblast (*Table 20.2*) [145, 155]. The beta-subunit of hCG, human placental lactogen (hPL), placental alkaline phosphatase (PLAP), inhibin, and low-molecular-weight cytokeratin are well-recognized markers of trophoblast. Recently, several other genes have been identified in human trophoblast. Antibodies against these markers, especially those that are commercially available and recognize the epitopes in formalin-fixed, paraffin-embedded tissue sections, have considerable value in the study and differential diagnosis of different types of GTD. For example, HSD3B1 is a newly characterized trophoblastic marker that is expressed almost exclusively in a few normal tissues including trophoblast and sebaceous glands. The commercially available antibody that reacts to HSD3B1 protein has been shown to be very useful to distinguish a trophoblastic from a non-trophoblastic lesion [93].

All forms of trophoblastic subpopulations and gestational trophoblastic lesions react strongly for cytokeratin when broad-spectrum antibodies (e.g., the AE1/AE3 antibody cocktail) are used. More specifically, trophoblast is positive for low-molecular-weight epithelium-type cytokeratins, including cytokeratins 7, 8, 18, and 19. In contrast, trophoblast is variably positive for cytokeratin 20 and is rarely positive for high-molecular-weight cytokeratin that is normally expressed by stratified squamous epithelium. Cytokeratin immunostaining is especially useful for demonstrating the presence of implantation site intermediate trophoblastic cells at the placental site since these cells are always admixed with the other cell types. The intermediate trophoblastic cells that are positive for low-molecular-weight cytokeratin are easily identified amid nonreactive decidual cells and smooth muscle cells. Myometrial smooth muscle cells can display punctate cytoplasmic cytokeratin immunoreactivity that is easily distinguished from the diffuse membrane staining of IT.

Cytotrophoblast is immunoreactive for a variety of antigens, including p63, cyclin E, leukemia inhibitory factor receptor, epidermal growth factor receptor, P2Y6 purinergic receptor, and a number of cell adhesion molecules including integrin and E-cadherin (*Table 20.2*). Unlike syncytiotrophoblast, cytotrophoblast fails to react with antibodies against a wide variety of steroid and pregnancy-associated hormones. Ki-67 proliferation-related antigen is highly expressed by cytotrophoblast (labeling index: 25–50%) especially in the region forming the trophoblastic columns (*Table 20.2*). These findings confirm that cytotrophoblast is a stem cell with a high level of proliferative activity and a limited functional role.

The differentiation of cytotrophoblast into syncytiotrophoblast is accompanied by dramatic changes in gene expression. For example, syncytiotrophoblast expresses several pregnancy-associated hormones, including beta-hCG, hPL, estradiol, progesterone, placental growth hormone, pregnancy-specific glycoprotein, relaxins, and inhibin. The immunodistribution of some of these hormones in syncytiotrophoblast is variable, depending on gestational age. For example, syncytiotrophoblast contains abundant beta-hCG from at least 12 days of gestation until approximately 8–10 weeks, after which

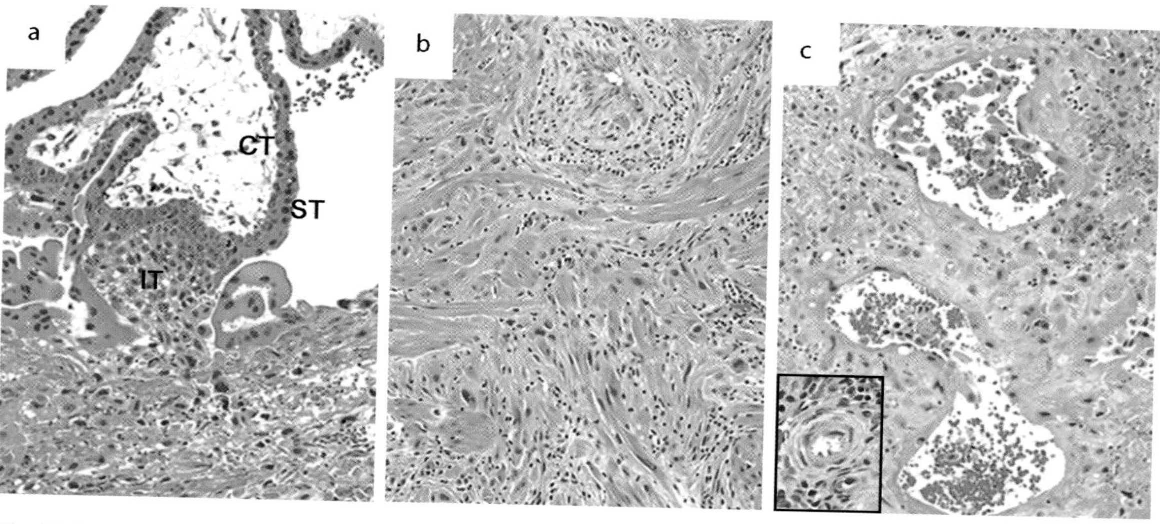

Fig. 20.4
Chorionic villus and implantation site. (**a**) An anchoring villus attaches to the implantation site. The villus is outlined by two trophoblastic layers – the inner cytotrophoblast (CT) and outer syncytiotrophoblast (ST). The intermediate trophoblast (IT) differentiates from the trophoblastic column and emanates from the distal column to the implantation site. (**b**) Intermediate trophoblastic cells infiltrate into endomyometrium and assume a distinctive pattern when they invade the myometrium. (**c**) Intermediate trophoblastic cells target the spiral arteries and transform them from small caliber and high resistant vascular channels (*inset*) into large caliber and low resistant arteries that direct blood into the intervillous space. Intermediate trophoblastic cells can be found in the lumen of the arteries and sometimes appear to occlude the entire lumen

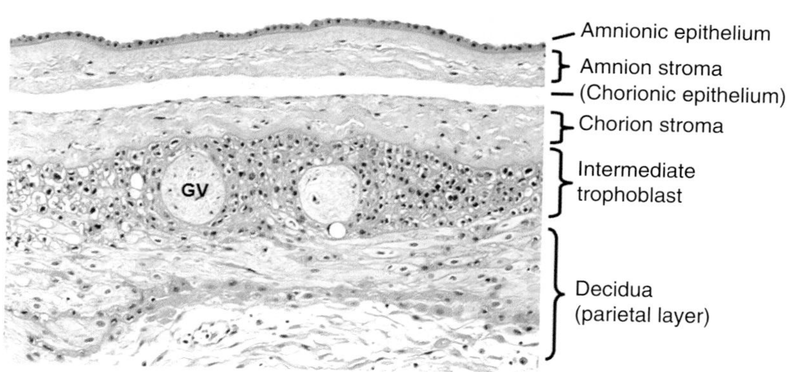

Fig. 20.5
Anatomy of chorion laeve (fetal membrane). The chorion epithelium is no longer present in chorion laeve because of fusion between the amnion and chorion. However, a cleft that represents the location where the chorionic epithelium resides before the fusion is always present due to tissue processing artifacts. The trophoblastic cells in the chorion laeve are termed "chorionic-type intermediate trophoblastic cells" and are characterized by distinct morphological and immunohistochemical features as compared to other trophoblastic subpopulations. GV: ghost villi

it diminishes. By 40 weeks it is present only focally. hPL is also localized in syncytiotrophoblast at 12 days but increases steadily thereafter. From late in the second trimester to term, hPL is diffusely distributed in the syncytiotrophoblast overlying the chorionic villi. Inhibin-α exhibits the highest expression in the first trimester and gradually decreases in immunointensity through the third trimester (Table 20.2) [152].

Table 20.2
Expression of trophoblastic markers in different trophoblastic subpopulations

Trophoblastic types	HSD3B1	HLA-G	hPL	β-hCG	cyclin E	p63	CD146*	HNK1	Muc4	β–cat
Cytotrophoblast										nuc
Syncytiotrophoblast										
IT in trophoblastic column	varied									memb
IT in implantation site				M						
IT in chorion laeve										

Immunointensity: Low — high

M : positive in multinucleated intermediate trophoblast (IT)

: increased expression toward the implantation site in a trophoblastic column

IT: intermediate trophoblastic cells; nuc: nuclear staining; memb: membrane staining; varied: variable staining pattern
*CD146 is a synonym of Mel-CAM

Syncytiotrophoblast also expresses placental alkaline phosphatase, leukemia inhibitory factor receptor, placental growth hormone, epidermal growth factor receptor, HSD3B1 (an enzyme involved in the synthesis of progesterone), p27^{kip1} (a negative regulator in cell cycle progression), c-fms oncoprotein CD10, and syncytin. Expression of syncytin has been shown to be involved in the fusion process of syncytiotrophoblast [102]. In contrast, several genes are down-regulated in syncytiotrophoblast as compared with cytotrophoblast. For example, syncytiotrophoblast fails to express E-cadherin and Ki-67 nuclear antigen. These findings are concordant with the view that syncytiotrophoblast is terminally differentiated and that its major functions are hormone production and molecular transport across the villous surface.

Among the various populations of trophoblast, the pattern of gene expression is most complex in intermediate trophoblast and depends on the differentiation status and anatomic location of the intermediate trophoblastic cells, i.e., the subpopulation of intermediate trophoblast (*Table 20.2*). The villous intermediate trophoblast in the trophoblastic columns uniquely expresses the HNK-1 carbohydrate epitope on glycosphingolipids, which is not present in other subpopulations of trophoblastic cells [157]. The genes that are upregulated as villous intermediate trophoblast differentiate into implantation site intermediate trophoblast including melanoma cell adhesion molecule (Mel-CAM or CD146; [149] inhibin-α [152], hPL [81], and cyclin E [94] (*Table 20.2*). The genes that are downregulated during differentiation of villous to implantation site intermediate trophoblast are Ki-67 nuclear antigen, epidermal growth factor (EGF) receptor, and E-cadherin. In terms of hormone production, implantation site intermediate trophoblast resembles syncytiotrophoblast. It contains abundant hPL, which appears as early as 12 days and reaches a peak at 11–15 weeks of gestation. Inhibin-α is also immunolocalized in the implantation site intermediate trophoblast after 10 weeks of gestation. In contrast, hCG is present only focally in implantation site intermediate trophoblast, appearing as early as 12 days and remaining until 6 weeks, after which it disappears. The so-called multinucleated trophoblastic giant cells exhibit an identical immunostaining pattern to the mononucleate counterparts except the former are negative for pregnancy-associated major basic protein [79]. Accordingly, these giant cells should be designated "multinucleated intermediate trophoblastic cells" rather than syncytiotrophoblastic giant cells [149].

The implantation site intermediate trophoblastic cells that invade the spiral arteries show the same staining pattern as those within the decidua and myometrium except that expression of neural cell adhesion molecule (NCAM; [15], E-cadherin, and beta-catenin are upregulated [147]. Implantation site intermediate trophoblast in both the endometrium and myometrium expresses leukemia inhibitory factor receptor [142], which interacts with leukemia inhibitory factor expressed by maternal decidual leukocytes. Although leukemia inhibitory factor plays an important role in implantation and placentation in several species, the paracrine role of leukemia inhibitory factor in the biology of human implantation site intermediate trophoblastic cells is not known. Those intermediate trophoblastic cells also express CD10, a neutral endopeptidase [64, 122].

In contrast to implantation site intermediate trophoblast, chorionic-type intermediate trophoblast is diffusely positive for p63 but is only focally positive for several trophoblast-associated antigens including hPL, Mel-CAM (CD146), mucin-4, and cyclin E (➲ *Table 20.2*). Chorionic-type intermediate trophoblastic cells exhibit mild proliferative activity as indicated by an increased Ki-67 labeling index (3–10%) in contrast to the absence of Ki-67 labeling in implantation site intermediate trophoblast.

The immunophenotype of trophoblastic cells in gestational trophoblastic lesions is similar to their normal counterparts. In routine pathology practice, HSD3B1, cytokeratin 18, hPL, p63, Ki-67, and cyclin E are particularly useful markers in the diagnosis of trophoblastic lesions. The practical application of immunohistochemistry in the differential diagnosis of gestational trophoblastic lesions is discussed under the section of immunohistochemistry application for differential diagnosis.

Functional Aspects of Trophoblast

Trophoblast plays a crucial role in implantation and embryonic development. The major functions of trophoblast are as follows. First, the villous trophoblast (syncytiotrophoblast and cytotrophoblast) provides a structural interface for molecular transport between the maternal and fetal compartments. Second, implantation site intermediate trophoblast establishes the fetomaternal circulation in the placental site (➲ *Fig. 20.4*). Third, syncytiotrophoblast secretes several pregnancy-associated hormones that are necessary for successful maintenance of the placenta and fetus. Finally, syncytiotrophoblast as well as chorionic-type intermediate trophoblast in the fetal membranes serve as an immunological barrier that prevents allograft rejection of the fetus by the maternal immune system. Functional abnormalities of trophoblast may account for several common gestational disorders including failure of implantation, which leads to spontaneous abortion, preeclampsia, and intrauterine growth retardation. The functions of specific trophoblastic subpopulations are discussed below.

Previllous Trophoblast

The previllous syncytiotrophoblast is responsible for the initial erosion of maternal tissues during the early stages of implantation. Subsequently, it appears that the previllous mononucleate trophoblastic cells are responsible for further invasion and expansion of the implantation site (➲ *Fig. 20.3*). At approximately 13 days of gestation, mesenchyme penetrates the trophoblastic mass and chorionic villi develop thus forming the rudimentary structure of the definitive placenta.

Cytotrophoblast

Cytotrophoblast is the trophoblastic stem cell and is located on the villous surface. Cytotrophoblast expresses epidermal growth factor receptor (EGF-R), which binds to EGF secreted by the decidua. It has been postulated that by a paracrine mechanism EGF-R and its ligand may provide persistent growth stimulation for cytotrophoblast. Cytotrophoblast differentiates along two main pathways. Along one pathway, cytotrophoblast continues to proliferate and fuses to form the overlying syncytiotrophoblast. This process results in expansion of the surface area of chorionic villi in the developing placenta. In the second pathway, cytotrophoblast differentiates into villous intermediate trophoblast in the trophoblastic columns and then into implantation site intermediate trophoblast in the placental site or chorionic-type intermediate trophoblast in the chorion laeve.

Syncytiotrophoblast

Syncytiotrophoblast is composed of terminally differentiated cells that synthesize and secrete a variety of pregnancy-associated hormones that are thought to be critical in the establishment and maintenance of pregnancy. Some of these secretory proteins may also have a paracrine function by regulating the local microenvironment of decidua cells, inflammatory cells, and smooth muscle cells at the placental site. In addition to its role as an endocrine organ, the syncytiotrophoblast is bathed in maternal blood and is responsible for the exchange of oxygen, nutrients, and a variety of metabolic products between the mother and fetus.

Villous Intermediate Trophoblast

Villous intermediate trophoblastic cells proliferate in the proximal portion of trophoblastic columns and serve as the source from which implantation site and chorionic-type intermediate trophoblast are derived. In addition, villous intermediate trophoblastic cells may play an important role in maintaining the structural integrity of the villi that anchor the placenta to the basal plate. HNK-1 carbohydrate moiety expressed on the surface of the villous intermediate trophoblast may contribute to the intercellular cohesion in the trophoblastic columns that counteract the mechanical sheering forces resulting from fetal movements and the turbulence created by the pulsatile blood flow in the placental bed [157].

Implantation Site Intermediate Trophoblast

The major function of implantation site intermediate trophoblast is to establish the maternal–fetal circulation by invading the spiral arteries in the basal plate during early pregnancy. The mechanisms underlying trophoblastic invasion are similar to those involved in tumor cell invasion. For example, proteases are responsible for matrix degradation and tissue remodeling, a prerequisite for trophoblastic migration and invasion. Loss of E-cadherin expression is closely associated with the infiltrative phenotype of implantation site intermediate trophoblast [147]. Expression of growth factors and their receptors constitutes a unique molecular mechanism regulating trophoblastic behavior and cell-to-cell communication (autocrine or paracrine) including cellular migration, proliferation, and differentiation. Expression of cell adhesion molecules is important for trophoblastic migration in different extracellular substrates and for cross-talk between trophoblastic cells and their microenvironment. It has been shown that implantation site intermediate trophoblastic cells produce hyperglycosylated hCG, a variant of hCG. This variant appears to be an autocrine factor, participating in the initiation and regulation of trophoblastic invasion [23].

Unlike malignant tumors, the invasion of implantation site intermediate trophoblast is tightly regulated, confined spatially to the implantation site and limited temporally to early pregnancy. While extensively infiltrating the endometrium of the basal plate, the implantation site intermediate trophoblast invade only the inner third of the myometrium in the first trimester, decreasing to less than 10% of the myometrium by term. Although the molecular mechanism underlying the control of trophoblastic invasion is currently unclear, the invasive process can be modulated by both the trophoblast and the local microenvironment. Fusion of mononucleate implantation site intermediate trophoblastic cells into multinucleated cells leads to the loss of their invasive and migratory phenotype. Although multinucleated implantation site intermediate trophoblastic cells can be seen in trophoblastic neoplasms such as PSTT, they are more frequently encountered in the normal or exaggerated placental site, a helpful morphological feature in distinguishing exaggerated placental site from PSTT.

Another feature that distinguishes non-neoplastic trophoblastic cells from tumor cells is their pattern of cellular proliferation. The differentiation of implantation site intermediate trophoblast is accompanied by a decrease in cellular proliferation in contrast to the uncontrolled proliferation in malignant neoplasms. Indeed, implantation site intermediate trophoblastic cells are negative for Ki-67, a proliferation marker, and are positive for several proteins which are involved in the arrest of cell cycle progression including $p21^{WAF1/CIP1}$ [19] and $p57^{kip-2}$ [21]. Accordingly, any proliferative activity (mitotic figures or Ki-67-positive trophoblastic cells) in the implantation site intermediate trophoblast should be considered abnormal and a neoplastic process must be considered.

Spiral arteries at the implantation site are the targets for invasion by implantation site intermediate trophoblast. The mechanisms that are responsible for the tropism of implantation site intermediate trophoblast to the spiral arteries, and not to other structures, are unclear; one postulate is that the oxygen gradient may be a guiding cue. The trophoblastic invasion into the vascular wall is associated with abundant deposition of extracellular matrix, which eventually replaces the entire smooth muscle layer of spiral arteries, resulting in the transformation of the arteries to large-caliber and low-resistant vascular channels. This unique feature of vascular invasion is not only observed in the normal placental site but also in the PSTT. Implantation site intermediate trophoblast replaces the lining endothelial cells and undergoes an epithelial–endothelial transdifferentiation characterized by the acquisition of several endothelial markers including VCAM-1, VE-cadherin, and beta-4 integrin, [186] and Mel-CAM (CD146) [143, 149], all of which are expressed by endothelial cells. Accordingly, the term "trophoblast pseudo-vasculogenesis" has been proposed to describe this unique differentiation pathway of implantation site intermediate trophoblast. Some of the implantation site intermediate trophoblastic cells that invade the spiral arteries migrate along the vascular wall in a retrograde fashion to reach the spiral arteries beyond the implantation site in the myometrium. The intravascular implantation site intermediate trophoblastic cells tend to form trophoblastic aggregates that act like valves or a sieve to control the blood flow in the trophoblast-modified spiral arteries. The process of aggregation is associated with the expression of NCAM and E-cadherin. These cell adhesion molecules may be responsible for the enhanced intercellular cohesion among cells in trophoblastic aggregates in the spiral arteries as NCAM and E-cadherin function as homotypic cell–cell adhesion molecules. This hypothesis has been supported by a recent study in which the E-cadherin gene was introduced into an E-cadherin negative implantation site intermediate trophoblastic cell line, IST-1, resulting in a stationary and cohesive phenotype of IST-1 cells in culture [147].

Chorionic-Type Intermediate Trophoblast

The functional role of chorionic-type intermediate trophoblastic cells is unknown. Unlike the implantation site intermediate trophoblast, the chorionic-type intermediate trophoblast proliferates throughout gestation as the total surface area of fetal membrane increases. Chorionic-type intermediate trophoblast may contribute to the synthesis of extracelluar matrix, which is required to maintain the tensile strength of the fetal membrane. It is also possible that chorionic-type intermediate trophoblast acts as a biological and mechanical barrier to the maternal immune system and is important for fetal allograft survival (see below).

Classification of Gestational Trophoblastic Disease

According to current WHO classification, GTD can be broadly divided into molar lesions and non-molar lesions. The molar lesions include partial and complete hydatidiform moles and invasive moles. The non-molar lesions include choriocarcinoma and lesions derived from implantation site intermediate trophoblast (exaggerated placental site and PSTT) and those from the chorionic-type intermediate trophoblast (placental site nodule and epithelioid trophoblastic tumor). In the past, exaggerated placental site and placental site nodule were classified as "unclassified GTD." Both lesions are benign and have distinct histogenesis and morphological features that justify their separate designation. The current classification also includes epithelioid trophoblastic tumor, which is a trophoblastic neoplasm distinct from choriocarcinoma, and PSTT.

General Features of Gestational Trophoblastic Disease

Epidemiology

The reported incidence of hydatidiform mole and choriocarcinoma varies widely throughout the world, being greatest in Asia, Africa, and Latin America and substantially lower in North America, Europe, and Australia. The incidence rates are difficult to compare, however, because of the limitations in the methodology of these studies. Furthermore, some studies of incidence rates have used hospital-based rather than population-based figures, which probably result in overreporting. There are no epidemiologic data on incidence or geographic distribution reported for the more recently described PSTT and epithelioid trophoblastic tumor. Despite the various incidence rates documented, the overall incidence of GTD has been decreasing in last few decades, especially in those geographic areas that have previously reported a high incidence [51, 76].

In North America and Europe, the frequency of hydatidiform moles is approximately 100 per 100,000 pregnancies. A higher frequency was reported in some areas of Asia and the Middle East, with an incidence rate from 100 to 1,000 per 100,000 pregnancies [3]. Choriocarcinoma occurs with a frequency of 1 in 20,000 to 1 in 40,000 pregnancies in the United States and Europe [123]. Estimates for the incidence in Asia, Africa, and Latin America generally are higher with incidence rates as high as 1 in 500 to 1,000 pregnancies reported [123]. As with molar disease, there are marked regional variations in incidence rates. In Nigeria, choriocarcinoma is the third most common malignant tumor in women at one institution, ranking behind breast and cervical carcinoma. Thus, despite methodological problems it appears that choriocarcinoma occurs at a substantially higher rate in developing countries than it does in North America and Europe. Similar to hydatidiform moles, the overall incidence of choriocarcinoma in recent years has dramatically decreased as socioeconomic conditions improve. These observations suggest that low socioeconomic conditions or dietary factors may contribute to the development of GTD. Recently, asbestos exposure has been reported to be associated with the development of GTD [135].

Gestational trophoblastic lesions are nearly always disorders of the reproductive years. Women who are sexually active are at risk for developing GTD, but the incidence is substantially higher in women before 20 and after 40 years. In rare cases, GTD can develop in a postmenopausal woman with a long interval between the diagnosis of GTD and the antecedent pregnancy. The absolute number of cases of mole or choriocarcinoma in women over 40 years is smaller because of their lower fertility. In contrast, maternal age has no effect on the risk of partial mole. Neither paternal age nor race seems to affect the risk of developing a hydatidiform mole. Malignant sequelae for hydatidiform mole occur more frequently in older patients. While hydatidiform mole, choriocarcinoma, exaggerated placental site, and placental site nodule are nearly always confined to reproductive age women, PSTT and epithelioid trophoblastic tumors occur infrequently in postmenopausal women.

Several studies reveal that a history of prior spontaneous abortions is more common in patients with hydatidiform mole and choriocarcinoma than with a normal pregnancy. Furthermore, women who have had one hydatidiform mole are at increased risk of having another [123]. Conversely, term pregnancy and live births have a protective effect, with GTD less common in patients who are parous [123]. The protective effect appears to increase with an increased number of live births.

Cytogenetics

Cytogenetic studies of complete and partial hydatidiform mole show that chromosomal abnormalities play an important role in their development [3, 175]. The karyotypic patterns of the two types of moles are considerably different. Complete hydatidiform moles have a normal DNA content and most complete moles have a karyotype of 46,XX and develop from the fertilization of an anuclear "empty" ovum by a single haploid (23X) sperm, in which the haploid genome duplicates (*Fig. 20.6*) [88]. The remaining group (4–15%) of complete moles are also androgenetic but are formed by dispermy, i.e., fertilization of an ovum lacking functional maternal chromosomes by two spermatozoa. Accordingly, the complete mole, being paternally derived, constitutes a total allograft in the mother. The opposite pathogenesis of a complete mole occurs in parthenogenesis, meaning that the maternal set of chromosomes duplicates itself in oocytes, and ovarian teratomas are believed to result from this process.

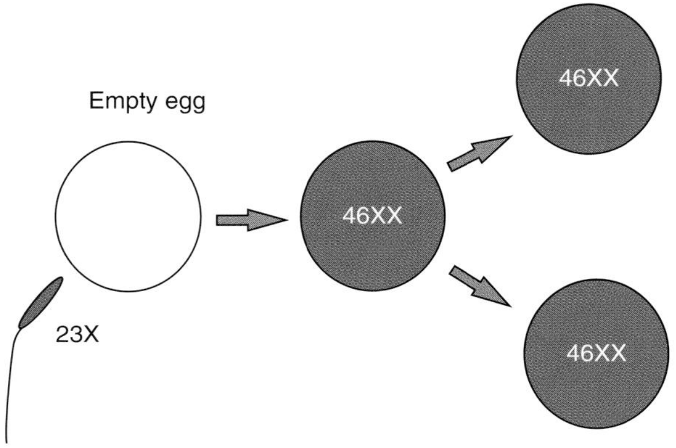

Fig. 20.6
Chromosomal origin of a complete hydatidiform mole. A single sperm fertilizes an empty egg. Reduplication of its 23X set results in a completely homozygous diploid genome of 46XX. A similar process follows fertilization of an empty egg by two sperms with two independent sets of 23X or 23Y. Note that both karyotypes 46XX and 46XY can ensue

The karyotype of a partial mole is nearly always triploid (69 chromosomes) (*Fig. 20.7*) with a maternal chromosome complement. Conversely, not all triploid conceptuses demonstrate histological features of a partial mole because the triploids are composed of different groups with distinct pathogenesis [46]. The percentage of partial moles among triploid conceptuses depends on the histologic criteria for the diagnosis and on the type of cytogenetic assays employed. When triploidy is present in a partial mole, the chromosomal complement usually is 69,XXY or 69,XXX and rarely 69,XYY. These abnormal conceptuses result from the fertilization of an egg with a haploid set of chromosomes by either two sperms, each with a set of haploid chromosomes, or by a single sperm with a diploid genome of 46,XY [88]. This condition is known as diandric or androgenetic (paternally derived) triploidy in which two of the three haploid sets are of paternal origin. Diandric triploids at early stages of development frequently show features of an early partial mole, but only a subgroup will go on to develop the complete phenotype of a partial mole. A conceptus with a diploid 46XX maternal genome due to failure of the first meiotic division and a haploid paternal set of chromosomes results in an abnormal, triploid (69XXX or 69XXY) fetus [134]. This is referred to as a digynic (maternally derived) conceptus in which two of the three haploid sets are of maternal origin. There is no agreement as to the percentage of digynic triploids among all triploid placentas,

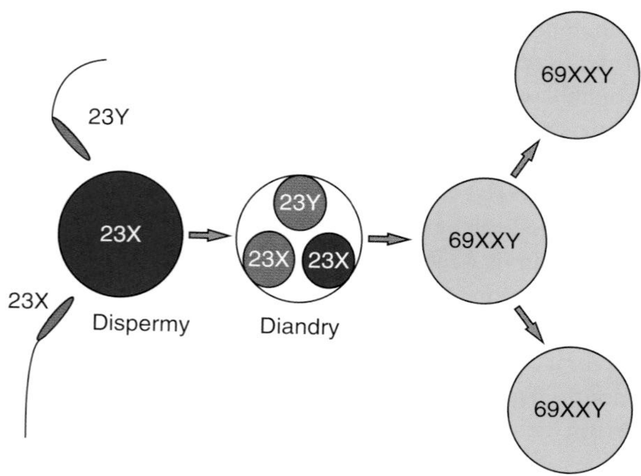

Fig. 20.7
Chromosomal origin of the triploid, partial hydatidiform mole. A normal egg with a 23X haploid set is fertilized by two sperm that carry either sex chromosome, to result in 69 chromosomes with a sex configuration of XXY, XXX, or XYY. A similar result can be obtained by fertilization of a sperm carrying the unreduced paternal genome 46XY (resulting sex complement, XXY only)

but it is believed that digynic triploids generally do not present as a molar pregnancy. In conclusion, most well-documented partial moles are (diandric) triploids, but not all triploid conceptuses are associated with partial moles.

Genetic studies of choriocarcinoma have shown that most choriocarcinomas are diploid [40], and that choriocarcinomas with aneuploidy may be associated with a poorer prognosis. Several studies have demonstrated the diandric (androgenetic) origin of choriocarcinoma following a complete hydatidiform mole [43, 88].

The cytogenetic studies of GTD other than molar pregnancy and choriocarcinoma such as PSTT and epithelioid trophoblastic tumor have not been as well studied because of the rarity of these neoplasms. However, new techniques such as fluorescence in situ hybridization, interphase cytogenetics, and polymorphism of oligonucleotide repeat sequences (microsatellites) have been performed on fixed tissue. Although the majority of GTD can be diagnosed by pathologists on morphological grounds alone, the application of these techniques may become more and more important in diagnosis and management of GTD. For example, microsatellite markers that differ in maternal or paternal origins have been used to confirm a complete mole. Both fluorescence in situ hybridization using chromosome-specific markers and polymerase chain reaction using polymorphic markers have been employed to assist in differentiating a hydropic abortus from a partial mole, and a partial mole from a complete mole [13, 97].

Serum Markers

Treatment of GTD is based on determining, if possible, the specific histological type of trophoblastic lesion, monitoring serum hCG titers, and instituting chemotherapy when appropriate. hCG has proved to be an ideal marker for all forms of GTD and measurement of serum hCG levels is an integral part of the management of this disease. hCG is a glycoprotein composed of two polypeptide chains, alpha and beta, attached to a carbohydrate moiety. The configuration of hCG is similar to other gonadotropins, particularly luteinizing hormone (LH). The α-polypeptide chain in all these hormones is identical; it is the difference in the beta chain that gives the hormones their unique immunologic specificity and biologic function. Accordingly, beta-hCG is the most specific marker for GTD. hCG is produced mainly by syncytiotrophoblast, and it is almost invariably detectable in the serum if trophoblastic tissue is present and when sensitive assays are used. In addition to syncytiotrophoblast, implantation site intermediate trophoblastic cells can also produce a variant of hCG that is hyperglycosylated. It has been reported that this hyperglycosylated hCG inhibits apoptosis in intermediate trophoblastic cells while promoting cell invasion and growth.

In normal pregnancy, beta-hCG peaks to 50,000–100,000 mIU/mL at about 10 weeks gestation and decreases to 10,000–20,000 mIU/mL by 20 weeks, remaining at that level until term. Levels as high as 600,000 mIU/mL have been reported in early pregnancy. In molar gestations, beta-hCG levels at diagnosis are variable, but most show a markedly elevated hCG titer, which is a useful diagnostic feature. Levels greater than 2 million mIU/mL have been reported. beta-hCG titers are generally higher in complete than partial moles [28]. Choriocarcinoma, almost invariably, produces very high level of beta-hCG and a case with a level of 11 million mIU/mL has been reported [59]. In contrast to the high levels in hydatidiform moles and choriocarcinoma, beta-hCG levels are much lower in PSTTs and epithelioid trophoblastic tumors [150]. Nevertheless, beta-hCG levels are very useful in monitoring patients with these tumors [25].

Beta-core fragment of hCG in urine has been reported to be an even more sensitive marker being detected in patients whose serum hCG levels are near to or below the limit of detection [136]. Also recently, a sensitive radioimmunoassay (RIA) and immunoradiometric assay

(IRMA) have been developed [22, 25] that can measure serum beta-hCG to a level of 0.5 mIU/mL. The assay can detect beta-hCG production from as few as 1,000 trophoblastic cells, thus permitting follow-up to complete disappearance of trophoblastic tissue. Disappearance of beta-hCG from the serum as measured by half-life shows two components, one with a half-life of 6 h and a slower component with a half-life of about 30 h. Since heterophilic antibodies are known to interfere with the measurement of serum analytes, concurrent serum, and urine testing for hCG has been recommended to be used as routine policy in the diagnosis and follow-up of the patients with GTD [138]. Except for hCG, the utilization of other trophoblastic markers including hPL, inhibin, activin, and progesterone in the detection and follow-up of GTD has not yet been established [141].

Staging and Prognostic Factors

Several systems including the modified International Federation of Gynecology and Obstetrics (FIGO) staging system, the World Health Organization (WHO) prognostic index score system, and the National Institute of Health (NIH) classification of metastatic GTD have been developed to predict prognosis and guide treatment (reviewed in [163]). The FIGO system uses an anatomic staging system, which is summarized in *Table 20.3*. Within each stage, patients with no risk factors are assigned to substage A, those with only one risk factor to substage B, and those with two risk factors are assigned to substage C. The NIH classification is a clinical classification and is based on a variety of clinical features and serum hCG levels that segregates patients into good and poor prognosis (*Table 20.4*). The WHO scoring system divides patients into low-, intermediate-, and high-risk groups based on the total score of a variety of prognostic features (*Table 20.5*). Based on the WHO system, patients with nonmetastatic (stage I) and low-risk metastatic (stages II and III, World Health Organization score < 7) gestational trophoblastic neoplasm (GTN) can be treated with single-agent chemotherapy, and the survival rate approaches 100%. In contrast, patients with high-risk metastatic GTN (stage IV, WHO score ≥ 7) requires initial multiagent chemotherapy with or without adjuvant radiation and surgery, and the survival rate is 80–90% [106, 114].

In addition to the diagnosis of choriocarcinoma, poor prognostic factors include metastatic disease at diagnosis, cerebral or hepatic metastases, symptoms for more than 4 months, failure of prior chemotherapy, and a pretreatment serum beta-hCG titer of more than 100,000 mIU/mL. More recently, the critical beta-hCG level has been reduced to 40,000 mIU/mL by some investigators. Metastatic disease limited to the lungs or vagina is not a poor prognostic sign. In contrast, although it is difficult to assess precisely the prognostic significance of extrapulmonary metastases, patients with CNS metastases have an approximately 50% remission rate compared with involvement of other visceral organs. Development of CNS metastases during the course of treatment confers an even worse prognosis. Patients with hepatic metastases also have a poor prognosis, but multiagent chemotherapy appears to increase the survival rate. Choriocarcinoma diagnosed after a term gestation has a worse prognosis than choriocarcinoma diagnosed after a mole.

Table 20.3
International Federation of Gynecology and Obstetrics (FIGO) staging of gestational trophoblastic disease

Stage	Definition
I	Confined to uterine corpus
II	Metastases to pelvis and vagina
III	Metastasis to lung
IV	Distant metastasis

Table 20.4
Clinical classification of malignant trophoblastic disease

Nonmetastatic GTD
Metastatic GTD
Good prognosis
Low hCG level (<40,000 mIU/ml serum beta-hCG) Symptoms present for less than 4 months No brain or liver metastasis No prior chemotherapy Pregnancy event is not term delivery (i.e., mole, ectopic, or spontaneous abortion)
Poor prognosis
High pretreatment hCG level (>40,000 mIU/ml serum beta-hCG) Symptoms present for more than 4 months Brain or liver metastasis Prior chemotherapeutic failure Antecedent term pregnancy

GTD, gestational trophoblastic disease; hCG, human chorionic gonadotropin.

Table 20.5
World Health Organization scoring system based on prognostic factors[a]

Prognostic factors	Score 0	1	2	4
Age (years)	$\leq$39	>39		
Antecedent pregnancy	Mole	Abortion	Term	
Interval[b]	4	4–6	7–12	>12
hCG (IU/L)	$<10^3$	103–10^4	10^4–10^5	$>10^5$
ABO groups (female × male)		O × A A × O	B AB	
Largest tumor (including uterine tumor)		3–5 cm	>5 cm	
Site of metastasis		Spleen, kidney	GI tract, liver	Brain
No. of metastases identified		1–4	4–8	>8
Prior chemotherapy			Single drug	Two or more drugs

[a]The total score for a patient is obtained by adding the individual scores for each prognostic factor. Total score: $\leq$4, low risk; 5–7, middle risk; and $\geq$8, high risk.
[b]Interval time (months) between end of antecedent pregnancy and start of chemotherapy.
hCG, human chorionic gonadotropin; GI tract, gastrointestinal tract.

Pathogenesis of Gestational Trophoblastic Disease

The pathogenesis of GTD is largely unknown as few molecular studies have been performed [155]. This is in part due to the relative rarity of GTD and the lack of appropriate experimental models. The most well-studied gestational trophoblastic lesion is hydatidiform mole and, to a lesser extent, choriocarcinoma [88]. Development of a hydatidiform mole appears to be associated with an excess of paternal haploid set of chromosomes. The higher the ratio of paternal/maternal chromosomes, the greater the molar change. Complete moles show a 2:0 paternal/maternal ratio, whereas partial moles show a 2:1 ratio. This hypothesis is best supported by the following two studies. First, a mouse model in which molecularly engineered mice that were either androgenetic or gynogenetic (parthenogenetic) were created by microtransfer of male or female pronuclei into enucleated oocytes. Androgenetic embryos transplanted to a foster mother developed a bulky, hypertrophic placenta similar to complete moles in humans, whereas the gynogenetic embryos developed only a small placenta with a secondarily stunted embryo. Another study using the mouse embryonic fibroblasts as the cell model demonstrates that paternal and maternal genomes confer opposite effects on proliferation, cell-cycle progression, senescence, and tumor formation [54]. In comparison with biparental fibroblasts, androgenetic fibroblasts whose genomic complement is exclusively from paternal origin exhibit highly proliferative activity, spontaneous transformation, and formation of tumors at low passage number, while the gynogenetic fibroblasts with exclusive maternal genomic complement show decreased proliferation and increased senescence. The molecular mechanism underlying this observation is the differential expression of imprinted genes. For example, the maternally expressed and paternally imprinted genes such as $p57^{kip2}$ decrease cellular proliferation. In contrast, the paternally expressed growth factor, Igf2, is essential for the long-term proliferation of all genotypes [54]. Therefore, it is likely that a similar mechanism is also involved in the pathogenesis of complete and partial hydatidiform moles. In rare familial/recurrent hydatidiform moles, which account for 2% of all molar cases, mutations have been detected in the maternal gene, NALP7, which plays a role in inflammation and apoptosis [108, 162].

As previously discussed (*Table 20.1*), there are at least three distinctive types of GTN including the most common type, choriocarcinoma, and the less common ones, PSTT and epithelioid trophoblastic tumor. Molecular analysis on GTN is largely based on the identification and characterization of trophoblastic markers in various types of GTN, and the reference of their unique gene expression patterns to different trophoblastic subpopulations in normal early placentas (reviewed in [145]). The main conclusion from those studies is that following neoplastic transformation of trophoblastic stem cells, presumably the cytotrophoblast, specific differentiation programs dictate the type of trophoblastic tumor that develops (*Fig. 20.8*). These patterns of differentiation in GTN recapitulate the stages of early placental development. For example, choriocarcinoma is composed of variable amounts of neoplastic cytotrophoblast, syncytiotrophoblast, and intermediate (extravillous) trophoblast, and resembles the previllous blastocyst, which is composed of a similar mixture of trophoblastic subpopulations. On the other hand, the neoplastic cytotrophoblast in PSTT differentiates mainly into intermediate (extravillous) trophoblastic cells in an implantation site, whereas the neoplastic cytotrophoblast in epithelioid trophoblastic tumor differentiates into

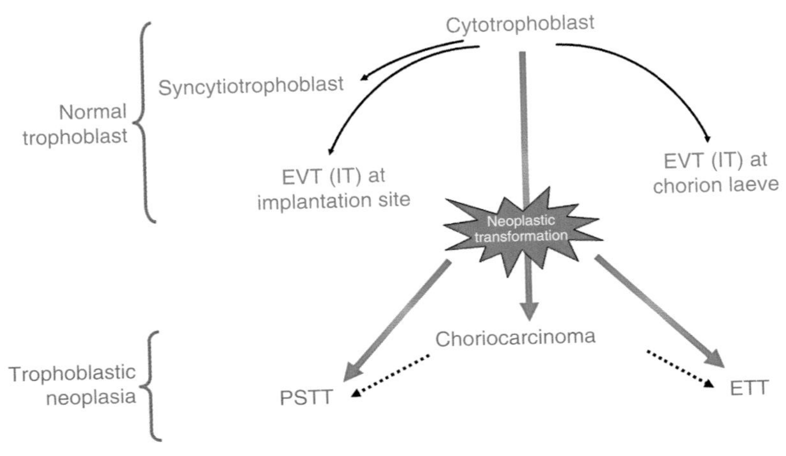

Fig. 20.8
Relationship of trophoblastic neoplasms to different subpopulations of intermediate trophoblastic cells. Exaggerated placental site and placental site trophoblastic tumor are related to the differentiation of implantation site intermediate trophoblast, whereas placental site nodule and epithelioid trophoblastic tumor are related to chorionic-type intermediate trophoblast. EVT: extravillous trophoblast (equivalent to intermediate trophoblast), PSTT: placental site trophoblastic tumor, ETT: epithelioid trophoblastic tumor

chorionic-type intermediate (extravillous) trophoblastic cells in chorion laeve. This model suggests that choriocarcinoma is the most primitive trophoblastic tumor, whereas PSTT and epithelioid trophoblastic tumor are relatively more differentiated. Furthermore, it explains the histologic mixture of choriocarcinoma and PSTT and/or epithelioid trophoblastic tumor in some GTNs.

Clinicopathological Features, Behavior, and Treatment of Molar Placentas

A hydatidiform mole is an abnormal placenta characterized by enlarged, edematous, and vesicular chorionic villi accompanied by villous trophoblastic hyperplasia. It is subdivided into complete hydatidiform mole and partial hydatidiform mole based on morphologic, cytogenetic, and clinicopathological features. Although typical complete and partial moles are easily distinguished on histologic examination, the routine use of ultrasound in pregnancy has led to the clinical diagnosis and evacuation of moles much earlier in gestation, often in the first trimester. As a result, the classical features of complete and partial moles that in the past were based on examination of specimens obtained in the second trimester are not as apparent, making the histopathologic diagnosis more difficult [43]. In addition, a variety of other genetic abnormalities such as trisomy and monosomy may be associated with abnormal placentas that display minor degrees of hydropic change and trophoblastic proliferation but do not qualify as moles. Although recent studies have proposed new and expanded criteria for the diagnosis of these early moles and abnormal placentas, the criteria are subtle and difficult to reproduce, making the histologic diagnosis somewhat subjective. Furthermore, with the recognition that the genetic alterations that underlie these various lesions are distinctly different, one can legitimately question whether the diagnosis should be based on genetic as well as morphologic assessment. At present there is insufficient data to provide a definitive answer. Genetic analysis is costly, labor-intensive, and is not available in most pathology laboratories. However as these techniques become cheaper and more widespread it is likely that genetic analysis will complement histopathologic evaluation in the diagnosis of difficult cases [13, 97]. The ratio of complete versus partial moles varies among studies and most reports show that complete moles outnumber partial moles [13, 28, 45, 65, 97, 121, 167]. Clinical, pathologic, and cytogenetic differences separate the two forms of hydatidiform mole, yet all molar pregnancies have the potential for persistent GTD [3], although the risk is much higher in complete than in partial hydatidiform moles.

Complete Hydatidiform Mole

Complete hydatidiform mole is characterized by hydropic swelling of the majority of villi, and a variable degree of trophoblastic proliferation and atypia. Fetal tissue usually is not present. Most complete hydatidiform moles have a 46, XX karyotype [43]. In a study analyzing 26 complete moles, all of them show diandric (paternal-only) genomes and the lesions include 24 homozygous and 2 heterozygous moles [13]. Early complete moles may lack hydropic swelling but trophoblastic proliferation and atypia are present.

Clinical Features

As discussed above, complete moles are being diagnosed now at an earlier gestational age than in the past (8.5–12 weeks versus 16–18 weeks) because of the routine use of sonography in pregnancy. Pelvic ultrasonic examination discloses a diagnostic snowstorm pattern but high resolution sonography typically reveals a complex intrauterine mass with many small cysts. This pattern, especially when associated with a markedly elevated beta-hCG level, is clinically diagnostic of molar pregnancy. Consequently, a complete mole now rarely presents with the classic signs and symptoms such as excessive uterine size, hyperemesis, theca lutein ovarian cysts, hyperthyroidism, or preeclampsia. The majority of patients present with vaginal bleeding or are discovered by sonography. While a presumptive diagnosis of an incomplete or missed abortion is usually made, serum beta-hCG levels greater than 100,000 mIU/mL should prompt the physician to consider the diagnosis of molar pregnancy. In the past, excessive uterine enlargement for the gestational age occurred in approximately two thirds of patients. Occasionally, the initial clinical manifestation is sudden passage of molar vesicles. Preeclampsia (pregnancy-induced hypertension with edema and proteinuria) occurs in up to one fourth of patients with complete mole. In contrast to nonmolar gestations, in which preeclampsia occurs typically in the last trimester, in molar gestations preeclampsia occurs in the first trimester. Thus, early onset of preeclampsia, especially when coupled with excessive uterine enlargement, suggests the presence of a molar pregnancy. Additional clinical signs of established molar pregnancy include hyperemesis gravidarum, hyperthyroidism, pulmonary embolization of trophoblast, and massive ovarian enlargement due to benign theca lutein cysts (hyperreactio luteinalis) [43]. Usually with complete mole the beta-hCG titer is markedly elevated.

Although these clinical signs and symptoms permit the diagnosis of a molar pregnancy before evacuation, the clinical presentation is quite variable. Up to 80% of cases are first diagnosed by histological study of spontaneously passed or curetted tissue. Hydatidiform moles also can be found unexpectedly in elective abortion specimens of asymptomatic patients and may be rarely detected in the fallopian tube and ovary. A primary mole involving the adnexa should be discriminated from the hydropic change that is frequent in an aborting ectopic pregnancy and from invasive mole with extension into the broad ligament.

Gross Findings

In typical cases, massively enlarged, edematous villi give the characteristic grape-like appearance to the placenta

a

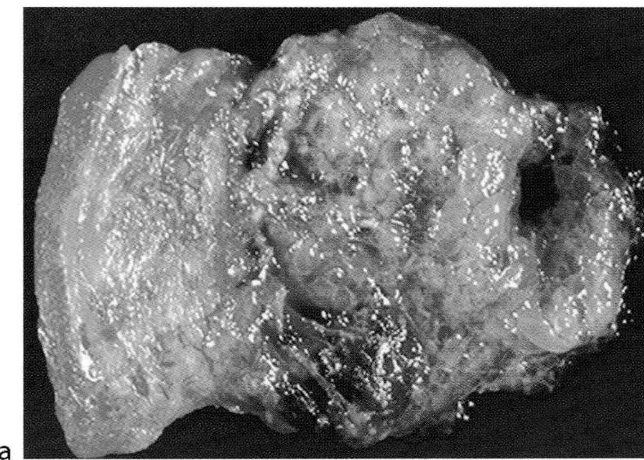

b

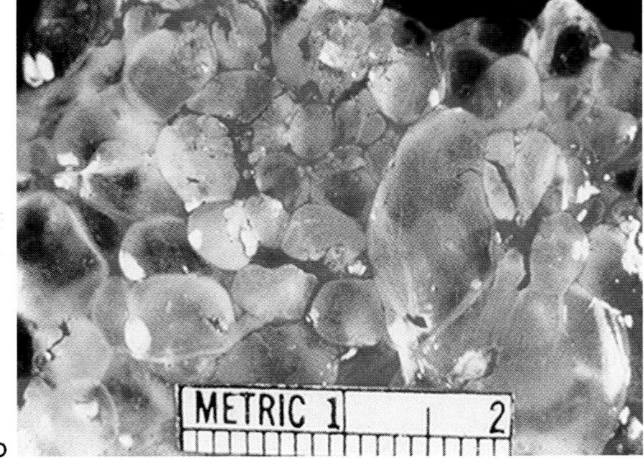

Fig. 20.9
Complete hydatidiform mole. **(a)** A hysterectomy specimen shows an enlarged uterus with molar tissue protruding into the uterine cavity. (Reprint from [146] with permission from Churchill Livingstone Elsevier.) **(b)** In a well-developed complete mole, the hydropic villi range from a few millimeters to more than 1 cm in diameter

(➲ *Fig. 20.9*). However, the specimen volume of contemporary complete moles is significantly less than in the past and in very early complete moles grossly hydropic change may be absent. In advanced mole, which is now rarely encountered, swollen villi may range from a few millimeters to as large as 3.0 cm in diameter but usually average about 1.5 cm. Rarely, fetal development may occur in complete mole. After suction curettage, molar villi may collapse and a large amount of bloody tissue may obscure the edematous villi, especially if a mole is extracted early in pregnancy when villous enlargement is less striking. In this instance, there may be no gross evidence of molar enlargement. Histological evaluation of the tissue adherent to the gauze that collects suctioned uterine contents is necessary to establish the diagnosis. Immersing the gross tissue in saline or formalin can resuspend collapsed villi.

Microscopic Findings

Complete moles have two key features: trophoblastic proliferation and villous edema. Many villi display central cistern formation characterized by a prominent central space that is entirely acellular (➲ *Fig. 20.10*). Smaller villi usually are present but these, too, are edematous. The villous stroma has a distinctive appearance with a pale blue-grey appearance having widely separated spindle cells beneath the villous surface, and edematous central cistern. Villous stroma of a complete mole contains numerous but inconspicuous CD34-positive blood vessels. All hydatidiform moles display some degree of haphazard trophoblastic proliferation on the villous surface. This trophoblastic proliferation in complete hydatidiform mole is circumferential around the villus (➲ *Fig. 20.11*). Columns and streamers of cells composed of a mixture of

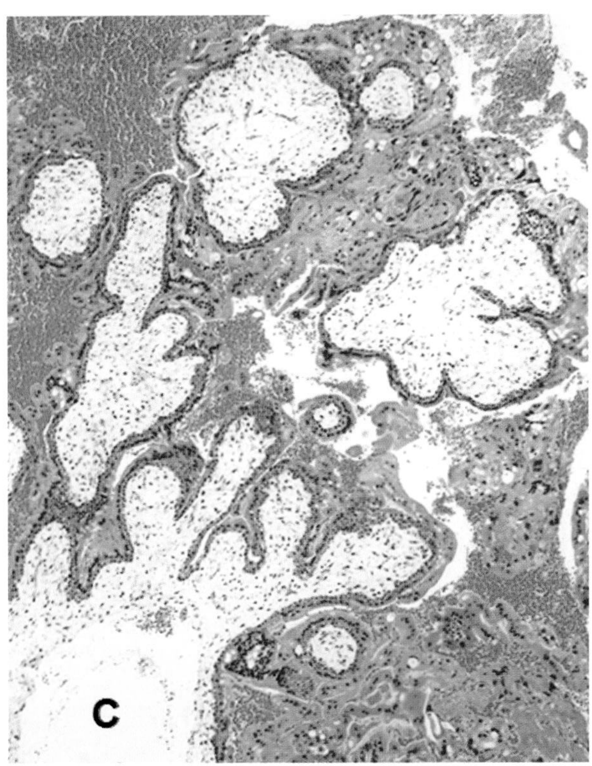

Fig. 20.10
Early complete hydatidiform mole. **Villi have extensive stromal edema with central cisterns (*C*). The periphery of the villi expands into bulbous projections with more prominent stromal cells. There is a large amount of proliferative trophoblast in this field (Courtesy of Dr. B. Ronnett)**

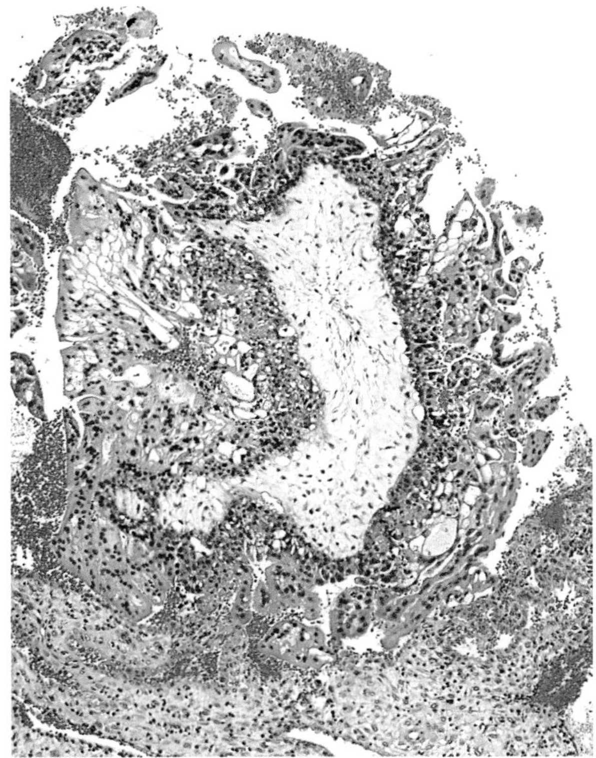

Fig. 20.11
Complete hydatidiform mole. **Enlarged villi with circumferential proliferation of trophoblast**

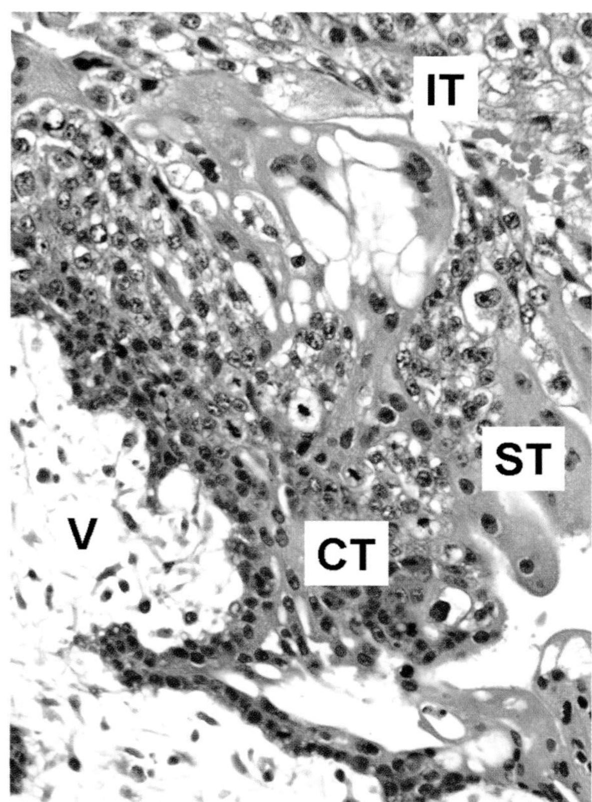

Fig. 20.12
Trophoblast in a complete mole. **A mixture of cytotrophoblast (CT), intermediate trophoblast (IT), and syncytiotrophoblast (ST) grows from the surface of a villus (V)**

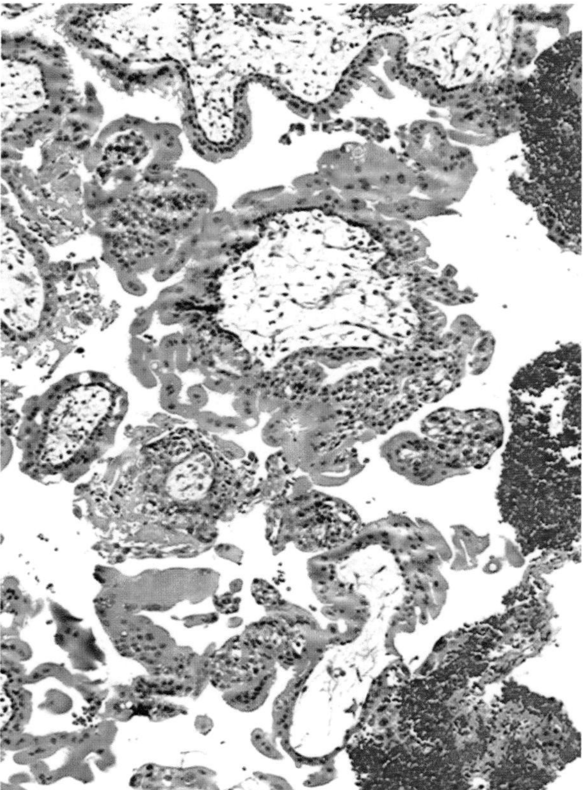

Fig. 20.13
An early complete hydatidiform mole. **The villi are not particularly hydropic and the trophoblastic hyperplasia and atypia are not marked. The circumferential proliferation of villous trophoblastic cells that project randomly from the villous surface is characteristic. This case has been molecularly confirmed as an androgenetic complete mole (Courtesy of Dr. B. Ronnett)**

cytotrophoblast, syncytiotrophoblast, and villous intermediate trophoblast project randomly from the villous surface (*Fig. 20.12*). The amount of proliferative trophoblast in moles varies greatly. It may be marked, affecting most villi, or it may be subtle and only focally present, emphasizing the need for thorough sampling. Large sheets of trophoblast including villous intermediate trophoblast that appear to be unattached to villi also may be present. These result from tangential sectioning, or they represent detached fragments of the trophoblast from the implantation site. Trophoblastic islands, structures seen in the normal early placentas, are rarely present in complete moles. The trophoblast of a complete mole always displays cytologic atypia. At times it may be as marked as in choriocarcinoma (*Fig. 20.12*). In addition, a linear distribution of atypical intermediate trophoblast overlying fibrin is a feature that occurs in trophoblastic lesions as opposed to an abortus.

As noted previously, the typical morphologic features of a complete mole may be absent or very subtle in molar specimens evacuated in the first trimester (*Fig. 20.13*). These complete moles are referred to as "early complete moles" that do not have the typical clinical presentation or classic sonogram appearance. The histologic features of an early complete mole are: (1) redundant or polypoid bulbous terminal villi; (2) hypercellular villous stroma with primitive stellate cells; (3) a labyrinthine network of villous stromal canaliculi; (4) focal hyperplasia of cytotrophoblast and syncytiotrophoblast on both villi and the undersurface of the chorionic plate; (5) atypical trophoblast lining the villi and in the implantation site [72, 107]; and (6) increased villous stromal apoptosis [75].

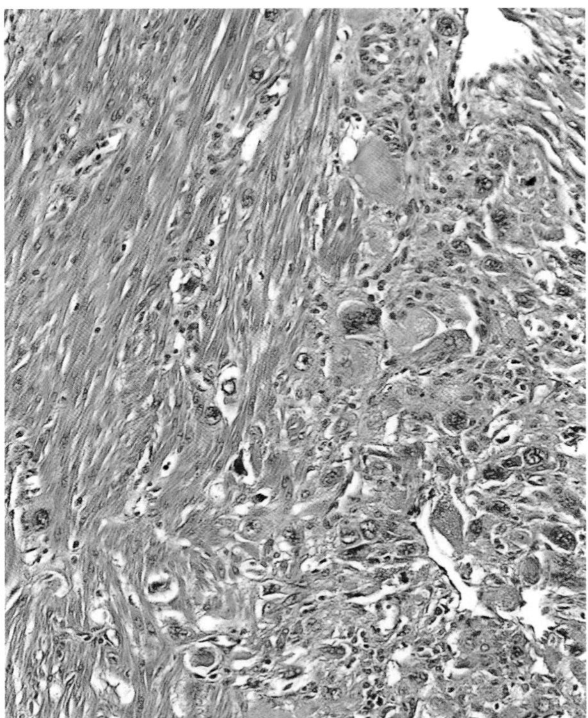

Fig. 20.14
Exaggerated placental site. **The lesion is associated with a complete hydatidiform mole. The intermediate trophoblastic cells extensively infiltrate the endomyometrium. The nuclei are enlarged and show cytologic atypia**

The implantation sites associated with a complete hydatidiform mole almost always show a morphological feature similar to an exaggerated placental site. As with the trophoblastic hyperplasia on the villous surface, the cells are more abundant and atypical than what is encountered with an abortus and for that matter an exaggerated placental site (*Fig. 20.14*). The immunostaining pattern for the markers of implantation site intermediate trophoblast is identical between the molar implantation site and an exaggerated placental site except the Ki-67 labeling index in a mole is elevated as compared to no Ki-67 labeling index in a nonmolar exaggerated placental site, suggesting that these two types of lesions are different despite their similar morphologic features [104, 151]. Interestingly, as compared with the normal placentas, complete moles exhibit a higher level of apoptosis in cytotrophoblast, indicating a complex but delicate regulation of the cell population in complete moles.

Differential Diagnosis (See section Partial Hydatidiform Mole)

The differential diagnosis of complete moles is discussed in the section of partial moles.

Behavior and Treatment

In the past, when the complete moles were not diagnosed early, 2 and 12% of patients experienced severe respiratory distress immediately after uterine evacuation of a hydatidiform mole. This phenomenon usually is attributed to massive deportation of trophoblast to the lungs, an exaggeration of a physiologic process occurring in normal pregnancy. The most serious complication after molar evacuation is persistent or metastatic GTD and the risk of developing choriocarcinoma. Postmolar trophoblastic disease may represent a persistent mole in the uterine cavity or it may be an invasive mole or a choriocarcinoma. Persistent GTD occurs in approximately 17–20% of women who have undergone evacuation [140] and in 3–5% of women who have undergone hysterectomy [44]. The risk of development of choriocarcinoma following a complete mole is about 2–5% in the United States [26, 33] and 13% in Japan [95]. Prediction of the behavior of complete hydatidiform moles based on biomarkers is notoriously difficult. The capricious nature of molar pregnancy should never be underestimated. In the past, a number of clinical, morphologic, and immunohistochemical studies have attempted to predict the prognosis of complete moles but no reliable features have emerged. More recently, Cheung et al. have found that higher mRNA and protein expression levels of Nanog, a transcription factor involved in embryonic stem cell development, are associated with worse clinical outcome in hydatidiform moles, i.e., increased risk for developing persistent GTD [148, 161]. Further studies including large case control studies or prospective cohorts are required to confirm this finding. It is recommended that follow-up with serial serum beta-hCG titers using sensitive assays and radiographic imaging remain the mainstay in managing patients with complete hydatidiform mole.

After treatment with chemotherapy there is minimal increase in the risk of spontaneous abortion or congenital anomalies and many patients have successful term pregnancies. In general, patients with molar pregnancy can be reassured that they can anticipate a normal future reproductive outcome after appropriate treatment [11]. A chest radiograph before treatment and 4 weeks later should be performed to exclude metastases. Following evacuation of a mole, careful beta-hCG monitoring is mandatory since it is the most reliable and sensitive method for the early detection of persistent GTD. The titers of beta-hCG should fall to normal between 10 and 170 days after evacuation of a mole, and most patients will have normal titers by 60 days postevacuation. Persistent GTD after molar pregnancy is heralded by plateauing beta-hCG titers for 2–4 weeks, rising beta-hCG titers, persistent uterine disease such as abnormal bleeding, or evidence of metastases. Initial therapy for persistent disease is usually methotrexate, dactinomycin, or a combination of the two. Multiagent chemotherapy that includes etoposide (VP-16) is used for the treatment of high-risk patients and for those who fail to respond to conventional forms of chemotherapy.

Partial Hydatidiform Mole

Partial hydatidiform mole features an intimate admixture of two populations of villi: enlarged, edematous villi and normal-sized villi that may be fibrotic. Partial molar pregnancies may have a grossly identifiable embryo or fetus with congenital anomalies.

Partial moles are usually the result of diandric triploidy; however, not all triploid conceptuses are partial moles. In a study analyzing 12 partial moles, all partial moles show diandric, monogenic genomes including 11 heterozygous and one homozygous lesions [13].

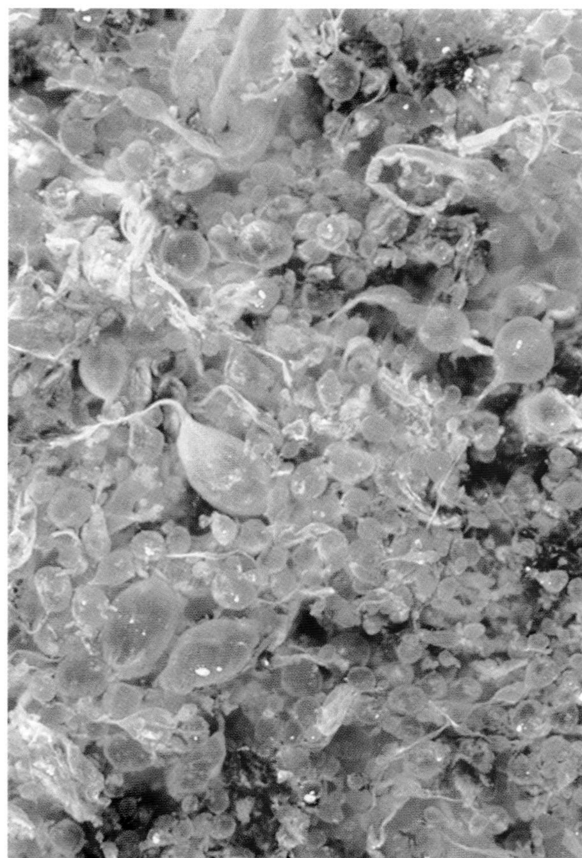

Fig. 20.15
Partial hydatidiform mole. **Hydropic villi mixed with smaller, "normal-appearing" villi**

Clinical Features

Patients with partial moles may have signs and symptoms similar to those seen in complete moles, but usually this is less likely. Uterine size is generally small for dates. Enlargement in excess of that expected for the gestational age is uncommon. Frequently, patients with partial moles appear to have a missed abortion, and vaginal bleeding is the main presenting symptom. Forty-two percent of patients with partial moles are at risk of pre-eclampsia, which tends to occur later than in complete mole but it can be equally severe [68]. Serum beta-hCG levels often are in the low or normal range for gestational age. Only a few patients with partial moles show markedly elevated beta-hCG titers such as those seen with complete moles.

Gross Findings

The volume of tissue is generally small, less than 100 or 200 mL. The villi may be grossly evident and recognizable as molar, yet are smaller than those found in a complete mole. For early partial moles, these gross features may not be apparent. In some cases a fetus or fetal membranes is present. When a fetus is found, it often shows gross congenital anomalies.

Microscopic Findings

Partial mole shows features in some villi that are similar to those seen in complete moles, but the molar change is focal (*Fig. 20.15*). By definition, there should be a mixture of edematous villi and small, relatively normal-sized villi. Central cisterns are less conspicuous than in complete moles. Smaller villi usually show stromal fibrosis similar to that seen in missed abortions (*Fig. 20.16*). Trophoblastic hyperplasia is less marked than in complete

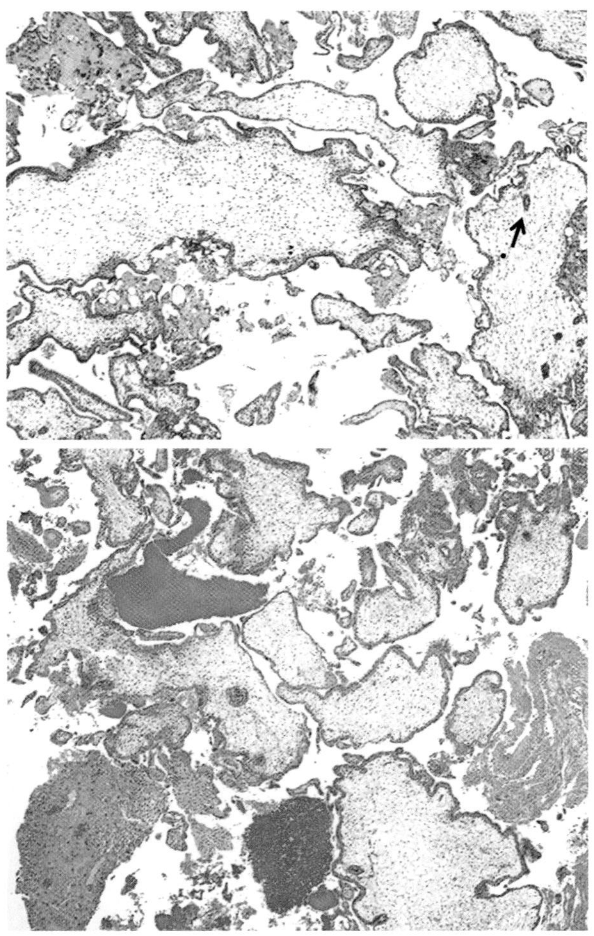

Fig. 20.16
Partial hydatidiform mole. **A mixture of enlarged villi and small, normal-sized, and fibrotic villi. There is mild haphazard trophoblastic hyperplasia and a scalloped villous surface with trophoblastic infoldings forming inclusions (arrow)**

mole. Generally it is focal and shows little, if any, atypia, consisting of small, haphazard tufts of trophoblast, often syncytiotrophoblast, emanating from the surface of some of the abnormal villi. Another feature commonly encountered in partial mole is a scalloped outline of the enlarged villi, yielding a pattern of trophoblastic invaginations into the villous stroma. When the invaginations do not show continuity with the surface trophoblast, they appear as inclusions within the stroma (*Figs. 20.15* and *20.16*). Invaginations are not exclusive for partial moles and may, on occasion, be found in other conditions including complete mole and nonmolar hydropic abortus.

Partial moles with triploidy often are associated with the presence of a fetus (usually abnormally formed) or its amnion, in contrast to the absence of fetal structures in most complete moles. Fetal demise with subsequent degeneration of fetal structures may make identification of fetal tissue difficult. A subtle clue is the presence of a functioning villous circulation containing nucleated red cells, a feature that requires fetal development. In contrast, the embryo associated with a complete mole usually dies before organogenesis and, therefore, fetal structures are not present in the specimen, and fetal erythrocytes are not present within placental vessels. One concern in the diagnosis of an apparent partial mole is that the specimen represents a twin gestation with a fetus and a complete mole. Such twin pregnancies may occur [82], but probably are an infrequent occurrence relative to singleton gestations of a partial mole. In summary, a partial mole is optimally diagnosed when the following four microscopic features are present: (1) two populations of villi (one hydropic and one small and fibrotic, (2) enlarged villi with central cavitation, (3) irregular villi with geographic, scalloped borders with trophoblast inclusions, and (4) minimal trophoblast hyperplasia (usually focal and involving syncytiotrophoblast) [44, 168].

Differential Diagnosis

In a practical sense, the most important diagnostic issue when encountering specimens with abnormal villous morphology is recognition of complete hydatidiform mole since this lesion has a higher risk to develop persistent GTD than partial hydatidiform moles and hydropic abortus. However, diagnosis of hydatidiform moles by histology can be complicated by overlap of morphological criteria for complete mole, partial mole, and a nonmolar hydropic abortus. Nevertheless, the diagnosis of complete versus partial moles is usually relatively straightforward, although it can be difficult when an early complete hydatidiform mole is encountered. The pathological features of partial as compared to complete moles are summarized in *Table 20.6*. Evidence of a fetus or embryo including villous erythrocytes strongly favors the diagnosis of partial mole, although the rare event of a twin gestation with one conceptus being a complete mole should be borne in mind.

Morphological distinction of a hydatidiform mole from an abortus with abnormal villous morphology may be problematic, and there is a considerable degree of interobserver variance in making this distinction [20]. Placentas with genetic abnormalities other than triplody,

Table 20.6
Pathologic features and behavior of complete and partial moles

Feature	Complete	Partial
Karyotype	46,XX, 46,XY	69,XXY, 69,XXX
Embryo/fetus	Absent	Present
Villous outline	Round	Scalloped
Villous stromal apoptosis	Prominent	Limited
Hydropic swelling	Marked; cisterns present	Less pronounced and focal
	All villi involved	Cisterns less prominent
		Small fibrotic villi can be present
Trophoblastic proliferation	Circumferential; Variable, may be marked	Focal and minimal
Trophoblastic atypia	Often present	Absent
Implantation site	Exaggerated[a]	Normal or occasionally exaggerated
P57 (kip2) staining	Negative	Diffusely positive
Behavior	17–20% develop pGTD	<4% develop pGTD

[a]Exaggerated implantation site indicates an increase in the number and the extent of intermediate trophoblastic cells.
pGTD, persistent gestational trophoblastic disease.

such as trisomy, can display morphologic changes suggestive of partial mole and can be misinterpreted as such by morphologic diagnosis alone [20]. However, some clues may be useful in assisting the differential diagnosis. Spontaneous abortions often are associated with failure of development or early demise of the embryo, the so-called blighted ovum or hydropic abortus. These specimens show some villous edema with hydropic swelling, features shared with molar placentas. The hydropic abortus usually is a smaller specimen, however. The villi in a hydropic abortus are enlarged only slightly and do not assume the large dimensions found in complete or partial moles. Cisterns can be seen in nonmolar abortions but they are focally distributed. Hyperplasia of villous trophoblast is not evident in these cases. The proliferative trophoblast on the villous surface of early pregnancy also must be distinguished from the trophoblastic hyperplasia of molar pregnancy. The trophoblast proliferating from the villous surface of an abortus shows polar distribution characterized by proliferation of trophoblast at the distal end of the villus that implants into the basal plate. Similarly, villi with trophoblastic islands can be regarded as polarized villi that are also associated with a nonmolar abortus. This directional orientation contrasts with the irregular or circumferential proliferation of molar trophoblast. In comparing abortion specimens with a non-molar etiology to partial mole it was found that partial moles display at least three of the following histologic features: two discrete populations of villi, circumferential mild trophoblastic hyperplasia, trophoblastic inclusions, prominent scalloping of villi, or cistern formation. In contrast, a non-triploid abortus villi display at most two of these features of partial moles [20]. Irregular trophoblastic hyperplasia from the villous surface is an especially critical feature for diagnosing molar pregnancy.

When large aggregates of atypical or proliferating trophoblast are encountered without any villi, the differential diagnosis should include choriocarcinoma or PSTT. Care must be taken to be certain that sampling is adequate since villi may be sparse and fragmented. Even complete mole can have limited villi in the sections if much of the tissue has been spontaneously aborted or if dealing with repeated curettage following primary evacuation. The entire specimen should be processed. Limited examination of a uterine, vaginal, or pulmonary lesion may show only trophoblast, but deeper sectioning may reveal molar villi.

Immunohistochemical stains with the p57^{kip2} antibody can be helpful in the differential diagnosis of complete hydatidiform moles. Expression of p57^{kip2}, a paternally imprinted gene, is either absent or low in trophoblast in cases of complete moles in contrast to diffuse staining in partial moles and non-molar placentas (*Figs. 20.17–20.19*) [17, 21]. Importantly, assessment of p57 immunoreactivity should be performed only in villous trophoblast and stroma cells rather than intermediate trophoblastic cells in the endomyometrium as the latter may reexpress p57 due to a mechanism related to "epigenetic relaxation" in a complete mole. The accuracy of p57 staining in the diagnosis of complete moles has been recently validated by molecular genetic studies [97, 132]. Besides the p57 expression pattern, the stromal apoptotic index has been shown to be significantly higher in very early complete mole than in very early partial mole or normal placental tissues, which can be potentially useful in differential diagnosis [75].

Given the fact that complete and partial moles are characterized by distinct molecular genetic features, ploidy

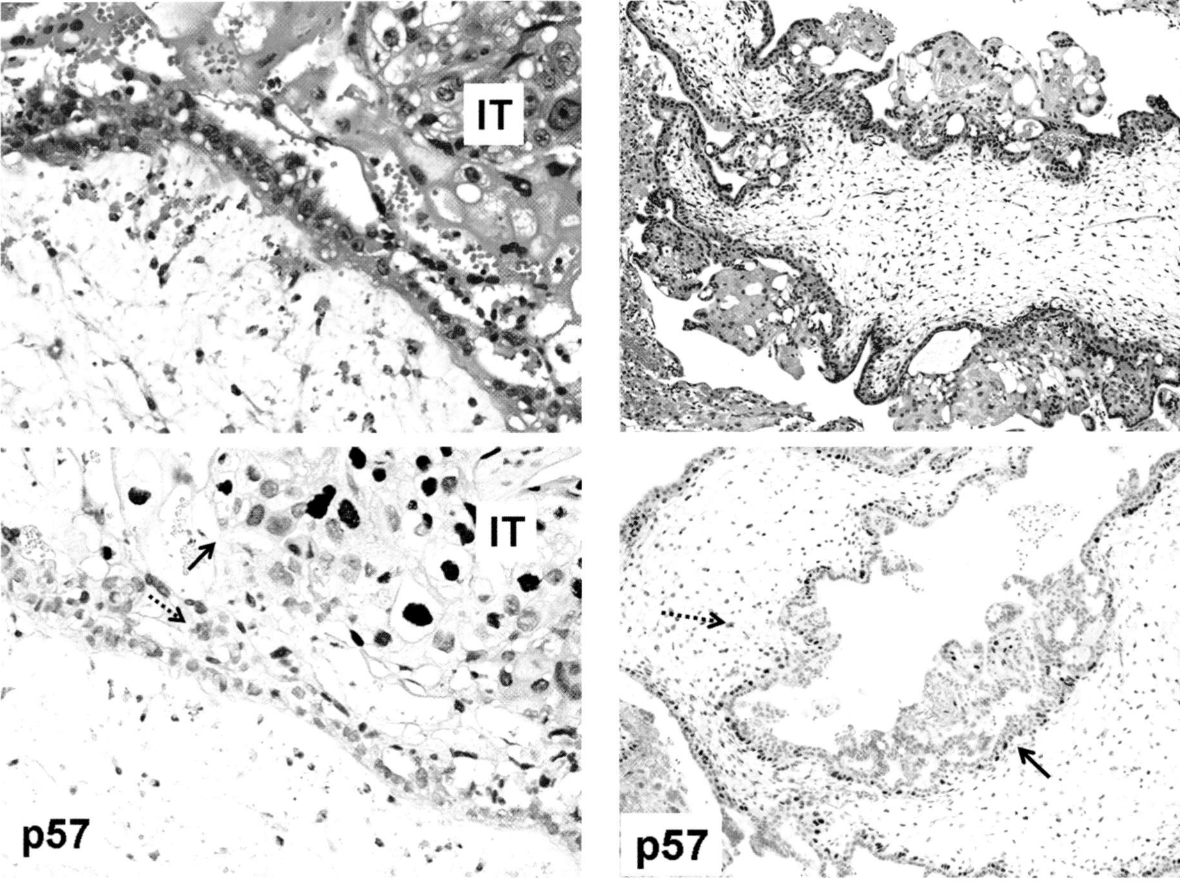

■ Fig. 20.17
p57 immunostaining of a complete hydatidiform mole. **The villous stromal cells and cytotrophoblastic cells (dashed arrow) do not show p57 immunoreactivity while the intermediate trophoblastic cells (IT) (arrow) are positive for p57**

■ Fig. 20.18
p57 immunostaining of a partial hydatidiform mole. **The villous stromal cells (*dashed arrow*) and cytotrophoblastic cells (*arrow*) demonstrate diffuse p57 immunoreactivity**

analysis has proven valuable in distinguishing a diploid complete mole from a triploid partial mole and diploid hydropic abortus from a triploid partial mole [175]. Flow cytometry and digital imaging systems are frequently employed to analyze ploidy; however, ploidy assays cannot be used to diagnose hydatidiform moles per se or to distinguish a diploid complete mole from a diploid hydropic abortus. Recently, the multiplex short tandem repeats (microsatellite markers) DNA analysis has gained wide acceptance in genotyping products of conception with abnormal villous morphology [89]. The assay can be performed using commercially available kits such as those used in practicing forensic medicine and the genomic DNA from villi and maternal tissues can be conveniently prepared from paraffin sections. Analyzing microsatellite markers provides a useful adjunct tool in the differential diagnosis among complete mole, partial mole, and nonmolar hydropic abortus.

In summary, it has been well known that diagnosis based solely on morphology suffers from unsatisfied interobserver reproducibility in distinguishing hydatidiform moles from nonmolar specimens with hydropic villi and subclassification of hydatidiform moles as complete hydatidiform mole, partial hydatidiform mole, or early complete hydatidiform mole. Moreover, chorionic villi associated with chromosomal abnormalities that are not triploid, such as trisomy, may display hydropic change and abnormal villous morphology that mimic a partial mole [20]. These abnormal placentas associated with hydropic abortus are not associated with an increased risk of GTD and therefore the

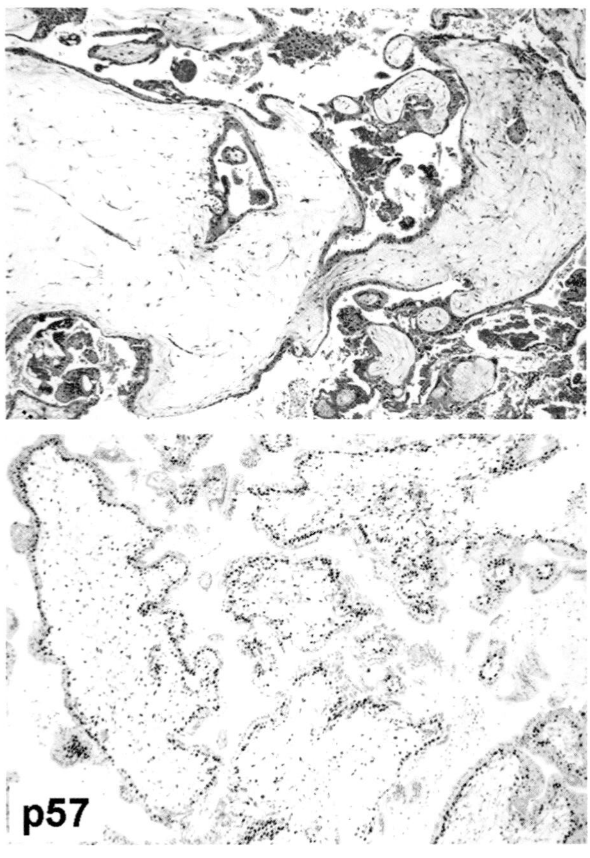

Fig. 20.19
Abnormal villous morphology. **The H&E shows irregularly shaped and variably sized villi with a trophoblastic inclusion, suggesting a partial hydatidiform mole (PHM). Similar to a PHM, the villous stromal cells and cytotrophoblast are diffusely positive for p57. However, genotyping analysis demonstrated biparental diploidy, consistent with a non-molar abortus (Courtesy of Dr. B. Ronnett)**

differential diagnosis is clinically important. A logistic approach in differential diagnosis of specimens with abnormal villous morphology has been proposed [97]. In that study, it is recommended that morphologically abnormal villi should be assessed for p57 immunostaining, which serves as a triage assay for the diagnosis of complete hydatidiform moles. When the diagnosis by routine morphology is equivocal, morphologic features together with a negative p57 result indicate a complete hydatidiform mole with a rare exception that the complete hydatidiform mole retains the maternal allele of chromosome 11 in which the *p57* gene resides. Molecular genotyping is then applied to validate a diagnosis of complete hydatidiform mole by demonstrating androgenetic diploidy and to resolve p57-positive cases into diandric triploid partial hydatidiform mole, biparental diploid nonmolar specimens, and the rare complete hydatidiform mole with aberrant p57 expression [98]. All genotyped nonmolar specimens demonstrated biparental diploidy, while partial hydatidiform moles demonstrated diandric triploidy.

Behavior and Treatment

Several studies have shown that partial moles are rarely followed by persistent or metastatic GTD with risk estimates ranging from 0 to 4% [9, 12, 47, 50, 82, 95, 100, 115, 140, 183]. Misinterpretation of complete moles as partial moles is a major factor contributing to the overestimated frequency of persistent GTD after partial mole in previous studies. Although the risk to develop persistent GTD or GTN is relatively low in partial mole, there are several case reports demonstrating the association of a partial mole and GTN. For example, invasive mole and metastatic pulmonary lesions have been reported in association with a partial mole [50], and choriocarcinomas have been reported in 3 of 3,000 patients with partial moles. In addition, an in situ or intraplacental choriocarcinoma arising in a partial mole have also been reported [99]. The magnitude of the risk of repeated partial moles is not known, although repetitive partial moles do occur. Therefore, despite the fact that development of persistent GTD following a partial mole is uncommon, follow-up of patients after evacuation of a partial mole is warranted.

Invasive Mole

Invasive mole is a hydatidiform mole in which hydropic villi invade the myometrium or blood vessels or, more rarely, are deported to extrauterine sites. Although invasive mole is not a true neoplastic disease, it is often clinically considered to be malignant since the lesion can invade the myometrium and metastasize.

Clinical Features

Invasive mole is a possible sequela of a hydatidiform mole, complete or partial. It is unusual for invasive mole to present primarily, although invasive mole may occur simultaneously with intracavitary molar pregnancy. Pathological diagnosis requires demonstration of molar villi invading the myometrium or deported to extrauterine sites. In histologically verified cases the lesion most often is confined to the uterus, with distant spread occurring in 20–40% of cases. Typically this involves the lungs, but the vagina, vulva, and broad ligament are also well recognized. Rare examples of spread to other sites such as the paraspinal soft tissue have been reported. The diagnosis usually is made on a hysterectomy specimen. However, invasive mole is rarely confirmed histologically since hysterectomy is rarely performed in patients with persistent beta-hCG titers after removal of an intrauterine mole and since metastatic lesions of GTD usually are treated successfully with cytotoxic chemotherapy without biopsy.

Gross Findings

In the uterus, invasive mole is an erosive, hemorrhagic lesion extending from the uterine cavity into the myometrium. Invasion can range from superficial penetration to extension through the wall, with perforation or involvement of the broad ligament. Molar vesicles often are grossly apparent.

Microscopic Findings

Microscopically, the diagnostic feature is the presence of molar villi along with trophoblast in the myometrium or at an extrauterine site (*Fig. 20.20*). Trophoblastic proliferation with atypia accompanies the enlarged villi and is as variable as in noninvasive mole, ranging from slightly proliferative with minimal atypia to marked trophoblastic proliferation with extreme atypia. Hydropic swelling tends not to be as marked as in noninvasive mole. Molar villi usually are no more than 4–5 mm in diameter. In metastatic sites, the diagnosis is based on the presence of villi. Careful searching may be necessary to identify villi within a lesion seemingly composed entirely of highly proliferative trophoblast. Lesions at distant sites usually are composed of molar villi confined within blood vessels without invasion into adjacent tissue. The molar villi at the extrauterine sites are the result of intravascular deportation.

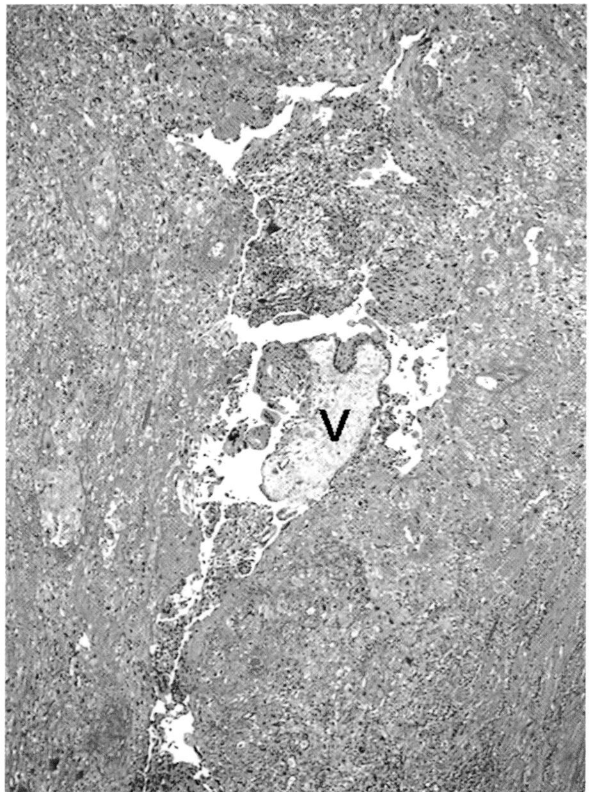

Fig. 20.20
Invasive mole. **A hydropic villus invades the myometrium. Intermediate trophoblastic cell proliferation is present in the myometrium**

Differential Diagnosis

Since the pathological diagnosis of invasive moles requires identification of molar villi and trophoblast either within the myometrium or at an extrauterine site, there are few lesions that enter into the differential. Recurettage of the endometrium after diagnosis of a mole may show proliferative trophoblast with villi but this does not represent an invasive mole unless myometrial invasion is found. If post-molar curettage yields only trophoblast, the diagnosis of invasive mole is not established. Two forms of placenta accreta, specifically placenta increta or percreta, represent normal placenta that has implanted without an intervening decidual layer and invaded myometrium. In contrast to invasive mole, however, the villi in accreta are not hydropic and the trophoblast does not show the proliferative activity found in a mole.

Invasive mole must be discriminated from choriocarcinoma. Both invasive mole and choriocarcinoma after a hydatidiform mole are manifested by a plateau or elevation in the beta-hCG titer. Furthermore, both can give rise to secondary lesions. Consequently, it is often not possible clinically to distinguish between these lesions. A repeat curettage may yield more molar tissue, obvious choriocarcinoma, or scant fragments of trophoblast unaccompanied by villi but lacking unequivocal features of choriocarcinoma. In the latter instance a diagnosis of atypical trophoblast is appropriate, accompanied by a description and the reasons why a diagnosis of residual mole or choriocarcinoma was not made. When more molar tissue is found, a diagnosis of persistent hydatidiform mole is made.

Behavior and Treatment

Invasive mole is the most common form of persistent or metastatic GTD after hydatidiform mole, which occurs six to ten times more frequently than choriocarcinoma. Using modern chemotherapy, death from invasive mole is unusual. Most patients, even with distant spread survive. The risk of progression to choriocarcinoma is no greater than that after complete mole.

Invasive mole is the clinical diagnosis given to many patients with extrauterine disease or abnormally persistent beta-hCG titers after molar pregnancy and no residual hydatidiform mole within the uterine cavity. In such instances, there is, however, a possibility that persistent beta-hCG levels may be due to choriocarcinoma. In these cases, the clinical term persistent GTD or gestational trophoblastic neoplasia is used without attempting to discriminate between invasive mole and choriocarcinoma.

Clinicopathological Features, Behavior, and Treatment of Trophoblastic Tumors and Tumor-like Lesions

Choriocarcinoma

Gestational choriocarcinoma is a highly malignant epithelial tumor arising from the trophoblast of any type of gestational event, most often a hydatidiform mole. Choriocarcinoma is for all practical purposes limited to reproductive-age women but rare examples in postmenopausal women have been reported. It consists predominantly of a biphasic proliferation of mononucleate trophoblast and syncytiotrophoblast that morphologically recapitulates the primitive trophoblast of the previllous stage during placental development. Chorionic villi are not a component of this tumor with an exception of intraplacental choriocarcinoma (see below). Molecular genetic study based on restriction fragment length polymorphism analysis using a minisatellite DNA probe suggests that the pathogenesis of choriocarcinoma varies, some being androgenetic and some gynogenetic [6]. However, the case number in that study is limited to permit from conclusions. The absence of Y chromosome has been demonstrated in the vast majority of choriocarcinomas, indicating that the shortfall of Y chromosomal complements in choriocarcinomas may simply be due to the genetic basis of their precursor lesions, complete hydatidiform moles in which most of cases had the genotype of XX [178].

Clinical Features

Theoretically, choriocarcinoma may arise in the trophoblast of the primitive blastocyst during implantation, but most cases of choriocarcinoma appear to follow a recognizable gestational event. Indeed, "in situ" or intraplacental choriocarcinoma can be found in a third-trimester placenta [29, 38] with a transition from normal-appearing cytotrophoblast to choriocarcinoma. The more abnormal the pregnancy, the more likely that choriocarcinoma may supervene. Hertig and Mansell found an incidence of 1 in 160,000 normal gestations, 1 in 15,386 abortions, 1 in 5,333 ectopic pregnancies, and 1 in 40 molar pregnancies [55]. In that series, one half of the cases of choriocarcinoma were preceded by hydatidiform mole, with 25% following abortion, 22.5% following normal pregnancy, and 2.5% following ectopic pregnancy [55].

The signs and symptoms of choriocarcinomas are protean. Abnormal uterine bleeding is one of the most frequent presentations of choriocarcinoma, but uterine lesions may be restricted to the myometrium and remain asymptomatic. Not all patients have a demonstrable lesion in the uterus after an intrauterine gestation. Many examples of metastatic choriocarcinoma without a primary uterine tumor have been described and in those cases, it is highly likely that the neoplasm undergoes regression in the uterus. Although the majority of choriocarcinomas develop shortly after the preceding gestation (➲ *Table 20.7*), long latency (>10 years) between the gestation and diagnosis can occur [127, 165]. Because of its rarity, the diagnosis of a postpartum choriocarcinoma can be delayed and the mean duration from onset of symptoms to treatment is 7 weeks [117]. Sometimes, symptoms related to metastases are the first indication that a choriocarcinoma is present, and the lungs are the most frequent sites for metastasis. Thyrotoxicosis and hemorrhagic events in the central nervous system, liver, and gastrointestinal or urinary tracts also occurs in choriocarcinoma. Although rare, gestational choriocarcinoma may coexist with an intrauterine

Table 20.7
Clinical features of gestational trophoblastic tumors

Features	Choriocarcinoma	PSTT	ETT
Clinical presentation	Persistent GTD after hydatidiform mole	Missed abortion	Abnormal vaginal bleeding
Last known pregnancy or GTD	Usually within months	Variable, can be remote	Variable, can be remote
History of mole	∼50% of cases	∼10%–50% of cases	∼10%–50% of cases
Serum beta-hCG	High (>10,000 IU/mL)	Low (<2,000 IU/mL)	Low (<2,000 IU/mL)
Clinical behavior	Aggressive if untreated, curable in most patients after treatment	Self-limited, persistent, or aggressive	Self-limited, persistent, or aggressive
Response to chemotherapy	Excellent	Variable	Variable
Primary treatment	Chemotherapy	Hysterectomy or local resection	Hysterectomy or local resection

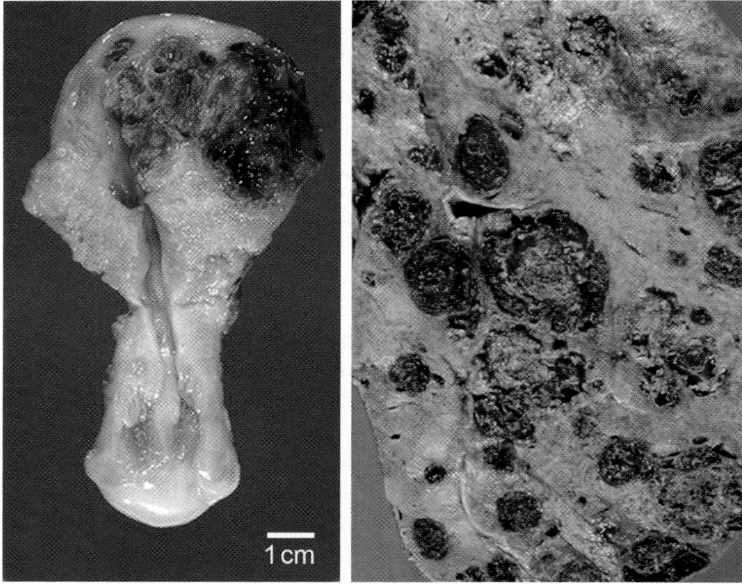

Fig. 20.21
Choriocarcinoma. ***Left***: **Choriocarcinoma in the uterus. The tumor forms a large, hemorrhagic mass that involves the endometrium and myometrium. (Reprint from [146] with permission from Churchill Livingstone Elsevier.)** ***Right***: **Liver metastasis from choriocarcinoma. Multiple, circumscribed, and hemorrhagic masses are evident**

pregnancy, either as an incidental microscopic finding or a concurrent disease with the diagnosis of choriocarcinoma during pregnancy. Gestational choriocarcinoma also may be primary in the fallopian tube, and in this extremely rare instance, the tumor probably is a sequela of an ectopic pregnancy.

Gross Findings

Uterine choriocarcinoma generally is a dark red, hemorrhagic mass with a shaggy, irregular surface and variable amounts of necrosis (*Fig. 20.21*). Occasionally, a lesion may lack significant hemorrhage and appear as a fleshy,

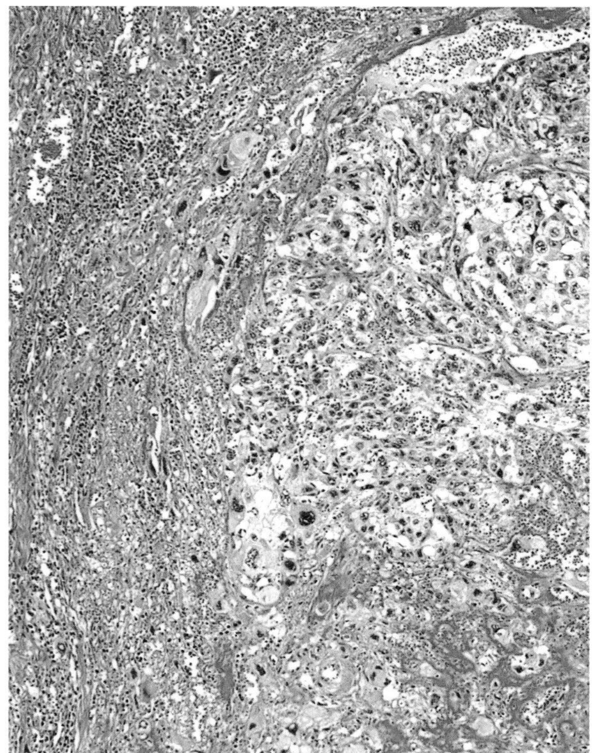

■ Fig. 20.22
Choriocarcinoma. **The tumor forms a circumscribed mass within the myometrium. Hemorrhage is present in the right lower corner**

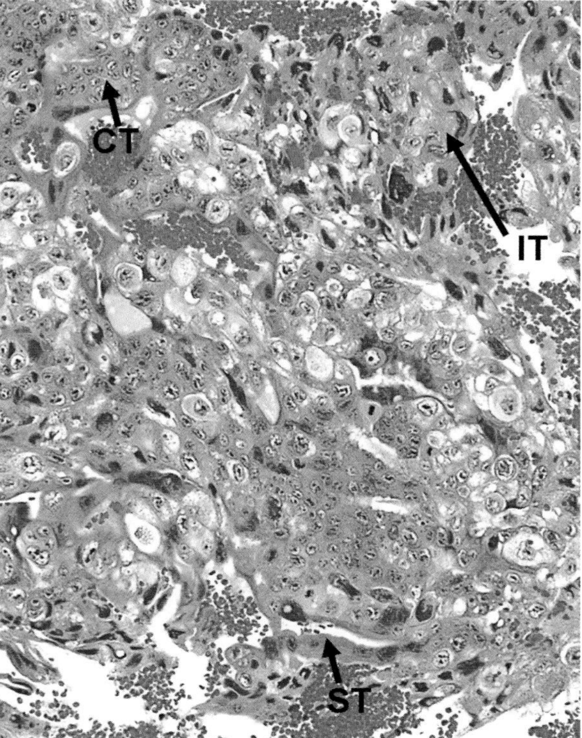

■ Fig. 20.23
Choriocarcinoma. **Syncytiotrophoblast (ST) lining vascular spaces and capping cytotrophoblast (CT) and intermediate trophoblast (IT). There is an alternating arrangement of multinucleated ST with intervening clusters of mononucleate IT and CT**

tan-gray mass with necrosis. The size of uterine lesions varies greatly, ranging from tiny, microscopic foci to huge, necrotic tumors. Metastases beyond the uterus appear well circumscribed and hemorrhagic. For the rare intraplacental choriocarcinoma, the diagnosis based on gross specimens is very difficult as the lesion may be very small and can mimic non-malignant conditions, such as placental infarction or even an old blood clot.

Microscopic Findings

Choriocarcinoma is characterized by masses and sheets of trophoblastic cells that invade surrounding tissue and permeate vascular spaces (*Figs. 20.22–20.26*). Choriocarcinoma is generally not associated with chorionic villi with the rare exception of choriocarcinoma arising within a placenta. Central hemorrhage and necrosis with viable tumor constituting only a thin peripheral rim is a characteristic feature. The interface with normal tissue, if preserved, is circumscribed and appears expansile or pushing (*Fig. 20.22*).

An intimate mixture of cytotrophoblast, intermediate trophoblast, and syncytiotrophoblast forms the cellular population of choriocarcinoma (*Fig. 20.23*) [92]. The cytotrophoblast and intermediate trophoblast tend to grow in clusters and sheets, separated by syncytiotrophoblast, forming the characteristic dimorphic growth pattern (*Fig. 20.23*). These patterns of growth recapitulate the relationship of the trophoblast to the maternal–placental circulation of the early implanting previllous blastocyst. A network of syncytiotrophoblast intimately admixed with cytotrophoblast and intermediate trophoblast comprises the plexiform pattern of trophoblast in many cases. The percentage of intermediate trophoblast in choriocarcinomas is highly variable ranging from 1 to 90%

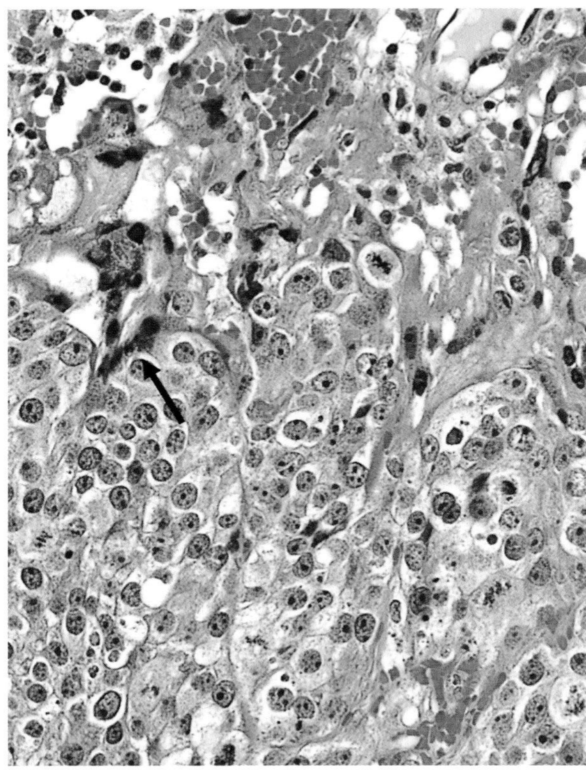

Fig. 20.24
Choriocarcinoma with inconspicuous syncytiotrophoblast. **Occasionally, choriocarcinoma is composed predominately of cytotrophoblast and intermediate trophoblast with indistinct or attenuated syncytiotrophoblast (*arrow*) forming monotonous and cohesive sheets. Although syncytiotrophoblast is inconspicuous, these cells have dense, eosinophilic cytoplasm and pyknotic nuclei. This pattern may simulate a poorly differentiated carcinoma**

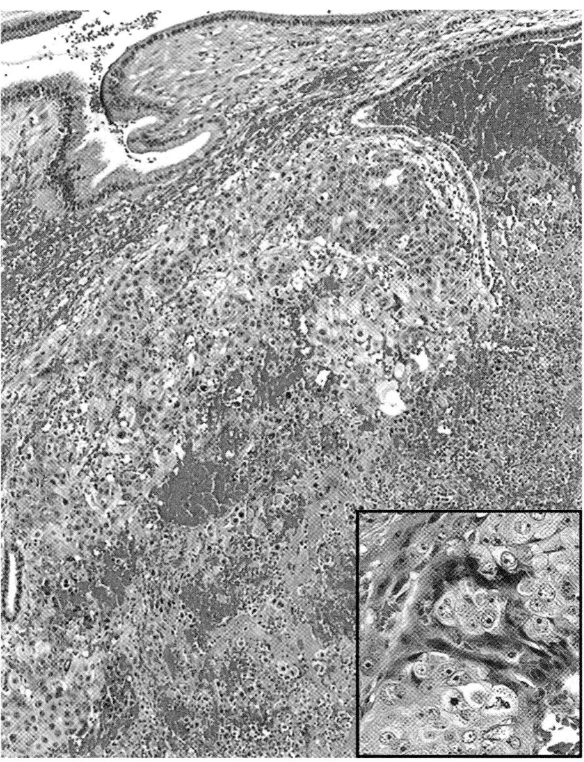

Fig. 20.25
Monomorphic choriocarcinoma in the cervix. **Mononucleate trophoblast (cytotrophoblast and intermediate trophoblast) is present and syncytiotrophoblast is indistinct in this section. However, syncytiotrophoblast appears in deeper sections and displays an alternating (biphasic) pattern of syncytiotrophoblast and mononucleate trophoblast (*inset*)**

of the mononucleate trophoblastic cellular population [149], and a recent study has demonstrated that choriocarcinoma is composed predominantly of a mixture of syncytiotrophoblast and intermediate trophoblast with only a small proportion of cytotrophoblast [92]. The intermediate trophoblastic cells in a choriocarcinoma tend to be larger with more abundant cytoplasm (*Fig. 20.23*). They are usually located adjacent to the cytotrophoblast, assuming a zonal pattern of differentiation from cytotrophoblast. Occasionally, choriocarcinoma appears predominately composed of cytotrophoblast and intermediate trophoblast forming a monotonous and cohesive sheet or mass with indistinct or attenuated syncytiotrophoblast (*Figs. 20.24* and *20.25*). This monomorphic variant may cause a problem in the differential diagnosis. Careful search for syncytiotrophoblast, deeper sectioning of the paraffin blocks, and immunostaining for beta-hCG may reveal syncytiotrophoblast in focal areas. Beta-hCG staining can be very useful in demonstrating attenuated or indistinct syncytiotrophoblast.

One of the unique morphological features of choriocarcinoma is the lack of new blood vessel formation (angiogenesis) in the center of the tumor (*Fig. 20.26*) although blood vessels stemming from the surrounding stroma can be detected in the periphery of a choriocarcinoma. Instead, the tumor cells within a choriocarcinoma establish intricate pseudovascular network and blood-lakes that are lined by trophoblastic cells rather than by endothelial cells. Those trophoblast-lined pseudovascular channels likely communicate with true blood vessels outside the

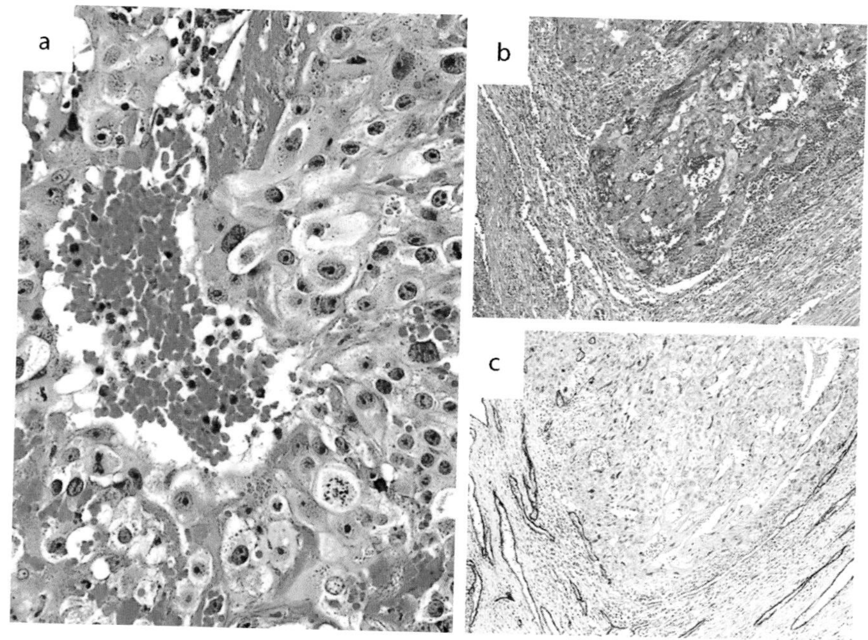

Fig. 20.26
Choriocarcinoma. **(a)** H&E stain shows high magnification of choriocarcinoma cells. **(b)** Trichrome stain demonstrates almost undetectable connective tissue within the choriocarcinoma. **(c)** CD34 staining reveals no evidence of endothelium-lined blood vessels in the tumor except in the tumor–stroma interface. The blood supply of choriocarcinoma in this specimen is derived from trophoblastic cells creating blood-filled channels and lakes that communicate with the circulation in the soft tissue surrounding the tumor

choriocarcinoma. The generation of microvascular-like channels by neoplastic cells was termed "vasculogenic mimicry," a term used to underscore their de novo generation without involvement by endothelial cells [37]. The vasculogenic mimicry can only be seen in a sizable choriocarcinoma usually obtained from a hysterectomy specimen (*Fig. 20.26*) and may not be obvious in small biopsy samples. In contrast to angiogenesis occurring in other solid tumors, the pseudovascular channels in choriocarcinoma are devoid of adequate stromal support, which contributes to hemorrhage and necrosis in the center of the tumor. Accordingly, it is not uncommon that only a small amount of viable choriocarcinoma tissue remains in a lesion and thus extensive sampling and sectioning may be required to identify the typical morphological features of choriocarcinoma.

There may be considerable cytological atypia in the trophoblast with pleomorphic-enlarged nuclei, abnormal mitotic figures, and bizarre cellular configurations. Nuclear chromatin is coarsely granular, with an uneven distribution, and nucleoli may be present (*Fig. 20.26*). Enlarged, multinucleated intermediate trophoblastic cells with two or several nuclei also occur, and they are distinguished from syncytiotrophoblast by their cytoplasm, which lacks the dense eosinophilia and vacuolization and by positive CD146 (Mel-CAM) immunostaining [149].

It is not uncommon for choriocarcinoma to display focal differentiation of a PSTT and/or an epithelioid trophoblastic tumor. The choriocarcinoma component can be discrete or it can merge imperceptibly with areas of PSTT or epithelioid trophoblastic tumor. To report those mixed GTN, we recommend using a term of "choriocarcinoma with PSTT or epithelioid trophoblastic tumor" to accentuate the clinical importance in recognizing the choriocarcinoma component, which requires cytotoxic chemotherapy. Further studies are required to determine the treatment response and clinical outcome in the mixed GTNs.

Differential Diagnosis

In general, the diagnosis of choriocarcinoma requires the presence of the biphasic pattern of trophoblastic growth (syncytiotrophoblast and mononucleate trophoblast) and invasion of the tumor typically associated with necrosis

Table 20.8
Morphological features of gestational trophoblastic tumors

Features	Choriocarcinoma	PSTT	ETT
Cellular population	Dimorphic; syncytiotrophoblast alternating with mononucleate trophoblast	Monomorphic; implantation site intermediate trophoblastic	Monomorphic; chorionic-type intermediate trophoblastic
Cell size and shape	Irregular, highly variable	Large and pleiomorphic	Smaller, round, and uniform
Cytoplasm	Variable pale to amphophilic	Abundant and eosinophilic	Eosinophilic or clear
Growth pattern	Circumscribed mass with central necrosis/ hemorrhage	Confluent sheets, masses or infiltrating single cells	Epithelioid nests or cords or solid masses
Tumor border	Circumscribed; pushing	Infiltrating	Circumscribed; expansile
Cellular necrosis	Extensive	Usually absent	Extensive
Calcification	Absent	Absent	Usually present
Vascular invasion	Tumor thrombi	From periphery to lumen	Absent
Fibrinoid change	Absent	Present	Present
Mitosis	High; 2–22/10 HPF	Variable; 0–6/10 HPF	Variable; 1–10/10 HPF
Associated chorionic villi	Absent	Absent	Absent

into the endomyometrium. The presence of detached fragments of biphasic trophoblastic tissue alone may be insufficient to diagnose choriocarcinoma unless very early placentas and trophoblastic hyperplasia associated with a complete hydatidiform mole can be excluded. Assessment of endomyometrial invasion should be thoroughly evaluated and deeper sections may be needed to demonstrate the invasive pattern associated with choriocarcinoma. Thus, choriocarcinoma must be distinguished from the normal trophoblast of early gestation, from molar pregnancies, as well as from PSTT, epithelioid trophoblastic tumor, and from other forms of epithelial malignancy. The differential diagnosis is primarily based on morphological grounds (*Table 20.8*). Occasionally, normal trophoblast of an early gestation is found in curettings without associated villi. In this circumstance, the trophoblast should be present only in small quantities and deeper sections may reveal chorionic villi. Normal trophoblast of an early gestation, although proliferative, does not show atypical features including marked cellular enlargement and nuclear abnormalities found in choriocarcinoma (*Fig. 20.27*). Thus, large amounts of trophoblast showing atypia should be viewed suspiciously for choriocarcinoma. Most importantly, fragments of normal trophoblast in curettings do not show tumor necrosis or destructive invasion. As a general rule, choriocarcinoma should not be diagnosed in the presence of villi. Proliferative trophoblast in association with villi usually indicates either an abortion or hydatidiform mole. The differential diagnosis of these lesions is discussed under "Hydatidiform mole." Rarely, gestational choriocarcinoma arises within a normally developing placenta, with the neoplasm intimately associated with well-formed, mature nonmolar villi [184]. If the diagnosis is in doubt, a chest radiograph and careful monitoring of beta-hCG levels should help resolve the problem.

Discriminating choriocarcinoma from other carcinomas either within the uterus or at other sites usually is not a problem. On occasion a biopsy may show a few syncytiotrophoblastic cells, or the entire lesion is composed of mononucleate trophoblastic cells, a pattern that can mimic a poorly differentiated carcinoma (*Figs. 20.24* and *20.25*). When this differential diagnosis arises, the clinical history may reveal a previous molar pregnancy or another suspicious pregnancy event that can assist in the diagnosis. Serum beta-hCG levels and immunohistochemical localization of beta-hCG, hPL, and HSD3B1 in syncytiotrophoblast can be useful (*Fig. 20.28*; *Table 20.2*).

Choriocarcinoma has been described as a primary tumor arising in a number of different sites besides the uterus and gonads. In women of reproductive age, however, pure choriocarcinoma that appears to be an extrauterine primary tumor probably represents

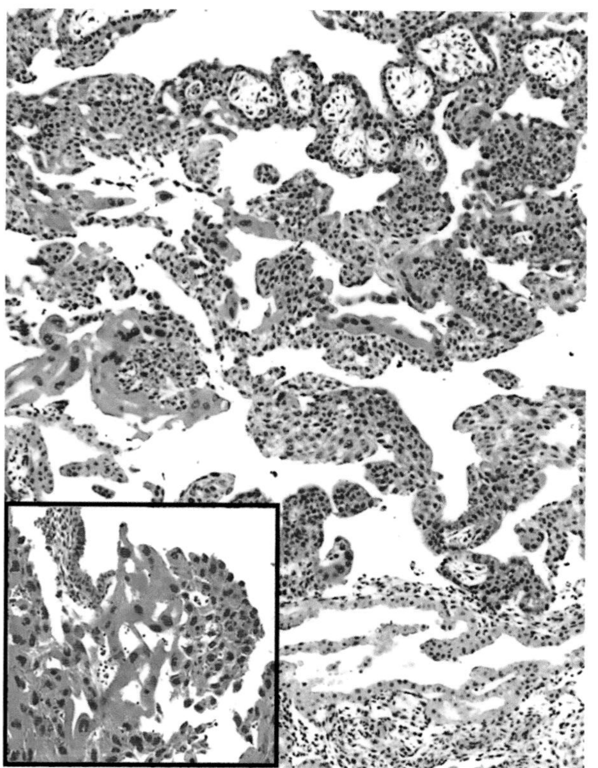

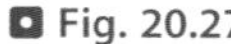 Fig. 20.27
Normal trophoblast in an early gestation. **The trophoblastic cells in an early placenta may exhibit "biphasic" growth as seen in choriocarcinoma (*inset*). Unlike choriocarcinoma, the normal trophoblastic cells, although proliferative, do not show atypical features including marked cellular enlargement and nuclear abnormalities. Normal trophoblast does not display tumor cell necrosis or destructive invasion. Large amounts of trophoblast with atypia should be viewed suspiciously for choriocarcinoma. Moreover, the presence of chorionic villi is important to establish the diagnosis of an early gestation. Deeper sections can be useful in identifying villi if they are absent in the original sections**

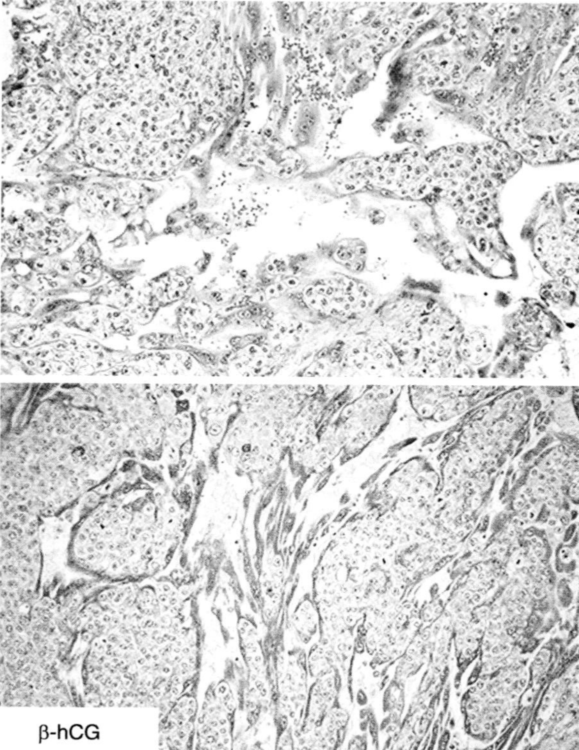

Fig. 20.28
Syncytiotrophoblast in choriocarcinoma. **Syncytiotrophoblast surrounds nests of mononucleate trophoblastic cells. In this case, syncytiotrophoblast is strongly positive for beta-hCG. In choriocarcinoma with inconspicuous syncytiotrophoblast, immunostaining with an anti-hCG antibody can be very useful in establishing the diagnosis by highlighting syncytiotrophoblast**

gestational choriocarcinoma in which the index pregnancy is undetected. True primary choriocarcinoma at an unusual site may be an extragonadal germ cell tumor, or it may be derived from dedifferentiation of an ordinary carcinoma [1]. Primary somatic tumors of the gastrointestinal tract, bladder, breast, lung, or endometrium rarely show choriocarcinomatous differentiation, and these show transitions from ordinary carcinoma to the trophoblastic component. Since somatic tumors also may produce beta-hCG without showing choriocarcinoma histology, the classic biphasic growth pattern should be present before rendering the diagnosis of choriocarcinoma.

The differential diagnosis of choriocarcinoma and PSTT and epithelioid trophoblastic tumor will be discussed in the following specific sections and is summarized in *Tables 20.7* and *20.8*.

Clinical Behavior and Treatment

Metastasis of choriocarcinoma most frequently occurs in brain and liver, and the majority of therapeutic failures have liver and/or brain metastases. High beta-hCG level is a risk factor for predicting the occurrence of brain and liver metastases [182]. Kidney and abdomen, including intestinal tract, are the other common sites of spread, but almost any organ, including the skin, may be involved. Lymph nodes contain tumor on occasion, often as tertiary metastatic lesions from other organs. Vaginal involvement has been reported in 16–32% of patients. There have been a few isolated reports of metastatic choriocarcinoma occurring in the mother and child of a term pregnancy [39, 184]. In most cases, the infant is disease-free, however.

In untreated cases, death from choriocarcinoma most commonly results from hemorrhage or pulmonary insufficiency. Fatal hemorrhage usually occurs in the central nervous system or lungs, but intraperitoneal and gastrointestinal hemorrhages also can cause death. Exsanguination may occur after biopsy of a vaginal metastasis. Pulmonary insufficiency can be due either to a large tumor burden or to the effects of irradiation and cytotoxic chemotherapy. An interval of less than 4 months since the antecedent pregnancy, a pretreatment beta-hCG level <40,000 mIU/mL, and absence of brain or liver metastases appear to be the significant predictors of a favorable outcome in postterm choriocarcinoma [137].

In the past, gestational choriocarcinoma usually was fatal. Before cytotoxic chemotherapy was available, hysterectomy and, in some instances, irradiation were the only forms of treatment. The absolute 5-year survival for patients treated by hysterectomy alone was 32%. Survival rates have improved dramatically since the introduction of cytotoxic chemotherapy combined with accurate and sensitive assays for beta-hCG to monitor the course of the disease. The chemotherapy regimens such as EMA/CO (etoposide, methotrexate, actinomycin D, cyclophosphamide, and vincristine) are highly effective in eradicating choriocarcinoma cells and, thus, choriocarcinoma represents one of the few cancers that are potentially curable by chemotherapeutic agents alone. The overall survival for choriocarcinoma at the present time approaches 100% [63], although some patients develop non-operable diseases with recurrent and chemoresistant choriocarcinoma. New therapeutic regimens have been proposed to salvage these unfortunate patients [145, 172].

The principles of management of choriocarcinoma are similar to those for GTD after hydatidiform mole; beta-hCG monitoring and chemotherapy are essential. In following the patients with beta-hCG, a measurement of urinary hCG is important due to the possible false-positive serum hCG titers [138]. Hysterectomy can reduce the length of hospitalization and the amount of chemotherapy needed to induce remission. Resection of pulmonary metastases may have therapeutic value in patients with persistent but limited pulmonary disease, if there is no evidence of tumor at other sites and the hCG titer is low. Irradiation combined with chemotherapy will give a 50% remission rate for cerebral metastases but irradiation to other sites generally is not useful.

Placental Site Trophoblastic Tumor

The PSTT is a relatively uncommon form of GTD accounting for less than 3% of GTD cases [53, 125]. The tumor is composed of neoplastic implantation site intermediate trophoblastic cells that resemble those infiltrating into the endometrium and myometrium of the placental site during early pregnancy. Molecular genetic data together with immunohistochemical findings support the trophoblastic nature of PSTT [120, 160]. The neoplasm lacks the biphasic pattern seen in choriocarcinoma, and the epithelial-like growth pattern of epithelioid trophoblastic tumor. The PSTT was originally termed atypical chorioepithelioma by Marchand in 1895, but because of its rarity, it was periodically rediscovered and renamed. Terms that have been used include atypical choriocarcinoma, syncytioma, chorioepitheliosis, and trophoblastic pseudotumor [80]. PSTT has been thought to develop as a result of neoplastic transformation of cytotrophoblastic cells and the transformed cells assume the differentiation toward implantation site intermediate trophoblast [145]. Both benign and malignant PSTTs do not demonstrate significant karyotypic abnormalities [62, 177]. Interestingly, more than 85% of patients with PSTT have had a female antecedent gestation either by history or genetic analysis. Furthermore, PSTTs lack Y chromosomes based on a molecular genetic analysis, suggesting a role of the paternally derived X chromosome in the pathogenesis of PSTT [36, 61, 77, 83, 178]. Alternatively, this shortfall of Y-chromosomal complements in PSTTs may reinforce the notion that the majority of PSTTs are derived from previous molar gestations.

Clinical Features

Patients usually are in the reproductive age group (19–62 years with an average of 30 years) and can present with either amenorrhea or abnormal bleeding, often accompanied by uterine enlargement [53, 80, 180] and frequently are thought to be pregnant. When uterine enlargement ceases, the diagnosis of a missed abortion is made. Serum levels of beta-hCG are generally low (<1,000 mIU/mL). Rarely, PSTT is associated with virilization, nephrotic syndrome, and erythrocytosis [14, 181]. In contrast to choriocarcinoma, which is preferentially associated with a complete mole, PSTT occurs commonly following a normal pregnancy but spontaneous abortions and hydatidiform moles have preceded the diagnosis of PSTT [32, 105, 125]. Usually, the relationship to the previous gestation is uncertain, because the PSTT can be diagnosed long after the last known pregnancy. Patients with PSTT can present either with amenorrhea or with abnormal bleeding [125, 153]. Rare examples of primary tubal and ovarian PSTT have been reported [5, 164], and metastasis to ovary has been documented [103]. The clinical features of PSTT as compared with choriocarcinoma and epithelioid trophoblastic tumor are summarized in *Table 20.7.*

Gross Findings

Most of the tumors are well circumscribed, and they can be polypoid, projecting into the uterine cavity or may predominantly involve the myometrium. The sectioned surface is usually soft and tan, containing only focal areas of hemorrhage or necrosis, if present. Invasion frequently extends to the uterine serosa and, in rare instances, to the adnexal structures including broad ligament [7].

Microscopic Findings

The predominant cell type in PSTT is the implantation site intermediate trophoblast. The microscopic features of PSTT are summarized in *Table 20.8.* Most of the cellular population is monomorphic in contrast to the mixture of cell types in choriocarcinoma (*Fig. 20.29–20.33*). PSTT is composed of large, polygonal implantation site intermediate trophoblastic cells with irregular, hyperchromatic

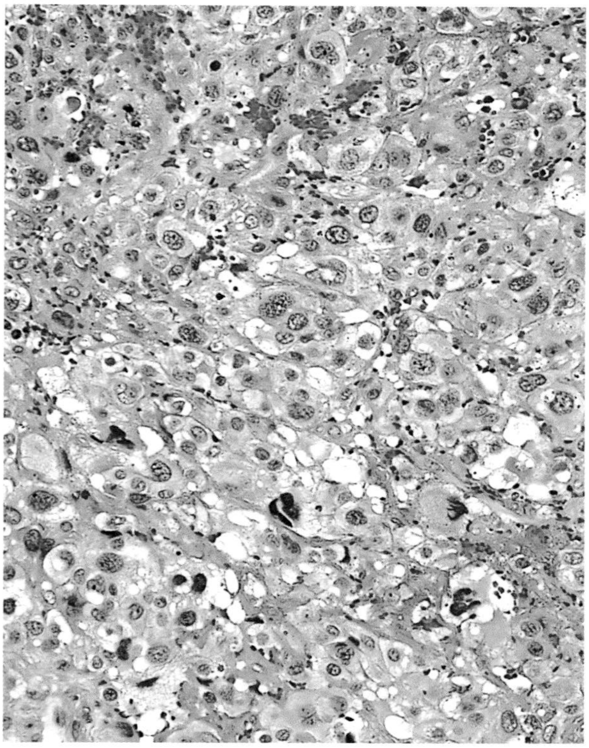

Fig. 20.29
Placental site trophoblastic tumor. **The tumor is composed of a confluent mass of large, polygonal implantation site intermediate trophoblastic cells with irregular, hyperchromatic nuclei and dense eosinophilic to amphophilic cytoplasm with occasional vacuoles**

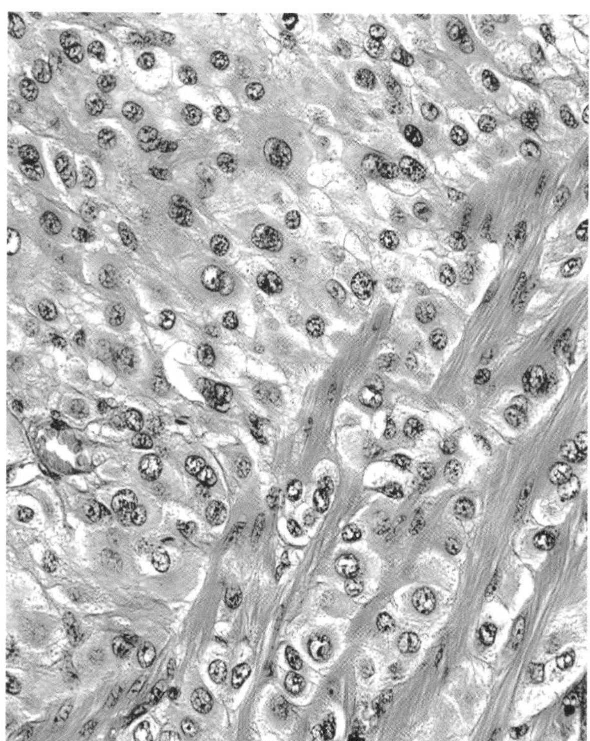

Fig. 20.30
Placental site trophoblastic tumor. **Tumor is composed of a confluent mass of a monomorphic intermediate trophoblast in contrast to the mixture of cytotrophoblast, syncytiotrophoblast, and intermediate trophoblast in choriocarcinoma. The implantation site intermediate trophoblastic cells characteristically separate muscle bundles as they invade the myometrium**

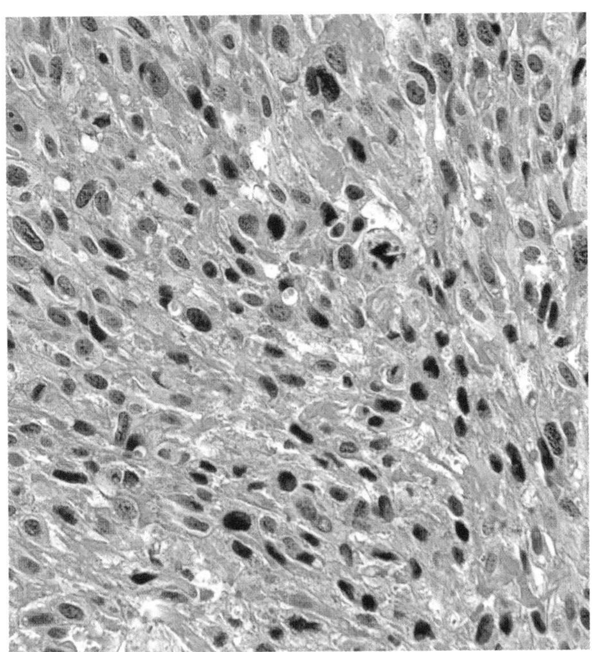

Fig. 20.31
Placental site trophoblastic tumor. **Implantation site intermediate trophoblastic cells may assume a spindle shape and, therefore, can be confused with leiomyosarcoma**

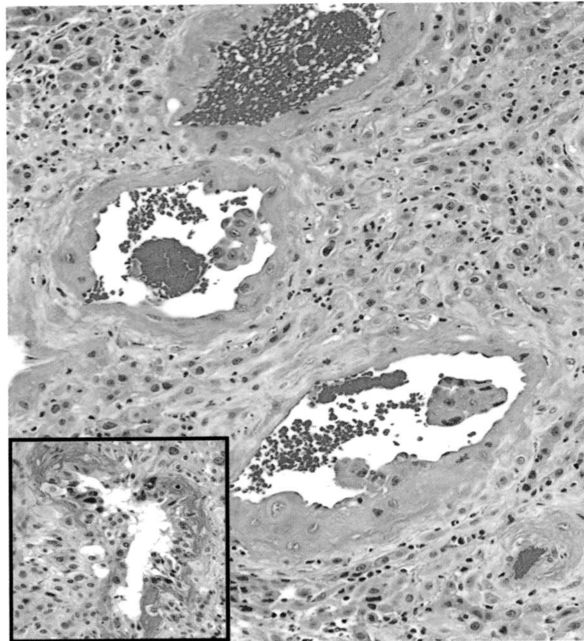

Fig. 20.32
Placental site trophoblastic tumor. **Vascular invasion by implantation site intermediate trophoblast resembles that of the normal implantation site. The neoplastic cells surround and invade a blood vessel, extending into the vascular lumen. The vessel wall has been replaced by fibrin. In some vessels, a dense eosinophilic fibrionoid deposit can be identified in the vascular wall (*inset*)**

nuclei and dense eosinophilic to amphophilic cytoplasm with occasional vacuoles (*Fig. 20.29*). PSTT also contains scattered multinucleated implantation site intermediate trophoblastic cells that can be mistaken for syncytiotrophoblast. The tumor cells often aggregate into confluent sheets; however, at the periphery of the tumor the trophoblast cells invade singly or in cords and nests, characteristically separating individual muscle fibers and groups of fibers (*Fig. 20.30*). Although most of the implantation site intermediate cells are polyhedral, many of them assume a spindle shape especially where they are closely apposed to myometrial cells (*Fig. 20.31*). Occasionally, PSTT is composed almost entirely of single cells or small nests of cells without forming sheets or masses. The individual neoplastic cells extensively infiltrate the endomyometrium and penetrate the uterine wall deeply. Although some tumors appear to cause relatively little tissue destruction, others are associated with extensive necrosis, a microscopic feature that is often associated with malignant behavior (see below). It is not uncommon for a PSTT to also exhibit histological features of choriocarcinoma and epithelioid trophoblastic tumor, and these tumors are termed mixed choriocarcinoma and PSTT or mixed PSTT and epithelioid trophoblastic tumor. Too few of these mixed cases have been studied to determine their clinical behavior.

As in the normal placental site, abundant extracellular eosinophilic fibrinoid material is present in the tumor. The neoplasm displays a characteristic form of vascular invasion in which blood vessel walls are extensively replaced by trophoblastic cells and fibrinoid material (*Fig. 20.32*), as observed in the normal placental site (*Fig. 20.4c*). These "transformed" blood vessels are unique among all human solid tumors and are diagnostic for PSTT. Decidua or an Arias-Stella reaction may be present in the adjacent, uninvolved endometrium. Villi are almost never identified.

PSTT is immunoreactive to the protein markers expressed in implantation site intermediate trophoblast

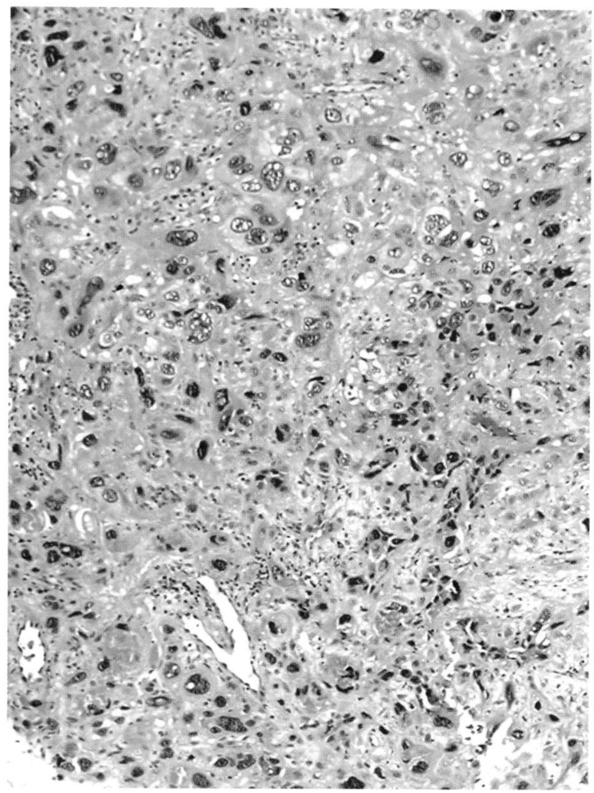

Fig. 20.33
Malignant placental site trophoblastic tumor. **As in a benign PSTT, malignant PSTT grows in masses and sheets and the cells are large with abundant eosinophilic cytoplasm. However, the tumor cells in a malignant PSTT exhibits a higher level of nuclear atypia**

(*Table 20.2*), because the tumor may likely arise from transformation of trophoblastic stem cells, presumably cytotrophoblast, undergoing differentiation toward the implantation site trophoblast (*Fig. 20.6*). For example, PSTT is diffusely positive for hPL, CD146 (Mel-CAM), HLA-G, CD10, and Mucin-4 that are expressed in normal implantation site intermediate trophoblastic cells [84, 92, 149]. Expression of these markers can be useful in the differential diagnosis of PSTT from other mimickers.

Differential Diagnosis

The differential diagnosis of PSTT includes exaggerated placental site, choriocarcinoma, epithelioid trophoblastic tumor, and epithelioid smooth muscle tumor. The most difficult differential diagnosis is that of an exaggerated placental site. Both lesions are characterized by an exuberant infiltration of implantation site intermediate trophoblastic cells. Moreover, the immunophenotype of both lesions is similar. The histologic features that favor the diagnosis of PSTT include confluent masses of trophoblastic cells, unequivocal mitotic figures, and absence of chorionic villi (*Table 20.8*). In contrast, the exaggerated placental site is microscopic in size, lacks mitotic activity, is composed of intermediate trophoblastic cells separated by masses of hyaline, and usually is admixed with decidua and chorionic villi (*Table 20.8*). In addition, an exaggerated placental site contains larger numbers of multinucleated trophoblastic cells than PSTT. Immunostaining for Ki-67 to assess proliferation activity in the implantation site intermediate trophoblastic cells has been shown to be superior to the mitotic index as a diagnostic adjunct in the differential diagnosis of an exaggerated placental site versus a PSTT [151]. The use of immunohistochemistry in the differential diagnosis of PSTT is discussed in the section Immunohistochemical Approach for Differential Diagnosis and in *Fig. 20.53*. Briefly, the Ki-67 labeling index is significantly elevated (>10%) in PSTT but is near zero in the normal and exaggerated implantation site. A diagnosis of a PSTT should be strongly considered if there are Ki-67-labeled implantation site intermediate trophoblastic cells. Although the Ki-67 index in molar implantation site, which is morphologically indistinguishable with exaggerated placental site, can be 10% or higher, the diagnosis of a PSTT versus a complete hydatidiform mole usually is not a problem. The Ki-67 labeling in the implantation site intermediate trophoblastic cells should be carefully assessed using stringent morphologic criteria since implantation site intermediate trophoblastic cells can closely resemble other cell types in a placental site. Many Ki-67-positive cells in the placental site or PSTT are natural killer cells and activated T lymphocytes, which can be positive for Ki-67. A double-staining technique utilizing MIB-1 antibody to determine the Ki-67 proliferative index and markers to identify implantation site intermediate trophoblastic cells such as HSD3B1, HLA-G, and Mel-CAM (CD146) can be very useful in distinguishing an exaggerated placental site from a PSTT [93, 144].

In contrast to the biphasic pattern of choriocarcinoma, PSTT is composed of a relatively monomorphic population of trophoblast. The multinucleated intermediate trophoblastic cells in PSTT should not be confused with syncytiotrophoblast in choriocarcinoma. In contrast to the interlacing pattern of elongated syncytiotrophoblast in choriocarcinoma, the multinucleated intermediate trophoblastic cells in PSTT are usually polygonal or round. Additionally, PSTT is diffusely (>50%) positive for hPL, but only focally positive for beta-hCG (mostly confined to the multinucleated intermediate trophoblastic cells). Ki-67 labeling index in intermediate trophoblastic cells is also helpful in the differential diagnosis of PSTT versus choriocarcinoma [151]. The Ki-67 index in intermediate trophoblastic cells of PSTT is significantly lower (<30%) than choriocarcinoma (>40%).

The differential diagnosis of epithelioid smooth muscle tumor can at times present a problem because of the infiltrative pattern of PSTT within the myometrium (➲ *Fig. 20.31*). The distinctive pattern of vascular invasion and the deposition of fibrinoid material in PSTT are helpful morphological clues (➲ *Fig. 20.32*). Positive staining for HSD3B1, cytokeratin 18, and hPL as well as the negative staining for smooth muscle markers are helpful in this differential diagnosis [93, 144]. The use of immunohistochemistry in the differential diagnosis of PSTT is discussed in the last section (➲ Immunohistochemical Approach for Differential Diagnosis) of this chapter.

Poorly differentiated carcinoma and metastatic melanoma can sometimes be confused with PSTT. The pattern of prominent blood vessel invasion, characteristic myometrial invasion, and extensive deposition of fibrinoid material (➲ *Figs. 20.30* and ➲ *20.32*) are key diagnostic features of PSTT. Immunohistochemical stains for HSD3B1, hPL, and HMB-45 help to distinguish PSTT from poorly differentiated carcinoma and melanoma (see section ➲ Immunohistochemical Approach for Differential Diagnosis). Typically, in choriocarcinoma the serum beta-hCG levels are high, ranging from 1,000 mIU/mL to over 1,000,000 mIU/mL, whereas in PSTT the levels are significantly lower, often less than 1,000 mIU/mL. A recent study further demonstrates that the percentage of hCG free beta-subunit is a reliable serum marker for PSTTs and can be used to rule out other trophoblastic neoplasms and non-trophoblastic tumors that produce hCG [25].

The differential diagnosis of PSTT from epithelioid trophoblastic tumor is considered in the section describing the latter lesion.

Behavior and Treatment

PSTTs often invade through the myometrium to the serosa, and therefore perforation at the time of curettage may occur. These tumors may also directly invade into the broad ligament and ovary. Despite deep myometrial invasion, most cases of PSTT are self-limited [18, 53, 125] and some patients have been cured by curettage alone. Approximately 10–15% of PSTT are clinically malignant, and patients have died despite intensive multiagent chemotherapy. The mortality rate in patients with PSTT is about 15–30%, which may be overestimated because benign cases are generally not reported [53, 58, 125]. The outcomes of patients with FIGO stage I–II disease after hysterectomy are excellent; while those with FIGO stage III–IV diseases have a 30% survival [18]. A recent large retrospective study demonstrates that the probabilities of overall and recurrence-free survival 10 years after first treatment are 70% and 73%, respectively. Patients with stage I disease had a 10-year probability of overall survival of 90% and the probability of overall survival at 10 years was 52% for patients with stage II disease and 49% for stage III and IV disease [139]. In one report, metastases at presentation occur in more than 30% of cases and recurrences develop in more than 30% of cases [35]. The overtly malignant tumors have had widely disseminated metastases resembling choriocarcinoma in their distribution with lung, liver, abdominal cavity, and brain involved. Metastases have the same histological appearance as the primary tumor and may develop several years after the initial diagnosis, as one fatal case recurred 5 years after hysterectomy. In general, PSTTs with multiple metastases have poor prognosis.

Because these tumors are composed of neoplastic implantation site intermediate trophoblastic cells that contain only small amounts of beta-hCG, serum levels of beta-hCG are usually in the range of 1,000 to 2,000 mIU/mL. These levels are much lower than those in choriocarcinoma. Despite the low level of serum beta-hCG in patients with PSTT, it is the best available marker to monitor the course of the disease [130]. Of note, the marker cannot be used to diagnose PSTT versus other trophoblastic diseases [52]. It is important to emphasize that the disease may still progress even if beta-hCG levels are low [58]. For those patients with undetectable or very low serum levels of beta-hCG, urinary or serum beta-core fragment of beta-hCG may be a better method to monitor treatment as the percentage is much higher in PSTTs than in choriocarcinoma and other carcinomas that produce beta-hCG [23].

It is difficult to predict with certainty the behavior of PSTT [154]. However, some studies have found that several clinical parameters may be associated with a poor clinical outcome in PSTT patients and they include FIGO stage [18, 56, 131], metastatic involvement [125], long interval from the antecedent pregnancy [8, 53, 56, 125], age > 35, hCG > 1,000 mIU/mL, depth of invasion [8, 131], and p53 immunoreactivity [109]. For example, based on multivariate analysis, investigators have found that the only significant independent predictor of overall and recurrence-free survival is time since antecedent pregnancy. In that report, a cutoff point of 48 months since antecedent pregnancy could differentiate between patients' probability of survival (<48 months) or death (≥48 months) with 93% specificity and 100% sensitivity, and with a positive predictive value of 100% and a negative predictive value of 98% [139]. Some studies showed that a high mitotic count was an adverse prognostic indicator in PSTT patients [8, 56] but it has also been shown that there is no correlation between clinical outcome and DNA ploidy, histopathological features, immunohistochemical features, and S-phase fraction [40, 41]. In our experience, malignant PSTTs as compared with benign cases generally are composed of larger masses and sheets of cells, many with clear instead of amphophilic cytoplasm. They have more extensive necrosis, prominent nuclear atypia and higher mitotic activity (➋ *Fig. 20.33*). Our preliminary findings suggest that the Ki-67 labeling index may be a reliable indicator of prognosis as the index is usually higher than 50% in malignant tumors.

The treatment of choice for patients whose disease is confined to the uterus is hysterectomy [35, 58, 131]. In some patients with localized PSTT who desire preservation of fertility, more conservative surgical therapy may be considered [85, 91, 118, 128]. Curettage and local excision may be therapeutic, but if uterine disease persists, as evidenced by persistently elevated serum beta-hCG levels, hysterectomy is indicated. For patients with more extensive or metastatic disease, chemotherapy in addition to surgery is indicated although the clinical outcome is variable [18, 30, 35, 112, 166, 171]. Combination chemotherapy usually results in a high response rate and long-term remission even in patients with recurrent, metastatic PSTT, but only a few patients achieve a complete response [10, 18, 67, 133]. In general, EMA/CO is the first line chemotherapy regimen and EMA/EP can be used in EMA/CO refractory cases [113]. In conclusion, with the use of dose-intensive chemotherapy, imaging techniques to define disease spread, surgery for localized disease, and the close surveillance with serologic measurement of the beta-hCG level, most patients with PSTT can be cured.

Epithelioid Trophoblastic Tumor

The term "epithelioid trophoblastic tumor" was introduced to describe an unusual type of trophoblastic tumor that is distinct from PSTT and choriocarcinoma with features resembling a carcinoma. The tumor was originally termed "atypical choriocarcinoma" and was described in the lungs of patients with antecedent choriocarcinoma following intensive chemotherapy [70, 96]. Similar lesions referred to as "multiple nodules of intermediate trophoblast" were subsequently reported in the uteri of patients following evacuation of hydatidiform moles [159]. Subsequently, similar tumors were observed in the uterus without history of antecedent GTD [150]. The relatively recent recognition of epithelioid trophoblastic tumor as a distinctive form of trophoblastic disease is in part due to its rarity and because many of the morphologic features of epithelioid trophoblastic tumor are more reminiscent of a carcinoma than of a trophoblastic tumor [150]. Epithelioid trophoblastic tumor is very rare, and experience with this tumor has been limited to approximately 59 cases reported so far [27, 49, 70, 78, 87, 90, 94, 96, 101, 109, 110, 119, 126, 150, 159, 170, 173, 174]. The trophoblastic nature of this tumor has been confirmed using molecular approaches [120, 160]. Based on morphologic, ultrastructural, and immunohistochemical studies, epithelioid trophoblastic tumor appears to develop from neoplastic transformation of cytotrophoblastic cells that differentiate toward chorionic-type intermediate trophoblastic cells [96, 145, 155].

Clinical Features

Based on an analysis of published 52 cases, Palmer et al. reported that 67% of patients present with abnormal vaginal bleeding, 36% had evidence of antecedent molar pregnancy, and 35% presented with metastases [124]. Mean age at diagnosis is 38 years and the mean interval between the preceding gestation and the diagnosis of epithelioid trophoblastic tumor is 76 months. hCG levels are usually low (<1,000 mIU/mL) [49, 150], but high levels of hCG can be present in some cases. Extrauterine epithelioid trophoblastic tumor without an identifiable trophoblastic lesion in the uterus has also been described, [49, 86, 150], and the origin of such tumors is not clear. It is well recognized that choriocarcinoma can develop after a long latent period without evidence of disease in the uterus, thus it is conceivable that extrauterine epithelioid trophoblastic tumors develop in a similar fashion. Rarely, epithelioid trophoblastic tumor can occur in an extrauterine site including broad ligament [78], gall bladder [90], and (para)adenxal tissue [116, 126]. Epithelioid trophoblastic tumor can be seen in association with choriocarcinoma and PSTT [150, 159]. Like PSTT, a recent molecular genetic study on a small series of epithelioid trophoblastic tumors demonstrates a balanced chromosomal profile without detectable gain or loss in the genome, suggesting that DNA copy number alterations as seen in most solid tumors are not a characteristic feature of this tumor [176].

Gross Findings

In one study, 30% of 14 epithelioid trophoblastic tumors were located in the uterine corpus, 50% in the lower uterine segment or endocervix, and the remaining 20% in extrauterine sites including the small bowel and lungs [150]. In cases in which a hysterectomy was performed, tumor size varied from 0.5 to 4.0 cm. All were solitary, discrete nodules that deeply invaded the cervix or myometrium. The cut surface was solid or cystic. Solid areas were typically tan to brown with varying amounts of hemorrhage and necrosis (*Fig. 20.33*). Metastatic epithelioid trophoblastic tumors show similar gross features (*Figs. 20.34* and *20.35*).

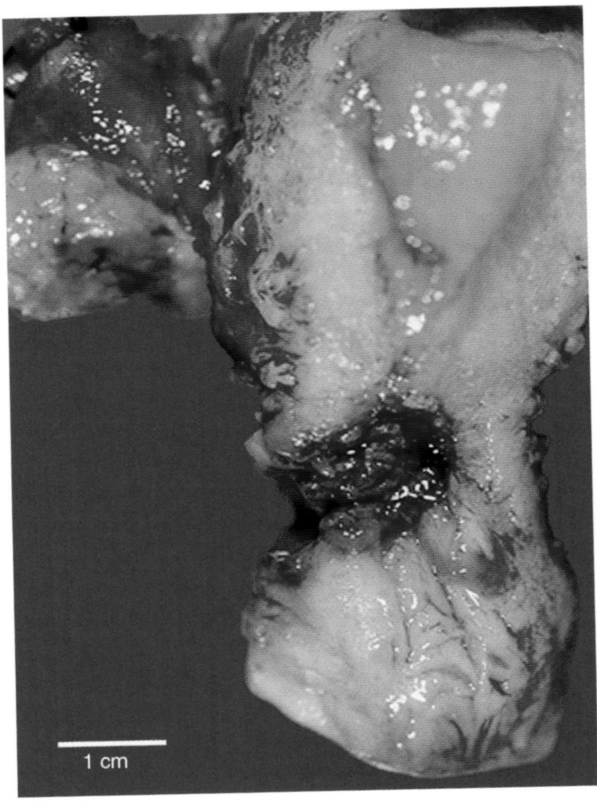

Fig. 20.34
Epithelioid trophoblastic tumor in the endocervical canal. It is well circumscribed and ulcerated with hemorrhage and necrosis (Reprinted by permission of [150])

Microscopic Findings

Epithelioid trophoblastic tumors are nodular and generally well circumscribed although focal infiltrative features can be present at the periphery. The tumors are composed of a relatively uniform population of mononucleate trophoblastic cells typically arranged in nests and cords and masses of cells that are intimately associated with an eosinophilic, fibrillar, hyaline-like material, and necrotic debris (*Figs. 20.36–20.40*). This hyaline-like material, composed of type IV collagen and fibronectin of oncofetal and adult types, is either located within the nests or surrounds them, coalescing to form large aggregates. This dense eosinophilic material and necrotic debris can simulate keratin (*Figs. 20.38–20.40*). The extensive areas of necrosis that surround islands of viable tumor cells create a “geographic” pattern (*Fig. 20.36*). Typically, a small blood vessel is located within the center of tumor nests. Blood vessels within the tumor are preserved with occasional deposition of amorphous fibrinoid material in the wall. A lymphocytic infiltrate often surrounds the tumor (*Fig. 20.38*). In most cases, apoptotic cells are diffusely distributed throughout the tumor.

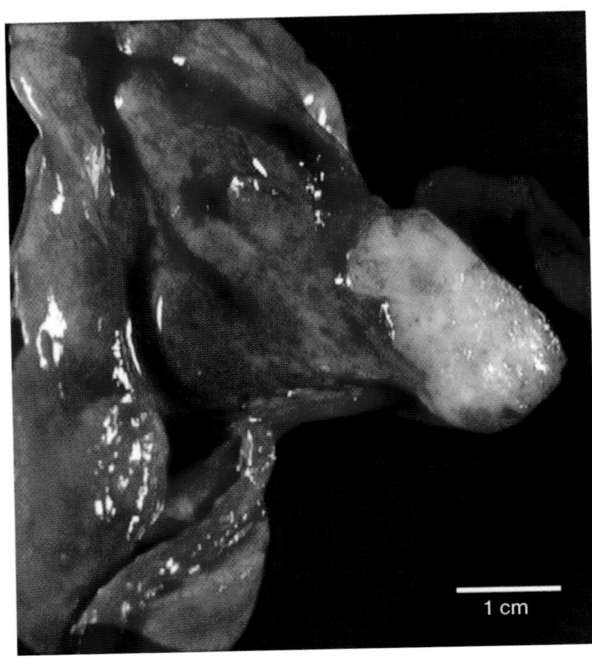

Fig. 20.35
Metastatic epithelioid trophoblastic tumor in the lung. A lobectomy specimen shows a discrete nodule with yellowish and necrotic cut surface

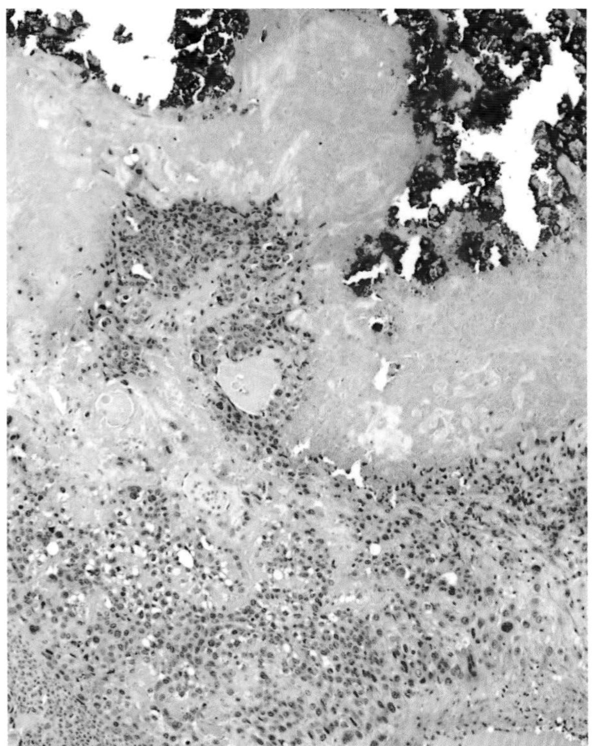

Fig. 20.36
Epithelioid trophoblastic tumor. **Tumor in a hysterectomy specimen contains nests of atypical mononucleate trophoblastic cells. Large areas of genographic necrosis and extensive calcification are characteristic features of the tumor, which lacks the typical dimorphic pattern of choriocarcinoma**

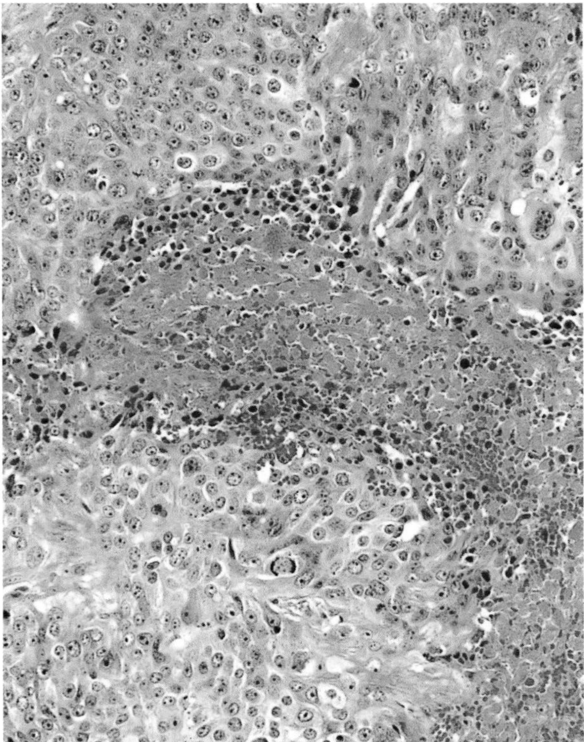

Fig. 20.37
Epithelioid trophoblastic tumor. **Relatively monotonous tumor cells are present in this section surrounded by necrosis. Occasional mitotic figures can be seen**

Calcification is common in epithelioid trophoblastic tumors but not in PSTT or choriocarcinoma, and this morphological feature is unique among all GTDs (➋ *Fig. 20.36*).

Chorionic-type intermediate trophoblast is the predominant cell population in the epithelioid trophoblastic tumor [145,150]. These cells contain round, uniform nuclei and eosinophilic or clear (glycogen-rich) cytoplasm surrounded by a well-defined cell membrane, morphological features characteristic of the intermediate trophoblastic cells in fetal membrane (chorion laeve; ➋ *Fig. 20.5*). For the most part, the cells are larger than cytotrophoblastic cells but smaller than the implantation site intermediate trophoblastic cells. The tumor cell nuclei have finely dispersed chromatin and prominent or inconspicuous nucleoli. Ultrastructurally these cells are transitional between cytotrophoblast and syncytiotrophoblast but differ from the implantation site intermediate trophoblast [96]. Occasionally, larger cells resembling implantation site intermediate trophoblastic cells can be found among the smaller tumor cells or embedded in the extracellular hyaline matrix. The mitotic index varies from 0 to 9 mitoses per 10 high power fields ($\times 40$) with an average of 2 mitoses per 10 high power fields [150]. Although most epithelioid trophoblastic tumors display a uniform architectural pattern, focal areas resembling placental site nodule, PSTT, and choriocarcinoma can occasionally be identified within the tumor. Furthermore, epithelioid trophoblastic tumor can be associated with a concurrent germ cell tumor such as teratoma [2], indicating epithelioid trophoblastic tumor may arise, although rarely, from a non-gestational event.

A unique feature of epithelioid trophoblastic tumor, among all GTDs, is its ability to replace and re-epithelialize the endocervical and/or endometrial surface epithelium (➋ *Fig. 20.41*) [34, 150]. When this tumor involves the

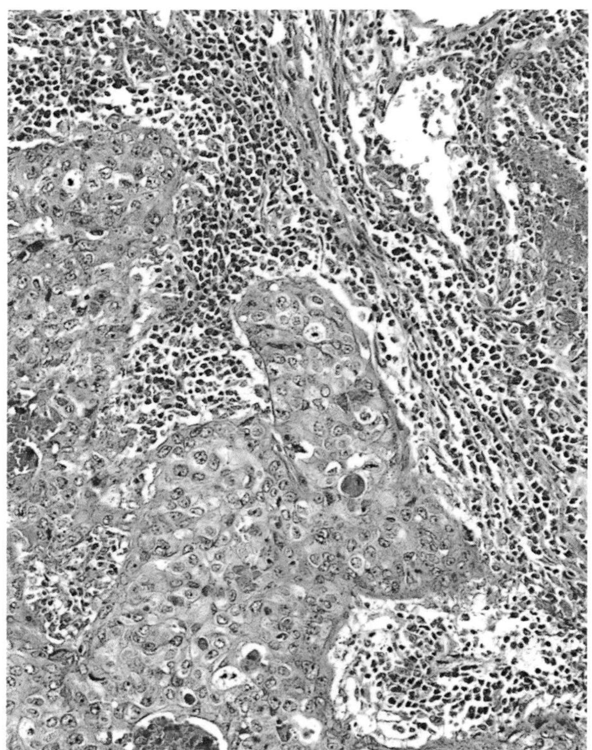

Fig. 20.38
Epithelioid trophoblastic tumor. **A solitary lung metastasis after chemotherapy for typical choriocarcinoma. The tumor cells form a cohesive sheet with scattered dense eosinophilic debris, resembling a keratinizing squamous cell carcinoma**

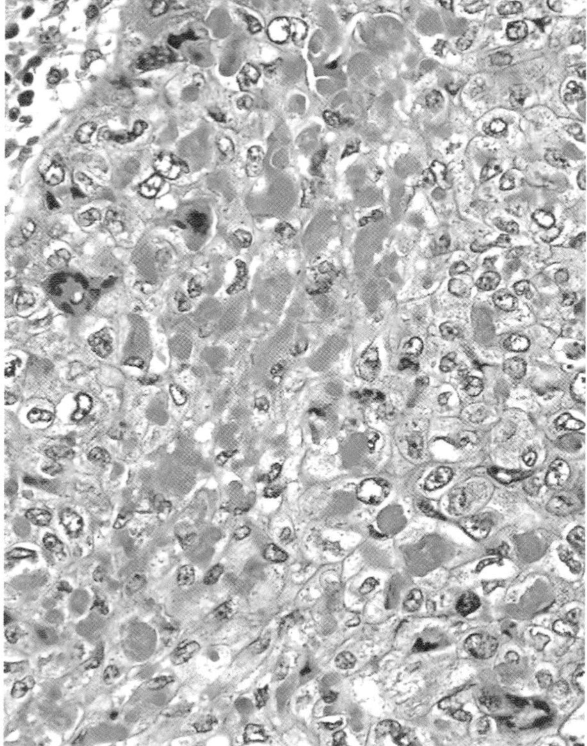

Fig. 20.39
Epithelioid trophoblastic tumor. **At high magnification, the dense eosinophilic debris is prominent within the tumor**

lower uterine segment and endocervix, the intraepithelial extension can mimic squamous carcinoma in situ. The tumor cells usually stratify into two to three layers, however, and are larger than cervical squamous cells with abundant eosinophilic cytoplasm and large hyperchromatic, pleomorphic nuclei.

The immunohistochemical features of the epithelioid trophoblastic tumor are similar to those of chorionic-type intermediate trophoblast (*Table 20.2*). The "classic" implantation site intermediate trophoblastic markers including hPL and CD146 (Mel-CAM) are only focally expressed. The immunophenotype of the epithelioid trophoblastic tumor contrasts with the PSTT, which is diffusely positive for CD146 (Mel-CAM) and hPL. Furthermore, epithelioid trophoblastic tumor exhibits similar morphological features and gene expression profile to the intermediate trophoblastic cells in a placental site nodule [153, 158], suggesting that the epithelioid trophoblastic tumor represents the neoplastic counterpart of the placental site nodule. Indeed, synchronous epithelioid trophoblastic tumor and placental site nodule in the same specimens can be occasionally observed [150, 158] and transformation of a placental site nodule into a malignant epithelioid trophoblastic tumor has been recently documented [170]. The morphological and immunohistochemical features of extrauterine epithelioid trophoblastic tumors are similar to those in the uterus [49].

Like PSTT, epithelioid trophoblastic tumor can present as a mixed lesion containing either a PSTT or a choriocarcinoma (*Fig. 20.42*). It has been proposed that these mixed tumors can result from aberration in the trophoblastic differentiation program in which the neoplastic cytotrophoblast (stem) cells differentiate into implantation site intermediate trophoblastic cells to form the PSTT component, and into chorionic-type intermediate trophoblastic cells to form the epithelioid trophoblastic component, or they remain relatively undifferentiated to form the choriocarcinoma component [145]. According to this model (*Fig. 20.8*), choriocarcinoma

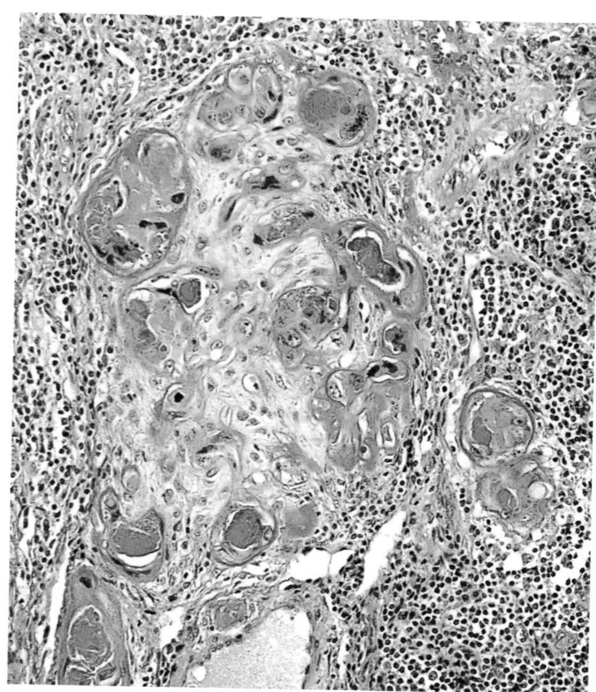

Fig. 20.40
Epithelioid trophoblastic tumor. **Dense eosinophilic material surrounds nests of tumor cells. The tumor is frequently accompanied by an abundant lymphocytic infiltration**

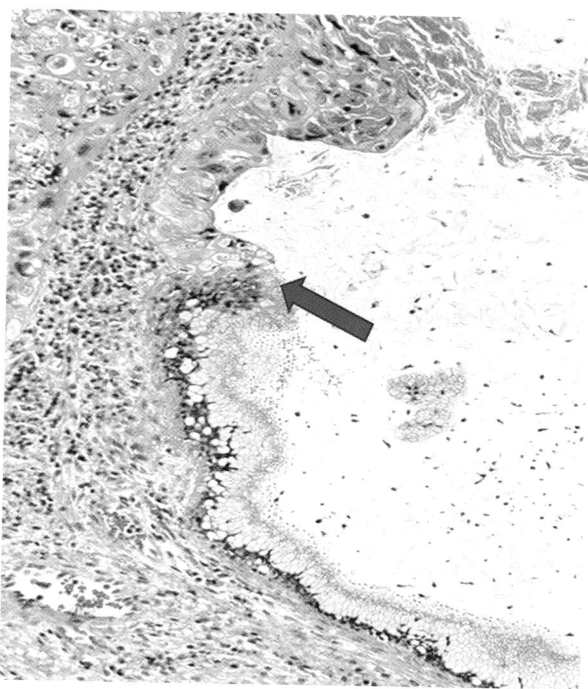

Fig. 20.41
Epithelioid trophoblastic tumor. **An endocervical gland is replaced by epithelium from an epithelioid trophoblastic tumor. There is an abrupt transition between the tumor and the endocervical epithelium (*arrow*) (Reprinted by permission of [150])**

is the most primitive trophoblastic tumor, whereas PSTT and epithelioid trophoblastic tumor are relatively more differentiated. This hypothesis explains the existence of trophoblastic tumors with a mixed histological pattern including choriocarcinoma and PSTT and/or epithelioid trophoblastic tumor. This new model also helps to explain the findings previously reported by Mazur who originally described epithelioid trophoblastic tumor as tumors after intense chemotherapy of metastatic choriocarcinomas in the lung. In these cases, it is plausible that chemotherapeutic agents direct choriocarcinoma cells to differentiate into an epithelioid trophoblastic tumor phenotype, which is more refractory to chemotherapy than the original choriocarcinoma. As a result, the epithelioid trophoblastic tumor outgrew the choriocarcinoma after chemotherapy.

Differential Diagnosis

The differential diagnosis of epithelioid trophoblastic tumor includes PSTT, placental site nodule, choriocarcinoma, epithelioid smooth muscle tumor, and keratinizing squamous cell carcinoma of the cervix [150, 174]. Epithelioid trophoblastic tumors exhibit a nodular growth pattern, and the border between the tumor and the myometrium is expansile. In contrast, the cells of PSTT infiltrate the myometrium by insinuating themselves between muscle bundles and fibers. In addition, the cells in epithelioid trophoblastic tumor are smaller than in PSTT (*Fig. 20.43*) and tend to grow in nests and cords, a pattern usually not observed in PSTT. In epithelioid trophoblastic tumors, there is extensive geographic necrosis accompanied by dystrophic calcification and the tumor cells are surrounded by fibrillar eosinophilic material instead of the more homogeneous fibrinoid material found in PSTT. Blood vessels in epithelioid trophoblastic tumor are often surrounded by tumor cells but vascular invasion is not a striking feature in contrast to the vascular invasion in PSTT, where tumor cells and hyaline material replace the vessel walls (*Fig. 20.32*). If calcification is detected, the lesion is most likely an epithelioid trophoblastic tumor rather than a PSTT. Finally, immunostains can be useful in difficult cases

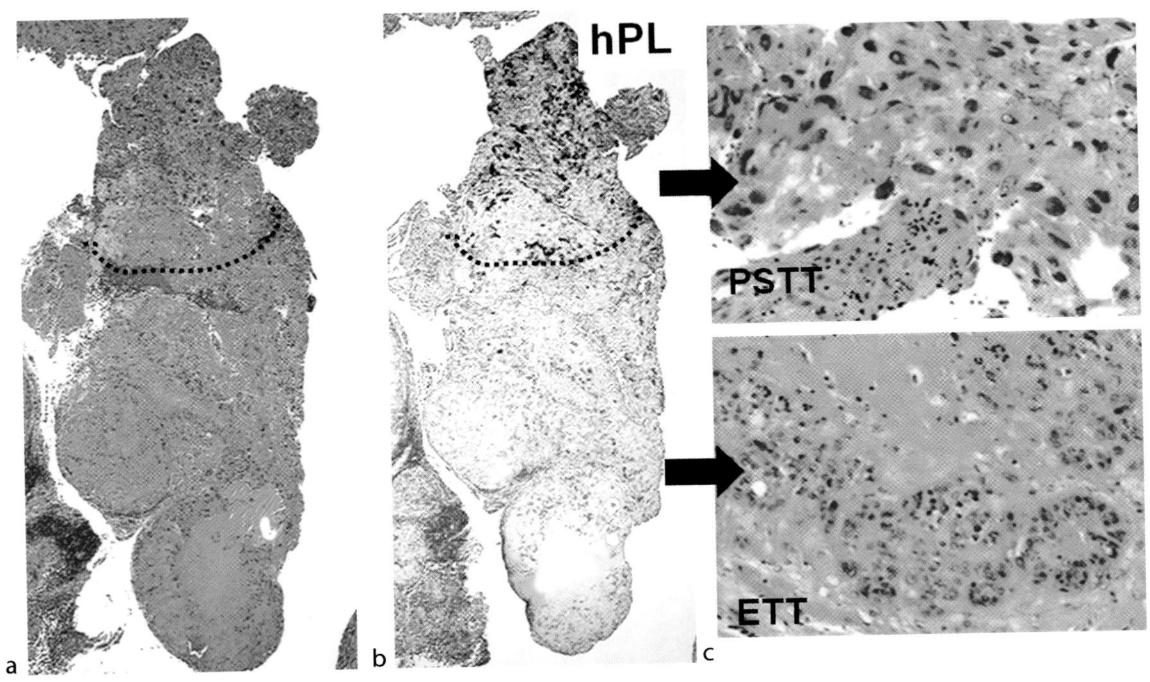

Fig. 20.42
A mixed PSTT and epithelioid trophoblastic tumor. (a) H&E stain. PSTT area (*above the dash line*) has higher cellularity than the epithelioid trophoblastic tumor component (*below the dashed line*) that shows geographic necrosis and abundant eosinophilic matrix deposition. (b) Immunostain with an anti-hPL antibody. hPL immunoreactivity is confined to the PSTT area. (c) Histological features from PSTT and epithelioid trophoblastic tumor (ETT) areas

(see section Immunohistochemical Approach for Differential Diagnosis and *Fig. 20.53* for details).

The differential diagnosis of placental site nodule versus epithelioid trophoblastic tumor is considered in the section of placental site nodule.

As compared with choriocarcinoma, the cells in an epithelioid trophoblastic tumor are aggregated into nests and cords. In addition, epithelioid trophoblastic tumor is not associated with marked hemorrhage as is the case with choriocarcinoma. Immunostains for beta-hCG can be helpful in the differential diagnosis. Beta-hCG immunostains highlight the dimorphic trophoblastic population of cells in choriocarcinoma with hCG-negative cytotrophoblast and intermediate trophoblast alternating with beta-hCG-positive syncytiotrophoblast. In contrast, beta-hCG-positive cells are randomly distributed as single mononucleate cells or small clusters of cells in epithelioid trophoblastic tumor.

Epithelioid smooth muscle tumors usually display areas composed of typical smooth muscle cells in addition to epithelioid areas. In addition, epithelioid smooth muscle tumors are positive for muscle markers including desmin and smooth muscle actin, which are not expressed by epithelioid trophoblastic tumors. Conversely, epithelioid trophoblastic tumors are positive for HSD3B1 and cytokeratin 18, which are not expressed in smooth muscle tumors [93].

Distinction between an epithelioid trophoblastic tumor and a keratinizing squamous cell carcinoma of the cervix can be challenging [129, 150]. The differential diagnosis is particularly difficult because of the tendency of epithelioid trophoblastic tumor to grow in the lower uterine segment and cervix and involve the endocervical epithelium. In this situation, immunostains are particularly helpful. The application of commercially available antibodies in the differential diagnosis is described in the section Immunohistochemical Approach for Differential Diagnosis and *Fig. 20.54*.

The morphological distinction between a pulmonary epithelioid trophoblastic tumor and a primary squamous cell carcinoma of the lung can be extremely difficult, especially in a postmenopausal patient [49, 86, 150]. Useful clues that support the diagnosis of epithelioid trophoblastic tumor include (1) lack of cytoplasmic eosinophilia

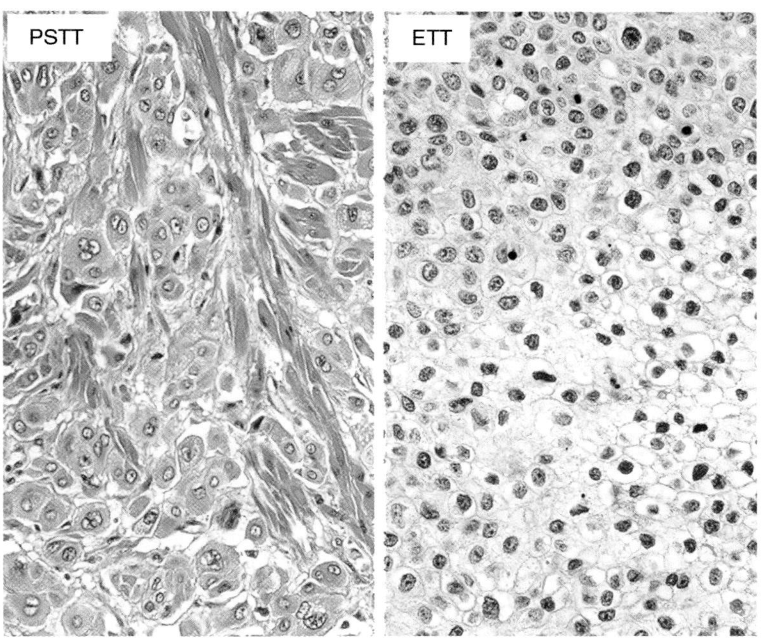

Fig. 20.43
Comparison of cytological features of PSTT and epithelioid trophoblastic tumor. **PSTT (*left*) is composed of implantation site intermediate trophoblastic cells. The epithelioid trophoblastic tumor (ETT) (*right*) is comprised of chorionic-type intermediate trophoblastic cells which are smaller and have round, uniform nuclei, eosinophilic to clear cytoplasm, and a well-defined cell membrane. The cells in PSTT are larger and polygonal with atypical nuclei. They infiltrate into smooth muscle**

and intercellular bridges that are frequently observed in differentiated squamous cell carcinoma; and (2) infiltration of alveolar spaces by highly atypical tumor cells and preservation of the alveolar septa, features not frequently seen in squamous cell carcinoma [49]. As in squamous cell carcinomas of the cervix, primary squamous cell carcinoma of the lung rarely reacts with antibodies to HSD3B1 and cytokeratin 18 [93].

Behavior and Treatment

Experience with epithelioid trophoblastic tumor is limited because only 59 cases have been reported to date. Generally, the behavior of epithelioid trophoblastic tumor is similar to that of PSTT. For the most part, epithelioid trophoblastic tumors behave in a benign fashion. Although most reported cases lack long-term follow-up, metastasis occurs in approximately 25% of patients and death in 13% [124]. Because the number of tumors that have behaved in an aggressive fashion is small and follow-up for many cases has been short, we have been unable to identify any feature that predicts outcome.

Although serum beta-hCG levels are variable and generally low in patients with epithelioid trophoblastic tumors, serum beta-hCG levels have been used successfully to monitor treatment. For those patients with undetectable or very low serum levels of beta-hCG, urinary beta-core fragment of beta-hCG may be useful [136]. Hysterectomy and lung resection have been used successfully, but the effectiveness of curettage of early lesions requires further evaluation. Unlike choriocarcinoma, epithelioid trophoblastic tumor appears to be only partially responsive to chemotherapy since tumors may recur or metastasize despite intensive chemotherapy [90, 96, 150, 159]. Recurrent disease can be late and complex [90]. Nonetheless, combined chemotherapy regimen such as EMA/CO has been used successfully in treating metastatic epithelioid trophoblastic tumor [170].

Exaggerated Placental Site (Reaction)

This lesion is defined as an exuberant infiltration of the myometrium by implantation site intermediate trophoblast. The distinction between a normal and exaggerated placental site is somewhat arbitrary since there are no reliable data quantifying the amount and extent of trophoblastic infiltration at different stages of normal gestation. The exaggerated placental site can occur in a normal pregnancy or an abortion from the first trimester. The incidence is approximately 1.6% of spontaneous and elective abortions from the first trimester based on a review of the surgical pathology files at the Johns Hopkins Hospital. In normal pregnancy and abortion, the apparent exaggerated placental site may actually only represent a fortuitous increase in the amount of placental site removed by curettage. Nonetheless, it is an important entity since it can mimic proliferative trophoblast seen in trophoblastic neoplasms.

The exaggerated placental site is characterized by an extensive infiltration of the endometrium and myometrium by implantation site intermediate trophoblastic cells, many of which are multinucleated (➋ *Figs. 20.44* and ➋ *20.45*). Despite the massive infiltration by trophoblastic cells, the overall architecture of the placental site is not disturbed. Endometrial glands and spiral arteries may be completely engulfed by trophoblastic cells but there is no necrosis. Similarly, the smooth muscle cells of the myometrium are separated by cords, nests, and individual trophoblastic cells that diffusely infiltrate the myometrium without producing necrosis (➋ *Fig. 20.44*). Cytologically, the trophoblastic cells in an exaggerated placental site are identical to the implantation site intermediate trophoblastic cells in the normal placental site. They contain abundant eosinophilic cytoplasm with hyperchromatic and irregular nuclei (➋ *Fig. 20.45*). In many cases, there are large numbers of multinucleated implantation site intermediate trophoblastic cells (➋ *Fig. 20.45*). Mitotic activity is absent. The associated chorionic villi are morphologically unremarkable.

The trophoblastic cells in the exaggerated placental site display an identical immunophenotypic profile to the implantation site intermediate trophoblastic cells found in the normal placental site (➋ *Table 20.2*). These findings indicate that the differentiation of implantation site intermediate trophoblastic cells is unaltered in an exaggerated placental site, and suggests that an exaggerated placental site is a normal variation of an implantation site. Despite the profuse infiltration of implantation site intermediate trophoblast in an exaggerated placental site, the Ki-67 indices of implantation site intermediate trophoblast are near zero [151]. Complete hydatidiform moles are always accompanied by exaggerated placental sites in which the implantation site intermediate trophoblastic cells are often more atypical than those in the exaggerated placental sites that are not associated with complete moles.

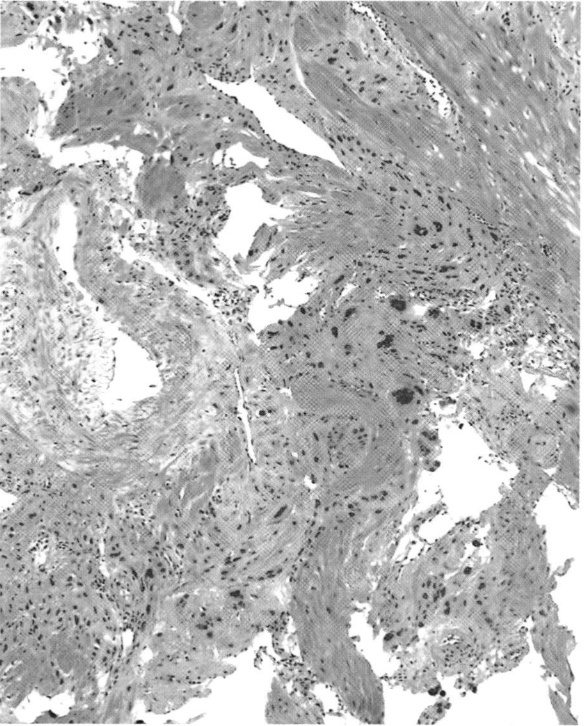

■ Fig. 20.44
Exaggerated placental site. **The lesion is characterized by an increased number of implantation site intermediate trophoblast exceeding that normally seen in the implantation site. Note large number of multinucleated giant cells, characteristic of this lesion**

Based on our previous study [151] and recent experience, the Ki-67 labeling index in molar exaggerated placental site ranges widely from 5% to 30% or even higher. It is debatable whether the molar exaggerated placental site with high Ki-67 labeling index represents trophoblastic hyperplasia associated with a complete mole or it is a PSTT arising from a complete mole. The answer depends on future molecular genetic studies to demonstrate the clonal event of implantation site intermediate trophoblast in molar exaggerated placental site.

The most important differential diagnosis of an exaggerated implantation site is PSTT, which is discussed in the section describing that entity. Although exaggerated placental site and PSTT share similar morphological and immunohistochemical features, the lack of genetic link between both lesions has been documented [31]. Occasionally, implantation site intermediate trophoblastic cells that infiltrate the myometrium may resemble the atypical smooth muscle cells found in symplastic leiomyomas.

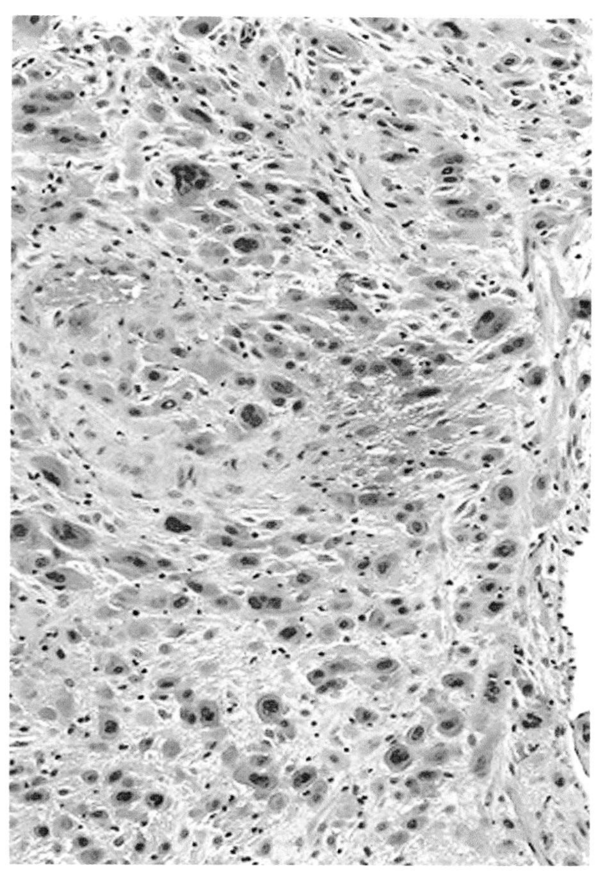

Fig. 20.45
Exaggerated placental site. **Mixture of mononucleate and multinucleated implantation site intermediate trophoblastic cells. The latter are more commonly seen in an exaggerated placental site than in a PSTT. Unlike PSTT, the trophoblastic cells in an exaggerated placental site are widely spaced, lacking confluent growth or necrosis. There is no mitotic activity**

The presence of chorionic villi, the infiltrative growth pattern of the trophoblastic cells, characteristic vascular invasion pattern, and positive stains for HSD3B1, cytokeratin, and hPL support the diagnosis of an exaggerated implantation site.

Exaggerated placental site probably represents a physiologic process that resolves spontaneously after curettage. Exaggerated placental site that is not associated with a hydatidiform mole does not carry an increased risk of persistent GTD. No specific treatment or follow-up is required. Thus, to distinguish an exaggerated placental site from a normal placental site may not be critical in routine pathology practice because of the subjective morphological criteria in defining this condition and the lack of clinical significance of exaggerated placental site. However, the report of an exaggerated placental site in curettage specimens may indicate that PSTT has been considered as a differential diagnosis in those cases.

Placental Site Nodule

Placental site nodules (or plaques) are small, well-circumscribed nodular aggregates of chorionic-type intermediate trophoblastic cells that are embedded in a hyalinized stroma. Placental site nodules have been thought to represent a portion of uninvoluted placental site from remote gestations in the uterus. However, the constituent cells in placental site nodules are more closely related to the intermediate trophoblast of chorion laeve (chorionic-type intermediate trophoblast) than to the intermediate trophoblast of a placental site (implantation site intermediate trophoblastic cells) [158]. Based on morphological and immunohistochemical studies, the placental site nodule appears to represent the benign counterpart of the epithelioid trophoblastic tumor.

Patients are in the reproductive age group. Placental site nodules are typically incidental findings in uterine or endocervical curettings, cervical biopsies, and occasionally in hysterectomy specimens. In addition, placental site nodules can also be detected in fallopian tubes, presumably a consequence of prior tubal pregnancy [7, 42, 66, 111]. In one study, 40% of placental site nodules were present in the endocervix, 56% in the endometrium, and 4% in the fallopian tube [158]. The diagnosis of placental site nodule has been made in a variety of clinical settings including evaluation of cervical intraepithelial neoplasia following an abnormal cervical smear (35%), dysmenorrhea and metromenorrhagia (30%), recurrent spontaneous abortion (5%), retained products of conception (5%), postcoital bleeding (2.5%), and infertility (2.5%) [158]. Many patients have a prior history of therapeutic abortion and cesarean section. A significant number of patients have had a history of a tubal ligation [16, 60, 158]. The antecedent pregnancy has been reported to have been as short as 2 months to as long as 108 months prior to the diagnosis, suggesting that these lesions can persist in the uterus for a long period of time.

Placental site nodules are usually small, ranging from 1 to 14 (average 2.1) mm. Occasionally, multiple and sizable (>5 mm) placental site nodules can be found. When grossly visible, placental site nodules appear as a yellow-white and necrotic-appearing nodule in the endometrium or superficial myometrium [74].

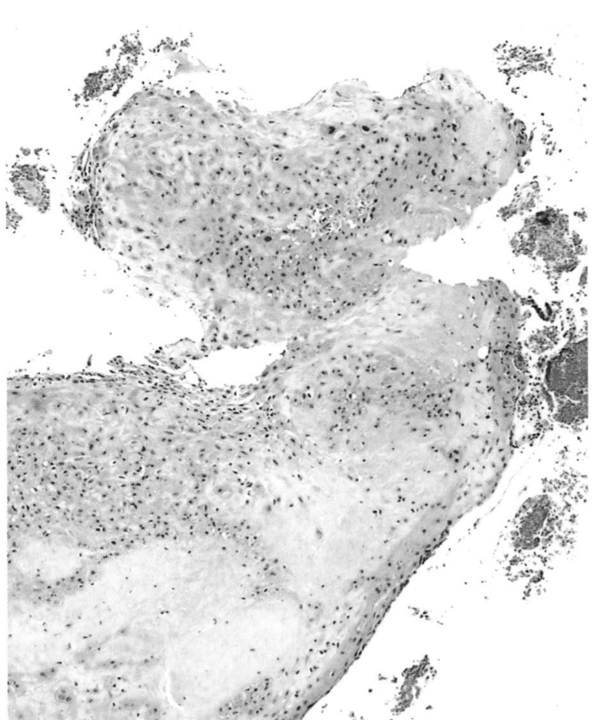

Fig. 20.46
Placental site nodule in endometrial curettings. **The lesion is well circumscribed and contains eosinophilic acellular material**

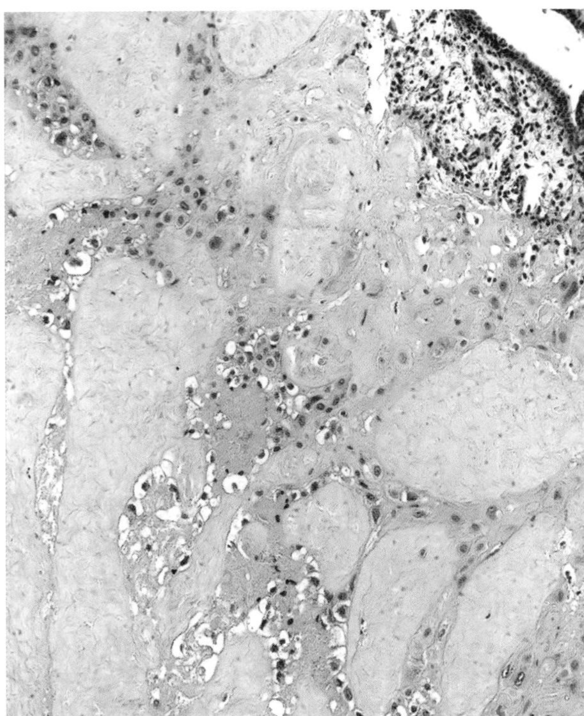

Fig. 20.47
Placental site nodule. **The nodule is composed of hyalin material that contains scattered chorionic-type intermediate trophoblast. There are two distinct populations of trophoblastic cells, one with eosinophilic cytoplasm and one with clear or vacuolated cytoplasm**

Microscopically, placental site nodules are small nodular or plaque-like lesions with rounded, well-circumscribed borders (Figs. *20.46–20.50*). The nodules are surrounded by a thin rim of chronic inflammatory cells and, occasionally, decidualized stroma. The nodules typically are composed of chorionic-type intermediate trophoblast (*Fig. 20.5*). The trophoblastic cells are arranged in a haphazard pattern, dispersed singly, in small clusters and cords, or occasionally diffusely throughout the nodule (*Fig. 20.50*). Mitotic figures are absent or rare. Often these cells occupy the outer portion of the nodule with a central hyalinized extracellular matrix (*Figs. 20.46–20.48*). The trophoblastic cells within the placental site nodule share several features with chorionic-type intermediate trophoblast in normal fetal membranes (*Fig. 20.49*) [158]. They are haphazardly distributed in an eosinophilic hyaline matrix with scattered large hyperchromatic nuclei easily visible at low magnification. The cells vary in size; many have relatively small uniform nuclei and a few have large, irregular, and hyperchromatic nuclei. Multinucleated cells are occasionally present. The cytoplasm of the larger trophoblastic cells is abundant and eosinophilic to amphophilic, whereas the smaller cells contain glycogen-rich clear cytoplasm (*Fig. 20.49*).

Rarely, placental site nodules demonstrate morphologic and immunostaining features suggestive of an epithelioid trophoblastic tumor but they are quantitatively and qualitatively insufficient to render the diagnosis of epithelioid trophoblastic tumor [94, 158, 170]. We have tentatively used "atypical placental site nodules" to describe and report those lesions. Although there are no criteria and quantitative measures in defining what is "atypical," atypical placental site nodules usually contain more abundant lesional tissues in curettage or biopsy specimens and appear more cellular than placental site nodules [94, 158, 170]. Specifically, these lesions are intermediate in size between placental site nodules, which rarely exceed 4 mm in diameter and the larger epithelioid trophoblastic tumors. Atypical placental site nodules tend to have higher cellularity and the trophoblastic cells are arranged in more cohesive nests and cords than the typical placental site nodules (Fig. 20.51) [146, 153, 154]. Also, the Ki-67 labeling index in usual placental site nodules is higher. These findings suggest that atypical placental site nodules are intermediate between a placental site nodule and an epithelioid trophoblastic tumor and may represent a transition from a benign placental site nodule to an epithelioid trophoblastic tumor. Based on the histologic and immunohistochemical features as well as the intimate association of some epithelioid trophoblastic tumors with placental site nodules, we have speculated that the epithelioid trophoblastic tumor represents the neoplastic counterpart of the placental site nodule [94, 170]. The clinical behavior of atypical placental site nodules is currently not known because only a few cases have been reported so far but the few cases in which we have follow-up information have behaved in a benign fashion.

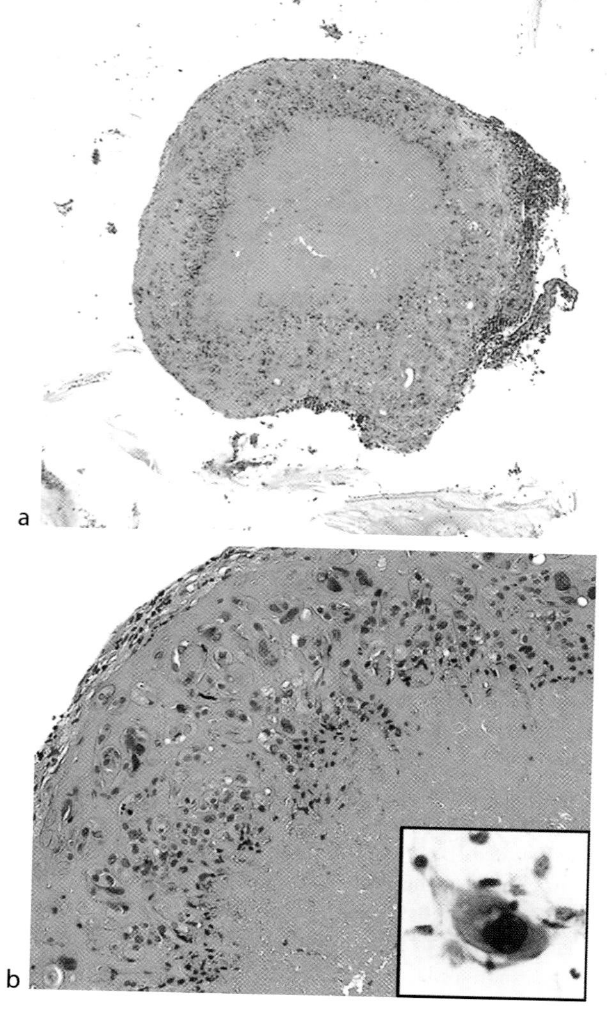
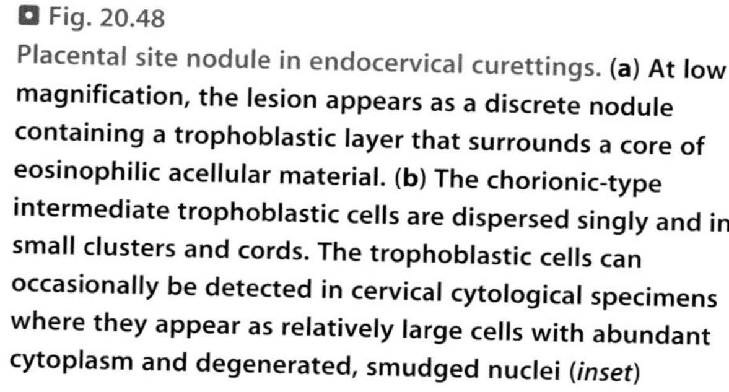

Fig. 20.48
Placental site nodule in endocervical curettings. (**a**) At low magnification, the lesion appears as a discrete nodule containing a trophoblastic layer that surrounds a core of eosinophilic acellular material. (**b**) The chorionic-type intermediate trophoblastic cells are dispersed singly and in small clusters and cords. The trophoblastic cells can occasionally be detected in cervical cytological specimens where they appear as relatively large cells with abundant cytoplasm and degenerated, smudged nuclei (*inset*)

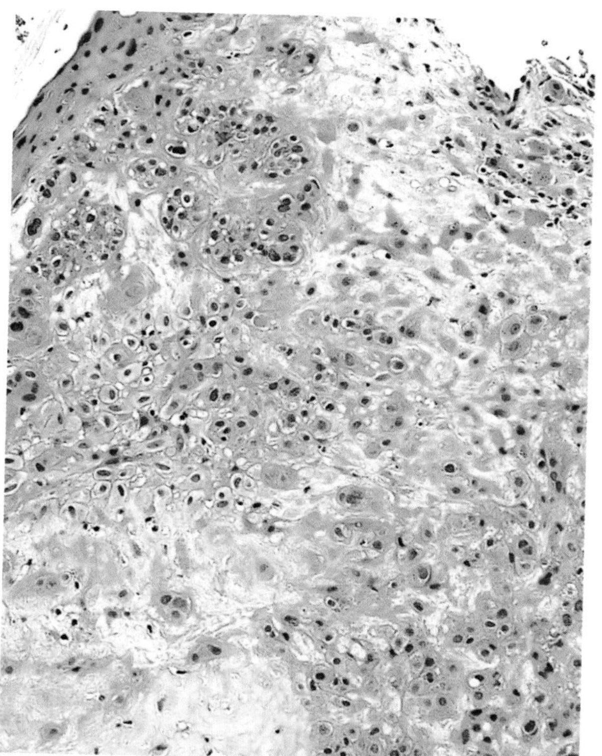

Fig. 20.49
Placental site nodule. Chorionic-type intermediate trophoblastic cells form small nests and cords with distinct cell borders. Mitotic figures are rare but can be seen

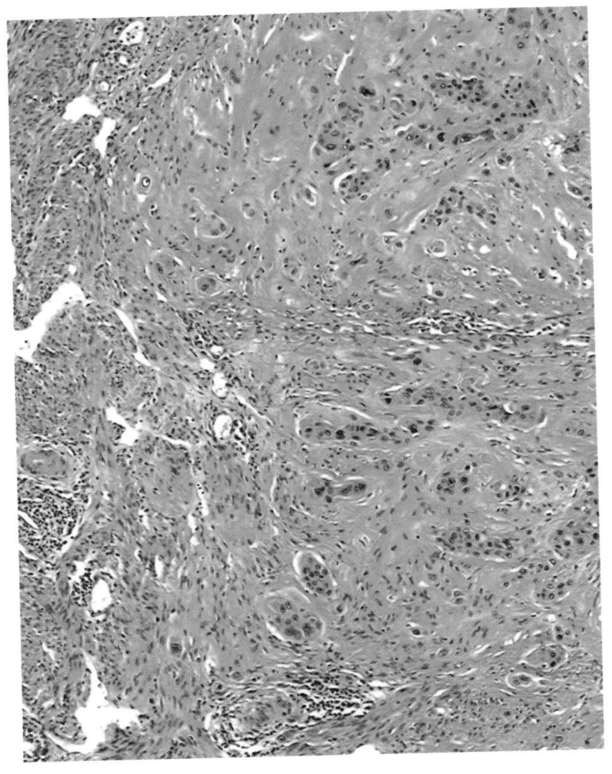

■ Fig. 20.50
Placental site nodule. **On some occasions, the trophoblastic cells are arranged in a haphazard pattern, dispersed in small clusters and cords, or sometimes diffusely throughout the nodule. The eosinophilic extracellular matrix is not prominent in this case (compared to ➲ *Figs. 20.47* and ➲ *20.46*). Each nest is accompanied by hyalinized material, a characteristic finding in placental site nodules**

The trophoblastic cells in the placental site nodule exhibit an immunophenotype similar to that of trophoblastic cells in the chorion laeve (fetal membrane; ➲ *Fig. 20.5*) but distinct from the implantation site intermediate trophoblast (➲ *Table 20.2*). For example, they are only focally positive for hPL and CD146 (Mel-CAM), and are negative for mucin-4, in contrast to the intermediate trophoblastic cells in the implantation site, where these antigens are highly and diffusely expressed [92, 146, 149, 153]. Immunoreactivity for beta-hCG is usually absent. In contrast to implantation site intermediate trophoblastic cell in the first trimester, the chorionic-type intermediate trophoblastic cells in placental site nodules are positive for p63 [84, 156]. Similar to the chorionic-type intermediate trophoblastic cells found in chorion laeve (fetal membrane) of normal pregnancy, there is a low level of proliferation in the cells of placental site nodules as indicated by a few scattered Ki-67-labeled nuclei [158]. In contrast, in the normal implantation site and even in exaggerated placental sites the Ki-67 index of implantation site intermediate trophoblastic cells is zero [151].

A placental site nodule may be confused with a PSTT, epithelioid trophoblastic tumor, and a non-trophoblastic lesion, notably invasive squamous carcinoma of the cervix [153, 179]. Their microscopic size, circumscription, extensive hyalinization, and paucicellularity are features that separate them from PSTT. In difficult cases, immunostaining is helpful. The application of immunohistochemistry in assisting the diagnosis of placental site nodule is described in the section ➲ Immunohistochemical Approach for Differential Diagnosis. As previously mentioned, the differential diagnosis between placental site nodule and cervical squamous carcinoma may arise in cervical biopsies from patients who are being evaluated for cervical neoplasia. Circumscription of the lesion, abundant eosinophilic extracellular deposit, and lack of mitotic activity favor a placental site nodule. Immunoreactivity for HSD3B1 and p16 are particularly useful in the differential diagnosis [93, 94]. Specifically, placental site nodule is positive for HSD3B1 but is negative for p16, while cervical squamous intraepithelial lesion and carcinoma are positive for p16 and is always negative for HSD3B1.

The distinction of an epithelioid trophoblastic tumor from a placental site nodule is usually not difficult as placental site nodules are microscopic lesions with sharply circumscribed borders [158]. Epithelioid trophoblastic tumors are larger and display substantial necrosis. The placental site nodule is much less cellular than epithelioid trophoblastic tumor (➲ *Fig. 20.52*). In addition, the lesional cells in a placental site nodule in contrast to an epithelioid trophoblastic tumor are bland and mitotic activity is low or absent. If calcification is present, the lesion is most likely an epithelioid trophoblastic tumor rather than a placental site nodule. Moreover, cyclin E is usually expressed in an epithelioid trophoblastic tumor but rarely in a placental site nodule (➲ *Fig. 20.52*) [94].

Placental site nodules are benign non-neoplastic lesions. Because of their small size and circumscription, the lesions are usually removed completely by the surgical procedure that led to their discovery. Neither local recurrence nor progression to persistent GTD has been documented in placental site nodules [153, 179]. Accordingly, no specific treatment or follow-up is necessary for this lesion. The behavior of atypical placental site nodules has not yet been studied.

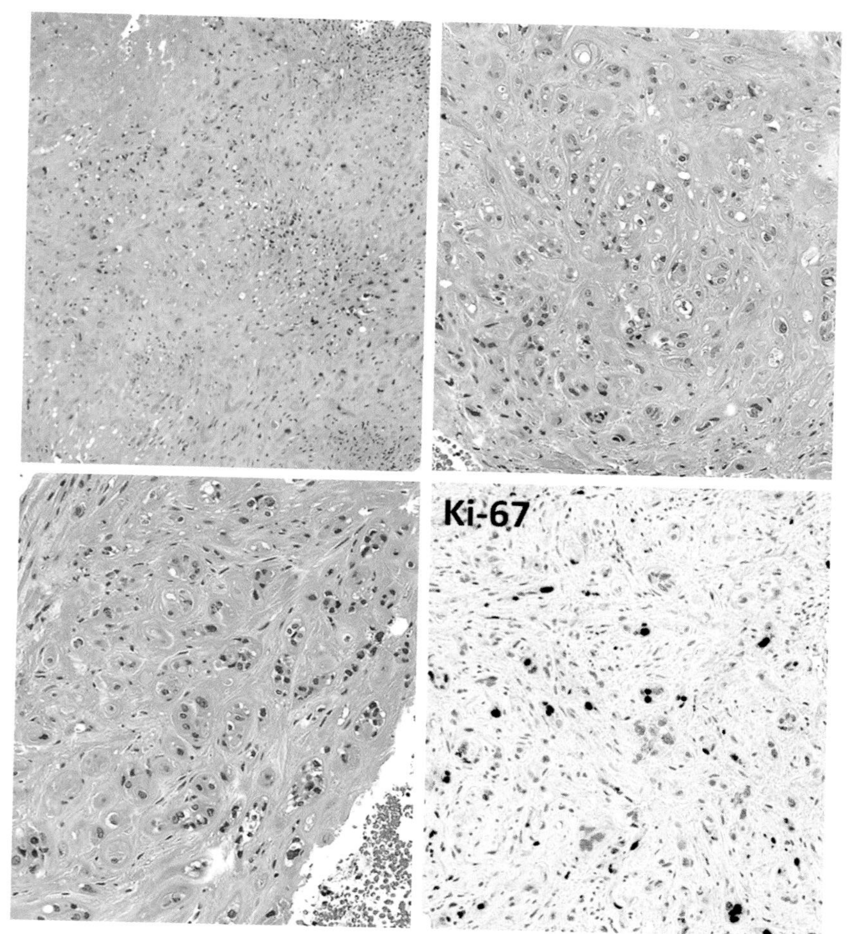

Fig. 20.51
Atypical placental site nodule. **The lesion is intermediate between a placental site nodule and an epithelioid trophoblastic tumor. These atypical placental site nodules tend to have higher cellularity and the trophoblastic cells are arranged in more cohesive nests and cords than the typical placental site nodule. The Ki-67 labeling index in this case is approximately 15–20%, which is higher than in a conventional placental site nodule**

Chorangiocarcinoma

Chorangiocarcinoma is discussed in this chapter because this lesion is likely of trophoblastic origin. Chorangiocarcinoma is an exceedingly rare placental lesion and only four cases have been reported so far in the literature [4, 48, 69, 169]; it has argued that the incidence is actually higher [73]. The tumor is usually an incidental finding in a term or a near-term placenta. Grossly, it is a discrete intraplacental lesion resembling a placental infarct. Microscopically it is a lesion characterized by an abnormal trophoblastic proliferation in conjunction with a hypervascular chorangiosis (or chorangioma) in the stroma of chorionic villi (*Fig. 20.53*). The unique morphologic feature of a proliferation in both epithelial and vascular components of chorionic villi distinguishes chorangiocarcinoma from other trophoblastic tumors and tumor-like lesions. The cells in the epithelial compartment form solid masses with massive central coagulation necrosis surrounded by a few (three to six) layers of viable epithelial tumor cells. At low magnification, the necrotic areas may occupy most of the tumor. The epithelial cells are highly proliferative with frequent mitotic figures. They express low-molecular-weight cytokeratin (such as cytokeratin 18), beta-hCG, and HSD3B1, supporting their trophoblastic origin [93]. The vascular component is similar to chorangiosis or a chorangioma with numerous intercalated vascular channels in the villous stroma.

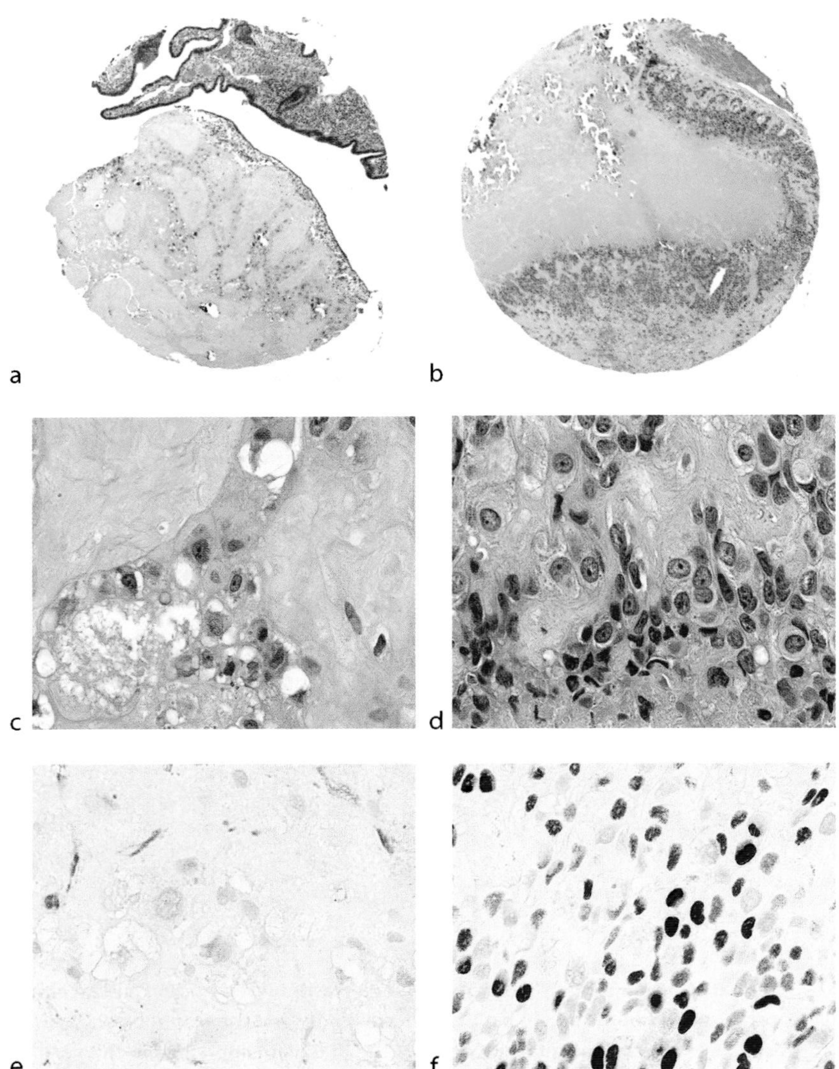

Fig. 20.52
Comparison of a placental site nodule (a, c, e) and an epithelioid trophoblastic tumor (b, d, f). (a, b): H&E sections at low magnification. (c, d) H&E sections at higher magnification. (e, f) Cyclin E immunostain (Reprinted by permission from [94])

The pathogenesis in the development of chorangiocarcinoma is undetermined. The lesion may represent a chorangioma with associated trophoblastic hyperplasia, a true trophoblastic neoplasm with a reactive chorangiosis response, a reactive lesion of trophoblastic cells and villous vascular channels, or a collision tumor of chorangioma and choriocarcinoma. The clinical experience with chorangiocarcinoma is very limited but the available data from the reported cases reveal that patients have an uneventful postpartum course and do not develop persistent GTD [48, 69, 73, 169].

Immunohistochemical Approach for Differential Diagnosis

Diagnosis of trophoblastic tumors and tumor-like lesions is usually straightforwardly based on clinical and morphological features (*Tables 20.7* and *20.8*). However; the diagnosis can be challenging in certain cases, especially in small biopsy and curettage specimens [110]. To assist in differential diagnosis, we have developed an algorithmic approach, termed "trophogram," using a three-tiered stepwise immunohistochemical staining procedure [144]

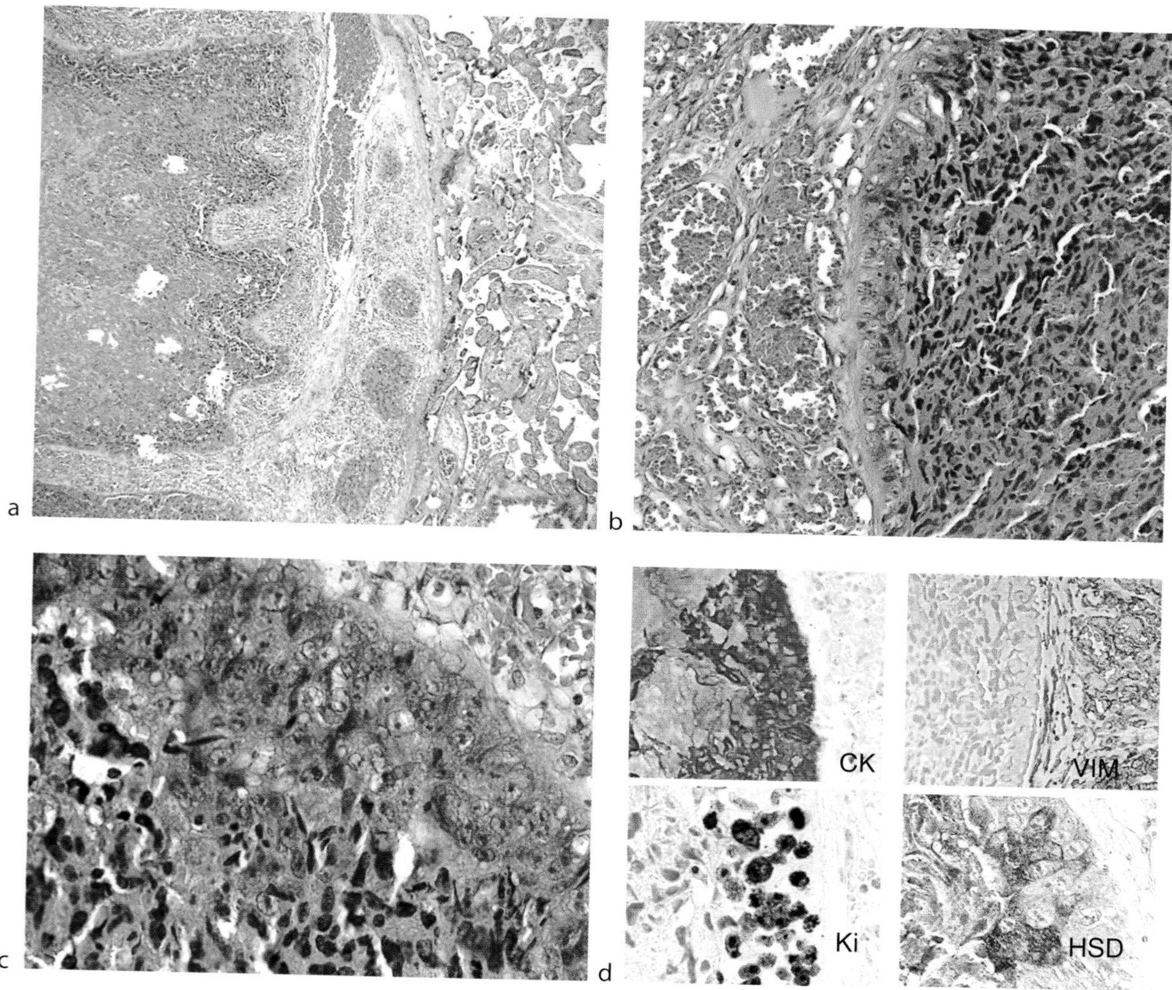

Fig. 20.53
Chorangiocarcinoma. **(a)** The tumor is characterized by an abnormal trophoblastic proliferation (*left*) and hypervascular chorangiosis (*right*) in the stroma of the chorionic villi. **(b, c)** The cells in the epithelial compartment form solid masses with massive central coagulative necrosis which is surrounded by a few (three to six) layers of viable epithelial (presumable trophoblastic) tumor cells. **(d)** Immunohistochemical features of chorangiocarcinoma. The viable tumor cells in the epithelial component are positive for low-molecular-weight cytokeratin (such as cytokeratin 18) and HSD3B1 (a trophoblast-associated marker), a finding supporting the tumor cells are of trophoblastic origin. The percentage of Ki-67 labeled epithelial cells is high (>90%) in the viable epithelial cells. In contrast, the vascular/chorangiosis component is negative for cytokeratin and HSD3B1 but is positive for vimentin

(➋ *Fig. 20.54*). The antibodies utilized in the algorithm are all commercially available and are listed in ➋ *Table 20.9*. The first tier in the algorithm discriminates a trophoblastic versus a non-trophoblastic lesion. The second tier determines if the lesion is related to implantation site intermediate trophoblast (i.e., exaggerated placental site and PSTT), to chorionic-type intermediate trophoblastic cells (i.e., placental site nodule and epithelioid trophoblastic tumor), or a choriocarcinoma. The third tier distinguishes a benign tumor-like lesion versus a trophoblastic neoplasm (➋ *Fig. 20.54*). An example of how the algorithm can be used in the diagnosis of a PSTT is illustrated in ➋ *Fig. 20.55*.

Using the algorithm, immunoreactivity of HSD3B1 and low-molecular-weight cytokeratin (e.g., cytokeratin 8 or 18) should first be assessed to determine if the lesion

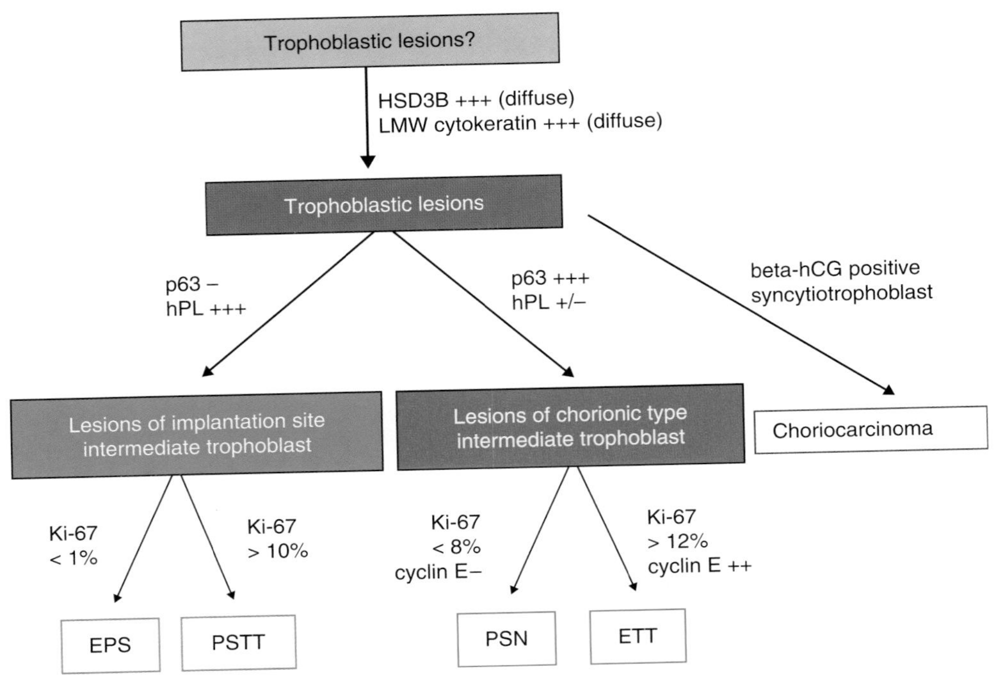

Fig. 20.54

Trophogram is an immunohistochemistry algorithm designed to assist in the differential diagnosis of trophoblastic tumors and tumor-like lesions. **A three-tier sequential staining procedure that utilizes a panel of commercially available antibodies listed in *Table 20.9*. The first tier discriminates a trophoblastic versus a non-trophoblastic lesion. The second determines if the lesion is a choriocarcinoma, a lesion related to implantation site intermediate trophoblast or a lesion related to chorionic-type intermediate trophoblastic cells. The third tier distinguishes a benign tumor-like lesion versus a true trophoblastic neoplasm. EPS, exaggerated placental site; PSTT, placental site trophoblastic tumor; PSN, placental site nodule; ETT, epithelioid trophoblastic tumor; LMW, low molecular weight**

Table 20.9

Commercial antibodies used in the trophogram

Marker	Antibody source	Application
HSD3B1	Abnova (3C11-D4[a])	Distinguish GTD from most non-GTD
Cytokeratin	Ventana (CAM5.2)	Exclude mimickers of mesenchymal origin
p63	Neomarker (4A4)	Distinguish ETT vs. PSTT
hPL	Dako (polyclonal)	Distinguish PSTT vs. ETT
beta-hCG	Dako (polyclonal)	Highlight ST in choriocarcinoma
Cyclin E	Zymed (HE12)	Distinguish ETT vs. PSN
Ki-67	Dako (MIB-1)	Distinguish ETT vs. PSN; PSTT vs. EPS

[a]Clone or name for the monoclonal antibody which may be obtained from other commercial sources.
GTD, gestational trophoblastic disease; ETT, epithelioid trophoblastic tumor; PSTT, placental site trophoblastic tumor; PSN, placental site nodule; EPS, exaggerated placental site; ST, syncytiotrophoblast.

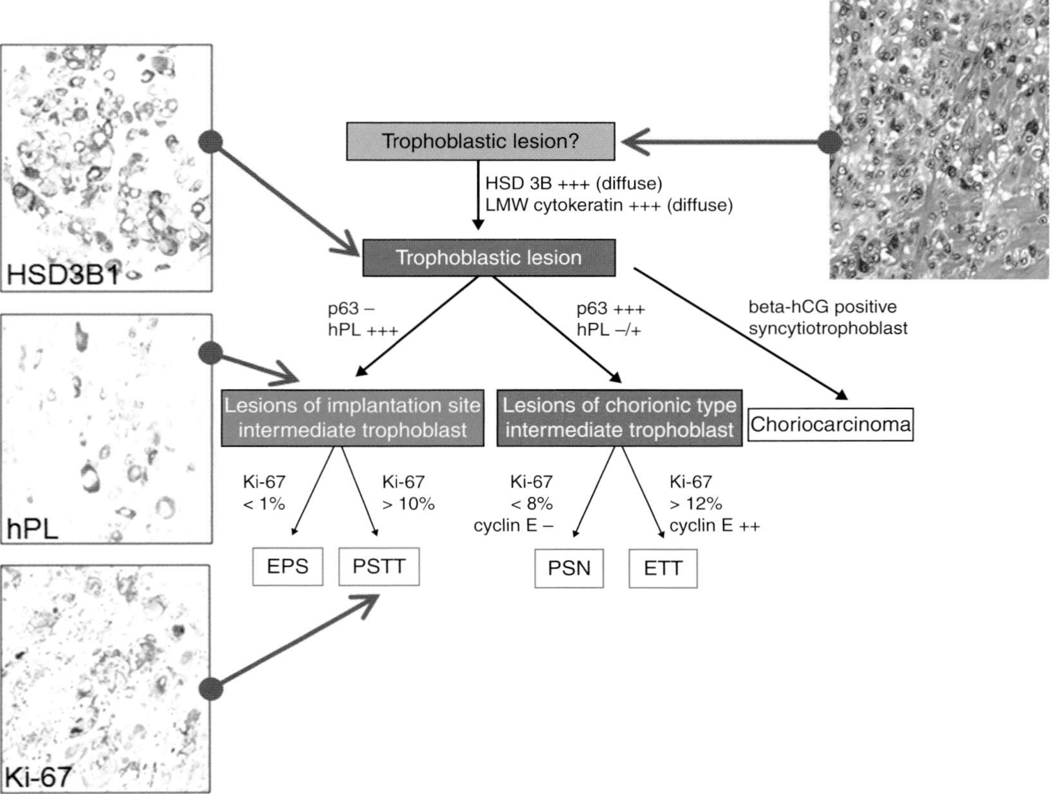

Fig. 20.55
The algorithm in the diagnosis of a PSTT. **Hematoxylin-and-eosin section shows a tumor composed of large, atypical cells forming confluent masses and cords. The differential diagnosis includes PSTT, exaggerated placental site, epithelioid trophoblastic tumor, smooth muscle neoplasm, and poorly differentiated carcinoma. Immunohistochemistry demonstrates that the tumor cells are diffusely positive for HSD3B1, indicating trophoblastic origin. The trophoblastic lesion was then stained with hPL followed by Ki-67 and is diffusely positive for hPL, indicating that it is derived from the implantation site intermediate trophoblastic cells. The Ki-67 labeling index is approximately 15%, confirming its neoplastic nature. The combination of morphologic and immunohistochemical findings indicate that the case is a PSTT. EPS, exaggerated placental site; PSTT, placental site trophoblastic tumor; PSN, placental site nodule; ETT, epithelioid trophoblastic tumor; LMW, low molecular weight**

in question is trophoblastic. Diffuse and intense HSD3B1 and low-molecular-weight cytokeratin immunoreactivity strongly suggests trophoblast origin [93]. It should be noted that HSD3B1 must be used in conjunction with low-molecular-weight cytokeratins because the latter are expressed in a wide variety of adenocarcinomas. Thus, cytokeratin should be used to further support the diagnosis of a trophoblastic lesion in HSD3B1-positive cases. Once the diagnosis of a trophoblastic lesion is established and hydatidiform mole is excluded, choriocarcinoma should be considered because it is the most common malignant trophoblastic neoplasm. The presence of beta-hCG-stained syncytiotrophoblast supports the diagnosis of choriocarcinoma. In choriocarcinomas where the syncytiotrophoblastic component is attenuated, beta-hCG-positive syncytiotrophoblast tends to lie between or envelop masses of mononucleate trophoblastic cells. Syncytiotrophoblast in choriocarcinoma should not be mistaken for beta-hCG positive multinucleated intermediate trophoblastic cells in PSTT and epithelioid trophoblastic tumor. The multinucleated intermediate trophoblastic cells are usually polygonal or round in shape with centrally located nuclei, whereas syncytiotrophoblast have an irregular often serpentine shape with dense, amphophilic cytoplasm and multiple hyperchromatic nuclei. A beta-hCG immunostaining can help demonstrate the characteristic growth pattern. Furthermore, choriocarcinoma has very high proliferative activity and accordingly the Ki-67 labeling index in mononucleate tumor cells in choriocarcinoma (Ki-67 index usually >40%) is significantly higher than that in most PSTTs and epithelioid trophoblastic tumors (Ki-67 index usually <30%). Of note, some malignant PSTTs and epithelioid trophoblastic tumors may have unusually high Ki-67 labeling index and thus the Ki-67 index is useful but not diagnostic of choriocarcinoma. Other immunohistochemical markers including HLA-G, Mel-CAM, p63, cytokeratin, and inhibin are not useful in the differential diagnosis of choriocarcinoma versus other trophoblastic tumors [71].

If choriocarcinoma has been ruled out, both hPL and p63 antibodies should be applied to determine if the lesion is related to implantation site intermediate trophoblast or chorionic-type intermediate trophoblast. hPL is diffusely positive (usually >50% of lesional cells) and p63 is always negative (or very focally positive) in PSTT and exaggerated placental site. In contrast, hPL is either negative or focally positive in epithelioid trophoblastic tumors and placental site nodules but p63 is diffusely positive (usually >50% of lesional cells) [84, 156, 185]. Of note, the antibody to p63 should be the one that recognizes all the p63 isoforms. If necessary, the Ki-67 labeling index can be used to distinguish an epithelioid trophoblastic tumor from a placental site nodule or a PSTT from an exaggerated placental site. The Ki-67 index in placental site nodule is generally low (<8%), while the index in epithelioid trophoblastic tumor is above 12%. Similarly, the Ki-67 index is near zero (<1%) in exaggerated placental site while it is usually above 10% in PSTT. One important pitfall in determining Ki-67 labeling index is that presence of NK cells and lymphocytes in the endomyometrium, which are proliferative and can result in an apparent increased Ki-67 labeling index [151]. Accordingly, it is important that the Ki-67 labeling index be exclusively evaluated in trophoblastic cells. Morphologically, trophoblastic cells tend to have enlarged and highly pleomorphic (degenerated) nuclei, whereas inflammatory cells usually have smaller and uniform nuclei, but at times distinction between trophoblastic cells and inflammatory cells may be difficult. The Ki-67 labeling index is more reliable in distinguishing PSTT from exaggerated placental site rather than epithelioid trophoblastic tumor from placental site nodule because the diagnostic margin of Ki-67 labeling index between epithelioid trophoblastic tumor and placental site nodule is relatively narrow in some cases. To address this potential concern, Mao et al. has recently reported that cyclin E immunoreactivity is useful in the discrimination between epithelioid trophoblastic tumors and placental site nodules [94]. Cyclin E is expressed in the nuclei of many epithelioid trophoblastic tumors but rarely in placental site nodules.

It should be emphasized that the sequence in applying the immunostaining scheme outlined in ➔ *Fig. 20.54* should be followed when applying the trophogram in the differential diagnosis of trophoblastic tumors and tumor-like lesions. For example, p63 immunoreactivity is informative only in the context of distinguishing trophoblastic tumors and tumor-like lesions that are related to either implantation site intermediate trophoblastic cells (PSTT and exaggerated placental site) or chorionic-type intermediate trophoblastic cells (epithelioid trophoblastic tumor and placental site nodule). p63 immunostaining is not useful in distinguishing trophoblastic versus non-trophoblastic lesions because it is expressed in several types of squamous carcinomas [57]. Likewise, cyclin E immunoreactivity is applicable only for distinguishing epithelioid trophoblastic tumors from placental site nodules. It is not useful in other diagnostic settings because a variety of neoplastic diseases express cyclin E.

References

1. Akbulut M, Tosun H, Soysal ME, Oztekin O (2008) Endometrioid carcinoma of the endometrium with choriocarcinomatous differentiation: a case report and review of the literature. Arch Gynecol Obstet 278:79–84
2. Allan RW, Algood CB, Shih Ie M (2009) Metastatic epithelioid trophoblastic tumor in a male patient with mixed germ-cell tumor of the testis. Am J Surg Pathol 33:1902–1905
3. Altieri A, Franceschi S, Ferlay J, Smith J, La Vecchia C (2003) Epidemiology and aetiology of gestational trophoblastic diseases. Lancet Oncol 4:670–678
4. Ariel I, Boldes R, Weintraub A, Reinus C, Beller U, Arbel R (2009) Chorangiocarcinoma: a case report and review of the literature. Int J Gynecol Pathol 28:267–271
5. Arroyo MR, Podda A, Cao D, Rodriguez MM (2008) Placental site trophoblastic tumor in the ovary of a young child with isosexual precocious puberty. Pediatr Dev Pathol 12:73–76
6. Azuma C, Saji F, Nobunaga T, Kamiura S, Kimura T, Tokugawa Y, Koyama M, Tanizawa O (1990) Studies on the pathogenesis of choriocarcinoma by analysis of restriction fragment length polymorphisms. Cancer Res 50:488–491
7. Baergen RN, Rutgers J, Young RH (2003) Extrauterine lesions of intermediate trophoblast. Int J Gynecol Pathol 22:362–367
8. Baergen RN, Rutgers JL, Young RH, Osann K, Scully RE (2006) Placental site trophoblastic tumor: A study of 55 cases and review of the literature emphasizing factors of prognostic significance. Gynecol Oncol 100:511–520
9. Bagshawe KD, Lawler SD, Paradinas FJ, Dent J, Brown P, Boxer GM (1990) Gestational trophoblastic tumours following initial diagnosis of partial hydatidiform mole. Lancet 335:1074–1076

10. Behtash N, Ghaemmaghami F, Hasanzadeh M (2005) Long term remission of metastatic placental site trophoblastic tumor (PSTT): case report and review of literature. World J Surg Oncol 3:34
11. Berkowitz RS, Im SS, Bernstein MR, Goldstein DP (1998) Gestational trophoblastic disease. Subsequent pregnancy outcome, including repeat molar pregnancy. J Reprod Med 43:81–86
12. Berkowitz LW, Lage JM (1990) Persistent gestational trophoblastic tumor after partial hydatidiform mole. Gynecol Oncol 36:358–362
13. Bifulco C, Johnson C, Hao L, Kermalli H, Bell S, Hui P (2008) Genotypic analysis of hydatidiform mole: an accurate and practical method of diagnosis. Am J Surg Pathol 32:445–451
14. Brewer CA, Adelson MD, Elder RC (1992) Erythrocytosis associated with a placental-site trophoblastic tumor. Obstet Gynecol 79: 846–849
15. Burrows TD, King A, Loke YW (1994) Expression of adhesion molecules by endovascular trophoblast and decidual endothelial cells: implications for vascular invasion during implantation. Placenta 15:21–33
16. Carinelli SG, Verdola N, Zanotti F (1989) Placental site nodule: a report of 17 cases. Pathol Res Pract 185:30–34
17. Castrillon DH, Sun D, Weremowicz S, Fisher RA, Crum CP, Genest DR (2001) Discrimination of complete hydatidiform mole from its mimics by immunohistochemistry of the paternally imprinted gene product p57KIP2. Am J Surg Pathol 25:1225–1230
18. Chang YL, Chang TC, Hsueh S, Huang KG, Wang PN, Liu HP, Soong YK (1999) Prognostic factors and treatment for placental site trophoblastic tumor: report of 3 cases and analysis of 88 cases. Gynecol Oncol 73:216–222
19. Cheung AN, Shen DH, Khoo US, Wong LC, Ngan HY (1998) p21WAF1/CIP1 expression in gestational trophoblastic disease: correlation with clinicopathological parameters, and Ki67 and p53 gene expression. J Clin Pathol 51:159–162
20. Chew SH, Perlman EJ, Williams R, Kurman RJ, Ronnett BM (2000) Morphology and DNA content analysis in the evaluation of first trimester placentas for partial hydatidiform mole (PHM). Hum Pathol 31:914–924
21. Chilosi M, Piazzola E, Lestani M, Benedetti A, Guasparri I, Granchelli G, Aldovini D, Leonardi E, Pizzolo G, Doglioni C et al (1998) Differential expression of p57kip2, a maternally imprinted cdk inhibitor, in normal human placenta and gestational trophoblastic disease. Lab Invest 78:269–276
22. Cole LA (1998) hCG, its free subunits and its metabolites. Roles in pregnancy and trophoblastic disease. J Reprod Med 43:3–10
23. Cole LA (2009) New discoveries on the biology and detection of human chorionic gonadotropin. Reprod Biol Endocrinol 7:8
24. Cole ME, Broaddus R, Thaker P, Landen C, Freedman RS (2008) Placental-site trophoblastic tumors: a case of resistant pulmonary metastasis. Nat Clin Pract Oncol 5:171–175
25. Cole LA, Khanlian SA, Muller CY, Giddings A, Kohorn E, Berkowitz R (2006) Gestational trophoblastic diseases: 3. Human chorionic gonadotropin-free beta-subunit, a reliable marker of placental site trophoblastic tumors. Gynecol Oncol 102:160–164
26. Coukos G, Makrigiannakis A, Chung J, Randall TC, Rubin SC, Benjamin I (1999) Complete hydatidiform mole. A disease with a changing profile [In Process Citation]. J Reprod Med 44:698–704
27. Coulson LE, Kong CS, Zaloudek C (2000) Epithelioid trophoblastic tumor of the uterus in a postmenopausal woman: a case report and review of the literature. Am J Surg Pathol 24:1558–1562
28. Czernobilsky B, Barash A, Lancet M (1982) Partial moles: a clinicopathologic study of 25 cases. Obstet Gynecol 59:75–77
29. Datta T, Banerjee AK, Adeyemo AK, McCullough WL, Duncan A (2007) Intraplacental choriocarcinoma associated with pregnancy continuum: a diagnostic dilemma. J Obstet Gynaecol 27:731–732
30. Denny LA, Dehaeck K, Nevin J, Soeters R, van Wijk AL, Megevand E, Bloch B (1995) Placental site trophoblastic tumor: three case reports and literature review. Gynecol Oncol 59:300–303
31. Dotto J, Hui P (2008) Lack of genetic association between exaggerated placental site reaction and placental site trophoblastic tumor. Int J Gynecol Pathol 27:562–567
32. Eckstein RP, Paradinas FJ, Bagshawe KD (1982) Placental site trophoblastic tumour (trophoblastic pseudotumour): a study of four cases requiring hysterectomy including one fatal case. Histopathology 6:211–226
33. Elston C (1995) Gestational trophoblastic disease, 4th edn. New York, Churchill Linvingstone
34. Fadare O, Parkash V, Carcangiu ML, Hui P (2006) Epithelioid trophoblastic tumor: clinicopathological features with an emphasis on uterine cervical involvement. Mod Pathol 19:75–82
35. Feltmate CM, Genest DR, Goldstein DP, Berkowitz RS (2002) Advances in the understanding of placental site trophoblastic tumor. J Reprod Med 47:337–341
36. Fisher RA, Paradinas FJ, Newlands ES, Boxer GM (1992) Genetic evidence that placental site trophoblastic tumours can originate from a hydatidiform mole or a normal conceptus. Br J Cancer 65:355–358
37. Folberg R, Hendrix MJ, Maniotis AJ (2000) Vasculogenic mimicry and tumor angiogenesis. Am J Pathol 156:361–381
38. Fox H, Laurini RN (1988) Intraplacental choriocarcinoma: a report of two cases. J Clin Pathol 41:1085–1088
39. Fraser GC, Blair GK, Hemming A, Murphy JJ, Rogers P (1992) The treatment of simultaneous choriocarcinoma in mother and baby. J Pediatr Surg 27:1318–1319
40. Fukunaga M, Ushigome S (1993) Malignant trophoblastic tumors: immunohistochemical and flow cytometric comparison of choriocarcinoma and placental site trophoblastic tumors. Hum Pathol 24:1098–1106
41. Fukunaga M, Ushigome S (1993) Metastasizing placental site trophoblastic tumor. An immunohistochemical and flow cytometric study of two cases. Am J Surg Pathol 17:1003–1010
42. Garg R, Russell J, Shih I-M, Bristow RE (2004) Have you ruled out a placental site nodule? Contempory Obst Gyn 49:18–20
43. Garner EI, Goldstein DP, Feltmate CM, Berkowitz RS (2007) Gestational trophoblastic disease. Clin Obstet Gynecol 50:112–122
44. Genest DR (2001) Partial hydatidiform mole: clinicopathological features, differential diagnosis, ploidy and molecular studies, and gold standards for diagnosis. Int J Gynecol Pathol 20:315–322
45. Golfier F, Raudrant D, Frappart L, Mathian B, Guastalla JP, Trillet-Lenoir V, Vaudoyer F, Hajri T, Schott AM (2007) First epidemiological data from the French Trophoblastic Disease Reference Center. Am J Obstet Gynecol 196(172):e171–e175
46. Golubovsky MD (2003) Postzygotic diploidization of triploids as a source of unusual cases of mosaicism, chimerism and twinning. Hum Reprod 18:236–242
47. Goto S, Yamada A, Ishizuka T, Tomoda Y (1993) Development of postmolar trophoblastic disease after partial molar pregnancy. Gynecol Oncol 48:165–170
48. Guschmann M, Schulz-Bischof K, Vogel M (2003) Incidental chorangiocarcinoma. Case report, immunohistochemistry and theories of possible histogenesis. Pathologe 24:124–127
49. Hamazaki S, Nakamoto S, Okino T, Tsukayama C, Mori M, Taguchi K, Okada S (1999) Epithelioid trophoblastic tumor:

morphological and immunohistochemical study of three lung lesions. Hum Pathol 30:1321–1327
50. Hancock BW, Nazir K, Everard JE (2006) Persistent gestational trophoblastic neoplasia after partial hydatidiform mole incidence and outcome. J Reprod Med 51:764–766
51. Hando T, Ohno M, Kurose T (1998) Recent aspects of gestational trophoblastic disease in Japan. Int J Gynaecol Obstet 60(Suppl 1): S71–S76
52. Harvey RA, Pursglove HD, Schmid P, Savage PM, Mitchell HD, Seckl MJ (2008) Human chorionic gonadotropin free beta-subunit measurement as a marker of placental site trophoblastic tumors. J Reprod Med 53:643–648
53. Hassadia A, Gillespie A, Tidy J, Everard RGNJ, Wells M, Coleman R, Hancock B (2005) Placental site trophoblastic tumour: clinical features and management. Gynecol Oncol 99:603–607
54. Hernandez L, Kozlov S, Piras G, Stewart CL (2003) Paternal and maternal genomes confer opposite effects on proliferation, cell-cycle length, senescence, and tumor formation. Proc Natl Acad Sci USA 100:13344–13349
55. Hertig AT (1956) Tumors of the female sex organs. Part 1. Hydatidifrom mole and choriocarcinoma. In: Atlas of tumor pathology, section 9, fascicle 33. Armed Forces Institute of Pathology, Washington DC
56. Hoekstra AV, Keh P, Lurain JR (2004) Placental site trophoblastic tumor: a review of 7 cases and their implications for prognosis and treatment. J Reprod Med 49:447–452
57. Houghton O, McCluggage WG (2009) The expression and diagnostic utility of p63 in the female genital tract. Adv Anat Pathol 16:316–321
58. How J, Scurry J, Grant P, Sapountzis K, Ostor A, Fortune D, Armes J (1995) Placental site trophoblastic tumor. Report of three cases and review of the literature. Int J Gynecol Cancer 5:241–249
59. Hsieh TY, Hsu KF, Kuo PL, Huang SC (2008) Uterine choriocarcinoma accompanied by an extremely high human chorionic gonadotropin level and thyrotoxicosis. J Obstet Gynaecol Res 34:274–278
60. Huettner PC, Gersell DJ (1994) Placental site nodule: a clinicopathologic study of 38 cases. Int J Gynecol Pathol 13:191–198
61. Hui P, Parkash V, Perkins AS, Carcangiu ML (2000) Pathogenesis of placental site trophoblastic tumor may require the presence of a paternally derived X chromosome. Lab Invest 80:965–972
62. Hui P, Riba A, Pejovic T, Johnson T, Baergen RN, Ward D (2004) Comparative genomic hybridization study of placental site trophoblastic tumour: a report of four cases. Mod Pathol 17:248–251
63. Ilancheran A (1998) Optimal treatment in gestational trophoblastic disease. Ann Acad Med Singapore 27:698–704
64. Ino K, Suzuki T, Uehara C, Nagasaka T, Okamoto T, Kikkawa F, Mizutani S (2000) The expression and localization of neutral endopeptidase 24.11/CD10 in human gestational trophoblastic diseases. Lab Invest 80:1729–1738
65. Jacobs PA, Hunt PA, Matsuura JS, Wilson CC, Szulman AE (1982) Complete and partial hydatidiform mole in Hawaii: cytogenetics, morphology and epidemiology. Br J Obstet Gynaecol 89:258–266
66. Jacques SM, Qureshi F, Ramirez NC, Lawrence WD (1997) Retained trophoblastic tissue in fallopian tubes: a consequence of unsuspected ectopic pregnancies. Int J Gynecol Pathol 16:219–224
67. Janni W, Hantschmann P, Rehbock J, Braun S, Lochmueller E, Kindermann G (1999) Successful treatment of malignant placental site trophoblastic tumor with combined cytostatic-surgical approach: case report and review of literature. Gynecol Oncol 75:164–169
68. Jauniaux E (1999) Partial moles: from postnatal to prenatal diagnosis. Placenta 20:379–388
69. Jauniaux E, Zucker M, Meuris S, Verhest A, Wilkin P, Hustin J (1988) Chorangiocarcinoma: an unusual tumour of the placenta. The missing link? Placenta 9:607–613
70. Jones WB, Romain K, Erlandson RA, Burt ME, Lewis JL Jr (1993) Thoracotomy in the management of gestational choriocarcinoma. A clinicopathologic study. Cancer 72:2175–2181
71. Kalhor N, Ramirez PT, Deavers MT, Malpica A, Silva EG (2009) Immunohistochemical studies of trophoblastic tumors. Am J Surg Pathol 33:633–638
72. Keep D, Zaragoza MV, Hassold T, Redline RW (1996) Very early complete hydatidiform mole. Hum Pathol 27:708–713
73. Khong TY (2000) Chorangioma with trophoblastic proliferation. Virchows Arch 436:167–171
74. Kim SY, Chang AS, Ratts VS (2005) Radiographic and hysteroscopic findings of a placental site nodule. Fertil Steril 83:213–215
75. Kim MJ, Kim KR, Ro JY, Lage JM, Lee HI (2006) Diagnostic and pathogenetic significance of increased stromal apoptosis and incomplete vasculogenesis in complete hydatidiform moles in very early pregnancy periods. Am J Surg Pathol 30:362–369
76. Kim JH, Park DC, Bae SN, Namkoong SE, Kim SJ (1998) Subsequent reproductive experience after treatment for gestational trophoblastic disease. Gynecol Oncol 71:108–112
77. Kodama S, Kase H, Aoki Y, Yahata T, Tanaka K, Motoyama T, Dewa K (1996) Recurrent placental site trophoblastic tumor of the uterus: clinical, pathologic, ultrastructural, and DNA fingerprint study. Gynecol Oncol 60:89–93
78. Kuo K-T, Chen M-J, Lin M-C (2004) Epithelioid trophoblastic tumor of the broad ligament. Am J Surg Pathol 28:405–409
79. Kurman RJ (1991) The morphology, biology, and pathology of intermediate trophoblast: a look back to the present. Hum Pathol 22:847–855
80. Kurman RJ, Scully RE, Norris HJ (1976) Trophoblastic pseudotumor of the uterus: an exaggerated form of "syncytial endometritis" simulating a malignant tumor. Cancer 38:1214–1226
81. Kurman RJ, Young RH, Norris HJ, Main CS, Lawrence WD, Scully RE (1984) Immunocytochemical localization of placental lactogen and chorionic gonadotropin in the normal placenta and trophoblastic tumors, with emphasis on intermediate trophoblast and the placental site trophoblastic tumor. Int J Gynecol Pathol 3:101–121
82. Lage JM, Mark SD, Roberts DJ, Goldstein DP, Bernstein MR, Berkowitz RS (1992) A flow cytometric study of 137 fresh hydropic placentas: correlation between types of hydatidiform moles and nuclear DNA ploidy. Obstet Gynecol 79:403–410
83. Lathrop JC, Lauchlan S, Nayak R, Ambler M (1988) Clinical characteristics of placental site trophoblastic tumor (PSTT). Gynecol Oncol 31:32–42
84. Lee Y, Kim KR, McKeon F, Yang A, Boyd TK, Crum CP, Parast MM (2007) A unifying concept of trophoblastic differentiation and malignancy defined by biomarker expression. Hum Pathol 38:1003–1013
85. Leiserowitz GS, Webb MJ (1996) Treatment of placental site trophoblastic tumor with hysterotomy and uterine reconstruction. Obstet Gynecol 88:696–699
86. Lewin SN, Aghajanian C, Moreira AL, Soslow RA (2009) Extrauterine epithelioid trophoblastic tumors presenting as primary lung carcinomas: morphologic and immunohistochemical features to resolve a diagnostic dilemma. Am J Surg Pathol 33:1809–1814
87. Li J, Shi Y, Wan X, Qian H, Zhou C, Chen X (2010) Epithelioid trophoblastic tumor: a clinicopathological and immunohistochemical study of seven cases. Med Oncol (in press)

88. Li HW, Tsao SW, Cheung AN (2002) Current understandings of the molecular genetics of gestational trophoblastic diseases. Placenta 23:20–31
89. Lipata F, Parkash V, Talmor M, Bell S, Chen S, Maric V, Hui P (2010) Precise DNA genotyping diagnosis of hydatidiform mole. Obstet Gynecol 115:784–794
90. Macdonald MC, Palmer JE, Hancock BW, Tidy JA (2008) Diagnostic challenges in extrauterine epithelioid trophoblastic tumours: a report of two cases. Gynecol Oncol 108:452–454
91. Machtinger R, Gotlieb WH, Korach J, Fridman E, Apter S, Goldenberg M, Ben-Baruch G (2005) Placental site trophoblastic tumor: outcome of five cases including fertility preserving management. Gynecol Oncol 96:56–61
92. Mao TL, Kurman RJ, Huang CC, Lin MC, Shih I-M (2007) Immunohistochemistry of choriocarcinoma: an aid in differential diagnosis and in elucidating pathogenesis. Am J Surg Pathol 31:1726–1732
93. Mao TL, Kurman RJ, Jeng YM, Huang W, Shih I-M (2008) HSD3B1 as a novel trophoblast-associated marker that assists in the differential diagnosis of trophoblastic tumors and tumorlike lesions. Am J Surg Pathol 32:236–242
94. Mao TL, Seidman JD, Kurman RJ, Shih I-M (2006) Cyclin E and p16 immunoreactivity in epithelioid trophoblastic tumor–an aid in differential diagnosis. Am J Surg Pathol 30:1105–1110
95. Matsui H, Iizuka Y, Sekiya S (1996) Incidence of invasive mole and choriocarcinoma following partial hydatidiform mole. Int J Gynaecol Obstet 53:63–64
96. Mazur MT (1989) Metastatic gestational choriocarcinoma. Unusual pathologic variant following therapy. Cancer 63:1370–1377
97. McConnell TG, Murphy KM, Hafez M, Vang R, Ronnett B (2009) Diagnosis and subclassification of hydatidiform moles using p57 immunohistochemistry and molecular genotyping: validation and prospective analysis in routine and consultation practice settings with development of an algorithmic approach. Am J Surg Pathol 33:805–817
98. McConnell TG, Norris-Kirby A, Hagenkord JM, Ronnett BM, Murphy KM (2009) Complete hydatidiform mole with retained maternal chromosomes 6 and 11. Am J Surg Pathol 33:1409–1415
99. Medeiros F, Callahan MJ, Elvin JA, Dorfman DM, Berkowitz RS, Quade BJ (2008) Intraplacental choriocarcinoma arising in a second trimester placenta with partial hydatidiform mole. Int J Gynecol Pathol 27:247–251
100. Menczer J, Girtler O, Zajdel L, Glezerman M (1999) Metastatic trophoblastic disease following partial hydatidiform mole: case report and literature review. Gynecol Oncol 74:304–307
101. Meydanli MM, Kucukali T, Usubutun A, Ataoglu O, Kafkasli A (2002) Epithelioid trophoblastic tumor of the endocervix: a case report. Gynecol Oncol 87:219–224
102. Mi S, Lee X, Li X-P, Veldman GM, Finnerty H, Racie L, LaVallie E, Tang X-Y, Edouard P, Howes S et al (2000) Syncytin is a captive retroviral envelope protein involved in human placental morphogenesis. Nature 403:785–789
103. Milingos D, Doumplis D, Savage P, Seckl M, Lindsay I, Smith JR (2007) Placental site trophoblastic tumor with an ovarian metastasis. Int J Gynecol Cancer 17:925–927
104. Montes M, Roberts D, Berkowitz RS, Genest DR (1996) Prevalence and significance of implantation site trophoblastic atypia in hydatidiform moles and spontaneous abortions. Am J Clin Pathol 105:411–416
105. Moore-Maxwell CA, Robboy SJ (2004) Placental site trophoblastic tumor arising from antecedent molar pregnancy. Gynecol Oncol 92:708–712
106. Morgan JM, Lurain JR (2008) Gestational trophoblastic neoplasia: an update. Curr Oncol Rep 10:497–504
107. Mosher R, Goldstein DP, Berkowitz R, Bernstein M, Genest DR (1998) Complete hydatidiform mole. Comparison of clinicopathologic features, current and past. J Reprod Med 43:21–27
108. Murdoch S, Djuric U, Mazhar B, Seoud M, Khan R, Kuick R, Bagga R, Kircheisen R, Ao A, Ratti B et al (2006) Mutations in NALP7 cause recurrent hydatidiform moles and reproductive wastage in humans. Nat Genet 38:300–302
109. Nagai Y, Kamoi S, Matsuoka T, Hata A, Jobo T, Ogasawara T, Aoki Y, Ohira S, Okamoto T, Nakamoto T et al (2007) Impact of p53 immunostaining in predicting advanced or recurrent placental site trophoblastic tumors: a study of 12 cases. Gynecol Oncol 106:446–452
110. Narita F, Takeuchi K, Hamana S, Ohbayashi C, Ayata M, Maruo T (2003) Epithelioid trophoblastic tumor (ETT) initially interpreted as cervical cancer. Int J Gynecol Cancer 13:551–554
111. Nayar R, Snell J, Silverberg SG, Lage JM (1996) Placental site nodule occurring in a fallopian tube. Hum Pathol 27:1243–1245
112. Newlands ES, Bower M, Fisher RA, Paradinas FJ (1998) Management of placental site trophoblastic tumors. J Reprod Med 43:53–59
113. Newlands ES, Mulholland PJ, Holden L, Seckl MJ, Rustin GJ (2000) Etoposide and cisplatin/etoposide, methotrexate, and actinomycin D (EMA) chemotherapy for patients with high-risk gestational trophoblastic tumors refractory to EMA/cyclophosphamide and vincristine chemotherapy and patients presenting with metastatic placental site trophoblastic tumors. J Clin Oncol 18:854–859
114. Ngan S, Seckl MJ (2007) Gestational trophoblastic neoplasia management: an update. Curr Opin Oncol 19:486–491
115. Niemann I, Hansen ES, Sunde L (2007) The risk of persistent trophoblastic disease after hydatidiform mole classified by morphology and ploidy. Gynecol Oncol 104:411–415
116. Noh HT, Lee KH, Lee MA, Ko YB, Hwang SH, Son SK (2008) Epithelioid trophoblastic tumor of paracervix and parametrium. Int J Gynecol Cancer 18:843–846
117. Nugent D, Hassadia A, Everard J, Hancock BW, Tidy JA (2006) Postpartum choriocarcinoma presentation, management and survival. J Reprod Med 51:819–824
118. Numnum TM, Kilgore LC, Conner MG, Straughn JM Jr (2006) Fertility sparing therapy in a patient with placental site trophoblastic tumor: a case report. Gynecol Oncol 103:1141–1143
119. Ohira S, Yamazaki T, Hatano H, Harada O, Toki T, Konishi I (2000) Epithelioid trophoblastic tumor metastatic to the vagina: an immunohistochemical and ultrastructural study. Int J Gynecol Pathol 19:381–386
120. Oldt RJ 3rd, Kurman RJ, Shih I-M (2002) Molecular genetic analysis of placental site trophoblastic tumors and epithelioid trophoblastic tumors confirms their trophoblastic origin. Am J Pathol 161: 1033–1037
121. Olsen JH, Mellemkjaer L, Gridley G, Brinton L, Johansen C, Kjaer SK (1999) Molar pregnancy and risk for cancer in women and their male partners. Am J Obstet Gynecol 181:630–634
122. Ordi J, Romagosa C, Tavassoli FA, Nogales F, Palacin A, Condom E, Torne A, Cardesa A (2003) CD10 expression in epithelial tissues and tumors of the gynecologic tract: a useful marker in the diagnosis of mesonephric, trophoblastic, and clear cell tumors. Am J Surg Pathol 27:178–186
123. Palmer JR (1994) Advances in the epidemiology of gestational trophoblastic disease. J Reprod Med 39:155–162
124. Palmer JE, Macdonald M, Wells M, Hancock BW, Tidy JA (2008) Epithelioid trophoblastic tumor: a review of the literature. J Reprod Med 53:465–475

125. Papadopoulos AJ, Foskett M, Seckl MJ, McNeish I, Paradinas FJ, Rees H, Newlands ES (2002) Twenty-five years' clinical experience with placental site trophoblastic tumors. J Reprod Med 47:460–464
126. Parker A, Lee V, Dalrymple C, Valmadre S, Russell P (2003) Epithelioid trophoblastic tumour: report of a case in the fallopian tube. Pathology 35:136–140
127. Patten DK, Lindsay I, Fisher R, Sebire N, Savage PM, Seckl MJ (2008) Gestational choriocarcinoma mimicking a uterine adenocarcinoma. J Clin Oncol 26:5126–5127
128. Pfeffer PE, Sebire N, Lindsay I, McIndoe A, Lim A, Seckl MJ (2007) Fertility-sparing partial hysterectomy for placental-site trophoblastic tumour. Lancet Oncol 8:744–746
129. Phippen NT, Lowery WJ, Leath CA 3rd, Kost ER (2010) Epithelioid trophoblastic tumor masquerading as invasive squamous cell carcinoma of the cervix after an ectopic pregnancy. Gynecol Oncol 117:387–388
130. Piura B (2006) Placental site trophoblastic tumor–a challenging rare entity. Eur J Gynaecol Oncol 27:545–551
131. Piura B, Rabinovich A, Meirovitz M, Shaco-Levy R (2007) Placental site trophoblastic tumor: report of four cases and review of literature. Int J Gynecol Cancer 17:258–262
132. Popiolek DA, Yee H, Mittal K, Chiriboga L, Prinz MK, Caragine TA, Budimlija ZM (2006) Multiplex short tandem repeat DNA analysis confirms the accuracy of p57(KIP2) immunostaining in the diagnosis of complete hydatidiform mole. Hum Pathol 37:1426–1434
133. Randall TC, Coukos G, Wheeler JE, Rubin SC (2000) Prolonged remission of recurrent, metastatic placental site trophoblastic tumor after chemotherapy. Gynecol Oncol 76:115–117
134. Redline RW, Hassold T, Zaragoza MV (1998) Prevalence of the partial molar phenotype in triploidy of maternal and paternal origin. Hum Pathol 29:505–511
135. Reid A, Heyworth J, de Klerk N, Musk AW (2009) Asbestos exposure and gestational trophoblastic disease: a hypothesis. Cancer Epidemiol Biomarkers Prev 18:2895–2898
136. Rinne K, Shahabi S, Cole L (1999) Following metastatic placental site trophoblastic tumor with urine b-core fragment. Gynecol Oncol 74:302–303
137. Rodabaugh KJ, Bernstein MR, Goldstein DP, Berkowitz RS (1998) Natural history of postterm choriocarcinoma. J Reprod Med 43:75–80
138. Rotmensch S, Cole LA (2000) False diagnosis and needless therapy of presumed malignant disease in women with false-positive human chorionic gonadotropin concentrations. Lancet 355:712–715
139. Schmid P, Nagai Y, Agarwal R, Hancock B, Savage PM, Sebire NJ, Lindsay I, Wells M, Fisher RA, Short D et al (2009) Prognostic markers and long-term outcome of placental-site trophoblastic tumours: a retrospective observational study. Lancet 374:48–55
140. Seckl MJ, Fisher RA, Salerno G, Rees H, Paradinas FJ, Foskett M, Newlands ES (2000) Choriocarcinoma and partial hydatidiform moles. Lancet 356:36–39
141. Seki K, Matsui H, Sekiya S (2004) Advances in the clinical laboratory detection of gestational trophoblastic disease. Clin Chim Acta 349:1–13
142. Sharkey AM, King A, Clark DE, Burrows TD, Loke YW (1999) Localization of leukemia inhibitory factor and its receptor in human placenta throughout pregnancy. Biol Reprod 60:355–364
143. Shih I-M (1999) The role of CD146 (Mel-CAM) in biology and pathology. J Pathol 189:4–11
144. Shih I-M (2007) Trophogram, an immunohistochemistry-based algorithmic approach, in the differential diagnosis of trophoblastic tumors and tumorlike lesions. Ann Diagn Pathol 11:228–234
145. Shih I-M (2007) Gestational trophoblastic neoplasia—pathogenesis and potential therapeutic targets. Lancet Oncol 8:642–650
146. Shih I-M (2009) Gestational trophoblastic lesions. In: Nucci MR, Oliva E (eds) Gynecologic pathology. Churchill Livingstone Elsevier, London, pp 645–665
147. Shih I-M, Hsu MY, Oldt RJ, Herlyn M, Gearhart JD, Kurman RJ (2002) The role of E-cadherin in the motility and invasion of implantation site intermediate trophoblast. Placenta 23:706–715
148. Shih I-M, Kuo KT (2008) Power of the eternal youth: Nanog expression in the gestational choriocarcinoma. Am J Pathol 173:911–914
149. Shih I-M, Kurman RJ (1996) Expression of melanoma cell adhesion molecule in intermediate trophoblast. Lab Invest 75:377–388
150. Shih I-M, Kurman RJ (1998) Epithelioid trophoblastic tumor: a neoplasm distinct from choriocarcinoma and placental site trophoblastic tumor simulating carcinoma. Am J Surg Pathol 22:1393–1403
151. Shih I-M, Kurman RJ (1998) Ki-67 labeling index in the differential diagnosis of exaggerated placental site, placental site trophoblastic tumor, and choriocarcinoma: a double immunohistochemical staining technique using Ki-67 and Mel-CAM antibodies. Hum Pathol 29:27–33
152. Shih I-M, Kurman RJ (1999) Immunohistochemical localization of inhibin-alpha in the placenta and gestational trophoblastic lesions. Int J Gynecol Pathol 18:144–150
153. Shih I-M, Kurman RJ (2001) The pathology of intermediate trophoblastic tumors and tumor-like lesions. Int J Gynecol Pathol 20:31–47
154. Shih I-M, Kurman RJ (2001) Placental site trophoblastic tumor–past as prologue. Gynecol Oncol 82:413–414
155. Shih I-M, Kurman RJ (2002) Molecular basis of gestational trophoblastic diseases. Curr Mol Med 2:1–12
156. Shih I-M, Kurman RJ (2004) p63 expression is useful in the distinction of epithelioid trophoblastic and placental site trophoblastic tumors by profiling trophoblastic subpopulations. Am J Surg Pathol 28:1177–1183
157. Shih I-M, Schnaar RL, Gearhart JD, Kurman RJ (1997) Distribution of cells bearing the HNK-1 epitope in the human placenta. Placenta 18:667–674
158. Shih I-M, Seidman JD, Kurman RJ (1999) Placental site nodule and characterization of distinctive types of intermediate trophoblast. Hum Pathol 30:687–694
159. Silva EG, Tornos C, Lage J, Ordonez NG, Morris M, Kavanagh J (1993) Multiple nodules of intermediate trophoblast following hydatidiform moles. Int J Gynecol Pathol 12:324–332
160. Singer G, Kurman RJ, McMaster M, Shih I-M (2002) HLA-G immunoreactivity is specific for intermediate trophoblast in gestational trophoblastic disease and can serve as a useful marker in differential diagnosis. Am J Surg Pathol 26(7):914–920
161. Siu MKY, Wong ESY, Chan H-Y, Ngan HYS, Chan KYK, Cheung ANY (2008) Overexpression of Nanog in gestational trophoblastic diseases. Effect on apoptosis, cell invasion and clinical outcome. Am J Pathol 173:1165–1172
162. Slim R, Mehio A (2007) The genetics of hydatidiform moles: new lights on an ancient disease. Clin Genet 71:25–34
163. Soper JT (2006) Gestational trophoblastic disease. Obstet Gynecol 108:176–187
164. Su YN, Cheng WF, Chen CA, Lin TY, Hsieh FJ, Cheng SP, Hsieh CY (1999) Pregnancy with primary tubal placental site trophoblastic

tumor–A case report and literature review. Gynecol Oncol 73:322–325
165. Suzuki T, Goto S, Nawa A, Kurauchi O, Saito M, Tomoda Y (1993) Identification of the pregnancy responsible for gestational trophoblastic disease by DNA analysis. Obstet Gynecol 82:629–634
166. Swisher E, Drescher CW (1998) Metastatic placental site trophoblastic tumor: long-term remission in a patient treated with EMA/CO chemotherapy. Gynecol Oncol 68:62–65
167. Szulman AE, Surti U (1982) The clinicopathologic profile of the partial hydatidiform mole. Obstet Gynecol 59:597–602
168. Tavassoli FA, Devilee P (2003) WHO classification of tumors. In: Pathology and genetics tumors of the breast and female genital organs, IARC Press, Lyon, pp 113–161
169. Trask C, Lage JM, Roberts DJ (1994) A second case of "chorangiocarcinoma" presenting in a term asymptomatic twin pregnancy: choriocarcinoma in situ with associated villous vascular proliferation. Int J Gynecol Pathol 13:87–91
170. Tsai HW, Lin CP, Chou CY, Li CF, Chow NH, Shih I-M, Ho CL (2008) Placental site nodule transformed into a malignant epithelioid trophoblastic tumour with pelvic lymph node and lung metastasis. Histopathology 53:601–604
171. Twiggs LB, Hartenbach E, Saltzman AK, King LA (1998) Metastatic placental site trophoblastic tumor. Int J Gynaecol Obstet 60(Suppl 1):S51–S55
172. Ueda SM, Mao TL, Kuhajda FP, Vasoontara C, Giuntoli RL, Bristow RE, Kurman RJ, Shih Ie M (2009) Trophoblastic neoplasms express fatty acid synthase, which may be a therapeutic target via its inhibitor C93. Am J Pathol 175:2618–2624
173. Urabe S, Fujiwara H, Miyoshi H, Arihiro K, Soma H, Yoshihama I, Mineo S, Kudo Y (2007) Epithelioid trophoblastic tumor of the lung. J Obstet Gynaecol Res 33:397–401
174. Vencken PM, Ewing PC, Zweemer RP (2006) Epithelioid trophoblastic tumour: a case report and review of the literature. J Clin Pathol 59:1307–1308
175. Wells M (2007) The pathology of gestational trophoblastic disease: recent advances. Pathology 39:88–96
176. Xu ML, Yang B, Carcangiu ML, Hui P (2009) Epithelioid trophoblastic tumor: comparative genomic hybridization and diagnostic DNA genotyping. Mod Pathol 22:232–238
177. Xue WC, Guan XY, Ngan HY, Shen DH, Khoo US, Cheung AN (2002) Malignant placental site trophoblastic tumor: a cytogenetic study using comparative genomic hybridization and chromosome in situ hybridization. Cancer 94:2288–2294
178. Yap KL, Hafez MJ, Mao TL, Kurman RJ, Murphy KM, Shih Ie M (2010) Lack of a y-chromosomal complement in the majority of gestational trophoblastic neoplasms. J Oncol 2010:364508
179. Young RH, Kurman RJ, Scully RE (1990) Placental site nodules and plaques. A clinicopathologic analysis of 20 cases. Am J Surg Pathol 14:1001–1009
180. Young RH, Scully RE (1984) Placental-site trophoblastic tumor: current status. Clin Obstet Gynecol 27:248–258
181. Young RH, Scully RE, McCluskey RT (1985) A distinctive glomerular lesion complicating placental site trophoblastic tumor: report of two cases. Hum Pathol 16:35–42
182. Yuan CC, Wang PH, Ng HT (1999) High hCG level is a risk factor for predicting the occurrence of brain and/or liver metastases from gestational choriocarcinoma. Int J Gynaecol Obstet 65:67–69
183. Zalel Y, Dgani R (1997) Gestational trophoblastic disease following the evacuation of partial hydatidiform mole: a review of 66 cases. Eur J Obstet Gynecol Reprod Biol 71:67–71
184. Zanetta G, Maggi R, Colombo M, Bratina G, Mangioni C (1997) Choriocarcinoma coexistent with intrauterine pregnancy: two additional cases and a review of the literature. Int J Gynecol Cancer 7:66–77
185. Zhang H-J, Xue W-C, Siu M, Liao X-Y, Ngan HY-S, Cheung AN-Y (2009) P63 expression in gestational trophoblastic disease: correlation with proliferation and apoptotic dynamics. Int J Gynecol Pathol 28:172–178
186. Zhou Y, Fisher SJ, Janatpour M, Genbacev O, Kdjana E, Wheelock M, Damsky CH (1997) Human cytotrophoblasts adopt a vascular phenotype as they differentiate: a strategy for successful endovascular invasion? J Clin Invest 99:2139–2151

21 Hematologic Neoplasms and Selected Tumor-Like Lesions Involving the Female Reproductive Organs

Judith A. Ferry

From the James Homer Wright Pathology Laboratories of the Massachusetts General Hospital and the Department of Pathology, Harvard Medical School, Boston, MA

R. J. Kurman, L. Hedrick Ellenson, B. M. Ronnett (eds.), *Blaustein's Pathology of the Female Genital Tract (6th ed.)*, DOI 10.1007/978-1-4419-0489-8_21,

A variety of hematologic neoplasms involves the female reproductive organs, including a number of different types of lymphomas and lymphoid leukemias, myeloid sarcomas and myeloid leukemias, and rare histiocytic neoplasms. When the female reproductive organs are affected by one of these disorders in the setting of widespread disease, the diagnosis is usually straightforward, but in the uncommon instance in which the female genital tract is the presenting site of a hematologic neoplasm, diagnosis may be problematic, and special problems in differential diagnosis may arise.

Lymphoid Neoplasms of the Female Reproductive Organs

Lymphoma rarely presents with involvement of the female reproductive organs. When it does, the ovaries are most commonly affected, followed by the uterine cervix, uterine corpus, vagina, vulva, and fallopian tubes. Nearly all cases are non-Hodgkin's lymphoma of B-lineage, with diffuse large B-cell lymphoma being the most common type throughout the female reproductive organs. T-cell lymphoma is very uncommon and the natural killer (NK)-cell lymphoma and Hodgkin's lymphoma are exceptional [21, 40]. Rare cases of lymphoma arising in the setting of HIV infection or iatrogenic immunosuppression [37, 42, 58] and a few cases of women with a family history of hematologic neoplasia have been described [23]. Endemic Burkitt's lymphoma is known to have a tendency to involve the ovaries.

Ovarian Lymphoma

Primary Ovarian Lymphoma

Overall, fewer than 1% of lymphomas present with ovarian involvement [14, 21, 22] and fewer than 1.5% of neoplasms arising in the ovary are lymphomas. However, in countries where Burkitt's lymphoma is endemic, approximately 50% of malignant ovarian neoplasms in childhood are Burkitt's lymphoma [78].

Clinical Features

Patients range in age from 18 months to 74 years [21], with a peak incidence in the thirties or forties [14, 21, 90]. Occasionally lymphoma develops during pregnancy [21, 49]. Rare patients have been HIV+ [42]. The presenting complaints are generally nonspecific symptoms related to the presence of a mass [14, 61, 90]. A minority have fatigue, weight loss, fever, or abnormal vaginal bleeding [14]. Rarely the lymphoma is an incidental finding [90].

Pathologic Features

Ovarian lymphomas range from microscopic [90] to large masses up to 25 cm in diameter with an average size of 11–14 cm [21, 90]. The external surfaces are usually intact and may be smooth or nodular. On sectioning, the tumors may be soft and fleshy or firm and rubbery, depending on the degree of cellularity and associated sclerosis. They are usually white, tan, or gray-pink and a minority has cystic degeneration, hemorrhage or necrosis [21]. Very rare cases of lymphoma in association with, possibly arising from, a teratoma have been described [53].

The most common lymphoma is diffuse large B-cell type, followed by Burkitt's lymphoma and follicular lymphoma [14]. Adolescents and children almost always have diffuse, aggressive lymphomas, including Burkitt's lymphoma, B lymphoblastic lymphoma and diffuse large B-cell lymphoma [40] while adults may have indolent or aggressive lymphomas. Ovarian lymphoma may preferentially spare corpora lutea, corpora albicantia, follicles, and a peripheral rim of cortical tissue but otherwise typically obliterates normal ovarian parenchyma. Lymphoma is rarely associated with hyperplasia and luteinization of the adjacent stroma [21].

Diffuse Large B-Cell Lymphoma

Diffuse large B-cell lymphoma in the ovary, as in other sites is composed of centroblasts, immunoblasts, multilobated cells, or a mixture of these. In the ovary, associated sclerosis is common and tumor cells may grow in cords and nests, simulating carcinoma [78], or be elongate and grow in a storiform pattern, mimicking a sarcoma (➋ *Fig. 21.1a–c*). A few diffuse large B-cell lymphomas have a component of follicular lymphoma [61, 90]. Tumor cells are CD20+, and in the few cases studied, expression of bcl6, CD10, and bcl2 is common [90].

Burkitt's Lymphoma

Ovarian Burkitt's lymphoma is most commonly encountered among children and adolescents [40]. Burkitt's lymphoma is more often bilateral than other ovarian lymphomas [41]. It is hypothesized that Burkitt's lymphoma occurring in pregnancy has a tendency to involve hormonally stimulated organs, such as the ovary [49].

Both sporadic and endemic Burkitt's lymphoma may present with ovarian involvement [13, 43], and ovarian

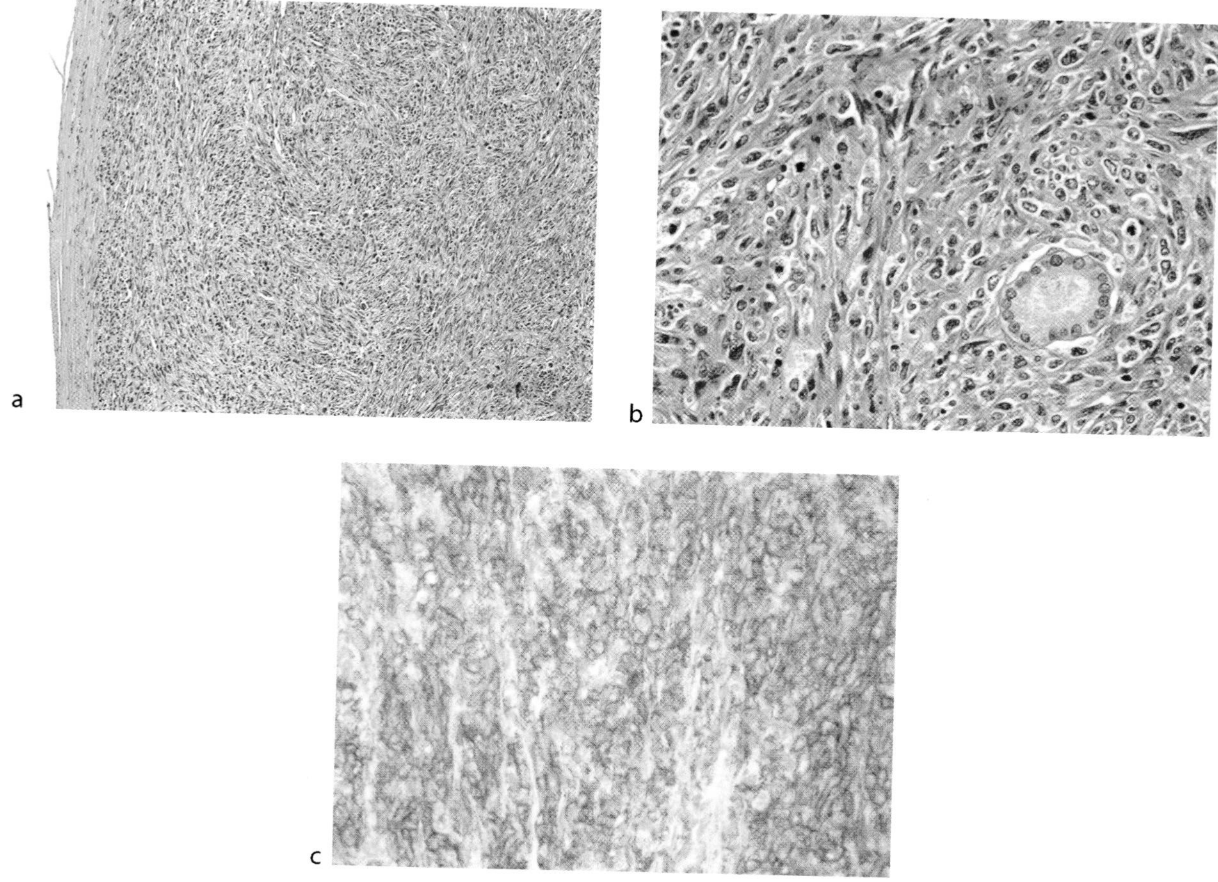

Fig. 21.1

Ovary, diffuse large B-cell lymphoma with spindle neoplastic cells. (a) Low power shows a thin layer of uninvolved tissue at the surface of the ovary. The neoplastic cells grow in a storiform pattern. (b) High power shows atypical cells with elongate, usually blunt-ended nuclei admixed with cells with round or lobated nuclei; there is interstitial sclerosis. The neoplastic proliferation spares a small epithelial inclusion gland. (c) Neoplastic cells are CD20+ confirming B lineage; they also expressed CD45, the leukocyte common antigen (not shown) (immunoperoxidase technique on a paraffin section)

involvement in the setting of immunodeficiency (HIV infection) has been described [42]. The histologic features are the same as those found in other sites. There is a diffuse proliferation of medium-sized, uniform cells with round nuclei containing stippled chromatin and several small nucleoli per cell in each nucleus. A moderate quantity of cytoplasm which is deep blue with Giemsa or Wright stain is present. Mitoses are numerous. Many scattered pale tingible body macrophages in a background of dark neoplastic cells impart a starry sky pattern at low power (*Fig. 21.2a and b*). Occasionally, neoplastic cells are somewhat more pleomorphic, chromatin may be more vesicular, and there is only a single nucleolus within each nucleus. In some cases, designated Burkitt's lymphoma with plasmacytoid differentiation, there is slightly more cytoplasm and tumor cells contain monotypic cytoplasmic immunoglobulin [13, 43]. Children with Burkitt's lymphoma usually have typical morphology, while Burkitt's lymphoma with plasmacytoid differentiation is usually found in the setting of immunodeficiency. As in other sites, the characteristic immunophenotype is monotypic IgM+, CD20+, CD10+, CD5–, bcl6+, bcl2–, Ki67 ~100% +, and the neoplastic cells harbor a translocation involving c-myc [10, 13, 40, 43]. Endemic Burkitt's lymphoma typically

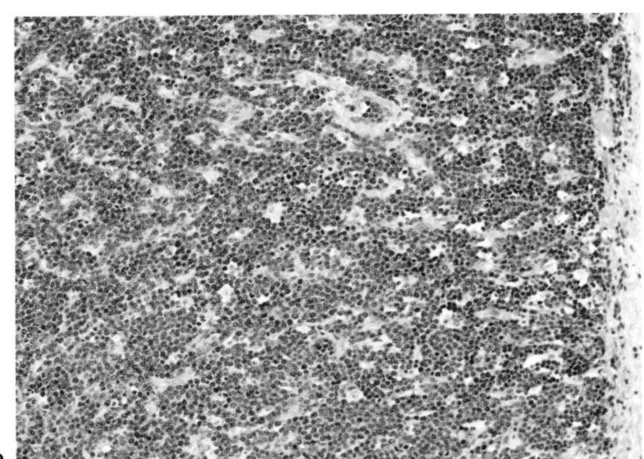

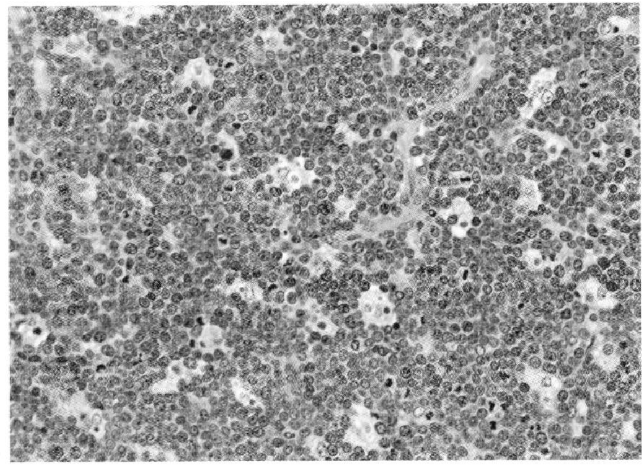

Fig. 21.2
Ovary, Burkitt's lymphoma. **(a) Low power shows scattered pale tingible body macrophages in a background of dark neoplastic cells, creating a "starry sky" pattern. (b) High power shows fairly uniform, medium-sized lymphoid cells with round nuclei, stippled chromatin, and numerous mitoses; the appearance is typical of Burkitt's lymphoma**

contains Epstein-Barr virus (EBV), while a minority of cases of sporadic Burkitt's lymphoma and immunodeficiency-associated Burkitt's lymphoma in HIV+ patients are positive for EBV [13, 43].

Follicular Lymphoma

Ovarian follicular lymphoma mainly affects older patients. They may be entirely follicular or may have conspicuous diffuse areas. They are composed of a variable admixture of centrocytes (small cleaved cells) and centroblasts (large non-cleaved cells). Follicular lymphomas of all three grades (grade 1: 0–5 centroblasts/average high power field (HPF); grade 2: 6–15 centroblasts/average HPF; grade 3: >15 centroblasts/average HPF) occur in the ovary (*Fig. 21.3a–d*) [41, 90].

Rare Lymphomas

Rare cases of CD30+ anaplastic large cell lymphoma of T lineage, and B and T lymphoblastic lymphoma presenting with ovarian involvement have been reported [33, 40, 76, 90]. Morphology, in conjunction with expression of terminal deoxynucleotidyl transferase (TdT) distinguishes precursor B and T-cell neoplasms from mature B and T-cell lymphomas.

Staging, Treatment and Outcome

At laparotomy there is involvement of one or both ovaries with approximately equal frequency. Staging discloses extraovarian spread in most cases, often involving pelvic or paraaortic lymph nodes and occasionally peritoneum, other genital organs, or distant sites [14, 21]. Ovarian lymphoma has traditionally been considered an aggressive tumor with a poor outcome, but improvements in therapy in recent years appear to be associated with a prognosis similar to that of lymph nodal lymphomas of comparable stage and histologic type [14, 51, 90].

Secondary Ovarian Lymphoma

Among patients with disseminated lymphoma and lymphoid leukemias, the ovary is a relatively common site of involvement, although it may be asymptomatic. Seven to twenty five percent of women dying with lymphoma have ovarian involvement [3, 21]. Any type of lymphoma may spread to the ovary, but mediastinal large B-cell lymphoma has a distinct tendency to involve the ovary (*Fig. 21.4a and b*) [12, 79, 97]. Acute lymphoblastic leukemia that relapsed in the ovaries during bone marrow remission has been reported [7, 93]. The ovaries were usually not the only site of relapse; there is frequent involvement of the peritoneum, omentum, fallopian tubes, lymph nodes, and central nervous system [7, 93].

Differential Diagnosis

The differential diagnosis of ovarian lymphoma is broad; it includes dysgerminoma, metastatic carcinoma, and primary small cell carcinoma of hypercalcemic and pulmonary types, adult granulosa cell tumor [61], spindle cell

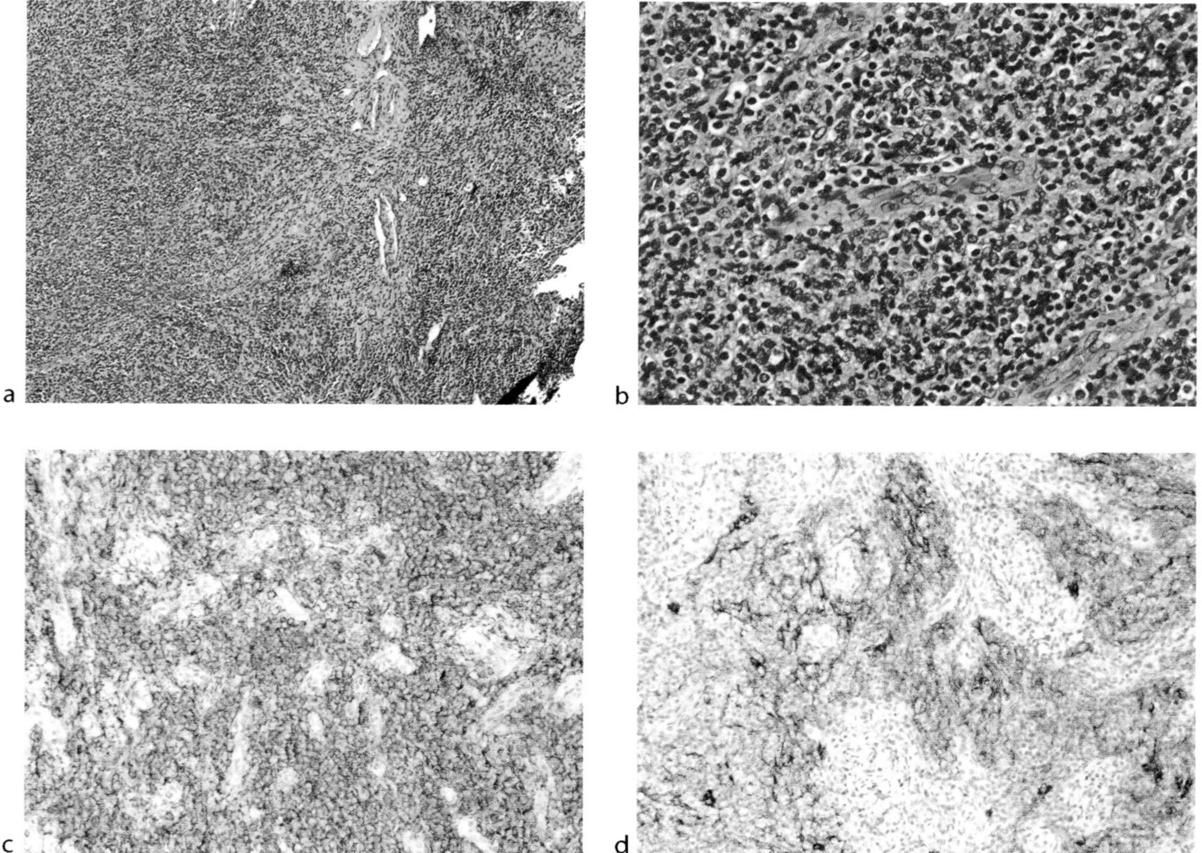

Fig. 21.3
Ovary, follicular lymphoma. **(a) The ovary is replaced by a vaguely nodular-appearing proliferation of atypical lymphoid cells. (b) The atypical cells are mostly small with irregular nuclei; very few large cells are present. (c) The atypical cells are B cells (CD20+); they also expressed the follicle center-associated antigen bcl6 (not shown). (d) CD21 highlights follicular dendritic meshworks; the follicular architecture is more readily appreciated than on routinely stained sections (c, d, immunoperoxidase technique on paraffin sections)**

sarcoma, undifferentiated carcinoma, and myeloid sarcoma [21]. Immunohistochemical studies readily confirm or exclude lymphoma. In contrast to lymphomas in the lower genital tract (see below), the differential diagnosis with inflammatory processes is only rarely problematic.

The main problem in differential diagnosis is distinguishing diffuse large B-cell lymphoma from nonlymphoid neoplasms because large lymphoid cells can have varying morphology and may overlap in size and shape with other types of neoplastic cells. Burkitt's lymphoma is a highly cellular tumor with a characteristic histologic appearance. Recognition of follicular lymphoma is facilitated by its, at least, partially follicular growth pattern. Selected features that aid in differential diagnosis are presented in *Table 21.1.*

Lymphoma of the Fallopian Tube

Primary Lymphoma of the Fallopian Tube

One case of primary tubal marginal zone B-cell lymphoma associated with salpingitis [63], one possible case of primary tubal follicular lymphoma (*Fig. 21.5a and b*), [20] and a bilateral primary tubal peripheral T-cell lymphoma [24] have been described.

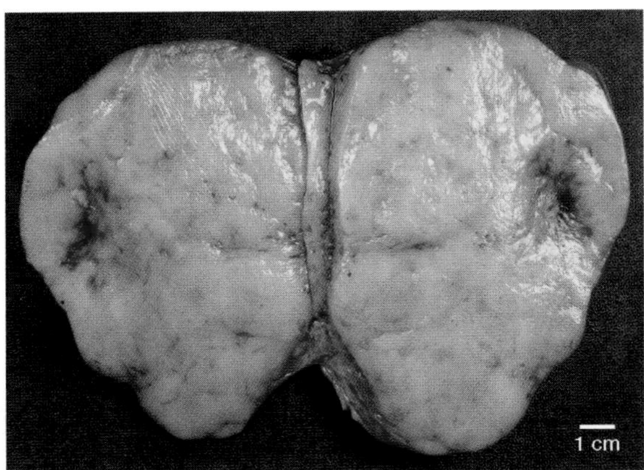

a

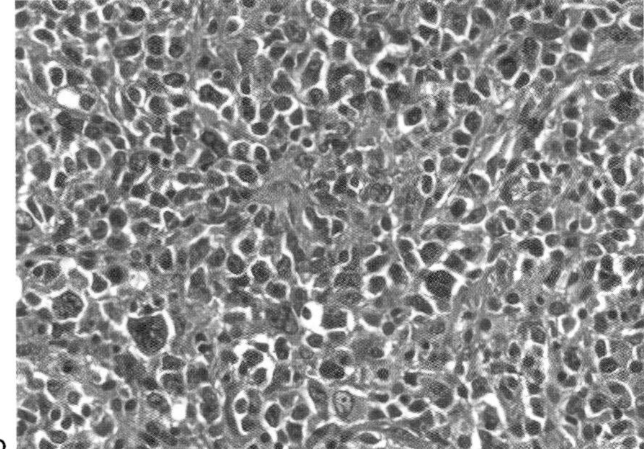

b

Fig. 21.4

Ovarian involvement by mediastinal large B-cell lymphoma. **(a)** Gross examination of the bisected ovarian tumor shows fleshy white tissue. **(b)** High power shows discohesive neoplastic cells with round or irregular nuclei and scant cytoplasm. A few cells are multilobated and rare cells are multinucleated

Table 21.1

Differential diagnosis of ovarian diffuse large B-cell lymphoma

Non-lymphoid tumor	Problem	Differential features	Usual immunophenotype of non-lymphoid tumor
Dysgerminoma	DLBCL composed of IBs: IBs have size, shape and prominent nucleoli, similar to cells of dysgerminoma	Dysgerminoma: Sheets and nests of tumor cells, fibrous trabeculae with lymphocytes, and histiocytes; nuclei flattened along one side, fine chromatin, abundant clear PAS+ cytoplasm, distinct cell borders: not seen in DLBCL	PLAP+, Oct4+, CD117+, CD45–, CD20–
Carcinoma	DLBCL with sclerosis can have cord-like or nested pattern resembling carcinoma	Cohesive growth, nuclear molding, lumen formation, mucin production favor carcinoma; follicles favor small cell carcinoma, hypercalcemic variant	Cytokeratin+, CD45–, CD20–
Spindle cell sarcoma	DLBCL with sclerosis can have spindle cell morphology	Sarcoma lacks admixed CBs and IBs; tumor cells usually more elongate	Mesenchymal markers (varied)+, CD45–, CD20–
Adult granulosa cell tumor	CBs and IBs have large pale vesicular nucleoli that could mimic cells of AGCT; AGCT can have a diffuse pattern, like DLBCL	Trabecular, insular, micro- or macrofollicular pattern, Call-Exner bodies, more pale, evenly dispersed chromatin, and nuclear grooves favor AGCT	Inhibin+, calretinin+, CD45–, CD20–
Myeloid sarcoma	Large lymphoid cells and primitive myeloid cells overlap morphologically; their patterns of growth are similar	Myeloblasts are slightly smaller than large lymphoid cells; they have more finely dispersed chromatin and usually smaller nucleoli. Some cells may have pink cytoplasm, suggesting myeloid differentiation. Bone marrow exam may show myeloid leukemia. Eosinophilic myelocytes may be present	Lysozyme+, MPO+/–, CD68+/–, CD34+/–, CD117+

DLBCL, diffuse large B-cell lymphoma; *IB*, immunoblast; *CB*, centroblast; *AGCT*, adult granulosa cell tumor; *MPO*, myeloperoxidase.

Secondary Tubal Involvement by Lymphoma

Tubal involvement is relatively common among patients with lymphoma of the ovaries [61]. Most are diffuse large B-cell lymphoma or Burkitt's lymphoma [86]; follicular lymphoma, peripheral T-cell lymphoma and lymphoblastic lymphoma/leukemia have also been reported [7, 61, 67, 86]. Tubal infiltration is also seen at autopsy in cases of disseminated lymphoma [30].

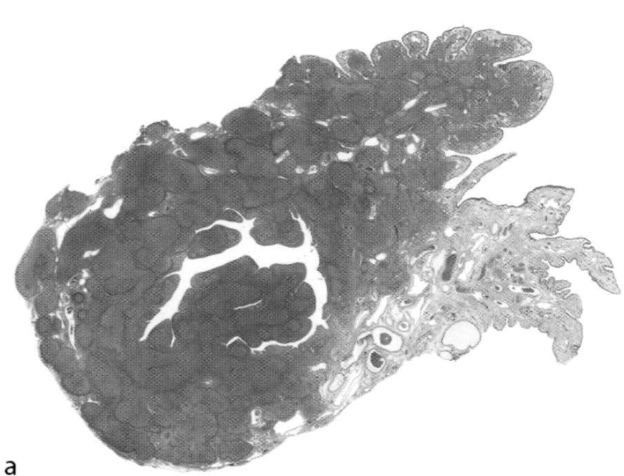

a

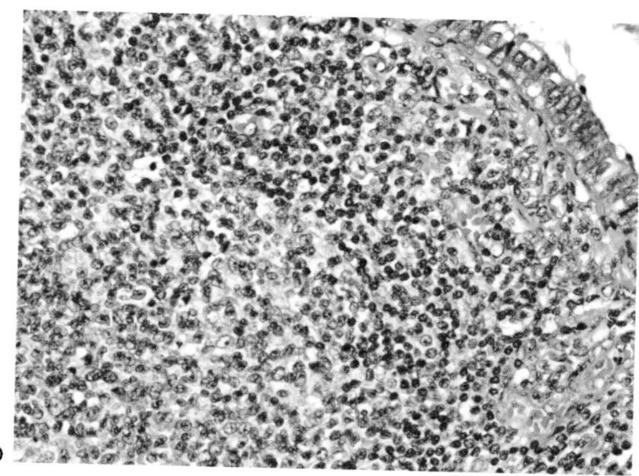

b

Fig. 21.5
Fallopian tube, follicular lymphoma. **(a)** Whole mount section shows tube with transmural involvement by crowded lymphoid follicles. **(b)** High power shows a portion of one of the neoplastic follicles; it is composed of small cleaved cells (centrocytes) with few admixed large non-cleaved cells (centroblasts). Small lymphocytes are present at the periphery of the follicle

Uterine Lymphoma

Primary Uterine Lymphoma

Less than 1% of extranodal lymphomas arise in this site [22]. Lymphoma arises more often in the cervix than in the corpus, with a 10:1 ratio in one series [87], although other series have not shown such a striking excess of cervical lymphomas [40].

Clinical Features

Uterine lymphoma affects adults over a broad age range [28], with a mean and a median age in the fifth decade [17, 23, 28, 50, 71]. The most common presenting symptom is abnormal vaginal bleeding [1, 8, 9, 11, 21, 23, 28, 50, 86]. Less common complaints are dyspareunia, perineal, pelvic, or abdominal pain. A few patients have systemic symptoms such as fever or weight loss [17, 21, 71]. Because lymphomas are typically not associated with ulceration, uterine lymphoma is only occasionally detected on a Papanicolaou smear.

Pathologic Features

Cervical lymphomas typically produce bulky lesions identifiable on pelvic examination. The classic appearance is diffuse, circumferential enlargement of the cervix ("barrel-shaped" cervix) (Fig. 21.6). The lymphoma may also form a discrete submucosal tumor [8, 28], a polypoid or multinodular lesion [9, 25, 28], or a fungating, exophytic mass; ulceration is unusual [28]. The tumors have been variously described as fleshy, rubbery, or firm, and white-tan to yellow [28]. Extensive local spread to sites such as vagina, parametria, or even pelvic side walls is common [9, 11, 23, 28] and invasion into the urinary bladder is described [38]. Patients commonly exhibit hydronephrosis secondary to ureteral obstruction [11, 21, 28]. Lymphomas of the uterine corpus are usually fleshy or soft, pale gray, yellow, or cream-colored. They may form a polypoid mass or diffusely infiltrate the endometrium, sometimes with deep invasion of the myometrium [21, 28].

The microscopic appearance of the lymphomas is similar to that of the same types of lymphoma seen in nodal and other extranodal sites. In the cervix, there is often a band of uninvolved normal tissue just beneath the surface epithelium, and the overlying epithelium is usually intact. In a large biopsy or hysterectomy specimen, deep invasion of the cervical wall is usually seen. In small biopsies, squeeze artifact is often prominent.

Diffuse Large B-Cell Lymphoma

Diffuse large B-cell lymphoma is the most common type of primary uterine lymphoma by far, in both the corpus and the cervix [1, 9, 23, 25, 38, 86, 87], accounting for about 70% of cases [17, 86]. Neoplastic cells may be centroblasts, immunoblasts, or multilobated large lymphoid cells, or a combination of these. Cervical lymphomas are frequently associated with prominent sclerosis [25, 41, 86], which may be associated with a cord-like arrangement or spindle-shaped tumor cells [28]. The spindle cell pattern may be sufficiently prominent to mimic a sarcoma resulting in usage of the terms "spindle cell variant" [5] and "sarcomatoid variant" [35]. Rare examples of intravascular large B-cell lymphoma presenting with involvement of the uterus and adnexa have been described [81, 94]. Microscopic examination revealed large atypical lymphoid cells filling the lumens of blood vessels (➲ *Fig. 21.7a and b*). One case had the unusual feature of CD5 co-expression by the large atypical CD20+, CD79a+ B cells; neoplastic cells were also positive for EBV [94].

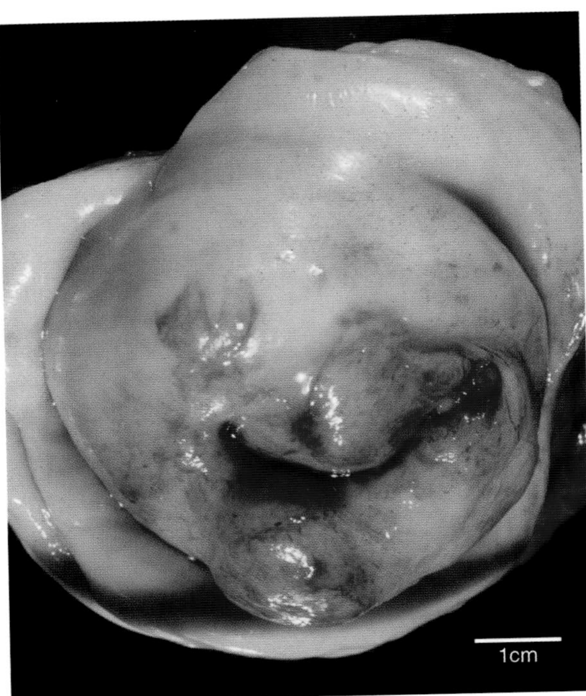

Fig. 21.6
Uterine cervix, lymphoma. **Gross examination shows circumferential expansion of the cervix, so-called barrel-shaped cervix**

Follicular Lymphoma

Follicular lymphoma is the second most common type of uterine lymphoma; follicular lymphomas of all three grades have been reported [40]. These are also often associated with sclerosis. Neoplastic follicles are often found in a perivascular location as they invade into the wall of the cervix (➲ *Fig. 21.8a–f*) [28].

Extranodal Marginal Zone Lymphoma (MALT Lymphoma)

A few cases of marginal zone B cell lymphoma arising in the endometrium or in the cervix have been described [21, 23, 40, 84, 86, 87].

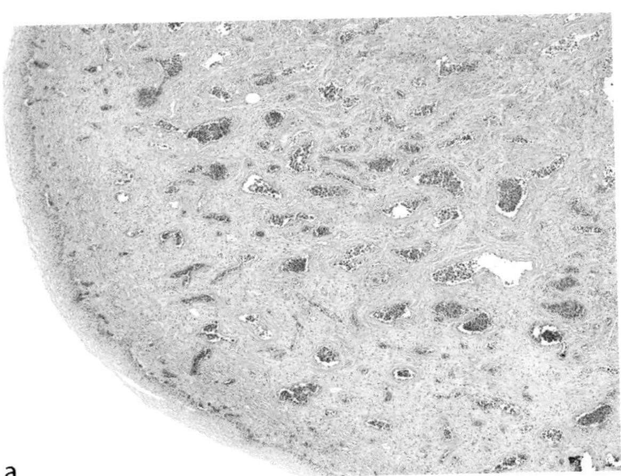

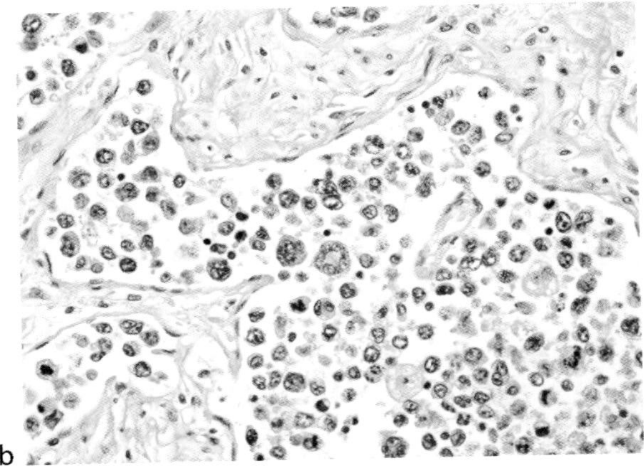

Fig. 21.7
Uterine cervix, intravascular large B-cell lymphoma. **(a) The exocervix has multiple blood vessels containing neoplastic cells. (b) High power shows a dilated blood vessel filled by large, atypical, pleomorphic lymphoid cells. The neoplastic cells were CD20+ and CD3− (not shown), consistent with B-lineage**

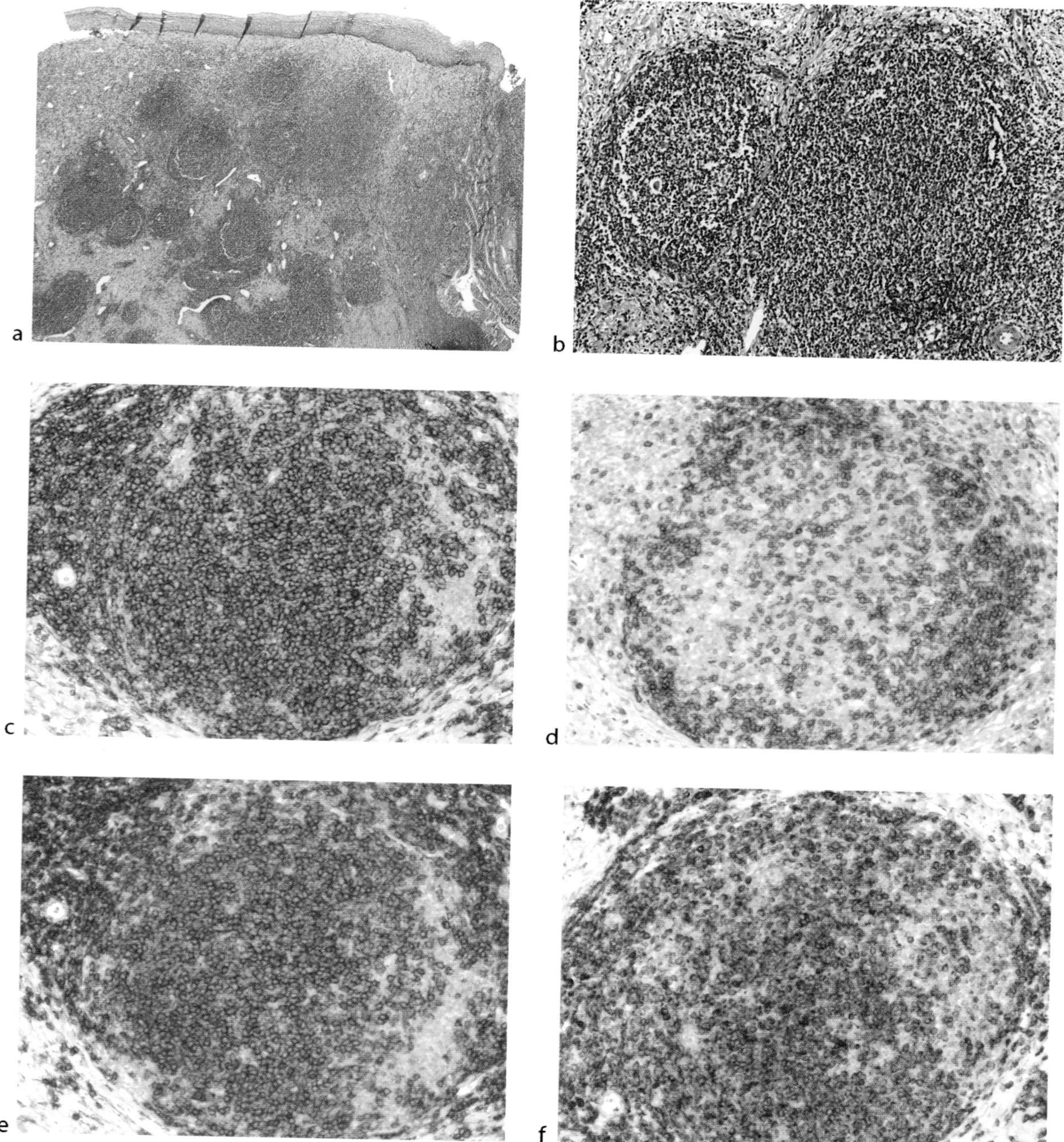

Fig. 21.8
Uterine cervix, follicular lymphoma. (**a**) Low power shows atypical lymphoid follicles invading deep into the wall of the cervix. The surface epithelium is intact and uninvolved by the lymphoid infiltrate. (**b**) Higher power shows crowded, ill-defined follicles composed of a monotonous population of small atypical lymphoid cells. Immunostains show follicles composed of B cells (**c**, CD20+) surrounded by T cells (**d**, CD3+). B cells co-express the follicle center-associated marker CD10 (**e**) as well as bcl2 (**f**); these immunohistochemical results confirm a diagnosis of follicular lymphoma (c–f, immunoperoxidase technique on paraffin sections)

In 1997 three cases of a distinctive type of low-grade endometrial B-cell lymphoma was described [84]. All affected women were in their sixties and the lymphomas were all incidental findings and confined to the uterus. On microscopic examination all were composed of large nodules with a monotonous population of small lymphoid cells with slightly irregular nuclei and scant cytoplasm adjacent to and sometimes surrounding endometrial glands. Immunohistochemical analysis showed B cells with aberrant co-expression of CD43. The immunoglobulin heavy chain genes were clonally rearranged. Follow-up, when available, was uneventful. The authors were reluctant to subclassify these lymphomas as marginal zone type because of lack of certain features that would support that diagnosis including absence of conspicuous lymphoepithelial lesions, lack of a marginal zone pattern, and lack of reactive follicle centers. In addition, only limited immunophenotyping could be performed. Subsequently, a case with identical histologic features was reported in which neoplastic cells were CD20+, bcl2+, without expression of CD5, bcl6, or cyclin D1. The cellular nodules were associated with altered CD21+ follicular dendritic cell meshworks [33]. This case was interpreted as an endometrial marginal zone lymphoma. These cases are best classified as endometrial marginal zone lymphomas, albeit with distinctive clinical and pathologic features (Fig. 21.9a–c).

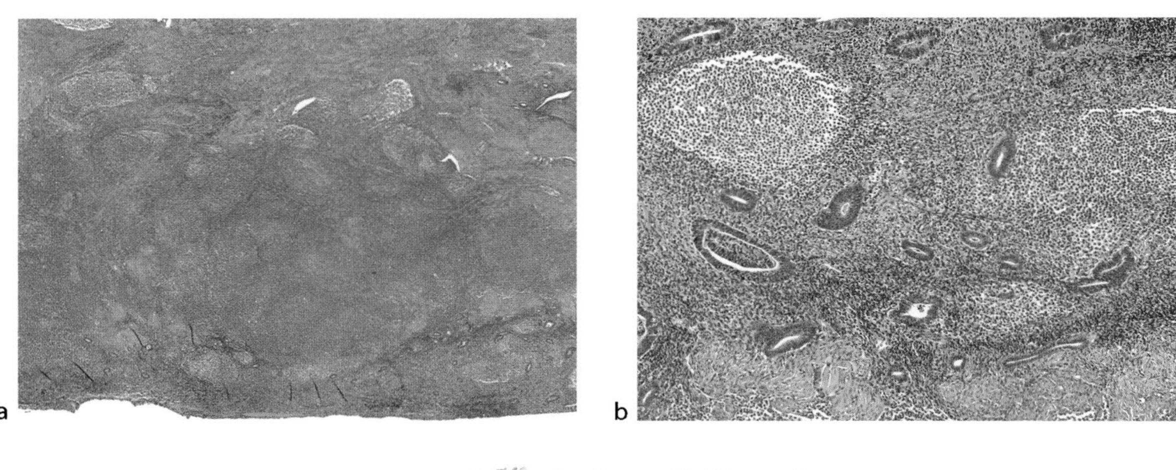

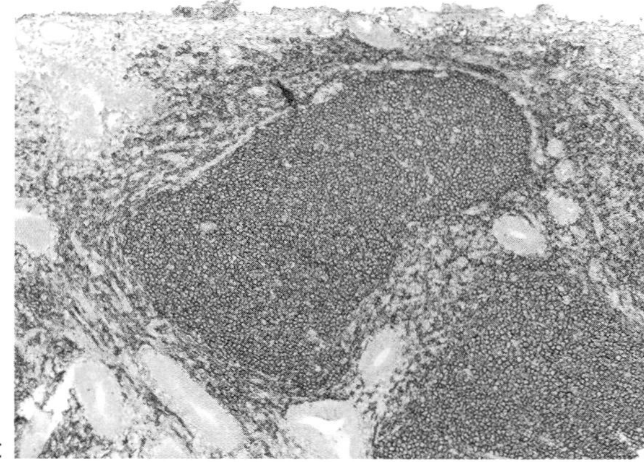

Fig. 21.9
Endometrium, marginal zone lymphoma. **(a) Crowded nodules of small lymphoid cells extensively replace the endometrium and extend superficially into the myometrium. (b) Nodules of small, bland lymphoid cells scattered among endometrial glands. (c) Lymphoid cells are predominantly B cells (CD20+). B cells co-expressed CD43 and were associated with CD21+ follicular dendritic meshworks (not shown) crowded nodules of small lymphoid cells (immunoperoxidase technique on a paraffin section)**

Rare Lymphomas

A few cases of Burkitt's lymphoma [40, 64] and rare cases of B lymphoblastic lymphoma [40], peripheral T cell lymphoma [39], and cervical extranodal NK/T-cell lymphoma [86] have been reported. The uterus is rarely the site of involvement by B-cell post-transplantation lymphoproliferative disorder [58]. Although Hodgkin's lymphoma in the female genital organs is vanishingly rare, a case of classical Hodgkin's lymphoma, lymphocyte depletion type, confirmed with immunophenotyping showing CD15 and CD30 expression by the neoplastic cells, has been reported [40].

Staging, Treatment, and Outcome

Although most uterine lymphomas are large at the time of diagnosis (the primary endometrial marginal zone lymphomas are an exception), the majority are localized (Ann Arbor stage I or stage II), with stage I more frequent than stage II [8, 87]. The type of therapy has varied. In a few cases, young women have been successfully treated using combination chemotherapy and some have preserved fertility [21, 25]. Uterine lymphoma has a relatively good prognosis [9, 21, 59, 86]. Between 70% and 90% of patients are alive and free of disease at last follow-up [8, 17]. Most prognostic information on uterine lymphoma is related to lymphoma arising in the cervix. The 5-year survival for cervical lymphoma is estimated to be approximately 80% [50, 87]. There is not enough information to draw definite conclusions about the prognosis of the rare endometrial lymphomas. However, those with localized disease tend to do well, including, in particular, the endometrial marginal zone lymphomas [23, 84]. Those with advanced disease presenting with endometrial involvement have a worse prognosis [28].

Secondary Uterine Lymphoma

Secondary involvement of the uterus in cases of disseminated lymphoma or lymphoid leukemia is not unusual; it may be asymptomatic or accompanied by vaginal bleeding or discharge [21, 40, 86]. In contrast to primary uterine lymphoma, in which the cervix is much more often involved than the corpus, when the uterus is secondarily involved, the corpus is involved at least as often as the cervix. Lymphomas secondarily involving the uterus are also of more varied types than in primary cases, with less of a predominance of diffuse large B-cell lymphoma. They include diffuse large B-cell lymphoma, follicular lymphoma, chronic lymphocytic leukemia, lymphoblastic lymphoma [21, 40, 86], T lymphoblastic leukemia [46] and extranodal NK/T-cell lymphoma [57]. The prognosis is much less favorable than that of primary uterine lymphoma [57, 87].

Uterine involvement is relatively common in patients dying with lymphoid leukemias. In one autopsy study, 25% of patients with acute lymphoblastic leukemia and 14% with chronic lymphocytic leukemia had involvement of the uterus [3].

Placental Involvement by Lymphoid Neoplasms

Approximately 0.1% of women have a malignancy during pregnancy, subsets of which are lymphomas or leukemias. Rarely, lymphoma or leukemia may be detected in the placenta of these patients [6, 34, 52, 54, 62]. Some of the women have been treated successfully, while others have succumbed to their disease. In most instances placental involvement does not lead to spread of the neoplasm to the fetus, although rarely this does occur [6, 52], sometimes with fatal consequences for the newborn [6].

On gross examination, white nodules or white granular areas or infarcts may be present [54, 62]. On microscopic examination, there is a variably dense infiltrate of neoplastic cells in the intervillous space (maternal circulation). In very rare cases, neoplastic cells are also found within the chorionic villi, involving blood vessels (fetal circulation) [6, 52] or the cord blood [85]; involvement of fetal circulation has rarely been associated with spread of the malignancy to the fetus, resulting in death within a few months of delivery [6]. This underscores the importance of careful gross and microscopic examination of the placenta in the setting of maternal malignancy.

The lymphomas and lymphoid leukemias have been of a variety of types, sometimes classified with older nomenclature [34]. Aggressive lymphomas of B and T lineage have been documented to involve the placenta [54]. Rare cases of mediastinal large B-cell lymphoma [62], anaplastic large cell lymphoma (ALK-positive) [54], and Epstein–Barr virus-positive aggressive NK-cell leukemia/lymphoma involving the placenta have been described [6]. An example of B-lymphoblastic leukemia, in which neoplastic cells were detected in cord blood, has been reported [85].

Vaginal Lymphoma

Primary Vaginal Lymphoma

Clinical Features

Lymphoma rarely arises in the vagina [21, 71, 89]. As in other parts of the female reproductive organs, primary vaginal lymphoma affects patients over a broad age range; their mean age is in the forties. Patients present with vaginal bleeding, discharge, pain, dyspareunia or urinary frequency. Some note a mass. The lesion may compress the urethra and cause anuria [95] or bladder distension [89]. The tumors typically result in ill-defined thickening or induration of the vaginal wall, often with invasion of adjacent structures such as the cervix and the rectovaginal septum [89]. As in the uterine cervix, surface epithelium is usually intact, so that Papanicolaou smears are generally negative [72].

Pathologic Features

The pathologic features are similar to those of cervical lymphoma. Nearly all of the lymphomas are diffuse large B-cell type [21, 40, 89]. Rare cases of follicular lymphoma [11, 28, 40], Burkitt's lymphoma, lymphoplasmacytic lymphoma [40], T-cell lymphoma [21, 72], and marginal zone lymphoma [95] have been reported. As in the cervix, vaginal diffuse large B-cell lymphomas are often associated with marked sclerosis and may be "sarcomatoid." Only a few of these cases have been studied in detail, but they have been CD20+, CD5–, CD10–, bcl6+, MUM1–, CD138–, Epstein–Barr virus (EBV)–, HHV-8–, with somatic mutation of both immunoglobulin and bcl6 genes. These features suggest that the so-called spindle cell variant of diffuse large B-cell lymphoma corresponds to an early germinal center stage of B cell maturation [5]. Rare primary vaginal lymphomas positive for EBV have been reported [15].

Staging, Treatment, and Outcome

Primary vaginal lymphoma typically presents with localized disease (Ann Arbor stage IE or IIE). Treatment has not been uniform, but vaginal lymphoma appears to have a favorable prognosis [11, 15, 71, 72, 89, 95]. In one series of eight cases of diffuse large B-cell lymphoma, for example, only one patient died of lymphoma [89].

Secondary Vaginal Lymphoma

Secondary involvement of the vagina by malignant lymphoma, including relapse of lymphoma in the vagina and involvement of the vagina in the setting of widespread disease, is more common than primary vaginal lymphoma [21]. The prognosis is much less favorable than for primary disease [72, 89].

Vulvar Lymphoma

Primary Vulvar Lymphoma

Primary vulvar lymphoma is exceedingly rare. Patients are adults who present with a nodule, swelling, or induration of the vulva [21, 88]. In rare cases the lymphoma has presented as a mass in the region of Bartholin's gland [82], or as a clitoral mass [40]. Patients appear to be, on average, older than patients with lymphoma arising in other parts of the reproductive tract [40]. A few patients have been HIV+ or iatrogenically immunosuppressed [21, 36, 37, 88]. Diffuse large B-cell lymphoma is the most common type [21, 48, 82, 88]. Other types are rare. Several cases of lymphoplasmacytic lymphoma have been reported [40] and a case of T-cell post-transplantation lymphoproliferative disorder has been described [37]. Vulvar lymphoma is, overall, relatively aggressive, but occasional patients have long disease-free survival.

Secondary Vulvar Lymphoma

Secondary involvement of the vulva by lymphoma at relapse or in the setting of widespread disease is rare. The lymphomas have been of various types [40]. Mycosis fungoides may involve the vulva but, typically, skin elsewhere is also involved [86].

Nonneoplastic Lymphoid Proliferations

Two entities, so-called lymphoma-like lesion and leiomyoma with lymphoid infiltration, stand out as distinctive nonneoplastic lymphoid proliferations that because of their typically extensive, tumor-like nature may mimic lymphoma.

Lymphoma-Like Lesions

In a small proportion of cases of inflammation of the lower reproductive tract, the lymphoid component is dense and extensive and contains numerous large lymphoid cells, potentially raising the question of malignant lymphoma. The cervix, and less often the endometrium and the vulva can be involved by these "lymphoma-like lesions" [27, 47, 96]. Lymphoma-like lesions almost always occur in women of reproductive age, and may be associated with abnormal vaginal bleeding. They are superficially located, and are often associated with erosion or ulceration of the overlying epithelium. In the cervix, they typically extend no more than 3 mm into the wall, and only rarely extend beyond the deepest endocervical glands. Large masses are very uncommon. The lesions are composed of a polymorphous cellular infiltrate composed of small and large lymphoid cells including immunoblasts, often with admixed plasma cells, and neutrophils. Lymphoma-like lesions involving the cervix or endometrium, typically, are found in a background of usual-appearing chronic cervicitis or endometritis, respectively. Large cells (CD20+ B cells) may form aggregates, which may represent follicle centers. Sclerosis is absent (*Fig. 21.10*). When follicle centers are present, they are CD20+, CD10+, bcl6+, and bcl2–, consistent with reactive follicles. Plasma cells are polytypic (mixture of κ+ and λ+). A few cases have occurred in the setting of Epstein-Barr virus infection or pelvic inflammatory disease [27, 47, 96]. In contrast, lymphoma of the lower reproductive tract usually produces a gross abnormality of the involved organ often with extension of the process into adjacent structures. On microscopic examination, lymphomas are composed of a monomorphous population of lymphoid cells (often with sclerosis), tend to invade deeply, sparing a narrow subepithelial zone, and often spread in proximity to blood vessels [96]. In some cases it may be difficult to distinguish between lymphoma-like lesions and lymphoma. In such cases rebiopsy may be helpful, as lymphoma-like lesions may resolve spontaneously.

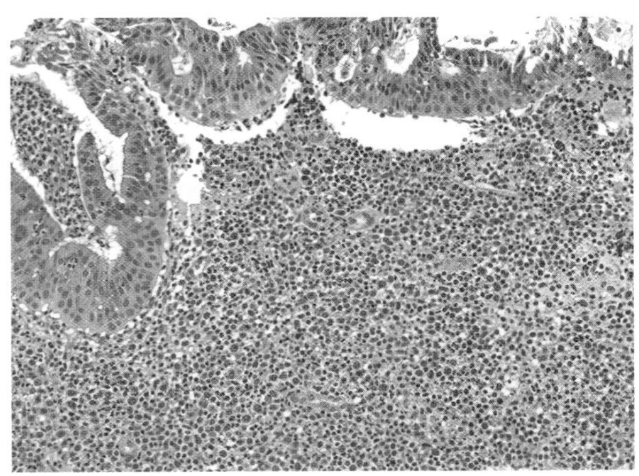

Fig. 21.10
Uterine cervix, lymphoma-like lesion. **The infiltrate involves the surface epithelium and is composed of loose aggregates of large cells with admixed small lymphocytes, plasma cells, and neutrophils. The large cells were mostly CD20+ B cells; small cells were mostly CD3+ T cells (not shown)**

Leiomyoma with Lymphoid Infiltration

Uterine leiomyoma with lymphoid infiltration is a rare lesion that has been described in women between 25 and 53 years of age. On gross examination, the myomas range from 2 to 12 cm in diameter; they may be grossly typical [75], while others are described as soft (*Fig. 21.11a*)

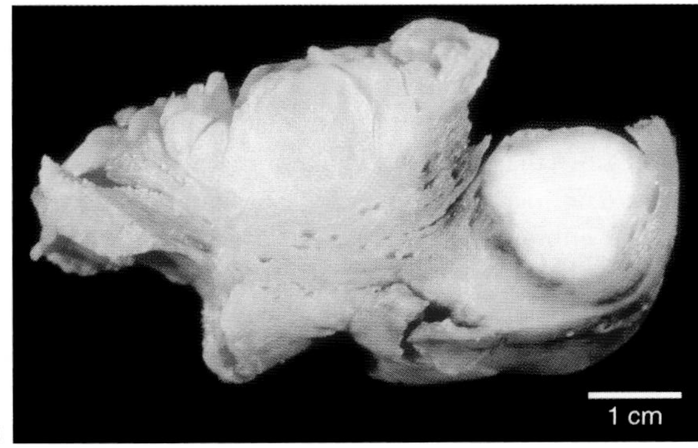

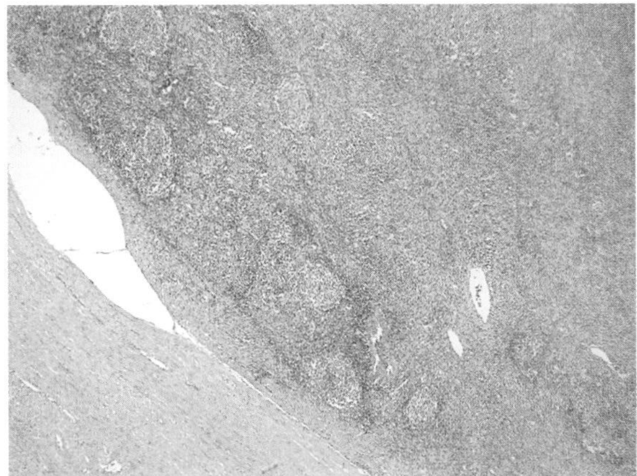

Fig. 21.11
Leiomyoma with lymphoid infiltrate. **(a) Gross examination of a cross section of the uterus shows one small, white, discrete typical leiomyoma (*right*) and one yellow-tan leiomyoma with lymphoid infiltration (*left*). (b) The leiomyoma is extensively involved by a lymphoid infiltrate; the adjacent myometrium is uninvolved. The infiltrate contains multiple lymphoid follicles, mainly near the periphery of the leiomyoma**

[65, 69]. On microscopic examination a moderate or marked infiltrate of small lymphocytes with scattered larger lymphoid cells, histiocytes, variable numbers of plasma cells and rarely eosinophils, is present. In some cases, reactive follicles may be observed. The infiltrate does not contain neutrophils [19, 65, 69, 75] and is typically confined to the leiomyoma (➲ *Fig. 21.11b*), but occasionally extends for a short distance into the adjacent myometrium [19, 75]. Immunohistochemical analysis has shown B cells (CD20+, CD79a+) in follicles and T cells (CD3+, CD45RO+) outside follicles. In several cases, there is a predominance of CD8+ or TIA-1+ T cells, consistent with a cytotoxic phenotype [69, 75]. In a single case, molecular analysis revealed clonal rearrangement of the T-cell receptor gamma chain gene [75]; the significance of this is uncertain as the patient was well with no evidence of lymphoma 3 years later. Occasionally, clonal B or T-cell populations may be found in inflammatory processes, and they are not necessarily indicative of lymphoma.

The etiology of this reactive process is not known, but several patients have had an intrauterine contraceptive device that could have played a role in initiating a chronic inflammatory process [19]. One patient had clinical features suggesting an underlying autoimmune disease [75]. Several patients had been treated with gonadotropin-releasing hormone (GnRH) agonists [75]. Prominent vascular damage within the leiomyomas in addition to lymphoid infiltration has been described in association with luteinizing hormone-releasing hormone therapy [65]. It is possible that the degenerative changes associated with such therapy may elicit an inflammatory response within leiomyomas [65, 69].

In all cases of leiomyoma with lymphoid infiltration follow-up, when reported, has been uneventful [19, 75]. One of the patients in the original series [19] had a large lipoma excised several months after the diagnosis of leiomyoma with lymphoid infiltration; the lipoma had multiple lymphoid aggregates. This patient was well with no evidence of lymphoma 8 years later (unpublished data).

The differential diagnosis of leiomyoma with lymphoid infiltration includes uterine lymphoma, but the polymorphous nature of the infiltrate and its confinement to the leiomyoma help to distinguish it from lymphoma. Inflammatory pseudotumor produces a mass lesion within the uterus, but it is composed of fibroblasts and myofibroblasts, rather than smooth muscle cells, and has an infiltrate that includes neutrophils. Pyomyomas are leiomyomas with marked neutrophilic infiltrate with suppurative necrosis and should not be confused with leiomyoma with lymphoid infiltration.

Differential Diagnosis of Lymphoma of the Lower Reproductive Tract

The differential diagnosis of lymphoma of the lower reproductive tract includes chronic inflammatory processes, carcinoma, sarcomas, and others. Lymphomas, particularly lymphomas with sclerosis, are prone to artifactual distortion by crush artifact, compounding the difficulty in reaching the correct diagnosis. Like many cervical lymphomas, idiopathic retroperitoneal fibrosis is a sclerosing process that may result in ureteral obstruction; the presence of many B cells outside follicles and atypical lymphoid cells favor lymphoma, but recognizing atypical lymphoid cells may be difficult if crush artifact is extensive. Features useful in differential diagnosis of selected entities are presented in ➲ *Table 21.2*.

Myeloid Neoplasms of the Female Reproductive Organs

The female reproductive organs are rarely involved by myeloid sarcoma, a mass-forming lesion composed of primitive myeloid elements. Myeloid sarcoma was initially described with the name of chloroma, because there was sometimes a sufficiently high myeloperoxidase content to impart a green color to the neoplasm. Subsequently, the term granulocytic sarcoma was put forward, to encompass those tumors that lacked a green color [74]. The WHO Classification uses the term myeloid sarcoma for tumor masses composed of myeloblasts or immature myeloid cells, present in extramedullary sites and in bone. The designation monoblastic sarcoma is used for the uncommon myeloid sarcomas composed of monoblasts [4].

Clinical Features

Myeloid sarcomas involve the reproductive organs in patients from early childhood to advanced age, with a median age of approximately 40 years [26]. It occurs in three settings: (1) known acute myelogenous leukemia; (2) chronic myeloproliferative diseases or related disorders; and (3) with no other evidence of hematopoietic disease [60]. Nearly half of the patients have a prior history of a myeloid neoplasm, which is usually acute myeloid leukemia, but which has occasionally been a chronic myeloproliferative disease or a myelodysplastic syndrome/myeloproliferative disorder; these cases thus represent relapse or progression of the patients' prior myeloid neoplasms. Myeloid sarcoma in a patient with a chronic

Table 21.2

Differential diagnosis of lower female genital tract lymphoma

Diagnosis	Features against lymphoma	Features supporting lymphoma
Lymphoma-like lesion	Absence of mass	Mass present
	Superficial location	Deep extension
	Erosion	Subepithelial sparing, no erosion
	Mixed infiltrate	Monomorphous infiltrate
	Absence of sclerosis	Presence of sclerosis
	Evidence of PID or EBV infection	
Carcinoma, especially small cell carcinoma and lymphoepithelial cell carcinoma	Cohesive growth, nuclear molding in best preserved areas	Discohesive tumor cells
	Obliteration of normal structures, e.g., endometrial or endocervical glands	Tumor cells: CBs, IBs, or multilobated cells
	Presence of SCIS or ACIS	Sparing of normal structures
	Cytokeratin+ atypical cells	No SCIS or ACIS
		CD45+, CD20+ neoplastic cells (for B-cell lymphoma)
Spindle cell sarcoma	Absence of admixed CBs, IBs, multilobated cells	CBs, IBs, or multilobated cells admixed with spindle cells
	CD45–, CD20– neoplastic cells	CD45+, CD20+ neoplastic cells (for B-cell lymphoma)
Endometrial stromal sarcoma, low-grade	Characteristic tongue-like growth	Closely packed tumor cells
	Evenly but loosely distributed cells	Blood vessels usually not prominent
	Small arterioles conspicuous	CD45+, CD20+, CD10–/+ (for B-cell lymphoma)
	Foam cells may be admixed	
	CD45–, CD20–, CD10+	
Embryonal rhabdomyosarcoma	Pediatric patient	Adult patient
	Alternating hyper- and hypocellular areas	Even distribution of atypical cells
	Myxoid background	Sclerotic background
	Desmin+, myogenin+, Myo-D1+ neoplastic cells	CD45+, CD20+ neoplastic cells (for B-cell lymphoma)
Extramedullary hematopoiesis, especially with erythroid predominance	Homogeneous dark chromatin characteristic of erythroid elements	Vesicular or stippled chromatin characteristic of lymphoid cells
	Presence of megakaryocytes and maturing myeloid elements	Absence of other hematopoietic cell lines
	Evidence of concurrent myeloproliferative disorder	

PID, pelvic inflammatory disease; *EBV*, Epstein-Barr virus; *SCIS*, squamous cell carcinoma in situ; *ACIS*, adenocarcinoma in situ; *IB*, immunoblast; *CB*, centroblast.

myeloproliferative disorder often coincides with blast crisis [60]. In the FAB classification, the leukemias have included M1, M2, M3, M4 [26], and M5 types [29]. Several have been associated with acute myeloid leukemia with abnormal marrow eosinophilia (AML, M4 eo) [16, 26]. Nearly all patients with myeloid sarcoma and no evidence of bone marrow disease will eventually develop overt leukemia [60]. However, in a few patients with isolated myeloid sarcoma who are treated aggressively with a combination of chemotherapy and radiation, there may be long survival without the development of acute leukemia [31, 55]. In general, patients have not had conditions predisposing to the development of myeloid neoplasia, although one patient had prior chemotherapy for breast cancer [73]. A few patients with acute myeloid leukemia and myeloid sarcoma involving the reproductive organs were exposed to radiation at Hiroshima or Nagasaki [45]. Most cases involve either the ovaries or the uterus. Vaginal and vulvar myeloid sarcomas are rare [26, 66].

Pathologic Features

Microscopic examination reveals a diffuse infiltrate of discohesive atypical cells that may spare certain normal structures, such as endometrial glands, or developing follicles in the ovary. A single-file pattern of growth is common. Mitoses are frequent. The neoplastic cells are medium-sized, with oval to irregular, sometimes distinctly indented nuclei with fine chromatin and small nucleoli. Cytoplasm ranges from very scant to moderate in quantity, sometimes with a pink color, reflecting the presence of myeloid granules. Scattered apoptotic cells are often present. A minority of cases show geographic necrosis. Scattered eosinophil precursor cells may be identified [26, 66]. The lesions may be subclassified as blastic, immature or differentiated based on the degree of cellular differentiation [4, 26]. The blastic type is composed mainly of myeloblasts, the immature type contains promyelocytes in addition to myeloblasts, and the differentiated type contains, in addition, more mature cells in the neutrophil series [4].

Immunophenotyping on paraffin sections typically shows neoplastic cells that are positive for myeloperoxidase, lysozyme, CD117, CD43, and often for CD34 and CD68. CD45 (leukocyte common antigen) is usually positive, but may be dimly expressed or even negative on paraffin sections, potentially leading to difficulty in recognizing such lesions as hematologic [4, 26, 70]. B and T-cell specific antigens are not expressed. Tumor cells are also positive for chloroacetate esterase. Monoblastic sarcomas are lysozyme+, CD68+, but do not express myeloperoxidase [4].

Ovarian Involvement by Myeloid Neoplasia

Leukemia rarely presents initially in the ovary, but infiltration of the ovary at autopsy is quite common. In an autopsy study of 1,206 patients with leukemia who died between 1958 and 1982, there was ovarian involvement by acute myelogenous leukemia in 11% and by chronic myelogenous leukemia in 9% [3] The authors noted a significant reduction in extramedullary tumor during the later years of the study and attributed this to more aggressive therapy.

The diagnosis of ovarian myeloid sarcoma is appropriate when immature myeloid cells form an ovarian tumor. Among patients with clinically evident myeloid sarcoma, the ovary is rarely involved. None of the 21 women with myeloid sarcoma studied by Neiman et al. [60] and only 1 of 9 women studied by Meis et al. [55] had involvement of the adnexa.

A few women and very rarely children have had what apparently was isolated ovarian myeloid sarcoma or ovarian myeloid sarcoma as the first manifestation of acute myeloid leukemia [16, 20, 66, 67]. The ovary can also be a clinically apparent, but usually not an isolated, site of relapse following chemotherapy for acute myelogenous leukemia [66].

The tumors can be unilateral or bilateral and range up to 19 cm in diameter (mean, 10–12 cm). They are typically solid, soft, and white or red-brown, but cystic degeneration, hemorrhage, or necrosis may be seen [20, 67]. A few cases have had a distinct green color on gross inspection [66], thus warranting a designation of chloroma.

Uterine Involvement by Myeloid Neoplasia

Myeloid sarcoma of the uterus is uncommon [66]. In two combined series of patients with myeloid sarcoma from a variety of sites, one of 30 women had myeloid sarcoma involving the corpus, and one had cervical involvement [55, 60]. Patients have been adults, with a mean age in the sixth decade, who typically present with abnormal vaginal bleeding, sometimes accompanied by abdominal pain [28, 29, 70, 73, 80]. Several patients had cervical smears positive for malignancy, although a specific diagnosis was not made [20, 80]. One was considered positive for malignant lymphoma or leukemia [80] and in one, the diagnosis of lymphoma was suggested [20]. The cervix is involved more often than the corpus, but both may be involved simultaneously [28, 73]. In only a minority of cases is tumor confined to the uterus [28]. In most cases tumor involved other reproductive organs, including the vagina [20, 80], vulva [80], ovaries, or fallopian tubes [26, 29], sometimes with parametrial involvement [20], with or without extension to the pelvic side walls [70]. Bulky pelvic masses may be associated with hydroureter [73]. Staging in some cases has revealed concurrent involvement of sites outside the reproductive tract, including lymph nodes [26, 28, 80], gastrointestinal tract [80], breast [26], or mediastinum [26]. Bone marrow examination may reveal acute myeloid leukemia [26]. Among those without acute myeloid leukemia at presentation, progression to acute myeloid leukemia is common [20, 28, 29]. One woman with chronic myelogenous leukemia developed granulocytic sarcomas of the breast and the endometrium, shortly after blast crisis [80]. One patient with a history of breast cancer treated with chemotherapy developed an isolated therapy-related uterine monoblastic sarcoma expressing CD45, CD43, CD68, and lysozyme associated with a translocation of the mixed – lineage leukemia gene at 11q23 [73]; acute myeloid leukemia with 11q23 abnormalities can arise as a complication of chemotherapy that includes DNA topoisomerase II inhibitors.

On gross examination, the lesions appear as nodules, ulcers, or large masses, often extending into the vagina or paracervical soft tissue [20]. The tumors range from gray-tan or gray-blue to green [28]. On microscopic examination, the immature granulocytes tend to infiltrate around, rather than destroy normal structures, a pattern that is also seen in cases of lymphoma. The histological appearance is similar to myeloid sarcoma in other sites.

The correct diagnosis was often not rendered on initial biopsy, particularly in earlier reports, when routine immunophenotyping was less prevalent and fewer antibodies were available for paraffin section immunohistochemistry. The most common misdiagnosis was malignant lymphoma [28]. One cervical biopsy was initially interpreted as small-cell squamous cell carcinoma and in another, the tumor was not recognized [20].

Involvement of the uterus in other forms of myeloproliferative disorders is very unusual. Extramedullary hematopoiesis may be seen in the endometrium, involving the endometrial stroma, or less often elsewhere in the reproductive tract. In approximately half of the cases, there is an associated hematologic neoplasm [83]. This author has seen an unpublished case of chronic idiopathic myelofibrosis in which there was extensive extramedullary hematopoiesis ("myeloid metaplasia") in the endometrium (*Fig. 21.12*).

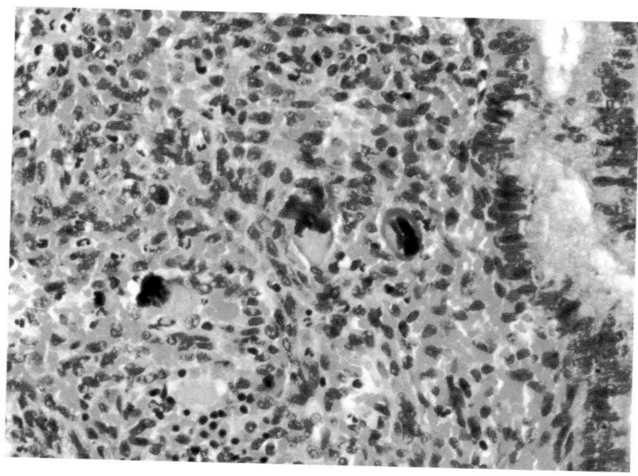

Fig. 21.12
Endometrium, extramedullary hematopoiesis. Several megakaryocytes with large, dark, atypical nuclei are scattered in the endometrial stroma. A loose cluster of nucleated red blood cells is present near the bottom of the image

Vaginal and Vulvar Involvement by Myeloid Neoplasia

Patients with acute myelogenous leukemia occasionally have leukemic infiltration of the vagina [20]. In addition, a handful of cases of myeloid sarcoma of the vagina have been documented (*Fig. 21.13a and b*). Oliva and coworkers described three cases in women aged 66, 73, and 76 years, presenting with postmenopausal bleeding, an abnormal Papanicolaou smear and the presence of a mass. One of them had a prior history of acute myeloid leukemia, one presented with vaginal myeloid sarcoma, but was found to have acute myeloid leukemia when a marrow biopsy was performed, and one had apparently isolated myeloid sarcoma. At last follow-up, one was alive with disease, and two had died [66]. Another case was described in a 48-year-old woman who presented with vaginal pain and leukorrhea; physical examination revealed an isolated vaginal mass that was green. Evaluation revealed a tumor that was CAE+, CD43+, CD45+, lysozyme+, and negative for CD20, CD3, S100, and cytokeratin. Despite treatment, the patient rapidly developed overt leukemia, classified as acute myeloid leukemia, M5a. Cytogenetic analysis revealed a complex karyotype. The patient developed myeloid sarcomas in other sites, including the breast and thigh, and she died of leukemia 10 months after presentation [29]. One 39-year-old patient with Down's syndrome presented with symptoms related to a myeloid sarcoma of the cervix and vagina [20]. Another case is presented without details in the large series of myeloid sarcomas reported by Neiman et al. [60].

A myeloid sarcoma presenting as a mass in the vulva of an elderly woman has been described; additional work-up showed that she had acute myeloid leukemia [18]. In another case, a woman with a myelodysplastic/myeloproliferative disorder developed what appeared to be a rash of the clitoris, but that proved to be myeloid sarcoma; acute myeloid leukemia developed two months later [26].

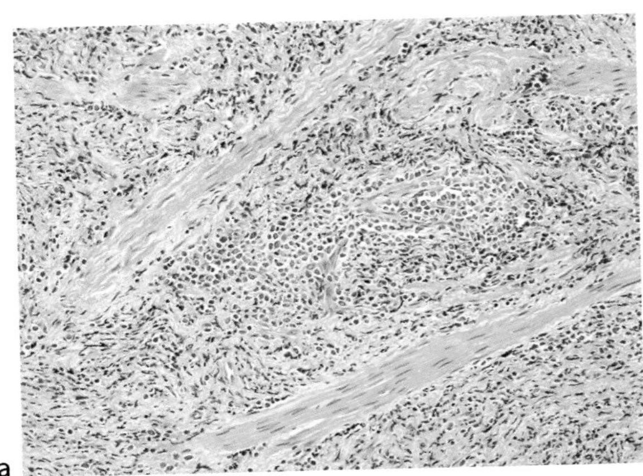
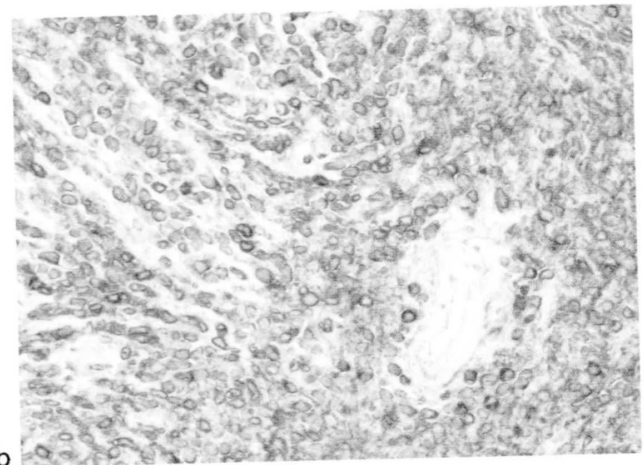

Fig. 21.13
Vagina, myeloid sarcoma. **(a)** An infiltrate of primitive, discohesive neoplastic cells with finely dispersed chromatin and scant cytoplasm permeates the fibromuscular stroma. **(b)** The neoplastic cells are positive for myeloperoxidase (immunoperoxidase technique on a paraffin section)

The prognosis of myeloid sarcoma in the reproductive tract is difficult to assess because only small numbers of patients have been studied over many years and treatment has varied. There are only a few sizable series [26, 66], and follow-up has often been short. Among patients presenting initially with isolated myeloid sarcoma, progression to acute myeloid leukemia is common [26] even among patients who are treated aggressively [29]. In general, patients with myeloid sarcoma of the female reproductive organs have had a poor prognosis, which will likely improve with advances in therapy for acute myeloid leukemia. Occasional patients, including those with isolated myeloid sarcoma and those with more widespread disease at presentation do achieve long-term disease-free survival [26, 66].

Differential Diagnosis

The majority of cases of myeloid sarcoma in some large series were initially misdiagnosed, most often as malignant lymphoma [55, 60]. This occurs less often currently because of greater use of immunophenotyping and larger number of antibodies available for paraffin section immunohistochemistry. Compared to lymphoma, myeloid sarcoma is generally composed of cells with more finely dispersed chromatin, often with more cytoplasm than a lymphoid cell with the same size nucleus. The cytoplasm may have a distinct red color. The identification of eosinophilic myelocytes in some cases is very helpful in making a diagnosis of a tumor of primitive myeloid origin. Establishing a diagnosis of myeloid sarcoma is not difficult in a patient who has been previously diagnosed with an acute myeloid leukemia that has been well characterized by flow cytometry. In those cases in which a myeloid sarcoma represents the first presentation with disease, it is essential to confirm this unusual diagnosis with immunohistochemistry. Using a panel of antibodies to myeloid-associated antigens, such as lysozyme, myeloperoxidase, CD68, CD34, and CD117, in conjunction with markers of B cells (such as CD20), T cells (such as CD3), and in selected cases, markers of non-hematolymphoid cells, such as cytokeratin and S-100. It should be noted that certain T-lineage-associated antigens, such as CD43, are not lineage-specific and may be expressed in myeloid sarcomas. Monoblastic sarcomas may express CD4 (usually more faintly than mature T helper cells), as well as CD56, usually considered an NK cell marker, so that judicious interpretation of unusual or unexpected immunophenotypic results is required (See *Table 21.1*).

Differentiating pyometra from myeloid sarcoma of the endometrium can at times be difficult. Some myeloid sarcomas show differentiation to mature forms. In the setting of severe acute inflammation degenerated neutrophils may have nuclei that lose their distinctive lobation and appear round, and thus may potentially be mistaken for primitive cells. A diagnosis of myeloid sarcoma should only be made if there is a convincing population of well-preserved primitive myeloid elements.

Histiocytic Neoplasms of the Female Reproductive Organs

Langerhans Cell Histiocytosis

Clinical Features

Langerhans cell histiocytosis, previously known as histiocytosis X, occurs in one of the three clinical syndromes: (1) eosinophilic granuloma, which is characterized by unifocal disease; (2) Hand–Schüller–Christian disease which is a chronic progressive multifocal disease typically involving one organ system, and (3) Letterer–Siwe disease, an aggressive, fulminant disorder with multifocal, multisystem involvement by Langerhans cell histiocytosis [56, 92].

Langerhans cell histiocytosis occasionally involves the reproductive organs, most often the vulva and infrequently the vagina or cervix [32, 44]. Endometrial and ovarian involvement has also been reported rarely [2]. Uterine involvement is almost always accompanied by vulvar or vaginal lesions, or both [20, 32]. There appears to be a strong association between diabetes insipidus and the presence of mucocutaneous lesions of Langerhans cell histiocytosis, particularly in the female reproductive tract [32]. Langerhans cell histiocytosis frequently has manifestations in other sites, prior to, or subsequent to, the reproductive organ involvement [2], in particular, in the form of bony lesions [32, 68]. Isolated Langerhans cell histiocytosis involving the reproductive organs is rare [77].

Langerhans cell histiocytosis in the reproductive tract falls into one of the four patterns [2, 68]:

1. Isolated genital disease, some with local recurrence but no distant involvement.
2. Isolated genital disease with subsequent dissemination to other sites most often bone, accompanied in some cases by diabetes insipidus.
3. Initial presentation with oral or skin disease, and subsequent genital and multiorgan disease.
4. Initial presentation with diabetes insipidus and subsequent genital and multiorgan disease.

Patients with Langerhans cell histiocytosis involving the reproductive tract range from 1 to 85 years; most have been young adults [2, 32]. The presenting complaints are usually vulvar pruritus or dyspareunia [32, 44]. The lesions can be single or multiple [32, 77] They are white or yellow-brown ulcers, papules, ulcerated nodules [32, 91], erythematous plaques, red papules [77], or irregular friable masses [20] and may mimic primary syphilis, squamous cell carcinoma, lymphogranuloma venereum [32], herpes simplex viral infection, or melanoma [20]. The lesions in the cervix are yellow-brown, brown or red papules [20, 32].

Pathologic Features

Microscopically they consist of submucosal nodules or sheets of Langerhans cells with pale, deeply creased, or folded nuclei with delicate nuclear membranes, pale chromatin and relatively abundant pale pink cytoplasm. There is often an admixture of eosinophils and lymphocytes in some areas, as well as neutrophils in some cases (➋ *Fig. 21.14a and b*). The cellular infiltrate is often associated with ulceration and a scale crust [32]. On microscopic examination, Langerhans cell histiocytosis can be confused with an inflammatory disorder, lymphoma, or carcinoma, but the presence of numerous Langerhans cells admixed with eosinophils should suggest the correct diagnosis. The Langerhans cells have a distinctive immunophenotype: they express both S-100 protein and CD1a. They are also variably positive for CD45, CD68, and lysozyme and negative for CD30, myeloperoxidase, and B- and T-cell specific markers. Like other histiocytes and monocytes, they may be CD4+. Immunohistochemical studies thus play an important role in confirming the diagnosis [68, 92]. It is uncertain whether Langerhans cell histiocytosis derives from neoplastic transformation of mature Langerhans cells in squamous epithelium or other tissues, or whether Langerhans cell histiocytosis is derived from an abnormal marrow-derived cell that assumes characteristics of Langerhans cells [56].

Treatment and Outcome

The behavior of Langerhans cell histiocytosis involving the reproductive organs is difficult to predict. Because of their rarity and variable behavior, uniform therapy has not been employed. Occasionally, small vulvar lesions may remit spontaneously, although nodular lesions do not [32]. The lesions may be treated initially with simple excision or with topical hydrocortisone. If these methods are unsuccessful, local radiation therapy may be effective, but may be followed by recurrences. In a few cases, systemic steroids or chemotherapy (methotrexate, vincristine, vinblastine, and others) have been used [2, 32, 44]. Since Langerhans cells

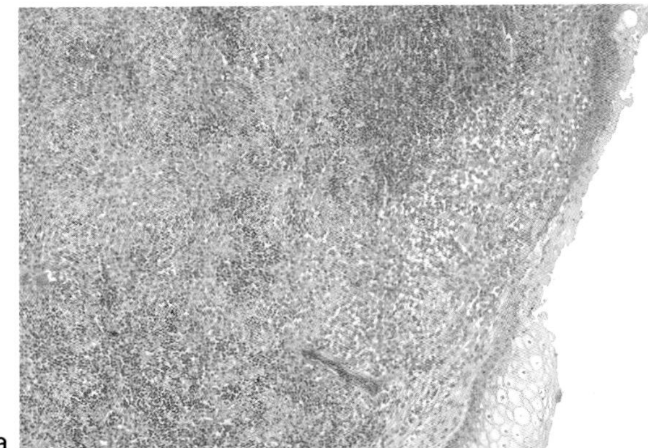

a

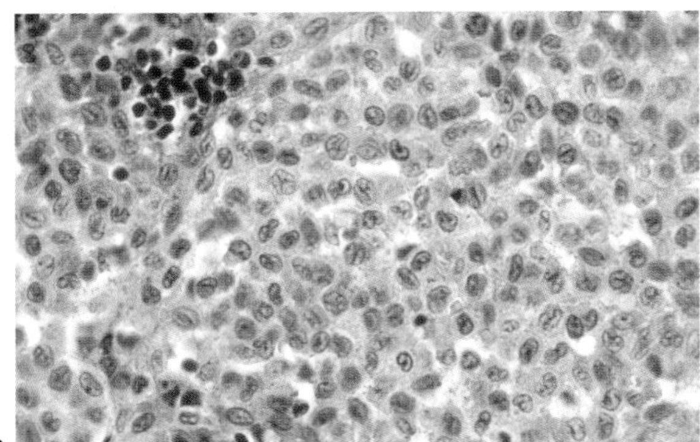

b

Fig. 21.14
Vulva, Langerhans cell histiocytosis. **(a) Low power shows sheets of pale histiocytes, aggregates of small lymphocytes and occasional eosinophils beneath squamous mucosa. (b) High power shows Langerhans cells with large, oval nuclei with nuclear folds and abundant pale pink cytoplasm, with a few admixed small lymphocytes and eosinophils**

play an important role as antigen-presenting cells in the immune response, immunomodulatory agents such as interferons have been tested as treatment for Langerhans cell histiocytosis. Dramatic responses of cutaneous and anogenital Langerhans cell histiocytosis have been described with interferons and thalidomide [56], although response is not always sustained. Thalidomide may be effective because it is an inhibitor of tumor necrosis factor (TNF), which plays a role in generating Langerhans cells from marrow precursors [77]. Whatever the therapy, incomplete responses, local recurrences, and distant relapses are common [68, 77, 91].

References

1. Alvarez A, Ortiz J, Sacristan F (1997) Large B-cell lymphoma of the uterine corpus: case report with immunohistochemical and molecular study. Gynecol Oncol 65:534–538
2. Axiotis C, Merino M, Duray P (1991) Langerhans cell histiocytosis of the female genital tract. Cancer 67:1650–1660
3. Barcos M, Lane W, Gomez GA et al (1987) An autopsy study of 1206 acute and chronic leukemias (1958–1982). Cancer 60:827–837
4. Brunning R, Matutes E, Flandrin G et al (2001) Acute myeloid leukemia not otherwise categorised. In: Jaffe E et al (eds) Pathology and genetics: tumours of haematopoietic and lymphoid tissues. IARC Press, Lyon, pp 91–105
5. Carbone A, Gloghini A, Libra M et al (2006) A spindle cell variant of diffuse large B-cell lymphoma possesses genotypic and phenotypic markers characteristic of a germinal center B-cell origin. Mod Pathol 19(2):299–306
6. Catlin EA, Roberts JD Jr, Erana R et al (1999) Transplacental transmission of natural-killer-cell lymphoma. N Engl J Med 341(2):85–91
7. Cecalupo AJ, Frankel LS, Sullivan MP (1982) Pelvic and ovarian extramedullary leukemic relapse in young girls. Cancer 50:587–593
8. Chan JK, Loizzi V, Magistris A et al (2005) Clinicopathologic features of six cases of primary cervical lymphoma. Am J Obstet Gynecol 193(3 Pt 1):866–872
9. Chandy L, Kumar L, Dawar R (1998) Non-Hodgkin's lymphoma presenting as a primary lesion in uterine cervix: case report. J Obstet Gynaecol Res 24(3):183–187
10. Chishima F, Hayakawa S, Ohta Y et al (2006) Ovarian Burkitt's lymphoma diagnosed by a combination of clinical features, morphology, immunophenotype, and molecular findings and successfully managed with surgery and chemotherapy. Int J Gynecol Cancer 16(Suppl 1):337–343
11. Cohn DE, Resnick KE, Eaton LA et al (2007) Non-Hodgkin's lymphoma mimicking gynecological malignancies of the vagina and cervix: a report of four cases. Int J Gynecol Cancer 17(1):274–279
12. de Leval L, Ferry J, Falini B et al (2001) Expression of bcl-6 and CD10 in primary mediastinal large cell lymphoma: evidence for derivation from germinal center B cells? Am J Surg Pathol 25(10):1277–1282
13. Diebold J, Jaffe E, Raphael M et al (2001) Burkitt's lymphoma. In: Jaffe E et al (eds) Pathology and genetics: tumours of haematopoietic and lymphoid tissues. IARC Press, Lyon, pp 181–184
14. Dimopoulos MA, Daliani D, Pugh W et al (1997) Primary ovarian non-Hodgkin's lymphoma: outcome after treatment with combination chemotherapy. Gynecol Oncol 64:446–450
15. Domingo S, Perales A, Torres V et al (2004) Epstein-Barr virus positivity in primary vaginal lymphoma. Gynecol Oncol 95(3):719–721
16. Drinkard LC, Waggoner S, Stein RN et al (1995) Acute myelomonocytic leukemia with abnormal eosinophils presenting as an ovarian mass: a report of two cases and a review of the literature. Gynecol Oncol 56:307–311
17. Dursun P, Gultekin M, Bozdag G et al (2005) Primary cervical lymphoma: report of two cases and review of the literature. Gynecol Oncol 98(3):484–489
18. Ersahin C, Omeroglu G, Potkul RK et al (2007) Myeloid sarcoma of the vulva as the presenting symptom in a patient with acute myeloid leukemia. Gynecol Oncol 106(1):259–261
19. Ferry JA, Harris NL, Scully RE (1989) Leiomyomas with lymphoid infiltration simulating lymphoma. A report of 7 cases. Int J Gynecol Pathol 8:263–270

20. Ferry JA, Young RH (1991) Malignant lymphoma, pseudolymphoma and hematopoietic disorders of the female genital tract. Pathol Annu 26(Pt 1):227–263
21. Ferry J, Young R (1997) Malignant lymphoma of the genitourinary tract. Curr Diagn Pathol 4:145–169
22. Freeman C, Berg J, Cutler S (1972) Occurrence and prognosis of extranodal lymphomas. Cancer 29(1):252–260
23. Frey NV, Svoboda J, Andreadis C et al (2006) Primary lymphomas of the cervix and uterus: the University of Pennsylvania's experience and a review of the literature. Leuk Lymphoma 47(9):1894–1901
24. Gaffan J, Herbertson R, Davis P et al (2004) Bilateral peripheral T-cell lymphoma of the fallopian tubes. Gynecol Oncol 95(3):736–738
25. Garavaglia E, Taccagni G, Montoli S et al (2005) Primary stage I-IIE non-Hodgkin's lymphoma of uterine cervix and upper vagina: evidence for a conservative approach in a study on three patients. Gynecol Oncol 97(1):214–218
26. Garcia MG, Deavers MT, Knoblock RJ et al (2006) Myeloid sarcoma involving the gynecologic tract: a report of 11 cases and review of the literature. Am J Clin Pathol 125(5):783–790
27. Hachisuga T, Ookuma Y, Fakuda K et al (1992) Detection of Epstein-Barr virus DNA from a lymphoma-like lesion of the uterine cervix. Gynecol Oncol 46:69–73
28. Harris NL, Scully RE (1984) Malignant lymphoma and granulocytic sarcoma of the uterus and vagina. A clinicopathologic analysis of 27 cases. Cancer 53:2530–2545
29. Hernandez JA, Navarro JT, Rozman M et al (2002) Primary myeloid sarcoma of the gynecologic tract: a report of two cases progressing to acute myeloid leukemia. Leuk Lymphoma 43(11):2151–2153
30. Iliya FA, Muggia FM, O'Leary JA et al (1968) Gynecologic manifestations of reticulum cell sarcoma. Obstet Gynecol 31:266–269
31. Imrie KR, Kovass MJ, Selby D et al (1995) Isolated chloroma: the effect of early antileukemic therapy. Ann Intern Med 123(5):351–353
32. Issa PY, Salem PA, Brihi E et al (1980) Eosinophilic granuloma with involvement of the female genitalia. Am J Obstet Gynecol 137:608–612
33. Iyengar P, Deodhare S (2004) Primary extranodal marginal zone B-cell lymphoma of MALT type of the endometrium. Gynecol Oncol 93(1):238–241
34. Jackisch C, Louwen F, Schwenkhagen A et al (2003) Lung cancer during pregnancy involving the products of conception and a review of the literature. Arch Gynecol Obstet 268(2):69–77
35. Kahlifa M, Buckstein R, Perez-Ordonez B (2003) Sarcomatoid variant of B-cell lymphoma of the uterine cervix. Int J Gynecol Pathol 22(3):289–293
36. Kaplan EJ, Chadburn A, Caputo TA (1996) Case report. HIV-related primary non-Hodgkin's lymphoma of the vulva. Gynecol Oncol 61:131–138
37. Kaplan MA, Jacobson JO, Ferry JA et al (1993) T cell lymphoma of the vulva with erythrophagocytosis in a renal allograft recipient. Am J Surg Pathol 17:842–849
38. Kawauchi S, Fukuma F, Morioka H et al (2002) Malignant lymphoma arising as a primary tumor of the uterine corpus. Pathol Int 52(5–6):423–424
39. Kirk CM, Naumann RW, Hartmann CJ et al (2001) Primary endometrial T-cell lymphoma. A case report. Am J Clin Pathol 115(4):561–566
40. Kosari F, Daneshbod Y, Parwaresch R et al (2005) Lymphomas of the female genital tract: a study of 186 cases and review of the literature. Am J Surg Pathol 29(11):1512–1520
41. Lagoo AS, Robboy SJ (2006) Lymphoma of the female genital tract: current status. Int J Gynecol Pathol 25(1):1–21
42. Lanjewar D, Dongaonkar D (2006) HIV-associated primary non-Hodgkin's lymphoma of ovary: a case report. Gynecol Oncol 102(3):590–592
43. Leoncini L, Raphael M, Stein H et al (2008) Burkitt's lymphoma. In: Swerdlow S et al (eds) WHO classification of tumours of haematopoietic and lymphoid tissues. IARC Press, Lyon, pp 262–264
44. Lieberman PH, Jones CR, Steinman RM et al (1996) Langerhans cells (eosinophilic) granulomatosis. Am J Surg Pathol 20:519–552
45. Liu PI, Ishimaru T, McGregor DH et al (1973) Autopsy study of granulocytic sarcoma (chloroma) in patients with myelogenous leukemia, Hiroshima-Nagasaki 1949–1969. Cancer 31:948–955
46. Lyman MD, Neuhauser TS (2002) Precursor T-cell acute lymphoblastic leukemia/lymphoma involving the uterine cervix, myometrium, endometrium, and appendix. Ann Diagn Pathol 6(2):125–128
47. Ma J, Shi Q, Zhou X et al (2007) Lymphoma-like lesion of the uterine cervix: report of 12 cases of a rare entity. Int J Gynecol Pathol 26(2):194–198
48. Macleod C, Palmer A, Findlay M (1998) Primary non-Hodgkin's lymphoma of the vulva: a case report. Int J Gynecol Cancer 8:504–508
49. Magloire LK, Pettker CM, Buhimschi CS et al (2006) Burkitt's lymphoma of the ovary in pregnancy. Obstet Gynecol 108(3 Pt 2):743–745
50. Makarewicz R, Kuzminska A (1995) Non-Hodgkin's lymphoma of the uterine cervix: a report of three patients. Clin Oncol (R Coll Radiol) 7:198–199
51. Mansouri H, Sifat H, Gaye M et al (2000) Primary malignant lymphoma of the ovary: an unusual presentation of a rare disease. Eur J Gynaec Oncol 21(6):616–618
52. Maruko K, Maeda T, Kamitomo M et al (2004) Transplacental transmission of maternal B-cell lymphoma. Am J Obstet Gynecol 191(1):380–381
53. McKelvey A, McKenna D, McManus D et al (2003) A case of lymphoma occurring in an ovarian teratoma. Gynecol Oncol 90(2):474–477
54. Meguerian-Bedoyan Z, Lamant L, Hopfner C et al (1997) Anaplastic large cell lymphoma of maternal origin involving the placenta: case report and literature survey. Am J Surg Pathol 21(10):1236–1241
55. Meis JM, Butler JJ, Osborne BM et al (1986) Granulocytic sarcoma in nonleukemic patients. Cancer 58:2697–2709
56. Montero AJ, Diaz-Montero CM, Malpica A et al (2003) Langerhans cell histiocytosis of the female genital tract: a literature review. Int J Gynecol Cancer 13(3):381–388
57. Murase T, Inagaki H, Takagi N et al (2002) Nasal NK-cell lymphoma followed by relapse in the uterine cervix. Leuk Lymphoma 43(1):203–206
58. Nagarsheth NP, Kalir T, Rahaman J (2005) Post-transplant lymphoproliferative disorder of the cervix. Gynecol Oncol 97(1):271–275
59. Nasu K, Yoshimatsu J, Urata K et al (1998) A case of primary non-Hodgkin's lymphoma of the uterine cervix treated by combination chemotherapy (THP-COP). J Obstet Gynaecol Res 24(2):157–160
60. Neiman RS, Barcos M, Berard C et al (1981) Granulocytic sarcoma: a clinicopathologic study of 61 biopsied cases. Cancer 48:1426–1437
61. Neuhauser TS, Tavassoli FA, Abbondanzo SL (2000) Follicle center lymphoma involving the female genital tract: a morphologic and molecular genetic study of three cases. Ann Diagn Pathol 4(5):293–299
62. Nishi Y, Suzuki S, Otsubo Y et al (2000) B-cell-type malignant lymphoma with placental involvement. J Obstet Gynaecol Res 26(1):39–43
63. Noack F, Lange K, Lehmann V et al (2002) Primary extranodal marginal zone B-cell lymphoma of the fallopian tube. Gynecol Oncol 86(3):384–386

64. Nomura S, Ishii K, Shimamoto Y et al (2006) Burkitt's lymphoma of the uterus in a human T lymphotropic virus type-1 carrier. Intern Med 45(4):215–217
65. Ohmori T, Wakamoto R, Lu LM et al (2002) Immunohistochemical study of a case of uterine leiomyoma showing massive lymphoid infiltration and localized vasculitis after LH-RH derivant treatment. Histopathology 41(3):276–277
66. Oliva E, Ferry JA, Young RH et al (1997) Granulocytic sarcoma of the female genital tract. A clinicopathologic study of 11 cases. Am J Surg Pathol 21:1156–1165
67. Osborne BM, Robboy SJ (1983) Lymphomas or leukemia presenting as ovarian tumors. An analysis of 42 cases. Cancer 52:1933–1943
68. Padula A, Medeiros LJ, Silva EG et al (2004) Isolated vulvar Langerhans cell histiocytosis: report of two cases. Int J Gynecol Pathol 23(3):278–283
69. Paik SS, Oh YH, Jang KS et al (2004) Uterine leiomyoma with massive lymphoid infiltration: case report and review of the literature. Pathol Int 54(5):343–348
70. Pathak B, Bruchim I, Brisson ML et al (2005) Granulocytic sarcoma presenting as tumors of the cervix. Gynecol Oncol 98(3):493–497
71. Perren T, Farrant M, McCarthy K et al (1992) Lymphomas of the cervix and upper vagina: a report of five cases and a review of the literature. Gynecol Oncol 44:87–95
72. Prevot S, Hugol D, Audouin J et al (1992) Primary non Hodgkin's malignant lymphoma of the vagina. Report of 3 cases with review of the literature. Path Res Pract 188:78–85
73. Pullarkat V, Veliz L, Chang K et al (2007) Therapy-related, mixed-lineage leukaemia translocation-positive, monoblastic myeloid sarcoma of the uterus. J Clin Pathol 60(5):562–564
74. Rappaport H (1966) Tumors of the hematopoietic system, Atlas of tumor pathology, Series I, Fascicle 8. Washington, DC, Armed Forces Institute of Pathology
75. Saglam A, Guler G, Taskin M et al (2005) Uterine leiomyoma with prominent lymphoid infiltrate. Int J Gynecol Cancer 15(1):167–170
76. Sakurai N, Tateoka K, Taguchi J et al (2008) Primary precursor B-cell lymphoblastic lymphoma of the ovary: case report and review of the literature. Int J Gynecol Pathol 27(3):412–417
77. Santillan A, Montero AJ, Kavanagh JJ et al (2003) Vulvar Langerhans cell histiocytosis: a case report and review of the literature. Gynecol Oncol 91(1):241–246
78. Scully RE (1979) Tumors of the ovary and maldeveloped gonads, Atlas of tumor pathology, Series 2, Fascicle 16. Armed Forces Institute of Pathology, Washington, DC, pp 117–127
79. Shulman LN, Hitt RA, Ferry JA (2008) Case records of the Massachusetts General Hospital. Case 4-2008. A 33-year-old pregnant woman with swelling of the left breast and shortness of breath. N Engl J Med 358(5):513–523
80. Spahr J, Behm FG, Schneider V (1982) Preleukemic granulocytic sarcoma of cervix and vagina. Initial manifestation by cytology. Acta Cytol 26:55–60
81. Sur M, Ross C, Moens F et al (2005) Intravascular large B-cell lymphoma of the uterus: a diagnostic challenge. Int J Gynecol Pathol 24(2):201–203
82. Tjalma W, Van de Velde A, Schroyens W (2002) Primary non-Hodgkin's lymphoma in Bartholin's gland. Gynecol Oncol 87(3): 308–309
83. Valeri RM, Ibrahim N, Sheaff MT (2002) Extramedullary hematopoiesis in the endometrium. Int J Gynecol Pathol 21(2):178–181
84. van de Rijn M, Kamel O, Chang P et al (1997) Primary low grade endometrial B-cell lymphoma. Am J Surg Pathol 21:187–194
85. van der Velden VH, Willemse MJ, Mulder MF et al (2001) Clearance of maternal leukaemic cells in a neonate. Br J Haematol 114(1): 104–106
86. Vang R, Medeiros LJ, Fuller GN et al (2001) Non-Hodgkin's lymphoma involving the gynecologic tract: a review of 88 cases. Adv Anat Pathol 8(4):200–217
87. Vang R, Medeiros LJ, Ha CS et al (2000) Non-Hodgkin's lymphomas involving the uterus: a clinicopathologic analysis of 26 cases. Mod Pathol 13(1):19–28
88. Vang R, Medeiros L, Malpica A et al (2000) Non-Hodgkin's lymphoma involving the vulva. Int J Gynecol Pathol 19(3):236–242
89. Vang R, Medeiros L, Silva E et al (2000) Non-Hodgkin's lymphoma involving the vagina. A clinicopathologic analysis of 14 patients. Am J Surg Pathol 24(5):719–725
90. Vang R, Medeiros L, Warnke R et al (2001) Ovarian non-Hodgkin's lymphoma: a clinicopathologic study of eight primary cases. Mod Pathol 14(11):1093–1099
91. Venizelos ID, Mandala E, Tatsiou ZA et al (2006) Primary Langerhans cell histiocytosis of the vulva. Int J Gynecol Pathol 25(1):48–51
92. Weiss L, Grogan T, Muller-Hermelink HK et al (2001) Langerhans cell histiocytosis. In: Jaffe E et al (eds) Pathology and genetics: tumours of haematopoietic and lymphoid tissues. IARC Press, Lyon, pp 280–282
93. Wyld PH, Lilleyman JS (1983) Ovarian disease in childhood lymphoblastic leukemia. Acta Haematol 69:278–280
94. Yamada N, Uchida R, Fuchida S et al (2005) CD5+ Epstein-Barr virus-positive intravascular large B-cell lymphoma in the uterus co-existing with huge myoma. Am J Hematol 78(3):221–224
95. Yoshinaga K, Akahira J, Niikura H et al (2004) A case of primary mucosa-associated lymphoid tissue lymphoma of the vagina. Hum Pathol 35(9):1164–1166
96. Young RH, Harris NL, Scully RE (1985) Lymphoma-like lesions of the lower female genital tract: a report of 16 cases. Int J Gynecol Pathol 4:289–299
97. Zinzani P, Martelli M, Bertini M et al (2002) Induction chemotherapy strategies for primary mediastinal large B-cell lymphoma with sclerosis: a retrospective multinational study on 426 previously untreated patients. Haematologica 87:1258–1264

22 Soft Tissue Lesions Involving Female Reproductive Organs

John F. Fetsch · William B. Laskin

The views expressed in this chapter are those of the authors and do not necessarily reflect official policy or position of the Armed Forces Institute of Pathology, the Department of the Army, the Department of Defense, or any other Department or Agency within the U.S. Government.

R. J. Kurman, L. Hedrick Ellenson, B. M. Ronnett (eds.), *Blaustein's Pathology of the Female Genital Tract (6th ed.)*, DOI 10.1007/978-1-4419-0489-8_22,

The most common benign mesenchymal tumor of the gynecologic tract is a leiomyoma. The most frequent malignant mesenchymal neoplasms of this anatomic region in pediatric and adult patients are rhabdomyosarcoma and leiomyosarcoma, respectively. Because these entities are well-recognized and expertly covered elsewhere in this textbook, they are not discussed in this chapter. Instead, this section concentrates on the myriad of other less common mesenchymal processes that occasionally affect the female reproductive organs. We attempt to cover the better documented and most relevant entities as comprehensively as space allows, and include brief comments and/or references for rarer lesions. Supplemental data from the Armed Forces Institute of Pathology Tumor Registry is included for selected topics. It is important to remember that some of the entities under discussion have only recently been recognized and remain works in progress. Readers are directed to standard soft tissue tumor texts for additional reading.

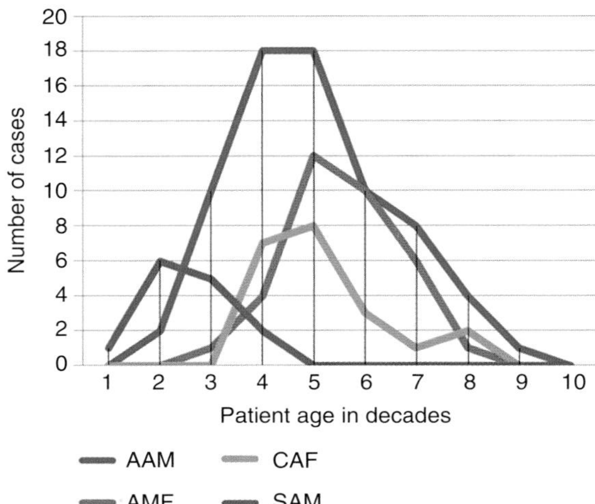

Fig. 22.1
Age distribution for patients with AAM (aggressive angiomyxoma), AMF (angiomyofibroblastoma), CAF (cellular angiofibroma), and SAM (superficial angiomyxoma/cutaneous myxoma), AFIP data

Soft Tissue Tumors and Tumor-like Lesions with Benign Behavior

Aggressive (Deep) Angiomyxoma

Aggressive angiomyxoma was characterized as a distinct clinicopathologic entity in 1983 [292]. In earlier literature, examples were sometimes classified as myxomas, vascular myxomas, or edematous or soft fibromas.

Clinical Features

Aggressive angiomyxoma has a predilection for adult females, with a peak incidence in the 4th and 5th decades (*Fig. 22.1*) [44, 92]. However, a recent review of 71 examples in the AFIP files revealed a broader age range than has generally been appreciated for this entity. Women 60 years of age and older comprised 18% of the total cases. This is a surprisingly high figure and probably reflects case referral bias, but it nonetheless stresses the point that postmenopausal status does not strongly militate against the diagnosis. In contrast, a diagnosis of aggressive angiomyxoma in a prepubertal girl should be viewed with suspicion. One purported example in an 11-year-old is more consistent with a superficial angiomyxoma [229, 323].

Most patients present with a slow-growing pelvicoperineal mass that is either asymptomatic or associated with dull regional pain, a pressure-like sensation, or dyspareunia. Tumor size is often significantly underestimated by physical examination, and preoperative clinical impressions generally revolve around a Bartholin gland cyst, vaginal cyst, hernia, or lipoma. The bulk of the process is frequently concealed within the deep soft tissues, and more than 50% of resected neoplasms in the AFIP files are ≥10 cm in size.

CT imaging demonstrates a hypo- or iso-attenuated mass that tends to grow around pelvic floor structures and generally does not cause significant disruption of the vaginal or rectal musculature [247]. T1-weighted MR images show a hypo- to iso-intense mass, whereas high signal intensity is evident in T2-weighted images [51, 64, 247]. Both T2-weighted MR and enhanced CT images often demonstrate a distinctive swirled or layered internal architecture [247]. These imaging techniques can accurately assess tumor extent and determine whether the pelvic diaphragm has been traversed, information critical for selecting an optimal surgical approach [247].

Pathologic Findings

Gross examination usually reveals a large mass, commonly >10 cm and not infrequently >20 cm. Small tumors under 5 cm make up <10% of examples in the AFIP files. The lesions often have a lobular gross appearance with adherence to fat, muscle, and other regional structures. A soft to moderately firm or rubbery consistency is often present, and the cut surface is generally described as glistening or myxedematous with a pink or reddish-tan color. Focal hemorrhage and cystic change are sometimes noted.

Aggressive angiomyxomas generally have fairly uniform, low to moderate cellularity, and they contain relatively small, stellate-shaped and spindled cells, set in a loosely collagenous, myxedematous matrix with scattered vessels of varying caliber and a variety of entrapped regional structures (*Figs. 22.2* and *22.3*). The tumor cells have scant eosinophilic cytoplasm with poorly-defined borders and relatively bland nuclei with an open chromatin pattern and a small, central nucleolus. Multinucleated tumors cells are sometimes present. Mitotic figures are infrequent. A characteristic finding, evident in most cases, is the presence of loosely organized collections of well-developed myoid (myofibroblastic vs. true smooth muscle) cells situated around larger nerve segments and vessels [92, 123, 285]. These cells are generally immunohistochemically distinct from the smooth muscle of vessel walls (see *Figs. 22.4e* and *22.4f*) [92]. While the tumor name implies the presence of abundant myxoid matrix, aggressive angiomyxomas are typically only weakly positive for mucosubstances, and edema appears to be a major component of the noncollagenous stroma [92, 292].

The neoplastic cells often have moderate to diffuse nuclear immunoreactivity for estrogen and progesterone receptor proteins (*Fig. 22.4*) [92, 206]. The cells have diffuse cytoplasmic reactivity for vimentin and variable levels of reactivity for desmin and actins. CD34 expression is less frequently observed and generally only a focal finding. Immunoreactivity for S100 protein is absent. In our experience, the small, stellate-shaped and spindled tumor cells typically have greater reactivity for the D33 desmin antibody (DAKO) than the DE-R-11 antibody (DAKO). The larger well-developed myoid cells, noted above, that often reside around nerves and vessels have stronger and more uniform immunoreactivity for both actins and desmin than the more prevalent population of smaller tumor cells with less abundant cytoplasm. Most, but not all, conventional cytogenetic analyses of aggressive angiomyxoma have demonstrated aberrations involving chromosome 12, and in several studies, its *HMGA2* (*HMGIC*) gene has been implicated [211, 239, 308]. In some tumors (the exact percentage is unresolved), this results in aberrant nuclear HMGA2 (HMGIC) protein expression, a finding that has also been noted in several other soft tissue entities (including uterine leiomyomas) but is reportedly absent in normal vulvovaginal soft tissue, as well as several key soft tissue tumors (e.g., angiomyofibroblastoma) that enter into the differential diagnosis [211, 235, 239].

Differential Diagnosis

The differential diagnosis for aggressive angiomyxoma includes superficial angiomyxoma, angiomyofibroblastoma,

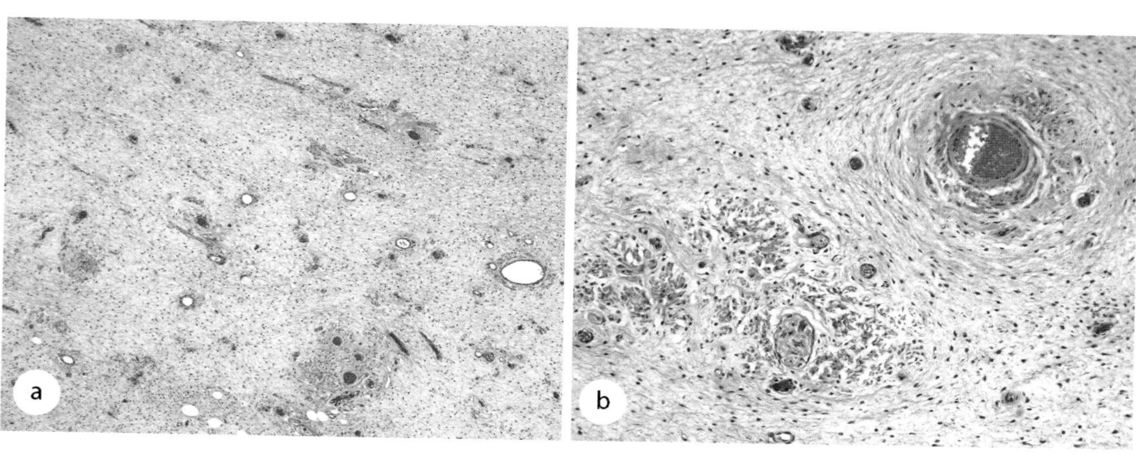

Fig. 22.2
Aggressive angiomyxoma. **Low (a) and medium (b) power views. Note the evenly spaced, small delicate tumor cells embedded in loosely collagenous matrix, the scattered larger vessels, and the proliferation of eosinophilic myoid cells around some of the nerves and vessels**

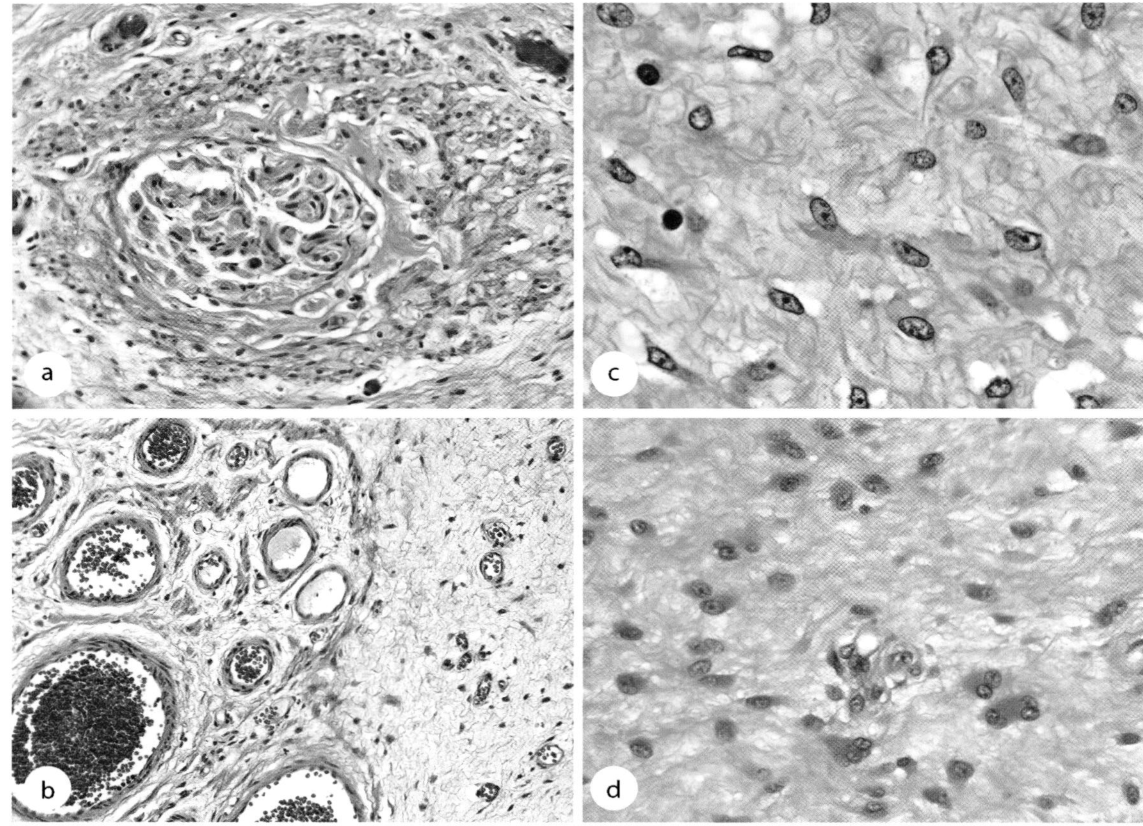

Fig. 22.3
Aggressive angiomyxoma. **A proliferation of well-developed myoid cells is present around a nerve segment (a) and several vessels (b). Figures (c) and (d) are high power views of the small neoplastic cells of aggressive angiomyxoma. Note the scant cytoplasm, indistinct cell borders and nuclei with small but distinct nucleoli. Two lymphocytes are present as a size reference in figure (c). Multinucleated tumor cells are illustrated in figure (d)**

cellular angiofibroma, myxoid and edematous smooth muscle tumors, pelvic fibromatosis, and low-grade myxofibrosarcoma (myxoid malignant fibrous histiocytoma). A detailed review of most of these entities is provided elsewhere in this chapter. Hydropic (edematous) and myxoid smooth muscle tumors usually feature larger tumor cells with spindled morphology, abundant eosinophilic cytoplasm (in which longitudinal cytoplasmic striations may be highlighted with a Masson trichrome stain), and sometimes, juxtanuclear vacuoles. True myxoid smooth muscle tumors contain abundant hyaluronic acid, a feature not seen in aggressive angiomyxoma. Myxofibrosarcoma (myxoid malignant fibrous histiocytoma) predominantly affects adults in the later decades of life. This entity has more pronounced mitotic activity and cytologic atypia, even in lower grade examples, than is present in aggressive angiomyxoma. Also, myxoid sarcomas usually contain a complex microvascular network with branching and curvilinear capillaries that is notably absent in most benign soft tissue tumors.

Sometimes physiologic conditions, such as childhood asymmetric labium majus enlargement (a.k.a., prepubertal vulvar fibroma or fibrous hyperplasia) [8, 155, 317] and vulvar hypertrophy with lymphedema [313], can also be confused with aggressive angiomyxoma, especially when one is confronted with a biopsy sample unaccompanied by relevant clinical information. Recognition that these poorly-demarcated processes are largely centered in the superficial soft tissues and the absence of many characteristic features of aggressive angiomyxoma, such as a perivascular/perineural myoid proliferation, are important

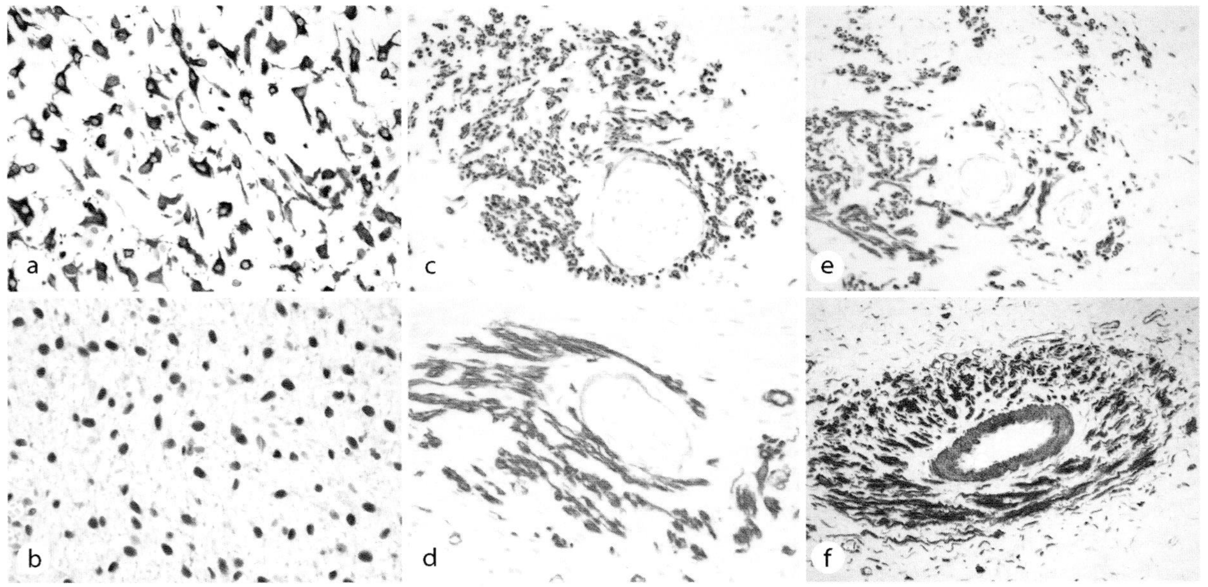

Fig. 22.4
Aggressive angiomyxoma immunohistochemistry. **(a)** desmin reactivity in the small neoplastic cells; **(b)** nuclear immunoreactivity for estrogen receptor protein; **(c, d)** desmin expression in perineural myoid cells; **(e)** desmin expression in perivascular myoid cells (note the actual vessel walls are negative); and **(f)** α-smooth muscle actin is expressed by the perivascular myoid cells and the smooth muscle cells of the vessel wall

first steps in their identification. Additional helpful features include the presence of immunoreactivity for CD34 and absence of desmin expression by the fibroblastic element in childhood asymmetric labial enlargement and the presence of dilated tortuous lymphatics in vulvar hypertrophy with lymphedema.

Behavior and Treatment

Aggressive angiomyxoma has a local recurrence rate that exceeds 35% [44, 92, 123]. As a result, complete excision is preferable if this can be accomplished without undo morbidity. In instances where complete removal would be associated with high morbidity or when preservation of fertility is desired, incomplete removal may be acceptable if the risks of recurrence and additional surgical intervention are understood [44]. All patients require long-term follow-up with periodic imaging analysis, because the tumors are generally slow growing and recurrences are difficult to detect by physical examination. Adjuvant radiation and chemotherapy have no proven role in the management of this tumor. There are anecdotal reports of dramatic responses to hormonal therapy [gonadotropin-releasing hormone (GnRH) agonist] and this may have a role in selected instances, but additional investigation is needed [94, 205].

There are two reports of metastasizing aggressive angiomyxomas. We do not regard the comments and illustrations accompanying the initial case report [280] as convincing, and suspect this patient's pelvic tumor is an unrelated myxoid sarcoma [229]. The most recent case report [25] is more difficult to dismiss, but in the absence of additional similar observations, its significance remains unclear. Certainly, the vast majority of aggressive angiomyxomas do not appear to have metastatic potential.

Superficial Angiomyxoma

Clinical Features

Superficial angiomyxoma (cutaneous myxoma) is a benign mesenchymal neoplasm of the dermis and subcutis that has potential for local recurrence [7, 37, 41, 93]. The process has a wide anatomic distribution and a broad age range, with an overall peak incidence in the 4th to early 5th decade [7, 37]. However, female patients with genital lesions commonly present in their late teens and early 20s [93]. On rare occasion, this tumor is associated with skin pigmentation abnormalities, endocrine overactivity, cardiac myxoma, psammomatous melanotic schwannoma, and other tumor types (Carney complex) [28, 293]. The process has been underrecognized in the vulvoperineal region. In AFIP files, approximately 13% of all cases of superficial angiomyxoma diagnosed in female patients involved this region.

Pathologic Findings

The tumors involve the dermis and subcutis, where they form lobular or multinodular masses that are usually ≤2.5 cm and only rarely >5 cm [41]. They contain abundant hyaluronic acid and a sparse to moderately cellular population of stellate-shaped and spindled cells with pale eosinophilic cytoplasm and mildly pleomorphic nuclei with "smudgy" chromatin and occasional cytoplasmic-nuclear invaginations (➋ *Figs. 22.5* and ➋ *22.6*). Focal multinucleation is common. The myxoid matrix disrupts the mesenchymal element, forming paucicellular pools and cleft-like spaces. The degree of vascularity is variable, but large caliber vessels as seen in aggressive angiomyxoma are typically absent. Scattered inflammatory cells (e.g., polymorphonuclear leukocytes, lymphocytes and plasma cells) are a frequent finding. Adnexal epithelial inclusions, sometimes with cystic change and peripheral buds of basaloid epithelium, are occasionally encountered [7, 41, 93].

The neoplastic cells are vimentin and CD34 positive [93]. Some weak cytoplasmic reactivity for S100 protein can be seen, and there may be limited actin expression. This entity lacks nuclear reactivity for estrogen and progesterone receptor proteins [93]. Negative results are obtained for glial fibrillary acidic protein and desmin.

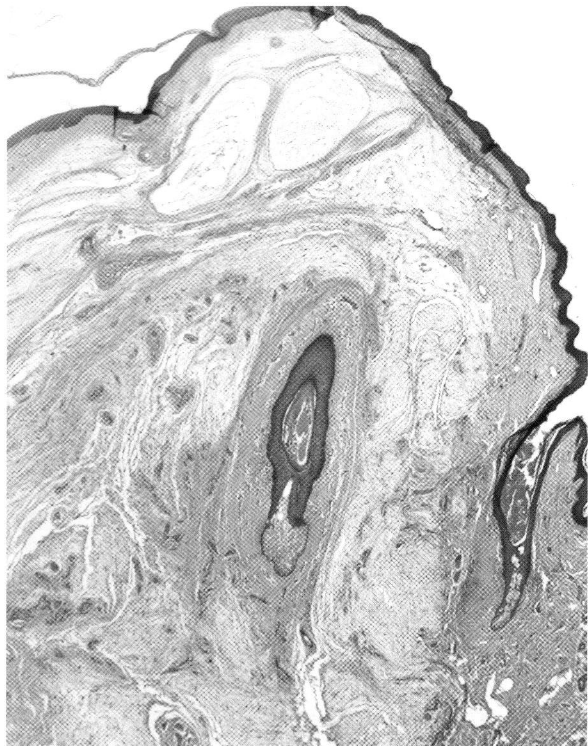

Fig. 22.5
Superficial angiomyxoma (cutaneous myxoma). **Note the multinodular growth pattern, abundant myxoid matrix and presence of paucicellular cleft-like spaces**

Differential Diagnosis

Superficial angiomyxoma has similarity to aggressive angiomyxoma only in name. It is easily distinguished from the latter by its superficial location, small size, abundant alcian blue (pH 2.5)-positive hyaluronic acid content, different tumor cell morphology and immunoprofile.

Behavior and Treatment

Superficial angiomyxoma has a documented recurrence rate of >30%, so complete excision with attention to margins is advisable. There are no reports of metastases. When this process is multifocal, encountered in childhood, or evident in a patient with other unusual clinical findings (e.g., prominent facial skin pigmentation, cardiac symptoms or endocrine abnormalities), evaluation for the Carney complex is recommended.

Angiomyofibroblastoma

Clinical Features

Angiomyofibroblastoma is a benign soft tissue tumor that primarily occurs in the subcutaneous tissue of the vulva. Rare examples have involved the vagina, usually near the introitus [101, 106, 183]. Affected individuals are frequently in the 4th through 7th decades of life, with a peak incidence in the 5th decade [106, 183, 229]. Patients usually present with a relatively small, painless mass.

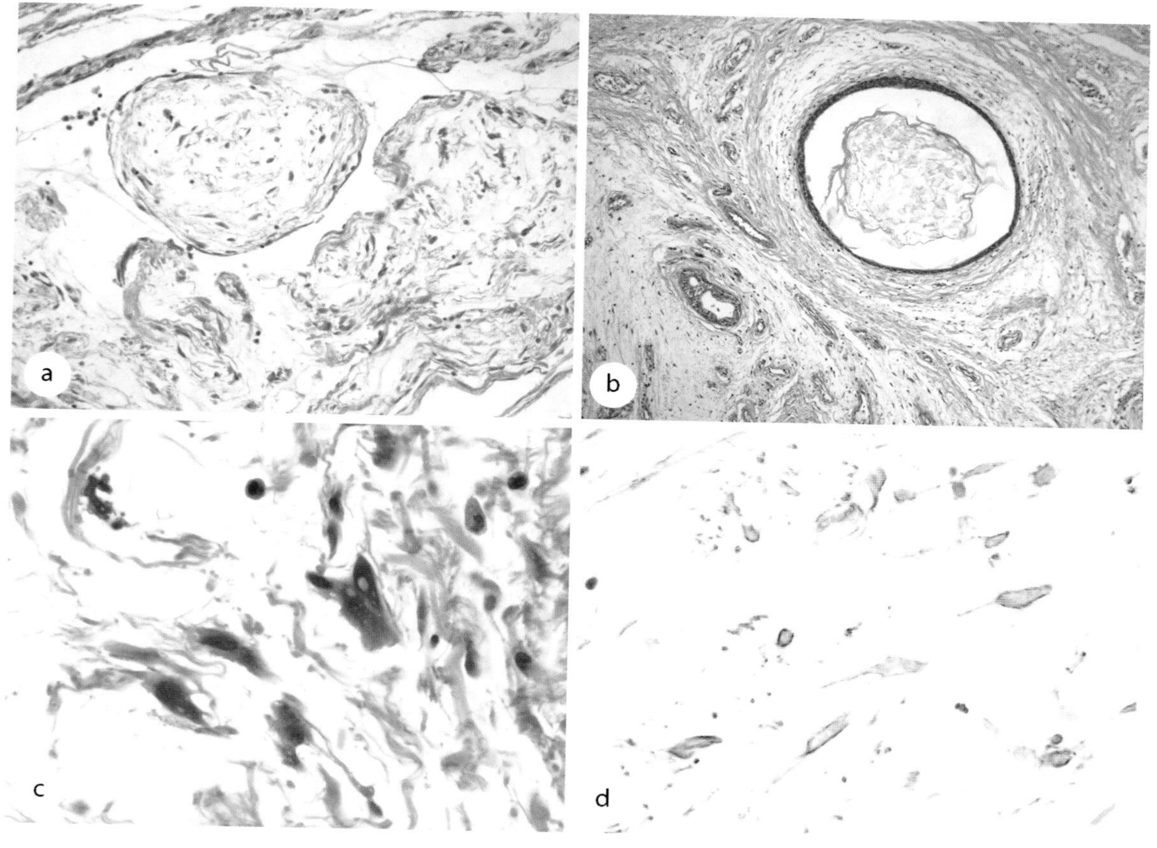

Fig. 22.6
Superficial angiomyxoma. (**a**) tumor nodules often have peripheral cleft-like spaces filled with hyaluronic acid; (**b**) cystic epithelial inclusions may be present; (**c**) tumor cells frequently have smudgy chromatin, and multinucleation and cytoplasmic-nuclear invaginations are common; and (**d**) tumor cells often express CD34

Pathologic Findings

Gross examination generally reveals a well-demarcated mass under 5 cm in size with a soft to rubbery consistency, pinkish tan to yellow color, and mucoid or myxedematous cut surface. Areas grossly consistent with fat may be present.

Microscopic features include relatively sharp margination, low to moderate cellularity, and abundant vasculature that consists predominantly of small capillary-sized vessels and venous segments, sometimes with focal hyalinization (*Figs. 22.7a* and *22.7b*). The cellularity often varies from one region to the next, and some areas may contain abundant myxedematous, loosely collagenized stroma. A polymorphic population of epithelioid, spindled, and multinucleated tumor cells with low level nuclear atypia and a low mitotic rate is typically present. Some epithelioid cells may have abundant eosinophilic cytoplasm, imparting a plasmacytoid appearance. There is a tendency for tumor cells to exhibit focal corded, nested, and trabecular growth patterns and for the cells to aggregate around the vasculature. Adipose tissue is present in >50% of AFIP cases, and in a small percentage, this is a prominent or even dominant feature, as documented in the lipomatous variant of angiomyofibroblastoma (*Figs. 22.7c* and *22.7d*) [38, 183]. Large caliber vessels and medium-sized nerve segments, as seen in aggressive angiomyxoma, are typically absent.

Angiomyofibroblastomas are immunoreactive for vimentin, and they usually express desmin [101, 106, 183, 226] and estrogen and progesterone receptor proteins [183]. There is variable, but generally minimal, reactivity for actins. CD34 expression is notably uncommon in conventional examples, but it is encountered with some

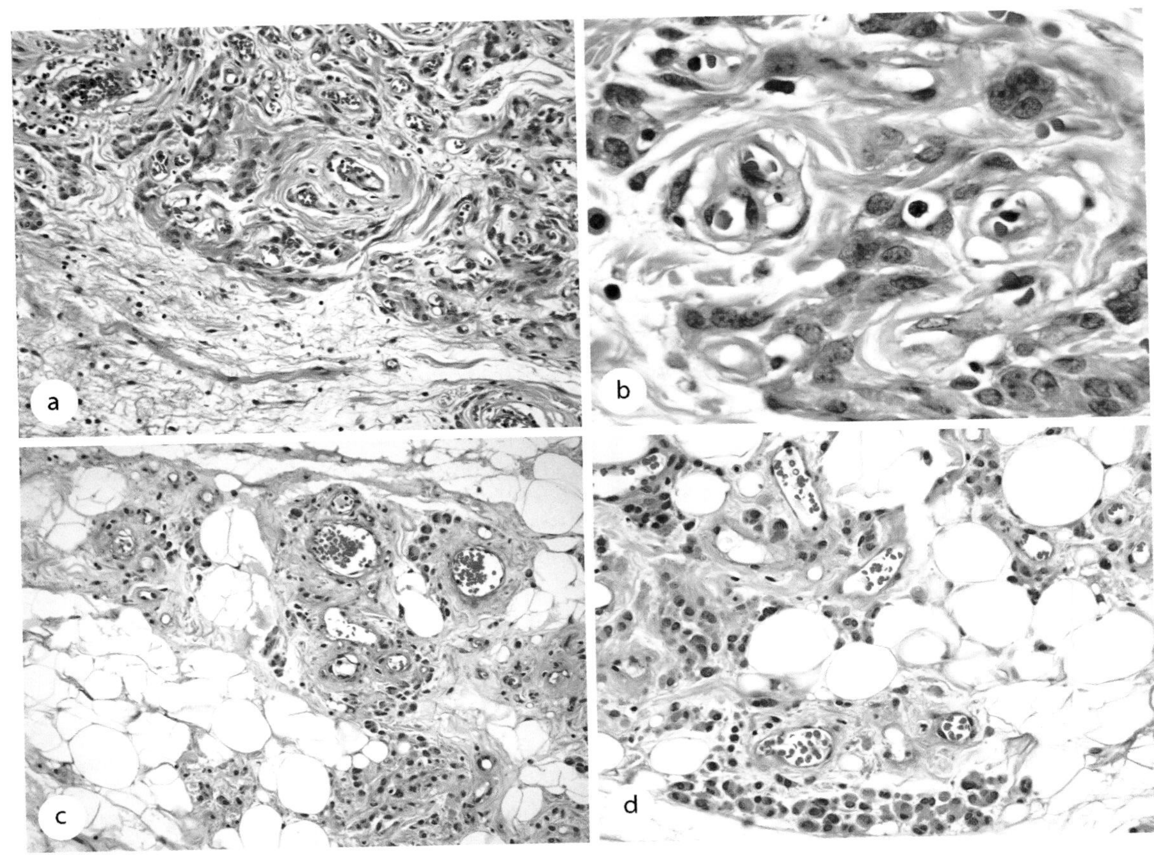

Fig. 22.7
Angiomyofibroblastoma. **Medium and high power views of a conventional (a, b) and lipomatous (c, d) angiomyofibroblastoma. Note a tendency for epithelioid tumor cells to aggregate around the vasculature**

frequency in the lipomatous variant [38, 183]. Some vaginal tumors with desmin and CD34 expression that have been reported as angiomyofibroblastomas are, in our opinion, more consistent with superficial cervicovaginal myofibroblastomas [108, 184, 226]. S100 protein expression and nuclear immunoreactivity for HMGA2 (HMGIC) are absent [235].

Differential Diagnosis

The differential diagnosis for angiomyofibroblastoma revolves primarily around aggressive angiomyxoma and cellular angiofibroma. Aggressive angiomyxomas typically present as large deep-seated masses with a "pushing" infiltrative border. They incorporate a variety of regional structures, including large vessels and nerves that are sometimes bordered by loosely organized collections of spindled myoid (smooth muscle-like) cells. The small neoplastic cells of aggressive angiomyxoma are generally more monomorphic and uniformly distributed than the cells of angiomyofibroblastoma. Although it has been stated in the literature that there are tumors with hybrid features of aggressive angiomyxoma and angiomyofibroblastoma [123], we have yet to encounter a resection specimen where distinction between the two was not possible.

Angiomyofibroblastoma and cellular angiofibroma have some overlapping features, as both present as relatively small superficial masses with high vascularity, both may be dominated by spindled cells, and both can contain fat. However, cellular angiofibroma lacks a prominent epithelioid tumor cell population with a tendency to aggregate around vessels, it can have more pronounced mitotic activity, it often has more notable perivascular hyalinization, and it is much less likely to have desmin expression.

Behavior and Treatment

Angiomyofibroblastoma is typically cured by simple local excision. There is a single unique case report of an angiomyofibroblastoma with sarcomatous transformation (angiomyofibrosarcoma) in an elderly female [230]. The sarcomatous component resembled myxofibrosarcoma (myxoid malignant fibrous histiocytoma).

Cellular Angiofibroma

Clinical Features

Cellular angiofibroma [156, 229, 237] (angiomyofibroblastoma-like tumor) [182] is a recently described benign superficial soft tissue tumor of the vulvoperineal and inguinal regions. Vaginal examples have been reported, but in our experience, these are usually located at the introitus. The process generally affected individuals in the 4th through 8th decades of life, with a median age in the 40s [156]. Most lesions are painless.

Pathologic Findings

Gross examination usually reveals a small (often <3 cm) well-demarcated mass with a cut surface similar to angiomyofibroblastoma.

Histologically, the tumors are generally well-circumscribed, and they contain a moderately cellular spindle cell population associated with numerous, rather uniformly distributed, small to medium sized vessels, oftentimes with perivascular hyaline fibrosis (➋ *Fig. 22.8*). Myxedematous matrix associated with wispy collagen, foci with thick eosinophilic collagen bundles, variable amounts of fat

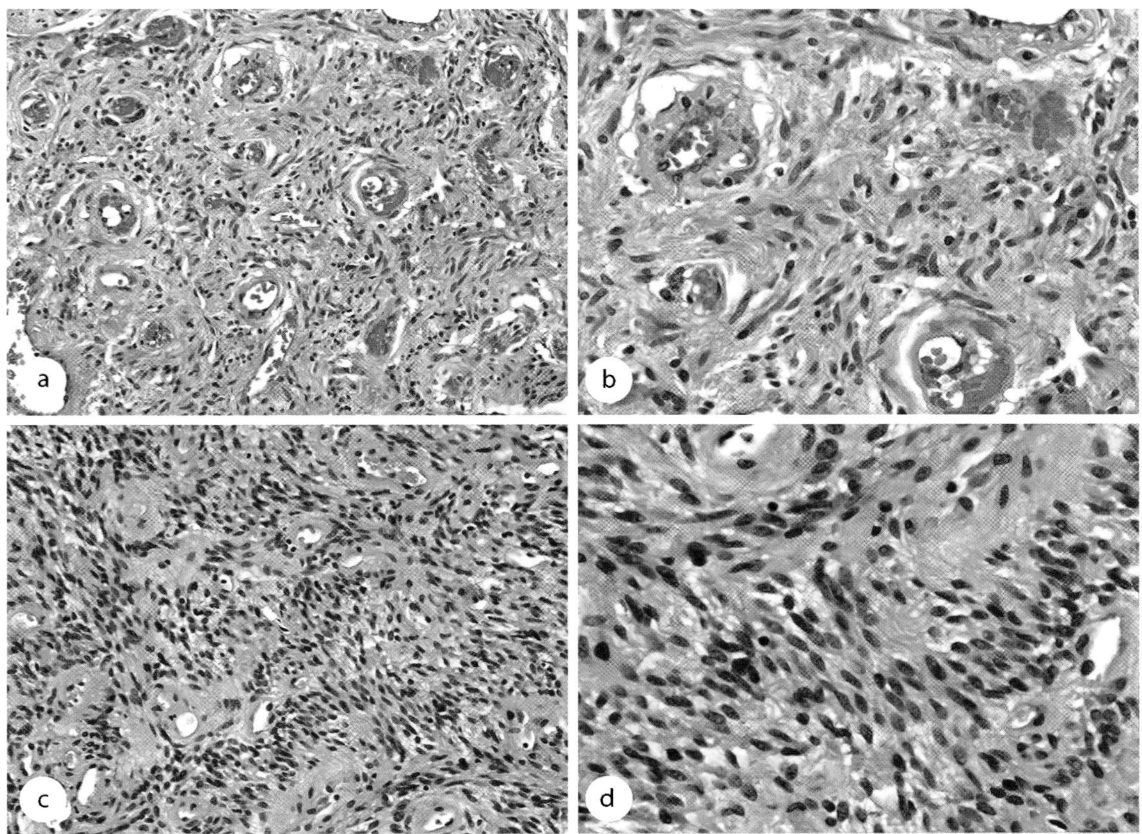

Fig. 22.8
Cellular angiofibroma. **Medium (a, c) and high (b, d) power views of two different cases. Note the appearance of the spindled tumor cells and numerous thick-walled vessels**

(present in up to 50% of cases), and a variety of degenerative changes (including hemorrhagic, cystic, and pseudoangiomatous stromal changes) may be present. Mitotic activity is usually sparse, but in exceptional cases, it can be relatively brisk [156]. Atypical mitotic figures are not present. Tumor cell nuclei generally have minimal or only low level atypia, but rare examples may have small areas where atypia is more pronounced. Tumor necrosis is absent.

There are notable differences in the reported immunoprofile for this tumor, and further study is needed to resolve some of these discrepancies. Strong diffuse reactivity is consistently present for vimentin, and CD34 expression has been reported in close to half of the cases [63, 156, 182]. Actin and desmin expression are seen in <20% and <10% of tumors, respectively. Estrogen and progesterone receptor proteins have been documented in up to 50% of cases.

Differential Diagnosis

Cellular angiofibroma has some morphologic overlap with both angiomyofibroblastoma and spindle cell lipoma, and these are the key considerations in the differential diagnosis of this entity [156, 182, 237]. Features that aid in distinguishing angiomyofibroblastoma from cellular angiofibroma are documented in the preceding text. Spindle cell lipoma is notably uncommon in the vulvar region. It generally features a greater adipocytic component, less pronounced vasculature, and more ropy collagen than cellular angiofibroma. Its spindle cell component also more consistently expresses CD34.

Behavior and Treatment

Cellular angiofibroma is optimally managed by complete local excision. Special attention to margins is advisable for those rare examples with a high mitotic rate and more pronounced atypia. Local recurrences are very uncommon [182, 207], and there are no reports of metastasis.

Granular Cell Tumor

In the older medical literature, this entity is often referred to as "granular cell myoblastoma." A few recent publications use the designation "granular cell schwannoma," reflecting the currently accepted cell of origin, but most authors continue to favor the above terminology.

Clinical Features

It has been estimated that 5–16% of all granular cell tumors occur in the vulvar region [52, 190, 223, 229]. The labia majus are most frequently involved, but other areas, including the mons pubis, clitoris, perineum and perianal region, may also be affected [148, 223, 329]. Approximately 70–80 cases arising in the female genital region are documented in the literature, and AFIP files contain an additional 62 examples (5.1% of all cases diagnosed in females). We have encountered an age range of 14–73 years, with a peak incidence in the 4th decade. Patients usually present with an asymptomatic mass, though occasionally pain or pruritus are present. The process is commonly misdiagnosed clinically, and in some instances, it can grossly resemble squamous cell carcinoma. Granular cell tumors occur with increased frequency in African-Americans, they are multifocal in 3–20% of cases, and rarely, they may be familial [178, 190, 198, 223, 255, 261]. Once a diagnosis has been rendered, some authors advocate a detailed clinical history and thorough physical examination to rule out the presence of other clinically occult lesions, as they can sometimes affect anatomically sensitive sites, such as the airways [9, 52, 190, 191]. Rarely, granular cell tumors have been reported to involve the vagina, uterine cervix and ovaries [107, 114, 261]. The vast majority of granular cell tumors are benign, with malignant behavior documented in no more than 1–2% of cases [89, 148, 190, 261, 266].

Pathologic Findings

More than 75% of gynecologic-related granular cell tumors in the AFIP files are <2 cm in size; examples ≥5 cm are exceptional. Epidermal or mucosal ulceration is occasionally present. The lesions have a firm consistency, and the cut surface often demonstrates a radially symmetrical, circumscribed or stellate-shaped, whitish-tan to yellowish mass.

Histologically, granular cell tumors feature large epithelioid and focally spindled neoplastic cells with abundant coarsely granular eosinophilic cytoplasm (➋ *Fig. 22.9*). Nuclei are hyperchromatic and generally fairly uniform in size, but foci with mild to moderate pleomorphism are occasionally encountered. Nucleoli may be present or inconspicuous. Usually, mitotic figures are only rarely encountered. The tumors may form relatively well-demarcated masses with little stromal reaction, or they can have an infiltrative, stellate-shaped appearance with prominent

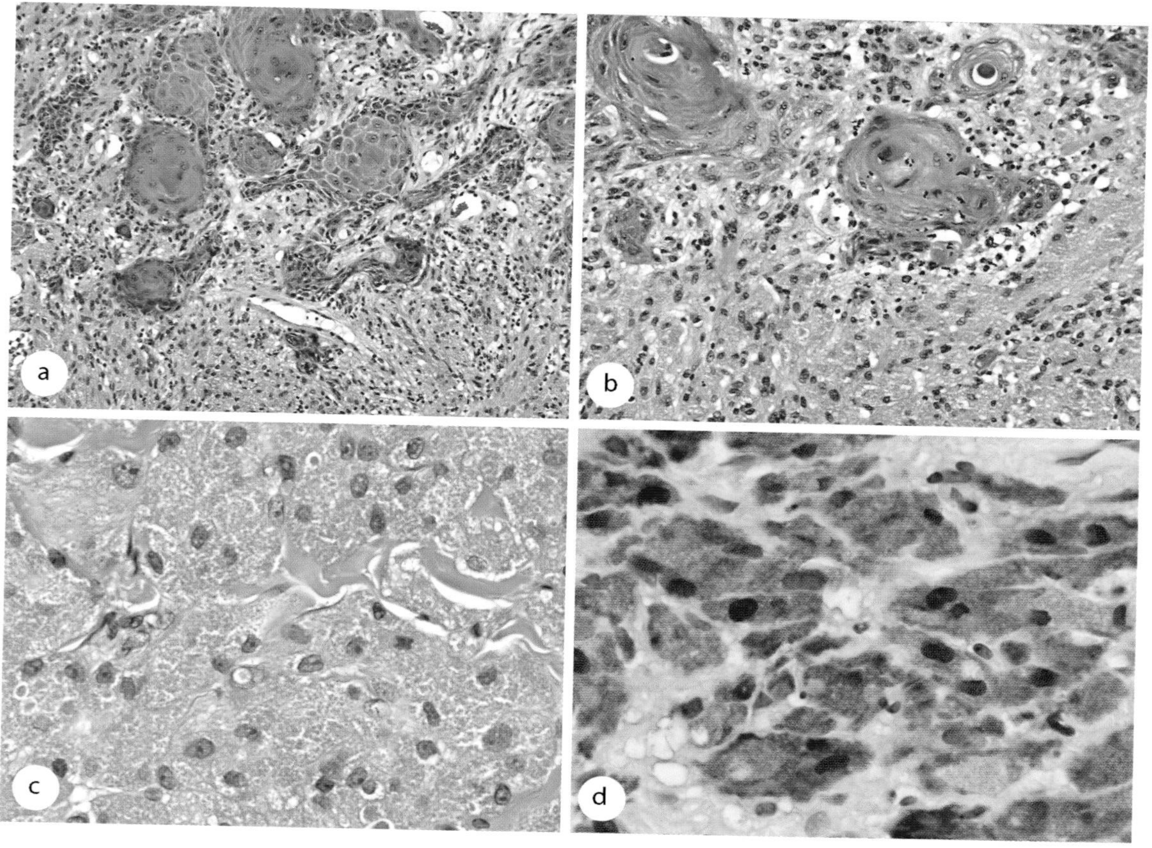

Fig. 22.9
Granular cell tumor. (**a**, **b**) medium and high power views of a granular cell tumor with pseudoepitheliomatous hyperplasia of the overlying squamous epithelium; (**c**) a high power view of the neoplastic Schwann cells demonstrating granular cytoplasm and nuclei with small nucleoli and scattered cytoplasmic-nuclear invaginations; and (**d**) both nuclear and cytoplasmic immunoreactivity for S100 protein is present

desmoplasia. Some examples are intimately associated with small nerve trunks. The bulk of cases involve the dermis and subcutis, and >25% of cases induce pseudoepitheliomatous hyperplasia of the overlying squamous epithelium. This can be misinterpreted as an invasive squamous cell carcinoma, especially in undersampled or superficially biopsied lesions where the granular cell population is not readily apparent [295, 329].

Attention should be paid to the tumor growth pattern and margins [9]. Although data are limited, there is some evidence suggesting gynecologic granular cell tumors with a well-defined nodular appearance and "pushing" border may have little potential for local recurrence when marginally excised. In contrast, tumors with an infiltrative edge seem to carry substantial risk for local recurrence.

Malignant granular cell tumors are often large, and they usually have extensive and conspicuous cytologic abnormality, not merely focal atypia. Rarely, the malignant potential of a granular cell tumor can be difficult to predict, because prominent atypia may be absent. However, in most instances, a combination of the following histologic features help with prognostication: tumor necrosis, *prominent* spindling of the tumor cells, *prominent* nuclear pleomorphism, *many* large vesicular nuclei with *macro*nucleoli, *many* cells with a high n/c ratio, and >2 mitoses/10 HPFs (especially if mitotic activity is widespread and accompanied by atypical mitotic figures). Fanburg-Smith et al. [89] regard the presence of three or more of these findings as an indication of malignant potential. Granular cell tumors meeting one or two of these criteria were interpreted as atypical, but no atypical tumors (only nine examples with follow-up) were demonstrated to have metastatic potential.

Granular cell tumors have immunoreactivity for S100 protein (nuclear and cytoplasmic), CD68, calretinin, and vimentin. They are nonreactive for keratins, EMA, actins, desmin, chromogranin, and HMB-45.

Differential Diagnosis

The differential diagnosis for granular cell tumor includes true histiocytic, "fibrohistiocytic," melanocytic, myogenic and epithelial tumors with granular cytoplasm. Most of these tumors can be easily ruled out with the immunoresults noted above. Histiocytic tumors often feature mononucleated cells with reniform nuclei, as well as multinucleated giant cells. When histiocytes are present en masse, "windowing" may be noted between the cells due to abundant surface pilopodia. Histiocytic proliferations commonly express CD68 and CD163, and some have immunoreactivity for CD45RB and other markers, such as CD1a or S100 protein. Benign fibrohistiocytic tumors are usually superficial (most are dermal-based), they commonly have a stellate configuration, and they feature a more heterogenous population of cells than granular cell tumor. The scattered S100 protein-positive cells randomly distributed in some fibrohistiocytic tumors are usually nonlesional dendritic cells.

Behavior and Treatment

The vast majority (≥98%) of granular cell tumors are benign. Many gynecologic authors recommend conservative wide local excision for these tumors to minimize the risk of local recurrence. However, simple local excision may prove adequate for examples with well-defined nodular growth. The most important prognostic factor for malignant granular cell tumors is tumor size [89]. These neoplasms tend to affect older patients than benign granular cell tumors, and they often behave as high-grade malignancies with a tendency to metastasize to regional lymph nodes, the lungs and bones. As a result, they warrant aggressive intervention. The possibility of multiple independent lesions should always be considered before assuming metastasis in the setting of granular cell tumor.

Schwannoma (Neurilemoma)

While there are rare reports of schwannoma involving the vulva [137, 325], vagina [78], uterine cervix [135, 189], uterine body, fallopian tubes [77], broad and round ligaments, and ovaries, most schwannomas occurring in the vicinity of genital organs arise in the pelvic retroperitoneum [151, 167, 309]. Vulvar schwannomas most commonly affect the labia [271], but other sites including the clitoris [54, 150] may be affected. Most schwannomas are of the classical type, but infrequent examples are plexiform [54, 271, 331, 333] (usually superficial) or cellular [325] (usually deep-seated).

Clinical Features

Superficial schwannomas often present as a firm, well-demarcated, nodular mass. Retroperitoneal examples may be incidentally discovered during evaluation for unrelated problems. Central degeneration and cystic change are frequent imaging findings [151]. Plexiform schwannomas may have a multinodular, "bag of worms" appearance when imaged. Symptoms are often absent, but sometimes patients report pain radiating along the course of the affected nerve segment.

Pathologic Findings

The lesions are sharply demarcated and moderately firm. The cut surface ranges from gray-white to yellow. Hemorrhagic foci and cystic areas with brownish liquid are sometimes present. These tumors lack the whorled cut surface common to smooth muscle neoplasms.

Histologically, the process is encapsulated. Deep-seated examples may be bordered by a thick rind of fibrous tissue with patchy chronic inflammation, and there may be adherence to adjacent structures. The lesions contain spindled Schwann cells with alternating patterns of growth (➲ *Fig. 22.10*). Antoni A areas have minimal myxoid matrix and more pronounced cellularity. These areas can have fascicular growth, as well as foci with nuclear palisading and Verocay body formations. Antoni B foci have myxoid matrix, lower cellularity and less ordered growth. Thick-walled vessels and perivascular xanthoma cells are frequent findings in schwannomas, and central cystic and hemorrhagic degeneration may be noted. Varying degrees of nuclear atypia (often viewed as "degenerative") can be present. Mitotic figures are generally uncommon, but they may be evident. Mitotic activity has much less clinical significance in a schwannoma than in a neurofibroma.

Cellular schwannomas are usually deep-seated, and they tend to be larger than conventional schwannomas [325].

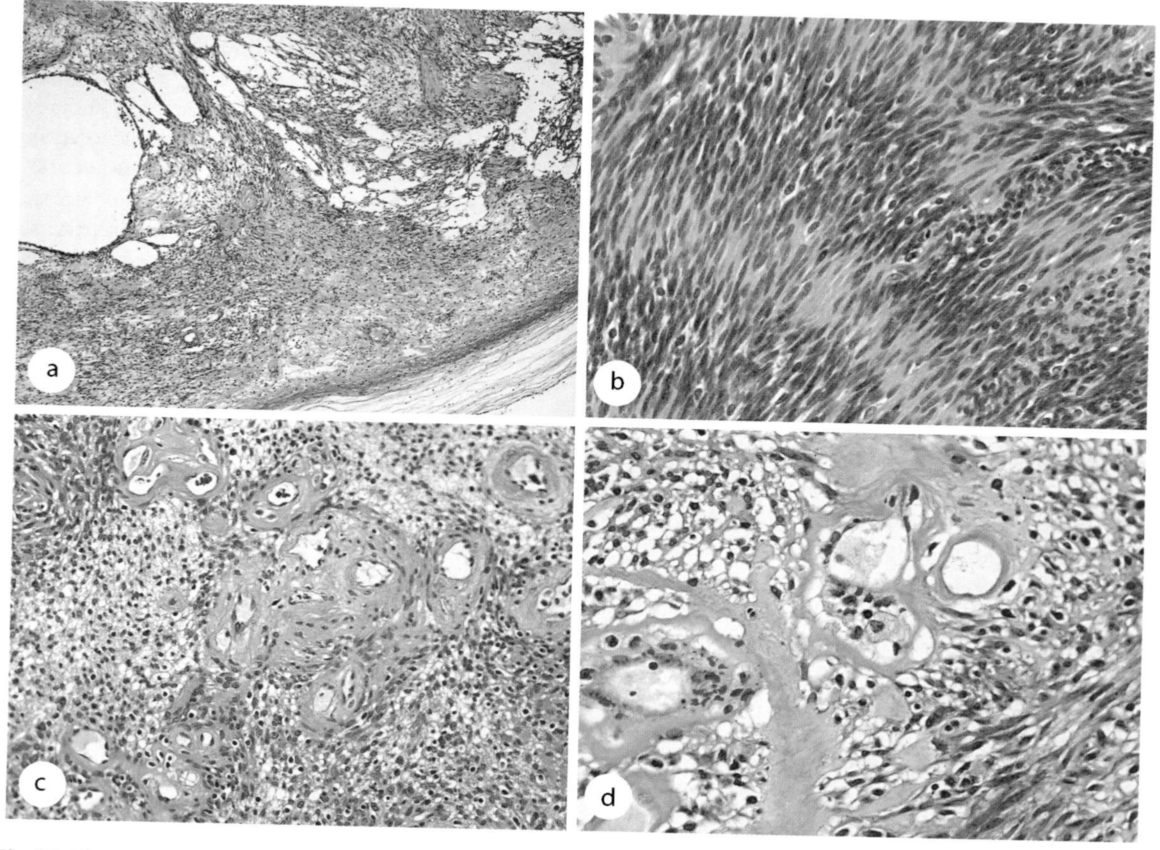

Fig. 22.10
Schwannoma. **(a)** a low power view demonstrating encapsulation and central cystic degeneration; **(b)** neoplastic Schwann cells with tapered nuclei and prominent nuclear palisading; **(c)** thick-walled vessels and **(d)** perivascular xanthoma cells

These tumors feature a prominent Antoni A component, and oftentimes, they have ≤10% Antoni B growth. Verocay bodies are generally absent. Because of high cellularity, focal nuclear atypia, and mitotic activity (usually ≤4 mitoses/10 HPFs), cellular schwannomas can be confused with sarcomas [325].

All schwannomas should have extensive nuclear and cytoplasmic immunoreactivity for S100 protein. Some examples also express GFAP. Infrequently, focal keratin expression is noted and is thought to be due to keratin antibodies crossreacting with GFAP epitopes. Schwann cells are nonreactive for actins and desmin.

Behavior and Treatment

Schwannomas are usually cured by local excision, and recurrences are very uncommon (<5%). Deep-seated examples can be difficult to excise because of proximity and adherence to regional structures, such as major vessels and the ureters, and removal is sometimes complicated by substantial blood loss [167, 325]. Malignant transformation of a true schwannoma is an extremely rare event.

Neurofibroma and Neurofibromatosis-1

Clinical Features

Neurofibromatosis-1 (NF1) is an autosomal dominant disorder that affects approximately 1 in 3,000 individuals [264]. The process has virtually 100% penetrance, and it is progressive, but there is marked variation in expressivity [264]. Approximately half of the patients have an affected parent, and the other half represent new mutations. Excellent reviews [134, 264] that include a summary of diagnostic criteria for this disorder are included in our references [134]. Six to eighteen percent of female patients with NF1 are reported to develop neurofibromas in the vulvar region [32, 47, 112, 276]. However, <1% are documented to have vaginal involvement. While there are a few reports of neurofibromas involving the uterine cervix [36, 47, 112, 122, 321], other sites, such as the uterine body [122, 335], fallopian tubes and ovaries [122, 138], are only very rarely affected.

Clitoral and preputial neurofibromas are often congenital, and in many cases, they are the presenting sign of NF1 in the pediatric population [26, 138, 297]. These lesions may be clinically confused with ambiguous genitalia, but they have a firmer consistency than hormonally-induced phallus enlargement [26, 297]. Careful examination often reveals the patients to have multiple cutaneous café-au-lait spots, but other diagnostic manifestations of NF1 may be absent in this age group and may not become evident until at or around the time of puberty [26, 32, 233, 265, 276, 297]. For many pediatric patients, clinical confirmation of NF1 hinges on documentation of an affected first degree relative [297].

Vaginal and cervical neurofibromas are usually diagnosed in early adulthood and are rarely seen outside of the setting of NF1. Approximately 30% of vaginal neurofibromas are detected during pregnancy or manifest as an obstructive complication during delivery [269]. Many patients with vaginal neurofibromas have co-existing bladder and/or vulvar disease [26, 47, 119, 265, 297]. For some individuals, urinary tract signs or symptoms are the presenting feature [47].

Localized cutaneous neurofibromas of the vulva are encountered throughout life but are uncommon before the age of 20. These tumors may be sporadic, or they may be associated with NF1.

Pathologic Findings

Localized, plexiform, and diffuse neurofibromas have all been reported in the genital region (➲ *Fig. 22.11*). Most clitoral and deep-seated genitourinary tract neurofibromas associated with NF1 are either plexiform neurofibromas or neurofibromas with an admixture of diffuse and plexiform features. Plexiform neurofibromas grossly distort nerve segments and impart a macroscopic "bag of worms" appearance. Diffuse neurofibromas form ill-defined, typically large, expansile masses with an off-white color. Localized neurofibromas may be ill-defined or discrete, depending on how much of the process is intraneural. These latter lesions may form a solid mass with a rubbery consistency or they may be soft and fluctuant due to abundant myxoid matrix. Very rarely, neurofibromas may be pigmented.

Neurofibromas contain neoplastic S100 protein-positive Schwann cells admixed with other nerve sheath elements (i.e., neurofilament protein-positive neuraxons, CD34-positive intraneural fibroblasts, and occasional EMA-positive perineurial cells). The Schwann cells usually have elongate bipolar cytoplasmic processes and wavy, tapered, dark-staining nuclei. Growth tends to be more random than in a schwannoma, and myxoid matrix is often more widely distributed. Nuclear palisading and Verocay bodies are usually not present. Mitotic figures are absent or extremely sparse in almost all instances. When high cellularity or significant nuclear atypia is accompanied by notable mitotic activity and/or necrosis, malignancy warrants strong consideration.

Diffuse neurofibromas often have Schwann cells with shorter cytoplasmic processes and less tapered (more ovoid) nuclei than are encountered in most other neurofibroma types. These cells tend to grow in a permeative, diffuse fashion with random or sometimes vague storiform orientation. Entrapment of regional structures is characteristic, and many examples contain small abnormal nerve twigs that give rise to Wagner-Meissner-like bodies (➲ *Fig. 22.11d*). As noted above, this neurofibroma variant can be seen in association with a plexiform neurofibroma. When a diffuse neurofibroma involves skin, it can sometimes be confused with dermatofibrosarcoma protuberans (DFSP), an error compounded by the fact that both processes contain cells with immunoreactivity for CD34 (➲ *Fig. 22.12*). However, in diffuse neurofibroma, there is a dual population of cells, delicate CD34-positive fibroblast-like cells and S100 protein-positive Schwann cells, and the latter component is absent in DFSP.

The postpartum microneuroma is a form of traumatic neuroma linked to parturition and should not be confused with a true neurofibroma [304]. These small (usually ≤1 mm) incidental cervical lesions consist of disorganized, but otherwise relatively unremarkable, nerve twigs that often satellite around a larger nerve segment.

Behavior and Treatment

Localized neurofibromas that cause cosmetic concern or are subject to constant irritation are generally managed by conservative resection. The recommended treatment for clitoral neurofibromas is clitoroplasty with preservation of the neurovascular bundle and glandular tissue [297]. When neurofibromas are extensive, functionally

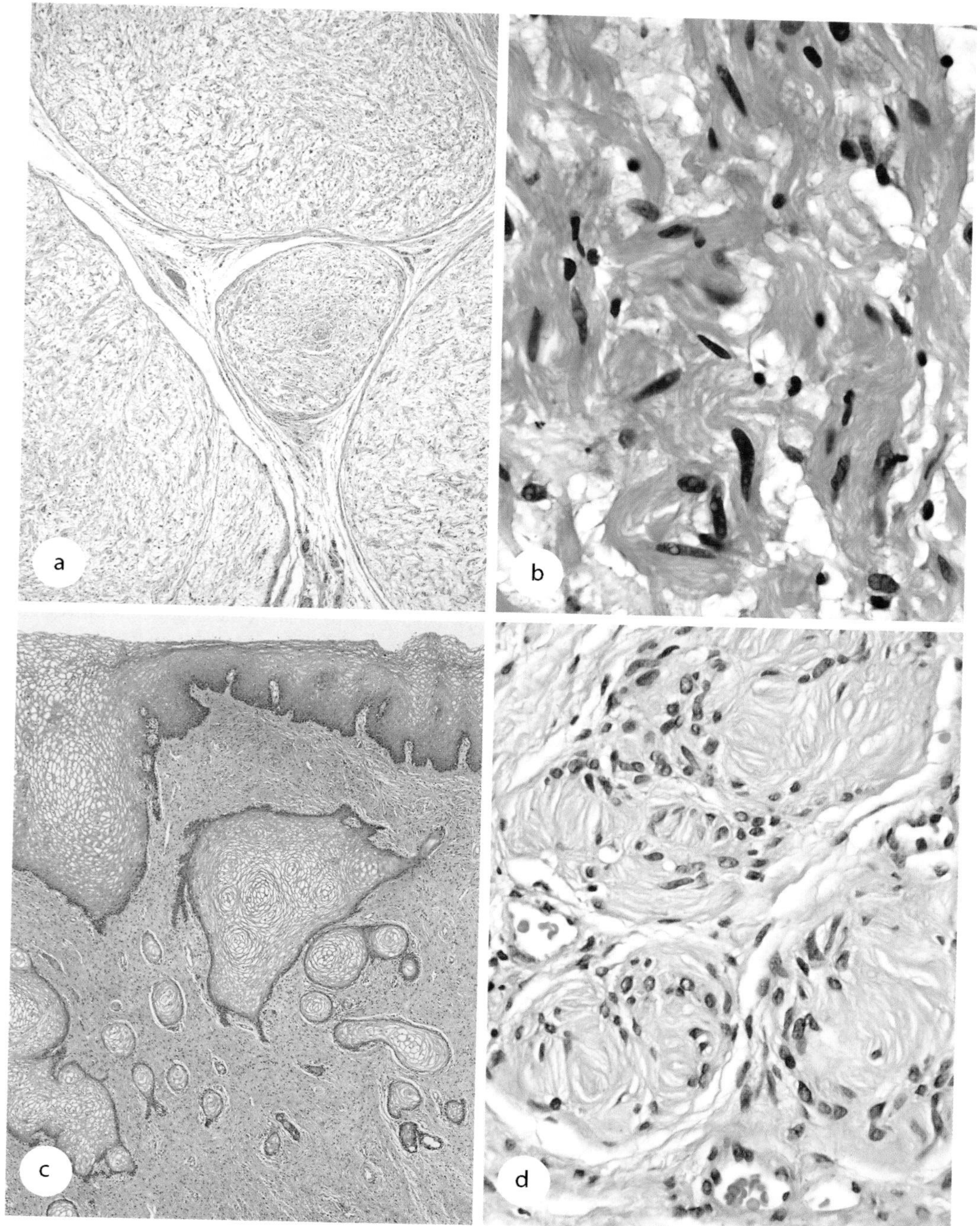

Fig. 22.11
Neurofibromas. Figures (**a**, **b**) depict an intraneural neurofibroma with abundant myxoid matrix. Note the dark staining, tapered and focally undulating, Schwann cell nuclei in figure (b). Figures (**c**, **d**) illustrate a diffuse neurofibroma from the vagina of an NF1 patient. Note vaginal epithelial changes in figure (c) reminiscent of that encountered with granular cell tumors, and the presence of Wagner-Meissner-like bodies (d)

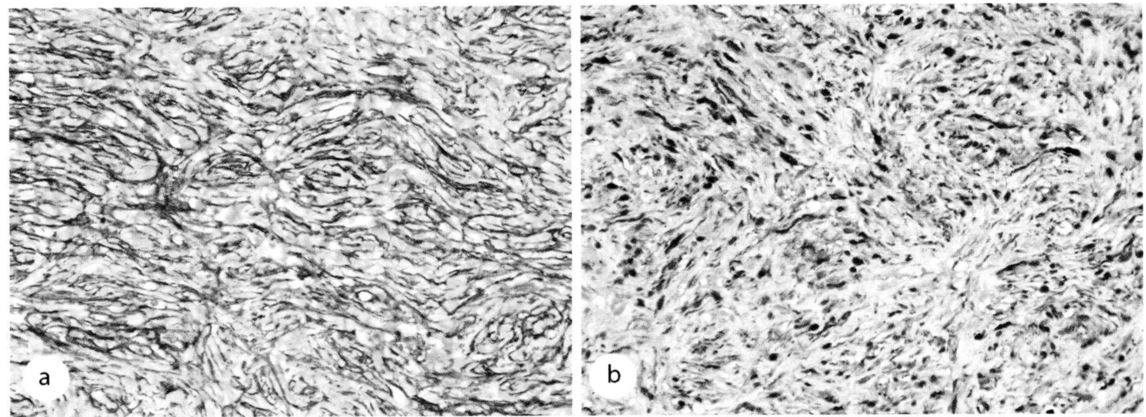

Fig. 22.12
Neurofibroma. **CD34 (a) and S100 protein (b) results for a diffuse neurofibroma. CD34 highlights numerous delicate fibroblast-like spindled cells, and S100 protein highlights the neoplastic Schwann cell population**

compromising and symptomatic, more aggressive intervention may be required. However, complete excision can be very difficult to achieve and may be impossible for many large plexiform neurofibromas of the genitourinary region [49]. Sudden growth in a pre-existing neurofibroma warrants immediate attention because of the risk of malignant transformation.

Nodular Fasciitis

Clinical Features

Nodular fasciitis typically presents as a rapidly growing mass of less than 2 months duration. The process may be asymptomatic or accompanied by mild pain or tenderness. The number of reported examples involving the vulva is small, totaling only 12 cases through 1998 [13, 240]. However, 26 examples of vulvar nodular fasciitis are present in the AFIP files (1.1% of cases diagnosed in females). A predilection for the labia, especially the labia majus, has been noted. Patients documented in the literature have ranged in age from 7 to 51 years. AFIP patients have ranged from 8 to 58 years with a peak incidence in the 4th decade and a median age of 34 years.

Pathologic Findings

Nodular fasciitis generally forms a well-circumscribed mass, usually <3 cm and almost always <5 cm in size. The median size for AFIP cases is 1.9 cm. The lesions have a cut surface that varies in appearance from myxoid, sometimes with focal cystic change, to fibrous.

Histologically, nodular fasciitis tends to form a lobulated mass with a relatively uniform population of plump "activated" (myo)fibroblasts with minimal atypia and no pleomorphism (*Fig. 22.13*). These spindle cells tend to be arranged in a loose, "feathery," tissue-culture-like growth pattern with scattered small areas of mucoid degeneration. More compact growth is sometimes present, especially at the tumor periphery. A sprinkling of intralesional lymphocytes is common, and occasional osteoclast-like giant cells may be encountered in the areas with mucoid degeneration. Mitotic figures can be abundant, but they are not atypical. Some later stage examples have central hyalinized (keloid-like) collagen.

The spindle cell population is usually immunoreactive for α-smooth muscle actin and muscle-specific actin, and it is generally negative for desmin [218]. No reactivity is present for S100 protein, CD34, or keratins. The osteoclast-like giant cells are readily highlighted with CD68 (KP-1).

Differential Diagnosis

Because of cellularity and mitotic activity, nodular fasciitis can be misinterpreted as a spindle cell sarcoma. However, helpful clues to correct classification are the small size and lobular contour of the mass, presence of areas with mucoid degeneration, lack of significant nuclear atypia or pleomorphism, and absence of atypical mitotic figures.

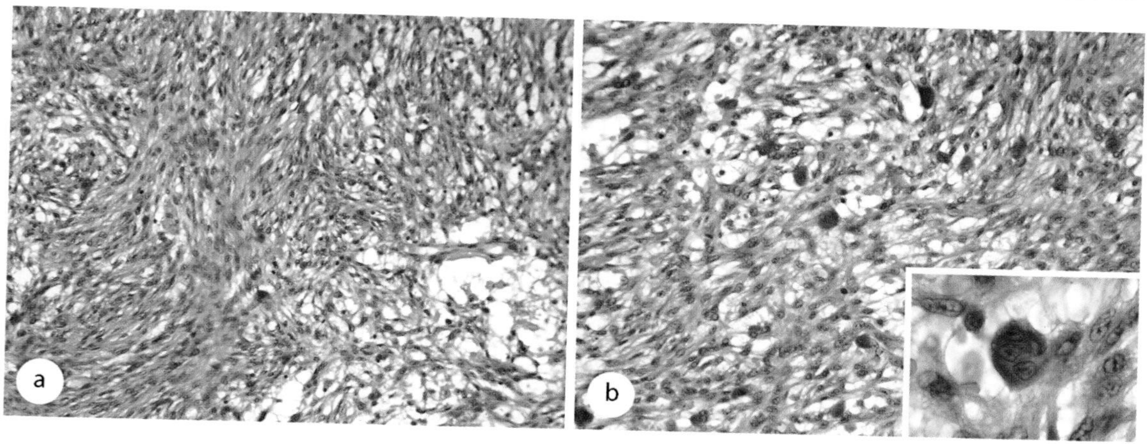

Fig. 22.13
Nodular fasciitis. **Note the loose tissue culture-like growth pattern and areas with mucoid degeneration (a). Scattered osteoclast-like giant cells are present in figure (b) and its inset**

Behavior and Treatment

Nodular fasciitis is a benign self-limiting condition, usually cured by simple local excision. Local recurrence is encountered in no more than 1–2% of cases and usually occurs shortly after an incomplete initial procedure. When a recurrence develops at the site of a previously diagnosed nodular fasciitis, the original specimen should be reevaluated to insure accuracy of the initial interpretation.

Desmoid Tumor (Musculoaponeurotic Fibromatosis)

Clinical Features

Desmoid tumors are rare with an estimated incidence of 2.4–4.3 new cases per 10^6 population per year [262]. These lesions have a wide anatomic distribution, but the single most common location is the anterior abdominal wall. Tumors at this site have a very strong female predilection (in AFIP files, the F:M ratio is >8:1). They usually occur between the ages of 18 and 40 and often develop during gestation or within the first year after childbirth. As a result, desmoids are one of the more common fibrogenic neoplasms encountered by gynecologists. Much more rarely, gynecologists may also be confronted with pelvic desmoids located in the iliac fossa or lower pelvic region [61, 100, 169, 200, 202, 228, 281]. These tumors also have a female predominance and occur over the same age range as abdominal wall desmoids. However, in AFIP files, they are more than 20 times rarer than abdominal wall desmoids. Although no clear link between pelvic desmoids and pregnancy or childbirth has been established in the literature, on recent review of in-house material, we noted a possible association with gestation in up to 40% of cases. Most desmoid tumors are sporadic, but some cases are associated with familial adenomatous polyposis/Gardner syndrome.

Pathologic Findings

Regardless of the anatomic site, desmoid tumors share certain gross and microscopic findings. They form poorly-circumscribed, firm masses that are often intimately associated with fascia and muscle. On cut section, they have a coarsely trabeculated off-white appearance. Histologically, the process is moderately cellular, infiltrative and composed of spindled cells with only mild nuclear atypia and no significant pleomorphism (*Fig. 22.14a*). The neoplastic cells often have small, but distinct, central nucleoli. Mitotic activity is variable but usually low. Abundant collagenous or myxocollagenous matrix is present, and the lesional cells are generally arranged in loose fascicular and broad storiform growth patterns. The vasculature tends to consist of evenly spaced, thin-walled vessels with slit-like or rounded lumens. Immunoreactivity is typically present for α-smooth muscle actin and muscle-specific actin, and some cases may have a small amount of reactivity for desmin. The vast majority of tumors also have at least focal nuclear staining for β-catenin (*Fig. 22.14b*) [23, 40].

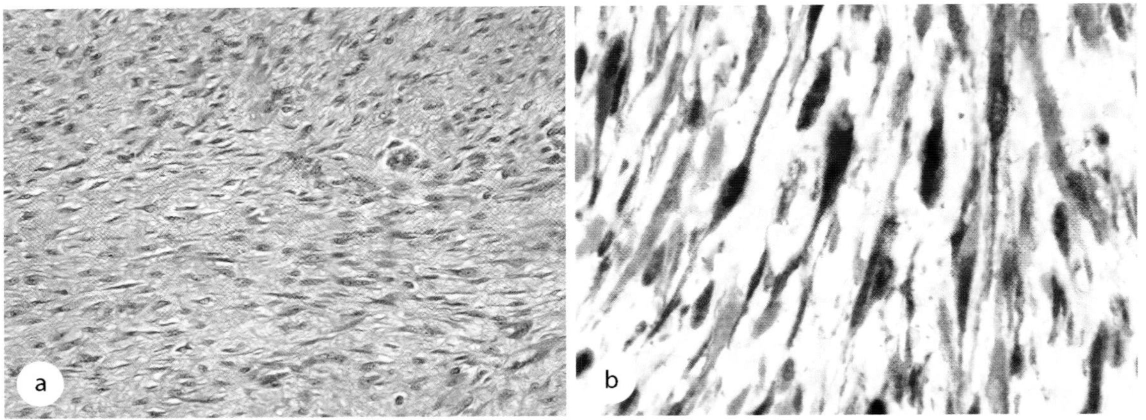

Fig. 22.14
Desmoid tumor. **A medium power view (a) of a desmoid tumor illustrating broad fascicular growth, and a high power view (b) demonstrating nuclear and cytoplasmic immunoreactivity for β-catenin**

Behavior and Treatment

Desmoid tumors have a strong propensity for local recurrence and are optimally managed by complete excision with wide tumor-free margins. In instances where this cannot be achieved without undo morbidity, lesser intervention is often advocated, because desmoid tumors do not metastasize [202]. In cases where tumor-free margins are not achieved, radiation therapy may be beneficial [158]. Other forms of therapy, including hormonal therapy [326], have also been tried with varying degrees of success. Radical surgery is generally reserved for cases where all other reasonable treatment options have been exhausted.

Genital Rhabdomyoma

In the past, genital rhabdomyomas were often regarded as a subtype of fetal rhabdomyoma. However, most soft tissue experts now view them as a separate and distinct tumor type.

Clinical Features

Approximately 39 genital rhabdomyomas have been documented in the literature [19, 73, 121, 154, 160, 175, 296]. More than 80% of tumors have involved the vagina, where they form an asymptomatic polypoid mass, typically in the 1–3 cm size range. The remaining cases are equally divided between the portio vaginalis/uterine cervix and vulva. Patients have ranged in age from 8 to 54 years, but the overwhelming majority present in their 4th and 5th decades. Tumors involving the vulva tend to manifest much earlier in life (age range: 8–24 years) [154].

Pathologic Findings

Gross examination typically reveals a polypoid or cauliflower-like mass with a mucosal surface. The average tumor size is approximately 2 cm. Histologic examination reveals fibrous stroma with interlacing collections of large strap-like cells admixed with scattered plump epithelioid cells with abundant eosinophilic cytoplasm (➲ *Fig. 22.15*). Close inspection usually reveals occasional tumor cells with cytoplasmic cross-striations (➲ *Fig. 22.15b* inset), highlightable with Masson trichrome and phosphotungstic acid-hematoxylin (PTAH) stains. The neoplastic cells usually have one large centrally located nucleus with a vesicular chromatin pattern and a prominent central nucleolus. Occasional multinucleated cells may be present. Anaplasia and mitotic activity are absent. No subepithelial "cambium" layer effect, as seen with botryoid rhabdomyosarcomas, is present.

Immunoreactivity is present for muscle-specific actin, desmin, myoglobin, and nuclear regulatory proteins for skeletal muscle differentiation (especially myogenin, personal observation). No reactivity is present for epithelial markers.

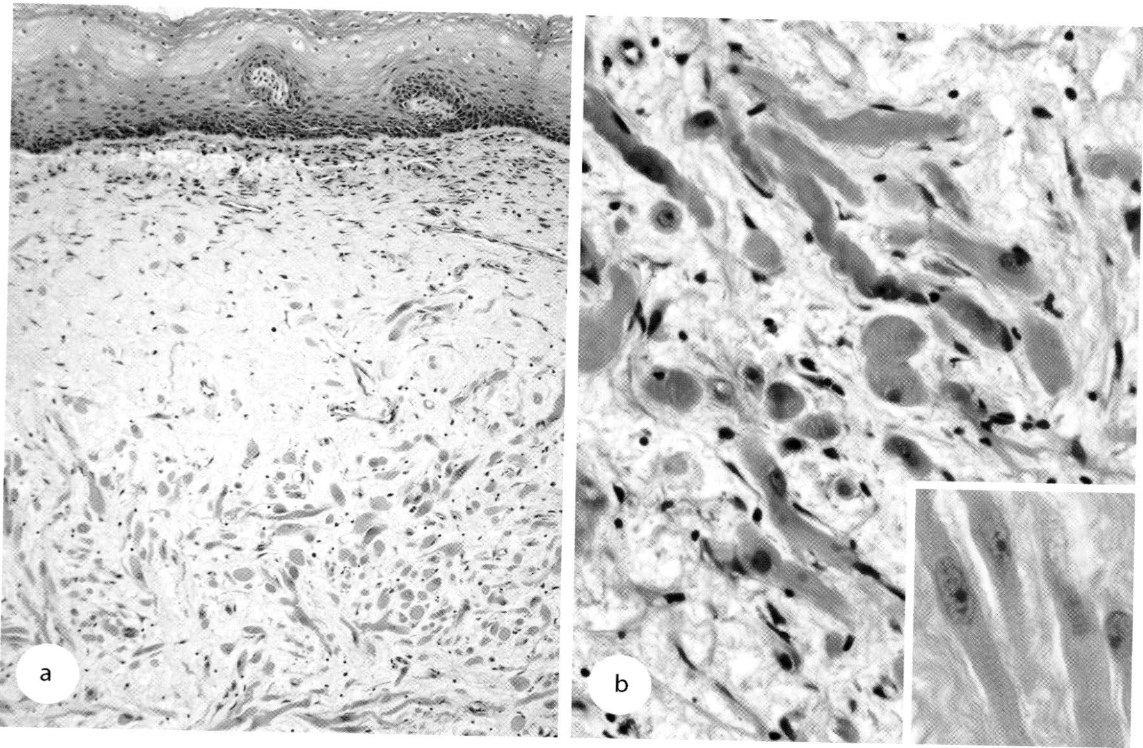

Fig. 22.15
Vaginal rhabdomyoma. **Low (a) and high (b) power views. Note the abundant eosinophilic cytoplasm and nuclear features. Cross striations are evident in the figure (b) inset**

Differential Diagnosis

In childhood, the key consideration in the differential diagnosis is the botryoid variant of embryonal rhabdomyosarcoma. This tumor classically contains a hypercellular subepithelial cambium-like layer of neoplastic cells. The process has infiltrative growth, significant nuclear atypia and mitotic activity. In older patients, a mesodermal stromal polyp would commonly be a leading consideration until skeletal muscle differentiation is confirmed. When the myogenic features become apparent, fleeting consideration might be given to a heterologous element from an adenosarcoma or carcinosarcoma, but no epithelial component is present and the mesenchymal cells lack malignant cytomorphologic features.

Behavior and Treatment

Genital rhabdomyomas are benign tumors, typically cured by simple local excision.

Glomus Tumor

There are rare reports of glomus tumor involving the labia minus [163, 174], clitoris [157, 290], periurethral area [290], and uterine cervix [6], and AFIP files contain an additional four examples. Patients have ranged in age from 27 to 67 years. The lesions are usually solitary and $\leq$1 cm in size, but rarely, they may be multifocal or measure up to 3 cm. The classic clinical scenario for vulvar examples is intense (sometimes incapacitating) nonradiating pain, unrelated to the menstrual cycle and localized to a specific "trigger" spot. Overlying erythema may be noted.

Histologic examination reveals a well-demarcated nodular mass composed of epithelioid and sometimes focally spindled (modified/specialized) smooth muscle cells organized around numerous vascular spaces (*Fig. 22.16*). The epithelioid cells often have a "fried egg" appearance with a central, hyperchromatic, round nucleus and pale to eosinophilic cytoplasm with a distinct cell border. So-called "degenerative" atypia is occasionally present. Mitotic figures are rarely encountered. The tumor cells

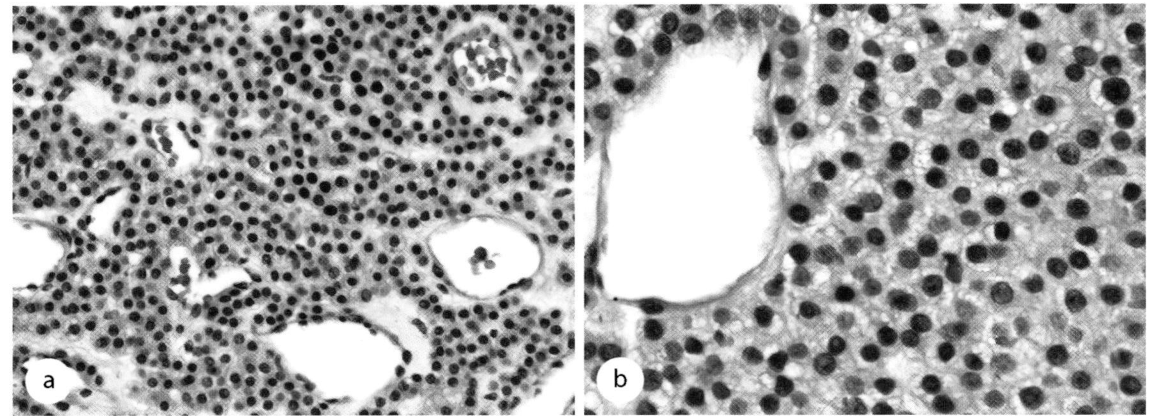

Fig. 22.16
Glomus tumor. **Medium (a) and high (b) power views. Note a tendency for aggregation around the vasculature. Also note the "fried egg" appearance of the tumor cells, with round, centrally located, nuclei and distinct cell borders**

have strong immunoreactivity for muscle-specific actin and α-smooth muscle actin, but they are usually negative for desmin. Many S100 protein-positive nerve twigs may be present in the background, but tumor cells are negative for this marker. There is no immunoreactivity for keratins, synaptophysin or chromogranin.

Complete local excision is curative.

Benign Tumors and Tumefactions of Blood Vessels

A wide variety of benign vascular lesions may affect the gynecologic tract. Lesions of the vulva, ranging from reactive vascular tumefactions secondary to infection (e.g., bacillary angiomatosis) [194] to vascular malformations and neoplasms [91], are similar in appearance to those encountered in other cutaneous sites and are not included in this chapter. Many of the more common vulvar lesions (e.g., juvenile hemangioma, lobular capillary hemangioma/pyogenic granuloma and angiokeratoma) [57] are discussed elsewhere in this textbook.

Vaginal angiomas are usually classified as capillary or cavernous hemangiomas, and much less frequently, are arteriovenous in nature [60, 65, 79, 132, 144, 263]. Most vaginal hemangiomas are small, isolated lesions that are detected incidentally. However, infrequently, they may be more extensive with coexisting vulvar, urethral, cervical or pelvic involvement. When widespread, the process is often classified as an angiomatosis. As with other vascular lesions of the gynecologic tract, rapid growth can occur during pregnancy.

The most common benign vascular lesions of the uterine cervix are also capillary and cavernous hemangiomas [5, 65, 87, 133]. These lesions may be incidentally discovered (e.g., during colposcopy or in a hysterectomy specimen for an unrelated medical condition), or they may cause abnormal vaginal bleeding. Grossly, they are usually <4 cm in size and have a red-purple color and soft to spongy consistency. Cervical hemangiomas have been reported over a wide age range, but the peak incidence is in the 3rd decade of life. Only rarely are they identified before puberty. We are aware of one report of bacillary angiomatosis affecting the uterine cervix [194].

Benign vascular lesions of the uterus proper can be asymptomatic or they may be associated with abnormal vaginal bleeding, infertility, spontaneous abortions, and fetal wastage. They can cause life-threatening complications during pregnancy, delivery and surgical procedures (e.g., myomectomy) [50, 67, 109, 303, 322]. Most vascular lesions of the uterus are detected in the 3rd through 5th decades and generally are either cavernous hemangiomas (a.k.a. cavernous angiomatosis of the uterus) [59, 67, 109, 173, 303, 310, 322] or arteriovenous malformations [199]. The former are often viewed as congenital and commonly exhibit widespread involvement of the uterus. The latter are either congenital or acquired (usually post-traumatic) and tend to be more localized ("tumor-like") in their distribution [109]. The distinction can have clinical relevance, because bleeding from arteriovenous malformations can be more difficult to control [59]. Spectral Doppler analysis is a valuable clinical tool in distinguishing the two processes [59].

Ovarian hemangiomas occur over a wide age range and fall into two general groups: those associated with abdominopelvic (hem)angiomatosis[185] and those occurring as localized lesions [10]. The former are often symptomatic, whereas the latter are frequently asymptomatic. Localized ovarian hemangiomas are usually unilateral, and they most commonly involve the medullary and hilar regions. They generally exhibit cavernous, or less commonly, capillary features. A small number of cases have been associated with ascites, an elevated serum CA-125, stromal luteinization and hormonal function [110, 126, 272, 334]. We are aware of one report of an infantile cellular hemangioma ("hemangioendothelioma") of the ovary in a newborn [257].

Patients with vascular abnormalities of the gynecologic tract may have other important physical findings that aid in their recognition. Some patients may have coexisting hemangiomas or vascular malformations involving the skin, deep soft tissue, or other organ systems [67, 109, 144, 303], and a few individuals have been documented to have Klippel-Trénaunay-Weber syndrome [59], tuberous sclerosis [109], hereditary hemorrhagic telangiectasia [109], and blue rubber bleb nevus syndrome [289].

Benign vascular lesions of the gynecologic tract have been treated in a variety of ways, ranging from clinical observation to local ablative therapy to resection of the affected organ. The treatment approach is influenced by the type, size and location of the vascular lesion, symptomatology, a desire to preserve fertility, and other factors.

Other Benign Soft Tissue Lesions Involving the Gynecologic Tract

Other benign soft tissue tumors and tumor-like lesions reported to involve the gynecologic tract include proliferative fasciitis, ischemic fasciitis [273], massive localized lymphedema as encountered in morbid obesity [229], lipoma [31, 72, 220], lymphangioma, and ganglioneuroma [95]. Rosai-Dorfman disease, which usually follows an indolent course, has also been documented [224].

Borderline/Low-Grade Soft Tissue Neoplasms and Mesenchymal Tumors with Varying Behavior

Dermatofibrosarcoma Protuberans

Dermatofibrosarcoma protuberans (DFSP) commonly develops in early to mid adult life and initially manifests as a small cutaneous plaque-like lesion that over time progresses to form a protuberant, multinodular mass. The rate of growth can be quite variable with long intervals of relative stasis, separated by periods of slow or more rapid enlargement. This process has a strong predilection for the trunk and limb girdle regions (old-fashioned bathing suit distribution), and more than two dozen examples have been reported to affect the vulva [11, 27, 113, 118, 232, 277, 316, 332]. Patients with vulvar involvement have ranged in age from 19 to 83 years with a median age in the early to mid 40s.

Most examples of DFSP arise in the dermis and subsequent spread to the subcutis, and occasionally, deeper structures. Histologically, the tumor is composed of relatively uniform spindled fibroblast-like cells arranged in a monotonous, tight storiform pattern (➋ *Figs. 22.17* and ➋ *22.18*). Other cellular elements such as lymphocytes, giant cells, and xanthoma cells are rarely seen. Hemorrhage, hemosiderin deposition, and necrosis are uncommon in conventional examples that have not been previously manipulated. The overlying epidermis is usually attenuated, as opposed to the acanthotic appearance commonly associated with fibrous histiocytomas. A frequent finding of diagnostic importance is the entrapment of fat and adnexa within the tumor. Myxoid matrix is present in some examples, though this is usually a focal finding, and rare cases (approximately 1–5%) may contain scattered melanin-laden spindled, epithelioid and dendritic cells (so-called Bednar tumors) (➋ *Fig. 22.18c*). There is generally minimal cellular pleomorphism. While mitotic activity can be quite variable, the overall mitotic rate is often relatively low.

A small percentage of DFSPs contain areas with solid fascicular growth, morphologically indistinguishable from classic adult-type fibrosarcoma (➋ *Fig. 22.18d*). These lesions are referred to as DFSP with fibrosarcomatous transformation (DFSP-FS) [1, 213, 332]. Criteria for diagnosis have varied considerably in the literature. Some authors require the fibrosarcomatous element to comprise 5–10% of the tumor area (without stipulating a minimum size in cm, but with the notation it must be more than a rare microscopic focus), whereas others require the fibrosarcomatous element to make up 25–30% of the tumor area or for it to be $\geq$1 cm in size. Histologically, the fibrosarcomatous component often arises in the subcutis, and it frequently (though not always) has increased cytologic atypia, greater cellularity, and more mitotic activity than adjacent areas of DFSP with storiform growth. Very rarely, DFSP can also harbor foci with substantial pleomorphism, mimicking malignant fibrous histiocytoma (pleomorphic undifferentiated sarcoma).

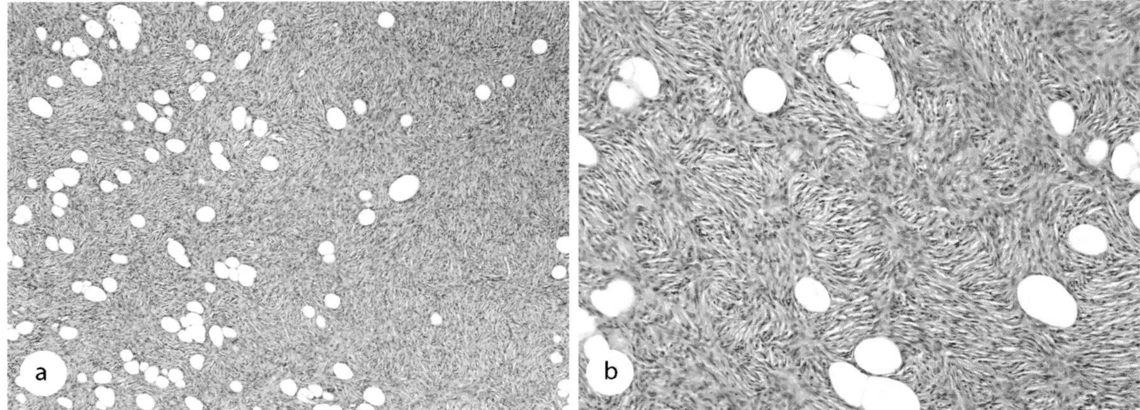

Fig. 22.17
Dermatofibrosarcoma protuberans (DFSP). **These low (a) and medium (b) power views demonstrate a well-developed storiform growth pattern and infiltration and entrapment of fat**

The typical spindled tumor cells of DFSP are immunoreactive for CD34 (*Fig. 22.18b*) and negative for S100 protein. Focal actin expression is sometimes observed. Areas with fibrosarcomatous transformation often have diminished expression of CD34. The melanin-laden spindled and dendritic cells encountered in pigmented DFSP (Bednar tumor) are immunoreactive for S100 protein, HMB-45, and Melan A (best observed with a red chromogen if the cells have not been bleached).

DFSP generally harbors either a supernumerary ring chromosome with low level amplification of sequences from chromosomes 17 and 22, or it contains a linear t(17;22) [197, 284]. The former is more common in adults, whereas the latter is common in pediatric patients. Both genetic events produce a *COL1A1/PDGFß* chimeric gene. There is wide variation in the break point on the *COL1A1* gene (from chromosome 17) but consistent involvement of exon 2 of the *PDGFß* gene (from chromosome 22). The resultant chimeric protein product is processed to mature PDGF-ßß, which leads to continuous autocrine and paracrine activation of the PDGFRß protein-tyrosine kinase, promoting cell proliferation and tumor growth [278].

DFSP is a tumor of "indeterminate" or low malignant potential. Less than 3% of conventional examples give rise to metastases. However, when fibrosarcomatous transformation is present, the risk of metastasis increases to 10–15% [1, 213]. The risk of metastasis is also believed higher when malignant fibrous histiocytoma-like areas are present, though this has not, to date, been adequately studied. A wide local excision is generally recommended, because invasion beyond grossly apparent margins is common, and there is a very strong propensity for recurrence [210, 268]. A 3 cm margin of normal-appearing tissue, with the inclusion of underlying fascia, has been advocated by some to minimize the risk of recurrence. However, using this approach, skin grafting may be required to cover the surgical defect, so management needs to be individualized. A growing number of patients have been successfully treated with Mohs' micrographic surgery [75, 116, 204, 288]. Long-term follow-up is required for all cases, and periodic screening for metastases (chest x-ray, etc.) is indicated when increased risk is documented. Imatanib mesylate, a potent inhibitor of several protein-tyrosine kinases, including PDGF receptors, has had a beneficial effect for some patients with locally advanced or metastatic disease [204].

Solitary Fibrous Tumor/ Hemangiopericytoma

The term "hemangiopericytoma" was originally used to describe a neoplasm of purported pericytic lineage composed of plump epithelioid or ovoid cells intimately associated with numerous thin-walled, branching (staghorn-like) vessels [81]. However, features diagnostic of pericytes are not faithfully reproduced in most of these tumors, and the above morphologic pattern can be encountered in a variety of other mesenchymal neoplasms, making the diagnosis one of exclusion. Solitary fibrous tumor shares many clinicopathological features with hemangiopericytoma [139] and many experts use the two terms synonymously [111]. Others continue to attempt to separate these

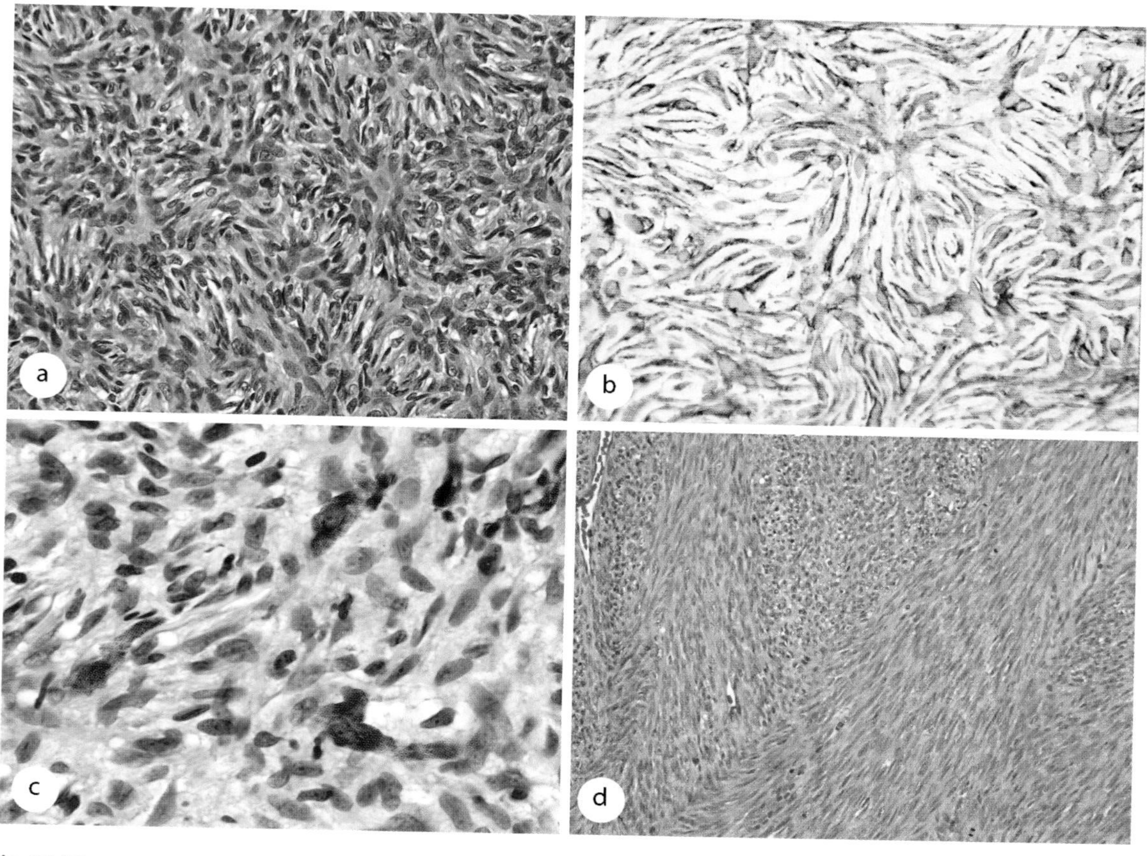

Fig. 22.18
Dermatofibrosarcoma protuberans. **Figure (a) is a high power view of the spindled neoplastic cells with a monotonous, tight, storiform growth pattern. Figure (b) illustrates immunoreactivity for CD34. Figure (c) contains scattered melanin-laden cells, as encountered in pigmented DFSP (Bednar tumor). Figure (d) demonstrates the fascicular growth that characterizes fibrosarcomatous transformation of DFSP**

processes, pointing out that classic solitary fibrous tumors tend to have more spindle cells, a greater amount of collagen, and less pronounced vascularity than classic hemangiopericytomas. That said, it is clear there are tumors where the morphologic distinction is blurred, and since the criteria for assessing malignant potential are essentially identical for the two lesions, this debate presently has little clinical relevance.

Clinical Features

Female genital tract hemangiopericytomas/solitary fibrous tumors (HPC/SFT) have been documented primarily in the vulvovaginal region [105], with rare examples noted in the uterus [53, 318], cervix, broad ligament, paraovarian tissue, and fallopian tube [24, 336]. Age range at presentation is wide, but most patients are in the 4th through 8th decades of life. Vulvovaginal tumors usually present as asymptomatic, slow-growing masses, while pain or bleeding typically herald the presence of a uterine or cervical tumor. One high-molecular-weight insulin-like growth factor II-secreting uterine tumor caused hypoglycemia [318]. HPC/SFTs also arise in the soft tissue of the pelvic fossa and retroperitoneum [81, 82, 139] and because of proximity to the gynecologic tract, they may also be encountered in gynecologic practices.

Pathologic Findings

There is considerable variation in tumor size, with most examples measuring between 3 and 15 cm in greatest dimension [24, 81]. Macroscopically, HPC/SFTs tend to form well-circumscribed, nodular masses that typically have a firm consistency and gray-white, whorled cut surface. Hemorrhage or myxoid change is sometimes observed. Histologically, the cellular variant of SFT (classic HPC) consists of ovoid to fusiform cells with round to oval nuclei and scanty, pale eosinophilic cytoplasm with ill-defined cell borders (➲ *Fig. 22.19a*). The neoplastic cells are intimately arranged around a myriad of thin-walled, partially collapsed, branching capillaries. Scattered larger vessels within the lesion often have a staghorn-like appearance. Perivascular collagen deposition is a common finding. The conventional SFT (fibrous HPC) (➲ *Fig. 22.19b*) characteristically exhibits hyper- and hypocellular areas. Hypercellular regions feature bland fusiform and elongated spindle cells (+/– some epithelioid cells) arranged haphazardly around hemangiopericytomatous vessels, in short fascicles or vague storiform arrays. The mitotic rate is generally low. Paucicellular regions contain abundant hyalinized collagen or myxoid matrix. Perivascular collagenization can be a prominent feature. Lipomatous HPC (fat-forming variant of SFT) [82] and giant cell angiofibroma (giant-cell-rich variant of SFT) [128, 139] have features of both conventional and cellular SFT [111]. The former, however, has a variable number of mature adipocytes, whereas the latter possesses multinucleated stromal giant cells found within the interstitium or lining ectatic pseudovascular spaces. Immunohistochemically, conventional SFT shows strong reactivity for CD34, bcl-2, and CD99 and variable reactivity in a small percentage of cases for EMA, smooth muscle actin, and nuclear beta-catenin [40, 139]. Keratin, desmin and S100 protein are usually absent. Tumors with classic HPC morphology are also usually CD34-positive, but less consistently so than conventional SFTs [82, 336]. There is a trend for atypical/malignant HPC/SFTs to have diminished CD34 expression.

Differential Diagnosis

HPC/SFT warrants separation from a number of highly vascular, site-specific, spindle cell lesions of the vulvovaginal region. Cellular angiofibroma shares with HPC/SFT perivascular collagen deposition, the occasional presence of some hemangiopericytoma-like vessels, and CD34-positive tumor cells. However, multipatterned architecture, *prominent* hemangiopericytomatous vasculature, and pericellular collagen deposition are not features common to cellular angiofibroma. Angiomyofibroblastoma typically lacks hemangiopericytomatous vessels and its spindle and epithelioid tumor cells (which often express desmin) have a notable tendency to concentrate around lesional vessels in corded and nested arrays. Endometrial stromal sarcoma and synovial sarcoma (especially monophasic fibrous and poorly-differentiated examples) can contain a hemangiopericytoma-like vascular component. However, both of these tumors tend to be more infiltrative than HPC/SFT, and they often have more pronounced nuclear atypia and mitotic activity. Additionally, concentration of tumor cells around arterioles is a distinct feature of endometrial stromal sarcoma. In comparison with HPC/SFT, endometrial stromal sarcoma

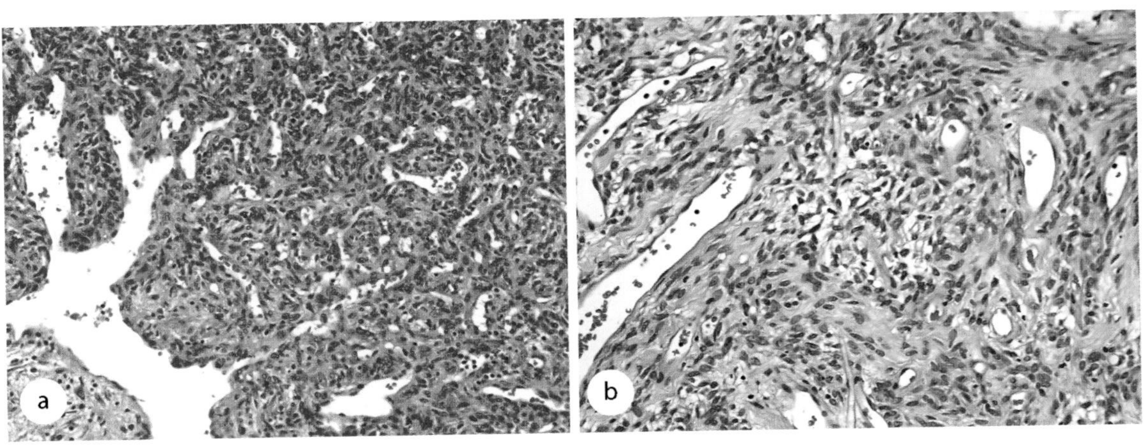

Fig. 22.19
Hemangiopericytoma (a) and Solitary fibrous tumor (b). **It is now widely recognized that these tumor types can sometimes have overlapping histologic features**

shows stronger expression of CD10 and progesterone receptor protein, and it is estrogen receptor protein-positive and CD34-negative [22]. Synovial sarcomas typically have focal keratin and EMA expression, and they are usually CD34-negative. Synovial sarcomas also feature an t(X;18) with SYT/SSX fusion transcripts.

Behavior and Treatment

Most HPC/SFTs behave in a benign fashion [81, 82, 120]. Recurrent or metastatic disease is reported in 6–15% of cases overall [81, 311], and the 5-year survival rate is >85% [82]. Histologic criteria for assessing malignant potential are imprecise and prognostication can be problematic, so complete excision with negative margins and long-term follow-up are generally recommended [311]. Features associated with aggressive behavior include large tumor size (>5 cm vs. >10 cm), infiltrative margins, high cellularity, nuclear pleomorphism, ≥4 mitoses/10 HPFs and necrosis [81, 120, 311]. Patients with large tumors containing a histologically malignant component should be considered for additional therapeutic intervention beyond surgery alone, as they may benefit from adjuvant therapy.

Inflammatory Myofibroblastic Tumor

This rare mesenchymal lesion has also been referred to in the literature as an inflammatory pseudotumor, plasma cell granuloma and plasma cell pseudotumor. It has been documented in a wide variety of anatomic sites, including the uterus [20, 97, 115, 161, 258, 279]. Recent evidence that the process often harbors clonal chromosomal aberrations involving 2p23 with various associated fusion gene transcripts (including *TPM3-ALK*, *TPM4-ALK* and others) supports the view this is a neoplastic rather than reactive process [33, 125, 186].

Reported examples in the uterus have affected individuals ranging in age from 6 to 60. Patients may present with findings related to mass effect, or the clinical picture can be dominated by constitutional signs or symptoms, including fever, weight loss, erythema of the face and extremities, malaise and fatigue.

Gynecologic examples have ranged in size from 1 to 12 cm and have exhibited polypoid growth within the endometrial cavity or diffuse involvement of the uterine wall. The cut surface can have a white, fibrous, whorled appearance similar to a smooth muscle tumor, or it can be smooth, soft and fish flesh-like or even gelatinous.

Histologically, the process features spindled and stellate-shaped cells with amphophilic or eosinophilic cytoplasm and a prominent nucleus with an "open" chromatin pattern and conspicuous central nucleolus (➲ *Fig. 22.20*). The lesional cells should lack significant hyperchromasia and pleomorphism. The mitotic rate is variable, but generally low, and bizarre mitotic figures are absent. The tumor cells may be loosely arranged due to a moderate amount of myxoid matrix, widely dispersed due to abundant fibrosclerotic stroma, or closely packed with broad storiform and fascicular growth. A prominent lymphoplasmacytic inflammatory infiltrate is a nearly universal finding.

Immunohistochemical results vary in the literature and may reflect methodological differences or case heterogeneity. In general, at least focal actin expression is common. Desmin expression is more variable, and when present, it is often observed in only a small percentage of cells. While there is inconsistency in ALK-1 expression amongst purported inflammatory myofibroblastic tumors (IMTs) from various anatomic sites [97, 219], uterine examples are typically positive for this marker [258]. Focal keratin reactivity has been noted in many IMTs, but to our knowledge, it has not yet been reported in a uterine tumor. IMTs are negative for CD34 and S100 protein, and they are usually negative for CD117 and estrogen receptor protein [258].

ALK (anaplastic lymphoma kinase) gene locus rearrangement can often be detected with FISH, and RT-PCR can be used to detect the *ALK* gene fusion partners that include, but are not limited to, *TPM3* (tropomyosin 3), *TPM4* (tropomyosin 4), and *CLTC* (clathrin heavy-chain gene).

In the past, most IMTs of the uterus were classified as smooth muscle tumors, often a myxoid leiomyoma or leiomyosarcoma. Clues for recognition as an IMT lay in the nuclear features of the neoplastic cells (i.e., the open chromatin pattern and distinct central nucleolus), the prominent lymphoplasmacytic inflammatory infiltrate, and a more blunted expression of myogenic markers than would generally be expected in a true smooth muscle neoplasm.

IMTs can be locally aggressive, and they have a documented propensity for local recurrence if incompletely excised, so complete surgical excision is generally advocated. While there are rare reports of IMTs outside of the gynecologic tract giving rise to metastases [219], this appears to be a very uncommon event, and the process is usually viewed as being more of a local problem, so radical intervention should be avoided whenever possible. There is some evidence to suggest that *rare* examples of IMT may, over time,

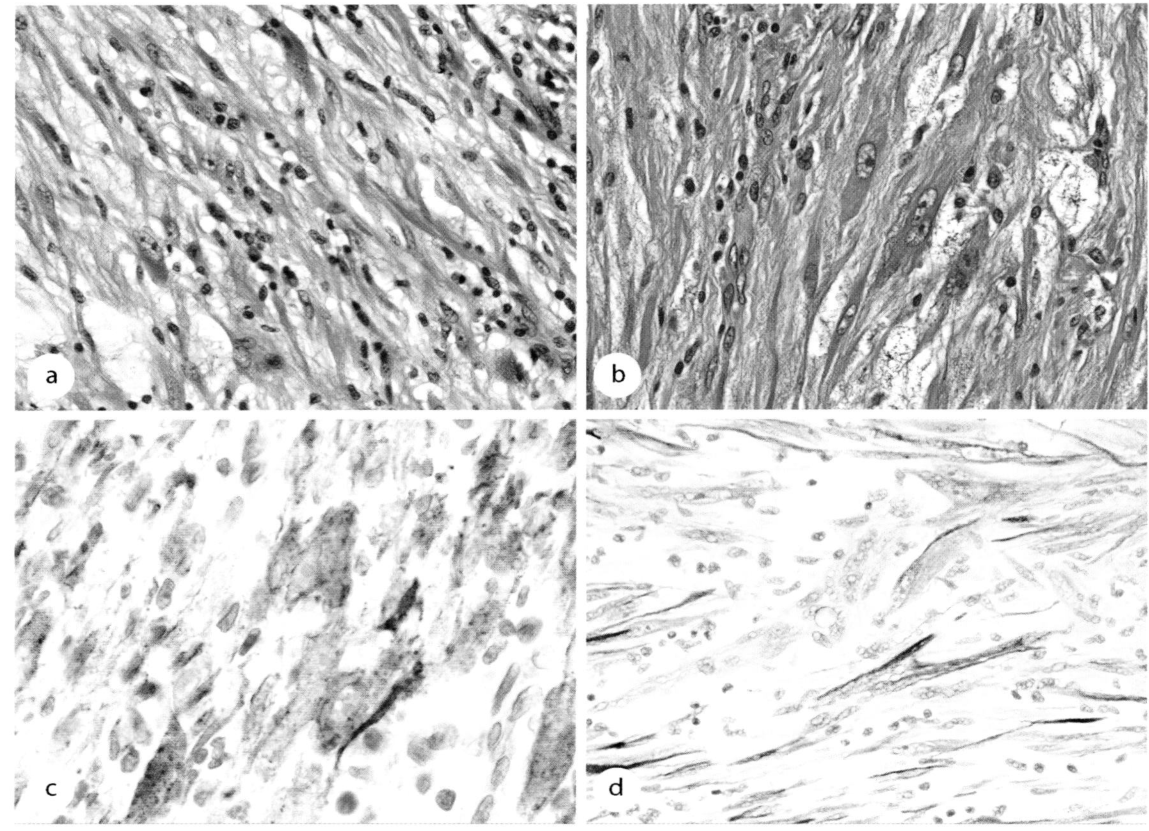

Fig. 22.20
Inflammatory myofibroblastic tumor of the uterus. **Medium (a) and high (b) power views demonstrating the loose growth pattern, lymphocytic infiltrate, and spindled neoplastic cells with amphophilic cytoplasm and large nuclei with an "open" chromatin pattern and prominent nucleoli. Figures (c) and (d) illustrate immunoreactivity for ALK-1 and desmin, respectively**

transform to fully malignant neoplasms, but at present, it is difficult to predict in which cases this will occur.

Postoperative Spindle Cell Nodule

Controversy exists as to whether postoperative spindle cell nodules (POSCN) [56, 165, 201, 256] are a unique (reactive versus neoplastic) exuberant fibroblastic/myofibroblastic proliferation or part of the morphologic spectrum of inflammatory myofibroblastic tumor (IMT). Current data, in our opinion, are insufficient to definitively resolve this issue. By definition, POSCNs are temporally associated with some type of local trauma, including instrumentation. They usually occur in middle-aged and elderly patients, and they often present as polypoid or nodular, mucosal-based masses, sometimes with substantial infiltration of underlying stroma. The fibroblastic/myofibroblastic population has many morphologic and immunohistochemical similarities to that encountered in IMTs, including occasional ALK-1 expression. Inconsistently reported differences from IMTs include more substantial mitotic activity, more prominently edematous stroma, less plasma cells, and a lack of ganglion-like myofibroblastic cells. POSCNs of the gynecologic tract have generally responded well to conservative local excision.

Perivascular Epithelioid Cell Tumor (Myomelanocytic Tumor)

Perivascular epithelioid cell tumors (PEComas) are a family of mesenchymal neoplasms with shared cytomorphologic and immunohistochemical features, namely the presence of epithelioid and spindled cells with lightly eosinophilic to clear cytoplasm, that may have an intimate relationship with vasculature and characteristically co-express melanocytic and myoid markers [84, 85, 103]. The prototypic tumors of this group are angiomyolipoma (renal and extrarenal variants), lymphangiomyomatosis, and clear cell "sugar" tumor of the lungs. PEComa, not otherwise specified (NOS), is a more recent addition to this family. This latter tumor has been documented in a wide variety of sites, but the single most common location is the uterus. A striking female predilection has been noted for all perivascular epithelioid cell tumor variants. Whereas angiomyolipoma and lymphangiomyomatosis have a strong association with the tuberous sclerosis complex (TSC), <10% of patients with PEComas, NOS, of gynecologic and soft tissue origin have clinical evidence of tuberous sclerosis.

Clinical Features

Within the gynecologic tract, the uterine corpus is by far the most commonly affected site with 37 cases documented, to date. PEComas in this location have affected patients ranging in age from 7 to 79 years (median, 37 years). Abnormal uterine bleeding is the most frequent presenting feature, but pain and hemoperitoneum have also been reported. There are four published examples of PEComa involving the uterine cervix (age range: 25–48 years), and rare examples have also occurred in the pelvis, vulva, vagina, broad ligament and ovary.

Pathologic Findings

The tumors have ranged in size from 1 to 30 cm. They often have a well-circumscribed appearance, but they may be frankly infiltrative, sometimes possessing tonguelike extensions reminiscent of an endometrial stromal sarcoma [314]. Histologically, the process features epithelioid and varying numbers of spindled cells with pale eosinophilic to clear (sometimes described as "moth-eaten") cytoplasm (➋ *Fig. 22.21a*). In some instances, the eosinophilic cytoplasm condenses around the nucleus and retracts from portions of the cell membrane, leaving skeins of cytoplasm that impart a spider-like appearance. Tumor cell nuclei are round to oval in epithelioid cells and more elongate in the spindle cell population. In most instances, the nuclei are relatively uniform with only low level atypia, but some tumors have significant atypia and pleomorphism. Scattered multinucleated giant cells may be encountered. Mitotic figures are often difficult to find, but they may be abundant and atypical in malignant examples.

The tumors characteristically feature a diffuse, intrinsic network of small capillaries, and some examples have hyalinized arterioles or other thick-walled vessels. Intimate growth of tumor cells around the vessels may be observed. The neoplastic cells exhibit a combination of nested, fascicular and sheetlike growth patterns. Occasional examples may have abundant fibrotic or hyalinized stroma.

Immunoreactivity is always present for HMB-45 (➋ *Fig. 22.21b*) or Melan A (a definitional characteristic with the former being more frequently expressed than the latter), and there is usually reactivity for α-smooth muscle actin (70–80%) [84, 85, 103]. Immunoreactivity may also

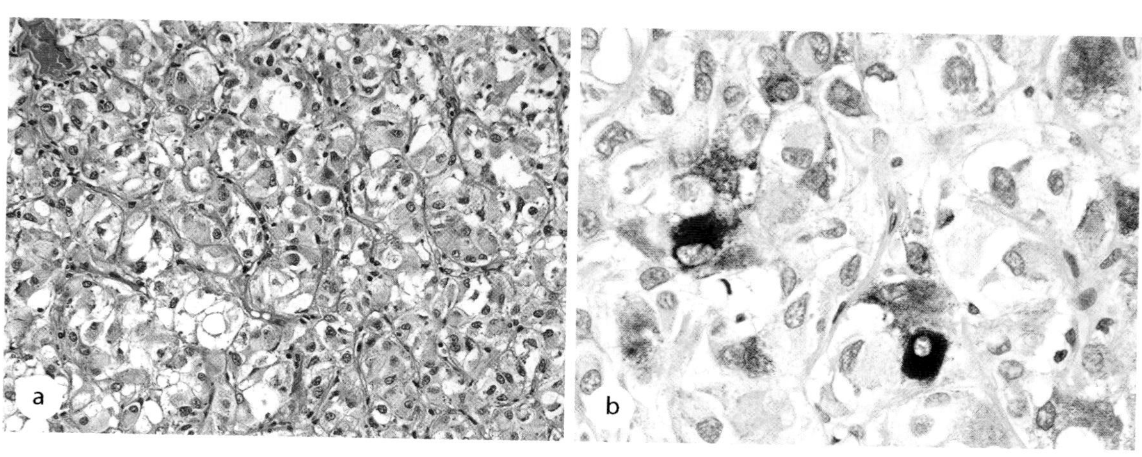

■ **Fig. 22.21**
Perivascular epithelioid cell tumor (PEComa) of the uterine cervix. **The neoplastic cells (a) and cytoplasmic immunoreactivity for HMB-45 (b) are depicted**

be present for h-caldesmon, desmin (≈50%), muscle-specific actin (>30%), microphthalmia transcription factor, and estrogen and progesterone receptor proteins. A small percentage of cases have been reported to express S100 protein, TFE-3, and rarely, keratins [84, 85, 103]. Negative results are usually obtained for CD34 and CD117.

Differential Diagnosis

The main considerations in the differential diagnosis are a uterine epithelioid smooth muscle tumor, and to a lesser extent, an unusual metastatic malignant melanoma or clear cell sarcoma. While most experts acknowledge some morphologic and immunohistochemical overlap between uterine smooth muscle tumors and PEComas, true epithelioid smooth muscle tumors typically lack the rather distinctive vascular network encountered in PEComas, and they usually contain some foci with conventional smooth muscle morphology (e.g., well-defined spindling, prominent and more homogeneous cytoplasmic eosinophilia, elongate cigar-shaped nuclei, and juxtanuclear vacuoles). Since HMB-45 expression has been documented in "normal" myometrium, as well as subsets of smooth muscle (and endometrial-type stromal) tumors [282], and because clear cell change is not unique to PEComas, some experts have argued that the presence of either of these findings in an otherwise *conventional* smooth muscle tumor is insufficient evidence to warrant classification as a PEComa [84, 85].

Metastatic malignant melanoma and clear cell sarcoma feature widespread nuclear atypia with prominent macronucleoli, notable mitotic activity, and often, strong nuclear and cytoplasm reactivity for S100 protein. Oftentimes, these tumors have more widespread reactivity for melanocytic markers than PEComas. Additionally, clinical history can be very helpful, and from a genetic standpoint, only clear cell sarcoma has a t(12;22)(q13;q13) with an *EWS-ATF1* fusion gene.

Discussion with Comments on Behavior and Treatment

There is debate amongst experts as to whether gynecologic PEComas warrant separate classification from smooth muscle tumors [84, 282, 314]. Support for this separation includes morphologic, immunohistochemical (including elevated phospho-p70S6K and decreased phospho-AKT expression, consistent with loss of TSC1/2 function), and genetic (evidence of the tuberous sclerosis complex in a small percent of patients)[29, 85, 314] findings that more closely linked these tumors to other members of the perivascular epithelioid cell tumor family than true smooth muscle neoplasms [168]. Additionally, current evidence suggests that the histopathologic criteria (e.g., the mitotic threshold) for prognosticating gynecologic-related PEComas differs from that presently used for epithelioid smooth muscle tumors.

Criteria for distinguishing benign from malignant PEComas of the gynecologic tract are still in a state of evolution. Folpe et al. [103] proposed classifying soft tissue and gynecologic PEComas as malignant when two or more of the following features were present: tumor size >5 cm, infiltrative growth, high nuclear grade and cellularity, coagulative tumor necrosis, vascular invasion, and mitotic activity >1 mitotic figure/50 HPFs. Tumors were considered of uncertain malignant potential if either large size or nuclear pleomorphism was encountered without other worrisome features. Tumors with no worrisome features were considered to have very low risk for aggressive behavior and were provisionally labeled benign. A more recent comprehensive review [84] restricted to gynecologic PEComas suggests the most reproducible criteria for defining malignancy in this location are: large size (as a continuous variable with the most effective threshold being 5 cm and the probability of malignancy increasing through 10 cm), coagulative necrosis, and mitotic activity (benign tumors usually have ≤1 mitosis/50 HPFs and almost always have ≤1 mitosis/10 HPFs). Other criteria, such as significant nuclear pleomorphism, are probably also relevant but require additional study. It is important to note that the absence of mitotic activity does not guarantee benignancy. When PEComas metastasize, they generally spread to the lungs, liver, bones and lymph nodes. Ovarian and omental metastases are also documented. Multifocal, morphologically benign, disease (a.k.a., PEComatosis) has been reported [88].

Recent observations consistent with mTOR activation and loss of TSC1/2 function in some PEComas, presents an avenue for further study to see if mTOR inhibitors, such as rapamycin, have a role in the treatment of these tumors [85, 168].

Malignant Soft Tissue Tumors

Alveolar Soft Part Sarcoma

Alveolar soft part sarcoma is a rare malignancy that usually arises in sites other than the gynecologic tract [246]. In children, it often affects the head and neck region, and in adolescents and adults (peak incidence: 3rd decade), the thigh and buttock are the most common locations. To date, approximately 30 cases have been diagnosed as primary tumors in the vulva, vagina [39, 46, 241], uterine cervix [2, 83, 102, 104, 142, 176, 270], uterine corpus [35, 129, 162, 234, 259], and broad ligament [124, 225, 267]. AFIP files contain an additional 7 unpublished gynecologic examples, as well as slides from two published cases, representing 7.4% of our female accessions for this entity.

Clinical Features

Most gynecologic examples of alveolar soft part sarcoma involve the uterine cervix or uterine corpus, these two sites being affected with nearly equal frequency. A smaller number of cases are documented in the vagina, and other locations are only rarely affected. Patients have ranged in age from 8 to 62 years, and their tumors have varied in size from 0.2 to 9.8 cm. The average patient age is in the early 30s, and the average tumor size approximates 3 cm. The most common clinical signs are a mass lesion, abnormal intermenstrual bleeding, and menometrorrhagia. Some examples have been incidentally noted in hysterectomy specimens removed for other reasons.

Pathologic Findings

The lesions tend to be well-circumscribed and solid with a grayish-white to yellowish-tan color, occasionally punctuated with foci of hemorrhage. Some examples are polypoid.

Histologically, the tumors contain numerous vessels, and the larger examples may have occasional well-developed fibrous septa (➲ *Fig. 22.22*). The neoplastic cells have epithelioid morphology with relatively abundant granular eosinophilic to focally clear, glycogen-rich, cytoplasm. In up to 80% of cases overall and approximately 65% of gynecologic examples, PAS-positive, diastase-resistant cytoplasmic crystals can be found (➲ *Fig. 22.22c*), and in most of the remaining cases, globular or granular cytoplasmic material with similar staining properties may be evident [225, 259]. Tumor cell nuclei are large and vesicular with prominent central macronucleoli. This process typically has a very low mitotic rate, often <1 mitotic figure/10 high power fields. The neoplastic cells may be present individually, in small aggregates, or in classic, large, alveolar-like nests.

The characteristic cytoplasmic crystals have recently been demonstrated to consist of a complex of monocarboxylate transporter 1 (MCT1) and its chaperone, CD147 [179]. By ultrastructural analysis, the crystals have an internal lattice pattern with a periodicity of ≈100 Å. They are usually membrane-bound, but occasionally, they may be free floating in the cytosol.

Alveolar soft part sarcoma has been shown to have a nonreciprocal translocation involving the *TFE3* gene of Xp11.2 and the *ASPL* gene of 17q25 [142, 180]. With the exception of nuclear immunoreactivity for TFE3 (the result of aberrant ASPL/TFE3 fusion protein accumulating in the nucleus) (➲ *Fig. 22.22d*) [16, 162, 267], immunostaining has little value in the diagnosis of alveolar soft part sarcoma, except to rule out other potential considerations in the differential diagnosis. The neoplastic cells are reported to be variably positive for vimentin, desmin, and actins. They are negative for chromogranin, synaptophysin, myogenin, Myo-D1, and with rare exception, S100 protein, keratins (focal +/– dot-like reactivity reported in two cases) and HMB-45 (focally positive with a negative S100 protein result in two cases) [225, 246, 267].

Differential Diagnosis

The differential diagnosis for alveolar soft part sarcoma includes paraganglioma, metastatic renal cell carcinoma, malignant melanoma, an epithelioid smooth muscle tumor, and PEComa. Paragangliomas are glycogen-poor, and they have immunoreactivity for chromogranin and synaptophysin. Rare renal cell carcinomas (encountered primarily in pediatric and adolescent patients) have the same *ASPL-TFE3* gene fusion and nuclear TFE3 immunoreactivity as seen in alveolar soft part sarcoma, but in this setting, the t(X;17) is balanced, and the tumors commonly have pseudopapillary growth, psammoma bodies, renal cell carcinoma antigen expression, and in approximately half of the cases, focal reactivity for EMA or keratin [14–16]. Malignant melanomas have greater anaplasia, more obvious mitotic activity, and frequent immunoreactivity for S100 protein, Melan-A and HMB-45. Epithelioid smooth muscle tumors often have (at least focally) a spindle cell component that is lacking in alveolar soft part sarcoma, and they generally have strong reactivity for α-smooth muscle actin. Perivascular epithelioid cell tumors (PEComas) tend to have an admixture of spindled and epithelioid cells with pale to clear "moth-eaten" cytoplasm, and they generally co-express melanocytic and smooth muscle markers. None of the considerations in the differential diagnosis have the characteristic cytoplasmic crystals encountered in most examples of alveolar soft part sarcoma.

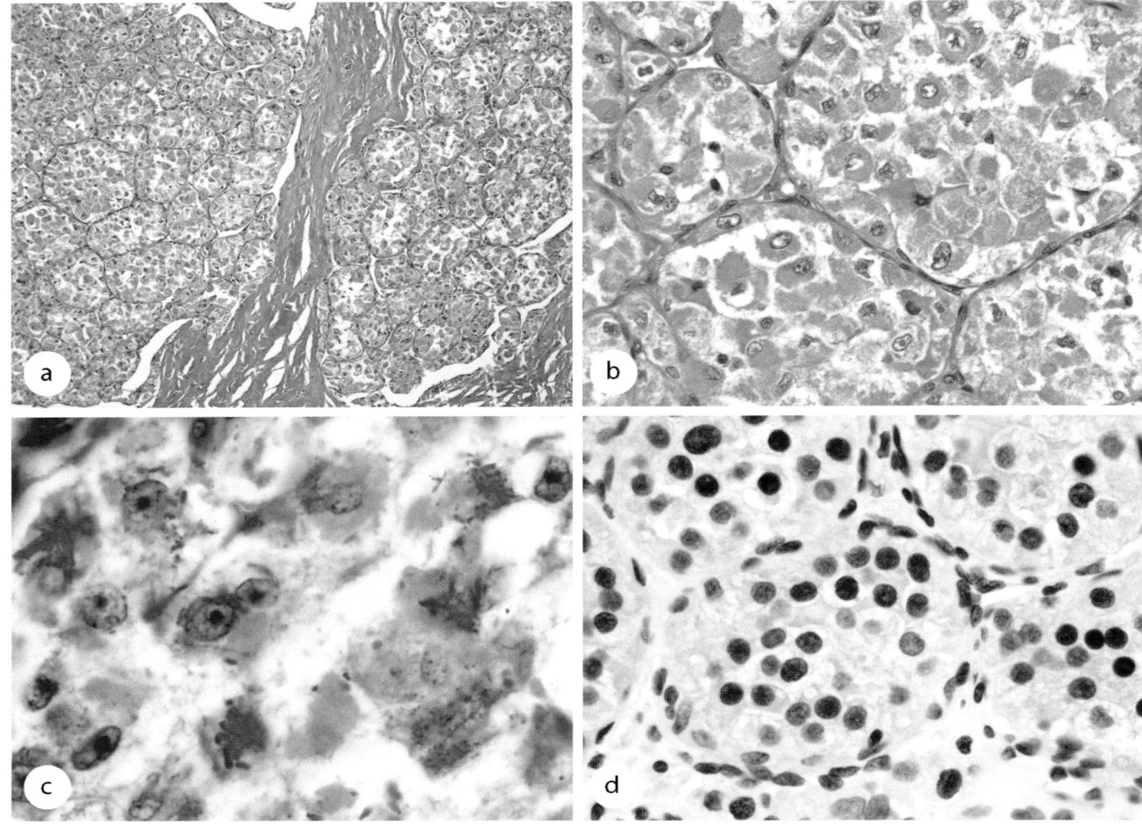

Fig. 22.22
Alveolar soft part sarcoma. **Note the nested growth pattern, high vascularity, and fibrous septa in figure (a). Figure (b) is a high power view demonstrating large alveolar-like nests of tumor cells. Note the granular eosinophilic cytoplasm with focal clearing and the large nuclei with distinct nucleoli. These tumors typically have a low mitotic rate. Figure (c) illustrates the characteristic PAS/D positive cytoplasmic crystals. Figure (d) demonstrates nuclear immunoreactivity for TFE-3**

Behavior and Treatment

In most instances, alveolar soft part sarcoma is a slowly progressive disease that ultimately metastasizes to the lungs, brain and skeleton and usually proves fatal. However, there is a suggestion in the literature that examples arising in the uterine body or cervix (but not other gynecologic sites) may have a much more favorable prognosis (only one metastasis thus far reported), perhaps related to small tumor size (<5 cm) and resectability [162, 225, 267]. Before a definite statement can be made in this regard, longer follow-up is required, because for patients presenting with a localized soft tissue primary, the median interval to first metastasis in one large series was 6 years, and almost 40% of these patients did not present with metastatic disease until ≥10 years after initial diagnosis [192]. Before accepting an alveolar soft part sarcoma as primary in the gynecologic tract, careful clinical evaluation to rule out a metastasis is recommended. Treatment should be directed at complete resection. Evaluation of regional lymph nodes is advisable, although nodal metastases are a relatively uncommon event. The value of adjuvant therapy is uncertain.

Epithelioid Sarcoma

Defined as a distinct clinicopathologic entity by Enzinger in 1970, the classical (or "distal-type") epithelioid sarcoma is a neoplasm of uncertain histogenesis that primarily affects individuals in the 2nd through 4th decades (mean age: 27 years) and has a strong predilection for the extremities (upper > lower), especially the distal portions [48, 80]. The tumor characteristically features an admixture of epithelioid and spindled cells with a notable tendency for pseudogranulomatous growth. More recently, a "proximal-type" variant of epithelioid sarcoma has been proposed [130, 140]. These tumors have a predilection for the truncal, pelvicoperineal and genital regions of a somewhat older age group, and they feature large atypical epithelioid or rhabdoid cells, with little tendency for pseudogranulomatous growth. Tumors in this latter category often have more aggressive clinical behavior than conventional ("distal-type") epithelioid sarcomas, and some examples have been interpreted in the literature as "atypical" epithelioid sarcomas or malignant extrarenal rhabdoid tumors [130, 252].

Clinical Features

Female genital tract epithelioid sarcomas present over a wide age range, but the peak incidence is in the 3rd through 5th decades of life [17, 130, 215, 254, 301, 305]. The tumors most commonly affect the labia majus, followed in frequency by the labia minus, clitoris, and Bartholin gland region. Clinically, the process often manifests as an asymptomatic nodular mass with a variable growth rate. Some examples mimic a Bartholin gland cyst or abscess.

Pathologic Findings

Macroscopically, the process presents as a single or multinodular fleshy, whitish mass. Foci of necrosis and hemorrhage are sometimes observed. Superficial tumors usually measure <5 cm in size, while deep-seated examples may be larger. Microscopically, classical examples of epithelioid sarcoma consist of a variable admixture of mild to moderately atypical, medium to large-sized epithelioid and plump spindled cells with a strong tendency to aggregate around zones of necrosis, necrobiosis, hyalinization or myxoid change, producing a rather characteristic multinodular, garland-like (pseudogranulomatous) growth pattern (➋ *Figs. 22.23a* and ➋ *22.23b*) [48, 80]. The cytoplasm of the cells is often eosinophilic and glassy, and the nuclei are round to oval and somewhat hyperchromatic, but with a relative abundance of euchromatin. A single, relatively small but distinct, central nucleolus is often present. Pleomorphism is usually not pronounced, but occasionally, it is evident. Some examples contain neoplastic cells with focal rhabdoid, or rarely, signet ring-like (mucin-negative) morphology. Mitotic activity varies but is generally low. Dystrophic calcification or metaplastic bone formation is noted in <20% of cases.

In contrast, most proximal-type ("large-cell" variant) epithelioid sarcomas (➋ *Figs. 22.23c* and ➋ *22.23d*) feature large epithelioid cells with abundant amphophilic or eosinophilic cytoplasm and prominent, markedly atypical, nuclei. The nuclei may be pleomorphic and hyperchromatic with small or inconspicuous nucleoli, or they may be large and vesicular with macronucleoli [130]. Some examples contain numerous cells with a rhabdoid appearance due to large hyaline cytoplasmic inclusions that laterally displace the nucleus. Multinodular and sheetlike growth patterns predominate. Necrosis is common, but pseudogranulomatous architecture is seldom observed. When intralesional hemorrhage is prominent, a pseudoangiosarcomatous pattern may be present. While rhabdoid cells can be encountered in both types of epithelioid sarcoma, they are a much more common component of the "large-cell" variant. A very rare "fibroma-like" variant of epithelioid sarcoma with relatively bland morphology, abundant collagen, and focal storiform or whorled (fibrous histiocytoma-like) growth has also been described.

Epithelioid sarcomas are usually immunoreactive for vimentin, keratins (especially CK 8 and 19), and EMA, and 1/2 to 2/3 of cases express CD34 [214]. Some examples also have focal reactivity for muscle-specific actin. Classical epithelioid sarcomas are usually negative for S100 protein and desmin. Proximal-type epithelioid sarcomas immunohistochemically differ from classical (distal-type) tumors in that they occasionally have desmin expression (primarily encountered in the rhabdoid cells), and by one account, they more commonly lack nuclear immunoreactivity for INI1. [130, 217]

Differential Diagnosis

The differential diagnosis for epithelioid sarcoma revolves primarily around a granulomatous inflammatory reaction, squamous and adnexal carcinomas, malignant melanoma, and malignant extrarenal rhabdoid tumor. Epithelioid sarcoma is usually readily distinguished from a granulomatous reaction, because the latter has less pronounced mitotic activity and considerably less cytologic atypia. Mononuclear histiocytes are generally smaller in size than the tumor cells of epithelioid sarcoma, and they often have reniform nuclei and finely vacuolated or granular cytoplasm.

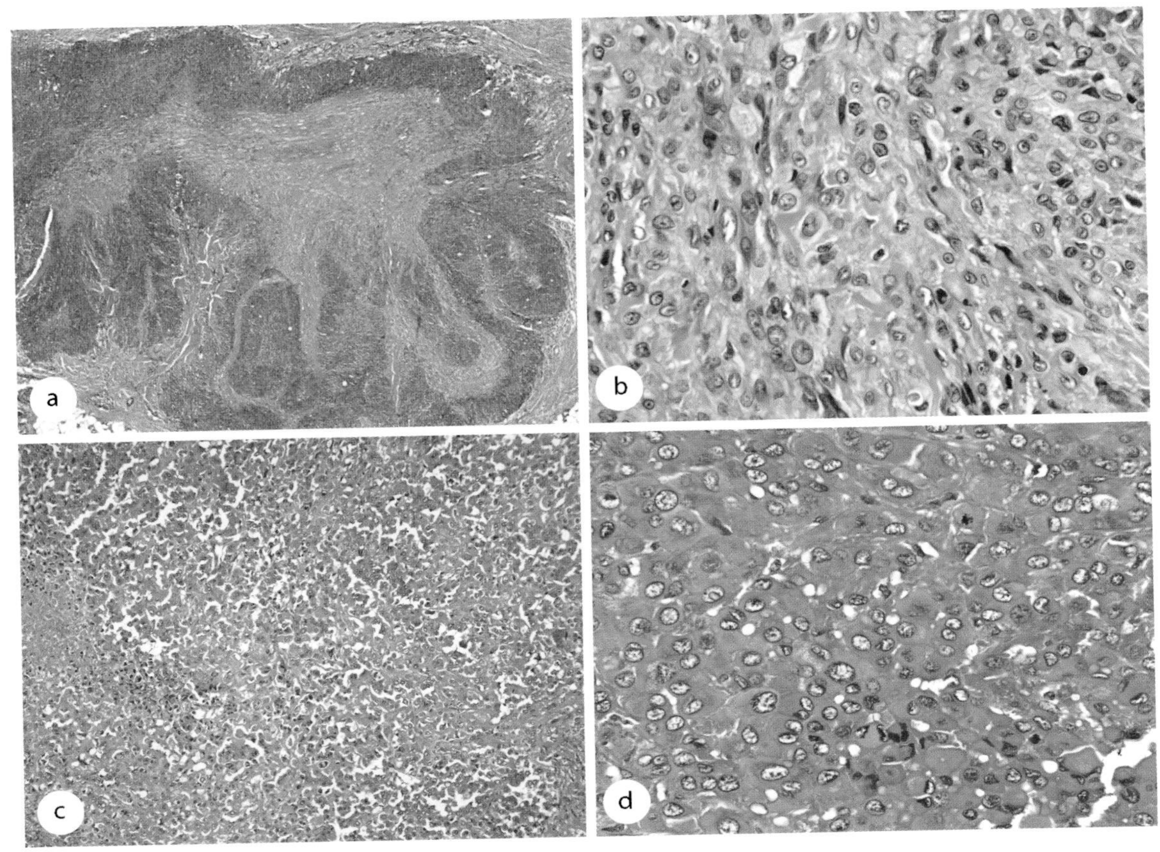

Fig. 22.23
Epithelioid sarcoma. **Figures (a) and (b) illustrate a conventional epithelioid sarcoma with a garland-like growth pattern (a) and an admixture of spindled and epithelioid tumor cells with low to moderate nuclear atypia (b). Figures (c) and (d) depict a proximal-type epithelioid sarcoma with sheet-like growth and focal necrosis. The tumor cells have abundant cytoplasm (with focal rhabdoid morphology). There is increased nuclear atypia, but nucleolar prominence was not a notable finding in this example**

Multinucleated giant cells are commonly encountered in granulomatous reactions but are uncommon in epithelioid sarcomas. While epithelioid sarcomas typically express keratins and EMA, histiocytic cells (for practical purposes) lack these markers and often have reactivity for CD163, CD68 (KP-1), lysozyme and/or CD45RB.

Distinguishing epithelioid sarcoma from carcinoma can be difficult in some instances. The presence of surface epithelial dysplasia and malignant change, cytoplasmic keratinization and intercellular bridge formation, and immunoreactivity for CK5/6 (especially if widespread) and p63 are features that can help support a diagnosis of squamous carcinoma [98]. Similarly, cytologic and architectural atypia within adjacent adnexa and the identification of a tumor component with a myoepithelial immunophenotype (e.g., a combination of keratin, GFAP, actins, calponin, S100 protein and p63) can help support classification as an adnexal neoplasm. Intracellular mucin is not a feature of epithelioid sarcoma and implies glandular differentiation. Lastly, immunoreactivity for CD34 is uncommon in carcinomas but is expressed in many epithelioid sarcomas.

Malignant melanomas usually have nuclear and cytoplasmic immunoreactivity for S100 protein, and many express HMB45, Melan A, tyrosinase, and/or microphthalmia transcription factor. Malignant melanomas only rarely express keratin. Since focal, weak, cytoplasmic-only, S100 protein expression is, on rare occasion, encountered in epithelioid sarcoma, this antibody should not be used as a sole discriminator between the two entities, but instead, it should be included as one component of an immunohistochemical panel.

Malignant extrarenal rhabdoid tumor (MERT) is characterized by the presence of: (1) round or polygonal cells with abundant globular eosinophilic cytoplasm and vesicular nuclei with prominent nucleoli, (2) PAS-positive hyaline or globoid intracytoplasmic inclusions, (3) immunoreactivity for keratin, EMA, and vimentin, and (4) absence of immunostaining for S100 protein (usually), desmin, MyoD1, myogenin, GFAP, and neurofilament protein. However, most experts do not regard these criteria as sufficient to define a specific clinicopathologic entity, because all of the above features may be encountered in carcinomas, mesotheliomas, and a variety of sarcomas, including synovial sarcoma and epithelioid sarcoma. It is our view that MERTs, as diagnosed in the adult segment of the population, are a heterogenous group of biologically aggressive neoplasms united by a common end-stage morphologic pattern. As a result, we rarely render this diagnosis, and only when all other alternate considerations have been exhausted. Distinguishing this process from a proximal-type epithelioid sarcoma can be extremely difficult, as there are many shared morphologic and immunohistochemical features (including loss of nuclear reactivity for INI1) [147], and this has occasionally led to the same tumor being diagnosed differently by different experts. While criteria for separating these entities are soft, the following findings favor a diagnosis of proximal-type epithelioid sarcoma: the presence of foci bearing a strong resemblance to classical-type epithelioid sarcoma and cytoplasmic immunoreactivity for CD34 and desmin [130, 243].

Behavior and Treatment

Classical (distal-type) epithelioid sarcoma often follows a rather slow but relentless clinical course punctuated by local recurrences and eventual regional lymph node and distant metastases, if incompletely excised. In the largest series to date [48], 77% of tumors recurred, 45% metastasized (most commonly to the lungs, followed in frequency by the regional lymph nodes, scalp, and bones), and 31% of patients died of disease. Factors implicated in aggressive behavior include proximal location, older age and male sex, increased tumor size and depth, high mitotic rate, necrosis, vascular invasion, and inadequate excision [30, 48, 98, 136]. Based on our review, between 40% and 50% of reported vulvar epithelioid sarcomas (most exhibited proximal-type morphology) have recurred or metastasized, and nearly 45% of patients died of disease.

For classical epithelioid sarcoma, a wide or radical resection with careful evaluation of regional lymph nodes is often advocated. Encouraging results are reported in several series when surgical treatment is combined with adjuvant radiation therapy [30, 48, 136]. The role of multiagent chemotherapy is more ambiguous.

Proximal (large-cell)-type epithelioid sarcomas often behave more aggressively than classical epithelioid sarcomas [98, 130, 140]. These tumors are frequently resistant to multimodal therapy, and early tumor-related deaths are common. As such, the behavior of this tumor has notable similarities to malignant extrarenal rhabdoid tumor, and this has led some experts to regard distinction between the two as being largely academic [17].

Synovial Sarcoma

Synovial sarcomas have been documented in a wide variety of anatomic sites and organ systems, and recognition has been enhanced in recent years by the identification of a characteristic t(X;18), detectable in >90% of cases. Rare examples have involved the vulva [12, 146, 227, 324], vagina [251], fallopian tube [216], ovary [286] and true pelvis [99]. Patients with gynecologic-related tumors have ranged in age from 23 to 72 years old. Individuals with vulvar primaries usually presented in their 4th decade. These neoplasms are histologically similar to synovial sarcomas in other sites (➋ *Fig. 22.24*). They are generally classified as biphasic, monophasic fibrous, or poorly-differentiated. Tumors in the last category may be pure, but more often, they are admixed with one of the first two patterns. Biphasic examples contain epithelial cells, spindled fibroblast-like cells, and often, small numbers of epithelioid or "transitional" cells. The epithelial cells vary in appearance from cuboidal to columnar and exhibit corded, nested, or glandular growth. Monophasic fibrous tumors feature an abundance of delicate spindled cells and rare to scattered epithelioid cells, but they lack a clearly defined epithelial component. Poorly-differentiated synovial sarcomas represent a form of tumor progression, encountered in <20% of cases [312]. Relatively large epithelioid cells with increased nuclear atypia and mitotic activity usually predominate, but some poorly-differentiated tumors exhibit a small cell (Ewing sarcoma/PNET-like) pattern or a high-grade spindle cell pattern reminiscent of a malignant peripheral nerve sheath tumor [312]. Poorly-differentiated synovial sarcomas characteristically have a high mitotic index with >10 mitoses/10 HPFs.

Synovial sarcomas are usually immunoreactive for keratins (e.g., AE1/AE3, CK7, CK19), EMA, and vimentin,

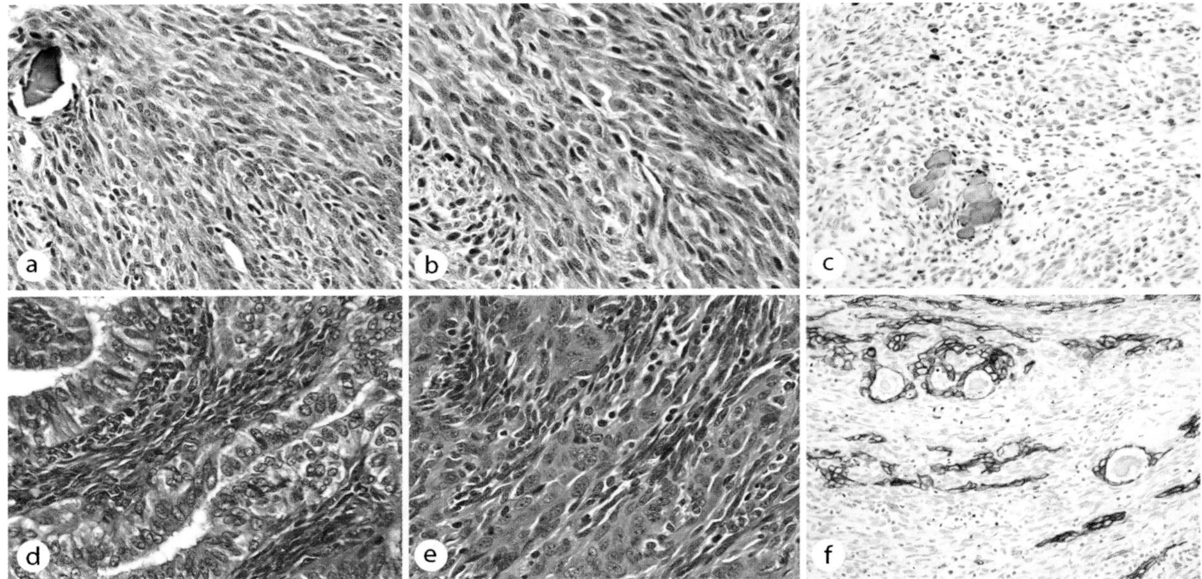

Fig. 22.24
Synovial sarcoma, monophasic fibrous (a–c) and biphasic (d–f) types. **Note the microcalcifications in figures (a) and (c) and an admixture of spindled and epithelioid ("transitional") neoplastic cells in figure (b). The epithelioid cells typically have strong immunoreactivity for keratins (c). There is considerable variation in the morphology of the epithelial component in biphasic synovial sarcomas (d, e), but the spindled neoplastic element tends to look the same from one case to the next. Figure (f) is a keratin cocktail immunostain**

and many examples express calretinin. They are typically negative for CD34. In problematic cases, FISH can be used to document gene rearrangement, and RT-PCR can be used to identify SYT-SSX fusion transcripts. Care should be taken not to confuse this neoplasm with benign processes such as endometriosis or hidradenoma papilliferum, or other malignancies of the gynecologic tract, including carcinosarcoma and adenosarcoma.

Synovial sarcomas range from intermediate to high grade. The most frequent sites of metastases are the lungs, lymph nodes, and bone. Treatment decisions are influenced by a variety of factors, including tumor size, tumor grade, patient age, and resectability [21, 127, 242]. This is one of the more chemotherapy sensitive soft tissue sarcomas [146, 216].

Angiosarcoma

Angiosarcomas only rarely affect the gynecologic tract. These tumors tend to fall into three clinicopathologic subgroups: those of vulvar and vaginal origin, uterine examples, and tumors primary to the ovaries. Angiosarcomas of the vulva/lower abdominal wall [43, 117, 131, 170, 187, 195, 248] and vagina [45, 203, 221, 306] are usually postirradiation tumors, developing 4–29 years after treatment for a carcinoma of the vulva, uterine cervix, or endometrium. Most patients are in the 7th and 8th decades of life, and they often present with a painless, purplish-red lesion in an area with radiodermatitis. The tumors may form ill-defined patches or plaques, they may be papulonodular, and some examples may be ulcerated. Sometimes there is accompanying lymphedema.

Uterine angiosarcomas primarily affect peri- and postmenopausal women (peak incidence: 6th decade), and they present with vaginal bleeding, anemia, weight loss, and a pelvic/abdominal mass [212, 222, 244, 274, 328]. There is usually no history of prior radiotherapy. A few examples have occurred in association with benign smooth muscle proliferations [74, 300]. The tumors are typically large and deeply invasive on presentation.

In contrast with the other two groups, ovarian angiosarcomas primarily affect young patients between the ages of 20 and 40 years (peak incidence: 3rd decade) [62, 193, 231, 238, 244]. Abdominal pain and distention and intraabdominal hemorrhage are the key presenting features. There are no recognized predisposing factors, although rare cases have occurred in association with dermoid cysts, as well as mucinous and serous tumors [70, 159, 231, 244].

Angiosarcomas have a broad morphologic spectrum (➋ *Fig. 22.25*), but almost all cases will contain some areas with interanastomosing vasoformative channels featuring atypical endothelial cells with mitotic activity and architectural disarray (including the piling and detachment of neoplastic cells). Destructive growth and necrosis are common. Some examples feature endothelial cells with prominent epithelioid morphology, and others may have frank spindling. Immunoreactivity is usually present for CD31 and factor VIIIrAg, whereas CD34 expression is more variable. Focal keratin reactivity may be encountered, especially in epithelioid angiosarcomas.

The prognosis for angiosarcoma is generally poor, with survival time often measured in months. The best chance for cure is with small, low-stage lesions.

Malignant Peripheral Nerve Sheath Tumor (Malignant Schwannoma, Neurofibrosarcoma)

Malignant peripheral nerve sheath tumors (MPNST) have been reported in the vulva [181, 196, 302], uterine cervix [83, 166], uterine corpus, and ovaries. However, it is difficult to substantiate some of these cases, due to lack of an association with a nerve, absence of S100 protein expression and no clinical history of NF1. Without fulfilling at least one of these often used criteria, the diagnosis of MPNST is, at best, presumptive. In general, 40–50% of MPNSTs occur in the setting of NF1, although <5% of all patients with this disorder ultimately develop a MPNST [76, 149]. MPNSTs in NF1 patients arise on average more than a decade earlier than in patients without NF1 [76, 291, 319, 330], and tumors occurring in the former group are often more aggressive [76, 291, 330]. Five to ten percent of MPNSTs are radiation-induced [149, 291, 330], and this patient group also has a poorer prognosis. Most MPNSTs are associated with a major nerve trunk or arise within a large, long-standing plexiform neurofibroma. MPNSTs have a strong tendency to metastasize to the lungs, but regional lymph node metastases are very uncommon [76, 149, 330].

In the setting of NF1, MPNSTs are often heralded by rapid growth or the onset of pain in a pre-existing neurofibroma. MPNSTs of the uterine cervix may present as polypoid masses associated with abnormal vaginal bleeding.

Histologically, these tumors are either spindled or spindled and epithelioid cell neoplasms with high cellularity, nuclear atypia, and mitotic activity. Many high-grade examples have areas with geographic necrosis. Some tumors contain a peculiar glomeruloid-like vascular proliferation, and up to 10–15% of cases (all anatomic sites) are reported to have foci with divergent (usually chondro-osseous, rhabdomyoblastic, or rarely, angiosarcomatous) differentiation [76, 149]. At least half of cases are reported to express S100 protein, but this is often a focal finding [149].

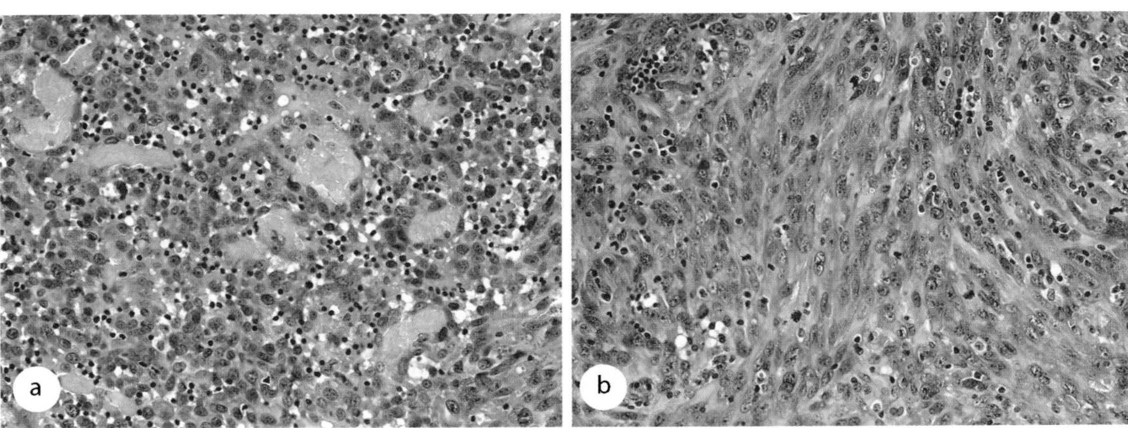

Fig. 22.25
Angiosarcoma. **These tumors can vary considerably in appearance, even within a given tumor, as illustrated in this example. Note the presence of vasoformative growth in figure (a) and more solid fascicular growth in figure (b)**

Most MPNSTs require aggressive surgical intervention with wide margins, because they have a very high local recurrence rate when incompletely excised, a low salvage rate when allowed to recur, a resistance to adjuvant radiotherapy (especially when total dosage is <60Gy) and chemotherapy, and a high mortality rate [76, 149, 291, 302, 330].

Ewing Family Tumors (EFT): Ewing sarcoma (EWS)/Peripheral Primitive Neuroectodermal Tumor (pPNET)

EFTs have been reported as primary neoplasms in the vulva [208, 275, 315], vagina [208, 315], uterine cervix [3, 42, 83, 250, 287, 307], uterine body [249, 283], ovaries [96, 164, 171], broad ligament [188], and rectovaginal septum [253]. Some of the cases are very well documented with a combination of immunohistochemistry and either molecular genetics or cytogenetic studies. Some are less well documented but contain solid presumptive evidence for the diagnosis. However, others are not convincing. A major point of confusion has been the misinterpretation of uterine and ovarian tumors with CNS-type neural differentiation as being part of this category. Classic peripheral (bone/soft tissue-type) PNET/EWSs do not exhibit mats of neuropil or ganglion cell, ependymal, astrocytic or medulloepithelial differentiation. In addition, for practical purposes (extremely rare exceptions noted), these tumors do not contain areas with frank epithelial differentiation, although there are now several molecularly confirmed pPNET/EWSs associated with small composite areas of endometrioid adenocarcinoma in uterine and ovarian sites. Most uterine primitive neuroectodermal tumors with CNS-type differentiation that present as polypoid intracavitary masses in postmenopausal women are thought to have a Mullerian derivation [68, 143], whereas most ovarian neuroectodermal tumors with similar differentiation (especially those associated with teratoma) have a germ cell origin [164, 172, 315]. Primitive neuroectodermal tumors with CNS-type differentiation are usually CD99-negative, and they lack the characteristic cytogenetic abnormalities detected in peripheral (bone/soft tissue-type) PNET/EWSs [164, 188].

EFTs of the gynecologic tract become clinically apparent through abnormal vaginal bleeding or mass effect. The better documented cases of vulvar origin have occurred at or below the age of 40, with most examples occurring between 10 and 30 years of age. Vaginal tumors have generally been diagnosed in patients in their early to mid 30s. Cervical tumors often occur between the ages of 20 and 45. Uterine body and ovarian tumors have affected individuals from 2nd to 8th decades, but classic examples often occur before 40 years of age. Some EFTs in postmenopausal women have been associated with a minor element of (usually low grade) endometrioid adenocarcinoma [96, 283].

EFTs are typically composed of a rather monomorphic population of small epithelioid cells that vary somewhat in appearance depending on the degree of neuroectodermal differentiation (➲ *Fig. 22.26*). The more primitive

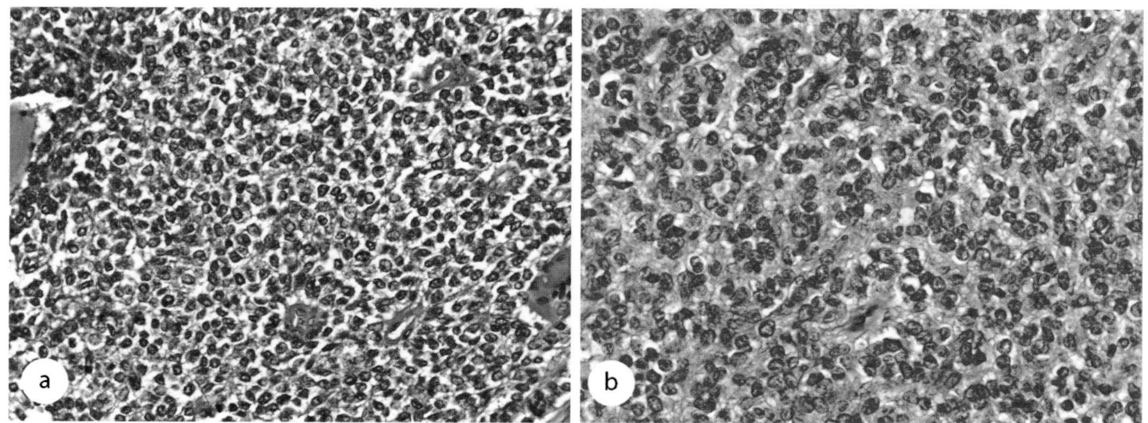

Fig. 22.26
Two tumors from the Ewing sarcoma/peripheral primitive neuroectodermal tumor family. **Tumors in this group form a morphologic continuum with the less differentiated neoplasms conforming to classical Ewing sarcoma morphology (a) and the more differentiated tumors with focal (pseudo)rosette formation showing progression to pPNET morphology (b)**

examples with classical EWS morphology are composed of sheets of round cells with scant, clear to lightly eosinophilic, glycogen-rich, cytoplasm. Examples with classical pPNET morphology often contain slightly larger cells that may have focal tapered cytoplasmic processes or spindling and can be glycogen-poor or glycogen-negative. These latter tumors have a notable tendency to form occasional Homer Wright (pseudo)rosettes, and much more rarely, Flexner-Wintersteiner rosettes. Mitotic activity is quite variable and can be either low or high. The neoplastic cells usually exhibit strong membranous reactivity for CD99, nuclear reactivity for FLI-1, and cytoplasmic reactivity for vimentin. There can be some reactivity for synaptophysin, Leu-7, and S100 protein (especially at the pPNET end of the spectrum), and a small amount of patchy reactivity for keratins is present in >30% of cases overall. The tumor cells are typically negative for chromogranin, GFAP, desmin, and actins. Approximately 85–90% of cases harbor a t(11;22) (q24;q12) translocation (usually type 1 or 2) that fuses the *EWS* gene on chromosome 22 to the *FLI-1* gene on chromosome 11 [188, 208]. This translocation can be detected in fresh tissue with cytogenetics. Indirect evidence of the gene fusion can also be detected in processed tissue via RT-PCR. Fluorescence in situ hybridization provides an alternate investigative approach and is of special value for the 10–15% of cases containing a variant translocation (e.g., t(21;22) (q22;q12)) that may not be detected with some RT-PCR tests. In the gynecologic tract, demonstration of one of the characteristic translocation abnormalities is the gold standard for EFT diagnosis [208].

There is speculation that EFTs of the vulva and vagina may have a better prognosis than similar tumors arising elsewhere in the gynecologic tract [208]. However, there are too few cases with too limited follow-up for any conclusive statement in this regard. EFTs are typically both chemo- and radiation therapy sensitive, and some gynecologic examples have shown dramatic response to conventional pPNET/EWS multimodality therapy [3, 253, 307].

Other Malignant or Potentially Malignant Soft Tissue Tumors that May Arise in the Gynecologic Tract

Additional soft tissue tumors that very rarely arise in the gynecologic tract include pleomorphic undifferentiated sarcoma/malignant fibrous histiocytoma [66, 232, 320], liposarcoma [34, 236, 298], osteosarcoma [69, 86, 145], chondrosarcoma [55, 299], and pleomorphic rhabdomyosarcoma [90, 245]. Before accepting any of the above as pure primary tumors, the possibility of a metastasis, direct extension from adjacent anatomy, or origin within another type of gynecologic neoplasm (e.g., a malignant mixed Mullerian tumor, teratoma, etc.) must be strongly considered. Other reported tumors include paraganglioma [58, 141, 209], (psammomatous) melanotic schwannoma [71], Kaposi sarcoma [4, 18, 177, 260], epithelioid hemangioendothelioma [294], and Langerhans cell histiocytosis [153]. In our opinion, all gastrointestinal stromal tumors (GISTs) involving the gynecologic tract must be assumed to be direct extensions from adjacent bowel or metastases [152, 327].

References

1. Abbott JJ, Oliveira AM, Nascimento AG (2006) The prognostic significance of fibrosarcomatous transformation in dermatofibrosarcoma protuberans. Am J Surg Pathol 30:436–443
2. Abeler V, Nesland JM (1989) Alveolar soft-part sarcoma in the uterine cervix. Arch Pathol Lab Med 113:1179–1183
3. Afenyi-Annan A, Paulino AF (2001) Abnormal uterine bleeding. Arch Pathol Lab Med 125:1389–1390
4. Agarossi A, Vago L, Lazzarin A et al (1991) Vulvar Kaposi's sarcoma. A case report. Ann Oncol 2:609–610
5. Ahern JK, Allen NH (1978) Cervical hemangioma: a case report and review of the literature. J Reprod Med 21:228–231
6. Albores-Saavedra J, Gilcrease M (1999) Glomus tumor of the uterine cervix. Int J Gynecol Pathol 18:69–72
7. Allen PW, Dymock RB, MacCormac LB (1988) Superficial angiomyxomas with and without epithelial components. Report of 30 tumors in 28 patients. Am J Surg Pathol 12:519–530
8. Altchek A, Deligdisch L, Norton K et al (2007) Prepubertal unilateral fibrous hyperplasia of the labium majus: report of eight cases and review of the literature. Obstet Gynecol 110:103–108
9. Althausen AM, Kowalski DP, Ludwig ME et al (2000) Granular cell tumors: a new clinically important histologic finding. Gynecol Oncol 77:310–313
10. Alvarez M, Cerezo L (1986) Ovarian cavernous hemangioma. Arch Pathol Lab Med 110:77–78
11. Alvarez-Canas MC, Mayorga M, Fernandez F et al (1996) Dermatofibrosarcoma protuberans of the vulva: clinico- pathological, immunohistochemical and flow cytometric study of a case. Acta Obstet Gynecol Scand 75:82–85
12. Ambani DS, White B, Kaplan AL et al (2006) A case of monophasic synovial sarcoma presenting as a vulvar mass. Gynecol Oncol 100:433–436
13. Aranda FI, Laforga JB (1998) Nodular fasciitis of the vulva. Report of a case with immunohistochemical study. Pathol Res Pract 194:805–807
14. Argani P, Antonescu CR, Illei PB et al (2001) Primary renal neoplasms with the *ASPL-TFE3* gene fusion of alveolar soft part sarcoma: a distinctive tumor entity previously included among renal cell carcinomas of children and adolescents. Am J Pathol 159:179–192
15. Argani P, Ladanyi M (2003) Recent advances in pediatric renal neoplasia. Adv Anat Pathol 10:243–260

16. Argani P, Lal P, Hutchinson B et al (2003) Aberrant nuclear immunoreactivity for TFE3 in neoplasms with *TFE3* gene fusions: a sensitive and specific immunohistochemical assay. Am J Surg Pathol 27:750–761
17. Argenta PA, Thomas S, Chura JC (2007) "Proximal-type" epithelioid sarcoma vs. malignant rhabdoid tumor of the vulva: a case report, review of the literature, and an argument for consolidation. Gynecol Oncol 107:130–135
18. Audouin AF, Lopes P, Lenne Y (1988) Sarcoma de Kaposi du col utérin associé á un condylome atypique chez une femme transplantée cardiaque (lors du post-partum). Arch Anat Cytol Path 36:226–228
19. Autio-Harmainen H, Apaja-Sarkkinen M, Martikainen J et al (1986) Production of basement membrane laminin and type IV collagen by tumors of striated muscle: an immunohistochemical study of rhabdomyosarcomas of different histologic types and a benign vaginal rhabdomyoma. Hum Pathol 17:1218–1224
20. Azuno Y, Yaga K, Suehiro Y et al (2003) Inflammatory myoblastic tumor of the uterus and interleukin-6. Am J Obstet Gynecol 189:890–891
21. Bergh P, Meis-Kindblom JM, Gherlinzoni F et al (1999) Synovial sarcoma: identification of low and high risk groups. Cancer 85:2596–2607
22. Bhargava R, Shia J, Hummer AJ et al (2005) Distinction of endometrial stromal sarcomas from "hemangiopericytomatous" tumors using a panel of immunohistochemical stains. Mod Pathol 18:40–47
23. Bhattacharya B, Dilworth HP, Iacobuzio-Donahue C et al (2005) Nuclear beta-catenin expression distinguishes deep fibromatosis from other benign and malignant fibroblastic and myofibroblastic lesions. Am J Surg Pathol 29:653–659
24. Biedrzycki OJ, Singh N, Habeeb H et al (2007) Solitary fibrous tumor of the female genital tract a case report and review of the literature. Int J Gynecol Pathol 26:259–264
25. Blandamura S, Cruz J, Faure Vergara L et al (2003) Aggressive angiomyxoma: a second case of metastasis with patient's death. Hum Pathol 34:1072–1074
26. Blickstein I, Lurie S (1990) The gynaecological problems of neurofibromatosis. Aust N Z Obstet Gynaecol 30:380–382
27. Bock JE, Andreasson B, Thorn A et al (1985) Dermatofibrosarcoma protuberans of the vulva. Gynecol Oncol 20:129–135
28. Boikos SA, Stratakis CA (2006) Carney complex: pathology and molecular genetics. Neuroendocrinology 83:189–199
29. Bonetti F, Martignoni G, Colato C et al (2001) Abdominopelvic sarcoma of perivascular epithelioid cells. Report of four cases in young women, one with tuberous sclerosis. Mod Pathol 14:563–568
30. Bos GD, Pritchard DJ, Reiman HM et al (1988) Epithelioid sarcoma. An analysis of fifty-one cases. J Bone Joint Surg Am 70:862–870
31. Brandfass RT, Everts-Suarez EA (1955) Lipomatous tumors of the uterus: a review of the world's literature with report of a case of true lipoma. Am J Obstet Gynecol 70:359–367
32. Brasfield RD, Das Gupta TK (1972) Von Reckinghausen's disease: a clinicopathological study. Ann Surg 175:86–104
33. Bridge JA, Kanamori M, Ma Z et al (2001) Fusion of the *ALK* gene to clathrin heavy chain gene, *CLTC*, in inflammatory myofibroblastic tumor. Am J Pathol 159:411–415
34. Brooks JJ, LiVolsi VA (1987) Liposarcoma presenting on the vulva. Am J Obstet Gynecol 156:73–75
35. Burch DJ, Hitchcock A, Masson GM (1994) Alveolar soft part sarcoma of the uterus: case report and review of the literature. Gynecol Oncol 54:91–94
36. Busby JG (1952) Neurofibromatosis of the cervix. Am J Obstet Gynecol 63:674–675
37. Calonje E, Guerin D, McCormick D et al (1999) Superficial angiomyxoma: clinicopathologic analysis of a series of distinctive but poorly recognized cutaneous tumors with tendency for recurrence. Am J Surg Pathol 23:910–917
38. Cao D, Srodon M, Montgomery EA et al (2005) Lipomatous variant of angiomyofibroblastoma: report of two cases and review of the literature. Int J Gynecol Pathol 24:196–200
39. Carinelli SG, Giudici MN, Brioschi D et al (1990) Alveolar soft part sarcoma of the vagina. Tumori 76:77–80
40. Carlson JW, Fletcher CD (2007) Immunohistochemistry for beta-catenin in the differential diagnosis of spindle cell lesions: analysis of a series and review of the literature. Histopathology 51:509–514
41. Carney JA, Headington JT, Su WP (1986) Cutaneous myxomas. A major component of the complex of myxomas, spotty pigmentation, and endocrine overactivity. Arch Dermatol 122:790–798
42. Cenacchi G, Pasquinelli G, Montanaro L et al (1998) Primary endocervical extraosseous Ewing's sarcoma/PNET. Int J Gynecol Pathol 17:83–88
43. Cerri A, Gianni C, Corbellino M et al (1998) Lymphangiosarcoma of the pubic region: a rare complication arising in congenital non-hereditary lymphedema. Eur J Dermatol 8:511–514
44. Chan IM, Hon E, Ngai SW et al (2000) Aggressive angiomyxoma in females: is radical resection the only option? Acta Obstet Gynecol Scand 79:216–220
45. Chan WW, SenGupta SK (1991) Postirradiation angiosarcoma of the vaginal vault. Arch Pathol Lab Med 115:527–528
46. Chapman GW, Benda J, Williams T (1984) Aleolar soft-part sarcoma of the vagina. Gynecol Oncol 18:125–129
47. Char G, Hanchard B, Manjoo RB (1982) Neurofibromatosis of the cervix uteri. West Indian Med J 31:90–92
48. Chase DR, Enzinger FM (1985) Epithelioid sarcoma. Diagnosis, prognostic indicators, and treatment. Am J Surg Pathol 9:241–263
49. Cheng L, Scheithauer BW, Leibovich BC (1999) Neurofibroma of the urinary bladder. Cancer 1999:505–513
50. Chestnut DH, Szpak CA, Fortier KJ et al (1988) Uterine hemangioma associated with infertility. South Med J 81:926–928
51. Chien AJ, Freeby JA, Win TT et al (1998) Aggressive angiomyxoma of the female pelvis: sonographic, CT, and MR findings. AJR Am J Roentgenol 171:530–531
52. Chiodi NE, Siegel IA, Guerin PF et al (1957) Granular-cell myoblastoma of the vulva and lower respiratory tract: report of a case. Obstet Gynecol 9:472–480
53. Chu PW, Liu JY, Peng YJ et al (2006) Solitary fibrous tumor of the uterus. Taiwan J Obstet Gynecol 45:350–352
54. Chuang WY, Yeh CJ, Jung SM et al (2007) Plexiform schwannoma of the clitoris. APMIS 115:889–890
55. Clement PB (1978) Chondrosarcoma of the uterus: report of a case and review of the literature. Hum Pathol 9:726–732
56. Clement PB (1988) Postoperative spindle-cell nodule of the endometrium. Arch Pathol Lab Med 112:566–568
57. Cohen PR, JR YAW, Tovell HM (1989) Angiokeratoma of the vulva: diagnosis and review of the literature. Obstet Gynecol Surv 44:339–346
58. Colgan TJ, Dardick I, O'Connell G (1991) Paraganglioma of the vulva. Int J Gynecol Pathol 10:203–208
59. Comstock CH, Monticello ML, Johnson TW et al (2005) Cavernous hemangioma: diffuse enlarged venous spaces within the myometrium in pregnancy. Obstet Gynecol 106:1212–1214
60. Cook CL, Sanfilippo JS, Verdi GD et al (1989) Capillary hemangioma of the vagina and urethra in a child: response to short-term steroid therapy. Obstet Gynecol 73:883–885

61. Cormio G, Cormio L, Marzullo A et al (1997) Fibromatosis of the female pelvis. Ann Chir Gynaecol 86:84–86
62. Cunningham MJ, Brooks JS, Noumoff JS (1994) Treatment of primary ovarian angiosarcoma with ifosfamide and doxorubicin. Gynecol Oncol 53:265–268
63. Curry JL, Olejnik JL, Wojcik EM (2001) Cellular angiofibroma of the vulva with DNA ploidy analysis. Int J Gynecol Pathol 20:200–203
64. Davani M, Chablani VN, Saba PR (1998) Aggressive angiomyxoma of pelvic soft tissues: MR imaging appearance. AJR Am J Roentgenol 170:1113–1114
65. Davis GD, Patton WS (1983) Capillary hemangioma of the cervix and vagina: management with carbon dioxide laser. Obstet Gynecol 62:95S–96S
66. Davos I, Abell MR (1976) Sarcomas of the vagina. Obstet Gynecol 47:342–350
67. Dawood MY, Teoh ES, Ratnam SS (1972) Ruptured haemangioma of a gravid uterus. J Obstet Gynaecol Br Commonw 79:474–475
68. Daya D, Lukka H, Clement PB (1992) Primitive neuroectodermal tumors of the uterus: a report of four cases. Hum Pathol 23:1120–1129
69. De Young B, Bitterman P, Lack EE (1992) Primary osteosarcoma of the uterus: report of a case with immunohistochemical study. Mod Pathol 5:212–215
70. den Bakker MA, Ansink AC, Ewing-Graham PC (2006) "Cutaneous-type" angiosarcoma arising in a mature cystic teratoma of the ovary. J Clin Pathol 59:658–660
71. Devaney K, Tavassoli FA (1991) Immunohistochemistry as a diagnostic aid in the interpretation of unusual mesenchymal tumors of the uterus. Mod Pathol 4:225–231
72. Dharkar DD, Kraft JR, Gangadharam D (1981) Uterine lipomas. Arch Pathol Lab Med 105:43–45
73. Di Sant'Agnese PA, Knowles DM 2nd (1980) Extracardiac rhabdomyoma: a clinicopathologic study and review of the literature. Cancer 46:780–789
74. Drachenberg CB, Faust FJ, Borkowski A et al (1994) Epithelioid angiosarcoma of the uterus arising in a leiomyoma with associated ovarian and tubal angiomatosis. Am J Clin Pathol 102:388–389
75. DuBay D, Cimmino V, Lowe L et al (2004) Low recurrence rate after surgery for dermatofibrosarcoma protuberans: a multidisciplinary approach from a single institution. Cancer 100:1008–1016
76. Ducatman BS, Scheithauer BW, Piepgras DG et al (1986) Malignant peripheral nerve sheath tumors: a clinicopathologic study of 120 cases. Cancer 57:2006–2021
77. Duran B, Guvenal T, Yildiz E et al (2004) An unusual cause of adnexal mass: fallopian tube schwannoma. Gynecol Oncol 92:343–346
78. Ellison DW, MacKenzie IZ, McGee JO (1992) Cellular schwannoma of the vagina. Gynecol Oncol 46:119–121
79. Emoto M, Tamura R, Izumi H et al (1997) Sonodynamic changes after transcatheter arterial embolization in a vaginal hemangioma: case report. Ultrasound Obstet Gynecol 10:66–67
80. Enzinger FM (1970) Epithelioid sarcoma. A sarcoma simulating a granuloma or a carcinoma. Cancer 26:1029–1041
81. Enzinger FM, Smith BH (1976) Hemangiopericytoma. An analysis of 106 cases. Hum Pathol 7:61–82
82. Espat NJ, Lewis JJ, Leung D et al (2002) Conventional hemangiopericytoma: modern analysis of outcome. Cancer 95:1746–1751
83. Fadare O (2006) Uncommon sarcomas of the uterine cervix: a review of selected entities. Diagn Pathol 1:30
84. Fadare O (2008) Perivascular epithelioid cell tumor (PEComa) of the uterus: an outcome-based clinicopathologic analysis of 41 reported cases. Adv Anat Pathol 15:63–75
85. Fadare O (2008) Uterine PEComa: appraisal of a controversial and increasingly reported mesenchymal neoplasm. Int Semin Surg Oncol 5:7
86. Fadare O, Bossuyt V, Martel M et al (2006) Primary osteosarcoma of the ovary: a case report and literature review. Int J Gynecol Pathol 26:21–25
87. Fadare O, Ghofrani M, Stamatakos MD et al (2006) Mesenchymal lesions of the uterine cervix. Pathol Case Rev 11:140–152
88. Fadare O, Parkash V, Yilmaz Y et al (2004) Perivascular epithelioid cell tumor (PEComa) of the uterine cervix asociated with intraabdominal "PEComatosis": A clinicopathologic study with comparative genomic hybridization analysis. World J Surg Oncol 2:35
89. Fanburg-Smith JC, Meis-Kindblom JM, Fante R et al (1998) Malignant granular cell tumor of soft tissue: diagnostic criteria and clinicopathologic correlation. Am J Surg Pathol 22:779–794
90. Ferguson SE, Gerald W, Barakat RR et al (2007) Clinicopathologic features of rhabdomyosarcoma of gynecologic origin in adults. Am J Surg Pathol 31:382–389
91. Fernández-Aguilar S, Fayt I, Noel JC (2004) Spindle cell vulvar hemangiomatosis associated with enchondromatosis: a rare variant of Maffucci's syndrome. Int J Gynecol Pathol 23:68–70
92. Fetsch JF, Laskin WB, Lefkowitz M et al (1996) Aggressive angiomyxoma: a clinicopathologic study of 29 female patients. Cancer 78:79–90
93. Fetsch JF, Laskin WB, Tavassoli FA (1997) Superficial angiomyxoma (cutaneous myxoma): a clinicopathologic study of 17 cases arising in the genital region. Int J Gynecol Pathol 16:325–334
94. Fine BA, Munoz AK, Litz CE et al (2001) Primary medical management of recurrent aggressive angiomyxoma with a gonadotrophin-releasing hormone agonist. Gynecol Oncol 81:120–122
95. Fingerland A (1938) Ganglioneuroma of the cervix uteri. J Pathol Bacteriol 47:631–634
96. Fischer G, Odunsi K, Lele S et al (2006) Ovarian primary primitive neuroectodermal tumor coexisting with endometroid adenocarcinoma: a case report. Int J Gynecol Pathol 25:151–154
97. Fisher C (2004) Myofibroblastic malignancies. Adv Anat Pathol 11:190–201
98. Fisher C (2006) Epithelioid sarcoma of Enzinger. Adv Anat Pathol 13:114–121
99. Fisher C, Folpe AL, Hashimoto H et al (2004) Intra-abdominal synovial sarcoma: a clinicopathological study. Histopathology 45:245–253
100. Fishman A, Girtanner RE, Kaplan AL (1996) Aggressive fibromatosis of the female pelvis. A case report and review of the literature. Eur J Gynaecol Oncol 17:208–211
101. Fletcher CD, Tsang WY, Fisher C et al (1992) Angiomyofibroblastoma of the vulva. A benign neoplasm distinct from aggressive angiomyxoma. Am J Surg Pathol 16:373–382
102. Flint A, Gikas PW, Roberts JA (1985) Alveolar soft part sarcoma of the uterine cervix. Gynecol Oncol 22:263–267
103. Folpe AL, Mentzel T, Lehr HA et al (2005) Perivascular epithelioid cell neoplasms of soft tissue and gynecologic origin: a clinicopathologic study of 26 cases and review of the literature. Am J Surg Pathol 29:1558–1575
104. Foschini MP, Eusebi V, Tison V (1989) Alveolar soft part sarcoma of the cervix uteri. A case report. Pathol Res Pract 184:354–358
105. Fukunaga M (2000) Atypical solitary fibrous tumor of the vulva. Int J Gynecol Pathol 19:164–168
106. Fukunaga M, Nomura K, Matsumoto K et al (1997) Vulval angiomyofibroblastoma. Clinicopathologic analysis of six cases. Am J Clin Pathol 107:45–51

107. Gal R, Dekel A, Ben-David M et al (1988) Granular cell myoblastoma of the cervix. Case report. Br J Obstet Gyneacol 95:720–722
108. Ganesan R, McCluggage WG, Hirschowitz L et al (2005) Superficial myofibroblastoma of the lower female genital tract: report of a series including tumours with a vulvar location. Histopathology 46:137–143
109. Gantchev S (1997) Vascular abnormalities of the uterus, concerning a case of diffuse cavernous angiomatosis of the uterus. Gen Diagn Pathol 143:71–74
110. Gehrig PA, Fowler WC Jr, Lininger RA (2000) Ovarian capillary hemangioma presenting as an adnexal mass with massive ascites and elevated CA-125. Gynecol Oncol 76:130–132
111. Gengler C, Guillou L (2006) Solitary fibrous tumour and haemangiopericytoma: evolution of a concept. Histopathology 48:63–74
112. Gersell DJ, Fulling KH (1989) Localized neurofibromatosis of the female genitourinary tract. Am J Surg Pathol 13:873–878
113. Ghorbani RP, Malpica A, Ayala AG (1999) Dermatofibrosarcoma protuberans of the vulva: clinicopathologic and immunohistochemical analysis of four cases, one with fibrosarcomatous change, and review of the literature. Int J Gynecol Pathol 18:366–373
114. Gifford RR, Birch HW (1973) Granular cell myoblastoma of multicentric origin involving the vulva: a case report. Am J Obstet Gynecol 117:184–187
115. Gilks CB, Taylor GP, Clement PB (1987) Inflammatory pseudotumor of the uterus. Int J Gynecol Pathol 6:275–286
116. Gloster HM Jr, Harris KR, Roenigk RK (1996) A comparison between Mohs micrographic surgery and wide surgical excision for the treatment of dermatofibrosarcoma protuberans. J Am Acad Dermatol 35:82–87
117. Goette DK, Detlefs RL (1985) Postirradiation angiosarcoma. J Am Acad Dermatol 12:922–926
118. Gökden N, Dehner LP, Zhu X et al (2003) Dermatofibrosarcoma protuberans of the vulva and groin: detection of COL1A1-PDGFB fusion transcripts by RT-PCR. J Cutan Pathol 30:190–195
119. Gold BM (1972) Neurofibromatosis of the bladder and vagina. Am J Obstet Gynecol 113:1055–1056
120. Gold JS, Antonescu CR, Hajdu C et al (2002) Clincopathologic correlates of solitary fibrous tumors. Cancer 94:1057–1068
121. Gold JH, Bossen EH (1976) Benign vaginal rhabdomyoma: a light and electron microscopic study. Cancer 37:2283–2294
122. Gordon MD, Weilert M, Ireland K (1996) Plexiform neurofibromatosis involving the uterine cervix, endometrium, myometrium, and ovary. Obstet Gynecol 88:699–701
123. Granter SR, Nucci MR, Fletcher CD (1997) Aggressive angiomyxoma: reappraisal of its relationship to angiomyofibroblastoma in a series of 16 cases. Histopathology 30:3–10
124. Gray GF Jr, Glick AD, Kurtin PJ et al (1986) Alveolar soft part sarcoma of the uterus. Hum Pathol 17:297–300
125. Griffin CA, Hawkins AL, Dvorak C et al (1999) Recurrent involvement of 2p23 in inflammatory myofibroblastic tumors. Cancer Res 59:2776–2780
126. Gücer F, Özyilmaz F, Balkanli-Kaplan P et al (2004) Ovarian hemangioma presenting with hyperandrogenism and endometrial cancer: a case report. Gynecol Oncol 94:821–824
127. Guillou L, Benhattar J, Bonichon F et al (2004) Histologic grade, but not SYT-SSX fusion type, is an important prognostic factor in patients with synovial sarcoma: a multicenter, retrospective analysis. J Clin Oncol 22:4040–4050
128. Guillou L, Gebhard S, Coindre JM (2000) Orbital and extraorbital giant cell angiofibroma: a giant cell-rich variant of solitary fibrous tumor? Clinicopathologic and immunohistochemical analysis of a series in favor of a unifying concept. Am J Surg Pathol 24:971–979
129. Guillou L, Lamoureux E, Masse S et al (1991) Alveolar soft-part sarcoma of the uterine corpus: histological, immunocytochemical, and ultrastructural study of a case. Vircows Archiv A Pathol Anat 418:467–471
130. Guillou L, Wadden C, Coindre JM et al (1997) "Proximal-type" epithelioid sarcoma, a distinctive aggressive neoplasm showing rhabdoid features. Clinicopathologic, immunohistochemical, and ultrastructural study of a series. Am J Surg Pathol 21:130–146
131. Guirguis A, Kanbour-Shakir A, Kelley J (2007) Epithelioid angiosarcoma of the mons after chemoradiation for vulvar cancer. Int J Gynecol Pathol 26:265–268
132. Gupta R, Singh S, Nigam S et al (2006) Benign vascular tumors of the female genital tract. Int J Gynecol Cancer 16:1195–1200
133. Gusdon JP (1965) Hemangioma of the cervix: four new cases and a review. Am J Obstet Gynecol 91:204–209
134. Gutmann DH, Aylsworth A, Carey JC et al (1997) The diagnostic evaluation and multidisciplinary management of neurofibromatosis 1 and neurofibromatosis 2. JAMA 278:51–57
135. Gwavava NJ, Traub AI (1980) A neurilemmoma of the cervix. Br J Obstet Gynaecol 87:444–446
136. Halling AC, Wollan PC, Pritchard DJ et al (1996) Epithelioid sarcoma: a clinicopathologic review of 55 cases. Mayo Clin Proc 71:636–642
137. Hanafy A, Lee RM, Peterson CM (1997) Schwannoma presenting as a Bartholin's gland abscess. Aust N Z J Obstet Gynaecol 37:483–484
138. Haraoka M, Naito S, Kumazawa J (1988) Clitoral involvement by neurofibromatosis: a case report and review of the literature. J Urol 139:95–96
139. Hasagawa T, Matsuno Y, Shimoda T et al (1999) Extrathoracic solitary fibrous tumors: their histological variability and potentially aggressive behavior. Hum Pathol 30:1464–1473
140. Hasegawa T, Matsuno Y, Shimoda T et al (2001) Proximal-type epithelioid sarcoma: a clinicopathologic study of 20 cases. Mod Pathol 14:655–663
141. Hassan A, Bennet A, Bhalla S et al (2003) Paraganglioma of the vagina: report of a case, including immunohistochemical and ultrastructural findings. Int J Gynecol Pathol 22:404–406
142. Heimann P, Devalck C, Debusscher C et al (1998) Alveolar soft-part sarcoma: further evidence by FISH for involvement of chromosome band 17q25. Genes Chromosomes Cancer 23:194–197
143. Hendrickson MR, Scheithauer BW (1986) Primitive neuroectoermal tumor of the endometrium: report of two cases, one with electron microscopic observations. Int J Gynecol Pathol 5:249–259
144. Herszkowicz L, dos Santos RG, Alves EV et al (2001) Benign neonatal hemangiomatosis with mucosal involvement. Arch Dermatol 137:828–829
145. Hines JF, Compton DM, Stacy CC et al (1990) Pure primary osteosarcoma of the ovary presenting as an extensively calcified adnexal mass: a case report and review of the literature. Gynecol Oncol 39:259–263
146. Holloway CL, Russell AH, Muto M et al (2007) Synovial cell sarcoma of the vulva: multimodality treatment incorporating preoperative external-beam radiation, hemivulvectomy, flap reconstruction, interstitial brachytherapy, and chemotherapy. Gynecol Oncol 104:253–256
147. Hoot AC, Russo P, Judkins AR et al (2004) Immunohistochemical analysis of hSNF5/INI1 distinguishes renal and extra-renal malignant rhabdoid tumors from other pediatric soft tissue tumors. Am J Surg Pathol 28:1485–1491

148. Horowitz IR, Copas P, Majmudar B (1995) Granular cell tumors of the vulva. Am J Obstet Gynecol 173:1710–1714
149. Hruban RH, Shiu MH, Senie RT et al (1990) Malignant peripheral nerve sheath tumors of the buttock and lower extremity. A study of 43 cases. Cancer 66:1253–1265
150. Huang HJ, Yamabe T, Tagawa H (1983) A solitary neurilemmoma of the clitoris. Gynecol Oncol 15:103–110
151. Inoue T, Kato H, Yoshikawa K et al (2004) Retroperitoneal schwannoma bearing at the right vaginal wall. J Obstet Gynaecol Res 30:454–457
152. Irving JA, Lerwill MF, Young RH (2005) Gastrointestinal stromal tumors metastatic to the ovary: a report of five cases. Am J Surg Pathol 29:920–926
153. Issa PY, Salem PA, Brihi E et al (1980) Eosinophilic granuloma with involvement of the female genitalia. Am J Obstet Gynecol 137:608–612
154. Iversen UM (1996) Two cases of benign vaginal rhabdomyoma. Case reports. APMIS 104:575–578
155. Iwasa Y, Fletcher CD (2004) Distinctive prepubertal vulvar fibroma: a hitherto unrecognized mesenchymal tumor of prepubertal girls: analysis of 11 cases. Am J Surg Pathol 28:1601–1608
156. Iwasa Y, Fletcher CD (2004) Cellular angiofibroma: clinicopathologic and immunohistochemical analysis of 51 cases. Am J Surg Pathol 28:1426–1435
157. Jagadha V, Srinivasan K, Panchacharam P (1985) Glomus tumor of the clitoris. N Y State J Med 85:611
158. Jelinek JA, Stelzer KJ, Conrad E et al (2001) The efficacy of radiotherapy as postoperative treatment for desmoid tumors. Int J Radiation Oncology Biol Phys 50:121–125
159. Jylling AM, Jørgensen L, Hølund B (1999) Mucinous cystadenocarcinoma in combination with hemangiosarcoma in the ovary. Pathol Oncol Res 5:318–319
160. Kapadia SB, Norris HJ (1993) Rhabdomyoma of the vagina. Mod Pathol 6:75A
161. Kargi HA, Özer E, Gökden N (1995) Inflammatory pseudotumor of the uterus: a case report. Tumori 81:454–456
162. Kasashima S, Minato H, Kobayashi M et al (2007) Alveolar soft part sarcoma of the endometrium with expression of CD10 and hormone receptors. APMIS 115:861–865
163. Katz VL, Askin FB, Bosch BD (1986) Glomus tumor of the vulva: a case report. Obstet Gynecol 67:43S–45S
164. Kawauchi S, Fukuda T, Miyamoto S et al (1998) Peripheral primitive neuroectodermal tumor of the ovary confirmed by CD99 immunostaining, karyotypic analysis, and RT-PCR for EWS/FLI-1 chimeric mRNA. Am J Surg Pathol 22:1417–1422
165. Kay S, Schneider V (1985) Reactive spindle cell nodule of the endocervix simulating uterine sarcoma. Int J Gynecol Pathol 4:255–257
166. Keel SB, Clement PB, Prat J et al (1998) Malignant schwannoma of the uterine cervix: a study of three cases. Int J Gynecol Pathol 17:223–230
167. Kemmann E, Conrad P, Chen CK et al (1977) Pelvic neurilemmoma. Report of a case, electron microscopic studies, and review of the literature. Gynecol Oncol 5:387–395
168. Kenerson H, Folpe AL, Takayama TK et al (2007) Activation of the mTOR pathway in sporadic angiomyolipomas and other perivascular epithelioid cell neoplasms. Hum Pathol 38:1361–1371
169. Kim DH, Goldsmith HS, Quan SH et al (1971) Intra-abdominal desmoid tumor. Cancer 27:1041–1045
170. Kim MK, Huh SJ, Kim DY et al (1998) Secondary angiosarcoma following irradiation – Case report and review of the literature. Radiat Med 16:55–60
171. Kim KJ, Jang BW, Lee SK et al (2004) A case of peripheral primitive neuroectodermal tumor of the ovary. Int J Gynecol Cancer 14:370–372
172. Kleinman GM, Young RH, Scully GM (1993) Primary neuroectodermal tumors of the ovary. A report of 25 cases. Am J Surg Pathol 17:764–778
173. Kobayashi T, Yamazaki T, Takahashi M (1999) Characteristic radiologic findings for cavernous hemangioma of the uterus. AJR Am J Roentgenol 172:1147–1148
174. Kohorn EL, Merino MJ, Goldenhersh M (1986) Vulvar pain and dyspareunia due to glomus tumor. Obstet Gynecol 67:41S–42S
175. Konrad EA, Meister P, Hübner G (1982) Extracardiac rhabdomyoma: report of different types with light microscopic and ultrastructural studies. Cancer 49:898–907
176. Kopolovic J, Weiss DB, Dolberg L et al (1987) Alveolar soft-part sarcoma of the female genital tract. Case report with ultrastructural findings. Arch Gynecol 240:125–129
177. Laartz BW, Cooper C, Degryse A et al (2005) Wolf in sheep's clothing: advanced Kaposi sarcoma mimicking vulvar abscess. South Med J 98:475–477
178. Lack EE, Worsham GF, Callihan MD et al (1980) Granular cell tumor: a clinicopathologic study of 110 patients. J Surg Oncol 13:301–316
179. Ladanyi M, Antonescu CR, Drobnjak M et al (2002) The precrystalline cytoplasmic granules of alveolar soft part sarcoma contain monocarboxylate transporter 1 and CD147. Am J Pathol 160:1215–1221
180. Ladanyi M, Lui MY, Antonescu CR et al (2001) The der(17)t(X;17)(p11;q25) of human alveolar soft part sarcoma fuses the *TFE3* transcription factor gene to *ASPL*, a novel gene at 17q25. Oncogene 4:48–57
181. Lambrou NC, Mirhashemi R, Wolfson A et al (2002) Malignant peripheral nerve sheath tumor of the vulva: a multimodal treatment approach. Gynecol Oncol 85:365–371
182. Laskin WB, Fetsch JF, Mostofi FK (1998) Angiomyofibroblastomalike tumor of the male genital tract: analysis of 11 cases with comparison to female angiomyofibroblastoma and spindle cell lipoma. Am J Surg Pathol 22:6–16
183. Laskin WB, Fetsch JF, Tavassoli FA (1997) Angiomyofibroblastoma of the female genital tract: analysis of 17 cases including a lipomatous variant. Hum Pathol 28:1046–1055
184. Laskin WB, Fetsch JF, Tavassoli FA (2001) Superficial cervicovaginal myofibroblastoma: fourteen cases of a distinctive mesenchymal tumor arising from the specialized subepithelial stroma of the lower female genital tract. Hum Pathol 32:715–725
185. Lawhead RA, Copeland LJ, Edwards CL (1985) Bilateral ovarian hemangiomas associated with diffuse abdominopelvic hemangiomatosis. Obstet Gynecol 65:597–599
186. Lawrence B, Perez-Atayde A, Hibbard MK et al (2000) *TPM3-ALK* and *TPM4-ALK* oncogenes in inflammatory myofibroblastic tumors. Am J Pathol 157:377–384
187. Leborgne F, Falconi LM (1980) Lymphangiosarcoma of the anterior abdominal wall: a case report. Cancer 46:1228–1230
188. Lee KM, Wah HK (2005) Primary Ewing's sarcoma family of tumors arising from the broad ligament. Int J Gynecol Pathol 24:377–381
189. LeMaire WJ, Kreiss C, Commodore A et al (2002) Neurilemmoma: an unusual benign tumor of the cervix. Alaska Med 44:63–65
190. Levavi H, Sabah G, Kaplan B et al (2006) Granular cell tumor of the vulva: six new cases. Arch Gynecol Obstet 273:246–249
191. Lieb SM, Gallousis S, Freedman H (1979) Granular cell myoblastoma of the vulva. Gynecol Oncol 8:12–20

192. Lieberman PH, Brennan MF, Kimmel M et al (1989) Alveolar soft-part sarcoma. A clinico-pathologic study of half a century. Cancer 63:1–13
193. Lifschitz-Mercer B, Leider-Trejo L, Messer G et al (1998) Primary angiosarcoma of the ovary: A clinicopathologic, immunohistochemical and electronmicroscopic study. Pathol Res Pract 194: 183–187
194. Long SR, Whitfeld MJ, Eades C et al (1996) Bacillary angiomatosis of the cervix and vulva in a patient with AIDS. Obstet Gynecol 88:709–711
195. Maddox JC, Evans HL (1981) Angiosarcoma of skin and soft tissue: a study of forty-four cases. Cancer 48:1907–1921
196. Maglione MA, Tricarico OD, Calandria L (2002) Malignant peripheral nerve sheath tumor of the vulva. A case report. J Reprod Med 47:721–724
197. Maire G, Martin L, Michalak-Provost S et al (2002) Fusion of *COL1A1* exon 29 with *PDGFB* exon 2 in a der(22)t(17;22) in a pediatric giant cell fibroblastoma with a pigmented Bednar tumor component. Evidence for age-related chromosomal pattern in dermatofibrosarcoma protuberans and related tumors. Cancer Genet Cytogenet 134:156–161
198. Majmudar B, Castellano PZ, Wilson RW et al (1990) Granular cell tumors of the vulva. J Reprod Med 35:1008–1014
199. Majmudar B, Ghanee N, Horowitz IR et al (1998) Uterine arteriovenous malformation necessitating hysterectomy with bilateral salpingo-oophorectomy in a young pregnant patient. Arch Pathol Lab Med 122:842–845
200. Manetta A, Abt AB, Mamourian AC et al (1989) Pelvic fibromatosis: case report and review of literature. Gynecol Oncol 32:91–94
201. Manson CM, Hirsch PJ, Coyne JD (1995) Post-operative spindle cell nodule of the vulva. Histopathology 26:571–574
202. Mariani A, Nascimento AG, Webb MJ et al (2000) Surgical management of desmoid tumors of the female pelvis. J Am Coll Surg 191:175–183
203. McAdam JA, Stewart F, Reid R (1998) Vaginal epithelioid angiosarcoma. J Clin Pathol 51:928–930
204. McArthur G (2006) Dermatofibrosarcoma protuberans: recent clinical progress. Ann Surg Oncol 14:2876–2886
205. McCluggage WG, Jamieson T, Dobbs SP et al (2006) Aggressive angiomyxoma of the vulva: Dramatic response to gonadotropin-releasing hormone agonist therapy. Gynecol Oncol 100:623–625
206. McCluggage WG, Patterson A, Maxwell P (2000) Aggressive angiomyxoma of pelvic parts exhibits oestrogen and progesterone receptor positivity. J Clin Pathol 53:603–605
207. McCluggage WG, Perenyei M, Irwin ST (2002) Recurrent cellular angiofibroma of the vulva. J Clin Pathol 55:477–479
208. McCluggage WG, Sumathi VP, Nucci MR et al (2007) Ewing family of tumours involving the vulva and vagina: report of a series of four cases. J Clin Pathol 60:674–680
209. McCluggage WG, Young RH (2006) Paraganglioma of the ovary: report of three cases of a rare ovarian neoplasm, including two exhibiting inhibin positivity. Am J Surg Pathol 30:600–605
210. McPeak CJ, Cruz T, Nicastri AD (1967) Dermatofibrosarcoma protuberans: an analysis of 86 cases—five with metastasis. Ann Surg 166:803–816
211. Medeiros F, Erickson-Johnson MR, Keeney GL et al (2007) Frequency and characterization of *HMGA2* and *HMGA1* rearrangements in mesenchymal tumors of the lower genital tract. Genes Chromosomes Cancer 46:981–990
212. Mendez LE, Joy S, Angioli R et al (1999) Primary uterine angiosarcoma. Gynecol Oncol 75:272–276
213. Mentzel T, Beham A, Katenkamp D et al (1998) Fibrosarcomatous ("high-grade") dermatofibrosarcoma protuberans: clinicopathologic and immunohistochemical study of a series of 41 cases with emphasis on prognostic significance. Am J Surg Pathol 22:576–587
214. Miettinen M, Fanburg-Smith JC, Virolainen M et al (1999) Epithelioid sarcoma: an immunohistochemical analysis of 112 classical and variant cases and a discussion of the differential diagnosis. Hum Pathol 30:934–942
215. Miettinen M, Virtanen I, Damjanov I (1985) Coexpression of keratin and vimentin in epithelioid sarcoma. Am J Surg Pathol 9:460–462
216. Mitsuhashi A, Nagai Y, Suzuka K et al (2006) Primary synovial sarcoma in fallopian tube: case report and literature review. Int J Gynecol Pathol 26:34–37
217. Modena P, Lualdi E, Facchinetti F et al (2005) *SMARCB1/INI1* tumor suppressor gene is frequently inactivated in epithelioid sarcomas. Cancer Res 65:4012–4019
218. Montgomery EA, Meis JM (1991) Nodular fasciitis. Its morphologic spectrum and immunohistochemical profile. Am J Surg Pathol 15:942–948
219. Montgomery EA, Shuster DD, Burkart AL et al (2006) Inflammatory myofibroblastic tumors of the urinary tract: a clinicopathologic study of 46 cases, including a malignant example inflammatory fibrosarcoma and a subset associated with high-grade urothelial carcinoma. Am J Surg Pathol 30:1502–1512
220. Moreno-Rodríguez M, Pérez-Sicilia M, Delinois R (1999) Lipoma of the endocervix. Histopathology 35:483–484
221. Morgan MA, Moutos DM, Pippitt CH Jr et al (1989) Vaginal and bladder angiosarcoma after therapeutic irradiation. South Med J 82:1434–1436
222. Morrel B, Mulder AF, Chadha S et al (1993) Angiosarcoma of the uterus following radiotherapy for squamous cell carcinoma of the cervix. Eur J Obstet Gynecol Reprod Biol 49:193–197
223. Moscovic EA, Azar HA (1967) Multiple granular cell tumors ("myoblastomas'). Case report with electron microscopic observations and review of the literature. Cancer 20:2032–2047
224. Murray J, Fox H (1991) Rosai-Dorfman disease of the uterine cervix. Int J Gynecol Pathol 10:209–213
225. Nielsen GP, Oliva E, Young RH et al (1995) Alveolar soft-part sarcoma of the female genital tract: a report of nine cases and review of the literature. Int J Gynecol Pathol 14:283–292
226. Nielsen GP, Rosenberg AE, Young RH et al (1996) Angiomyofibroblastoma of the vulva and vagina. Mod Pathol 9:284–291
227. Nielsen GP, Shaw PA, Rosenberg AE et al (1996) Synovial sarcoma of the vulva: a report of two cases. Mod Pathol 9:970–974
228. Nielsen GP, Young RH (1997) Fibromatosis of soft tissue type involving the female genital tract: a report of two cases. Int J Gynecol Pathol 16:383–386
229. Nielsen GP, Young RH (2001) Mesenchymal tumors and tumor-like lesions of the female genital tract: a selective review with emphasis on recently described entities. Int J Gynecol Pathol 20:105–127
230. Nielsen GP, Young RH, Dickersin GR et al (1997) Angiomyofibroblastoma of the vulva with sarcomatous transformation ("angiomyofibrosarcoma"). Am J Surg Pathol 21:1104–1108
231. Nielsen GP, Young RH, Prat J et al (1997) Primary angiosarcoma of the ovary: a report of seven cases and review of the literature. Int J Gynecol Pathol 16:378–382
232. Nirenberg A, Östör AG, Slavin J et al (1995) Primary vulvar sarcomas. Int J Gynecol Pathol 14:55–62
233. Nishimura K, Sugao H, Sato K et al (1991) Neurofibroma of the clitoris. A case report. Urol Int 46:109–111

234. Nolan NP, Gaffney EF (1990) Alveolar soft part sarcoma of the uterus. Histopathology 16:97–99
235. Nucci MR, Castrillon DH, Bai H et al (2003) Biomarkers in diagnostic obstetric and gynecologic pathology: a review. Adv Anat Pathol 10:55–68
236. Nucci MR, Fletcher CD (1998) Liposarcoma (atypical lipomatous tumor) of the vulva: a clinicopathologic study of six cases. Int J Gynecol Pathol 17:17–23
237. Nucci MR, Granter SR, Fletcher CD (1997) Cellular angiofibroma: a benign neoplasm distinct from angiomyofibroblastoma and spindle cell lipoma. Am J Surg Pathol 21:636–644
238. Nucci MR, Krausz T, Lifschitz-Mercer B et al (1998) Angiosarcoma of the ovary: clinicopathologic and immunohistochemical analysis of four cases with a broad morphologic spectrum. Am J Surg Pathol 22:620–630
239. Nucci MR, Weremowicz S, Neskey DM et al (2001) Chromosomal translocation t(8;12) induces aberrant HMGIC expression in aggressive angiomyxoma of the vulva. Genes Chromosomes Cancer 32:172–176
240. O'Connell JX, Young RH, Nielsen GP et al (1997) Nodular fasciitis of the vulva: a study of six cases and literature review. Int J Gynecol Pathol 16:117–123
241. O'Toole RV, Tuttle SE, Lucas JG et al (1985) Alveolar soft part sarcoma of the vagina: an immunohistochemical and electron microscopic study. Int J Gynecol Pathol 4:258–265
242. Oda Y, Hashimoto H, Tsuneyoshi M et al (1993) Survival in synovial sarcoma. A multivariate study of prognostic factors with special emphasis on the comparison between early death and long-term survival. Am J Surg Pathol 17:35–44
243. Oda Y, Tsuneyoshi M (2006) Extrarenal rhabdoid tumors of soft tissue: clinicopathological and molecular genetic review and distinction from other soft-tissue sarcomas with rhabdoid features. Pathol Int 56:287–295
244. Ongkasuwan C, Taylor JE, Tang CK et al (1982) Angiosarcomas of the uterus and ovary: clinicopathologic report. Cancer 49:1469–1475
245. Ordi J, Stamatakos MD, Tavassoli FA (1997) Pure pleomorphic rhabdomyosarcomas of the uterus. Int J Gynecol Pathol 16:369–377
246. Ordóñez NG (1999) Alveolar soft part sarcoma: A review and update. Adv Anat Pathol 6:125–139
247. Outwater EK, Marchetto BE, Wagner BJ et al (1999) Aggressive angiomyxoma: findings on CT and MR imaging. AJR 172:435–438
248. Paik HH, Komorowski R (1976) Hemangiosarcoma of the abdominal wall following irradiation therapy of endometrial carcinoma. Am J Clin Pathol 66:810–814
249. Park JY, Lee S, Kang HJ et al (2007) Primary Ewing's sarcoma-primitive neuroectodermal tumor of the uterus: a case report and literature review. Gynecol Oncol 106:427–432
250. Pauwels P, Ambros P, Hattinger C et al (2000) Peripheral primitive neuroectodermal tumour of the cervix. Virchows Arch 436:68–73
251. Pelosi G, Luzzatto F, Landoni F et al (2007) Poorly differentiated synovial sarcoma of the vagina: first reported case with immunohistochemical, molecular and ultrastructural data. Histopathology 50:808–810
252. Perrone T, Swanson PE, Twiggs L et al (1989) Malignant rhabdoid tumor of the vulva: is distinction from epithelioid sarcoma possible? Am J Surg Pathol 13:848–858
253. Petković M, Zamolo G, Muhvić D et al (2002) The first report of extraosseous Ewing's sarcoma in the rectovaginal septum. Tumori 88:345–346
254. Piver MS, Tsukada Y, Barlow J (1972) Epithelioid sarcoma of the vulva. Obstet Gynecol 40:839–842
255. Pressoir R, Chung EB (1980) Granular cell tumor in black patients. J Natl Med Assoc 72:1171–1175
256. Proppe KH, Scully RE, Rosai J (1984) Postoperative spindle cell nodules of genitourinary tract resembling sarcomas. Am J Surg Pathol 8:101–108
257. Prus D, Rosenberg AE, Blumenfeld A et al (1997) Infantile hemangioendothelioma of the ovary: a monodermal teratoma or a neoplasm of ovarian somatic cells? Am J Surg Pathol 21:1231–1235
258. Rabban JT, Zaloudek CJ, Shekitka KM et al (2005) Inflammatory myofibroblastic tumor of the uterus: a clinicopathologic study of 6 cases emphasizing distinction from aggressive mesenchymal tumors. Am J Surg Pathol 29:1348–1355
259. Radig K, Buhtz P, Roessner A (1998) Alveolar soft part sarcoma of the uterine corpus. Report of two cases and review of the literature. Pathol Res Pract 194:59–63
260. Rajah SB, Moodley J, Pudifin DJ et al (1990) Kaposi's sarcoma associated with acquired immunodeficiency syndrome presenting as a vulval papilloma. A case report. S Afr Med J 77:585–586
261. Ramos PC, Kapp DS, Longacre TA et al (2000) Malignant granular cell tumor of the vulva in a 17-year-old: Case report and literature review. Int J Gynecol Cancer 10:429–434
262. Reitamo JJ, Häyry P, Nykyri E et al (1982) The desmoid tumor. I. Incidence, sex-, age-, and anatomic distribution in the Finnish population. Am J Clin Pathol 77:665–673
263. Rezvani FF (1997) Vaginal cavernous hemangioma in pregnancy. Obstet Gynecol 89:824–825
264. Riccardi VM (1981) Von Recklinghausen neurofibromatosis. N Engl J Med 305:1617–1627
265. Rink RC, Mitchell ME (1983) Genitourinary neurofibromatosis in childhood. J Urol 130:1176–1179
266. Robertson AJ, McIntosh W, Lamont P et al (1981) Malignant granular cell tumor (myoblastoma) of the vulva: report of a case and review of the literature. Histopathology 5:69–79
267. Roma AA, Yang B, Senior ME et al (2005) TFE3 immunoreactivity in alveolar soft part sarcoma of the uterine cervix: case report. Int J Gynecol Pathol 24:131–135
268. Roses DF, Valensi Q, LaTrenta G et al (1986) Surgical treatment of dermatofibrosarcoma protuberans. Surg Gynecol Obstet 162:449–452
269. Saha SC, Dogra M, Malhotra S (1993) Pelvic plexiform neurofibroma—an obstetric dilemma. Int J Gynecol Obstet 43:61–62
270. Sahin AA, Silva EG, Ordonez NG (1989) Alveolar soft part sarcoma of the uterine cervix. Mod Pathol 2:676–680
271. Santos LD, Currie BG, Killingsworth MC (2001) Case report: plexiform schwannoma of the vulva. Pathology 33:526–531
272. Savargaonkar PR, Wells S, Graham I et al (1994) Ovarian haemangiomas and stromal luteinization. Histopathology 25: 185–188
273. Scanlon R, Kelehan P, Flannelly G et al (2003) Ischemic fasciitis: an unusual vulvovaginal spindle cell lesion. Int J Gynecol Pathol 23:65–67
274. Schammel DP, Tavassoli FA (1998) Uterine angiosarcoma: a morphologic and immunohistochemical study of four cases. Am J Surg Pathol 22:246–250
275. Scherr GR, d'Ablaing G 3rd, Ouzounian JG (1994) Peripheral primitive neuroectodermal tumor of the vulva. Gynecol Oncol 54:254–258
276. Schreiber MM (1963) Vulvar von Recklinghausen's disease. Arch Dermatol 88:320–321
277. Schwartz BM, Kuo DY, Goldberg GL (1999) Dermatofibrosarcoma protuberans of the vulva: a rare tumor presenting during pregnancy in a teenager. J Lower Genital Tract Dis 3:139–142

278. Shimizu A, O'Brien KP, Sjöblom T et al (1999) The dermatofibrosarcoma protuberans-associated collagen type Ialpha1/platelet-derived growth factor (PDGF) B-chain fusion gene generates a transforming protein that is processed to functional PDGF-BB. Cancer Res 59:3719–3723
279. Shintaku M, Fukushima A (2006) Inflammatory myofibroblastic tumor of the uterus with prominent myxoid change. Pathol Int 56:625–628
280. Siassi RM, Papadopoulos T, Matzel KE (1999) Metastasizing aggressive angiomyxoma. N Engl J Med 341:1772
281. Simon NL, Mazur MT, Shingleton HM (1985) Pelvic fibromatosis: an unusual gynecologic tumor. Obstet Gynecol 65:767–769
282. Simpson KW, Albores-Saavedra J (2007) HMB-45 reactivity in conventional uterine leiomyosarcomas. Am J Surg Pathol 31:95–98
283. Sinkre P, Albores-Saavedra J, Miller DS et al (2000) Endometrial endometroid carcinomas associated with Ewing sarcoma/peripheral primitive neuroectodermal tumor. Int J Gynecol Pathol 19:127–132
284. Sirvent N, Maire G, Pedeutour F (2003) Genetics of dermatofibrosarcoma protuberans family of tumors: from ring chromosome to tyrosine kinase inhibitor treatment. Genes Chromosomes Cancer 37:1–19
285. Skálová A, Michal M, Hušek K et al (1993) Aggressive angiomyxoma of the pelvioperineal region. Immunohistochemical and ultrastructural study of seven cases. Am J Dermatopathol 15:446–451
286. Smith CJ, Ferrier AJ, Russell P et al (2005) Primary synovial sarcoma of the ovary: first reported case. Pathology 37:385–387
287. Snijders-Keilholz A, Ewing P, Seynaeve C et al (2005) Primitive neuroectodermal tumor of the cervix uteri: a case report – changing concepts in therapy. Gynecol Oncol 98:516–519
288. Snow SN, Gordon EM, Larson PO et al (2004) Dermatofibrosarcoma protuberans: a report on 29 patients treated by Mohs micrographic surgery with long-term follow-up and review of the literature. Cancer 101:28–38
289. Sobottka Ventura AC, Remonda L, Mojon DS (2001) Intermittent visual loss and exophthalmos due to the blue rubber bleb nevus syndrome. Am J Ophthalmol 132:132–135
290. Sonobe H, Ro JY, Ramos M et al (1994) Glomus tumor of the female external genitalia: a report of two cases. Int J Gynecol Pathol 13:359–364
291. Sordillo PP, Helson L, Hajdu SI et al (1981) Malignant schwannoma – clinical characteristics, survival, and response to therapy. Cancer 47:2503–2509
292. Steeper TA, Rosai J (1983) Aggressive angiomyxoma of the female pelvis and perineum. Report of nine cases of a distinctive type of gynecologic soft-tissue neoplasm. Am J Surg Pathol 7:463–475
293. Stratakis CA, Kirschner LS, Carney JA (2001) Clinical and molecular features of the Carney complex: diagnostic criteria and recommendations for patient evaluation. J Clin Endocrinol Metab 86:4041–4046
294. Strayer SA, Yum MN, Sutton GP (1992) Epithelioid hemangioendothelioma of the clitoris: a case report with immunohistochemical and ultrastructural findings. Int J Gynecol Pathol 11:234–239
295. Strong EW, McDivitt RW, Brasfield RD (1970) Granular cell myoblastoma. Cancer 25:415–422
296. Suarez Vilela D, Gimenez Pizarro A, Rio Suarez M (1990) Vaginal rhabdomyoma and adenosis. Histopathology 16:393–394
297. Sutphen R, Galán-Goméz E, Kousseff BG (1995) Clitoromegaly in neurofibromatosis. Am J Med Genet 55:325–330
298. Takeuchi K, Murata K, Funaki K et al (2000) Liposarcoma of the uterine cervix: case report. Eur J Gynaecol Oncol 21:290–291
299. Talerman A, Auerbach WM, van Meurs AJ (1981) Primary chondrosarcoma of the ovary. Histopathology 5:319–324
300. Tallini G, Price FV, Carcangiu ML (1993) Epithelioid angiosarcoma arising in uterine leiomyomas. Am J Clin Pathol 100:514–518
301. Tan GW, Lim-Tan SK, Salmon YM (1989) Epithelioid sarcoma of the vulva. Sing Med J 30:308–310
302. Terada KY, Schmidt RW, Roberts JA (1988) Malignant schwannoma of the vulva. A case report. J Reprod Med 33:969–972
303. Thanner F, Suetterlin M, Kenn W et al (2001) Pregnancy-associated diffuse cavernous hemangioma of the uterus. Acta Obstet Gynecol Scand 80:1150–1151
304. Tiltman AJ, Duffield MS (1996) Postpartum microneuromas of the uterine cervix. Histopathology 28:153–156
305. Tjalma WA, Hauben EI, Deprez SM et al (1999) Epithelioid sarcoma of the vulva. Gynecol Oncol 73:160–164
306. Tohya T, Katabuchi H, Fukuma K et al (1991) Angiosarcoma of the vagina. A light and electronmicroscopy study. Acta Obstet Gynecol Scand 70:169–172
307. Tsao AS, Roth LM, Sandler A et al (2001) Cervical primitive neuroectodermal tumor. Gynecol Oncol 83:138–142
308. Tsuji T, Yoshinaga M, Inomoto Y et al (2007) Aggressive angiomyxoma of the vulva with a sole t(5;8)(p15;q22) chromosome change. Int J Gynecol Pathol 26:494–496
309. Ueda M, Okamoto Y, Ueki M (1996) A pelvic retroperitoneal schwannoma arising in the right paracolpium. Gynecol Oncol 60:480–483
310. Uzunlar AK, Yilmaz F, Kilinç N et al (2002) Cavernous hemangioma of the uterus (a case report). Eur J Gynaecol Oncol 23:72–73
311. Vallat-Decouvelaere A-V, Dry SM, Fletcher CD (1998) Atypical and malignant solitary fibrous tumors in extrathoracic locations: evidence of their comparability to intra-thoracic tumors. Am J Surg Pathol 22:1501–1511
312. van de Rijn M, Barr FG, Xiong QB et al (1999) Poorly differentiated synovial sarcoma: an analysis of clinical, pathologic, and molecular genetic features. Am J Surg Pathol 23:106–112
313. Vang R, Connelly JH, Hammill HA et al (2000) Vulvar hypertrophy with lymphedema. A mimicker of aggressive angiomyxoma. Arch Pathol Lab Med 124:1697–1699
314. Vang R, Kempson RL (2002) Perivascular epithelioid cell tumor ('PEComa') of the uterus: a subset of HMB-45-positive epithelioid mesenchymal neoplasms with an uncertain relationship to pure smooth muscle tumors. Am J Surg Pathol 26:1–13
315. Vang R, Taubenberger JK, Mannion CM et al (2000) Primary vulvar and vaginal extraosseous Ewing's sarcoma/peripheral neuroectodermal tumor: diagnostic confirmation with CD99 immunostaining and reverse transcriptase-polymerase chain reaction. Int J Gynecol Pathol 19:103–109
316. Vanni R, Faa G, Dettori T et al (2000) A case of dermatofibrosarcoma protuberans of the vulva with a *COL1A1/PDGFB* fusion identical to a case of giant cell fibroblastoma. Virchows Arch 437:95–100
317. Vargas SO, Kozakewich HP, Boyd TK et al (2005) Childhood asymmetric labium majus enlargement: mimicking a neoplasm. Am J Surg Pathol 29:1007–1016
318. Wakami K, Tateyama H, Kawashima H et al (2005) Solitary fibrous tumor of the uterus producing high-molecular-weight insulin-like growth factor II and associated with hypoglycemia. Int J Gynecol Pathol 24:79–84
319. Wanebo JE, Malik JM, VandenBerg SR et al (1993) Malignant peripheral nerve sheath tumors: a clinicopathologic study of 28 cases. Cancer 71:1247–1253

320. Webb MJ, Symmonds RE, Weiland LH (1974) Malignant fibrous histiocytoma of the vagina. Am J Obstet Gynecol 119:190–192
321. Wei EX, Albores-Saavedra J, Fowler MR (2005) Plexiform neurofibroma of the uterine cervix: a case report and review of the literature. Arch Pathol Lab Med 129:783–786
322. Weissman A, Talmon R, Jakobi P (1993) Cavernous hemangioma of the uterus in a pregnant woman. Obstet Gynecol 81:825–827
323. White J, Chan YF (1994) Aggressive angiomxyoma of the vulva in an 11-year-old girl. Pediatr Pathol 14:27–37
324. White BE, Kaplan A, Lopez-Terrada DH et al (2008) Monophasic synovial sarcoma arising in the vulva: a case report and review of the literature. Arch Pathol Lab Med 132:698–702
325. White W, Shiu MH, Rosenblum MK et al (1990) Cellular schwannoma. A clinicopathologic study of 57 patients and 58 tumors. Cancer 66:1266–1275
326. Wilcken N, Tattersall MH (1991) Endocrine therapy for desmoid tumors. Cancer 68:1384–1388
327. Wingen CB, Pauwels PA, Debiec-Rychter M et al (2005) Uterine gastrointestinal stromal tumour (GIST). Gynecol Oncol 97:970–972
328. Witkin GB, Askin FB, Geratz JD et al (1987) Angiosarcoma of the uterus: a light microscopic, immunohistochemical, and ultrastructural study. Int J Gynecol Pathol 6:176–184
329. Wolber RA, Talerman A, Wilkinson EJ et al (1991) Vulvar granular cell tumors with pseudocarcinomatous hyperplasia: a comparative analysis with well-differentiated squamous carcinoma. Int J Gynecol Pathol 10:59–66
330. Wong WW, Hirose T, Scheithauer BW et al (1998) Malignant peripheral nerve sheath tumor: analysis of treatment outcome. Int J Radiation Oncology Biol Phys 42:351–360
331. Woodruff JM, Marshall ML, Godwin TA et al (1983) Plexiform (multinodular) schwannoma. A tumor simulating the plexiform neurofibroma. Am J Surg Pathol 7:691–697
332. Wrotnowski U, Cooper PH, Shmookler BM (1988) Fibrosarcomatous change in dermatofibrosarcoma protuberans. Am J Surg Pathol 12:287–293
333. Yamashita Y, Yamada T, Ueki K et al (1996) A case of vulvar schwannoma. J Obstet Gynaecol Res 22:31–34
334. Yamawaki T, Hirai Y, Takeshima N et al (1996) Ovarian hemangioma associated with concomitant stromal luteinization and ascites. Gynecol Oncol 61:438–441
335. Yousem HL, Dorfman HD (1962) Myometrial involvement in von Recklinghausen's disease: report of a case. Obstet Gynecol 20:781–784
336. Zubor P, Kajo K, Szunyogh N et al (2007) A solitary fibrous tumor in the broad ligament of the uterus. Pathol Res Pract 203:555–560

Index

A

B

H

I

M

P

Q

R

S

T

U

V

W

X